PHARMACIST'S DRUG HANDBOOK

PHARMACIST'S DRUG HANDBOOK

American Society of Health-System Pharmacists
Bethesda, Maryland

Springhouse Corporation
Springhouse, Pennsylvania

Staff

Senior Publisher
Donna O. Carpenter

Editorial Director
William J. Kelly

Clinical Director
Ann M. Barrow, RN, MSN

Design Director
John Hubbard

Art Director
Elaine Kasmer Ezrow

Drug Information Editors
Tracy A. Roux, PharmD;
Lisa Truong, RPh, PharmD

Senior Editor
Cindy Laufenberg

Clinical Project Editor
Theresa P. Fulginiti, RN, BSN, CEN

Editors
Peter H. Johnson, Patricia Nale

Clinical Editors
Nancy LaPlante, RN, BSN; Pamela S. Messer, RN, MSN; Kimberly A. Zalewski, RN, MSN, CEN

Copy Editors
Louise Quinn, Jane R. Smith

Designers
Arlene Putterman (associate design director), Joseph John Clark, Donald G. Knauss

Electronic Production Services
Diane Paluba (electronic production services manager), Joy Rossi Biletz (electronic production technician), Val Molettiere (electronic production technician)

Manufacturing
Deborah Meiris (director), Patricia K. Dorshaw (manager), Otto Mezei (book production manager)

Editorial Assistants
Carol A. Caputo, Arlene Claffee

Indexer
Barbara Hodgson

The clinical information in this product is based on research and consultation with medical, pharmaceutical, nursing, and legal authorities. To the best of our knowledge, this information reflects currently accepted practice; nevertheless, it can't be considered absolute and universal. For individual application, all recommendations must be considered in light of the patient's clinical condition and, before the administration of new or infrequently used drugs, in light of the latest package-insert information. The authors and publisher disclaim responsibility for adverse effects resulting directly or indirectly from the information presented, from undetected errors, or from the reader's misunderstanding of the text.

Visit www.eDrugInfo.com and www.ashp.org

PharmDH—D N O
03 02 01 00 10 9 8 7 6 5 4 3 2 1
ISBN 1-58255-093-X

American Society of Health-System Pharmacists Consultants

Gerald K. McEvoy, PharmD
Editor

Kathy Litvak, MS
Senior Editor, Drug Information Development

Olin H. Welsh, PharmD
Associate Editor, Editorial Development

Elaine K. Snow, BS
Assistant Editor

Donald R. Dewey, BS
Senior Drug Information Analyst

Phillip A. Fong, PharmD
Senior Drug Information Analyst

Anne O'Rourke, BS
Senior Drug Information Analyst

Laura A. Bollinger, MS
Drug Information Analyst

Laura K. Brady, PharmD
Drug Information Analyst

Janie Kim, PharmD
Drug Information Analyst

Tran Le, PharmD
Drug Information Analyst

Gerald Scott Melton, DVM
Drug Information Analyst

Barbara F. Young, PharmD, MHA
Drug Information Analyst

Jeffery Shick, BS
Director, Database Services

P.M. Douglas, RN, BSc
Associate Editor, Drug Information Services

M.E. Ford, MD, MPH
Contributing Editor

Linda Kester, MS
Contributing Editor

Linda Bedford Arcuri, PharmD
Contributor

Marjorie Kay Fredrickson, BS
Contributor

Susan Braun, PharmD
Contributor

Contents

Clinical consultants

Paul Amato, BS Pharmacy
Clinical Drug Information Pharmacist
Hartford Hospital
Hartford, Conn.

Daniel A. Behrens, RPh, PharmD
Medical Information Projects Manager
Zeneca Pharmaceuticals
Wilmington, Del.

Lawrence Carey, PharmD
Clinical Pharmacist Supervisor
Jefferson Home Infusion Service
Philadelphia

David M. DiPersio, PharmD, BCPS
Clinical Pharmacist, Critical Care
Vanderbilt University Medical Center
Nashville, Tenn.

Ronald L. Greenberg, PharmD, BCPS
Clinical Pharmacy Coordinator
Fairview Ridges Hospital
Burnsville, Minn.

Edgar R. Gonzalez, PharmD
Associate Professor of Emergency Medicine
Medical College of Virginia
Richmond

Mildred D. Gottwald, PharmD
Assistant Clinical Professor
University of California
San Francisco

Bridget A. Haupt, PharmD
Director of Pharmacy
Children's Seashore House
Philadelphia

Barbara S. Kannewurf, PharmD, BSPh
Clinical Pharmacist, Cardiology
Clinical Instructor
University of Washington Medical Center
Seattle

Patricia A. Keys, PharmD
Associate Professor of Clinical Pharmacy
Duquesne University School of Pharmacy
Pittsburgh

Thomas E. Lackner, PharmD, CGP, FASCP
Professor, Director of Clinical Services
University of Minnesota College of Pharmacy
Institute for the Study of Geriatric Pharmacotherapy
Minneapolis

Jan E. Markind, RPh, PharmD
Drug Information Specialist
Clinical Assistant Professor
University of Illinois
Chicago

Steven B. Meisel, PharmD
Assistant Director of Pharmacy
Fairview Southdale Hospital
Edina, Minn.

Susan W. Sard, PharmD
Clinical Pharmacist
Anne Arundel Medical Center
Annapolis, Md.

Joel Shuster, PharmD
Clinical Associate Professor
School of Pharmacy, Temple University
Clinical Pharmacist
Medical College of Pennsylvania
Philadelphia

Foreword

To provide excellent pharmaceutical care, pharmacists must have the most complete, up-to-date drug information available. The need for drug information has intensified because of the increased rate of new drug approvals, the publication of many consensus therapeutic guidelines, and the recognition of the complex nature of the interactions of drugs with other drugs, nutrients, and herbal medicines. The responsibilities of pharmacists continue to expand, particularly because health care consumers, who are more educated about drugs than ever before, expect their medication regimens to be as safe as possible. Pharmacists are challenged with assembling a diverse array of facts about drugs, incorporating these facts into a rational approach, and individualizing a therapeutic regimen in light of patient-specific factors, while maximizing therapeutic benefits and reducing the risk of adverse effects. To do this effectively, pharmacists need access to the most current drug information available along with drug-use guidelines that have been constructed from knowledgeable and authoritative sources.

The *Pharmacist's Drug Handbook* provides a unique and valuable reference for pharmacists and other health care professionals by effectively combining drug information with therapeutic monitoring guidelines. Designed specifically for pharmacists, it includes comprehensive information in a portable, easy-to-read format. This concise and informative handbook is a joint publishing effort by Springhouse Corporation and the American Society of Health-System Pharmacists (ASHP), who also publish the well-established and continually updated reference source *AHFS Drug Information*. The *Pharmacist's Drug Handbook* gives you comprehensive profiles of more than 780 generic and 2,000 brand-name drugs as well as valuable information on 39 pharmacologic classes.

The book also features 10 informative appendices that every pharmacist should have but that weren't found in such a readily accessible format until now. The appendices on cancer chemotherapy acronyms; subcutaneous, intramuscular, and intravenous injection techniques; cytochrome P-450 enzymes and common drug interactions; and herbal medicines are particularly useful in addressing common issues that arise in health care settings. The appendix on therapeutic drug monitoring guidelines provides a useful, drug-focused structure for monitoring individual drugs. And there are also guidelines for using selected antimicrobials, a list of selected analgesic combination products, an immunization schedule, a guide to selected antidotes, and creatinine clearance calculations.

Another useful feature of this resource is a handy 16-page photoguide featuring full-color, actual-size photos of 300 of the most commonly prescribed tablets and capsules. And you can easily access changes and updates to the drug information by visiting www.eDrugInfo.com.

Pharmacists need a comprehensive resource that gives them all the up-to-date information they need in an easy-to-use format. The *Pharmacist's Drug Handbook* is a valuable tool for any pharmacist looking to ensure positive therapeutic outcomes while providing the highest quality of pharmaceutical care.

Joseph T. DiPiro, PharmD
Panoz Professor of Pharmacy
University of Georgia
College of Pharmacy
Clinical Professor of Surgery
Medical College of Georgia
Augusta, Georgia

How to use this book

The *Pharmacist's Drug Handbook* provides up-to-date information on virtually every drug in current clinical use. It covers aspects of drug information from fundamental pharmacology to specific management of toxicity and overdose. It also includes several indispensable features — individual entries that describe major pharmacologic classes; interactions categorized as drug-drug, drug-food, drug-lifestyle, and drug-herb; special guidance for drug therapy in pregnant, breast-feeding, pediatric, and geriatric patients; and therapeutic management guidelines. If you need more detailed information on a particular drug, consult *AHFS Drug Information.*

Pharmacologic class entries

Listed alphabetically as a separate section, 39 entries describe the pharmacology, clinical indications and actions, adverse effects, and special implications of drugs in major pharmacologic groups. This allows the reader to compare the effects and uses of drugs within each class. Pharmacologic class entries list special considerations common to all generic members of the class, including geriatric, pediatric, and breast-feeding considerations. If specific considerations are unknown, these headings are omitted.

Representative combinations appear at the end of each class entry. These lists show combinations of generic drugs in the class with other generics of the same or another class, followed by trade names of products that contain each combination of generics.

Generic drug entries

The individual drug entries provide detailed information on virtually all drugs in current clinical use, arranged alphabetically by generic name for easy access. A guide word at the top of each page identifies the generic drug presented on that page. Each generic entry is complete where it falls alphabetically and doesn't require cross-referencing to other sections of the book.

In each drug entry, the **generic name,** with alternative generic names following in parentheses, precedes an alphabetically arranged list of current trade names (an asterisk signals products available only in Canada). Several drugs available solely as combinations — such as acetaminophen and oxycodone hydrochloride (Percocet) — are listed in an appendix.

The **pharmacologic and therapeutic classifications** identify the pharmacologic or chemical category of the drug and its major clinical uses. Listing both classifications helps the reader grasp the multiple, varying, and sometimes overlapping uses of drugs within a single pharmacologic class and among different classes. If appropriate, the next line identifies any drug that the Drug Enforcement Agency (DEA) lists as a controlled substance and specifies the schedule of control as II, III, IV, or V.

The **pregnancy risk category** identifies the potential risk to the fetus. Categories listed were determined by application of the FDA definitions to available clinical data in order to define the potential of a drug to cause birth defects or fetal death. These categories, labeled A, B, C, D, and X, are explained below. Drugs in category A usually are considered safe to use in pregnancy; drugs in category X usually are contraindicated.

Pregnancy risk category A: Adequate studies in pregnant women have failed to show a risk to the fetus in the first trimester of pregnancy — and there's no evidence of risk in later trimesters.

Pregnancy risk category B: Animal studies haven't shown an adverse effect on the fetus, but there are no adequate clinical studies in pregnant women.

Pregnancy risk category C: Animal studies have shown an adverse effect on the fetus, but there are no adequate studies in humans. The drug may be useful in pregnant women despite its potential risks.

Pregnancy risk category D: There is evidence of risk to the human fetus, but the potential benefits of use in pregnant women may be acceptable despite potential risks.

Pregnancy risk category X: Studies in animals or humans show fetal abnormalities, or adverse reaction reports indicate evidence of fetal risk. The risks involved clearly outweigh potential benefits.

Pregnancy risk category NR: Not rated.

Pregnancy risk classifications were assigned for all generic drugs according to the above criteria.

Each drug entry is then broken down into the following subheads:

- **How supplied** lists the preparations available for each drug, such as tablets, capsules, solution, or injection, specifying available dosage forms and strengths. Its prescription or nonprescription status is also indicated.

▪ **Indications and dosages** presents all clinically accepted indications for use with general dosage recommendations for adults and children; dosage adjustments for specific patient groups, such as the elderly or patients with renal or hepatic impairment, are included when appropriate. (Note that additional information may be found in the *Clinical considerations* section.) A preceding open diamond signals a clinically accepted but unlabeled use. Dosage instructions reflect current clinical trends in therapeutics and shouldn't be considered as absolute and universal recommendations. For individual application, dosage must be considered according to the patient's conditions.

▪ **Pharmacodynamics** explains the mechanism and effects of the physiologic action of the drug.

▪ **Pharmacokinetics** describes absorption, distribution, metabolism, and excretion of the drug; it specifies peak levels and half-life as appropriate. A chart outlining the route, onset, peak, and duration of action is also included.

▪ **Contraindications and precautions** lists conditions associated with special risks in patients who receive the drug.

▪ **Interactions** specifies the clinically significant additive, synergistic, or antagonistic effects that result from combined use of the drug with other drugs. Interactions are broken down into four categories: drug-drug, drug-herb, drug-food, and drug-lifestyle. The interacting agent is italicized.

▪ **Effects on diagnostic tests** lists significant interference with a diagnostic test or its result by direct effects on the test itself or by systemic drug effects that lead to misleading test results.

▪ **Adverse reactions** lists the undesirable effects that may follow use of the drug; these effects are arranged by body systems (CNS, CV, EENT, GI, GU, Hematologic, Hepatic, Metabolic, Musculoskeletal, Respiratory, Skin, and Other). Local effects occur at the site of drug administration (by application, infusion, or injection); adverse reactions not specific to a single body system (for example, the effects of hypersensitivity) are listed under Other. The most common adverse reactions (those experienced by at least 10% of all people taking the drug in clinical trials) are in *italic* type; less common reactions are in roman type; life-threatening reactions are in ***bold italic*** type; and reactions that are both common and life-threatening are in **BOLD CAPITAL** letters. At the end of this section, Note signals a list of severe and hazardous reactions that mandate discontinuation of the drug.

▪ **Overdose and treatment** summarizes the signs and symptoms of drug overdose and recommends specific treatment as appropriate. Usually, this segment recommends emesis or gastric lavage, followed by activated charcoal to reduce the amount of drug absorbed and possibly a cathartic to eliminate the toxin. This section specifies antidotes, drug therapy, and other special care, if known. It also specifies the effects of hemodialysis or peritoneal dialysis for dialyzable drugs.

▪ **Clinical considerations** offers recommendations specific to the drug for preparation and administration, and for care and teaching of the patient during therapy. This section includes pointers for preventing and treating adverse reactions, for promoting patient comfort, and for storing the drug. Recommendations common to all members of the pharmacologic class of the drug are listed only in the relevant pharmacologic class entry. An ***ALERT*** logo points out drugs that are likely to cause medication errors, such as those with sound-alike drug names.

▪ **Therapeutic monitoring** provides recommendations for monitoring the effects of drug therapy.

▪ **Special populations** offers recommendations for drug therapy in pregnant, breast-feeding, pediatric, and geriatric patients.

▪ **Patient counseling** lists patient teaching guidelines to use during drug therapy.

Photoguide

This section provides full-color photographs of more than 320 of the most commonly prescribed tablets and capsules in the United States. They are shown actual size and organized alphabetically for quick reference. A page reference to drug information appears with each drug shown.

Appendices

The appendices include a review of subcutaneous, intramuscular, and intravenous injection techniques; therapeutic drug monitoring guidelines; guidelines for use of selected antimicrobials; a summary of selected analgesic combination products; a chart of cancer chemotherapy acronyms; an immunization schedule; a table of cytochrome P-450 enzymes and common drug interactions; a guide to selected antidotes; calculations for creatinine clearance; and a guide to herbal medicines.

Index

The index lists both the generic and trade names, diseases, and pharmacologic classes. Generic drugs and pharmacologic classes appear alphabetically within the main text.

Common abbreviations

AIDS	acquired immunodeficiency syndrome
ALT	alanine aminotransferase
AST	aspartate aminotransferase
ATP	adenosine triphosphate
AV	atrioventricular
b.i.d.	twice a day
BPH	benign prostatic hyperplasia
BUN	blood urea nitrogen
cAMP	cyclic 3', 5' adenosine monophosphate
CBC	complete blood count
CK	creatine kinase
CNS	central nervous system
COPD	chronic obstructive pulmonary disease
CPR	cardiopulmonary resuscitation
CSF	cerebrospinal fluid
CV	cardiovascular
CVA	cerebrovascular accident
CVP	central venous pressure
DIC	disseminated intravascular coagulation
DNA	deoxyribonucleic acid
ECG	electrocardiogram
EEG	electroencephalogram
FDA	Food and Drug Administration
g	gram
G	gauge
GGT	gamma glutamyltransferase
G6PD	glucose-6-phosphate dehydrogenase
GI	gastrointestinal
GU	genitourinary
HIV	human immunodeficiency virus
h.s.	at bedtime
I.D.	intradermal
I.M.	intramuscular
INR	international normalized ratio
IU	International Unit
I.V.	intravenous
kg	kilogram
L	liter
LD	lactate dehydrogenase
m^2	square meter
mm^3	cubic millimeter
MAO	monoamine oxidase
mcg	microgram
mEq	milliequivalent
mg	milligram
MI	myocardial infarction
ml	milliliter
ng	nanogram (millimicrogram)
NSAID	nonsteroidal anti-inflammatory drug
OTC	over-the-counter
P.O.	by mouth
P.R.	per rectum
p.r.n.	as needed
PT	prothrombin time
PVC	premature ventricular contraction
q	every
q.i.d.	four times a day
RBC	red blood cell
RNA	ribonucleic acid
SA	sinoatrial
S.C.	subcutaneous
SIADH	syndrome of inappropriate antidiuretic hormone
S.L.	sublingually
T_3	triiodothyronine
T_4	thyroxine
t.i.d.	three times a day
WBC	white blood cell

Pharmacologic classes

adrenergics, direct and indirect acting

albuterol sulfate, arbutamine hydrochloride, bitolterol mesylate, brimonidine tartrate, dobutamine hydrochloride, dopamine hydrochloride, ephedrine, ephedrine hydrochloride, ephedrine sulfate, epinephrine, epinephrine bitartrate, epinephrine hydrochloride, epinephryl borate, isoetharine hydrochloride, isoetharine mesylate, isoproterenol, isoproterenol hydrochloride, isoproterenol sulfate, metaproterenol sulfate, metaraminol bitartrate, naphazoline hydrochloride, norepinephrine bitartrate, phenylephrine hydrochloride, pirbuterol acetate, pseudoephedrine hydrochloride, pseudoephedrine sulfate, ritodrine hydrochloride, salmeterol xinafoate, terbutaline sulfate, tetrahydrozoline hydrochloride, xylometazoline hydrochloride

Beta-receptor activation is associated with the activation of adenylate cyclase and the accumulation of cAMP; the cellular consequences of alpha-receptor activation are less well understood.

Alpha$_1$ receptors are located on smooth muscle and glands and are excitatory; alpha$_2$ receptors are prejunctional regulatory receptors in the CNS and postjunctional receptors in many peripheral tissues. Beta$_1$ receptors are located in cardiac tissues and are excitatory; beta$_2$ receptors are located primarily on smooth muscle and glands and are inhibitory.

Adrenergic drugs may mimic the naturally occurring catecholamines norepinephrine, epinephrine, and dopamine or may function by stimulating the release of norepinephrine.

Pharmacology

Most actions of clinically useful adrenergic agents involve peripheral excitatory actions on glands and vascular smooth muscle; cardiac and CNS excitatory actions; peripheral inhibitory actions on smooth muscle of the bronchial tree and blood vessels supplying skeletal muscles and gut; and metabolic and endocrine effects. Because different tissues respond in varying degrees to adrenergic agonists, differences in the actions of catecholamines are attributed to the presence of different receptor types within the tissues (alpha and beta).

Clinical indications and actions

Most agents act on two or more receptor sites; the net effect is the sum of alpha and beta activity. Dopaminergic and serotonergic activity may occur, possibly stimulating receptors in the CNS to release histamine.

Temporary appetite suppression is another effect, often resulting in a reboundlike weight gain after tolerance to the anorexic effect develops or after withdrawal of the drug. Other uses include support of blood pressure, suppression of urinary incontinence and enuresis, and relief from pain of dysmenorrhea.

Hypotension

Alpha agonists, such as norepinephrine, metaraminol, phenylephrine, and pseudoephedrine, cause arteriolar and venous constriction, resulting in increased blood pressure. This action helps support blood pressure in hypotension and in management of serious allergic conditions. Topical formulations are used to induce local vasoconstriction (decongestion), arrest superficial hemorrhage (styptic), stimulate radial smooth muscle of the iris (mydriasis), and, with local anesthetics, localize anesthesia and prolong duration of action. Ophthalmic preparations reduce aqueous humor production and increase uveoscleral outflow.

Cardiac stimulation

Beta$_1$ agonists, such as dobutamine, act primarily in the heart, producing a positive inotropic effect. Because they increase heart rate, enhance AV conduction, and increase the strength of the heartbeat, beta$_1$ agonists may be used to restore heartbeat in cardiac arrest and for heart block in syncopal seizures, which isn't a treatment of choice, or to treat acute heart failure and cardiogenic or other types of shock. Their use in shock is somewhat controversial, because beta$_1$ agonists induce lipolysis (increase of free fatty acids in plasma), which promotes a metabolic acidosis, and because they favor arrhythmias, which pose a special threat in cardiogenic shock.

Bronchodilation

Beta$_2$ agonists, such as albuterol, bitolterol, isoetharine, metaproterenol, salmeterol, pirbuterol, and terbutaline, act primarily on smooth muscle of the bronchial tree, vasculature, intestines, and uterus. They also induce hepatic and muscle glycogenolysis, which results in hyperglycemia (sometimes useful in insulin overdose) and hyperlactic acidemia.

Some are used as bronchodilators, some as vasodilators. They're also used to relax the uterus, to delay delivery in premature labor, and for dysmenorrhea. Some degree of cardiostimulation may occur, because all beta$_2$ agonists have some degree of beta$_1$ activity.

Renal vasodilation
Dopamine is currently the only commercially available sympathomimetic with significant dopaminergic activity, although some other sympathomimetics appear to act on dopamine receptors in the CNS. Dopamine receptors are prominent in the periphery (splanchnic and renal vasculature), where they mediate vasodilation, which is useful in inducing diuresis in patients with acute renal failure, heart failure, and shock.

Overview of adverse reactions
Geriatric patients, infants, and patients with thyrotoxicosis or CV disease are more sensitive to the effects of these drugs.

Alpha agonists commonly produce CV reactions. An excessive increase in blood pressure is a major adverse reaction of systemically administered alpha agonists. Exaggerated pressor response may occur in hypertensive or geriatric patients, which may evoke vagal reflex responses and result in bradycardia and AV block. Alpha agonists also interfere with lactation and may cause nausea, vomiting, sweating, piloerection, rebound congestion or miosis, difficult urination, and headache. Ophthalmic use may cause mydriasis, photophobia, burning, stinging, and blurring.

Beta agonists most frequently cause tachycardia, palpitations, and other arrhythmias. Their other effects include premature atrial and ventricular contractions; tachyarrhythmias, and myocardial necrosis. Reflex tachycardia and palpitations occur with $beta_2$ agonists because of decreased blood pressure.

Metabolic reactions to beta agonists include hyperglycemia, increased metabolic rate, hyperlactic acidosis, and local and systemic acidosis (decreased bronchodilator response).

Respiratory reactions include increased perfusion of nonfunctioning portions of lungs (COPD); mucous plugs may develop as a result of increased mucus secretion. Other reactions include tremors, vertigo, insomnia, sweating, headache, nausea, vomiting, and anxiety.

Centrally acting adrenergics have similar effects, which may also be associated with dry mouth, flushing, diarrhea, impotence, hyperthermia (excessive doses), agitation, anorexia, dizziness, dyskinesia, and changes in libido. Chronic use of adrenergics in children may cause endocrine disturbances that arrest growth; however, growth usually rebounds after withdrawal of drug.

Clinical considerations
Parenteral preparations
- If used as a pressor agent, recommend correcting fluid volume depletion before administration. Adrenergics aren't a substitute for blood, plasma, fluid, or electrolytes.
- Recommend carefully monitoring blood pressure, pulse, and respiratory and urinary output during therapy.
- Tachyphylaxis or tolerance may develop after prolonged or excessive use.

Inhalation therapy
- The preservative sodium bisulfite is present in many adrenergic formulations. Patients with a history of allergy to sulfites should avoid drugs that contain this preservative.
- Recommend administering when patient arises in morning and before meals, to reduce fatigue by improving ventilation.
- For unknown reasons, paradoxical airway resistance, manifested by sudden increase in dyspnea, may result from repeated excessive use of isoetharine. If this occurs, tell patient to discontinue drug and use alternative therapy, such as epinephrine.
- Adrenergic inhalation may be alternated with other drug administration (steroids, other adrenergics), if necessary, but avoid giving simultaneously because of danger of excessive tachycardia.
- Don't use discolored or precipitated solutions.
- Protect solutions from light, freezing, and heat. Store at controlled room temperature.
- Systemic absorption, although infrequent, can follow applications to nasal and conjunctival membranes. Advise patient to stop drug if symptoms of systemic absorption occur.
- Prolonged or too-frequent use may cause tolerance to bronchodilating and cardiac stimulant effect. Rebound bronchospasm may follow end of drug effect.

Special populations
Pregnant patients. Pregnancy risk categories range from B to D in this group. Refer to specific package insert for manufacturer recommendations.

Breast-feeding patients. The use of adrenergics during breast-feeding usually isn't recommended.

Pediatric patients. Lower doses of adrenergics are recommended.

Geriatric patients. May be more sensitive to therapeutic and adverse effects of some adrenergics and may require lower doses.

Patient counseling
Inhalation therapy
- Instruct patient in correct use of nebulizer and warn to use lowest effective dose.
- Explain that overuse of adrenergic bronchodilators may cause tachycardia, headache, nausea and dizziness, loss of effectiveness, possible paradoxical reaction, and cardiac arrest.
- Tell patient to contact his health care provider if bronchodilator causes dizziness, chest pain, or lack of therapeutic response to usual dose.
- Advise patient to avoid other adrenergic medications unless they're prescribed.

■ Inform patient that saliva and sputum may appear pink after inhalation treatment.
■ Instruct patient to begin treatment with first symptoms of bronchospasm.
■ Caution patient to keep spray away from eyes.
■ Tell patient not to discard drug applicator. Refill units are available.

Nasal therapy

■ Instruct patient to blow nose gently, with both nostrils open, to clear nasal passages before administration of medication.
■ Instruct patient on proper method of instillation, as follows:
— Drops: Tilt head back while sitting or standing up, or lie on bed with head over side. Stay in position a few minutes to permit medication to spread through nose.
— Spray: With head upright, squeeze bottle quickly and firmly to produce 1 or 2 sprays into each nostril; wait 3 to 5 minutes, blow nose, and repeat dose.
— Jelly: Place in each nostril and sniff it well back into nose.
■ Tell patient not to use nasal decongestant for longer than 3 to 5 days.

Ophthalmic therapy

■ Tell patient to apply pressure to lacrimal sac during and for 1 to 2 minutes after instillation of drops to avoid excessive systemic absorption.
■ Inform patient that after instillation of ophthalmic preparation, pupils of eyes will be very large and eyes may be more sensitive to light than usual. Advise patient to wear dark glasses until pupils return to normal.
■ Warn patient to use drug only as directed.
■ Instruct patient to contact his health care provider if no relief occurs or condition worsens.
■ Tell patient to store drug away from heat and light and out of reach of children.
■ Advise patient not to use drug for longer than 48 to 72 hours without consulting a doctor.

Representative combinations

Ephedrine sulfate with guaifenesin and theophylline: Bronkolixir; with guaifenesin, theophylline, and phenobarbital: Bronkotabs; with belladonna extract, boric acid, zinc oxide, beeswax, and cocoa butter: Wyanoids Relief Factor.

Epinephrine with benzalkonium chloride: Glaucon; with pilocarpine: E-Pilo.

Isoproterenol hydrochloride with phenylephrine bitartrate: Duo-Medihaler.

Naphazoline with antazoline phosphate, boric acid, phenylmercuric acetate, and carbonate anhydrous: Vasocon-A Solution; with pheniramine maleate: Naphcon-A; with phenylephrine hydrochloride, pyrilamine maleate, and phenylpropanolamine hydrochloride: 4-Way Long Lasting Spray; with polyvinyl alcohol: Albalon.

Pseudoephedrine with chlorpheniramine maleate: Chlor-Trimeton; with codeine phosphate and guaifenesin: Alamine Expectorant, Deproist Expectorant with Codeine, Guiatussin DAC, Isoclor Expectorant, Novahistine Expectorant, Robitussin-DAC; with dextromethorphan and acetaminophen: Contac Severe Cold and Flu Nighttime; with dextromethorphan, acetaminophen, and guaifenesin: Vicks 44M Cough, Cold, and Flu Relief; with dexbrompheniramine: Disophrol, Drixoral; with dexchlorpheniramine: Polaramine; with guaifenesin: Robitussin-PE, Zephrex; with hydrocordone bitartrate: De-Tuss, Detussin Liquid, Entuss-D, Tussend; with triprolidine: Actagen, Actamin, Actifed, Allerfrim Tablets, Aprodine, Cenafed Plus, Triposed.

See also *antihistamines, barbiturates, and xanthine derivatives.*

adrenocorticoids (nasal and oral inhalation)

Nasal: beclomethasone dipropionate, budesonide, flunisolide, fluticasone propionate, triamcinolone acetonide

Oral: beclomethasone dipropionate, budesonide, flunisolide, fluticasone propionate, triamcinolone acetonide

Topical administration through oral aerosol and nasal spray delivers adrenocorticoids to sites of inflammation in the nasal passages or the tracheobronchial tree. Because smaller doses are administered, less drug is absorbed systemically, with fewer systemic adverse effects.

Pharmacology

Inhaled glucocorticoid is absorbed through the nasal mucosa or through the trachea, bronchi, and alveoli. The anti-inflammatory effects of glucocorticoids depend on the direct local action of the steroid. Glucocorticoids stimulate transcription of messenger RNA in individual cell nuclei to synthesize enzymes that decrease inflammation. These enzymes stimulate biochemical pathways that decrease the inflammatory response by stabilizing leukocyte lysosomal membranes, which prevent the release of destructive acid hydrolases from leukocytes; inhibiting macrophage accumulation in inflamed areas; reducing leukocyte adhesion to the capillary endothelium; reducing capillary wall permeability and edema formation; decreasing complement components; antagonizing histamine activity and release of kinin from substrates; reducing fibroblast proliferation, collagen deposition, and scar tissue formation; and by other unknown mechanisms.

NASAL ADRENOCORTICOIDS FOR INFLAMMATION DUE TO ALLERGIC RHINITIS

Drug	Pediatric daily dose*	Adult daily dose*
beclomethasone dipropionate	**Nasal aerosol:** Under age 6: not recommended Ages 6-12: 84 mcg b.i.d. to q.i.d. Maximum dose: 168-336 mcg/day **Nasal solution** Under age 6: not recommended Ages 6-12: 84 mcg t.i.d. Maximum dose: 252 mcg/day	**Nasal aerosol:** 84 mcg b.i.d. to q.i.d. Maximum dose: 168-336 mcg/day **Nasal solution:** 84-168 mcg b.i.d. Maximum dose: 336 mcg/day
budesonide	**Nasal powder:** Under age 6: not recommended Ages 6-12: 200-400 mcg/day Maximum dose: 400 mcg/day **Nasal solution:** Under age 6: not recommended Ages 6-12: 64-256 mcg/day Maximum dose: 256 mcg/day	**Nasal powder:** 200-400 mcg/day Maximum dose: 800 mcg/day **Nasal solution:** 64-256 mcg/day Maximum dose: 256 mcg/day
flunisolide	**Nasal solution:** Under age 6: not recommended Ages 6-14: 50-100 mcg b.i.d. Maximum dose: 200 mcg/day	**Nasal solution:** 50-100 mcg b.i.d. to t.i.d. Maximum dose: 400 mcg/day
fluticasone propionate	**Nasal solution:** Under age 4: not recommended Ages 4-12: 100-200 mcg once daily Maximum dose: 200 mcg/day	**Nasal solution:** 100-200 mcg once daily Maximum dose: 200 mcg daily
triamcinolone acetonide	**Nasal aerosol:** Under age 5: not recommended Ages 6-12: 110-220 mcg once daily Maximum dose: 220 mcg/day **Nasal solution:** Under age 6: not recommended Ages 6-12: 110-220 mcg/day Maximum dose: 220 mcg/day	**Nasal aerosol:** 110-220 mcg once daily Maximum dose: 440 mcg/day **Nasal solution:** 110-220 mcg/day Maximum dose: 220 mcg/day

* Total doses to both nostrils.

Clinical indications and actions

Nasal inflammation

Nasal solutions are used to relieve symptoms of seasonal or perennial rhinitis when antihistamines and decongestants are ineffective, to treat inflammatory conditions of the nasal passages, and to prevent recurrence after surgical removal of nasal polyps. (See *Nasal adrenocorticoids for inflammation due to allergic rhinitis.*)

Chronic bronchial asthma

Aerosols treat chronic bronchial asthma not controlled by bronchodilators and other nonsteroidal drugs. (See *Oral inhalation adrenocorticoids for chronic bronchial asthma.*)

Overview of adverse reactions

Nasal: Local sensations of nasal burning and irritation occur in about 10% of patients; sneezing attacks occur immediately after nasal application in about 10% of patients; transient mild nosebleeds occur in 10% to 15% of patients. It's unknown whether these are effects of the nasal solution or of the dryness it induces in the nasal passages. Localized candidal infections of the nose or pharynx rarely occur.

Oral: Localized infections with *Candida albicans* or *Aspergillus niger* occur commonly in the mouth and pharynx and occasionally in the larynx.

Systemic: Systemic absorption may occur, potentially leading to hypothalamic-pituitary-adrenal (HPA) axis suppression. This is more likely to occur with large doses or with combined nasal and oral corticosteroid therapy.

Other: Hypersensitivity reactions are possible. Some patients may be intolerant of the fluorocarbon propellants in the preparations.

Clinical considerations

- Full therapeutic benefit requires regular use and is usually evident within a few days, although a few patients may require up to 3 weeks of therapy for maximum benefit. Discontinue therapy in the absence of significant sympto-

ORAL INHALATION ADRENOCORTICOIDS FOR CHRONIC BRONCHIAL ASTHMA

Drug	Pediatric daily dose	Adult daily dose
beclomethasone dipropionate	**Inhalation aerosol:** Under age 6: not recommended Ages 6-12: 42-84 mcg t.i.d. to q.i.d. or 168 mcg b.i.d. Maximum dose: 420 mcg/day	**Inhalation aerosol:** 84 mcg t.i.d. to q.i.d. or 168 mcg b.i.d. Maximum dose: 840 mcg/day
budesonide	**Inhalation powder:** Under age 6: not recommended Ages 6-12: 200-400 mcg b.i.d. Maximum dose: 800 mcg/day	**Inhalation powder:** 200-400 mcg b.i.d. Maximum dose: 1600 mcg/day
flunisolide	**Inhalation aerosol:** Under age 6: not recommended Over age 6: 500 mcg b.i.d. Maximum dose: 1 mg/day	**Inhalation aerosol:** 500 mcg b.i.d. Maximum dose: 2 mg/day
fluticasone propionate	**Inhalation aerosol:** Under age 12: not recommended **Inhalation powder:** Under age 4: not recommended Ages 4-11: 50 mcg b.i.d. Maximum dose: 200 mcg/day	**Inhalation aerosol:** 88-440 mcg b.i.d. Maximum dose: 1,760 mcg/day **Inhalation powder:** 100-500 mcg b.i.d. Maximum dose: 2 mg/day
triamcinolone acetonide	**Inhalation aerosol:** Under age 6: not recommended Ages 6-12: 100-200 mcg t.i.d. or q.i.d., or 200-400 mcg b.i.d. Maximum dose: 1,200 mcg/day	**Inhalation aerosol:** 200 mcg t.i.d. or q.i.d., or 400 mcg b.i.d. Maximum dose: 1,600 mcg/day

matic improvement within recommended time frame (varies with drug used).

■ Use of nasal or oral inhalation therapy may allow a patient to discontinue systemic corticosteroid therapy.

■ After the desired clinical effect is obtained, reduce maintenance dosage to the smallest amount necessary to control symptoms.

■ Discontinue drug if signs of systemic absorption (such as Cushing's syndrome, hyperglycemia, or glucosuria), mucosal irritation or ulceration, hypersensitivity, or infection develop. If antifungals or antibiotics are being used with corticosteroids and the infection doesn't respond immediately, discontinue corticosteroids until the infection is controlled.

Special populations

Pregnant patients. Corticosteroids shouldn't be used, especially in large doses or for long periods of time. They should only be used when the potential benefits outweigh the potential risks.

Breast-feeding patients. Use with caution. Corticosteroids may cause growth suppression in infants if drug is secreted in breast milk.

Pediatric patients. Nasal or oral inhalant corticosteroid therapy may be successfully substituted for systemic corticosteroid therapy. However, the risk of HPA axis suppression and Cushing's syndrome still exists.

Geriatric patients. Many geriatric patients have conditions that could be aggravated by the excessive use of corticosteroid inhalant therapy. Geriatric patients have a reduced ability to metabolize and eliminate drugs; monitor patient closely for adverse effects.

Patient counseling

Nasal therapy

■ Instruct patient to use only as directed. Inform him that full therapeutic effect isn't immediate but requires regular use of inhaler.

■ Encourage patient with blocked nasal passages to use an oral decongestant 30 minutes before intranasal corticosteroid administration to ensure adequate penetration. Advise patient to clear nasal passages of secretions before using the inhaler.

■ Instruct patient to clean inhaler according to manufacturer's instructions.

Oral therapy

■ Instruct patient to use only as directed.

■ Advise patient receiving bronchodilators by inhalation to use the bronchodilator before the corticosteroid to enhance penetration of the corticosteroid into the bronchial tree. He should wait several minutes to allow time for the bronchodilator to relax the smooth muscle.

■ Instruct patient to hold his breath for a few seconds to enhance placement and action of the drug and to wait 1 minute before taking subsequent puffs of medication.

■ Tell patient to rinse mouth with water after using the inhaler to decrease the chance of oral fungal infections. Tell him to check nasal and oral mucous membranes frequently for signs of fungal infection.

- Instruct patient to clean inhaler properly.
- Warn asthmatic patient not to increase use of corticosteroid inhaler during a severe asthma attack, but to call for adjustment of therapy, possibly by adding a systemic steroid.
- Inform patient that medication is for preventative therapy, not to abort an acute attack.

Nasal or oral therapy

- Tell patient to report decreased response; dosage adjustment or discontinuation of drug may be needed.
- Instruct patient to observe for adverse effects and, if fever or local irritation develops, to discontinue use and report the effect promptly.

Representative combinations

None.

adrenocorticoids (systemic)

Glucocorticoids: **betamethasone, betamethasone sodium phosphate, betamethasone sodium phosphate and betamethasone acetate, cortisone acetate, dexamethasone, dexamethasone acetate, dexamethasone sodium phosphate, hydrocortisone, hydrocortisone acetate, hydrocortisone cypionate, hydrocortisone sodium phosphate, hydrocortisone sodium succinate, methylprednisolone, methylprednisolone acetate, methylprednisolone sodium succinate, prednisolone, prednisolone acetate, prednisolone sodium phosphate, prednisolone tebutate, prednisone, triamcinolone, triamcinolone acetonide, triamcinolone diacetate, triamcinolone hexacetonide**

Mineralocorticoid: **fludrocortisone acetate**

Active adrenocortical extracts were first prepared in 1930; by 1942, chemists had isolated 28 steroids from the adrenal cortex.

Adrenocortical hormones are classified according to their activity into two groups: mineralocorticoids and glucocorticoids. Mineralocorticoids regulate electrolyte homeostasis. Glucocorticoids regulate carbohydrate, lipid, and protein metabolism; inflammation; and the body's immune responses to diverse stimuli. Many corticosteroids exert both kinds of activity. (See *Comparing systemic glucocorticoids.*)

Pharmacology

Corticosteroids dramatically affect almost all body systems. They control the rate of protein synthesis, reacting with receptor proteins in the cytoplasm of sensitive cells to form a steroid-receptor complex. Steroid receptors have been identified in many tissues. The steroid-receptor complex migrates into the nucleus of the cell, where it binds to chromatin. Information carried by the steroid of the receptor protein directs the genetic apparatus to transcribe RNA, resulting in the synthesis of specific proteins that serve as enzymes in various biochemical pathways. Because the maximum pharmacologic activity lags behind peak blood levels, the effects of corticosteroids may result from modification of enzyme activity rather than from direct action by the drugs.

Glucocorticoids stimulate transcription of messenger RNA in individual cell nuclei to synthesize enzymes that decrease inflammation. These enzymes stimulate biochemical pathways that decrease the inflammatory response by stabilizing leukocyte lysosomal membranes, which prevent the release of destructive acid hydrolases from leukocytes; inhibiting macrophage accumulation in inflamed areas; reducing leukocyte adhesion to the capillary endothelium; reducing capillary wall permeability and edema formation; decreasing complement components; antagonizing histamine activity and release of kinin from substrates; reducing fibroblast proliferation, collagen deposition, and scar tissue formation; and by other unknown mechanisms.

Mineralocorticoids act renally at the distal tubules to enhance the reabsorption of sodium ions, and thus water, from the tubular fluid into the plasma, and the urinary excretion of both potassium and hydrogen ions. The primary features of excess mineralocorticoid activity are positive sodium balance and expansion of the extracellular fluid volume, normal or slight increase in the level of sodium in the plasma, hypokalemia, and alkalosis. In contrast, deficiency of mineralocorticoids produces sodium loss, hyponatremia, hyperkalemia, contraction of the extracellular fluid volume, and cellular dehydration.

Clinical indications and actions

Asthma

Treatment of status asthmaticus and acute asthma episodes. Therapy is combined with sympathomimetics and aminophylline.

Sarcoidosis

Therapy is aimed at the management of ocular, CNS, glandular, myocardial, or severe pulmonary involvement. Systemic glucocorticoids may also be used for hypercalcemia or severe skin lesions.

Advanced pulmonary or extrapulmonary tuberculosis

Systemic glucocorticoids have been used to help decrease inflammation caused by *Mycobacterium tuberculosis.*

COMPARING SYSTEMIC GLUCOCORTICOIDS

Drug	Approximate equivalent dose (mg)	Relative glucocorticoid (anti-inflammatory) potency	Relative mineralocorticoid potency	Plasma half-life (hr)	Biological half-life (hr)
betamethasone, oral	0.6-0.75	20-30	0	> 5	36-54
betamethasone acetate	0.6-0.75	20-30	0	> 5	36-54
betamethasone sodium phosphate	0.6-0.75	20-30	0	> 5	36-54
cortisone acetate	25	0.8	2	½	8-12
dexamethasone, oral	0.5-0.75	20-30	0	2-3½	36-54
dexamethasone acetate	0.5-0.75	20-30	0	2-3½	36-54
dexamethasone sodium phosphate	0.5-0.75	20-30	0	2-3½	36-54
hydrocortisone, oral	20	1	2	1½-2	8-12
hydrocortisone acetate	20	1	2	1½-2	8-12
hydrocortisone cypionate	20	1	2	1½-2	8-12
hydrocortisone sodium phosphate	20	1	2	1½-2	8-12
hydrocortisone sodium succinate	20	1	2	1½-2	8-12
methylprednisolone, oral	4	5	0	1-3	18-6
methylprednisolone acetate	4	5	0	1-3	18-36
methylprednisolone sodium succinate	4	5	0	1-3	18-36
prednisolone, oral	5	4	1	2¼-3½	18-36
prednisolone acetate	5	4	1	2¼-3½	18-36
prednisolone sodium phosphate	5	4	1	2¼-3½	18-36
prednisolone tebutate	5	4	1	2¼-3½	18-36
prednisone	5	4	1	1	18-36
triamcinolone, oral	4	5	0	>3⅓	18-36
triamcinolone acetonide	4	5	0	>3⅓	18-36
triamcinolone diacetate	4	5	0	>3⅓	18-36
triamcinolone hexacetonide	4	5	0	>3⅓	18-36

Pericarditis
Unlabeled use for systemic glucocorticoids for the treatment of pain, fever, and inflammation of pericarditis.

Inflammation
A major pharmacologic use of glucocorticoids is treatment of inflammation. The anti-inflammatory effects depend on the direct local action of the steroids. Glucocorticoids decrease the inflammatory response by stabilizing leukocyte lysosomal membranes, which prevent the release of destructive acid hydrolases from leukocytes; inhibiting macrophage accumulation in inflamed areas; reducing leukocyte adhesion to the capillary endothelium; reducing capillary wall permeability and edema formation; decreasing complement components; antagonizing histamine activity and release of kinin from substrates; reducing fibroblast proliferation, collagen deposition, and subsequent scar tissue formation; and by other unknown mechanisms.

Immunosuppression
The full mechanisms of immunosuppressive actions are unknown. Glucocorticoids reduce activity and volume of the lymphatic system, producing lymphocytopenia, decreasing immunoglobulin and complement concentrations, decreasing passage of immune complexes through basement membranes, and possibly depressing reactivity of tissue to antigen-antibody interaction.
Adrenal insufficiency
Combined mineralocorticoid and glucocorticoid therapy is used in treating adrenal insufficiency and in salt-losing forms of congenital adrenogenital syndrome.
Rheumatic and collagen diseases; other severe diseases
Glucocorticoids are used to treat rheumatic and collagen diseases, such as arthritis, polyarteritis nodosa, and systemic lupus erythematosus; thyroiditis; severe dermatologic diseases, such as pemphigus, exfoliative dermatitis, lichen planus, and psoriasis; allergic reactions; ocular disorders, such as inflammations; respiratory diseases, such as asthma, sarcoidosis, and lipid pneumonitis; hematologic diseases, such as autoimmune hemolytic anemia and idiopathic thrombocytopenia; neoplastic diseases, such as leukemias and lymphomas; and GI diseases, such as ulcerative colitis, regional enteritis, and celiac disease. Other indications include myasthenia gravis, organ transplantation, nephrotic syndrome, and septic shock.
Antenatal use in preterm labor
Dexamethasone and betamethasone have been used as short-course I.M. therapy in women with preterm labor to hasten fetal maturation of lungs and cerebral blood vessels.
Hypercalcemia
Glucocorticoids are used to treat hypercalcemia secondary to sarcoidosis, vitamin D intoxication, multiple myeloma, and breast cancer in postmenopausal women.
Cerebral edema
High-dose parenteral glucocorticoid administration may decrease cerebral edema in brain tumors and during neurosurgery.
Acute spinal cord injury
Large I.V. doses of glucocorticoids, when given shortly after injury, may improve motor and sensory function in patients with acute spinal cord injury.

Overview of adverse reactions

Suppression of the hypothalamic-pituitary-adrenal (HPA) axis is the major effect of systemic therapy with corticosteroids. When administered in high doses or for prolonged therapy, glucocorticoids suppress release of corticotropin from the pituitary gland; subsequently, the adrenal cortex stops secreting endogenous corticosteroids. The degree and duration of HPA axis suppression produced by the drugs is highly variable among patients and depends on the dose, frequency and time of administration, and duration of therapy.

Patients with a suppressed HPA axis resulting from exogenous glucocorticoid administration who abruptly discontinue therapy may experience severe withdrawal symptoms, such as fever, myalgia, arthralgia, malaise, anorexia, nausea, desquamation of skin, orthostatic hypotension, dizziness, fainting, dyspnea, and hypoglycemia. Therefore, corticosteroid therapy should always be withdrawn gradually.

Adrenal suppression may persist for as long as 12 months in patients who have received large doses for prolonged periods. Until complete recovery occurs, patients subjected to stress may show signs and symptoms of adrenal insufficiency and may need glucocorticoid and mineralocorticoid replacement therapy.

Cushingoid symptoms, the effects of excessive glucocorticoid therapy, may develop in patients receiving large doses of glucocorticoids over several weeks or longer. These include moon face, central obesity, striae, hirsutism, acne, ecchymoses, hypertension, osteoporosis, muscle atrophy, sexual dysfunction, diabetes, cataracts, hyperlipidemia, peptic ulcer, increased susceptibility to infection, and fluid and electrolyte imbalances.

Other adverse reactions to normal or high doses of corticosteroids may include CNS effects (euphoria, insomnia, psychotic behavior, pseudotumor cerebri, mental changes, nervousness, restlessness); CV effects (heart failure, hypertension, edema); GI effects (peptic ulcer, irritation, increased appetite); metabolic effects (hypokalemia, sodium retention, fluid retention, weight gain, hyperglycemia, osteoporosis); musculoskeletal effects (acute tendon rupture, muscle wasting and pain, myopathy); skin effects (delayed wound healing, acne, skin eruptions, muscle atrophy, striae, Kaposi's sarcoma); and immunosuppression (increased susceptibility to infection, activation of latent infection, exacerbation of intercurrent infections).

Clinical considerations

- The patient may experience sudden weight gain, edema, change in blood pressure, or change in electrolyte status.
- During times of physiologic stress, such as trauma, surgery, and infection, the patient may require additional steroids and may experience signs of steroid withdrawal; patients who were previously steroid-dependent may need systemic corticosteroids to prevent adrenal insufficiency.
- Reduce drug gradually in long-term therapy; rapid reduction may cause withdrawal symptoms.
- Caregivers should be aware of patient's psychological history and watch for behavioral changes.
- Observe patient for infection or delayed wound healing.

Special populations

Pregnant patients. Glucocorticoids may cause fetal abnormalities; avoid use if possible.

Breast-feeding patients. Women taking pharmacologic doses of corticosteroids shouldn't breast-feed.

Pediatric patients. Long-term administration of pharmacologic doses of glucocorticoids may retard bone growth. Signs and symptoms of adrenal suppression include retardation of linear growth, delayed weight gain, low plasma cortisol levels, and lack of response to corticotropin stimulation. Alternate-day therapy is recommended to minimize growth suppression. Benefits of therapy should strongly outweigh side effects.

Geriatric patients. Many geriatric patients have conditions that could easily be aggravated by corticosteroid therapy. Geriatric patients have a reduced ability to metabolize and eliminate drugs; monitor patient closely.

Patient counseling

- Explain the need to take the adrenocorticoid as prescribed. Give patient instructions on what to do if a dose is inadvertently missed.
- Warn patient not to stop drug abruptly.
- Inform patient of therapeutic and adverse effects of drug and tell him to report complications right away.
- Tell patient to carry a medical identification card noting the need for more adrenocorticoids during stress.

Representative combinations

Betamethasone sodium phosphate with betamethasone acetate: Celestone Soluspan.

Dexamethasone sodium phosphate with lidocaine hydrochloride: Decadron with Xylocaine.

adrenocorticoids (topical)

alclometasone dipropionate, amcinonide, betamethasone benzoate, betamethasone dipropionate, betamethasone valerate, clobetasol propionate, clocortolone pivalate, desonide, desoximetasone, dexamethasone, dexamethasone sodium phosphate, diflorasone diacetate, fluocinolone acetonide, fluocinonide, flurandrenolide, fluticasone propionate, halcinonide, halobetasol propionate, hydrocortisone, hydrocortisone acetate, hydrocortisone butyrate, hydrocortisone valerate, methylprednisolone acetate, triamcinolone acetonide

Since topical hydrocortisone was introduced in the 1950s, numerous analogues have been developed to provide a wide range of potencies in creams, ointments, lotions, and gels.

Pharmacology

The anti-inflammatory effects of topical glucocorticoids depend on the direct local action of the steroid. Although the exact mechanism of action is unclear, many researchers believe that glucocorticoids stimulate transcription of messenger RNA in individual cell nuclei to synthesize enzymes that decrease inflammation. These enzymes stimulate biochemical pathways that decrease the inflammatory response by stabilizing leukocyte lysosomal membranes, which prevents the release of destructive acid hydrolases from leukocytes, inhibiting macrophage accumulation in inflamed areas; reducing leukocyte adhesion to the capillary endothelium; reducing capillary wall permeability and edema formation; decreasing complement components; antagonizing histamine activity and release of kinin from substrates; and reducing fibroblast proliferation, collagen deposition, and subsequent scar tissue formation; and by other unknown mechanisms.

Topical corticosteroids are minimally absorbed systemically and cause fewer adverse effects than systemically administered corticosteroids. Fluorinated derivatives are absorbed to a greater extent than are other topical steroids. The degree of absorption depends on the site of application, the amount applied, the relative potency, the presence of an occlusive dressing (may increase penetration by 10%), the condition of the skin, and the vehicle carrying the drug. Topical corticosteroids are used to relieve pruritus, inflammation, and other signs of corticosteroid-responsive dermatoses.

Ointments are preferred for dry, scaly areas; solutions, gels, aerosols, and lotions for hairy areas. Creams can be used for most areas except those in which dampness may cause maceration. Gels and lotions can be used for moist lesions; however, gels may contain alcohol, which can dry and irritate the skin. The topical preparations are classified by potency into six groups: group I is the most potent and group VI the least potent. (See *Potencies of topical corticosteroids,* page 10.)

Clinical indications and actions

Inflammatory disorders of skin and mucous membranes

Topical adrenocorticoids relieve inflammatory and pruritic skin disorders, including localized neurodermatitis, psoriasis, atopic or seborrheic dermatitis, the inflammatory phase of xerosis, anogenital pruritus, discoid lupus erythematosus, lichen planus, granuloma annulare, and lupus erythematosus.

These drugs may also relieve irritant or allergic contact dermatitis; however, relief of acute dermatosis may require systemic adrenocorticoids.

Rectal disorders responsive to this class of drugs include ulcerative colitis, cryptitis, in-

POTENCIES OF TOPICAL CORTICOSTEROIDS

Topical corticosteroid preparations can be grouped according to relative anti-inflammatory activity. The following list arranges groups of topical corticosteroids in decreasing order of potency (based mainly on vasoconstrictor assay or clinical effectiveness in psoriasis). Preparations within each group are approximately equivalent.

Group	Drug	Concentration (%)
I	betamethasone dipropionate (Diprolene)	0.05
	betamethasone dipropionate (Diprolene AF)	0.05
	clobetasol propionate (Temovate)	0.05
	diflorasone diacetate (Psorcon)	0.05
II	amcinonide (Cyclocort)	0.1
	betamethasone dipropionate ointment (Diprosone)	0.05
	desoximetasone (Topicort)	0.05, 0.25
	diflorasone diacetate (Florone, Maxiflor)	0.05
	fluocinonide (Lidex)	0.05
	fluocinonide gel	0.05
	halcinonide (Halog)	0.1
III	betamethasone benzoate gel	0.025
	betamethasone dipropionate cream (Diprosone)	0.05
	betamethasone valerate ointment (Valisone)	0.1
	diflorasone diacetate cream (Florone, Maxiflor)	0.05
	triamcinolone acetonide cream (Aristocort)	0.5
IV	desoximetasone (Topicort LP)	0.05
	fluocinolone acetonide (Synalar-HP)	0.2
	fluocinolone acetonide ointment (Synalar)	0.025
	flurandrenolide (Cordran)	0.05
	fluticasone propionate (Cutivate)	0.005, 0.05
	triamcinolone acetonide ointment (Aristocort, Kenalog)	0.1
V	betamethasone benzoate cream	0.025
	betamethasone dipropionate lotion (Diprosone)	0.05
	betamethasone valerate cream or lotion (Valisone)	0.1
	fluocinolone acetonide cream (Synalar)	0.025
	flurandrenolide (Cordran)	0.05
	hydrocortisone butyrate (Locoid)	0.1
	hydrocortisone valerate (Westcort)	0.2
	triamcinolone acetonide cream or lotion (Kenalog)	0.1
VI	alclometasone dipropionate (Aclovate)	0.05
	desonide (Tridesilon)	0.05
	fluocinolone acetonide solution (Synalar)	0.01

flamed hemorrhoids, postirradiation or factitial proctitis, and pruritus ani.

Oral lesions, such as nonherpetic oral inflammatory and ulcerative lesions and routine gingivitis, may respond to treatment with topical adrenocorticoids.

OTC formulations of topical corticosteroids are indicated for minor skin irritation such as itching; rash caused by eczema, dermatitis, insect bites, poison ivy, poison oak, or poison sumac; or dermatitis caused by exposure to soaps, detergents, cosmetics, and jewelry.

Overview of adverse reactions

Local effects include burning, itching, irritation, dryness, folliculitis, striae, miliaria, acne, perioral dermatitis, hypopigmentation, hypertrichosis, allergic contact dermatitis, secondary infection, and atrophy.

Systemic absorption may occur, leading to hypothalamic-pituitary-adrenal (HPA) axis suppression.

The risk of adverse reactions increases with the use of occlusive dressings or more potent steroids, in patients with liver disease, and in children (because of their greater ratio of skin surface to body weight).

Prolonged application around the eyes may lead to cataracts or glaucoma.

Clinical considerations

- Wash hands before and after applying the drug.
- Gently clean the area of application. Washing or soaking the area before application may increase drug penetration.
- Apply sparingly in a light film; rub in lightly. Avoid contact with eyes, unless using an ophthalmic product.

- Avoid prolonged application of drug in areas near the eyes, genitals, rectum, face, and skin folds. High-potency topical corticosteroids are more likely to cause striae and atrophy in these areas because of their higher rates of absorption.
- Monitor response. Observe area of inflammation.
- Don't apply occlusive dressings over topical steroids.
- Stop drug if signs of systemic absorption develop.

Special populations

Pregnant patients. Safe use of topical steroids during pregnancy hasn't been established. It's unknown if topical steroids affect fertility.
Breast-feeding patients. Use topical corticosteroids with caution.
Pediatric patients. Limit topical corticosteroid therapy to the minimum amount necessary for therapeutic efficacy. Advise parents not to use tight-fitting diapers or plastic pants on a child whose diaper area is being treated, because such garments may act as occlusive dressings. Pediatric patients may be more susceptible to topical corticosteroid-induced HPA-axis suppression and Cushing's syndrome than adults because of a greater skin surface area-to-body weight ratio.
Geriatric patients. Loss of collagen may lead to friable and transparent skin with increased epidermal permeability to water and certain chemicals. Topically applied drugs such as steroid creams may have a greater effect locally than in younger patients. Geriatric patients also have a reduced ability to metabolize and eliminate drugs and may have higher plasma drug levels and more adverse reactions. Monitor closely.

Patient counseling

- Instruct patient on use of drug.
- Advise patient to discontinue drug and report local or systemic adverse reactions, worsening condition, or persistent symptoms.
- Warn patient not to use OTC topical products other than those specifically recommended.
- Tell patient to apply a missed dose as soon as it's remembered and to continue with his regular schedule of application. However, if it's almost time for the next application, tell him to wait and continue his regular schedule. He shouldn't apply a double dose.

Representative combinations

Betamethasone dipropionate with clotrimazole: Lotrisone.

Dexamethasone with neomycin sulfate: NeoDecadron Cream; with neomycin sulfate and polymyxin B sulfate: Dexacidin Ointment.

Fluocinolone acetonide with neomycin: Neo-Synalar.

Flurandrenolide with neomycin: Cordran.

Hydrocortisone with iodoquinol: Vytone Cream; with iodochlorhydroxyquin: Vioform-Hydrocortisone Cream, AP, Corque Cream, Hysone; with neomycin: Hydrocortisone-Neomycin, Neo-Cortef; with pramoxine: Pramosone, Zone-A Forte; with neomycin and polymyxin B: Cortisporin Cream; with neomycin, bacitracin, and polymyxin B sulfate: Cortisporin Ointment; with neomycin sulfate and polymyxin B sulfate: Cortisporin; with dibucaine: Corticaine; with pyrilamine maleate and chlorpheniramine maleate: HC Derma-Pax; with benzoyl peroxide and mineral oil: Vanoxide-HC; with lidocaine and glycerin: Lida-Mantle-HC; with sulfur and salicylic acid: Therac Lotion.

Methylprednisolone with neomycin: Neo-Medrol Acetate.

Triamcinolone acetonide with nystatin: Mykacet, Myco II, Myco-Biotic II, Mycogen II, Mycolog-II, Myco-Triacet II, Mytrex, Nystatin-Triamcinolone Acetonide, N.G.T.; with neomycin, gramicidin, and nystatin: Myco-Triacet II, Tri-Statin II.

alpha blockers

carvedilol, dihydroergotamine mesylate, doxazosin mesylate, ergotamine tartrate, phentolamine mesylate, prazosin hydrochloride, tamsulosin hydrochloride, terazosin hydrochloride, tolazoline hydrochloride

Drugs that block the effects of peripheral neurohormonal transmitters (such as norepinephrine, epinephrine, and related sympathomimetic amines) on adrenergic receptors in various effector systems are designated as adrenergic-blocking agents. Just as adrenoreceptors are classified into two subtypes—alpha and beta—so too are the blocking agents. Essentially, those agents that antagonize mydriasis, vasoconstriction, nonvascular smooth muscle excitation, and other adrenergic responses caused by alpha receptor stimulation are termed alpha blockers.

Pharmacology

Nonselective alpha blockers

Ergotamine, phentolamine, and tolazoline antagonize both $alpha_1$ and $alpha_2$ receptors. Generally, alpha blockade results in tachycardia, palpitations, and increased secretion of renin caused by the abnormally large amounts of norepinephrine (transmitter "overflow") released from adrenergic nerve endings as a result of the concurrent blockade of $alpha_1$ and $alpha_2$ receptors. The effects of norepinephrine are clinically counterproductive to the major uses of nonselective alpha blockers, which include treating peripheral vascular disorders such as Raynaud's disease, acrocyanosis, frostbite, acute atrial occlusion, phlebitis, phlebothrombosis, diabetic gangrene, shock, and pheochromocytoma.

Selective alpha blockers

$Alpha_1$ blockers have readily observable effects and are currently the only alpha-adrenergic agents with known clinical uses. They decrease vascular resistance and increase venous capacitance, thereby lowering blood pressure and causing pink warm skin, nasal and scleroconjunctival congestion, ptosis, orthostatic and exercise hypotension, mild to moderate miosis, and interference with ejaculation. They also relax nonvascular smooth muscle, notably in the prostate capsule, reducing urinary symptoms in men with BPH. Because $alpha_1$ blockers don't block $alpha_2$ receptors, they don't cause transmitter overflow. In theory, $alpha_1$ blockers should be useful in the same conditions as nonselective alpha blockers; however, doxazosin, prazosin, and terazosin are approved for treating hypertension. Terazosin and doxazosin are approved in treatment of prostatic outflow obstruction secondary to BPH.

$Alpha_2$ blockers produce more subtle physiologic effects and currently have no therapeutic applications. Yohimbine is one such agent.

Clinical indications and actions

Peripheral vascular disorders

Alpha blockers are indicated for treating peripheral vascular disorders, including Raynaud's disease, acrocyanosis, frostbite, acute atrial occlusion, phlebitis, and diabetic gangrene. Dihydroergotamine and ergotamine have been used to treat vascular headaches. Prazosin has been used to treat Raynaud's disease. Phentolamine is indicated to treat dermal necrosis caused by extravasation of norepinephrine, dopamine, or phenylephrine (alpha agonists).

Hypertension

Tolazoline is indicated to treat persistent pulmonary hypertension in neonates. Prazosin, carvedilol, doxazosin, and terazosin are used in managing essential hypertension. Phentolamine is used to control hypertension and is a useful adjunct in surgical treatment of pheochromocytoma.

BPH

Terazosin, tamsulosin, and doxazosin are used to control mild to moderate urinary obstructive symptoms in men with BPH.

Overview of adverse reactions

Nonselective alpha blockers typically cause orthostatic hypotension, tachycardia, palpitations, fluid retention (from excess renin secretion), nasal and ocular congestion, and aggravation of the signs and symptoms of respiratory infection. Use of these agents is contraindicated in patients with severe cerebral and coronary atherosclerosis and in those with renal insufficiency.

Selective alpha blockers may cause severe orthostatic hypotension and syncope, especially with the first dose; the most common adverse effects of alpha blockade are dizziness, headache, and malaise.

Clinical considerations

- Recommend monitoring vital signs, especially blood pressure.
- Advise administering dose at bedtime to reduce potential of dizziness or light-headedness.
- To avoid first-dose syncope, begin with a small dose.

Special populations

Pregnant patients. Avoid use in pregnant women.

Breast-feeding patients. Women taking these medications shouldn't breast feed their infants.

Pediatric patients. Safety and efficacy of many of these medications haven't been established for use in children. Refer to specific drug monograph for more information.

Geriatric patients. Hypotensive effects may be more pronounced.

Patient counseling

- Warn patient about orthostatic hypotension. Tell him to avoid suddenly moving to an upright position.
- Tell patient to promptly report dizziness or irregular heartbeat.
- Advise patient to take dose at bedtime to reduce potential for dizziness or light-headedness.
- Warn patient to avoid driving and other hazardous tasks that require mental alertness until effects of medication are established.
- Reassure patient that adverse effects, including dizziness, should lessen after several doses.
- Tell patient that alcohol use, excessive exercise, prolonged standing, and exposure to heat will intensify adverse effects.
- Advise patient of the reason for taking the medication.

Representative combinations

None.

aminoglycosides

amikacin sulfate, gentamicin sulfate, kanamycin sulfate, neomycin sulfate, paromycin, streptomycin sulfate, tobramycin sulfate

Aminoglycoside antibiotics were discovered during the search for drugs to treat serious penicillin-resistant, gram-negative infections. Streptomycin, derived from soil actinomycetes, was the first therapeutically useful aminoglycoside. Bacterial resistance to this prototype and adverse reactions soon led to the development of kanamycin, gentamicin, neomycin, netilmicin, tobramycin, and amikacin.

The basic structure of aminoglycosides is an aminocyclitol nucleus joined with one to two amino sugars by glycosidic linkage, hence the name aminoglycosides.

Aminoglycosides share certain pharmacokinetic properties, such as poor oral absorption, poor CNS penetration, and renal excretion, as well as serious adverse reactions and toxicity; their clinical use may require close monitoring of serum levels.

Pharmacology

Aminoglycosides are bactericidal. Although the exact mechanism of action isn't fully known, the drugs appear to bind directly and irreversibly to 30S ribosomal subunits, inhibiting bacterial protein synthesis. Bacterial resistance to aminoglycosides may be from decreased bacterial cell wall permeability, low affinity of the drug for ribosomal binding sites, or enzymatic degradation by microbial enzymes.

Aminoglycosides are active against many aerobic gram-negative organisms and some aerobic gram-positive organisms; they don't kill fungi, viruses, or anaerobic bacteria.

Gram-negative organisms susceptible to aminoglycosides include *Acinetobacter, Citrobacter, Enterobacter, Escherichia coli, Klebsiella*, indole-positive and indole-negative *Proteus, Providencia, Pseudomonas aeruginosa, Salmonella, Serratia*, and *Shigella*. Streptomycin is active against *Brucella, Calymmatobacterium granulomatis, Francisella tularensis, Haemophilus influenzae, Haemophilus ducreyi, Pasteurella multocida*, and *Yersinia pestis*.

Susceptible aerobic gram-positive organisms include *Staphylococcus aureus* and *S. epidermidis*. Streptomycin is active against *Nocardia, Erysipelothrix, Enterococcus faecalis*, and some mycobacteria, including *Mycobacterium tuberculosis, Mycobacterium marinum*, and certain strains of *Mycobacterium kansasii* and *Mycobacterium leprae*.

Paromycin is active against protozoa, especially *Entamoeba histolytica* and is somewhat effective against *Taenia saginata, Hymenolepsis nana, Diphyllobothrium latum*, and *Taenia solium*. Neomycin and paromycin have some activity against *Acanthamoeba*.

Aminoglycosides aren't systemically absorbed after oral administration in patients with intact GI mucosa and usually are used parenterally for systemic infections; intraventricular or intrathecal administration is necessary for CNS infections. Kanamycin and neomycin are given orally for bowel sterilization.

Aminoglycosides are distributed widely throughout the body after parenteral administration; CSF concentrations are minimal even in patients with inflamed meninges. Over time, aminoglycosides accumulate in body tissue, especially the kidney and inner ear, causing drug saturation. The drug is released slowly from these tissues. Most aminoglycosides are minimally protein-bound and aren't metabolized. They don't penetrate abscesses well.

Aminoglycosides are excreted primarily in urine, chiefly by glomerular filtration; neomycin is chiefly excreted unchanged in feces when taken orally. Elimination half-life ranges between 2 and 4 hours and is prolonged in patients with decreased renal function. (See *Aminoglycosides: Renal function and half-life*, page 14.)

Clinical indications and actions

Infection caused by susceptible organisms

Aminoglycosides are used as sole therapy for:

- infections caused by susceptible aerobic gram-negative bacilli, including septicemia; postoperative, pulmonary, intra-abdominal, and serious, recurrent urinary tract infections; and infections of skin, soft tissue, bones, and joints
- infections from aerobic gram-negative bacillary meningitis (not susceptible to other antibiotics); because of poor CNS penetration, drugs are given intrathecally or intraventricularly (in ventriculitis)
- kanamycin or paromycin is used orally and neomycin is used orally or as a retention enema as an adjunct therapy to inhibit ammonia-forming bacteria in the GI tract of patients with hepatic encephalopathy
- gentamicin encapsulated in liposomes is being evaluated for the treatment of disseminated *Mycobacterium avium* complex infections.

Aminoglycosides are combined with other antibacterials in many other types of infection, including:

- serious staphylococcal infections (with an antistaphylococcal penicillin)
- serious *P. aeruginosa* infections (with such drugs as an antipseudomonal penicillin or cephalosporin)
- enterococcal infections, including endocarditis (with such drugs as penicillin G, ampicillin, or vancomycin)
- as initial empiric therapy in febrile, leukopenic compromised host (with an antipseudomonal penicillin or cephalosporin)
- serious *Klebsiella* infections (with a cephalosporin)
- nosocomial pneumonia (with a cephalosporin)
- anaerobic infections involving *Bacteroides fragilis* (with such drugs as clindamycin, metronidazole, cefoxitin, doxycycline, chloramphenicol, or ticarcillin)
- tuberculosis (use of parenteral amikacin, kanamycin or streptomycin with other antitubercular agents)
- treatment of pelvic inflammatory disease (PID) (gentamicin with clindamycin).

AMINOGLYCOSIDES: RENAL FUNCTION AND HALF-LIFE

As the table shows, aminoglycosides, which are excreted by the kidneys, have significantly prolonged half-lives in patients with end-stage renal disease. Knowing this can help you assess the patient's potential for drug accumulation and toxicity. Nephrotoxicity, a major hazard of therapy with aminoglycosides, is linked to serum levels that exceed the therapeutic levels listed below. Therefore, monitoring peak and trough levels is essential for safe use of these drugs.

	Half-life (hr)		Therapeutic levels (mcg/ml)	
Drug and route	**Normal renal function**	**End-stage renal disease**	**Peak**	**Trough**
amikacin I.M., I.V.	2 to 3	24 to 60	16 to 32	< 10
gentamicin I.M., I.V., topical	2	24 to 60	4 to 8	< 2
kanamycin I.M., I.V., topical	2 to 3	24 to 60	15 to 40	< 10
neomycin oral, topical	2 to 3	12 to 24	Not applicable	Not applicable
netilmicin I.M., I.V.	2 to 2½	< 10	6 to 10	< 2
streptomycin I.M., I.V.	2½	100	20 to 30	Not applicable
tobramycin I.M., I.V., topical	2 to 2½	24 to 60	4 to 8	< 2

Overview of adverse reactions

Systemic: Ototoxicity and nephrotoxicity are the most serious complications of aminoglycoside therapy. Ototoxicity involves both vestibular and auditory functions and usually is related to persistently high serum drug levels. Damage is reversible only if detected early and if drug is discontinued promptly.

Any aminoglycoside may cause usually reversible nephrotoxicity. The damage results in tubular necrosis. Mild proteinuria and casts are early signs of declining renal function; elevated serum creatinine levels follow several days after the decline has begun. Nephrotoxicity usually begins on day 4 to 7 of therapy and appears to be dose-related.

Neuromuscular blockade results in skeletal weakness and respiratory distress similar to that seen with the use of neuromuscular-blocking agents, such as tubocurarine and succinylcholine.

Oral aminoglycoside therapy most often causes nausea, vomiting, and diarrhea. Less common adverse reactions include hypersensitivity reactions (ranging from mild rashes, fever, and eosinophilia to fatal anaphylaxis) and hematologic reactions (hemolytic anemia, transient neutropenia, leukopenia, and thrombocytopenia). Transient elevations of liver function values also occur.

Local: Parenterally administered forms of aminoglycosides may cause vein irritation, phlebitis, and sterile abscess.

Clinical considerations

- Don't give an aminoglycoside to a patient with history of hypersensitivity reactions to any aminoglycoside.
- Culture and sensitivity tests should be done before first dose.
- Recommend monitoring of vital signs, electrolyte levels, and renal function studies before and during therapy; be sure patient is well hydrated to minimize chemical irritation of renal tubules; watch for signs of declining renal function.
- Keep peak serum levels and trough serum levels at recommended concentrations, especially in patients with decreased renal function. Blood is drawn for peak level 1 hour after I.M. injection (30 minutes to 1 hour after I.V. infusion); for trough level, sample is drawn just before the next dose. Time and date all blood samples. Don't use heparinized tube to collect blood samples; it interferes with results.
- Recommend that patient's hearing be evaluated before and during therapy; monitor for complaints of tinnitus, vertigo, or hearing loss.
- Avoid use of aminoglycosides with other ototoxic or nephrotoxic drugs.

- Usual duration of therapy is 7 to 10 days; if no response occurs in 3 to 5 days, discontinue drug and repeat cultures for reevaluation of therapy.
- Recommend that patients on long-term therapy be closely monitored—especially geriatric and debilitated patients and others receiving immunosuppressant or radiation therapy—for possible bacterial or fungal superinfection; monitor especially for fever.
- Don't add or mix other drugs with I.V. infusions, particularly penicillins, which inactivate aminoglycosides; the two groups are chemically and physically incompatible. If other drugs must be given I.V., temporarily stop infusion of primary drug.
- Oral aminoglycosides may be absorbed systemically in patients with ulcerative GI lesions; significant absorption may endanger patients with decreased renal function.

Oral and parenteral administration

- Rapid I.V. administration may cause neuromuscular blockade. Infuse I.V. drug continuously or intermittently over 30 to 60 minutes for adults, 1 to 2 hours for infants; dilution volume for children is determined individually.
- Solutions should always be clear, colorless to pale yellow (in most cases, darkening indicates deterioration), and free of particles; don't give solutions containing precipitates or other foreign matter.
- Amikacin, gentamicin (without preservatives), kanamycin, and tobramycin have been administered intrathecally or intraventricularly. Some clinicians prefer intraventricular administration to ensure adequate CSF levels in the treatment of ventriculitis.

Special populations

Pregnant patients. Pregnancy risk category is D; drugs cross the placenta, creating the potential for fetal toxicity and possibly causing congenital deafness.
Breast-feeding patients. Small amounts of drugs are secreted in breast milk; recommend an alternative feeding method during therapy.
Pediatric patients. Half-life of aminoglycosides is prolonged in neonates and premature infants because of immaturity of their renal systems; dosage alterations may be necessary.
Geriatric patients. Geriatric patients often have decreased renal function and are at greater risk for nephrotoxicity; they often require lower drug dose and longer dosing intervals. They're also susceptible to ototoxicity and superinfection.

Patient counseling

- Tell patient signs and symptoms of hypersensitivity and other adverse reactions to aminoglycosides.
- Teach signs and symptoms of bacterial or fungal superinfection to geriatric patients, debilitated patients, and patients with low resistance from immunosuppressants or irradiation; emphasize the need to report them promptly.

Representative combinations

Neomycin with polymyxin B sulfates and bacitracin: Neosporin, Mycitracin, Foille Plus; with polymyxin B sulfates and gramicidin: Neosporin; with polymyxin B sulfates and hydrocortisone: Cortisporin, Drotic, Octicair, Otocort; with dexamethasone sodium phosphate: Neo-Decadron; with flurandrenolide: Cordran SP.

See also *adrenocorticoids (topical).*

androgens

danazol, fluoxymesterone, methyltestosterone, testosterone, testosterone cypionate, testosterone enanthate, testosterone propionate, testosterone transdermal system

Testosterone is the endogenous androgen, or male sex hormone. The testosterone esters (cypionate, enanthate, propionate), methyltestosterone, and fluoxymesterone are synthetic derivatives with greater potency or longer duration of action than testosterone.

Pharmacology

Testosterone promotes maturation of the male sexual organs and the development of secondary sexual characteristics (facial and body hair and vocal cord thickening). Testosterone also causes the growth spurt of adolescence and terminates growth of the long bones by closing the epiphyses (growth plates at the ends of bones). Testosterone promotes retention of calcium, nitrogen, phosphorus, sodium, and potassium and enhances anabolism (tissue building). Through negative feedback on the pituitary, exogenously administered testosterone (and other androgenic drugs) decreases endogenous testosterone production and to some degree inhibits spermatogenesis in men. Androgens repeatedly stimulate production of erythrocytes, apparently by enhancing the production of erythropoietic stimulating factor.

Clinical indications and actions

Androgen deficiency

Androgens (testosterone, all testosterone esters, methyltestosterone, fluoxymesterone) are indicated to treat androgen deficiency resulting from testicular failure or castration, or gonadotropin or luteinizing hormone-releasing hormone deficiency of pituitary origin. Methyltestosterone and testosterone cypionate are also indicated to treat male climacteric symptoms and impotence when these are caused by androgen deficiency.

Delayed male puberty
All androgens may be used to stimulate the onset of puberty when it's significantly delayed and psychological support proves insufficient.
Breast cancer
Testosterone, all testosterone esters, and fluoxymesterone are indicated for palliative treatment of metastatic breast cancer in women during the first 5 postmenopausal years. Androgens also may be used in premenopausal women with metastatic disease if the tumor is hormone-responsive.
Postpartum breast engorgement
Fluoxymesterone, testosterone, methyltestosterone, and testosterone propionate are indicated to treat painful postpartum breast engorgement in non-breast-feeding women.
Hereditary angioedema
Danazol is indicated in the prophylaxis of angioedema attacks.
Endometriosis
Danazol is indicated for palliative treatment of endometriosis. Danazol relieves pain and helps resolve endometrial lesions in 30% to 80% of patients who receive it. Endometriosis usually recurs 8 to 12 months after danazol is discontinued.
Fibrocystic breast disease
Danazol is indicated for palliative treatment of fibrocystic breast disease that's unresponsive to simple therapy. It usually relieves pain before it reduces nodularity. Fibrocystic breast disease recurs in about half of patients who have undergone successful treatment with danazol, usually 1 year after discontinuing the drug.

Danazol has been used for palliative treatment of virginal breast hypertrophy, for gynecomastia, and excessive menstrual blood loss; for contraception in men (in combination with testosterone) and women; for treatment of $alpha_1$-antitrypsin deficiency, systemic lupus erythematosus, gynecomastia in men, and Melkersson-Rosenthal syndrome; and for management of patients with hemophilia A (factor VIII deficiency, classic hemophilia), hemophilia B (factor IX deficiency, Christmas disease), and idiopathic thrombocytopenic purpura (ITP).

Overview of adverse reactions

The most common adverse effects associated with androgen therapy are extensions of the hormonal action. In men, frequent and prolonged erections, bladder irritability (causing frequent urination), and gynecomastia (swelling or tenderness of breast tissue) may occur. In women, clitoral enlargement, deepening of the voice, growth of facial or body hair, unusual hair loss, and irregular or absent menses may occur. Note that virilization, including hirsutism, deepening of voice, or clitoral enlargement may be irreversible even with prompt discontinuation of the drug. Oily skin or acne occurs commonly in both sexes.

Metabolic adverse effects include retention of fluid and electrolytes (occasionally resulting in edema), increased serum calcium levels (hypercalcemia may occur, especially in women receiving the drug for breast cancer metastatic to bone), decreased blood glucose levels, and increased serum cholesterol levels.

Long-term administration of androgens may cause loss of libido and suppression of spermatogenesis in men. Although rare, serious hepatic dysfunction, including hepatic necrosis and hepatocellular carcinoma, has been reported in prolonged androgen administration.

Clinical considerations

- Don't administer androgens to men with breast or prostatic cancer or with symptomatic prostatic hypertrophy; to patients with severe cardiac, renal, or hepatic disease; or to patients with undiagnosed abnormal genital bleeding.
- Hypercalcemia symptoms may be difficult to distinguish from symptoms of the condition being treated unless anticipated and thought of as a cluster. Hypercalcemia is most likely to occur in women with breast cancer, particularly when metastatic to bone.
- Priapism indicates that dose is excessive.
- Yellowing of the sclera of the eyes or of skin may indicate hepatic dysfunction resulting from administration of androgens.

Special populations

Pregnant patients. Don't administer androgens during pregnancy because they may cause masculinization of a female fetus or other fetal harm.
Breast-feeding patients. The degree of androgen excretion in breast milk is unknown. Because androgens may induce premature sexual development in boys or virilization in girls, women receiving androgens shouldn't breastfeed.
Pediatric patients. Observe children receiving androgens carefully for excessive virilization and precocious puberty. Androgen therapy may cause premature epiphyseal closure and short stature. Regular X-ray examinations of hand bones may be used to monitor skeletal maturation during therapy.
Geriatric patients. Elderly men receiving androgens may be at increased risk for prostatic hypertrophy and prostatic carcinoma. Androgens can aggravate prostatic hypertrophy with obstruction and are contraindicated in these cases.

Patient counseling

- Warn patient against using androgens to improve athletic performance. Androgens are classified as Schedule III controlled substances and their distribution is regulated by the Drug Enforcement Agency.
- Advise patient to report GI upset.

- Tell patient that virilization, including hirsutism, deepening of voice, or clitoral enlargement, may not be reversible.
- Explain to women that medication may cause menstrual cycle irregularities in premenopausal women and withdrawal bleeding in postmenopausal women.

Representative combinations

Fluoxymesterone with ethinyl estradiol: Halodrin.

Testosterone cypionate with estradiol cypionate: De-Comberol, depAndrogyn, Depo-Testadiol, Depotestogen, Duo-Cyp, Duratestin, Menoject-L.A., Test-Estro Cypionate.

Testosterone enanthate with estradiol valerate: Andrest 90-4, Andro-Estro 90-4, Androgyn L.A., Duo-Gen L.A., Duogex L.A.*, Neo-Pause*, Teev, Valertest No. 1

angiotensin-converting enzyme (ACE) inhibitors

benazepril hydrochloride, captopril, enalapril maleate, fosinopril sodium, lisinopril, moexipril hydrochloride, perindopril erbumine, quinapril hydrochloride, ramipril, trandolapril

ACE inhibitors are used to manage hypertension, and most are used to treat heart failure. Captopril is indicated for the prevention of diabetic nephropathy, and captopril and lisinopril are useful in improving survival rate in patients after an MI.

Pharmacology

ACE inhibitors prevent the conversion of angiotensin I to angiotensin II, a potent vasoconstrictor. Besides decreasing vasoconstriction, and thus reducing peripheral arterial resistance, inhibition of angiotensin II decreases adrenocortical secretion of aldosterone. This results in decreased sodium and water retention and extracellular fluid volume.

Clinical indications and actions

Hypertension, heart failure

ACE inhibitors are used to treat hypertension; their antihypertensive effects are secondary to decreased peripheral resistance and decreased sodium and water retention.

ACE inhibitors are used to manage heart failure; they decrease systemic vascular resistance (afterload) and pulmonary capillary wedge pressure (preload). They're also used after MI to decrease mortality rate and to prevent diabetic nephropathy. (See *Comparing doses of angiotensin-converting enzyme inhibitors,* page 18.)

Overview of adverse reactions

The most common adverse effects of therapeutic doses of ACE inhibitors are headache, fatigue, hypotension, tachycardia, dysgeusia, proteinuria, hyperkalemia, rash, cough, and angioedema of the face and extremities. Severe hypotension may occur at toxic drug levels. ACE inhibitors should be used cautiously in patients with impaired renal function or serious autoimmune disease, and in patients taking other drugs known to depress WBC count or immune response.

Clinical considerations

- Diuretic therapy should be discontinued 2 to 3 days before starting ACE inhibitor therapy to reduce risk of hypotension; if drug doesn't adequately control blood pressure, reinstate diuretics. If diuretics can't be discontinued, begin ACE inhibitor at lowest dose.
- Recommend periodic monitoring of WBC counts.
- Lower doses are necessary in patients with impaired renal function.
- Use potassium supplements with caution because ACE inhibitors may cause potassium retention.

Special populations

Pregnant patients. Discontinue ACE inhibitors if pregnancy is detected. Drug may harm or cause fetal death during the second or third trimesters.

Breast-feeding patients. Captopril and enalapril are distributed into breast milk. An alternative feeding method is recommended during therapy.

Pediatric patients. Safety and efficacy of ACE inhibitors in children haven't been established; use only if potential benefit outweighs risk.

Geriatric patients. Geriatric patients may need lower doses because of impaired drug clearance. These patients may be more sensitive to hypotensive effects.

Patient counseling

- Tell patient that the agents may cause a dry, persistent, tickling cough, which is reversible when therapy is discontinued.
- Tell patient to report feelings of light-headedness, especially in the first few days, so dose can be adjusted; signs of infection such as sore throat and fever because drugs may decrease WBC count; facial swelling or difficulty breathing because drugs may cause angioedema; and loss of taste, which may necessitate discontinuation of drug.
- Advise patient to avoid sudden position changes to minimize orthostatic hypotension.
- Warn patient to seek medical approval before taking OTC cold preparations.
- Tell patient to call if troublesome cough develops.
- Instruct patient to promptly report pregnancy.

COMPARING DOSES OF ANGIOTENSIN-CONVERTING ENZYME INHIBITORS

Drug	Target adult daily dose	Dosage adjustments
benazepril	10-40 mg in single or divided doses	Creatinine clearance < 30 ml/min or on concurrent diuretic: initially, 5 mg per day
captopril	25-150 mg in single or divided doses	Renal impairment, hyponatremia or hypovolemia: 6.25 to 12.5 mg b.i.d. or t.i.d.
enalapril	P.O.: 10-40 mg in single or divided doses I.V.: 1.25 mg (≥ 5 minutes) q 6 hours	Creatinine clearance ≤ 30 ml/min or on concurrent diuretic: initially, 2.5 mg per day
fosinopril	20-40 mg in single or divided doses	Use cautiously if on concurrent diuretic: initially, 10 mg per day
lisinopril	20-40 mg in a single dose	Creatinine clearance ≤ 10-30 ml/min or concurrent diuretic: initially, 5 mg per day Creatinine clearance < 10 ml/min: initially, 2.5 mg per day
moexipril	7.5-30 mg in single or divided doses	Creatinine clearance < 40 ml/min: initially, 3.75 mg per day
perindopril	4-8 mg in single or divided doses	Creatinine clearance OF 30-60 ml/min: initially, 2 mg per day
quinapril	20-80 mg in single or divided doses	Creatinine clearance of 30-60 ml/min or on concurrent diuretic: initially, 5 mg per day Creatinine clearance of 10-30 ml/min: initially, 2.5 mg per day
ramipril	2.5-20 mg in single or divided doses	Creatinine clearance < 40 ml/min or serum creatinine > 2.5 mg/dl: initially, 1.25 mg per day
trandolapril	1-4 mg in a single dose	Creatinine clearance < 30 ml/min, on concurrent diuretic, hepatic cirrhosis: initially, 0.5 mg per day

Tell patient not to take potassium-containing salt substitutes without medical approval.

Representative combinations

Captopril with hydrochlorothiazide: Capozide.

Benazepril hydrochloride with amlodipine: Lotrel; with hydrochlorothiazide: Lotensin HCT.

Enalapril with hydrochlorothiazide: Vaseretic.

Lisinopril with hydrochlorothiazide: Prinzide, Zestoretic.

angiotensin II receptor antagonists

candesartan cilexetil, irbesartan, losartan potassium, telmisartan, valsartan

Angiotensin II receptor antagonists (AIIRAs) are a class of antihypertensive drugs that exert their therapeutic effects by selectively blocking the binding of angiotensin II to the angiotensin II type 1 (AT_1) receptor. They're indicated as monotherapy and in combination with other antihypertensive agents. In comparison to ACE inhibitors, AIIRAs are associated with fewer side effects, such as cough and angioedema.

Pharmacology

Angiotensin II is a potent vasoconstrictor that's formed from angiotensin I by the enzyme ACE. Angiotensin II causes vasoconstriction, increased aldosterone secretion, cardiac stimulation, and reabsorption of sodium by the kidney. AIIRAs selectively block the binding of angiotensin II to the AT_1 receptor. AT_1 receptors are found in many tissues throughout the body including vascular smooth muscle and the adrenal gland. Blockade of AT_1 receptors by the AIIRAs results in vasodilation, decreased aldosterone secretion , a 2- to 3-fold increase in plasma renin activity, and an increase in angiotensin II. The increase in renin and angiotensin II is due to removal of the negative feedback of angiotensin II and isn't enough to overcome the antihypertensive effects of AIIRAs. Another type of receptor is called the AT_2 receptor. The role of the AT_2 receptor isn't known, but it doesn't appear to be involved

COMPARING ANGIOTENSIN II RECEPTOR ANTAGONISTS

Drug	Oral bio-availability (%)	Effect of food	Prodrug	Metabolized by cytochrome P-450 isoenzymes	Protein binding (%)	Half-life (hr)
candesartan	15	No effect	Yes	Unknown	>99	9
irbesartan	60-80	No effect	No	Yes CYP2C9	90	11-15
losartan	33	↓AUC ~10%	Yes	Yes CYP2C9 and CYP3A4	~ 99	2 (6-9 for active metabolite)
telmisartan	42-58	↓AUC 6%-20%	No	No	>99.5	24
valsartan	25	↓AUC ~ 40%	No	Unknown	95	6

in cardiovascular homeostasis. AIIRAs are 1,000- to 20,000-fold more selective for the AT_1 than the AT_2 receptor. (See *Comparing angiotensin II receptor antagonists.)*

Clinical indications and actions

Hypertension

All AIIRAs are indicated for hypertension, either as monotherapy or in combination with other agents. AIIRAs act by selectively blocking the binding of angiotensin II to the AT_1 receptor, resulting in vasodilation.

Heart failure

Heart failure is associated with elevated levels of angiotensin II and aldosterone. ACE inhibitors have been shown to decrease mortality rates in patients with heart failure and to increase quality of life related to their inhibition of the renin-angiotensin-aldosterone-system (RAAS). Whether AIIRAs will have similar effects on mortality rates as ACE inhibitors in patients with heart failure is being studied. Until more information is available, reserve AIIRAs for patients unable to tolerate ACE inhibitors.

Overview of adverse reactions

AIIRAs are well tolerated, with side effects similar to those of placebos. Adverse effects include dizziness, insomnia, headache, fatigue, anxiety, nervousness, diarrhea, dyspepsia, heartburn, nausea, vomiting, arthralgia, back or leg pain, muscle cramps, myalgia, upper respiratory infection, cough, nasal congestion, sinusitis, pharyngitis, rhinitis, influenza, bronchitis, viral infection, edema, chest pain, rash, tachycardia, urinary tract infection, peripheral edema, and albuminuria.

Symptomatic hypotension may occur in patients who are volume- or salt-depleted (such as patients taking diuretics). AIIRAs can cause deterioration in renal function, including oliguria, acute renal failure, and progressive azotemia. Decreased hemoglobin and hematocrit; increased serum potassium levels, and occasional increases in liver function tests (LFTs) have occurred in patients receiving valsartan.

Clinical considerations

- Use extreme caution when using AIIRAs in combination with potassium supplements or potassium-sparing diuretics.
- Use caution in volume-depleted patients (such as patients taking diuretics); correct volume depletion before administration and use a lower starting dose.
- Use caution in patients with hepatic dysfunction; losartan requires dosing adjustment.
- Use with caution in patients whose renal function may be dependent on the RAAS; a worsening of renal function may occur (such as heart failure or renal artery stenosis).
- Telmisartan increases peak digoxin levels by 49% and troughs by 20%. Monitor digoxin levels more frequently.

Special populations

Pregnant patients. AIIRAs are pregnancy risk category C in the first trimester and category D in the second and third trimester. Drugs that act on the RAAS have been associated with fetal and neonatal injury, and death when intrauterine exposure occurred during the second and third trimester of pregnancy. Patients taking AIIRAs who become pregnant should have the drug discontinued by their doctor unless use is considered life-saving.

Breast-feeding patients. It isn't known if AIIRAs are excreted in breast milk; because of potential risk to the nursing infant, a decision should be made regarding drug discontinuation.

Pediatric patients. The safety and efficacy of AIIRAs haven't been established in patients under age 18.

Geriatric patients. No dosing adjustments are required.

Patient counseling

- Inform women about the risks associated with exposure to AIIRAs during the second and third trimester of pregnancy; adverse effects on the fetus don't appear to occur when intrauterine exposure is limited to the first trimester.
- Tell patient to report pregnancy to her doctor as soon as possible.
- Advise patient to continue taking drugs unless a doctor instructs her to stop.
- Instruct patient to take missed doses as soon as they're remembered unless it's almost time for the next dose.
- Tell patient to call his doctor if signs of allergy or dizziness develop.

Representative combinations

Hydrochlorothiazide and losartan: Hyzaar.

Hydrochlorothiazide and irbesartan: Avapro HCT.

Hydrochlorothiazide and valsartan: Diovan HCT.

anticholinergics

***Belladonna alkaloids*: atropine sulfate, hyoscyamine sulfate, scopolamine hydrobromide**

***Synthetic quaternary anticholinergics:* clidinium bromide, glycopyrrolate, ipratropium bromide, mepenzolate bromide, methoscopalamine bromide, propantheline bromide**

***Tertiary synthetic and semi-synthetic (antispasmodic) derivatives:* dicyclomine hydrochloride, homatropine, oxybutynin chloride, tolterodine tartrate**

***Antiparkinsonian agents:* benztropine mesylate, biperiden hydrochloride, biperiden lactate, trihexyphenidyl hydrochloride**

Anticholinergics are used to treat various spastic conditions, including acute dystonic reactions, muscle rigidity, parkinsonism, and extrapyramidal disorders. They're also used to reverse neuromuscular blockade, prevent nausea and vomiting resulting from motion sickness, as adjunctive treatment for peptic ulcer disease and other GI disorders, and preoperatively to decrease secretions and block cardiac reflexes. Belladonna alkaloids are naturally occurring anticholinergics that have been used for centuries. Many semisynthetic alkaloids and synthetic anticholinergic compounds are available; however, most offer few advantages over naturally occurring alkaloids. (See *Comparing systemic anticholinergics.*)

Pharmacology

Anticholinergics competitively antagonize the actions of acetylcholine and other cholinergic agonists at muscarinic and nicotinic receptors within the parasympathetic nervous system and smooth muscles that lack cholinergic innervation. Lack of specificity for site of action increases the hazard of adverse effects in association with therapeutic effects.

Antispasmodics are structurally similar to anticholinergics; however, their anticholinergic activity usually occurs only at high doses. Their mechanism of action is unknown, but they're believed to directly relax smooth muscle.

Clinical indications and actions

Hypersecretory conditions

Many anticholinergics, such as atropine, belladonna leaf, glycopyrrolate, hyoscyamine, levorotatory alkaloids of belladonna, and mepenzolate, are used therapeutically for their antisecretory properties. These properties derive from competitive blockade of cholinergic receptor sites, causing decreased gastric acid secretion, salivation, bronchial secretions, and sweating.

GI tract disorders

Some anticholinergics, such as atropine, belladonna leaf, glycopyrrolate, hyoscyamine, levorotatory alkaloids of belladonna, mepenzolate, and propantheline, as well as the antispasmodics such as dicyclomine, are used to treat spasms and other GI tract disorders. These drugs competitively block the actions of acetylcholine at cholinergic receptor sites. Antispasmodics presumably act by a nonspecific, direct spasmolytic action on smooth muscle. These agents are useful in treating pylorospasm, ileitis, and irritable bowel syndrome. Transdermal scopolamine is used to prevent nausea and vomiting associated with recovery from anesthesia and surgery. Atropine may be useful in treating nausea and vomiting associated with morphine used in treatment of a myocardial infarction.

Sinus bradycardia

Atropine is used to treat sinus bradycardia caused by drugs, poisons, or sinus node dysfunction. It blocks normal vagal inhibition of the SA node and causes an increase in heart rate. Atropine may be used for the treatment of sustained bradycardia and hypotension associated with nitroglycerine used in treatment of a myocardial infarction.

Dystonia and parkinsonism

Biperiden, benztropine, and trihexyphenidyl hydrochloride are used to treat acute dystonic reactions and drug-induced extrapyramidal adverse effects. They act centrally by blocking cholinergic receptor sites, balancing cholinergic activity with dopamine.

Perioperative use

Atropine, glycopyrrolate, and hyoscyamine are used postoperatively with anticholinesterase agents to reverse nondepolarizing neuromus-

COMPARING SYSTEMIC ANTICHOLINERGICS

Drug	Plasma half-life (hr)	Onset of action	Duration of action
atropine, oral	2½	Inhibition of saliva occurs in 30-60 min	4-6 hr
atropine, parenteral	2½	Peak increase in heart rate occurs after 2-4 min	Brief
benztropine	Unknown	P.O.: 1-2 hr I.V., I.M.: 15 min	24 hr
clidinium	Biphasic with initial half-life of 2½ and terminal half-life of 20	1 hr	3 hr
dicyclomine	9-10	Unknown	Unknown
glycopyrrolate	½-4½ I.V. 15-30 min I.M.	1 min I.V.	2-7 hr
homatropine	Unknown	40-60 min	1-3 days
hyoscyamine, oral	3½	20-30 min	4-6 hr
hyoscyamine, parenteral	3½	2-3 min	4-6 hr
mepenzolate	Unknown	Unknown	Unknown
methoscopolamine	Unknown	1 hr	6-8 hr
oxybutynin	Unknown	30-60 min	6-10 hr
propantheline	1½	1½ hr	6 hr
scopolamine, oral	1 hr	4-6 hr	
scopolamine, parenteral	30 min	4 hr	
tolterodine	Unknown	1 hr	5 hr
trihexyphenidyl	Unknown	Within 1 hr	6-12 hr

cular blockade. These agents block muscarinic effects of anticholinesterase agents by competitively blocking muscarinic receptor sites.

Atropine, glycopyrrolate, and scopolamine are used preoperatively to decrease secretions and block cardiac vagal reflexes. They diminish secretions by competitively inhibiting muscarinic receptor sites; they block cardiac vagal reflexes by preventing normal vagal inhibition of the SA node.

Bronchospasm

Atropine and ipratropium are potent bronchodilators and are used to treat antigen-, methacholine-, histamine-, or exercise-induced bronchospasm (oral inhalation and I.M. atropine); oral inhalation of atropine or ipratropium is effective in the treatment of chronic bronchitis and asthma; oral inhalation of atropine sulfate has been used for the short-term treatment and prevention of bronchospasm associated with chronic bronchial asthma, bronchitis, and chronic obstructive pulmonary disease.

Genitourinary tract disorders

Atropine, oxybutynin, tolterodine, and propantheline have been used to treat reflex neurogenic bladder.

Poisoning

Atropine is used to reverse the cholinergic effects of toxic exposure to organophosphate, carbamate anticholinesterase pesticides, and ingestion of cholinomimetic plants and fungi.

Motion sickness

Scopolamine is effective in preventing nausea and vomiting associated with motion sickness. Its exact mechanism of action is unknown, but it's thought to affect neural pathways originating in the labyrinth of the ear.

Overview of adverse reactions

Dry mouth, decreased sweating or anhidrosis, headache, mydriasis, blurred vision, cycloplegia, xerophthalmia, dry skin, urinary hesitancy and retention, constipation, palpitations, and tachycardia most commonly occur with therapeutic doses and usually disappear once the drug is discontinued. Signs of drug toxicity include CNS signs resembling psychosis (disorientation, confusion, hallucinations, delusions, anxiety, agitation, and restlessness) and such peripheral effects as dilated, nonreactive pupils; blurred vision; hot, dry, flushed skin; dry mucous membranes; dysphagia; stupor, seizures, decreased or absent bowel sounds; urine retention; hyperthermia; tachycardia; hypertension; and increased respiration.

Clinical considerations

- Recommend monitoring patient's vital signs, urine output, visual changes, and signs of impending toxicity.
- Constipation may be relieved by stool softeners or bulk laxatives.

Special populations

Pregnant patients. The safety of anticholinergic therapy during pregnancy hasn't been determined. Use by pregnant women is indicated only when the benefits of drug outweigh potential risks to the fetus.
Breast-feeding patients. Some anticholinergics may be excreted in breast milk, possibly resulting in infant toxicity; breast-feeding women should avoid these drugs. Anticholinergics may decrease milk production.
Pediatric patients. Safety and efficacy haven't been established.
Geriatric patients. Administer cautiously. Lower doses are usually indicated. Patients over age 40 may be more sensitive to the effects of these drugs.

Patient counseling

- Teach patient how and when to take drug.
- Warn patient to avoid driving and other hazardous tasks if he experiences dizziness, drowsiness, or blurred vision.
- Advise patient to avoid alcoholic beverages, because they may cause additive CNS effects.
- Advise patient to consume plenty of fluids and dietary fiber to help avoid constipation.
- Tell patient to promptly report dry mouth, blurred vision, rash, eye pain, or significant changes in urine volume, or pain or difficulty on urination.
- Warn patient that drug may cause increased sensitivity or intolerance to high temperatures, resulting in dizziness.
- Instruct patient to report confusion and rapid or pounding heartbeat.
- Advise women to report pregnancy or intent to conceive.
- Warn patient to avoid OTC agents such as Benadryl or Nytol, which also have anticholinergic activity.

Representative combinations

Atropine with meperidine: Atropine/Demerol injection; with scopolamine hydrobromide (hyoscine hydrobromide), hyoscyamine sulfate, and phenobarbital: Antispasmodic Elixir, Donnatal No. 2, Phenobarbital with Belladonna Alkaloids Elixir, Bellalphen, Donnatal, Haponal, Kinesed, Spasmolin; with scopolamine hydrobromide (hyoscine hydrobromide), hyoscyamine sulfate, kaolin, pectin, sodium benzoate, alcohol, and powdered opium: Donnagel-PG; with phenazopyridine, hyoscyamine, and scopolamine: Urogesic; with hyoscyamine, methenamine, phenyl salicylate, methylene blue, and benzoic acid: Urised; with scopolamine hydrobromide, hyoscyamine hydrobromide, and phenobarbital: Barbidonna No. 2 Tablets, Barbidonna Tablets, Belladonna Alkaloids with Phenobarbital Tablets, Barophen, Donnamor, Donnapine, Donnatal Extentabs, Hyosophen Tablets, Malatal Tablets, Spasmophen, Spasquid, Susano.

Belladonna alkaloids with ergotamine tartrate, caffeine, and phenacetin: Wigraine; with phenobarbital: Chardonna-2, Butibel Elixir; with powdered opium: B&O Supprettes No. 15A, B&O Supprettes No. 16A.

Belladonna extract with butabarbital: Butibel.

Hyoscyamine sulfate with phenobarbital: Levsin with Phenobarbital Tablets, Levsin-PB, Bellacane Tablets.

antihistamines

azelastine hydrochloride, brompheniramine maleate, cetirizine hydrochloride, chlorpheniramine maleate, clemastine fumarate, cyclizine hydrochloride, cyclizine lactate, cyproheptadine hydrochloride, dimenhydrinate, diphenhydramine hydrochloride, fexofenadine hydrochloride, loratadine, meclizine hydrochloride, promethazine hydrochloride, tripelennamine hydrochloride, triprolidine hydrochloride

Antihistamines, synthetically produced H_1-receptor antagonists, were discovered in the late 1930s and proliferated rapidly during the next decade. They have many applications related specifically to chemical structure, their widespread use testifying to their versatility and relative safety. Some antihistamines are used primarily to treat rhinitis or pruritus, whereas others are used more often for their antiemetic and antivertigo effects; still others are used as sedative-hypnotics, local anesthetics, and antitussives.

Pharmacology

Antihistamines are structurally related chemicals that compete with histamine for H_1-receptor sites on the smooth muscle of the bronchi, GI tract, uterus, and large blood vessels, binding to the cellular receptors and preventing access and subsequent activity of histamine. They don't directly alter histamine or prevent its release. Also, antihistamines antagonize the action of histamine that causes increased capillary permeability and resultant edema and suppress flare and pruritus associated with the endogenous release of histamine.

Clinical indications and actions

Allergy

Most antihistamines (azelastine, brompheniramine, chlorpheniramine, clemastine, cyproheptadine, diphenhydramine, promethazine, and triprolidine) are used to treat allergic symptoms, such as rhinitis and urticaria. By preventing access of histamine to H_1-receptor sites, they suppress histamine-induced allergic symptoms.

Pruritus

Cyproheptadine and hydroxyzine are used systemically. It's believed that these drugs counteract histamine-induced pruritus by a combination of peripheral effects on nerve endings and local anesthetic and sedative activity.

Tripelennamine and diphenhydramine are used topically to relieve itching associated with minor skin irritation. Structurally related to local anesthetics, these compounds prevent initiation and transmission of nerve impulses.

Vertigo, nausea, and vomiting

Cyclizine, dimenhydrinate, and meclizine are used only as antiemetic and antivertigo agents; their antihistaminic activity hasn't been evaluated. Diphenhydramine and promethazine are used as antiallergic and antivertigo agents and as antiemetics and antinauseants. Although the mechanisms aren't fully understood, antiemetic and antivertigo effects probably result from central antimuscarinic activity.

Sedation

Diphenhydramine and promethazine are used for their sedative action; the mechanism of antihistamine-induced CNS depression is unknown.

Suppression of cough

Diphenhydramine syrup is used as an antitussive. The cough reflex is suppressed by a direct effect on the medullary cough center.

Dyskinesia

The central antimuscarinic action of diphenhydramine reduces drug-induced dyskinesias and parkinsonism through inhibition of acetylcholine (anticholinergic effect).

Overview of adverse reactions

At therapeutic dosage levels, all antihistamines except astemizole and loratadine are likely to cause drowsiness and impaired motor function during initial therapy. Also, their anticholinergic action usually causes dry mouth and throat, blurred vision, and constipation. Antihistamines that are also phenothiazines, such as promethazine, may cause other adverse effects, including cholestatic jaundice (thought to be a hypersensitivity reaction), and may predispose patients to photosensitivity; patients taking such drugs should avoid prolonged exposure to sunlight.

Toxic doses elicit a combination of CNS depression and excitation as well as atropine-like symptoms, including sedation, reduced mental alertness, apnea, CV collapse, hallucinations, tremors, seizures, dry mouth, flushed skin, and fixed, dilated pupils. Toxic effects reverse when medication is discontinued. Used appropriately, in correct doses, antihistamines are safe for prolonged use.

Clinical considerations

- Don't use antihistamines during an acute asthma attack because they may not alleviate the symptoms, and antimuscarinic effects can cause thickening of secretions.
- Use antihistamines with caution in geriatric patients and in those with increased intraocular pressure, hyperthyroidism, CV or renal disease, diabetes, hypertension, bronchial asthma, urine retention, prostatic hypertrophy, bladder neck obstruction, or stenosing peptic ulcers.
- Recommend monitoring blood counts during long-term therapy; watch for signs of blood dyscrasias.
- Recommend giving antihistamines with food to reduce GI distress; recommend sugarless gum, sour hard candy, or ice chips to relieve dry mouth; increase fluid intake (if allowed) or humidify air to decrease adverse effect of thickened secretions.
- If tolerance develops to one antihistamine, another may be substituted.
- Some antihistamines may mask ototoxicity from high doses of aspirin and other salicylates.

Special populations

Pregnant patients. Safe use of antihistamines during pregnancy hasn't been established. Some manufacturers recommend that drugs not be used during the third trimester of pregnancy because of the risk of severe reactions, such as seizures, in neonates and premature infants.

Breast-feeding patients. Antihistamines shouldn't be used during breast-feeding.

Pediatric patients. Children, especially those under age 6, may experience paradoxical hyperexcitability with restlessness, insomnia, nervousness, euphoria, tremors, and seizures.

Geriatric patients. Geriatric patients are usually more sensitive to adverse effects of antihistamines and are especially likely to experience a greater degree of dizziness, sedation, hypotension, and urine retention.

Patient counseling

- Advise patient to take drug with meals or snacks to prevent gastric upset and to use any of the following measures to relieve dry mouth: warm water rinses, artificial saliva, ice chips, or sugarless gum or candy. The patient should avoid overusing mouthwash, which may add

to dryness (alcohol content) and destroy normal flora.
- Warn patient to avoid hazardous activities, such as driving a car or operating machinery, until extent of CNS effects are known and to seek medical approval before using alcoholic beverages, tranquilizers, sedatives, pain relievers, or sleeping medications.
- Warn patient to stop taking antihistamines 4 days before diagnostic skin tests to preserve accuracy of tests.

Representative combinations

Carbinoxamine maleate with pseudoephedrine and dextromethorphan: Carbodec DM, Pseudo-Car DM, Rondec-DM, Tussafed; with pseudoephedrine hydrochloride: Rondec, Rondec-TR; with pseudoephedrine and guaifenesin: Brexin L.A.

Chlorpheniramine with phenylephrine and phenylpropanolamine: Naldecon; with dextromethorphan: Vicks Formula 44 Cough Mixture; with codeine and guaifenesin: Tussar SF; with acetaminophen: Coricidin Tablets; with pseudoephedrine and dextromethorphan: Rhinosyn-DM; with pseudoephedrine, dextromethorphan, and acetaminophen: Co-Apap; with phenylpropanolamine: Contac 12-hour, Ornade, Resaid S.R., Triaminic-12, Dura-Vent; with pseudoephedrine hydrochloride: Cophene No. 2, Rescon Capsules, Chlordrine S.R., Chlorphendrine SR, Colfed-A, Duralex, Klerist-D, Kronofed-A, N-D Clear, Pseudo-Clor, Rescon-ED, Time-Hist, Chlorpheniramine Maleate/Pseudoephedrine HCl.

Diphenhydramine with pseudoephedrine: Benadryl Decongestant, Benylin DM; with acetaminophen: Tylenol Severe Allergy.

Promethazine with codeine: Phenergan with codeine; with dextromethorphan: Phenergan with Dextromethorphan; with phenylephrine: Phenergan VC; with phenylephrine and codeine: Phenergan VC with codeine.

Pyrilamine maleate with codeine: Tricodene Cough and Cold; with phenylephrine and codeine: Codimal; with phenylephrine and dextromethorphan: Codimal DM; with phenylephrine, dextromethorphan, and acetaminophen: Robitussin Night Relief; with phenylephrine and hydrocodone: Codimal; with phenylpropanolamine, chlorpheniramine maleate, and dextromethorphan: Tricodene Forte, Tricodene NN, Triminol Cough.

Triprolidine with pseudoephedrine and codeine: Actifed with Codeine, CoActifed*, Pseudodine C Cough; with pseudoephedrine: Actagen, Actifed, Allerfrin, Novafed, Triacin-C, Triafed with Codeine, Trifed-C, Trifed-C Cough, Triofed, Triposed.

barbiturates

amobarbital, amobarbital sodium, aprobarbital, butabarbital sodium, mephobarbital, metharbital, phenobarbital, pentobarbital sodium, phenobarbital sodium, primidone, secobarbital sodium

Barbituric acid was compounded in 1864. The first hypnotic barbiturate, barbital, was introduced into medicine in 1903. Although barbiturates have been used extensively as sedative-hypnotics and antianxiety agents, benzodiazepines are the current drugs of choice for sedative-hypnotic effects. Phenobarbital, mephobarbital, and metharbital remain effective for anticonvulsant therapy. A few short-acting barbiturates are used as general anesthetics.

Pharmacology

Barbiturates are structurally related compounds that act throughout the CNS, particularly in the mesencephalic reticular activating system, which controls the CNS arousal mechanism. Barbiturates induce an imbalance in central inhibitory and facilitatory mechanisms, which, in turn, influence the cerebral cortex and the reticular formation. Barbiturates decrease both presynaptic and postsynaptic membrane excitability.

The exact mechanisms of action of barbiturates at these sites aren't known, nor is it clear which cellular and synaptic actions result in sedative-hypnotic effects. Barbiturates can produce all levels of CNS depression, from mild sedation to coma to death. Barbiturates exert their effects by facilitating the actions of gamma-aminobutyric acid (GABA). Barbiturates also exert a central effect, which depresses respiration and GI motility. Barbiturates have no analgesic action and may increase the reaction to painful stimuli at subanesthetic doses. The principal anticonvulsant mechanism of action is reduction of nerve transmission and decreased excitability of the nerve cell. Barbiturates also raise the seizure threshold.

Clinical indications and actions

Seizure disorders

Phenobarbital is used in the prophylactic treatment and acute management of seizure disorders. It's used mainly in tonic-clonic (grand mal) and partial seizures. At anesthetic doses, all barbiturates have anticonvulsant activity. Phenobarbital is an effective parenteral agent for status epilepticus (with airway support). Mephobarbital and metharbital may also be used.

Barbiturates suppress the spread of seizure activity produced by epileptogenic foci in the cortex, thalamus, and limbic systems by enhancing the effects of GABA.

Sedation, hypnosis
Most currently available barbiturates are used as sedative-hypnotics for short-term (up to 2 weeks) treatment of insomnia because of their nonspecific CNS effects.

Barbiturates aren't used routinely as sedatives. Barbiturate-induced sleep differs from physiologic sleep in that rapid-eye-movement sleep cycles are reduced.

Preanesthesia sedation
Barbiturates are also used as preanesthetic sedatives and for relief of anxiety.

Psychiatric use
Barbiturates (especially amobarbital) have been used parenterally in narcoanalysis and narcotherapy and in identifying schizophrenia.

Overview of adverse reactions
Drowsiness, lethargy, vertigo, headache, and CNS depression are common with barbiturates. After hypnotic doses, a hangover effect, subtle distortion of mood, and impairment of judgment or motor skills may continue for many hours. After a decrease in dose or discontinuation of barbiturates used for hypnosis, rebound insomnia or increased dreaming or nightmares may occur. Barbiturates cause hyperalgesia in subhypnotic doses. Hypersensitivity reactions (rash, fever, serum sickness) aren't common and are more likely to occur in patients with a history of asthma or allergies to other drugs; reactions include urticaria, rash, angioedema, and Stevens-Johnson syndrome. Barbiturates can cause paradoxical excitement at low doses, confusion in geriatric patients, and hyperactivity in children. High fever, severe headache, stomatitis, conjunctivitis, or rhinitis may precede skin eruptions. Because of the potential for fatal consequences, discontinue barbiturates if dermatologic reactions occur.

Withdrawal symptoms may occur after as little as 2 weeks of uninterrupted therapy. Symptoms of abstinence usually occur within 8 to 12 hours after the last dose, but may be delayed up to 5 days. They include weakness, anxiety, nausea, vomiting, insomnia, hallucinations, and possibly seizures.

Clinical considerations
- Doses of barbiturates must be individualized.
- Don't use barbiturates in patients with porphyria, liver impairment, severe respiratory disease, or previous addiction to barbiturates or in nephritic patients.
- Use barbiturates cautiously, if at all, in patients who are mentally depressed or have suicidal tendencies or history of drug abuse.
- Avoid administering barbiturates to patients with status asthmaticus.
- Parenteral solutions are highly alkaline and contain organic solvents (propylene glycol); infuse at 100 mg/min or less; avoid extravasation, which may cause local tissue damage and tissue necrosis; inject I.V. or deep I.M. only. Don't exceed 5 ml per I.M. injection site to avoid tissue damage.
- Rapid I.V. administration of barbiturates may cause respiratory depression, apnea, laryngospasm, or hypotension. Have resuscitative measures available. I.V. site should be assessed for signs of infiltration or phlebitis.
- Drug may be given P.R. if oral or parenteral route is inappropriate; it shouldn't be given intra-arterially or S.C.
- Recommend assessment of level of consciousness before and frequently during therapy to evaluate effectiveness of drug. Recommend monitoring of neurologic status for possible alterations or deteriorations and monitoring of seizure character, frequency, and duration for changes.
- Vital signs must be checked frequently, especially during I.V. administration.
- Assess patient's sleeping patterns before and during therapy to ensure effectiveness of drug.
- Recommend safety measures—side rails, assistance when out of bed, call light within reach—to prevent falls and injury.
- Consider airway support during I.V. administration.
- Anticipate possible rebound confusion and excitatory reactions in patient.
- Monitor patient for complaints of constipation. Advise diet high in fiber, if indicated.
- Carefully monitor PT and INR in patients taking anticoagulants; dose of anticoagulant may require adjustment to counteract possible interaction.
- Abrupt discontinuation may cause withdrawal symptoms; discontinue slowly.
- Death is common with an overdose of 2 to 10 g; it may occur at much smaller doses if alcohol is also ingested.

Special populations
Pregnant patients. Barbiturates may cause fetal harm. Postpartum hemorrhage and hemorrhagic disease of the newborn has occurred. The latter can be reversed with vitamin K therapy. If a woman is taking these medications in the last trimester of pregnancy, neonates may exhibit withdrawal symptoms.

Breast-feeding patients. Barbiturates are excreted in breast milk and may result in infant CNS depression. Use with caution.

Pediatric patients. Premature infants are more susceptible to the depressant effects of barbiturates because of immature hepatic metabolism. Children receiving barbiturates may experience hyperactivity, excitement, or hyperalgia.

Geriatric patients. Geriatric patients and patients receiving subhypnotic doses may experience hyperactivity, excitement, confusion, depression, or hyperalgesia. Use with caution.

Patient counseling

- Warn patient to avoid use of other drugs with CNS depressant effects, such as antihistamines, analgesics, and alcohol, because they have additive effects and result in increased drowsiness. Instruct patient to seek medical approval before taking OTC cold or allergy preparations.
- Caution patient not to change dose or frequency without medical approval; abrupt discontinuation of medication may trigger rebound insomnia, with increased dreaming, nightmares, or seizures.
- Warn patient against driving and other hazardous tasks that require alertness while taking barbiturates. Instruct him in safety measures to prevent injury.
- Be sure women understand that barbiturates are capable of causing physical or psychological dependence (addiction), and that these effects may be transmitted to a fetus; withdrawal symptoms can occur in neonates whose mothers took barbiturates in the third trimester.
- Instruct patient to report skin eruption or other marked adverse effect.
- Explain that a morning hangover is common after therapeutic use of barbiturates.

Representative combinations

Amobarbital with secobarbital: Tuinal 100 mg Pulvules, Tuinal 200 mg Pulvules.

Butabarbital with acetaminophen: Sedapap; with belladonna: Butibel.

Phenobarbital with CNS stimulants: Bronkolixir, Bronkotabs, Quadrinal; with ergotamine tartrate: Bellergal-S; with phenytoin: Dilantin Kapseals; with aminophylline and ephedrine hydrochloride: Mudrane; with belladonna: Chardonna-2, Butibel, Butibel Elixir; with atropine: Antrocol; with hyoscyamine: Levsin-PB, Levsin and Phenobarbital, Bellacane; with ASA and codeine phosphate: Phenaphen with Codeine No. 3, Phenaphen with Codeine No. 4; with atropine, hyoscyamine, and scopolamine hydrobromide: Donnatal, Donnatol No. 2, Donnamor, Donnapine, Donnatal Extentabs, Barbidonna, Barophen, Hyosophen, Kinesed, Spasmophen, Spasquid, Susano, Barbidonna No. 2, Belladonna Alkoids with Phenobarbital Tablets, Malatal, Antispasmodic Elixir, Hyoscyamine Compound, Phenobarbital with Belladonna Alkaloids Elixir.

Pentobarbital sodium with ephedrine: Ephedrine and Nembutal Sodium; with ergotamine tartrate and caffeine: Cafergot-PB.

See also *anticholinergics (belladonna alkaloids).*

benzodiazepines

alprazolam, chlordiazepoxide hydrochloride, clonazepam, clorazepate dipotassium, diazepam, estazolam, flurazepam hydrochloride, lorazepam, midazolam hydrochloride, oxazepam, quazepam, temazepam, triazolam

Benzodiazepines, synthetically produced sedative-hypnotics, gained popularity in the early 1960s, replacing barbiturates as the treatment of choice for anxiety, convulsive disorders, and sedation. These drugs are preferred over barbiturates because therapeutic doses produce less drowsiness, respiratory depression, and impairment of motor function, and toxic doses are less likely to be fatal.

Pharmacology

Benzodiazepines are a group of structurally related chemicals that selectively act on polysynaptic neuronal pathways throughout the CNS. Their precise sites and mechanisms of action aren't completely known. However, the benzodiazepines enhance or facilitate the action of gamma-aminobutyric acid (GABA), an inhibitory neurotransmitter in the CNS. The drugs appear to act at the limbic, thalamic, and hypothalamic levels of the CNS. These drugs produce anxiolytic, sedative, hypnotic, skeletal muscle relaxant, and anticonvulsant effects. All of the benzodiazepines have CNS-depressant activities; however, individual derivatives act more selectively at specific sites, allowing them to be subclassified into five categories based on their predominant clinical use.

Clinical indications and actions

Seizure disorders

Four of the benzodiazepines (diazepam, clonazepam, clorazepate, and parenteral lorazepam) are used as anticonvulsants. Their anticonvulsant properties are derived from an ability to suppress the spread of seizure activity produced by epileptogenic foci in the cortex, thalamus, and limbic systems by enhancing presynaptic inhibition. Clonazepam is useful in the adjunctive treatment of petit mal variant (Lennox-Gastaut syndrome), myoclonic, or akinetic seizures. Benzodiazepines are also useful adjuncts for the prophylactic management of partial seizures with elementary symptoms (Jacksonian seizures), psychomotor seizures, and petit mal seizures. Parenteral diazepam is indicated to treat status epilepticus.

Anxiety, tension, and insomnia

Most benzodiazepines (alprazolam, chlordiazepoxide, clorazepate, diazepam, estazolam, flurazepam, lorazepam, oxazepam, quazepam, temazepam, and triazolam) are useful as antianxiety agents or sedative-hypnotic agents. They have a similar mechanism of action; they're believed to facilitate the effects of GABA in the ascending reticular activating system, increasing inhibition and blocking both cortical and limbic arousal.

They're used to treat anxiety and tension that occur alone or as an adverse effect of a primary disorder. They aren't recommended for tension associated with everyday stress. The choice of a specific benzodiazepine depends on individual metabolic characteristics of the drug. For instance, in patients with depressed renal or hepatic function, alprazolam, lorazepam, or oxazepam may be selected because they have a relatively short duration of action and have no active metabolites.

The sedative-hypnotic properties of chlordiazepoxide, clorazepate, diazepam, lorazepam, and oxazepam make these the drugs of choice as preoperative medication and as an adjunct in the rehabilitation of alcoholics.

Surgical adjuncts for conscious sedation or amnesia

Diazepam, midazolam, and lorazepam have amnesic effects. The mechanism of such action isn't known. Parenteral administration before such procedures as endoscopy or elective cardioversion causes impairment of recent memory and interferes with the establishment of memory trace, producing anterograde amnesia.

Skeletal muscle spasm, tremor

Because oral forms of diazepam and chlordiazepoxide have skeletal muscle relaxant properties, they're often used to treat neurologic conditions involving muscle spasms and tetanus. The mechanism of such action is unknown, but they're believed to inhibit spinal polysynaptic and monosynaptic afferent pathways.

Delirium

Benzodiazepines may be beneficial alone or in combination with antipsychotic agents to treat delirium. However, caution should be used because benzodiazepines can also exacerbate delirium.

◇ ***Schizophrenia***

Benzodiazepines have been used as an adjunct to antipsychotic drugs in the management of schizophrenia.

◇ ***Cancer chemotherapy-induced nausea and vomiting***

Benzodiazepines have been used as an adjunct to control nausea and vomiting associated with emetogenic cancer chemotherapy.

◇ ***Neonatal opiate withdrawal***

Parenteral diazepam has been used to relieve agitation associated with neonatal opiate withdrawal.

Overview of adverse reactions

Therapeutic dosage of the benzodiazepines usually causes drowsiness and impaired motor function, which should be monitored early in treatment. It may or may not be persistent. GI discomfort, such as constipation, diarrhea, vomiting, and changes in appetite, with urinary alterations, also have been reported. Visual disturbances and CV irregularities also are common. Continuing problems with short-term memory, confusion, severe depression, shakiness, vertigo, slurred speech, staggering, bradycardia, shortness of breath or difficulty breathing, and severe weakness usually indicate a toxic dose level. Prolonged or frequent use of benzodiazepines can cause physical dependency and withdrawal syndrome when use is discontinued.

Clinical considerations

- Benzodiazepines shouldn't be used in patients with chronic pulmonary insufficiency, sleep apnea, depressive neuroses or psychotic reactions without predominant anxiety, or acute alcohol intoxication.
- Recommend assessing level of consciousness and neurologic status before and frequently during therapy for changes. Health care professionals should monitor for paradoxical reactions, especially early in therapy.
- Recommend observing sleep patterns and quality, and for changes in seizure character, frequency, or duration.
- Recommend assessing vital signs frequently during therapy. Significant changes in blood pressure and heart rate may indicate impending toxicity.
- Recommend administering dose with milk or immediately after meals to prevent GI upset. Give antacid, if needed, at least 1 hour before or after dose to prevent interaction and ensure maximum drug absorption and effectiveness.
- Periodically monitor renal and hepatic function to ensure adequate drug removal and prevent cumulative effects.
- Recommend safety measures be instituted—raised side rails and ambulatory assistance—to prevent injury. Anticipate possible rebound excitement reactions.
- After prolonged use, abrupt discontinuation may cause withdrawal symptoms; discontinue gradually.

Special populations

Pregnant patients. Benzodiazepines can cause fetal harm if administered during pregnancy. There's an increased risk of congenital malformation if given during the first trimester. Use of benzodiazepines during labor may cause neonatal flaccidity. Use should be determined if benefits outweigh risks.

Breast-feeding patients. The breast-fed infant of a mother who uses a benzodiazepine drug may show sedation, feeding difficulties, and weight loss. Safe use hasn't been established.

Pediatric patients. Because children, particularly very young ones, are sensitive to the

CNS depressant effects of benzodiazepines, exercise caution. A neonate whose mother took a benzodiazepine during pregnancy may exhibit withdrawal symptoms.
Geriatric patients. Because they're sensitive to CNS effects, geriatric patients receiving benzodiazepines require lower doses; use with caution.

Parenteral administration of these drugs is more likely to cause apnea, hypotension, bradycardia, and cardiac arrest.

Geriatric patients may show prolonged elimination of benzodiazepines, except possibly of oxazepam, lorazepam, temazepam, and triazolam.

Patient counseling

- Warn patient to avoid use of alcohol or other CNS depressants, such as antihistamines, analgesics, MAO inhibitors, antidepressants, and barbiturates, to prevent additive depressant effects.
- Caution patient to take drug as prescribed and not to give medication to others. Tell him not to change the dose or frequency and to call before taking OTC cold or allergy preparations that may potentiate CNS depressant effects.
- Warn patient to avoid activities requiring alertness and good psychomotor coordination until the CNS response to the drug is determined. Instruct him in safety measures to prevent injury.
- Tell patient to avoid using antacids, which may delay drug absorption, unless prescribed.
- Be sure patient understands that benzodiazepines are capable of causing physical and psychological dependence with prolonged use.
- Warn patient not to stop taking the drug abruptly to prevent withdrawal symptoms after prolonged therapy.
- Tell patient that smoking decreases the effectiveness of the drug. Encourage patient to stop smoking during therapy.
- Tell patient to report adverse effects. These are often dose-related and can be relieved by dosage adjustments.
- Inform a woman of child-bearing age who is taking drug to report if she suspects pregnancy or intends to become pregnant during therapy.

Representative combinations

Chlordiazepoxide with amitriptyline hydrochloride: Limbitrol DS; with clidinium bromide: Librax; with esterified estrogens: Menrium.

beta blockers

beta$_1$ blockers: **acebutolol, atenolol, betaxolol hydrochloride, bisoprolol, esmolol, metoprolol tartrate**

beta$_1$ and beta$_2$ blockers: **carteolol hydrochloride, carvedilol, labetalol, levobunolol hydrochloride, metipranolol hydrochloride, nadolol, penbutolol sulfate, pindolol, propranolol, sotalol, timolol maleate**

Beta blockers were first used in the early 1960s; they're currently widely used to treat hypertension, angina pectoris, and arrhythmias. These agents are well tolerated by most patients.

Pharmacology

Beta blockers are chemicals that compete with beta agonists for available beta-receptor sites; individual agents differ in their ability to affect beta receptors. Some available agents are considered nonselective; that is, they block both beta$_1$ receptors in cardiac muscle and beta$_2$ receptors in bronchial and vascular smooth muscle. Several agents are cardioselective and in lower doses primarily inhibit beta$_1$ receptors. Some beta blockers have intrinsic sympathomimetic activity and simultaneously stimulate and block beta receptors, decreasing cardiac output; still others also have membrane-stabilizing activity, which affects cardiac action potential. (See *Comparing beta blockers*.)

Clinical indications and actions

Hypertension

Most beta blockers are used to treat hypertension. Although the exact mechanism of their antihypertensive effect is unknown, the action is thought to result from decreased cardiac output, decreased sympathetic outflow from the CNS, and suppression of renin release.

Angina

Propranolol, atenolol, nadolol, and metoprolol are used to treat angina pectoris; they decrease myocardial oxygen requirements through the blockade of catecholamine-induced increases in heart rate, blood pressure, and the extent of myocardial contraction.

Arrhythmias

Propranolol, acebutolol, sotalol, and esmolol are used to treat arrhythmias; they prolong the refractory period of the AV node and slow AV conduction.

Glaucoma

The mechanism by which betaxolol, levobunolol, metipranolol, and timolol reduce intraocular pressure is unknown, but the drug effect is at least partially caused by decreased production of aqueous humor.

COMPARING BETA BLOCKERS

Drug	Half-life (hr)	Lipid solubility	Membrane-stabilizing activity	Intrinsic sympathomimetic activity
Nonselective				
carteolol	6	low	0	++
carvedilol	7 to 10	high	not known	0
labetalol	6 to 8	moderate	0	0
metipranolol	4	low to moderate	0	0
nadolol	20	low	0	0
penbutolol	5	high	0	+
pindolol	3 to 4	moderate	+	+++
propranolol	4	high	++	0
timolol	4	low to moderate	0	0
$Beta_1$-selective				
acebutolol	3 to 4	low	+	+
atenolol	6 to 7	low	0	0
betaxolol	14 to 22	low	+	0
bisoprolol	9 to 12	low	0	0
esmolol	0.15	low	0	0
metoprolol	3 to 7	moderate	♦	0

♦ Only in higher-than-usual doses.
+ Activity that drug possesses in comparison to other beta blockers.

MI
Timolol, propranolol, atenolol, and metoprolol are used to prevent MI in susceptible patients.

Migraine prophylaxis
Propranolol and timolol are used to prevent recurrent attacks of migraine and other vascular headaches. The exact mechanism by which propranolol and timolol decrease the incidence of migraine headache attacks is unknown, but it's thought to result from inhibition of vasodilation of cerebral vessels.

Other uses
Some beta blockers have been used as antianxiety agents, for managing subaortic stenosis, as adjunctive therapy of bleeding esophageal varices or pheochromocytomas, and to treat portal hypertension or essential tremors. Carvedilol is used to treat heart failure with cardiac glycosides, diuretics, or ACE inhibitors.

Overview of adverse reactions
Therapeutic doses may cause bradycardia, fatigue, and dizziness; some cause other CNS disturbances, such as nightmares, depression, memory loss, or hallucinations. Impotence, cold extremities, and elevated cholesterol levels may also occur. Severe hypotension, bradycardia, heart failure, or bronchospasm usually indicates toxic dose levels.

Clinical considerations
- Recommend monitoring of BP, ECG, and apical heart rate and rhythm frequently; be alert for progression of AV block or severe bradycardia.
- Patients with heart failure must be weighed regularly; watch for gains of more than 5 lb (2.27 kg) per week.
- Signs of hypoglycemic shock are masked; watch diabetic patients for sweating, fatigue, and hunger. Tachycardia in hyperthyroidism is also masked.
- Don't discontinue these drugs before surgery for pheochromocytoma; before any surgical procedure, notify anesthesiologist that patient is taking a beta blocker.
- Glucagon may be prescribed to reverse signs and symptoms of beta blocker overdose.
- Don't dispense to patients with asthma, sinus bradycardia, first-degree heart block, cardiogenic shock, or overt cardiac failure.

Special populations
Pregnant patients. Pregnancy risk category is C/D. Avoid beta blocker therapy in pregnant women. Atenolol has been associated with intrauterine growth retardation.
Breast-feeding patients. Beta blockers are distributed into breast milk. Recommendations for breast-feeding vary with individual drugs.
Pediatric patients. Safety and efficacy of beta blockers in children haven't been established; they should be used only if potential benefit outweighs risk.
Geriatric patients. Geriatric patients may require lower maintenance dosages of beta blockers; they also may experience enhanced adverse effects.

Patient counseling

- Explain rationale for therapy, and emphasize importance of taking drug as prescribed, even when feeling well.
- Warn patient that abrupt discontinuation can exacerbate angina or precipitate MI.
- Teach patient to minimize dizziness from orthostatic hypotension by taking dose at bedtime, and by rising slowly and avoiding sudden position changes.
- Advise patient to seek medical approval before taking OTC cold preparations.

Representative combinations

Atenolol with chlorthalidone: Tenoretic.

Bisoprolol with hydrochlorothiazide: Ziac Tablets.

Metoprolol with hydrochlorothiazide: Lopressor HCT.

Pindolol with hydrochlorothiazide: Viskazide.

Propranolol hydrochloride with hydrochlorothiazide: Inderide, Inderide LA.

Timolol with hydrochlorothiazide: Timolide.

calcium channel blockers

amlodipine besylate, bepridil hydrochloride, diltiazem hydrochloride, felodipine, isradipine, nicardipine hydrochloride, nifedipine, nimodipine, nisoldipine, verapamil hydrochloride

Calcium channel blockers (also called slow channel calcium antagonists or slow channel blockers) were introduced in the United States in the early 1980s. They have become increasingly popular as a treatment for classic and variant angina and have come to be the preferred drugs for Prinzmetal's variant angina (vasospastic angina). They have been used as antihypertensives. Verapamil has proved effective in the acute treatment of supraventricular tachycardias (SVTs). (See *Comparing oral calcium channel blockers.)*

Pharmacology

The main physiologic action of calcium channel blockers is to inhibit calcium influx across the slow channels of myocardial and vascular smooth muscle cells. By inhibiting calcium influx into these cells, calcium channel blockers reduce intracellular calcium concentrations. This, in turn, dilates coronary arteries, peripheral arteries, and arterioles, and slows cardiac conduction.

When used to treat Prinzmetal's variant angina, calcium channel blockers inhibit coronary spasm, increasing oxygen delivery to the heart. Peripheral artery dilation leads to a decrease in total peripheral resistance; this reduces afterload, which, in turn, decreases myocardial oxygen consumption. Inhibition of calcium influx into the specialized cardiac conduction cells (specifically, those in the SA and AV nodes) slows conduction through the heart. This effect is most pronounced with verapamil and diltiazem.

Clinical indications and actions

Angina

Calcium channel blockers are useful in managing Prinzmetal's variant angina, chronic stable angina, and unstable angina. In Prinzmetal's variant angina, they inhibit spontaneous and ergonovine-induced coronary spasm, thereby increasing coronary blood flow and maintaining myocardial oxygen delivery. In unstable and chronic stable angina, their effectiveness presumably stems from their ability to reduce afterload.

Arrhythmias

Of the calcium channel blockers, verapamil and diltiazem have the greatest effect on the AV node, slowing the ventricular rate in atrial fibrillation or flutter and converting SVT to normal sinus rhythm.

Hypertension

Because they dilate systemic arteries, most of these agents are useful in mild to moderate hypertension.

Other uses

Calcium channel blockers (especially verapamil) may also prove to be effective as a hypertrophic cardiomyopathy therapy adjunct by improving left ventricular outflow as a result of negative inotropic effects and possibly improved diastolic function. They've been used to treat migraine headaches, peripheral vascular disorders, subarachnoid hemorrhage (nimodipine) and as adjunctive therapy in the treatment of esophageal spasm.

Overview of adverse reactions

Verapamil may cause adverse effects on the conduction system, including bradycardia and various degrees of heart block, exacerbate heart failure, and cause hypotension after rapid I.V. administration. Prolonged oral verapamil therapy may cause constipation.

Adverse effects of nifedipine include hypotension, reflex tachycardia, peripheral edema, flushing, light-headedness, and headache.

Diltiazem most commonly causes anorexia, nausea, various degrees of heart block, bradycardia, heart failure, and peripheral edema.

Clinical considerations

- Recommend monitoring of cardiac rate and rhythm and blood pressure carefully when initiating therapy or increasing dose.
- Use of calcium supplements may decrease the effectiveness of calcium channel blockers.

COMPARING ORAL CALCIUM CHANNEL BLOCKERS

Drug	Onset of action	Peak serum level	Half-life	Therapeutic serum level
bepridil	1 hr	2 to 3 hr	24 hr	1 to 2 ng/ml
diltiazem	15 min	30 min	3 to 4 hr	50 to 200 ng/ml
felodipine	2 to 5 hr	2.5 to 5 hr	11 to 16 hr	unknown
nicardipine	20 min	1 hr	8.6 hr	28 to 50 ng/ml
nifedipine	5 to 30 min	30 min to 2 hr	2 to 5 hr	25 to 100 ng/ml
nimodipine	unknown	<1 hr	1 to 2 hr	unknown
nisoldipine	unknown	6 to 12 hr	7 to 12 hr	unknown
verapamil	30 min	1 to 2.2 hr	6 to 12 hr	80 to 300 ng/ml

- Use cautiously in patients with impaired left ventricular function.

Special populations

Pregnant patients. Pregnancy risk category is C. Avoid use in pregnant women.
Breast-feeding patients. Calcium channel blocking agents (verapamil and diltiazem) may be excreted in breast milk. To avoid possible adverse effects in infants, discontinue breast-feeding during therapy with these drugs.
Pediatric patients. Adverse hemodynamic effects of parenteral verapamil have been observed in neonates and infants. Safety and effectiveness of diltiazem and nifedipine haven't been established.
Geriatric patients. Use with caution because the half-life of calcium channel blockers may be increased as a result of decreased clearance.

Patient counseling

- Tell patient not to abruptly discontinue drug; gradual dose reduction may be necessary.
- Instruct patient to report irregular heartbeat, shortness of breath, swelling of hands and feet, pronounced dizziness, constipation, nausea, or hypotension.
- Warn patient not to double the dose.

Representative combinations

Amlodipine and benazepril hydrochloride: Lotrel.

cephalosporins

First-generation cephalosporins: **cefadroxil, cefazolin sodium, cephalexin monohydrate, cephalothin sodium, cephradine**

Second-generation cephalosporins: **cefaclor, cefamandole nafate, cefmetazole sodium, cefonicid sodium, cefotetan disodium, cefoxitin sodium, cefprozil, ceftibuten, cefuroxime axetil, cefuroxime sodium**

Third-generation cephalosporins: **cefdinir, cefixime, cefoperazone sodium, cefotaxime sodium, cefpodoxime proxetil, ceftazidime, ceftizoxime sodium, ceftriaxone sodium**

Fourth-generation cephalosporin: **cefepime hydrochloride**

Cephalosporins are beta-lactam antibiotics first isolated in 1948 from the fungus *Cephalosporium acremonium.* Their mechanism of action is similar to that of penicillins, but their antibacterial spectra differ.

Pharmacology

Cephalosporins are chemically and pharmacologically similar to penicillin; their structure contains a beta-lactam ring, a dihydrothiazine ring, and side chains, and they act by inhibiting bacterial cell wall synthesis, causing rapid cell lysis. (See *Comparing cephalosporins,* page 32.)

The sites of action for cephalosporins are enzymes known as penicillin-binding proteins (PBP). The affinity of certain cephalosporins for PBP in various microorganisms helps explain the differing spectra of activity in this class of antibiotics.

COMPARING CEPHALOSPORINS

Drug and route	Elimination half-life (hr)		Sodium (mEq/g)	CSF Penetration
	Normal renal function	End-stage renal disease		
cefaclor oral	0.5 to 1	3 to 5.5	Unknown	No
cefadroxil oral	1 to 2	20 to 25	Unknown	No
cefamandole I.M., I.V.	0.5 to 2	12 to 18	3.3	No
cefazolin I.M., I.V.	1.2 to 2.2	3 to 7	2.0 to 2.1	No
cefdinir P.O.	1.5	16	Unknown	Unknown
cefepime I.M., I.V.	2	17 to 21	Unknown	Yes
cefixime oral	3 to 4	11.5	Unknown	Unknown
cefmetazole I.V.	1.2	Unknown	2	Unknown
cefonicid I.M., I.V.	3.5 to 5.8	11	3.7	No
cefoperazone I.M., I.V.	1.5 to 2.5	1.3 to 2.9	1.5	Sometimes
cefotaxime I.M., I.V.	1 to 1.5	3 to 11	2.2	Yes
cefotetan I.M., I.V.	2.8 to 4.6	13 to 35	3.5	No
cefoxitin I.M., I.V.	0.5 to 1	6.5 to 21.5	2.3	No
cefpodoxime oral	2 to 3	9.8	Unknown	Unknown
cefprozil oral	1 to 1.5	5.2 to 5.9	Unknown	Unknown
ceftazidime I.M., I.V.	1.5 to 2	35	2.3	Yes
ceftibuten oral	2.4	13.4 to 22.3	Unknown	Unknown
ceftizoxime I.M., I.V.	1.5 to 2	30	2.6	Yes
ceftriaxone I.M., I.V.	5.5 to 11	15.7	3.6	Yes
cefuroxime I.M., I.V.	1 to 2	15 to 22	2.4	Yes
cephalexin oral	0.5 to 1	19 to 22	Unknown	No
cephalothin I.M., I.V.	0.5 to 1	19	2.8	No
cephapirin I.M., I.V.	0.5 to 1	1.0 to 1.5	2.4	No
cephradine oral, I.M., I.V.	0.5 to 2	8 to 15	6	No

Bacterial resistance to beta-lactam antibiotics is conferred most significantly by production of beta-lactamase enzymes (by both gram-negative and gram-positive bacteria) that destroy the beta-lactam ring and thus inactivate cephalosporins; decreased cell wall permeability and alteration in binding affinity to PBP also contribute to bacterial resistance.

Cephalosporins are bactericidal; they act against many gram-positive and gram-negative bacteria, and some anaerobic bacteria; they don't kill fungi or viruses.

First-generation cephalosporins act against many gram-positive cocci, including penicillinase-producing *Stapylococcus aureus* and *Staphylococcus epidermidis; Streptococcus pneumoniae, Streptococcus agalactiae* (group B streptococci), and *Streptococcus pyogenes* (group A beta-hemolytic streptococci); susceptible gram-negative organisms include *Klebsiella pneumoniae, Escherichia coli, Proteus mirabilis,* and *Shigella.*

Second-generation cephalosporins are effective against all organisms attacked by first-generation drugs and have additional activity against *Branhamella catarrhalis, Haemophilus influenzae, Enterobacter, Citrobacter, Providencia, Acinetobacter, Serratia,* and *Neisseria; Bacteroides fragilis* is susceptible to cefotetan and cefoxitin.

Third-generation cephalosporins are less active than first- and second-generation drugs against gram-positive bacteria, but more active against gram-negative organisms, including those resistant to first- and second-generation drugs; they have the greatest stability against beta-lactamases produced by gram-negative bacteria. Susceptible gram-negative organisms *include E. coli, Klebsiella, Enterobacter, Providencia, Acinetobacter, Serratia, Proteus, Morganella,* and *Neisseria;* some third-generation drugs are active against *B. fragilis* and *Pseudomonas.*

The fourth-generation cephalosporin cefepime is active against a wide range of gram-positive and gram-negative bacteria. Susceptible gram-negative organisms *include Enterobacter spp., E. coli, K. pneumoniae, P. mirabilis,* and *Pseudomonas aeruginosa;* susceptible gram-positive organisms include *S. aureus* (methicillin-susceptible strains only), *S. pneumoniae,* and *S. pyogenes* (Lancefield's group A streptococci).

Oral absorption of cephalosporins varies widely; many must be given parenterally. Most are distributed widely into the body, the actual amount varying with individual drugs. CSF penetration by first- and second-generation drugs is minimal; third-generation drugs achieve much greater penetration, and although the fourth-generation drug cefepime is known to cross the blood-brain barrier, it isn't known to what degree. Cephalosporins cross the placenta. Degree of metabolism varies with individual drugs; some aren't metabolized at all, whereas others are extensively metabolized.

Cephalosporins are excreted primarily in urine, chiefly by renal tubular effects; elimination half-life ranges from 30 minutes to 10 hours in patients with normal renal function. Some drug is excreted in breast milk. Most cephalosporins can be removed by hemodialysis or peritoneal dialysis. Patients on dialysis may require dosage adjustment.

Clinical indications and actions

Infection caused by susceptible organisms

Parenteral cephalosporins: Cephalosporins are used to treat serious infections of the lungs, skin, soft tissue, bones, joints, urinary tract, blood (septicemia), abdomen, and ◇heart (endocarditis).

Third-generation cephalosporins (except moxalactam and cefoperazone) and the second-generation drug cefuroxime are used to treat CNS infections caused by susceptible strains *of N. meningitidis, H. influenzae,* and *S. pneumoniae;* meningitis caused by *E. coli* or *Klebsiella* can be treated with ceftriaxone, cefotaxime, or ceftizoxime.

First-generation and some second-generation cephalosporins also can be given prophylactically to reduce postoperative infection after surgical procedures classified as contaminated or potentially contaminated; third-generation drugs aren't usually indicated.

Penicillinase-producing *N. gonorrhoeae* can be treated with cefoxitin, cefotaxime, ceftriaxone, ceftizoxime, or cefuroxime.

Oral cephalosporins: Cephalosporins can be used to treat otitis media and infections of the respiratory tract, urinary tract, and skin and soft tissue.

◇Ceftriaxone, cefotaxime, or cefuroxime axetil has been used in the treatment of Lyme disease.

Cefepime, ceftazidime, and ceftriaxone have been used parenterally for empiric anti-infective therapy of probable bacterial infections in febrile neutropenic patients.

Overview of adverse reactions

Hypersensitivity reactions range from mild rash, fever, and eosinophilia to fatal anaphylaxis, and are more common in patients with penicillin allergy. Hematologic reactions include positive direct and indirect antiglobulin (Coombs' test), thrombocytopenia or thrombocythemia, transient neutropenia, and reversible leukopenia. Adverse renal effects, nausea, vomiting, diarrhea, abdominal pain, glossitis, dyspepsia, tenesmus, and minimal elevation of liver function test results have occurred. Hemolytic anemia with extravascular hemoysis and some fatalities have occurred in patients receiving cefotaxime, ceftizoxime, ceftriaxone, and cerotetan.

Local venous pain and irritation are common after I.M. injection; such reactions occur more often with higher doses and long-term therapy.

Disulfiram-type reactions occur when cefamandole, cefoperazone, moxalactam, cefonicid, or cefotetan are administered within 48 to 72 hours of alcohol ingestion.

Bacterial and fungal superinfection results from suppression of normal flora.

Clinical considerations

- Review patient's history of allergies.
- Recommend monitoring continuously for possible hypersensitivity reactions or other untoward effects.
- Monitor renal function studies; doses of certain cephalosporins must be lowered in patients with severe renal impairment. In decreased renal function, monitor BUN levels, serum creatinine levels, and urine output for significant changes.
- Recommend monitoring PT and platelet counts and assessing patient for signs of hypoprothrombinemia, which may occur, with or without bleeding, during therapy with cefamandole, cefepime, cefoperazone, cefonicid, or cefotetan, usually in geriatric, debilitated, or malnourished patients.
- Recommend monitoring patients on long-term therapy for possible bacterial and fungal superinfection, especially geriatric and debilitated patients, and others receiving immunosuppressants or radiation therapy.
- Recommend monitoring susceptible patients receiving sodium salts of cephalosporins for possible fluid retention; consult individual drug entry for sodium content.
- Cephalosporins cause false-positive results in urine glucose tests using cupric sulfate solutions (Benedict's reagent or Clinitest); glucose oxidase tests aren't affected. Consult individual drug entries for other possible test interactions.

Administration

- Give cephalosporins at least 1 hour before giving bacteriostatic antibiotics (tetracyclines, erythromycins, and chloramphenicol); these drugs inhibit bacterial cell growth, decreasing cephalosporin uptake by bacterial cell walls.
- Give oral cephalosporin at least 1 hour before or 2 hours after meals for maximum absorption.
- Refrigerate oral suspensions; shake well before administering to assure correct dose.
- Recommend administering I.M. dose deep into large muscle mass (gluteal or midlateral thigh); rotate injection sites.
- Don't add or mix other drugs with I.V. infusions, particularly aminoglycosides, which are inactivated if mixed with cephalosporins; if other drugs must be given I.V., temporarily stop infusion of primary drug.
- Adequate dilution of I.V. infusion and rotation of the site every 48 hours help minimize local vein irritation; use of small-gauge needle in larger available vein may be helpful.

Special populations

Pregnant patients. Safety in pregnancy hasn't been established. Use only when clearly needed.

Breast-feeding patients. Cephalosporins are excreted in breast milk; use with caution in breast-feeding women.

Pediatric patients. Serum half-life is prolonged in neonates and in infants up to age 1.

Geriatric patients. Use with caution; geriatric patients are susceptible to superinfection and to coagulopathies. Geriatric patients commonly have renal impairment and may require lower doses of cephalosporins.

Patient counseling

- Explain the disease process and rationale for therapy.
- Teach patient signs and symptoms of hypersensitivity and other adverse reactions, and emphasize need to report any unusual effects.
- Teach patient signs and symptoms of bacterial and fungal superinfection to geriatric and debilitated patients and others with low resistance from immunosuppressants or irradiation; emphasize need to report them promptly.
- Warn patient not to ingest alcohol in any form within 72 hours of treatment with cefamandole, cefoperazone, moxalactam, cefonicid, or cefotetan.
- Suggest patient add yogurt or buttermilk to diet to prevent intestinal superinfection resulting from suppression of normal intestinal flora.
- Advise diabetic patients to monitor urine glucose level with Diastix, Chemstrip uG, or glucose enzymatic test strip and not to use Clinitest.
- Tell patient to take oral drug with food if GI irritation occurs.
- Be sure patient understands how and when to take drug; urge patient to complete entire prescribed regimen, to comply with instructions for around-the-clock dosing, and to keep follow-up appointments.
- Counsel patient to check expiration date of drug, how to store drug, and to discard unused drug.

Representative combinations

None.

diuretics, loop

bumetanide, ethacrynate sodium, ethacrynic acid, furosemide, torsemide

Loop diuretics are sometimes referred to as high-ceiling diuretics because they produce a peak diuresis greater than that produced by other

COMPARING LOOP DIURETICS

Drug and route	Onset (min)	Peak (hr)	Duration (hr)	Usual dosage
bumetanide				
I.V.	≤ 5	¼ to ¾	4 to 6	0.5 to 1 mg ≤ t.i.d
P.O.	30 to 60	1 to 2	½ to 1	0.5 to 2 mg/day
ethacrynic acid				
I.V.	≤ 5	¼ to ½	2	50 mg/day
P.O.	≤ 30	2	6 to 8	50 to 100 mg/day
furosemide				
I.V.	≤ 5	⅓ to 1	2	20 to 40 mg q 2 hr, p.r.n.
P.O.	30 to 60	1 to 2	6 to 8	20 to 80 mg ≤ b.i.d.
torsemide				
I.V.	≤ 10	≤ 1	6 to 8	5 to 20 mg/day
P.O.	≤ 60	1 to 2	6 to 8	5 to 20 mg/day

agents. Loop diuretics are particularly useful in edema associated with heart failure, hepatic cirrhosis, and renal disease. Ethacrynic acid was synthesized during the search for compounds that might interact with renal sulfhydryl groups like mercurial diuretics. However, ethacrynic acid is associated with ototoxicity and a higher incidence of GI reactions and is therefore used less frequently. Structurally similar to furosemide, bumetanide is about 40 times more potent. Torsemide is the newest loop diuretic. (See *Comparing loop diuretics.*)

Pharmacology
Loop diuretics inhibit sodium and chloride reabsorption in the ascending loop of Henle, thus increasing renal excretion of sodium, chloride, and water; like thiazide diuretics, loop diuretics increase excretion of potassium. Loop diuretics produce greater maximum diuresis and electrolyte loss than thiazide diuretics.

Clinical indications and actions
Edema
Loop diuretics effectively relieve edema associated with heart failure. They may be useful in patients refractory to other diuretics; because furosemide and bumetanide may increase glomerular filtration rate, they're useful in patients with renal impairment. I.V. loop diuretics are used adjunctively in acute pulmonary edema to decrease peripheral vascular resistance. Loop diuretics also are used to treat edema associated with hepatic cirrhosis and nephrotic syndrome.

Hypertension
Loop diuretics are used in patients with mild to moderate hypertension, although thiazides are the initial diuretics of choice in most patients. Loop diuretics are preferred in patients with heart failure or renal impairment; used I.V., they're a helpful adjunct in managing hypertensive crises.

◇Loop diuretics have been used to increase excretion of calcium in patients with hypercalcemia.

Loop diuretics have been used to enhance the elimination of drugs and toxic substances following intoxication.

Overview of adverse reactions
The most common adverse effects associated with therapeutic doses of loop diuretics are metabolic and electrolyte disturbances (particularly potassium depletion), hypochloremic alkalosis, hyperglycemia, hyperuricemia, and hypomagnesemia. Rapid parenteral administration of loop diuretics may cause hearing loss (including deafness) and tinnitus. High doses may produce profound diuresis, leading to hypovolemia and CV collapse.

Clinical considerations
- Advise safety measures for all ambulatory patients until response to the diuretic is known.
- Patients taking digitalis glycosides are at increased risk of digitalis toxicity from potassium depletion.
- Patients with hepatic disease are especially susceptible to diuretic-induced electrolyte imbalance; in extreme cases, stupor, coma, and death can result.
- Consider possible dosage adjustment in the following circumstances: reduced doses for patients with hepatic dysfunction; increased doses in patients with renal impairment, oliguria, or decreased diuresis (inadequate urine output may result in circulatory overload, causing water intoxication, pulmonary edema, and heart failure); increased doses of insulin or oral hy-

poglycemics in diabetic patients; and reduced doses of other antihypertensive agents.

- Recommend monitoring of blood pressure and pulse rate (especially during rapid diuresis), establish baseline values before therapy, and watch for significant changes.
- Recommend establishing baseline and periodically reviewing CBC, including WBC count; serum electrolytes; carbon dioxide; magnesium; BUN and creatinine levels; and results of liver function tests.
- Recommend administering diuretics in the morning so major diuresis occurs before bedtime. To prevent nocturia, don't prescribe diuretics for use after 6 p.m.
- Recommend monitoring for signs of excessive diuresis: hypotension, tachycardia, poor skin turgor, and excessive thirst.
- Recommend monitoring patient for edema and ascites.

Special populations

Pregnant patients. There are no adequately controlled studies for use of loop diuretics in pregnant women. Avoid use if possible.
Breast-feeding patients. Don't use loop diuretics in breast-feeding women.
Pediatric patients. Use loop diuretics with caution in neonates; don't use ethacrynic acid and ethacrynate sodium in infants. The usual pediatric dose can be used, but extend dose intervals.
Geriatric patients. Geriatric and debilitated patients require close observation, because they're more susceptible to drug-induced diuresis. Excessive diuresis can quickly lead to dehydration, hypovolemia, hypokalemia, and hyponatremia and may cause circulatory collapse. Reduced doses may be indicated.

Patient counseling

- Explain to patient the rationale for therapy and diuretic effect of these drugs (increased volume and frequency of urination).
- Teach patient signs of adverse effects, especially hypokalemia (weakness, fatigue, muscle cramps, paresthesias, confusion, nausea, vomiting, diarrhea, headache, dizziness, or palpitations), and importance of reporting such symptoms promptly.
- Advise patient to eat potassium-rich foods.
- Tell patient to report increased edema or weight or excess diuresis (more than 2-lb. [0.9-kg] weight loss per day).
- With initial doses, caution patient to change position slowly, especially when rising to upright position, to prevent dizziness from orthostatic hypotension.
- Instruct patient to call at once if he experiences chest, back, or leg pain; shortness of breath; or dyspnea.
- Inform patient that photosensitivity may occur in some patients. Caution patient to take protective measures, such as using sunscreens and protective clothing, against exposure to ultraviolet light or sunlight.

Representative combinations

None.

diuretics, potassium-sparing

amiloride hydrochloride, spironolactone, triamterene

Potassium-sparing diuretics are less potent than many others; in particular, amiloride and triamterene have little clinical effect when used alone. However, they protect against potassium loss and are used with more potent diuretics. Spironolactone, an aldosterone antagonist, is particularly useful in patients with edema and hypertension associated with hyperaldosteronism.

Pharmacology

Amiloride and triamterene act directly on the distal renal tubules, inhibiting sodium reabsorption and potassium excretion, thereby reducing potassium loss. Spironolactone competitively inhibits aldosterone at the distal renal tubules, also promoting sodium excretion and potassium retention.

Clinical indications and actions

Edema
All potassium-sparing diuretics are used to manage edema associated with hepatic cirrhosis, nephrotic syndrome, and heart failure.
Hypertension
Amiloride and spironolactone are used to treat mild and moderate hypertension; the exact mechanism is unknown. Spironolactone may block the effect of aldosterone on arteriolar smooth muscle.
Diagnosis of primary hyperaldosteronism
Because spironolactone inhibits aldosterone, correction of hypokalemia and hypertension is presumptive evidence of primary hyperaldosteronism.
Other uses
Amiloride has been used to correct metabolic alkalosis produced by thiazide and other kaliuretic diuretics, and in combination with hydrochlorothiazide in patients with recurrent calcium nephrolithiasis. It has also been used to manage lithium-induced polyuria secondary to lithium-induced nephrogenic diabetes insipidus.

Spironolactone has been used to aid in the treatment of hypokalemia and for prophylaxis of hypokalemia in patients taking cardiac glycosides. It has also been used in the treatment of precocious puberty, female hirsutism, and as an adjunct to treatment in myasthenia gravis and familial periodic paralysis.

Overview of adverse reactions

Hyperkalemia is the most important adverse reaction; it may occur with all drugs in this class and could lead to arrhythmias. Other adverse reactions include nausea, vomiting, headache, weakness, fatigue, bowel disturbances, cough, and dyspnea.

Potassium-sparing diuretics are contraindicated in patients with serum potassium levels above 5.5 mEq/L, in those receiving other potassium-sparing diuretics or potassium supplements, and in patients with anuria, acute or chronic renal insufficiency, diabetic nephropathy, or known hypersensitivity to the drug. They should be used cautiously in patients with severe hepatic insufficiency because electrolyte imbalance may precipitate hepatic encephalopathy, and in patients with diabetes, who are at increased risk of hyperkalemia.

Clinical considerations

- Administer diuretics in the morning to ensure that major diuresis occurs before bedtime. To prevent nocturia, don't prescribe diuretics for use after 6 p.m.
- Establish safety measures for ambulatory patients until response is known; diuretics may cause orthostatic hypotension, weakness, ataxia, and confusion.
- Consider possible dosage adjustments in the following circumstances: reduced doses for patients with hepatic dysfunction and for those taking other antihypertensive agents; increased doses in patients with renal impairment; and changes in insulin requirements in diabetic patients.
- Recommend monitoring for hyperkalemia and arrhythmias; measuring serum potassium and other electrolyte levels frequently, and checking for significant changes. Recommend monitoring the following at baseline and periodic intervals: CBC including WBC count, carbon dioxide, BUN, and creatinine levels and, especially, liver function studies.
- Recommend monitoring vital signs, intake and output, weight, and blood pressure daily; also checking patient for edema, oliguria, or lack of diuresis, which may indicate drug tolerance.
- Recommend monitoring patient with hepatic disease in whom mild drug-induced acidosis may be hazardous; watch for mental confusion, lethargy, or stupor. Patients with hepatic disease are especially susceptible to diuretic-induced electrolyte imbalance; in extreme cases, coma and death can result.
- Recommend monitoring for other signs of toxicity.

Special populations

Pregnant patients. There are no adequately controlled studies for use in pregnant women.
Breast-feeding patients. Safety hasn't been established; drug may be excreted in breast milk.
Pediatric patients. If indicated, use drugs with caution; children are more susceptible to hyperkalemia.
Geriatric patients. Geriatric and debilitated patients require close observation because they're more susceptible to drug-induced diuresis and hyperkalemia. Reduced doses may be indicated.

Patient counseling

- Explain to patient the signs and symptoms of possible adverse effects and the importance of reporting unusual effects.
- Tell patient to report increased edema or weight loss (more than 2-lb. [0.9-kg] per day) or excess diuresis and to record weight each morning after voiding and before dressing and breakfast, using the same scale.
- Teach patient how to minimize dizziness from orthostatic hypotension by avoiding sudden postural changes.
- Advise patient to avoid potassium-rich food and potassium-containing salt substitutes or supplements, which increase the hazard of hyperkalemia.
- Tell patient to take drug at same time each morning to avoid interrupted sleep from nighttime diuresis.
- Advise patient to take drug with or after meals to minimize GI distress.
- Caution patient to avoid hazardous activities, such as driving or operating machinery, until response to drug is known.
- Tell patient to seek medical approval before taking OTC drugs; many contain sodium and potassium and can cause electrolyte imbalance.

Representative combinations

Amiloride with hydrochlorothiazide: Moduretic.

Spironolactone with hydrochlorothiazide: Aldactazide.

Triamterene with hydrochlorothiazide: Dyazide, Maxzide.

diuretics, thiazide

bendroflumethiazide, chlorothiazide, chlorothiazide sodium, hydrochlorothiazide, hydroflumethiazide, methyclothiazide, polythiazide, trichlormethiazide

diuretics, thiazide-like

chlorthalidone, indapamide, metolazone

Thiazide diuretics were discovered and synthesized as an outgrowth of studies on carbonic anhydrase inhibitors. Until the 1950s, organic mercurials were the only effective diuretics available; though potent, they were also toxic.

COMPARING THIAZIDES

Drug	Equivalent dose (mg)	Onset (hr)	Peak (hr)	Duration (hr)
bendroflumethiazide	5	within 2	4	6-12
chlorothiazide	500	within 2	4	6-12
hydrochlorothiazide	50	within 2	4-6	6-12
methyclothiazide	5	within 2	4-6	24

Introduction of thiazides in 1957 proved a major advance because these were the first potent, and safe, diuretics.

Pharmacology

Thiazide diuretics interfere with sodium transport across tubules of the cortical diluting segment of the nephron, thereby increasing renal excretion of sodium, chloride, water, potassium, and calcium. Bicarbonate, magnesium, phosphate, bromide, and iodide excretion are also increased. These drugs may also decrease excretion of ammonia, causing increased serum ammonia levels. Long-term thiazide therapy can cause mild metabolic alkalosis associated with hypokalemia and hypochloremia.

The exact mechanism of thiazides' antihypertensive effect is unknown; however, it's thought to be partially caused by direct arteriolar dilatation. Thiazides initially decrease extracellular fluid volume, plasma volume, and cardiac output; extracellular fluid volume and plasma volume revert to near baseline levels in several weeks but remain slightly below normal. Cardiac output returns to normal or slightly above. Total body sodium level remains slightly below pretreatment levels. Peripheral vascular resistance is initially elevated but falls below pretreatment levels with chronic diuretic therapy. (See *Comparing thiazides.*)

In patients with diabetes insipidus, thiazides cause a paradoxical decrease in urine volume and increase in renal concentration of urine, possibly because of sodium depletion and decreased plasma volume, which leads to an increase in renal water and sodium reabsorption. In addition, thiazides can cause hyperglycemia, exacerbation of diabetes mellitus, or precipitation of diabetes mellitus.

Clinical indications and actions

Edema

Thiazide diuretics are used to treat edema associated with congestive heart failure and nephrotic syndrome and, with spironolactone, to treat edema and ascites secondary to hepatic cirrhosis. Thiazides may also be used to control edema during pregnancy except if caused by renal disease. This treatment isn't indicated for mild edema.

Efficacy and toxicity profiles of thiazide and thiazide-like diuretics are equivalent at comparable doses; the single exception is metolazone, which may be more effective in patients with impaired renal function. Usually, thiazide diuretics are less effective than loop diuretics in patients with renal insufficiency.

Hypertension

Thiazide diuretics are commonly used for initial management of all degrees of hypertension. Used alone, they reduce mean blood pressure by only 10 to 15 mm Hg; in mild hypertension, thiazide diuresis alone will usually reduce blood pressure to desired levels. However, in moderate to severe hypertension that doesn't respond to thiazides alone, combination therapy with another antihypertensive agent is necessary.

◊***Diabetes insipidus***

In diabetes insipidus, thiazides cause a paradoxical decrease in urine volume; urine becomes more concentrated, possibly because of sodium depletion and decreased plasma volume. Thiazides are particularly effective in nephrogenic diabetes insipidus.

Other uses

Prophylaxis of renal calculi formation associated with hypercalciuria and in the treatment of electrolyte disturbances associated with renal tubular necrosis.

Overview of adverse reactions

Therapeutic doses of thiazide diuretics cause electrolyte and metabolic disturbances, the most common being potassium depletion; patients may require dietary supplementation.

Other abnormalities include hypochloremic alkalosis, hypomagnesemia, hyponatremia, hypercalcemia, hyperuricemia, elevated cholesterol levels, and hyperglycemia. Overdose of thiazides may produce lethargy that can progress to coma within a few hours.

Clinical considerations

- Thiazides and thiazide-like diuretics (except metolazone) are ineffective in patients with a glomerular filtration rate below 25 ml per minute.

■ Because thiazides may cause adverse lipid effects, consider an alternative agent in patients with significant hyperlipidemia.
■ Recommend monitoring intake and output, weight, and serum electrolyte levels regularly.
■ Recommend monitoring serum potassium levels and consulting a dietitian to provide high-potassium diet. Foods rich in potassium include citrus fruits, tomatoes, bananas, dates, and apricots. Watch for signs of hypokalemia, such as muscle weakness or cramps. Patients also taking a cardiac glycoside have an increased risk of digitalis toxicity from the potassium-depleting effect of these diuretics.
■ Thiazides may be used with potassium-sparing diuretics or potassium supplements to prevent potassium loss.
■ Recommend monitoring blood glucose values in diabetic patients. Thiazides may cause hyperglycemia and a need to adjust insulin or oral hypoglycemic doses.
■ Recommend monitoring serum creatinine and BUN levels regularly. Drug isn't as effective if these levels are more than twice normal.
■ Recommend monitoring blood uric acid levels, especially in patients with history of gout; these agents may cause an increase in uric acid levels.
■ Antihypertensive effects persist for about 1 week after discontinuation of drug.

Special populations

Pregnant patients. Thiazides cross the placenta and appear in cord blood. Risks and benefits must be evaluated. There are some reports of teratogenic effects, but they're inconclusive. Some clinicians recommend avoiding use in the first trimester. Routine use isn't recommended with mild edema.
Breast-feeding patients. Thiazides are distributed in breast milk; safety and effectiveness in breast-feeding women haven't been established.
Pediatric patients. Safety and effectiveness in children haven't been established for all thiazide diuretics. Indapamide and metolazone aren't recommended for use in children.
Geriatric patients. Geriatric and debilitated patients require close observation and may require reduced doses. They're more sensitive to excess diuresis because of age-related changes in CV and renal function. In geriatric patients, excess diuresis can quickly lead to dehydration, hypovolemia, hyponatremia, hypomagnesemia, and hypokalemia.

Patient counseling

■ Explain rationale of therapy and diuretic effects of these drugs (increased volume and frequency of urination).
■ Instruct patient to report joint swelling, pain, or redness; these signs may indicate hyperuricemia.
■ Warn patient to call immediately if signs of electrolyte imbalance occur; these include weakness, fatigue, muscle cramps, paresthesia, confusion, nausea, vomiting, diarrhea, headache, dizziness, and palpitations.
■ Tell patient to report increased edema, excess diuresis, or weight loss (more than a 2-lb. [0.9-kg] per day); advise him to record weight each morning after voiding and before dressing and breakfast, using the same scale.
■ Advise patient to take drug in the morning to prevent nocturia.
■ Instruct patient to take drug with food to minimize gastric irritation; to eat potassium-rich foods; and not to add salt to other foods. Recommend use of salt substitutes.
■ Counsel patient to avoid smoking because nicotine increases blood pressure.
■ Tell patient to seek medical approval before taking OTC drugs.
■ Warn patient about photosensitivity reactions.

With initial doses

■ Caution patient to change position slowly, especially when rising to upright position, to prevent dizziness from orthostatic hypotension.
■ Instruct patient to call immediately if he experiences chest, back, or leg pain; shortness of breath; or dyspnea.
■ Tell patient to take drug only as prescribed and at the same time each day, to prevent nighttime diuresis and interrupted sleep.

Representative combinations

Chlorthalidone with atenolol: Tenoretic, Atenolol/Chlorthalidone Tablets; with reserpine: Regroton.

Hydrochlorothiazide with bisoprolol: Ziac Tablets; with deserpidine: Oreticyl; with guanethidine monosulfate: Esimil; with hydralazine: Apresazide, Hydrochlorothiazide/Hydralazine Caps; with hydralazine hydrochloride and reserpine: Hydrap-ES Tablets, Marpres Tablets, Tri-Hydroserpine Tablets; with methyldopa: Aldoril, Methyldopa and Hydrochlorothiazide Tablets; with propranolol: Inderide, Propranolol/Hydrochlorothiazide Tablets; with reserpine: Hydrochlorothiazide/Reserpine Tablets, Hydropine, Hydropres, Hydro-Serp, Hydroserpine, Hydrotensin, Mallopres; with hydralazine and reserpine: Ser-Ap-Es, Unipres; with spironolactone: Aldactazide; with timolol maleate: Timolide; with triamterene: Dyazide, Maxzide; with amiloride hydrochloride: Moduretic.

Hydroflumethiazide with reserpine: Salutensin Tablets.

estrogens

dienestrol, diethylstilbestrol, diethylstilbestrol diphosphate, esterified estrogens, estradiol, estradiol cypionate, estradiol valerate, estrogen and progestin, estrogenic substances (conjugated), estropipate, ethinyl estradiol

Estrogens were first discovered in the urine of humans and animals in 1930. Since that time, numerous synthetic modifications of naturally occurring estrogen molecules and completely synthetic estrogenic compounds have been developed.

Estrogens have several uses: in treating the symptoms of menopause, atrophic vaginitis, breast cancer, and other diseases; in the prophylaxis of osteoporosis; and as contraceptives when used in combination with progestins.

Pharmacology

Estrogens are hormones secreted by ovarian follicles and also by the adrenals, corpeus luteum, placenta, and testes. Conjugated estrogens and estrogenic substances are normally obtained from the urine of pregnant mares. Other estrogens are manufactured synthetically. Of the six naturally occurring estrogens, three (estradiol, estrone, and estriol) are present in significant quantities.

Estrogens promote the development and maintenance of the female reproductive system and secondary sexual characteristics. Estrogens inhibit the release of pituitary gonadotropins and also have various metabolic effects, including retention of fluid and electrolytes, retention and deposition in bone of calcium and phosphorus, and mild anabolic activity. They also increase high-density lipoproteins and decrease low-density lipoproteins.

Estrogens and estrogenic substances administered as drugs have effects related to endogenous estrogen's mechanism of action. They can mimic the action of endogenous estrogen when used as replacement therapy or produce such useful effects as inhibiting ovulation or inhibiting growth of certain hormone-sensitive cancers.

Use of estrogens isn't without risk. Long-term use is associated with an increased incidence of endometrial cancer, gallbladder disease, and thromboembolic disease. Elevations in blood pressure often occur as well.

Clinical indications and actions

Moderate to severe vasomotor symptoms of menopause

Endogenous estrogens are markedly reduced in concentration after menopause. This commonly results in vasomotor symptoms, such as hot flashes and dizziness. Diethylstilbestrol, estradiol cypionate, and ethinyl estradiol serve to mimic the action of endogenous estrogens in preventing these symptoms.

Atrophic vaginitis; kraurosis vulvae

Diethylstilbestrol stimulates development, cornification, and secretory activity in vaginal tissues.

Carcinoma of the breast

Conjugated estrogens, diethylstilbestrol, esterified estrogens, estradiol, and ethinyl estradiol inhibit the growth of hormone-sensitive cancers in certain carefully selected men and postmenopausal women.

Carcinoma of the prostate

Conjugated estrogens, diethylstilbestrol, esterified estrogens, estradiol, estradiol valerate, and ethinyl estradiol inhibit growth of hormone-sensitive cancer tissue in men with advanced disease.

Cardiovascular risk prevention

Although somewhat controversial, estrogen and estrogen/progestin has shown to reduce the risk of ischemic heart disease by 50%. Therapy initiation should be highly individualized.

Prophylaxis of postmenopausal osteoporosis

Conjugated estrogens replace or augment activity of endogenous estrogen in causing calcium and phosphate retention and preventing bone decalcification.

Contraception

Estrogens are also used in combination with progestins for ovulation control to prevent conception.

Overview of adverse reactions

Acute reactions include changes in menstrual bleeding patterns (spotting, prolongation or absence of bleeding), abdominal cramps, swollen feet or ankles, bloated sensation (fluid and electrolyte retention), breast swelling and tenderness, weight gain, nausea, loss of appetite, headache, photosensitivity, loss of libido.

With chronic administration, adverse reactions include increased blood pressure (sometimes into the hypertensive range), thromboembolic disease, cholestatic jaundice, benign hepatomas, endometrial carcinoma (rare). Risk of thromboembolic disease increases markedly with cigarette smoking, especially in women over age 35. Increased risk of thromboembolic events also seen in postmenopausal women, women undergoing surgery, and those with fractures or who are immobilized.

Clinical considerations

- Some clinicians recommend that women discontinue estrogen replacement therapy during immobilization due to fracture, stroke, or severe illness; estrogen replacement therapy can be restarted when normal activity is resumed.
- Don't use estrogens in patients with thrombophlebitis or thromboembolic disorders; can-

cer of the breast, reproductive organs, or genitals; or undiagnosed abnormal genital bleeding.
■ Use with caution in patients with hypertension, asthma, mental depression, bone disease, blood dyscrasias, gallbladder disease, migraine, seizures, diabetes mellitus, amenorrhea, heart failure, hepatic or renal dysfunction, or a family history of breast or genital tract cancer. Development or worsening of these conditions may require discontinuation of the drug.
■ Give patient package insert describing estrogen adverse reactions, and also provide verbal explanation.
■ Recommend closely monitoring patients with diabetes mellitus for loss of diabetes control.
■ If patient is receiving a warfarin-type anticoagulant, recommend monitoring PT and INR for anticoagulant dosage adjustment.
■ Estrogen therapy is usually administered cyclically. The drugs are usually given once daily for 3 weeks, followed by 1 week without the drugs; this regimen is repeated as necessary.

Special populations

Pregnant patients. Estrogens are contraindicated for use in pregnancy.
Breast-feeding patients. Estrogens are contraindicated in breast-feeding women.
Pediatric patients. Because of the effects of estrogen on epiphyseal closure, use estrogens with caution in adolescents whose bone growth isn't complete. Estrogens aren't used in children.
Geriatric patients. Postmenopausal women with long-term estrogen use have an increased risk of endometrial cancer if they have a uterus. This risk can be reduced by adding a progestin to the regimen.

Patient counseling

■ Warn patient to report adverse reactions immediately.
■ Tell men on long-term therapy about possible gynecomastia and impotence.
■ Explain to patient on cyclic therapy for postmenopausal symptoms that, although withdrawal bleeding may occur in week off drug, fertility hasn't been restored; ovulation doesn't occur.
■ Diabetic patients should report symptoms of hyperglycemia or glycosuria.
■ Tell women who are planning to breast-feed not to take estrogens.

Representative combinations

Estradiol cypionate with testosterone cypionate and chlorobutanol: Depo-testadiol, Duo-cyp, Menoject, testosterone cypionate and estradiol cypionate, depAndrogyn, Depotestogen, Duratestrin, T-E Cypionates, Test-Estro Cypionate.

Estradiol valerate with testosterone enanthate: Deladumone, Delatestadiol, Teev, Testosterone Enanthate and Estradiol Valerate Injection, Valertest.

Estrogen with methyltestosterone: Estratest, Estratest H.S.

Estrogenic substances (conjugated) with meprobamate: Milprem, PMB; with methyltestosterone: Premarin with methyltestosterone; with medroxyprogesterone: Premphase, Prempro.

Esterified estrogens with chlordiazepoxide: Menrium.

Ethinyl estradiol with norethindrone: Brevicon, Genora 1/35, Jenest, Loestrin Fe 1.5/30, ModiCon, Nelova1/35E, Ortho-Novum 1/35, Ortho-Novum 7/7/7, Ortho-Novum 10/11; with norgestimate: Cyclen; with ethynodiol diacetate: Demulen 1/35, Demulen 1/50; with desogestrel: Desogen, Marvelon; with norgestrel: Lo/Ovral, Ovral; with levonorgestrel: Levlen, Min-Ovral, Nordette, Tri-Levlen, Triphasil, Triquilar.

Ethynodiol diacetate with ethinyl estradiol: Demulen 1/35, Demulen 1/50.

fluoroquinolones

ciprofloxacin, enoxacin, levofloxacin, lomefloxacin hydrochloride, norfloxacin, ofloxacin, sparfloxacin, trovafloxacin mesylate/alatrofloxacin mesylate

Fluoroquinolones are broad-spectrum, systemic antibacterial agents active against a wide range of aerobic gram-positive and gram-negative organisms. Gram-positive aerobic bacteria include *Staphlococcus aureus, S. epidermis, S. saprophyticus, S. hemolyticus,* penicillinase- and non-penicillinase-producing staphlococci as well as some methicillin-resistant strains, *Streptococcus pneumoniae*, group A (beta) hemolytic streptococci *(S. pyogenes)*, group B streptococci *(S. agalactiae), viridans streptococci*, groups C, F, and G streptococci and nonenterococcal group D streptococci, *Enterococcus faecalis.* These drugs are active against gram-positive aerobic bacilli including *Corynebacterium, Listeria monocytogenes,* and *Nocardia asteroides*

Fluoroquinolones are effective against gram-negative aerobic bacteria including, but not limited to, *Neisseria meningitidis* and most strains of penicillinase- and non-penicillinase-producing *Neisseria gonorrhoeae, Haemophilus influenzae, Haemophilus parainfluenzae, Haemophilus ducreyi, Moraxella catarrhalis*, and most clinically important Enterobacteriaceae, *P. aeruginosa, Vibrio cholerae,* and *Vibrio parahaemolyticus*. Certain fluoroquinolones are active against *Chlamydia trachomatis, Mycoplasma hominis, Mycoplasma pneumoniae, Legionella pneumophila,* and *Mycobacterium avium-intracellulare.*

COMPARING FLUOROQUINOLONES

Drug	Oral bioavailability (%)	Plasma protein binding (%)	Half-life (hr)
ciprofloxacin	70-80	20-40	Normal renal function: 4-6 Severe renal failure: 6-8
enoxacin	90	40	Normal renal function: 3-6 Severe renal failure: 9-10
levofloxacin	100 (without regard to food)	50	Normal renal function: 6
lomefloxacin	78-86 (may take with or without food)	10	Normal renal function: not stated Severe renal failure: 21-45
norfloxacin	Not stated	10-15	Normal renal function: 3-4 Severe renal failure: 9-10
ofloxacin	Not stated	20-25	Normal renal function: 4½-7 Severe renal failure: 15-16
sparfloxacin	92	45	Normal renal function: 16-30
trovafloxacin/ alatrofloxacin	88 (without regard to food)	76	Normal renal function: 9-11¼

Pharmacology

Fluoroquinolones produce a bactericidal effect by inhibiting intracellular DNA topoisomerase II (DNA gyrase) or topoisomerase IV. These enzymes are essential catalysts in the duplication, transcription, and repair of bacterial DNA. (See *Comparing fluoroquinolones.)*

Clinical indications and actions

Fluoroquinolones are indicated for the treatment of the following infections when caused by susceptible organisms: bone and joint infections, bacterial bronchitis, endocervical and urethral chlamydial infections, bacterial gastroenteritis, endocervical and urethral gonorrhea, intra-abdominal infections, empiric therapy for febrile neutropenia, pelvic inflammatory disease, bacterial pneumonia, bacterial prostatitis, acute sinusitis, skin and soft tissue infections, typhoid fever, bacterial urinary tract infections, chancroid, meningococcal carriers, and bacterial septicemia. Fluoroquinolones may be used for the prevention of bacterial urinary tract infections.

Overview of adverse reactions

The following side effects are observed rarely with fluoroquinolones, but require medical attention: CNS stimulation (acute psychosis, agitation, hallucinations, tremors); hepatotoxicity; hypersensitivity reactions; interstitial nephritis; phlebitis; pseudomembranous colitis; and tendinitis or tendon rupture. The following side effects don't require medical attention unless they persist or become intolerable: CNS adverse effects (dizziness, headache, nervousness, drowsiness, insomnia); gastrointestinal reactions; and photosensitivity.

Clinical considerations

- Consider the risk-benefit ratio of therapy with fluoroquinolones on an individual basis when any of the following conditions is present: seizure disorders, cerebral ischemia, severe hepatic dysfunction, or renal insufficiency.
- Recommend that renal and liver function tests be monitored in patients with impaired renal or hepatic function.
- Achilles and other tendon ruptures have been reported. Discontinue drug if patient experiences pain, inflammation, or rupture of a tendon.

Special populations

Pregnant patients. Pregnancy risk category is C. Adequate, well-controlled trials haven't been completed, but these drugs cross the placenta and may cause arthropathies.

Breast-feeding patients. Whether fluoroquinolones are readily distributed into breast milk is unknown. Therefore, their use in nursing mothers isn't recommended because these drugs may cause arthropathies in newborns and infants.

Pediatric patients. Fluoroquinolones aren't recommended because they can cause joint problems.

Geriatric patients. Because renal function deteriorates over time, geriatric patients may require a reduction in their daily dose.

Peak concentration (hr)	Elimination	Dosage adjustment	Dialyzability
1-2	40-70% of drug is cleared unchanged by the kidneys in 24 hr	Renal failure	< 10% removed by hemodialysis
1-3	40-60% of drug is cleared unchanged by the kidneys in 48 hr	Renal failure	< 5% removed by hemodialysis
1	Almost entirely eliminated unchanged in the urine	Renal failure	Not defined
1½	60-80% of drug is cleared unchanged by the kidneys in 48 hr	Renal failure	< 3% removed by hemodialysis
1-2	26% of drug is cleared unchanged by the kidneys in 24 hr	Renal failure	< 10% removed by hemodialysis
1-2	70-90% of drug is cleared unchanged by the kidneys in 36 hr	Renal failure	< 10-30% removed by hemodialysis
3-6	10% is excreted unchanged in the urine	Renal failure	Not defined
1-2	50% of oral dose (43% in feces and 6% in urine) excreted as unchanged drug	Cirrhosis	Not efficiently removed by dialysis.

Patient counseling
- Instruct patient to take this medication as prescribed and to finish the full course of therapy.
- Tell patient to take the medication with an 8-oz glass of water.
- Enoxacin and norfloxacin should be taken on an empty stomach
- Instruct patient that if a dose is missed, the next dose should be taken as soon as possible; don't double the dose.
- Avoid concurrent use of antacids or sucralfate and orally administered fluoroquinolones.
- Don't take other medications concurrently without first checking with a pharmacist or doctor.

Representative combinations
None.

histamine$_2$ (H_2)-receptor antagonists

cimetidine, famotidine, nizatidine, ranitidine, ranitidine bismuth citrate

The introduction of H_2-receptor antagonists has revolutionized the treatment of peptic ulcer disease. These drugs structurally resemble histamine and competitively inhibit the action of histamine on gastric H_2 receptors. Cimetidine, approved for clinical use in 1977, is the prototype of this class. (See *Adult dosages of histamine$_2$-receptor antagonists,* page 44.)

Pharmacology
All H_2-receptor antagonists inhibit the action of histamine at H_2 receptors in gastric parietal cells, reducing gastric acid output and concentration regardless of the stimulatory agent (histamine, food, insulin, caffeine, betazole, pentagastrin) or basal conditions.

Clinical indications and actions
Duodenal ulcer
Cimetidine, famotidine, nizatidine, and ranitidine are used to treat acute duodenal ulcer and to prevent ulcer recurrence. Ranitidine bismuth citrate is used in combination with clarithromycin to treat active duodenal ulcer associated with *Helicobacter pylori* infection.
Gastric ulcer
Cimetidine famotidine, nizatidine, and ranitidine are indicated for acute gastric ulcer. However, the benefits of long-term therapy (over 8 weeks) with these drugs remain unproven.
Hypersecretory states
Cimetidine, famotidine, nizatidine, and ranitidine are used to treat hypersecretory states such as Zollinger-Ellison syndrome. Because patients with these conditions require much higher doses than patients with peptic ulcer disease, they may experience more pronounced adverse effects.
Reflux esophagitis
Cimetidine, famotidine, nizatidine, and ranitidine are used to provide short-term relief from gastroesophageal reflux in patients who don't respond to conventional therapy (lifestyle changes, antacids, diet modification). They act by raising the stomach pH. Some clinicians pre-

ADULT DOSAGES OF HISTAMINE$_2$-RECEPTOR ANTAGONISTS

Indication	cimetidine	famotidine	nizatidine	ranitidine
Duodenal ulcer	P.O. 800 mg h.s. or 300 mg q.i.d. with meals and h.s. or 400 mg b.i.d.	P.O. 40 mg h.s. or 20 mg b.i.d..	P.O. 300 mg h.s. or 150 mg b.i.d..	P.O. 150 mg b.i.d. or 300 mg once per day after evening meal or h.s.
Duodenal ulcer maintenance	P.O. 400 mg h.s.	P.O. 20 mg h.s.	P.O. 150 mg h.s.	P.O. 150 mg h.s.
Gastric ulcer	P.O. 800 mg h.s. or 300 mg q.i.d. with meals and h.s.	P.O. 4 0 mg h.s.	P.O. 300 mg h.s. or 150 mg b.i.d.	P.O. 150 mg b.i.d.
Gastric ulcer maintenance	NA	NA	NA	P.O. 150 mg h.s.
Gastroesophageal reflux disease	P.O. 400 mg q.i.d. or 800 mg b.i.d.	P.O. 20 mg b.i.d.	P.O. 150 mg b.i.d.	P.O. 150 mg b.i.d.
Erosive esophagitis	P.O. 400 mg q.i.d. or 800 mg b.i.d.	P.O. 20-40 mg b.i.d.	P.O. 150 mg b.i.d.	P.O. 150 mg q.i.d.
Erosive esophagitis healing maintenance	NA	NA	NA	P.O. 150 mg b.i.d.
Pathological hypersecretory conditions	P.O. 300 mg q.i.d. with meals and h.s.	P.O. 20 mg Q 6 hours	NA	P.O. 150 mg b.i.d.
Prevention of upper GI bleeding	I.V.: 50 mg/hr continuous infusion	NA	NA	NA
Heartburn,acid indigestion,sour stomach	P.O. 200 mg, p.r.n., up to 200 mg b.i.d.	P.O. 10 mg, p.r.n., up to 10 mg b.i.d.	P.O. 75 mg, p.r.n., up to 75 mg b.i.d.	P.O. 75 mg p.r.n., up to 75 mg b.i.d.
Product information	Tablet: 100 mg (OTC), 200 mg, 300 mg, 400 mg, 800 mg Liquid: 300 mg/5 ml Injection: 300 mg/2 ml Injection, premixed: 300 mg/50 ml normal saline, 300 mg/2 ml	Tablet: 10 mg (OTC), 20 mg, 40 mg Oral suspension: 40 mg/5 ml Injection: 10 mg/ml Injection, premixed: 20 mg/50 ml in normal saline	Capsule: 75 mg (OTC), 150 mg, 300 mg	Tablet: 75 mg (OTC), 150 mg, 300 mg Effervescent tablet: 150 mg Effervescent granule: 150 mg Capsule: 150 mg, 300 mg Syrup: 15 mg/ml Injection: 0.5 mg/ml, 25 mg/ml

NA: Not FDA-approved.

fer to combine the H_2-receptor antagonist with metoclopramide, but further study is necessary to confirm effectiveness of the combination.

◊ ***Stress ulcer prophylaxis***

Cimetidine, famotidine, nizatidine, and ranitidine are used to prevent stress ulcers in critically ill patients, particularly those in intensive care units. However, this remains an unlabeled (FDA-unapproved) indication; some health care providers prefer intensive antacid therapy for such patients.

◊ ***Other uses***

H_2-receptor antagonists have been used for a number of other unlabeled indications, including short-bowel syndrome, prophylaxis for allergic reactions to I.V. contrast medium, and to eradicate *Helicobacter pylori* in treatment of peptic ulcers. Ranitidine bismuth citrate in combination with clarithromycin is used to treat *H. pylori* infection.

Other uses include relief of occasional heartburn, acid indigestion, or sour stomach.

Overview of adverse reactions

H_2-receptor antagonists rarely cause adverse reactions. However, mild transient diarrhea, neutropenia, dizziness, fatigue, arrhythmias, and gynecomastia have been reported.

HISTAMINE$_2$-RECEPTOR ANTAGONISTS: DOSAGE ADJUSTMENTS FOR RENAL IMPAIRMENT

Drug	Estimated creatinine clearance (ml/min)	Recommended dosage adjustment
cimetidine	20-40	q 8 hr or 75% of normal dose
famotidine	< 10	q 24 hr or 50% of normal dose
nizatidine	20-50	150 mg/day (active treatment) or 150 mg q other day (maintenance)
ranitidine	< 50	150 mg q 24 hr; increase to every 12 hr as tolerated

Cimetidine may inhibit hepatic enzymes, thereby impairing the metabolism of certain drugs. Ranitidine may also produce this effect, but to a lesser extent. Famotidine and nizatidine haven't been shown to inhibit hepatic enzymes or drug clearance.

Clinical considerations

- Give a single daily dose at bedtime, twice-daily doses morning and evening, and multiple doses with meals and at bedtime. Most clinicians prefer the once-daily dose at bedtime regimen for improved compliance.
- Recommend that when administering drugs I.V., not to exceed recommended infusion rates because this may increase the risk of adverse CV effects. Continuous I.V. infusion may yield better suppression of acid secretion.
- Advise that because antacids may decrease drug absorption, give them at least 1 hour apart from H_2-receptor antagonists.
- Patients with renal disease may require a modified schedule. (See *Histamine$_2$-receptor antagonists: Dosage adjustments for renal impairment.)*
- Avoid discontinuing these drugs abruptly.
- Many investigational uses for these drugs (particularly cimetidine) are being evaluated. Ranitidine bismuth citrate shouldn't be prescribed alone for the treatment of active duodenal ulcers.
- Symptomatic response to therapy doesn't rule out gastric malignancy.

Special populations

Pregnant patients. There are no adequate controlled studies in pregnant women. Cimetidine may potentially result in reversible decreased sperm concentrations in men.

Breast-feeding patients. H_2-receptor antagonists may be secreted in breast milk. Ratio of risk to benefit must be considered.

Pediatric patients. Safety and efficacy in children haven't been established.

Geriatric patients. Use caution when administering these drugs to geriatric patients because of the increased risk of adverse reactions, particularly those affecting the CNS. Dosage adjustment is required in patients with impaired renal function.

Patient counseling

Instruct patient to avoid smoking during drug therapy because smoking stimulates gastric acid secretion and worsens the disease.

Representative combinations

None.

HMG-CoA reductase inhibitors

atorvastatin, cerivastatin sodium, fluvastatin sodium, lovastatin, pravastatin sodium, simvastatin

HMG-CoA reductase inhibitors, also known as statins, are a highly effective class of medications that have become first line pharmacologic therapy for the management of hypercholesterolemia.

Pharmacology

Statins lower cholesterol by competitively inhibiting the enzyme 3-hydroxy-3-methylglutaryl-coenzyme A (HMG-CoA) reductase. This enzyme catalyzes the conversion of HMG-CoA to mevalonate, which is an early rate-limiting step in cholesterol biosynthesis. Statins decrease low-density lipoproteins cholesterol (LDL-C), total cholesterol (total-C), apoprotein B (apo-B), very low-density lipoprotein (VLDL) cholesterol, and plasma triglycerides, and increase high-density lipoprotein cholesterol (HDL-C). Coronary artery disease may be caused by increased levels of total cholesterol, apo-B, and LDL-C, as well as by decreased levels of HDL-C. In addition, cardiovascular morbidity and mortality rates vary directly with the level of total-C and LDL-C, and inversely with the level of HDL-C. The mechanism by which statins lower LDL-C may be related to both a reduction of VLDL cholesterol and an induction of the LDL receptor,

COMPARING HMG-CoA REDUCTASE INHIBITORS

Drug	Usual dose	Absolute bioavailability (%)	Metabolism Enzymes	Active Metabolite	Excretion (%)
atorvastatin	10-80 mg/day	14	CYP3A4	Yes	< 2 (urine)
cerivastatin	0.2-0.3 mg/day in evening	60	CYP3A4	Yes	24 (urine) 70 feces
fluvastatin	20-80 mg/day at bedtime	24	CYP2C9	Yes	< 6 (urine) ~90 (feces)
lovastatin	20-80 mg/day with evening meal	< 5	CYP3A4	No	10 (urine) 83 (feces)
pravastatin	10-40 mg/day at bedtime	17	not reported	No	~ 20 (urine) 70 (feces)
simvastatin	10-80 mg/day in evening	< 5	CYP3A4	No	13 (urine) 60 (feces)

which results in reduced synthesis or increased breakdown of LDL-C.

Statins are highly effective at lowering total and LDL-C in patients with heterozygous familial and nonfamilial forms of hypercholesterolemia. Initial cholesterol-lowering effects are seen within 1 to 2 weeks, with maximum lowering effects observed within 4 to 6 weeks. Because cholesterol synthesis occurs mainly at night, single daily doses of all the agents except atorvastatin should be given in the evening or at bedtime. Lovastatin should be taken with the evening meal because food increases its absorption. (See *Comparing HMG-CoA reductase inhibitors.*)

Clinical indications and actions

Cardiovascular events

All statins are indicated for the treatment of primary hypercholesterolemia and mixed dyslipidemia. Atorvastatin is indicated for hypertriglyceridemia and primary dysbetalipoproteinemia. Atorvastatin and simvastatin are indicated for homozygous familial hyperlipidemia. Pravastatin is indicated for the primary prevention of coronary events. All statins except atorvastatin and cerivastatin are indicated for the secondary prevention of cardiovascular events.

◇ ***Unlabeled uses***

Lovastatin: diabetic dyslipidemia; nephrotic hyperlipidemia; neck artery disease; familial beta dysbetalipoproteinemia; and familial combined hyperlipidemia

Pravastatin: heterozygous familial hypercholesterolemia; diabetic dyslipidemia in non-insulin-dependent diabetes; hypercholesterolemia secondary to the nephrotic syndrome; homozygous hypercholesterolemia in patients with reduced LDL receptor activity.

Simvastatin: heterozygous familial hypercholesterolemia, familial combined hyperlipidemia, diabetic dyslipidemia in type II diabetes, hyperlipidemia secondary to the nephrotic syndrome, and homozygous familial hypercholesterolemia in patients with defective LDL receptors.

Overview of adverse reactions

Statins are well tolerated and have very few side effects. Adverse reactions include photosensitivity, hepatotoxicity, defined as an increase in transaminase levels to greater than 3 times normal; mild, nonspecific GI complaints; transient and mild increase in creatine phosphokinase (CPK) levels; myopathy, characterized by myalgia; and muscle weakness associated with CPK values greater than 10 times the upper limit of normal. Lovastatin and simvastatin may cause insomnia.

A rare hypersensitivity syndrome has been reported. It's characterized by at least one of the following features: anaphylaxis, angioedema, lupus erythematosus-like syndrome, polymyalgia rheumatica, vasculitis, purpura, thrombocytopenia, leukopenia, hemolytic anemia, positive ANA, increased ESR, eosinophilia, arthritis; asthenia, photosensitivity, fever, chills, flushing, malaise, dyspnea, toxic epidermal necrolysis, erythema multiforme, and dermatomyositis.

Clinical considerations

- Statins are contraindicated in pregnancy and lactation, as well as in patients with active liver disease or unexplained persistent elevations of LFTs.
- Use statins with caution in patients who consume large quantities of alcohol.
- Monitor LFTs before the initiation of statins and at 6 and 12 weeks following initiation of treatment or increasing the dose, and periodically (such as semiannually) thereafter. Dis-

Protein binding (%)	Half-life (hr)	% LDL-C lowering
≥ 98	~ 14	↓26.5-60
> 99	2-3	↓25.3-28.2
98	< 1	↓18.9-35
> 95	3-4	↓21-40
~ 50	1¾	↓22-34
~ 95	3	↓14-47

continue drug if AST increases more than 3 times upper limits of normal.

- Closely monitor patients taking pravastatin with renal insufficiency.
- The absorption of lovastatin is increased when taken with food, and it should be taken with the evening meal. All other statins, except atorvastatin, may be taken without regard to meals, but should be taken in the evening or at bedtime, because most cholesterol synthesis occurs at night.
- The risk of myopathy is increased when statins are taken with cyclosporine, erythromycin, gemfibrozil, fibric acid derivatives, azole antifungals, or lipid-lowering doses of niacin.
- Because of increased risk of myopathy, avoid concurrent use of statins with fibrates.
- Consider myopathy in any patient with diffuse myalgias, muscle tenderness, weakness, or CPK increases greater than 10 times the upper limit of normal. Discontinue drug if markedly elevated CPK levels occur or if myopathy is suspected. Don't exceed 20 mg/day of lovastatin or 10 mg/day of simvastatin in patients taking cyclosporine or itraconazole.
- Suggest withholding or discontinuing statins in patients with risk factors for renal failure secondary to rhabdomyolysis including: severe acute infection; sepsis; hypotension; major surgery; trauma; severe metabolic, endocrine, or electrolyte disorders; and uncontrolled seizures.

Special populations

Pregnant patients. Statin drugs are pregnancy category X and are contraindicated during pregnancy. Cholesterol is essential for fetal development and drugs that inhibit cholesterol synthesis may have adverse effects on the developing fetus. If patients become pregnant while taking a statin, discontinue the drug immediately.

Breast-feeding patients. Some statins are secreted in breast milk. Because of the potential adverse effects, women shouldn't take statins while breast-feeding.

Pediatric patients. Safety and efficacy in patients under age 18 haven't been established; use isn't recommended.

Geriatric patients. Plasma concentrations don't vary with age for cervastatin, fluvastatin, and atorvastatin. In patients over age 70, the AUC is increased with lovastatin and simvastatin. For pravastatin, patients over age 65 show a greater effect on LDL-C, total-C, and LDL:HDL ratio compared to patients under age 65.

Patient counseling

- Tell patient that statin drugs may cause photosensitivity and to avoid prolonged exposure to sun and other sources of ultraviolet light. Recommend wearing protective clothing and sunscreens.
- Instruct a woman of child-bearing age on the potential hazards of statin drugs in pregnancy. Tell her to discontinue drug immediately if she becomes pregnant and to notify her doctor.
- Instruct patient to promptly notify his doctor if he experiences any unexplained muscle pain, tenderness, or weakness, especially if accompanied by malaise or fever.
- Instruct patient on the importance of adhering to dietary recommendations.
- Tell patient to take lovastatin with the evening meal; fluvastatin, pravastatin, and simvastatin may be taken without regard to meals but should be taken in the evening or at bedtime for best results; atorvastatin may be taken without regard to meals and at any time of the day.

Representative combinations

None.

nitrates

amyl nitrite, isosorbide dinitrate, isosorbide mononitrate, nitroglycerin, pentaerythritol tetranitrate

Nitrates have been recognized as effective vasodilators for more than 100 years. The best-known drug of this group, nitroglycerin, remains the therapeutic mainstay for classic and variant angina. With the availability of a commercial I.V. nitroglycerin form, use of the drug in reducing afterload and preload in various cardiac disorders has generated renewed enthusiasm. Various other dosage forms of nitroglycerin and of other nitrates also are available, thereby improving and extending their clinical usefulness.

Pharmacology

The major pharmacologic property of nitrates is vascular smooth muscle relaxation, resulting in generalized vasodilation. Venous effects predominate; however, nitroglycerin produces dose-dependent dilatation of both arterial and venous beds. Nitrates are metabolized to a free radical nitric oxide, which is thought to be an endothelium-derived relaxing factor (EDRF), which is usually impaired in patients with coronary artery disease. Decreased peripheral venous resistance results in venous pooling of blood and decreased venous return to the heart (preload); decreased arteriolar resistance reduces systemic vascular resistance and arterial pressure (afterload). These vascular effects lead to reduction of myocardial oxygen consumption, promoting a more favorable oxygen supply:demand ratio. Although nitrates reflexively increase heart rate and myocardial contractility, reduced ventricular wall tension results in a net decrease in myocardial oxygen consumption. In the coronary circulation, nitrates redistribute circulating blood flow along collateral channels and preferentially increase subendocardial blood flow, improving perfusion to the ischemic myocardium.

Nitrates relax all smooth muscle—not just vascular smooth muscle—regardless of autonomic innervation, including bronchial, biliary, GI, ureteral, and uterine smooth muscle.

Clinical indications and actions

Angina pectoris

By relaxing vascular smooth muscle in both the venous and arterial beds, nitrates cause a net decrease in myocardial oxygen consumption; by dilating coronary vessels, they lead to redistribution of blood flow to ischemic tissue. Although systemic and coronary vascular effects may vary slightly, depending on which nitrate is used, both smooth muscle relaxation and vasodilation probably account for the value of nitrates in treating angina. Because individual nitrates have similar pharmacologic and therapeutic properties, the best nitrate to use in a specific situation depends mainly on the onset of action and duration of effect required.

Sublingual nitroglycerin is considered the drug of choice to treat acute angina pectoris because of its rapid onset of action, relatively low cost, and well-established effectiveness. Lingual or buccal nitroglycerin and other rapidly acting nitrates, such as amyl nitrite and sublingual or chewable isosorbide dinitrate, also may be useful for this indication. Amyl nitrite is rarely used because it's expensive, inconvenient, and carries a high risk of adverse effects. Sublingual, lingual, or buccal nitroglycerin or sublingual or chewable isosorbide dinitrate or mononitrate typically are effective in circumstances likely to provoke an angina attack.

Beta blockers usually are considered the drug of choice in the prophylactic management of angina pectoris. Nitrates with a relatively long duration of effect include oral preparations of isosorbide mononitrate and isosorbide dinitrate, and oral or topical nitroglycerin. Combination treatment of beta blockers and nitrates appears to be the therapy of choice.

The effectiveness of oral nitrates is debatable, although isosorbide dinitrate, isosorbide mononitrate, and nitroglycerin generally are considered effective. However, the effectiveness of topical nitroglycerin preparations haven't been fully determined. Some experts believe oral nitrates are ineffective or less effective than rapidly acting I.V. nitrates in reducing frequency of angina and increasing exercise tolerance. Also, prolonged use of oral nitrates may cause cross-tolerance to sublingual nitrates.

I.V. nitroglycerin may be used to treat unstable angina pectoris, Prinzmetal's angina, and angina pectoris in patients who haven't responded to recommended doses of nitrates or a beta blocker.

Sedatives may be useful in the adjunctive management of angina pectoris associated with psychogenic factors. However, if combination therapy is required, each drug should be adjusted individually; fixed combinations of oral nitrates and sedatives should be avoided.

Acute MI

The hemodynamic effects of I.V., sublingual, or topical nitroglycerin may prove beneficial in treating left ventricular failure and pulmonary congestion associated with acute MI. However, the effects of the drug on morbidity and mortality in patients with these conditions is controversial.

I.V., sublingual, and topical nitroglycerin and isosorbide dinitrate are effective adjunctive agents in managing acute and chronic heart failure. Sublingual administration can quickly reverse the signs and symptoms of pulmonary congestion in acute pulmonary edema; however, the I.V. form may control hemodynamic status more accurately.

Other uses

I.V. nitroglycerin is used to control perioperative hypertension, hypertensive emergencies, congestive heart failure (CHF), and pulmonary edema associated with MI.

◊I.V. nitroglycerin has been used to treat severe hypertension and hypertensive crises; other forms have been used to treat refractory CHF. Nitroglycerin also has been used for relief of pain, dysphagia, and spasm in patients with diffuse esophageal spasm without gastroesophageal reflux.

Overview of adverse reactions

Headache is most common early in therapy; it may be severe, but usually diminishes rapidly. Orthostatic hypotension, dizziness, weakness, and transient flushing may occur. In patients sensitive to hypotensive effects, nausea, vomiting, weakness, restlessness, pallor, cold sweats, tachycardia, syncope, or CV collapse may occur. Dose reduction may control GI upset; discontinue therapy if blurred vision, dry mouth, or rash develops. Tolerance and dependence can occur with repeated, prolonged use.

Tolerance to both the vascular and antianginal effects of the drugs can develop, and cross-tolerance between the nitrates and nitrites has been demonstrated. Tolerance is associated with a high or sustained plasma drug level and occurs with oral, I.V., and topical therapy. It rarely occurs with intermittent sublingual use. However, patients taking oral isosorbide dinitrate or topical nitroglycerin haven't exhibited cross-tolerance to sublingual nitroglycerin.

To prevent tolerance, the lowest effective dose and an intermittent dosing schedule should be used. A nitrate-free interval of 10 to 12 hours daily may also be helpful.

Clinical considerations

Oral dosage form

- Provide a dosage regimen that incorporates a 10- to 12-hour nitrate-free interval.
- Best absorption occurs when taken on an empty stomach (1 hour before or 2 hours after meals) and with a full glass of water.
- Adjust dosage to patient response. Patient should avoid switching brands after they are stabilized on a particular formulation.

Buccal dosage form

- Place the tablet between the upper lip or cheek and gum.
- Dissolution rate varies, but usually ranges from 3 to 5 hours. Hot liquids increase dissolution rate and should be avoided.
- Patient shouldn't use buccal form at bedtime because of risk of aspiration.

Sublingual dosage form

- Only the sublingual and translingual forms should be used to relieve acute angina attack. Although a burning sensation was formerly an indication of the potency of a drug, many current preparations don't produce this sensation.

Translingual spray

- Only the sublingual and translingual forms should be used to relieve acute angina attack. Spray the translingual form onto or under the tongue. Patient shouldn't inhale the spray.

Topical dosage form

- To apply ointment, spread in uniform thin layer to any hairless part of the skin except distal parts of arms and legs, because absorption isn't maximal at these sites. Don't rub in. Cover with plastic film to aid absorption and to protect clothing. If using Tape-Surrounded Appli-Ruler (TSAR) system, keep TSAR on skin to protect clothing and ensure that ointment remains in place. If serious adverse reactions develop in patients using ointment or transdermal system, remove product at once or wipe ointment from skin. Be sure to avoid contact with ointment.
- Be sure to remove transdermal patch before defibrillation. Because of the aluminum backing of the patch, electric current may cause patch to explode.
- Don't administer with sildenafil (Viagra).

Special populations

Pregnant patients. Pregnancy risk category is C. There are no adequate controlled studies in pregnant women. Use only if clearly indicated.

Breast-feeding patients. Excretion into breast milk is unknown. Use with caution.

Pediatric patients. Safety and effectiveness of nitrates in children haven't been established.

Patient counseling

- Advise patient to avoid alcohol while taking nitrates, because severe hypotension and CV collapse may occur.
- Instruct patient to sit or lie down when taking nitrates, to prevent injury from transient episodes of dizziness, syncope, or other signs of cerebral ischemia that the drug may cause.
- Advise patient to treat headache with aspirin or acetaminophen.
- Tell patient to report blurred vision, dry mouth, or persistent headache.
- Warn patient not to stop taking drug abruptly because this may cause withdrawal symptoms.
- Advise patient that nitrates and sildenafil can't be taken together because the combination can produce life-threatening hypotension.

Representative combinations

None.

nonsteroidal anti-inflammatory drugs (NSAIDs)

celecoxib, choline magnesium salicylate, diclofenac potassium, diclofenac sodium, diflunisal, etodolac, fenoprofen calcium, flurbiprofen sodium, ibuprofen, indomethacin, indomethacin sodium trihydrate, ketoprofen, ketorolac meclofenamate, mefenamic acid, tromethamine, nabumetone, naproxen, naproxen sodium, oxaprozin, piroxicam, rofecoxib, salsalate, sulindac, tolmetin sodium

NSAIDs are a growing class of drugs prescribed widely for their analgesic and anti-inflammatory effects; some members of this class have an antipyretic effect.

Pharmacology

The analgesic effect of NSAIDs may result from interference with the prostaglandins involved in pain. Prostaglandins appear to sensitize pain receptors to mechanical stimulation or to other chemical mediators (such as bradykinin and histamine). NSAIDs inhibit synthesis of prostaglandins peripherally and possibly centrally. Their anti-inflammatory action may also contribute indirectly to their analgesic effect.

Like the salicylates, the anti-inflammatory effects of NSAIDs may result in part from inhibition of prostaglandin synthesis and release during inflammation. The exact mechanism hasn't been established, but the anti-inflammatory effect of NSAIDs correlates with their ability to inhibit prostaglandin synthesis. Selective inhibition of the cyclo-oxygenase 2 (COX-2) enzyme by the COX-2 inhibitors results in the anti-inflammatory efficacy and pain relief equivalent to other NSAIDs but with improved safety in that these newer NSAIDs don't result in gastric and renal adverse effects resulting from the lack of inhibition of the COX-1 enzyme.

The antipyretic effect may be due to suppression of prostaglandin synthesis in the CNS (probably the hypothalamus).

Clinical indications and actions

Pain, inflammation, and fever

NSAIDs are used principally for symptomatic relief of mild to moderate pain and inflammation. These agents usually provide temporary relief of mild to moderate pain, especially that associated with inflammation. NSAIDs are used to treat low-intensity pain of headache, arthralgia, myalgia, neuralgia, and mild to moderate pain from dental or surgical procedures or dysmenorrhea.

Oral NSAIDs are also used for long-term treatment of rheumatoid arthritis, juvenile arthritis, and osteoarthritis. In osteoarthritis, NSAIDs are used primarily for analgesia. NSAIDs offer only symptomatic treatment for rheumatoid conditions, and don't reverse or arrest the disease process. NSAIDs reduce pain, stiffness, swelling, and tenderness. COX-2 inhibitors such as celecoxib and rofecoxib are new NSAIDs which also exhibit anti-inflammatory and analgesic actions.

Overview of adverse reactions

Adverse reactions to oral NSAIDs chiefly involve the GI tract, particularly erosion of the gastric mucosa. Most common symptoms are dyspepsia, heartburn, epigastric distress, nausea, and abdominal pain. GI symptoms usually occur in the first few days of therapy, and often subside with continuous treatment. They can be minimized by administering NSAIDs with meals or food, antacids, or large quantities of water or milk.

CNS adverse effects (headache, dizziness, drowsiness) may also occur. Flank pain with other signs and symptoms of nephrotoxicity has occasionally been reported. Fluid retention may aggravate preexisting hypertension or heart failure. NSAIDs shouldn't be used in patients with renal insufficiency.

Clinical considerations

- Use NSAIDs cautiously in patients with history of GI disease, increased risk of GI bleeding, or decreased renal function.
- Patients with known "triad" symptoms (aspirin hypersensitivity, rhinitis or nasal polyps, and asthma) are at high risk of bronchospasm.
- NSAIDs may mask the signs and symptoms of acute infection.
- Administer oral NSAIDs with a full 8-oz (240-ml) glass of water to ensure adequate passage into stomach.
- Tablets may be crushed and mixed with food or fluids to aid swallowing, and with antacids to minimize gastric upset.
- Recommend monitoring for signs and symptoms of bleeding. Assess bleeding time if surgery is required.
- Recommend monitoring ophthalmic and auditory function before and periodically during therapy to prevent toxicity.
- Recommend monitoring CBC, platelets, PT, and hepatic and renal function studies periodically to detect abnormalities.
- Use of an NSAID with an opioid analgesic has an additive effect. Use of lower doses of the opioid analgesic may be possible.

Special populations

Pregnant patients. Pregnant women should avoid using all NSAIDs, especially during the third trimester, when prostaglandin inhibition may cause prolonged gestation, dystocia, and delayed parturition.

Breast-feeding patients. Most NSAIDs are distributed into breast milk; NSAID therapy isn't recommended during breast-feeding.

Pediatric patients. Don't use long-term NSAID therapy in children under age 14; safety hasn't been established.

Geriatric patients. Patients over age 60 may be more susceptible to the toxic effects of NSAIDs because of decreased renal function, resulting in NSAID accumulation.

The effects of NSAIDs on renal prostaglandins may cause fluid retention and edema, a significant drawback for geriatric patients, especially those with heart failure.

Patient counseling

- Tell patient to take medication with 8 oz (240 ml) of water 30 minutes before or 2 hours after meals, or with food or milk if gastric irritation occurs.
- Explain to patient that taking drug as directed is necessary to achieve the desired effect; 2 to

4 weeks of treatment may be needed before benefit is seen.

- Advise patient on chronic NSAID therapy to arrange for monitoring of laboratory parameters, especially BUN, serum creatinine, liver function tests, and CBC.
- Warn patient with current rectal bleeding or history of rectal bleeding to avoid using rectal NSAID suppositories. Because they must be retained in the rectum for at least 1 hour, they may cause irritation and bleeding.
- Warn patient that use of alcoholic beverages while on NSAID therapy may cause increased GI irritation and, possibly, GI bleeding.

Representative combinations

Diclofenac sodium and misoprostil: Arthrotec.

nucleoside reverse transcriptase inhibitors

abacavir sulfate, didanosine, lamivudine, stavudine, zalcitidine, zidovudine

These antiviral agents act specifically against human immunodeficiency virus (HIV) through inhibition of HIV DNA polymerase (reverse transcriptase).

Pharmacology

Nucleoside reverse transcriptase inhibitors suppress HIV replication by inhibition of HIV DNA polymerase. Competitive inhibition of nucleoside reverse transcriptase inhibits DNA viral replication by chain termination, competitive inhibition of reverse transcriptase, or both. (See *Comparing nucleoside reverse transcriptase inhibitors,* pages 52 and 53.)

Clinical indications and actions

Nucleoside reverse transcriptase inhibitors are indicated for the treatment of HIV infection and acquired immunodeficiency syndrome (AIDS). Note that two drug regimens containing only nucleoside reverse transcriptase inhibitors are now considered suboptimal. Combination therapy including protease inhibitors or nonnucleoside reverse transcriptase inhibitors are recommended. These agents may also be used for the prevention of maternal-fetal HIV transmission and in the prevention of HIV infection after occupational exposure (such as needlesticks or other parenteral exposures).

Overview of adverse reactions

Because of the complexity of HIV infection, it's often difficult to distinguish between disease-related symptoms and adverse drug reactions. The most frequently reported side effects of nucleoside reverse transcriptase inhibitors include anemia, leukopenia, and neutropenia. Less frequent side effects include thrombocytopenia. Rare side effects of nucleoside reverse transcriptase inhibitors include hepatotoxicity, myopathy, and neurotoxicity. The occurrence of any of the aforementioned side effects requires prompt medical attention. The following side effects don't require medical attention unless they persist or are bothersome: headache, severe insomnia, myalgias, nausea, or hyperpigmentation of nails.

Clinical considerations

- Consider the risk-benefit ratio of therapy with nucleoside reverse transcriptase inhibitors on an individual basis when any of the following conditions is present: alcoholism, cardiac disease, hypertriglyceridemia, pancreatitis, bone marrow suppression, fluid overload, folic acid or vitamin B_{12} deficiency, liver dysfunction, peripheral neuropathy, or renal or hepatic dysfunction. These conditions may predispose the patient to adverse drug reactions during treatment with nucleoside reverse transcriptase inhibitors.
- The bone marrow suppressant action of the nucleoside reverse transcriptase inhibitors may cause increased susceptibility to certain microbial infections; this effect may be accentuated by other medications that also cause bone marrow suppression.

Special populations

Pregnant patients. Pregnancy risk category is C (didanosine is category B). Adequate, well-controlled trials haven't been completed, but the risk of HIV transmission to the fetus is decreased with the use of nucleoside reverse transcriptase inhibitors during pregnancy. Teratogenicity or ill effects haven't been seen in neonates. This drug crosses the placenta and decreases the perinatal transmission of HIV. Doctors are encouraged to contact the registry at 1-800-258-4263 to report pregnant women on therapy.

Breast-feeding patients. The rate and extent of excretion of nucleoside reverse transcriptase inhibitors into breast milk is unknown. Therefore, their use in breast-feeding women isn't recommended. However, the risks and benefits to both the woman and infant must be considered in each case.

Pediatric patients. Nucleoside reverse transcriptase inhibitors may be used in children age 3 months or older. The half-life of these agents may be prolonged in neonates, but otherwise the pharmacokinetic and safety profile of nucleoside reverse transcriptase inhibitors is similar in children and adults.

Geriatric patients. Safety and efficacy of nucleoside reverse transcriptase inhibitors in geriatric patients are unknown. Anecdotal evidence suggests that geriatric patients respond well to this therapy, but that they may experience a more prolonged half-life of elimination.

COMPARING NUCLEOSIDE REVERSE TRANSCRIPTASE INHIBITORS

Drug	Oral bioavailability	Plasma protein binding (%)	Half-life (hr)	Elimination
abacavir sulfate	83%; may be taken with or without food	About 50	1½	Renal clearance accounts for 82.2%; fecal elimination is 16%
didanosine	Acid labile, variable absorption, take on an empty stomach	< 5	Adults: ¾-2¾ Children: ½-1¼ Severe renal failure: 4½	Renal clearance by glomerular filtration and active tubular secretion accounts for 50% of total body clearance
lamivudine	60%-88%; food reduces the rate but not the extent of absorption	36	Adults: 2-11 Children: 1¾-2 CrCl 10-40 ml/min: 13½ CrCl < 10 ml/min: 19½	Renal clearance by glomerular filtration and active tubular secretion accounts for 68%-71% of total body clearance
stavudine	78%-86%; may take with or without food	Negligible	Adults: 1-1½ Children: 1-1¼ CrCl < 25 ml/min: 4¾	Renal clearance by glomerular filtration and active tubular secretion; 40% is excreted unchanged in 6-24 hr
zalcitidine	80% in adults; 54% in children. Food decreases bioavailability by 14%	< 4	Adults: 1-3 Children: ¾ CrCl < 55 ml/min: 8½	70% excreted unchanged in urine
zidovudine	65%; unknown effect of food on bioavailability	34-38	Adults: 1 CrCl < 20 ml/min: 1½	90% excreted in urine

Patient counseling

- Tell the patient to take the medication as prescribed, that it's important not to take more or less medication than instructed, and to finish the full course of therapy.
- Instruct patient not to miss a dose but, if a dose is missed, to take the next dose as soon as possible; don't double the dose.
- Advise patient to adhere to scheduled doctor's appointments because important blood tests are needed to evaluate the response to this drug.
- Tell patient not to take other medications concurrently without first checking with the pharmacist or doctor.
- Instruct patient to floss and brush teeth carefully to prevent unnecessary bleeding from the gums.
- Tell patient to avoid sexual intercourse or to use a condom to decrease the risk of HIV transmission.

Representative combinations

Lamivudine and zidovudine combination (Combivir).

opioids

alfentanil hydrochloride, codeine phosphate, codeine sulfate, difenoxin hydrochloride, diphenoxylate hydrochloride, fentanyl citrate, hydromorphone hydrochloride, levomethadyl acetate hydrochloride, meperidine hydrochloride, methadone hydrochloride, morphine sulfate, oxycodone hydrochloride, oxymorphone hydrochloride, propoxyphene hydrochloride, propoxyphene napsylate, remifentanil hydrochloride, sufentanil citrate

Opioids, previously called narcotic agonists, are usually understood to include natural and semisynthetic alkaloid derivatives from opium and their synthetic surrogates, whose actions mimic those of morphine. Most of these drugs are classified as Schedule II by the Federal Drug Enforcement Agency because they have a high potential for addiction and abuse. In the past, opioids were used indiscriminately for analgesia and sedation and to control diarrhea and cough. (See *Comparing opioids,* page 54.)

Dosage adjustment	Dialyzability	Dosage
Not known	Not known	Adults: 300 mg b.i.d. Children: 8 mg/kg b.i.d. up to a maximum of 300 mg b.i.d.
No adjustment for renal or hepatic failure.	20% loss following a 4-hr dialysis	Adults > 132 lb (60 kg): 200 mg (tablets) q 12 hr, or 250 mg (buffered powder) q 12 hr Adults < 132 lb (60 kg): 125 mg (tablets) q 12 hr, or 167 mg (buffered powder) q 12 hr Children: 31 to 125 mg q 8-12 hr based on body surface area
Patients 16 or older with renal impairment require dosage adjustment.	Not known	Adults > 110 lb (50 kg): 150 mg b.i.d. Adults < 110 lb (50 kg): 2 mg/kg b.i.d. Children: 4 mg/kg b.i.d. to maximum of 150 mg q 12 hr
Patients with CrCl < 50 ml/min may require dosage adjustment.	Not known	Adults < 132 lb (60 kg): 30 mg q 12 hr Adults ≥ 132 lb (60 kg): 40 mg q 12 hr Children 66-132 lb (30-60 kg): 30 mg q 12 hr Children < 66 lb (30 kg): 1 mg/kg q 12 hr
Patients with CrCl < 50 ml/min may require dosage adjustment.	Not known	Adults ≥ 66 lb (30 kg): 0.75 mg q 8 hr
Anemia, neutropenia, renal disease patients may require adjustment.	Negligible effect	Adults: 600 mg/day in divided doses Children: 3 months to 12 years: 180 mg/m^2 q 6 hr (720 mg/m^2/day), not to exceed 200 mg q 6 hr

Pharmacology

Opioids act as agonists at specific opiate receptor binding sites in the CNS and other tissues; these are the same receptors occupied by endogenous opioid peptides (enkephalins and endorphins) to alter CNS response to painful stimuli. Opiate agonists don't alter the cause of pain, but only the patient's perception of the pain; they relieve pain without affecting other sensory functions. Opiate receptors are present in highest concentrations in the limbic system, thalamus, striatum, hypothalamus, midbrain, and spinal cord.

Opioids produce respiratory depression by a direct effect on the respiratory centers in the brain stem, resulting in decreased sensitivity and responsiveness to increases in carbon dioxide tension. The antitussive effects of these drugs are mediated by a direct suppression of the cough reflex center. They cause nausea, probably by stimulation of the chemoreceptor trigger zone in the medulla oblongata; through orthostatic hypotension, which causes dizziness; and possibly by increasing vestibular sensitivity.

Opioids also cause drowsiness, sedation, euphoria, dysphoria, mental clouding, and EEG changes; higher than usual analgesic doses cause anesthesia. Most opioids cause miosis, although meperidine and its derivatives may also cause mydriasis or no pupillary change.

Because opioids decrease gastric, biliary, and pancreatic secretions and delay digestion, constipation is a common adverse reaction. At the same time, these drugs increase tone in the biliary tract and may cause biliary spasms. Some patients may have no biliary effects, whereas others may have biliary spasms that increase plasma amylase and lipase levels up to 15 times normal values.

Opioids increase smooth muscle tone in the urinary tract and induce spasms, causing urinary urgency. These drugs have little CV effect in a supine patient, but may cause orthostatic hypotension when the patient assumes upright posture. These drugs are also associated with manifestations of histamine release or peripheral vasodilation, including pruritus, flushing, red eyes, and sweating. These effects are often mistakenly attributed to allergy and should be evaluated carefully.

Opiates can be divided chemically into three groups: phenanthrenes (codeine, hydrocodone, hydromorphone, morphine, oxycodone, and oxymorphone); diphenylheptanes (levomethadyl, methadone, and propoxyphene); and phenylpiperidines (alfentanil, diphenoxylate,

COMPARING OPIOIDS

Drug	Route	Onset (min)	Peak	Duration (hr)
alfentanil	I.V.	Immediate	Not available	Not available
codeine	I.M., P.O., S.C.	15 to 30	30 to 60 min	4 to 6
fentanyl	I.M., I.V.	7 to 8	Not available	1 to 2
hydrocodone	P.O.	30	60 min	4 to 6
hydromorphone	I.M., I.V., S.C. P.O., rectal	15 30	30 min 60 min	4 to 5 4 to 5
meperidine	I.M. P.O. S.C.	10 to 15 15 to 30 10 to 15	30 to 50 min 60 min 40 to 60 min	2 to 4 2 to 4 2 to 4
methadone	I.M., P.O., S.C.	30 to 60	30 to 60 min	4 to 6 †
morphine	I.M. P.O., rectal S.C.	≤ 20 ≤ 20 ≤ 20	30 to 60 min ≤ 60 min 50 to 90 min	3 to 7 3 to 7 3 to 7
oxycodone	P.O.	15 to 30	30 to 60 min	4 to 6
oxymorphone	I.M., S.C. I.V. rectal	10 to 15 5 to 10 15 to 30	30 to 60 min 30 to 60 min 30 to 60 min	3 to 6 3 to 6 3 to 6
propoxyphene	P.O.	20 to 60	2 to 2½ hr	4 to 6
remifentanil	I.V.	Immediate	Not available	Not available
sufentanil	I.V.	1.3 to 3	Not available	Not available

† Due to cumulative effects, duration of action increases with repeated doses.

fentanyl, meperidine, and remifentanil, sufentanil). If a patient is hypersensitive to an opioid, agonist-antagonist, or antagonist of a given chemical group, use extreme caution in considering the use of another agent from the same chemical group; however, a drug from the other groups might be well tolerated.

Some opioids are well absorbed after oral or rectal administration; others must be administered parenterally. I.V. dosing is the most rapidly effective and reliable; absorption after I.M. or S.C. dosing may be erratic. Opioids vary in onset and duration of action; they are removed rapidly from the bloodstream and distributed, in decreasing order of concentration, into skeletal muscle, kidneys, liver, intestinal tract, lungs, spleen, and brain; they readily cross the placenta.

Opioids are metabolized mainly in the microsomes in the endoplasmic reticulum of the liver (first-pass effect) and also in the CNS, kidneys, lungs, and placenta. They undergo conjugation with glucuronic acid, hydrolysis, oxidation, or N-dealkylation. They are excreted primarily in the urine; small amounts are excreted in the feces.

Clinical indications and actions

The opioids produce varying degrees of analgesia and have antitussive, antidiarrheal, and sedative effects. Clinical response is dose-related and varies with each patient.

Analgesia

Opioids may be used in the symptomatic management of moderate to severe pain associated with acute and some chronic disorders, including renal or biliary colic, MI, acute trauma, postoperative pain, or terminal cancer. They also may be used to provide analgesia during diagnostic and orthopedic procedures and during labor. Drug selection, route of administration, and dose depend on a variety of factors. For example, in mild pain, oral therapy with codeine or oxycodone usually suffices. In acute pain of known short duration, such as that associated with diagnostic procedures or orthopedic manipulation, a short-acting drug such as meperidine or fentanyl is effective. These drugs are often given to alleviate postoperative pain, but because they influence CNS function, special care should be taken to monitor the course of recovery and to detect early signs of complications. Opioids are commonly used to manage severe, chronic pain associated with terminal cancer; this requires careful evaluation and titration of drug used, dose, and route of administration.

Pulmonary edema

Morphine, meperidine, oxymorphone, hydromorphone, and other similar drugs have been used to relieve anxiety in patients with dyspnea associated with acute pulmonary edema and acute left ventricular failure. These drugs shouldn't be used to treat pulmonary edema resulting from a chemical respiratory stimulant. Opioids decrease peripheral resistance, causing pooling of blood in the extremities and decreased venous return, cardiac workload, and pulmonary venous pressure; blood is shifted from the central to the peripheral circulation.

Preoperative sedation
Routine use of opioids for preoperative sedation in patients without pain isn't recommended because it may cause complications during and after surgery. To allay preoperative anxiety, a barbiturate or benzodiazepine is equally effective, with a lower incidence of postoperative vomiting.

Anesthesia
Certain opioids, including alfentanil, fentanyl, remifentanil, and sufentanil, may be used for induction of anesthesia, as an adjunct in the maintenance of general and regional anesthesia, or as a primary anesthetic agent in surgery.

Cough suppression
Some opioids, most commonly codeine and its derivative, hydrocodone, are used as antitussives to relieve dry, nonproductive cough.

Diarrhea
Diphenoxylate and other opioids are used as antidiarrheal agents. All opioids cause constipation to some degree; however, only a few are indicated for this use. Usually, opiate antidiarrheals are empirically combined with antacids, absorbing agents, and belladonna alkaloids in commercial preparations.

Overview of adverse reactions

Respiratory depression and, to a lesser extent, circulatory depression (including orthostatic hypotension) are the major hazards of treatment with opioids. Rapid I.V. administration increases the incidence and severity of these serious adverse effects. Respiratory arrest, shock, and cardiac arrest have occurred. It's likely that equianalgesic doses of individual opiates produce a comparable degree of respiratory depression, but its duration may vary. Other adverse CNS effects include dizziness, visual disturbances, mental clouding or depression, sedation, coma, euphoria, dysphoria, weakness, faintness, agitation, restlessness, nervousness, seizures, and, rarely, delirium and insomnia. Adverse effects seem to be more prevalent in ambulatory patients and those not experiencing severe pain. Adverse GI effects include nausea, vomiting, and constipation, as well as increased biliary tract pressure that may result in biliary spasm or colic. Tolerance, psychological dependence, and physical dependence (addiction) may follow prolonged, high-dose therapy (more than 100 mg of morphine daily for more than 1 month).

Use opiate agonists with extreme caution during pregnancy and labor, because they readily cross the placenta. Premature infants appear especially sensitive to their respiratory and CNS depressant effects when used during delivery.

Opiate agonists have a high potential for addiction and should always be administered with caution in patients susceptible to physical or psychological dependence. The agonist-antagonists have a lower potential for addiction and abuse, but the liability still exists.

Clinical considerations

- Administer with extreme caution to patients with head injury, increased intracranial pressure, seizures, asthma, COPD, alcoholism, prostatic hypertrophy, severe hepatic or renal disease, acute abdominal conditions, arrhythmias, hypovolemia, or psychiatric disorders, and to geriatric or debilitated patients. Reduced doses may be necessary.
- Advise that resuscitative equipment and a narcotic antagonist (naloxone) be available. Health care providers should be prepared to provide support of ventilation and gastric lavage.
- Parenteral administration of opiates provides better analgesia than oral administration. Give I.V. administration by slow injection, preferably in diluted solution. Rapid I.V. injection increases the incidence of adverse effects.
- Give parenteral injections by I.M. or S.C. route cautiously to patients who are chilled, hypovolemic, or in shock, because decreased perfusion may lead to accumulation of the drug and toxic effects. Rotate I.M. or S.C. injection sites to avoid induration.
- A regular dosing schedule (rather than "as needed for pain") is preferred to alleviate the symptoms and anxiety that accompany pain.
- Duration of respiratory depression may be longer than the analgesic effect. Monitor patient closely with repeated dosing.
- With chronic administration, advise that the patient's respiratory status be evaluated before each dose. Because severe respiratory depression may occur (especially with accumulation from chronic dosing), watch for respiratory rate below the patient's baseline level. Evaluate the patient for restlessness, which may be a sign of compensatory response for hypoxia.
- Opiates or agonist-antagonists may cause orthostatic hypotension in ambulatory patients. The patient should sit or lie down to relieve dizziness or fainting.
- Because opiates depress respiration when used postoperatively, encourage patient turning, coughing, and deep breathing to avoid atelectasis.
- Recommend that if gastric irritation occurs, give oral products with food; food delays absorption and onset of analgesia.
- Opiates may obscure the signs and symptoms of an acute abdominal condition or worsen gallbladder pain.

■ The antitussive activity of opiates is used to control persistent, exhausting cough or dry, nonproductive cough.
■ The first sign of tolerance to the therapeutic effect of opioid agonists or agonist-antagonists is usually a shortened duration of effect.
■ Preservative-free morphine (Astramorph, Duramorph) is available for epidural or intrathecal use.

Special populations

Pregnant patients. Meperidine and oxymorphone hydrochloride are classified as pregnancy risk category B, but D if used for a prolonged time or for high doses used at term. Most opioids are listed as pregnancy risk category C. Administration of an opiate to a woman shortly before delivery may cause respiratory depression in the neonate. Monitor closely and be prepared to resuscitate.
Breast-feeding patients. Codeine, meperidine, methadone, morphine, and propoxyphene are excreted in breast milk and should be used with caution in breast-feeding women. Methadone has been shown to cause physical dependence in breast-feeding infants of women maintained on methadone.
Pediatric patients. Safety and efficacy in children haven't been established. Use care when administering to children.
Geriatric patients. Lower doses are usually indicated for geriatric patients, who may be more sensitive to the therapeutic and adverse effects of drug.

Patient counseling

■ Instruct patient to use drug with caution and to avoid hazardous activities that require full alertness and coordination.
■ Tell patient to avoid drinking alcohol when taking opioid agonists, because alcohol causes additive CNS depression.
■ Explain that constipation may result from taking an opiate. Suggest measures to increase dietary fiber content, or recommend a stool softener.
■ If patient's condition allows, instruct patient to breathe deeply, cough, and change position every 2 hours to avoid respiratory complications.
■ Encourage patient to void at least every 4 hours to avoid urine retention.
■ Tell the patient to take drug as prescribed and to call if significant adverse effects occur.
■ Tell patient not to increase dose if he isn't experiencing the desired effect, but to call for prescribed dosage adjustment.
■ Instruct the patient not to double the dose. Tell him to take a missed dose as soon as he remembers unless it's almost time for the next dose. If this is the case, he should skip the missed dose and go back to the regular dosing schedule.
■ Tell patient to call immediately for emergency help if he thinks he or someone else has taken an overdose.
■ Explain signs of overdose to patient and his family.

Representative combinations

Codeine with acetaminophen: Phenaphen with codeine, Tylenol with codeine, Capital with codeine, Aceta with codeine, Acetaminophen with Codeine Oral Solution, Acetaminophen with Codeine Tablets, Margesic No. 3, Tylenol with Codeine No. 4, Phenaphen with Codeine No. 4; with caffeine: Fioricet with codeine; with calcium iodide and alcohol: Calcidrine.

Codeine phosphate with guaifenesin: Cheracol, Guiatuss AC, Guiatussin with Codeine Liquid, Mytussin AC, Robitussin A-C, Tolu-Sed Cough; with iodinated glycerol: Tussi-Organidin NR; with triprolidine hydrochloride and pseudoephedrine hydrochloride: Actifed with Codeine.

Codeine with aspirin: Empirin with codeine, Aspirin with Codeine No. 3, Aspirin with Codeine No. 4.

Codeine and aspirin with caffeine and butalbital: Fiorinal with Codeine; with carisoprodol: Soma Compound with Codeine.

Dihydrocodeine with acetaminophen and caffeine: Synalgos-DC.

Fentanyl with droperidol: Innovar, Fentanyl Citrate and Droperidol.

Hydrocodone bitartrate with acetaminophen: Anexsia 5/500 Tablets, Anexsia 7.5/650 Tablets, Anexsia 10/660 Tablets, Bancap HC, Dolacet, Duocet, Hydrocet, Lorcet-HD, Lorcet Plus, Zydone, Lortab, Lortab Elixir, Co-Gesic, Damason-P, Hydrogesic, Hy-Phen, Vicodin, Vicodin ES, Hydrocodone Bitartrate and Acetaminophen Tablets; with aspirin: Lortab ASA, Panasal 5/500; with aspirin and caffeine: Damason-P; with aspirin, acetaminophen, and caffeine: Hyco-Pap; with guaifenesin: Hycotuss Expectorant Syrup (with alcohol); with guaifenesin and pseudoephedrine hydrochloride: Detussin Expectorant, Entuss-D; with guaifenesin and phenindamine tartrate: P-V-Tussin tablets; with guaifenesin and phenylephrine: Donatussin DC; with potassium guaiacosulfonate: Codiclear DH, Entuss-D Liquid; with pseudoephedrine hydrochloride: Detussin Liquid; with homatropine methylbromide: Hycodan; with phenylephrine hydrochloride and pyrilamine maleate: Codimal DH; with phenylpropanolamine hydrochloride: Hycomine; with phenylephrine hydrochloride, pyrilamine maleate, chlorpheniramine maleate salicylamide, citric acid, and caffeine: Citra Forte; with pheniramine maleate, pyrilamine maleate, potassium citrate, and ascorbic acid: Citra forte; with phenylephrine hydrochloride, phenylpropanolamine hydrochloride, pheniramine maleate, pyrilamine maleate, and alcohol: Ru-Tuss with hydrocodone; with guaifenesin and alcohol: S-T forte; with phenyltoloxamine: Tussionex.

Hydromorphone with guaifenesin: Dilaudid Cough.

Meperidine with promethazine: Mepergan, Mepergan Fortis; with atropine sulfate: Atropine and Demerol Injection.

Oxycodone hydrochloride with acetaminophen: Tylox, Roxicet, Roxicet 5/500 Caplets, Roxicet Oral Solution, Oxycodone with Acetaminophen Capsules, Roxilox Capsules, Oxycocet*, Percocet, Percocet-Demi; with aspirin: Oxycodone with Aspirin Tablets, Roxiprin Tablets; with oxycodone terephthalate and aspirin: Percodan, Percodan-Demi.

Propoxyphene with acetaminophen: Lorcet, Wygesic, Darvocet-N, Propacet 100, Propoxyphene Napsylate and Acetaminophen, E-Lor Tablets, Genagesic.

Propoxyphene napsylate with acetaminophen: Darvocet-N 50, Darvocet-N 100, Propocet 100; with aspirin: Propoxyphene HCl Compound Capsules; with aspirin and caffeine: Darvon Compound, Propoxyphene Compound, PC-CAP.

opioid (narcotic) agonist-antagonists

buprenorphine hydrochloride, butorphanol tartate, nalbuphine hydrochloride, pentazocine hydrochloride

The term "opioid (or narcotic) agonist-antagonist" is somewhat imprecise. This class of drugs has varying degrees of agonist and antagonist activity. These drugs are potent analgesics, with somewhat less addiction potential than the pure narcotic agonists.

Pharmacology

The detailed pharmacology of these drugs is poorly understood. Each agent is believed to act on different opiate receptors in the CNS to a greater or lesser degree, thus yielding slightly different effects. Like the opioid agonists, these drugs can be divided into related chemical groups. Buprenorphine, butorphanol, and nalbuphine are phenanthrenes, like morphine, whereas pentazocine falls into a unique class, the benzmorphans.

Clinical indications and actions

Pain

Opioid agonist-antagonists are primarily used as analgesics, particularly in patients at high risk for drug dependence or abuse. Some are used as preoperative or preanesthetic medication, to supplement balanced anesthesia, or to relieve prepartum pain.

Other uses

◇ Buprenorphine has been used to reverse fentanyl-induced anesthesia. Buprenorphine and naloxone have been used to reduce opiate consumption in patients who are physically dependent on opiates.

Overview of adverse reactions

Major hazards of agonist-antagonists are respiratory depression, apnea, shock, and cardiopulmonary arrest, possibly causing death. All opioid agonist-antagonists can cause respiratory depression, but the severity of such depression each drug can cause has a "ceiling"; for example, each drug depresses respiration to a certain point, but increased doses don't depress it further. All opioid agonist-antagonists have been reported to cause withdrawal symptoms after abrupt discontinuation of long-term use; they appear to have some addiction potential, but less than that of the pure opioid agonists.

CNS effects are the most common adverse reactions and may include drowsiness, sedation, light-headedness, dizziness, hallucinations, disorientation, agitation, euphoria, dysphoria, insomnia, confusion, headache, tremor, miosis, seizures, and psychological dependence. CV reactions may include tachycardia, bradycardia, palpitations, chest wall rigidity, hypertension, hypotension, syncope, and edema. GI reactions may include nausea, vomiting, and constipation (most common), dry mouth, anorexia, and biliary spasms (colic). Other effects include urine retention or hesitancy, decreased libido, flushing, rash, pruritus, and pain at the injection site.

Opioid agonist-antagonists can produce morphine-like dependence and thus have abuse potential. Psychological and physiologic dependence with drug tolerance can develop upon chronic repeated administration. Patients with dependence or tolerance to narcotic agonist-antagonists usually present with an acute abstinence syndrome or withdrawal signs and symptoms, of which the severity is related to the degree of dependence, abruptness of withdrawal, and the drug used.

Common signs and symptoms of withdrawal are yawning, lacrimation, and sweating (early); mydriasis, piloerection, flushing of face, tachycardia, tremor, irritability, and anorexia (intermediate); and muscle spasms, fever, nausea, vomiting, and diarrhea (late).

Clinical considerations

- Opioid agonist-antagonists are contraindicated in patients with known hypersensitivity to any drug of the same chemical group. Use these drugs with extreme caution in patients with supraventricular arrhythmias; avoid or administer drug with extreme caution in patients with head injury or increased intracranial pressure, because neurologic parameters are ob-

scured; during pregnancy and labor, because drug crosses placenta readily (premature infants are especially sensitive to respiratory and CNS depressant effects of opioid agonist-antagonists).
■ Use opioid agonist-antagonists cautiously in patients with renal or hepatic dysfunction, because drug accumulation or prolonged duration of action may occur; in patients with pulmonary disease (asthma, COPD) because drug depresses respiration and suppresses cough reflex; in patients undergoing biliary tract surgery because drug may cause biliary spasm; in patients with convulsive disorders because drug may precipitate seizures; in geriatric and debilitated patients, who are more sensitive to both therapeutic and adverse drug effects; and in patients susceptible to physical or psychological addiction because of the high risk of addiction to this drug.
■ Opioid agonist-antagonists have a lower potential for abuse than do opioid agonists, but the risk still exists.
■ Before administration, visually inspect all parenteral products for particles and discoloration and note the strength of the solution.
■ Parenteral administration of opioid agonist-antagonists provides better analgesia than does oral dosing. Give I.V. dosing by very slow injections, preferably in diluted solution. Rapid I.V. injection increases the incidence of adverse effects.
■ Give I.M. or S.C. injections cautiously to patients who are chilled, hypovolemic, or in shock, because decreased perfusion may lead to accumulation.
■ Opioid agonist-antagonists, as well as opioid antagonists, can reverse the desired effects of opioids; thus, members of different pharmacologic groups (such as meperidine and buprenorphine) shouldn't be prescribed at the same time.
■ Recommend that resuscitative equipment be on hand and an opioid antagonist (naloxone) available. Health care providers should be prepared to provide ventilation and gastric lavage.
■ Patient tolerance may develop to the opiate agonist activity but doesn't develop to opiate antagonist activity.
■ A regular dosing schedule (rather than an "as needed for pain" regimen) is preferable to alleviate the symptoms and anxiety that accompany pain.
■ The duration of respiratory depression may be longer than the analgesic effect. Monitor patient closely with repeated dosing.
■ During chronic administration, regularly evaluate the patient's respiratory status. Because severe respiratory depression may occur (especially with accumulation on chronic dosing), watch for a respiratory rate that's less than the patient's baseline respiratory rate. Also evaluate patient for restlessness, which may be a compensatory response to hypoxia.
■ Opioid agonist-antagonists may cause orthostatic hypotension in ambulatory patients. Advise patient to sit or lie down to relieve dizziness or fainting.
■ Because opioid agonist-antagonists can depress respiration when used postoperatively, strongly encourage patient turning, coughing, and deep breathing to avoid atelectasis. Monitor respiratory status.
■ Oral opioid agonist-antagonists may be taken with food to prevent gastric irritation. Food delays absorption and the onset of analgesia.
■ Opioid agonist-antagonists may obscure the signs and symptoms of an acute abdominal condition or worsen gallbladder pain.
■ The first sign of tolerance to the therapeutic effect of opioid agonist-antagonists is usually a reduced duration of effect.

Special populations

Pregnant patients. Most drugs in this class are pregnancy risk category C. Administering an opiate agonist-antagonist to a woman shortly before delivery may cause respiratory depression in the neonate. The infant must be closely monitored and staff should be prepared to resuscitate.
Breast-feeding patients. These drugs aren't recommended for use in breast-feeding women.
Pediatric patients. Neonates may be more susceptible to the respiratory depressant effects of opiate agonist-antagonists.
Geriatric patients. Lower doses are usually indicated for geriatric patients, who may be more sensitive to the therapeutic and adverse effects of these drugs.

Patient counseling

■ Advise ambulatory patients to be cautious when performing tasks that require alertness, such as driving, if they're taking an opioid agonist-antagonist.
■ Warn patient not to stop taking an opioid agonist-antagonist abruptly if he's been taking it for a prolonged period or at a high dose.
■ Tell patient not to increase dose if it isn't producing the desired effect, but to call for prescribed dosage adjustment.
■ Advise patient to avoid drinking alcohol when taking opioid agonist-antagonists because additive CNS depression will occur.
■ Tell patient that constipation may result. Suggest measures to increase dietary fiber content or recommend a stool softener.
■ Instruct patient not to double the dose. Tell him to take a missed dose as soon as he remembers unless it's almost time for the next dose. If this is the case, tell him to skip the missed dose and go back to regular dosing schedule.
■ Tell patient to call for emergency help if he thinks he or someone else has taken an overdose.
■ Explain signs of overdose to patient and to his family.
■ Instruct patient to breathe deeply, cough, and change position every 2 hours to avoid respi-

ratory complications.

- Encourage patient to void at least every 4 hours to avoid urine retention.
- Tell patient to take the drug as prescribed and to promptly report any significant adverse effects.
- Inform a woman taking an opioid agonist-antagonist to call promptly if she is planning or suspects pregnancy; warn her that her fetus may become addicted to drug.

Representative combinations

Pentazocine with acetaminophen: Talacen; with aspirin: Talwin Compound; with naloxone: Talwin Nx.

Buprenorphine and naloxone.

penicillins

Natural penicillins: **penicillin G benzathine, penicillin G potassium, penicillin G procaine, penicillin G sodium, penicillin V potassium**

Aminopenicillins: **amoxicillin trihydrate with clavulanate potassium, ampicillin, ampicillin sodium with sulbactam sodium, ampicillin trihydrate**

Penicillinase-resistant penicillins: **cloxacillin sodium, dicloxacillin sodium, nafcillin sodium, oxacillin sodium**

Extended spectrum penicillins: **carbenicillin indanyl sodium, mezlocillin sodium, piperacillin sodium, piperacillin sodium with tazobactam sodium, ticarcillin disodium, ticarcillin with clavulanate potassium**

Penicillins are very effective antibiotics with low toxicity. Their activity was first discovered by Sir Alexander Fleming in 1928, but they weren't developed for use against systemic infections until 1940. Penicillin is naturally derived from a mold, *Penicillium chrysogenum.* New synthetic derivatives are created by chemical reactions that modify their structure, resulting in increased GI absorption, resistance to destruction by beta-lactamase (penicillinase), and a broader spectrum of susceptible organisms.

Pharmacology

The basic structure of penicillin is a thiazolidine ring connected to a beta-lactam ring that contains a side chain. This nucleus is the main structural requirement for antibacterial activity; modifications of the side chain alter the antibacterial and pharmacologic effects of penicillin.

Penicillins are generally bactericidal. They inhibit synthesis of the bacterial cell wall, causing rapid cell lysis, and are most effective against fast-growing susceptible bacteria.

The sites of action for penicillins are enzymes known as penicillin-binding proteins (PBPs). The affinity of certain penicillins for PBPs in various microorganisms helps explain differing spectra of activity in this class of antibiotics.

Bacterial resistance to beta-lactam antibiotics is conferred most significantly by bacterial production of beta-lactamase enzymes, which destroy the beta-lactam ring and thus inactivate penicillin; decreased cell wall permeability and alteration in binding affinity to PBP also contribute to such resistance.

Oral absorption of penicillin varies widely; the most acid labile is penicillin G. Side-chain modifications in penicillin V, ampicillin, amoxicillin, and other orally administered penicillins are more stable in gastric acid and permit better absorption from the GI tract. (See *Comparing penicillins,* page 60.)

Penicillins are distributed widely throughout the body; CSF penetration is minimal but is enhanced in patients with inflamed meninges. Most penicillins are only partially metabolized. With the exception of nafcillin, penicillins are excreted primarily in urine, chiefly through renal tubular effects; nafcillin undergoes enterohepatic circulation and is excreted chiefly through the biliary tract.

Clinical indications and actions

Infection caused by susceptible organisms

Natural penicillins. Penicillin G is the prototype of this group; derivatives such as penicillin V are more acid stable and thus better absorbed by the oral route. All natural penicillins are vulnerable to inactivation by beta-lactamase-producing bacteria. Natural penicillins act primarily against gram-positive organisms.

Clinical indications for natural penicillins include streptococcal pneumonia, enterococcal and nonenterococcal group D endocarditis, diphtheria, anthrax, meningitis, tetanus, botulism, actinomycosis, syphilis, relapsing fever, Lyme disease, rat-bite fever, Whipple's disease, and others. Natural penicillins are used prophylactically against pneumococcal infections, rheumatic fever, bacterial endocarditis, and neonatal group B streptococcal disease.

Susceptible aerobic gram-positive cocci include nonpenicillinase-producing *Staphylococcus aureus, Staphylococcus epidermis;* nonenterococcal group D streptococci, groups A, B, C, D, G, H, K, L, and M streptococci, *Streptococcus viridans*; and enterococcus (usually in combination with an aminoglycoside). Susceptible aerobic gram-negative cocci include *Neisseria meningitidis* and nonpenicillinase–producing *N. gonorrhoeae.*

Susceptible aerobic gram-positive bacilli include *Corynebacterium* (both diphtheria and

COMPARING PENICILLINS

Drug	Route	Adult dosage	Frequency	Penicillinase-resistant
amoxicillin	P.O.	250 to 500 mg 3 g with 1 g probenecid for gonorrhea	q 8 hr single dose	No
amoxicillin/ clavulanate potassium	P.O.	250 mg 500 mg	q 8 hr q 12 hr	Yes
ampicillin	I.M., I.V. P.O.	2 to 14 g daily 250 to 500 mg 2.5 g with 1 g probenecid (for gonorrhea)	divided doses given q 4 to 6 hr q 6 hr single dose	No
ampicillin sodium/ sulbactam sodium	I.M., I.V.	1.5 to 3 g	q 6 to 8 hr	Yes
carbenicillin	P.O.	382 to 764 mg	q 6 hr	No
cloxacillin	P.O.	250 mg to 1 g	q 6 hr	Yes
dicloxacillin	P.O.	125 to 500 mg	q 6 hr	Yes
mezlocillin	I.M., I.V.	3 to 4 g	q 4 to 6 hr	No
nafcillin	I.M., I.V. P.O.	250 mg to 2 g 500 mg to 1 g	q 4 to 6 hr q 6 hr	Yes
oxacillin	I.M., I.V. P.O.	250 mg to 2 g 500 mg to 1 g	q 4 to 6 hr q 6 hr	Yes
penicillin G benzathine	I.M.	1.2 to 2.4 million units	single dose	No
penicillin G potassium	I.M., I.V.	200,000 to 4 million units	q 4 hr	No
penicillin G procaine	I.M.	600,000 to 1.2 million units 4.8 million units with 1 g probenecid (for syphilis)	q 1 to 3 days single dose for primary, secondary, and early latent syphilis; weekly for 3 weeks for late latent syphilis	No
penicillin G sodium	I.M., I.V.	200,000 to 4 million units	q 4 hr	No
penicillin V potassium	P.O.	250 to 500 mg	q 6 to 8 hr	No
piperacillin	I.M., I.V.	100 to 300 mg/kg daily	divided dose given q 4 to 6 hr	No
piperacillin sodium/ tazobactam sodium	I.V.	3.375 g	q 6 hr	Yes
ticarcillin	I.M., I.V.	150 to 300 mg/kg daily	divided doses given q 3 to 6 hr	No
ticarcillin/ clavulanate potassium	I.V.	3.1 g	q 4 to 6 hr	Yes

opportunistic species), *Listeria,* and *Bacillus anthracis.* Susceptible anaerobes include *Peptococcus, Peptostreptococcus, Actinomyces, Clostridium, Fusobacterium, Veillonella,* and non-beta-lactamase-producing strains of *Streptococcus pneumoniae.* The drugs are also active against some gram-negative aerobic bacilli including some strains of *Haemophilus influenzae, Pasturella multocida, Streptobacillus moniliformis,* and *Spirillum minus.*

Susceptible spirochetes include *Treponema pallidum, Treponema pertenue, Leptospira,* and *Borrelia recurrentis* and possibly *Borrelia burgdorferi.*

Aminopenicillins (amoxicillin and ampicillin) offer a broader spectrum of activity including many gram-negative organisms. Like natural penicillins, aminopenicillins are vulnerable to inactivation by penicillinase. They are primarily used to treat septicemia, gynecologic infections, and infections of the urinary, respiratory, and GI tracts, and skin, soft tissue, bones, and joints. Their activity spectrum includes *Escherichia coli, Proteus mirabilis, Shigella, Salmonella, S. pneumoniae, N. gonorrhoeae, H. influenzae, S. aureus, S. epidermidis* (non-penicillinase-producing *Staphylococcus*), and *Listeria monocytogenes.*

Penicillinase-resistant penicillins (cloxacillin, dicloxacillin, oxacillin, and nafcillin) are semisynthetic penicillins designed to remain stable against hydrolysis by most staphylococcal penicillinases and thus are the drugs of choice against susceptible penicillinase-producing staphylococci. They also retain activity against most organisms susceptible to natural penicillins. Clinical indications are much the same as for aminopenicillins.

Extended-spectrum penicillins (carbenicillin, mezlocillin, piperacillin, and ticarcillin), as their name implies, offer a wider range of bactericidal action than the other three classes, are used in hard-to-treat gram-negative infections, and are usually given in combination with aminoglycosides. They are used most often against susceptible strains of *Enterobacter, Klebsiella, Citrobacter, Serratia, Bacteroides fragilis, and Pseudomonas aeruginosa;* their gram-negative spectrum also includes *Proteus vulgaris, Proteus mirabilis, Providencia rettgeri, Salmonella, Shigella,* and *Morganella morganii.* These penicillins are also vulnerable to destruction by beta-lactamase or penicillinases.

Overview of adverse reactions

Systemic: Hypersensitivity reactions range from mild rash, fever, and eosinophilia to fatal anaphylaxis. Hematologic reactions include hemolytic anemia, transient neutropenia, leukopenia, and thrombocytopenia.

Certain adverse reactions are more common with specific classes of penicillin: bleeding episodes are usually seen at high-dose levels of extended-spectrum penicillins; acute interstitial nephritis is reported most often with methicillin; GI adverse effects are most common with but not limited to ampicillin. High doses, especially of penicillin G, irritate the CNS in patients with renal disease, causing confusion, twitching, lethargy, dysphagia, seizures, and coma. Hepatotoxicity is most common with penicillinase-resistant penicillins; hyperkalemia, and hypernatremia with extended-spectrum penicillins.

Jarisch-Herxheimer reaction can occur when penicillin G is used in secondary syphilis; signs and symptoms are chills, fever, headache, myalgia, tachycardia, malaise, sweating, hypotension, and sore throat—attributed to release of endotoxin following spirochete death.

Local: Local irritation from parenteral therapy may be severe enough to require discontinuation of the drug or administration by subclavian catheter if drug therapy is to continue.

Clinical considerations

- Assess patient's history of allergies.
- Keep in mind that a negative history for penicillin hypersensitivity doesn't preclude future allergic reactions; monitor patient continuously for possible allergic reactions or other untoward effects.
- Reduce dose in patients with renal impairment based on creatinine clearance and manufacturer's guidelines.
- Recommend assessing level of consciousness, neurologic status, and renal function when high doses are used, because excessive blood levels can cause CNS toxicity.
- Recommend monitoring vital signs, electrolytes, and renal function studies; monitor body weight for fluid retention with extended-spectrum penicillins for possible hypokalemia or hypernatremia.
- Coagulation abnormalities, even frank bleeding, can follow high doses, especially of extended-spectrum penicillins. Monitor PT and platelet counts, and assess patient for signs of occult or frank bleeding.
- Monitor patients on long-term therapy for possible superinfection, especially geriatric and debilitated patients and others receiving immunosuppressants or radiation therapy; monitor closely, especially for fever.

Oral and parenteral administration

- Give penicillins at least 1 hour before giving bacteriostatic antibiotics (tetracyclines, erythromycins, and chloramphenicol); these drugs inhibit bacterial cell growth, decreasing rate of penicillin uptake by bacterial cell walls.
- Refrigerate oral suspensions; shake well before administering to ensure correct dose.
- Give oral penicillin at least 1 hour before or 2 hours after meals to enhance gastric absorption; food may or may not decrease absorption.
- Administer I.M. dose deep into large muscle mass (gluteal or midlateral thigh); rotate injection sites to minimize tissue injury; don't

inject more than 2 g of drug per injection site. Apply ice to injection site for pain.
■ Don't add or mix other drugs with I.V. infusions, particularly aminoglycosides, which are inactivated if mixed with penicillins; they're chemically and physically incompatible. If other drugs must be given I.V., temporarily stop infusion of primary drug.
■ Infuse I.V. drug continuously or intermittently (over 30 minutes) and assess I.V. site frequently to prevent infiltration or phlebitis; rotate infusion site every 48 hours; intermittent I.V. infusion may be diluted in 50 to 100 ml sterile water, normal saline solution, D_5W, D_5W and 0.45% saline, or lactated Ringer's solution.

Special populations

Pregnant patients. Safe use of penicillins in pregnancy hasn't been definitely established. However, penicillin G has been used for the treatment of syphilis without adverse effects, and amoxicillin and ampicillin have been used for the treatment of urinary tract infections without adverse effects.
Breast-feeding patients. Consult individual drug recommendations.
Pediatric patients. Specific dosage recommendations have been established for most penicillins.
Geriatric patients. Use with caution; geriatric patients are susceptible to superinfection.

Many geriatric patients have renal impairment, which decreases excretion of penicillins; lower the dose in geriatric patients with diminished creatinine clearance.

Patient counseling

■ Explain to patient disease process and rationale for therapy.
■ Teach patient signs and symptoms of hypersensitivity and other adverse reactions; emphasize need to report unusual reactions.
■ Teach patient signs and symptoms of bacterial and fungal superinfection to patients, especially geriatric and debilitated patients and others with low resistance from immunosuppressants or irradiation; emphasize need to report signs of infection.
■ Be sure patient understands how and when to take drugs; urge him to complete entire prescribed regimen, to comply with instructions for around-the-clock dosing, and to keep follow-up appointments.
■ Counsel patient to check expiration date of drug and to discard unused drug and not give it to family members or friends.

Representative combinations

Amoxicillin with clavulanate potassium: Augmentin.

Ampicillin with probenecid: Polycillin-PRB, Probampacin.

Ampicillin sodium with sulbactam sodium: Unasyn.

Ampicillin trihydrate with probenecid: Polycillin-PRB, Principen with Probenecid, Probampacin.

Penicillin G benzathine with penicillin G procaine: Bicillin C-R, Bicillin C-R 900/300.

Piperacillin sodium with tazobactam sodium: Zosyn.

Ticarcillin disodium with clavulanate potassium: Timentin.

phenothiazines

***Aliphatic derivatives:* chlorpromazine hydrochloride, promethazine hydrochloride, trimeprazine, triflupromazine**

***Piperazine derivatives:* fluphenazine hydrochloride, perphenazine, prochlorperazine, trifluoperazine hydrochloride**

***Piperidine derivatives:* mesoridazine besylate, thioridazine**

***Thioxanthene:* thiothixene**

Phenothiazines were originally synthesized by European scientists seeking aniline-like dyes in the late 1800s. Several decades later, in the 1930s, promethazine was identified and found to have sedative, antihistaminic, and narcotic-potentiating effects. Chlorpromazine was synthesized in the 1950s; this drug has many effects, among them strong antipsychotic activity.

Pharmacology

Phenothiazines are classified in terms of chemical structure: the aliphatic agent (chlorpromazine) has a greater sedative, hypotensive, and allergic activity. Piperazines (perphenazine, prochlorperazine, fluphenazine, and trifluoperazine) are more likely to produce extrapyramidal symptoms. Piperidines (thioridazine and mesoridazine) have intermediate effects. Thioxanthenes are chemically similar to phenothiazines and are pharmacologically similar to piperazine phenothiazines. Promethazine is a derivative that has antihistamine qualities.

All antipsychotics have fundamentally similar mechanisms of action; they're believed to function as dopamine antagonists, blocking postsynaptic dopamine receptors in various parts of the CNS; their antiemetic effects result from blockage of the chemoreceptor trigger zone. They also produce varying degrees of anticholinergic and alpha-adrenergic receptor blocking actions. The drugs are structurally similar to tricyclic antidepressants (TCAs) and share many adverse reactions.

All antipsychotics have equal clinical efficacy when given in equivalent doses; choice of specific therapy is determined primarily by the individual patient's response and adverse reaction profile. A patient who doesn't respond to one drug may respond to another.

Onset of full therapeutic effects requires 6 weeks to 6 months; therefore, dosage adjustment is recommended at not less than weekly intervals.

Clinical indications and actions

Psychoses

Phenothiazines (except promethazine) and thiothixene are indicated to treat agitated psychotic states. They're especially effective in controlling hallucinations in schizophrenic patients, the manic phase of manic-depressive illness, and excessive motor and autonomic activity.

Nausea and vomiting

Chlorpromazine, perphenazine, promethazine, and prochlorperazine are effective in controlling severe nausea and vomiting induced by CNS disturbances. They don't prevent motion sickness or vertigo.

◇***Anxiety***

Chlorpromazine, mesoridazine, promethazine, prochlorperazine, and trifluoperazine also may be used for short-term treatment of moderate anxiety in selected nonpsychotic patients, for example, to control anxiety before surgery.

Severe behavior problems

Chlorpromazine and thioridazine are indicated to control combativeness and hyperexcitability in children with severe behavior problems. They're also used in hyperactive children for short-term treatment of excessive motor activity with labile moods, impulsive behavior, aggressiveness, attention deficit, and poor tolerance of frustration. Mesoridazine is used to manage hypersensitivity and to promote cooperative behavior in patients with mental deficiency and chronic brain syndrome.

Tetanus

Chlorpromazine is an effective adjunct in treating tetanus.

Porphyria

Because of its effects on the autonomic nervous system, chlorpromazine is effective in controlling abdominal pain in patients with acute intermittent porphyria.

Delirium

Phenothiazines have been used in the treatment of delirium. Antipsychotics remain first-line therapy.

Intractable hiccups

Chlorpromazine has been used to treat patients with intractable hiccups. The mechanism is unknown.

Neurogenic pain

Fluphenazine is a useful adjunct, managing selected chronic pain states.

Allergies and pruritus

Because of their potent antihistaminic effects, many of these drugs (including promethazine and trimeprazine) are used to relieve itching or symptomatic rhinitis.

Overview of adverse reactions

Phenothiazines may produce extrapyramidal symptoms (dystonic movements, torticollis, oculogyric crises, parkinsonian symptoms) from akathisia during early treatment, to tardive dyskinesia after long-term use.

In rare cases, a neuroleptic malignant syndrome resembling severe parkinsonism may occur; it consists of rapid onset of hyperthermia, muscular hyperreflexia, marked extrapyramidal and autonomic dysfunction, arrhythmias, and sweating.

Other adverse reactions are similar to those seen with TCAs, including sedative and anticholinergic effects, orthostatic hypotension, reflex tachycardia, fainting, dizziness, arrhythmias, anorexia, nausea, vomiting, abdominal pain, local gastric irritation, seizures, endocrine effects, hematologic disorders, ocular changes, skin eruptions, and photosensitivity. Allergic manifestations are usually marked by elevation of liver enzymes progressing to obstructive jaundice.

Piperidine derivatives have the most pronounced CV effects; piperazine derivatives have the least. Parenteral administration is often associated with CV effects because of more rapid absorption. Seizures are common with aliphatic derivatives.

Clinical considerations

- Phenothiazines are contraindicated in patients with known hypersensitivity to phenothiazines and related compounds.
- Use with caution in patients with cardiac disease (arrhythmias, heart failure, angina pectoris, valvular disease, or heart block).
- Use cautiously in patients with encephalitis, Reye's syndrome, head injury, epilepsy, or other seizure disorders.
- Use phenothiazines cautiously in patients with glaucoma, prostatic hypertrophy, paralytic ileus, urine retention, hepatic or renal dysfunction, Parkinson's disease, pheochromocytoma, and hypocalcemia.
- Recommend that vital signs be checked regularly for decreased blood pressure (especially before and after parenteral therapy) or tachycardia; observe patient carefully for other adverse reactions.
- Recommend monitoring of intake and output for urine retention or constipation, which may require dose reduction.
- Recommend monitoring bilirubin levels weekly for first 4 weeks; monitor CBC, ECG (for quinidine-like effects), liver and renal function studies, electrolyte levels (especially potassium), and eye examinations at baseline and periodically thereafter, especially in patients on long-term therapy.
- Recommend observing patient for mood changes to monitor progress; benefits may not be apparent for several weeks.

- Recommend monitoring patient for involuntary movements. Check patient receiving prolonged treatment at least once every 6 months.
- Advise that drug not be withdrawn abruptly; although physical dependence doesn't occur with antipsychotic drugs, rebound exacerbation of psychotic symptoms may occur, and many drug effects persist.
- Carefully follow manufacturer's instructions regarding drug color for reconstitution, dilution, administration, and storage of drugs; slightly discolored liquids may or may not be usable.

Special populations

Pregnant patients. Safety of phenothiazine use during pregnancy hasn't been established.
Breast-feeding patients. If possible, patient shouldn't breast-feed while taking antipsychotics; most phenothiazines are excreted in breast milk and have a direct effect on prolactin levels. Benefit to mother must outweigh hazard to infant.
Pediatric patients. Unless otherwise specified, antipsychotics aren't recommended for children under age 12; be careful when using phenothiazines for nausea and vomiting because acutely ill children (suffering from chickenpox, measles, CNS infections, dehydration) are at greatly increased risk of dystonic reactions.
Geriatric patients. Lower doses are indicated in geriatric patients, who are more sensitive to therapeutic and adverse effects, especially cardiac toxicity, tardive dyskinesia, and other extrapyramidal effects. Adjust dose to patient response.

Patient counseling

- Explain to patient rationale and anticipated risks and benefits of therapy, and that full therapeutic effect may not occur for several weeks.
- Teach patient signs and symptoms of adverse reactions and importance of reporting unusual effects, especially involuntary movements.
- Tell patient to avoid beverages and drugs containing alcohol, and not to take other drugs (especially CNS depressants) including OTC products without medical approval.
- Instruct diabetic patient to monitor blood glucose because drug may alter insulin needs.
- Teach patient how and when to take drug, not to increase dose without medical approval, and never to discontinue drug abruptly; suggest taking full dose at bedtime if daytime sedation is troublesome.
- Advise patient to lie down for 30 minutes after first dose (1 hour if I.M.) and to rise slowly from sitting or supine position to prevent orthostatic hypotension.
- Warn patient to avoid tasks requiring mental alertness and psychomotor coordination such as driving until full effects of drug are established; emphasize that sedative effects will lessen after several weeks.
- Advise patient to take drug with milk or food to minimize GI distress because drugs are locally irritating. Warn that oral concentrates and solutions will irritate skin, and tell patient not to crush or open sustained-release products, but to swallow them whole.
- Warn patient that photosensitivity reactions, such as burns and abnormal hyperpigmentation, may occur.
- Tell patient to avoid exposure to extremes of heat or cold, because of risk of hypothermia or hyperthermia induced by alteration in thermoregulatory function.
- Explain to patient that phenothiazines may cause pink to brown discoloration of urine.

Representative combinations

None.

progestins

hydroxyprogesterone caproate, medroxyprogesterone acetate, megestrol acetate, norethindrone, norethindrone acetate, norgestrel, progesterone

Progesterone is the endogenous progestin, secreted by the corpus luteum within the female ovary. Several synthetic progesterone derivatives with greater potency or duration of action have been synthesized. Some of these derivatives also possess weak androgenic or estrogenic activity. Progestins are used to treat dysfunctional uterine bleeding and certain cancers. They're also used as contraceptives, either alone or in combination with estrogens.

Pharmacology

Progesterone is formed from steroid precursors in the ovary, testis, adrenal cortex, and placenta. Luteinizing hormone stimulates the synthesis and secretion of progesterone from the corpus luteum. Progesterone causes secretory changes in the endometrium, changes in the vaginal epithelium, increases in body temperature, relaxation of uterine smooth muscle, stimulation of growth of breast alveolar tissue, inhibition of gonadotropin release from the pituitary, and withdrawal bleeding (in the presence of estrogens). Synthetic progesterone derivatives have these properties as well.

Clinical indications and actions

Hormonal imbalance, female

Hydroxyprogesterone, medroxyprogesterone, norethindrone, and progesterone are indicated to treat amenorrhea and dysfunctional uterine bleeding resulting from hormonal imbalance. Hydroxyprogesterone also is indicated to produce desquamation and a secretory endometrium.

Endometriosis
Norethindrone and norethindrone acetate are used to treat endometriosis.

Carcinoma
Hydroxyprogesterone, medroxyprogesterone, and megestrol are used in the adjunctive and palliative treatment of certain types of metastatic tumors. They're not considered primary therapy. See individual agents for specific indications.

Contraception
Norethindrone, medroxyprogesterone acetate, and norgestrel are approved for use with estrogens or alone as oral contraceptives.

Progestins are no longer indicated to detect pregnancy (because of teratogenicity) or to treat threatened or habitual abortion, for which they're not effective.

Overview of adverse reactions
The most common adverse effect is a change in menstrual bleeding pattern, ranging from spotting or breakthrough bleeding to complete amenorrhea. Other reactions include breast tenderness and secretion, weight changes, increases in body temperature, edema, nausea, acne, somnolence, insomnia, hirsutism, hair loss, depression, cholestatic jaundice, and allergic reactions (rare). Some patients taking parenteral progestins have also suffered localized reactions at the injection site.

Clinical considerations
- Progestins are contraindicated during pregnancy and in patients with thromboembolic disorders, breast cancer, undiagnosed abnormal vaginal bleeding, or severe hepatic disease.
- Use cautiously in patients with diabetes mellitus, cardiac or renal disease, seizure disorder, migraine, or mental depression.
- Advise giving oil injections deep I.M. in gluteal muscles. I.M. injections may be painful; observe injection site for sterile abscess formation.
- Glucose tolerance may be altered in diabetic patients. Monitor patient closely because antidiabetic medication may need to be adjusted.
- When used as an oral contraceptive, progestins are administered daily without interruption, regardless of menstrual cycle.
- Use of progestins may lead to gingival bleeding and hyperplasia.
- A patient who is exposed to progestins during the first 4 months of pregnancy or who becomes pregnant while receiving the drug should be informed of the potential risks to the fetus.
- Because oral contraceptive combinations contain progestins, consider the precautions associated with oral contraceptives in patients receiving progestins.

Special populations
Pregnant patients. Progestins are listed as pregnancy category X. Potential adverse effects include masculinization of the female fetus, hypospadias in males, and potential cardiovascular and limb defects.

Breast-feeding patients. Don't use progestins in breast-feeding women, except for Depo-Provera, which may be used in breast-feeding women after 6 weeks.

Patient counseling
- Tell patient that GI distress may subside with use, after a few cycles.
- Instruct patient receiving progestins to have a full physical examination, including a gynecologic examination and a Papanicolaou test, every 6 to 12 months.
- Advise patient to discontinue therapy and call immediately if migraine or visual disturbances occur, or if sudden severe headache or vomiting develops.
- Teach patient how to perform breast self-examination.
- Tell patient to call promptly if period is missed or unusual bleeding occurs; and to call and discontinue drug immediately if pregnancy is suspected.
- Advise patient who misses a dose to take the missed dose as soon as possible or omit it.
- Advise patient who misses consecutive doses when used as a contraceptive to discontinue the drug and use an alternative contraception method until period begins or pregnancy is ruled out.
- Inform patient that drug may cause possible dental problems (tenderness, swelling, or bleeding of gums). Advise patient to brush and floss teeth, massage gums, and have dentist clean teeth regularly. She should check with dentist if there are questions about care of teeth or gums or if tenderness, swelling, or bleeding of gums is noticed.
- Advise patient to use extra care to avoid pregnancy when starting use of drug as an oral contraceptive and for at least 3 months after discontinuing it.
- Advise patient to keep an extra 1-month supply available.
- Tell patient to keep tablets in original container.
- Emphasize to patient the importance of not giving medication to anyone else.

Representative combinations
Hydroxyprogesterone caproate with estradiol valerate: Hylutin.

Norethindrone acetate with ethinyl estradiol: Brevicon, Loestrin 1.5/30, Loestrin Fe 1.5/30, Loestrin 21 1/20, Loestrin Fe 1/20, Modicon, Norinyl 1 + 35, Ortho 1/35*, Ortho 7/7/7*, Ortho 10/11*, Ortho-Novum 7/7/7, Ovcon-35, Ovcon-50, Tri-Norinyl; with mestranol: Norinyl 1/50, Ortho-Novum 0.5/35*, Ortho-Novum 1/50, Ortho-Novum 1/35.

Norgestrel with ethinyl estradiol: Lo/Ovral, Ovral.

COMPARING PROTEASE INHIBITORS

Drug	Oral bioavailability	Plasma protein binding (%)	Half-life (hr)	Peak concentration (hr)
imprenavir	May be taken without food, but shouldn't be taken with a high-fat meal, which reduces absorption. Absolute bioavailability hasn't been established.	90	Adults: 7-10½	1-2
indinavir	Meals rich in fats, proteins, or calories reduce bioavailability by 77%.	60	Adults: 1¾	Fasting: ¾
nelfinavir	Food produces 2- to 3-fold increase in bioavailability.	>98	Adults: 3½-5	Fed: 2 to 4
ritonavir	Food produces 15% increase in bioavailability.	98-99	Adults: 3-5	Fasted: 2 Fed: 4
saquinavir	High fat meals produce a 4% increase in bioavailability of Invirase. Soft gelatin capsule formulation (Fortovase) has a 33% increase in bioavailability.	98	Not defined	Not defined

protease inhibitors

amprenavir, indinavir sulfate, nelfinavir mesylate, ritonavir, saquinavir, saquinavir mesylate

These antiviral agents act specifically against human immunodeficiency virus (HIV) through inhibition of HIV protease.

Pharmacology

Protease inhibitors bind to the protease active site and inhibit the activity of HIV protease. This enzyme is required for the proteolysis of viral polyprotein precursors into individual functional proteins found in infectious HIV. The net effect is formation of noninfectious, immature viral particles. Note that two drug regimens containing only nucleoside reverse transcriptase inhibitors are now considered suboptimal. Combination therapy including protease inhibitors or nonnucleoside reverse transcriptase inhibitors are recommended. (See *Comparing protease inhibitors.*)

Clinical indications and actions

Protease inhibitors are used as monotherapy or in combination with nucleoside analogues for the treatment of HIV infection and acquired immunodeficiency syndrome (AIDS).

◊Protease inhibitors may be used in conjunction with zidovudine and lamivudine for postexposure prophylaxis of HIV infection.

Overview of adverse reactions

The most frequently reported side effects of protease inhibitors, for which immediate medical attention should be sought, include kidney stones, diabetes or hyperglycemia, ketoacidosis, or paresthesias. Frequently reported side effects that don't require medical attention unless they persist or are bothersome include generalized weakness, GI disturbances, headache, insomnia, and taste perversion. Less frequent side effects include dizziness and somnolence.

Clinical considerations

- Consider the risk-benefit ratio of therapy with protease inhibitors on an individual basis when either hemophilia or liver dysfunction is present.
- Indinavir may cause nephrolithiasis. Advise increasing fluid intake.

Special populations

Pregnant patients. Pregnancy risk categories are B and C. Adequate, well-controlled trials haven't been completed, because the drug can produce hyperbilirubinemia; exercise caution in pregnant women to prevent ill effects in neonates. Doctors are encouraged to contact the registry at 1-800-258-4263 to report pregnant women on therapy.

Breast-feeding patients. The rate and extent of excretion of protease inhibitors into breast milk is unknown. Therefore, their use in breast-feeding women isn't recommended. However, the risks and benefits to both the woman and infant must be considered in each case.

Pediatric patients. Refer to specific drug monographs for dosing information.

Geriatric patients. Safety and efficacy haven't been evaluated systemically.

Elimination	Dosage adjustment	Dosage
14% renal, 75% fecal elimination	Reduce dose with impaired hepatic function.	Adults: 1,200 mg b.i.d. Children: 20-22.5 mg/kg b.i.d.
83% hepatic; 19% renal	Reduce dose in cirrhosis	Adults: 800 mg q 8 hr Adults with cirrhosis: 600 mg q 8 hr
87% fecal elimination; 78% as metabolites; 1%-2% recovered unchanged in urine	None	Adults: 750 mg t.i.d. with food Children: 20-30 mg/kg t.i.d. with food
88% fecal elimination; 34% as unchanged drug; 11% excreted in urine; 4% as unchanged drug	None	Adults: 600 mg b.i.d. with food Children > 2: 250 mg/m²-400 mg/m² b.i.d. with food
88% fecal elimination as unchanged drug and metabolites; 1% recovered unchanged in urine	None	Fortovase: 1,200 mg t.i.d. with food or within 2 hr of a meal Invirase: 600 mg t.i.d. with food or within 2 hr of a meal

Patient counseling

- Instruct patient to take drug as prescribed and to finish the full course of therapy.
- Tell patient to take the next dose as soon as possible after a missed dose, but not to double the dose.
- Tell patient that drug should be taken with plenty of water, 1 or 2 hours before meals, and he should drink about 48 oz of water daily.
- Instruct patient not to take other medications concurrently without first checking with the pharmacist or doctor.

Representative combinations

None.

selective serotonin reuptake inhibitors

citalopram hydrobromide, fluoxetine, fluvoxamine maleate, sertraline hydrochloride, paroxetine

These drugs are antidepressant, antiobsessional, antipanic agents that selectively inhibit the reuptake of serotonin with little or no effects on other neurotransmitters such as norepinephrine or dopamine. (See *Comparing selective serotonin reuptake inhibitors,* pages 68 and 69.)

Pharmacology

The antidepressant, antiobsessional, antipanic actions of fluoxetine, fluvoxamine maleate, sertraline, and paroxetine are thought to be related to the potent and selective inhibition of serotonin uptake, but not of norepinephrine or dopamine uptake, in the central nervous system. These agents lack affinity for alpha-adrenergic receptors and muscarinic receptors.

Clinical indications and actions

Selective serotonin reuptake inhibitors are used in the treatment of major depression, obsessive-compulsive disorder (OCD), bulimia nervosa, premenstrual dysphoric disorders, and panic disorders. Sertraline is the first drug approved for the treatment of posttraumatic stress disorder (PTSD).

◊Fluoxetine has been used for the treatment of bipolar disorder, symptomatic management of cataplexy, and management of alcohol dependence.

◊Paroxetine and sertraline have been used for the treatment of premature ejaculation and chronic headache; paroxetine for the symptoms of diabetic neuropathy.

Overview of adverse reactions

Frequent side effects include headache, tremor, dizziness, sleep disturbances, GI disturbances, and sexual dysfunction. Less frequent side effects include bleeding (red spots on skin, nose bleeds), akathesia (restlessness), breast tenderness or enlargement, extrapyramidal effects, dystonia, fever, hyponatremia, mania or hypomania, palpitations, serotonin syndrome, weight gain or loss, skin rash, hives, or itching.

Clinical considerations

- Hyponatremia is usually due to inappropriate secretion of antidiuretic hormone. This prob-

COMPARING SELECTIVE SEROTONIN REUPTAKE INHIBITORS

Drug	Oral bioavailability	Plasma protein binding (%)	Half-life (hr)	Onset of action (wk)
citalopram	No food effect	80	35	1-4
fluoxetine	Well absorbed; no food effect	94½	2-3 days for fluoxetine and 7-9 days for norfluoxetine	1-3, may be 5 for OCD
fluvoxamine	No food effect	80	13½-15½	4-5
paroxetine	50%-100%, no food effect	95	Average of 21-24	1-3
sertraline	Food increase rate and extent of absorption	98	Sertraline: 24-26 N-desmethyl-sertraline: 62-104	2-4

lem is most often seen in geriatric patients and those treated with diuretics.

■ Diarrhea, fever, palpitations, mood swings or behavioral changes, restlessness, shaking, and shivering characterize serotonin syndrome. Hypertension and seizures may accompany the serotonin syndrome. This syndrome is most commonly seen within days following dosage increases or concurrent administration of a serotonergic agent.

Special populations

Pregnant patients. Pregnancy risk category is C. Data haven't shown evidence of teratogenicity or ill effects in neonates of women given SSRIs during the first trimester of pregnancy or throughout gestation. The effects of SSRIs on labor and delivery aren't known.

Breast-feeding patients. SSRIs distribute into breast milk and may cause diarrhea and sleep disturbance in neonates. Use of SSRIs in breast-feeding women isn't recommended. However, the risks and benefits to both the woman and infant must be considered in each case.

Pediatric patients. There's insufficient information to establish the safety and efficacy of SSRIs in children, but there's evidence of beneficial response following SSRI treatment for depression or OCD in this population. Pediatric patients appear to be more susceptible than adults to the behavioral adverse reactions of SSRIs (mania, social inhibition, irritability, restlessness, and insomnia).

Geriatric patients. The use of SSRIs is safe and effective in geriatric patients. Geriatric patients are more sensitive to the insomniac effects of SSRIs. Plasma concentration of sertraline may be decreased in these patients.

Patient counseling

■ Tell patient that drug may take 4 to 5 weeks to produce its full-intended benefit. Drug should be taken as prescribed. If a dose is missed, dose shouldn't be doubled.

■ Instruct patient to stop taking medication and contact a doctor or pharmacist as soon as possible if a rash or hives develops.

■ Avoid alcoholic beverages and use of medications or substances that have serotonergic activity.

■ Tell patient to use caution when driving or doing jobs requiring alertness since this medication may cause drowsiness or impairment of judgment or motor skills.

Representative combinations

None.

sulfonamides

co-trimoxazole (trimethoprim-sulfamethoxazole), sulfadiazine, sulfamethoxazole, sulfasalazine, sulfisoxazole

Sulfonamides were the first effective drugs used to treat systemic bacterial infections. The prototype, sulfanilamide, was discovered in 1908 and first used clinically in 1933. Since then, many derivatives have been synthesized, and many therapeutic milestones have been reached, including improved solubility of sulfonamides in urine (which reduces renal toxicity) and discovery of the advantages of combinations such as triple sulfa and, especially, of combined trimethoprim and sulfamethoxazole (co-trimoxazole). Development of other major antibiotics has reduced the clinical impact of sulfonamides; however, introduction of

Peak concentration (hr)	Elimination	Dosage adjustment	Adult dosage
4 (after a single dose)	35% excreted in urine; 65% in feces	Lower dosing recommended in the elderly	20-40 mg/day
6-8 (after a single dose)	80% excreted in urine; 15% in feces	No adjustment for renal or hepatic failure	20-60 mg/day in single or divided doses
3-8	94% renal excretion	Reduction of initial dosage and modification of subsequent doses in renal and hepatic impairment	50-300 mg/day at h.s. Total daily dose of >100 mg/day should be given in two divided doses
2-8	64% excreted in urine; 36% in feces	Maximum dose of 40 mg/day in severe renal or hepatic failure	20 to 60 mg/day in single or divided doses
4½-8½	45% renal; 45% in feces	Reduce dose or increase interval in severe hepatic failure	25-50 mg once daily

the combination agent co-trimoxazole has increased their usefulness in certain infections.

Pharmacology

Sulfonamides are bacteriostatic. Their mechanism of action correlates directly with the structural similarities they share with para-aminobenzoic acid. They inhibit biosynthesis of folic acid, which is needed for cell growth; susceptible bacteria are those that synthesize folic acid.

Sulfonamides are well absorbed from the GI tract after oral administration, except for sulfasalazine, which is absorbed minimally by the oral route. Sulfonamides are distributed widely into tissues and fluids, including pleural, peritoneal, synovial, and ocular fluids; some, including sulfisoxazole, penetrate CSF. Sulfonamides readily cross the placenta and are found in low concentrations in breast milk. Sulfonamides are metabolized by the liver and the parent drug and metabolites are excreted in urine by glomerular filtration. Hemodialysis removes both sulfamethoxazole and sulfisoxazole, but peritoneal dialysis removes only sulfisoxazole.

Clinical indications and actions

Bacterial infections

When first introduced, sulfonamides were active against many gram-positive and gram-negative organisms; over time, many bacteria have become resistant. Currently, sulfonamides are active against some strains of staphylococci, streptococci, *Nocardia asteroides, Nocardia brasiliensis, Clostridium tetani, Clostridium perfringens, Bacillus anthracis, Escherichia coli, Neisseria gonorrhoeae,* and *Neisseria meningitidis.* Resistance to sulfonamides is common if therapy continues beyond 2 weeks; resistance to one sulfonamide usually means cross-resistance to others.

Sulfonamides are used to treat urinary tract infections caused by *E. coli, Proteus mirabilis, Proteus vulgaris, Klebsiella, Enterobacter,* and *Staphylococcus aureus,* and genital lesions caused by *Haemophilus ducreyi* (chancroid). They're the drugs of choice in nocardiosis, usually with surgical drainage or combined with other antibiotics, including ampicillin, erythromycin, cycloserine, or minocycline. Sulfonamides also are used to treat otitis media. Sulfadiazine is used to eradicate meningococci from the nasopharynx of asymptomatic carriers of *N. meningitidis.*

Co-trimoxazole is used to treat infections of the urinary tract, respiratory tract, and ear; to treat chronic bacterial prostatitis; and to prevent recurrent urinary tract infection in women and "traveler's diarrhea."

Co-trimoxazole is also used to treat *Pneumocystis carinii* pneumonia.

Parasitic infections

Sulfonamides combined with pyrimethamine are used to treat toxoplasmosis; certain sulfonamides are combined with quinine and pyrimethamine to treat chloroquine-resistant *Plasmodium falciparum* malaria.

Inflammation

Sulfasalazine, used to treat inflammatory bowel disease, is cleaved in the intestine to sulfapyridine and 5-aminosalicylic acid.

Plague

Co-trimazole is recommended by the CDC for anti-infective prophylaxis in adults 18 and over and children 2 months or over who are at high risk for exposure to pneumonic plague.

Overview of adverse reactions

Sulfonamides cause adverse reactions affecting many organs and systems. Many are considered to be caused by hypersensitivity, including the following: rash, fever, pruritus, erythema multiforme, erythema nodosum, Stevens-Johnson syndrome, Lyell's syndrome, exfoliative dermatitis, photosensitivity, joint pain, conjunctivitis, leukopenia, and bronchospasm. Hematologic reactions include granulocytopenia, thrombocytopenia, agranulocytosis, hypoprothrombinemia, and, in G6PD deficiency, hemolytic anemia. Renal effects usually result from crystalluria (precipitation of the sulfonamide in the renal system). GI reactions include anorexia, stomatitis, pancreatitis, diarrhea, and folic acid malabsorption. Oral therapy commonly causes nausea and vomiting. Hepatotoxicity and CNS reactions (dizziness, confusion, headache, ataxia, drowsiness, and insomnia) are rare.

Clinical considerations

- Assess patient's history of allergies; don't give a sulfonamide to patient with history of hypersensitivity reactions to sulfonamides or to other drugs containing sulfur.
- Sulfonamides are also contraindicated in patients with severe renal or hepatic dysfunction, or porphyria; during pregnancy at term, and during breast-feeding. Sulfonamides may cause kernicterus in infants, because they displace bilirubin at the binding site, cross the placenta, and are excreted in breast milk. Don't use in infants under age 2 months (except in the treatment of congenital toxoplasmosis as adjunctive therapy with pyrimethamine).
- Administer sulfonamides with caution in patients with the following conditions: mild to moderate renal or hepatic impairment; urinary obstruction, because of the risk of drug accumulation; severe allergies; asthma; blood dyscrasia; or G6PD deficiency.
- Continuously monitor patient for possible hypersensitivity reactions or other untoward effects; patients with AIDS have a much higher incidence of adverse reactions.
- Obtain cultures and sensitivity tests before giving first dose, but therapy may begin before laboratory tests are complete; check test results periodically to assess drug efficacy. Recommend monitoring urine cultures, CBCs, and urinalysis before and during therapy.
- Recommend monitoring patients on prolonged therapy for superinfection, especially geriatric and debilitated patients and others receiving immunosuppressants or radiation therapy.
- Sulfonamides may interact with other drugs (oral anticoagulants, cyclosporine, digoxin, folic acid, hydantoins, methotrexate, and sulfonylureas) and may alter test results; consult individual drug entries for possible test interactions.

Administration

- Give oral dose with full 8-oz (240-ml) glass of water, and force fluids to 12 to 16 glasses per day, depending on the agent; patient's urine output should be at least 1,500 ml/day.
- Follow manufacturer's directions for reconstitution, dilution, and storage of drugs; check expiration dates.
- Give oral sulfonamide at least 1 hour before or 2 hours after meals for maximum absorption.
- Shake oral suspensions well before administering to ensure correct dose.

Special populations

Pregnant patients. Safe use during pregnancy hasn't been established. There is potential for cleft palate, other bony abnormalities, and kernicterus in the infant.

Breast-feeding patients. Because sulfonamides are excreted in breast milk, a decision should be made whether to discontinue breast-feeding or to discontinue the drug, taking into account the importance of the drug to the woman. Premature infants, infants with hyperbilirubinemia, and those with G6PD deficiency are at risk for kernicterus.

Pediatric patients. Sulfonamides are contraindicated in infants under age 2 months, unless there's no therapeutic alternative.

Give sulfonamides with caution to children with fragile X chromosome associated with mental retardation because they're vulnerable to psychomotor depression from folate depletion.

Geriatric patients. Use with caution; geriatric patients are susceptible to bacterial and fungal superinfection, are at greater risk of folate deficiency anemia after sulfonamide therapy, and commonly are at greater risk of renal and hematologic effects because of diminished renal function.

Patient counseling

- Teach patient the signs and symptoms of hypersensitivity and other adverse reactions, and emphasize the need to report these; specifically, urge patient to report bloody urine, difficulty breathing, rash, fever, chills, or severe fatigue.
- Teach patient the signs and symptoms of bacterial and fungal superinfection to geriatric and debilitated patients and others with low resistance from immunosuppressants or irradiation; emphasize the need to report them.
- Advise diabetic patient that sulfonamides may increase effects of oral hypoglycemic and not to monitor urine glucose levels with Clinitest; sulfonamides alter results of tests using cupric sulfate.
- Advise patient to avoid exposure to direct sunlight because of risk of photosensitivity reaction.
- Tell patient to take oral drug with a full glass of water and to drink at least 12 to 16 8-oz (240-ml) glasses of water daily depending on the agent; explain that tablet may be crushed

and swallowed with water to ensure maximal absorption.

- Be sure patient understands how and when to take drugs; urge him to complete entire prescribed regimen, to comply with instructions for around-the-clock dosing, and to keep follow-up appointments.
- Teach patient to check expiration date of drug and how to store drug, and to discard unused drug.
- For sulfasalazine, inform patient to take with food if GI irritation occurs and tell him that it may cause an orange-yellow discoloration of the urine or skin and may permanently stain soft contact lenses yellow.
- Photosensitization may occur; therefore, caution patient to take protective measures (such as wearing sunscreen and protective clothing) against exposure to ultraviolet light or sunlight until tolerance is determined.

Representative combinations

Sulfadiazine with sulfamerazine and sulfamethazine: Triple Sulfa.

Sulfamethizole with oxytetracycline hydrochloride and phenazopyridine: Urobiotic-250; with sulfathiazole, sulfacetamide, sulfabenzamide, and urea: Triple Sulfa, V.V.S., Trysul, Gyne-Sulf, Sultrin.

Sulfamethoxazole with phenazopyridine hydrochloride: Azo Gantanol, Azo-Sulfamethoxazole; with trimethoprim: Bactrim, Cotrim, Co-Trimoxazole, Septra, SMZ-TMP.

Sulfisoxazole with erythromycin ethylsuccinate: Pediazole; with phenazopyridine hydrochloride: Azo Gantrisin.

Sulfadoxine with pyrimethamine: Fansidar.

sulfonylureas

acetohexamide, chlorpropamide, glimepiride, glipizide, glyburide, tolazamide, tolbutamide

In 1942, sulfonamide, an antibacterial agent, was discovered to have hypoglycemic effects. Subsequent experiments showed that this drug didn't exert similar effects in pancreatectomized animals. Later, tolbutamide was introduced and became popular for managing certain diabetic patients. Sulfonylureas are useful only in patients with mild to moderately severe type 2, or non-insulin-dependent diabetes mellitus (NIDDM). These drugs can be used only in patients with functioning beta cells of the pancreas.

Pharmacology

Sulfonylurea antidiabetic agents are sulfonamide derivatives that exert no antibacterial activity.

Sulfonylureas lower blood glucose levels by stimulating insulin release from the pancreas. These agents work only in the presence of functioning beta cells in the islet tissue of the pancreas. After prolonged administration, they produce hypoglycemia through significant extrapancreatic effects, including reduction of hepatic glucose production and enhanced peripheral sensitivity to insulin. The latter may result from an increase in the number of insulin receptors or from changes in events after insulin binding. (See *Comparing sulfonylureas,* page 72.)

Sulfonylureas are divided into first-generation agents (chlorpropamide) and second-generation agents (glyburide, glipizide, and glimepiride). Although their mechanisms of action are similar, the second-generation agents carry a more lipophilic side chain, are more potent, and cause fewer adverse reactions. Their most important differences are their durations of action.

Clinical indications and actions

Diabetes mellitus, non-insulin-dependent

Sulfonylureas are used to manage mild to moderately severe, stable, nonketotic NIDDM that can't be controlled by diet alone. Sulfonylureas stimulate insulin release from the pancreas. After long-term therapy, extrapancreatic hypoglycemic effects include reduced hepatic glucose production, an increased number of insulin receptors, and changes in insulin binding.

◇***Neurogenic diabetes insipidus***

Although an unlabeled indication, chlorpropamide has been used in selected patients to treat neurogenic diabetes insipidus. The drug appears to potentiate the effect of minimal levels of antidiuretic hormone.

Overview of adverse reactions

Dose-related adverse effects, which usually aren't serious and respond to decreased doses, include headache, nausea, vomiting, anorexia, heartburn, weakness, and paresthesia. Hypoglycemia may follow excessive doses, increased exercise, decreased food intake, or consumption of alcohol. Signs and symptoms of overdose include anxiety, chills, cold sweats, confusion, cool pale skin, difficulty concentrating, drowsiness, excessive hunger, headache, nausea, nervousness, rapid heartbeat, shakiness, unsteady gait, weakness, and unusual fatigue.

Clinical considerations

- Recommend administering sulfonylureas 30 minutes before the morning meal for once-daily dosing, or 30 minutes before the morning and evening meals for twice-daily dosing.
- Contraindicated in patients with juvenile-onset, brittle, or severe diabetes; diabetes mellitus adequately controlled by diet; and maturity-onset diabetes complicated by ketosis, acidosis, diabetic coma, Raynaud's gangrene, renal or hepatic impairment, or thyroid or other endocrine dysfunction.

COMPARING SULFONYLUREAS

Typically, sulfonylureas have similar actions and produce similar effects. They differ mainly in duration of action and dosage.

Drug	Usual daily dosage	Onset (hr)	Peak (hr)	Duration (hr)
First generation				
acetohexamide	500 mg once daily or b.i.d.	1	2	12 to 24
chlorpropamide	250 mg once daily	1	3 to 6	24 to 60
tolazamide	250 mg once daily or b.i.d.	4 to 6	6 to 10	12 to 24
tolbutamide	1,000 mg b.i.d. or t.i.d.	½ to 1	4 to 8	6 to 12
Second generation				
glimepiride	1 to 4 mg once daily	1	2 to 3	24
glipizide	5 mg once daily	1 to 3	2 to 3	10 to 24
glyburide	5 mg once daily	2	3 to 4	12 to 24

- Use cautiously in patients with sulfonamide hypersensitivity.
- Advise close monitoring of patients transferring from insulin therapy to a sulfonylurea agent for urine glucose and ketones at least three times daily, before meals; emphasize the need for testing a double-voided specimen. Patients may require hospitalization during such changes in therapy.
- Patients transferring from another sulfonylurea (except chlorpropamide) usually need no transition period.
- NIDDM patients may require insulin therapy during periods of increased stress, such as infection, fever, surgery, or trauma. Monitor patients closely for hyperglycemia in these situations.

Special populations

Pregnant patients. Don't use sulfonylurea antidiabetic agents in pregnant women because of prolonged, severe hypoglycemia lasting from 4 to 10 days in neonates born to women taking these drugs. Also, use of insulin permits more rigid control of blood glucose levels, which should reduce the incidence of congenital abnormalities, mortality, and morbidity caused by abnormal glucose levels.

Breast-feeding patients. Oral antidiabetic agents are excreted in breast milk in minimal amounts and may cause hypoglycemia in the breast-feeding infant.

Pediatric patients. Oral antidiabetic agents aren't effective in insulin-dependent (type 1, juvenile-onset) diabetes mellitus.

Geriatric patients. Geriatric patients and those with renal insufficiency may be more sensitive to these agents because of decreased metabolism and excretion. They usually require lower doses and should be closely monitored.

Hypoglycemia may be more difficult to recognize in geriatric patients, although it usually causes neurologic symptoms in such patients. Avoid agents with prolonged duration of action in geriatric patients.

Patient counseling

- Teach patient about the nature of his disease.
- Emphasize the importance of following therapeutic regimen and adhering to specific diet, weight reduction, exercise, and personal hygiene recommendations. Teach patient how to avoid infections, test for glycosuria and ketonuria, and know signs and symptoms of hypoglycemia (fatigue, excessive hunger, profuse sweating, numbness of extremities) and hyperglycemia (excessive thirst or urination, excessive urine glucose or ketones).
- Be sure patient knows that therapy relieves symptoms but doesn't cure the disease.
- Discourage patient from consuming moderate to large amounts of alcohol while taking sulfonylureas; disulfiram-type reactions are possible.

Representative combinations

None.

tetracyclines

demeclocycline hydrochloride, doxycycline hyclate, minocycline hydrochloride, oxytetracycline hydrochloride, tetracycline hydrochloride

Tetracycline antibiotics were discovered during the random screening of soil samples for antibiotic-producing microorganisms. The prototype, chlortetracycline, was discovered in 1948; tetracycline was developed in 1952. Structural modifications that enhanced both antibacterial activity and pharmacokinetic parameters led to development of doxycycline in 1966 and minocycline in 1972.

Usually well-tolerated with few serious adverse effects, tetracyclines have an unusually broad spectrum of antibacterial activity, including gram-negative and gram-positive anaerobic and aerobic bacteria, *Chlamydia,* and protozoa; longer-acting tetracyclines have enhanced activity against *Chlamydia* and *Legionella.*

Demeclocycline has a higher incidence of severe photosensitivity reactions; also, because of its renal effects, it's rarely prescribed for clinical use, although it's used investigationally to treat SIADH secretion.

Pharmacology

Tetracyclines are bacteriostatic but may be bactericidal against certain organisms. They bind reversibly to 30S and 50S ribosomal subunits, inhibiting bacterial protein synthesis. Bacterial resistance to tetracyclines is usually mediated by plasmids (R-factor resistance), which decrease bacterial cell wall permeability; this is the most important cause of resistance by staphylococci, streptococci, most aerobic gram-negative organisms, and *Pseudomonas aeruginosa.* With two exceptions, cross-resistance occurs with all tetracyclines; doxycycline is active against *Bacteroides fragilis,* and minocycline is active against *Staphylococcus aureus, Acinetobacter, and Enterobacteriaceae.*

Tetracyclines attack many pathogens; they aren't antifungal or antiviral.

Susceptible gram-positive organisms include *Bacillus anthracis, Actinomyces israelii, Clostridium perfringens, Clostridium tetani, Listeria monocytogenes,* and *Nocardia.* Initial but transient activity exists against staphylococci and streptococci; infections caused by these organisms are usually treated with other drugs.

Susceptible gram-negative organisms include *Bartonella bacilliformis, Calymmatobacterium granulomatis, Francisella tularensis, Leptotrichia buccalis, Neisseria gonorrhoeae, N. meningitidis, Pasteurella multocida, Legionella pneumophila, Brucella, Vibrio cholerae, Yersinia enterocolitica, Vibrio parahaemolyticus, Yersinia pestis, Bordetella pertussis, Haemophilus influenzae, H.ducreyi, Campylobacter fetus, Spirillum minus, Streptobacillus moniliformis, Shigella,* and many other common pathogens.

Other susceptible organisms include *Rickettsia akari, Rickettsia typhi, Rickettsia prowazekii, Rickettsia tsutsugamushi, Coxiella burnetii, Chlamydia trachomatis, Chlamydia psittaci, Mycoplasma pneumoniae, Mycoplasma hominis, Leptospira, Treponema pallidum, Treponema pertenue,* and *Borrelia recurrentis.*

Tetracyclines are absorbed systemically after oral administration, chiefly from the duodenum; with the exception of doxycycline and minocycline, absorption is decreased by food, milk, and divalent and trivalent cations. Oral absorption of tetracyclines is affected by chelation with certain minerals such as calcium (doxycycline is least involved); chelation causes tetracyclines to localize in bones and teeth. Because of hepatotoxicity and thrombophlebitis, only doxycycline and, to a lesser extent, minocycline, are used I.V.

Tetracyclines occur widely into body tissues and fluid, but CSF penetration is minimal; lipid-soluble minocycline and doxycycline penetrate fluids and tissues better; all tetracyclines cross the placenta.

Tetracyclines are excreted primarily in urine, chiefly by glomerular filtration; some drug is excreted in breast milk, and some inactivated drug is excreted in feces. Unlike other tetracyclines, minocycline undergoes enterohepatic circulation and is excreted in feces.

Oxytetracycline is moderately hemodialyzable; other tetracyclines are removed only minimally by hemodialysis or peritoneal dialysis.

Clinical indications and actions

Bacterial, antiprotozoal, rickettsial, and fungal infections

Tetracyclines are used as first-line therapy for chlamydial infections and are the drugs of choice for lymphogranuloma venereum, nonlymphogranuloma venereum strains *of C. trachomatis* in sexually transmitted diseases, psittacosis, and nongonococcal urethritis if the primary pathogen is probably *M. hominis* or *C. trachomatis.* They're also the drugs of choice for rickettsial infections (Rocky Mountain spotted fever, scrub and endemic typhus, rickettsial pox, and Q fever) and brucellosis. Tetracyclines also are used to treat infections caused by *Campylobacter,* mycoplasma pneumonia (after Legionnaire's disease is ruled out), pertussis, cholera (in United States only), leprosy, and gonorrhea.

Tetracyclines are second-line drugs in therapy of syphilis, actinomycosis, listeriosis, chancroid, and infections caused by *P. multocida* and *Y. pestis.* They also provide economic prophylaxis in chronic pulmonary disease.

Tetracyclines are used orally to treat inflammatory acne vulgaris, topically for mild to moderate inflammatory acne, and as eyedrops for superficial eye infections, inclusion conjunctivitis, and prophylaxis of ophthalmia neonatorum.

Individual tetracyclines are more effective against certain species or strains of a particular organism.

◇***Diuretic agent in SIADH***
Demeclocycline causes diuresis by blocking antidiuretic hormone-induced reabsorption of water in the distal convoluted tubules and collecting ducts of the kidney.

Sclerosing agent
Parenteral tetracycline hydrochloride has been administered by intracavitary injection as a sclerosing agent in pleural or pericardial effusion. Parenteral doxycycline hyclate has been used as a sclerosing agent to control pleural effusions associated with metastatic tumors.

Other uses
◇Oral doxycycline and oral tetracycline have been used to treat Lyme disease.

Tetracyline is used as an adjunct to therapy for *H. pylori* infection.

◇Tetracyline is used to treat various GI infections including balantidiasis caused by *Balantidium coli,* Whipple's disease, blind-loop syndrome, and tropical sprue.

Doxycycline is used for the suppression or prophylactic treatment of malaria caused by *Plasmodium falciparum* (chloroquine-resistant or sulfadoxine- and pyrimethamine-resistant) in individuals traveling for less than 4 months.

Overview of adverse reactions

The most common adverse effects of tetracyclines involve the GI tract and are dose related. Among them are anorexia, flatulence, nausea, vomiting, bulky and loose stools, epigastric burning, and abdominal discomfort.

Hypersensitivity reactions are infrequent; they manifest as urticaria, rash, pruritus, eosinophilia, and exfoliative dermatitis.

Photosensitivity reactions may be severe; they commonly occur with demeclocycline, rarely with minocycline.

Renal effects are minor and include occasional elevations in BUN levels (without increase in serum creatinine level) and a reversible diabetes insipidus syndrome (reported only with demeclocycline); renal failure has been attributed to Fanconi's syndrome after use of outdated tetracycline.

Rare adverse effects include hepatotoxicity (often in pregnant women receiving more than 2 g/day I.V.), leukocytosis, thrombocytopenia, hemolytic anemia, leukopenia, neutropenia, and atypical lymphocytes. There have also been reports of vaginal candidiasis, microscopic thyroid discoloration (after chronic use), light-headedness, dizziness, drowsiness, vein irritation (after I.V. use), and permanent discoloration of teeth in children under age 8.

Drug use with oral contraceptives can decrease the effectiveness of the contraceptive and increase risk of pregnancy.

Clinical considerations

- Assess patient's allergic history; don't give tetracycline antibiotics to patient with history of hypersensitivity reactions to other tetracyclines; monitor patient continuously for this and other adverse reactions.
- Recommend results of cultures and sensitivity tests be obtained before giving first dose, but don't delay therapy; check cultures periodically to assess drug efficacy.
- Recommend monitoring vital signs, electrolytes, and renal function studies before and during therapy.
- Check expiration dates. Outdated tetracyclines may cause nephrotoxicity.
- Recommend monitoring for bacterial and fungal superinfection, especially in geriatric, debilitated, and other patients receiving immunosuppressants or radiation therapy; watch especially for oral candidiasis. If symptoms occur, discontinue drug.
- Tetracyclines may interfere with certain laboratory tests; consult individual drug entry.

Administration

- Give oral drugs 1 hour before or 2 hours after meals for maximum absorption; don't give with food, milk or other dairy products, sodium bicarbonate, iron compounds, or antacids, which may impair absorption.
- Give water with and after oral drug to facilitate passage to stomach because incomplete swallowing can cause severe esophageal irritation; don't administer within 1 hour of bedtime, to prevent esophageal reflux.
- Follow manufacturer's directions for reconstitution and storage; keep product refrigerated and out of light.
- Avoid I.V. use of drug in patients with decreased renal function.
- I.V. use of tetracyclines in pregnancy or in patients with renal impairment, especially when dose exceeds 2 g/day, can cause hepatic failure.
- Monitor I.V. injection sites and rotate routinely to reduce local irritation. I.V. use may cause severe phlebitis.

Special populations

Pregnant patients. Tetracyclines may cause fetal toxicity in pregnant women.

Breast-feeding patients. Avoid use of tetracyclines by breast-feeding women.

Pediatric patients. Don't use in children under age 8 unless there's no alternative. Tetracyclines can cause permanent discoloration of teeth, enamel hypoplasia, and a reversible decrease in bone calcification.

Geriatric patients. Some geriatric patients have decreased esophageal motility; use tetracyclines cautiously and monitor for local irritation from slowly passing oral dosage forms. Geriatric patients are more susceptible to superinfection.

Patient counseling

- Explain to patient the disease process and rationale for therapy.
- Teach patient signs and symptoms of adverse reactions, and emphasize need to report these promptly; urge patient to report unusual effects.
- Teach patient signs and symptoms of bacterial and fungal superinfection to geriatric and debilitated patients and others with low resistance from immunosuppressants or irradiation.
- Advise patient using oral contraceptives to use a backup method of contraception during drug therapy.
- Advise patient to avoid direct sunlight and to use a sunscreen to prevent photosensitivity reactions.
- Tell patient to take oral tetracyclines with a full 8-oz (240-ml) glass of water (to facilitate passage to the stomach) 1 hour before or 2 hours after meals for maximum absorption, and not less than 1 hour before bedtime (to prevent irritation from esophageal reflux).
- Emphasize that taking drug with food, milk or other dairy products, sodium bicarbonate, or iron compounds may interfere with absorption. Tell patient to take antacids 3 hours after tetracycline.
- Stress importance of completing prescribed regimen exactly as ordered and keeping follow-up appointments.
- Tell patient that doxycycline and monocycline may be taken with food.
- Instruct patient to check expiration date before use.

Representative combinations

Oxytetracycline with polymyxin B sulfate: Terramycin with polymyxin B, Terramycin topical ointment.

Oxytetracycline hydrochloride with phenazopyridine hydrochloride and sulfamethizole: Urobiotic-250.

Tetracycline hydrochloride with citric acid: Achromycin V.

thrombolytic enzymes

alteplase, anistreplase, reteplase (recombinant), streptokinase, urokinase

When a thrombus obstructs a blood vessel, permanent damage to the ischemic area may occur before the body can dissolve the clot. Thrombolytic agents were developed in the hope that speeding lysis of the clot would prevent permanent ischemic damage. Thrombolytic activity attributable to streptokinase was described in 1933; the effects of this compound have since been studied on various kinds of clots. It isn't clear whether such agents significantly reduce thrombosis-induced ischemic damage in all situations for which the drugs are currently used. (See *Comparing thrombolytic enzymes,* page 76.)

Pharmacology

Streptokinase is a protein-like substance produced by group C beta-hemolytic streptococci; urokinase is an enzyme isolated from human kidney tissue cultures. Alteplase is a tissue-type plasminogen activator synthesized by recombinant DNA technology. Anistreplase is anisoylated streptokinase-plasminogen activated complex; it's a fibrinolytic enzyme (plasminogen) plus activator complex (streptokinase) with the activator temporarily blocked by an anisoyl group. Reteplase is a recombinant-plasminogen activator. Thrombolytic enzymes act to lyse clots chiefly by converting plasminogen to plasmin; in contrast, anticoagulants act by preventing thrombi from developing. Thrombolytics are more likely to produce clinical bleeding than are oral anticoagulants.

Clinical indications and actions

Thrombosis, thromboembolism

Alteplase, streptokinase, and urokinase are used to treat acute pulmonary thromboembolism; streptokinase and urokinase are used to treat deep vein thrombosis, acute arterial thromboembolism, or acute coronary arterial thrombosis and to clear arteriovenous cannula occlusion and venous catheter obstruction. Anistreplase, alteplase, reteplase, streptokinase, and urokinase are indicated in acute MI. These agents are administered in an attempt to lyse coronary artery thrombi, which may result in improved ventricular function and decreased risk of heart failure. Alteplase is used in the management of acute ischemic stroke.

Overview of adverse reactions

Adverse reactions to these agents are essentially an extension of their actions; hemorrhage is the most common adverse effect. These agents cause bleeding twice as often as does heparin. Streptokinase is more likely to cause an allergic reaction than urokinase. Information regarding hypersensitivity to alteplase is limited.

Clinical considerations

- Thrombolytic therapy requires medical supervision with continuous clinical and laboratory monitoring.
- Thrombolytics act only on fibrin clots, not those formed by a precipitated drug.

COMPARING THROMBOLYTIC ENZYMES

Thrombolytic enzymes dissolve clots by accelerating the formation of plasmin by activated plasminogen. Plasminogen activators, found in most tissues and body fluids, help plasminogen (an inactive enzyme) convert to plasmin (an active enzyme), which dissolves the clot.

Doses of five enzymes listed below may vary according to the patient's condition.

Drug	Action	Initial dose	Maintenance therapy
alteplase	Directly converts plasminogen to plasmin	I.V. bolus: 6 to 10 mg over 1 to 2 min	I.V. infusion: 60 mg/hr in the 1st hr; then 20 mg/hr for the next 2 hr for a total of 100 mg
anistreplase	Directly converts plasminogen to plasmin	I.V. push: 30 units over 2 to 5 min	Not necessary
reteplase	Enhances the cleavage of plasminogen to generate plasmin	Double I.V. bolus injection of 10 + 10 units	Not necessary
streptokinase	Indirectly activates plasminogen, which converts to plasmin	Intracoronary bolus: 15,000 to 20,000 IU	Intracoronary infusion: 2,000 to 4,000 IU/min over 1 hr; total dose 140,000 IU
		I.V. bolus: none needed	I.V. infusion: 1,500,000 units over 1 hr
urokinase	Directly converts plasminogen to plasmin	Intracoronary bolus: none needed	Intracoronary infusion: 2,000 units/lb/hr (4,400 units/kg/hr); rate of 15 ml of solution/hr for total of 12 hr (total volume shouldn't exceed 200 ml)

- Follow instructions for reconstitution precisely and pass solution through a filter 0.45 microns or smaller to remove filaments in the solution; don't use with dextran because it can interfere with coagulation as well as blood typing and crossmatching.
- Advise obtaining pretherapy baseline determinations of thrombin time, activated partial thromboplastin time, PT, INR, hematocrit, and platelet count for subsequent blood monitoring. During systemic thrombolytic therapy, as in pulmonary embolism or venous thrombosis, PT, INR, or thrombin time after 4 hours of therapy should be about twice the pretreatment value.
- Administer drugs by infusion pump to ensure accuracy; I.M. injections are contraindicated during therapy because of increased risk of bleeding at the injection site.
- Recommend checking vital signs frequently, monitoring for blood pressure alterations in excess of 25 mm Hg and any change in cardiac rhythm; checking pulses, color, and sensitivity of extremities every hour; monitoring for excessive bleeding every 15 minutes for first hour, every 30 minutes for second through eighth hours; then at least once every 8 hours. Advise stopping therapy if bleeding is evident; pretreatment with heparin or drugs affecting platelets increases risk.
- Recommend monitoring for hypersensitivity as well as hemorrhage; keep available typed and crossmatched packed RBCs and whole blood, aminocaproic acid to treat bleeding, and corticosteroids to treat allergic reactions.
- Advise keeping involved extremity in straight alignment to prevent bleeding from infusion site. Establish precautions to prevent injury and avoid unnecessary handling of patient because bruising is likely.
- At end of infusion, flush remaining dose from pump tubing with I.V. 5% dextrose or normal saline solution.
- Continuous heparin infusion usually is started with the prescribed thrombolytic.
- Before using thrombolytic to clear an occluded catheter, try to gently aspirate or flush with heparinized saline solution. Avoid forcible flushing or vigorous suction, which could rupture the catheter or expel the clot into the circulation.
- When treating MI or CVA, the sooner treatment is administered, the greater the benefit.

Special populations

Pregnant patients. Thrombolytics should only be used in pregnancy if clearly indicated.
Breast-feeding patients. Safety in breast-feeding women hasn't been established.
Pediatric patients. Safety in children hasn't been established.

Geriatric patients. Patients age 75 or over are at greater risk of cerebral hemorrhage, because they're more apt to have preexisting cerebrovascular disease.

Patient counseling

- Explain to patient the rationale for treatment and procedure, and necessity for bed rest.
- Ask patient to be alert for signs of bleeding.
- When using these drugs to clear catheter, tell patient to exhale and hold breath at any time catheter isn't connected, to prevent air entering the open catheter.

Representative combinations

None.

tricyclic antidepressants (TCAs)

amitriptyline hydrochloride, amoxapine, clomipramine hydrochloride, desipramine hydrochloride, doxepin hydrochloride, imipramine hydrochloride, imipramine pamoate, nortriptyline hydrochloride, protriptyline, trimipramine maleate

The inherent mood-elevating activity of tricyclic antidepressants (TCAs) was discovered during research with iminodibenzyl, a compound originally investigated for sedative, analgesic, antihistaminic, and antiparkinsonian effects. Clinical trials in 1958 with the class prototype, imipramine, found no antipsychotic activity, but showed marked mood-elevating effects.

Pharmacology

Although the precise mechanism of their CNS effects isn't established, TCAs may exert their effects by inhibiting reuptake of the neurotransmitters norepinephrine and serotonin in CNS nerve terminals (presynaptic neurons), resulting in increased concentration and enhanced activity of neurotransmitters in the synaptic cleft. TCAs also have antihistaminic, sedative, anticholinergic, vasodilatory, and quinidine-like effects; the drugs are structurally similar to phenothiazines and share similar adverse reactions.

Individual TCAs differ somewhat in their degree of CNS inhibitory effect. The tertiary amines (amitriptyline, doxepin, imipramine, and trimipramine) exert greater sedative effects; tertiary amines and protriptyline have more profound effects on cardiac conduction, whereas desipramine has the least anticholinergic activity. All of the currently available TCAs have equal clinical efficacy when given in equivalent therapeutic doses; choice of specific therapy is determined primarily by pharmacokinetic properties and the patient's adverse reaction profile. Patients may respond to some TCAs and not others; if patient doesn't respond to one drug, another should be tried.

Clinical indications and actions

Depression

TCAs are used to treat major depression and dysthymic disorder. Depressed patients who are also anxious are helped most by the more sedating agents: doxepin, imipramine, and trimipramine. Protriptyline has a stimulant effect that evokes a favorable response in withdrawn depressed patients; only maprotiline has FDA approval for use in depression mixed with anxiety.

Obsessive-compulsive disorder (OCD)

Clomipramine is used in the treatment of OCD.

Enuresis

Imipramine is used for enuresis in children over age 6.

Severe, chronic pain

TCAs, especially amitriptyline, desipramine, doxepin, imipramine, and nortriptyline, are useful in the management of severe chronic pain.

Other psychiatric disorders

◇TCAs have been used to treat phobic disorders with panic attacks, eating disorders (bulimia nervosa), and in the short-term treatment of duodenal or gastric ulcer.

Overview of adverse reactions

Adverse reactions to TCAs are similar to those seen with phenothiazine antipsychotic agents, including varying degrees of sedation, anticholinergic effects, and orthostatic hypotension. The tertiary amines have the strongest sedative effects; tolerance to these effects usually develops in a few weeks. Protriptyline has the least sedative effect (and may be stimulatory), but shares with the tertiary amines the most pronounced effects on blood pressure and cardiac tissue. Maprotiline and amoxapine are most likely to cause seizures, especially in overdose situations. Desipramine has a greater margin of safety in patients with prostatic hypertrophy, paralytic ileus, glaucoma, and urine retention because of its relatively low level of anticholinergic activity.

Clinical considerations

- TCAs impair ability to perform tasks requiring mental alertness, such as driving a car.
- Recommend checking vital signs regularly for decreased blood pressure or tachycardia; observe patient carefully for adverse reactions and report changes. Obtain ECG in patients over age 40 before initiating therapy.
- Advise having the patient take the first dose in the office to allow close observation for adverse reactions.
- Suggest checking for anticholinergic adverse reactions, which may require dose reduction.

- Caregiver should be sure patient swallows each dose of drug when given; as depressed patients begin to improve, they may hoard pills for suicide attempt.
- Recommend observing patients for mood changes to monitor progress; benefits may not occur for several (3 to 6) weeks.
- Don't withdraw full dose of drug abruptly; gradually reduce dose over a period of weeks to avoid rebound effect or other adverse reactions.
- Carefully follow manufacturer's instructions for reconstitution, dilution, and storage of drugs.
- Investigational uses include treating peptic ulcer, migraine prophylaxis, and allergy. Potential toxicity has, to date, outweighed most advantages.
- Because suicidal overdose with TCAs is usually fatal, prescribe only small amounts. If possible, entrust a reliable family member with the drug and warn him to store drug safely away from children.

Special populations

Pregnant patients. Safe use of tricyclic antidepressants in pregnancy hasn't been established. Fetal malformations, urinary retention, CNS effects (lethargy), developmental delay, and withdrawal symptoms have occurred in neonates born to women taking TCAs during pregnancy.
Breast-feeding patients. Safety in breast-feeding women hasn't been established.
Pediatric patients. TCAs aren't advised for children under age 12.
Geriatric patients. Use lower doses because these patients are more sensitive to both therapeutic and adverse effects of TCAs.

Patient counseling

- Explain to patient the rationale for therapy and anticipated risks and benefits; also explain that full therapeutic effect may not occur for several weeks.
- Teach patient the signs and symptoms of adverse reactions and the importance of reporting them.
- Tell patient to avoid beverages and drugs containing alcohol and not to take other drugs (including OTC products) without medical approval.
- Teach patient how and when to take drug, not to increase dose without medical approval, and never to discontinue drug abruptly.
- Tell patient to lie down for 30 minutes after first dose and to rise slowly to avoid orthostatic hypotension.
- Advise taking drug with milk or food to minimize GI distress; suggest taking full dose at bedtime if daytime sedation is troublesome.
- Urge diabetic patients to monitor blood glucose, as drug may alter insulin needs.
- Advise patient to avoid tasks that require mental alertness until full effect of drug is determined.
- Warn patient that excessive exposure to sunlight, heat lamps, or tanning beds may cause burns and abnormal hyperpigmentation.
- Recommend sugarless gum or hard candy, artificial saliva, or ice chips to relieve dry mouth.
- Advise patient that unpleasant adverse effects (except dry mouth) generally diminish over time.

Representative combinations

Amitriptyline hydrochloride with perphenazine: Etrafon, Triavil; with chlordiazepoxide: Limbitrol.

vitamins

***Fat-soluble:* vitamin A (retinol), vitamin A acid (retinoic acid), vitamin D, vitamin D_2 (ergocalciferol), vitamin D_3 (calcipotriene), vitamin E, vitamin K (phytonadione)**

***Water-soluble:* vitamin B_1 (thiamine), vitamin B_2 (riboflavin), vitamin B_3 (niacin), vitamin B_6 (pyridoxine), vitamin B_9 (folic acid, folacin), vitamin B_{12} (cyanocobalamin), vitamin C (ascorbic acid)**

Vitamins are chemically unrelated organic compounds that are required for normal growth and maintenance of metabolic functions. Because the body is unable to synthesize many vitamins, it must obtain them from exogenous sources. Vitamins don't furnish energy and aren't essential building blocks for the body; however, they're essential for the transformation of energy and for the regulation of metabolic processes.

Vitamins are classified as fat-soluble or water-soluble, and the Food and Nutrition Board of the National Research Council determines the RDAs for each. These allowances represent amounts that will provide adequate nutrition in most healthy persons; they're not minimum requirements. Note that a diet that includes ample intake of the major food groups provides sufficient amounts of vitamins. If needed, vitamins should be used as an adjunct to a regular diet and not as a food substitute.

Controversy has existed for years over the vitamin issue. Some argue that vitamin supplementation is unnecessary; some advise moderate supplementation; still others advocate the use of megavitamins.

Pharmacology

Vitamins are available as single drugs or in combination with several other vitamins with or without minerals, trace elements, iron, flu-

RECOMMENDED DAILY ALLOWANCES FOR ADULTS AGES 23 TO 50

Vitamin	Men	Women	Pregnant women†	Lactating women†
A	1,000 mcg	800 mcg	800 mcg	1,300 mcg
B_1	1.5 mg	1.1 mg	1.5 mg	1.6 mg
B_2	1.7 mg	1.3 mg	1.6 mg	1.8 mg
B_6	2 mg	1.6 mg	2.2 mg	2.1 mg
B_{12}	2 mcg	2 mcg	2.2 mcg	2.6 mcg
C	60 mg	60 mg	70 mg	95 mg
D	200 IU	200 IU	400 IU	400 IU
E	15 IU	12 IU	15 IU	18 IU
K	80 mcg	65 mcg	65 mcg	65 mcg
folic acid	200 mcg	180 mcg	400 mcg	280 mcg
niacin	19 mg	15 mg	17 mg	20 mg

†First 6 months.

oride, or other nutritional supplements. Often, diets deficient in one vitamin are also deficient in other vitamins of similar dietary source. Malabsorption syndromes also affect the usage of several vitamins as do certain disease states that increase metabolic rates. Therefore, multiple vitamin therapy may be useful in these situations.

Fat-soluble vitamins are absorbed with dietary fats and stored in the body in moderate amounts; they aren't normally excreted in urine. Chronic ingestion leads to excessive build-up of these agents and toxicity.

Water-soluble vitamins aren't stored in the body in any appreciable amounts and are excreted in urine. These agents seldom cause toxicity in patients with normal renal function.

Both types of vitamins are needed for the maintenance of normal structure and metabolic functions of the body. (See *Recommended daily allowances for adults ages 23 to 50.)*

Clinical indications and actions

Vitamin deficiency or malabsorption; conditions of metabolic stress

Vitamin supplementation is required when deficiencies exist, in malabsorption syndrome, in hypermetabolic disease states, during pregnancy and lactation, and in the elderly, alcoholics, or dieters. Multiple vitamins may be indicated for patients taking oral contraceptives, estrogens, prolonged antibiotic therapy, isoniazid, or for patients receiving prolonged total parenteral nutrition.

Persons with increased metabolic requirements such as infants and those suffering severe injury, trauma, major surgery, or severe infection also require supplementation. Prolonged diarrhea, severe GI disorders, malignancy, surgical removal of sections of GI tract, obstructive jaundice, cystic fibrosis, and other conditions leading to reduced or poor absorption are indications for multiple vitamin therapy. Refer to individual agents for specific indications.

Overview of adverse reactions

Common adverse reactions seen with both fat-soluble and water-soluble vitamins include nausea, vomiting, diarrhea, tiredness, weakness, headache, loss of appetite, rash, and itching.

Clinical considerations

- Monitoring may be required. See specific vitamin entries for details.
- Vitamins containing iron may cause constipation and black, tarry stools.
- Excessive fluoride supplements can result in hypocalcemia and tetany.
- Recommend giving with food or after meals to reduce GI distress associated with vitamin therapy.

Special populations

Pregnant patients. Vitamin supplementation in pregnancy should be regulated by a health care provider.

Breast-feeding patients. RDAs may be increased in breast-feeding women.

Pediatric patients. RDAs vary with age. Excessive amounts of vitamins, particularly in neonates, may be toxic.

Patient counseling

- Stress to patient the importance of adequate dietary intake. Vitamins aren't food substitutes.
- Tell patient to take vitamins only as directed, not to exceed RDA, and to take with food, milk, or after meals to reduce chance of stomach upset.
- Store vitamins away from heat and light, and out of the reach of small children.
- Warn patient that vitamins with iron may cause constipation and black, tarry stools.
- Tell patient to read all label directions. Warn him not to take large doses unless prescribed.
- Inform patient that liquid vitamins may be mixed with food or juice.
- Advise patient not to refer to vitamins or other drugs as candy and to avoid taking them indiscriminately.

Representative combinations

The following list includes selected combinations that are available only by prescription.

B vitamins (oral) niacin (B_3), pantothenic acid (B_5), pyridoxine (B_6), and cyanocobalamin (B_{12}), with folic acid (B_9), iron, manganese, zinc, and 13% alcohol: Megaton Elixir; with thiamine (B_1), riboflavin (B_2), ferric pyrophosphate, and 15% alcohol: Senilezol Liquid; with thiamine (B_1), riboflavin (B_2), ascorbic acid, and folic acid: Berocca, B-Plex, Strovite, B-C with folic acid; with thiamine (B_1), riboflavin (B_2), ascorbic acid, folic acid, and biotin: Nephrocaps.

B vitamins (parenteral) with riboflavin (B_2), niacin (B_3), pantothenic acid (B_5), pyridoxine (B_6), and ascorbic acid: Becomject-100.

Multivitamins (oral) vitamins E, thiamine (B_1), riboflavin (B_2), niacin (B_3), pantothenic acid (B_5), pyridoxine (B_6), cyanocobalamin (B_{12}), ascorbic acid, and folic acid: Cefol Filmtabs; with vitamins A, D, E, thiamine (B_1), riboflavin (B_2), niacin (B_3), pantothenic acid (B_5), pyridoxine (B_6), cyanocobalamin (B_{12}), ascorbic acid, iron, and folic acid: Unicomplex-T&M Tablets, Cerovite Jr., Quintabs-M, Centrum Jr. with Iron, Monocaps, Unicap Sr., Hi-Po-Vites.

Multivitamins (parenteral) vitamins A, D, E, thiamine (B_1), riboflavin (B_2), niacin (B_3), pantothenic acid (B_5), pyridoxine (B_6), anocobalamin (B_{12}), ascorbic acid, biotin, and folic acid: Berocca Parenteral Nutrition, M.V.I.-12.

Multivitamins with fluoride (oral) vitamins A, D, thiamine (B_1), riboflavin (B_2), niacin (B_3), pantothenic acid (B_5), pyridoxine (B_6), cyanocobalamin (B_{12}), ascorbic acid, folic acid, and fluoride: Polyvitamin Fluoride, Mulvidren-F Softab Tablets, Polytabs-F; vitamins A, D, E, thiamine (B_1), riboflavin (B_2), niacin (B_3), pyridoxine (B_6), cyanocobalamin (B_{12}), ascorbic acid, folic acid, and fluoride: Poly-Vi-Flor, Florvite, Vi-Daylin/F.

A

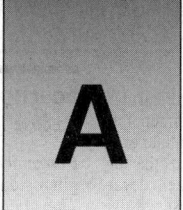

abacavir sulfate

Ziagen

Pharmacologic classification: nucleoside analogue reverse transcriptase inhibitor (NRTI)
Therapeutic classification: antiviral
Pregnancy risk category C

How supplied

Available by prescription only
Tablets: 300 mg
Oral solution: 20 mg/ml

Indications and dosages

Human immunodeficiency virus type 1 (HIV-1) infection
Adults: 300 mg P.O. twice daily in combination with other antiretroviral agents.
Children age 3 months to 16 years: 8 mg/kg P.O. twice daily (up to maximum of 300 mg P.O. twice daily) in combination with other antiretroviral agents.

Pharmacodynamics

Antiviral action: Converted intracellularly to an active metabolite, carbovir triphosphate, which inhibits the activity of HIV-1 reverse transcriptase by competing with the natural substrate deoxyguanosine-5'-triphosphate (dGTP) and by incorporation into viral DNA.

Pharmacokinetics

Absorption: Rapidly and extensively absorbed after oral administration; the mean absolute bioavailability of the tablet was 83%.
Distribution: Distributed in the extravascular space. About 50% of drug binds to plasma proteins.
Metabolism: Primarily metabolized by alcohol dehydrogenase and glucuronyl transferase to form two metabolites that lack antiviral activity.
Excretion: Primarily excreted in urine; about 16% of dose is excreted in feces. Elimination half-life in single-dose studies was 1 to 2 hours.

Route	Onset	Peak	Duration
P.O.	Unknown	Unknown	Unknown

Contraindications and precautions

Contraindicated in patients with hypersensitivity to the drug or its components. Use cautiously in patients with known risk factors for liver disease.

Interactions

Drug-lifestyle. *Alcohol use:* Reduces elimination of abacavir, increasing overall exposure to drug. Monitor alcohol consumption. Use together cautiously.

Effects on diagnostic tests

None reported.

Adverse reactions

CNS: insomnia and sleep disorders, headache.
GI: *nausea, vomiting,* diarrhea, loss of appetite (anorexia).
Skin: rash.
Other: ***hypersensitivity reaction,*** fever.

Overdose and treatment

There's no known antidote, and it isn't known whether the drug is removed by peritoneal dialysis or hemodialysis.

Clinical considerations

- Abacavir should always be used in combination with other antiretroviral agents and shouldn't be added as a single agent when antiretroviral regimens are changed as a result of loss of virologic response.
- Because the drug is absorbed equally well from both dosage forms, solution and tablets can be used interchangeably.
- The drug has caused fatal hypersensitivity reactions. If signs or symptoms of hypersensitivity (fever, skin rash, fatigue, GI symptoms such as nausea, vomiting, diarrhea, or abdominal pain) develop, discontinue drug as soon as a reaction is suspected and seek immediate medical attention.

□ ***ALERT*** Drug shouldn't be started following a hypersensitivity reaction because more severe symptoms will recur within hours and may include life-threatening hypotension and death. Symptoms usually appear within the first 6 weeks of treatment, but may occur at any time.

- To facilitate reporting of hypersensitivity reactions and collection of information on each case, an abacavir hypersensitivity registry has been established at 1-800-270-0425.

Therapeutic monitoring

■ Lactic acidosis and severe (even fatal) hepatomegaly with steatosis have been reported with use of nucleoside analogues alone or in combination, including abacavir and other antiretrovirals. Stop treatment if a patient develops clinical or laboratory findings suggestive of lactic acidosis or pronounced hepatotoxicity (which may include hepatomegaly and steatosis even in the absence of marked transaminase elevations).
■ Monitor patient for hypersensitivity reactions.

Special populations

Pregnant patients. There are no adequate controlled studies in pregnant women. Report maternal-fetal outcomes of pregnant women exposed to drug to the Antiretroviral Pregnancy Registry at 1-800-258-4263.
Breast-feeding patients. Because of the potential for HIV transmission through breastfeeding and because of the possible adverse effects of abacavir, women shouldn't breastfeed if receiving this drug.
Pediatric patients. Safety and efficacy haven't been established in children age 3 months to 13 years.
Geriatric patients. Generally, dose selection for a geriatric patient should be cautious, taking into account greater frequency of decreased hepatic, renal, or cardiac function, and of concomitant disease or other drug therapy in this age group.

Patient counseling

■ Advise patient of the risk of a life-threatening hypersensitivity reaction with this drug.
■ Tell patient to immediately contact the prescriber if signs or symptoms of hypersensitivity (fever; skin rash; severe tiredness; GI symptoms such as nausea, vomiting, diarrhea or stomach pain; achiness; or generally ill feeling) develop.
■ Instruct patient to always carry a medical alert card summarizing the symptoms of the hypersensitivity reaction.
■ Explain that this drug isn't a cure for HIV infection nor does it reduce the risk of transmission of HIV to others through sexual contact or blood contamination. Advise patient to remain under a doctor's care throughout drug therapy and to use safe sex practices.
■ Inform patient that long-term effects of this drug are unknown.
■ Advise patient to take drug exactly as prescribed.
■ Urge patient to read the medication guide that comes with each new prescription and refill.
■ Tell patient that the drug may be taken without regard to meals.

acarbose

Precose

Pharmacologic classification: alpha-glucosidase inhibitor
Therapeutic classification: antidiabetic
Pregnancy risk category B

How supplied

Available by prescription only
Tablets: 25 mg, 50 mg, 100 mg

Indications and dosages

Dietary adjunct to lower blood glucose levels in patients with type 2 (non-insulin-dependent) diabetes mellitus whose hyperglycemia can't be managed by diet alone or by diet and a sulfonylurea
Adults: Initially, 25 mg P.O. t.i.d. with the first bite of each main meal. Subsequent dosage adjustment made at 4- to 8-week intervals based on 1-hour postprandial glucose levels and tolerance. Maintenance dosage is 50 to 100 mg P.O. t.i.d. depending on patient's weight. Maximum dose for patients weighing 132 lb (60 kg) or less is 50 mg P.O. t.i.d.; for patients weighing over 132 lb, maximum dose is 100 mg P.O. t.i.d.
Adjunct to insulin or metformin therapy in patients with type 2 (non-insulin-dependent) diabetes mellitus whose hyperglycemia can't be managed by diet, exercise, and insulin or metformin alone
Adults: Initially, 25 mg P.O. t.i.d. with first bite of each main meal. Adjust dosage at 4- to 8-week intervals based on 1-hour postprandial glucose levels and tolerance to determine minimum effective dosage of each drug. Maintenance dosage is 50 to 100 mg P.O. t.i.d. based on patient's weight. Maximum dose for patients weighing 132 lb (60 kg) or less is 50 mg P.O. t.i.d.; for patients weighing over 132 lb, maximum dose is 100 mg P.O. t.i.d.

Pharmacodynamics

Antidiabetic action: The ability of acarbose to lower blood glucose results from a competitive, reversible inhibition of pancreatic alpha-amylase and membrane-bound intestinal alpha-glucoside hydrolase enzymes. In diabetic patients, this enzyme inhibition results in delayed glucose absorption and a lowering of postprandial hyperglycemia. The drug doesn't enhance insulin secretion.

Pharmacokinetics

Absorption: Minimally absorbed.
Distribution: Acts locally within the GI tract.
Metabolism: Metabolized exclusively within the GI tract, principally by intestinal bacteria with some metabolized action caused by digestive enzymes.

Excretion: Within 96 hours, 51% of dose is excreted in feces as unabsorbed drug. The fraction of drug absorbed is almost completely excreted by the kidneys. Plasma elimination half-life of acarbose is about 2 hours. Drug accumulation doesn't occur with t.i.d. oral dosing.

Route	Onset	Peak	Duration
P.O.	Unknown	1 hr	2-4 hr

Contraindications and precautions
Contraindicated in patients with hypersensitivity to drug, diabetic ketoacidosis, cirrhosis, inflammatory bowel disease, colonic ulceration, or partial intestinal obstruction and in those predisposed to intestinal obstruction. Also contraindicated in patients with chronic intestinal diseases associated with marked disorders of digestion or absorption and in those with conditions that may deteriorate because of increased gas formation in the intestine. Avoid using drug in patients with serum creatinine levels exceeding 2 mg/dl and in breast-feeding or pregnant women.

Use cautiously in patients with mild to moderate renal impairment.

Interactions
Drug-drug. *Calcium channel blocking agents, corticosteroids, estrogens, isoniazid, nicotinic acid, oral contraceptives, phenothiazines, phenytoin, sympathomimetics, thiazides, other diuretics, and thyroid products:* May cause hyperglycemia or hypoglycemia when withdrawn. Monitor patient's blood glucose levels.

Intestinal adsorbents (activated charcoal), digestive enzyme preparations containing carbohydrate-splitting enzymes (amylase, pancreatin): May reduce the effect of acarbose. Don't administer together.

Sulfonylureas or insulin: When used with acarbose, the hypoglycemic potential of these agents may be increased. Monitor patient's blood glucose level closely.

Effects on diagnostic tests
None reported.

Adverse reactions
GI: *abdominal pain, diarrhea, flatulence.*
Hepatic: elevated serum transaminase levels.

Overdose and treatment
Unlike sulfonylureas or insulin, acarbose overdose doesn't result in hypoglycemia. An overdose may result in transient increases in flatulence, diarrhea, and abdominal discomfort, which quickly subside.

Clinical considerations
- Advise maintaining exercise and diet control in addition to acarbose therapy.
- Acarbose isn't effective as sole therapy in patients with diabetes mellitus complicated by acidosis, ketosis, or coma; management of these conditions requires the use of insulin.
- Because of its mechanism of action, acarbose shouldn't cause hypoglycemia when administered alone in the fasted or postprandial state.

Therapeutic monitoring
- Acarbose alone doesn't cause hypoglycemia. However, when given in combination with a sulfonylurea or insulin, it may increase the hypoglycemic potential of the sulfonylurea. Closely monitor patient receiving both drugs. If hypoglycemia occurs, treat with oral glucose (dextrose), whose absorption isn't inhibited by acarbose, rather than sucrose (cane sugar). Severe hypoglycemia may require I.V. glucose infusion or glucagon administration. Dosage adjustment in acarbose and sulfonylurea may be required to prevent further episodes of hypoglycemia.
- During periods of increased stress, such as infection, fever, surgery, or trauma, patient may require insulin therapy. Recommend monitoring patient closely for hyperglycemia in these situations.
- Recommend monitoring patient's 1-hour postprandial plasma glucose levels to determine therapeutic effectiveness of acarbose and to identify appropriate dose. Thereafter, measure glycosylated hemoglobin every 3 months. Treatment goals include decreasing both postprandial plasma glucose and glycosylated hemoglobin levels to normal or near normal by using the lowest effective dose of acarbose either as monotherapy or in combination with sulfonylureas.
- Recommend monitoring serum transaminase levels every 3 months during first year of therapy and then periodically thereafter in patients receiving doses exceeding 50 mg t.i.d. Abnormalities may require dosage adjustment or withdrawal of drug.

Special populations
Breast-feeding patients. It isn't known if drug is excreted in breast milk. Acarbose shouldn't be given to breast-feeding women.
Pediatric patients. Safety and efficacy in pediatric patients under age 18 haven't been established.

Patient counseling
- Tell patient to take drug with the first bite of each of three main meals daily.
- Make sure patient understands that therapy relieves symptoms but doesn't cure disease.
- Stress the importance of adhering to specific diet, reducing weight, exercising, and following personal hygiene programs. Explain how and when to perform self-monitoring of blood glucose level, and teach recognition of and intervention for hyperglycemia.

■ Teach patient to recognize and intervene for hypoglycemia if a sulfonylurea agent is also taken. Tell patient to treat symptoms of low blood glucose with a form of dextrose instead of products containing table sugar.
■ Advise patient to carry medical identification regarding diabetic status.

acebutolol

Sectral

Pharmacologic classification: beta blocker
Therapeutic classification: antihypertensive, antiarrhythmic
Pregnancy risk category B

How supplied

Available by prescription only
Capsules: 200 mg, 400 mg

Indications and dosages

Hypertension
Adults: 400 mg P.O. either as a single daily dose or 200 mg b.i.d. Patients may receive as much as 1,200 mg divided b.i.d.
Ventricular arrhythmias
Adults: 200 mg P.O. b.i.d. Increase dosage to provide an adequate clinical response. Usual daily dose is 600 to 1,200 mg.
◊***Angina***
Adults: Initially, 200 mg b.i.d. Increase up to 800 mg daily until angina is controlled. Patients with severe angina may require higher doses.
≡***Dosage adjustment.*** Reduce dosage in geriatric patients and in those with impaired renal function. If creatinine clearance is 25 to 49 ml/minute, decrease dose by 50%. If creatinine clearance is less than 25 ml/minute, decrease dose by 75%. Avoid doses over 800 mg/day in geriatric patients.

Pharmacodynamics

Antihypertensive action: Exact mechanism of antihypertensive $beta_1$-adrenergic blocker effect is unknown. Drug has cardioselective beta blocking properties and mild intrinsic sympathomimetic activity.
Antiarrhythmic action: Drug decreases heart rate and prevents exercise-induced increases in heart rate; it also decreases myocardial contractility, cardiac output, and SA and AV nodal conduction velocity.

Pharmacokinetics

Absorption: Well absorbed after oral administration.
Distribution: About 26% protein-bound; minimal quantities are detected in CSF.
Metabolism: Undergoes extensive first-pass metabolism in the liver; peak levels of its major active metabolite, diacetolol, occur at about 3½ hours.
Excretion: From 30% to 40% of a given dose is excreted in urine; remainder occurs in feces and bile. Half-life of acebutolol is 3 to 4 hours; half-life of diacetolol is 8 to 13 hours.

Route	Onset	Peak	Duration
P.O.	1½ hr	2½ hr	24 hr

Contraindications and precautions

Contraindicated in patients with persistent severe bradycardia, second- and third-degree heart block, overt cardiac failure, and cardiogenic shock. Use cautiously in patients at risk for heart failure and in patients with bronchospastic disease, diabetes, hyperthyroidism, and peripheral vascular disease, and in patients with impaired hepatic function

Interactions

Drug-drug. *Other antihypertensive agents:* Acebutolol may potentiate hypotensive effects. Monitor blood pressure.
Insulin or oral antidiabetics: Dosage requirements in stable diabetic patients may be altered. Recommend monitoring blood glucose levels.
Indomethacin, NSAIDs, and alpha-adrenergic stimulants such as those in OTC cold remedies: Hypotensive effects of acebutolol may be antagonized by these drugs. Use together cautiously.

Effects on diagnostic tests

Acebutolol may cause positive antinuclear antibody titers.

Adverse reactions

CNS: depression, dizziness, fatigue, headache, hyperesthesia, hypoesthesia, impotence, insomnia.
CV: bradycardia, chest pain, edema, ***heart failure,*** hypotension.
GI: abdominal pain, constipation, diarrhea, dyspepsia, flatulence, nausea, vomiting.
Musculoskeletal: arthralgia, myalgia.
Respiratory: ***bronchospasm,*** cough, dyspnea.
Skin: rash.

Overdose and treatment

Signs of overdose include severe hypotension, bradycardia, heart failure, and bronchospasm.

After acute ingestion, empty stomach by emesis or gastric lavage; follow with activated charcoal to reduce absorption. Then provide symptomatic and supportive treatment.

Clinical considerations

Consider the following recommendations in addition to those relevant to all beta blockers:
■ Store capsules in well-closed containers, protected from light at room temperature.

- Adjust drug dose every 1 to 2 months if blood pressure control is inadequate.
- Don't discontinue drug abruptly because it may exacerbate angina symptoms or precipitate MI in patients with coronary artery disease. Discontinue gradually over 2 weeks.

Therapeutic monitoring
Carefully monitor blood pressure during dosage adjustment.

Special populations
Pregnant patients. There are no adequate and controlled studies in pregnant women. Infants born to women receiving acebutolol during pregnancy had lower birth weights, decreased systolic blood pressures and heart rates during the first 72 hours after delivery.
Breast-feeding patients. Both acebutolol and its metabolite, diacetolol, are excreted in breast milk; breast-feeding isn't recommended.
Pediatric patients. Safety and efficacy in children under age 12 haven't been established.
Geriatric patients. Avoid doses over 800 mg.

Patient counseling
Advise patient to promptly report wheezing.

acetaminophen
Acephen, Anacin-3, Bromo-Seltzer, Feverall, Panadol, Tempra, Tylenol

Pharmacologic classification: para-aminophenol derivative
Therapeutic classification: nonnarcotic analgesic, antipyretic
Pregnancy risk category B

How supplied
Available without a prescription
Tablets: 325 mg, 500 mg, 650 mg
Tablets (chewable): 80 mg, 160 mg
Tablets (extended-release): 650 mg
Capsules: 500 mg
Suppositories: 80 mg, 120 mg, 125 mg, 325 mg, 650 mg
Solution: 48 mg/ml, 80 mg/ml*, 100 mg/ml, 80 mg/5 ml, 120 mg/5 ml, 160 mg/5 ml, 167 mg/5 ml, 500 mg/15 ml
Suspension: 80 mg/ml*, 100 mg/ml, 80 mg/5 ml*, 160 mg/5 ml
Caplets: 160 mg, 500 mg, 325 mg
Syrup: 16 mg/ml
Sprinkle capsules: 80 mg, 160 mg

Indications and dosages
Mild pain, fever
Adults and children over age 12: 325 to 650 mg P.O. or P.R. q 4 to 6 hours p.r.n. Maximum dose shouldn't exceed 4 g daily. Maximum dose for long-term therapy is 2.6 g daily; alternatively, two 650-mg extended-release tablets every 8 hours p.r.n., not to exceed 4 g per day.
Children age 11 to 12: 480 mg/dose P.O. or P.R. q 4 to 6 hours.
Children age 9 to 10: 400 mg/dose P.O. or P.R. q 4 to 6 hours.
Children age 6 to 8: 320 mg/dose P.O. or P.R. q 4 to 6 hours.
Children age 4 to 5: 240 mg/dose P.O. or P.R. q 4 to 6 hours.
Children age 2 to 3: 160 mg/dose P.O. or P.R. q 4 to 6 hours.
Children age 12 to 23 months: 120 mg/dose P.O. or P.R. q 4 to 6 hours.
Children age 4 to 11 months: 80 mg/dose P.O. or P.R. q 4 to 6 hours.
Children age 3 months or less: 40 mg/dose P.O or P.R. q 4 to 6 hours.
Osteoarthritis
Adults: Up to 1 g P.O. q.i.d.; doses of 3 to 4 g per day common in these patients.

Pharmacodynamics
Mechanism and site of action may be related to inhibition of prostaglandin synthesis in CNS.
Analgesic action: Analgesic effect may be related to an elevation of the pain threshold.
Antipyretic action: Drug may exert antipyretic effect by direct action on hypothalamic heat-regulating center to block effects of endogenous pyrogen. This results in increased heat dissipation through sweating and vasodilation.

Pharmacokinetics
Absorption: Absorbed rapidly and completely via the GI tract.
Distribution: 25% protein-bound. Plasma levels don't correlate well with analgesic effect, but do correlate with toxicity.
Metabolism: About 90% to 95% is metabolized in the liver.
Excretion: Excreted in urine. Average elimination half-life ranges from 1 to 4 hours. In acute overdose, prolongation of elimination half-life is correlated with toxic effects. Half-life over 4 hours is associated with hepatic necrosis; over 12 hours is associated with coma.

Route	Onset	Peak	Duration
P.O., P.R.	Unknown	1-3 hr	3-4 hr

Contraindications and precautions
No known contraindications. Use cautiously in patients with history of chronic alcohol abuse because hepatotoxicity has occurred after therapeutic doses. Also use cautiously in patients with hepatic or CV disease, renal function impairment, or viral infection.

Interactions
Drug-drug. *Anticoagulants and thrombolytic drugs:* May potentiate effects of these drugs, but this appears to be clinically insignificant.
Antacids: Delay and decrease the absorption of acetaminophen. Separate administration times.

Anticonvulsants and isoniazid: Increased risk of hepatotoxicity. Use together cautiously.
Phenothiazines: If used with acetaminophen in large doses, hypothermia may result. Use together cautiously.
Drug-herb. *Watercress:* May inhibit oxidative metabolism of acetaminophen. Avoid use together.
Drug-food. *Foods:* Delay and decrease absorption of acetaminophen. Advise taking drug on an empty stomach.
Caffeine: May enhance therapeutic effect of acetaminophen. Avoid use together.
Drug-lifestyle. *Alcohol use:* Increases the risk of liver toxicity. Discourage alcohol use.

Effects on diagnostic tests
Acetaminophen may cause a false-positive test result for urinary 5-hydroxyindoleacetic acid.

Adverse reactions
Hematologic: hemolytic anemia, ***neutropenia, leukopenia, pancytopenia, thrombocytopenia*** (rare).
Hepatic: jaundice, ***severe liver damage*** (with toxic doses).
Metabolic: hypoglycemia.
Skin: rash, urticaria.

Overdose and treatment
In all cases of suspected acetaminophen overdose, a regional poison center or the Rocky Mountain Poison Center (1-800-525-6115) may be called for assistance. In acute overdose, plasma levels of 300 mcg/ml 4 hours postinjection or 50 mcg/ml 12 hours postinjection are associated with hepatotoxicity. Signs and symptoms of overdose include cyanosis, anemia, jaundice, skin eruptions, fever, emesis, CNS stimulation, delirium, methemoglobinemia progressing to depression, coma, vascular collapse, seizures, and death. Acetaminophen poisoning develops in stages:
Stage 1 (12 to 24 hours after ingestion): nausea, vomiting, diaphoresis, anorexia
Stage 2 (24 to 48 hours after ingestion): clinically improved but elevated liver function tests
Stage 3 (72 to 96 hours after ingestion): peak hepatotoxicity
Stage 4 (7 to 8 days after ingestion): recovery.

To treat toxic overdose of acetaminophen, empty stomach immediately by inducing emesis with ipecac syrup if patient is conscious or by gastric lavage. Administer activated charcoal by way of nasogastric tube. Oral acetylcysteine (Mucomyst) is a specific antidote for acetaminophen poisoning and is most effective if started within 10 to 12 hours after ingestion, but it can help if started within 24 hours after ingestion. Administer a Mucomyst loading dose of 140 mg/kg P.O., followed by maintenance dosages of 70 mg/kg P.O. every 4 hours for an additional 17 doses. Doses vomited within 1 hour of administration must be repeated. Remove charcoal before giving acetylcysteine because it may interfere with absorption of this antidote.

Acetylcysteine minimizes hepatic injury by supplying sulfydryl groups that bind with acetaminophen metabolites. Hemodialysis may be helpful to remove acetaminophen from the body. Monitor laboratory parameters and vital signs closely. Provide symptomatic and supportive measures (respiratory support, correction of fluid and electrolyte imbalances). Determine plasma acetaminophen levels at least 4 hours after overdose. If plasma acetaminophen levels indicate hepatotoxicity, perform liver function tests every 24 hours for at least 96 hours.

Clinical considerations
- Acetaminophen has no significant anti-inflammatory effect. Even so, studies have shown substantial benefit in patients with osteoarthritis of the knee. Therapeutic benefits may stem from the analgesic effects of the drug.
- Many OTC products contain acetaminophen. Be aware of this when dispensing this drug.

☐ **ALERT** Be aware of patient's total daily intake of acetaminophen, especially if he is also prescribed other drugs containing this component, such as Percocet. Toxicity can occur.

- Patients unable to tolerate aspirin may be able to tolerate acetaminophen.
- When buffered acetaminophen effervescent granules are prescribed, consider sodium content for sodium-restricted patients.
- Advise patients with phenylketonuria that many preparations contain aspartame.
- Many acetaminophen preparations contain sulfites.
- The extended-release tablet shouldn't be crushed, chewed, or dissolved in liquid.
- Store rectal acetaminophen suppositories in refrigerator.

Therapeutic monitoring
- Address patient's level of pain and response before and after drug administration.
- Recommend monitoring vital signs, especially temperature, to evaluate effectiveness of drug.
- Recommend monitoring PT and INR values in patients receiving oral anticoagulants and sustained acetaminophen therapy.

Special populations
Breast-feeding patients. Drug is excreted in breast milk in low concentrations. No adverse effects have been reported.
Pediatric patients. Children shouldn't take more than five doses per day or take drug for more than 5 days unless prescribed. Instruct caregivers on weight-based acetaminophen dosing, to use the provided calibrated measuring device with the preparation, and not to give more than the recommended dose. Also,

caution caregivers not to use other OTC preparations that contain acetaminophen.
Geriatric patients. Geriatric patients are more sensitive to drug. Use with caution.

Patient counseling

- Instruct patient in proper administration of prescribed form of drug.
- Advise patient on chronic high-dose drug therapy to arrange for monitoring of laboratory parameters, especially BUN, serum creatinine, liver function tests, and CBC.
- Warn patient with current or past rectal bleeding to avoid using rectal acetaminophen suppositories. If they're used, they must be retained in the rectum for at least 1 hour.
- Warn patient that high doses or unsupervised chronic use of acetaminophen can cause liver damage. Use of alcoholic beverages increases the risk of liver toxicity.
- Tell patient to avoid use with temperature of more than 103° F (39° C), a fever persisting longer than 3 days, or a recurrent fever.
- Tell patient not to take NSAIDs with acetaminophen on a regular basis.
- Warn patient to avoid taking tetracycline antibiotics within 1 hour after taking buffered acetaminophen effervescent granules.
- Tell patient not to use drug for arthritic or rheumatic conditions without medical approval. Drug may relieve pain but not other symptoms.
- Advise adult patient not to take drug for more than 10 days without medical approval.
- Tell patient on high-dose or long-term therapy that regular follow-up visits are essential.

acetazolamide

acetazolamide sodium

Dazamide, Diamox, Diamox Sequels

Pharmacologic classification: carbonic anhydrase inhibitor
Therapeutic classification: antiglaucoma agent, anticonvulsant, diuretic, altitude sickness agent (prevention and treatment)
Pregnancy risk category C

How supplied

Available by prescription only
Tablets: 125 mg, 250 mg
Capsules (extended-release): 500 mg
Injection: 500 mg

Indications and dosages

Secondary glaucoma and preoperative management of acute angle-closure glaucoma
Adults: 250 mg P.O. q 4 hours, or 250 mg P.O. b.i.d. for short-term therapy. In acute cases, 500 mg P.O. followed by 125 to 250 mg P.O. q 4 hours. To rapidly lower intraocular pressure, 500 mg I.V., which may be repeated in 2 to 4 hours, if necessary, followed by 125 to 250 mg P.O. q 4 hours.
Children: 5 to 10 mg/kg I.V. q 6 hours.
Edema in heart failure
Adults: 250 to 375 mg P.O. daily in morning.
Children: 5 mg/kg or 150 mg/m^2 P.O. or I.V. daily in morning.
Drug-induced edema
Adults: 250 to 375 mg (5 mg/kg) P.O. as single daily dose for 1 to 2 days alternating with 1 drug-free day.
Chronic open-angle glaucoma
Adults: 250 mg to 1 g P.O. daily in divided doses, or 500 mg (extended-release) P.O. once daily or b.i.d. Doses over 1 g daily don't produce an increased effect.
Children: 8 to 30 mg/kg P.O. or 300 to 900 mg/m^2 daily in three divided doses.
Prevention or amelioration of acute mountain sickness
Adults: 500 mg to 1 g P.O. daily in divided doses (such as 250 mg q 8 to 12 hours) or 500 mg (extended-release) P.O. q 12 to 24 hours, taken preferably 48 hours before ascent and continued for at least 48 hours after arrival at high altitude.
Myoclonic seizures, refractory generalized tonic-clonic (grand mal) or absence (petit mal) seizures, mixed seizures
Adults and children: 8 to 30 mg/kg P.O. daily, divided into one to four doses. The optimum dose range is 375 mg to 1 g P.O. daily. When given with other anticonvulsants, the initial dose is 250 mg daily.
Periodic paralysis
Adults: 250 mg P.O. b.i.d. or t.i.d. Maximum dose, 1.5 g daily.

Pharmacodynamics

Antiglaucoma action: In open-angle glaucoma and perioperatively for acute angle-closure glaucoma, acetazolamide and acetazolamide sodium decrease the formation of aqueous humor, lowering intraocular pressure.
Anticonvulsant action: Inhibition of carbonic anhydrase in the CNS appears to slow down abnormal paroxysmal discharge from the neurons.
Diuretic action: Acetazolamide and acetazolamide sodium act by noncompetitive reversible inhibition of the enzyme carbonic anhydrase, which is responsible for formation of hydrogen and bicarbonate ions from carbon dioxide and water. This inhibition results in decreased hydrogen concentration in the renal tubules, promoting excretion of bicarbonate, sodium, potassium, and water; systemic acidosis may occur because carbon dioxide isn't eliminated as rapidly.
Altitude sickness agent: Acetazolamide shortens the period of high-altitude acclimatization; by inhibiting conversion of carbon dioxide to bicarbonate, it may increase carbon dioxide

tension in tissues and decrease it in the lungs. The resultant metabolic acidosis may also increase oxygenation during hypoxia.

Pharmacokinetics

Absorption: Well absorbed from the GI tract after oral administration.
Distribution: Distributed throughout body tissues.
Metabolism: None.
Excretion: Excreted primarily in urine via tubular secretion and passive reabsorption.

Route	Onset	Peak	Duration
P.O.	1-1½ hr	2-4 hr	8-12 hr
P.O. (extended)	2 hr	3-6 hr	18-24 hr
I.V.	2 min	15 min	1-5 hr

Contraindications and precautions

Contraindicated in patients with hypersensitivity to drug; in long-term therapy for chronic noncongestive angle-closure glaucoma; and in those with hyponatremia or hypokalemia, renal or hepatic disease or dysfunction, adrenal gland failure, and hyperchloremic acidosis. Use cautiously in patients with respiratory acidosis, emphysema, diabetes, or COPD and in those receiving other diuretics.

Interactions

Drug-drug. *Amphetamines, flecainide, procainamide, and quinidine:* Acetazolamide alkalinizes urine and thus may decrease excretion of these drugs. Monitor patient closely.
Salicylates, phenobarbital, and lithium: Increased excretion of these drugs causes low plasma levels, possibly necessitating dosage adjustments.

Effects on diagnostic tests

Because it alkalinizes urine, acetazolamide may cause false-positive proteinuria in Albustix or Albutest.

Adverse reactions

CNS: confusion, drowsiness, paresthesia.
EENT: hearing dysfunction, transient myopia, tinnitus.
GI: anorexia, altered taste, diarrhea, nausea, vomiting.
GU: hematuria, polyuria.
Hematologic: ***aplastic anemia,*** hemolytic anemia, ***leukopenia.***
Metabolic: asymptomatic hyperuricemia, hyperchloremic acidosis, hypokalemia, decreased thyroid iodine uptake.
Skin: rash.

Overdose and treatment

Specific recommendations are unavailable. Treatment is supportive and symptomatic. Acetazolamide increases bicarbonate excretion and may cause hypokalemia and hyperchloremic acidosis. Induce emesis or perform gastric lavage. Don't induce catharsis because this may exacerbate electrolyte disturbances. Monitor fluid and electrolyte levels.

Clinical considerations

- Suspensions containing 250 mg/5 ml of syrup are the most palatable and can be made by the pharmacist. These remain stable for about 1 week. Tablets don't dissolve in fruit juice.
- Reconstitute powder by adding at least 5 ml sterile water for injection.
- Direct I.V. administration is preferred if drug must be given parenterally.

Therapeutic monitoring

- Recommend monitoring electrolytes and serum glucose.
- Recommend monitoring patient for hepatic coma or precoma in patients with hepatic cirrhosis, hypokalemia, or elevations in blood ammonia concentrations caused by drug therapy.

Special populations

Pregnant patients. Acetazolamide may cause fetal toxicity when administered to pregnant women.
Breast-feeding patients. Safety of drug in breast-feeding women hasn't been established.
Geriatric patients. Observe geriatric and debilitated patients closely because they're more susceptible to drug-induced diuresis. Excessive diuresis promotes rapid dehydration, leading to hypovolemia, hypokalemia, and hyponatremia and may cause circulatory collapse. Reduced dosages may be indicated.

Patient counseling

Warn patient to use caution while driving or performing tasks that require alertness, coordination, or physical dexterity because drug may cause drowsiness.

acetylcysteine

Mucomyst, Mucosil, Parvolex*

Pharmacologic classification: amino acid (L-cysteine) derivative
Therapeutic classification: mucolytic, antidote for acetaminophen overdose
Pregnancy risk category B

How supplied

Available by prescription only
Solution: 10%, 20%
Injection:* 200 mg/ml

Indications and dosages

Acute and chronic bronchopulmonary disease, tracheostomy care, pulmonary com-

plications of surgery, diagnostic bronchial studies
Administer by nebulization, direct application, or intratracheal instillation.
Adults and children: 1 to 2 ml of 10% or 20% solution by direct instillation into trachea as often as hourly; or 3 to 5 ml of 20% solution or 6 to 10 ml of 10% solution administered by nebulizer q 2 to 3 hours. For instillation via percutaneous intratracheal catheter, administer 1 to 2 ml of 20% solution or 2 to 4 ml of 10% solution q 1 to 4 hours; via tracheal catheter to treat a specific bronchopulmonary tree segment, administer 2 to 5 ml of 20% solution. For diagnostic bronchial studies (administered before procedure), administer 1 to 2 ml of 20% solution or 2 to 4 ml of 10% solution for two or three doses.
Acetaminophen toxicity
Adults and children: Initially, 140 mg/kg P.O., followed by 70 mg/kg q 4 hours for 17 doses (a total of 1,330 mg/kg) or until acetaminophen assay reveals nontoxic level.

Alternatively, drug may be administered I.V.: Loading dose 150 mg/kg I.V. in 200 ml D_5W over 15 minutes, followed by 50 mg/kg I.V. in 500 ml D_5W over 4 hours, followed by 100 mg/kg I.V. in 1,000 ml D_5W over 16 hours.

Pharmacodynamics
Mucolytic action: Drug produces its mucolytic effect by splitting the disulfide bonds of mucoprotein, the substance responsible for increased viscosity of mucus secretions in the lungs; thus, pulmonary secretions become less viscous and more liquid.
Acetaminophen antidote: Mechanism by which acetylcysteine reduces acetaminophen toxicity isn't fully understood; it's thought that acetylcysteine restores hepatic stores of glutathione or inactivates the toxic metabolite of acetaminophen via a chemical interaction, thereby preventing hepatic damage.

Pharmacokinetics
Absorption: Most inhaled acetylcysteine acts directly on mucus in the lungs; the remainder is absorbed by pulmonary epithelium. After oral administration, drug is absorbed from the GI tract.
Distribution: Unknown.
Metabolism: Metabolized in the liver.
Excretion: Unknown.

Route	Onset	Peak	Duration
P.O., I.V., inhalation	Unknown	Unknown	Unknown

Contraindications and precautions
Contraindicated in patients hypersensitive to drug. Use cautiously in geriatric or debilitated patients with severe respiratory insufficiency.

Interactions
Drug-drug. *Activated charcoal:* Absorbs orally administered acetylcysteine, preventing its absorption. Remove charcoal before acetylcysteine administration.
Oxytetracycline, tetracycline, chlortetracycline, erythromycin lactobionate, amphotericin B, ampicillin, iodized oil, chymotrypsin, trypsin, and hydrogen peroxide: Incompatible with these medications. Administer drugs separately.

Effects on diagnostic tests
None reported.

Adverse reactions
CV: chest tightness, hypotension, hypertension, tachycardia.
EENT: *rhinorrhea.*
GI: *nausea, stomatitis, vomiting.*
Respiratory: ***bronchospasm*** (especially in asthmatic patients).
Other: clamminess, fever.

Overdose and treatment
No information available.

Clinical considerations
- Acetylcysteine solutions release hydrogen sulfide and discolor on contact with rubber and some metals (especially iron, nickel, and copper); drug tarnishes silver (this doesn't affect drug potency).
- Solution may turn light purple; this doesn't affect safety or efficacy of the drug. Use plastic, stainless steel, or other inert metal when administering drug by nebulization. Don't use hand-held bulb nebulizers; output is too small and particle size too large.
- After opening, store in refrigerator or use within 96 hours.
- When used orally for acetaminophen overdose, dilute with cola, fruit juice, or water to a 5% concentration and administer within 1 hour.
- Don't place directly in the chamber of a heated (hot pot) nebulizer.
- Optimal results occur when acetylcysteine is administered within 16 hours of acetaminophen ingestion, but preferably 8 hours; however, drug may be administered up to 24 hours after acetaminophen ingestion. A regional poison center or the Rocky Mountain Poison Center may be contacted at 1-800-525-6115 for assistance for use of acetylcysteine as an antidote.

Therapeutic monitoring
- Recommend monitoring cough type and frequency; for maximum effect, instruct patient to clear airway by coughing before aerosol administration. Many clinicians pretreat with bronchodilators before administration of acetylcysteine. Keep suction equipment available; if patient has insufficient cough to clear increased

secretions, suction will be needed to maintain open airway.

- If encephalopathy develops as a result of hepatic failure, stop acetylcysteine therapy to prevent further accumulation of nitrogenous substances.
- Recommend obtaining a 4-hour postingestion acetaminophen level (for peak concentration); the results are used in combination with a nomogram to estimate the potential for hepatotoxicity. This guides the administration of acetylcysteine.

Special populations

Pregnant patients. There are no adequate studies in pregnant women. Use only if clearly indicated.
Breast-feeding patients. It's unknown if drug is excreted in breast milk.
Pediatric patients. Drug may be given by tent or croupette. Use a sufficient volume (up to 300 ml) of a 10% or 20% solution to maintain a heavy mist in the tent for the time prescribed. Administration may be continuous or intermittent.
Geriatric patients. Geriatric patients may have inadequate cough and be unable to clear airway completely of mucus. Keep suction equipment available and monitor patient closely.

Patient counseling

Warn patient of unpleasant odor (rotten egg odor of hydrogen sulfide), and explain that increased amounts of liquefied bronchial secretion plus unpleasant odor may cause nausea and vomiting; have patient rinse mouth with water after nebulizer treatment.

activated charcoal

Actidose-Aqua, Charco Aid, Charco Caps, Insta-Char Pediatric

Pharmacologic classification: adsorbent
Therapeutic classification: antidote, antidiarrheal, antiflatulent
Pregnancy risk category NR

How supplied

Available without a prescription
Tablets: 325 mg, 650 mg
Tablets with 40 mg simethicone (delayed-release): 200 mg
Tablets (delayed-release) with 80 mg simethicone: 250 mg
Capsules: 260 mg
Powder: 30 g, 50 g
Suspension: 0.625 g/5 ml, 0.7 g/5 ml (50 g), 1 g/5 ml, 1.25 g/5 ml
Hemoperfusion system: 300 g

Indications and dosages

Flatulence or dyspepsia
Adults: 600 mg to 5 g P.O. as a single dose, or 975 mg to 3.9 g t.i.d. after meals.
Poisoning
Adults and children: Five to ten times the estimated weight of drug or chemical ingested. Dose is 30 to 100 g in 250 ml water to make a slurry.

Give orally, preferably within 30 minutes of ingestion. Larger doses are necessary if food is in the stomach. Drug is used adjunctively in treating poisoning or overdose with acetaminophen, amphetamines, antimony, aspirin, atropine, arsenic, barbiturates, camphor, cocaine, cardiac glycosides, glutethimide, ipecac, malathion, morphine, opium, oxalic acid, parathion, phenol, phenothiazines, phenytoin, poisonous mushrooms, potassium permanganate, propoxyphene, quinine, strychnine, sulfonamides, or tricyclic antidepressants.

Activated charcoal may be given 20 to 60 g q 4 to 12 hours (gastric dialysis) to enhance removal of some drugs from the bloodstream. Monitor serum drug level.

◇ ***To relieve GI disturbances (halitosis, anorexia, nausea, vomiting) in uremic patients***
Adults: 20 to 50 g PO. daily.

Pharmacodynamics

Antidote action: Drug adsorbs ingested toxins, thereby inhibiting GI absorption.
Antidiarrheal action: Activated charcoal adsorbs toxic and nontoxic irritants that cause diarrhea or GI discomfort.
Antiflatulent action: Activated charcoal adsorbs intestinal gas to relieve discomfort.

Pharmacokinetics

Absorption: Not absorbed from the GI tract.
Distribution: None.
Metabolism: None.
Excretion: Excreted in feces.

Route	Onset	Peak	Duration
P.O.	Immediate	Unknown	Unknown

Contraindications and precautions

No known contraindications.

Interactions

Drug-drug. *Syrup of ipecac, orally administered acetylcysteine:* Activated charcoal inactivates these medications and many other orally administered medications. Charcoal should be removed by gastric lavage before acetylcysteine is administered.
Drug-food. *Milk products:* Decrease the effectiveness of activated charcoal. Don't dilute drug with dairy products.

Effects on diagnostic tests

None reported.

Adverse reactions
GI: black stools, constipation, nausea.

Overdose and treatment
No information available.

Clinical considerations
☐ ***ALERT*** Don't use activated charcoal if poisoning involves corrosive agents, cyanide, iron, mineral acids, or organic solvents.
- Don't give activated charcoal by mouth to a semiconscious or unconscious patient; instead, administer the drug through a nasogastric tube.
- Because activated charcoal adsorbs and inactivates syrup of ipecac, give only after emesis is complete.
- Dose may need to be repeated if patient vomits shortly after administration.
- Activated charcoal is most effective when used within 30 minutes of toxin ingestion; a cathartic is commonly administered with or after activated charcoal to speed removal of the toxin/charcoal complex.
- Powder form is most effective. Mix with tap water to form consistency of thick syrup. A small amount of fruit juice or flavoring may be added to make mixture more palatable.
- If administering drug for indications other than poisoning, be sure to give other medications 1 hour before or 2 hours after activated charcoal.
- Activated charcoal may be used orally to decrease colostomy odor.

Therapeutic monitoring
- Advise monitoring of patient's nutritional status; prolonged use (over 72 hours) may impair patient's nutritional status.
- Recommend monitoring serum electrolytes if repeated dosing of charcoal with sorbitol or in children who may be more sensitive to sorbitol.

Special populations
Pediatric patients. Don't use charcoal with sorbitol in children under 1 year old.

Patient counseling
- Tell patient to call poison information center or hospital emergency department before taking activated charcoal as an antidote.
- If patient is using activated charcoal as an antidiarrheal or antiflatulent, instruct him to take medications 1 hour before or 2 hours after activated charcoal. For antidiarrheal use, advise patient to report diarrhea that persists after 2 days of therapy; fever; or flatulence that persists after 7 days.
- Warn patient that activated charcoal turns stools black.
- Advise patient not to mix drug with milk products, which may lessen its effectiveness.

acyclovir (acycloguanosine)

acyclovir sodium
Zovirax

Pharmacologic classification: synthetic purine nucleoside
Therapeutic classification: antiviral
Pregnancy risk category C

How supplied
Available by prescription only
Tablets: 400 mg, 800 mg
Capsules: 200 mg
Oral suspension: 200 mg/5 ml
Injection: 500 mg/vial, 1 g/vial
Ointment: 5%
Injection concentrate for I.V. infusion: 25 mg/ml, 50 mg/ml
Redi-infusion: 5 mg/ml in sodium chloride 0.9%

Indications and dosages
Initial and recurrent mucocutaneous herpes simplex virus (HSV type 1 and HSV type 2) or severe initial genital herpes or herpes simplex in immunocompromised patient
Adults and children over age 12: 5 mg/kg, given at a constant rate over 1 hour by I.V. infusion q 8 hours for 7 days (5 days for genital herpes).
Children under age 12: 10 mg/kg infused at a constant rate over 1 hour by I.V. infusion q 8 hours for 7 days (5 days for genital herpes).
◇ ***Mucocutaneous herpes simplex virus (HSV type 1 and HSV type 2) in immunocompromised patient***
Adults: 400 mg P.O. q 4 hours while awake (5 times daily).
Children: 1 g P.O. daily divided into three to five doses for 7 to 14 days; dose shouldn't exceed 80 mg/kg daily.
◇ ***Disseminated herpes zoster***
Adults: 5 to 10 mg/kg I.V. q 8 hours for 7 to 10 days. Infuse over at least 1 hour.
Initial genital herpes
Adults: 200 mg P.O. q 4 hours while awake (a total of five capsules daily). Treatment should continue for 10 days. Alternatively, 400 mg P.O. t.i.d. for 7 to 10 days.
◇ ***Genital herpes in the immunocompromised patient***
Adults: 400 mg P.O. 3 to 5 times daily.
◇ ***Rectal herpes infection***
Adults: 400 mg P.O. 5 times daily for 10 days or until resolution; alternatively, 800 mg P.O. q 8 hours for 7 to 10 days for initial infections.
Acute herpes zoster infections
Adults: 800 mg P.O. five times daily for 7 to 10 days. Initiate therapy within 48 hours of rash onset.

Intermittent therapy for recurrent genital herpes
Adults: 200 mg P.O. q 4 hours while awake (a total of five capsules daily). Continue treatment for 5 days. Initiate therapy at first sign of recurrence.
Chronic suppressive therapy for recurrent genital herpes
Adults: 400 mg P.O. b.i.d. for up to 1 year, followed by reevaluation.
Genital herpes; non-life-threatening herpes simplex infection in immunocompromised patients
Adults and children: Apply sufficient quantity of ointment to adequately cover all lesions q 3 hours, six times daily for 7 days.
Neonatal herpes simplex virus infection
Neonates and infants up to 3 months: 10 mg/kg I.V. every 8 hours for 10 days.
Preterm neonates: 10 mg/kg I.V. q 12 hours.
Primary or recurrent HSV infections in patients with HIV
Adults: 200 to 800 mg P.O. 5 times daily.
◊ ***Chronic suppressive or maintenance prophylaxis therapy for recurrent HSV infections in patients with HIV***
Adults and adolescents: 200 mg P.O. t.i.d. or 400 mg P.O. b.i.d.
Infants and children: 600 to 1,000 mg P.O. daily in three to five divided doses; alternatively, 80 mg/kg in 3 to 4 divided doses.
Acute varicella (chickenpox) infections
Adults and children age 2 and older weighing over 88 lb (40 kg): 800 mg P.O. q.i.d. for 5 days.
Children age 2 or over weighing under 88 lb: 20 mg/kg P.O. q.i.d. for 5 days.
◊***Acute herpes zoster ophthalmicus***
Adults: 600 mg P.O. q 4 hours 5 times daily for 10 days; preferably within 72 hours of rash onset, but no more than 7 days.
Varicella in the immunocompromised patient
Adults and children over age 12: 10 mg/kg I.V. over 1 hour q 8 hours for 7 days.
Children under age 12: 20 mg/kg I.V. over 1 hour q 8 hours for 7 days.
Herpes simplex encephalitis
Adults and children over age 12: 10 mg/kg I.V. over 1 hour q 8 hours for 10 days.
Children age 3 months to 12 years: 20 mg/kg q 8 hours I.V. over at least 1 hour for 10 days.
≡ ***Dosage adjustment.*** In patients with renal failure, adjust normal oral dose (200 to 400 mg) to 200 mg q 12 hours if creatinine clearance drops below 10 ml/minute/1.73 m^2. For normal doses exceeding 400 mg, refer to package insert.

In patients with renal failure, give 100% of the I.V. dose q 8 hours if creatinine clearance exceeds 50 ml/minute/1.73 m^2; 100% of the dose q 12 hours if it ranges between 25 and 50 ml/minute/1.73 m^2; 100% of the dose q 24 hours if it ranges between 10 and 25 ml/minute/1.73 m^2; and 50% of the dose q 24 hours if it falls below 10 ml/minute/1.73 m^2.

Pharmacodynamics

Antiviral action: Acyclovir is converted by the viral cell into its active form (triphosphate) and inhibits viral DNA polymerase.

In vitro, acyclovir is active against herpes simplex virus type 1, herpes simplex virus type 2, varicella-zoster virus, Epstein-Barr virus, and cytomegalovirus. In vivo, acyclovir may reduce the duration of acute infection and speed lesion healing in initial genital herpes episodes. Patients with frequent herpes recurrences (more than six episodes a year) may receive oral acyclovir prophylactically to prevent recurrences or reduce their frequency.

Pharmacokinetics

Absorption: With oral administration, absorbed slowly and incompletely (15% to 30%). Absorption isn't affected by food. With topical administration, absorption is minimal.
Distribution: Distributed widely to organ tissues and body fluids. CSF levels equal about 50% of serum levels. About 9% to 33% of a dose binds to plasma proteins.
Metabolism: Metabolized inside the viral cell to its active form. About 10% of dose is metabolized extracellularly.
Excretion: Up to 92% of systemically absorbed acyclovir is excreted as unchanged drug by the kidneys by glomerular filtration and tubular secretion. In patients with normal renal function, half-life is 2 to 3½ hours. Renal failure may extend half-life to 19 hours.

Route	Onset	Peak	Duration
P.O.	Unknown	2-5 hr	Unknown
I.V.	Immediate	Immediate	Unknown
Topical	Unknown	Unknown	Unknown

Contraindications and precautions

Contraindicated in patients with hypersensitivity to drug. Use cautiously in patients with underlying neurologic problems, renal disease, or dehydration and in those receiving nephrotoxic drugs.

Interactions

Drug-drug. *Probenecid:* May result in reduced renal tubular secretion of acyclovir, leading to increased drug half-life, reduced elimination rate, and decreased urine excretion. This reduced clearance causes more sustained serum drug levels. Avoid use together.
Methotrexate: Possible reaction in patients who have had a previous neurologic reaction to intrathececal methotrexate administration. Use I.V. acyclovir with caution in these patients.
Zidovudine: May result in increased levels of acyclovir, causing toxicity. Monitor acyclovir levels closely.

Effects on diagnostic tests
None reported.

Adverse reactions
CNS: *encephalopathic changes (lethargy, obtundation, tremor, confusion, hallucinations, agitation,* ***seizures, coma****)*, headache, malaise.
GI: diarrhea, *nausea, vomiting.*
GU: hematuria, *transient elevations of serum creatinine and BUN levels.*
Hematologic: ***bone marrow hypoplasia, leukopenia,*** megaloblastic hematopoiesis, thrombocytosis, ***thrombocytopenia.***
Skin: itching, rash, transient burning and stinging, pruritus, urticaria, vulvitis.
Other: *inflammation, phlebitis* (at injection site).

Overdose and treatment
Overdose has followed I.V. bolus administration in patients with unmonitored fluid status or in patients receiving inappropriately high parenteral dosages. Acute toxicity hasn't been reported after high oral dosage. Hemodialysis results in 60% decrease in plasma level of the drug.

Clinical effects of overdose include signs of nephrotoxicity, including elevated serum creatinine and BUN levels, progressing to renal failure.

Clinical considerations
- Drug shouldn't be administered S.C., I.M., by I.V. bolus, or ophthalmically.
- Reconstitute drug by adding 10 to 20 ml of sterile water for injection to a 500 mg or 1 g acyclovir vial, respectively, to provide a solution containing 50 mg/mL. Don't use bacteriostatic water for injection. Use reconstituted solution within 12 hours. Further dilute in 50 to 125 mL of a compatible I.V. solution to a concentration of no more than 7 mg/mL.
- Infuse I.V. dose over at least 1 hour to prevent renal tubular damage.
- Solubility of acyclovir in urine is low. Ensure that patient taking the systemic form of drug is well hydrated to prevent nephrotoxicity.
- Don't apply topical preparation to vagina or cervix.

Therapeutic monitoring
- Monitor serum creatinine level. If level doesn't return to normal within a few days after therapy begins, increase hydration, adjust dose, or discontinue drug.
- Recommend monitoring for encephalopathic signs; they're more likely in patients who have experienced neurologic reactions to cytotoxic drugs.

Special populations
Pregnant patients. Use only if benefits outweigh the risks.
Pediatric patients. Safety and effectiveness of oral and topical acyclovir in children haven't been established. I.V. acyclovir has been used in only a few children. To reconstitute acyclovir for children, don't use bacteriostatic water for injection that contains benzyl alcohol.
Geriatric patients. Administer drug cautiously to geriatric patients because they may suffer from renal dysfunction or dehydration.

Patient counseling
- Warn patient that although drug helps manage the disease, it doesn't cure it or prevent its spread to others.
- Tell patient to begin taking drug when early infection symptoms, such as tingling, itching, or pain, occur.
- Instruct patient taking ointment to use a finger cot or rubber glove and to apply about a ½" ribbon of ointment for every 4 square inches of area to be covered. Ointment should thoroughly cover each lesion. Warn patient to avoid getting ointment in the eye.
- Instruct patient to avoid sexual intercourse during active genital infection.

adenosine
Adenocard

Pharmacologic classification: nucleoside
Therapeutic classification: antiarrhythmic
Pregnancy risk category C

How supplied
Available by prescription only
Injection: 3 mg/ml in 2-ml and 5-ml vials

Indications and dosages
Conversion of paroxysmal supraventricular tachycardia (PSVT) to sinus rhythm
Adults: 6 mg I.V. by rapid bolus injection (over 1 to 2 seconds). If PSVT isn't eliminated in 1 to 2 minutes, give 12 mg by rapid I.V. push. Repeat 12-mg dose if necessary. Single doses over 12 mg aren't recommended.

Pharmacodynamics
Antiarrhythmic action: Adenosine is a naturally occurring nucleoside. In the heart, it acts on the AV node to slow conduction and inhibit reentry pathways. Adenosine is also useful for the treatment of PSVT associated with accessory bypass tracts (Wolff-Parkinson-White syndrome).

Pharmacokinetics
Absorption: Administered by rapid I.V. injection.
Distribution: Rapidly taken up by erythrocytes and vascular endothelial cells.

Metabolism: Metabolized within tissues to inosine and adenosine monophosphate.
Excretion: Unknown; circulating plasma half-life is less than 10 seconds.

Route	Onset	Peak	Duration
I.V.	Immediate	Immediate	Unknown

Contraindications and precautions
Contraindicated in patients with hypersensitivity to drug and in those with second- or third-degree heart block or sick sinus syndrome, unless an artificial pacemaker is present, because adenosine decreases conduction through the AV node and may produce first-, second-, or third-degree heart block. These effects are usually transient; however, patients in whom significant heart block develops after a dose of adenosine shouldn't receive additional doses.

Don't use in atrial fibrillation or atrial flutter. Use cautiously in patients with asthma because bronchoconstriction may occur.

Interactions
Drug-drug. *Carbamazepine:* Higher degrees of heart block occur in patients receiving concurrent therapy. Avoid use together.
Dipyridamole: May potentiate the effects of the drug; smaller doses may be necessary.
Methylxanthines: Antagonize effects of adenosine. Therefore, patients receiving theophylline may require higher doses or may not respond to adenosine therapy.
Drug-herb. *Guarana:* May decrease response of adenosine. Monitor patient closely.
Drug-food. *Caffeine:* May antagonize the effects of adenosine. Patient may require higher doses or may not respond to adenosine therapy.

Effects on diagnostic tests
None reported.

Adverse reactions
CNS: apprehension, back pain, blurred vision, burning sensation, dizziness, heaviness in arms, light-headedness, neck pain, numbness, tingling in arms.
CV: chest pain, *facial flushing,* headache, hypotension, palpitations, diaphoresis.
GI: metallic taste, nausea.
Respiratory: *chest pressure, dyspnea, shortness of breath,* hyperventilation.
Other: *throat tightness, groin pressure.*

Overdose and treatment
Because the half-life of adenosine is less than 10 seconds, the adverse effects of overdose usually dissipate rapidly and are self-limiting. Treat lingering adverse effects symptomatically.

Clinical considerations
- Advise caution in using Adenocard in patients with previous history of ventricular fibrillation or those taking digoxin and verapamil.
- Rapid I.V. injection is necessary for drug action. Administer directly into a vein if possible; if an I.V. line is used, use the most proximal port and follow with a rapid sodium chloride flush to ensure that drug reaches the systemic circulation rapidly.
- Check solution for crystals, which may occur if solution is cold. If crystals are visible, gently warm solution to room temperature. Don't use solutions that aren't clear.
- Discard unused drug because it contains no preservatives.

☐ ***ALERT*** Don't confuse adenosine phosphate with adenosine (Adenocard).

Therapeutic monitoring
- Recommend monitoring ECG rhythm during administration; drug may cause short-lasting first-, second-, or third-degree heart block or asystole.

Special populations
Pediatric patients. There have been no controlled studies.

Patient counseling
Warn patient of adverse reactions.

albumin, human (normal serum albumin, human)
Albuminar-5, Albuminar-25, Albutein 5%, Albutein 25%, Buminate 5%, Buminate 25%, Plasbumin-5, Plasbumin-25

Pharmacologic classification: blood derivative
Therapeutic classification: plasma protein
Pregnancy risk category C

How supplied
Injection: 5% (50 mg/ml) in 50-ml, 250-ml, 500-ml, 1,000-ml vials; 25% (250 mg/ml) in 20-ml, 50-ml, 100-ml vials

Indications and dosages
Shock
Adults: Initially, 500 ml (5% solution) by I.V. infusion, may repeat after 30 minutes. Dosage varies with patient's condition and response. Don't exceed 250 g in 48 hours.
Children: 10 to 20 ml/kg (5% solution) by I.V. infusion, at a rate up to 5 to 10 ml/minute.
Hypoproteinemia
Adults: 1,000 to 1,500 ml 5% solution by I.V. infusion daily, maximum rate 5 to 10 ml/minute; or 200 to 300 ml of 25% solution by I.V. infusion daily, maximum rate 3 ml/minute. Dosage varies with patient's condition and response.

Burns
Adults and children: Dosage varies based on extent of burn and patient's condition. Usually maintain plasma albumin level at 2 to 3 g/dl.
Hyperbilirubinemia
Infants: 1 g/kg albumin (4 ml/kg of 25% solution) by I.V. infusion 1 to 2 hours before transfusion.
◊ *High-risk neonates with low serum protein concentration:* 1.4 to 1.8 ml/kg by I.V. infusion of 25% solution.

Pharmacodynamics
Plasma volume-expanding action: Albumin 5% supplies colloid to the blood and expands plasma volume. Albumin 25% provides intravascular oncotic pressure at 5:1, causing fluid to shift from interstitial space to circulation and slightly increasing plasma protein level.

Pharmacokinetics
Absorption: Not adequately absorbed from the GI tract.
Distribution: Accounts for about 50% of plasma proteins; distributed into the intravascular space and extravascular sites, including skin, muscle, and lungs. In patients with reduced circulating blood volume, hemodilution secondary to albumin administration persists for many hours; in patients with normal blood volume, excess fluid and protein are lost.
Metabolism: Although synthesized in the liver, liver isn't involved in clearance of albumin from plasma in healthy individuals.
Excretion: Little is known about excretion in healthy individuals. Administration of albumin decreases hepatic albumin synthesis and increases albumin clearance if plasma oncotic pressure is high. In certain pathologic states, the liver, kidneys, or intestines may provide elimination mechanisms for albumin.

Route	Onset	Peak	Duration
I.V.	< 15 min	< 15 min	Several hr

Contraindications and precautions
Contraindicated in patients with hypersensitivity to drug. Use with extreme caution in patients with hypertension, cardiac disease, severe pulmonary infection, severe chronic anemia, or hypoalbuminemia with peripheral edema.

Interactions
Drug-drug. *ACE inhibitors:* Atypical reactions when used with plasma exchange of large volumes of albumin. Withhold ACE inhibitors for 24 hours before plasma exchange.

Effects on diagnostic tests
None significant.

Adverse reactions
CNS: headache.
CV: hypotension, tachycardia, *vascular overload after rapid infusion.*
GI: increased salivation, nausea, vomiting.
Metabolic: increased serum alkaline phosphatase level, slightly increased plasma albumin level.
Respiratory: altered respiration, dyspnea, ***pulmonary edema.***
Skin: urticaria, rash.
Other: chills, fever, back pain.

Overdose and treatment
Symptoms of overdose include signs of circulatory overload, such as increased venous pressure and distended neck veins, or pulmonary edema; slow flow to a keep-vein-open rate and reevaluate therapy.

Clinical considerations
- Solution should be a clear amber color; don't use if cloudy or contains sediment. Store at room temperature; freezing may break bottle.
- Use opened solution promptly, discarding unused portion after 4 hours; solution contains no preservatives and becomes unstable.
- One volume of 25% albumin produces the same hemodilution and relative anemia as five volumes of 5% albumin; reference to "1 unit" albumin usually indicates 50 ml of the 25% concentration containing 12.5 g of albumin.
- Dilute if necessary with normal saline solution or 5% dextrose injection. Use 5-micron or larger filter; don't give through 0.22-micron I.V. filter.
- Be certain patient is properly hydrated before starting infusion; product may be administered without regard to blood typing and crossmatching.
- Avoid rapid I.V. infusion; rate is individualized based on patient's age, condition, and diagnosis. In patients with hypovolemic shock, infuse 5% solution at a rate not exceeding 2 to 4 ml/minute, and 25% solution (diluted or undiluted) at a rate not exceeding 1 ml/minute; in patients with normal blood volume, infuse 5% solution at a rate not exceeding 5 to 10 ml/minute, and 25% solution (diluted or undiluted) at a rate not exceeding 2 to 3 ml/minute. Don't give more than 250 g in 48 hours.
- Each liter contains 130 to 160 mEq of sodium before dilution with any additional I.V. fluids; a 50-ml bottle of solution contains 7 to 8 mEq sodium. This preparation was once known as "salt-poor albumin".

Therapeutic monitoring
- Vital signs must be monitored carefully and the patient observed for adverse reactions.
- Monitor intake and output, hematocrit, serum protein, hemoglobin, and electrolyte levels to help determine continuing dosage.
- The goal is to maintain plasma albumin concentrations at 2 to 3 g/dl or an oncotic pres-

sure of 20 (total serum protein concentration of 5.2 g/dl).

Special populations

Pediatric patients. Premature infants with low serum protein concentrations may receive 1.4 to 1.8 ml/kg of a 25% albumin solution/kg by I.V. infusion (350 to 450 mg albumin).

albuterol sulfate

Airet, Proventil, Proventil HFA, Proventil Repetabs, Proventil Syrup, Ventolin, Ventolin Syrup, Volmax

Pharmacologic classification: adrenergic
Therapeutic classification: bronchodilator
Pregnancy risk category C

How supplied

Available by prescription only
Tablets: 2 mg, 4 mg
Tablets (sustained-release): 4 mg, 8 mg
Syrup: 2 mg/5 ml
Aerosol inhaler: 90 mcg/metered spray
Solution for nebulization: 0.083%, 0.5%
Capsules for inhalation: 200 mcg microfine

Indications and dosages

Bronchospasm in patients with reversible obstructive airway disease
Adults and children age 12 and older: Tablets: give 2 to 4 mg (immediate-release) P.O. t.i.d. or q.i.d.; maximum dose, 8 mg q.i.d. Alternatively, use sustained-release tablets. Usual starting dose is 4 mg q 12 hours. Increase to 8 mg q 12 hours if patient fails to respond. Cautiously increase stepwise as needed and tolerated to 16 mg q 12 hours.
Children age 6 to 14: Oral solution: 2 mg P.O. t.i.d. to q.i.d.; may increase to 24 mg/day in divided doses.
Adults and children age 4 and older: Aerosol inhalation: One to two inhalations q 4 to 6 hours. More frequent administration or a greater number of inhalations isn't usually recommended. However, because deposition of inhaled medications is variable, higher doses are occasionally used, especially in patients with acute bronchospasm.
Adults: Solution for inhalation: 2.5 mg t.i.d. or q.i.d. by nebulizer.
Children ages 2 to 12: 0.1 mg/kg to 0.15 mg/kg to maximum of 2.5 mg t.i.d. to q.i.d.
Adults and children age 4 and older: Capsules for inhalation: 200 mcg inhaled q 4 to 6 hours using a Rotahaler inhalation device.
Children age 6 to 11: Administer 2 mg P.O. t.i.d. or q.i.d. or 4 mg extended-release preparation q 12 hours
Children age 2 to 5: Administer 0.1 mg/kg P.O. t.i.d., not to exceed 2 mg t.i.d.
≡***Dosage adjustment.*** In adults over age 65, give 2 mg P.O. t.i.d. or q.i.d.
To prevent exercise-induced bronchospasm
Adults and children age 4 and older: Two inhalations 15 minutes before exercise.

Pharmacodynamics

Bronchodilator action: Selectively stimulates beta-adrenergic receptors of the lungs, uterus, and vascular smooth muscle. Bronchodilation results from relaxation of bronchial smooth muscles, which relieves bronchospasm and reduces airway resistance.

Pharmacokinetics

Absorption: After oral inhalation, appears to be absorbed gradually, over several hours, from the respiratory tract; however, dose is mostly swallowed and absorbed through the GI tract.
Distribution: Doesn't cross the blood-brain barrier.
Metabolism: Extensively metabolized in the liver to inactive compounds.
Excretion: Rapidly excreted in urine and feces. After oral inhalation, 70% of dose is excreted in urine unchanged and as metabolites within 24 hours; 10% in feces. Elimination half-life is about 4 hours. After oral administration, 75% of dose is excreted in urine within 72 hours as metabolites; 4% in feces.

Route	Onset	Peak	Duration
P.O.	15-30 min	2-3 hr	6-12 hr
I.V.	Variable	Unknown	4-6 hr
Inhalation	5-15 min	½-2 hr	2-6 hr

Contraindications and precautions

Contraindicated in patients with hypersensitivity to drug or any component of its formulation. Use cautiously in patients with CV disorders, including coronary insufficiency and hypertension; in patients with hyperthyroidism or diabetes mellitus; and in those who are unusually responsive to adrenergics.

Interactions

Drug-drug. *Epinephrine and other orally inhaled sympathomimetic amines:* May increase sympathomimetic effects and risk of toxicity. Avoid use together.
MAO inhibitors and tricyclic antidepressants: Serious CV effects may follow use. Avoid use together.
Propranolol and other beta blockers: May antagonize the effects of albuterol. Exercise caution when used together.

Effects on diagnostic tests

Albuterol may decrease the sensitivity of spirometry used for the diagnosis of asthma.

Adverse reactions

CNS: *tremor, nervousness,* dizziness, insomnia, *headache, hyperactivity,* weakness, CNS stimulation, malaise, hypesthesia, migraine, hypertonia.
CV: *tachycardia, palpitations,* hypertension.
EENT: dry and irritated nose and throat (with inhaled form), nasal congestion, epistaxis, hoarseness, taste perversion.
GI: heartburn, *nausea, vomiting,* anorexia.
Metabolic: hypokalemia (with high doses).
Musculoskeletal: muscle cramps.
Respiratory: ***bronchospasm,*** cough, wheezing, dyspnea, bronchitis, increased sputum.
Other: increased appetite, ***hypersensitivity reactions.***

Overdose and treatment

Signs and symptoms of overdose include exaggeration of common adverse reactions, particularly angina, hypertension, hypokalemia, and seizures. Cardiac arrest may occur.

To treat, use selective beta blockers (such as metoprolol) with extreme caution; they may induce asthmatic attack. Dialysis isn't appropriate. Monitor vital signs and electrolyte levels closely.

Clinical considerations

Orally inhaled albuterol has been used investigationally to prevent or alleviate episodes of muscle paralysis in the treatment of some patients with hyperkalemic familial periodic paralysis.

Therapeutic monitoring

- Small, transient increases in blood glucose levels may occur after oral inhalation.
- Serum potassium levels may decrease after I.V. and inhalation therapy administration, but potassium supplementation is usually unnecessary.
- Effectiveness of treatment is measured by periodic monitoring of patient's pulmonary function. Monitor for worsening symptoms or loss of control.

Special populations

Pregnant patients. The potential exists for cleft palate and limb defects, however, there's no consistent pattern of congenital abnormalities.
Breast-feeding patients. Because it's unknown if albuterol is excreted in breast milk, alternative feeding methods are recommended.
Pediatric patients. Safety and efficacy of extended-release tablets or immediate-release tablets in children under age 6 haven't been established.
Geriatric patients. Lower doses may be required because geriatric patients are more sensitive to sympathomimetic amines.

Patient counseling

- Instruct patient in proper use of inhaler. Tell him to read directions before use, that dryness of mouth and throat may occur, and that rinsing with water after each dose may help.
Administration by metered-dose nebulizers: Instruct patient to shake canister thoroughly to activate; place mouthpiece well into mouth, aimed at back of throat. Close lips and teeth around mouthpiece. Exhale through nose as completely as possible, then inhale through mouth slowly and deeply while actuating the nebulizer to release dose. Hold breath 10 seconds (count "1-100, 2-100, 3-100," until "10-100" is reached). Remove mouthpiece, and exhale slowly.
Administration by metered powder inhaler: Caution patient not to take forced deep breath, but to breathe with normal force and depth. Observe patient closely for exaggerated systemic drug action.
Administration by oxygen aerosolization: Administer over 15- to 20-minute period, with oxygen flow rate adjusted to 4 L/minute. Turn on oxygen supply before patient places nebulizer in mouth. Lips don't have to be closed tightly around nebulizer opening. Placement of Y tube in rubber tubing permits patient to control administration. Advise patient to rinse mouth immediately after inhalation therapy to help prevent dryness and throat irritation. Rinse mouthpiece thoroughly with warm running water at least once daily to prevent clogging (it isn't dishwasher-safe.) After cleaning, wait until mouthpiece is completely dry before storing. Don't place near artificial heat, such as a dishwasher or oven. Replace reservoir bag every 2 to 3 weeks or as needed; replace mouthpiece every 6 to 9 months or as needed.
Note: Replacement of bags or mouthpieces may require a prescription.
- Advise patient that repeated use may result in paradoxical bronchospasm. In such a case, patient should discontinue drug and contact his health care provider immediately.
- Tell patient to contact his health care provider if troubled breathing persists 1 hour after using medication, if symptoms return within 4 hours, if condition worsens, or if new (refill) canister is needed within 2 weeks.
- Advise patient to wait 15 minutes after using inhaled albuterol before using adrenocorticoids (beclomethasone, dexamethasone, flunisolide, or triamcinolone).
- Warn patient to use only as directed and not to use more than prescribed amount or more often than prescribed.

alclometasone dipropionate

Aclovate

Pharmacologic classification: topical adrenocorticoid
Therapeutic classification: anti-inflammatory
Pregnancy risk category C

How supplied

Available by prescription only
Cream, ointment: 0.05%

Indications and dosages

Inflammation of corticosteroid-responsive dermatoses
Adults: Apply a thin film to affected areas b.i.d. or t.i.d. Gently massage until medication disappears, or apply a thick layer and cover with an occlusive dressing and tape and leave in place overnight or at least 6 hours. Course of treatment may last 2 to 6 weeks. Use occlusive dressing for severe or resistant dermatomes.

Pharmacodynamics

Anti-inflammatory action: Drug stimulates the synthesis of enzymes needed to decrease the inflammatory response. Alclometasone is a group VI nonfluorinated topical glucocorticoid with less anti-inflammatory activity than hydrocortisone 0.2% or greater. It's similar in potency to desonide 0.05% and fluocinolone acetonide 0.01%. Applied topically, alclometasone may be used for refractory lesions of psoriasis and other deep-seated dermatoses such as localized neurodermatitis.

Pharmacokinetics

Absorption: Amount absorbed depends on amount of drug applied and on nature of the skin at the application site. It ranges from about 1% in areas with thick stratum corneum (such as the palms, soles, elbows, and knees) to as high as 36% in areas of the thinnest stratum corneum (face, eyelids, and genitals). Absorption increases in areas of skin damage, inflammation, or occlusion. Some systemic absorption of topical steroids may occur, especially through the oral mucosa.
Distribution: After topical application, distributed throughout the local skin. If absorbed into the circulation, is rapidly removed from the blood and distributed into muscle, liver, skin, intestines, and kidneys.
Metabolism: After topical administration, metabolized primarily in the skin. The small amount absorbed into systemic circulation is metabolized primarily in the liver to inactive compounds.
Excretion: Inactive metabolites are excreted by the kidneys, primarily as glucuronides and sulfates, but also as unconjugated products. Small amounts of the metabolites are also excreted in feces.

Route	Onset	Peak	Duration
Topical	Unknown	Unknown	Unknown

Contraindications and precautions

Contraindicated in patients hypersensitive to corticosteroids.

Interactions

None reported.

Effects on diagnostic tests

None reported.

Adverse reactions

EENT: cataracts, glaucoma (if used around eyes for a prolonged period).
Metabolic: hyperglycemia, glycosuria.
Skin: burning, pruritus, irritation, dryness, erythema, folliculitis, acneiform eruptions, perioral dermatitis, hypopigmentation, hypertrichosis, allergic contact dermatitis; *secondary infection,* maceration, atrophy, striae, miliaria (with occlusive dressings).
Other: ***hypothalamic-pituitary-adrenal axis suppression, Cushing's syndrome.***

Overdose and treatment

No information available.

Clinical considerations

- Recommendations for use of alclometasone and care and teaching of patient during therapy are the same as those for all topical adrenocorticoids.
- Alclometasone isn't for use in the treatment of acne, rosacea, or perioral dermatitis.

Therapeutic monitoring

Monitor for worsening or improved condition.

Special populations

Pregnant patients. The potential exists for maternal toxicity as with other adrenocorticoids.
Breast-feeding patients. Recommendations for use of alclometasone in breast-feeding women are the same as those for all topical adrenocorticoids.
Pediatric patients. Alcometasone has been used safely and effectively in pediatric patients; observe usual precautions involving topical steroid therapy in children.
Geriatric patients. Recommendations for use of alclometasone in geriatric patients are the same as those for all topical adrenocorticoids.

Patient counseling

- Tell patient to use drug as directed.
- Advise patient to contact health care provider if condition worsens.

aldesleukin (interleukin-2, IL-2)

Proleukin

Pharmacologic classification: lymphokine
Therapeutic classification: immunoregulatory
Pregnancy risk category C

How supplied

Available by prescription only
Injection: 22 million IU/vial

Indications and dosages

Metastatic renal cell carcinoma, metastatic melanoma

Adults: 600,000 IU/kg (0.037 mg/kg) I.V. q 8 hours for 5 days (a total of 14 doses). After a 9-day rest, repeat sequence for another 14 doses. Repeat courses may be administered after a rest period of at least 7 weeks from hospital discharge.
◊*Adults:* Continuous I.V. infusion of 18 million IU/m^2 for two 5-day cycles with a 5- to 8-day rest between cycles.
◊*Adults:* 18 million IU S.C. daily for 5 days, followed by 2-day rest period.

Pharmacodynamics

Immunoregulatory action: Aldesleukin is a lymphokine, a highly purified immunoregulatory protein synthesized using genetically engineered *Escherichia coli*. The drug produced is similar to human IL-2: it enhances lymphocyte mitogenesis, stimulates long-term growth of IL-2-dependent cell lines, enhances lymphocyte cytotoxicity, induces both lymphokine-activated and natural killer cell activity, and induces the production of interferon gamma.

Pharmacokinetics

Absorption: Onset is rapid after I.V. administration.
Distribution: Peak serum levels are proportional to dose. About 30% is rapidly distributed in plasma; the balance is rapidly distributed to the liver, kidneys, and lungs. Initial studies indicate that the distribution half-life is 13 minutes after a 5-minute I.V. infusion.
Metabolism: Metabolized by the kidneys to amino acids within the cells lining the proximal convoluted tubules.
Excretion: Excreted through the kidneys by peritubular extraction and glomerular filtration. Peritubular extraction ensures drug clearance as renal function diminishes and serum creatinine increases. Elimination half-life is 85 minutes.

Route	Onset	Peak	Duration
I.V.	4 wk	Unknown	< 12 mo

Contraindications and precautions

Contraindicated in patients hypersensitive to drug or any component of the formulation and in those with abnormal cardiac (thallium) stress test or pulmonary function tests or organ allografts. Retreatment is contraindicated in patients who experience the following adverse effects: pericardial tamponade; respiratory dysfunction requiring intubation; disturbances in cardiac rhythm that were uncontrolled or unresponsive to intervention; sustained ventricular tachycardia (five beats or more); chest pain accompanied by ECG changes, indicating MI or angina pectoris; renal dysfunction requiring dialysis for 72 hours or more; coma or toxic psychosis lasting 48 hours or more; seizures that are repetitive or difficult to control; ischemia or perforation of the bowel; GI bleeding requiring surgery.

Use with extreme caution in patients with cardiac or pulmonary disease or seizure disorders.

Interactions

Drug-drug. *Antihypertensives:* May increase risk of hypotension. Use together cautiously.
Corticosteroids: May decrease antitumor effectiveness of aldesleukin. Recommend monitoring drug effect.
Hepatotoxic, nephrotoxic, cardiotoxic, or myelotoxic drugs: May enhance the toxicity of these drugs. Use together cautiously.
Psychotropic agents: Altered CNS function. Use together cautiously.

Effects on diagnostic tests

None reported.

Adverse reactions

CNS: *malaise, headache, mental status changes, dizziness, sensory dysfunction, special senses disorders, syncope, motor dysfunction,* ***coma,*** fatigue, ***seizures.***
CV: *hypotension, sinus tachycardia,* ***arrhythmias, bradycardia,*** *PVCs, premature atrial contractions,* chest pain, ***MI, heart failure, cardiac arrest,*** myocarditis, endocarditis, ***CVA,*** pericardial effusion, thrombosis, ***capillary leak syndrome (CLS).***
EENT: conjunctivitis.
GI: *nausea, vomiting, diarrhea,* abdominal pain, *stomatitis, anorexia, bleeding, dyspepsia, constipation,* ***bowel perforation/infarction.***
GU: *elevated BUN and serum creatinine levels, oliguria, anuria, proteinuria, hematuria, dysuria,* urine retention, urinary frequency, urinary tract infection (UTI).
Hematologic: *anemia,* **THROMBOCYTOPENIA, LEUKOPENIA,** *coagulation disorders,* leukocytosis, eosinophilia.
Hepatic: *jaundice,* ascites, hepatomegaly, *elevated bilirubin, serum transaminase, and alkaline phosphatase levels.*
Metabolic: *hypomagnesemia; acidosis; hypocalcemia; hypophosphatemia; hypokalemia;*

hyperuricemia; hypoalbuminemia; hypoproteinemia; hyponatremia; hyperkalemia.
Musculoskeletal: arthralgia; myalgia, back pain.
Respiratory: pulmonary congestion, dyspnea, ***pulmonary edema, respiratory failure, pleural effusion, apnea***, pneumothorax, tachypnea.
Skin: pruritus, erythema, rash, dryness, exfoliative dermatitis, purpura, alopecia, petechiae.
Other: fever; chills; weakness; edema; infections of catheter tip or injection site; phlebitis; **SEPSIS;** weight gain or loss, ***gangrene.***

Overdose and treatment

Administration of high doses produces rapid onset of expected adverse reactions, including cardiac, renal, and hepatic toxicity.

Drug toxicity is dose-related. Treatment is supportive. Because of short serum half-life of drug, discontinuation may ameliorate many of the adverse effects. Dexamethasone may decrease the toxicity of drug but may also impair effectiveness.

Clinical considerations

- Patients should be neurologically stable with a negative computed tomography scan for CNS metastases. Drug may exacerbate symptoms in patients with unrecognized or undiagnosed CNS metastases.
- Renal and hepatic impairment occur during treatment. Avoid administering other hepatotoxic or nephrotoxic drugs because toxicity may be additive. Be prepared to adjust dosage of other drugs to compensate for this impairment. Dosage modification because of toxicity is usually accomplished by holding a dose or interrupting therapy rather than by reducing the dose to be administered.
- Severe anemia or thrombocytopenia may occur. Packed RBCs or platelets may be necessary.
- Treat previous infections before initiating therapy.
- Treat CLS with careful monitoring of fluid status, pulse, mental status, urine output, and organ perfusion. Central venous pressure monitoring is necessary.
- Because fluid management or administration of pressor agents may be essential to treat CLS, use cautiously in patients who require large volumes of fluid (such as patients with hypercalcemia).
- Reconstitute and dilute carefully to avoid altering the pharmacologic properties of drug; follow manufacturer's recommendations. Don't mix with other drugs.
- Reconstitute vial containing 22 million IU (1.3 mg) with 1.2 ml sterile water for injection. Don't use bacteriostatic water or normal saline injection because these diluents cause increased aggregation of drug. Direct the stream at the sides of the vial and gently swirl to reconstitute. Don't shake.
- Reconstituted solution will have a concentration of 18 million IU (1.1 mg)/ml. Reconstituted drug should be particle-free and colorless to slightly yellow.
- Add the correct dose of reconstituted drug to 50 ml D_5W and infuse over 15 minutes. Don't use an in-line filter. Plastic infusion bags are preferred because they provide consistent drug delivery.
- Vials are for single-use only and contain no preservatives. Discard unused drug.
- Powder for injection or reconstituted solutions must be stored in the refrigerator. After reconstitution and dilution, drug must be administered within 48 hours. Be sure that solutions are returned to room temperature before administering drug to patient.
- Preliminary studies indicate that a high percentage of patients (over 75%) develop nonneutralizing antibodies to aldesleukin when treated with the every-8-hour dosing regimen. Neutralizing antibodies develop in less than 1%. The clinical significance of this finding isn't yet known.
- Aldesleukin has been investigated for various cancers, including Kaposi's sarcoma, metastatic melanoma, colorectal cancer, and malignant lymphoma.

Therapeutic monitoring

- Recommend performing standard hematologic tests, including CBC, differential, and platelet counts; serum electrolytes; and renal and hepatic function tests before therapy. Also recommend obtaining chest X-ray. This should be repeated daily during drug administration.
- Recommend monitoring CNS effects of drug and discontinuing drug if moderate to severe lethargy or somnolence develops because continued administration can result in coma.
- Advise taking vital signs including patient's temperature q 4 hours and weighing patient daily.

Special populations

Pregnant patients. It's unknown if drug causes fetal harm in pregnant women. Don't use in pregnancy if possible.
Breast-feeding patients. It's unknown if drug is excreted in breast milk. Consider risk and benefit and decide whether to discontinue drug or breast-feeding because of risk of serious adverse effects to the infant.
Pediatric patients. Safety and efficacy haven't been established in children under age 18.

Patient counseling

- Make sure patient understands the serious toxicity associated with drug. Adverse effects are expected with normal doses, and serious toxicity may occur despite close clinical monitoring.

alendronate sodium

Fosamax

Pharmacologic classification: osteoclast-mediated bone resorption inhibitor
Therapeutic classification: antiosteoporotic
Pregnancy risk category C

How supplied

Available by prescription only
Tablets: 5 mg, 10 mg, 40 mg

Indications and dosages

Osteoporosis in postmenopausal women
Adults: 10 mg P.O. daily taken with water at least 30 minutes before first food, beverage, or medication of the day.
Prevention of osteoporosis in postmenopausal women
Adults: 5 mg P.O. daily taken with water at least 30 minutes before first food, beverage, or medication of the day.
Conjunction with calcium and vitamin D supplementation in the treatment of corticosteroid-induced osteoporosis
Adults: 5 mg P.O. daily. In postmenopausal women not receiving estrogen replacement therapy, dose is 10 mg P.O. daily.
Paget's disease of bone
Adults: 40 mg P.O. daily for 6 months taken with water at least 30 minutes before first food, beverage, or medication of the day.

Pharmacodynamics

Antiosteoporotic action: At the cellular level, alendronate suppresses osteoclast activity on newly formed resorption surfaces, which reduces bone turnover. Bone formation exceeds bone resorption at bone remodeling sites and thus leads to progressive gains in bone mass.

Pharmacokinetics

Absorption: Absorbed from the GI tract. Food or beverages can decrease bioavailability significantly.
Distribution: Distribution is to soft tissues but is then rapidly redistributed to bone or excreted in urine. Protein binding is about 78%.
Metabolism: Doesn't appear to be metabolized.
Excretion: Excreted in urine.

Route	Onset	Peak	Duration
P.O.	Unknown	Unknown	Unknown

Contraindications and precautions

Contraindicated in patients with hypersensitivity to any component of drug, hypocalcemia, or severe renal insufficiency (creatinine clearance below 35 ml/minute).

Use cautiously in patients with active upper GI problems, such as dysphagia, symptomatic esophageal diseases, gastritis, duodenitis, or ulcers, and in patients with mild to moderate renal insufficiency (creatinine clearance between 35 and 60 ml/minute).

Interactions

Drug-drug. *Antacids and calcium supplements:* Interfere with absorption of alendronate. Instruct patient to wait at least 30 minutes after taking alendronate before consuming other drugs.
Aspirin and NSAIDs: Increase risk of upper GI adverse reactions with alendronate doses above 10 mg daily. Monitor patient closely.
Hormone replacement therapy: Not recommended when used in treatment of osteoporosis with alendronate because of lack of clinical evidence regarding effectiveness.

Effects on diagnostic tests

None reported.

Adverse reactions

CNS: headache.
EENT: taste perversion.
GI: abdominal pain, nausea, dyspepsia, constipation, diarrhea, flatulence, acid regurgitation, esophageal ulcer, vomiting, dysphagia, abdominal distention, gastritis.
Metabolic: musculoskeletal pain.

Overdose and treatment

Hypocalcemia, hypophosphatemia, and upper GI adverse effects, such as upset stomach, heartburn, esophagitis, gastritis, or ulcer, may result from oral overdose. Specific information isn't available, but consider administration of milk or antacids (to bind alendronate). Dialysis isn't beneficial.

Clinical considerations

- Hypocalcemia must be corrected before drug therapy begins. Other disturbances of mineral metabolism (such as vitamin D deficiency) should also be corrected before initiating therapy.
- When drug is used to treat osteoporosis in postmenopausal women, disease is confirmed by low bone mass findings on diagnostic studies or history of an osteoporotic fracture.
- Drug is indicated for patients with Paget's disease who have alkaline phosphatase levels at least twice the upper limit for normal, in those who are symptomatic, or in those at risk for future complications from the disease.

□ ***ALERT*** Advise patient to take with a full glass of water and sit upright for 30 minutes to avoid esophageal ulcer formation.

Therapeutic monitoring

- Monitor patient's serum calcium and phosphate levels throughout therapy.

- Recommend assessing for dysphagia, odynophagia, or retrosternal pain.
- Monitor patient's renal function tests. Manufacturer doesn't recommend using medication in patients with creatinine clearance less than 35ml/minute.

Special populations
Breast-feeding patients. Because drug may be excreted in breast milk, don't give to breast-feeding women.
Pediatric patients. Safety and efficacy in children haven't been established.
Geriatric patients. Although no overall differences in efficacy or safety were observed in clinical trials between geriatric and younger patients, greater sensitivity of some older individuals can't be ruled out. Use cautiously in this age group.

Patient counseling
- Stress importance of taking each tablet with a glass of plain water (not mineral water or other beverage) first thing in the morning at least 30 minutes before ingesting food, beverages, or other drugs. Tell patient that waiting longer than 30 minutes improves absorption of drug.
- Warn patient not to lie down for at least 30 minutes after taking drug to facilitate delivery to stomach and to reduce the potential for esophageal irritation.
- Tell patient to take supplemental calcium and vitamin D if daily dietary intake is inadequate.
- Inform patient about the benefit of weight-bearing exercises in increasing bone mass and the importance of modifying excessive cigarette smoking and alcohol consumption, if these factors are part of patient's lifestyle.

alitretinoin
Panretin

Pharmacologic classification: retinoid
Therapeutic classification: anti-Kaposi's sarcoma lesions
Pregnancy risk category D

How supplied
Available by prescription only
Gel: 0.1%

Indications and dosages
Cutaneous lesions in patients with Kaposi's sarcoma related to AIDS
Adults: Initially, apply generous coating of gel twice daily to lesions only. Frequency may be increased to 3 to 4 times daily based on patient tolerance. If site toxicity occurs, frequency may be reduced. If severe irritation occurs, drug may be temporarily discontinued for a few days until symptoms subside.

Pharmacodynamics
Anti-Kaposi's sarcoma lesion action: Binds to and activates all known intracellular retinoid receptor subtypes. Once activated, these receptors function as transcription factors that regulate the expression of genes that control the process of cellular differentiation and proliferation in both normal and neoplastic cells. Alitretinoin inhibits the growth of Kaposi's sarcoma cells in vitro.

Pharmacokinetics
No information available.

Route	Onset	Peak	Duration
Topical	Unknown	Unknown	Unknown

Contraindications and precautions
Contraindicated in women with childbearing potential and in patients with known hypersensitivity to retinoids or drug or its components.

Gel shouldn't be used on patients requiring systemic anti-Kaposi's sarcoma therapy, such as those with more than 10 new Kaposi's sarcoma lesions in the prior month, symptomatic lymphedema, symptomatic pulmonary Kaposi's sarcoma, or symptomatic visceral involvement.

Interactions
Drug-lifestyle: *Sun exposure:* Photosensitization may result. Minimize exposure of treated areas to sunlight and sunlamps during use.
DEET (N,N-diethyl-m-toluamide), a common component of insect repellent products: Increases DEET toxicity. Don't use insect repellent products containing DEET while using this gel.

Effects on diagnostic tests
None reported.

Adverse reactions
CNS: paresthesia.
Skin: rash, burning pain at application site, pruritus, exfoliative dermatitis, skin disorder (excoriation, drainage, fissures, cracking, scabbing, crusting, oozing), edema.

Overdose and treatment
There has been no experience with acute overdose of Panretin gel in humans. Systemic toxicity following acute overdose with topical application of Panretin is unlikely because of limited systemic plasma levels observed with normal therapeutic doses. There is no specific antidote for overdose.

Clinical considerations
- For severe irritation, application of drug can be temporarily discontinued for a few days until symptoms subside.

■ Although effects of medication may be evident after 2 weeks, most patients require longer application time.
■ Don't apply an occlusive dressing to the site.

Therapeutic monitoring

If application site toxicity occurs, advise reduced frequency of use.

Special populations

Pregnant patients. Significant systemic absorption could cause fetal harm.
Breast-feeding patients. It's unknown if alitretinoin or its metabolites are excreted in breast milk. Because many drugs are excreted in breast milk and because of the potential for adverse reactions from Panretin in nursing infants, women should discontinue nursing before using the drug.
Pediatric patients. Safety and effectiveness in pediatric patients haven't been established.
Geriatric patients. Safety and effectiveness in patients age 65 or over haven't been established.

Patient counseling

■ Inform the patient that a response may be seen as soon as 2 weeks after starting treatment but most patients require longer application. Some patients need more than 14 weeks to respond.
■ Tell patient to continue the drug as long as there is benefit.
■ Advise patient to avoid photosensitivity reaction by limiting exposure to sunlight and sunlamps.
■ Tell patient to allow the gel to dry for 3 to 5 minutes before covering with clothing. Because unaffected skin may become irritated, avoid application of the gel to normal skin surrounding the lesions. In addition, tell patient not to apply gel on or near mucosal surfaces of the body.

allopurinol

Purinol*, Zyloprim

allopurinol sodium

Aloprim

Pharmacologic classification: xanthine oxidase inhibitor
Therapeutic classification: antigout
Pregnancy risk category C

How supplied

Available by prescription only
Tablets (scored): 100 mg, 200 mg*, 300 mg
Injection: 500 mg/30 ml vials

Indications and dosages

Gout, primary or secondary hyperuricemia
Gout may be secondary to diseases such as acute or chronic leukemia, polycythemia vera, multiple myeloma, or psoriasis or after administration of chemotherapeutic agents. Dosage varies with severity of disease; it can be given as single dose or divided, but divide doses larger than 300 mg.
Adults: Mild gout, 200 to 300 mg P.O. daily; severe gout with large tophi, 400 to 600 mg P.O. daily. Same dose for maintenance in secondary hyperuricemia.
Hyperuricemia secondary to malignancies
Children age 6 to 10: 300 mg P.O. daily (100 mg t.i.d.).
Children under age 6: 150 mg P.O. daily (50 mg t.i.d.).
Prevention of acute gouty attacks
Adults: 100 mg P.O. daily; increase at weekly intervals by 100 mg without exceeding maximum dose (800 mg) until serum uric acid level decreases to 6 mg/dl or less.
Prevention of uric acid nephropathy during cancer chemotherapy
Adults: 600 to 800 mg P.O. daily for 2 to 3 days in conjunction with high fluid intake. In those who can't tolerate oral therapy, 200 to 400 mg/m^2 I.V. daily as a single infusion or in divided infusions at 6-, 8-, or 12-hour intervals. Maximum I.V. dose is 600 mg/day.
Children: 200 mg/m^2 I.V. daily as a single infusion or in divided infusions at 6-, 8-, or 12-hour intervals.
≡***Dosage adjustment.*** For I.V. allopurinol sodium in patients with a creatinine clearance of less than 3 ml/minute, give 100 mg/day at extended intervals; for creatinine clearance of 3 to 10 ml/minute, give 100 mg/day; for 10 to 20 ml/minute, give 200 mg/day.
Recurrent calcium oxalate calculi
Adults: 200 to 300 mg P.O. daily in single dose or divided doses.
≡***Dosage adjustment.*** In adults with creatinine clearance up to 9 ml/minute, give 100 mg q 3 days; for creatinine clearance of 10 to 19 ml/minute, give 100 mg every other day; for 20 to 39 ml/minute, give 100 mg daily; for 40 to 59 ml/minute, give 150 mg daily; for 60 to 79 ml/minute, give 200 mg daily; for 80 ml/minute, give 250 mg daily.

Pharmacodynamics

Antigout action: Allopurinol inhibits xanthine oxidase, the enzyme catalyzing the conversion of hypoxanthine to xanthine, and the conversion of xanthine to uric acid. By blocking this enzyme, allopurinol and its metabolite, oxypurinol, prevent the conversion of oxypurines (xanthine and hypoxanthine) to uric acid, thus decreasing serum and urine levels of uric acid. Drug has no analgesic, anti-inflammatory, or uricosuric action.

Pharmacokinetics

Absorption: After oral administration, about 80% to 90% of dose is absorbed.
Distribution: Distributed widely throughout the body except in the brain, where drug concentrations are 50% of those found in the rest of the body. Allopurinol and oxypurinol aren't bound to plasma proteins.
Metabolism: Metabolized to oxypurinol by xanthine oxidase. Half-life of allopurinol is 1 to 2 hours; half-life of oxypurinol, about 15 hours.
Excretion: 5% to 7% of allopurinol dose is excreted in the urine unchanged within 6 hours of ingestion. Afterward, it's excreted by the kidneys as oxypurinol, allopurinol, and oxypurinol ribonucleosides. About 70% of the administered daily dose is excreted in the urine as oxypurinol and an additional 2% appears in the feces as unchanged drug within 48 to 72 hours.

Route	Onset	Peak	Duration
P.O.	Unknown	½-2 hr	1-2 wk
I.V.	Unknown	½ hr	Unknown

Contraindications and precautions

Contraindicated in patients with hypersensitivity to drug and in those with idiopathic hemochromatosis.

Interactions

Drug-drug. *Thiazide diuretics:* In patients with decreased renal function, the use of allopurinol with a thiazide diuretic may increase the risk of allopurinol-induced hypersensitivity reactions. Use together cautiously.
Azathioprine and mercaptopurine: May increase the toxic effects of these drugs, particularly bone marrow depression. Combined use of these drugs requires reduction of initial doses of azathioprine or mercaptopurine to 25% to 33% of the usual dose, with subsequent doses adjusted according to patient response and toxic effects.
Cyclophosphamide: May increase the incidence of bone marrow depression through an unknown mechanism. Advise monitoring patient for this effect.
Dicumarol: Allopurinol inhibits hepatic microsomal metabolism of this drug, thus increasing the half-life of dicumarol; observe patients receiving both drugs for increased anticoagulant effects.
Ampicillin or amoxicillin: May increase the incidence of rash. Advise monitoring patient for this effect.
Chlorpropamide: Because allopurinol or its metabolites may compete with chlorpropamide for renal tubular secretion, observe patients who receive these drugs together for signs of excessive hypoglycemia.
Co-trimoxazole: Use with allopurinol has been associated with thrombocytopenia. Recommend monitoring CBC with platelets.
Theophylline: Theophylline clearance can decrease with large doses (600 mg/day), leading to increased plasma theophylline levels. Recommend monitoring drug levels.

Effects on diagnostic tests

None reported.

Adverse reactions

CNS: drowsiness, headache, paresthesia, peripheral neuropathy, neuritis.
CV: hypersensitivity vasculitis, necrotizing angitis.
EENT: epistaxis, taste loss or perversion.
GI: nausea, vomiting, diarrhea, abdominal pain, gastritis, dyspepsia.
GU: ***renal failure,*** uremia.
Hematologic: ***agranulocytosis,*** anemia, ***aplastic anemia, thrombocytopenia, leukopenia,*** leukocytosis, eosinophilia.
Hepatic: altered liver function studies, ***hepatitis, hepatic necrosis,*** hepatomegaly, cholestatic jaundice.
Musculoskeletal: arthralgia, myopathy.
Skin: alopecia, ecchymoses, *rash* (usually maculopapular); ***exfoliative, urticarial, and purpuric lesions; Stevens-Johnson syndrome (erythema multiforme);*** severe furunculosis of nose; ichthyosis, ***toxic epidermal necrolysis.***
Other: fever, chills.

Overdose and treatment

No information available.

Clinical considerations

- Rash occurs mostly in patients taking diuretics and in those with renal disorders.
- If renal insufficiency occurs during treatment, reduce allopurinol dose.
- Acute gouty attacks may occur in first 6 weeks of therapy; concurrent use of colchicine or another anti-inflammatory agent may be prescribed prophylactically.
- Minimize GI adverse reactions by administering drug with meals or immediately after. Tablets may be crushed and administered with fluid or food.
- Allopurinol may predispose patient to ampicillin-induced rash if taken together.
- Allopurinol-induced rash may occur weeks after discontinuation of drug.
- When allopurinol is added to a therapeutic regimen of colchicine, uricosuric agents, or anti-inflammatory agents, it may take months to discontinue the latter drugs.
- Allopurinol has been used to reduce hyperuricemia resulting from G6PD deficiency, Lesch-Nyhan syndrome, polycythemia vera, sarcoidosis, and administration of thiazides or ethambutol.

■ Preparation of allopurinol sodium includes reconstitution and dilution. Dissolve each 30-ml vial with 25 ml of sterile water for injection. Dilute this solution to a desired concentration (no greater than 6 mg/ml) with normal saline injection or 5% dextrose for injection. Sodium-bicarbonate-containing solutions shouldn't be used. Store at 68° to 77° F (20° to 25° C) and use within 10 hours. Don't use if particulate matter or discoloration is present. Refer to package insert for a full list of drugs with which Aloprim is incompatible in solution.

Therapeutic monitoring

■ Monitor patient's intake and output. Daily urine output of at least 2 L and maintenance of neutral or slightly alkaline urine is desirable.
■ Recommend monitoring CBC, serum uric acid levels, and hepatic and renal function at start of therapy and periodically thereafter.

Special populations

Breast-feeding patients. Because oxypurinol and allopurinol are distributed in breast milk, use allopurinol with extreme caution in breast-feeding women.
Pediatric patients. Don't use drug in children except to treat hyperuricemia resulting from malignancies.
Geriatric patients. Follow dosage recommendations for adults. Watch for renal disorders or impaired renal function and treat according to dosage recommendations for patients with impaired renal function.

Patient counseling

■ Encourage patient to drink 10 to 12 8-oz (240-ml) glasses of water daily while taking drug unless otherwise contraindicated.
■ When using drug to treat recurrent calcium oxalate stones, advise patient to reduce dietary intake of animal protein, sodium, refined sugars, vitamin C, oxalate-rich foods, and calcium.
■ Advise patient to avoid hazardous activities requiring alertness until CNS response to drug is known, because drowsiness may occur.
■ Advise patient to avoid alcohol because it decreases effectiveness of allopurinol.
■ Tell patient to report all adverse reactions immediately.
■ Advise patient to take a missed dose when it's remembered unless it's time for next scheduled dose; he shouldn't double the dose.
■ Tell patient to discontinue drug and contact his health care provider at first sign of rash or other allergic reaction.

alprazolam

Alprazolam Intensol, Apo-Alpraz*, Novo-Alprazol*, Xanax

Pharmacologic classification: benzodiazepine
Therapeutic classification: antianxiety
Controlled substance schedule IV
Pregnancy risk category D

How supplied

Available by prescription only
Tablets: 0.25 mg, 0.5 mg, 1 mg, 2 mg
Oral solution: 0.1 mg/1 ml, 1 mg/1 ml

Indications and dosages

Anxiety
Adults: Usual starting dose is 0.25 to 0.5 mg P.O. t.i.d. Increase dose p.r.n. q 3 to 4 days. Maximum total daily dose, 4 mg in divided doses.
≡***Dosage adjustment.*** In geriatric or debilitated patients or those with hepatic impairment, initial dose is 0.25 mg P.O. b.i.d. or t.i.d.
Panic disorder
Adults: Initially, 0.5 mg P.O. t.i.d. Increase as needed and tolerated at intervals of 3 to 4 days in increments of 1 mg daily. Most patients require more than 4 mg daily; however, doses from 1 to 10 mg daily have been reported.

Pharmacodynamics

Anxiolytic action: Alprazolam depresses the CNS at the limbic and subcortical levels of the brain. It produces an antianxiety effect by enhancing the effect of the neurotransmitter gamma-aminobutyric acid on its receptor in the ascending reticular activating system, which increases inhibition and blocks both cortical and limbic arousal.

Pharmacokinetics

Absorption: Well absorbed when administered orally.
Distribution: Distributed widely throughout the body. About 80% to 90% of an administered dose is bound to plasma protein.
Metabolism: Metabolized in the liver equally to alpha-hydroxyalprazolam and inactive metabolites.
Excretion: Excreted in urine. Half-life of alprazolam is 12 to 15 hours.

Route	Onset	Peak	Duration
P.O.	15-30 min	1-2 hr	Unknown

Contraindications and precautions

Contraindicated in patients with hypersensitivity to drug or other benzodiazepines or acute angle-closure glaucoma. Use cautiously in patients with hepatic, renal, or pulmonary disease.

Interactions

Drug-drug. *Phenothiazines, narcotics, barbiturates, general anesthetics, antihistamines, MAO inhibitors, and antidepressants:* Alprazolam potentiates the CNS depressant effects of these drugs. Avoid use together.
Cimetidine and possibly disulfiram: Diminished hepatic metabolism of alprazolam, increasing its plasma level. Monitor patient carefully.
Haloperidol: Benzodiazepines may decrease serum levels of haloperidol.
Digoxin: Plasma levels of digoxin may increase. Monitor serum digoxin levels.
Rifampin: The effects of alprazolam may decrease with use of rifampin. Recommend monitoring for clinical effect.
Theophylline: May increase the sedative effects of alprazolam. Use together cautiously.
Drug-herb. *Kava:* May induce coma if taken with alprazolam. Avoid use together.
Drug-lifestyle. *Heavy smoking:* Accelerates alprazolam metabolism, thus lowering clinical effectiveness. Advise patient to avoid smoking.
Alcohol use: Alprazolam potentiates the CNS depressant effects of alcohol. Avoid use together.

Effects on diagnostic tests

None reported.

Adverse reactions

CNS: *drowsiness, light-headedness,* minor changes in EEG patterns, headache, confusion, tremor, dizziness, syncope, *depression,* insomnia, nervousness.
CV: hypotension, tachycardia.
EENT: blurred vision, nasal congestion.
GI: *dry mouth,* nausea, vomiting, *diarrhea, constipation.*
Hepatic: elevated liver function test.
Musculoskeletal: muscle rigidity.
Skin: dermatitis.
Other: weight gain or loss.

Overdose and treatment

Signs and symptoms of overdose include somnolence, confusion, coma, hypoactive reflexes, dyspnea, labored breathing, hypotension, bradycardia, slurred speech, unsteady gait, and impaired coordination.

Support blood pressure and respiration until drug effects subside; monitor vital signs. Flumazenil, a specific benzodiazepine antagonist, may be useful. Mechanical ventilatory assistance via endotracheal tube may be required to maintain a patent airway and support adequate oxygenation. As needed, use I.V. fluids and vasopressors, such as dopamine and phenylephrine, to treat hypotension. If the patient is conscious, induce emesis. Use gastric lavage if ingestion was recent, but only if an endotracheal tube is in place to prevent aspiration. After emesis or lavage, administer activated charcoal with a cathartic as a single dose. Dialysis is of limited value. Don't use barbiturates if excitation occurs because of possible exacerbation of excitation or CNS depression.

Clinical considerations

Consider the recommendations relevant to all benzodiazepines as well as the following:
- Lower doses are effective in geriatric patients and patients with renal or hepatic dysfunction.
- Anxiety associated with depression is also responsive to alprazolam but may require more frequent dosing.
- Store drug in a cool, dry place away from direct light.

Therapeutic monitoring

- Recommend monitoring patients receiving prolonged therapy with high doses because they should be weaned from the drug gradually to prevent withdrawal symptoms. A 2- to 3-month withdrawal may be necessary at a decreasing rate of no more than 0.5 mg q 3 days.

Special populations

Breast-feeding patients. The breast-fed infant of a woman taking alprazolam may become sedated, have feeding difficulties, or lose weight. Avoid use in breast-feeding women.
Pediatric patients. Closely observe neonate for withdrawal symptoms if mother took alprazolam during pregnancy. Use of alprazolam during labor may cause neonatal flaccidity. Safety hasn't been established in children or adolescents under age 18.
Geriatric patients. Lower doses are usually effective in geriatric patients because of decreased elimination. During initiation of therapy or after an increase in dose, geriatric patients who receive drug require supervision with ambulation and activities of daily living.

Patient counseling

- Be sure patient understands potential for physical and psychological dependence with chronic use of alprazolam.
- Instruct patient not to alter drug regimen.
- Warn patient that sudden changes in position can cause dizziness. Advise him to dangle legs for a few minutes before getting out of bed to prevent falls and injury.

alprostadil

Prostin VR Pediatric

Pharmacologic classification:
prostaglandin
Therapeutic classification:
prostaglandin derivative
Pregnancy risk category NR

How supplied

Available by prescription only
Injection: 500 mcg/ml

Indications and dosages

Temporary maintenance of patency of ductus arteriosus until surgery can be performed

Infants: Initial I.V. infusion of 0.05 to 0.1 mcg/kg/minute via infusion pump. After satisfactory response is achieved, reduce infusion rate to the lowest dose that will maintain response. Maintenance dosages vary. Infusion rate should be the lowest possible dose and is usually achieved by progressively halving the initial dose. Rates as low as 0.002 to 0.005 mcg/kg/minute have been effective.

Pharmacodynamics

Ductus arteriosus patency adjunct action: Alprostadil, also known as prostaglandin E_1 or PGE_1 is a prostaglandin that relaxes or dilates the rings of smooth muscle of the ductus arteriosus and maintains patency in neonates when infused before natural closure.

Pharmacokinetics

Absorption: Administered I.V.
Distribution: Distributed rapidly throughout the body.
Metabolism: 68% of dose is metabolized in one pass through the lung, primarily by oxidation; 100% is metabolized within 24 hours.
Excretion: Excreted in urine within 24 hours.

Route	Onset	Peak	Duration
I.V.	20 min	1-2 hr	Length of infusion

Contraindications and precautions

Contraindicated in neonates with respiratory distress syndrome. Use cautiously in neonates with bleeding disorders.

Interactions

None reported.

Effects on diagnostic tests

None reported.

Adverse reactions

CNS: ***seizures.***
CV: ***bradycardia***, hypotension, tachycardia, ***cardiac arrest,*** edema.
GI: diarrhea.
Hematologic: ***DIC.***
Metabolic: *hypokalemia.*
Respiratory: **APNEA.**
Other: *flushing, fever,* ***sepsis.***

Overdose and treatment

Signs and symptoms are similar to the adverse reactions and include apnea, bradycardia, pyrexia, hypotension, and flushing. Apnea most commonly occurs in neonates weighing under 4.4 lb (2 kg) at birth and usually develops during the first hour of drug therapy.

Treatment of apnea or bradycardia requires discontinuance of the infusion and appropriate supportive therapy, including mechanical ventilation as needed. Pyrexia or hypotension may be treated by reducing the infusion rate. Correct flushing by repositioning the intra-arterial catheter.

Clinical considerations

- Adding a 500-mcg solution to 50 ml of D_5W or normal saline solution provides a concentration of 10 mcg/ml. At this concentration, a 0.01-ml/kg/minute infusion rate delivers 0.1 mcg/kg/minute of alprostadil. During dilution, take care to avoid direct contact of the concentrate with the wall of the plastic volumetric infusion chamber; if a hazy solution develops, discard the chamber and solution.

□ ***ALERT*** Dilute drug before administration. Discard prepared solution after 24 hours.

- In infants with restricted pulmonary blood flow, measure effectiveness of drug by monitoring blood oxygenation. In infants with restricted systemic blood flow, measure effectiveness of drug by monitoring systemic blood pressure and blood pH.
- Apnea and bradycardia may reflect drug overdose. Stop the infusion immediately if they occur.
- Peripheral arterial vasodilation (flushing) may respond to repositioning of the catheter.
- Drug should be administered only by personnel trained in pediatric intensive care.
- Store ampules in refrigerator.

Therapeutic monitoring

- Assess all vital functions closely and frequently to prevent adverse effects.
- Recommend monitoring arterial pressure by umbilical artery catheter, auscultation, or Doppler transducer. Slow the rate of infusion if arterial pressure decreases significantly.
- Advise close monitoring of respiratory status during treatment, and have ventilatory assistance immediately available.

Special populations

This drug isn't for use in pregnant, breast-feeding, or geriatric adults.

alprostadil

Caverject, Muse, Edex

Pharmacologic classification: prostaglandin
Therapeutic classification: corrective agent for impotence
Pregnancy risk category NR

How supplied

Available by prescription only
Sterile powder for intracavernosal injection for intracavernosal use: 6.15-mcg, 6.225-mcg, 10.75 mcg, 11.9-mcg, 12.45-mcg, 21.5 mcg, 23.2-mcg, 24.9-mcg, 43 mcg, 49.8-mcg vials

Injection (frozen) intracavitary: 10.2 mcg/ml, 20.2 mcg/ml, 40.4 mcg/mL
Urethral suppository pellet: 125 mcg, 250 mcg, 500 mcg, 1,000 mcg

Indications and dosages

Erectile dysfunction of vasculogenic, psychogenic, or mixed etiology
Adults: Dosages are highly individualized. For injection: Initial dose is 2.5 mcg intracavernously. If partial response occurs, increase second dose by 2.5 to 5 mcg, and then increase dose further in increments of 5 to 10 mcg until patient achieves an erection (suitable for intercourse but not lasting over 1 hour). If initial dose isn't effective, increase second dose to 7.5 mcg within 1 hour; then increase dose further in 5- to 10-mcg increments until patient achieves an erection. Patient must remain in doctor's office until complete detumescence occurs. If patient responds, don't repeat procedure for 24 hours. For pellet, start initially with lower doses (125 or 250 mcg). Increases or decreases should be made on separate occasions in a stepwise manner until patient achieves an erection that's sufficient for sexual intercourse.
Erectile dysfunction of pure neurologic etiology (spinal cord injury)
Adults: Dosages are highly individualized. Initial dose is 1.25 mcg intracavernously. If partial response occurs, give second dose of 1.25 mcg and then a third dose of 2.5 mcg; increase dose further in 5-mcg increments until patient achieves an erection (suitable for intercourse but not lasting over 1 hour). If initial dose isn't effective, increase second dose to 2.5 mcg within 1 hour; then increase further in 5-mcg increments until patient achieves an erection. Patient must remain in doctor's office until complete detumescence occurs. No more than two doses administered 1 hour apart should be given in 1 day. If patient responds, don't repeat procedure for 24 hours.

Pharmacodynamics

Corrective action in impotence: A prostaglandin derivative that induces erection by relaxation of trabecular smooth muscle and by dilation of cavernosal arteries. This leads to expansion of lacunar spaces and entrapment of blood by compressing the venules against the tunica albuginea, a process referred to as the corporal veno-occlusive mechanism.

Pharmacokinetics

Absorption: Absolute bioavailability hasn't been determined.
Distribution: Bound in plasma protein primarily to albumin (81%).
Metabolism: Rapidly converted to compounds that are further metabolized before excretion.
Excretion: Excreted primarily in urine, the remainder in feces.

Route	Onset	Peak	Duration
Intracavernous	Unknown	2-5 min	2 hr
P.R.	10 min	16 min	1-2 hr

Contraindications and precautions

Contraindicated in patients with hypersensitivity to drug, conditions associated with disposition to priapism (sickle cell anemia or trait, multiple myeloma, or leukemia), or penile deformation (angulation, cavernosal fibrosis, or Peyronie's disease). Don't administer to men with penile implants or when sexual activity is contraindicated. Also avoid use in women, children, and neonates. Muse shouldn't be used for sexual intercourse with a pregnant woman unless the couple uses a condom barrier.

Interactions

Drug-drug. *Anticoagulants:* Increased risk of bleeding from intracavernosal injection site. Monitor patient closely.
Cyclosporine: Decreased cyclosporine level. Use together cautiously.
Vasoactive agents: Safety and efficacy of use with other agents hasn't been studied and, therefore, isn't recommended.

Effects on diagnostic tests

None reported.

Adverse reactions

CNS: headache, dizziness, fainting.
CV: hypertension, hypotension, swelling of leg veins.
GU: *penile pain,* prolonged erection, penile fibrosis, penis disorder, penile rash, penile edema, prostatic disorder, testicular and perineal aching, burning of urethra, minor urethral burning.
Musculoskeletal: back pain.
Respiratory: upper respiratory infection, flu syndrome, sinusitis, nasal congestion, cough.
Other: injection site hematoma, injection site ecchymosis, localized trauma, localized pain.

Overdose and treatment

If intracavernous overdose of drug occurs, patient should be under medical supervision until systemic effects have resolved or penile detumescence has occurred. Symptomatic treatment of systemic symptoms is appropriate.

Clinical considerations

- Patient must have underlying treatable medical causes of erectile dysfunction diagnosed and treated before initiation of therapy.
- Regular follow-up of patient with careful examination of the penis is strongly recommended to detect signs of penile fibrosis. Discontinue drug in patient in whom penile angulation, cav-

ernosal fibrosis, or Peyronie's disease develops.
■ Female partners of users of Muse may experience vaginal itching and burning.
■ Intercavernosal alprostadil has been used as an adjunct to different diagnoses of erectile dysfunction and in evaluating hemodynamic status of erectile tissue.

Therapeutic monitoring
■ Recommend monitoring for hypotension; adjust drug to the lowest effective dose.
■ Advise monitoring for adverse effects and discontinue immediately if penile angulation, cavernosal fibrosis, or Peyronie's disease develops.

Special populations
Breast-feeding patients. Drug isn't indicated for use in women.
Pediatric patients. Drug isn't indicated for use in neonates or children.

Patient counseling
■ To ensure safe and effective use, thoroughly instruct patient how to prepare and administer alprostadil before beginning intracavernosal treatment at home. Stress importance of following instructions carefully.
■ Tell patient to discard vials with precipitates or discoloration. Reconstituted vial is designed for one use only and should be discarded after withdrawal of proper volume of the solution.
■ Instruct patient not to shake the contents of reconstituted vial.
■ Stress importance of not reusing or sharing needles or syringes as well as not sharing medication.
■ Ensure that patient has the manufacturer's instructions for administration included in each package of alprostadil.
■ Tell patient that desirable dose will be established in the doctor's office. Patient shouldn't change the dose without medical approval.
■ Inform patient that he can expect an erection to occur within 5 to 20 minutes after drug administration and that standard treatment goal is to produce an erection not lasting over 1 hour.
■ Warn patient that an erection lasting over 6 hours has been known to occur after alprostadil injection. If this occurs, instruct patient to seek medical attention immediately.
■ Tell patient that drug shouldn't be used more than three times weekly, with at least 24 hours between each use. The maximum frequency use of Muse is two administrations per 24-hour period.
■ Review possible adverse reactions with patient. Tell patient to immediately report priapism, penile pain that wasn't present before or that's increased in intensity, and the occurrence of nodules or hard tissue in the penis.
■ Instruct patient to inspect penis daily for signs or symptoms of redness, swelling, tenderness, or curvature of the erect penis, which might suggest an infection. The patient should contact his health care provider if he suspects infection.
■ Remind patient that regular follow-up visits are necessary to evaluate effectiveness and safety of therapy.
■ Inform patient that drug doesn't offer protection from transmission of sexually transmitted diseases and that protective measures continue to be necessary.
■ Warn patient that a small amount of bleeding can occur at the injection site. This can increase the risk of transmitting blood-borne diseases, if present, to his sexual partner.
■ Caution patient using Muse to use a condom when having sexual intercourse with a pregnant partner; this will also prevent potential vaginal burning and itching in female partner.

alteplase (recombinant alteplase, tissue plasminogen activator)
Activase

Pharmacologic classification: enzyme
Therapeutic classification: thrombolytic enzyme
Pregnancy risk category C

How supplied
Available by prescription only
Injection: 20-mg (11.6 million IU), 50-mg (29 million IU), 100-mg (58 million IU) vials

Indications and dosages
Lysis of thrombi obstructing coronary arteries in management of acute MI
Three-hour infusion
Adults weighing over 143 lb (65 kg): 60 mg in first hour, with 6 to 10 mg I.V. bolus over first 1 to 2 minutes; then 20 mg/hour for an additional 2 hours. Total dose, 100 mg.
Adults weighing 143 lb or less: 1.25 mg/kg given over 3 hours as described above.
Accelerated infusion
Adults weighing over 148 lb (67 kg): 15 mg I.V. push, 50 mg over 30 minutes, then 35 mg over 60 minutes.
Adults weighing 148 lb or less: 15 mg I.V. push, 0.75 mg/kg over 30 minutes (not to exceed 50 mg), then 0.50 mg/kg over 60 minutes (not to exceed 35 mg).
◊ ***Prevention of reocclusion after thrombolysis for acute MI***
Adults: 3.3 mcg/kg/min by I.V. infusion for 4 hours together with heparin therapy immediately after initial thrombolytic infusion.
Pulmonary embolism
Adults: 100 mg by I.V. infusion over 2 hours. Initiate heparin therapy at the end of infusion.

◊*Adults:* 30 to 50 mg infused via the intrapulmonary artery over 1½ or 2 hours, respectively, in conjunction with heparin therapy.
◊***Lysis of arterial occlusion in a peripheral vessel or bypass graft***
Adults: 0.5 to 0.1 mg/kg/hour infused via the intrapulmonary artery for 1 to 8 hours.
Acute ischemic stroke
Adults: 0.9 mg/kg (maximum dose, 90 mg). Administer 10% of dose as an I.V. bolus over 1 minute; remaining 90% over 1 hour.

Pharmacodynamics
Thrombolytic action: Alteplase is an enzyme that catalyzes the conversion of tissue plasminogen to plasmin in the presence of fibrin. This fibrin specificity produces local fibrinolysis in the area of recent clot formation, with limited systemic proteolysis. In patients with acute MI, this allows for reperfusion of ischemic cardiac muscle and improved left ventricular function with a decreased incidence of heart failure after an MI.

Pharmacokinetics
Absorption: Must be given I.V.
Distribution: Rapidly cleared from the plasma by the liver; 80% of dose is cleared within 10 minutes after infusion is discontinued.
Metabolism: Primarily hepatic.
Excretion: Over 85% of drug is excreted in urine; 5% in feces. Plasma half-life is under 10 minutes.

Route	Onset	Peak	Duration
I.V.	Immediate	45 min	4 hr

Contraindications and precautions
Contraindicated in patients with history or evidence of intracranial hemorrhage, suspected subarachnoid hemorrhage, seizure at the onset of stroke, active internal bleeding, intracranial neoplasm, arteriovenous malformation, aneurysm, and severe uncontrolled hypertension (more than 185 mm Hg systolic or 110 mm Hg diastolic). Also contraindicated in patients with a history of CVA, recent (within 2 months) intraspinal or intracranial trauma or surgery, or known bleeding diathesis (see package insert).

Use cautiously in patients with recent (within 10 days) major surgery; in pregnancy and first 10 days postpartum; organ biopsy; trauma (including cardiopulmonary resuscitation); GI or GU bleeding; cerebrovascular disease; hypertension; likelihood of left-sided heart thrombus; hemostatic defects, including those secondary to severe hepatic or renal disease; hepatic dysfunction; occluded AV cannula; severe neurologic deficit (NIH Stroke Scale over 22); signs of major early infarct on a computed tomographic (CT) scan; mitral stenosis; atrial fibrillation; acute pericarditis or subacute bacterial endocarditis; septic thrombophlebitis; diabetic hemorrhagic retinopathy or other hemorrhagic ophthalmic conditions; in those receiving anticoagulants; and in patients age 75 and older.

Interactions
Drug-drug. *Drugs that antagonize platelet function (abciximab, aspirin, dipyridamole):* May increase risk of bleeding if given before, during, or after alteplase therapy. Use together cautiously.

Effects on diagnostic tests
Altered results may be expected in coagulation and fibrinolytic tests. The use of aprotinin (150 to 200 U/ml) in the blood sample may attenuate this interference.

Adverse reactions
CNS: ***cerebral hemorrhage,*** fever.
CV: hypotension, ***arrhythmias,*** edema.
GI: nausea, vomiting.
Hematologic: ***severe, spontaneous bleeding (cerebral, retroperitoneal, GU, GI).***
Other: bleeding at puncture sites, ***hypersensitivity reactions (anaphylaxis).***

Overdose and treatment
No information is available regarding accidental ingestion.

Excessive I.V. dosage can lead to bleeding problems. Doses of 150 mg have been associated with an increased incidence of intracranial bleeding. Discontinue infusion immediately if signs or symptoms of bleeding are observed.

Clinical considerations
- Expect to begin alteplase infusions as soon as possible after onset of MI symptoms, such as angina pain or equivalent greater than 30 minutes' duration; angina that's unresponsive to nitroglycerin; or ECG evidence of MI.
- Administer drug within 3 hours after onset of stroke symptoms after exclusion of intracranial hemorrhage by CT scan or other diagnostic imaging methods capable of detecting presence of hemorrhage. Treatment should only be performed in facilities that can provide appropriate evaluation and management of intracranial hemorrhage.
- Heparin is usually administered during or after alteplase as part of the treatment regimen for acute MI or pulmonary embolism. The use of anticoagulant or antiplatelet therapy for 24 hours is contraindicated when alteplase is used for acute ischemic stroke.
- Discontinue drug therapy for acute ischemic stroke in patients who haven't recently used oral anticoagulants or heparin if pretreatment PT exceeds 15 seconds or if an elevated activated partial PT is identified.
- Staff should avoid I.M. injections, venipuncture, and arterial puncture during therapy. Use

pressure dressings or ice packs on recent puncture sites to prevent bleeding. If arterial puncture is necessary, select a site on the arm and apply pressure for 30 minutes afterward.

- Prepare solution using supplied sterile water for injection. Don't use bacteriostatic water for injection.
- Don't mix other drugs with alteplase. Use 18G needle for preparing solution—aim water stream at lyophilized cake. Expect a slight foaming to occur. Don't use if vacuum isn't present.
- Drug may be further diluted with normal saline solution injection or D_5W to yield a concentration of 0.5 mg/ml. Reconstituted or diluted solutions are stable for up to 8 hours at room temperature.

Therapeutic monitoring

- Advise monitoring for bleeding or hemorrhage.
- Recommend monitoring ECG for transient arrhythmias (sinus bradycardia, ventricular tachycardia, accelerated idioventricular rhythm, ventricular premature depolarizations) associated with reperfusion after coronary thrombolysis. Antiarrhythmic agents should be available.

Special populations

Pediatric patients. Safety and efficacy for use in children haven't been established, but the drug has been used investigationally in children with some success.
Geriatric patients. Due to the potential of CV side effects, use cautiously in patients over age 75.

Patient counseling

- Teach patient signs and symptoms of internal bleeding and tell him to report these immediately.
- Advise patient about proper dental care to avoid excessive gum trauma resulting from vigorous brushing; drug increases chances of bleeding.

aluminum carbonate

Basaljel

Pharmacologic classification: inorganic aluminum salt
Therapeutic classification: antacid, hypophosphatemic agent
Pregnancy risk category NR

How supplied

Available without a prescription
Tablets or capsules: aluminum hydroxide equivalent 500 mg
Suspension: aluminum hydroxide equivalent 400 mg/5 ml

Indications and dosages

Antacid
Adults: 10 ml suspension P.O. q 2 hours p.r.n. or 1 to 2 tablets or capsules q 2 hours p.r.n.
Hyperphosphatemia and prevention of urinary phosphate stones formation (with low-phosphate diet)
Adults: 1 g P.O. t.i.d. or q.i.d.; adjust to lowest possible dose after therapy is initiated, monitoring diet and serum levels.

Pharmacodynamics

Antacid action: Exerts its antacid effect by neutralizing gastric acid; this increases pH, thereby decreasing pepsin activity.
Hypophosphatemic action: Aluminum carbonate reduces serum phosphate levels by complexing with phosphate in the gut. This results in formation of insoluble, nonabsorbable aluminum phosphate, which is then excreted in feces. Calcium absorption increases secondary to reduced phosphate absorption.

Pharmacokinetics

Absorption: Largely unabsorbed; small amounts may be absorbed systemically.
Distribution: None.
Metabolism: None.
Excretion: Excreted in feces; some may be excreted in breast milk.

Route	Onset	Peak	Duration
P.O.	20 min	Unknown	20-180 min

Contraindications and precautions

No known contraindications. Use cautiously in patients with chronic renal disease.

Interactions

Drug-drug. *Tetracycline, quinolones, coumarin anticoagulants, phenothiazines (especially chlorpromazine), chenodiol, antimuscarinics, diazepam, chlordiazepoxide, indomethacin, isoniazid, vitamin A, digoxin, iron salts, and sodium or potassium phosphate:* Aluminum carbonate may decrease absorption of many drugs, thereby lessening their effectiveness. Recommend separate administration by at least 2 hours.
Enterically coated drugs: Premature drug release; these drugs shouldn't be taken together.

Effects on diagnostic tests

Aluminum carbonate may interfere with imaging techniques using sodium pertechnetate Tc99m and thus impair evaluation of Meckel's diverticulum. It may also interfere with reticuloendothelial imaging of liver, spleen, or bone marrow using technetium Tc99m sulfur colloid. It may antagonize the effect of pentagastrin during gastric acid secretion tests.

Adverse reactions

CNS: encephalopathy.

GI: *constipation,* intestinal obstruction increase serum gastrin levels.
Metabolic: hypophosphatemia.
Musculoskeletal: osteomalacia.

Overdose and treatment
No information available. Patients with impaired renal function are at a higher risk of aluminum toxicity to brain, bone, and parathyroid glands.

Clinical considerations
- When administering suspension, shake well and give with small amounts of water or fruit juice.
- After administration through a nasogastric tube, flush tube with water to prevent obstruction.
- When administering drug as an antiurolithic, encourage increased fluid intake to enhance drug effectiveness.
- Constipation may be managed with stool softeners or bulk laxatives, or administer alternately with magnesium-containing antacids (unless patient has renal disease).
- Long-term aluminum carbonate use can lead to calcium resorption and subsequent bone demineralization.

Therapeutic monitoring
Recommend monitoring serum calcium and phosphate levels periodically; reduced serum phosphate levels may lead to increased serum calcium levels.

Special populations
Pediatric patients. Use cautiously in children under age 6. Safety and efficacy haven't been established in children, but drug has been used in a few cases.
Geriatric patients. Because geriatric patients commonly have decreased GI motility, they may become constipated from this drug.

Patient counseling
- Advise patient to take drug only as directed and not to take more than 24 capsules or tablets or 120 ml (24 tsp) of regular suspension in a 24-hour period. Instruct patient to shake suspension well.
- As needed, advise patient to restrict sodium intake, to drink plenty of fluids, and to follow a low-phosphate diet.
- Advise patient not to switch antacids without medical approval.

aluminum hydroxide
ALterna-GEL, Alu-Cap, Alu-Tab, Amphojel, Dialume, Nephrox

Pharmacologic classification: aluminum salt
Therapeutic classification: antacid, hypophosphatemic agent
Pregnancy risk category C

How supplied
Available without a prescription
Tablets: 300 mg, 500 mg, 600 mg
Capsules: 475 mg, 500 mg
Liquid: 600 mg/5 ml
Suspension: 320 mg/5 ml, 450 mg/5 ml, 675 mg/5 ml

Indications and dosages
Antacid; hyperphosphatemia
Adults: 500 to 1,500 mg P.O. (tablet or capsule) 1 hour after meals and h.s.; or 5 to 30 ml of suspension p.r.n. 1 hour after meals and h.s.

Pharmacodynamics
Antacid action: Aluminum hydroxide neutralizes gastric acid, reducing the direct acid irritant effect. This increases pH, thereby decreasing pepsin activity.
Hypophosphatemic action: Aluminum hydroxide reduces serum phosphate levels by complexing with phosphate in the gut, resulting in insoluble, nonabsorbable aluminum phosphate, which is then excreted in feces. Calcium absorption increases as a result of decreased phosphate absorption.

Pharmacokinetics
Absorption: Absorbed minimally; small amounts may be absorbed systemically.
Distribution: None.
Metabolism: None.
Excretion: Excreted in feces; some may be excreted in breast milk.

Route	Onset	Peak	Duration
P.O.	Variable	Unknown	20-180 min

Contraindications and precautions
No known contraindications. Use cautiously in patients with renal disease.

Interactions
Drug-drug. *Quinolones, tetracycline, phenothiazines (especially chlorpromazine), coumarin anticoagulants, chenodiol, antimuscarinics, diazepam, chlordiazepoxide, isoniazid, vitamin A, digoxin, iron salts, and sodium or potassium phosphate:* Aluminum hydroxide may decrease absorption of many drugs, thereby decreasing their effectiveness; separate administration by at least 2 hours.

Enterically coated drugs: Aluminum hydroxide causes premature release of these drugs. Advise separation of doses by 1 hour.

Effects on diagnostic tests

Drug therapy may interfere with imaging techniques using sodium pertechnetate Tc99m and thus impair evaluation of Meckel's diverticulum. It may also interfere with reticuloendothelial imaging of liver, spleen, and bone marrow using technetium Tc99m sulfur colloid. It may antagonize the effect of pentagastrin during gastric acid secretion tests.

Adverse reactions

CNS: encephalopathy.
GI: *constipation,* intestinal obstruction, elevated serum gastrin levels.
Metabolic: hypophosphatemia.
Musculoskeletal: osteomalacia.

Overdose and treatment

No information available. Patients with impaired renal function are at a higher risk of aluminum toxicity to brain, bone, and parathyroid glands.

Clinical considerations

- Shake suspension well (especially extra-strength suspension) and give with small amounts of water or fruit juice.
- After administering through nasogastric tube, flush tube with water to prevent obstruction.
- When drug is used as an antiurolithic, encourage increased fluid intake to enhance drug effectiveness.
- Constipation may be managed with stool softeners or bulk laxatives. Suggest alternating aluminum hydroxide with magnesium-containing antacids (unless patient has renal disease).

Therapeutic monitoring

- Recommend periodically monitoring serum calcium and phosphate levels; decreased serum phosphate levels may lead to increased serum calcium levels.
- Observe patient for hypophosphatemia signs and symptoms (anorexia, muscle weakness, and malaise).

Special populations

Breast-feeding patients. Although drug may be excreted in breast milk, no problems have been associated with its use in breast-feeding women.
Pediatric patients. Use with caution in children under age 6.
Geriatric patients. Because geriatric patients commonly have decreased GI motility, they may become constipated from this drug.

Patient counseling

- Caution patient to take drug only as directed; to shake suspension well or chew tablets thoroughly; and to follow with sips of water or juice.
- As indicated, instruct patient to restrict sodium intake, drink plenty of fluids, or follow a low-phosphate diet.
- Advise patient not to switch to another antacid without medical approval.

amantadine hydrochloride

Symmetrel

Pharmacologic classification: synthetic cyclic primary amine
Therapeutic classification: antiviral, antiparkinsonian
Pregnancy risk category C

How supplied

Available by prescription only
Capsules: 100 mg
Syrup: 50 mg/5 ml
Tablets: 100 mg

Indications and dosages

Prophylaxis or symptomatic treatment of influenza type A virus, respiratory tract illnesses in geriatric or debilitated patients
Adults up to age 64 and children age 10 and older weighing over 88 lb (40 kg): 200 mg P.O. daily in a single dose or divided b.i.d.
Children age 1 to 9: 4.4 to 8.8 mg/kg P.O. daily up to a maximum of 150 mg/day. To reduce toxicity, 5 mg/kg/day given in one or two divided doses (up to a maximum of 150 mg/day) is recommended.
Adults over age 64: 100 mg P.O. once daily. Continue treatment for 24 to 48 hours after symptoms disappear. Prophylaxis should start as soon as possible after initial exposure and continue for at least 10 days after exposure. Prophylactic treatment may be continued up to 90 days for repeated or suspected exposures if influenza virus vaccine is unavailable. If used with influenza virus vaccine, continue dose for 2 to 4 weeks until protection from vaccine develops.
Drug-induced extrapyramidal reactions
Adults: 100 to 300 mg/day P.O. in divided doses.
Idiopathic parkinsonism, parkinsonian syndrome
Adults: 100 mg P.O. b.i.d.; in patients who are seriously ill or receiving other antiparkinsonian drugs, 100 mg/day for at least 1 week, then 100 mg b.i.d., p.r.n. Patient may benefit from as much as 400 mg/day, but doses over 200 mg must be closely supervised.

≡ ***Dosage adjustment.*** In patients with renal dysfunction, base maintenance dosage on creatinine clearance value, as follows:

For syrup, give 200 mg P.O. on the first day; for capsules, give 200 mg P.O the first day, and then 100 mg daily if creatinine clearance is between 30 and 50 ml/minute/1.73 m^2; 200 mg on the first day and 100 mg q alternating day if it ranges between 15 to 29 ml/minute/1.73 m^2; and 200 mg q 7 days if it's below 15 ml/minute/1.73 m^2.

Note: Patients on chronic hemodialysis should receive 200 mg P.O. q 7 days.

Pharmacodynamics

Antiviral action: Amantadine interferes with viral uncoating of the RNA in lysosomes. In vitro, amantadine is active only against influenza type A virus. (However, spontaneous resistance commonly occurs.) In vivo, amantadine may protect against influenza type A virus in 70% to 90% of patients; when administered within 24 to 48 hours of onset of illness, it reduces duration of fever and other systemic symptoms.

Antiparkinsonian action: Amantadine is thought to cause the release of dopamine in the substantia nigra.

Pharmacokinetics

Absorption: Well absorbed from the GI tract with oral administration. Usual serum level is 0.2 to 0.9 mcg/ml. (Neurotoxicity may occur at levels exceeding 1.5 mcg/ml.)

Distribution: Distributed widely throughout body; crosses the blood-brain barrier.

Metabolism: About 10% of dose is metabolized.

Excretion: About 90% of dose is excreted unchanged in urine, primarily by tubular secretion. Portion of drug may be excreted in breast milk. Excretion rate depends on urine pH (acidic pH enhances excretion). Elimination half-life in patients with normal renal function is about 24 hours; in those with renal dysfunction, it may be prolonged to 10 days.

Route	Onset	Peak	Duration
P.O.	Unknown	1-4 hr	Unknown

Contraindications and precautions

Contraindicated in patients with hypersensitivity to drug. Don't use in patients with untreated angle-closure glaucoma. Use cautiously in patients with seizure disorders, heart failure, peripheral edema, hepatic disease, mental illness, eczematoid rash, renal impairment, orthostatic hypotension, and CV disease, and in the elderly.

Interactions

Drug-drug. *Trihexyphenidyl and benztropine (when these drugs are given in high doses):* When used together, amantadine may potentiate anticholinergic adverse effects, possibly causing confusion and hallucinations.

Hydrochlorothiazide and triamterene: A combination of these drugs may decrease urinary amantadine excretion, resulting in increased serum amantadine levels and possible toxicity. Avoid use together.

CNS stimulants: May cause additive stimulation. Avoid use together.

Co-trimoxazole: Decreased renal clearance of amantadine with the potential for toxic delirium. Avoid use together.

Drug-herb. *Jimson weed:* May adversely affect cardiovascular system function. Avoid use together.

Drug-lifestyle. *Alcohol use*: May result in lightheadedness, confusion, fainting, and hypotension. Discourage use together.

Effects on diagnostic tests

None reported.

Adverse reactions

CNS: depression, fatigue, confusion, *dizziness,* hallucinations, anxiety, *irritability,* ataxia, *insomnia,* headache, *light-headedness.*

CV: peripheral edema, orthostatic hypotension, ***heart failure.***

GI: anorexia, *nausea,* constipation, vomiting, dry mouth.

Skin: livedo reticularis (with prolonged use).

Overdose and treatment

Clinical effects of overdose include nausea, vomiting, anorexia, hyperexcitability, tremors, slurred speech, blurred vision, lethargy, anticholinergic symptoms, seizures, and possible ventricular arrhythmias, including torsades de pointes and ventricular fibrillation. CNS effects result from increased levels of dopamine in the brain.

Treatment includes immediate gastric lavage or emesis induction along with supportive measures, forced fluids, and, if necessary, I.V. administration of fluids. Urine acidification may be used to increase drug excretion. Physostigmine may be given (1 to 2 mg by slow I.V. infusion at 1- to 2-hour intervals) to counteract CNS toxicity. Seizures or arrhythmias may be treated with conventional therapy. Monitor patient closely.

Clinical considerations

- To prevent orthostatic hypotension, advise patient to move slowly when changing position (especially when rising to standing position).
- If patient experiences insomnia, administer dose several hours before bedtime.
- Prophylactic drug use is recommended for selected high-risk patients who can't receive influenza virus vaccine. Manufacturer recommends prophylactic therapy lasting up to 90 days with possible repeated or unknown exposure.

Therapeutic monitoring

Recommend monitoring patient's blood pressure if dizziness or lightheadedness occurs.

Special populations

Pregnant patients. There are no adequate controlled studies in pregnant women. Use drug only when benefits outweigh the risks.
Breast-feeding patients. Excreted in breast milk. Avoid breast-feeding during therapy with amantadine.
Pediatric patients. Safety and effectiveness of drug in children under age 1 haven't been established.
Geriatric patients. Geriatric patients are more susceptible to adverse neurologic effects; dividing daily dosage into two doses may reduce risk.

Patient counseling

- Warn patient that drug may impair mental alertness.
- Advise patient to take drug after meals to ensure best absorption.
- Caution patient to avoid abrupt position changes because these may cause light-headedness or dizziness.
- If drug is being taken to treat parkinsonism, warn patient not to discontinue it abruptly because that might precipitate a parkinsonian crisis.
- Warn patient to avoid alcohol while taking drug.
- Instruct patient to report adverse effects promptly, especially dizziness, depression, anxiety, nausea, and urine retention.

amikacin sulfate

Amikin

Pharmacologic classification: aminoglycoside
Therapeutic classification: antibiotic
Pregnancy risk category D

How supplied

Available by prescription only
Injection: 50 mg/ml, 250 mg/ml
Injection for I.V. infusion: 5 mg/ml

Indications and dosages

Serious infections caused by susceptible organisms
Adults and children with normal renal function: 15 mg/kg/day divided q 8 to 12 hours I.M. or I.V. (in 100 to 200 ml D_5W or normal saline administered over 30 to 60 minutes). Don't exceed 1.5 g/day or 15 mg/kg.
◇*Adults:* 4 to 20 mg given intrathecally or intraventricularly as a single dose in conjunction with I.M. or I.V. administration.
Neonates with normal renal function: Initially, 10 mg/kg I.M. or I.V. (in D_5W or normal saline administered over 1 to 2 hours), then 7.5 mg/kg q 12 hours.
Uncomplicated urinary tract infections
Adults: 250 mg I.M. or I.V. b.i.d.
◇***Clinical tuberculosis***
Adults, children, and older infants: 15 mg/kg I.M. daily, 5 times weekly as an adjunct to other antitubercular drugs.
≡***Dosage adjustment.*** In renal failure, initially, 7.5 mg/kg. Subsequent doses and frequency determined by blood amikacin levels and renal function studies. One method is to administer additional 7.5 mg/kg doses and alter dosing interval based on steady state serum creatinine. 7.5 mg/kg doses can be given at intervals (in hours) calculated by multiplying the patient's steady state serum creatinine (in mg/dL) by 9.

Keep peak serum levels between 15 and 35 mcg/ml; trough serum levels shouldn't exceed 5 to 10 mcg/ml.

Pharmacodynamics

Antibiotic action: Amikacin is bactericidal; it binds directly to the 30S ribosomal subunit, thus inhibiting bacterial protein synthesis. Its spectrum of activity includes many aerobic gram-negative organisms (including most strains of *Pseudomonas aeruginosa*) and some aerobic gram-positive organisms. Amikacin may act against some organisms resistant to other aminoglycosides, such as *Proteus, Pseudomonas,* and *Serratia;* some strains of these may be resistant to amikacin. Drug is ineffective against anaerobes.

Pharmacokinetics

Absorption: Poorly absorbed after oral administration and is given parenterally.
Distribution: Distributed widely after parenteral administration; intraocular penetration is poor. Factors that increase volume of distribution (burns, peritonitis) may increase dosage requirements. CSF penetration is low, even in patients with inflamed meninges. Intraventricular administration produces high concentrations throughout the CNS. Protein binding is minimal. Amikacin crosses the placenta.
Metabolism: Not metabolized.
Excretion: Excreted primarily in urine by glomerular filtration; small amounts may be excreted in bile and breast milk. Elimination half-life in adults is 2 to 3 hours. In patients with severe renal damage, half-life may extend to 30 to 86 hours. Over time, amikacin accumulates in inner ear and kidneys; urine concentrations approach 800 mcg/ml 6 hours after a 500-mg I.M. dose.

Route	Onset	Peak	Duration
I.V.	Immediate	Immediate	8-12 hr
I.M.	Unknown	1 hr	8-12 hr

Contraindications and precautions
Contraindicated in patients with hypersensitivity to drug or other aminoglycosides. Use cautiously in patients with impaired renal function or neuromuscular disorders, in neonates and infants, and in the elderly.

Interactions
Drug-drug. *Amphotericin B, loop diuretics, methoxyflurane, polymyxin B, capreomycin, cisplatin, cephalosporins, vancomycin, and other aminoglycosides:* Concurrent use may increase the hazard of nephrotoxicity, ototoxicity, and neurotoxicity. Use together cautiously.
Ethacrynic acid, furosemide, bumetanide, urea, or mannitol: Increased hazard of ototoxicity. Use together cautiously.
Dimenhydrinate, other antiemetics, and antivertigo drugs: May mask amikacin-induced ototoxicity. Monitor patient closely.
General anesthetics or neuromuscular blocking agents such as succinylcholine and tubocurarine: Amikacin may potentiate neuromuscular blockade. Monitor patient closely.
Penicillins: Results in a synergistic bactericidal effect against *Pseudomonas aeruginosa, Escherichia coli, Klebsiella, Citrobacter, Enterobacter, Serratia,* and *Proteus mirabilis.* However, the drugs are physically and chemically incompatible and are inactivated when mixed or given together. Avoid use together.

Effects on diagnostic tests
None reported.

Adverse reactions
CNS: ***neuromuscular blockade.***
EENT: *ototoxicity.*
GU: *nephrotoxicity, azotemia.*
Musculoskeletal: arthralgia, acute muscular paralysis.

Overdose and treatment
Clinical signs of overdose include ototoxicity, nephrotoxicity, and neuromuscular toxicity. Drug can be removed by hemodialysis or peritoneal dialysis. Treatment with calcium salts or anticholinesterases reverses neuromuscular blockade.

Clinical considerations
Consider the recommendations relevant to all aminoglycosides as well as the following:
- Because drug is dialyzable, patients undergoing hemodialysis need dosage adjustments.
- Recommendations for care and teaching of patients during therapy and use in geriatric patients and breast-feeding women are the same as for all aminoglycosides.

□ ***ALERT*** Amikacin may be mistaken as Amicar.
- Prepare I.V. infusion by adding 500 mg of amikacin to 100 to 200 ml of I.V. infusion fluid. Alternatively, prepare ADD-Vantage vials per manufacturer instructions. Infuse over 30 to 60 minutes. For infants, dilute enough to allow an infusion period of 1 to 2 hours.

Therapeutic monitoring
Recommend monitoring peak and trough levels. Peak serum concentrations should be no more than 35 mcg/ml and trough serum concentrations no more than 10 mcg/ml.

Special populations
Pediatric patients. Because potential for ototoxicity is unknown, use amikacin in infants only when other drugs are ineffective or contraindicated. Monitor patient closely during therapy.

Patient counseling
- Instruct patient to report adverse reactions promptly.
- Encourage adequate fluid intake.

amiloride hydrochloride
Midamor

Pharmacologic classification: potassium-sparing diuretic
Therapeutic classification: diuretic, antihypertensive
Pregnancy risk category B

How supplied
Available by prescription only
Tablets: 5 mg

Indications and dosages
Hypertension; edema associated with heart failure, usually in patients who are also taking thiazide or other potassium-wasting diuretics
Adults: Usually 5 mg P.O. daily. Dose may be increased to 10 mg daily, if necessary. Don't exceed 20 mg daily.
◊ ***Lithium-induced polyuria***
Adults: 5 to 10 mg P.O. b.i.d.

Pharmacodynamics
Diuretic action: Amiloride acts directly on the distal renal tubule to inhibit sodium reabsorption and potassium excretion, thereby reducing potassium loss.
Antihypertensive action: Amiloride is commonly used in combination with more effective diuretics to manage edema associated with heart failure, hepatic cirrhosis, and hyperaldosteronism. Mechanism of amiloride's hypotensive effect is unknown.

Pharmacokinetics
Absorption: About 50% is absorbed from GI tract. Food decreases absorption to 30%.
Distribution: Wide extravascular distribution.
Metabolism: Insignificant.

Excretion: Most is excreted in urine; half-life is 6 to 9 hours in patients with normal renal function.

Route	Onset	Peak	Duration
P.O.	2 hr	6-10 hr	24 hr

Contraindications and precautions
Contraindicated in patients with elevated serum potassium level (over 5.5 mEq/L). Don't administer to patients receiving other potassium-sparing diuretics, such as spironolactone and triamterene. Also contraindicated in patients with anuria, acute or chronic renal insufficiency, diabetic nephropathy, and hypersensitivity to drug.

Use with extreme caution in patients with diabetes mellitus.

Interactions
Drug-drug. *Antihypertensive agents:* Amiloride may potentiate hypotensive effects. This may be used to therapeutic advantage.
Digoxin: Renal clearance of digoxin may be decreased, along with the inotropic effect. Use together cautiously.
Lithium: Amiloride may reduce renal clearance of lithium and increase lithium blood levels. Use together cautiously.
NSAIDs, such as indomethacin or ibuprofen: May alter renal function and thus affect potassium excretion. Use together cautiously.
Potassium-sparing diuretics, angiotensin-converting enzyme inhibitors, or potassium-containing medications (parenteral penicillin G): Amiloride increases the risk of hyperkalemia when administered with other drugs. Use together cautiously.
Drug-food. *Potassium-containing salt substitutes:* Increase risk of hyperkalemia. Avoid use together.

Effects on diagnostic tests
Amiloride therapy causes severe hyperkalemia in diabetic patients following I.V. glucose tolerance testing; discontinue drug at least 3 days before testing.

Adverse reactions
CNS: *headache,* weakness, dizziness, encephalopathy.
CV: orthostatic hypotension.
GI: *nausea, anorexia, diarrhea, vomiting,* abdominal pain, constipation, appetite changes.
GU: impotence, abnormal renal function tests.
Hematologic: ***aplastic anemia, neutropenia.***
Hepatic: abnormal hepatic function tests.
Metabolic: hyperkalemia.
Musculoskeletal: muscle cramps.
Respiratory: dyspnea.
Other: fatigue.

Overdose and treatment
Signs and symptoms of overdose are consistent with dehydration and electrolyte disturbance.

Treatment is supportive and symptomatic. In acute ingestion, empty stomach by emesis or lavage. In severe hyperkalemia (6.5 mEq/L or more), reduce serum potassium levels with I.V. sodium bicarbonate or glucose with insulin. A cation exchange resin, sodium polystyrene sulfonate (Kayexalate), given orally or as a retention enema, may also reduce serum potassium levels.

Clinical considerations
Recommendations for use of amiloride and for care and teaching of the patient during therapy are the same as those for all potassium-sparing diuretics.

Therapeutic monitoring
Advise monitoring for signs of hyperkalemia including paresthesia, muscular weakness, fatigue, flaccid paralysis of the extremities, bradycardia, shock, and ECG abnormalities.

Special populations
Pregnant patients. There are no adequate studies involving pregnant women.
Breast-feeding patients. Amiloride is excreted in breast milk in animals; no human data are available.
Pediatric patients. Safety and efficacy in children haven't been established, but a dose of 0.625 mg/kg/day has been used in children weighing 13 to 44 lb (6 to 20 kg).
Geriatric patients. Geriatric and debilitated patients require close observation because they're more susceptible to drug-induced diuresis and hyperkalemia. Reduced dosages may be indicated.

Patient counseling
- Tell patient to take drug with food because it may cause stomach upset.
- Advise patient to avoid consumption of large quantities of foods that are high in potassium.
- Tell patient to notify doctor if symptoms of dehydration occur.

aminocaproic acid
Amicar

Pharmacologic classification: carboxylic acid derivative
Therapeutic classification: fibrinolysis inhibitor
Pregnancy risk category C

How supplied
Available by prescription only
Tablets: 500 mg
Syrup: 250 mg/ml

Injection: 5 g/20 ml for dilution; 24 g/96 ml for infusion

Indications and dosages

Excessive acute bleeding from hyperfibrinolysis

Adults: 4 to 5 g I.V. or P.O. over first hour, followed with constant infusion of 1 g/hour for about 8 hours or until bleeding is controlled. Maximum dose, 30 g/24 hours.

Children: 100 mg/kg I.V., or 3 g/m^2 I.V. first hour, followed by constant infusion of 33.3 mg/kg/hour or 1 g/m^2/hour. Maximum dose, 18 g/m^2 for 24 hours.

Chronic bleeding tendency

Adults: 5 to 30 g/day P.O. in divided doses at 3- to 6-hour intervals.

◊***Antidote for excessive thrombolysis due to administration of streptokinase or urokinase***

Adults: 4 to 5 g I.V. in first hour, followed by continuous infusion of 1 g/hour. Continue treatment for 8 hours or until hemorrhage is controlled.

◊***Secondary ocular hemorrhage in nonperforating traumatic hyphema***

Adults: 100 mg/kg P.O. q 4 hours for 5 days; maximum, 5 g/dose and 30 g/day.

◊***Hereditary hemorrhagic telangiectasia***

Adults: 1 to 1.5 g P.O. b.i.d. for 1 to 2 months followed by 1 to 2 g daily.

Pharmacodynamics

Hemostatic action: Aminocaproic acid inhibits plasminogen activators; to a lesser degree, it blocks antiplasmin activity by inhibiting fibrinolysis.

Pharmacokinetics

Absorption: Rapidly and completely absorbed from GI tract.

Distribution: Readily permeates human blood cells and other body cells; not protein-bound.

Metabolism: Insignificant.

Excretion: 40% to 60% of a single oral dose is excreted unchanged in urine in 12 hours.

Route	Onset	Peak	Duration
P.O.	1 hr	2 hr	Unknown
I.V.	1 hr	Unknown	3 hr

Contraindications and precautions

Contraindicated in patients with active intravascular clotting or presence of DIC unless heparin is used concomitantly. Injectable form is contraindicated in neonates. Use cautiously in patients with cardiac, renal, or hepatic disease.

Interactions

Drug-drug. *Estrogens and oral contraceptives containing estrogen:* Increases risk of hypercoagulability. Use with caution.

Effects on diagnostic tests

None reported.

Adverse reactions

CNS: dizziness, malaise, headache, delirium, ***seizures,*** hallucinations, weakness.

CV: hypotension, bradycardia, ***arrhythmias*** (with rapid I.V. infusion), generalized thrombosis.

EENT: tinnitus, nasal congestion, conjunctival suffusion.

GI: nausea, cramps, diarrhea.

GU: ***acute renal failure.***

Hepatic: increased AST, ALT.

Metabolic: ***hyperkalemia.***

Musculoskeletal: myopathy.

Skin: rash.

Overdose and treatment

Signs and symptoms of overdose include nausea, diarrhea, delirium, thrombotic episodes, and cardiac and hepatic necrosis. Discontinue drug immediately. Animal studies have demonstrated subendocardial hemorrhagic lesions after long-term high-dose administration.

Clinical considerations

- Aminocaproic acid has been used investigationally to treat missed abortion, allergic reaction, dermatitides, prophylaxis for blood transfusion reaction, connective tissue disease, and rheumatoid arthritis.

□ ***ALERT*** Bulk doses and bulk packages must be further diluted.

- To prepare an I.V. infusion, use normal saline injection, D_5W injection, or lactated Ringer's injection for dilution. Dilute doses up to 5 g with 250 ml of solution, doses of 5 g or greater with at least 500 ml.

□ ***ALERT*** Avoid rapid I.V. infusion to minimize risk of CV adverse reactions, such as hypotension, bradycardia, and arrythmias; use infusion pump to ensure constancy of infusion.

Therapeutic monitoring

- Recommend monitoring coagulation studies, heart rhythm, and blood pressure. Chronic use of drug requires routine creatine kinase determinations.
- Be alert for signs of phlebitis. If skeletal myopathy occurs, consider cardiomyopathy.

Special populations

Pediatric patients. Safety and efficacy in children haven't been established.

Patient counseling

- Advise patient to change positions slowly to minimize dizziness.
- Tell patient that routine CK determinations will be necessary with long-term use.
- Teach patient signs and symptoms of thrombophlebitis, and advise him to report them promptly.

aminophylline

Phyllocontin, Truphylline

Pharmacologic classification: xanthine derivative
Therapeutic classification: bronchodilator
Pregnancy risk category C

How supplied

Available by prescription only
Tablets: 100 mg, 200 mg
Tablets (controlled-release): 225 mg
Liquid: 105 mg/5 ml
Injection: 250-mg, 500-mg vials and ampules
Rectal suppositories: 250 mg, 500 mg

Indications and dosages

Symptomatic relief of acute bronchospasm
Patients not currently receiving theophylline who require rapid relief of symptoms: Loading dose is 6 mg/kg (equivalent to 4.7 mg/kg anhydrous theophylline) I.V. slowly (25 mg/minute or less), then maintenance infusion.

Maintenance infusions
Adults (nonsmokers): 0.7 mg/kg/hour I.V. for 12 hours, then 0.5 mg/kg/hour I.V.; or 3 mg/kg P.O. q 6 hours for two doses, then 3 mg/kg P.O. q 8 hours.
Otherwise healthy adult smokers: 1 mg/kg/hour I.V. for 12 hours, then 0.8 mg/kg/hour I.V.; or 3 mg/kg P.O. q 4 hours for three doses, then 3 mg/kg P.O. q 6 hours.
Older patients; adults with cor pulmonale: 0.6 mg/kg/hour I.V. for 12 hours, then 0.3 mg/kg/hour I.V.; or 2 mg/kg P.O. q 6 hours for two doses, then 2 mg/kg P.O. q 8 hours.
Adults with heart failure or liver disease: 0.5 mg/kg/hour I.V. for 12 hours, then 0.1 to 0.2 mg/kg/hour I.V.; or 2 mg/kg P.O. q 8 hours for two doses, then 1 to 2 mg/kg P.O. q 12 hours.
Children age 9 to 16 years: 1 mg/kg/hour I.V. for 12 hours, then 0.8 mg/kg/hour I.V.; or 3 mg/kg P.O. q 4 hours for three doses, then 3 mg/kg P.O. q 6 hours.
Children age 6 months to 9 years: 1.2 mg/kg/hour I.V. for 12 hours, then 1 mg/kg/hour I.V.; or 4 mg/kg P.O. q 4 hours for three doses, then 4 mg/kg P.O. q 6 hours.
Patients currently receiving theophylline: Aminophylline loading infusions of 0.63 mg/kg (0.5 mg/kg anhydrous theophylline) will increase plasma levels of theophylline by 1 mcg/ml, after serum levels have been evaluated. Some clinicians recommend a loading dose of 3.1 mg/kg I.V. (2.5 mg/kg anhydrous theophylline) if no obvious signs of theophylline toxicity are present, then maintenance infusion.

Chronic bronchial asthma
Adults and children: 16 mg/kg or 400 mg (whichever is less) P.O. daily in three or four divided doses q 6 to 8 hours if using rapidly absorbed dosage forms. Dosage may be increased, if tolerated, in increments of 25% q 2 to 3 days. Alternatively, if using extended-release preparations, 12 mg/kg or 400 mg (whichever is less) P.O. daily in two or three divided doses q 8 to 12 hours. Dosage may be increased, if tolerated, by 2 to 3 mg/kg daily q 3 days.

Regardless of dosage form, the following are recommended maximum doses. For adults and children age 16 and older, 13 mg/kg daily or 900 mg/day (whichever is less); children age 12 to 16, 18 mg/kg daily; children age 9 to 12, 20 mg/kg daily; and children age 1 to 9, 24 mg/kg daily.

When recommended maximum dose is reached, dosage adjustment is based on peak serum theophylline concentrations. Monitor serum levels to ensure that theophylline concentrations range from 10 to 20 mcg/ml.

Note: Rectal dose is the same as that recommended for oral dose.

◇***Periodic apnea associated with Cheyne-Stokes respirations, promote diuresis, paroxysmal nocturnal dyspnea***
Adults: 200 to 400 mg I.V. bolus.

◇***Reduction of severe bronchospasm in infants with cystic fibrosis***
Infants: 10 to 12 mg/kg I.V. daily.

Pharmacodynamics

Bronchodilating action: Aminophylline acts at the cellular level after it's converted to theophylline. (Aminophylline [theophylline ethylenediamine] is 79% theophylline). Theophylline acts by either inhibiting phosphodiesterase or blocking adenosine receptors in the bronchi, thereby relaxing smooth muscle. Drug also stimulates the respiratory center in the medulla and prevents diaphragmatic fatigue.

Pharmacokinetics

Absorption: Most dosage forms are absorbed well; absorption of the suppository, however, is unreliable and slow. Rate and onset of action also depend on the dosage form selected. Food may alter the rate, but not the extent of absorption, of oral doses.
Distribution: Distributed in all tissues and extracellular fluids except fatty tissue.
Metabolism: Converted to theophylline, then metabolized to inactive compounds.
Excretion: Excreted in urine as theophylline (10%).

Route	Onset	Peak	Duration
P.O.	15-60 min	1-7 hr	Variable
I.V.	15 min	Immediate	Variable
P.R.	Unknown	Unknown	Unknown

Contraindications and precautions

Contraindicated in patients with hypersensitivity to xanthine compounds (caffeine, theobromine) and ethylenediamine and in patients with active peptic ulcer disease and seizure disorders (unless adequate anticonvulsant therapy is given). Rectal suppositories are also contraindicated in patients who have an irritation or infection of the rectum or lower colon.

Use cautiously in neonates and infants under age 1, young children, the elderly, and patients with heart failure, CV disorders, COPD, cor pulmonale, renal or hepatic disease, hyperthyroidism, diabetes mellitus, peptic ulcer, severe hypoxemia, or hypertension.

Interactions

Drug-drug. *Alkali-sensitive drugs:* Reduce activity of aminophylline. Don't add these drugs to I.V. fluids containing aminophylline.
Cimetidine, allopurinol (high dose), propranolol, erythromycin, quinolones, or troleandomycin: May increase serum concentration of aminophylline by decreasing hepatic clearance. Use together cautiously.
Lithium: Aminophylline increases the excretion of lithium. Recommend monitoring lithium levels.
Phenobarbital, rifampin, phenytoin, carbamazepine, tobacco, marijuana, and aminoglutethimide: Decreased effects of aminophylline. Use together cautiously.
Drug-lifestyle. *Tobacco and marijuana use:* Decreases effects of aminophylline. Discourage use.

Effects on diagnostic tests

Aminophylline may alter the assay for uric acid, depending on method used. Theophylline levels are falsely elevated in the presence of furosemide, phenylbutazone, probenecid, theobromine, caffeine, tea, chocolate, cola beverages, and acetaminophen, depending on type of assay used. These substances don't interfere with levels if measured using high-pressure liquid chromatography.

Adverse reactions

CNS: *nervousness, restlessness,* headache, *insomnia,* ***seizures,*** muscle twitching, irritability.
CV: *palpitations, sinus tachycardia,* extrasystoles, flushing, marked hypotension, ***arrhythmias.***
GI: *nausea, vomiting,* diarrhea, epigastric pain, hematemesis.
Respiratory: tachypnea, ***respiratory arrest.***
Skin: urticaria.
Other: irritation (with rectal suppositories), hyperglycemia, fever, increased plasma-free fatty acids and urinary catecholamines.

Overdose and treatment

Signs and symptoms of overdose include nausea, vomiting, insomnia, irritability, tachycardia, extrasystoles, tachypnea, and tonic-clonic seizures. Onset of toxicity may be sudden and severe; arrhythmias and seizures are the first signs. Induce emesis, except in patients with seizures, then use activated charcoal and cathartics. Charcoal hemoperfusion may be beneficial. Treat arrhythmias with lidocaine and seizures with I.V. benzodiazepine; support respiratory and CV systems.

Clinical considerations

- Check that patient hasn't had recent theophylline therapy before giving loading dose.
- Don't combine in fluids for I.V. infusion with ascorbic acid, chlorpromazine, codeine phosphate, dimenhydrinate, dobutamine, epinephrine, erythromycin gluceptate, hydralazine, insulin, levorphanol tartrate, meperidine, methadone, methicillin, morphine sulfate, norepinephrine bitartrate, oxytetracycline, penicillin G potassium, phenobarbital, phenytoin, prochlorperazine, promazine, promethazine, tetracycline, vancomycin, or vitamin B complex with vitamin C.
- Don't crush controlled-release tablets.
- I.V. drug administration includes I.V. push at a very slow rate or an infusion with 100 to 200 ml of 5% dextrose or normal saline.
- GI symptoms may be relieved by taking oral drug with full glass of water at meals, although food in stomach delays absorption. Enteric-coated tablets may also delay absorption. There's no evidence that antacids reduce GI adverse reactions.
- Suppositories are slowly and erratically absorbed; retention enemas may be absorbed more rapidly. Rectally administered preparations can be given when patient can't take drug orally. Schedule after evacuation, if possible; may be retained better if given before meal. Advise patient to remain recumbent 15 to 20 minutes after insertion.

Therapeutic monitoring

- Individuals metabolize xanthines at different rates. Adjust dose by monitoring response, tolerance, pulmonary function, and theophylline blood levels. Therapeutic level is 10 to 20 mcg/ml, but some patients may respond at lower levels; toxicity occurs at levels over 20 mcg/ml.
- Monitor serum theophylline levels. Plasma clearance may be decreased in patients with heart failure, hepatic dysfunction, or pulmonary edema. Smokers show accelerated clearance. Dose adjustments are necessary.

Special populations

Breast-feeding patients. Drug is excreted in breast milk and may cause irritability, insomnia, or fretfulness in the breast-fed infant.
Pediatric patients. Drug isn't recommended for use in infants under age 6 months.
Geriatric patients. Use reduced doses and monitor patient closely. Warn geriatric patients

of dizziness, a common adverse reaction at start of therapy.

Patient counseling

- Teach patient rationale for therapy and importance of compliance with prescribed regimen; if a dose is missed, patient should take it as soon as possible, but should not double the dose.
- Advise patient of adverse effects and possible signs of toxicity.
- Tell patient not to eat or drink large quantities of xanthine-containing foods and beverages.
- Warn patient that OTC remedies may contain ephedrine in combination with theophylline salts; excessive CNS stimulation may result. Tell patient to seek medical approval before taking any other medications.

amiodarone hydrochloride

Cordarone

Pharmacologic classification: benzofuran derivative
Therapeutic classification: ventricular and supraventricular antiarrhythmic
Pregnancy risk category D

How supplied

Available by prescription only
Tablets: 100 mg*, 200 mg
Injection: 50 mg/ml

Indications and dosages

Recurrent ventricular fibrillation and unstable ventricular tachycardia; ◇atrial fibrillation; ◇angina; ◇hypertrophic cardiomyopathy
Adults: Loading dose of 800 to 1,600 mg P.O. daily for 1 to 3 weeks until initial therapeutic response occurs. Reduce to 600-800 mg per day for 1 month. Maintenance dosage, 200 to 600 mg P.O. daily. Alternatively, for first 24 hours, 150 mg I.V. over 10 minutes (mixed in 100 ml D_5W); then 360 mg I.V. over 6 hours (mix 900 mg in 500 ml D_5W); then maintenance dosage of 540 mg I.V. over 18 hours at a rate of 0.5 mg/minute. After first 24 hours, continue a maintenance infusion of 0.5 mg/minute in a 1 to 6 mg/ml concentration. For infusions greater than 1 hour, concentrations shouldn't exceed 2 mg/ml unless a central venous catheter is used. Don't use for more than 3 weeks.
Children: 10 to 15 mg/kg P.O. daily or 600 to 800 mg/1.73 m^2 P.O. daily for 4 to 14 days or until response is seen. Then 5 mg/kg or 200 to 400 mg/1.73 m^2; usual maintenance dosage is 2.5 mg/kg or 200 mg/1.73 m^2/day.

◇Supraventricular arrhythmias
Adults: 600 to 800 mg P.O. for 1 to 4 weeks or until supraventricular tachycardia is controlled. Maintenance dosage is 100 to 400 mg daily.
Conversion from I.V. to P.O.
Adults: Daily dose of 720 mg (rate 0.5 mg/minute): for 1 week, 800 to 1,600 mg daily; 1 to 3 weeks, 600 to 800 mg daily; more than 3 weeks, 400 mg daily.

Pharmacodynamics

Ventricular antiarrhythmic action: Although generally considered a class III agent, amiodarone hydrochloride has activity in each of the four Vaughn-Williams antiarrhythmic classes. It increases the action potential duration (repolarization inhibition). With prolonged therapy, the effective refractory period increases in the atria, ventricles, AV node, His-Purkinje system, and bypass tracts, and conduction slows in the atria, AV node, His-Purkinje system, and ventricles; sinus node automaticity decreases. Amiodarone also noncompetitively blocks beta-adrenergic receptors. Clinically, it has little, if any, negative inotropic effect. Coronary and peripheral vasodilator effects may occur with long-term therapy. Amiodarone is among the most effective antiarrhythmic agents, but its therapeutic applications are somewhat limited by its severe adverse reactions.

Pharmacokinetics

Absorption: Slow, variable absorption. Bioavailability is about 22% to 86%. Onset of action may be delayed from 2 to 3 days to 2 to 3 months—even with loading doses.
Distribution: Distributed widely because it accumulates in adipose tissue and in organs with marked perfusion, such as the lungs, liver, and spleen. It is also highly protein-bound (96%). The therapeutic serum level isn't well defined but may range from 1 to 2.5 mcg/ml.
Metabolism: Metabolized extensively in the liver to a pharmacologically active metabolite, desethyl amiodarone.
Excretion: Main excretory route is hepatic through the biliary tree (with enterohepatic recirculation). Because no renal excretion occurs, patients with impaired renal function don't require dosage reduction. Terminal elimination half-life is 25 to 110 days, the longest of any antiarrhythmic; in most patients, half-life ranges from 40 to 50 days.

Route	Onset	Peak	Duration
P.O.	2 days-3 weeks	3-7 hr	Variable
I.V.	Unknown	Unknown	Variable

Contraindications and precautions

Contraindicated in patients with hypersensitivity to drug and in those with severe SA node disease resulting in preexisting bradycardia. Unless an artificial pacemaker is present, drug is contraindicated in patients with second- or third-degree AV block and in those in whom bradycardia has caused syncope. Use with caution in patients already receiving antiarrhythmics, beta blockers, and calcium channel blockers. Use of amidoraone and ritonavir is contraindicated. Use cautiously with amprenavir.

Interactions

Drug-drug. *Beta-adrenergic and calcium channel blocking agents:* Using amiodarone with these drugs may cause sinus bradycardia, sinus arrest, and AV block. Avoid use together.
Cholestyramine: Increased elimination of amiodarone. Avoid use together.
Cimetidine: Increases amiodarone levels. Avoid use together.
Digoxin, flecainide, theophylline, cyclosporine, lidocaine, quinidine, phenytoin, or procainamide: May lead to increased serum levels of these drugs, resulting in enhanced effects. Recommend monitoring drug levels.
General anesthetics: Serious cardiac and CV effects may occur. Close perioperative monitoring of patient is needed.
Phenytoin: Decreased amiodarone levels. Recommend monitoring patient for clinical effect.
Quinidine, disopyramide, tricyclic antidepressants, cisapride, pimozide, phenothiazines, or sparfloxacin: May cause additive effects that lead to a prolonged QT interval, possibly resulting in torsades de pointes ventricular tachycardia. Use together very cautiously.
Warfarin: May cause prolonged PT, as a result of enhanced drug displacement from protein-binding sites. Monitor patient closely and decrease warfarin dosage.
Drug-herb. *Pennyroyal:* Amiodarone may change the rate of formation of toxic metabolites of pennyroyal. Avoid use together.
Drug-lifestyle. *Sunlight exposure:* Photosensitivity reactions may result. Encourage precautions.

Effects on diagnostic tests

None reported.

Adverse reactions

CNS: peripheral neuropathy, ataxia, paresthesia, tremor, insomnia, sleep disturbances, headache, *malaise, fatigue.*
CV: bradycardia, hypotension, ***arrhythmias, heart failure, heart block, sinus arrest, asystole.***
EENT: *corneal microdeposits,* visual disturbances.
GI: *nausea, vomiting,* constipation, abdominal pain.
Hepatic: *altered liver enzymes,* hepatic dysfunction, ***hepatic failure.***
Respiratory: SEVERE PULMONARY TOXICITY (PNEUMONITIS, ALVEOLITIS), hemoptysis, bronchiolitis obliterans, ***organizing pneumonia*** (may be fatal), pleuritis.
Skin: *photosensitivity,* blue-gray skin pigmentation, solar dermatitis.
Other: hypothyroidism, hyperthyroidism, edema, coagulation abnormalities, ***pancytopenia, neutropenia.***

Overdose and treatment

Clinical effects of overdose include bradyarrhythmias. Treatment may involve beta-adrenergic agonists, such as isoproterenol, or artificial pacing to help restore an acceptable heart rate. To treat hypotension, positive inotropic agents, such as dopamine or dobutamine, or vasopressors, such as epinephrine or norepinephrine, may be administered. General supportive measures should be used, as necessary. Drug can't be removed by dialysis.

Clinical considerations

- Drug is effective in treating arrhythmias resistant to other drug therapy. However, its high incidence of adverse effects limits its use.
- Divide loading dose into three equal doses, and give with meals to minimize GI intolerance. Maintenance dosage may be given once daily but may be divided into two doses taken with meals if GI intolerance occurs.
- Decrease digoxin, quinidine, phenytoin, and procainamide doses during amiodarone therapy to avoid toxicity.
- Adverse effects are more prevalent with high doses but usually resolve within about 4 months after drug therapy stops.

☐ ***ALERT*** Don't confuse amrinone, an inotrope, with amiodarone, an antiarrhythmic with negative chronotropic effects. Don't confuse drug with amiloride.

- When mixed in D_5W, amiodarone is incompatible with aminophylline, cefamandole nafate, cefazolin sodium, mezlocillin, heparin sodium, and sodium bicarbonate.
- To produce the solution required for the first loading infusion or for supplemental infusions, add 3 ml of amiodarone concentrate to 100 ml of 5% dextrose, resulting in a concentration of 1.5 mg/ml. To produce the solution for slow infusion or maintenance infusion, add 18 ml of amiodarone concentrate to 500 ml of 5% dextrose, resulting in a concentration of 1.8 mg/ml. Subsequent maintenance infusions may contain 1 to 6 mg/ml of amiodarone. Administer solutions containing 2 mg/ml or more via a central venous catheter. Use an in-line filter. Infusions are administered in a three-step process; a rapid loading dose, a slow loading dose, and a maintenance infusion.
- Administer amiodarone I.V. infusions exceeding 2 hours in glass or polyolefin bottles containing D_5W.
- Store tablets and injection at room temperature and protected from light and excessive

heat. Protect diluted solutions from light during administration.

Therapeutic monitoring

- Recommend monitoring blood pressure and heart rate and rhythm frequently for significant change.
- Advise periodically monitoring hepatic and thyroid function tests. Perform periodic eye exams to assess for corneal microdeposits.
- Patient needs monitoring for signs and symptoms of pneumonitis, such as exertional dyspnea, nonproductive cough, pleuritic chest pain, pulmonary function tests, and chest X-ray (pulmonary toxicity is more common with daily doses exceeding 600 mg). Pulmonary complications require discontinuation of amiodarone and possibly treatment with corticosteroids.
- Patient needs close monitoring during general anesthesia.

Special populations

Pregnant patients. Possible embryotoxic effects in pregnant women. Avoid use.
Breast-feeding patients. Drug is excreted in breast milk and shouldn't be used in breast-feeding women.
Pediatric patients. Drug has been used in children for refractory SVT and ventricular tachycardia. Children receiving amiodarone with digoxin may experience more acute effects of interaction. Children may experience faster onset of action and shorter duration of effect than adults.
Geriatric patients. Use cautiously in geriatric patients because ataxia may occur.

Patient counseling

- Advise patient to use sunscreen to prevent photosensitivity reactions to sunlight and UV light, which may cause sunburn and blistering.
- Although corneal microdeposits typically appear 1 to 4 months after therapy begins, only 2% to 3% of patients have actual visual disturbances. To minimize this complication, recommend frequent instillation of methylcellulose ophthalmic solution.

amitriptyline hydrochloride

Amitriptyline, Elavil, Levate*, Novotriptyn*

Pharmacologic classification: tricyclic antidepressant
Therapeutic classification: antidepressant
Pregnancy risk category NR

How supplied

Available by prescription only
Tablets: 10 mg, 25 mg, 50 mg, 75 mg, 100 mg, 150 mg
Injection: 10 mg/ml

Indications and dosages

Depression, ◇anorexia or bulimia associated with depression, ◇adjunctive treatment of neurogenic pain
Adults: Initial outpatient, 75 to 100 mg/day P.O. in divided doses or 50 to 150 mg h.s.; inpatient, 100 to 300 mg/day. I.M. dosage is 20 to 30 mg q.i.d., which should be changed to oral route as soon as possible. Maintenance dosage is 50 to 100 mg/day.
≡ ***Dosage adjustment.*** In geriatric or adolescent patients, 10 mg P.O. t.i.d. and 20 mg h.s.

Pharmacodynamics

Antidepressant action: Amitriptyline is thought to exert its antidepressant effects by inhibiting reuptake of norepinephrine and serotonin in CNS nerve terminals (presynaptic neurons), resulting in increased concentrations and enhanced activity of these neurotransmitters in the synaptic cleft. Amitriptyline more actively inhibits reuptake of serotonin than norepinephrine; it carries a high incidence of undesirable sedation, but tolerance to this effect usually develops within a few weeks.

Pharmacokinetics

Absorption: Absorbed rapidly from the GI tract after oral administration and from muscle tissue after I.M. administration.
Distribution: Distributed widely into the body, including the CNS and breast milk; 96% protein-bound.
Metabolism: Metabolized by the liver to the active metabolite nortriptyline; a significant first-pass effect may account for variability of serum concentrations in different patients taking the same dosage.
Excretion: Excreted mostly in urine.

Route	Onset	Peak	Duration
P.O., I.M.	Unknown	2-12 hr	Unknown

Contraindications and precautions

Contraindicated during acute recovery phase of MI, in patients with hypersensitivity, and in patients who have received an MAO inhibitor within the past 14 days.

Use cautiously in patients with recent history of MI and in those with unstable heart disease or renal or hepatic impairment.

Interactions

Drug-drug. *Atropine or other anticholinergic drugs, including phenothiazines, antihistamines, meperidine, and antiparkinsonian agents:* May cause oversedation, paralytic ileus, visual changes, and severe constipation. Recommend monitoring clinical effects closely.
Barbiturates: Induce metabolism and decrease therapeutic efficacy. Recommend monitoring clinical effects closely.
Centrally acting antihypertensive drugs, such as *guanethidine, guanabenz, guanadrel, cloni-*

dine, methyldopa, and reserpine: May decrease hypotensive effects of these drugs. Monitor blood pressure.
CNS depressants, including analgesics, barbiturates, narcotics, tranquilizers, and anesthetics: Oversedation. Recommend monitoring clinical effects closely.
Disulfiram or ethchlorvynol: May cause delirium and tachycardia. Avoid use together.
Methylphenidate, cimetidine, oral contraceptives, propoxyphene, selective serotonin reuptake inhibitors (such as Prozac), and beta blockers: May inhibit amitriptyline metabolism, increasing plasma levels and toxicity. Use together cautiously.
Metrizamide: Increased risk of seizures. Avoid use together.
Phenothiazines and haloperidol: Decrease amitriptyline's metabolism, decreasing therapeutic efficacy. Avoid use together.
Sympathomimetics, including epinephrine, phenylephrine, phenylpropanolamine, and ephedrine (commonly found in nasal sprays): May increase blood pressure. Recommend monitoring BP.
Thyroid hormones, pimozide, or antiarrhythmic agents (quinidine, disopyramide, procainamide): May increase incidence of arrhythmias and conduction defects. Avoid use together.
Warfarin: May increase PT and cause bleeding. Recommend monitoring PT and INR and decreasing warfarin.
Drug-lifestyle. *Alcohol use:* Additive effects are likely after use. Don't use together.
Heavy smoking: Induces amitriptyline metabolism and decreases therapeutic efficacy. Discourage use together.
Sun exposure: Photosensitivity reactions may result. Advise patient to take precautions.

Effects on diagnostic tests
None reported.

Adverse reactions
CNS: ***coma, seizures,*** hallucinations, delusions, disorientation, ataxia, tremor, peripheral neuropathy, anxiety, insomnia, restlessness, drowsiness, dizziness, weakness, fatigue, headache, extrapyramidal reactions.
CV: ***MI, stroke, arrhythmias,*** heart block, *orthostatic hypotension, tachycardia, ECG changes,* hypertension.
EENT: *blurred vision,* tinnitus, mydriasis, increased intraocular pressure elevate liver function test results.
GI: *dry mouth,* nausea, vomiting, anorexia, epigastric distress, diarrhea, constipation, paralytic ileus.
GU: urine retention.
Hematologic: ***agranulocytosis, thrombocytopenia, leukopenia,*** eosinophilia.
Skin: rash, urticaria, photosensitivity, decrease or increase in serum glucose levels.
Other: *diaphoresis,* hypersensitivity reaction, edema.
After abrupt withdrawal of long-term therapy: nausea, headache, malaise (doesn't indicate addiction).

Overdose and treatment
The first 12 hours after acute ingestion are a stimulatory phase characterized by excessive anticholinergic activity (agitation, irritation, confusion, hallucinations, hyperthermia, parkinsonian symptoms, seizure, urine retention, dry mucous membranes, pupillary dilation, constipation, and ileus). This is followed by CNS depressant effects, including hypothermia, decreased or absent reflexes, sedation, hypotension, cyanosis, and cardiac irregularities, including tachycardia, conduction disturbances, and quinidine-like effects on the ECG.

Severity of overdose is best indicated by widening of the QRS complex and usually represents a serum level in excess of 1,000 mg/ml; metabolic acidosis may follow hypotension, hypoventilation, and seizures. Delayed cardiac anomalies and death may occur.

Treatment is symptomatic and supportive, including maintaining airway, stable body temperature, and fluid and electrolyte balance. Induce emesis with ipecac if gag reflex is intact; follow with gastric lavage and activated charcoal to prevent further absorption. Dialysis is of little use. Physostigmine may be cautiously used to reverse the symptoms of tricyclic antidepressant poisoning in life-threatening situations. Treatment of seizures may include parenteral diazepam or phenytoin; treatment of arrhythmias, parenteral phenytoin or lidocaine; and treatment of acidosis, sodium bicarbonate. Don't give barbiturates; these may enhance CNS and respiratory depressant effects.

Clinical considerations
Consider the following recommendations along with those relevant to all tricyclic antidepressants:
- Drug may be used to prevent migraine and cluster headaches, intractable hiccups and post-therapeutic neuralgia.
- Amitriptyline causes a high incidence of sedative effects. Tolerance to sedative effects may develop over several weeks.
- The full dose may be given at bedtime to help offset daytime sedation.
- Substitute oral administration route for parenteral route as soon as possible.

☐ ***ALERT*** Parenteral form of drug is for I.M. administration only. Drug shouldn't be given I.V.
- I.M. administration may result in a more rapid onset of action than oral administration.
- Don't withdraw drug abruptly.
- Discontinue drug at least 48 hours before surgical procedures.

■ Sugarless chewing gum, hard candy or ice may alleviate dry mouth. Stress the importance of regular dental hygiene because dry mouth can increase the incidence of dental caries.
■ Depressed patients, particularly those with known manic depressive illness, may experience a shift to mania or hypomania.

Therapeutic monitoring

■ Recommend checking vital signs regularly for decreased blood pressure or tachycardia; observe patient carefully for adverse reactions and report changes. Obtain ECG in patients over age 40 before initiating therapy. Advise having patient take the first dose in the office to allow close observation for adverse reactions.
■ Advise checking for anticholinergic adverse reactions, which may require dose reduction.
■ Recommend observing patients for mood changes to monitor progress; benefits may not occur for several (3 to 6) weeks.

Special populations

Breast-feeding patients. Drug is excreted in breast milk in concentrations equal to or greater than those in maternal serum. About 1% of the ingested dose appears in the breast-fed infant's serum. The potential benefit to the woman should outweigh the possible adverse reactions in the infant.
Pediatric patients. Drug isn't recommended for children under age 12.
Geriatric patients. Geriatric patients may be at greater risk for adverse cardiac effects.

Patient counseling

■ Tell patient to take drug exactly as prescribed and not to double the dose for missed ones.
■ Advise patient that full dose may be taken at bedtime to alleviate daytime sedation. Alternatively, it may be taken in the early evening to avoid morning hangover.
■ Explain that full effects of drug may not become apparent for up to 4 weeks after initiation of therapy.
■ Warn patient that drug may cause drowsiness or dizziness. Tell him to avoid hazardous activities that require alertness until full effects of drug are known.
■ Warn patient not to drink alcoholic beverages while taking drug.
■ Suggest taking drug with food or milk if it causes stomach upset and using sugarless gum or candy to relieve dry mouth.
■ After initial doses, advise patient to lie down for about 30 minutes and rise to upright position slowly to prevent dizziness or fainting.
■ Warn patient not to stop taking drug suddenly.
■ Encourage patient to report troublesome or unusual effects, especially confusion, movement disorders, rapid heartbeat, dizziness, fainting, or difficulty urinating.

amlodipine besylate

Norvasc

Pharmacologic classification: dihydropyridine calcium channel blocker
Therapeutic classification: antianginal, antihypertensive
Pregnancy risk category C

How supplied

Available by prescription only
Tablets: 2.5 mg, 5 mg, 10 mg

Indications and dosages

Chronic stable angina, vasospastic angina (Prinzmetal's or variant angina)
Adults: Initially, 5 to 10 mg P.O. daily.
Hypertension
Adults: Initially, 2.5 to 5 mg P.O. daily. Adjust dosage based on patient response and tolerance every 7 to 14 days. Maximum daily dose, 10 mg.
≡ ***Dosage adjustment.*** In small, frail, or geriatric patients, those receiving other antihypertensives, or those with hepatic insufficiency, give 2.5 mg daily.

Pharmacodynamics

Antianginal and antihypertensive actions: Contractility of cardiac muscle and vascular smooth muscle depends on movement of extracellular calcium ions into cardiac and smooth-muscle cells through specific ion channels. Amlodipine inhibits the transmembrane influx of calcium ions into vascular smooth muscle and cardiac muscle, thus decreasing myocardial contractility and oxygen demand. As a peripheral arterial vasodilator, the drug acts directly on vascular smooth muscle to reduce peripheral vascular resistance and blood pressure. It also dilates coronary arteries and arterioles.

Pharmacokinetics

Absorption: After oral administration of therapeutic doses of amlodipine. Absolute bioavailability has been estimated to be between 64% and 90%.
Distribution: About 93% of the circulating drug is bound to plasma proteins in hypertensive patients.
Metabolism: Extensively metabolized in the liver, with about 90% converted to inactive metabolites.
Excretion: Excreted primarily in urine.

Route	Onset	Peak	Duration
P.O.	Unknown	6-12 hr	24 hr

Contraindications and precautions

Contraindicated in patients with hypersensitivity to drug. Use cautiously in patients receiving other peripheral dilators and in those with aortic stenosis, heart failure, or severe hepatic disease.

Interactions
None reported.

Effects on diagnostic tests
None reported.

Adverse reactions
CNS: *headache,* somnolence, fatigue, dizziness, light-headedness, paresthesia.
CV: *edema,* flushing, palpitations.
GI: nausea, abdominal pain.
Musculoskeletal: muscle pain.
Respiratory: dyspnea.
Skin: rash, pruritus.

Overdose and treatment
Symptoms of overdose include nausea, weakness, dizziness, drowsiness, confusion, and slurred speech. Overdose also can cause excessive peripheral vasodilation with marked hypotension and bradycardia, both of which may reduce cardiac output. Junctional rhythms and second- or third-degree AV block also can occur. Massive overdose warrants active cardiac and respiratory monitoring and frequent blood pressure measurements. Treatment of hypotension consists of CV support, including elevation of the extremities and judicious administration of fluids. If hypotension remains unresponsive to these conservative measures, consider administration of vasopressors (such as phenylephrine), with attention to circulating volume and urine output. I.V. calcium gluconate may help reverse the effects of calcium entry blockade. Because amlodipine is highly protein-bound, hemodialysis isn't likely to benefit the patient.

Clinical considerations
Because the vasodilation induced by amlodipine is gradual in onset, acute hypotension has rarely been reported after oral administration of amlodipine. However, exercise caution when administering drug, particularly in patients with severe aortic stenosis.

Therapeutic monitoring
- Monitor patient carefully.
- Some patients, especially those with severe obstructive coronary artery disease, have developed increased frequency, duration, or severity of angina or even acute MI after initiation of calcium channel blocker therapy or at a time of dosage increase.
- Blood pressure must be monitored closely, especially at the initiation of therapy.

Special populations
Breast-feeding patients. Because it isn't known if amlodipine is excreted in human milk, breast-feeding isn't recommended during amlodipine therapy.
Pediatric patients. Safety and efficacy in children haven't been established.
Geriatric patients. Geriatric patients may require a smaller dosage of amlodipine.

Patient counseling
- Tell patient to take nitroglycerin S.L. as needed for acute anginal symptoms. If patient continues nitrate therapy during titration of amlodipine dosage, urge continued compliance.
- Caution patient to continue taking amlodipine even when feeling better.
- Tell patient to notify doctor about signs of heart failure, such as swelling of hands and feet or shortness of breath.

amoxapine
Asendin

Pharmacologic classification: dibenzoxazepine, tricyclic antidepressant
Therapeutic classification: antidepressant
Pregnancy risk category C

How supplied
Available by prescription only
Tablets: 25 mg, 50 mg, 100 mg, 150 mg

Indications and dosages
Depression
Adults: Initial dose is 50 mg P.O. b.i.d. or t.i.d; may increase to 100 mg b.i.d. or t.i.d. by end of first week. Increases above 300 mg daily should be made only if this dose has been ineffective during a trial period of at least 2 weeks. When effective dose is established, entire dose (not exceeding 300 mg) may be given h.s. No more than 400 mg/day for outpatients. Maximum dose in hospitalized patients, 600 mg.

Note: Don't give more than 300 mg in a single dose.

≡ ***Dosage adjustment.*** In geriatric patients, recommended starting dose is 25 mg P.O. b.i.d. to t.i.d.

Pharmacodynamics
Antidepressant action: Drug is thought to exert its antidepressant effects by inhibiting reuptake of norepinephrine and serotonin in CNS nerve terminals (presynaptic neurons), which results in increased levels and enhanced activity of these neurotransmitters in the synaptic cleft. Amoxapine has a greater inhibitory effect on norepinephrine reuptake than on serotonin. Drug also blocks CNS dopamine receptors, which may account for the higher incidence of movement disorders during therapy.

Pharmacokinetics

Absorption: Absorbed rapidly and completely from the GI tract after oral administration.
Distribution: Distributed widely into the body, including the CNS and breast milk. Drug is 92% protein-bound. Steady state is reached within 2 to 7 days. Proposed therapeutic plasma levels (parent drug and metabolite) range from 200 to 500 ng/ml.
Metabolism: Metabolized by the liver to the active metabolite 8-hydroxyamoxapine; a significant first-pass effect may explain variability of serum levels in different patients taking the same dosage.
Excretion: Excreted in urine and feces (7% to 18%); about 60% of a given dose is excreted as the conjugated form within 6 days.

Route	Onset	Peak	Duration
P.O.	Unknown	1½ hr	Unknown

Contraindications and precautions

Contraindicated in patients with hypersensitivity, during acute recovery phase of MI, and in those who have received an MAO inhibitor within the past 14 days.

Use cautiously in patients with history of urine retention, CV disease, angle-closure glaucoma, or increased intraocular pressure. Use extremely cautiously in patients with history of seizures.

Interactions

Drug-drug. *Atropine or other anticholinergic drugs, including phenothiazines, antihistamines, meperidine, and antiparkinsonian agents:* Oversedation, paralytic ileus, visual changes, and severe constipation. Use together cautiously.
Barbiturates: Induce amoxapine metabolism and decrease therapeutic efficacy. Recommend monitoring for clinical effects.
Centrally acting antihypertensive drugs such as guanethidine, guanabenz, guanadrel, clonidine, methyldopa, and reserpine: Amoxapine decreases hypotensive effects. Monitor clinical response.
CNS depressants, including analgesics, barbiturates, narcotics, tranquilizers, and anesthetics: Increased sedation. Use together cautiously.
Disulfiram or ethchlorvynol: May cause delirium and tachycardia. Use together cautiously.
Methylphenidate, cimetidine, oral contraceptives, propoxyphene, and beta blockers: May inhibit amoxapine metabolism, increasing plasma levels. Monitor for toxicity.
Metrizamide: Increased risk of seizures. Avoid use together.
Phenothiazines and haloperidol: Decreased metabolism, decreasing therapeutic efficacy. Recommend monitoring for clinical effects.
Sympathomimetics, including epinephrine, phenylephrine, phenylpropanolamine, and ephedrine (commonly found in nasal sprays): May increase blood pressure. Avoid use together.
Thyroid medication, pimozide, and antiarrhythmic agents (quinidine, disopyramide, procainamide): Increased incidence of arrhythmias and conduction defects. Avoid use together.
Warfarin: Increased PT and INR, and bleeding. Recommend monitoring laboratory values and decreasing warfarin.
Drug-lifestyle. *Alcohol use:* Increased sedation. Avoid use together.
Heavy smoking: Induces amoxapine metabolism and decreases therapeutic efficacy. Discourage use together.
Sun exposure: Photosensitivity reactions may result. Advise patient to take precautions.

Effects on diagnostic tests

None reported.

Adverse reactions

CNS: *drowsiness, dizziness,* excitation, tremor, weakness, confusion, anxiety, insomnia, restlessness, nightmares, ataxia, fatigue, headache, nervousness, *tardive dyskinesia, EEG changes,* ***seizures,*** extrapyramidal reactions (rare), ***neuroleptic malignant syndrome (high fever, tachycardia, tachypnea, profuse diaphoresis).***
CV: *orthostatic hypotension, tachycardia,* hypertension, palpitations, prolonged conduction time (elongation of QT and PR intervals, flattened T waves on ECG).
EENT: *blurred vision.*
GI: *dry mouth, constipation,* nausea, excessive appetite.
GU: *urine retention, acute renal failure* (with overdose).
Hematologic: decreased WBC counts.
Hepatic: elevated liver function test results.
Metabolic: decreased or increased serum glucose levels.
Skin: rash, edema.
Other: *diaphoresis.*
After abrupt withdrawal of long-term therapy: nausea, headache, malaise (doesn't indicate addiction).

Overdose and treatment

The first 12 hours after acute ingestion are a stimulatory phase characterized by excessive anticholinergic activity (agitation, irritation, confusion, hallucinations, hyperthermia, parkinsonian symptoms, seizures, urine retention, dry mucous membranes, pupillary dilation, constipation, and ileus). This is followed by CNS depressant effects, including hypothermia, decreased or absent reflexes, sedation, hypotension, cyanosis, and cardiac irregularities, including tachycardia, conduction disturbances, and quinidine-like effects on the ECG.

Overdose with amoxapine produces a much higher incidence of CNS toxicity than do other antidepressants. Acute deterioration of renal function (evidenced by myoglobin in urine) occurs in 5% of overdosed patients; this is most likely to occur in patients with repeated seizures after the overdose. Seizures may progress to status epilepticus within 12 hours.

Severity of overdose is best indicated by widening of the QRS complex, which generally represents a serum level in excess of 1,000 ng/ml; serum levels aren't usually helpful. Metabolic acidosis may follow hypotension, hypoventilation, and seizures.

Treatment is symptomatic and supportive, including maintaining airway, stable body temperature, and fluid and electrolyte balance; monitor renal status because of the risk of renal failure. Induce emesis with ipecac if patient is conscious; follow with gastric lavage and activated charcoal to prevent further absorption. Dialysis is of little use. Treat seizures with parenteral diazepam or phenytoin (the value of physostigmine is less certain); arrhythmias, with parenteral phenytoin or lidocaine; and acidosis, with sodium bicarbonate. Don't give barbiturates; these may enhance CNS and respiratory depressant effects.

Clinical considerations

Consider the recommendations relevant to all tricyclic antidepressants as well as the following:

☐ ***ALERT*** Be aware of sound-alikes: amoxicillin and amoxapine.

- Amoxapine is associated with a high incidence of seizures.
- Antidepressants can cause manic episodes during the depressed phase in patients with bipolar disorder.
- The full dose may be given at bedtime to help reduce daytime sedation.
- The full dose shouldn't be withdrawn abruptly.
- Tolerance to sedative effects usually develops over the first few weeks of therapy.
- Discontinue drug at least 48 hours before surgical procedures.
- Sugarless chewing gum, hard candy, or ice may alleviate dry mouth.

Therapeutic monitoring

- Recommend monitoring for tardive dyskinesia and other extrapyramidal effects may occur because of the dopamine-blocking activity of amoxapine.
- Recommend monitoring for gynecomastia in men and women because amoxapine may increase cellular division in breast tissue.

Special populations

Pregnant patients. Safe use of tricyclic antidepressants in pregnancy hasn't been established. Fetal malformations, urinary retention, CNS effects (lethargy), developmental delay, and withdrawal symptoms have occurred in neonates born to mothers taking tricyclic antidepressants during pregnancy.

Breast-feeding patients. Amoxapine is excreted in breast milk in concentrations of 20% of maternal serum as parent drug and 30% as metabolites. The potential benefits to the woman should outweigh the possible adverse reactions in the infant.

Pediatric patients. Drug isn't recommended for patients under age 16.

Geriatric patients. Lower doses are indicated because older patients are more sensitive to the therapeutic and adverse effects of drug. Geriatric patients are much more susceptible to tardive dyskinesia and extrapyramidal symptoms.

Patient counseling

- Explain that full effects of drug may not become apparent for at least 2 weeks or more after therapy begins, perhaps not for 4 to 6 weeks.
- Tell patient to take drug exactly as prescribed; however, full dose may be taken at bedtime to alleviate daytime sedation. Patient shouldn't double the dose for missed ones.
- Warn patient that hazardous activities that require alertness should be avoided until the full effects of the drug are known because drug may cause drowsiness or dizziness.
- Tell patient not to drink alcoholic beverages while taking drug.
- Suggest that patient take drug with food or milk if it causes stomach upset; dry mouth can be relieved with sugarless gum or hard candy.
- After initial doses, tell patient to lie down for about 30 minutes and rise slowly to prevent dizziness.
- Warn patient not to discontinue drug suddenly.
- Encourage patient to report unusual or troublesome reactions immediately, especially confusion, movement disorders, rapid heartbeat, dizziness, fainting, or difficulty urinating.
- Inform patient that exposure to sunlight, sunlamps, or tanning beds may cause burning of the skin or abnormal pigmentary changes.

amoxicillin/clavulanate potassium

Augmentin, Clavulin*

Pharmacologic classification: aminopenicillin and beta-lactamase inhibitor
Therapeutic classification: antibiotic
Pregnancy risk category B

How supplied

Available by prescription only
Tablets (chewable): 125 mg amoxicillin trihydrate, 31.25 mg clavulanic acid; 200 mg amoxicillin trihydrate, 28.5 mg clavulanic acid; 250

mg amoxicillin trihydrate, 62.5 mg clavulanic acid; 400 mg amoxicillin trihydrate, 57 mg clavulanic acid
Tablets: 250 mg amoxicillin trihydrate, 125 mg clavulanic acid; 500 mg amoxicillin trihydrate, 125 mg clavulanic acid; 875 mg amoxicillin trihydrate, 125 mg clavulanic acid
Oral suspension: 125 mg amoxicillin trihydrate and 31.25 mg clavulanic acid/5 ml (after reconstitution); 200 mg amoxicillin trihydrate and 28.5 mg clavulanic acid/5 ml (after reconstitution); 250 mg amoxicillin trihydrate and 62.5 mg clavulanic acid/5 ml (after reconstitution); 400 mg amoxicillin trihydrate and 57 mg clavulanic acid/5 ml (after reconstitution)

Indications and dosages

Lower respiratory infections, otitis media, sinusitis, skin and skin structure infections, and urinary tract infections caused by susceptible organisms
Adults and children weighing over 88 lb (40 kg): 250 mg (based on amoxicillin component) P.O. q 8 hours or one 500-mg tablet q 12 hours. For more severe infections, 500 mg q 8 hours or 875 mg q 12 hours.
Children weighing under 88 lb: 25 to 45 mg/kg/day P.O. (based on amoxicillin component) given in divided doses q 8 to 12 hours.
Neonates and infants under 12 weeks: 30 mg/kg daily in divided doses q 12 hours.

Dosage adjustment. In patients with creatinine clearance of 15 to 30 ml/min, usual dose q 12 to 18 hours; 5 to 15 ml/min, usual dose q 20 to 36 hours; less than 5 ml/min, usual dose every 48 hours. Some clinicians recommend not using if creatinine clearance is less than 30 ml/min.

In hemodialysis patients, give 500 mg P.O. midway through treatment and then 500 mg P.O. at the end of treatment.

Pharmacodynamics

Antibiotic action: Amoxicillin is bactericidal; it adheres to bacterial penicillin-binding proteins, thus inhibiting bacterial cell wall synthesis.

Clavulanate has only weak antibacterial activity and doesn't affect mechanism of action of amoxicillin. However, clavulanic acid has a beta-lactam ring and is structurally similar to penicillin and cephalosporins; it binds irreversibly with certain beta-lactamases and prevents them from inactivating amoxicillin, enhancing its bactericidal activity.

This combination acts against penicillinase- and non-penicillinase-producing gram-positive bacteria, *Neisseria gonorrhoeae, Neisseria meningitidis, Haemophilus influenzae, Moraxella catarrhalis, Escherichia coli, Proteus mirabilis, Citrobacter diversus, Klebsiella pneumoniae, Proteus vulgaris, Salmonella,* and *Shigella, Clostridium, Peptococcus,* and *Peptostreptococcus.*

Pharmacokinetics

Absorption: Well absorbed after oral administration.
Distribution: Distributes into pleural fluid, lungs, and peritoneal fluid; high urine concentrations are attained. Amoxicillin also distributes into synovial fluid, liver, prostate, muscle, and gallbladder; and penetrates into middle ear effusions, maxillary sinus secretions, tonsils, sputum, and bronchial secretions. Amoxicillin and clavulanate cross the placenta and low concentrations are excreted in breast milk. Amoxicillin and clavulanate potassium have minimal protein-binding of 17% to 20% and 22% to 30%, respectively.
Metabolism: Amoxicillin is metabolized only partially. The metabolic fate of clavulanate potassium isn't completely identified, but it appears to undergo extensive metabolism.
Excretion: Amoxicillin is excreted principally in urine by renal tubular secretion and glomerular filtration; drug is also excreted in breast milk.

Clavulanate potassium is excreted by glomerular filtration. Elimination half-life of amoxicillin in adults is 1 to 1½ hours; it is prolonged to 7½ hours in patients with severe renal impairment. Half-life of clavulanate in adults is about 1 to 1½ hours, prolonged to 4½ hours in patients with severe renal impairment.

Both drugs are removed readily by hemodialysis and minimally removed by peritoneal dialysis.

Route	Onset	Peak	Duration
P.O.	Unknown	1-2½ hr	6-8 hr

Contraindications and precautions

Contraindicated in patients with hypersensitivity to drug or other penicillins and in those with a previous history of amoxicillin-associated cholestatic jaundice or hepatic dysfunction. An oral penicillin shouldn't be used in patients with severe pneumonia, empyema, bacteremia, pericarditis, meningitis, and purulent or septic arthritis. Use with caution in patients with mononucleosis.

Interactions

Drug-drug. *Allopurinol:* Appears to increase incidence of rash from both drugs. Avoid use together.
Probenecid: Blocks tubular secretion of amoxicillin, raising its serum levels; it has no effect on clavulanate. Avoid use together.
Methotrexate: Large doses of penicillins may interfere with renal tubular secretion of methotrexate , thus delaying elimination and prolonging elevated serum levels of methotrex-

ate. Recommend monitoring for adverse effects.
Oral contraceptives: Effectiveness of oral contraceptives may be reduced. Advise using alternative barrier method.

Effects on diagnostic tests

Amoxicillin/potassium clavulanate alters results of urine glucose tests that use cupric sulfate (Benedict's reagent or Clinitest). Make urine glucose determinations with glucose oxidase methods (Chemstrip uG or Diastix or glucose enzymatic test strip). Positive Coombs' tests have been reported with other clavulanate combinations. Amoxicillin/potassium clavulanate may produce a positive direct antiglobulin test (DAT).

Adverse reactions

CNS: agitation, anxiety, insomnia, confusion, behavioral changes, dizziness.
GI: *nausea,* vomiting, *diarrhea,* indigestion, gastritis, stomatitis, glossitis, black "hairy" tongue, enterocolitis, pseudomembranous colitis.
GU: vaginitis.
Hematologic: anemia, ***thrombocytopenia,*** thrombocytopenic purpura, eosinophilia, ***leukopenia, agranulocytosis.***
Other: hypersensitivity reactions (erythematous maculopapular rash, urticaria, ***anaphylaxis***), overgrowth of nonsusceptible organisms.

Overdose and treatment

Clinical signs of overdose include neuromuscular sensitivity or seizures. After recent ingestion (4 hours or less), empty the stomach by induced emesis or gastric lavage; follow with activated charcoal to reduce absorption. Amoxicillin/clavulanate potassium can be removed by hemodialysis.

Clinical considerations

Consider the recommendations relevant to all penicillins as well as the following:
- Amoxicillin/clavulanate potassium has been used to treat infections caused by *Eikenella corrodens* or *Pasteurella multocida* and infections caused by anaerobic and mixed aerobic-anaerobic bacterial infections.

☐ ***ALERT*** Both 250-mg and 500-mg film-coated tablets contain the same amount of clavulanic acid (125 mg). Therefore, two 250-mg tablets aren't equivalent to one 500-mg tablet.

- Oral dosage is maximally absorbed from an empty stomach, but food doesn't cause significant impairment of absorption.
- For reconstitution, add specified water in 2 parts and agitate well after each addition.
- Suspension is stable for 10 days in refrigerator after reconstitution.
- Commercial products containing aspartame shouldn't be used in pediatric patients with phenylketonuria.
- Because amoxicillin/clavulanate potassium is dialyzable, patients undergoing hemodialysis may need dosage adjustments.

Therapeutic monitoring

- Monitor renal, hepatic, and hematologic function periodically.
- Recommend testing for *Clostridium difficile* in patients with diarrhea.

Special populations

Pregnant patients. There are no adequate and controlled studies of use of this drug in pregnant women. Only use in pregnant women if clearly needed.
Breast-feeding patients. Both amoxicillin and potassium clavulanate are excreted in breast milk; use with caution in breast-feeding women.
Geriatric patients. In geriatric patients, diminished renal tubular secretion may prolong half-life of amoxicillin.

Patient counseling

- Tell patient to chew chewable tablets thoroughly or crush before swallowing and wash down with liquid to ensure adequate absorption of drug; capsule may be emptied and contents swallowed with water.
- Instruct patient to report diarrhea promptly.
- Inform patient to complete full course of medication.

amoxicillin trihydrate

Amoxil, Polymox, Trimox

Pharmacologic classification: aminopenicillin
Therapeutic classification: antibiotic
Pregnancy risk category B

How supplied

Available by prescription only
Tablets (chewable): 125 mg, 200 mg, 250 mg, 400 mg
Tablets (film-coated): 500 mg, 875 mg
Capsules: 250 mg, 500 mg
Suspension: 125 mg/5 ml, 250 mg/5 ml
Pediatric drops: 50 mg/ml (after reconstitution)

Indications and dosages

Systemic infections, acute and chronic urinary or respiratory tract infections caused by susceptible organisms, uncomplicated urinary tract infections caused by susceptible organisms
Adults: 250 mg P.O. q 8 hours or 500 mg q 12 hours. In adults who have severe infections or those caused by susceptible organisms, 500 mg

q 8 hours or 875 mg q 12 hours may be needed.
Children: 20 to 40 mg/kg P.O. daily, divided into doses given q 8 hours.
Neonates and infants up to 12 weeks: 30 mg/kg P.O. daily in divided doses q 12 hours

Pediatric drops: children under 13 lb (6 kg), 0.75 ml q 8 hours; 13 to 15 lb (6 to 7 kg), 1 ml q 8 hours; 16 to 18 lb (7 to 8 kg), 1.25 ml q 8 hours. Children with lower respiratory tract infection only weighing under 13 lb, 1.25 ml q 8 hours; 13 to 15 lb, 1.75 ml q 8 hours; 16 to 18 lb, 2.25 ml q 8 hours.

Uncomplicated gonorrhea
Adults: 3 g P.O. as a single dose.
Children over age 2: 50 mg/kg given with 25 mg/kg probenecid as a single dose.

Chlamydial and mycoplasmal infections during pregnancy
Adults: 500 mg P.O. t.i.d. for 7 to 10 days.

◊ ***Lyme disease***
Adults: 250 to 500 mg P.O. t.i.d. to q.i.d. for 10 to 30 days.
Children: 25 to 50 mg/kg daily (maximum 1 to 2 g daily) P.O. in three divided doses for 10 to 30 days.

◊ ***Acute uncomplicated urinary tract infection in nonpregnant women***
3 g P.O. as one single dose

≡ ***Dosage adjustment.*** In renal failure, patients who require repeated doses may need adjustment of dosing interval. If creatinine clearance is 10 to 30 ml/minute, increase interval to q 12 hours; if creatinine clearance is less than 10 ml/minute, administer q 24 hours. Supplemental doses may be necessary after hemodialysis.

Oral prophylaxis of bacterial endocarditis
Consult current American Heart Association recommendations before administering drug.
Adults: 2 g 1 hour before procedure.
Children: 50 mg/kg 1 hour before procedure.

Pharmacodynamics

Antibacterial action: Amoxicillin is bactericidal; it adheres to bacterial penicillin-binding proteins, thus inhibiting bacterial cell wall synthesis.

Spectrum of action of amoxicillin includes non-penicillinase-producing gram-positive bacteria, *Streptococcus* group B, *Neisseria gonorrhoeae, Proteus mirabilis, Salmonella,* and *Haemophilus influenzae.* It's also effective against non-penicillinase-producing *Staphylococcus aureus, Streptococcus pyogenes, Streptococcus bovis, Streptococcus pneumoniae, Streptococcus viridans, N. meningitidis, Escherichia coli, Salmonella typhi, Bordetella pertussis, Peptococcus,* and *Peptostreptococcus.*

Pharmacokinetics

Absorption: About 80% absorbed after oral administration.
Distribution: Distributes into pleural peritoneal and synovial fluids and into the lungs, prostate, muscle, liver, and gallbladder; it also penetrates middle ear, maxillary sinus and bronchial secretions, tonsils, and sputum. Amoxicillin readily crosses the placenta; about 17% to 20% is protein-bound.
Metabolism: Metabolized only partially.
Excretion: Excreted principally in urine by renal tubular secretion and glomerlar filtration; also excreted in breast milk. Elimination half-life in adults is about 1 to 1¼ hours; severe renal impairment increases half-life to 7¼ hours.

Route	Onset	Peak	Duration
P.O.	Unknown	1-2 hr	6-8 hr

Contraindications and precautions

Contraindicated in patients with hypersensitivity to drug or other penicillins. Use with caution in patients with mononucleosis.

Interactions

Drug-drug. *Allopurinol:* Increased incidence of rash from both drugs. Monitor patient.
Clavulanate potassium: Enhances effect of amoxicillin against certain beta-lactamase-producing bacteria. Recommend therapeutic benefits.
Methotrexate: Large doses of penicillins may interfere with renal tubular secretion of methotrexate, thus delaying elimination and prolonging elevated serum levels of methotrexate. Recommend monitoring patient for toxicity.
Oral contraceptives: Effectiveness of oral contraceptives may be decreased. Advise using alternative barrier method.
Probenecid: Blocks renal tubular secretion of amoxicillin, raising its serum concentrations. Probenecid may be used for this purpose.

Effects on diagnostic tests

Amoxicillin may alter results of urine glucose tests that use cupric sulfate (Benedict's reagent or Clinitest). Make urine glucose determinations with glucose oxidase methods (Chemstrip uG, Diastix, or glucose enzymatic test strip).

Adverse reactions

CNS: lethargy, hallucinations, ***seizures,*** anxiety, confusion, agitation, depression, dizziness, fatigue.
GI: *nausea,* vomiting, *diarrhea,* glossitis, stomatitis, gastritis, abdominal pain, enterocolitis, pseudomembranous colitis, black "hairy" tongue.
GU: interstitial nephritis, nephropathy, vaginitis.
Hematologic: anemia, ***thrombocytopenia,*** thrombocytopenic purpura, eosinophilia, ***leukopenia, hemolytic anemia, agranulocytosis.***

Other: ***hypersensitivity reactions*** (erythematous maculopapular rash, urticaria, ***anaphylaxis***), overgrowth of nonsusceptible organisms.

Overdose and treatment
Clinical signs of overdose include neuromuscular sensitivity or seizures. After recent ingestion (4 hours or less), empty the stomach by induced emesis or gastric lavage; follow with activated charcoal to reduce absorption. Drug can be removed by hemodialysis.

Clinical considerations
Consider the recommendations relevant to all penicillins as well as the following:
- 200 mg and 400 mg chewable Amoxil tablets contain aspartame and shouldn't be given to patients with phenylketonuria.
- Oral dosage is maximally absorbed from an empty stomach, but food doesn't cause significant loss of potency.
- Pediatric drops may be placed on child's tongue or added to formula, milk, fruit juice, or soft drink. Be sure child ingests all of prepared dose.
- Suspension and drops are stable for 14 days in refrigerator after reconstitution.
- Amoxicillin may cause less diarrhea than ampicillin.

Therapeutic monitoring
If prolonged therapy, recommend monitoring renal, hepatic, and hematologic tests.

Special populations
Pregnant patients. There are no adequate controlled studies in pregnant women, but drug has been used effectively without evidence of adverse effects.
Breast-feeding patients. Drug is distributed readily into breast milk; safe use in breast-feeding women hasn't been established. Alternative feeding method is recommended during therapy.
Geriatric patients. Because of diminished renal tubular secretion, half-life may be prolonged in geriatric patients.

Patient counseling
- Tell patient to chew tablets thoroughly or crush before swallowing and wash down with liquid to ensure adequate absorption of drug; capsule may be emptied and contents swallowed with water.
- Tell patient to report diarrhea promptly.
- Instruct patient to complete full course of medication.

amphetamine sulfate

Pharmacologic classification: amphetamine
Therapeutic classification: CNS stimulant, short-term adjunctive anorexigenic agent, sympathomimetic amine
Controlled substance schedule II
Pregnancy risk category C

How supplied
Available by prescription only
Tablets: 5 mg, 10 mg

Indications and dosages
Attention deficit disorder with hyperactivity
Children age 6 and older: 5 mg P.O. daily. Increase at 5-mg increments weekly until desired response. Dose rarely exceeds 40 mg/day. Give first dose upon awakening; give additional doses at 4- to 6-hour intervals.
Children age 3 to 5: 2.5 mg P.O. daily, increase at 2.5-mg increments weekly until desired response is achieved.
Narcolepsy
Adults: 5 to 60 mg P.O. daily in divided doses or a single dose.
Children over age 12: 10 mg P.O. daily, with 10-mg increments weekly, p.r.n.
Children age 6 to 12: 5 mg P.O. daily, with 5-mg increments weekly, p.r.n.
Short-term adjunct in exogenous obesity
Adults: 5 to 30 mg daily in divided doses of 5 to 10 mg.

Pharmacodynamics
CNS stimulant action: Amphetamines are sympathomimetic amines with CNS stimulant activity; in hyperactive children, they have a paradoxical calming effect.

Amphetamines are used to treat narcolepsy and as adjuncts to psychosocial measures in attention deficit disorder in children. The cerebral cortex and reticular activating system appear to be their primary sites of activity; amphetamines release nerve terminal stores of norepinephrine, promoting nerve impulse transmission. At high doses, effects are mediated by dopamine.

Anorexigenic action: Anorexigenic effects are thought to occur in the hypothalamus, where decreased smell and taste acuity decreases the appetite. Amphetamines may be tried for short-term control of refractory obesity, with caloric restriction and behavior modification.

Pharmacokinetics
Absorption: Absorbed completely within 3 hours after oral administration; therapeutic effects persist for 4 to 24 hours.

Distribution: Distributed widely throughout body, with high concentrations in the brain. Therapeutic plasma levels are 5 to 10 mcg/dl.
Metabolism: Metabolized by hydroxylation and deamination in the liver.
Excretion: Excreted in urine.

Route	Onset	Peak	Duration
P.O.	Unknown	Unknown	4 to 24 hr

Contraindications and precautions

Contraindicated in patients with hypersensitivity or idiosyncrasy to the sympathomimetic amines, symptomatic CV disease, hyperthyroidism, moderate to severe hypertension, glaucoma, advanced arteriosclerosis, or history of drug abuse; within 14 days of MAO inhibitor therapy; and in agitated patients.

Use cautiously in geriatric, debilitated, or hyperexcitable patients or in those with suicidal or homicidal tendencies.

Interactions

Drug-drug. *Ammonium chloride or ascorbic acid*: Enhances amphetamine excretion or shortens duration of action. Recommend monitoring for clinical effect.
Antacids, sodium bicarbonate, or acetazolamide: May enhance reabsorption of amphetamine and prolong its duration of action. Recommend monitoring for clinical effect.
Antihypertensives: May antagonize their hypertensive effects. Avoid use together.
Barbiturates: Counteract amphetamine by CNS depression; other CNS stimulants produce additive effects: Avoid use together.
Guanethidine: May decrease the effectiveness of guanethidine. Recommend monitoring for clinical effect.
Insulin: Amphetamines may alter insulin requirements. Recommend monitoring blood glucose.
MAO inhibitors (or drugs with MAO-inhibiting effects such as furazolidone) or within 14 days of such therapy: May cause hypertensive crisis. Avoid use together.
Phenothiazines or haloperidol: Decreases amphetamine effects. Recommend monitoring for clinical effect.
Drug-food. *Caffeine:* Produces additive effects. Avoid use together.

Effects on diagnostic tests

Amphetamines may interfere with urinary steroid determinations.

Adverse reactions

CNS: *restlessness,* tremor, *hyperactivity, talkativeness, insomnia,* irritability, dizziness, headache, chills, dysphoria, euphoria.
CV: *tachycardia, palpitations,* hypertension, ***arrhythmias.***
GI: dry mouth, metallic taste, diarrhea, constipation, anorexia, weight loss.
GU: impotence, altered libido.
Metabolic: elevated plasma corticosteroid levels.
Skin: urticaria.

Overdose and treatment

Signs and symptoms of acute overdose include increasing restlessness, irritability, insomnia, tremor, hyperreflexia, diaphoresis, mydriasis, flushing, confusion, hypertension, tachypnea, fever, delirium, self-injury, arrhythmias, seizures, coma, circulatory collapse, and death.

Treat overdose symptomatically and supportively: If ingestion is recent (within 4 hours) use gastric lavage or emesis; activated charcoal, sodium chloride catharsis, and urinary acidification may enhance excretion. Forced fluid diuresis may help. In massive ingestion, hemodialysis or peritoneal dialysis may be needed. Keep patient in a cool room, monitor temperature, and minimize external stimulation. Haloperidol may be used for psychotic symptoms; diazepam, for hyperactivity.

Clinical considerations

- Avoid administration late in the day (after 4 p.m.) to prevent insomnia.
- Amphetamine capsules shouldn't be used for initial or subsequent titration of dosage; however, once dosage has been established, capsules can be substituted if once-daily dosing is required.
- If therapy is prolonged, don't withdraw suddenly.

Therapeutic monitoring

- Recommend monitoring for adverse cardiac effects in susceptible patients.
- Recommend monitoring of patient diet and calorie count when used as adjunct to weight reduction.

Special populations

Pregnant patients. Drug shouldn't be used during pregnancy, especially during first trimester.
Pediatric patients. Amphetamines aren't recommended for weight reduction in children under age 12; use of amphetamines for hyperactivity is contraindicated in children under age 3.

Patient counseling

Instruct patient about the potential for drowsiness and to avoid activities such as driving that require alertness.

amphotericin B
Fungizone

Pharmacologic classification: polyene antibiotic
Therapeutic classification: antifungal
Pregnancy risk category B

How supplied
Available by prescription only
Oral suspension: 100 mg/ml
Powder for injection: 50 mg
Cream: 3%
Lotion: 3%
Ointment: 3%

Indications and dosages
Systemic (potentially fatal) fungal infections caused by susceptible organisms, ◇fungal endocarditis, fungal septicemia
Adults and children: Some clinicians recommend an initial dose of 1 mg I.V. in 20 ml D_5W infused over 20 minutes. If test dose is tolerated, then give daily doses of 0.25 to 0.30 mg/kg, gradually increasing by 5 to 10 mg/day until daily dose is 1 mg/kg/day or 1.5 mg/kg q alternate day. Duration of therapy is dependent upon the severity and nature of infection.
Sporotrichosis: 0.4 to 0.5 mg/kg amphotericin B daily I.V. for up to 9 months. Total I.V. dosage of 2.5 g over 9 months.
Aspergillosis: Total I.V. dosage of 1.5 to 4.0 g over 11 months. Initially, 0.5 to 0.6 mg/kg/day.
◇Fungal meningitis
Adults: Intrathecal injection of 25 mcg/0.1 ml diluted with 10 to 20 ml of CSF and administered by barbotage two or three times weekly. Initial dose shouldn't exceed 50 mcg.
◇Candidal cystitis
Adults: Bladder irrigations in concentrations of 5 to 50 mcg/ml instilled periodically or continuously for 5 to 7 days.
Oropharyngeal candidiasis
Adults and children: 100 mg/ml oral suspension q.i.d. swish and swallow.
Topical fungal infections (3% cream, lotion, ointment)
Adults and children: Apply liberally and rub well into affected area b.i.d. to q.i.d.
Cutaneous or mucocutaneous candidal infections
Adults and children: Apply topical product b.i.d., t.i.d., or q.i.d. for 1 to 3 weeks; apply up to several months for interdigital or paronychial lesions.
◇Sinus irrigation
Adults: 1 mg/ml
◇Histoplasmal pulmonary and intrapleural effusion
Adults: 15 to 20 mg with 25 mg hydrocortisone sodium succinate.
◇Pulmonary coccidioidomycosis
Adults: Via intermittent positive pressure breathing device, 5 to 10 mg q.i.d.
◇Ophthalmic candidal infection
Adults: 0.1 to 1 mg/ml drop suspension q 30 minutes.

Note: Intrathecal and intra-articular uses are unapproved.
◇Empiric therapy of presumed fungal infections in febrile, neutropenic patients including cancer patients and bone marrow transplant (BMT) or solid organ transplant recipients
Adults: 0.8 mg/kg daily for 8 days.

Pharmacodynamics
Antifungal action: Amphotericin B is *fungistatic* or *fungicidal,* depending on the concentrations available in body fluids and on the susceptibility of the fungus. It binds to sterols in the fungal cell membrane, increasing membrane permeability of fungal cells, causing subsequent leakage of intracellular components; it also may interfere with some human cell membranes that contain sterols.

Spectrum of activity includes *Histoplasma capsulatum, Coccidioides immitis, Blastomyces dermatitidis, Cryptococcus neoformans, Candida* species, *Aspergillus fumigatus, Mucor* species, *Rhizopus* species, *Absidia* species, *Entomophthora* species, *Basidiobolus* species, *Paracoccidioides brasiliensis, Sporothrix schenckii,* and *Rhodotorula* species.

Pharmacokinetics
Absorption: Absorbed poorly from the GI tract.
Distribution: Distributes well into inflamed pleural cavities and joints; in low concentrations into aqueous humor, bronchial secretions, pancreas, bone, muscle, and parotids. CSF concentrations reach about 3% of serum concentrations. Drug is 90% to 95% bound to plasma proteins; it reportedly crosses the placenta.
Metabolism: Not well defined.
Excretion: Elimination is biphasic: initial serum half-life of 24 hours, followed by a second phase half-life of about 15 days. About 2% to 5% of drug is excreted unchanged in urine. Amphotericin B isn't readily removed by hemodialysis.

Route	Onset	Peak	Duration
P.O.	Unknown	Unknown	Unknown
I.V.	Immediate	Unknown	Unknown
Topical	Unknown	Unknown	Unknown

Contraindications and precautions
Contraindicated in patients with hypersensitivity to drug. Use cautiously in patients with renal impairment.

Interactions

Drug-drug. *Aminoglycosides, cisplatin, pentamidine, and other nephrotoxic drugs:* Added nephrotoxic effects. Avoid use together.
Clotrimazole, fluconazole, itraconazole, ketoconazole, miconazole: May antagonize amphotericin B. Monitor patient closely.
Corticosteroids, corticotropin: Electrolyte imbalances. Requires careful monitoring of serum electrolyte levels and cardiac function.
Digoxin: Increases the risk of digitalis toxicity. Recommend monitoring serum digoxin level if drugs are used together.
Flucytosine and other antibiotics: Potentiated effects. Use together cautiously.
Skeletal muscle relaxants: Amphotericin B-induced hypokalemia may enhance effects of skeletal muscle relaxants. Use together cautiously.
Zidovudine: Increased myelotoxicity and nephrotoxicity. Recommend monitoring renal and hematologic function.
Drug-herb. *Gossypol:* May increase risk of renal toxicity. Avoid use together.

Effects on diagnostic tests

None reported.

Adverse reactions

CNS: *malaise, headache,* peripheral neuropathy, ***seizures*** (with systemic form).
CV: hypotension, ***arrhythmias, asystole,*** hypertension (with systemic form).
EENT: hearing loss, tinnitus, transient vertigo, blurred vision, diplopia (with systemic form).
GI: *anorexia, weight loss, nausea, vomiting, dyspepsia, diarrhea, epigastric pain, cramping,* melena, ***hemorrhagic gastroenteritis*** (with systemic form), increased alkaline phosphatase, and bilirubin levels.
GU: *abnormal renal function with hypokalemia, azotemia, hyposthenuria, renal tubular acidosis, nephrocalcinosis;* with large doses, ***permanent renal impairment,*** anuria, oliguria (with systemic form).
Hematologic: *normochromic, normocytic anemia,* ***thrombocytopenia, leukopenia, agranulocytosis,*** eosinophilia, leukocytosis (with systemic form).
Hepatic: hepatitis, jaundice, ***acute liver failure*** (with systemic form).
Metabolic: hypokalemia and hypomagnesemia.
Musculoskeletal: arthralgia, myalgia.
Respiratory: dyspnea, tachypnea, bronchospasm, wheezing (with systemic form).
Skin: maculopapular rash, pruritus without rash (with systemic form); possible dryness, contact sensitivity, erythema, burning, pruritus (with topical administration).
Other: tissue damage with extravasation, *phlebitis, thrombophlebitis, pain at injection site, fever, chills, generalized pain,* flushing, ***anaphylactoid reactions*** (with topical administration).

Overdose and treatment

Overdose may affect CV and respiratory function. Treatment is largely supportive. Hemodialysis isn't effective. Correction of electrolyte imbalances is usually necessary.

Clinical considerations

☐ ***ALERT*** Different amphotericin B preparations aren't interchangeable and dosages will vary.

- Cultures and histologic and sensitivity testing must be completed and diagnosis confirmed before starting therapy in nonimmunocompromised patient.
- Prepare infusion as manufacturer directs, with strict aseptic technique, using only 10 ml of sterile water to reconstitute. To avoid precipitation, don't mix with solutions containing sodium chloride, other electrolytes, or bacteriostatic agents such as benzyl alcohol.
- Don't use if reconstituted solution contains a precipitate or other foreign particles. Store the dry form at 35.6° to 46.4° F (2° to 8° C). Protect drug from light, and check expiration date.
- For I.V. infusion, use an in-line membrane with a mean pore diameter larger than 1 micron.
- Infuse slowly; rapid infusion may cause CV collapse.
- Don't mix or piggyback antibiotics with amphotericin B infusion; the I.V. solution appears compatible with small amounts of heparin sodium, hydrocortisone sodium succinate, and methylprednisolone sodium succinate.
- Severity of some adverse reactions can be reduced by premedication with aspirin or acetaminophen, antihistamines, antiemetics, meperidine, or small doses of corticosteroids; by addition of phosphate buffer to the solution; and by alternate-day dosing. If reactions are severe, drug may have to be discontinued for varying periods.
- Use topical products for folds of groin, neck, or armpit; avoid occlusive dressing with ointment, and discontinue if signs of hypersensitivity develop.
- Store at room temperature. Solution is stable at room temperature and in indoor light for 24 hours or in the refrigerator for 1 week.

Therapeutic monitoring

- Advise giving in distal veins, and monitor site for discomfort or thrombosis; if thrombosis occurs, alternate-day therapy may be considered.
- Advise checking vital signs every 30 minutes for at least 4 hours after start of I.V. infusion; fever may appear in 1 to 2 hours but should subside within 4 hours of discontinuing drug.

- Recommend observing for first dose acute infusion reactions, which include fever, chills, hypotension, nausea, vomiting, headache, dyspnea, and tachycardia. Reaction may occur in 1 to 3 hours.
- Recommend monitoring intake and output and check for changes in urine appearance or volume; renal damage may be reversible if drug is stopped at earliest sign of dysfunction.
- Recommend monitoring potassium and magnesium levels closely; monitor calcium and magnesium levels twice weekly; perform liver and renal function studies and CBCs weekly.

Special populations

Pregnant patients. Safety during pregnancy hasn't been established, but the drug has been used without obvious adverse effects to the fetus.

Breast-feeding patients. Safety hasn't been established in breast-feeding women.

Patient counseling

- Teach patient signs and symptoms of hypersensitivity and other adverse reactions, especially those associated with I.V. therapy. Warn that fever and chills are likely to occur and can be severe when therapy is initiated. These symptoms usually subside with repeated doses. Encourage patient feedback during infusion.
- Warn patient that therapy may take several months; recommend personal hygiene and other measures to prevent spread and recurrence of lesions.
- Urge patient to adhere to regimen and to return, as instructed, for follow-up.
- Tell patient that topical products may stain skin and clothing; cream or lotion may be removed from clothing with soap and water.

amphotericin B cholesteryl sulfate complex

Amphotec

Pharmacologic classification: polyene antibiotic
Therapeutic classification: antifungal
Pregnancy risk category B

How supplied

Available by prescription only
Injection: 50 mg/20 ml, 100 mg/50 ml

Indications and dosages

Invasive aspergillosis in patients in whom renal impairment or unacceptable toxicity precludes use of conventional amphotericin B deoxycholate in effective doses and in those with invasive aspergillosis in whom prior amphotericin B deoxycholate therapy has failed ◇ **Candida** ***and*** **Cryptococcus** ***infections not responsive or tolerable to conventional amphotericin B***

Adults and children: 3 to 4 mg/kg/day I.V.; may increase to 6 mg/kg/day if no improvement occurs or if fungal infection has progressed. Administer by continuous infusion at 1 mg/kg/hour. Perform a test dose before commencing new courses of treatment; infuse a small amount of drug (10 ml of final preparation containing 1.6 to 8.3 mg of drug) over 15 to 30 minutes and monitor for next 30 minutes.

◇***Empiric therapy of presumed fungal infections in febrile, neutropenic patients including cancer patients and bone marrow transplant (BMT) or solid organ transplant recipients***

Adults: 4 mg/kg I.V. daily for 8 days.

Pharmacodynamics

Fungistatic and fungicidal actions: Depend on concentration of drug and susceptibility of fungal organism. Drug binds to sterols in cell membranes of sensitive fungi, resulting in leakage of intracellular contents and causing cell death due to changes in membrane permeability. Also binds to sterols in mammalian cell membranes, which is believed to account for human toxicity.

Spectrum of activity includes *Aspergillus fumigatus, Candida albicans, Coccidioides immitis,* and *Cryptococcus neoformans.*

Pharmacokinetics

Absorption: For an infusion rate of 1 mg/kg/hour and dosage ranges from 3 to 6 mg/kg/day, maximum plasma level at the end of an infusion ranges from 2.6 to 3.4 mcg/ml.
Distribution: Multicompartmental; steady-state volume increases with higher doses, possibly from uptake by tissues.
Metabolism: Unknown.
Excretion: Unclear; elimination half-life, 27 to 29 hours; increasing doses increase the elimination half-life. Drug may not be removed by dialysis.

Route	Onset	Peak	Duration
I.V.	Unknown	3 hr	Unknown

Contraindications and precautions

Contraindicated in patients with hypersensitivity to any component of drug unless the benefits outweigh the risk of hypersensitivity.

Interactions

No formal drug interaction studies have been done. However, the following drugs are known to interact with amphotericin B.

Drug-drug. *Antineoplastic agents:* Enhanced renal toxicity, bronchospasm, hypotension. Avoid use together.
Cardiac glycosides: Enhanced potassium excretion, which increases risk of digitalis toxi-

city. Recommend monitoring serum digoxin levels.
Corticosteroids, corticotropin: Enhanced potassium depletion, which could predispose patient to cardiac dysfunction. Monitor patient closely.
Cyclosporine and tacrolimus: May possibly increase serum creatinine levels. Recommend monitoring serum creatinine levels.
Flucytosine: May cause synergistic effect and cause increased toxicity of flucytosine. Avoid use together.
Imidazoles (ketoconazole, miconazole, fluconazole, clotrimazole): May cause antagonistic effects. Recommend monitoring for adverse effects.
Nephrotoxic drugs (such as aminoglycosides, pentamidine): May enhance renal toxicity. Recommend monitoring renal function closely.
Skeletal muscle relaxants (such as tubocurarine): Amphotericin B-induced hypokalemia may enhance curariform effects of skeletal muscle relaxants due to hypokalemia. Use together cautiously.
Zidovudine: Increased myelotoxicity and nephrotoxicity. Recommend monitoring renal and hematologic function.
Drug-herb. *Gossypol:* Increases risk of renal toxicity. Avoid use together.

Effects on diagnostic tests
None reported.

Adverse reactions
CNS: abnormal thoughts, anxiety, agitation, confusion, depression, dizziness, hallucinations, headache, hypertonia, neuropathy, paresthesia, *seizures,* somnolence, stupor, asthenia.
CV: ***arrhythmias,*** *atrial fibrillation,* ***bradycardia, cardiac arrest, heart failure, hemorrhage,*** hypertension, *hypotension,* phlebitis, syncope, orthostatic hypotension, ***shock, supraventricular tachycardia,*** *tachycardia,* ***ventricular extrasystoles.***
EENT: eye hemorrhage, tinnitus, mucous membrane disorder.
GI: anorexia, GI disorder, GI hemorrhage, hematemesis, melena, *nausea,* stomatitis, *vomiting.*
GU: abnormal renal function, hematuria, ***renal failure.***
Hematologic: anemia, agranulocytosis, coagulation disorders, hypochromic anemia, increased PT, leukocytosis, ***leukopenia, thrombocytopenia.***
Hepatic: jaundice, abnormal liver function test results, ***hepatic failure.***
Metabolic: *hypokalemia,* hypocalcemia, hyperglycemia, hypervolemia, hypophosphatemia, hyponatremia, hyperkalemia, *increased creatinine, bilirubinemia,* hypomagnesemia, alkaline phosphatase, BUN, AST, ALT, LD levels.
Musculoskeletal: arthralgia, myalgia, abdominal, chest, or back pain.
Respiratory: ***apnea,*** asthma, dyspnea, epistaxis, hemoptysis, hyperventilation, hypoxia, increased cough, lung or respiratory disorders, *pulmonary edema.*
Skin: pruritus, rash, sweating, skin disorder.
Other: ***allergic reaction; anaphylaxis;*** *chills;* edema; *fever;* peripheral or facial edema; infection; pain or reaction at injection site; ***sepsis.***

Overdose and treatment
Amphotec isn't dialyzable. Amphotericin B deoxycholate overdose has been reported to result in cardiorespiratory arrest. If overdose is suspected, discontinue therapy, monitor clinical status, and administer supportive therapy.

Clinical considerations
- Pretreatment with antihistamines and corticosteroids or reducing the rate of infusion (or both) may reduce acute infusion-related reactions.

□ ***ALERT*** Note the differences in amphotericin B products. Don't interchange.
- Dilute in D_5W and administer by continuous infusion at 1 mg/kg/hour. If drug is well tolerated, can shorten infusion time to 2 hours or lengthen infusion time based on patient tolerance.
- Drug is incompatible with saline, electrolyte solutions, and bacteriostatic agents.
- Infuse drug over at least 2 hours.
- Don't mix with other drugs. If administered through an existing I.V. line, flush line with D_5W before infusion or use a separate line.
- Store vials at room temperature. Reconstitute 50-mg vial with rapid addition of 10 ml of sterile water for injection, and 100-mg vial with rapid addition of 20 ml sterile water with a sterile syringe and 20G needle. Shake vial gently. Don't use diluent other than sterile water for injection.
- Reconstituted drug is clear or opalescent liquid and is stable for 24 hours refrigerated. Discard partially used vials.
- Don't filter or use an in-line filter and don't freeze.

Therapeutic monitoring
- Recommend monitoring vital signs every 30 minutes during initial therapy. Acute infusion-related reactions (fever, chills, hypotension, nausea, tachycardia) usually occur 1 to 3 hours after starting I.V. infusion. These reactions are usually more severe after initial doses and usually diminish with subsequent doses. If severe respiratory distress occurs, stop infusion immediately and don't treat further with drug.
- Patient monitoring includes intake and output, and reporting changes in urine appearance or volume.
- Recommend monitoring renal and hepatic function tests, serum electrolytes (especially

potassium, magnesium, and calcium), CBCs, and PT and INR.

Special populations

Pregnant patients. Safe use during pregnancy hasn't been established, but the drug has been used without obvious adverse effects to the fetus.
Breast-feeding patients. It's unknown if drug is excreted in breast milk. Because of the potential for serious adverse reactions in breastfed infants, a decision should be made to discontinue breast-feeding or to stop treatment, taking into account the importance of drug to the woman.
Pediatric patients. No unexpected adverse events have been reported.
Geriatric patients. No unexpected adverse events have been reported.

Patient counseling

- Instruct patient to report symptoms of hypersensitivity immediately.
- Warn patient of possible discomfort at I.V. site.
- Advise patient of potential adverse effects, such as fever, chills, nausea, and vomiting. Tell him that these can be severe with initial treatment but usually subside with repeated doses.

amphotericin B lipid complex

Abelcet

Pharmacologic classification: polyene antibiotic
Therapeutic classification: antifungal
Pregnancy risk category B

How supplied

Available by prescription only
Suspension for injection: 100 mg/20-ml vial

Indications and dosage

Invasive fungal infections, including Aspergillus sp. and Candida sp., in patients who are refractory to or intolerant of conventional amphotericin B therapy
Adults and children: 5 mg/kg daily I.V. as a single infusion administered at rate of 2.5 mg/kg/hour.

Pharmacodynamics

Antifungal activity: The active component of Abelcet, amphotericin B, binds to sterols in fungal cell membranes, resulting in enhanced cellular permeability and cell damage. Amphotericin B has fungistatic or fungicidal effects depending on fungal susceptibility.

Pharmacokinetics

Absorption: Administered I.V.
Distribution: Well distributed. The distribution volume increases with increasing dose. Abelcet yields measurable amphotericin B levels in spleen, lung, liver, lymph nodes, kidney, heart, and brain.
Metabolism: Unknown.
Excretion: Although rapidly cleared from blood, Abelcet has a long terminal half-life (173.4 hr), probably due to slow elimination from tissues.

Route	Onset	Peak	Duration
I.V.	Unknown	Unknown	Unknown

Contraindications and precautions

Contraindicated in patients with hypersensitivity to amphotericin B or its components. Use cautiously in patients with renal impairment.

Interactions

Drug-drug. *Antineoplastics:* Increased risk of renal toxicity, bronchospasm, and hypotension. Use cautiously.
Cardiac glycosides: Increased risk of digitalis toxicity due to amphotericin B-induced hypokalemia. Recommend monitoring serum potassium levels closely.
Clotrimazole, fluconazole, itraconazole, ketoconazole, miconazole: May antagonize amphotericin B. Monitor patient closely.
Corticosteroids, corticotropin: Enhanced hypokalemia, which may lead to cardiac toxicity. Recommend monitoring serum electrolyte levels and cardiac function.
Cyclosporine: Increased renal toxicity. Monitor patient closely.
Flucytosine: Increased risk of flucytosine toxicity due to increased cellular uptake or impaired renal excretion. Use cautiously.
Nephrotoxic drugs (such as aminoglycosides, pentamidine): Increased risk of renal toxicity. Use cautiously. Recommend monitoring renal function closely.
Skeletal muscle relaxants: Enhanced effects of skeletal muscle relaxants resulting from amphotericin B-induced hypokalemia. Recommend monitoring serum potassium levels closely.
Zidovudine: Increased myelotoxicity and nephrotoxicity. Recommend monitoring renal and hematologic function.

Effects on diagnostic tests

None reported.

Adverse reactions

CNS: headache, pain.
CV: chest pain, ***cardiac arrest,*** hypertension, hypotension.
GI: abdominal pain, diarrhea, ***GI hemorrhage,*** nausea, vomiting.
GU: *increased serum creatinine level,* ***kidney failure.***

Hematologic: anemia, ***leukopenia, thrombocytopenia.***
Hepatic: bilirubinemia.
Metabolic: hypokalemia.
Respiratory: dyspnea, respiratory disorder, ***respiratory failure.***
Skin: rash.
Other: *chills, fever,* infection, **MULTIPLE ORGAN FAILURE,** ***sepsis.***

Overdose and treatment
Overdose has been associated with cardiorespiratory arrest. Doses as high as 7 to 13 mg/kg haven't produced serious acute toxicity. If overdose is suspected, discontinue therapy, monitor patient's clinical condition, and provide supportive treatment as needed. Drug isn't removed by hemodialysis.

Clinical considerations
□ ***ALERT*** The different amphotericin B preparations aren't interchangeable and dosages will vary.
- Premedication with acetaminophen, antihistamines, and corticosteroids can prevent or lessen severity of infusion-related reactions, such as fever, chills, nausea, and vomiting, which occur 1 to 2 hours after start of infusion.
- If severe respiratory distress occurs, discontinue infusion, provide supportive therapy for anaphylaxis, and notify prescriber. Drug shouldn't be reinstituted in this situation.
- Leukocyte transfusions shouldn't be given with drug because acute pulmonary toxicity has been reported with concurrent administration.
- To prepare, shake vial gently until there's no yellow sediment. Using aseptic technique, withdraw calculated dose into one or more 20-ml syringes, using an 18-gauge needle. More than one vial will be required. Attach a 5-micron filter needle to the syringe and inject the dose into an I.V. bag of D_5W. One filter needle can be used for up to four vials of amphotericin B lipid complex. The volume of D_5W should be sufficient to yield a final concentration of 1 mg/ml.
- Drug has an unlabeled use for empiric therapy in febrile neutropenic patients.
- For pediatric patients and patients with cardiovascular disease, recommended final concentration is 2 mg/ml.
- Don't mix with saline or infuse in same I.V. line as other drugs. Don't use an in-line filter.
- Discard any unused drug; it doesn't contain a preservative.
- Use an infusion pump and administer by continuous infusion at a rate of 2.5 mg/kg/hour. If infusion time exceeds 2 hours, mix contents by shaking infusion bag every 2 hours.
- If infusing through an existing I.V. line, flush first with D_5W.
- Infusions are stable for up to 48 hours if refrigerated at 36° to 46° F (2° to 8° C) and up to 6 hours at room temperature.

Therapeutic monitoring
- Vital signs should be taken frequently. Fever, shaking chills, and hypotension may appear within 2 hours of initiating infusion. Slowing infusion rate may decrease incidence of infusion-related reactions.
- Monitor serum creatinine and electrolyte levels (especially magnesium and potassium), liver function, and CBC during therapy.
- The need for dosage adjustment should be based on the overall clinical status of the patient. Renal toxicity is more common at higher doses.

Special populations
Breast-feeding patients: It's unknown if drug is excreted in breast milk. The decision to administer Abelcet to a lactating woman should be based on the risk of adverse reactions in the infant compared to the benefits of treatment.
Pediatric patients: No unexpected adverse reactions have been reported in children age 16 or under when given 5 mg/kg/day.
Geriatric patients: No unexpected adverse reactions have been reported when treated with 5 mg/kg/day.

Patient counseling
- Inform patient that fever, chills, nausea, and vomiting may occur during infusion and that these reactions usually subside with subsequent doses.
- Instruct patient to report any redness or pain at infusion site.
- Teach patient to recognize and report any symptoms of acute hypersensitivity such as respiratory distress.
- Warn patient that therapy may take several months.
- Tell patient to expect frequent laboratory testing to monitor kidney and liver function.

amphotericin B liposomal
AmBisome

Pharmacologic classification: polyene antibiotic
Therapeutic classification: antifungal
Pregnancy risk category B

How supplied
Available by prescription only
Injection: 50-mg vial

Indications and dosage
Empirical therapy for presumed fungal infection in febrile, neutropenic patients
Adults and children: 3 mg/kg I.V. infusion daily.

Systemic fungal infections due to* Aspergillus sp., Candida sp., *or* Cryptococcus sp. *refractory to amphotericin B deoxycholate or in patients in whom renal impairment or unacceptable toxicity precludes use of amphotericin B deoxycholate
Adults and children: 3 to 5 mg/kg I.V. infusion daily.
Visceral leishmaniasis in immunocompetent patients
Adults and children: 3 mg/kg I.V. infusion daily on days 1 to 5, 14, and 21. A repeat course of therapy may be beneficial if initial treatment fails to achieve parasitic clearance.
Visceral leishmaniasis in immunocompromised patients
Adults and children: 4 mg/kg I.V. infusion daily on days 1 to 5, 10, 17, 24, 31, and 38. Expert advice regarding further treatment is recommended if initial therapy fails or patient experiences relapse.

Pharmacodynamics
Antifungal activity: Amphotericin B, the active component of AmBisome, binds to the sterol component of a fungal cell membrane leading to alterations in cell permeability and cell death.

Pharmacokinetics
Absorption: Administered IV.
Distribution: Unknown.
Metabolism: Unknown.
Excretion: The initial half-life is 7 to 10 hours with 24 hour dosing; terminal elimination half-life is 100 to 153 hours.

Route	Onset	Peak	Duration
I.V.	Unknown	Unknown	Unknown

Contraindications and precautions
Contraindicated in patients with hypersensitivity to drug or its components. Use cautiously in patients with impaired renal function, in geriatric patients, and in pregnant women.

Interactions
Drug-drug. *Antineoplastics:* May enhance potential for renal toxicity, bronchospasm, and hypotension. Use cautiously.
Cardiac glycosides: Increased risk of digitalis toxicity due to amphotericin B-induced hypokalemia. Recommend monitoring serum potassium level closely.
Clotrimazole, fluconazole, ketoconazole, miconazole: May induce fungal resistance to amphotericin B. Use together cautiously.
Corticosteroids, corticotropin: May potentiate potassium depletion, which could result in cardiac dysfunction. Recommend monitoring serum electrolyte level and cardiac function.
Flucytosine: May increase flucytosine toxicity by increasing cellular reuptake or impairing renal excretion of flucytosine. Use cautiously.
Other nephrotoxic drugs, such as antibiotics, antineoplastics: May cause additive nephrotoxicity. Administer cautiously. Recommend monitoring renal function closely.
Skeletal muscle relaxants: Enhanced effects of skeletal muscle relaxants resulting from amphotericin B-induced hypokalemia. Recommend monitoring serum potassium levels.

Effects on diagnostic tests
None reported.

Adverse reactions
CNS: *anxiety, confusion, headache, insomnia, asthenia.*
CV: *chest pain, hypotension, tachycardia,* hypertension, *edema.*
EENT: *epistaxis, rhinitis.*
GI: *nausea, vomiting, abdominal pain, diarrhea,* ***GI hemorrhage.***
GU: *hematuria, elevated creatinine and BUN levels.*
Hepatic: *elevated ALT and AST levels, increased alkaline phosphatase level, bilirubinemia.*
Metabolic: *hyperglycemia,* hypernatremia, *hypocalcemia, hypokalemia, hypomagnesemia.*
Musculoskeletal: *back pain.*
Respiratory: *increased cough, dyspnea,* hypoxia, *pleural effusion, lung disorder,* hyperventilation.
Skin: *pruritus, rash, sweating.*
Other: *chills, infection, flushing,* ***anaphylaxis,*** *pain,* ***sepsis,*** *fever, blood product infusion reaction.*

Overdose and treatment
Repeated daily doses of up to 7.5 mg/kg have been given without toxicity. If overdose occurs, cease administration immediately. Symptomatic supportive measures should be instituted. Pay particular attention to monitoring renal function. The drug isn't hemodialyzable.

Clinical considerations
- Patients also receiving chemotherapy or bone marrow transplantation are at greater risk for additional adverse reactions, including seizures, arrhythmias, and thrombocytopenia.
- Leukocyte transfusions shouldn't be given with drug because acute pulmonary toxicity has been reported with concurrent administration.
- To lessen risk or severity of adverse reactions, premedication with antipyretics, antihistamines, antiemetics, or corticosteroids can be ordered.

□ ***ALERT*** The different amphotericin B preparations aren't interchangeable and dosages will vary.

- Patients given amphotericin B liposomal had a lower incidence of chills, elevated BUN, hypokalemia, hypertension, and vomiting than patients treated with conventional amphotericin B.

- Reconstitute each 50-mg vial of amphotericin B liposomal with 12 ml of sterile water for injection to yield a solution of 4 mg amphotericin B/ml.

□ *ALERT* Don't reconstitute with bacteriostatic water for injection and don't allow bacteriostatic agent in solution. Don't reconstitute with saline or add saline to reconstituted concentration or mix with other drugs.

- After reconstitution, shake vial vigorously for 30 seconds or until particulate matter is dispersed.
- Withdraw calculated amount of reconstituted solution into a sterile syringe and inject through a 5-micron filter into the appropriate amount of D_5W to further dilute to a final concentration of 1 to 2 mg/ml. Lower concentrations (0.2 to 0.5 mg/ml) may be appropriate for pediatric patients to provide sufficient volume of infusion.
- An existing I.V. line must be flushed with D_5W before infusion of drug. If this isn't feasible, administer drug through a separate line.
- Use a controlled infusion device and an in-line filter with a mean pore diameter larger than 1 micron. Initially, infuse drug over at least 2 hours. Infusion time may be reduced to 1 hour if treatment is well tolerated. If patient experiences discomfort during infusion, duration of infusion may be increased.
- Recommend clinician observe patient closely for adverse reactions during infusion. If anaphylaxis occurs, stop infusion immediately, provide supportive therapy, and notify prescriber.
- Unopened drug is stored under refrigeration at 36° to 46° F (2° to 8° C). Once reconstituted, vial of reconstituted concentrate may be stored for up to 24 hours at 36° to 46°F. Don't freeze.

Therapeutic monitoring

- Monitor BUN and serum creatinine and electrolyte levels (particularly magnesium and potassium), liver function, and CBC. Therapy may take several weeks to months.
- Patient requires close observation for signs of hypokalemia (ECG changes, muscle weakness, cramping, drowsiness).

Special populations

Breast-feeding patients. It's unknown if drug is excreted in human milk, but because of the potential for serious adverse reactions in breast-fed infants, a decision should be made whether to discontinue nursing or to discontinue the drug, taking into account the importance of the drug to the woman.

Pediatric patients. Safety and efficacy in pediatric patients under age 1 month haven't been established.

Geriatric patients. No dosage alteration is necessary. Carefully monitor geriatric patients.

Patient counseling

- Teach patient signs and symptoms of hypersensitivity, and stress importance of reporting them immediately.
- Warn patient that therapy may take several months; teach personal hygiene and other measures to prevent spread and recurrence of lesions.
- Instruct patient to report any adverse reactions that occur while receiving drug.
- Instruct patient to watch for and report signs of hypokalemia (muscle weakness, cramping, drowsiness)
- Advise patient that frequent laboratory testing will be necessary.

ampicillin

Apo-Ampi*, Novo-Ampicillin*, Omnipen, Penbritin*

ampicillin sodium

Ampicin*, Omnipen-N, Penbritin*

ampicillin trihydrate

Omnipen, Principen, Totacillin

Pharmacologic classification: aminopenicillin
Therapeutic classification: antibiotic
Pregnancy risk category B

How supplied

Available by prescription only
Capsules: 250 mg, 500 mg
Suspension: 125 mg/5 ml, 250 mg/5 ml, 500 mg/5 ml (after reconstitution)
Parenteral: 125 mg, 250 mg, 500 mg, 1 g, 2 g
Infusion: 500 mg, 1 g, 2 g

Indications and dosages

Systemic infections, acute and chronic urinary tract infections caused by susceptible organisms
Adults: 250 to 500 mg P.O. q 6 hours.
Children under 88 lb (40 kg): 25 to 100 mg/kg P.O. daily, divided into doses given q 6 hours; or 100 to 200 mg/kg I.V. daily for 3 days and then I.M., divided into doses given q 6 to 8 hours.

Meningitis
Adults: 8 to 14 g I.V. or 150 to 200 mg/kg/day divided q 3 to 4 hours for 3 days; then may give I.M. if desired.
Children age 2 months to 12 years: 200 to 400 mg/kg I.V. daily in divided doses q 4 to 6 hours. May be given along with chloramphenicol, pending culture results.

Neonates under 1 week old: 50 to 75 mg/kg I.V. q 12 hours (weight under 2 kg) or q 8 hours (weight over 2 kg).
Neonates over 1 week old: 50 mg/kg I.V. q 8 hours (weight under 2 kg) or q 6 hours (weight over 2 kg).
Neonatal group B streptococcal meningitis
Neonates age 7 days or under: 200 mg/kg/daily I.V. given in three divided doses.
Neonates age 7 days or over: 300 mg/kg/daily I.V. given in 4 to 6 divided doses.
Uncomplicated gonorrhea
Adults: 3.5 g P.O. with 1 g probenecid given as a single dose.
≡***Dosage adjustment.*** Increase dosing interval to q 12 hours in patients with severe renal impairment (creatinine clearance 10 ml/minute or less).
Prophylaxis for bacterial endocarditis before dental or minor respiratory procedures
Adults: 2 g (I.V. or I.M.) 30 minutes before procedure.
Children: 50 mg/kg I.V. or I.M. 30 minutes before procedure.
Treatment of enterococcal endocarditis
Adults: 12 g daily by continuous I.V. infusion or in six equally divided doses in conjunction with gentamicin for 4 to 6 weeks.
◇***Prophylaxis of neonatal group B streptococcus infections***
Adult: 2 g I.V. given to the mother 4 hours before delivery, then 1 to 2 g I.V. q 4 to 6 hours until delivery.

Pharmacodynamics

Antibiotic action: Ampicillin is bactericidal; it adheres to bacterial penicillin-binding proteins, inhibiting bacterial cell wall synthesis.

Spectrum of action includes non-penicillinase-producing gram-positive bacteria. It's also effective against many gram-negative organisms, including *Neisseria gonorrhoeae, Neisseria meningitidis, Haemophilus influenzae, Escherichia coli, Proteus mirabilis, Salmonella,* and *Shigella.* Ampicillin should be used in gram-negative systemic infections only when organism sensitivity is known.

Pharmacokinetics

Absorption: About 42% of ampicillin is absorbed after an oral dose.
Distribution: Distributes into pleural, peritoneal and synovial fluids, lungs, prostate, liver, and gallbladder; it also penetrates middle ear effusions, maxillary sinus and bronchial secretions, tonsils, and sputum. Readily crosses the placenta; minimally protein-bound (15% to 25%).
Metabolism: Only partially metabolized.
Excretion: Excreted in urine by renal tubular secretion and glomerular filtration. It's also excreted in breast milk. Elimination half-life is about 1 to 1½ hours; in patients with extensive renal impairment, half-life is extended to 10 to 24 hours.

Route	Onset	Peak	Duration
P.O.	Unknown	2 hr	6-8 hr
I.V.	Immediate	Immediate	Unknown
I.M.	Unknown	1 hr	Unknown

Contraindications and precautions

Contraindicated in patients with hypersensitivity to drug or other penicillins. Use with caution in patients with mononucleosis.

Interactions

Drug-drug. *Aminoglycoside antibiotic:* A synergistic bactericidal effect against some strains of enterococci and group B streptococci. However, the drugs are physically and chemically incompatible and are inactivated if mixed or given together. Don't mix together.
Allopurinol: Appears to increase incidence of rash from both drugs. Monitor patient closely.
Clavulanate: Results in increased bactericidal effects because clavulanic acid is a beta-lactamase inhibitor. Use drugs together for clinical effect.
Probenecid: Inhibits renal tubular secretion of ampicillin, raising its serum concentrations. Avoid use together.
Methotrexate: Large doses of penicillins may interfere with renal tubular secretion of methotrexate, delaying elimination and elevating serum levels of methotrexate. Recommend monitoring for methotrexate toxicity.
Oral contraceptives: Effects of oral contraceptives may be decreased. Advise using alternative barrier method.

Effects on diagnostic tests

Ampicillin alters results of urine glucose tests that use cupric sulfate (Benedict's reagent or Clinitest). Urine glucose determinations should be done with glucose oxidase methods (Chemstrip uG, Diastix, or glucose enzymatic test strip).

Adverse reactions

CNS: lethargy, hallucinations, ***seizures***, anxiety, confusion, agitation, depression, dizziness, fatigue.
GI: *nausea*, vomiting, *diarrhea*, glossitis, stomatitis, gastritis, abdominal pain, enterocolitis, pseudomembranous colitis, black "hairy" tongue.
GU: interstitial nephritis, nephropathy, vaginitis.
Hematologic: anemia, ***thrombocytopenia***, thrombocytopenic purpura, eosinophilia, ***leukopenia***, ***hemolytic anemia***, ***agranulocytosis.***
Other: ***hypersensitivity reactions*** (erythematous maculopapular rash, urticaria, ***anaphylaxis***), overgrowth of nonsusceptible organ-

isms, pain at injection site, vein irritation, thrombophlebitis.

Overdose and treatment

Clinical signs of overdose include neuromuscular sensitivity or seizures. After recent ingestion (within 4 hours), empty the stomach by induced emesis or gastric lavage; follow with activated charcoal to reduce absorption. Drug can be removed by hemodialysis.

Clinical considerations

- Consider the recommendations relevant to all penicillins.
- Obtain patient's allergy history before dispensing drug.
- Administer I.M. or I.V. only when patient is too ill to take oral drug.

Therapeutic monitoring

Recommend monitoring renal, hepatic, hematologic systems during prolonged therapy.

Special populations

Pregnant patients. Safe use during pregnancy hasn't been established, but drug has been used to treat urinary tract infections in pregnant women without affecting the fetus.
Breast-feeding patients. Use cautiously. Ampicillin is distributed readily into breast milk; safety in breast-feeding women hasn't been established.
Geriatric patients. Because of diminished renal tubular secretion in geriatric patients, half-life of drug may be prolonged.

Patient counseling

- Advise patient to report diarrhea promptly.
- Instruct patient to complete all of the prescribed drug.

ampicillin sodium/ sulbactam sodium

Unasyn

Pharmacologic classification: aminopenicillin/beta-lactamase inhibitor combination
Therapeutic classification: antibiotic
Pregnancy risk category B

How supplied

Available by prescription only
Injection: vials and piggyback vials containing 1.5 g (1 g ampicillin sodium with 500 mg sulbactam sodium) and 3 g (2 g ampicillin sodium with 1 g sulbactam sodium)

Indications and dosages

***Skin and skin-structure infections, intra-abdominal and gynecologic infections caused by susceptible gram positive bacteria, gram negative bacteria, beta-lactamase-producing strains of* Staphylococcus aureus, Escherichia coli, Klebsiella *(including* K. pneumoniae*),* Proteus mirabilis, Bacteroides *(including* B. fragilis*),* Enterobacter, Neisseria meningitidis, Neisseria gonorrhoeae, Moraxella catarrhalis, *and* Acinetobacter calcoaceticus**
Adults: 1.5 to 3 g I.M. or I.V. q 6 hours. Don't exceed 4 g/day sulbactam sodium.
For skin and skin structure infections caused by susceptible organisms
Children under 88 lb (40 kg): same as adult dose.
Children 1 year and older weighing less than 40 kg: 300 mg/kg I.V. daily in divided doses q 6 hours not to exceed 14 days of therapy.
≡ ***Dosage adjustment.*** For patients with renal impairment, give the usually recommended doses, but less frequently. Patients with creatinine clearances of 30 ml/min/1.73 m^2 or greater receive 1.5 to 3 g of the drug every 6 to 8 hours and patients with creatinine clearances of 15 to 29 ml/min/1.73 m^2 receive these doses every 12 to 24 hours.

Pharmacodynamics

Antibiotic action: Ampicillin is bactericidal; it adheres to bacterial penicillin-binding proteins, thus inhibiting bacterial cell wall synthesis. Sulbactam inhibits beta-lactamase, an enzyme produced by ampicillin-resistant bacteria that degrades ampicillin.

Pharmacokinetics

Absorption: Well absorbed after I.V. and I.M. administration.
Distribution: Both distribute into pleural, peritoneal and synovial fluids, lungs, prostate, liver, and gallbladder; they also penetrate middle ear effusions, maxillary sinus and bronchial secretions, tonsils, and sputum. Ampicillin readily crosses the placenta; it's minimally protein-bound at 15% to 25%; sulbactam is about 38% bound.
Metabolism: Both are metabolized only partially; only 15% to 25% of both are metabolized.
Excretion: Both are excreted in the urine by renal tubular secretion and glomerular filtration. It's also excreted in breast milk. Elimination half-life is 1 to 1¼ hours; in patients with extensive renal impairment, half-life can be as long as 10 to 24 hours.

Route	Onset	Peak	Duration
I.V.	15 min	Immediate	Unknown
I.M.	Unknown	Unknown	Unknown

Contraindications and precautions

Contraindicated in patients with hypersensitivity to drug or other penicillins. Use cautiously in patients with maculopapular rash.

Interactions

Drug-drug. *Probenecid*: Decreases excretion of both ampicillin and sulbactam. Recommend monitoring for toxicity.
Allopurinol: May lead to an increased incidence of rash. Monitor patient closely.
Aminoglycosides: The ampicillin component may cause in vitro inactivation of aminoglycosides if these antibiotics are mixed in the same infusion container. Don't mix together.
Anticoagulants: Large doses of I.V. penicillins can increase bleeding risks of anticoagulants because of a prolongation of bleeding times. Recommend monitoring PT and INR.

Effects on diagnostic tests

Ampicillin alters results of urine glucose tests that use cupric sulfate (Benedict's reagent or Clinitest). Make urine glucose determinations with glucose oxidase methods (Chemstrip uG, Diastix, or glucose enzymatic test strip).

In pregnant women, transient decreases in serum estradiol, conjugated estrone, conjugated estriol, and estriol glucuronide may occur.

Adverse reactions

GI: *nausea,* vomiting, *diarrhea,* glossitis, stomatitis, gastritis, black "hairy" tongue, enterocolitis, pseudomembranous colitis.
Hematologic: anemia, ***thrombocytopenia,*** thrombocytopenic purpura, eosinophilia, ***leukopenia, agranulocytosis.***
Other: ***hypersensitivity reactions*** (erythematous maculopapular rash, urticaria, ***anaphylaxis***), ***overgrowth of nonsusceptible organisms,*** pain at injection site, vein irritation, thrombophlebitis.

Overdose and treatment

Neurologic adverse reactions, including seizures, are likely. Treatment is supportive. Ampicillin and sulbactam are likely to be removed by hemodialysis.

Clinical considerations

☐ ***ALERT*** Give I.V. administration by slow injection over at least 10 to 15 minutes or infused in greater dilutions with 50 to 100 ml of a compatible diluent over 15 to 30 minutes to avoid risk for seizures.

- Store powder at 86° F (30° C) or colder.
- For I.V. use, reconstitute powder in piggyback units to desired concentrations with sterile water for injection, normal saline injection, 5% dextrose injection, lactated Ringer's injection, 1/6 M sodium lactate injection, 5% dextrose in 0.45% saline, or 10% invert sugar.
- For I.M. injection, reconstitute with sterile water for injection, or 0.5% or 2% lidocaine hydrochloride injection. To obtain 375 mg/ml solutions (250 mg ampicillin/125 mg sulbactam/ml), add contents of the 1.5-g vial to 3.2 ml of diluent to produce 4 ml withdrawal volume; add 3-g vial to 6.4 ml of diluent to produce 8 ml withdrawal volume.
- Reconstituted solutions are stable for varying periods (from 2 to 72 hours) depending on diluent used. Refer to package insert for specific information. For patients on sodium restriction, note that a 1.5-g dose of ampicillin sodium/sulbactam sodium yields 5 mEq of sodium.

Therapeutic considerations

- Recommend testing for *Clostridium difficile* in patients with persistent diarrhea.
- Recommend monitoring for overgrowth of nonsusceptible organisms.

Special populations

Pregnant patients. Safety in pregnant women hasn't been established.
Breast-feeding patients. Distributed readily into breast milk; safety in breast-feeding women hasn't been established. Alternative feeding method is recommended during therapy.
Pediatric patients. Safety in children under age 1 hasn't been established. Safety and efficacy for use in children for treatment of skin and skin structure infections has been established. Not for use for other infections or for I.M. use.
Geriatric patients. Because of diminished renal tubular secretion in geriatric patients, half-life of drug may be prolonged.

Patient counseling

- Tell patient to report a rash, fever, chills. A rash is the most frequent allergic reaction.
- Advise patient to report discomfort at insertion site.
- Warn patient that I.M. injection may cause pain at the injection site.

amprenavir

Agenerase

Pharmacologic classification: protease inhibitor
Therapeutic classification: antiretroviral
Pregnancy risk category C

How supplied

Available by prescription only
Capsules: 50 mg, 150 mg
Oral solution: 15 mg/ml

Indications and dosages

Treatment of HIV-1 infection in combination with other antiretroviral agents
Adults and children age 13 to 16 weighing over 110 lb (50 kg): 1,200 mg P.O. (eight 150-mg capsules) b.i.d. in combination with other antiretroviral agents.

Children age 4 to 12 or 13 to 16 weighing under 110 lb: Capsules: 20 mg/kg P.O. b.i.d. or 15 mg/kg P.O. t.i.d. (to a maximum daily dose of 2400 mg) in combination with other antiretroviral agents.
Oral Solution: 22.5 mg/kg P.O. (1.5 ml/kg) b.i.d. or 17 mg/kg P.O. (1.1 ml/kg) t.i.d. (to a maximum daily dose of 2800 mg) in combination with other antiretroviral agents.
≡ ***Dosage adjustment.*** Patients with moderate or severe hepatic impairment should receive reduced dosage.
Patients with Child-Pugh score of 5 to 8: 450 mg (capsules) P.O. b.i.d.
Patients with Child-Pugh score of 9 to 12: 300 mg (capsules) P.O. b.i.d.

Pharmacodynamics
Antiretroviral action: Amprenavir binds to the active site of HIV-1 protease and thereby prevents the processing of viral *gag* and *gag-pol* polyprotein precursors, resulting in the formation of immature noninfectious viral particles.

Pharmacokinetics
Absorption: Rapidly absorbed.
Distribution: About 90% bound to plasma proteins.
Metabolism: Metabolized in the liver by the cytochrome P-450 CYP3A4 enzyme system.
Excretion: Excretion of unchanged amprenavir in urine and feces is minimal. The plasma elimination half-life ranges from 7.1 to 10.6 hours.

Route	Onset	Peak	Duration
P.O.	Unknown	1-2 hr	Unknown

Contraindications and precautions
Contraindicated in patients with previously demonstrated clinically significant hypersensitivity to drug or any of its components. Use cautiously in patients with a known sulfonamide allergy, those with hepatic impairment, and those with hemophilia A and B.

Interactions
Drug-drug. *Antiarrhythmics such as amiodarone, lidocaine (systemic), quinidine; anticoagulants such as warfarin, and tricyclic antidepressants:* When used together, amprenavir serum levels may be affected. Monitor closely.
Macrolides: Increase amprenavir plasma levels. Dose adjustment may be required.
Psychotherapeutic agents: May cause increased CNS effects. Monitor patient closely.
Rifabutin: Decreased amprenavir levels and a substantial increase in rifabutin levels. Recommend reducing dosage.
Sildenafil: Substantially increased sildenafil levels, which may cause an increase in sildenafil-associated effects, including hypotension, visual changes, and priapism. Avoid use together.
Bepridil, cisapride, dihydroergotamine, midazolam, rifampin, and triazolam: Serious and life-threatening interactions may occur. Avoid use together.
Antacids: Advise nurse to separate administration of antacids and drug by at least 1 hour to avoid possible interference with absorption.
Drug-food. *High-fat meals:* Reduce drug absorption. Recommend not taking drug with a high-fat meal.

Effects on diagnostic tests
None reported.

Adverse reactions
CNS: *paresthesia*, depressive or mood disorders, headache.
GI: *nausea, vomiting, diarrhea or loose stools,* taste disorders.
Metabolic: *hyperglycemia, hypertriglyceridemia,* hypercholesterolemia.
Skin: *rash,* ***Stevens-Johnson syndrome.***

Overdose and treatment
No known antidote. It isn't known whether amprenavir can be removed by peritoneal lavage or hemodialysis. If overdose occurs, monitor patient for evidence of toxicity and give supportive treatment as needed.

Clinical considerations
- Drug is a sulfonamide. Patients with a known sulfonamide allergy should be treated with caution.
- Capsules and oral solution aren't interchangeable on milligram per milligram basis.
- Store capsules and oral solution at room temperature.

Therapeutic monitoring
- Monitor for adverse reactions. Drug may cause redistribution or accumulation of body fat including central obesity, dorsocervical fat enlargement (buffalo hump), peripheral wasting, breast enlargement, or cushingoid appearance. Severe and life-threatening reactions, including Stevens-Johnson syndrome, have occurred.
- Recommend performing CBC weekly and as clinically indicated to monitor for neutropenia in patients also receiving rifabutin.

Special populations
Pregnant patients. To monitor maternal-fetal outcomes of pregnant women exposed to drug, an Antiretroviral Pregnancy Registry has been established. Prescribers may call 1-800-258-4263 to register patients who have been exposed to drug during pregnancy.
Breast-feeding patients. It isn't known if drug is excreted in breast milk, so instruct breast-feeding women not to breast-feed if they're re-

ceiving drug. In addition, it's recommended that HIV-infected women not breast-feed their infants to avoid risking postnatal transmission of HIV.

Pediatric patients. An adverse event profile similar to that in adults is seen in pediatric patients. Safety, efficacy, and pharmacokinetics of drug haven't been evaluated in children under age 4.

Geriatric patients. Dosing in the elderly should be cautious, reflecting the greater frequency of decreased hepatic, renal, or cardiac function, and of concomitant disease or other drug therapy.

Patient counseling

- Inform patient that drug isn't a cure for HIV infection and opportunistic infections and other complications associated with the disease may continue to develop. The drug doesn't reduce the risk of transmitting HIV to others through sexual contact.
- Tell patient he may take drug without regard to meals but to avoid taking with high-fat meals because absorption may be decreased.
- Advise patient to take drug each day as prescribed. It must always be taken in combination with other antiretroviral drugs. Dose must not be altered or discontinued without consulting a doctor.
- Tell patient if a dose is missed to take the dose as soon as possible and then return to the normal schedule. However, if a dose is skipped, don't double the next dose.
- Instruct patients taking hormonal contraceptives to use alternate contraceptive measures during drug therapy.

amrinone lactate

Inocor

Pharmacologic classification: bipyridine derivative
Therapeutic classification: inotropic, vasodilator
Pregnancy risk category C

How supplied

Available by prescription only
Injection: 5 mg/ml

Indications and dosages

Short-term management of heart failure
Adults: Initially, 0.75 mg/kg I.V. bolus over 2 to 3 minutes; then begin maintenance infusion of 5 to 10 mcg/kg/minute. Additional bolus of 0.75 mg/kg may be given 30 minutes after therapy is initiated. Maximum daily dose is 10 mg/kg.

Cardiac life support in patients in whom other preferred drugs cannot be used for pump failure and acute pulmonary edema
Adults: 0.75 mg/kg I.V. bolus over 2 to 3 minutes, then 5 to 15 mcg/kg/minute.

Pharmacodynamics

Vasodilating action: The primary vasodilating effect of amrinone seems to stem from a direct effect on peripheral vessels.
Inotropic action: The mechanism of action responsible for the apparent inotropic effect isn't fully understood; however, it may be associated with inhibition of phosphodiesterase activity, resulting in increased cellular levels of adenosine 3',5'-cyclic phosphate; this, in turn, may alter intracellular and extracellular calcium levels. The role of calcium homeostasis hasn't been determined. Clinical effects include increased cardiac output mediated by reduced afterload and, possibly, inotropism.

Pharmacokinetics

Absorption: Rapidly absorbed.
Distribution: Distribution volume is 1.2 L/kg. Distribution sites are unknown. Protein binding ranges from 10% to 49%. Therapeutic steady-state serum levels range from 0.5 to 7 mcg/ml (ideal concentration: 3 mcg/ml).
Metabolism: Metabolized in the liver to several metabolites of unknown activity.
Excretion: In normal patients, amrinone is excreted in the urine, with a terminal elimination half-life of about 4 hours. Half-life may be prolonged slightly in patients with heart failure.

Route	Onset	Peak	Duration
I.V.	2-5 min	10 min	½-2 hr

Contraindications and precautions

Contraindicated in patients with hypersensitivity to amrinone or bisulfites. It shouldn't be used in patients with severe aortic or pulmonic valvular disease in place of surgical intervention or during an acute phase of MI.

Interactions

Drug-drug. *Disopyramide:* May cause severe hypotension. Avoid use together.
Cardiac glycosides: Increased inotropic effect. This is a benefit in certain conditions.

Effects on diagnostic tests

None reported.

Adverse reactions

CV: ***arrhythmias,*** hypotension, chest pain.
GI: nausea, vomiting, anorexia, abdominal pain.
Hematologic: ***thrombocytopenia*** (based on dose and duration of therapy).
Hepatic: elevated enzymes, hepatotoxicity (rare).
Metabolic: decreased serum potassium.

Other: burning at injection site, ***hypersensitivity reactions*** (pericarditis, ascites, myositis vasculitis, pleuritis), fever.

Overdose and treatment
Clinical effects of overdose include severe hypotension. Treatment may include administration of a potent vasopressor, such as norepinephrine, as well as other general supportive measures, including cautious fluid volume replacement.

Clinical considerations
☐ ***ALERT*** Don't confuse amrinone, an inotrope, with amiodarone, an antiarrhythmic with negative chronotropic effects.
- Dispense drug as supplied or dilute in normal or half-normal saline solution to concentration of 1 to 3 mg/ml. Don't dilute drug with solutions containing dextrose because a slow chemical reaction occurs over 24 hours. However, amrinone can be injected into running dextrose infusions through Y-connector or directly into tubing. Use diluted solution within 24 hours.
- Advise nurse not to administer furosemide in I.V. lines containing amrinone because a chemical reaction occurs immediately.
- Amrinone is prescribed primarily for patients who haven't responded to therapy with cardiac glycosides, diuretics, and vasodilators.
- Store at room temperature and protect from light.

Therapeutic monitoring
- Recommend monitoring blood pressure and heart rate throughout infusion. Slow or stop infusion if patient's blood pressure decreases or if arrhythmias (ventricular or supraventricular) occur. Dosage may need to be reduced.
- Monitor platelet counts. A count below 150,000/mm^3 usually necessitates dosage reduction. Thrombocytopenia usually occurs after prolonged treatment.
- Monitor electrolyte levels (especially potassium) because drug increases cardiac output, which may cause diuresis.
- Hemodynamic monitoring may be useful in guiding therapy.
- Recommend monitoring liver function tests to detect hepatic damage (rare).
- Observe for adverse GI effects (such as nausea, vomiting, and diarrhea); reduce dosage or discontinue drug.

Special populations
Pediatric patients. Safety and efficacy in children under age 18 haven't been established.
Breast-feeding patients. Drug may be excreted in breast milk. Safety in breast-feeding women hasn't been established.

Patient counseling
- Warn patient that burning may occur at the site of injection.
- Tell patient to report adverse reactions promptly.

anastrozole
Arimidex

Pharmacologic classification: nonsteroidal aromatase inhibitor
Therapeutic classification: antineoplastic
Pregnancy risk category D

How supplied
Available by prescription only
Tablets: 1 mg

Indications and dosages
Treatment of advanced breast cancer in postmenopausal women with disease progression following tamoxifen therapy
Adults: 1 mg P.O. daily.

Pharmacodynamics
Antineoplastic action: A potent and selective nonsteroidal aromatase inhibitor, anastrozole significantly lowers serum estradiol concentrations. Estradiol is the principal estrogen circulating in postmenopausal women that has the ability to stimulate breast cancer cell growth.

Pharmacokinetics
Absorption: Absorbed from the GI tract; food affects the extent of absorption.
Distribution: 40% bound to plasma proteins in the therapeutic range.
Metabolism: Metabolized in the liver.
Excretion: About 11% of anastrozole is excreted in urine as parent drug and about 60% is excreted in urine as metabolites. Half-life is about 50 hours.

Route	Onset	Peak	Duration
P.O.	< 24 hr	Unknown	< 6 days

Contraindications and precautions
Contraindicated in pregnant women.

Interactions
None reported.

Effects on diagnostic tests
None reported.

Adverse reactions
CNS: *asthenia, headache,* dizziness, depression, paresthesia.
CV: chest pain, edema, thromboembolic disease.
GI: dry mouth, *nausea,* vomiting, diarrhea, constipation, abdominal pain, anorexia.

GU: vaginal hemorrhage, vaginal dryness.
Musculoskeletal: *back pain,* bone pain, pelvic pain.
Respiratory: dyspnea, increased cough, pharyngitis.
Skin: *hot flashes,* rash, sweating.
Other: *pain,* peripheral edema, weight gain, increased appetite.

Overdose and treatment
A single dose of anastrozole that results in life-threatening symptoms hasn't been established. Single oral doses that exceeded 100 mg/kg were associated with severe irritation of the stomach (necrosis, gastritis, ulceration, and hemorrhage) in animals. There is no specific antidote to overdose and treatment must be symptomatic. Vomiting may be induced if the patient is alert. Dialysis may be helpful. General supportive care, including frequent monitoring of vital signs and close observation of the patient, is indicated.

Clinical considerations
- Pregnancy must be excluded before treatment is started with anastrozole.
- Administer drug under supervision of qualified staff experienced in the use of anticancer agents.
- Patients treated with drug don't require glucocorticoid or mineralocorticoid therapy.

Therapeutic monitoring
For patients with mild to moderate hepatic impairment, recommend monitoring for side effects.

Special populations
Breast-feeding patients. It isn't known if anastrozole is excreted in breast milk. Drug shouldn't be administered to breast-feeding women.
Pediatric patients. Safety and efficacy in pediatric patients haven't been established.

Patient counseling
- Instruct patient to report adverse reactions.
- Stress importance of follow-up care.

apraclonidine hydrochloride
Iopidine

Pharmacologic classification: alpha-adrenergic agonist
Therapeutic classification: ocular hypotensive
Pregnancy risk category C

How supplied
Available by prescription only
Ophthalmic solution: 0.5%, 1%

Indications and dosages
Prevention or control of intraocular pressure elevations after argon laser trabeculoplasty or iridotomy
Adults: Instill 1 drop (1% solution) in the eye 1 hour before initiation of laser surgery on the anterior segment, followed by 1 drop immediately upon completion of surgery.
Short-term adjunctive therapy in patients on maximally tolerated medical therapy who require additional intraocular pressure reduction
Adults: Instill 1 to 2 drops (0.5% solution) in the eye t.i.d.
◊ ***Open-angle glaucoma***
Adults: Instill 1 drop (0.5% solution) in the eye b.i.d. or t.i.d.

Pharmacodynamics
Ocular hypotensive action: Apraclonidine is an alpha-adrenergic agonist that reduces intraocular pressure, possibly by decreasing aqueous humor production.

Pharmacokinetics
Absorption: No information available.
Distribution: Onset of action is within 1 hour after instillation, and maximum effect on intraocular pressure reduction occurs in 3 to 5 hours.
Metabolism: No information available.
Excretion: No information available.

Route	Onset	Peak	Duration
Ophthalmic	1 hour	3-5 hours	12 hours

Contraindications and precautions
Contraindicated in patients hypersensitive to apraclonidine or clonidine and in those on concurrent MAO inhibitor therapy. Use cautiously in patients with severe cardiac disease, including hypertension and vasovagal attacks.

Interactions
Drug-drug: *Topical beta blockers or pilocarpine:* May produce additive lowering of intraocular pressure. Use together cautiously.

Effects on diagnostic tests
None reported.

Adverse reactions
CNS: insomnia, irritability, dream disturbances, headache, irritability, paresthesia.
CV: bradycardia, vasovagal attack, palpitations, hypotension, orthostatic hypotension.
EENT: upper eyelid elevation, conjunctival blanching and microhemorrhage, mydriasis, eye burning or discomfort, foreign body sensation in eye, eye dryness and *itching, hyperemia,* conjunctivitis, blurred vision, nasal burning or dryness or increased pharyngeal secretions.

GI: abdominal pain, discomfort, diarrhea, vomiting, taste disturbances, dry mouth.
Skin: pruritus not associated with rash, sweaty palms.
Other: body heat sensation, decreased libido, extremity pain or numbness, allergic response.

Overdose and treatment
No information available.

Clinical considerations
Protect stored drug from light and freezing.

Therapeutic monitoring
- Patients with severe systemic disease, including hypertension require close monitoring of cardiovascular status.
- Remind staff to observe closely for vasovagal attack during laser surgery.

Special populations
Breast-feeding patients. There is no information regarding the excretion of apraclonidine in breast milk. Consider discontinuing breast-feeding on the day of surgery.
Pediatric patients. Safety and efficacy in children haven't been established.

Patient counseling
Warn patient about the potential for dizziness and drowsiness.

ardeparin sodium
Normiflo

Pharmacologic classification: low-molecular-weight heparin
Therapeutic classification: anticoagulant
Pregnancy risk category C

How supplied
Available by prescription only
Injection: 5,000 anti-factor Xa U/0.5 ml, 10,000 anti-factor Xa U/0.5 ml

Indications and dosages
Prevention of deep venous thrombosis which may lead to pulmonary embolism following knee replacement surgery
Adults: 50 anti-factor Xa U/kg S.C. q 12 hours for 14 days or until patient is ambulatory, whichever is shorter. Give initial dose the evening of day of surgery or the following morning.

The manufacturer recommends using the Tubex containing 0.5 ml of ardeparin sodium 10,000 units/ml in patients weighing 220 lb (100 kg) or less and 0.5 ml of the 20,000 units /ml in patients weighing more than 100 kg. To calculate volume (in ml) to be administered in each dose:

For patients weighing 220 lb (100 kg) or less, multiply weight in kg x 0.005 ml/kg. For patients weighing 220 lb (100 kg) or more, multiply weight in kg x 0.0025 ml/kg.

Pharmacodynamics
Anticoagulant activity: Ardeparin is a low-molecular-weight heparin that binds to and accelerates the activity of antithrombin III. This results in an inactivation of factor Xa and thrombin, which prevents the formation of clots. Ardeparin also inhibits thrombin by binding to heparin cofactor II.

Pharmacokinetics
Absorption: Mean absolute bioavailability based on anti-factor Xa activity is 92%.
Distribution: Steady-state volume of distribution based on anti-factor Xa activity is about 99 ml/kg.
Metabolism: Information not available.
Excretion: Elimination half-life based on anti-factor Xa activity is about 3 hours.

Route	Onset	Peak	Duration
S.C.	Unknown	3 hr	Unknown

Contraindications and precautions
Contraindicated in patients with known hypersensitivity to drug, active bleeding, or thrombocytopenia associated with antiplatelet antibodies in the presence of drug. Don't use in patients with known hypersensitivity to pork products.

Use with extreme caution in patients with history of heparin-induced thrombocytopenia and in those with a known hypersensitivity to methylparaben, propylparaben, and sulfites. Use cautiously in patients at increased risk for hemorrhage (bacterial endocarditis) and in those with congenital or acquired bleeding disorders; active ulcerative disease; angiodysplastic GI disease; hemorrhagic stroke; recent eye, spinal, or brain surgery or procedures; severe uncontrolled hypertension; or in patients treated with platelet inhibitors. When epidural or spinal anesthesia or spinal puncture is used, patients who are anticoagulated or scheduled to be anticoagulated with low-molecular-weight heparins are at risk of development of epidural or spinal hematomas, which can result in long-term paralysis.

Interactions
Drug-drug. *Anticoagulants and antiplatelet agents (including aspirin, NSAIDs):* Increased risk of bleeding. Recommend decreasing doses of these agents and monitoring PT and INR.

Effects on diagnostic tests
None reported.

Adverse reactions
CNS: dizziness, headache, *CVA,* insomnia.
CV: chest pain, peripheral edema.
GI: nausea, vomiting.
Hematologic: anemia, ecchymosis, ***hemorrhage, thrombocytopenia,*** hematoma (at injection site)
Skin: pruritus, rash, local reaction.
Other: arthralgia, fever, pain, increase transaminase and serum triglyceride levels.

Overdose and treatment
Bleeding is the principal sign of ardeparin overdose. Most bleeding can be stopped by discontinuing the drug and applying pressure to the site and replacing hemostatic blood elements if necessary. Protamine sulfate can also be administered. Dose of protamine should be equal to the dose of ardeparin administered (1 mg of protamine neutralizes 100 anti-factor Xa U of ardeparin). If bleeding persists after 2 hours, draw blood and determine residual anti-factor Xa levels. Additional protamine can be administered if clinically important bleeding persists or anti-factor Xa levels remain high. Drug doesn't appear to be dialyzable.

Clinical considerations
- Base dosing on actual body weight.
- Ardeparin can't be used interchangeably (unit for unit) with heparin sodium or other low-molecular-weight heparins.
- Don't mix with other injections or infusions.
- Drug should be given with patient sitting or lying down, as a deep S.C. injection in the abdomen (avoiding the navel), outer aspect of upper arm, or anterior thigh. Extrude air and excess medication before administration. The full length of the needle should be introduced into the skin fold held between the thumb and forefinger. Hold skin fold throughout the injection. Rotate injection site.

□ ***ALERT*** Don't give drug I.M. to avoid possible occurrence of hematoma at the injection site.

Therapeutic monitoring
Recommend routine monitoring of CBC, platelet counts, urinalysis and occult blood in stools throughout therapy. Routine monitoring of coagulation parameters isn't required.

Special populations
Breast-feeding patients. It isn't known if drug is excreted in breast milk. Use cautiously when administering to breast-feeding women.
Pediatric patients. Safety and efficacy in children haven't been established.
Geriatric patients. No significant difference was seen in patients over age 65 compared with those under age 65.

Patient counseling
- Instruct patient to report abnormal bruising, bleeding, or dark stools.
- Instruct patient to observe for hematoma at injection site.
- Tell patient to avoid use of OTC medications such as aspirin or NSAIDs.

ascorbic acid (vitamin C)
Ascorbicap, Cebid Timecelles, Cecon, Cevalin, Cevi-Bid, Ce-Vi-Sol, Dull-C, Flavorcee

Pharmacologic classification: water-soluble vitamin
Therapeutic classification: vitamin
Pregnancy risk category A (C if exceeds RDA)

How supplied
Available by prescription only
Injection: 100 mg/ ml, 250 mg/ml in 2-ml ampules and 2-ml and 30-ml vials; 500 mg/ml in 2-ml and 5-ml ampules and 50-ml vials; 500 mg/ml (with monothioglycerol) in 1-ml ampules
Available without a prescription
Tablets: 25 mg, 50 mg, 100 mg, 250 mg, 500 mg, 1,000 mg
Tablets (chewable): 100 mg, 250 mg, 500 mg
Tablets (extended-release): 500 mg, 1,000 mg, 1,500 mg
Capsules (extended-release): 500 mg
Crystals: 100 g (4 g/tsp), 1,000 g (4 g/tsp, sugar-free)
Lozenges: 60 mg
Powder: 100 g (4 g/tsp), 500 g (4 g/tsp)
Liquid: 50 ml (35 mg/0.6 ml)
Solution: 50 ml (100 mg/ml)
Syrup: 20 mg/ml in 120 ml and 480 ml; 500 mg/5 ml in 5 ml, 10 ml, 120 ml, and 473 ml

Indications and dosages
Frank and subclinical scurvy
Adults: 100 to 250 mg, depending on severity, P.O., S.C., I.M., or I.V. daily or b.i.d., then at least 50 mg/day for maintenance.
Infants and children: 100 to 300 mg, depending on severity, P.O., S.C., I.M., or I.V. daily, then at least 35 mg/day for maintenance.
Prevention of ascorbic acid deficiency in those with poor nutritional habits or increased requirements
Adults: 45 to 60 mg P.O., S.C., I.M., or I.V. daily.
Pregnant or breast-feeding women: At least 60 to 80 mg P.O., S.C., I.M., or I.V. daily.
Children and infants over age 2 weeks: At least 20 to 50 mg P.O., S.C., I.M., or I.V. daily.
Potentiation of methenamine in urine acidification
Adults: 4 to 12 g daily in divided doses.

Adjunctive therapy in the treatment of idiopathic methemoglobinemia
Adults: 300 to 600 mg P.O. daily in divided doses.
Reduce tyrosinemia in premature infants on high-protein diets
Premature infants: 100 mg P.O. or I.M. daily.
To increase iron excretion resulting from deferoxamine administration
Adults: 100 to 200 mg P.O. q day.
Prevent and treat the common cold
Adults: 1 to 3 g or more P.O. per day.

Pharmacodynamics
Nutritional action: Ascorbic acid, an essential vitamin, is involved with the biologic oxidations and reductions used in cellular respiration. It's essential for the formation and maintenance of intracellular ground substance and collagen. In the body, ascorbic acid is reversibly oxidized to dehydroascorbic acid and influences tyrosine metabolism, conversion of folic acid to folinic acid, carbohydrate metabolism, resistance to infections, and cellular respiration. Ascorbic acid deficiency causes scurvy, a condition marked by degenerative changes in the capillaries, bone, and connective tissues. Restoring adequate ascorbic acid intake completely reverses symptoms of ascorbic acid deficiency. Data regarding use of ascorbic acid as a urinary acidifier are conflicting.

Pharmacokinetics
Absorption: After oral administration, ascorbic acid is absorbed readily. After very large doses, absorption may be limited because absorption is an active process. Absorption also may be reduced in patients with diarrhea or GI diseases. Normal plasma concentrations of ascorbic acid are about 10 to 20 mcg/ml. Plasma levels below 1.5 mcg/ml are associated with scurvy. However, leukocyte levels (although not usually measured) may better reflect ascorbic acid tissue saturation. About 1.5 g of ascorbic acid is stored in the body. Within 3 to 5 months of ascorbic acid deficiency, clinical signs of scurvy become evident.
Distribution: Distributed widely in the body, with large concentrations found in the liver, leukocytes, platelets, glandular tissues, and lens of the eye. Ascorbic acid crosses the placenta; cord blood levels are usually two to four times the maternal blood levels. Ascorbic acid is distributed into breast milk.
Metabolism: Metabolized in the liver.
Excretion: Reversibly oxidized to dehydroascorbic acid. Some is metabolized to inactive compounds that are excreted in urine. The renal threshold is about 14 mcg/ml. When the body is saturated and blood levels exceed the threshold, unchanged ascorbic acid is excreted in urine. Renal excretion is directly proportional to blood levels. Ascorbic acid is also removed by hemodialysis.

Route	Onset	Peak	Duration
P.O., I.V., I.M., S.C.	Unknown	Unknown	Unknown

Contraindications and precautions
No known contraindications. Use cautiously in patients with renal insufficiency.

Interactions
Drug-drug. *Acidic drugs in large doses (more than 2 g/day):* May lower urine pH, causing renal tubular reabsorption of acidic drugs. Recommend monitoring for clinical and adverse effects.
Basic drugs (such as amphetamines or tricyclic antidepressants): May cause decreased reabsorption and therapeutic effect. Recommend monitoring for clinical and adverse effects.
Sulfonamides: May cause crystallization. Avoid use together.
Iron: Ascorbic acid and iron maintains it in the ferrous state and increases iron absorption in the GI tract, but this increase may not be significant. A combination of 30 mg of iron with 200 mg of ascorbic acid is sometimes recommended.
Dicumarol: Influences the intensity and duration of the anticoagulant effect. Recommend monitoring PT and INR.
Warfarin: May inhibit the anticoagulant effect. Recommend monitoring PT and INR.
Ethinyl estradiol: May increase plasma levels of ethinyl estradiol. Recommend monitoring these levels.
Salicylates: Inhibit ascorbic acid uptake by leukocytes and platelets. Recommend observing for symptoms of ascorbic acid deficiency.
Drug-lifestyle. *Smoking:* May decrease serum ascorbic acid levels, thus increasing dosage requirements of this vitamin. Monitor patient closely.

Effects on diagnostic tests
Ascorbic acid is a strong reducing agent; it alters results of tests that are based on oxidation-reduction reactions. Large doses of ascorbic acid (over 500 mg) may cause false-negative glucose determinations using the glucose oxidase method, or false-positive results using the copper reduction method or Benedict's reagent.

Ascorbic acid shouldn't be used for 48 to 72 hours before an amine-dependent test for occult blood in the stool is conducted. A false-negative result may occur.

Depending on the reagents used, ascorbic acid may also cause interactions with other diagnostic tests.

Adverse reactions

CNS: faintness, dizziness (with too-rapid I.V. administration).
GI: diarrhea.
GU: acid urine, oxaluria, renal calculi.
Other: discomfort at injection site.

Overdose and treatment

Excessively high doses of parenteral ascorbic acid are excreted renally after tissue saturation and rarely accumulate. Serious adverse effects or toxicity are uncommon. Severe effects require discontinuation of therapy.

Clinical considerations

- Administer large doses of ascorbic acid (1,000 mg/day) in divided amounts because the body uses only a limited amount and excretes the rest in urine. Large doses may increase small intestine pH and impair vitamin B_{12} absorption. The recommended RDA of ascorbic acid is as follows:
Adults: 60 mg/day
Smokers: 100 mg/day
Pregnant women: 70 mg/day
Lactating women: 90 to 95 mg/day
Infants and children: 30 to 60 mg/day
Patients on chronic hemodialysis: 100 to 200 mg/day
- Administer oral solutions of ascorbic acid directly into the mouth or mix with food.
- Administer I.V. solution slowly.
- Conditions that elevate the metabolic rate (hyperthyroidism, fever, infection, burns and other severe trauma, postoperative states, neoplastic disease, and chronic alcoholism) significantly increase ascorbic acid requirements.
- Prolonged use of large doses results in increased metabolism of ascorbic acid; scurvy may result when reduced to normal.
- Reportedly, patients taking oral contraceptives require ascorbic acid supplements.
- Smokers appear to have increased requirements for ascorbic acid because the vitamin is oxidized and excreted more rapidly than in nonsmokers.
- Use ascorbic acid cautiously in patients with renal insufficiency because the vitamin is normally excreted in urine.
- Patients whose diets are chemically deficient in fruits and vegetables can develop subclinical ascorbic acid deficiency. Observe for such deficiency in elderly and indigent patients, patients on restricted diets, those receiving long-term treatment with I.V. fluids or hemodialysis, and drug addicts or alcoholics.
- Protect ascorbic acid solutions from light. Solution darkens upon exposure to light, but this doesn't impair the therapeutic activity of the drug. Drug is incompatible with many drugs.

Therapeutic monitoring

Recommend monitoring for symptoms of ascorbic acid deficiency include irritability; emotional disturbances; general debility; pallor; anorexia; sensitivity to touch; limb and joint pain; follicular hyperkeratosis (particularly on thighs and buttocks); easy bruising; petechiae; bloody diarrhea; delayed healing; loosening of teeth; sensitive, swollen, and bleeding gums; and anemia.

Special populations

Pregnant patients. Ingestion of large doses during pregnancy has resulted in scurvy in neonates.
Breast-feeding patients. Administer with caution to breast-feeding women because ascorbic acid is excreted in breast milk.
Pediatric patients. Infants fed on cow's milk alone require supplemental ascorbic acid.

Patient counseling

- Suggest good dietary sources of ascorbic acid, such as citrus fruits, leafy vegetables, tomatoes, green peppers, and potatoes.
- Inform patient to cover foods and fruit juices tightly and to use them promptly.
- Advise patients with ascorbic acid deficiency to decrease or stop smoking. Replacement ascorbic acid dosages are greater for the smoker.
- Tell patients who are prone to renal calculi, who have diabetes, who are undergoing tests for occult blood in stools, or who are on sodium-restricted diets or anticoagulant therapy to avoid high doses of ascorbic acid.

asparaginase

Elspar

Pharmacologic classification: enzyme (L-asparagine amidohydrolase) (cell cycle-phase specific, G1 phase)
Therapeutic classification: antineoplastic
Pregnancy risk category C

How supplied

Available by prescription only
Injection: 10,000-unit vials

Indications and dosages

Indications and dosages may vary. Check current literature for recommended protocol.
Acute lymphocytic leukemia
Adults and children: When used alone, 200 units/kg daily I.V. for 28 days. When used in combination with other chemotherapeutic agents, dosage is highly individualized.

Pharmacodynamics

Antineoplastic action: Asparaginase exerts its cytotoxic activity by inactivating the amino acid asparagine, which is required by tumor cells to synthesize proteins. Because the tumor cells can't synthesize their own asparagine, protein synthesis and eventually synthesis of DNA and RNA are inhibited.

Pharmacokinetics

Absorption: Not absorbed across the GI tract after oral administration; therefore, it must be given I.V. or I.M.
Distribution: Distributes primarily within the intravascular space, with detectable levels in the thoracic and cervical lymph. Crosses the blood-brain barrier to a minimal extent.
Metabolism: Metabolic fate of asparaginase is unclear; hepatic sequestration by the reticuloendothelial system may occur.
Excretion: Plasma elimination half-life, which isn't related to dose, sex, age, or hepatic or renal function, ranges from 8 to 30 hours.

Route	Onset	Peak	Duration
I.V.	Immediate	Immediate	23-33 days
I.M.	Unknown	14-24 hr	23-33 days

Contraindications and precautions

Contraindicated in patients with pancreatitis or history of pancreatitis and previous hypersensitivity unless desensitized. Use cautiously in patients with hepatic dysfunction.

Interactions

Drug-drug. *Methotrexate:* Decreases the effectiveness of methotrexate because asparaginase destroys the actively replicating cells that methotrexate requires for its cytotoxic action. Avoid use together.
Vincristine: Can cause additive neuropathy and disturbances of erythropoiesis. Avoid use together.
Prednisone: Hyperglycemia may result from an additive effect on the pancreas. Recommend monitoring serum blood glucose.

Effects on diagnostic tests

None reported.

Adverse reactions

CNS: confusion, drowsiness, depression, hallucinations, ***intracranial hemorrhage,*** fatigue, ***coma,*** agitation, headache, lethargy, somnolence.
CV: ***MI.***
GI: **HEMORRHAGIC PANCREATITIS,** *vomiting, anorexia, nausea,* cramps, weight loss.
GU: *azotemia,* ***renal failure,*** glycosuria, polyuria.
Hematologic: ***anemia, hypofibrinogenemia,*** depression of other clotting factors, ***leukopenia.***
Hepatic: elevated AST and ALT levels, *hepatotoxicity.*
Metabolic: *hyperglycemia,* alters the results of thyroid function tests.
Skin: *rash, urticaria,* hypersensitivity reactions.
Other: **ANAPHYLAXIS,** chills, ***death, fatal hyperthermia,*** fever.

Overdose and treatment

Signs and symptoms of overdose include nausea and diarrhea. Treatment is generally supportive and includes antiemetics and antidiarrheals.

Clinical considerations

- Reconstitute drug for I.M. administration with 2 ml unpreserved normal saline. Don't dispense if precipitate forms.
- I.M. injections shouldn't contain more than 2 ml per injection. Multiple injections may be used for each dose.
- For I.V. administration: Reconstitute with 5 ml of sterile water for injection or saline injection. Solution will be clear or slightly cloudy. May further dilute with saline injection or D_5W and administer I.V. over 30 minutes. Filtration through a 5-micron in-line filter during administration removes particulate matter that may develop on standing; filtration through a 0.22-micron filter results in a loss of potency. Don't use if precipitate forms.
- Shake vial gently when reconstituting. Vigorous shaking results in a decrease of potency.
- Refrigerate unopened dry powder. Use reconstituted solution within 8 hours.
- Don't use as sole agent to induce remission unless combination therapy is inappropriate. Not recommended for maintenance therapy.
- Administer drug only in hospital settings with close supervision.
- I.V. administration of asparaginase with or immediately before vincristine or prednisone may increase toxicity reactions.
- A skin test should be done before initial dose. Advise staff to observe site for 1 hour. Erythema and wheal formation indicate a positive reaction. Advise the following procedure: Withdraw 0.1 ml from reconstituted vial and inject into vial containing 9.9 ml of sodium chloride injection or sterile water. Inject 0.1 ml (2 units) intradermally and observe site for at least 1 hour.
- Risk of hypersensitivity increases with repeated doses. Patient may be desensitized, but this doesn't rule out risk of allergic reactions. Routine administration of 2-unit intradermal test dose may identify high-risk patients.
- Asparaginase has an unlabeled use as post induction intestification therapy for childhood acute myeloid leukemia.
- Because of vomiting, patient may need parenteral fluids for 24 hours or until oral fluids are tolerated.
- Tumor lysis can result in uric acid nephropathy. This can be prevented by increasing fluid intake. Allopurinol should be started before therapy begins.

- Epinephrine, diphenhydramine, and I.V. corticosteroids must be available for treatment of anaphylaxis.

Therapeutic monitoring

- Monitor CBC and bone marrow function. Bone marrow regeneration may take 5 to 6 weeks.
- Recommend obtaining frequent serum amylase determinations to check pancreatic status. If elevated, discontinue asparaginase.
- Monitor hepatic, renal, and CNS function.
- Monitor blood glucose and urine tests for glucose before and during therapy. Monitor for signs of hyperglycemia, such as glycosuria and polyuria.

Special populations

Pregnant patients. There are no adequate studies indicating safe use in pregnancy.
Breast-feeding patients. It isn't known if drug is excreted in breast milk. However, because of the potential for serious adverse reactions and carcinogenicity in the infant, breast-feeding isn't recommended.
Pediatric patients. Drug toxicity appears to be less severe in children than adults.

Patient counseling

- Encourage patient to maintain adequate intake of fluids to increase urine output and facilitate excretion of uric acid.
- Tell patient that because drowsiness may occur during therapy or for several weeks after treatment has ended, he should avoid hazardous activities requiring mental alertness.
- Advise patient to watch for signs of bleeding.

aspirin

A.S.A., Ascriptin, Aspergum, Bufferin, Ecotrin, Empirin, Halfprin, Novasen*, ZORprin

Pharmacologic classification: salicylate
Therapeutic classification: nonnarcotic analgesic, antipyretic, anti-inflammatory, antiplatelet
Pregnancy risk category D

How supplied

Available by prescription only
Tablets (enteric-coated): 975 mg
Tablets (extended-release): 800 mg
Available without a prescription
Tablets: 81 mg, 325 mg (5 grains), 500 mg, 650 mg
Tablets (enteric-coated): 81 mg, 162 mg,165 mg, 325 mg, 500 mg, 650 mg
Tablets (extended-release): 650 mg
Chewing gum: 227.5 mg
Suppositories: 60 mg, 120 mg, 125 mg, 200 mg, 300 mg, 600 mg

Indications and dosages

Arthritis
Adults: Initially, 2.4 to 3.6 g P.O. daily in divided doses. Increase 325 mg to 1.2 g daily no more frequently than at weekly intervals. Maintenance dosage is 3.6 to 5.4 g P.O. daily in divided doses.
Children: 60 to 130 mg/kg P.O. daily in divided doses.
Juvenile arthritis
Children weighing 55 lb (25 kg) or more: 2.4 to 3.6 g P.O. daily in divided doses.
Children weighing 55 lb (25 kg) or less: 60 to 130 mg/kg P.O. daily in divided doses.
Increase 10 mg/kg daily no more than at weekly intervals. Maintenance dosages usually range between 80 and 100 mg/kg daily; up to 130 mg/kg daily.
Mild pain or fever
Adults: 650 mg to 1.3 g extended-release tablets P.O. q 8 hours p.r.n. not to exceed 3.9 g daily.
Adults and children over age 11: 325 to 650 mg P.O. or P.R. q 4 hours, p.r.n. Not to exceed 4 g daily. Alternatively, 454 mg chewing gum piece chewed for 15 minutes and discarded p.r.n.; not to exceed 3.63 g daily.
Children age 6 to 11: 227 mg to 454 mg chewed for 15 minutes and discarded, p.r.n.; not to exceed 1.82 g daily.
Children age 3 to 5 years: 227 mg chewed for 15 minutes and discarded, p.r.n.; not to exceed 681 mg per day.
Mild pain
Children age 2 to 11: 65 mg/kg P.O. or P.R. daily divided q 4 to 6 hours, p.r.n. Not to exceed 2.5 g/m^2.
Transient ischemic attacks and thromboembolic disorders
Adults: 50 to 325 mg P.O. daily (prophylactic in men) and 160 mg to 325 mg (treatment) P.O. q day immediately or within 48 hours of stroke onset.
Treatment or reduction of the risk of heart attack in patients with previous MI or unstable angina
Adults: ◊Primary prevention; 75 to 325 mg P.O. daily.
Secondary prevention: 75 to 325 mg P.O. daily.
Treatment: 160 to 325 mg P.O. once daily.
Treatment of Kawasaki (mucocutaneous lymph node) syndrome
Adults: 80 to 100 mg/kg P.O. daily in four divided doses. Some patients may require up to 120 mg/kg daily to maintain acceptable serum salicylate levels of over 200 mcg/ml during the febrile phase. After the fever subsides, reduce dosage to 3 to 5 mg/kg once daily. Therapy is usually continued for 6 to 8 weeks.

◇ ***Rheumatic fever***
Adults: 4.9 to 7.8 g P.O. daily divided q 4 to 6 hours for 1 to 2 weeks; then decrease to 60 to 70 mg/kg daily for 1 to 6 weeks; then gradually withdraw over 1 to 2 weeks.
Children: 90 to 130 mg/kg P.O. daily divided q 4 to 6 hours.
◇ ***Pericarditis following acute MI***
160 to 325 mg P.O. daily.
Prevent reocclusion in coronary revascularization procedures
Adults: 325 mg P.O. 6 hours after surgery and continued for at least 1 year.
◇ ***Stent implantation***
Adults: 160 to 325 mg P.O. 2 hours before stent placement and continued indefinitely.

Pharmacodynamics

Analgesic action: Aspirin produces analgesia by an ill-defined effect on the hypothalamus (central action) and by blocking generation of pain impulses (peripheral action). The peripheral action may involve blocking of prostaglandin synthesis via inhibition of cyclo-oxygenase enzyme.
Anti-inflammatory action: Although the exact mechanism is unknown, aspirin is believed to inhibit prostaglandin synthesis; it may also inhibit the synthesis or action of other mediators of inflammation.
Antipyretic action: Aspirin relieves fever by acting on the hypothalamic heat-regulating center to produce peripheral vasodilation. This increases peripheral blood supply and promotes sweating, which leads to loss of heat and to cooling by evaporation.
Anticoagulant action: At low doses, aspirin appears to impede clotting by blocking prostaglandin synthetase action, which prevents formation of the platelet-aggregating substance thromboxane A_2. This interference with platelet activity is irreversible and can prolong bleeding time. However, at high doses, aspirin interferes with prostacyclin production, a potent vasoconstrictor and inhibitor of platelet aggregation, possibly negating its anticlotting properties.

Pharmacokinetics

Absorption: Absorbed rapidly and completely from the GI tract. Therapeutic blood salicylate concentrations for analgesia and anti-inflammatory effect are 150 to 300 mcg/ml; responses vary with the patient.
Distribution: Distributed widely into most body tissues and fluids. Protein-binding to albumin is concentration dependent, ranges from 75% to 90%, and decreases as serum level increases. Severe toxic effects may occur at serum levels greater than 400 mcg/ml.
Metabolism: Hydrolyzed partially in the GI tract to salicylic acid with almost complete metabolism in the liver.
Excretion: Excreted in urine as salicylate and its metabolites. Elimination half-life ranges from 15 to 20 minutes.

Route	Onset	Peak	Duration
P.O. tablet	5-30 min	25-40 min	1-4 hr
P.O. buffered	5-30 min	1-2 hr	1-4 hr
P.O. extended	5-30 min	1-4 hr	1-4 hr
P.O. enteric-coated	5-30 min	4-8 hr	1-4 hr
P.O. solution	5-30 min	15-40 min	1-4 hr
P.R.	Unknown	3-4 hr	1-4 hr

Contraindications and precautions

Contraindicated in patients with hypersensitivity to drug, G6PD deficiency, bleeding disorders such as hemophilia, von Willebrand's disease, or telangiectasia. Also contraindicated in patients with NSAID-induced sensitivity reactions or in children with chickenpox or flulike symptoms.

Use cautiously in patients with GI lesions, impaired renal function, hypoprothrombinemia, vitamin K deficiency, thrombotic thrombocytopenic purpura, or hepatic impairment.

Interactions

Drug-drug. *Anticoagulants and thrombolytic drugs:* May to some degree potentiate the platelet-inhibiting effects of aspirin. Recommend monitoring of PT and INR.
Phenytoin, sulfonylureas, warfarin: May cause displacement of either drug and adverse effects. Recommend monitoring therapy closely for both drugs.
Steroids, antibiotics, and other NSAIDs: May potentiate the adverse GI effects of the aspirin. Use together with caution.
Aminoglycosides, bumetanide, capreomycin, ethacrynic acid, furosemide, cisplatin, vancomycin, or erythromycin: May potentiate ototoxic effects. Monitor for this effect.
Lithium: Aspirin decreases renal clearance of lithium carbonate, thus increasing serum lithium levels and the risk of adverse effects. Recommend monitoring lithium levels.
Phenylbutazone, probenecid, and sulfinpyrazone: Aspirin is antagonistic to the uricosuric effect of these drugs. Avoid use together.
Ammonium chloride and other urine acidifiers: Increased aspirin blood levels. Recommend monitoring for aspirin toxicity.
Antacids in high doses, and other urine alkalizers: Decreased aspirin blood levels. Recommend monitoring for decreased salicylate effect.
Corticosteroids: Enhance aspirin elimination. Recommend monitoring for decreased salicylate effect.
Antacids: Delay and decrease absorption of aspirin. Recommend monitoring for decreased salicylate effect.

Drug-herb. *Horse chestnut, kelpware, prickly ash, red clover:* May increase risk of bleeding. Monitor patient closely.
Drug-food. *Food:* Delays and decreases absorption of aspirin. Recommend monitoring for decreased salicylate effect.
Drug-lifestyle. *Alcohol use*: May potentiate adverse GI effects of aspirin. Discourage use.

Effects on diagnostic tests

Aspirin interferes with urinary glucose analysis performed with Diastix, Chemstrip uG, glucose enzymatic test strip, Clinitest, and Benedict's solution, and with urinary 5-hydroxyindoleacetic acid and vanillylmandelic acid tests. Serum uric acid levels may be falsely increased. Aspirin may interfere with the Gerhardt test for urine acetoacetic acid.

Adverse reactions

EENT: *tinnitus, hearing loss.*
GI: *nausea, GI distress, occult bleeding, dyspepsia,* ***GI bleeding.***
Hematologic: ***leukopenia, thrombocytopenia,*** *prolonged bleeding time.*
Hepatic: abnormal liver function studies, hepatitis.
Skin: *rash,* bruising, urticaria, angioedema.
Other: ***hypersensitivity reactions (anaphylaxis,*** asthma), ***Reye's syndrome.***

Overdose and treatment

Signs and symptoms of overdose include GI discomfort, oliguria, acute renal failure, hyperthermia, EEG abnormalities, and restlessness as well as metabolic acidosis with respiratory alkalosis, hyperpnea, and tachypnea because of increased CO_2 production and direct stimulation of the respiratory center.

To treat aspirin overdose, empty the patient's stomach immediately by inducing emesis with ipecac syrup if patient is conscious, or by gastric lavage. Administer activated charcoal via nasogastric tube. Provide symptomatic and supportive measures (respiratory support and correction of fluid and electrolyte imbalances). Closely monitor laboratory parameters and vital signs. Enhance renal excretion by administering sodium bicarbonate to alkalinize urine. Use cooling blanket or sponging if patient's rectal temperature is more than 104° F (40° C). Hemodialysis is effective in removing aspirin, but is only used in severely poisoned individuals or those at risk for pulmonary edema.

Clinical considerations

- Salicylates must be used with caution in patients with history of GI disease (especially peptic ulcer disease), increased risk of GI bleeding, or decreased renal function.
- Tablets may be chewed, broken, or crumbled and administered with food or fluids to aid swallowing. Uncoated plain aspirin tablets allowed to remain in contact with mucous membranes of the mouth and aspirin chewing gum have produced mucosal erosions and mouth ulcerations.
- Enteric-coated products are absorbed slowly and are not suitable for acute therapy. They're ideal for long-term therapy, such as that for arthritis.
- There is no evidence that aspirin reduces the incidence of transient ischemic attacks in women.
- Stop aspirin therapy 1 week before elective surgery, if possible.
- Adults shouldn't use drug for self-medication for longer than 10 days.
- Moisture may cause aspirin to lose potency. Store in a cool, dry place, and avoid using if tablets smell like vinegar.
- Patient should take 8 oz (240 ml) of water or milk with salicylates to ensure passage into stomach. Advise patient to sit up for 15 to 30 minutes after taking salicylates to prevent lodging of salicylate in esophagus.
- Recommend dose reduction if fever or illness causes fluid depletion.

Therapeutic monitoring

- Recommend monitoring vital signs frequently, especially temperature.
- Salicylates may mask the signs and symptoms of acute infection (fever, myalgia, erythema); carefully evaluate patient at risk for infections, such as those with diabetes.
- Recommend monitoring CBC, platelets, PT, BUN, serum creatinine, and liver function studies periodically during salicylate therapy to detect abnormalities.
- Advise assessing for signs and symptoms of potential hemorrhage, such as petechiae, bruising, coffee ground vomitus, and black tarry stools.

Special populations

Pregnant patients. Aspirin has been used for the prevention of complications in pregnancy including preeclampsia, pregnancy loss with history of antiphospholipid syndrome, recurrent loss. Generally, avoid use in pregnancy.
Breast-feeding patients. Salicylates are distributed into breast milk; avoid use during breast-feeding.
Pediatric patients. Because of epidemiologic association with Reye's syndrome, the Centers for Disease Control and Prevention recommend that children with chickenpox or flulike symptoms not be given aspirin or other salicylates. Don't use long-term salicylate therapy in children under age 14; safety hasn't been established. Don't use more than 5 times per day or for more than 5 days.
Geriatric patients. Patients over age 60 may be more susceptible to the toxic effects of aspirin. Use with caution. Effects of aspirin on renal prostaglandins may cause fluid retention

and edema, a significant drawback for geriatric patients and those with heart failure.

Patient counseling

- Tell parents to keep aspirin out of children's reach; encourage use of child-resistant closures because aspirin is a leading cause of poisoning.
- Advise patients receiving high-dose, long-term aspirin therapy to watch for petechiae, bleeding gums, and signs of GI bleeding.
- Instruct patient to avoid use of aspirin if allergic to tartrazine dye.
- Tell patient to take drug with food or after meals to avoid GI upset.

atenolol

Tenormin

Pharmacologic classification: beta blocker
Therapeutic classification: antihypertensive, antianginal
Pregnancy risk category C

How supplied

Available by prescription only
Tablets: 25 mg, 50 mg, 100 mg
Injection: 5 mg/10 ml

Indications and dosages

Hypertension
Adults: Initially, 25 to 50 mg P.O. as a single daily dose. May increase dose to 100 mg/day after 7 to 14 days. Higher doses are unlikely to produce further benefit.
Chronic stable angina pectoris
Adults: 50 mg P.O. once daily; may be increased to 100 mg/day after 7 days for optimal effect. Maximum daily dose is 200 mg/day.
To reduce risk of CV mortality in patients with acute MI
Adults: 5 mg I.V. over 5 minutes, followed by another 5 mg I.V. 10 minutes later. Initiate oral therapy (50 mg) 10 minutes after the final dose in patients who tolerate the full I.V. dose. Thereafter, 50 mg P.O. 12 hours later. Then, 100 mg P.O. daily or 50 mg P.O. b.i.d. for 6 to 9 days or until discharged from the hospital.
◇ ***To slow rapid ventricular response to atrial tachyarrythmias following AMI without LVD and AV block***
Adults: 2.5 to 5 mg I.V. over 2 minutes, p.r.n., to control rate; no more than 10 mg over a 10 to 15 minute period.
≡ ***Dosage adjustment.*** In patients with renal failure, adjust dosage if creatinine clearance is below 35 ml/minute. In patients with creatinine clearance of 15 to 35 ml/minute/1.73 m^2, give 50 mg/day; in patients with creatinine clearance below 15 ml/minute/1.73 m^2, give 25 mg/day; in patients undergoing hemodialysis, dosage is 25 to 50 mg after each treatment under close supervision.

Pharmacodynamics

Antihypertensive action: Atenolol may reduce blood pressure by adrenergic receptor blockade, thereby decreasing cardiac output by decreasing the sympathetic outflow from the CNS and by suppressing renin release. At low doses, atenolol, like metoprolol, selectively inhibits cardiac $beta_1$-receptors; it has little effect on $beta_2$-receptors in bronchial and vascular smooth muscle.
Antianginal action: Atenolol aids in treating chronic stable angina by decreasing myocardial contractility and heart rate (negative inotropic and chronotropic effect), thus reducing myocardial oxygen consumption.
Cardioprotective action: The mechanism whereby atenolol improves survival in patients with MI is unknown. However, it does reduce the frequency of PVCs, chest pain, and enzyme elevation.

Pharmacokinetics

Absorption: About 50% to 60% of an atenolol dose is absorbed.
Distribution: Distributed into most tissues and fluids except the brain and CSF; about 5% to 15% is protein-bound.
Metabolism: Metabolized minimally.
Excretion: About 40% to 50% of a given dose is excreted unchanged in urine; remainder is excreted as unchanged drug and metabolites in feces. In patients with normal renal function, plasma half-life is 6 to 7 hours; half-life increases as renal function decreases.

Route	Onset	Peak	Duration
P.O.	1 hr	2-4 hr	24 hr
I.V.	5 min	5 min	12 hr

Contraindications and precautions

Contraindicated in patients with sinus bradycardia, greater than first-degree heart block, overt cardiac failure, or cardiogenic shock. Use cautiously in patients at risk for heart failure and in those with bronchospastic disease, diabetes, and hyperthyroidism.

Interactions

Drug-drug. *Other antihypertensive agents:* Atenolol may potentiate the antihypertensive effects of other antihypertensive agents. Recommend monitoring blood pressure.
Insulin or oral hypoglycemic: Altered dosage requirements in stable diabetic patients. Recommend monitoring serum glucose.
Indomethacin, NSAIDs, and alpha-adrenergic agents such as those found in OTC cold remedies: Antihypertensive effects of atenolol may be antagonized. Recommend monitoring for clinical effect.

Effects on diagnostic tests
None reported.

Adverse reactions
CNS: *fatigue,* lethargy, vertigo, drowsiness, *dizziness,* mental depression.
CV: ***bradycardia, hypotension,*** heart failure, intermittent claudication, changes in exercise tolerance and ECG.
GI: nausea, diarrhea, dry mouth.
GU: elevated BUN and creatinine.
Metabolic: hyperkalemia, hyperglycemia, hypoglycemia.
Hepatic: elevated transaminase, alkaline phosphatase, elevated bilirubin.
Respiratory: dyspnea, ***bronchospasm.***
Skin: rash.
Other: fever, leg pain, ***agrunulocytosis, nonthrombocytopenic or thrombocytopenic purpura..***

Overdose and treatment
Clinical signs of overdose include severe hypotension, bradycardia, heart failure, and bronchospasm.

After acute ingestion, empty stomach by emesis or gastric lavage; follow with activated charcoal to reduce absorption. Thereafter, treat symptomatically and supportively.

Clinical considerations
Consider the recommendations relevant to all beta blockers as well as the following:
- Patient should take oral single daily dose at same time each day.
- Drug may be taken without food.
- Dosage may need to be reduced in patients with renal insufficiency.
- I.V. atenolol affords a rapid onset of the protective effects of beta blockade against reinfarction.
- Patients who can't tolerate I.V. atenolol after an MI may be candidates for oral atenolol therapy. Some evidence suggests that gastric absorption of atenolol may be delayed in the early phase of MI. This may result from the physiologic changes that accompany MI or from the effects of morphine, which is commonly administered to treat chest pain. However, oral therapy alone may still provide benefits.
- I.V. atenolol may be given undiluted or diluted no more than 1 mg/minute.
- Protect medication from heat, direct light, and moisture and store at room temperature.
- Caution against abrupt withdrawal of medication; may precipitate MI, increased angina.

Therapeutic monitoring
Recommend monitoring blood pressure, heart rate and ECG during I.V. administration.

Special populations
Pregnant patients. Atenolol can cause fetal harm (intrauterine growth retardation).
Breast-feeding patients. Safety hasn't been established. An alternative feeding method is recommended during therapy.
Pediatric patients. Safety and efficacy in children haven't been established; use only if potential benefit outweighs risk.
Geriatric patients. Geriatric patients may require lower maintenance dosages of atenolol because of increased bioavailability or delayed metabolism; they also may experience enhanced adverse effects.

Patient counseling
- Stress importance of not missing doses, but tell patient not to double the dose if one is missed, especially if taking drug once daily.
- Advise patient to seek medical approval before taking OTC cold preparations.

atorvastatin calcium
Lipitor

Pharmacologic classification: 3-hydroxy-3-methylglutaryl-coenzyme A (HMG-CoA) reductase inhibitor
Therapeutic classification: antilipemic
Pregnancy risk category X

How supplied
Available by prescription only
Tablets: 10 mg, 20 mg, 40 mg

Indications and dosages
Adjunct to diet to reduce elevated low-density lipoprotein (LDL), total cholesterol, apo B, and triglyceride levels in patients with primary hypercholesterolemia and mixed dyslipidemia
Adults: Initially, 10 mg P.O. once daily. Increase dose, p.r.n., to maximum of 80 mg daily as single dose. Dosage based on blood lipid levels drawn within 2 to 4 weeks after starting therapy.
Alone or as an adjunct to lipid-lowering treatments such as LDL apheresis in patients with homozygous familial hypercholesterolemia
Adults and children over age 9: 10 to 80 mg P.O. once daily.

Pharmacodynamics
Antilipemic action: Inhibits HMG-CoA reductase, an early (and rate-limiting) step in cholesterol biosynthesis.

Pharmacokinetics
Absorption: Rapidly absorbed.
Distribution: Mean volume of distribution is approximately 565 L. Drug is 98% or more bound to plasma proteins with poor drug penetration into RBCs. Likely to be secreted in breast milk.

Metabolism: Extensively metabolized to orthohydroxylated and parahydroxylated derivatives and various beta-oxidation products. In vitro inhibition of HMG-CoA reductase by orthohydroxylated and parahydroxylated metabolites is equivalent to that of atorvastatin. About 70% of circulating inhibitory activity for HMG-CoA reductase is attributed to active metabolites. In vitro studies suggest the importance of atorvastatin metabolism by cytochrome P-450 CYP3A4.
Excretion: Eliminated primarily in bile following hepatic or extrahepatic metabolism; however, drug doesn't appear to undergo enterohepatic recirculation. Mean plasma elimination half-life of atorvastatin is about 14 hours, but the half-life of inhibitory activity for HMG-CoA reductase is 20 to 30 hours because of the contribution of active metabolites. Less than 2% of a dose of atorvastatin is recovered in urine following oral administration.

Route	Onset	Peak	Duration
P.O.	Unknown	1-2 hr	Unknown

Contraindications and precautions
Contraindicated in patients hypersensitive to drug or with active hepatic disease or conditions associated with unexplained persistent elevations of serum transaminase levels, in pregnant or breast-feeding women, and in women of childbearing age (except in women not at risk for becoming pregnant).

Use cautiously in patients with history of hepatic disease or heavy alcohol use.

Interactions
Drug-drug. *Azole antifungals, cyclosporine, erythromycin, fibric acid derivatives, and niacin:* May increase risk of rhabdomyolysis. Avoid use together.
Antacids: May cause decreased levels of atorvastatin. LDL-cholesterol reduction not affected. Monitor patient.
Digoxin: May increase plasma digoxin levels. Monitor serum digoxin levels.
Erythromycin: Increases plasma level of drug. Monitor patient.
Oral contraceptives: May increase levels of hormones. Consider when selecting an oral contraceptive.

Effects on diagnostic tests
None reported.

Adverse reactions
CNS: asthenia, *headache.*
GI: abdominal pain, constipation, diarrhea, dyspepsia, flatulence.
Hepatic: increased liver function test
Musculoskeletal: arthralgia, back pain, myalgia.
Respiratory: pharyngitis, sinusitis.
Skin: rash.
Other: accidental injury, ***allergic reaction***, flu-like syndrome, *infection.*

Overdose and treatment
There is no specific treatment for atorvastatin overdose. If overdose occurs, treat patient symptomatically, and provide supportive measures as required. Because of extensive drug binding to plasma proteins, hemodialysis isn't expected to significantly enhance drug clearance.

Clinical considerations
- Withhold or discontinue drug in patients with serious, acute conditions that suggest myopathy or those at risk for renal failure secondary to rhabdomyolysis as a result of trauma; major surgery; severe metabolic, endocrine, and electrolyte disorders; severe acute infection; hypotension; or uncontrolled seizures.
- Use drug only after diet and other nonpharmacologic treatments prove ineffective. Patient should follow a standard low-cholesterol diet before and during therapy.
- Drug may be given as a single dose at any time of day without regard for food.

Therapeutic monitoring
- Before initiating treatment, exclude secondary causes for hypercholesterolemia and perform a baseline lipid profile. Periodic liver function tests and lipid levels should be done before starting treatment, at 6 and 12 weeks after initiation, or after an increase in dosage and periodically thereafter.
- Watch for signs of myositis.

Special populations
Breast-feeding patients. Because of the potential for adverse reactions in breast-fed infants, women taking atorvastatin shouldn't breast-feed.
Pediatric patients. Experience in children is limited to drug doses up to 80 mg daily for 1 year in eight patients with homozygous familial hypercholesteremia. No clinical or biochemical abnormalities were reported in these patients. Safety and efficacy haven't been established in children under age 9.
Geriatric patients. Safety and efficacy in patients age 70 and older with drug doses up to 80 mg daily were similar to those of patients under age 70.

Patient counseling
- Teach patient proper dietary management, weight control, and exercise. Explain the importance of controlling elevated serum lipid levels.
- Warn patient to avoid alcohol.
- Tell patient to report adverse reactions, such as muscle pain, malaise, and fever.
- Warn women that drug is contraindicated during pregnancy because of potential danger

to the fetus. Advise her to call immediately if pregnancy occurs.

atracurium besylate

Tracrium

Pharmacologic classification: nondepolarizing neuromuscular blocker
Therapeutic classification: skeletal muscle relaxant
Pregnancy risk category C

How supplied

Available by prescription only
Injection: 10 mg/ml

Indications and dosages

Adjunct to general anesthesia, to facilitate endotracheal intubation, and to provide skeletal muscle relaxation during surgery or mechanical ventilation

Dosage depends on anesthetic used, individual needs, and response. Doses are representative and must be adjusted.

Adults and children over age 2: Initially, 0.4 to 0.5 mg/kg by I.V. bolus. Maintenance dosage of 0.08 to 0.10 mg/kg within 20 to 45 minutes of initial dose should be administered during prolonged surgical procedures. Maintenance dosages may be administered q 15 to 25 minutes in patients receiving balanced anesthesia.

Children age 1 month to 2 years: Initially, 0.3 to 0.4 mg/kg by I.V. bolus when under halothane anesthesia. Frequent maintenance dosages may be needed.

Pharmacodynamics

Skeletal muscle relaxant action: Atracurium produces skeletal muscle paralysis by causing a decreased response to acetylcholine (ACh) at the neuromuscular junction. Because of its high affinity to ACh receptor sites, atracurium competitively blocks access of ACh to the motor end-plate, thus blocking depolarization. At usual doses (0.45 mg/kg), atracurium produces minimal CV effects and doesn't affect intraocular pressure, lower esophageal sphincter pressure, barrier pressure, heart rate or rhythm, mean arterial pressure, systemic vascular resistance, cardiac output, or central venous pressure. CV effects such as decreased peripheral vascular resistance, usually seen at doses greater than 0.5 mg/kg, are caused by histamine release.

Pharmacokinetics

Absorption: Maximum neuromuscular blockade increases with increasing dose. Repeated administration doesn't appear to be cumulative, nor is recovery time prolonged.

Distribution: Distributed into the extracellular space after I.V. administration; about 82% protein-bound.

Metabolism: In plasma, is rapidly metabolized by Hofmann elimination and by nonspecific enzymatic ester hydrolysis. The liver doesn't appear to play a major role.

Excretion: Excreted in urine and feces by biliary elimination.

Route	Onset	Peak	Duration
I.V.	2 min	3-5 min	35-70 min

Contraindications and precautions

Contraindicated in patients with hypersensitivity to drug. Use cautiously in patients with CV disease; severe electrolyte disorder; bronchogenic carcinoma; hepatic, renal, or pulmonary impairment; neuromuscular disease; myasthenia gravis; and in geriatric or debilitated patients.

Interactions

Drug-drug. *Enflurane and isoflurane, aminoglycoside antibiotics, clindamycin, lincomycin, polymyxin antibiotics, furosemide, lithium, beta blockers, depolarizing neuromuscular blockers, other nondepolarizing neuromuscular blockers, parenteral magnesium salts, quinidine, quinine, procainamide, thiazide diuretics, and potassium-depleting drugs:* The neuromuscular blockade associated with atracurium may be enhanced by use with many general anesthetics. Carefully monitor patient.

Opioid analgesics: May cause additive respiratory depression. Recommend using with extreme caution during surgery and immediately postoperatively.

Effects on diagnostic tests

None reported.

Adverse reactions

CV: ***bradycardia,*** hypotension, tachycardia.
Respiratory: ***prolonged dose-related apnea,*** wheezing, increased bronchial secretions, dyspnea, ***bronchospasm, laryngospasm.***
Skin: *flushing,* erythema, pruritus, urticaria, rash.
Other: ***anaphylaxis.***

Overdose and treatment

Signs and symptoms of overdose include prolonged respiratory depression or apnea and CV collapse. A sudden release of histamine may also occur.

A peripheral nerve stimulator is recommended to monitor response and to determine the nature and degree of neuromuscular block. Maintain an adequate airway and manual or mechanical ventilation until patient can maintain respiration unassisted.

For treatment, administer cholinesterase inhibitors, such as edrophonium, neostigmine, or pyridostigmine, to reverse neuromuscular blockade; and atropine or glycopyrrolate to counteract muscarinic adverse effects of cholinesterase inhibitors. Monitor vital signs at least every 15 minutes until patient is stable, then every 30 minutes for next 2 hours. Observe airway until patient has fully recovered from drug effects. Note rate, depth, and pattern of respirations.

Clinical considerations

- Advise I.V. injection because I.M. injection causes tissue irritation.
- Dilute to desired concentration, usually 0.2 to 0.5 mg/ml.
- Reduce dose and administration rate in patients in whom histamine release may be hazardous.
- Prior administration of succinylcholine doesn't prolong duration of action of atracurium, but it quickens onset and may deepen neuromuscular blockade.
- Atracurium has a longer duration of action than succinylcholine and a shorter duration than tubocurarine or pancuronium.
- Drug has little or no effect on heart rate and doesn't counteract or reverse the bradycardia caused by anesthetics or vagal stimulation. Thus, bradycardia is seen more frequently with atracurium than with other neuromuscular blocking agents. Pretreatment with anticholinergics (atropine or glycopyrrolate) is advised.
- Alkaline solutions such as barbiturates shouldn't be mixed in the same syringe or given through the same needle with atracurium.
- Use drug only if endotracheal intubation, administration of oxygen under positive pressure, artificial respiration, and assisted or controlled ventilation are immediately available.
- Until head and neck muscles recover from blockade effects, patient may find speech difficult.
- If indicated, assess for need for pain medication or sedation. Drug doesn't affect consciousness or relieve pain.
- Store in refrigerator at 2° to 8° C. Use within 14 days after removing from refrigerator, even if returned for storage.
- Drug is stable for 24 hours when diluted in most solutions except lactated Ringer's (8 hours); spontaneous degradation occurs more rapidly.

Therapeutic monitoring

- Recommend monitoring for bradycardia during drug administration; patient may require I.V. atropine.
- Use a peripheral nerve stimulator to monitor responses during ICU administration; it may be used to detect residual paralysis during recovery and to avoid atracurium overdose.

Special populations

Pregnant patients. There are no adequate and controlled studies for use in this population.
Breast-feeding patients. It's unknown if drug is excreted in breast milk; therefore, use cautiously in breast-feeding women.
Pediatric patients. Safety and efficacy haven't been established for children under age 1 month.
Geriatric patients. Geriatric patients may be more sensitive to the effects of the drug.

Patient counseling

Remind staff to explain all events and procedures to patient because he can still hear.

atropine sulfate

Pharmacologic classification: anticholinergic, belladonna alkaloid
Therapeutic classification: antiarrhythmic, vagolytic
Pregnancy risk category C

How supplied

Available by prescription only
Tablets: 0.4 mg
Injection: 0.05 mg/ml, 0.1 mg/ml, 0.3 mg/ml, 0.4 mg/ml, 0.5 mg/ml, 0.8 mg/ml, and 1 mg/ml
Ophthalmic ointment: 1%
Ophthalmic solution: 0.5%, 1%, 2%

Indications and dosages

Symptomatic bradycardia, bradyarrhythmia (junctional or escape rhythm)
Adults: Usually 0.5 to 1 mg by I.V. push; repeat q 3 to 5 minutes, to maximum of 0.03 mg/kg in patients with mild bradycardia and or 2.5 mg (0.4 mg/kg) in patients with severe bradycardia or ventricular asystole. Lower doses (less than 0.5 mg) may cause bradycardia.
Children: 0.02 mg/kg I.V. up to maximum 1 mg; or 0.3 mg/m^2; may repeat q 5 minutes.

Note: Dose may be administered at 2½ times the I.V. dose and diluted in 10 ml of normal saline solution (adults) or 1 to 2 ml of half-normal or normal saline solution (child) and administered via the endotracheal tube during CPR if I.V. access unavailable.

Preoperatively for diminishing secretions and blocking cardiac vagal reflexes
Adults and children weighing over 44 lb (20 kg): 0.4 mg I.M. or S.C. 30 to 60 minutes before anesthesia.
Children weighing less than 44 lb: 0.1 mg I.M. for 6.6 lb (3 kg), 0.2 mg I.M. for 8.8 to 20 lb (4 to 9 kg), 0.3 mg I.M. for 22 to 44 lb (10 to 20 kg) 30 to 60 minutes before anesthesia.
To block adverse muscarinic effects of anticholinesterase agents when these agents are used to reverse neuromuscular blockade produced by curariform agents
Adults: 0.6 to 1.2 mg for each 0.5 to 2.5 mg of neostigmine or 10 to 20 mg of pyridostigmine administered; administer I.V. a few minutes before the anticholinesterase agent.

Antidote for anticholinesterase insecticide poisoning
Adults: 1 to 2 mg I.M. or I.V. repeated q 5 to 60 minutes until muscarinic symptoms disappear. In severe cases, 2 to 6 mg may be given initially, repeating doses every 5 to 60 minutes.
Children: 0.05 mg/kg I.V. or I.M. repeated every 10 to 30 minutes until muscarinic signs and symptoms disappear.
Hypotonic radiograph of the GI tract
Adults: 1 mg I.M.
Short-term treatment or prevention of bronchospasm
Adults: 0.025 mg/kg administered via nebulizer t.i.d. or q.i.d. to maximum dose of 2.5 mg.
Children: 0.05 mg/kg t.i.d. or q.i.d.
Acute iritis, uveitis
Adults: 1 to 2 drops (0.5% or 1% solution) into the eye t.i.d. (in children use 0.5% solution) or a small amount of ointment in the conjunctival sac t.i.d.
Cycloplegic refraction
Adults: 1 drop (1% solution) 1 hour before refraction.
Children: 1 to 2 drops (0.5% solution) into each eye b.i.d. for 1 to 3 days before eye examination and 1 hour before examination.

Pharmacodynamics

Antiarrhythmic action: An anticholinergic (parasympatholytic) agent with many uses, atropine remains the mainstay of pharmacologic treatment for bradyarrhythmias. It blocks the effects of acetylcholine on the SA and AV nodes, thereby increasing SA and AV node conduction velocity. It also increases sinus node discharge rate and decreases the effective refractory period of the AV node. These changes result in an increased heart rate (both atrial and ventricular).

Atropine has variable—and clinically negligible—effects on the His-Purkinje system. Small doses (below 0.5 mg) and occasionally larger doses may lead to a paradoxical slowing of the heart rate, which may be followed by a more rapid rate.
Anticholinergic action: As a cholinergic blocking agent, atropine decreases the action of the parasympathetic nervous system on certain glands (bronchial, salivary, and sweat), resulting in decreased secretions. It also decreases cholinergic effects on the iris, ciliary body, and intestinal and bronchial smooth muscle.
Antidote for cholinesterase poisoning: As an antidote for cholinesterase poisoning, atropine blocks the cholinomimetic effects of these pesticides.

Pharmacokinetics

Absorption: I.V. administration is the most common route for bradyarrhythmia treatment. With endotracheal administration, is well absorbed from the bronchial tree; drug has been used in 1-mg doses in acute bradyarrhythmia when an I.V. line hasn't been established.
Distribution: Well distributed throughout the body, including the CNS. Only 18% of drug binds with plasma protein (clinically insignificant).
Metabolism: Metabolized in the liver to several metabolites. About 30% to 50% of a dose is excreted by the kidneys as unchanged drug.
Excretion: Excreted primarily through the kidneys; however, small amounts may be excreted in the feces and expired air. Elimination half-life is biphasic, with an initial 2-hour phase followed by a terminal half-life of about 12¼ hours.

Route	Onset	Peak	Duration
P.O.	½-2 hr	1-2 hr	4 hr
I.V.	Immediate	2-4 min	4 hr
I.M.	5-40 min	20-60 min	4 hr
S.C.	Unknown	Unknown	Unknown
Ophthalmic	Unknown	½-3 hr	7-10 days

Contraindications and precautions

Contraindicated in patients with hypersensitivity to drug or sodium metabisulfite, acute angle-closure glaucoma, obstructive uropathy, obstructive disease of GI tract, paralytic ileus, toxic megacolon, intestinal atony, unstable CV status in acute hemorrhage, asthma, and myasthenia gravis.

Ophthalmic form is contraindicated in patients with glaucoma or hypersensitivity to drug or belladonna alkaloids and in those who have adhesions between the iris and lens. Atropine shouldn't be used during the first 3 months of life because of the possible association between cycloplegia produced and development of amblyopia.

Use cautiously in patients with Down syndrome. Ophthalmic form should be used with caution in patients with increased intraocular pressure and the elderly.

Interactions

Drug-drug. *Other anticholinergics or drugs with anticholinergic effects:* Additive effects. Monitor patient carefully.
Amantadine: May result in an increase in anticholinergic adverse effects. Monitor patient carefully.
Drug-herb: *The tannic acid in squaw vine:* May decrease metabolic breakdown of atropine. Monitor patient.
Betel palm: May cause reduced temperature elevating effects and enhanced CNS effects. Avoid use together.
Jaborandi tree products: May reduce effects of atropine. Monitor patient closely.
Jimson weed: May adversely affect CV function. Avoid use together.

Choline in pill-bearing spurge: May decrease effects of atropine. Use together cautiously.

Effects on diagnostic tests
None reported.

Adverse reactions
CNS: *headache, restlessness,* ataxia, disorientation, hallucinations, delirium, *insomnia, dizziness,* excitement, agitation, confusion, especially in geriatric patients (with systemic or oral form); confusion, somnolence, headache (with ophthalmic form).
CV: palpitations and bradycardia following low-dose atropine, tachycardia after higher doses (with systemic or oral form); tachycardia (with ophthalmic form).
EENT: photophobia, increased intraocular pressure, *blurred vision, mydriasis,* cycloplegia (with systemic or oral form), ocular congestion with long-term use, conjunctivitis, contact dermatitis of eye, ocular edema, eye dryness, transient stinging and burning, eye irritation, hyperemia (with ophthalmic form).
GI: *dry mouth,* thirst, *constipation,* nausea, vomiting (with systemic or oral form); dry mouth, abdominal distention in infants (with ophthalmic form).
GU: urine retention, impotence (with systemic or oral form).
Hematologic: leukocytosis (with systemic or oral form).
Skin: dryness (with ophthalmic form).
Other: severe allergic reactions, including ***anaphylaxis*** and urticaria (systemic or oral form).

Overdose and treatment
Signs of overdose reflect excessive anticholinergic activity, especially CV and CNS stimulation.

Treatment includes physostigmine administration to reverse excessive anticholinergic activity and general supportive measures, as necessary.

Clinical considerations
- With I.V. administration, drug may cause paradoxical initial bradycardia, which usually disappears within 2 minutes.
- High doses may cause hyperpyrexia, urinary retention, and CNS effects, including hallucinations and confusion (anticholinergic delirium). Other anticholinergic drugs may increase vagal blockage.
- Atropine sulfate injection is physically incompatible with norepinephrine bitartrate, mataraminol bitartrate, and sodium bicarbonate injection. A haze or precipitate will form within 15 minutes of mixing with methohexital solutions.
- Store drug at 59° to 86° F (15° to 30° C) and protect from heat, light, and air.

Therapeutic monitoring
- Recommend observing patient for tachycardia if he has cardiac disorder.
- Monitor patient's fluid intake and output; drug causes urine retention and hesitancy. If possible, patient should void before taking drug.

Special populations
Geriatric patients. Monitor closely for urine retention in elderly men with BPH.

Patient counseling
- Tell patient to report serious adverse reactions promptly.
- Teach patient how to instill eye medication.
- Warn patient to avoid hazardous activities until blurry vision subsides.
- Advise patient to ease photophobia by wearing dark glasses.

attapulgite
Children's Kaopectate, Diasorb, Donnagel, Fowler's*, Kaopectate, Kaopectate Advanced Formula, Kaopectate Maximum Strength, K-Pek, Parepectolin, Rheaban, Rheaban Maximum Strength

Pharmacologic classification: hydrated magnesium aluminum silicate
Therapeutic classification: antidiarrheal
Pregnancy risk category NR

How supplied
Available without a prescription
Tablets: 300 mg, 600 mg*, 630 mg*, 750 mg
Tablets (chewable): 600 mg
Oral suspension: 600 mg/15 ml, 750 mg/5 ml, 750 mg/15 ml*, 900 mg/15 ml*

Indications and dosages
Acute, nonspecific diarrhea
Adults and adolescents: 1.2 to 1.5 g (unless using Diasorb, in which case dosage can be as high as 3 g) P.O. after each loose bowel movement; don't exceed 9 g within 24 hours.
Children age 6 to 12: 600 mg (suspension) or 750 mg (tablet) P.O. after each loose bowel movement; don't exceed 4.2 g (suspension and chewable tablets) or 4.5 g (tablet) within 24 hours.
Children age 3 to 6: 300 mg P.O. after each loose bowel movement; don't exceed 2.1 g within 24 hours.

Pharmacodynamics
Antidiarrheal action: Although its exact action is unknown, it's believed that attapulgite absorbs large numbers of bacteria and toxins and reduces water loss in the GI tract.

Pharmacokinetics
Absorption: Not absorbed.
Distribution: Not applicable.
Metabolism: Not applicable.
Excretion: Excreted unchanged in feces.

Route	Onset	Peak	Duration
P.O.	Unknown	Unknown	Unknown

Contraindications and precautions
Contraindicated in patients with dysentery or suspected bowel obstruction. Use cautiously in dehydrated patients.

Interactions
Drug-drug. *Other medications:* Absorption of oral medications may be impaired if given together with attapulgite. Attapulgite must be given not less than 2 hours before or 3 to 4 hours after these medications, and monitor for decreased effectiveness.

Effects on diagnostic tests
None reported.

Adverse reactions
GI: constipation.

Overdose and treatment
Because attapulgite isn't absorbed, an overdose is unlikely to pose a significant health problem.

Clinical considerations
- Ensure that patient achieves adequate fluid intake to compensate for fluid loss from diarrhea.
- Drug shouldn't be used if diarrhea is accompanied by fever or blood or mucus in the stool. Discontinue drug if any of these signs occurs during treatment.

Therapeutic monitoring
Recommend monitoring patient for signs and symptoms of dehydration.

Special populations
Pediatric patients. Use only under medical supervision in children under age 3.
Geriatric patients. Use cautiously and only under medical supervision.

Patient counseling
- Tell patient to take drug after each loose bowel movement until diarrhea is controlled.
- Instruct patient to call if diarrhea isn't controlled within 48 hours or if fever develops.

auranofin
Ridaura

Pharmacologic classification: gold salt
Therapeutic classification: antiarthritic
Pregnancy risk category C

How supplied
Available by prescription only
Capsules: 3 mg

Indications and dosages
Rheumatoid arthritis, ◇psoriatic arthritis, ◇active systemic lupus erythematosus, ◇Felty's syndrome
Adults: 6 mg P.O. daily, administered either as 3 mg b.i.d. or 6 mg once daily. After 4 to 6 months, may be increased to 9 mg daily (3 mg t.i.d.). If response remains inadequate after 3 months at 9 mg daily, discontinue drug.

Pharmacodynamics
Antiarthritic action: Auranofin suppresses or prevents, but doesn't cure, adult or juvenile arthritis and synovitis. It is anti-inflammatory in active arthritis. This drug is thought to reduce inflammation by altering the immune system. Auranofin has been shown to decrease high serum levels of immunoglobulins and rheumatoid factors in patients with arthritis. However, the exact mechanism of action remains unknown.

Pharmacokinetics
Absorption: When administered P.O., 25% of the gold in auranofin is absorbed through the GI tract.
Distribution: 60% protein-bound and is distributed widely in body tissues. Oral gold from auranofin is bound to a higher degree than gold from the injectable form. Synovial fluid levels are about 50% of blood levels. No correlation between blood-gold levels and safety or efficacy has been determined.
Metabolism: The metabolic fate of auranofin isn't known, but it's believed that drug isn't broken down into elemental gold.
Excretion: 60% of absorbed auranofin (15% of the administered dose) is excreted in the urine and the remainder in the feces. Average plasma half-life is 26 days, compared with about 6 days for gold sodium thiomalate.

Route	Onset	Peak	Duration
P.O.	Unknown	2 hr	Unknown

Contraindications and precautions
Contraindicated in patients with history of severe gold toxicity, necrotizing enterocolitis, pulmonary fibrosis, exfoliative dermatitis, bone marrow aplasia, severe hematologic disorders,

or history of severe toxicity caused by previous exposure to other heavy metals.

Use cautiously with other drugs that cause blood dyscrasias or in patients with renal, hepatic, or inflammatory bowel disease; rash; or bone marrow depression. Use of drug in pregnant women isn't recommended.

Interactions
Drug-drug. *Other drugs that may cause blood dyscrasias:* May produce additive hematologic toxicity. Recommend monitoring hematologic studies.

Effects on diagnostic tests
Serum protein-bound iodine test, especially when done by the chloric acid digestion method, gives false readings during and for several weeks after gold therapy. TB skin test may have an enhanced response. Consider this when interpreting results.

Adverse reactions
CNS: confusion, hallucinations, ***seizures.***
EENT: conjunctivitis.
GI: *diarrhea, abdominal pain, nausea, stomatitis,* glossitis, anorexia, metallic taste, dyspepsia, flatulence, constipation, dysgeusia, *ulcerative colitis.*
GU: proteinuria, hematuria, *nephrotic syndrome,* glomerulonephritis, ***acute renal failure.***
Hematologic: ***thrombocytopenia*** (with or without purpura), ***aplastic anemia, agranulocytosis, leukopenia,*** eosinophilia, anemia.
Hepatic: jaundice, elevated liver enzymes.
Respiratory: interstitial pneumonitis.
Skin: *rash, pruritus, dermatitis,* exfoliative dermatitis, urticaria, erythema, alopecia.

Overdose and treatment
In acute overdose, empty gastric contents by induced emesis or gastric lavage. When severe reactions to gold occur, corticosteroids, dimercaprol (a chelating agent), or penicillamine may be given to aid recovery. Prednisone 40 to 100 mg daily in divided doses is recommended to manage severe renal, hematologic, pulmonary, or enterocolitic reactions to gold. Dimercaprol may be used together with steroids to facilitate the removal of the gold when steroid treatment alone is ineffective. Use of chelating agents is controversial, and caution is recommended. Appropriate supportive therapy is indicated as necessary.

Clinical considerations
- When switching from injectable gold, initial dose is 6 mg P.O. daily.
- To encourage patient compliance with follow up, initial prescription should be for 2 weeks and subsequent prescriptions for 1 month.

Therapeutic monitoring
- Discontinue drug if platelet count decreases to below 100,000/mm³.
- Recommend monitoring CBC, platelet count, urinalysis, and kidney and liver function tests before therapy for baseline and then monthly.
- Monitor for signs of toxicity which include leukocyte count less than 400/mm³, granulocyte count less than 1,500/mm³, decreased platelet count to 150,000/mm³, proteinuria, hematuria, pruritus, rash, stomatitis, persistent diarrhea.
- Advise monitoring for uncontrolled diarrhea; dose reduction or temporary discontinuance of drug may relieve diarrhea.

Special populations
Pregnant patients. There are no adequate and controlled studies, but clinical experience doesn't indicate evidence of adverse effects on the fetus.
Breast-feeding patients. Drug isn't recommended for use during breast-feeding.
Pediatric patients. Controlled clinical trials for the treatment of juvenile rheumatoid arthritis in children ages 4 to 16 is ongoing. Safe dosage hasn't been established; use in children currently isn't recommended.
Geriatric patients. Administer usual adult dose. Use cautiously in patients with decreased renal function.

Patient counseling
- Emphasize importance of monthly follow-up to monitor patient's platelet count.
- Reassure patient that beneficial drug effect may be delayed for 3 months. However, if response is inadequate after 6 to 9 months, auranofin will probably be discontinued.
- Encourage patient to take drug as prescribed and not to alter the dosage schedule.
- Diarrhea is the most common adverse reaction. Tell patient to continue taking drug if he experiences mild diarrhea; however, tell him to call immediately if blood occurs in stool.
- Tell patient to continue taking concomitant drug therapy, such as NSAIDs, if prescribed.
- Dermatitis is a common adverse reaction. Advise patient to report rash or other skin problems immediately.
- Stomatitis is another common adverse reaction. Tell patient that stomatitis is often preceded by a metallic taste and advise him to call his doctor immediately.

azathioprine

Imuran

azathioprine sodium

Imuran

Pharmacologic classification: purine antagonist
Therapeutic classification: immunosuppressive
Pregnancy risk category D

How supplied

Available by prescription only
Tablets: 50 mg
Injection: 100 mg per vial

Indications and dosages

Prevention of the rejection of kidney transplants
Adults and children: Initially, 3 to 5 mg/kg P.O. daily beginning on day of (or 1 to 3 days before) transplantation. After transplantation, dosage may be administered I.V., until patient is able to tolerate oral dosage. Usual maintenance dosage is 1 to 3 mg/kg daily. Dosage varies with patient response.
Severe, refractory rheumatoid arthritis
Adults: Initially, 1 mg/kg (about 50 to 100 mg) P.O. taken as a single dose or in divided doses. If patient response is unsatisfactory after 6 to 8 weeks, dose may be increased by 0.5 mg/kg daily (up to a maximum of 2.5 mg/kg daily) at 4-week intervals. If no response after 12 weeks, discontinue.

Pharmacodynamics

Immunosuppressant action: The mechanism of immunosuppressive activity is unknown; however, drug may inhibit RNA and DNA synthesis, mitosis, or (in patients undergoing renal transplantation) coenzyme formation and functioning. Azathioprine suppresses cell-mediated hypersensitivity and alters antibody production.

Pharmacokinetics

Absorption: Well absorbed orally.
Distribution: Drug and its major metabolite, mercaptopurine, are distributed throughout the body; both are 30% protein-bound. Azathioprine and its metabolites cross the placenta.
Metabolism: Metabolized primarily to mercaptopurine.
Excretion: Small amounts of azathioprine and mercaptopurine are excreted in urine intact; most of a given dose is excreted in urine as secondary metabolites.

Route	Onset	Peak	Duration
P.O., I.V.	4-8 wk	1-2 hr	Several days

Contraindications and precautions

Contraindicated in patients hypersensitive to drug and during pregnancy. Use cautiously in patients with impaired renal or hepatic function.

Interactions

Drug-drug. *Allopurinol:* The major metabolic pathway of azathioprine is inhibited by allopurinol, which competes for the oxidative enzyme xanthine oxidase. Azathioprine with allopurinol is potentially hazardous and should be avoided. If use together is unavoidable, reduce dose by one-third to one-fourth the usual dose.
Tubocurarine and pancuronium: Drug may reverse neuromuscular blockade resulting from use of the nondepolarizing muscle relaxants. Recommend monitoring for this effect.
Methotrexate: May increase plasma levels of the metabolite 6-MP. Recommend monitoring patient for toxicity.
Cyclosporine: Plasma levels of cyclosporine may be decreased. Recommend monitoring for clinical effect.
Angiotensin-converting enzyme inhibitors: Anemia and severe leukopenia have been reported with use of azathioprine. Use together cautiously.

Effects on diagnostic tests

None reported.

Adverse reactions

GI: *nausea, vomiting,* ***pancreatitis***, steatorrhea, diarrhea, abdominal pain.
Hematologic: LEUKOPENIA, ***bone marrow suppression***, anemia, ***pancytopenia, thrombocytopenia, immunosuppression*** (possibly profound).
Hepatic: ***hepatotoxicity,*** jaundice.
Musculoskeletal: arthralgia, myalgia.
Skin: rash.
Other: alopecia, ***infections***, fever, ***increased risk of neoplasia.***

Overdose and treatment

Signs and symptoms of overdose include nausea, vomiting, diarrhea, and extension of hematologic effects. Supportive treatment may include treatment with blood products if necessary.

Clinical considerations

- If used to treat rheumatoid arthritis, continue NSAIDs when azathioprine therapy is initiated.
- Chronic immunosuppression with azathioprine is associated with an increased risk of neoplasia.
- Reconstitute 100 mg vial with 10 ml of sterile water for injection. The resultant concentration is 10 mg/ml. Visually inspect for particles before use. Drug may be administered by

direct I.V. injection or further diluted in normal saline for injection or D_5W and infused over 30 to 60 minutes. Use only in patients who are unable to tolerate oral medications.

- If infection occurs, reduce drug dosage.
- If nausea and vomiting occur, dose may be divided or given with or after meals.

Therapeutic monitoring

- Recommend monitoring patient for signs of hepatic damage: clay-colored stools, dark urine, jaundice, pruritus, and elevated liver enzyme levels.
- Recommend monitoring for unusual bleeding or bruising, fever, or sore throat.
- Monitor hematologic status while patient is receiving azathioprine. CBCs, including platelet counts, should be taken at least weekly during the first month, twice monthly for the second and third months, then monthly.

Special populations

Pregnant patients. May cause fetal harm in pregnant women. Drug may also cause temporary depression of spermatogenesis.

Patient counseling

- Explain possible adverse effects of medication and importance of reporting them, especially unusual bleeding or bruising, fever, sore throat, mouth sores, abdominal pain, pale stools, or dark urine.
- Encourage compliance with therapy and follow-up visits.
- Advise patient to avoid pregnancy during therapy and for 4 months after stopping therapy.
- Tell patient with rheumatoid arthritis that clinical response may not be apparent for up to 12 weeks.
- Suggest taking drug with or after meals or in divided doses to prevent nausea.

azithromycin

Zithromax

Pharmacologic classification: azalide macrolide
Therapeutic classification: antibiotic
Pregnancy risk category B

How supplied

Available by prescription only
Tablets: 250 mg
Powder for oral suspension: 100 mg/5 ml, 200 mg/5 ml; 300 mg*, 600 mg*, 900 mg*, 1,000 mg/packet
Injection: 500 mg

Indications and dosages

***Acute bacterial exacerbations of chronic obstructive pulmonary disease caused by* Haemophilus influenzae, Moraxella (Branhamella) catarrhalis, *or* Streptococcus pneumoniae; *uncomplicated skin and skin structure infections caused by* Staphylococcus aureus, Streptococcus pyogenes, *or* Streptococcus agalactiae; *and second-line therapy of pharyngitis or tonsillitis caused by* S. pyogenes**

Adults and adolescents age 16 and older: Initially, 500 mg P.O. as a single dose on day 1, followed by 250 mg daily on days 2 through 5. Total cumulative dose is 1.5 g.

***Community-acquired pneumonia caused by* Chlamydia pneumoniae, H. influenzae, Mycoplasma pneumoniae, S. pneumoniae; *I.V. form can be used for above infections and those caused by* Legionella pneumophila, M. catarrhalis, *and* S. aureus**

Adults and adolescents age 16 and older: 500 mg P.O. as a single dose on day 1, followed by 250 mg P.O. daily on days 2 to 5. Total dose is 1.5 g. For those who require initial I.V. therapy, 500 mg I.V. as a single daily dose for 2 days, followed by 500 mg P.O. as a single daily dose to complete a 7- to 10-day course of therapy. The timing of the change from I.V. to P.O. therapy should be based on patient's clinical response.

***Nongonococcal urethritis or cervicitis caused by* Chlamydia trachomatis**

Adults and adolescents age 16 and older: 1 g P.O. as a single dose.

Pelvic inflammatory disease caused by* Chlamydia trachomatis, Neisseria gonorrhoeae, *or* Mycoplasma hominis *in patients requiring initial I.V. therapy

Adults: 500 mg I.V. as a single daily dose for 1 to 2 days, followed by 250 mg P.O. daily to complete a 7-day course of therapy. The timing of the change from I.V. to P.O. therapy should be directed by the health care provider based on patient's clinical response.

Otitis media

Children over age 6 months: 10 mg/kg dose P.O. on day 1; then 5 mg/kg once daily on days 2 to 5.

Tonsillitis

Children over age 2: 12 mg/kg P.O. daily for 5 days.

Chancroid

Adults: 1 g P.O. as a single dose.
◇*Infants and children:* 20 mg/kg (maximum of 1 g) as a single oral dose

Prevention of disseminated* Mycobacterium avium *complex (MAC) in patients with advanced infection with HIV

Adults: 1.2 g P.O. once weekly alone or in combination with rifabutin.
◇*Children:* 20 mg/kg P.O. (maximum of 1.2 g) weekly or 5 mg/kg (maximum of 250 mg) can be given P.O. daily.

◊ ***Prophylaxis of bacterial endocarditis in penicillin-allergic adults at moderate to high risk***
Adults: 500 mg 1 hour prior to the procedure.
◊ ***Chlamydial ophthalmia neonatorum***
Infants: 20 mg/kg once daily P.O. for 3 days.

Pharmacodynamics
Antibiotic action: Azithromycin, a derivative of erythromycin, binds to the 50S subunit of bacterial ribosomes, blocking protein synthesis. It is bacteriostatic or bactericidal, depending on concentration. Azithromycin is effective against many gram-positive and gram-negative aerobic and anaerobic bacteria in addition to *Borrelia burgdorferi, Chlamydia pneumoniae, C. trachomatis, Mycoplasma pneumoniae*, and *Mycobacterium avium* complex (MAC).

Pharmacokinetics
Absorption: Rapidly absorbed from the GI tract; food decreases both maximum plasma levels and amount of drug absorbed.
Distribution: Rapidly distributed throughout the body and readily penetrates cells; it doesn't readily enter the CNS. It concentrates in fibroblasts and phagocytes. Significantly higher levels of drug are reached in the tissues as compared with the plasma. Uptake and release of drug from tissues contributes to the long half-life. With a loading dose, peak and trough blood levels are stable within 48 hours. Without a loading dose, 5 to 7 days are required before steady state is reached.
Metabolism: Not metabolized.
Excretion: Excreted mostly in the feces after excretion into the bile. Less than 10% is excreted in the urine. Terminal elimination half-life is 68 hours.

Route	Onset	Peak	Duration
P.O.	Unknown	2½-4½ hr	Unknown
I.V.	Unknown	Unknown	Unknown

Contraindications and precautions
Contraindicated in patients with hypersensitivity to erythromycin or other macrolides. Use cautiously in patients with impaired hepatic function.

Interactions
Drug-drug. *Aluminum- and magnesium-containing antacids:* May result in lower peak plasma levels of azithromycin. Advise nurse to separate administration times by at least 2 hours.
Theophylline: Macrolides may increase plasma theophylline levels by decreasing theophylline clearance. Recommend monitoring theophylline levels carefully.
Drugs metabolized by the hepatic cytochrome P-450 system (such as phenytoin, barbiturates, carbamazepine, and cyclosporine): May result in impaired metabolism of these agents and increased risk of toxicity. Recommend monitoring patient for signs of drug toxicity.
Triazolam: Clearance of triazolam may be decreased, increasing the risk of triazolam toxicity. Recommend monitoring patient for signs of drug toxicity.
Ergotamine or dihydroergotamine: Acute ergot toxicity has been reported when macrolides have been administered with ergotamine or dihydroergotamine. Use together cautiously.
Warfarin: Other macrolides may increase PT and INR; effect of azithromycin is unknown. Recommend monitoring PT and INR carefully.

Effects on diagnostic tests
None reported.

Adverse reactions
CNS: dizziness, vertigo, headache, fatigue, somnolence.
CV: palpitations, chest pain.
GI: *nausea, vomiting, diarrhea, abdominal pain,* dyspepsia, flatulence, melena, cholestatic jaundice, pseudomembranous colitis.
GU: candidiasis, vaginitis, nephritis.
Skin: rash, photosensitivity.
Other: ***angioedema.***

Overdose and treatment
No information available. Treat symptomatically.

Clinical considerations
- Azithromycin has been used investigationally in *H. pylori* regimens, infections caused by *Bartonella*, Lyme disease caused by *Borrelia burgdorferi, Toxoplasma gondii* encephalitis, babesiosis, granuloma inguanale, and AIDS-related cryptosporidiosis.
- Obtain culture and sensitivity tests before giving first dose. Therapy can begin before results are obtained.
- Reconstitute 500-mg vial with 4.8 ml of sterile water for injection. Shake well until drug is dissolved (yields a concentration of 100 mg/ml). Dilute solution further in at least 250 ml of normal saline, 0.45% saline, D_5W, or lactated Ringer's solution to yield a concentration range of 1 to 2 mg/ml.

□ ***ALERT*** Recommend infusion of 500-mg dose of azithromycin I.V. over 1 or more hours. Don't give as a bolus or I.M. injection.

- Oral form shouldn't be used for moderate to severe pneumonia or when complicating risk factors exist.

Therapeutic monitoring
- Recommend monitoring liver enzymes, especially in patients with impaired renal function.
- Advise serologic tests for syphilis and cultures for gonorrhea in patients diagnosed with sexually transmitted urethritis or cervicitis.

Drug shouldn't be used to treat gonorrhea or syphilis.

- Drug may cause overgrowth of nonsusceptible bacteria or fungi. Watch for signs and symptoms of superinfection.

Special populations

Pregnant patients. Preliminary studies have proven drug to be safe for the treatment of chlamydial infection in pregnant women, but there is insufficient data for routine use.
Breast-feeding patients. It's unknown if drug is excreted in breast milk. Use cautiously in breast-feeding women.
Pediatric patients. Safety and efficacy in children age 16 and under for I.V. administration and 6 months and under for P.O. administration haven't been established.
Geriatric patients. In clinical trials of patients with normal hepatic and renal function, in using the 5-day dosage regimen, no significant pharmacokinetic differences were seen in those between ages 65 and 85.

Patient counseling

- Tell patient to take all of drug prescribed, even if he's feeling better.
- Remind patient that drug should always be taken on an empty stomach because food or antacids decrease absorption. Patient should take drug 1 hour before or 2 hours after a meal and shouldn't take antacids.
- Instruct patient to promptly report adverse reactions.

aztreonam

Azactam

Pharmacologic classification: monobactam
Therapeutic classification: antibiotic
Pregnancy risk category B

How supplied

Available by prescription only
Injection: 500-mg, 1-g, 2-g vials

Indications and dosages

Urinary tract, respiratory tract, intra-abdominal, gynecologic, or skin infections; septicemia caused by gram-negative bacteria; ◇adjunct therapy in pelvic inflammatory disease; ◇gonorrhea
Adults: 500 mg to 2 g I.V. or I.M. q 8 to 12 hours. For severe systemic or life-threatening infections, 2 g q 6 to 8 hours may be given. Maximum dose is 8 g daily. For gonorrhea, give 1 g I.M. single dose.
≡ ***Dosage adjustment.*** In patients with a creatinine clearance of 10 to 30 ml/minute/1.73 m^2, reduce dose by one half after an initial dose of 1 to 2 g. In patients with a creatinine clearance below 10 ml/minute/1.73 m^2, an initial dose of 500 mg to 2 g should be followed by one fourth of the usual dose at the usual intervals; give one eighth the initial dose after each session of hemodialysis.

Pharmacodynamics

Antibacterial action: Aztreonam is a monobactam that inhibits mucopeptide synthesis of the bacterial cell wall. It preferentially binds to penicillin-binding protein 3 (PBP3) of susceptible organisms and often causes cell lysis and cell death.

Aztreonam has a narrow spectrum of activity and is usually bactericidal in action. Aztreonam is effective against *Escherichia coli, Enterobacter, Klebsiella pneumoniae, Proteus mirabilis,* and *Pseudomonas aeruginosa.* It has limited activity against *Citrobacter, Haemophilus influenzae, K. oxytoca, Hafnia, Serratia marcescens, E. aerogenes, Morganella morganii, Providencia, Moraxella catarrhalis, Proteus vulgaris,* and *Neisseria gonorrhoeae.*

Pharmacokinetics

Absorption: Absorbed poorly from GI tract after oral administration but is absorbed rapidly and completely after I.M. or I.V. administration.
Distribution: Distributed rapidly and widely to all body fluids and tissues, including bile, breast milk, and CSF. It crosses the placental barrier and is found in fetal circulation.
Metabolism: From 6% to 16% is metabolized to inactive metabolites by nonspecific hydrolysis of the beta-lactam ring; 56% to 60% is protein-bound, less if renal impairment is present.
Excretion: Excreted principally in urine as unchanged drug by glomerular filtration and tubular secretion; 1½% to 3½% is excreted in feces as unchanged drug. Half-life averages 1¾ hours. Drug is excreted in breast milk; it may be removed by hemodialysis and peritoneal dialysis.

Route	Onset	Peak	Duration
I.V.	Unknown	Immediate	Unknown
I.M.	Unknown	<1 hr	Unknown

Contraindications and precautions

Contraindicated in patients with hypersensitivity to drug. Use cautiously in patients with impaired renal function and in the elderly.

Interactions

Drug-drug. *Probenecid*: May prolong the rate of tubular secretion of aztreonam. Avoid use together.
Aminoglycosides, or other beta-lactam antibiotics, including piperacillin, cefoperazone, cefotaxime, clindamycin, or metronidazole: Synergistic or additive effects occur. Avoid use together.

Potent inducers of beta-lactamase production (cefoxitin, imipenem): May inactivate aztreonam. Avoid use together.
Chloramphenicol: Antagonistic reaction. Advise staff to give the two preparations several hours apart.
Clavulanic acid: May be synergistic or antagonistic, depending on organism involved. Avoid use together.

Effects on diagnostic tests

Aztreonam therapy alters urinary glucose determinations using cupric sulfate (Clinitest or Benedict's solution) and gives false-positive Coombs' test results.

Adverse reactions

CNS: ***seizures***, headache, insomnia, confusion.
CV: hypotension.
GI: diarrhea, nausea, vomiting.
GU: transient elevation of creatinine.
Hematologic: ***neutropenia***, anemia, ***pancytopenia***, ***thrombocytopenia***, leukocytosis, thrombocytosis.
Hepatic: transient elevation of LD, Cr, ALT and AST.
Other: ***hypersensitivity reactions*** (rash, ***anaphylaxis***), thrombophlebitis (at I.V. site); discomfort, swelling (at I.M. injection site).

Overdose and treatment

No information is available on the symptoms of overdose. Hemodialysis or peritoneal dialysis increases elimination of aztreonam.

Clinical considerations

- Drug has also been used to treat bone and joint infection caused by susceptible aerobic, gram-negative bacteria.
- To reconstitute for I.M. use, dilute with at least 3 ml of sterile water for injection, bacteriostatic water for injection, normal saline solution, or bacteriostatic normal saline solution for each gram of aztreonam (15-ml vial).
- To reconstitute for I.V. use, add 6 to 10 ml of sterile water for injection to each 15-ml vial; for I.V. infusion, prepare as for I.M. solution. May be further diluted by adding to normal saline, Ringer's solution, lactated Ringer's solution, 5% or 10% dextrose, or other electrolyte-containing solutions. For I.V. piggyback (100-ml bottles), add at least 50 ml of diluent for each gram of aztreonam. Final concentration shouldn't exceed 20 mg/ml.
- I.V. route is preferred for doses larger than 1 g or in patients with bacterial septicemia, localized parenchymal abscesses, peritonitis, or other life-threatening infections; administer by direct I.V. push over 3 to 5 minutes or by intermittent infusion over 20 to 60 minutes.
- Solutions may be colorless or light straw yellow. On standing, they may develop a slight pink tint; potency isn't affected.
- Drug may be stored at room temperature for 48 hours or in refrigerator for 7 days.

Therapeutic monitoring

- Monitor renal and hepatic function tests. Reduced dose may be required in patients with impaired renal function, cirrhosis, or other hepatic impairment.
- Recommend testing for *Clostridium difficile* in patients with prolonged diarrhea.

Special populations

Pregnant patients. There are no adequate and controlled studies for use in pregnant women.
Breast-feeding patients. Although drug is excreted in breast milk, it isn't absorbed from infant's GI tract and is unlikely to cause any serious problems.
Pediatric patients. Manufacturer doesn't recommend use of drug in infants under age 1 month.
Geriatric patients. Studies in age 65 to 75 have shown that the half-life of aztreonam may be prolonged in geriatric patients because of their diminished renal function.

Patient counseling

Tell patient to call immediately if rash, redness, or itching develops.

B

bacillus Calmette-Guérin (BCG), live intravesical
TheraCys

Pharmacologic classification: bacterial
Therapeutic classification: antineoplastic
Pregnancy risk category C

How supplied
Available by prescription only
Suspension (powder form) for bladder instillation: 81 mg/vial

Indications and dosages
Treatment of in situ carcinoma of the urinary bladder (primary and relapsed)
Adults: Consult published protocols, specialized references, and manufacturer's recommendations.

Typical dose is 1 to 8 $\times$ 10^8 colony-forming units (CFUs). Be aware that FDA has reported errors in some treatment protocols giving 10 times the recommended dose.

Pharmacodynamics
Antitumor action: Exact mechanism unknown. Instillation of the live bacterial suspension causes a local inflammatory response. Local infiltration of histiocytes and leukocytes is followed by a decrease in the superficial tumors within the bladder.

Pharmacokinetics
No information available.

Route	Onset	Peak	Duration
Intravesical	Unknown	Unknown	Unknown

Contraindications and precautions
Contraindicated in immunocompromised patients, in those receiving immunosuppressive therapy, and in those with urinary tract infection or fever of unknown origin. If fever is caused by infection, withhold drug until patient recovers.

Interactions
Drug-drug. *Antimicrobial therapy for other infections:* May attenuate the response to BCG live. Avoid use together.
Drugs that depress the bone marrow, radiation therapy, and immunosuppressants: May impair the response to BCG intravesical because these treatments can decrease the patient's immune response. These treatments may also increase the risk of osteomyelitis or disseminated BCG infection. Avoid use together.

Effects on diagnostic tests
Tuberculin sensitivity may be rendered positive by BCG intravesical treatment. Determine patient's reactivity to tuberculin before initiating therapy.

Adverse reactions
GI: *nausea, vomiting, anorexia,* diarrhea.
GU: *dysuria, urinary frequency, hematuria, cystitis, urinary urgency,* nocturia, urinary incontinence, *urinary tract infection,* cramps, pain, decreased bladder capacity, renal toxicity, genital pain.
Hematologic: *anemia,* ***leukopenia.***
Hepatic: elevated liver enzyme levels.
Musculoskeletal: myalgia, arthralgia.
Other: ***hypersensitivity reaction****, malaise, fever, chills,* ***disseminated mycobacterial infection.***

Overdose and treatment
Closely monitor the patient for signs of systemic BCG infection and treat with antituberculosis medication.

Clinical considerations
- Reconstitute drug just before use, using only diluent provided. All persons handling drug should wear masks and gloves.
- Handle drug and all material used for instillation of the drug as infectious material because it contains live attenuated mycobacteria. Dispose of all associated materials (syringes, catheters, and containers) as biohazardous waste.
- The vial of TheraCys should be reconstituted with 3 ml of the supplied diluent. Don't remove the rubber stopper to prepare the solution. Further dilute in 50 ml of sterile, preservative-free saline (final volume, 53 ml). A urethral catheter is instilled into the bladder under aseptic conditions, the bladder is drained, and then the prepared solution is added by gravity feed. The catheter is then removed.
- Use strict aseptic technique to administer drug, thus minimizing the trauma to the GU

tract and preventing introduction of other contaminants to the area.

- If there's evidence of traumatic catheterization, don't administer drug and delay treatment for at least 1 week. Subsequent treatment may resume as if no interruption of the schedule has occurred.
- Bladder irritation can be treated symptomatically with phenazopyridine, acetaminophen, and propantheline bromide. Systemic adverse reactions that are caused by hypersensitivity can be treated with diphenhydramine hydrochloride.
- Protect drug from light and store at less than 41° F (5° C). Drug expires 1 year after date of issue if stored at this temperature.

Therapeutic monitoring

Recommend monitoring for cystitis and hematuria.

Special populations

Breast-feeding patients. It isn't known if drug is excreted in breast milk. Use with caution in breast-feeding women.

Pediatric patients. Safety in children hasn't been established.

Patient counseling

- After instillation, patient should retain the fluid in bladder for 2 hours (if possible). For the first hour, tell patient to lie 15 minutes prone, 15 minutes supine, and 15 minutes on each side. Patient may be up for the second hour.
- For safety, patient should be seated when voiding. Instruct patient to disinfect urine for 6 hours after instillation of drug. Tell patient to add undiluted household bleach (5% sodium hypochlorite solution) in equal volume to voided urine to the toilet; let stand for 15 minutes before flushing.
- Tell patient to call if symptoms worsen or if any of the following occur: blood in the urine, fever and chills, frequent urge to urinate or painful urination, nausea, vomiting, joint pain, rash, or cough.

bacitracin

AK-Tracin, Altracin, Baciguent, Baci-IM

Pharmacologic classification: polypeptide antibiotic
Therapeutic classification: antibiotic
Pregnancy risk category C

How supplied

Available without a prescription
Topical: ointment form (500 units/g) and in combination products containing neomycin, polymyxin B, and bacitracin

Available by prescription only
Injection: 50,000-unit vials
Ophthalmic ointment: 500 units/g

Indications and dosages

Topical infections, impetigo, abrasions, cuts, and minor wounds
Adults and children: Apply thin film to cleansed area once daily to t.i.d. for no more than 7 days.

Pneumonia and empyema caused by a staphylococcal infection
Children weighing under 5.5 lb (2.5 kg): Give 900 units/kg I.M. daily in two or three divided doses.
Children weighing over 5.5 lb: Give 1,000 units/kg I.M. daily in two or three divided doses.
◊*Adults:* 10,000 to 25,000 units I.M. q 6 hours not to exceed 100,000 units per day.

◊ ***Treatment of antibiotic-associated pseudomembranous colitis caused by* Clostridium difficile**
Adults: 20,000 to 25,000 units P.O. q 6 hours for 7 to 10 days.

Short-term topical treatment of superficial infections of the eye involving the conjunctiva and cornea caused by bacitracin-susceptible organisms
Adults and children: Apply ophthalmic ointment to affected area 1 or more times daily.

Pharmacodynamics

Antibacterial action: Bacitracin impairs bacterial cell wall synthesis, damaging the bacterial plasma membrane and making the cell more vulnerable to osmotic pressure. Drug is effective against many gram-positive organisms such as staphylococci, streptococci, anaerobic cocci, corynebacteria, and *C. difficile.* The drug is also effective against gonococci, meningococci, fusobacteria, *Actinomyces israelii, Treponema pallidum,* and *Treponema vincenti.* Drug is only minimally active against gram-negative organisms.

Pharmacokinetics

Absorption: With I.M. administration, is absorbed rapidly and completely; serum levels range from 0.2 to 2 mcg/ml. Drug isn't absorbed from the GI tract and isn't significantly absorbed from intact or denuded skin wounds or mucous membranes.
Distribution: Distributed widely throughout all body organs and fluids except CSF (unless meninges are inflamed). Binding to plasma protein is minimal.
Metabolism: Not significantly metabolized.
Excretion: When administered I.M., the kidneys excrete 10% to 40% of dose.

Route	Onset	Peak	Duration
I.M.	Unknown	1-2 hr	Unknown
Ophthalmic, topical	Unknown	Unknown	Unknown

Contraindications and precautions

Contraindicated in patients hypersensitive to drug and in atopic patients. Use cautiously in patients with myasthenia gravis and neuromuscular disease.

Interactions

Drug-drug. *Anesthetics or neuromuscular blocking agents:* Prolonged or increased neuromuscular blockade. Carefully monitor patient.
Other nephrotoxic drugs: Systemically administered bacitracin may induce additive damage when given with bacitracin. Administer together cautiously.

Effects on diagnostic tests

None reported.

Adverse reactions

CV: tightness in chest, hypotension.
EENT: slowed corneal wound healing, temporary visual haze (with ophthalmic form), ototoxicity (when topical form is used over large areas for prolonged periods or with systemic use).
GU: ***nephrotoxicity, renal failure.***
Skin: stinging, rash, other allergic reactions; pruritus, burning, swelling of lips or face (with topical form).
Other: ***hypersensitivity reactions***; overgrowth of nonsusceptible organisms (with ophthalmic form).

Overdose and treatment

With parenteral administration over several days, bacitracin may cause nephrotoxicity. Acute oral overdose may cause nausea, vomiting, and minor GI upset. Treatment is supportive.

Clinical considerations

- Bacitracin has been used orally as an intestinal antiseptic. Sterile solutions have been injected intrathecally for the treatment of meningitis, intraperitoneally for peritoneal infections, intrapleurally for staphylococcal empyema, and intrasynovially after surgical treatment of chronic osteomyelitis.
- Culture and sensitivity tests should be done before starting treatment.
- Patients allergic to neomycin may also be allergic to bacitracin.
- Injectable forms of drug may be used for I.M. administration only. I.V. administration may cause severe thrombophlebitis. Dilute injectable drug in solution containing sodium chloride and 2% procaine hydrochloride (if hospital policy permits). After reconstitution, bacitracin concentration should range from 5,000 to 10,000 units/ml. Inject deeply into upper outer quadrant of buttocks (may be painful). Don't give if patient is sensitive to procaine or para-aminobenzoic acid derivatives.
- Drug may be used orally with neomycin as bowel preparation or in solution as wound irrigating agent.

Therapeutic monitoring

- Recommend obtaining baseline renal function studies before starting therapy and monitoring results daily for signs of deterioration.
- Advise ensuring adequate fluid intake and monitoring output closely.
- Recommend monitoring patient's urine pH. It should be kept above 6 with good hydration, and alkalinizing agents (such as sodium bicarbonate) should be given, if necessary, to limit nephrotoxicity.

Special populations

Pregnant patients. Bacitracin shouldn't be used in pregnancy.

Patient counseling

- Advise patient to discontinue topical use of drug and to call promptly if condition worsens or doesn't respond to treatment.
- Warn patient with a skin infection to avoid sharing washcloths and towels with family members.
- Instruct patient to wash hands before and after applying ointment.
- Advise patient using ophthalmic ointment to clean eye area of excess exudate before applying ointment. Warn him not to touch tip of tube to any part of eye or surrounding tissue.
- Warn patient that ophthalmic ointment may cause blurred vision. Tell him to stop drug immediately and report symptoms of sensitivity, such as itchy eyelids or constant burning.
- Instruct patient to store ophthalmic ointment in tightly closed, light-resistant container.
- Caution patient not to share eye medications with other persons.

baclofen

Lioresal

Pharmacologic classification: chlorophenyl derivative
Therapeutic classification: skeletal muscle relaxant
Pregnancy risk category C

How supplied

Available by prescription only
Tablets: 10 mg, 20 mg
Intrathecal kit: 500 mcg/ml, 2,000 mcg/ml

Indications and dosages

Spasticity in multiple sclerosis and other spinal cord lesions
Adults: Initially, 5 mg P.O. t.i.d. for 3 days. Dosage may be increased (based on response) at 3-day intervals by 15 mg (5 mg/dose) daily

up to maximum of 80 mg daily. For geriatric patients, increase oral dose more gradually.
Intrathecal administration
Must be diluted with sterile preservative-free normal saline injection.
Adults: Initial intrathecal bolus of 50 mcg in 1 ml over not less than 1 minute. Observe patient for response over subsequent 4 to 8 hours. A positive response consists of a significant decrease in muscle tone or frequency or severity of spasm. If initial response is inadequate, repeat dose with 75 mcg in 1.5 ml 24 hours after last injection. Repeat observation of patient over 4 to 8 hours. If the response is still inadequate, repeat dosing at 100 mcg in 2 ml 24 hours later. If still no response, patient shouldn't be considered for an implantable pump for chronic baclofen administration. Ranges for chronic doses are 12 to 2,003 mcg/day.
Children under age 12: Test dose is the same as for adults (50 mcg); but for very small pediatric patients, an initial dose of 25 mcg may be given. Maintenance dosage averages 274 mcg daily (range 24 to 1200 mcg daily).
Postimplant dose titration
If the screening dose produced the desired effect for over 8 hours, the initial intrathecal dose is the same as the test dose; this dose is infused intrathecally for 24 hours. If the screening dose produced the desired effect for less than 8 hours, the initial intrathecal dose is twice the test dose, followed slowly by 10% to 30% increments at 24-hour intervals.

Pharmacodynamics
Skeletal muscle relaxant action: Precise mechanism of action is unknown, but drug appears to act at the spinal cord level to inhibit transmission of monosynaptic and polysynaptic reflexes, possibly through hyperpolarization of afferent fiber terminals. It may also act at supraspinal sites because baclofen at high doses produces generalized CNS depression. Baclofen decreases the number and severity of spasms and relieves associated pain, clonus, and muscle rigidity and therefore improves mobility.

Pharmacokinetics
Absorption: Rapidly and extensively absorbed from the GI tract, but is subject to individual variation. As dose increases, rate and extent of absorption decreases. Onset of therapeutic effect may not be immediately evident; varying from hours to weeks. Peak effect is seen at 2 to 3 hours.
Distribution: Studies indicate that baclofen is widely distributed throughout body, with small amounts crossing the blood-brain barrier. About 30% is plasma protein-bound.
Metabolism: About 15% is metabolized in the liver via deamination.
Excretion: 70% to 80% is excreted in urine unchanged or as its metabolites; remainder, in feces.

Route	Onset	Peak	Duration
P.O.	Hrs-wks	2-3 hr	Unknown
Intrathecal	½-1 hr	4 hr	4-8 hr

Contraindications and precautions
Contraindicated in patients with hypersensitivity to drug. Use cautiously in patients with renal impairment or seizure disorders or when spasticity is used to maintain motor function.

Interactions
Drug-drug. *Antidiabetic drugs or insulin:* Baclofen may increase blood glucose levels and require dosage adjustments of antidiabetic drug or insulin. Recommend monitoring serum glucose levels.
CNS depressant drugs, including, narcotics, antipsychotics, anxiolytics, and general anesthetics: May add to the CNS effects of drug. Use together cautiously.
Tricyclic antidepressants or MAO inhibitors: May cause CNS depression, respiratory depression, and hypotension. Avoid use together.
Drug-lifestyle. *Alcohol use:* May add to the CNS effects of drug. Discourage use.

Effects on diagnostic tests
None reported.

Adverse reactions
CNS: CNS depression ***(potentially life-threatening with intrathecal administration)***, *drowsiness, dizziness,* headache, *weakness, fatigue, hypotonia, confusion,* insomnia, dysarthria, SEIZURES.
CV: ***CV collapse*** (secondary to CNS depression), hypotension, hypertension.
EENT: blurred vision, nasal congestion, slurred speech.
GI: *nausea,* constipation, *vomiting.*
GU: urinary frequency.
Hepatic: increased AST and alkaline phosphatase levels.
Metabolic: hyperglycemia, weight gain.
Respiratory: ***respiratory failure*** (secondary to CNS depression), dyspnea.
Skin: rash, pruritus.
Other: excessive perspiration.

Overdose and treatment
Signs and symptoms of overdose include absence of reflexes, vomiting, muscular hypotonia, marked salivation, drowsiness, visual disorders, seizures, respiratory depression, and coma.

Treatment requires supportive measures, including endotracheal intubation and positive-pressure ventilation. If patient is conscious, remove drug by inducing emesis followed by gastric lavage.

If patient is comatose, don't induce emesis. Gastric lavage may be performed after endotracheal tube is in place with cuff inflated. Don't use respiratory stimulants. Monitor vital signs closely.

Clinical considerations

- Intrathecal administration should be performed only by qualified individuals familiar with administration techniques and patient management problems.
- Incidence of adverse reactions may be reduced by slowly decreasing the dosage. Abrupt withdrawal can result in hallucinations or seizures and acute exacerbation of spasticity.
- Baclofen is used investigationally to reduce choreiform movements in Huntington's chorea; to reduce rigidity in Parkinson's disease; to reduce spasticity in CVA, cerebral lesions, cerebral palsy, and rheumatic disorders; for analgesia in trigeminal neuralgia; and for treatment of unstable bladder.
- In some patients, smoother response may be obtained by giving daily dose in four divided doses.
- Patient may need supervision during walking. The initial loss of spasticity induced by baclofen may affect patient's ability to stand or walk. (In some patients, spasticity helps patient to maintain upright posture and balance.)
- Discontinue drug if signs of improvement don't occur within 1 to 2 months.
- Implantable pump or catheter failure can result in sudden loss of effectiveness of intrathecal baclofen.
- During prolonged intrathecal baclofen therapy for spasticity, about 10% of patients become refractory to baclofen therapy requiring a "drug holiday" to regain sensitivity to its effects.
- Store tablets in a tight container.
- Store baclofen at temperatures not exceeding 86° F (30° C). Don't freeze. Each vial is for individual use. Use only sterile, preservative-free normal saline for injection for dilution. Baclofen must be diluted to a concentration of 50 mcg/ml prior to injecting into the subarachnoid space.

Therapeutic monitoring

- Recommend routine monitoring of blood glucose levels in diabetic patients.
- Recommend observing patient's response to drug. Signs of effective therapy may appear in a few hours to 1 week and may include diminished frequency of spasms and severity of foot and ankle clonus, increased ease and range of joint motion, and enhanced performance of daily activities.
- Increased incidence of seizures may occur in patients with epilepsy. Closely monitor patients with epilepsy by EEG, clinical observation, and interview for possible loss of seizure control.

Special populations

Pregnant patients. There are no adequate and controlled studies in pregnant women.
Pediatric patients. Use of oral form isn't recommended for children under age 12. Safety of intrathecal administration in children under age 4 hasn't been established.
Geriatric patients. Geriatric patients are especially sensitive to drug. Observe carefully for adverse reactions, such as mental confusion, depression, and hallucinations. Lower doses are usually indicated.

Patient counseling

- Advise patient to report adverse reactions promptly. Most can be reduced by decreasing dosage. Reportedly, drowsiness, dizziness, and ataxia are more common in patients over age 40.
- Warn patient of additive effects with use of other CNS depressants, including alcohol.
- Caution patient to avoid hazardous activities that require mental alertness.
- Tell diabetic patient that baclofen may elevate blood glucose levels and may require adjustment of insulin dosage during treatment with baclofen. Urge patient to promptly report changes in urine or blood glucose tests.
- Caution patient against taking OTC drugs without medical approval. Explain that hazardous drug interactions are possible.
- Inform patient that drug should be withdrawn gradually over 1 to 2 weeks. Abrupt withdrawal after prolonged use of drug may cause anxiety, agitated behavior, auditory and visual hallucinations, severe tachycardia, and acute spasticity.

becaplermin

Regranex Gel

Pharmacologic classification: recombinant human platelet-derived growth factor (rhPDGF-BB)
Therapeutic classification: wound repair agent
Pregnancy risk category C

How supplied

Available by prescription only
Gel: 100 mcg/g in tubes of 2 g, 7.5 g, 15 g

Indications and dosages

Treatment of lower extremity diabetic neuropathic ulcers that extend into the subcutaneous tissue and beyond and have an adequate blood supply

Adults: Apply daily in 1/16" even thickness to entire surface of wound. Cover site with a saline-moistened dressing. Remove after 12 hours. Rinse gel from wound with saline or water and cover wound with moist dressing. Continue treatment until complete healing occurs.

When squeezing gel from tube, length of gel to be applied varies with tube size and ulcer area.

Tube size (g)	Inches	Centimeters
2	ulcer length × ulcer width × 1.3	(ulcer length × ulcer width) ÷ 2
7.5, 15	ulcer length × ulcer width × 0.6	(ulcer length × ulcer width) ÷ 4

Pharmacodynamics

Wound repair action: Recombinant of human platelet-derived growth factor that promotes the chemotactic recruitment and proliferation of cells involved in wound repair and enhances the formation of new granulation tissue.

Pharmacokinetics

Absorption: Minimal systemic absorption, less than 3% in rats.
Distribution: Unknown.
Metabolism: Unknown.
Excretion: Unknown.

Route	Onset	Peak	Duration
Topical	Unknown	Unknown	Unknown

Contraindications and precautions

Contraindicated in patients with known hypersensitivity to any component of product or in those with known neoplasms at site of application. Gel is for external use only. If an application site reaction occurs, consider possibility of sensitization or irritation caused by parabens or m-cresol.

Interactions

None reported.

Effects on diagnostic tests

None reported.

Adverse reactions

Skin: erythematous rash.

Overdose and treatment

No information available.

Clinical considerations

- When used as an adjunct to (not a substitute for) good ulcer care practices, including initial sharp debridement, pressure relief, and infection control, gel increases incidence of complete healing of diabetic ulcers. Its efficacy in treating diabetic neuropathic ulcers that don't extend through the dermis into subcutaneous tissue or ischemic diabetic ulcers hasn't been evaluated.
- Don't use gel in wounds that close by primary intention.
- To apply gel, squeeze the calculated length of gel onto a clean measuring surface, such as wax paper. Then transfer the measured gel from the measuring surface using an application aid.
- Use gel in addition to good ulcer care program, including a strict nonweight-bearing program.

Therapeutic monitoring

- Recommend monitoring for wound healing and application site reactions.
- Recalculate amount of gel to be applied weekly. If ulcer doesn't decrease in size by about one-third after 10 weeks or complete healing hasn't occurred by 20 weeks, reassess continued treatment.

Special populations

Breast-feeding patients. It isn't known if drug is excreted in breast milk. Use drug with caution when administering to breast-feeding patients.

Pediatric patients. Safety and efficacy in patients under age 16 haven't been established.

Patient counseling

- Instruct patient to wash hands thoroughly before applying gel.
- Advise patient not to touch tip of tube against ulcer or other surfaces.
- Inform patient to use a cotton swab, tongue blade, or other application aid to apply gel evenly over the surface of the ulcer, producing a thin (1/16") continuous layer.
- Tell patient to apply drug once daily in a carefully measured quantity. Quantity will change on a weekly basis.
- Tell patient to store gel in the refrigerator, and never to freeze it.
- Inform patient not to use gel after expiration date on the bottom, crimped end of the tube.

beclomethasone dipropionate

beclomethasone dipropionate monohydrate

Nasal inhalants
Beconase, Vancenase

Nasal sprays
Beconase AQ, Vancenase AQ, Vancenase AQ Double Strength

Oral inhalants
Beclovent, Becloforte*, Vanceril, Vanceril Double Strength

Pharmacologic classification: glucocorticoid
Therapeutic classification: anti-inflammatory, antiasthmatic
Pregnancy risk category C

How supplied

Available by prescription only
Nasal aerosol: 42 mcg/metered spray
Nasal spray: 42 mcg/metered spray, 84 mcg/metered spray
Oral inhalation aerosol: 42 mcg/metered spray, 84 mcg/metered spray

Indications and dosages

Steroid-dependent asthma
Oral inhalation
Adults and children over age 12: For regular strength formulation: Two inhalations t.i.d. or q.i.d. or four inhalations b.i.d. For severe asthma, start with 12 to 16 sprays per day and then reduce the dosage to the lowest effective level. Maximum of 20 inhalations daily. Double strength: 2 inhalations b.i.d.; in severe asthma start with 6 to 8 inhalations and adjust down. Don't exceed 10 inhalations/day.
Children age 6 to 12: For regular strength formulation: One to two inhalations t.i.d. or q.i.d. Maximum of 10 inhalations daily. Double strength: Two inhalations b.i.d.; don't exceed five inhalations/day.
Perennial or seasonal rhinitis; prevention of recurrence of nasal polyps after surgical removal
Nasal inhalation
Adults and children over age 12: One spray (42 mcg) in each nostril b.i.d. to q.i.d. Usual total dose is 168 to 336 mcg daily.
Children age 6 to 12: One spray in each nostril t.i.d. (252 mcg daily).
Nasal spray
Adults and children over age 6: One or two sprays of single strength (42 to 84 mcg) in each nostril b.i.d. If the double strength preparation is used, 1 or 2 sprays (84 to 168 mcg) into each nostril once daily (168 to 336 mcg). Maintenance dosage: 1 spray (42 mcg) into each nostril t.i.d.

Pharmacodynamics

Anti-inflammatory action: Beclomethasone stimulates the synthesis of enzymes needed to decrease the inflammatory response. The anti-inflammatory and vasoconstrictor potency of topically applied beclomethasone is, on a weight basis, about 5,000 times greater than that of hydrocortisone, 500 times greater than that of betamethasone or dexamethasone, and about 5 times greater than fluocinolone or triamcinolone.
Antiasthmatic action: Beclomethasone is used as a nasal inhalant to treat symptoms of seasonal or perennial rhinitis and to prevent the recurrence of nasal polyps after surgical removal, and as an oral inhalant to treat bronchial asthma in patients who require chronic administration of corticosteroids to control symptoms.

Pharmacokinetics

Absorption: After nasal inhalation, absorbed primarily through the nasal mucosa, with minimal systemic absorption. After oral inhalation, absorbed rapidly from the lungs and GI tract. Greater systemic absorption is associated with oral inhalation, but systemic effects don't occur at usual doses because of rapid metabolism in the liver and local metabolism of drug that reaches the lungs.
Distribution: Distribution after intranasal administration hasn't been described. There is no evidence of tissue storage of drug or its metabolites. About 10% to 25% of a nasal spray or orally inhaled dose is deposited in the respiratory tract. The remainder, deposited in the mouth and oropharynx, is swallowed. When absorbed, it is 87% bound to plasma proteins.
Metabolism: Swallowed drug undergoes rapid metabolism in the liver or GI tract to several metabolites, some of which have minor glucocorticoid activity. The portion inhaled into the respiratory tract is partially metabolized before absorption into systemic circulation. Mostly metabolized in the liver.
Excretion: Excretion of inhaled drug hasn't been described; however, when drug is administered systemically, its metabolites are excreted mainly in feces via biliary elimination and to a lesser extent in urine. Biological half-life of drug averages 15 hours.

Route	Onset	Peak	Duration
Nasal	5-7 days	3 wk	Unknown
Inhalation	1-4 wk	Unknown	Unknown

Contraindications and precautions

Contraindicated in patients hypersensitive to drug and in those experiencing status asthmaticus or other acute episodes of asthma. Use cautiously in patients with tuberculosis, fungal or bacterial infection, herpes, or systemic viral infection.

Interactions
None reported.

Effects on diagnostic tests
None reported.

Adverse reactions
CNS: headache.
EENT: *mild transient nasal burning and stinging,* nasal congestion, sneezing, burning, stinging, dryness, epistaxis, nasopharyngeal fungal infections, hoarseness, fungal infection of throat, throat irritation.
GI: dry mouth, fungal infection of mouth.
Respiratory: ***bronchospasm,*** wheezing.
Skin: hypersensitivity reactions (urticaria, rash).
Other: ***angioedema, suppression of hypothalamic-pituitary-adrenal function, adrenal insufficiency,*** facial edema.

Overdose and treatment
No information available.

Clinical considerations
- Use with extreme caution, if at all, in patients with tuberculosis, fungal or bacterial infections, ocular herpes simplex, or systemic viral infections.
- Don't use drug in patients with asthma controlled by bronchodilators or other noncorticosteroids alone or for those with nonasthmatic bronchial diseases.
- Use drug with caution in patients receiving systemic corticosteroid therapy.
- A spacer device may help ensure delivery of the proper dose and decrease local (oral) adverse effects.
- Therapy should last for no longer than 3 weeks, in the absence of substantial symptomatic improvement.
- Store Beconase inhalation at 36° to 86° F (2° to 30° C). Store Vancenase nasal inhaler at 59° to 86° F (15° to 30° C).
- During times of stress (trauma, surgery, or infection) systemic corticosteroids may be needed to prevent adrenal insufficiency in previously steroid-dependent patients.

ALERT Taper oral glucocorticoid therapy slowly. Acute adrenal insufficiency and death have occurred in asthmatics who changed abruptly from oral corticosteroids to beclomethasone.

Therapeutic monitoring
- Recommend monitoring for drug effectiveness.
- Periodic measurement of growth and development may be necessary during high-dose or prolonged therapy in children.

Special populations
Pregnant patients. Orally inhaled beclomethasone should only be used in pregnant women if the benefits outweigh the risks.
Pediatric patients. Drug isn't recommended for children under age 6.

Patient counseling
- Inform patient that drug doesn't provide relief for acute asthma attacks.
- Tell patient requiring a bronchodilator to use it several minutes before beclomethasone.
- Instruct patient to carry a medical identification card indicating his need for supplemental systemic glucocorticoids during stress.
- If patient uses a metered-dose inhaler, instruct him to shake canister well before use.
- Advise patient to allow 1 minute to elapse before taking subsequent puffs of medication and to hold his breath for a few seconds to enhance action of drug.
- Instruct patient to contact his prescriber if response to therapy decreases or if symptoms don't improve within 3 weeks; dosage may need to be adjusted. Tell him not to exceed recommended dosage on his own.
- Tell patient to keep inhaler clean and unobstructed. He should wash it with warm water and dry it thoroughly.
- Advise patient to prevent oral fungal infections by gargling or rinsing mouth with water after each use, but not to swallow the water.
- Tell patient to report symptoms associated with corticosteroid withdrawal, including fatigue, weakness, arthralgia, orthostatic hypotension, and dyspnea.
- Instruct patient to store medication between 59° and 86° F (15° and 30° C). Advise patient to ensure delivery of proper dose by gently warming canister to room temperature before using.

benazepril hydrochloride
Lotensin

Pharmacologic classification: ACE inhibitor
Therapeutic classification: antihypertensive
Pregnancy risk category C (D in second and third trimesters)

How supplied
Available by prescription only
Tablets: 5 mg, 10 mg, 20 mg, 40 mg

Indications and dosages
Hypertension
Adults: Initially, 10 mg P.O. daily. Adjust dosage as needed and tolerated; maintenance dosage range is 20 to 40 mg daily in one or two equally divided doses.

≡ ***Dosage adjustment.*** In patients with renal failure with creatinine clearance below 30 ml/minute/1.73 m^2 or serum creatinine levels exceeding 3 mg/dl, initial dose is 5 mg P.O. daily. Don't exceed 40 mg daily.

Note: Although rare, angioedema has been reported in patients receiving ACE inhibitors. Angioedema associated with laryngeal edema or shock may be fatal. If angioedema of the face, extremities, lips, tongue, glottis, or larynx occurs, discontinue treatment with benazepril and institute appropriate therapy immediately.

Pharmacodynamics

Antihypertensive action: Benazepril and its active metabolite, benazeprilat, inhibit ACE, preventing conversion of angiotensin I to angiotensin II, a potent vasoconstrictor. Reduced formation of angiotensin II decreases peripheral arterial resistance and aldosterone secretion, which reduces sodium and water retention and lowers blood pressure.

Although the primary mechanism through which benazepril lowers blood pressure is believed to be suppression of the renin-angiotensin-aldosterone system, benazepril has an antihypertensive effect even in patients with low renin levels.

Pharmacokinetics

Absorption: At least 37% of drug is absorbed.
Distribution: Serum protein binding of drug is about 96.7%; that of benazeprilat, 95.3%.
Metabolism: Almost completely metabolized in the liver to benazeprilat, which has much greater ACE inhibitory activity than benazepril, and to the glucuronide conjugates of benazepril and benazeprilat.
Excretion: Excreted primarily in the urine.

Route	Onset	Peak	Duration
P.O.	1 hr	2-4 hr	24 hr

Contraindications and precautions

Contraindicated in patients with hypersensitivity to ACE inhibitors. Use cautiously in patients with renal or hepatic impairment.

Interactions

Drug-drug. *Allopurinol:* Increased risk of hypersensitivity reaction. Monitor patient carefully.
Digoxin: Increased plasma digoxin levels. Recommend monitoring digoxin levels.
Diuretics and other antihypertensive agents: Increased risk of excessive hypotension. The diuretic may need to be discontinued or benazepril dose lowered.
Lithium: Increased serum lithium levels and lithium toxicity. Avoid use together.
Potassium-sparing diuretics and potassium supplements: Risk of hyperkalemia. Avoid use together.

Drug-food. *Sodium substitutes containing potassium:* Risk of hyperkalemia. Avoid use together.

Effects on diagnostic tests

None reported.

Adverse reactions

CNS: headache, dizziness, anxiety, fatigue, insomnia, nervousness, paresthesia.
CV: symptomatic hypotension, palpitations.
EENT: dysphagia, increased salivation.
GI: nausea, vomiting, abdominal pain, constipation.
GU: impotence.
Metabolic: hyperkalemia.
Musculoskeletal: arthralgia, arthritis, myalgia
Respiratory: dry, persistent, tickling, nonproductive cough; dyspnea.
Skin: ***hypersensitivity reactions*** (rash, pruritus), increased diaphoresis.
Other: ***angioedema.***

Overdose and treatment

Hypotension is the most common symptom of overdose. No data suggest physiologic maneuvers that might accelerate elimination of benazepril and its metabolite if an overdose occurs. Drug is only slightly dialyzable, but dialysis might be considered in overdosed patients with severely impaired renal function. Angiotensin II could presumably serve as a specific antagonist-antidote, but angiotensin II is essentially unavailable outside of scattered research facilities. Because the hypotensive effect of the drug is achieved through vasodilation and effective hypovolemia, treatment of benazepril overdose by I.V. infusion of normal saline solution is reasonable.

Clinical considerations

Excessive hypotension can occur when drug is given with diuretics. If possible, discontinue diuretic therapy 2 to 3 days before starting benazepril to decrease the potential for excessive hypotensive response. If benazepril doesn't adequately control blood pressure, diuretic therapy may be reinstituted with care. If the diuretic can't be discontinued, initiate benazepril therapy at 5 mg P.O. daily.

Therapeutic monitoring

- Measure blood pressure when drug levels are at peak (2 to 6 hours after a dose) and at trough (just before a dose) to verify adequate blood pressure control.
- Recommend assessing renal and hepatic function before and periodically throughout therapy. Also recommend monitoring serum potassium levels.
- Other ACE inhibitors have been associated with agranulocytosis and neutropenia. Recommend monitoring CBC with differential

counts before therapy, every 2 weeks for first 3 months of therapy, and periodically thereafter.

Special populations

Breast-feeding patients. Minimal amounts of unchanged benazepril and benazeprilat are excreted in breast milk. Use cautiously when administering to breast-feeding women.
Pediatric patients. Safety and efficacy in children haven't been established.

Patient counseling

- Advise patient to report signs or symptoms of infection (such as fever and sore throat); easy bruising or bleeding; swelling of tongue, lips, face, eyes, mucous membranes, or extremities; difficulty swallowing or breathing; and hoarseness.
- Because light-headedness can occur, especially during the first few days of therapy, tell patient to rise slowly to minimize this effect and to report symptoms. Patients who experience syncope should stop taking drug and call immediately.
- Tell patient to use caution in hot weather and during exercise. Inadequate fluid intake, vomiting, diarrhea, and excessive perspiration can lead to light-headedness and syncope.
- Tell patient to avoid sodium substitutes; these products may contain potassium, which can cause hyperkalemia in patients on drug therapy.
- Tell women of childbearing age about consequences of second- and third-trimester exposure to ACE inhibitors. Explain that these don't appear to result from exposure during the first trimester. Advise her to report suspected pregnancy as soon as possible.
- A persistent dry cough may occur and usually doesn't subside unless drug is stopped. Advise patient to call if this effect becomes bothersome.

benzocaine

Americaine, Dermoplast, Hurricaine, Lanacane, Maximum Strength Anbesol, Mouth Aid, Orabase Gel, Orajel, Solarcaine

Pharmacologic classification: local anesthetic (ester)
Therapeutic classification: anesthetic
Pregnancy risk category C

How supplied

Available without a prescription
Gel: 20%
Ointment, cream, and dental paste: 1% to 20%
Topical solution: 20%
Topical spray: 3%, 5%, 13.6%, 20%
Lotion: 0.5% to 8%
Lozenges: 5 mg, 10 mg, 15 mg
Solution: 2.1%, 20%

Indications and dosages

Local anesthetic for dental pain or dental procedures
Adults and children: Apply topical gel (20%) or dental paste to area, p.r.n. or as directed by prescriber.
Local anesthetic for pruritic dermatoses, pruritus, or other irritations
Adults: Apply topical preparation (1% to 20%) to affected area t.i.d. to q.i.d. or as directed by prescriber.
Relief of pain and pruritus in acute congestive and serous otitis media, acute swimmer's ear, and other forms of otitis externa
Adults: 4 to 5 drops (otic) in external auditory canal; insert cotton into meatus; repeat q 1 to 2 hours.
Temporary relief of minor sore throat pain
Adults and children over age 3: 1 lozenge dissolved slowly in the mouth and repeated, p.r.n. Don't use as self-medication for more than 2 days.
Male genital desensitization
Adults: Apply a small amount of a topical preparation containing 3% to 7.5% of benzocaine in water-soluble base to head and shaft of penis before intercourse. Patient should wash off any remaining benzocaine after intercourse to reduce potential for allergic reaction.

Pharmacodynamics

Analgesic action: Acts at sensory neurons to produce a local anesthetic effect.

Pharmacokinetics

No information available.

Route	Onset	Peak	Duration
Topical	Unknown	Unknown	Unknown

Contraindications and precautions

Contraindicated in patients with hypersensitivity to any component of the preparation or related substances and in those with secondary infection in the area or serious burns. Don't use in eyes or in ears with a perforated tympanic membrane or discharge. Use cautiously in patients with severely traumatized mucosa or local sepsis.

Interactions

None significant.

Effects on diagnostic tests

None reported.

Adverse reactions

Skin: urticaria, burning, stinging, tenderness, irritation, itching, erythema, rash.
Other: edema.

Note: Discontinue drug if symptoms of hypersensitivity occur.

Overdose and treatment
Maximum recommended dose is 5 g/day. Benzocaine overdose is unlikely; however, methemoglobinemia has been reported after topical application for teething pain. Treat symptomatically; if necessary, administer methylene blue 1% 0.1 ml/kg I.V. over at least 10 minutes.

Clinical considerations
- Use drug with antibiotic to treat underlying cause of pain because using alone may mask more serious condition.
- Keep container tightly closed and away from moisture.
- Drug is meant for temporary use, no more than 7 days.

Therapeutic monitoring
Monitor patient for worsening of condition.

Special populations
Pediatric patients. Excessive use may cause methemoglobinemia in infants. Don't use in children under age 2.

Patient counseling
- Tell patient to contact their health care provider if pain lasts longer than 48 hours, if burning or itching occurs, or if the condition persists.
- Instruct patient to keep container tightly closed and away from moisture.
- Advise patient not to eat or chew gum until effect of local anesthetic has worn off to avoid the risk of bite trauma.

benztropine mesylate
Cogentin

Pharmacologic classification: anticholinergic
Therapeutic classification: antiparkinsonian
Pregnancy risk category C

How supplied
Available by prescription only
Tablets: 0.5 mg, 1 mg, 2 mg
Injection: 1 mg/ml in 2-ml ampule

Indications and dosages
Parkinsonism
Adults: Range of 0.5 to 6 mg P.O. daily. Initially, 0.5 to 1 mg I.M. or P.O. increased 0.5 mg q 5 to 6 days. Adjust dosage to meet individual requirements. Maximum dose, 6 mg/day.
Drug-induced extrapyramidal reactions
Adults: 1 to 4 mg P.O. or I.M. daily or b.i.d. Adjust dosage to meet individual requirements. Maximum dose, 6 mg/day.
Acute dystonic reaction
Adults: 1 to 2 mg I.V. followed by 1 to 2 mg P.O. b.i.d. to prevent recurrence.

Pharmacodynamics
Antiparkinsonian action: Benztropine blocks central cholinergic receptors, helping to balance cholinergic activity in the basal ganglia. It may also prolong effects of dopamine by blocking dopamine reuptake and storage at central receptor sites.

Pharmacokinetics
Absorption: Absorbed from the GI tract.
Distribution: Largely unknown; however, drug crosses the blood-brain barrier and may cross the placenta.
Metabolism: Unknown.
Excretion: Like other muscarinics, benztropine is excreted in the urine as unchanged drug and metabolites. After oral therapy, small amounts are probably excreted in feces as unabsorbed drug.

Route	Onset	Peak	Duration
P.O.	1-2 hr	Unknown	24 hr
I.V., I.M.	15 min	Unknown	24 hr

Contraindications and precautions
Contraindicated in patients with hypersensitivity to drug or its components or acute angle-closure glaucoma and in children under age 3. Use cautiously in hot weather, in patients with mental disorders, and in children over age 3.

Interactions
Drug-drug. *Amantadine:* May amplify such adverse anticholinergic effects as confusion and hallucinations. Decrease benztropine dosage before giving amantadine.
Haloperidol and phenothiazines: May decrease their effect, possibly reflecting direct CNS antagonism. Recommend monitoring patient for clinical effect.
Phenothiazines: Increase the risk of adverse anticholinergic effects. Use reduced phenothiazine dose.
CNS depressants: Increase the sedative effects of benztropine. Use together cautiously.
Antacids and antidiarrheals: May decrease benztropine absorption. Administer benztropine at least 1 hour before administering these agents.
Drug-lifestyle. *Alcohol use*: Increases the sedative effects of benztropine. Discourage use.

Effects on diagnostic tests
None reported.

Adverse reactions
CNS: disorientation, hallucinations, depression, toxic psychosis, confusion, memory impairment, nervousness.

CV: tachycardia.
EENT: dilated pupils, blurred vision.
GI: dry mouth, *constipation,* nausea, vomiting, paralytic ileus.
GU: urine retention, dysuria.

Note: Some adverse reactions may result from atropine-like toxicity and are dose related.

Overdose and treatment

Signs and symptoms of overdose include central stimulation followed by depression and psychotic symptoms such as disorientation, confusion, hallucinations, delusions, anxiety, agitation, and restlessness. Peripheral effects may include dilated, nonreactive pupils; blurred vision; hot, flushed, dry skin; dryness of mucous membranes; dysphagia; decreased or absent bowel sounds; urine retention; hyperthermia; tachycardia; hypertension; and increased respiration.

Treatment is primarily symptomatic and supportive, as necessary. Maintain a patent airway. If patient is alert, induce emesis (or use gastric lavage) and follow with a sodium chloride cathartic and activated charcoal to prevent further absorption. In severe cases, physostigmine may be administered to block the antimuscarinic effects of benztropine. Give fluids as needed to treat shock, diazepam to control psychotic symptoms, and pilocarpine (instilled into the eyes) to relieve mydriasis. If urine retention occurs, catheterization may be necessary.

Clinical considerations

Consider the recommendations relevant to all anticholinergics as well as the following:

- To help prevent gastric irritation, administer drug after meals.
- Never discontinue drug abruptly.
- Store in well-sealed containers between 59° and 86° F (15° and 30° C). Avoid freezing injectable preparation.

Therapeutic monitoring

- Monitor patient for intermittent constipation and abdominal distention and pain, which may indicate paralytic ileus.
- Recommend periodic monitoring of patient since effects are cumulative, especially if patient is prone to tachycardia and prostatic hypertrophy.
- Recommend observing patients with mental disorders for worsening symptoms or toxic psychoses, especially initially and during drug dosage adjustment.

Special populations

Pregnant patients. Safe use during pregnancy hasn't been established.
Breast-feeding patients. Drug may be excreted in breast milk, possibly causing infant toxicity. Avoid use in breast-feeding women. Benztropine may decrease milk production.
Pediatric patients. Drug isn't recommended for use in children under age 3.

Patient counseling

- Explain to patient that the full effect of the drug may not occur for 2 to 3 days after therapy begins.
- Caution patient not to discontinue drug suddenly; dosage should be reduced gradually.
- Tell patient that drug may increase sensitivity of eyes to light.

bepridil hydrochloride

Vascor

Pharmacologic classification: calcium channel blocker
Therapeutic classification: antianginal
Pregnancy risk category C

How supplied

Available by prescription only
Tablets: 200 mg, 300 mg

Indications and dosages

Treatment of chronic stable angina (classic effort-associated angina) in patients who are unresponsive or inadequately responsive to other antianginals
Adults: Initially, 200 mg P.O. daily; after 10 days, adjust dosage based on patient tolerance and response. Most common maintenance dosage is 300 mg daily. Maximum daily dose, 400 mg.

Pharmacodynamics

Antianginal action: Precise mechanism of action is unknown. It inhibits calcium ion influx into cardiac and vascular smooth muscle and also inhibits the sodium inward influx, resulting in reductions in the maximal upstroke velocity and amplitude of the action potential. It's believed to reduce heart rate and arterial pressure by dilating peripheral arterioles and reducing total peripheral resistance (afterload). The effects are dose-dependent. Bepridil has dose-related class I antiarrhythmic properties affecting electrophysiologic changes, such as prolongation of QT and QTc intervals.

Pharmacokinetics

Absorption: Rapidly and completely absorbed after oral administration.
Distribution: Over 99% of drug is plasma protein-bound.
Metabolism: Metabolized in the liver.
Excretion: Elimination is biphasic. Bepridil has a distribution half-life of 2 hours. Over 10 days, 70% is excreted in urine, 22% in feces as metabolites. Terminal half-life after multi-

ple dosing averaged 42 hours (range, 26 to 64 hours).

Route	Onset	Peak	Duration
P.O.	1 hr	2-3 hr	24 hr

Contraindications and precautions
Contraindicated in patients with hypersensitivity to drug; uncompensated cardiac insufficiency, sick sinus syndrome or second- or third-degree AV block unless pacemaker is present; hypotension (below 90 mm Hg systolic); congenital QT interval prolongation; or history of serious ventricular arrhythmias. Also contraindicated in those receiving other drugs that prolong QT interval.

Use cautiously in patients with left bundle-branch block, sinus bradycardia, impaired renal or hepatic function, or heart failure. Drug isn't recommended for use in patients within 3 months of an MI.

Interactions
Drug-drug. *Beta blockers:* Excessive bradycardia and conduction abnormalities. Avoid use together.
Digoxin: Modest increases in steady-state serum digoxin levels. Recommend monitoring serum digoxin levels.
Potassium-wasting diuretics: Potential for causing hypokalemia, which increases risk of serious ventricular arrhythmias. Avoid use together.
Quinidine, procainamide, or tricyclic antidepressants: Additive prolongation of QT interval. Avoid use together.

Effects on diagnostic tests
None reported.

Adverse reactions
CNS: *dizziness,* drowsiness, *nervousness, headache,* insomnia, paresthesia, *asthenia,* tremor.
CV: edema, flushing, palpitations, tachycardia, ***ventricular arrhythmias, including torsades de pointes, ventricular tachycardia, ventricular fibrillation.***
EENT: tinnitus.
GI: *nausea, diarrhea,* constipation, abdominal discomfort, dry mouth, anorexia, increased ALT levels and abnormal liver function test.
Hematologic: ***agranulocytosis.***
Respiratory: dyspnea, shortness of breath.
Skin: rash.
Other: flu syndrome.

Overdose and treatment
Exaggerated adverse reactions, especially clinically significant hypotension, high-degree AV block, and ventricular tachycardia, have been observed. Treat with appropriate supportive measures, including gastric lavage, beta-adrenergic stimulation, parenteral calcium solutions, vasopressor agents, and cardioversion, as necessary. Close observation in a cardiac care facility for a minimum of 48 hours is recommended.

Clinical considerations
- Careful patient selection and monitoring are essential. Use the following selection criteria: Diagnosis of chronic stable angina with failure to respond or inadequate response to other therapies, QTc interval less than 0.44 second, absence of hypokalemia, hypotension, severe left ventricular dysfunction, serious ventricular arrhythmias, unpacked sick sinus syndrome, second- or third-degree AV block, and no use of other drugs that prolong the QT interval.
- Beta blockers, nitrates, digoxin, insulin, and oral antidiabetic agents may be used with bepridil.
- Food doesn't interfere with absorption of bepridil. Food may alleviate or prevent nausea.
- Use cautiously in patients with renal or hepatic disorders. No clinical data are available.

Therapeutic monitoring
- Monitor serum potassium levels and correct hypokalemia before initiating therapy. Use potassium-sparing diuretics for patients who require diuretic therapy.
- Recommend monitoring QTc interval before and during therapy. Reduced dosage is required if QTc prolongation is greater than 0.52 second or increases more than 25%. If prolongation of QTc interval persists, discontinue bepridil.
- Recommend monitoring for development of cough or dyspnea; consider pulmonary infiltrates or fibroses as a potential cause.

Special populations
Breast-feeding patients. Drug is excreted in breast milk; risk-benefit must be assessed.
Pediatric patients. Safety and efficacy in children under age 18 haven't been established.
Geriatric patients. Recommended starting dose is same as in adult patients; however, more frequent monitoring may be required.

Patient counseling
- Instruct patient to recognize signs and symptoms of hypokalemia and the importance of compliance with prescribed potassium supplements.
- Tell patient to report signs or symptoms of infection, such as sore throat and fever.
- Instruct patient to take drug with food or at bedtime if nausea occurs.

betamethasone (systemic)

Betnelan*, Celestone

betamethasone sodium phosphate

Betnesol*, Celestone Phosphate, Selestoject

betamethasone sodium phosphate and betamethasone acetate

Celestone Soluspan

Pharmacologic classification: glucocorticoid
Therapeutic classification: anti-inflammatory
Pregnancy risk category NR

How supplied

Available by prescription only
betamethasone
Tablets: 0.6 mg
Syrup: 0.6 mg/5 ml
betamethasone sodium phosphate
Tablets (effervescent): 500 mcg*
Injection: 4 mg (3 mg base)/ml in 5-ml vials
Enema:* 5 mg (base)
betamethasone sodium phosphate and betamethasone acetate suspension
Injection: betamethasone acetate 3 mg and betamethasone sodium phosphate (equivalent to 3 mg base) per ml (not for I.V. use)

Indications and dosages

Note: Betamethasone acetate suspension shouldn't be given I.V.

Severe inflammation or immunosuppression
Adults: 0.6 to 7.2 mg P.O. daily; usually 2.4 to 4.8 mg daily divided into two to four doses.
Children: 0.0175 to 0.25 mg/kg P.O. daily or 0.5 to 7.5 mg/m^2 daily in three to four divided doses.
betamethasone sodium phosphate
Adults: 0.5 to 9 mg I.M., I.V., or into joint or soft tissue daily.
betamethasone sodium phosphate and betamethasone acetate suspension
Adults: 0.25 to 2 ml into joint or soft tissue q 1 to 2 weeks, p.r.n. Effects may last a few days or 1 to 2 weeks depending on the joint condition being treated.

◊ ***Hyaline membrane disease***
Adults: Give 2 ml I.M. daily to expectant mothers for 2 to 3 days before delivery.

Pharmacodynamics

Anti-inflammatory action: Stimulates the synthesis of enzymes needed to decrease the inflammatory response. It's a long-acting steroid with an anti-inflammatory potency 25 times that of an equal weight of hydrocortisone. It has essentially no mineralocorticoid activity. Betamethasone tablets and syrup are used as oral anti-inflammatory agents.

Betamethasone sodium phosphate is highly soluble, has a prompt onset of action, and may be given I.V. Betamethasone sodium phosphate and betamethasone acetate (Celestone Soluspan) combine the rapid-acting phosphate salt and the slightly soluble, slowly released acetate salt to provide rapid anti-inflammatory effects with a sustained duration of action. It's a suspension and isn't to be given I.V. It's particularly useful as an anti-inflammatory agent in intra-articular, intradermal, and intralesional injections.

Pharmacokinetics

Absorption: Absorbed readily after oral administration. Systemic absorption occurs slowly following intra-articular injections.
Distribution: Removed rapidly from the blood and distributed to muscle, liver, skin, intestines, and kidneys. Betamethasone is bound weakly to plasma proteins (transcortin and albumin). Only the unbound portion is active. Adrenocorticoids are distributed into breast milk and through the placenta.
Metabolism: Metabolized in the liver to inactive glucuronide and sulfate metabolites.
Excretion: Inactive metabolites and small amounts of unmetabolized drug are excreted by the kidneys. Insignificant quantities of drug are also excreted in feces. Biological half-life of drug is 36 to 54 hours.

Route	Onset	Peak	Duration
P.O.	Prompt	Unknown	3-25 days
I.M.	Unknown	Unknown	7-14 days

Contraindications and precautions

Contraindicated in patients hypersensitive to drug and in those with viral or bacterial infections (except in life-threatening situations) or systemic fungal infections.

Use with caution in patients with renal disease, hypertension, osteoporosis, diabetes mellitus, hypothyroidism, cirrhosis, diverticulitis, nonspecific ulcerative colitis, recent intestinal anastomoses, thromboembolic disorders, seizures, myasthenia gravis, heart failure, tuberculosis, ocular herpes simplex, emotional instability, and psychotic tendencies.

Interactions

Drug-drug. *Oral anticoagulants:* Decrease the effects of oral anticoagulants (rarely). Recommend monitoring PT and INR.
Barbiturates, phenytoin, and rifampin: Decreased corticosteroid effects because of increased hepatic metabolism. Recommend monitoring for clinical effect.

Cardiac glycosides: Increased risk of toxicity in patients concurrently receiving cardiac glycosides. Use together cautiously.
Cholestyramine, colestipol, and antacids: Decreased effect of betamethasone by adsorbing the corticosteroid, decreasing the amount absorbed. Use together cautiously.
Diuretic or amphotericin B therapy: Betamethasone may enhance hypokalemia. Recommend monitoring serum potassium levels and observing patient carefully.
Estrogens: Reduced metabolism of corticosteroids by increasing the concentrations of transcortin. Recommend monitoring for adverse effects.
Insulin or oral antidiabetic agents: Hyperglycemia, requiring dosage adjustment in diabetic patients. Recommend monitoring serum glucose levels.
Isoniazid and salicylates: Increase the metabolism of these drugs. Recommend monitoring for clinical effect.
Ulcerogenic drugs such as NSAIDs: May increase the risk of GI ulceration. Use together cautiously.

Effects on diagnostic tests
Adrenocorticoid therapy suppresses reactions to skin tests; causes false-negative results in the nitroblue tetrazolium tests for systemic bacterial infections.

Adverse reactions
Most adverse reactions to corticosteroids are dose- or duration-dependent.
CNS: *euphoria, insomnia,* psychotic behavior, pseudotumor cerebri, vertigo, headache, paresthesia, ***seizures.***
CV: ***heart failure,*** hypertension, edema, ***arrhythmias,*** thrombophlebitis, ***thromboembolism.***
EENT: cataracts, glaucoma.
Endocrine: menstrual irregularities, cushingoid state (moonface, buffalo hump, central obesity).
GI: *peptic ulceration,* GI irritation, increased appetite, pancreatitis, nausea, vomiting.
Metabolic: hypokalemia, hyperglycemia, and carbohydrate intolerance; increased thyroxine, and triiodothyronine levels.
Musculoskeletal: muscle weakness, osteoporosis.
Skin: delayed wound healing, acne, various skin eruptions.
Other:, hirsutism, susceptibility to infections; growth suppression in children; ***acute adrenal insufficiency may follow increased stress (infection, surgery, or trauma) or abrupt withdrawal after long-term therapy.***

Note: After abrupt withdrawal: rebound inflammation, fatigue, weakness, arthralgia, fever, dizziness, lethargy, depression, fainting, orthostatic hypotension, dyspnea, anorexia, hypoglycemia. After prolonged use, sudden withdrawal may be fatal.

Overdose and treatment
Acute ingestion, even in massive doses, rarely occurs. Toxic signs and symptoms rarely occur if drug is used for less than 3 weeks, even at large doses. However, chronic use causes adverse physiologic effects, including suppression of the hypothalamic-pituitary-adrenal axis, cushingoid appearance, muscle weakness, and osteoporosis.

Clinical considerations
- Recommendations for use of betamethasone and for care and teaching of patients during therapy are the same as those for all systemic adrenocorticoids.
- Investigational use includes prevention of respiratory distress syndrome in premature infants (hyaline membrane disease). Give 6 mg (2 ml) of Celestone Soluspan I.M. once daily 24 to 36 hours before induced delivery.
- Gradually reduce dose after long-term use.
- Store tablets in a well-closed container and protected from light at temperatures of 36° to 86° F (2° to 30° C).
- Protect betamethasone sodium phosphate injection from light and store at a temperature between 59° and 86° F (15° and 30° C). Avoid freezing.
- Protect betamethasone sodium phosphate and betamethasone acetate sterile solution from light and store at 36° to 77° F (2° to 25° C); avoid freezing. Don't mix the sterile solution with diluents or local anesthetics containing preservatives because flocculation of the suspension may occur.

Therapeutic monitoring
Recommend continuous monitoring for effect and dosage adjustment, remissions, exacerbations, stress.

Special populations
Breast-feeding patients. Information is incomplete. Risk versus benefits must be determined and reviewed with patient.
Pediatric patients. Chronic use of betamethasone in children and adolescents may delay growth and maturation.

Patient counseling
- Warn patient not to stop drug abruptly.
- Instruct patient to take drug with food or milk.
- Tell patient to report symptoms associated with corticosteroid withdrawal including fatigue, weakness, arthralgia, orthostatic hypotension, and dyspnea.
- Instruct patient to carry a card indicating his need for supplemental glucocorticoid therapy during stress.

betamethasone dipropionate, augmented
Diprolene, Diprolene AF

betamethasone dipropionate
Alphatrex, Diprosone, Maxivate

betamethasone valerate
Betaderm*, Betatrex, Beta-Val, Betnovate*, Celestoderm-V*, Ectosone*, Luxig, Metaderm*, Novobetamet*, Valisone

Pharmacologic classification: topical glucocorticoid
Therapeutic classification: anti-inflammatory
Pregnancy risk category C

How supplied
Available by prescription only
betamethasone dipropionate, augmented
Cream, gel, lotion, ointment: 0.05%
betamethasone dipropionate
Lotion, ointment, cream: 0.05%
Aerosol: 0.1%
betamethasone valerate
Lotion, ointment: 0.1%
Cream: 0.01%, 0.1%,
Foam: 0.12%

Indications and dosages
Inflammation of corticosteroid-responsive dermatoses
betamethasone valerate
Adults and children: Apply cream, lotion, ointment, or gel in a thin layer once daily to q.i.d.
Relief of inflammatory and pruritic manifestations of corticosteroid-responsive dermatoses of scalp
Adults: Gently massage small amounts of foam into affected scalp areas twice daily (apply once in the morning and once at night) until control is achieved. If no improvement is seen within 2 weeks, reassess diagnosis.
betamethasone dipropionate
Adults and children over age 12: Apply cream, lotion, or ointment sparingly daily or b.i.d. Dosage of augmented 0.05% gels or lotions shouldn't exceed 50 g or 50 ml per week. Dosage of Diprolene ointments or creams 0.05% shouldn't exceed 45 g per week. To apply aerosol, direct spray onto affected area from a distance of 6 in. (15 cm) for only 3 seconds t.i.d. or q.i.d.

Pharmacodynamics
Anti-inflammatory action: Stimulates the synthesis of enzymes needed to decrease the inflammatory response. Betamethasone, a fluorinated derivative, has the advantage of availability in various bases to vary the potency for individual conditions.

Pharmacokinetics
Absorption: Amount absorbed depends on the potency of the preparation, amount applied, and nature of the skin at the application site. It ranges from about 1% in areas with a thick stratum corneum to as high as 36% in areas with a thin stratum corneum. Absorption increases in areas of skin damage, inflammation, or occlusion. Some systemic absorption of topical steroids occur.
Distribution: After topical application, distributed throughout the local skin. Drug absorbed into circulation is removed rapidly from the blood and distributed into muscle, liver, skin, intestines, and kidneys.
Metabolism: After topical administration, metabolized primarily in the skin. The small amount that's absorbed into systemic circulation is metabolized primarily in the liver to inactive compounds.
Excretion: Inactive metabolites are excreted by the kidneys, primarily as glucuronides and sulfates, but also as unconjugated products. Small amounts of the metabolites are also excreted in feces.

Route	Onset	Peak	Duration
Topical	Unknown	Unknown	Unknown

Contraindications and precautions
Contraindicated in patients hypersensitive to corticosteroids.

Interactions
None significant.

Effects on diagnostic tests
None reported.

Adverse reactions
Skin: burning, pruritus, irritation, dryness, erythema, folliculitis, acneiform eruptions, perioral dermatitis, hypopigmentation, hypertrichosis, allergic contact dermatitis; *secondary infection, maceration, atrophy, striae, miliaria* (with occlusive dressings).
Metabolic: hyperglycemia, glycosuria (with betamethasone dipropionate).
Other: ***hypothalamic-pituitary-adrenal axis suppression,*** Cushing's syndrome.

Overdose and treatment
No information available.

Clinical considerations
Consider the recommendations relevant to all topical adrenocorticoids as well as the following:
- Diprolene ointment may suppress the hypothalamic-pituitary-adrenal axis at doses as low as 7 g daily. Patient shouldn't use more than

45 g weekly and shouldn't use occlusive dressings.
- To apply, gently wash skin before applying. To prevent skin damage, rub medication in gently, leaving a thin coat. When treating hairy sites, part hair and apply directly to lesions.
- For application to the scalp, invert the can containing the foam. Dispense a small amount of drug onto a cool surface (but not directly to the hand because the drug will melt). Massage foam into scalp until foam disappears.

Therapeutic monitoring
Monitor for systemic adverse reactions if prolonged use or used on a large body surface area.

Special populations
Pediatric patients. Treatment with Diprolene ointment isn't recommended in children under age 12.

Patient counseling
- Teach patient how to apply drug.
- Tell patient to stop drug and report signs of systemic absorption, skin irritation or ulceration, hypersensitivity, or infection.

betaxolol hydrochloride
Betoptic, Betoptic S, Kerlone

Pharmacologic classification: beta blocker
Therapeutic classification: antiglaucoma, antihypertensive
Pregnancy risk category C

How supplied
Available by prescription only
Tablets: 10 mg, 20 mg
Ophthalmic solution: 5 mg/ml (0.5%) in 2.5-ml, 5-ml, 10-ml, 15-ml dropper bottles
Ophthalmic suspension: 2.5 mg/ml (0.25%) in 2.5-ml, 5-ml, 10-ml, 15-ml dropper bottles

Indications and dosages
Chronic open-angle glaucoma and ocular hypertension
Adults: Instill 1 to 2 drops in eyes b.i.d.
Management of hypertension (used alone or with other antihypertensives)
Adults: Initially, 10 mg P.O. once daily. After 7 to 14 days, full antihypertensive effect should be seen. If necessary, double the dose to 20 mg P.O. once daily. Doses up to 40 mg daily have also been used.
≡ ***Dosage adjustment.*** In patients with renal impairment or the elderly, initial dose is 5 mg P.O. daily. Increase by 5-mg/day increments q 2 weeks to maximum of 20 mg/day.

Pharmacodynamics
Antihypertensive action: Cardioselective adrenergic blocking effects of betaxolol slow heart rate and decrease cardiac output.
Ocular hypotensive action: Betaxolol hydrochloride is a cardioselective $beta_1$ blocker that reduces intraocular pressure (IOP), possibly by reducing production of aqueous humor when administered as an ophthalmic solution.

Pharmacokinetics
Absorption: Essentially complete after oral administration; minimal after ophthalmic use. A small first-pass effect reduces bioavailability by about 10%. Absorption isn't affected by food or alcohol.
Distribution: About 50% bound to plasma proteins.
Metabolism: Hepatic; about 85% of drug is recovered in the urine as metabolites. Elimination half-life is prolonged in patients with hepatic disease, but clearance isn't affected, so dosage adjustment is unnecessary.
Excretion: Primarily renal (about 80%). Plasma half-life is 14 to 22 hours.

Route	Onset	Peak	Duration
P.O.	3 hr	2-4 hr	24-48 hr
Ophthalmic	½-1 hr	2 hr	>12 hr

Contraindications and precautions
Contraindicated in patients with hypersensitivity to drug, severe bradycardia, greater than first-degree heart block, cardiogenic shock, or uncontrolled heart failure.

Interactions
Drug-drug. *Beta blockers:* Ophthalmic betaxolol may increase the systemic effect of oral beta blockers. Monitor patient closely.
Reserpine and catecholamine-depleting agents: Ophthalmic betaxolol enhances the hypotensive and bradycardiac effect of these drugs. Monitor patient closely.
Pilocarpine, epinephrine, and carbonic anhydrase inhibitors: Ophthalmic betaxolol enhances the lowering of IOP with these agents. Monitor for clinical effect.
Reserpine and catecholamine-depleting drugs: Use of oral betaxolol with these drugs may have an additive effect when administered with a beta blocker.
General anesthetics: May cause increased hypotensive effects. Recommend observing patient carefully for excessive hypotension, bradycardia, or orthostatic hypotension.
Calcium channel blocking agents: Increases risk of hypotension, left-sided heart failure, and AV conduction disturbances. Use I.V. calcium antagonists with caution.
Beta blockers: Betaxolol may increase the effects of lidocaine. Recommend monitoring for clinical effect.

Effects on diagnostic tests
None reported.

Adverse reactions
Ophthalmic form
CNS: insomnia, depressive neurosis.
EENT: *eye stinging on instillation causing brief discomfort,* photophobia, erythema, itching, keratitis, occasional tearing.
Systemic form
CNS: dizziness, fatigue, headache, insomnia, lethargy, anxiety.
CV: bradycardia, chest pain, ***heart failure,*** edema.
GI: nausea, diarrhea, dyspepsia.
GU: impotence.
Metabolic: altered results of glucose tolerance tests
Musculoskeletal: arthralgia.
Respiratory: dyspnea, pharyngitis, ***bronchospasm.***
Skin: rash.

Overdose and treatment
Signs and symptoms of overdose, which are extremely rare with ophthalmic use, may include diplopia, bradycardia, heart block, hypotension, shock, increased airway resistance, cyanosis, fatigue, sleepiness, headache, sedation, coma, respiratory depression, seizures, nausea, vomiting, diarrhea, hypoglycemia, hallucinations, and nightmares. Discontinue drug and flush eye with normal saline solution or water. For treatment of accidental substantial ingestion, emesis is most effective if initiated within 30 minutes, providing the patient isn't obtunded, comatose, or having seizures. Activated charcoal may be used. Treat bradycardia, conduction defects, and hypotension with I.V. fluids, glucagon, atropine, or isoproterenol; refractory bradycardia may require a transvenous pacemaker. Treat bronchoconstriction with I.V. aminophylline; seizures, with I.V. diazepam.

Clinical considerations
Ophthalmic use
- Betaxolol is a cardioselective beta blocker. Its pulmonary and systemic effects are considerably milder than those of timolol or levobunolol.
- Ophthalmic betaxolol is intended for twice-daily dosage. Encourage patient to comply with this regimen.

Systemic use
- Withdrawal of beta blocker therapy before surgery is controversial. Some clinicians advocate withdrawal to prevent any impairment of cardiac responsiveness to reflex stimuli and to prevent any decreased responsiveness to exogenous catecholamines.
- To withdraw drug, gradually reduce dosage over at least 2 weeks.

Therapeutic monitoring
- In some patients, a few weeks' treatment may be required to stabilize pressure-lowering response. Determine IOP during the first 4 weeks of drug therapy.
- Recommend monitoring blood pressure closely.
- Monitor serum glucose; signs of hypoglycemia may be masked in patients taking beta blockers.

Special populations
Breast-feeding patients. Use with caution. After oral administration, betaxolol is excreted in breast milk in sufficient amounts to exert an effect on the breast-feeding infant.
Pediatric patients. The ophthalmic preparation shouldn't be used in patients under age 18.
Geriatric patients. Use with caution in geriatric patients with cardiac or pulmonary disease.

Patient counseling
Ophthalmic use
- Tell patient to shake suspension well before use.
- Instruct patient to tilt head back and, while looking up, instill the drug into the lower lid.
- Warn patient not to touch dropper to eye or surrounding tissue.
- Instruct patient not to close eyes tightly or blink more than usual after instillation.
- Remind patient to wait at least 5 minutes before using other eyedrops.
- Advise patient to wear sunglasses or avoid exposure to bright lights.

Systemic use
- Instruct patient to take drug exactly as prescribed and warn against discontinuing it suddenly.
- Advise patient to report shortness of breath or difficulty breathing, unusually fast heartbeat, cough, or fatigue with exertion.

bethanechol chloride
Duvoid, Myotonachol, Urecholine

Pharmacologic classification: cholinergic agonist
Therapeutic classification: urinary tract and GI tract stimulant
Pregnancy risk category C

How supplied
Available by prescription only
Tablets: 5 mg, 10 mg, 25 mg, 50 mg
Injection: 5 mg/ml

Indications and dosages
Acute postoperative and postpartum nonobstructive (functional) urine reten-

tion, neurogenic atony of urinary bladder with retention
Adults: 10 to 50 mg P.O. b.i.d., t.i.d, or q.i.d. Or 2.575 to 5.15 mg S.C. (use 10 mg S.C. with extreme caution). Never give I.M. or I.V. When used for urine retention, some patients may require 50 to 100 mg P.O. per dose. Use such doses with extreme caution. Test dose: 2.5 mg S.C. repeated at 15- to 30-minute intervals to a maximum of four doses to determine the minimal effective dose, then use minimal effective dose three or four times daily. Adjust dosage to meet individual requirements.
Restore bladder function in patients with chronic neurogenic bladder
Adults: 7.5 to 10 mg S.C. q 4 hours around the clock. Dosage adjustments are made based on residual urine measurements.
◊ ***Bladder dysfunction caused by phenothiazines***
Adults: 50 to 100 mg P.O. q.i.d.
◊ ***Lessen the adverse effects of tricyclic antidepressants***
Adults: 25 mg P.O. t.i.d.
◊ ***Chronic gastric reflux***
Adults: 25 mg P.O. q.i.d.
◊ ***Familial dysautonomia***
Children: 0.2 to 0.4 mg/kg S.C. q.i.d. 30 minutes before meals with an oral antacid; then after 2 weeks, give 1 to 2 mg P.O. q.i.d.
◊ ***To diagnose flaccid or atonic neurogenic bladder***
Adults: 2.5 mg S.C.
◊ ***To diagnose cystic fibrosis***
Before administration, dilute 5 mg of drug in 3 ml of D_5W to yield a concentration of 1.25 mg/ml.
Children over age 1: 1 mg intradermally.
Children age 2 months to 1 year: 0.5 mg intradermally.
Infants from birth to age 2 months: 0.25 mg intradermally.

Pharmacodynamics
Urinary tract stimulant action: Bethanechol directly binds to and stimulates muscarinic receptors of the parasympathetic nervous system. This increases tone of the bladder detrusor muscle, usually resulting in contraction, decreased bladder capacity, and subsequent urination.
GI tract stimulant action: Bethanechol directly stimulates cholinergic receptors, leading to increased gastric tone and motility and peristalsis. Drug improves lower esophageal sphincter tone by directly stimulating cholinergic receptors, thereby alleviating gastric reflux.

Pharmacokinetics
Absorption: Poorly absorbed from the GI tract (absorption varies considerably among patients).
Distribution: Largely unknown; however, therapeutic doses don't penetrate the blood-brain barrier.
Metabolism: Unknown.
Excretion: Unknown.

Route	Onset	Peak	Duration
P.O.	30-90 min	1 hr	6 hr
S.C.	5-15 min	15-30 min	2 hr

Contraindications and precautions
Contraindicated for I.M. or I.V. use and in patients with hypersensitivity to drug or its components; uncertain strength or integrity of bladder wall; mechanical obstructions of GI or urinary tract; hyperthyroidism, peptic ulceration, latent or active bronchial asthma, pronounced bradycardia or hypotension, vasomotor instability, cardiac or coronary artery disease, seizure disorder, Parkinson's disease, spastic GI disturbances, acute inflammatory lesions of the GI tract, peritonitis, or marked vagotonia; or when increased muscular activity of GI or urinary tract is harmful. Use cautiously in pregnant women.

Interactions
Drug-drug. *Cholinergic drugs, especially cholinesterase inhibitors:* Additive effects may occur. Avoid use together.
Ganglionic blockers such as mecamylamine: May cause a critical blood pressure decrease; this effect is usually preceded by abdominal symptoms. Avoid use together.
Procainamide and quinidine: May reverse the cholinergic effect of bethanechol on muscle. Recommend monitoring patient for clinical effect.

Effects on diagnostic tests
None reported.

Adverse reactions
CNS: headache, malaise.
CV: hypotension, reflex tachycardia.
EENT: lacrimation, miosis.
GI: *abdominal cramps, diarrhea,* excessive salivation, nausea, belching, borborygmus.
GU: urinary urgency.
Hepatic: increased serum levels of amylase, lipase, bilirubin, and AST.
Respiratory: ***bronchoconstriction,*** increased bronchial secretions.
Skin: flushing, diaphoresis.

Overdose and treatment
Clinical signs and symptoms of overdose include nausea, vomiting, abdominal cramps, diarrhea, involuntary defecation, urinary urgency, excessive salivation, miosis, excessive tearing, bronchospasm, increased bronchial secretions, hypotension, excessive sweating, bradycardia or reflex tachycardia, and substernal pain.

Treatment requires discontinuation of drug and administration of atropine by S.C., I.M., or I.V. route. (Atropine must be administered cautiously; an overdose could cause bronchial plug formation.) Contact local or regional poison control center for more information.

Clinical considerations

- Atropine sulfate should be readily available to counteract toxic reactions that may occur during treatment with bethanechol.

□ ***ALERT*** Never give bethanechol I.M. or I.V. because that could cause circulatory collapse, hypotension, severe abdominal cramps, bloody diarrhea, shock, or cardiac arrest. Give only by S.C. route when giving parenterally.

- For administration to treat urine retention, bedpan should be readily available.
- Give drug on an empty stomach; eating soon after drug administration may cause nausea and vomiting.
- Store drug in tight container between 59° and 86° F (15° and 30° C). Avoid freezing. The injection may be autoclaved at 248° F (120° C) for 20 minutes without discoloration or loss of potency.

Therapeutic monitoring

Recommend monitoring blood pressure; patients with hypertension receiving bethanechol may experience a precipitous decrease in blood pressure.

Special populations

Pregnant patients. Bethanechol shouldn't be used in pregnant women.
Pediatric patients. Safety and efficacy haven't been established in children.

Patient counseling

Instruct patient to take oral form on an empty stomach and at regular intervals.

bicalutamide

Casodex

Pharmacologic classification: nonsteroidal antiandrogen
Therapeutic classification: antineoplastic
Pregnancy risk category X

How supplied

Available by prescription only
Tablets: 50 mg

Indications and dosages

Adjunct therapy for treatment of advanced prostate cancer
Adults: 50 mg P.O. once daily in morning or evening.

Pharmacodynamics

Antineoplastic action: Drug competitively inhibits the action of androgens by binding to cytosol androgen receptors in the target tissue. Prostatic carcinoma, known to be sensitive to androgens, responds to treatment that either counteracts the effect of androgen or removes its source.

Pharmacokinetics

Absorption: Well absorbed from GI tract.
Distribution: 96% is protein-bound.
Metabolism: Undergoes stereospecific metabolism. The S (inactive) isomer is metabolized primarily by glucuronidation. The R (active) isomer also undergoes glucuronidation but is predominantly oxidized to an inactive metabolite followed by glucuronidation.
Excretion: Excreted in urine and feces.

Route	Onset	Peak	Duration
P.O.	Unknown	Unknown	Unknown

Contraindications and precautions

Contraindicated in patients with hypersensitivity to drug or to any component in the tablet and during pregnancy. Use cautiously in patients with moderate to severe hepatic impairment (drug is extensively metabolized by the liver).

Interactions

Drug-drug. *Coumarin anticoagulants:* Bicalutamide displaces coumarin anticoagulants from their protein-binding sites. Recommend monitoring PT and INR closely. The anticoagulant dose may need adjustment.

Effects on diagnostic tests

None reported.

Adverse reactions

CNS: headache, dizziness, paresthesia, insomnia.
CV: *hot flashes, asthenia,* hypertension, chest pain, peripheral edema.
GI: *constipation, nausea, diarrhea,* abdominal pain, flatulence, increased liver enzymes, vomiting, weight loss.
GU: nocturia, hematuria, urinary tract infection, impotence, gynecomastia, urinary incontinence, increased BUN, and creatinine levels.
Hematologic: hypochromic anemia, iron-deficiency anemia.
Metabolic: hyperglycemia.
Musculoskeletal: *back or pelvic pain,* bone pain.
Respiratory: dyspnea.
Skin: rash, sweating.
Other: *general pain, infection,* flu syndrome.

Overdose and treatment

A single dose of bicalutamide that results in symptoms of an overdose considered to be life-threatening hasn't been established. There's no specific antidote; treatment of an overdose should be symptomatic. Vomiting may be induced if patient is alert. Dialysis isn't likely to be helpful because bicalutamide is highly protein-bound and is extensively metabolized.

Clinical considerations
- Bicalutamide is used in combination therapy with a luteinizing hormone-releasing hormone (LHRH) analogue for the treatment of advanced prostate cancer. Treatment should begin at the same time as that with the prescribed LHRH analogue.
- Administer bicalutamide at the same time each day.
- Drug isn't indicated for use in women.

Therapeutic monitoring
- Recommend monitoring serum prostate specific antigen (PSA) levels regularly. PSA levels help in assessing patient's response to therapy. Elevated levels require a reevaluation of patient to determine disease progression.
- Recommend monitoring liver function studies. Discontinue drug when a patient develops jaundice or exhibits laboratory evidence of liver injury in the absence of liver metastases. Abnormalities are usually reversible on drug discontinuation.

Special populations
Breast-feeding patients. Drug isn't indicated for use in women.
Pediatric patients. Safety and efficacy in children haven't been established.

Patient counseling
- Inform patient that drug may be taken without regard to meals.
- Advise patient to take drug at the same time each day.
- Tell patient that bicalutamide is used with other drug therapy. Stress importance of not interrupting or stopping any of these drugs without medical consultation.

biperiden hydrochloride

biperiden lactate
Akineton

Pharmacologic classification: anticholinergic
Therapeutic classification: antiparkinsonian
Pregnancy risk category C

How supplied
Available by prescription only
Tablets: 2 mg
Injection: 5 mg/ml in 1-ml ampule

Indications and dosages
Extrapyramidal disorders
Adults: 2 mg P.O. daily, b.i.d., or t.i.d., depending on severity. Usual dose is 2 mg daily. For treatment of extrapyramidal symptoms induced by drugs, give 2 mg I.M. or slow I.V. q 30 minutes, not to exceed 8 mg in a 24-hour period.
Parkinsonism
Adults: 2 mg P.O. t.i.d. or q.i.d. For prolonged therapy, adjust dose to maximum of 16 mg daily.
◇ ***Treatment of unrelated spastic disorders (such as spinal cord injury)***
Adults: 2 mg P.O. b.i.d. to q.i.d.

Pharmacodynamics
Antiparkinsonian action: Drug blocks central cholinergic receptors, helping to balance cholinergic activity in the basal ganglia. It may also prolong the effects of dopamine by blocking dopamine reuptake and storage at central receptor sites.

Pharmacokinetics
Absorption: Well absorbed from the GI tract.
Distribution: Minimally absorbed; is metabolized in the liver.
Metabolism: Exact metabolic fate is unknown.
Excretion: Excreted in the urine as unchanged drug and metabolites. After oral therapy, small amounts are probably excreted as unabsorbed drug.

Route	Onset	Peak	Duration
P.O.	1 hr	Unknown	6-12 hr
I.V.	< Few min	Unknown	1-8 hr
I.M.	10-30 min	Unknown	Unknown

Contraindications and precautions
Contraindicated in patients with hypersensitivity to drug, angle-closure glaucoma, bowel obstruction, or megacolon. Use cautiously in patients with prostatic hyperplasia, arrhythmias, or seizure disorders.

Interactions
Drug-drug. *Amantadine:* Increased anticholinergic adverse effects of biperiden, such as confusion and hallucinations. Decrease biperiden dosage before amantadine administration.
Haloperidol or phenothiazines: May decrease the antipsychotic effectiveness of these drugs, possibly by direct CNS antagonism. Recommend monitoring for clinical effect.
Phenothiazines: Increased risk of anticholinergic adverse effects. Avoid use together.
CNS depressants: Increased sedative effects of biperiden. Use together cautiously.
Antacids and antidiarrheals: Decreased biperiden absorption. Administer biperiden at least 1 hour before these drugs are administered.

Digoxin: Plasma levels of digoxin may be elevated. Recommend monitoring digoxin level.
Drug-lifestyle. *Alcohol use:* Increases sedative effects of biperiden. Discourage use.

Effects on diagnostic tests
None reported.

Adverse reactions
CNS: disorientation, euphoria, drowsiness, agitation.
CV: transient postural hypotension (with parenteral use).
EENT: blurred vision.
GI: dry mouth, *constipation.*
GU: urine retention.

Note: Adverse reactions are dose-related and may resemble atropine toxicity.

Overdose and treatment
Clinical effects of overdose include central stimulation followed by depression and psychotic symptoms, such as disorientation, confusion, hallucinations, delusions, anxiety, agitation, and restlessness. Peripheral effects may include dilated, nonreactive pupils; blurred vision; hot, dry, flushed skin; dry mucous membranes; dysphagia; decreased or absent bowel sounds; urine retention; hyperthermia; headache; tachycardia; hypertension; and increased respiration.

Treatment is primarily symptomatic and supportive, as necessary. Maintain patent airway. If the patient is alert, induce emesis (or use gastric lavage) and follow with a sodium chloride cathartic and activated charcoal to prevent further absorption of orally administered drug. In severe cases, physostigmine may be administered to block antimuscarinic effects of biperiden. Give fluids, as needed, to treat shock; diazepam to control psychotic symptoms; and pilocarpine (instilled into the eyes) to relieve mydriasis. If urine retention occurs, catheterization may be necessary.

Clinical considerations
Consider the recommendations relevant to all anticholinergics as well as the following:
- When giving drug parenterally, keep patient supine; parenteral administration may cause transient orthostatic hypotension and disturbed coordination.
- When giving biperiden I.V., inject drug slowly.
- Because biperiden may cause dizziness, patient may need assistance when walking.
- In patients with severe parkinsonism, tremors may increase when drug is administered to relieve spasticity.

Therapeutic monitoring
- Monitor for adverse reactions related to anticholinergics.
- Recommend monitoring for tolerance to drug and notifying prescriber.

Special populations
Breast-feeding patients. Drug may be excreted in breast milk, possibly resulting in infant toxicity. It may also decrease milk production. Avoid use of drug in breast-feeding women.
Pediatric patients. Drug isn't recommended for children.
Geriatric patients. Use cautiously in geriatric patients. Lower doses are indicated.

Patient counseling
- Tell patient that tolerance to therapeutic and adverse effects can occur with chronic drug use.
- Advise patient that drug may increase sensitivity of the eyes to light.
- Instruct patient to take drug with food to avoid GI upset.

bisacodyl
Bisco-Lax, Dulcagen, Dulcolax, Fleet Laxative

Pharmacologic classification: diphenylmethane derivative
Therapeutic classification: stimulant laxative
Pregnancy risk category B

How supplied
Available without a prescription
Tablets: 5 mg
Suppositories: 10 mg
Rectal suspension: 10 mg/30 ml

Indications and dosages
Constipation, preparation for delivery, surgery, or rectal or bowel examination
Adults and children over age 12: 5 to 15 mg P.O. daily. In adults, up to 30 mg may be used for thorough evacuation needed for examinations or surgery. Alternatively, give one suppository (10 mg) or 30 ml of rectal suspension P.R. daily.
Children age 3 to 12: 5 to 10 mg P.O. daily or 0.3 mg/kg daily.
Children age 2 to 11: ½ to 1 suppository (5 to 10 mg) or 15 ml of rectal suspension P.R. daily.
Children under age 2: ½ suppository (5 mg) P.R. daily.

Pharmacodynamics
Laxative action: Bisacodyl has a direct stimulant effect on the colon, increasing peristalsis and enhancing bowel evacuation.

Pharmacokinetics
Absorption: Minimal.
Distribution: Distributed locally.
Metabolism: Absorbed minimally; metabolized in the liver.

Excretion: Excreted primarily in feces; some in urine.

Route	Onset	Peak	Duration
P.O.	6-12 hr	Variable	Variable
P.R.	15-60 min	Variable	Variable

Contraindications and precautions

Contraindicated in patients with hypersensitivity, abdominal pain, nausea, vomiting, or other symptoms of appendicitis or acute surgical abdomen and in those with rectal bleeding, gastroenteritis, or intestinal obstruction.

Interactions

Drug-drug. *Antacids and drugs that increase gastric pH levels:* May cause premature dissolution of the enteric coating, resulting in intestinal or gastric irritation or cramping. Avoid use together.
Drug-food. *Milk*: May cause premature dissolution of the enteric coating, resulting in intestinal or gastric irritation or cramping. Avoid use together.

Effects on diagnostic tests

None reported.

Adverse reactions

CNS: muscle weakness with excessive use, dizziness, faintness.
GI: *nausea, vomiting, abdominal cramps,* diarrhea (with high doses), *burning sensation in rectum* (with suppositories), laxative dependence with long-term or excessive use.
Metabolic: alkalosis, hypokalemia, tetany, protein-losing enteropathy in excessive use, fluid and electrolyte imbalance.

Overdose and treatment

No cases of overdose have been reported.

Clinical considerations

Patient should swallow tablets whole rather than crushing or chewing them, to avoid GI irritation. Administer with 8 oz (240 ml) of fluid.

Therapeutic monitoring

Recommend monitoring patient for diarrhea, electrolyte abnormalities (hypokalemia), dehydration (with chronic use); drug is meant for short-term therapy.

Special populations

Breast-feeding patients. May be used by breast-feeding women.

Patient counseling

- Instruct patient not to take drug within 1 hour of milk or antacid consumption.
- Tell patient to take only as directed to avoid laxative dependence.

bismuth subsalicylate

Pepto-Bismol

Pharmacologic classification: adsorbent
Therapeutic classification: antidiarrheal
Pregnancy risk category C (D in third trimester)

How supplied

Available without a prescription
Tablets (chewable): 262 mg
Suspension: 262 mg/15 ml, 524 mg/15 ml

Indications and dosages

Mild, nonspecific diarrhea
Adults: 30 ml or 2 tablets P.O. q 30 minutes to 1 hour up to a maximum of eight doses and for no more than 2 days.
Children age 9 to 12: 15 ml or 1 tablet P.O.
Children age 6 to 9: 10 ml or ⅔ tablet P.O.
Children age 3 to 6: 5 ml or ⅓ tablet P.O.
Children's doses given q 30 minutes to 1 hour up to a maximum of eight doses in 24 hours and for no more than 2 days.

Pharmacodynamics

Antidiarrheal action: Bismuth adsorbs extra water in the bowel during diarrhea. It also adsorbs toxins and forms a protective coating for the intestinal mucosa.

Pharmacokinetics

Absorption: Absorbed poorly; significant salicylate absorption may occur after using bismuth subsalicylate.
Distribution: Distributed locally in the gut.
Metabolism: Metabolized minimally.
Excretion: Excreted in urine.

Route	Onset	Peak	Duration
P.O.	1 hr	Unknown	Unknown

Contraindications and precautions

Contraindicated in patients hypersensitive to salicylates. Use cautiously in patients already taking aspirin or aspirin-containing medications.

Interactions

Drug-drug. *Tetracycline:* Bismuth subsalicylate may impair tetracycline absorption. Separate administration times.
Sulfinpyrazone: Impaired uricosuric effect. Recommend monitoring for clinical effect.
Salicylates: Increased risk of aspirin toxicity. Monitor patient closely.

Effects on diagnostic tests

Because bismuth is radiopaque, it may interfere with radiologic examination of the GI tract.

Adverse reactions
GI: temporary darkening of tongue and stools.
Other: salicylism (with high doses).

Overdose and treatment
Overdose has not been reported. However, overdose is more likely with bismuth subsalicylate; probable clinical effects include CNS effects, such as tinnitus and fever.

Clinical considerations
- Bismuth subsalicylate has been used investigationally to treat peptic ulcer. Doses of 600 mg P.O. t.i.d. may be as effective as cimetidine 800 mg P.O. once daily.
- If giving drug by nasogastric tube, flush tube to clear it before administration to ensure drug delivery to stomach; flush afterward.
- If patient is also receiving tetracycline, administer bismuth at least 1 hour apart; to avoid decreased drug absorption, dosages or schedules of other medications may require adjustment.
- Don't administer drug to children or adolescents recovering from flu or chickenpox.
- Discontinue drug if tinnitus occurs.
- Drug is useful for indigestion without causing constipation; for nausea; and for relief of flatulence and abdominal cramps.

Therapeutic monitoring
Recommend monitoring hydration status and serum electrolyte levels, and recording number and consistency of stools.

Special populations
Breast-feeding patients. Small amounts of drug are excreted in breast milk. Patient should seek medical approval before use.

Patient counseling
- Advise patient taking anticoagulants or medication for diabetes or gout to seek medical approval before taking drug.
- Instruct patient to chew tablets well or to shake suspension well before using.
- Tell patient to report persistent diarrhea.
- Warn patient that bismuth may temporarily darken stools and tongue.

bisoprolol fumarate
Zebeta

Pharmacologic classification: beta blocker
Therapeutic classification: antihypertensive
Pregnancy risk category C

How supplied
Available by prescription only
Tablets: 5 mg, 10 mg

Indications and dosages
Hypertension (used alone or in combination with other antihypertensives)
Adults: Initially, 2.5 to 5 mg P.O. once daily. If response is inadequate, increase to 10 mg once daily. Maximum recommended dose, 20 mg daily.
≡ ***Dosage adjustment.*** In adults with renal impairment (creatinine clearance less than 40 ml/minute) or hepatic dysfunction, cirrhosis or hepatitis, start at 2.5 mg P.O.; then increase with caution.

Pharmacodynamics
Antihypertensive action: Mechanism of action has not been completely established. Possible antihypertensive factors include decreased cardiac output, inhibition of renin release by the kidneys, and diminution of tonic sympathetic outflow from the vasomotor centers in the brain.

Pharmacokinetics
Absorption: Bioavailability after a 10-mg oral dose is about 80%. Absorption isn't affected by the presence of food.
Distribution: About 30% binds to serum proteins.
Metabolism: The first-pass metabolism is about 20%.
Excretion: Eliminated equally by renal and nonrenal pathways, with about 50% of dose appearing unchanged in the urine and the remainder appearing as inactive metabolites. Less than 2% of dose is excreted in the feces. The plasma elimination half-life of drug is 9 to 12 hours (slightly longer in geriatric patients, in part because of decreased renal function in that population).

Route	Onset	Peak	Duration
P.O.	Unknown	1-4 hr	24 hr

Contraindications and precautions
Contraindicated in patients with hypersensitivity to drug and in those with cardiogenic shock, overt cardiac failure, marked sinus bradycardia, or second- or third-degree AV block. Use cautiously in patients with bronchospastic disease.

Interactions
Drug-drug. *Other beta blockers:* Bisoprolol shouldn't be used with other beta blockers.
Catecholamine-depleting drugs, such as reserpine or guanethidine: Excessively reduced sympathetic activity. Monitor patient closely.
Concurrent therapy with clonidine: Discontinue bisoprolol for several days before clonidine withdrawal. Monitor patient closely.

Effects on diagnostic tests
None reported.

Adverse reactions

CNS: asthenia, fatigue, dizziness, *headache,* hypesthesia, vivid dreams, depression, insomnia.
CV: ***bradycardia,*** peripheral edema, chest pain.
EENT: pharyngitis, rhinitis, sinusitis.
GI: nausea, vomiting, diarrhea, dry mouth.
Metabolic: hypoglycemia; interference with glucose or insulin tolerance tests.
Musculoskeletal: arthralgia.
Respiratory: cough, dyspnea.

Overdose and treatment

The most common signs of overdose from a beta blocker such as bisoprolol are bradycardia, hypotension, heart failure, bronchospasm, and hypoglycemia. If overdose occurs, discontinue drug therapy and provide supportive and symptomatic treatment.

Clinical considerations

- Patients with renal or hepatic dysfunction or bronchospastic disease unresponsive to or intolerant of other antihypertensive therapies should start therapy at 2.5 mg P.O. daily. A $beta_2$-adrenergic agonist (bronchodilator) should be made available to patients with bronchospastic disease.
- Treatment with a beta blocker for heart failure (unlabeled use) should be initiated at a very low dose (1.25 mg P.O. daily for 2 to 4 weeks), although this low-dose strength is not available in the U.S. If dose is tolerated, increase to 2.5 mg daily for 2 to 4 weeks. Subsequent doses can be doubled every 2 to 4 weeks if tolerated. May be adjusted up to 5 to 10 mg daily.
- Exacerbation of angina pectoris, MI, and ventricular arrhythmia has been observed in patients with coronary artery disease after abrupt cessation of therapy with beta blockers. It's advisable, even in patients without overt coronary artery disease, to taper therapy with bisoprolol over 1 week, with patient under careful observation. If withdrawal symptoms occur, reinstitute bisoprolol therapy, at least temporarily.

Therapeutic monitoring

- Recommend monitoring blood pressure closely.
- Recommend monitoring serum glucose; signs of hypoglycemia may be masked in patients taking beta blockers.
- Recommend monitoring patients with hyperthyroidism carefully; beta blockers mask symptoms (tachycardia).

Special populations

Breast-feeding patients. It isn't known if drug is excreted in breast milk. Use with caution when administering to breast-feeding women.
Pediatric patients. Safety and efficacy in children haven't been established.

Patient counseling

- Inform diabetic patients subject to spontaneous hypoglycemia or those requiring insulin or oral hypoglycemic agents that bisoprolol may mask some manifestations of hypoglycemia, particularly tachycardia.
- Warn patient not to drive, operate machinery, or perform any other task requiring alertness until reaction to bisoprolol has been established.
- Stress importance of taking drug as prescribed, even when feeling well. Advise patient not to discontinue drug abruptly because serious consequences can occur.
- Instruct patient to call if adverse reactions occur.
- Tell patient to seek medical approval before taking OTC medications.

bitolterol mesylate

Tornalate

Pharmacologic classification: adrenergic, $beta_2$ agonist
Therapeutic classification: bronchodilator
Pregnancy risk category C

How supplied

Available by prescription only
Aerosol inhaler: 370 mcg/metered spray
Solution for nebulization: 0.2%

Indications and dosages

To prevent and treat bronchial asthma and bronchospasm
Adults and children over age 12: For symptomatic relief of bronchospasm, 2 inhalations at an interval of at least 1 to 3 minutes followed by a third inhalation, if needed; to prevent bronchospasm, 2 inhalations q 8 hours. Usually, dose shouldn't exceed 3 inhalations q 6 hours or 2 inhalations q 4 hours.

Nebulizer: For intermittent flow, 1 mg t.i.d. For continuous flow, 2.5 mg t.i.d. However, because deposition of inhaled medications is variable, higher doses are occasionally used, especially in patients with acute bronchospasm. In some patients, higher doses (1.5 mg for intermittent flow and 3.5 mg for continuous flow nebulizer) or increased frequency may be required. The interval between treatments shouldn't be less than 4 hours. The maximum dose for intermittent flow is 8 mg and 14 mg for the continuous flow nebulizer system.

Pharmacodynamics

Bronchodilator action: Bitolterol selectively stimulates $beta_2$-adrenergic receptors of the lungs. Bronchodilation results from relaxation of bronchial smooth muscles, which relieves bronchospasm and reduces airway resistance. Some CV stimulation may occur as a result of beta$_2$-adrenergic stimulation, including mild tachycardia, palpitations, and changes in blood pressure or heart rate.

Pharmacokinetics

Absorption: After oral inhalation, bronchodilation results from local action on the bronchial tree, with most of the inhaled dose being swallowed.
Distribution: Widely distributed throughout body.
Metabolism: Hydrolyzed by esterases to active metabolites.
Excretion: After oral administration, excreted primarily in urine.

Route	Onset	Peak	Duration
Aerosol	3-5 min	½-2 hr	4-8 hr
Nebulizer	2-3 min	30-60 min	6-8 hr

Contraindications and precautions

Contraindicated in patients with hypersensitivity to drug. Use cautiously in patients with ischemic heart disease, hypertension, hyperthyroidism, diabetes mellitus, arrhythmias, seizure disorders, or history of unusual responsiveness to beta-adrenergic agonists.

Interactions

Drug-drug. *Other orally inhaled beta-adrenergic agonists:* Additive sympathomimetic effects. Use together cautiously.
Propranolol and other beta blockers: Antagonize the effects of bitolterol. Use together cautiously.
Theophylline salt such as aminophylline: Cardiotoxic effects may be increased. Recommend monitoring patient for these effects.

Effects on diagnostic tests

May render spirometry insensitive for the diagnosis of asthma.

Adverse reactions

CNS: *tremor,* nervousness, headache, dizziness, light-headedness.
CV: palpitations, chest discomfort, tachycardia.
EENT: throat irritation, cough.
GI: nausea, vomiting, increased AST levels.
GU: proteinuria.
Hematologic: decreased platelet or leukocyte count.
Respiratory: dyspnea.
Other: ***hypersensitivity reactions.***

Overdose and treatment

Signs and symptoms of overdose include exaggeration of common adverse reactions, especially arrhythmias, extreme tremor, nausea, and vomiting.

Treatment requires supportive measures. To reverse effects, use selective beta$_2$-adrenergic blockers (acebutolol, atenolol, metoprolol) with extreme caution (may induce asthmatic attack). Monitor vital signs and ECG closely.

Clinical considerations

Consider the recommendations relevant to all adrenergics as well as the following:

- Avoid excessive or prolonged use because it can lead to tolerance.
- Repeated use may result in paradoxical bronchospasm. Discontinue drug immediately if this occurs.
- Store at 59° to 86° F (15° to 30° C). Nebulizer solution shouldn't be mixed with other medications (such as cromolyn sodium and acetylcysteine) in the nebulizer because of incompatabilities.

Therapeutic monitoring

Recommend monitoring for decreased effectiveness. Don't increase frequency or dose; fatal reactions have occurred from excessive use of sympathomimetic amine oral inhalations.

Special populations

Pregnant patients. There are no adequate and controlled studies for use in pregnant women.
Breast-feeding patients. Administer cautiously to breast-feeding women. It's unknown if drug is excreted in breast milk.
Pediatric patients. Drug isn't recommended for use in children under age 12.
Geriatric patients. Lower doses are indicated in geriatric patients who may be more sensitive to the effects of the drug.

Patient counseling

- Tell patient to use drug only as directed and not to exceed the prescribed amount or shorten intervals between doses.
- Teach patient to use drug correctly. Tell patient to ensure proper delivery of dose by cleaning plastic mouthpiece with warm tap water and drying thoroughly at least once daily. Tell him that dryness of mouth and throat may occur, but that rinsing with water after each dose may help.
- Tell patient to call promptly if troubled breathing persists 1 hour after using drug, if symptoms return within 4 hours, if condition worsens, or if new (refill) canister is needed within 2 weeks.
- Advise patient to wait 15 minutes after use of bitolterol before using adrenocorticoid inhaler.
- Give patient instructions on proper use of inhaler, as follows:

Administration by metered-dose nebulizers: Shake canister to activate; place mouthpiece well into mouth, aimed at back of throat. Close lips and teeth around mouthpiece. Exhale through nose, then inhale through mouth slowly and deeply, while actuating the nebulizer, to release dose. Hold breath 10 seconds (count

"1-100, 2-100, 3-100" to "10-100"), remove mouthpiece, then exhale slowly.
Administration by metered powder inhaler: Caution patient not to take forced deep breaths, but to breathe normally. Observe patient closely for exaggerated systemic drug action. Patients requiring more than three aerosol treatments within 24 hours should be under close medical supervision.
Administration by oxygen aerosolization: Administer over 15 to 20 minutes, with oxygen flow rate adjusted to 4 L/minute. Turn on oxygen supply before patient places nebulizer in mouth. Patient need not close lips tightly around nebulizer opening. Placement of Y tube in rubber tubing permits patient to control administration. Advise patient to rinse mouth immediately after inhalation therapy to help prevent dryness and throat irritation. Rinse mouthpiece with warm running water at least once daily to prevent clogging; it's not dishwasher-safe. Wait until mouthpiece is dry before storing. Don't place near artificial heat, such as a dishwasher or oven. Replace reservoir bag every 2 to 3 weeks or p.r.n.; replace mouthpiece every 6 to 9 months or p.r.n. Replacement of bags or mouthpieces may require a prescription.

bleomycin sulfate

Blenoxane

Pharmacologic classification: antibiotic, antineoplastic (cell cycle-phase specific, G2 and M phase)
Therapeutic classification: antineoplastic
Pregnancy risk category D

How supplied

Available by prescription only
Injection: 15-unit, 30-unit vials

Indications and dosages

Dosage and indications may vary. Check literature for current protocol.
Hodgkin's disease, squamous cell carcinoma, malignant lymphoma, or testicular carcinoma
Adults: 10 to 20 units/m² (0.25 to 0.5 units/kg) I.V., I.M., or S.C., one or two times weekly. After 50% response in regression of tumor size in Hodgkin's disease, maintenance dosage of 1 unit daily or 5 units weekly.
Malignant pleural effusion; prevention of recurrent pleural effusions or ◊to manage pneumothorax associated with AIDS and* Pneumocystis carinii *pneumonia
Adults: 50 to 60 units in 50 to 100 ml of normal saline solution by intracavitary administration not to exceed 1 unit/kg.
≡ ***Dosage adjustment.*** For geriatric patients receiving intracavitary administration in the pleural space, don't exceed 40 units/m².
Tumors of the head and neck
Adults: 10 to 20 units/m² daily by I.V. or ◊regional arterial administration for 5 to 14 days.
◊AIDS-related Kaposi's sarcoma
Adults: 20 units/m² daily I.V. continuously over 72 hr every 3 weeks.

Pharmacodynamics

Antineoplastic action: The exact mechanism of cytotoxicity of bleomycin is unknown. Its action may be through scission of single- and double-stranded DNA and inhibition of DNA, RNA, and protein synthesis. Bleomycin also appears to inhibit cell progression out of the G2 phase.

Pharmacokinetics

Absorption: Poorly absorbed across the GI tract following oral administration. I.M. administration results in lower serum levels than those occurring after equivalent I.V. doses.
Distribution: Distributes widely into total body water, mainly in the skin, lungs, kidneys, peritoneum, and lymphatic tissue.
Metabolism: Metabolic fate of drug is undetermined; however, extensive tissue inactivation occurs in the liver and kidney and much less in the skin and lungs.
Excretion: Excreted primarily in urine. The terminal plasma elimination phase half-life is reported at 2 hours.

Route	Onset	Peak	Duration
I.V., S.C.	Unknown	Unknown	Unknown
I.M.	Unknown	½-1 hr	Unknown

Contraindications and precautions

Contraindicated in patients hypersensitive to drug. Use cautiously in patients with renal or pulmonary impairment.

Interactions

Drug-drug. *Phenytoin and digoxin:* Using together may decrease serum levels of these drugs. Recommend monitoring serum levels.

Effects on diagnostic tests

None reported.

Adverse reactions

GI: stomatitis, anorexia, nausea, vomiting, diarrhea.
Metabolic: increased blood and urine concentrations of uric acid.
Respiratory: ***pulmonary fibrosis***, pulmonary toxicity such as **PNEUMONITIS.**
Skin: *erythema, hyperpigmentation, acne, rash, reversible alopecia, striae, skin tenderness, pruritus.*
Other: *chills,* fever, weight loss, ***severe idiosyncratic reaction consisting of hypotension,***

mental confusion, fever, chills, and wheezing has occurred in about 1% of lymphoma patients.

Overdose and treatment

Signs and symptoms of bleomycin overdose include pulmonary fibrosis, fever, chills, vesiculation, and hyperpigmentation. Treatment is usually supportive and includes antipyretics for fever.

Clinical considerations

- To prepare solution for I.M. administration, reconstitute drug with 1 to 5 ml (15-unit vial) or 2 to 10 ml (30-unit vial) of normal saline solution, bacteriostatic water, or sterile water for injection. D_5W or dextrose containing diluents shouldn't be used.
- For I.V. administration, dilute with a minimum of 5 ml (15-unit vial) or 10 ml (30-unit vial) of diluent (concentration shouldn't exceed 3 units/ml) and administer over 10 minutes as I.V. push injection.
- For intrapleural administration, dissolve 60 units of bleomycin in 50 to 100 ml of normal saline injection and administer via thoracostomy tube.
- Use precautions in preparing and handling drug; wear gloves and wash hands after preparing and administering.
- Drug can be administered by intracavitary route (see manufacturer's recommendation), intra-arterially, or via intratumoral injection. It can also be instilled into bladder for bladder tumors.
- Cumulative lifetime dosage shouldn't exceed 400 units.
- Response to bleomycin therapy may take 2 to 3 weeks.
- Recommend administering a 1- to 2-unit test dose to lymphoma patients for the first two doses to assess hypersensitivity to bleomycin. If no reaction occurs, then follow the dosing schedule. The test dose can be incorporated as part of the total dose for the regimen.
- Recommend having epinephrine, diphenhydramine, I.V. corticosteroids, and oxygen available in case of anaphylactic reaction.
- Premedication with aspirin, steroids, and diphenhydramine may reduce drug fever and risk of anaphylaxis.
- Reduce dosage in patients with renal or pulmonary impairment.
- Lung damage may occur at lower oxygen levels than normal. This is an important consideration for patients undergoing surgery.
- Drug concentrates in keratin of squamous epithelium. To prevent linear streaking, don't use adhesive dressings on skin.
- Allergic reactions may be delayed, especially in patients with lymphoma.
- Investigational uses for the drug include treatment of AIDS-related Kaposi's sarcoma, renal carcinomas, soft tissue sarcomas, otorhinolaryngeal tumors, and mycosis fungoides.
- Bleomycin is stable for 24 hours at room temperature and 48 hours under refrigeration. Refrigerate unopened vials containing dry powder.

Therapeutic monitoring

- Pulmonary function tests may be useful in predicting fibrosis; they should be performed to establish a baseline and then monitored periodically.
- Recommend monitoring chest X-rays and auscultating the lungs to monitor for pulmonary toxicity.

Special populations

Pregnant patients. Drug may cause fetal toxicity in pregnant women.
Breast-feeding patients. It isn't known if drug occurs in breast milk. However, because of risk of serious adverse reactions, mutagenicity, and carcinogenicity in infants, breast-feeding isn't recommended.
Geriatric patients. Use with caution in patients over age 70 because they're at increased risk for pulmonary toxicity.

Patient counseling

Explain to patient that hair should grow back after treatment is discontinued.

bretylium tosylate

Bretylate*, Bretylol

Pharmacologic classification: adrenergic blocker
Therapeutic classification: ventricular antiarrhythmic
Pregnancy risk category C

How supplied

Available by prescription only
Injection: 50 mg/ml
Injection in dextrose: 500 mg, 1 g in 5 % dextrose; 2 mg/ml, 4 mg/ml

Indications and dosages

Ventricular fibrillation and hemodynamically unstable ventricular tachycardia
Adults: 5 mg/kg undiluted by rapid I.V. injection. If ventricular fibrillation persists, increase dosage to 10 mg/kg and repeat, p.r.n.(usually 5- to 30-minute intervals) to total of 30 to 35 mg/kg. For continuous suppression, administer diluted solution by continuous I.V. infusion at 1 to 2 mg/minute, or infuse diluted solution at 5 to 10 mg/kg over more than 8 to 10 minutes q 6 hours.
Other ventricular arrhythmias
Adults: Initially, 5 to 10 mg/kg I.M., undiluted, or I.V. diluted. Repeat in 1 to 2 hours if necessary. Maintenance dosage is 5 to 10 mg/kg

q 6 to 8 hours I.M. or I.V. or 1 to 2 mg/minute I.V. infusion.
◊ *Children:* For acute ventricular fibrillation, initially 5 mg/kg I.V., followed by 10 mg/kg q 15 to 30 minutes, with a maximum total dose of 30 mg/kg; maintenance dosage, 5 to 10 mg/kg q 6 hours. For other ventricular arrhythmias, 5 to 10 mg/kg q 6 hours or 2 to 5 mg/kg I.M. as a single dose.

Pharmacodynamics

Ventricular antiarrhythmic action: Bretylium is a class III antiarrhythmic used to treat ventricular fibrillation and tachycardia. Like other class III antiarrhythmics, it widens the action potential duration (repolarization inhibition) and increases the effective refractory period (ERP); it doesn't affect conduction velocity. These actions follow a transient increase in conduction velocity and shortening of the action potential duration and ERP.

Initial effects stem from norepinephrine release from sympathetic ganglia and postganglionic adrenergic neurons immediately after drug administration. Norepinephrine release also accounts for an increased threshold for successful defibrillation, increased blood pressure, and increased heart rate. This initial phase of drug's action is brief (up to 1 hour).

Bretylium also alters the disparity in action potential duration between ischemic and nonischemic myocardial tissue; its antiarrhythmic action may result from this activity.

Hemodynamic drug effects include increased blood pressure, heart rate, and possible cardiac irritability (all resulting from initial norepinephrine release). Drug-induced adrenergic blockade ultimately predominates, leading to vasodilation and a subsequent blood pressure drop (primarily orthostatic). This effect has been referred to as chemical sympathectomy.

Pharmacokinetics

Absorption: Incompletely and erratically absorbed from the GI tract; well absorbed after I.M. administration.
Distribution: Distributed widely throughout the body. Doesn't cross the blood-brain barrier. Only about 1% to 10% is plasma protein-bound.
Metabolism: No metabolites have been identified.
Excretion: Excreted in urine mostly as unchanged drug; half-life ranges from 5 to 10 hours (longer in patients with renal impairment).

Route	Onset	Peak	Duration
P.O.	Unknown	Unknown	Unknown
I.V.	Immediate	Immediate	6-24 hr
I.M.	5-40 min	1 hr	6-24 hr

Contraindications and precautions

Contraindicated in digitalized patients unless the arrhythmia is life-threatening, not caused by a cardiac glycoside, and unresponsive to other antiarrhythmics. Use with caution in patients with aortic stenosis and pulmonary hypertension.

Interactions

Drug-drug. *Other antiarrhythmic agents:* Additive toxic effects and additive or antagonistic cardiac effects. Avoid use if possible.
Cardiac glycosides: May exacerbate ventricular tachycardia associated with digitalis toxicity. Use together cautiously.
MAO inhibitors: May potentiate the bretylium-induced release of catecholamines from nerve endings. Use together cautiously.
Pressor amines (sympathomimetics): Bretylium may potentiate the action of these drugs. Monitor for the effects of these drugs.

Effects on diagnostic tests

None reported.

Adverse reactions

CNS: *vertigo, dizziness, light-headedness, syncope* (usually secondary to hypotension).
CV: SEVERE HYPOTENSION (especially orthostatic), ***bradycardia***, anginal pain, transient ***arrhythmias***, transient hypertension, increased PVCs.
GI: severe nausea, vomiting.
Other: hyperthermia.

Overdose and treatment

Clinical effects of overdose primarily involve severe hypotension.

Treatment includes administration of vasopressors to support blood pressure, and general supportive measures. Volume expanders and positional changes also may be effective.

Clinical considerations

- Administer I.V. infusion at appropriate rate to avoid or minimize adverse reactions.
- For I.M. injection, don't exceed 5-ml volume in any one site and rotate sites.
- Advise patient to remain supine and avoid sudden postural changes until tolerance to hypotension develops.
- Avoid simultaneous initiation of therapy with a cardiac glycoside and bretylium.
- Because bretylium is excreted exclusively by the kidneys, patients with renal impairment require dosage modification. Increase dosage interval because the elimination half-life increases three- to six-fold.
- Subtherapeutic doses (less than 5 mg/kg) may cause hypotension.
- Drug isn't a first-line agent, according to American Heart Association advanced cardiac life-support guidelines. With ventricular fibrillation, drug should follow lidocaine; with

ventricular tachycardia, drug should follow lidocaine and procainamide.
- Ventricular tachycardia and other ventricular arrhythmias respond to drug less rapidly than ventricular fibrillation.
- Drug is ineffective against atrial arrhythmias.
- Store bretylium between 59° and 86° F (15° and 30° C). Solutions in 5% dextrose should be protected from freezing and stored at room temperature. Following dilution of bretylium injection to 10 mg/ml, the drug is stable for 48 hours at room temperature or 7 days at 40° F (4° C). Drug is compatible with most standard I.V. solutions.

Therapeutic monitoring
- Recommend monitoring ECG and blood pressure throughout therapy.
- Monitor patient closely if he is receiving pressor amines (sympathomimetics) to correct hypotension; bretylium potentiates the effects of these drugs.
- Observe susceptible patients for increased anginal pain.

Special populations
Breast-feeding patients. Safety in breast-feeding women hasn't been established.
Pediatric patients. Safety and efficacy in children haven't been established.
Geriatric patients. Initiate dosing at lower end of dosing range. Geriatric patients are at greater risk for adverse effects and orthostatic hypotension.

Patient counseling
- Instruct patient to report adverse reactions immediately.
- Advise patient to avoid any sudden postural changes.

bromocriptine mesylate
Parlodel

Pharmacologic classification: dopamine receptor agonist
Therapeutic classification: semisynthetic ergot alkaloid, dopaminergic agonist, antiparkinsonian, inhibitor of prolactin release, inhibitor of growth hormone release
Pregnancy risk category B

How supplied
Available by prescription only
Tablets: 2.5 mg
Capsules: 5 mg

Indications and dosages
Amenorrhea and galactorrhea associated with hyperprolactinemia; female infertility
Adults: 1.25 to 2.5 mg P.O. daily, increased by 2.5 mg daily at 3- to 7-day intervals as tolerated until optimal therapeutic effects are achieved. Maintenance dosage is usually 5 to 7.5 mg daily (range, 2.5 to 15 mg daily). Up to 40 mg daily has been used.
Acromegaly
Adults: Initially, 1.25 to 2.5 mg P.O. daily h.s. for 3 days. An additional 1.25 to 2.5 mg may be added q 3 to 7 days until patient receives therapeutic benefit. Therapeutic dose range varies from 20 to 30 mg daily in most patients. Maximum dose shouldn't exceed 100 mg daily. Dosages of 20 to 60 mg daily have been administered as divided doses.
Parkinson's disease
Adults: Initially, 1.25 mg P.O. b.i.d. with meals. Dosage may be increased by 2.5 mg daily q 14 to 28 days, up to 100 mg daily or until a maximal therapeutic response is achieved. Safety in doses over 100 mg daily hasn't been established.
◇***Premenstrual syndrome***
Adults: 2.5 to 7.5 mg P.O. b.i.d. from day 10 of menstrual cycle until onset of menstruation.
◇***Cushing's syndrome***
Adults: 1.25 to 2.5 mg P.O. b.i.d. to q.i.d.
◇***Hepatic encephalopathy***
Adults: 1.25 mg P.O. daily, increased by 1.25 mg q 3 days until 15 mg is reached.
◇***Neuroleptic malignant syndrome associated with neuroleptic drug therapy***
Adults: 2.5 to 5 mg P.O. 2 to 6 times per day.

Pharmacodynamics
Prolactin-inhibiting action: Reduces prolactin concentrations by inhibiting release of prolactin from the anterior pituitary gland, a direct action on the pituitary. It may also stimulate postsynaptic dopamine receptors in the hypothalamus to release prolactin-inhibitory factor via a complicated catecholamine pathway. Drug reduces high serum prolactin levels and restores ovulation and ovarian function in amenorrheic women and suppresses puerperal or nonpuerperal lactation in women with adequate gonadotropin concentrations and ovarian function. The average time for reversing amenorrhea is 6 to 8 weeks, but it may take up to 24 weeks.
Antiparkinsonian action: Activates dopaminergic receptors in the neostriatum of the CNS, which may produce its antiparkinsonism activity. Dysregulation of brain serotonin activity also may occur. The precise role of bromocriptine in treating parkinsonism syndrome requires further study of its safety and efficacy in long-term therapy.

Pharmacokinetics
Absorption: 28% absorbed when given orally
Distribution: About 90% to 96% is bound to serum albumin.
Metabolism: First-pass metabolism occurs with over 90% of the absorbed dose. Metabolized completely in the liver, principally by hydrolysis, before excretion. The metabolites aren't active or toxic.
Excretion: Primarily excreted in bile. Only 2.5% to 5.5% of dose is excreted in urine. Almost all (85%) of dose is excreted in feces within 5 days.

Route	Onset	Peak	Duration
P.O.	2 hr	8 hr	24 hr

Contraindications and precautions
Contraindicated in patients with hypersensitivity to ergot derivatives, uncontrolled hypertension, or toxemia of pregnancy. Use cautiously in patients with renal or hepatic impairment and history of MI with residual arrhythmias.

Interactions
Drug-drug. *Amitriptyline, butyrophenones, imipramine, methyldopa, phenothiazines, and reserpine:* Increase prolactin levels. This may require increased dosage of bromocriptine.
Antihypertensive agents: Potentiation of effects. Reduced dosage prevents hypotension.
Drug-lifestyle. *Alcohol use:* Intolerance may result when high doses of bromocriptine are administered. Advise patient to limit ingestion of alcohol.

Effects on diagnostic tests
None reported.

Adverse reactions
CNS: *dizziness, headache,* fatigue, mania, lightheadedness, drowsiness, delusions, nervousness, insomnia, depression, ***seizures.***
CV: *hypotension,* ***stroke, acute MI.***
EENT: nasal congestion, blurred vision.
GI: *nausea,* vomiting, *abdominal cramps, constipation,* diarrhea, anorexia.
GU: urine retention, urinary frequency.
Skin: coolness and pallor of fingers and toes.

Overdose and treatment
Overdose of bromocriptine may cause nausea, vomiting, and severe hypotension. Treatment includes emptying the stomach by aspiration and lavage, and administering I.V. fluids to treat hypotension.

Clinical considerations
- Patient must be examined carefully for pituitary tumor (Forbes-Albright syndrome). Use of bromocriptine doesn't affect tumor size, although it may alleviate amenorrhea or galactorrhea.
- First-dose phenomenon occurs in 1% of patients. Sensitive patients may experience syncope for 15 to 60 minutes but can usually tolerate subsequent treatment without ill effects. Patient should begin therapy with lowest dosage, taken at bedtime.
- Administer drug with meals, milk, or snacks to diminish GI distress.
- Alcohol intolerance may occur, especially when high doses of bromocriptine are administered; therefore, advise patient to limit alcohol intake.
- As an antiparkinsonism agent, drug is usually given with either levodopa alone or levodopa-carbidopa combination. In treatment of Parkinsonism, if levodopa dosage must be decreased due to adverse effects, daily bromocriptine doses may be increased gradually in 2.5 mg increments.
- Adverse reactions are more common when drug is given in high doses, as in treating parkinsonism.

Therapeutic monitoring
- Monitor hepatic, hematopoietic, cardiovascular, and renal function in long-term use.
- Recommend monitoring blood pressure, especially during first few days of therapy.
- Monitor for pulmonary changes in long-term use.
- Monitor patient with acromegaly for cold-induced digital vasospasm and signs and symptoms of peptic ulcer.

Special populations
Pregnant patients. Discontinue drug if pregnancy occurs. Recommend regular checks of the visual field in patients with underlying prolactin-secreting pituitary tumors.
Breast-feeding patients. Because drug inhibits lactation, it shouldn't be used in women who intend to breast-feed.
Pediatric patients. Drug isn't recommended for children under age 15.
Geriatric patients. Use with caution, particularly in patients receiving long-term, high-dose therapy. Regular physical assessment is recommended, with particular attention toward changes in pulmonary function and blood pressure. Safety isn't established for long-term use at the doses required to treat Parkinson's disease. Therapy should be started at the low end of the dosage range.

Patient counseling
- Advise patient that it may take 6 to 8 weeks or longer for menses to resume and for galactorrhea to be suppressed.
- Tell patient to take first dose where and when she can lie down because drowsiness commonly occurs after initiation of therapy.

- Instruct patient to report visual problems, severe nausea and vomiting, or acute headaches.
- Tell patient to take drug with meals to avoid GI upset.
- Warn patient that the CNS effects of drug may impair ability to perform tasks that require alertness and coordination.
- Instruct patient to use a nonhormonal contraceptive during treatment because of potential amenorrheic adverse effects.
- Advise patient to limit use of alcohol during treatment.

brompheniramine maleate
Dimetapp Allergy

Pharmacologic classification: alkylamine antihistamine
Therapeutic classification: antihistamine (H_1-receptor antagonist)
Pregnancy risk category C

How supplied
Available with or without a prescription
Tablets: 4 mg
Tablets (extended-release): 8 mg, 12 mg
Elixir: 2 mg/5 ml
Injection: 10 mg/ml

Indications and dosages
Rhinitis, allergies
Adults and children age 12 and older: 4 mg P.O. q 4 to 6 hours. Don't exceed 24 mg in 24 hours. Alternatively, extended-release tablets of 8 or 12 mg q 8 to 12 hours.
Children age 7 to 11: 2 mg P.O. q 4 to 6 hours. Don't exceed 12 mg in 24 hours. Alternatively, extended-release tablets of 8 or 12 mg P.O. q 12 hours.
Children age 2 to 6: 1 mg P.O. q 4 to 6 hours. Don't exceed 6 mg in 24 hours.
Hypersensitivity
Adults and children age 12 and older: 5 to 20 mg S.C., I.M., or I.V. b.i.d. Don't exceed 40 mg in 24 hours.
Children under age 12: 0.5 mg/kg/day or 15 mg/m^2/day S.C., I.M., or I.V. in three to four divided doses.

Pharmacodynamics
Antihistamine action: Antihistamines compete with histamine for histamine$_1$-receptor sites on the smooth muscle of the bronchi, GI tract, uterus, and large blood vessels; by binding to cellular receptors, they prevent access of histamine and suppress histamine-induced allergic symptoms, even though they don't prevent its release.

Pharmacokinetics
Absorption: Absorbed readily from the GI tract.
Distribution: Distributed widely into the body.
Metabolism: About 90% to 95% is metabolized by the liver.
Excretion: Half-life of drug is about 22 hours. Brompheniramine and its metabolites are excreted primarily in urine; a small amount is excreted in feces. About 5% to 10% of an oral dose is excreted unchanged in urine.

Route	Onset	Peak	Duration
P.O.	15-60 min	2-5 hr	3-24 hr
I.V., I.M., S.C.	Unknown	Unknown	Unknown

Contraindications and precautions
Contraindicated in patients with hypersensitivity to drug's ingredients; in those with acute asthma, severe hypertension or coronary artery disease, angle-closure glaucoma, urine retention, and peptic ulcer; and within 14 days of MAO-inhibitor therapy. Use cautiously in patients with increased intraocular pressure, diabetes mellitus, ischemic heart disease, hyperthyroidism, hypertension, bronchial asthma, or prostatic hyperplasia and in the elderly.

Interactions
Drug-drug. *MAO inhibitors:* Interfere with the metabolism of brompheniramine and thus prolong and intensify their central depressant and anticholinergic effects. Don't use together.
Other CNS depressants, such as antianxiety agents, barbiturates, sleeping aids, and tranquilizers: Additive CNS depression. Use together cautiously.
Sulfonylureas: Diminished effects of sulfonylureas. Recommend monitoring clinical effectiveness.
Heparin: Partially counteract the anticoagulant effects. Recommend monitoring partial thromboplastin time.
Drug-lifestyle. *Alcohol use:* Additive CNS depression may occur. Discourage use.

Effects on diagnostic tests
Discontinue drug 4 days before performing diagnostic skin tests; it can prevent, reduce, or mask positive skin test response.

Adverse reactions
CNS: dizziness, tremors, irritability, insomnia, *drowsiness, stimulation.*
CV: hypotension, palpitations, syncope.
GI: anorexia, nausea, vomiting, *dry mouth and throat.*
GU: urine retention.
Hematologic: ***thrombocytopenia, agranulocytosis.***
Skin: urticaria, rash.
Other: (after parenteral administration) local stinging, diaphoresis.

Overdose and treatment
Signs and symptoms of overdose may include either those of CNS depression (sedation, re-

duced mental alertness, apnea, and CV collapse) or of CNS stimulation (insomnia, hallucinations, tremors, or seizures). Anticholinergic symptoms, such as dry mouth, flushed skin, fixed and dilated pupils, and GI symptoms, are common, especially in children.

Treat overdose by inducing emesis with ipecac syrup (in conscious patients), followed by activated charcoal to reduce further drug absorption. Use gastric lavage if patient is unconscious or ipecac fails. Treat hypotension with vasopressors, and control seizures with diazepam or phenytoin I.V. Don't give stimulants.

Clinical considerations

Consider the recommendations relevant to all antihistamines as well as the following:

- Drug causes less drowsiness than some antihistamines.
- In patients with phenylketonuria; be aware some products contain aspartame.
- Store parenteral solutions and elixirs away from light and freezing temperatures; solution may crystallize if stored below 32° F (0° C). Crystals dissolve when warmed to 86° F (30° C).
- Injectable form (10 mg/ml) may be given diluted or undiluted.

Therapeutic monitoring

Recommend monitoring CBC in long-term therapy.

Special populations

Pregnant patients. Drug is used during first and second trimesters only when benefits outweigh the potential risks to the fetus, but not during the third trimester because of the risk of seizures in neonates.

Breast-feeding patients. Antihistamines such as brompheniramine shouldn't be used during breast-feeding. Many of these drugs are excreted in breast milk, exposing the infant to risks of unusual excitability, especially premature infants and other neonates, who may experience seizures.

Pediatric patients. Drug isn't indicated for use in newborns; children, especially those under age 6, may experience paradoxical hyperexcitability.

Geriatric patients. Geriatric patients are usually more sensitive to adverse effects of antihistamines and are especially likely to experience a greater degree of dizziness, sedation, hyperexcitability, dry mouth, and urine retention than younger patients. Symptoms usually respond to a decrease in medication dosage.

Patient counseling

Instruct patients who self-medicate not to exceed 24 mg/day (for adults and children age 12 and older) or 12 mg/day (for children age 6 to 11).

budesonide

Pulmicort Turbuhaler, Rhinocort

Pharmacologic classification: corticosteroid
Therapeutic classification: anti-inflammatory
Pregnancy risk category C

How supplied

Available by prescription only
Nasal inhaler: 32 mcg/metered dose (200 doses per container)
Oral inhalation powder: 200 mcg/dose (200 doses per container)

Indications and dosages

Management of symptoms of seasonal or perennial allergic rhinitis or nonallergic perennial rhinitis

Adults and children over age 6: 2 sprays in each nostril in the morning and evening or 4 sprays in each nostril in the morning. Maintenance dosage should be the fewest number of sprays needed to control symptoms. Doses exceeding 256 mcg/day (4 sprays/nostril) aren't recommended.

Note: If improvement doesn't occur within 3 weeks, discontinue treatment.

Chronic asthma

Adults: 200 to 400 mcg oral inhalation b.i.d. when previously used bronchodilators alone or inhaled corticosteroids; 400 to 800 mcg oral inhalation b.i.d. when previously used oral corticosteroids.

Children age 6 or over: Initially, 200 mcg oral inhalation b.i.d. Maximum dose is 400 mg b.i.d.

Pharmacodynamics

Anti-inflammatory action: Precise mechanism of action of corticosteroids like budesonide on allergic and nonallergic rhinitis isn't known. Corticosteroids show a wide range of inhibitory activities against multiple cell types (such as mast cells, eosinophils, neutrophils, macrophages, and lymphocytes) and mediators (such as histamine, eicosanoids, leukotrienes, and cytokines) involved in allergic and nonallergic, irritant-mediated inflammatory processes.

Pharmacokinetics

Absorption: The amount of an intranasal dose that reaches systemic circulation is generally low (about 20%).

Distribution: 88% protein-bound in the plasma; volume of distribution is 200 L.

Metabolism: Rapidly and extensively metabolized in the liver.

Excretion: Eliminated in urine (about 67%) and feces (about 33%).

Route	Onset	Peak	Duration
Inhalation	24 hr	1-2 wk	Unknown
Nasal	Unknown	Unknown	Unknown

Contraindications and precautions

Contraindicated in patients hypersensitive to drug or its components and in those who have had recent septal ulcers, nasal surgery, or nasal trauma until total healing has occurred.

Use cautiously in patients with tuberculosis infections; untreated fungal, bacterial, or systemic viral infections; or ocular herpes simplex.

Interactions

Drug-drug. *Other inhaled corticosteroids or alternate-day prednisone therapy:* May increase the risk of hypothalamic-pituitary-adrenal suppression. Monitor patient closely.
Ketoconazole: May increase plasma levels of budesonide. Monitor patient.

Effects on diagnostic tests

None reported.

Adverse reactions

CNS: *headache,* nervousness.
EENT: *nasal irritation, epistaxis, pharyngitis, sinusitis,* reduced sense of smell, nasal pain, hoarseness.
GI: taste perversion, dry mouth, dyspepsia, nausea, vomiting.
Respiratory: *cough,* candidiasis, wheezing, dyspnea.
Musculoskeletal: myalgia.
Skin: facial edema, rash, pruritus, contact dermatitis.
Other: ***hypersensitivity reactions***, weight gain.

Overdose and treatment

Acute overdose is unlikely as a result of the limited amount of product in each container. Chronic overdose may produce signs and symptoms of hyperadrenocorticism.

Clinical considerations

- Replacing a systemic corticosteroid with a topical corticosteroid can result in signs of adrenal insufficiency; in addition, some patients may experience symptoms of withdrawal, such as joint or muscular pain, lassitude, and depression.
- In patients with asthma or other clinical conditions requiring long-term systemic treatment, a too-rapid decrease in systemic corticosteroids may severely exacerbate symptoms.
- Excessive doses of budesonide or use of drug with other inhaled corticosteroids may lead to signs or symptoms of hyperadrenocorticism.

Therapeutic monitoring

- Carefully monitor patients previously treated for prolonged periods with systemic corticosteroids who are subsequently given topical glucocorticosteroids for acute adrenal insufficiency in response to stress.
- Because corticosteroids can affect growth, monitor children closely, weighing benefits of therapy against the possibility of growth suppression.
- Patients using budesonide for several months or longer should be examined for evidence of *Candida* infection or other signs of adverse effects on the nasal mucosa.

Special populations

Breast-feeding patients. Use cautiously when administering drug to breast-feeding women.
Pediatric patients. Safety and efficacy of drug for treating seasonal or perennial allergic rhinitis in children under age 6 haven't been established. Drug isn't recommended for treatment of nonallergic rhinitis in children because adequate numbers of such children haven't been studied.

Patient counseling

- Warn patient not to exceed prescribed dosage or to use for long periods because of risk of hypothalamic-pituitary-adrenal axis suppression.
- Tell patient to follow these instructions for the nasal inhaler: After opening aluminum pouch, use within 6 minutes. Shake canister well before using. Blow nose to clear nasal passages. Tilt head slightly forward; insert nozzle into nostril, pointing away from septum; hold other nostril closed; inspire gently; and spray. Shake canister again and repeat in other nostril. Store with valve downward. Don't store in area of high humidity. Don't break, incinerate, or store canister in extreme heat; contents under pressure.
- Instruct patient to hold the inhaler upright when loading Pulmicort Turbuhaler, not to blow or exhale into the inhaler nor shake it while loaded, and to hold inhaler upright while orally inhaling the dose. Place the mouthpiece between the lips and inhale forcefully and deeply.
- Assure patient that drug rarely causes nasal irritation or burning; advise patient to call if such symptoms recur.
- Warn patient to avoid exposure to chickenpox or measles, if at risk for contacting these diseases, and to consult doctor immediately if exposed.
- Teach patient good nasal and oral hygiene.
- Tell patient to call if condition worsens or if symptoms don't improve within 3 weeks.
- Inform patient that effects aren't immediate; response requires regular use.
- Inform patient that with use of oral inhaler improvement in asthma control can occur within 24 hours, with maximum benefit anticipat-

ed between 1 to 2 weeks and possibly taking longer.

☐ *ALERT:* Advise patient that Pulmicort Turbohaler isn't indicated for relief of acute bronchospasm.

bumetanide

Bumex

Pharmacologic classification: loop diuretic
Therapeutic classification: diuretic
Pregnancy risk category C

How supplied

Available by prescription only
Tablets: 0.5 mg, 1 mg, 2 mg
Injection: 0.25 mg/ml

Indications and dosages

Edema (heart failure, hepatic and renal disease); ◇postoperative edema; ◇premenstrual syndrome; ◇disseminated cancer
Adults: 0.5 to 2 mg P.O. once daily. If diuretic response isn't adequate, give a second or third dose at 4- to 5-hour intervals. Maximum dose is 10 mg/day. Give parenterally when oral route isn't feasible. Usual initial dose is 0.5 to 1 mg I.V. over 1 to 2 minutes or I.M. If response isn't adequate, give a second or third dose at 2- to 3-hour intervals. Maximum dose is 10 mg/day.

◇Pediatric heart failure
Children: 0.015 mg/kg every other day to 0.1 mg/kg daily. Use with extreme caution in neonates.

◇Hypertension
Adults: 0.5 mg P.O. daily. Oral maintenance of 1 to 4 mg daily; a maximum of 5 mg has been used in patients with normal renal function

≡***Dosage adjustment.*** In patients with impaired renal function, oral or I.V. dosages up to 20 mg have been administered despite manufacturer recommendations for a maximum of 10 mg/day for the management of edema.

Pharmacodynamics

Diuretic action: Loop diuretics inhibit sodium and chloride reabsorption in the proximal part of the ascending loop of Henle, promoting the excretion of sodium, water, chloride, and potassium; bumetanide produces renal and peripheral vasodilation and may temporarily increase glomerular filtration rate and decrease peripheral vascular resistance.

Pharmacokinetics

Absorption: After oral administration, 85% to 95% of dose is absorbed; food delays oral absorption. I.M. bumetanide is completely absorbed.

Distribution: About 92% to 96% protein-bound; it's unknown whether bumetanide enters CSF or breast milk or crosses the placenta.

Metabolism: Metabolized by the liver to at least five metabolites.

Excretion: Excreted in urine (80%) and feces (10% to 20%). Half-life ranges from 1 to 1½ hours.

Route	Onset	Peak	Duration
P.O.	½-1 hr	1-2 hr	4-6 hr
I.V.	Within minutes	15-30 min	½-1 hr
I.M.	40 min	Unknown	5-6 hr

Contraindications and precautions

Contraindicated in patients with hypersensitivity to drug or sulfonamides (possible cross-sensitivity), in those with anuria or hepatic coma, and in patients in states of severe electrolyte depletion.

Use cautiously in patients with hepatic cirrhosis and ascites and in those with depressed renal function.

Interactions

Drug-drug. *Other antihypertensive agents and other diuretics:* Bumetanide potentiates the hypotensive effects. These actions are used to therapeutic advantage.
Potassium-sparing diuretics (spironolactone, triamterene, amiloride): May decrease bumetanide-induced potassium loss. Recommend monitoring serum potassium levels.
Other potassium-depleting drugs such as steroids and amphotericin B: May cause severe potassium loss. Use together cautiously.
Lithium: Reduced renal clearance of lithium and increased lithium levels. Lithium dosage may require adjustment.
Indomethacin and probenecid: May reduce the diuretic effect of bumetanide. Their combined use isn't recommended; however, if there's no therapeutic alternative, an increased dose of bumetanide may be required.
Ototoxic or nephrotoxic drugs: May result in enhanced toxicity. Use together cautiously.

Effects on diagnostic tests

None reported.

Adverse reactions

CNS: dizziness, headache, vertigo.
CV: volume depletion and dehydration, orthostatic hypotension, ECG changes, chest pain.
EENT: transient deafness, tinnitus.
GI: nausea, vomiting, upset stomach, dry mouth, diarrhea, pain.
GU: ***renal failure,*** premature ejaculation, difficulty maintaining erection, oliguria.
Hematologic: azotemia, ***thrombocytopenia.***
Metabolic: hypokalemia; hypochloremic alkalosis; asymptomatic hyperuricemia; fluid and electrolyte imbalances, including dilutional

hyponatremia, hypocalcemia, hyperglycemia, and glucose intolerance impairment.
Musculoskeletal: weakness; arthritic pain; muscle pain and tenderness.
Skin: rash, pruritus, diaphoresis.

Overdose and treatment

Signs and symptoms of overdose include profound electrolyte and volume depletion, which may cause circulatory collapse.

Treatment of drug overdose is primarily supportive; replace fluid and electrolytes as needed.

Clinical considerations

Consider the recommendations relevant to all loop diuretics; give I.V. bumetanide slowly, over 1 to 2 minutes, for I.V. infusion; dilute bumetanide in D_5W, normal saline solution, or lactated Ringer's solution; use within 24 hours.

Therapeutic monitoring

- Recommend monitoring for clinical effect in renally and hepatic-impaired patients.
- With increased dosage, monitor for ototoxicity.
- Monitor for electrolyte imbalance, especially hypokalemia.

Special populations

Breast-feeding patients. Drug shouldn't be used in breast-feeding women.
Pediatric patients. Safety and efficacy in children under age 18 haven't been established.
Geriatric patients. Geriatric and debilitated patients require close observation because they're more susceptible to drug-induced diuresis. Excessive diuresis promotes rapid dehydration, hypovolemia, hypokalemia, and hyponatremia in these patients, and may cause circulatory collapse. Reduced dosages may be indicated.

Patient counseling

- Tell patient to take drug in the morning to prevent nocturia, and if second dose is prescribed, to take it in early afternoon.
- Instruct patient to take drug with food or milk.
- Advise patient to stand up slowly to prevent dizziness, and to limit alcohol intake and strenuous exercise in hot weather to avoid exacerbating orthostatic hypertension.
- Instruct patient to weigh himself daily to monitor fluid status.

buprenorphine hydrochloride

Buprenex

Pharmacologic classification: narcotic agonist-antagonist, opioid partial agonist
Therapeutic classification: analgesic
Controlled substance schedule V
Pregnancy risk category C

How supplied

Available by prescription only
Injection: 0.3 mg/ml in 1-ml ampules

Indications and dosages

Moderate to severe pain
Adults and children over age 13: 0.3 mg I.M. or slow I.V. q 6 hours, p.r.n. May repeat 0.3 mg 30 to 60 minutes after initial dose or increase to 0.6 mg per dose if necessary. S.C. administration isn't recommended.
◊*Adults:* 25 to 250 mcg/hour via I.V. infusion. (over 48 hours for postoperative pain)
◊*Adults:* 60 to 180 mcg via epidural injection.
◊***Reverse fentanyl-induced anesthesia***
Adults: 0.3 to 0.8 mg, I.V. or I.M., 1 to 4 hours after the induction of anesthesia and about 30 minutes before the end of surgery.
◊***Circumcision***
Children age 9 months to 9 years: 3 mcg/kg I.M. along with surgical anesthesia.

Pharmacodynamics

Analgesic action: Exact mechanisms of action of buprenorphine are unknown. It's believed to be a competitive antagonist at some opiate receptors and an agonist at others, thus relieving moderate to severe pain.

Pharmacokinetics

Absorption: Absorbed rapidly after I.M. administration.
Distribution: About 96% is protein-bound.
Metabolism: Metabolized in the liver.
Excretion: Duration of action is 6 hours. Excreted primarily in the feces as unchanged drug with about 30% excreted in urine.

Route	Onset	Peak	Duration
I.V.	Immediate	2 min	6 hr
I.M.	15 min	1 hr	6 hr

Contraindications and precautions

Contraindicated in patients with hypersensitivity to drug. Use cautiously in geriatric or debilitated patients and in patients with head injuries, increased intracranial pressure, and intracranial lesions; respiratory, kidney, or hepatic impairment; CNS depression or coma; thyroid irregularities; adrenal insufficiency; prostatic hyperplasia; urethral stricture; acute alcoholism; delirium tremens; or kyphoscoliosis.

Interactions

Drug-drug. *Barbiturate anesthetics such as thiopental:* Buprenorphine may produce additive CNS and respiratory depressant effects and, possibly, apnea. Use together cautiously.
CNS depressants (narcotic analgesics, antihistamines; phenothiazines, barbiturates, benzodiazepines, sedative-hypnotics), tricyclic antidepressants, and muscle relaxants: Potentiate the respiratory and CNS depression, sedation, and hypotensive effects. Reduced doses of buprenorphine are usually necessary.
General anesthetics: Severe CV depression. Use together cautiously.
MAO inhibitors: Additive effects. Use together cautiously.
Diazepam: Potential for respiratory and CV collapse. Avoid use together.
Drug-lifestyle. *Alcohol use:* May potentiate the respiratory and CNS depression, sedation, and hypotensive effects of the drug. Discourage use.

Effects on diagnostic tests

None reported.

Adverse reactions

CNS: *dizziness, sedation, headache,* confusion, nervousness, euphoria, *vertigo,* ***increased intracranial pressure.***
CV: *hypotension,* bradycardia, tachycardia, hypertension.
EENT: *miosis,* blurred vision.
GI: *nausea,* vomiting, constipation, dry mouth.
GU: urine retention.
Respiratory: ***respiratory depression,*** hypoventilation, dyspnea.
Skin: pruritus, *diaphoresis.*

Overdose and treatment

Safety of buprenorphine in acute overdose is expected to be better than that of other opioid analgesics because of its antagonist properties at high doses. Overdose may cause CNS depression, respiratory depression, and miosis (pinpoint pupils). Other acute toxic effects might include hypotension, bradycardia, hypothermia, shock, apnea, cardiopulmonary arrest, circulatory collapse, pulmonary edema, and seizures.

To treat acute overdose, first establish adequate respiratory exchange via a patent airway and ventilation as needed; administer a narcotic antagonist (naloxone) to reverse respiratory depression. Because the duration of buprenorphine is longer than that of naloxone, repeated naloxone dosing is necessary. Naloxone shouldn't be given unless the patient has clinically significant respiratory or CV depression. Monitor vital signs closely.

Naloxone doesn't completely reverse buprenorphine-induced respiratory depression; mechanical ventilation and higher than usual doses of naloxone and doxaprane may be indicated.

Provide symptomatic and supportive treatment (continued respiratory support, correction of fluid or electrolyte imbalance). Closely monitor laboratory parameters, vital signs, and neurologic status.

Clinical considerations

Consider the recommendations relevant to all opioid (narcotic) agonist-antagonists as well as the following:

- Adverse effects of drug may not be as readily reversed by naloxone as are those of pure agonists.
- Patients who become physically dependent on this drug may experience acute withdrawal syndrome if given an antagonist. Use with caution and monitor closely.
- Buprenorphine 0.3 mg is equal to 10 mg morphine or 75 to 100 mg meperidine in analgesic potency; duration of analgesia is longer than either.
- Use I.M. injection in adults not at risk for respiratory depression.
- Buprenorphine has been diluted to a concentration of 15 mcg/ml in 0.9% sodium chloride for continuous I.V. infusion. For epidural injection, drug has been diluted to a concentration of 6 to 30 mcg/ml in 0.9% sodium chloride.
- Store ampules between 59° and 86° F (15° and 30° C) and protect from light. Drug is incompatible with diazepam and lorazepam.

Therapeutic monitoring

Recommend monitoring for respiratory depression. Avoid use in patients with pulmonary impairment or compromised respiratory function.

Special populations

Breast-feeding patients. It's unknown if drug is excreted in breast milk; use with caution.
Pediatric patients. Buprenorphine has an unlabeled use as a supplement to anesthesia for children. Safety and efficacy hasn't been established in children under age 2.
Geriatric patients. Administer with caution; lower doses are usually indicated for geriatric patients, who may be more sensitive to the therapeutic and adverse effects of these drugs.

Patient counseling

- Teach patient to avoid activities that require full alertness.
- Instruct patient to avoid alcohol and other CNS depressants.

bupropion hydrochloride

Wellbutrin, Wellbutrin SR

Pharmacologic classification: aminoketone
Therapeutic classification: antidepressant
Pregnancy risk category B

How supplied

Available by prescription only
Tablets: 75 mg, 100 mg
Tablets (sustained-release): 100 mg, 150 mg

Indications and dosages

Depression
Adults: Initially, 100 mg P.O. b.i.d. or 75 mg P.O. t.i.d. If necessary, increase after 3 days to usual dosage of 100 mg P.O. t.i.d. (maximum dose). If no response occurs after several weeks of therapy, consider increasing dosage to 150 mg t.i.d. For sustained-release tablets, start with 150 mg P.O. q morning; increase to target dose of 150 mg P.O. b.i.d. as tolerated as early as day 4 of dosing. Maximum dose is 400 mg/day.

Pharmacodynamics

Antidepressant action: Mechanism of action is unknown. Bupropion doesn't inhibit MAO; it's a weak inhibitor of norepinephrine, dopamine, and serotonin reuptake.

Pharmacokinetics

Absorption: Only 5% to 20% is bioavailable in animal studies.
Distribution: At plasma levels up to 200 mcg/ml, appears to be about 80% bound to plasma proteins.
Metabolism: Metabolism is probably hepatic; several active metabolites have been identified. With prolonged use, the active metabolites are expected to accumulate in the plasma and their level may exceed that of the parent compound. Appears to induce its own metabolism.
Excretion: Excretion is primarily renal; elimination half-life of parent compound in single-dose studies ranged from 8 to 24 hours.

Route	Onset	Peak	Duration
P.O.	Unknown	2 hr	Unknown
P.O. (sustained)	Unknown	3 hr	Unknown

Contraindications and precautions

Contraindicated in patients with hypersensitivity to drug or seizure disorders and who have taken MAO inhibitors within previous 14 days. Also contraindicated in patients taking the smoking cessation drug Zyban, or those with history of bulimia or anorexia nervosa because of a higher incidence of seizures. Use cautiously in patients with recent MI, unstable heart disease, and renal or hepatic impairment.

Interactions

Drug-drug. *Levodopa, phenothiazines, MAO inhibitors, or tricyclic antidepressants or recent and rapid withdrawal of benzodiazepines:* May increase the risk of adverse effects, including seizures. Monitor patient closely.

Effects on diagnostic tests

None reported.

Adverse reactions

CNS: *headache,* ***seizures,*** anxiety, *confusion,* delusions, euphoria, hostility, impaired sleep quality, *insomnia, sedation, tremor,* akinesia, akathisia, *agitation, dizziness,* fatigue.
CV: ***arrhythmias,*** hypertension, hypotension, palpitations, syncope, *tachycardia.*
EENT: *auditory disturbances,* blurred vision.
GI: *dry mouth,* taste disturbance, increased appetite, *constipation,* dyspepsia, *nausea, vomiting, weight loss, anorexia, weight gain,* diarrhea.
GU: impotence, menstrual complaints, urinary frequency, decreased libido, urine retention.
Musculoskeletal: arthritis.
Skin: pruritus, rash, cutaneous temperature disturbance, *excessive diaphoresis.*
Other: fever, chills, hyperglycemia.

Overdose and treatment

Signs of overdose include labored breathing, salivation, arched back, ptosis, ataxia, and seizures. If ingestion was recent, empty the stomach using gastric lavage or induce emesis with ipecac, as appropriate; follow with activated charcoal. Treatment should be supportive. Control seizures with I.V. benzodiazepines; stuporous, comatose, or convulsing patients may need intubation. There are no data to evaluate the benefits of dialysis, hemoperfusion, or diuresis.

Clinical considerations

- Consider the inherent risk of suicide until significant improvement of depressive state occurs. High-risk patients should have close supervision during initial drug therapy. To reduce risk of suicidal overdose, prescribe the smallest quantity of tablets consistent with good management.
- Gradual increase of drug (no more than 75 mg/day to 100 mg/day q 2 to 3 days) reduces the risk of seizures and occurrences of agitation, motor restlessness, and insomnia.
- Many patients experience a period of increased restlessness, especially at initiation of therapy. This may include agitation, insomnia, and anxiety. In clinical studies, these symptoms required sedative-hypnotic agents in some patients; about 2% had to discontinue drug.
- Antidepressants can cause manic episodes during the depressed phase in patients with bipolar disorder.

- Investigational uses of drug include treatment of bipolar depression and attention deficit hyperactivity disorder in children.

Therapeutic monitoring
Recommend monitoring renal and hepatic function during therapy.

Special populations
Pediatric patients. Safety in children under age 18 hasn't been established.
Pregnant patients. Safety hasn't been established in pregnant women. Use drug only when absolutely necessary and use registry for monitoring outcomes: Bupropion Pregnancy Registry, 800-336-2176.
Breast-feeding patients. Because of the potential for serious adverse reactions in the infant, breast-feeding during therapy isn't recommended.

Patient counseling
- Advise patient to take drug regularly as scheduled, and to take each day's dosage in three divided doses, preferably at 6-hour intervals, to minimize risk of seizures.
- Warn patient to avoid the use of alcohol, which may contribute to the development of seizures.
- Advise patient to avoid activities that require alertness and coordination until CNS effects of drug are known.
- Tell patient not to chew, divide, or crush sustained-release tablets.
- Instruct patient not to take Zyban in combination with Wellbutrin, nor should he take other medications, including OTC medications, without medical approval.

bupropion hydrochloride
Zyban

Pharmacologic classification: aminoketone
Therapeutic classification: nonnicotine aid to smoking cessation
Pregnancy risk category B

How supplied
Available by prescription only
Tablets (sustained-release): 150 mg

Indications and dosages
Aid to smoking cessation treatment
Adults: 150 mg daily P.O. for 3 days; increased to maximum of 300 mg daily P.O. given as two doses of 150 mg taken at least 8 hours apart.

Note: Therapy is started while patient is still smoking; approximately 1 week is needed to achieve steady-state blood levels of drug. Patient should set target cessation date during second week of treatment. Course of treatment is usually 7 to12 weeks.

Pharmacodynamics
Smoking cessation action: Bupropion is a relatively weak inhibitor of the neuronal uptake of norepinephrine, serotonin, and dopamine, and doesn't inhibit MAO. The mechanism by which drug enhances the ability to abstain from smoking is unknown.

Pharmacokinetics
Absorption: Well absorbed after oral administration.
Distribution: Volume of distribution from a single 150-mg dose is estimated to be 1,950 L. 84% bound to plasma proteins at concentrations up to 200 mcg/ml.
Metabolism: Extensively metabolized in the liver mainly by the P-450 2B6 isoenzyme system to three active metabolites.
Excretion: Mean elimination half-life is thought to be about 21 hours. Following oral administration, 87% of a dose is recovered in the urine and 10% in the feces. The fraction of a dose excreted unchanged is 0.5%.

Route	Onset	Peak	Duration
P.O.	Unknown	3 hr	Unknown

Contraindications and precautions
Contraindicated in patients with seizure disorders or with a current or prior diagnosis of bulimia or anorexia nervosa because of potential for seizures.

Concurrent administration of MAO inhibitors is contraindicated; at least 14 days must elapse between discontinuation of an MAO inhibitor and starting bupropion therapy. Concurrent administration of Wellbutrin, Wellbutrin SR, or others medications containing bupropion is contraindicated because of potential for seizures. Also contraindicated in patients known to be allergic to drug or to its formulation.

Interactions
Drug-drug. *Drugs that affect enzyme metabolism, such as orphenadrine and cyclophosphamide:* May cause an interaction because bupropion is metabolized to hydroxybupropion by the CYP2B6 isoenzyme. Closely monitor patient.
Carbamazepine, phenobarbital, and phenytoin: Induced metabolism of bupropion. Closely monitor patient.
Cimetidine: Inhibited metabolism of bupropion. Closely monitor patient.
MAO inhibitors, phenelzine: Enhanced acute toxicity of bupropion. Avoid use together.
Levodopa: Higher incidence of adverse reactions in patients receiving concurrent administration. If concurrent use is necessary, give small initial doses of bupropion and gradually increase dose.
Antipsychotics, antidepressants, theophylline, systemic steroids, or treatment regimens (abrupt

withdrawal of benzodiazepines): Lower seizure threshold. Use together cautiously.

Effects on diagnostic tests
None reported.

Adverse reactions
CNS: agitation, dizziness, hot flashes, *insomnia,* somnolence, tremor.
CV: ***complete AV block***, hypertension, hypotension, tachycardia.
EENT: *dry mouth,* taste perversion.
GI: anorexia, dyspepsia, increased appetite.
GU: impotence, polyuria, urinary frequency and urgency.
Metabolic: edema, weight gain.
Musculoskeletal: arthralgia, leg cramps and twitching, myalgia, neck pain.
Respiratory: bronchitis, ***bronchospasm.***
Skin: dry skin, pruritus, rash, urticaria.
Other: ***allergic reactions,*** hyperglycemia.

Overdose and treatment
Hospitalization is recommended for overdoses. If patient is conscious, induce vomiting with syrup of ipecac. Activated charcoal may also be administered every 6 hours for first 12 hours. Perform ECG and EEG monitoring for first 48 hours. Provide adequate fluid intake and obtain baseline tests.

If patient is stuporous, comatose, or experiencing seizures, airway intubation is recommended before undertaking gastric lavage. Gastric lavage may be beneficial within first 12 hours after ingestion because drug absorption may not be complete. Although diuresis, dialysis, or hemoperfusion is sometimes used to treat drug overdose, there is no experience with their use in managing bupropion overdose. Based on animal studies, seizures can be treated with an I.V. benzodiazepine and other supportive measures.

Clinical considerations
- Because drug use is associated with a dose-dependent risk of seizures, don't exceed 300 mg daily for smoking cessation.
- If patient hasn't made progress toward abstinence by week 7 of therapy, stop therapy because it's unlikely that he'll quit smoking.
- Dose doesn't have to be tapered when stopping treatment.

Therapeutic monitoring
- Recommend monitoring patient for development of hypertension when bupropion is used in combination with transdermal nicotine.
- Recommend monitoring renal and hepatic functions.

Special populations
Pregnant patients. Drug isn't for use in pregnant women.
Breast-feeding patients. Drug and its metabolites are secreted in breast milk. Because of the potential for serious adverse reactions in the infant, a choice must be made between breast-feeding and drug therapy.
Pediatric patients. Safety and efficacy in children haven't been established.
Geriatric patients. Experience in patients age 60 and older was similar to that in younger patients.

Patient counseling
- Stress importance of combining behavioral interventions, counseling, and support services with drug therapy.
- Explain to the patient that risk of seizures is increased if the patient has a seizure or eating disorder (bulimia or anorexia nervosa), exceeds the recommended dose, or takes other medications containing bupropion.
- Instruct patient to take doses at least 8 hours apart.
- Inform patient that drug is usually taken for 7 to 12 weeks.
- Advise patient that, although he may continue to smoke during drug therapy, it reduces his chance of breaking the smoking habit.
- Tell patient that drug and nicotine patch should only be used together under medical supervision because his blood pressure may increase.

buspirone hydrochloride
BuSpar

Pharmacologic classification: azaspirodecanedione derivative
Therapeutic classification: antianxiety
Pregnancy risk category B

How supplied
Available by prescription only
Tablets: 5 mg, 10 mg

Indications and dosages
Management of anxiety disorders
Adults: Initially, 5 mg P.O. t.i.d. Dosage may be increased at 3-day intervals. Usual maintenance dosage is 20 to 30 mg daily in divided doses. Don't exceed 60 mg/day.

Pharmacodynamics
Anxiolytic action: Buspirone is an azaspirodecanedione derivative with anxiolytic activity. It suppresses conflict and aggressive behavior and inhibits conditioned avoidance responses. Its precise mechanism of action hasn't been determined, but it appears to depend on simultaneous effects on several neurotransmitters and receptor sites: decreasing serotonin neuronal activity, increasing norepinephrine metabolism, and partial action as a presynaptic dopamine antagonist. Studies sug-

gest an indirect effect on benzodiazepine gamma-aminobutyric acid (GABA)-chloride receptor complex or GABA receptors, or on other neurotransmitter systems.

Buspirone isn't pharmacologically related to benzodiazepines, barbiturates, or other sedative and anxiolytic agents. It exhibits a nontraditional clinical profile and is uniquely anxiolytic. It has no anticonvulsant or muscle relaxant activity and doesn't appear to cause physical dependence or significant sedation.

Pharmacokinetics

Absorption: Absorbed rapidly and completely after oral administration, but extensive first-pass metabolism limits absolute bioavailability to 1% to 13% of the oral dose. Food slows absorption but increases the amount of unchanged drug in systemic circulation.
Distribution: 95% protein-bound; it doesn't displace other highly protein-bound medications such as warfarin.
Metabolism: Metabolized in the liver by hydroxylation and oxidation, resulting in at least one pharmacologically active metabolite, 1, pyrimidinylpiperazine (1-PP).
Excretion: 29% to 63% is excreted in urine in 24 hours, primarily as metabolites; 18% to 38% is excreted in feces.

Route	Onset	Peak	Duration
P.O.	Unknown	40-90 min	Unknown

Contraindications and precautions

Contraindicated in patients hypersensitive to drug or within 14 days of therapy with an MAO inhibitor. Use cautiously in patients with renal or hepatic impairment.

Interactions

Drug-drug. *MAO inhibitors:* Elevated blood pressure. Avoid use together.
Digoxin: Buspirone may displace digoxin from serum-binding sites when the drugs are used together. Recommend monitoring digoxin levels.
CNS depressants: Increased sedation. Avoid use together.
Haloperidol: Increased serum haloperidol levels. Recommend decreased doses of haloperidol.
Drug-lifestyle. *Alcohol use:* Increased sedation may result. Discourage alcohol use.

Effects on diagnostic tests

None reported.

Adverse reactions

CNS: *dizziness, drowsiness,* nervousness, insomnia, headache, light-headedness, fatigue, numbness.
EENT: blurred vision.
GI: dry mouth, nausea, diarrhea, abdominal distress.

Overdose and treatment

Signs of overdose include severe dizziness, drowsiness, unusual constriction of pupils, and stomach upset, including nausea and vomiting.

Treatment of overdose is symptomatic and supportive; empty stomach with immediate gastric lavage. Monitor respiration, pulse, and blood pressure. No specific antidote is known. Effect of dialysis is unknown.

Clinical considerations

- Buspirone has been used investigationally to treat nonmelancholic depression and parkinsonian syndrome.
- Patients previously given benzodiazepines may not show good clinical response to this agent.
- Although buspirone doesn't appear to cause tolerance or physical or psychological dependence, the possibility exists that a patient prone to drug abuse may experience these effects.
- Buspirone doesn't block the withdrawal syndrome associated with benzodiazepines or other common sedative and hypnotic agents; therefore, these agents should be withdrawn gradually before replacement with buspirone therapy.
- Store tablets in tight, light-resistant containers at temperatures less than 86° F (30° C).

Therapeutic monitoring

Recommend monitoring hepatic and renal function. Hepatic and renal impairment impedes metabolism and excretion of drug and may lead to toxic accumulation; dosage reduction may be necessary.

Special populations

Breast-feeding patients. Buspirone and its metabolites are excreted in the breast milk of rats; however, the extent of excretion in human milk is unknown. Avoid using buspirone in breast-feeding women.

Patient counseling

- Advise patient to take drug exactly as prescribed; explain that therapeutic effect may not occur for 2 weeks or more. Warn patient not to double the dose if one is missed, but to take a missed dose as soon as possible, unless it's almost time for next dose.
- Caution patient to avoid hazardous tasks requiring alertness until the effects of the drug are known. The effects of alcohol and other CNS depressants, such as antihistamines, sedatives, tranquilizers, sleeping aids, prescription pain medication, barbiturates, seizure medicine, muscle relaxants, anesthetics, and medicines for colds, coughs, hay fever, or allergies, may be enhanced by additive sedation and drowsiness caused by buspirone.
- Tell patient to store drug away from heat and light and out of the reach of children.

- Explain importance of regular follow-up visits to check progress. Urge patient to report adverse reactions immediately.
- Inform patient that results may not be seen in 3 to 4 weeks; however, an improvement may be noted within 7 to 10 days.

busulfan

Myleran, Busulfex

Pharmacologic classification: alkylating agent (cell cycle-phase nonspecific)
Therapeutic classification: antineoplastic
Pregnancy risk category D

How supplied

Available by prescription only
Tablets (scored): 2 mg
Injection for I.V. infusions: 6 mg/ml

Indications and dosages

Dosage and indications may vary. Check package insert for recommended protocol.

Chronic myelogenous leukemia
Adults: For remission induction, usual dosage is 4 to 8 mg P.O. daily; however, may range from 1 to 12 mg P.O. daily (0.06 mg/kg or 1.8 mg/m^2). For maintenance therapy, 1 to 3 mg P.O. daily.
Children: 0.06 to 0.12 mg/kg or 1.8 to 4.6 mg/m^2 P.O. daily. Dosage should be adjusted to maintain WBC count of about 20,000/mm^3.

◊***Myelofibrosis***
Adults: Initially, 2 to 4 mg P.O. daily then followed by the same dose two to three times weekly.

Allogenic hematopoietic stem cell transplantation
Adults: 0.8 mg/kg of ideal body weight or actual body weight (whichever is lower) I.V. q 6 hr for 4 consecutive days for a total of 16 doses. Give phenytoin for seizure prophylaxis.

Pharmacodynamics

Antineoplastic action: Busulfan is an alkylating agent that exerts its cytotoxic activity by interfering with DNA replication and RNA transcription, causing a disruption of nucleic acid function.

Pharmacokinetics

Absorption: Well absorbed from the GI tract.
Distribution: Distribution into the brain and CSF is unknown.
Metabolism: Metabolized in the liver.
Excretion: Cleared rapidly from the plasma. Drug and its metabolites are excreted in urine.

Route	Onset	Peak	Duration
P.O.	1-2 wk	Unknown	Unknown

Contraindications and precautions

Contraindicated in patients whose chronic myelogenous leukemia has demonstrated prior resistance to drug. Also contraindicated in patients with chronic lymphocytic leukemia or acute leukemia and in those in "blastic" crisis of chronic myelogenous leukemia.

Use cautiously in patients recently given other myelosuppressants or radiation treatment; in those with depressed neutrophil or platelet counts, head trauma, and seizures; or in patients taking other medications that reduce seizure threshold.

Interactions

None reported.

Effects on diagnostic tests

Drug-induced cellular dysplasia may interfere with interpretation of cytologic studies.

Adverse reactions

CNS: unusual tiredness or weakness, fatigue.
EENT: cataracts.
GI: cheilosis, dry mouth, anorexia.
GU: gynecomastia, profound hyperuricemia caused by increased cell lysis.
Hematologic: ***leukopenia*** (WBC count decreasing after about 10 days and continuing to decrease for 2 weeks after stopping drug), ***thrombocytopenia, anemia, severe pancytopenia.***
Respiratory: ***irreversible pulmonary fibrosis*** (commonly called *busulfan lung).*
Skin: alopecia, *transient hyperpigmentation,* rash, urticaria, anhidrosis, jaundice.
Other: Addison-like wasting syndrome.

Overdose and treatment

Signs and symptoms of overdose include hematologic manifestations, such as leukopenia and thrombocytopenia.

Treatment is supportive and includes transfusion of blood components and antibiotics for infections that may develop.

Clinical considerations

- Avoid all I.M. injections when platelets are less than 100,000/mm^3.
- Patient response (increased appetite, sense of well-being, decreased total leukocyte count, reduction in size of spleen) usually begins 1 to 2 weeks after initiating the drug.
- Pulmonary fibrosis may be delayed for 4 to 6 months.
- Persistent cough and progressive dyspnea with alveolar exudate may result from drug toxicity, not pneumonia. Instruct patient to report symptoms so dosage adjustments can be made.
- Minimize hyperuricemia by adequate hydration, alkalinization of urine, and administration of allopurinol.

Therapeutic monitoring

- Observe patient for signs or symptoms of infection, such as fever and sore throat.
- Monitor uric acid, CBC, and kidney function.
- Recommend monitoring serum alkaline phosphatase, bilirubin, and serum aminotransferase concentrations for potential hepatotoxicity
- Recommend monitoring leukocyte count; the manufacturer recommends discontinuing busulfan when the leukocyte count is 15,000/mm³ or less.

Special populations

Pregnant patients. Busulfan may cause fetal harm (malformations, bone marrow depression, fetal growth retardation, and fetal death). Also, drug may impair fertility. Avoid use.
Breast-feeding patients. It isn't known if drug is distributed into breast milk. However, potential for mutagenicity, carcinogenicity, and serious adverse reactions in the infant should be taken into consideration when a decision to breast-feed is made.

Patient counseling

- Advise patient to use caution when taking aspirin-containing products and to promptly report any sign of bleeding.
- Tell patient to take medication at the same time each day.
- Emphasize importance of continuing to take medication despite nausea and vomiting.
- Instruct patient about the signs and symptoms of infection and tell him to report them promptly if they occur.
- Advise patient to use contraceptive methods during therapy.

butoconazole nitrate

Femstat

Pharmacologic classification: synthetic imidazole derivative
Therapeutic classification: topical fungistat
Pregnancy risk category C

How supplied

Available by prescription only
Vaginal cream: 2% supplied with applicators

Indications and dosages

Vulvovaginal candidiasis (moniliasis)
Adults (nonpregnant): One applicatorful intravaginally h.s. for 3 days (may be extended to 6 days if necessary).
Adults (pregnant): One applicatorful intravaginally h.s. for 6 days. Use only during second or third trimester.

Pharmacodynamics

Antifungal action: Although the exact mechanism is unknown, it's thought that butoconazole controls or destroys fungi by disrupting the permeability of the cell membrane and reducing its osmotic pressure resistance. Drug is active against many fungi, including dermatophytes and yeasts. It's also active in vitro against some gram-positive bacteria.

Pharmacokinetics

Absorption: About 5.5% is absorbed through the vaginal walls.
Distribution: Unknown.
Metabolism: Systemically absorbed drug appears to be metabolized, probably in the liver.
Excretion: Systemically absorbed drug appears to be excreted in the urine and feces.

Route	Onset	Peak	Duration
Intravaginal	Unknown	Unknown	Unknown

Contraindications and precautions

Contraindicated in patients hypersensitive to drug.

Interactions

None reported.

Effects on diagnostic tests

None reported.

Adverse reactions

GU: vulvovaginal burning and itching, soreness, and swelling.
Skin: finger itching.

Overdose and treatment

No information available.

Clinical considerations

- Ascertain that patient understands directions for use and length of therapy.
- Drug may be used together with oral contraceptives and antibiotic therapy.
- Store drug at room temperature.

Therapeutic monitoring

Advise monitoring for recurrent infection; may be caused by resistant strains (*Candida albicans, Candida glabrata*) or underlying disease (HIV, diabetes mellitus), or pregnancy.

Special populations

Pregnant patients. Drug isn't for use during the first trimester.
Pediatric patients. Drug isn't for use in children under age 12 for self-medication.
Breast-feeding patients. Use drug with caution in breast-feeding women because it's unknown if it's excreted in breast milk.

Patient counseling

- Instruct patient to follow the directions enclosed in the package, to insert the applicator high into the vagina, and to wash hands after use.
- Tell patient to complete the full course of therapy, including through menstrual period. However, advise her to avoid using tampons during treatment.
- Advise patient to refrain from sexual contact or to have partner use a condom to avoid reinfection during therapy.
- Tell patient to use a sanitary napkin to prevent staining clothing and to absorb discharge.
- Tell patient to report symptoms that persist after full course of therapy.

butorphanol tartrate

Stadol, Stadol NS

Pharmacologic classification: narcotic agonist-antagonist; opioid partial agonist
Therapeutic classification: analgesic, adjunct to anesthesia
Controlled substance schedule IV
Pregnancy risk category C

How supplied

Available by prescription only
Injection: 1 mg/ml, 1-ml vials; 2 mg/ml, 1-ml, 2-ml, and 10-ml vials
Nasal spray: 10 mg/ml

Indications and dosages

Moderate to severe pain
Adults: 1 to 4 mg I.M. q 3 to 4 hours, p.r.n.; or 0.5 to 2 mg I.V. q 3 to 4 hours, p.r.n., or around-the-clock. Alternatively, give 1 mg by nasal spray (1 spray in one nostril). Repeat if pain relief is inadequate after 60 to 90 minutes. Repeat q 3 to 4 hours, p.r.n. For severe pain, an initial 2 mg by nasal spray (1 spray in each nostril). Repeat no more than q 3 to 4 hours, p.r.n.
Pain during labor
Adults: 1 to 2 mg I.M. or I.V. q 4 hours but not 4 hours before delivery.
Preoperative anesthesia
Adults: 2 mg I.M. 60 to 90 minutes before surgery or 2 mg I.V. shortly before induction.
≡***Dosage adjustment.*** Patients with hepatic or renal impairment and geriatric patients should receive one-half of the usual parenteral adult dose at 6 hour intervals as needed. For nasal spray, the initial dose (1 spray in 1 nostril) is the same, but repeat dose is in 90 to 120 minutes, if needed. Repeat doses thereafter q 6 hours, p.r.n.

Pharmacodynamics

Analgesic action: The exact mechanisms of action of butorphanol are unknown. Drug is believed to be a competitive antagonist at some, and an agonist at other, opiate receptors, thus relieving moderate to severe pain. Like narcotic agonists, it causes respiratory depression, sedation, and miosis.

Pharmacokinetics

Absorption: Well absorbed after I.M. administration.
Distribution: Rapidly crosses the placenta, and neonatal serum levels are 0.4 to 1.4 times maternal levels.
Metabolism: Metabolized extensively in the liver, primarily by hydroxylation, to inactive metabolites.
Excretion: Excreted in inactive form, mainly by the kidneys. About 11% to 14% of a parenteral dose is excreted in feces.

Route	Onset	Peak	Duration
I.V.	2-3 min	30-60 min	3-4 hr
I.M.	10-15 min	30-60 min	3-4 hr
Nasal	15 min	1-2 hr	4-5 hr

Contraindications and precautions

Contraindicated in patients receiving repeated doses of narcotic medications or with narcotic addiction; may precipitate withdrawal syndrome. Also contraindicated in patients with hypersensitivity to drug or to the preservative benzethonium chloride.

Use cautiously in emotionally unstable patients and in those with history of drug abuse, head injuries, increased intracranial pressure, acute MI, ventricular dysfunction, coronary insufficiency, respiratory disease or depression, and renal or hepatic dysfunction.

Interactions

Drug-drug. *Barbiturate anesthetics such as thiopental:* Additive CNS and respiratory depressant effects and, possibly, apnea. Closely monitor patient.
Cimetidine: May potentiate butorphanol toxicity, causing disorientation, respiratory depression, apnea, and seizures. Use cautiously and be prepared to administer a narcotic antagonist if toxicity occurs.
Other CNS depressants (narcotic analgesics, antihistamines, phenothiazines, barbiturates, benzodiazepines, sedative-hypnotics, tricyclic antidepressants, muscle relaxants): Potentiate respiratory and CNS depression, sedation, and hypotensive effects. Reduced doses of butorphanol are usually necessary.
General anesthetics: Severe CV depression. Avoid use together.

Rifampin, phenytoin, digitoxin: Drug accumulation and enhanced effects. Recommend reduced butorphanol dose.
Narcotic antagonists: Patients who become physically dependent on opioids may experience acute withdrawal syndrome. Use with caution and monitor patient closely.
Pancuronium: May increase conjunctival changes. Monitor patient.
Drug-lifestyle. *Alcohol use:* May potentiate respiratory and CNS depression, sedation, and hypotensive effects of the drug. Don't use together.

Effects on diagnostic tests
None reported.

Adverse reactions
CNS: *confusion,* nervousness, lethargy, headache, *somnolence, dizziness, insomnia,* anxiety, paresthesia, euphoria, hallucinations, flushing, ***increased intracranial pressure.***
CV: palpitations, vasodilation, hypotension.
EENT: blurred vision, *nasal congestion* (with nasal spray), tinnitus, taste perversion.
GI: *nausea, vomiting, constipation,* anorexia.
Respiratory: ***respiratory depression.***
Skin: rash, hives, *clamminess, excessive diaphoresis.*
Other: sensation of heat.

Overdose and treatment
No information available.

Clinical considerations
Consider the recommendations relevant to all opioid (narcotic) agonist-antagonists as well as the following:
- Patients using nasal formulation for severe pain may initiate therapy with 2 mg (one spray in each nostril) provided they remain recumbent. Dose isn't repeated for 3 to 4 hours.
- Mild withdrawal symptoms have been reported with chronic use of the injectable form.

Therapeutic monitoring
- Drug has the potential to be abused. Recommend close supervision in emotionally unstable patients and in those with history of drug abuse when long-term therapy is necessary.
- Recommend monitoring patient for respiratory depression.

Special populations
Pregnant patients. Safe use during pregnancy (except during labor) hasn't been established.
Breast-feeding patients. Use of drug in breast-feeding women isn't recommended.
Pediatric patients. Safety and efficacy in children under age 18 haven't been established.
Geriatric patients. Lower doses are usually indicated for geriatric patients because they may be more sensitive to the therapeutic and adverse effects of the drug. Plasma half-life is increased by 25% in patients over age 65.

Patient counseling
Teach patient how to use nasal spray. Patient should use one spray in one nostril unless otherwise directed.

C

calcipotriene
Dovonex

Pharmacologic classification: synthetic vitamin D_3 analogue
Therapeutic classification: topical antipsoriatic
Pregnancy risk category C

How supplied
Available by prescription only
Cream, ointment, solution: 0.005%

Indications and dosages
Moderate plaque psoriasis
Adults: Apply a thin layer to affected skin b.i.d. Rub in gently and completely.

Pharmacodynamics
Antipsoriatic action: Calcipotriene is a synthetic vitamin D_3 analogue that binds to vitamin D_3 receptors in skin cells (keratinocytes), regulating skin cell production and development.

Pharmacokinetics
Absorption: About 6% of the applied dose of calcipotriene is absorbed systemically when the ointment is applied topically to psoriasis plaques or 5% when applied to normal skin.
Distribution: Vitamin D and its metabolites are transported in the blood, bound to specific plasma proteins, to many parts of the body containing keratinocytes. (The scaly red patches of psoriasis are caused by the abnormal growth and production of keratinocytes.)
Metabolism: Drug metabolism after systemic uptake is rapid and occurs via a pathway similar to the natural hormone. The primary metabolites are much less potent than the parent compound.
Excretion: The active form of the vitamin, 1,25-dihydroxy vitamin D_3 (calcitriol), is recycled via the liver and excreted in bile.

Route	Onset	Peak	Duration
Topical	Unknown	Unknown	Unknown

Contraindications and precautions
Contraindicated in patients hypersensitive to drug or its components. Also contraindicated in patients with hypercalcemia or evidence of vitamin D toxicity. Use cautiously in breast-feeding patients and in the elderly. Drug shouldn't be used on the face.

Interactions
None reported.

Effects on diagnostic tests
None reported.

Adverse reactions
Metabolic: hypercalcemia.
Skin: *burning, pruritus, irritation,* atrophy, dermatitis, dry skin, erythema, folliculitis, hyperpigmentation, peeling, rash, worsening of psoriasis.

Overdose and treatment
Topically applied calcipotriene can be absorbed in sufficient amounts to produce systemic effects. Serum calcium levels may increase with excessive use.

Clinical considerations
- Drug is for topical dermatologic use only. It isn't intended for ophthalmic, oral, or intravaginal use.
- Improvement usually begins after 2 weeks of therapy and marked improvement occurs after 8 weeks; only about 10% of cases show complete clearing.
- Safety and effectiveness of topical calcipotriene in dermatoses other than psoriasis haven't been established.
- Use of calcipotriene may cause irritation of lesions and surrounding uninvolved skin. If irritation develops, discontinue drug.

Therapeutic monitoring
Transient, rapidly reversible elevation of serum calcium level may occur. If serum calcium level increases outside the normal range, discontinue treatment until normal calcium levels are restored.

Special populations
Breast-feeding patients. It isn't known if drug is excreted in breast milk. Use caution when administering calcipotriene ointment to a breast-feeding patient.
Pediatric patients. Safety and effectiveness in children haven't been established.
Geriatric patients. Adverse dermatologic effects of topical calcipotriene may be more severe in patients over age 65.

Patient counseling
■ Tell patient that drug is for external use only, as directed, and to avoid contact with the face or eyes.
■ Instruct patient to wash hands thoroughly after application.
■ Tell patient to report signs of local adverse reactions.

calcitonin
Calcimar (salmon), Miacalcin (salmon), Osteocalcin (salmon), Salmonine (salmon)

Pharmacologic classification: thyroid hormone
Therapeutic classification: hypocalcemic
Pregnancy risk category C

How supplied
Available by prescription only
Injection: 200-IU/ml, 2-ml vials (salmon)
Nasal spray: 200 IU/activation

Indications and dosages
Paget's bone disease (osteitis deformans)
Adults: Initially, 100 IU salmon calcitonin S.C. or I.M. daily. Maintenance dosage is 50 to 100 IU salmon calcitonin, three times weekly.
Hypercalcemia
Adults: 4 IU/kg calcitonin (salmon) I.M. or S.C. q 12 hours; increase by 8 IU/kg q 12 hours, or ◊ 2 to 16 IU/kg I.V. infusion q 12 hours.
Postmenopausal osteoporosis
Adults: 100 IU calcitonin (salmon) S.C. or I.M. daily, or 200 IU (one spray) daily in alternating nostril.
◊ ***Osteogenesis imperfecta***
Adults: 2 IU/kg calcitonin (salmon) three times weekly, with daily calcium supplementation.

Pharmacodynamics
Hypocalcemic action: Calcitonin directly inhibits the bone resorption of calcium. This effect is mediated by drug-induced increase of cAMP concentration in bone cells, which alters transport of calcium and phosphate across the plasma membrane of the osteoclast. A secondary effect occurs in the kidneys, where calcitonin directly inhibits tubular resorption of calcium, phosphate, and sodium, thereby increasing their excretion. A clinical effect may not be seen for several months in patients with Paget's disease.

Pharmacokinetics
Absorption: Drug can be administered parenterally or nasally. Plasma levels of 0.1 to 0.4 mg/ml are achieved within 15 minutes of a 200-IU S.C. dose. The maximum effect is seen in 2 to 4 hours; duration of action may be 8 to 24 hours for S.C. or I.M. doses, and ½ to 12 hours for I.V. doses. Peak plasma levels appear 31 to 39 minutes after using the nasal form.
Distribution: It's unknown if drug enters the CNS or crosses the placenta.
Metabolism: Rapid metabolism occurs in the kidney, with additional activity in the blood and peripheral tissues.
Excretion: Excreted in urine as inactive metabolites.

Route	Onset	Peak	Duration
I.M., S.C.	15 min	4 hr	8-24 hr
Intranasal	Rapid	½ hr	1 hr
I.V.	Immediate	2-4 hr	½-12 hr

Contraindications and precautions
Contraindicated in patients hypersensitive to salmon calcitonin.

Interactions
None reported.

Effects on diagnostic tests
None reported.

Adverse reactions
CNS: headache, weakness, dizziness, paresthesia.
CV: edema of feet, chills, chest pressure, shortness of breath.
EENT: eye pain, nasal congestion.
GI: *transient nausea,* unusual taste, diarrhea, anorexia, *vomiting,* epigastric discomfort, abdominal pain.
GU: *increased urinary frequency,* nocturia.
Skin: *facial flushing,* rash, pruritus of ear lobes, *inflammation at injection site.*
Other: hypersensitivity reactions ***(anaphylaxis),*** tender palms and soles.

Overdose and treatment
Signs and symptoms of overdose include hypocalcemia and hypocalcemic tetany. This usually occurs in patients at higher risk during the first few doses. Parenteral calcium will correct the symptoms and should be readily available.

Clinical considerations
S.C. route is the preferred method of administration.

Therapeutic monitoring
■ Consider a skin test using salmon calcitonin before initiating therapy with it. If patient has allergic reactions to foreign proteins, test for hypersensitivity before therapy. Systemic allergic reactions are possible because hormone is a protein. Keep epinephrine readily available.
■ Keep parenteral calcium available during the first doses in case of hypocalcemic tetany.
■ Periodically monitor serum calcium levels during therapy.
■ Observe patient for signs of hypocalcemic tetany during therapy (muscle twitching, tetan-

ic spasms, and convulsions if hypocalcemia is severe).

- Watch for signs of hypercalcemic relapse: Bone pain, renal calculi, polyuria, anorexia, nausea, vomiting, thirst, constipation, lethargy, bradycardia, muscle hypotonicity, pathologic fracture, psychosis, and coma. Patient with good initial clinical response to calcitonin who suffers relapse should be evaluated for antibody formation response to the hormone protein.
- Refrigerate solution. Once activated, store nasal spray upright at room temperature.

Special populations

Pregnant patients. Use with caution.
Breast-feeding patients. Use with caution.
Pediatric patients. There are inadequate data to support the use of calcitonin in pediatric patients.

Patient counseling

- Instruct patient on self-administration of drug and assist him until proper technique is achieved.
- Tell patient to handle missed doses as follows:

Daily dosing: Take as soon as possible; don't double the doses.
Every other day dosing: Take as soon as possible, then restart the alternate days from this dose.

- Stress importance of regular follow-up to assess progress.
- If given for postmenopausal osteoporosis, remind patient to take adequate calcium and vitamin D supplements.
- Instruct patient using the nasal spray to activate pump before using.
- Tell patient to report nasal irritation. Perform periodic nasal examination.

calcitriol

Calcijex, Rocaltrol

Pharmacologic classification: vitamin D analogue
Therapeutic classification: antihypocalcemic
Pregnancy risk category C

How supplied

Available by prescription only
Capsules: 0.25 mcg, 0.5 mcg
Injection: 1 mcg/ml, 2 mcg/ml
Oral solution: 1 mcg/ml

Indications and dosages

Management of hypocalcemia in patients undergoing chronic dialysis

Oral

Adults: Initially, 0.25 mcg P.O. daily. Dosage may be increased by 0.25 mcg daily at 4- to 8-week intervals. Maintenance dosage, 0.25 mcg every other day up to 0.5 to 1 mcg P.O. daily.

Parenteral

Adults: 0.5 mcg I.V. three times weekly, about every other day. Dosage may be increased by 0.25 to 0.5 mcg at 2- to 4-week intervals. Maintenance dosage, 0.5 to 3 mcg I.V. three times weekly.

Management of hypoparathyroidism and pseudohypoparathyroidism

Adults and children age 6 and older: Initially, 0.25 mcg P.O. daily in the morning. Dosage may be increased at 2- to 4-week intervals. Maintenance dosage, 0.5 to 2 mcg daily.
Children age 1 to 5 (hypoparathyroidism only): 0.25 to 0.75 mcg P.O. daily.

Prevention or management of secondary hyperparathyroidism and resultant metabolic bone disease in predialysis patients (moderate to severe chronic renal failure with creatinine clearance of 15 to 55 ml/minute)

Adults and children age 3 and older: Initially, 0.25 mcg P.O. daily. Dosage may be increased to 0.5 mcg/day if necessary.
Children under age 3: Initially, 10 to 15 ng/kg P.O. daily.

◊ ***Psoriasis vulgaris***

Adults: 0.5 mcg/day P.O. for 6 months and topically (0.5 mcg/g petroleum) daily for 8 weeks.

Pharmacodynamics

Antihypocalcemic action: Calcitriol is a vitamin D analogue (1,25-dihydroxycholecalciferol), or activated cholecalciferol. It promotes absorption of calcium from the intestine by forming a calcium-binding protein. It reverses the signs of rickets and osteomalacia in patients who can't activate or use ergocalciferol or cholecalciferol. In patients with renal failure, it reduces bone pain, muscle weakness, and parathyroid serum levels.

Pharmacokinetics

Absorption: Absorbed readily after oral administration.
Distribution: Distributed widely and is protein-bound.
Metabolism: Metabolized in the liver and kidney, with a half-life of 3 to 8 hours. No activation step is required.
Excretion: Excreted primarily in the feces.

Route	Onset	Peak	Duration
P.O.	2-6 hr	3-6 hr	3-5 days
I.V.	Immediate	Unknown	3-5 days

Contraindications and precautions

Contraindicated in patients with hypercalcemia or vitamin D toxicity. Withhold all preparations containing vitamin D.

Interactions

Drug-drug. *Cardiac glycosides:* Increased risk of arrhythmias. Avoid use together.

Orlistat: Decreases absorption of vitamin D. Give at least 2 hours apart.
Cholestyramine, mineral oil, and colestipol: May alter calcitriol absorption. Avoid use together.
Corticosteroids: May counteract the effects of vitamin D analogues. Don't use together.
Magnesium-containing antacids: May induce hypermagnesemia, especially in patients with chronic renal failure. Avoid use together.

Effects on diagnostic tests
None reported.

Adverse reactions
CNS: headache, somnolence, weakness, irritability, psychosis (rare).
CV: hypertension, ***arrhythmias.***
EENT: conjunctivitis, photophobia, rhinorrhea.
GI: nausea, vomiting, constipation, polydipsia, pancreatitis, metallic taste, dry mouth, anorexia.
GU: polyuria, nocturia.
Musculoskeletal: bone and muscle pain.
Skin: pruritus.
Other: weight loss, hyperthermia, nephrocalcinosis, decreased libido.

Note: Vitamin D intoxication is associated with hypercalcemia.

Overdose and treatment
Treatment of hypercalcemia (a sign of overdose) requires discontinuation of drug, institution of a low-calcium diet, increased fluid intake, and supportive measures. Calcitonin administration may help reverse hypercalcemia. In severe cases, death has followed CV and renal failure.

Clinical considerations
- Calcitriol therapy may falsely elevate cholesterol determinations made using the Zlatkis-Zak reaction. It also alters serum alkaline phosphatase concentrations and may alter electrolytes, such as magnesium, phosphate, and calcium in serum and urine.
- Protect drug from heat and light.

Therapeutic monitoring
- Monitor serum calcium levels several times weekly after initiating therapy.
- There is some evidence that monitoring urine calcium and urine creatinine is very helpful in screening for hypercalciuria. The ratio of urine calcium to urine creatinine should be less than or equal to 0.18. A value of more than 0.2 suggests hypercalciuria, and the dose should be decreased regardless of serum calcium level. The product of serum calcium times phosphate shouldn't be allowed to exceed 70.

Special populations
Breast-feeding patients. Very little drug is excreted in breast milk; however, the effect of vitamin D levels exceeding the recommended daily allowance in infants isn't known. Therefore, large doses shouldn't be administered to breast-feeding women.
Pediatric patients. Some infants may be hyperreactive to drug. Long-term treatment has been well-tolerated except for occasional episodes of electrolyte imbalance, which resolves with alteration of therapy.

Patient counseling
- Instruct patient on the importance of a calcium-rich diet.
- Tell patient that drug must not be taken by anyone for whom it wasn't prescribed. It's the most potent form of vitamin D.
- Advise patient to report adverse reactions immediately.
- Tell patient to avoid magnesium-containing antacids and other self-prescribed drugs.

calcium salts

calcium acetate
Phos-Ex, PhosLo

calcium carbonate
Alka-mints, Amitone, Calciday-667, Cal-Plus, Caltrate 600, Chooz, Os-Cal 500, Rolaids, Titralac, Tums, Tums E-X

calcium chloride

calcium citrate
Citracal

calcium glubionate
Neo-Calglucon

calcium gluceptate

calcium gluconate

calcium lactate

calcium phosphate, tribasic
Posture

Pharmacologic classification: calcium supplement
Therapeutic classification: therapeutic agent for electrolyte balance, cardiotonic
Pregnancy risk category C

How supplied
Available by prescription only
calcium chloride
Injection: 10% solution (1 g/10 ml; each ml of solution provides 27.2 mg or 1.36 mEq of calcium) in 10-ml ampules, vials, and syringes

calcium gluceptate
Injection: 1.1 g/5 ml ampules or 50-ml vials for preparation of I.V. admixtures (each ml of solution provides 18 mg or 0.9 mEq of calcium)
calcium gluconate
Injection: 10% solution (1 g/10 ml; each ml of solution provides 9.3 mg or 0.46 mEq of calcium) in 10-ml ampules and vials, or 20-ml vials

Available without a prescription
calcium acetate
Tablets: 250 mg (62.5 mg of calcium), 668 mg (167 mg of calcium), 1,000 mg (250 mg of calcium)
Capsules: 500 mg
calcium carbonate
Tablets: 500 mg, 650 mg, 667 mg, 1.25 g, 1.5 g
Tablets (chewable): 350 mg, 420 mg, 500 mg, 750 mg, 835 mg, 850 mg, 1.25 g
Oral suspension: 1.25 g (500 mg of calcium) per 5 ml
Capsules: 1.25 g (500 mg of calcium), 1.5 g (600 mg of calcium)
Powder: 6.5 g
calcium citrate
Tablets: 950 mg (contains 200 mg of elemental calcium/g)
Tablets (effervescent): 2,376 mg (500 mg of calcium)
calcium glubionate
Syrup: 1.8 g/5 ml (contains 115 mg of elemental calcium/g)
calcium gluconate
Tablets: 500 mg, 650 mg, 975 mg, 1 g (contains 90 mg of elemental calcium/g)
calcium lactate
Tablets: 325 mg, 650 mg (contains 130 mg of elemental calcium/g)
calcium phosphate, tribasic
Tablets: 600 mg

Indications and dosages

Emergency treatment of hypocalcemia
calcium chloride
Adults: 500 mg to 1 g I.V. slowly (not to exceed 1 ml/minute).
Children: 0.2 ml/kg I.V. slowly (not to exceed 1 ml/minute).
calcium gluconate
Adults: 7 to 14 mEq I.V. slowly (not to exceed 0.7 to 1.8 mEq/minute).
Children: 1 to 7 mEq I.V. slowly (not to exceed 0.7 to 1.8 mEq/minute).
Repeat above dosage based on clinical laboratory value.
Cardiotonic use
calcium chloride
Adults: 500 mg to 1 g I.V. slowly (not to exceed 1 ml/minute); or 200 to 800 mg intraventricularly as a single dose.
Hyperkalemia
calcium gluconate
Adults: 2.25 to 14 mEq I.V. slowly. Adjust administration based on ECG response.
Hypermagnesemia
calcium chloride
Adults: 500 mg I.V. initially, repeated based on clinical response.
calcium gluceptate
Adults: 2 to 5 ml I.M., or 5 to 20 ml I.V.
calcium gluconate
Adults: 4.5 to 9 mEq I.V. slowly.
During exchange transfusions
Adults: 1.35 mEq I.V. concurrently with each 100-ml citrated blood exchange.
Neonates: 0.45 mEq I.V. after every 100 ml of citrated blood exchange.
Hypocalcemia
calcium acetate
Adults: 2 to 4 tablets P.O. with meals.
calcium gluconate
Adults: For hypocalcemic tetany, 4.5 to 16 mEq I.V. until therapeutic response is obtained.
Children: For hypocalcemic tetany, 0.5 to 0.7 mEq/kg I.V. t.i.d. or q.i.d. or until tetany is controlled.
Neonates: 2.4 mEq/kg/day in divided doses until therapeutic response is obtained.
calcium lactate
Adults: 325 mg to 1.3 g P.O. t.i.d. with meals.
Osteoporosis prevention
Adults: 1 to 1.5 g P.O. daily of elemental calcium.
Hyperphosphatemia in end-stage renal failure
calcium acetate
Adults: 2 to 4 tablets P.O. with each meal.

Pharmacodynamics

Calcium replacement: Calcium is essential for maintaining the functional integrity of the nervous, muscular, and skeletal systems, and for cell membrane and capillary permeability. Calcium salts are used as a source of calcium cation to treat or prevent calcium depletion in patients in whom dietary measures are inadequate. Conditions associated with hypocalcemia are chronic diarrhea, vitamin D deficiency, steatorrhea, sprue, pregnancy and lactation, menopause, pancreatitis, renal failure, alkalosis, hyperphosphatemia, and hypoparathyroidism.

Pharmacokinetics

Absorption: I.M. and I.V. calcium salts are absorbed directly into the bloodstream. Oral dose is absorbed actively in the duodenum and proximal jejunum and, to a lesser extent, in the distal part of the small intestine. Calcium is absorbed only in the ionized form. Pregnancy and reduction of calcium intake may increase the efficiency of absorption. Vitamin D in its active form is required for calcium absorption.
Distribution: Enters the extracellular fluid and is incorporated rapidly into skeletal tissue. Bone contains 99% of the total calcium; 1% is distributed equally between the intracellular and extracellular fluids. CSF levels are about 50% of serum calcium levels.

Metabolism: None significant.
Excretion: Excreted mainly in the feces as unabsorbed calcium that was secreted through bile and pancreatic juice into the lumen of the GI tract. Most calcium entering the kidney is reabsorbed in the loop of Henle and the proximal and distal convoluted tubules. Only small amounts of calcium are excreted in the urine.

Route	Onset	Peak	Duration
P.O.	Unknown	Unknown	Unknown
I.V.	Immediate	Immediate	½-2 hr

Contraindications and precautions

Contraindicated in patients with ventricular fibrillation, hypercalcemia, hypophosphatemia, or renal calculi. Use cautiously in patients with sarcoidosis, renal or cardiac disease, cor pulmonale, respiratory acidosis, or respiratory failure and in digitalized patients.

Interactions

Drug-drug. *Atenolol, fluoroquinolones, tetracyclines:* Decreased bioavailability of these agents and calcium when oral preparations are taken together. Separate administration times.
Cardiac glycosides: Increase digitalis toxicity; administer calcium cautiously, if at all, to digitalized patients.
Calcium channel blocker drugs (*verapamil*): Decreased calcium effectiveness. Avoid use together.
Phenytoin: Decreases absorption of both drugs. Avoid use together. Monitor levels closely if use together is required.
Sodium polystyrene sulfonate: Risk of metabolic acidosis in patients with renal disease. Avoid use together.
Thiazide diuretics: Risk of hypercalcemia. Avoid use together.
Drug-lifestyle. *Tobacco use, alcohol use:* May affect calcium absorption. Discourage use together.
Drug-food. *Foods containing oxalic acid (rhubarb, spinach), phytic acid (bran, whole cereals), and phosphorus (milk, dairy products):* May interfere with calcium absorption. Avoid use together.
Caffeine: May affect calcium absorption. Advise patient to avoid caffeine-containing beverages.

Effects on diagnostic tests

I.V. calcium may produce transient elevation of plasma 11-hydroxycorticosteroid levels (Glen-Nelson technique) and false-negative values for serum and urine magnesium as measured by the Titan yellow method.

Adverse reactions

CNS: tingling sensations, sense of oppression or heat waves, headache, irritability, weakness (with I.V. use); syncope (with rapid I.V. injection).
CV: mild decrease in blood pressure; vasodilation, bradycardia, ***arrhythmias, cardiac arrest*** (with rapid I.V. injection).
GI: irritation, hemorrhage, *constipation* (with oral use); chalky taste, rebound hyperacidity, nausea (with I.V. use); hemorrhage, *nausea,* vomiting, thirst, abdominal pain (with oral calcium chloride).
GU: hypercalcemia, polyuria, renal calculi.
Skin: local reactions including burning, necrosis, tissue sloughing, cellulitis, soft tissue calcification (with I.M. use).
Other: pain and irritation (with S.C. injection); *vein irritation* (with I.V. use).

Overdose and treatment

Acute hypercalcemia syndrome is characterized by a markedly elevated plasma calcium level, lethargy, weakness, nausea and vomiting, and coma, and may lead to sudden death.

In case of overdose, discontinue calcium immediately. After oral ingestion of calcium overdose, treatment includes removal by emesis or gastric lavage followed by supportive therapy, as needed.

Clinical considerations

- Monitor ECG when giving calcium I.V. Give such injections slowly at a rate dependent on salt form used. Stop injection if patient complains of discomfort.
- Give calcium chloride I.V. only.
- I.V. route is recommended in children, but not by scalp vein because calcium salts can cause tissue necrosis.
- Administer I.V. calcium slowly through a small-bore needle into a large vein to avoid extravasation and necrosis.
- After I.V. injection, patient should be recumbent for 15 minutes to prevent orthostasis.
- If perivascular infiltration occurs, discontinue I.V. immediately. Venospasm may be reduced by administering 1% procaine hydrochloride and hyaluronidase to the affected area.
- Use I.M. route only in emergencies when no I.V. route is available. Give I.M. injections in the gluteal region in adults, lateral thigh in infants.

Therapeutic monitoring

- Monitor serum calcium levels frequently, especially in patients with renal impairment.
- Hypercalcemia may result when large doses are given to patients with chronic renal failure.
- Severe necrosis and tissue sloughing may occur after extravasation. Calcium gluconate is less irritating to veins and tissue than calcium chloride.
- Assess Chvostek's and Trousseau's signs periodically to check for tetany.
- If GI upset occurs with oral calcium, give 2 to 3 hours after meals.

- With oral product, patient may need laxatives or stool softeners to manage constipation.
- Monitor for symptoms of hypercalcemia (nausea, vomiting, headache, mental confusion, anorexia), and report them immediately. Calcium absorption of an oral dose is decreased in patients with certain disease states such as achlorhydria, renal osteodystrophy, steatorrhea, or uremia.

Special populations
Breast-feeding patients. Calcium passes into breast milk, but not in quantities large enough to affect the breast-feeding infant.
Pediatric patients. Administer calcium cautiously to children by I.V. route (usually not administered I.M.).
Geriatric patients. Calcium absorption (after oral administration) may be decreased in geriatric patients.

Patient counseling
- Tell patient not to exceed the manufacturer's recommended dosage of calcium.
- Warn patient not to use bone meal or dolomite as a source of calcium; they may contain lead.
- Advise patient to avoid tobacco and to limit intake of alcohol and caffeine-containing beverages.

candesartan cilexetil
Atacand

Pharmacologic classification: selective angiotensin II receptor antagonist
Therapeutic classification: antihypertensive
Pregnancy risk category C (D in second and third trimesters)

How supplied
Available by prescription only
Tablets: 4 mg, 8 mg, 16 mg, 32 mg

Indications and dosages
Treatment of hypertension (used alone or in combination with other antihypertensive agents)
Adults: Initially, 16 mg P.O. once daily when used as monotherapy; usual dosage range is 8 to 32 mg P.O. daily as a single dose or divided b.i.d.

Pharmacodynamics
Antihypertensive action: Inhibits the vasoconstrictor and aldosterone-secreting effects of angiotensin II by selectively blocking the binding of angiotensin II to the AT_1 receptor in many tissues, such as vascular smooth muscle and the adrenal gland.

Pharmacokinetics
Absorption: Rapidly and completely bioactivated during absorption from the GI tract.
Distribution: Highly bound to plasma proteins (more than 99%).
Metabolism: Undergoes minor hepatic metabolism.
Excretion: Primarily recovered in the urine and feces. Elimination half life is about 9 hours.

Route	Onset	Peak	Duration
P.O.	Unknown	3-4 hr	24 hr

Contraindications and precautions
Contraindicated in patients with hypersensitivity to drug or its ingredients.

Use cautiously in patients whose renal function depends on the renin-angiotensin-aldosterone system (such as patients with heart failure) because there's potential for oliguria and progressive azotemia with acute renal failure or death. Also use cautiously in patients who are volume- or salt-depleted because there is potential for symptomatic hypotension. Start therapy with a lower dosage range, as ordered, and monitor blood pressure carefully.

Interactions
None reported.

Effects on diagnostic tests
None reported.

Adverse reactions
CNS: dizziness, fatigue, headache.
CV: chest pain, peripheral edema.
EENT: pharyngitis, rhinitis, sinusitis.
GI: abdominal pain, diarrhea, nausea, vomiting.
GU: albuminuria.
Musculoskeletal: arthralgia, back pain.
Respiratory: coughing, bronchitis, upper respiratory tract infection.

Overdose and treatment
The most likely signs of overdose are hypotension, dizziness, and tachycardia; bradycardia could occur from parasympathetic (vagal) stimulation. Treatment should be supportive. Dialysis isn't effective.

Clinical considerations
- Drugs that act directly on the renin-angiotensin system (such as candesartan) can cause fetal and neonatal morbidity and death when administered to pregnant women. These problems haven't been detected when exposure was limited to first trimester. If pregnancy is suspected, discontinue drug immediately.

Therapeutic monitoring
- If hypotension occurs after a dose of candesartan, place patient in the supine position

and, if necessary, give an I.V. infusion of normal saline.

- Most of the antihypertensive effect is present within 2 weeks. Maximal antihypertensive effect is obtained within 4 to 6 weeks. Diuretic may be added if blood pressure isn't controlled by drug alone.

Special populations

Pregnant patients. Inform woman of childbearing age of the consequences of second and third trimester exposure to drug. Advise her to notify doctor immediately if pregnancy is suspected.
Breast-feeding patients. It isn't known if drug is excreted in breast milk; therefore, breastfeeding during drug therapy isn't recommended.
Pediatric patients. Safety and efficacy in pediatric patients haven't been established.
Geriatric patients. Serum levels of drug are higher in elderly persons than in younger adults; however, the drug and its inactive metabolite don't accumulate in the serum of geriatric patients after repeated once-daily dosing.

Patient counseling

- Instruct patient to store medication at room temperature and to keep container tightly sealed.
- Inform patient to report adverse reactions without delay.
- Tell patient that drug may be taken without regard to meals.

capecitabine

Xeloda

Pharmacologic classification: fluoropyrimidine carbamate
Therapeutic classification: antineoplastic
Pregnancy risk category D

How supplied

Available by prescription only
Tablets: 150 mg, 500 mg

Indications and dosages

Treatment of patients with metastatic breast cancer resistant to both paclitaxel and an anthracycline-containing chemotherapy regimen or resistant to paclitaxel and for whom further anthracycline therapy isn't indicated
Adults: 2,500 mg/m^2 P.O. daily in two divided doses (about 12 hours apart) at end of a meal for 2 weeks, followed by a 1-week rest period and given as 3-week cycles.
≡ ***Dosage adjustment.*** National Cancer Institute of Canada (NCIC) Common Toxicity Criteria:

NCIC grade 2: First appearance, interrupt treatment until resolved to grade 0 to 1, then restart at 100% of starting dose for next cycle; second appearance, interrupt treatment until resolved to grade 0 to 1 and use 75% of starting dose for next cycle; third appearance, interrupt treatment until resolved to grade 0 to 1 and use 50% of starting dose for next cycle; fourth appearance, discontinue treatment permanently.

NCIC grade 3: First appearance, interrupt treatment until resolved to grade 0 to 1 and use 75% of starting dose for next cycle; second appearance, interrupt treatment until resolved to grade 0 to 1 and use 50% of starting dose for next cycle; third appearance, discontinue treatment permanently.

NCIC grade 4: First appearance, discontinue treatment permanently or interrupt treatment until resolved to grade 0 to 1 and use 50% of starting dose for next cycle.

Note: Toxicity criteria relate to degrees of severity of diarrhea, nausea, vomiting, stomatitis, and hand/foot syndrome. Refer to capecitabine package insert for specific toxicity definitions.

Pharmacodynamics

Antineoplastic action: Capecitabine is converted to the active drug 5-fluorouracil (5-FU). 5-FU is metabolized by both normal and tumor cells to metabolites that cause cellular injury by way of two different mechanisms: interference with DNA synthesis to inhibit cell division and interference with RNA processing and protein synthesis.

Pharmacokinetics

Absorption: Readily absorbed from the GI tract. The rate and extent of absorption are decreased with food.
Distribution: About 60% is bound to plasma proteins.
Metabolism: Extensively metabolized to 5-FU (an active metabolite).
Excretion: Elimination half-life of the parent drug and the active moiety is about 45 minutes with 70% excreted in the urine.

Route	Onset	Peak	Duration
P.O.	Unknown	1½-2 hr	Unknown

Contraindications and precautions

Contraindicated in patients with known hypersensitivity to 5-FU. Severe diarrhea can occur; monitor electrolytes and proper hydration. Use cautiously in the elderly and in patients with history of coronary artery disease, mild-to-moderate hepatic dysfunction resulting from liver metastases, hyperbilirubinemia, and renal insufficiency. Capecitabine therapy may need to be interrupted or decreased if hand-and-foot syndrome (characterized by numbness, paresthesia, tingling, painless or painful swelling, erythema, desquamation, blistering, and severe pain of hands or feet, hyperbilirubinemia, and severe nausea) occurs.

Interactions

Drug-drug: *Leucovorin:* Increased concentration of 5-FU with enhanced toxicity. Patient requires close monitoring.
Antacids: Increased rate of absorption of capecitabine. Dosage change may be necessary.
Coumadin: Altered PT and bleeding with use together. Monitor patient closely.

Effects on diagnostic tests

None reported.

Adverse reactions

CNS: dizziness, *fatigue,* headache, insomnia, *paresthesia.*
CV: edema.
EENT: eye irritation.
GI: *diarrhea, nausea, vomiting, stomatitis, abdominal pain, constipation, anorexia,* intestinal obstruction, *dyspepsia.*
Hematologic: **NEUTROPENIA, THROMBOCYTOPENIA,** *anemia, lymphopenia.*
Hepatic: *hyperbilirubinemia.*
Musculoskeletal: myalgia, pain in limb.
Skin: *hand-and-foot syndrome, dermatitis,* nail disorder.
Other: *pyrexia,* dehydration.

Overdose and treatment

Overdose should be managed by supportive medical care aimed at correcting the clinical signs and symptoms. Dialysis may be of benefit in drug removal.

Clinical considerations

- Store tablets at room temperature. Keep container tightly closed.
- Tablets should be taken within 30 minutes after a meal.
- Inform doctor if patient is taking folic acid or warfarin.

Therapeutic monitoring

- Altered coagulation parameters and bleeding may occur within several days up to several months after initiating therapy and, rarely, within one month after stopping capecitabine therapy.
- Fluid and electrolyte replacement may be needed for severe diarrhea.
- Drug may need to be immediately interrupted until diarrhea resolves or decreases in intensity.
- Hyperbilirubinemia may require discontinuing drug.
- Monitor patient carefully for toxicity. Toxicity may be managed by symptomatic treatment, dose interruptions, and dosage adjustments.

Special populations

Pregnant patients. Due to teratogenic effects, women of child-bearing age should avoid becoming pregnant while taking capecitabine.
Breast-feeding patients. Patients should discontinue breast-feeding while on drug therapy.
Pediatric patients. Safety and efficacy in patients under 18 years of age haven't been established.
Geriatric patients. Patients over age 80 may experience a greater incidence of GI adverse effects.

Patient counseling

- Inform patient and caregiver of expected adverse effects of drug, especially nausea, vomiting, diarrhea, and hand-and-foot syndrome (pain, swelling or redness of hands or feet). Tell them that patient-specific dose adaptations during therapy are expected and necessary.
- Instruct patient to stop taking drug and contact health care provider immediately if the following adverse effects occur: diarrhea (more than four bowel movements daily or diarrhea at night), vomiting (two to five episodes in a 24-hour period), nausea, appetite loss or decrease in amount of food taken each day, stomatitis (pain, redness, swelling, or sores in mouth), hand-and-foot syndrome, temperature of 100.5° F (38° C) or greater, or other evidence of infection.
- Tell patient that most adverse effects improve within 2 to 3 days after stopping drug. If they don't improve, tell him to contact doctor.
- Tell patient how to take the drug. Drug is usually taken for 14 days followed by a 7-day rest period (no drug) given as a 21-day cycle. The doctor determines the number of treatment cycles.
- Instruct patient to take drug with water within 30 minutes after end of a meal (breakfast and dinner).
- If a combination of tablets is prescribed, teach patient importance of correctly identifying the tablets to avoid possible misdosing.
- For missed doses, instruct patient not to take the missed dose and not to double the next one. Instead, he should continue with regular dosing schedule and check with the doctor.
- Instruct patient to inform doctor if he's taking the vitamin folic acid.
- Advise women of childbearing age to avoid becoming pregnant while receiving treatment.

captopril

Capoten

Pharmacologic classification: ACE inhibitor
Therapeutic classification: antihypertensive, adjunctive treatment of heart failure
Pregnancy risk category C (D second and third trimesters)

How supplied

Available by prescription only
Tablets: 12.5 mg, 25 mg, 50 mg, 100 mg

Indications and dosages

Mild to severe hypertension; ◇ idiopathic edema; ◇ Raynaud's phenomenon

Adults: Initially, 25 mg P.O. b.i.d. or t.i.d.; if necessary, dosage may be increased to 50 mg b.i.d. or t.i.d. after 1 to 2 weeks; if control is still inadequate after 1 to 2 weeks more, a diuretic may be added. Dosage may be increased to a maximum of 150 mg t.i.d. (450 mg/day) while continuing the diuretic. Daily dose may be given b.i.d.

Heart failure

Adults: 25 mg P.O. t.i.d. If patient is on a diuretic, is hyponatremic or hypovolemic, an initial dose of 6.25 to 12.5 mg t.i.d. should be given. Maintenance dosage is 50 to 100 mg t.i.d.

Prevention of diabetic nephropathy

Adults: 25 mg P.O. t.i.d.

Left ventricular dysfunction after MI

Adults: Give 6.25 mg P.O. as a single dose 3 days after an MI; then 12.5 mg t.i.d., increasing dose to 25 mg t.i.d. Target dose is 50 mg t.i.d.

≡ ***Dosage adjustment.*** In the elderly and in patients with renal failure, use lower initial daily doses and smaller increments for adjustment.

Pharmacodynamics

Antihypertensive action: Captopril inhibits ACE, preventing conversion of angiotensin I to angiotensin II, a potent vasoconstrictor. Reduced formation of angiotensin II decreases peripheral arterial resistance, which results in decreased aldosterone secretion, thus reducing sodium and water retention and lowering blood pressure.

Cardiac load–reducing action: Captopril decreases systemic vascular resistance (afterload) and pulmonary capillary wedge pressure (preload), thus increasing cardiac output in patients with heart failure.

Pharmacokinetics

Absorption: 60% to 75% of an oral dose is absorbed through the GI tract; food may reduce absorption by up to 40%. Antihypertensive effect begins in 15 minutes. Maximum therapeutic effect may require several weeks.

Distribution: Distributed into most body tissues except CNS; drug is about 25% to 30% protein-bound.

Metabolism: About 50% is metabolized in the liver.

Excretion: Excreted primarily in urine; small amounts are excreted in feces. Duration of effect is usually 2 to 6 hours, increasing with higher doses. Elimination half-life is less than 3 hours. Duration of action may be increased in patients with renal dysfunction.

Route	Onset	Peak	Duration
P.O.	¼-1 hr	1-1½ hr	6-12 hr

Contraindications and precautions

Contraindicated in patients with hypersensitivity to drug or other ACE inhibitors. Use cautiously in patients with impaired renal function, renal artery stenosis, or serious autoimmune diseases (especially lupus erythematosus) and in those taking drugs that affect WBC counts or immune response.

Interactions

Drug-drug. *Antacids*: Decrease the effects of captopril and should be given at different dose intervals.

Digoxin: May increase serum digoxin concentration by 15% to 30%. Patient requires close monitoring.

Diuretics or other antihypertensive drugs: Risk of excessive hypotension. Diuretics may need to be discontinued or captopril dosage lowered.

Insulin, oral antidiabetic agents: Risk of hypoglycemia when captopril therapy is initiated. Monitor patient closely.

Lithium: Increased lithium levels and symptoms of toxicity may occur. Monitor patient closely.

NSAIDs: May decrease the antihypertensive effect of captopril. Monitor patient closely.

Potassium-sparing diuretics, potassium supplements: Increased risk of hyperkalemia. Avoid these agents unless hypokalemic blood levels are confirmed.

Drug-herb. *Black catechu* may cause additional hypotensive effects. Avoid use together.

Effects on diagnostic tests

Captopril may cause false-positive results for urinary acetone.

Adverse reactions

CNS: dizziness, fainting, headache, malaise, fatigue.

CV: *tachycardia, hypotension,* angina pectoris.

GI: anorexia, *dysgeusia,* nausea, vomiting, abdominal pain, constipation, dry mouth, transient elevated liver enzyme.

Hematologic: ***leukopenia, agranulocytosis, pancytopenia,*** anemia, ***thrombocytopenia.***

Hepatic: transient increase in hepatic enzymes.

Metabolic: hyperkalemia.

Respiratory: *dry, persistent, tickling, nonproductive cough,* dyspnea.

Skin: *urticarial rash, maculopapular rash,* pruritus, alopecia.

Other: fever, ***angioedema of face and extremities.***

Overdose and treatment

A sign of overdose is severe hypotension. After acute ingestion, stomach must be emptied by induced emesis or gastric lavage. Follow with activated charcoal to reduce absorption. Subsequent treatment is usually symptomatic and supportive. In severe cases, hemodialysis may be considered.

Clinical considerations

- Diuretic therapy is usually discontinued 2 to 3 days before beginning ACE inhibitor therapy, to reduce risk of hypotension; if drug doesn't adequately control blood pressure, diuretics may be reinstated.

Therapeutic monitoring

- WBC and differential counts should be done before treatment, every 2 weeks for 3 months, and periodically thereafter; serum potassium levels must be checked because of potassium retention.
- Lower dosage or reduced dosing frequency is necessary in patients with impaired renal function. Adjust drug to effective levels over a 1- to 2-week interval, then reduce dosage to lowest effective level.
- Several weeks of therapy may be required before the beneficial effects of captopril are seen.
- Proteinuria and nephrotic syndrome may occur in patients.

Special populations

Pregnant patients. Because ACE inhibitors can cause fetal harm or death, discontinue drug use as soon as pregnancy is detected.
Breast-feeding patients. Captopril is distributed into breast milk, but its effect on breast-feeding infants is unknown; use drug with caution in breast-feeding women.
Pediatric patients. Safety and efficacy in children haven't been established; use only if potential benefit outweighs risk.
Geriatric patients. Geriatric patients may need lower doses because of impaired drug clearance. They also may be more sensitive to the hypotensive effects of captopril.

Patient counseling

- Instruct patient to call doctor immediately if pregnancy occurs.
- Tell patient to report feelings of light-headedness, especially in first few days, so dosage can be adjusted; signs of infection, such as sore throat or fever, because drug may decrease WBC count; facial swelling or difficulty breathing, because drug may cause angioedema; and loss of taste, which may necessitate discontinuing drug.
- Instruct patient to take captopril 1 hour before meals to prevent decreased absorption.
- Advise patient to avoid sudden position changes to minimize orthostatic hypotension.
- Warn patient to seek medical approval before taking OTC cold preparations.
- Tell patient that a persistent, dry cough may occur and usually doesn't subside until medication is stopped. Call prescriber if this effect becomes bothersome.

carbamazepine

Atretol, Carbatrol, Epitol, Tegretol

Pharmacologic classification: iminostilbene derivative; chemically related to tricyclic antidepressants
Therapeutic classification: anticonvulsant, analgesic
Pregnancy risk category D

How supplied

Available by prescription only
Tablets: 200 mg
Tablets (chewable): 100 mg
Tablets (extended-release): 100 mg, 200 mg, 400 mg
Capsules (extended-release): 200 mg, 300 mg
Oral suspension: 100 mg/5 ml

Indications and dosages

Generalized tonic-clonic, complex-partial, mixed seizure patterns
Adults and children over age 12: 200 mg P.O. b.i.d., or 100 mg P.O. q.i.d. of suspension, on day 1. May increase by 200 mg/day P.O. at weekly intervals, in divided doses at 6- to 8-hour intervals. Adjust to minimum effective level when control is achieved; don't exceed 1,000 mg/day in children age 12 to 15, or 1,200 mg/day in those over age 15. In rare instances, doses up to 1,600 mg/day have been used in adults.

For extended-release capsules, initial dose, 200 mg P.O. b.i.d. Increase at weekly intervals by up to 200 mg/day until optimal response is obtained. Dose shouldn't exceed 1,000 mg/day in children age 12 to 15 and 1,200 mg/day in patients over age 15. Some adult doses may be up to 1,600 mg/day. Maintenance dosage is usually 800 to 1,200 mg/day.
Children age 6 to 12: Initially, 100 mg P.O. b.i.d., or 50 mg P.O. q.i.d. of suspension. Increase at weekly intervals by adding 100 mg P.O. daily, first using a t.i.d. schedule and then q.i.d. if necessary. Adjust dosage based on patient response. Generally, dose shouldn't exceed 1,000 mg/day. Children taking total daily dose of immediate-release form of 400 mg or more may be converted to same total daily dose of extended-release capsules using a b.i.d. regimen.
Children under age 6: Initially, 10 to 20 mg/kg/day P.O. b.i.d. or t.i.d. as tablets or q.i.d. as suspension. Increase weekly to achieve optimal clinical response administered t.i.d. or q.i.d. There is no recommendation for safe administration at doses of more than 35 mg/kg/day. If optimal clinical response hasn't been achieved at a dose less than 35 mg/kg/day, check plasma levels to determine whether it's within the therapeutic range.

Oral loading dose for rapid seizure control
Adults and children over age 12: 8 mg/kg P.O. of oral suspension.
◇ ***Bipolar affective disorder, intermittent explosive disorder***
Adults: Initially, 200 mg P.O. b.i.d.; increase, p.r.n., q 3 to 4 days. Maintenance dosage may range from 600 to 1,600 mg/day.
Trigeminal neuralgia
Adults: 100 mg P.O. b.i.d. with meals on day 1. Increase by 100 mg q 12 hours until pain is relieved. Don't exceed 1.2 g daily. Maintenance dosage is 200 to 1,200 mg P.O. daily. For extended-release capsules, 200 mg P.O. day 1. Daily dose may be increased by up to 200 mg/day q 12 hours, p.r.n., to achieve freedom from pain. Maintenance dosage is usually 400 to 800 mg/day.
◇ ***Chorea***
Children: 15 to 25 mg/kg P.O. per day.
◇ ***Restless leg syndrome***
Adults: 100 to 300 mg P.O. h.s.

Pharmacodynamics

Anticonvulsant action: Carbamazepine is chemically unrelated to other anticonvulsants and its mechanism of action is unknown. The anticonvulsant activity appears principally to involve limitations of seizure propagation by reduction of posttetanic potentiation (PTP) of synaptic transmissions.
Analgesic action: In trigeminal neuralgia, carbamazepine is a specific analgesic through its reduction of synaptic neurotransmission.

Pharmacokinetics

Absorption: Absorbed slowly from the GI tract.
Distribution: Distributed widely throughout body; it crosses the placenta and accumulates in fetal tissue. About 75% is protein-bound. Therapeutic serum levels in adults are 4 to 12 mcg/ml; nystagmus can occur at serum levels of more than 4 mcg/ml, and ataxia, dizziness, and anorexia can occur at serum levels of 10 mcg/ml or more. Serum levels may be misleading because an unmeasured active metabolite also can cause toxicity. Carbamazepine levels in breast milk approach 60% of serum levels. There is poor correlation between plasma levels and dose in children.
Metabolism: Metabolized by the liver to an active metabolite. It may also induce its own metabolism; over time, higher doses are needed to maintain plasma levels. Half-life is initially 25 to 65 hours and 12 to 17 hours with multiple dosing.
Excretion: Excreted in urine (70%) and feces (30%).

Route	Onset	Peak	Duration
P.O.	Unknown	1½-12 hr	Unknown

Contraindications and precautions

Contraindicated in patients with history of previous bone marrow suppression or hypersensitivity to drug or tricyclic antidepressants and in patients who have taken an MAO inhibitor within 14 days of therapy. Use cautiously in patients with mixed-type seizure disorders.

Interactions

Drug-drug. *Cimetidine, danazol, diltiazem, fluoxetine, fluvoxamine, isoniazid, macrolides (such as erythromycin), propoxyphene, valproic acid, verapamil:* May increase carbamazepine blood levels. Use cautiously.
Doxycycline, felbamate, haloperidol, oral contraceptives, phenytoin, theophylline, warfarin: May decrease blood levels of these drugs. Monitor patient for decreased effect.
Lithium: Increased CNS toxicity of lithium. Avoid use together.
MAO inhibitors: Increased depressant and anticholinergic effects. Don't use together.
Phenobarbital, phenytoin, primidone: May decrease carbamazepine levels. Monitor patient for decreased effect.
Drug-herb. *Psyllium seed:* May inhibit GI absorption; avoid use together.

Effects on diagnostic tests

None reported.

Adverse reactions

CNS: *dizziness, vertigo, drowsiness,* fatigue, *ataxia,* ***worsening of seizures*** (usually in patients with mixed-type seizure disorders, including atypical absence seizures), confusion, headache, syncope.
CV: ***heart failure***, hypertension, hypotension, aggravation of coronary artery disease, ***arrhythmias, AV block.***
EENT: conjunctivitis, dry mouth and pharynx, blurred vision, diplopia, nystagmus.
GI: *nausea, vomiting,* abdominal pain, diarrhea, anorexia, stomatitis, glossitis.
GU: urinary frequency, urine retention, impotence, albuminuria, glycosuria, elevated BUN.
Hematologic: ***aplastic anemia, agranulocytosis,*** eosinophilia, leukocytosis, ***thrombocytopenia.***
Hepatic: abnormal liver function test results, ***hepatitis.***
Respiratory: pulmonary hypersensitivity.
Skin: rash, urticaria, ***erythema multiforme, Stevens-Johnson syndrome.***
Other: excessive diaphoresis, fever, chills, SIADH, decrease values of thyroid function tests.

Overdose and treatment

Symptoms of overdose may include irregular breathing, respiratory depression, tachycardia, blood pressure changes, shock, arrhythmias, impaired consciousness (ranging to deep coma), seizures, restlessness, drowsiness, psychomotor disturbances, nausea, vomiting, anuria, or oliguria.

Treat overdose with repeated gastric lavage, especially if patient ingested alcohol concurrently. Oral charcoal and laxatives may hasten excretion. Carefully monitor vital signs, ECG, and fluid and electrolyte balance. Diazepam may control seizures but can exacerbate respiratory depression.

Clinical considerations

- Adjust drug dosage based on individual response.
- Chewable tablets are available for children.
- Unlabeled uses of carbamazepine include hypophyseal diabetes insipidus, certain psychiatric disorders, and management of alcohol withdrawal.
- For administering through a nasogastric tube, mix with an equal volume of diluent (D_5W or normal saline solution) and administer; then flush with 100 ml of diluent.

Therapeutic monitoring

- Hematologic toxicity is rare but serious. Hematologic and liver functions must be checked. Periodic eye examinations are recommended.

Special populations

Breast-feeding patients. Significant amounts of drug are excreted in breast milk; alternative feeding method is recommended during therapy.
Pediatric patients. Safety and efficacy haven't been established for children under age 6 in doses higher than 35 mg/kg/day.
Geriatric patients. Drug may activate latent psychosis, confusion, or agitation in geriatric patients; use with caution.

Patient counseling

- Remind patient to store drug in a cool, dry place, and not in the medicine cabinet. Reduced bioavailability has been reported with use of improperly stored tablets.
- Tell patient that drug may cause GI distress. Patient should take drug with food at equally spaced intervals.
- Warn patient not to stop drug abruptly.
- Encourage patient to promptly report unusual bleeding, bruising, jaundice, dark urine, pale stools, abdominal pain, impotence, fever, chills, sore throat, mouth ulcers, edema, or disturbances in mood, alertness, or coordination.
- Warn patient that drug may cause drowsiness, dizziness, and blurred vision. Patient should avoid hazardous activities that require alertness, especially during first week of therapy and when dosage is increased.
- Remind patient to shake suspension well before using.
- Tell patient, if necessary, that the Carbatrol capsule can be opened and its contents sprinkled over food (such as a teaspoon of applesauce), but the capsule or its contents should never be crushed or chewed.
- Emphasize importance of follow-up laboratory tests and continued medical supervision.

carbamide peroxide

Auro Ear Drops, Debrox, Gly-Oxide Liquid, Murine Ear, Orajel, Orajel Perioseptic, Proxigel

Pharmacologic classification: urea hydrogen peroxide
Therapeutic classification: ceruminolytic, topical antiseptic
Pregnancy risk category C

How supplied

Available without a prescription
Otic solution: 6.5% carbamide in glycerin or glycerin and propylene glycol
Oral solution: 10% carbamide with glycerin and propylene glycol; 15% with anhydrous glycerin, methylparaben, and propylene glycol
Oral gel: 10% carbamide in water-free gel base

Indications and dosages

Impacted cerumen
Adults and children age 12 and older: 5 to 10 drops otic solution into ear canal b.i.d. for 3 to 4 days.
Inflammation or irritation of lips, mouth, gums
Adults and children over age 3: Apply several drops of undiluted oral solution to affected area or place 10 drops on tongue (mix with saliva, swish for 1 to 3 minutes, then expectorate) after meals and h.s.
Children: Apply undiluted gel to affected area (massage into area with finger or swab) q.i.d.

Pharmacodynamics

Ceruminolytic action: Emulsifies and disperses accumulated cerumen.
Antiseptic action: Releases oxygen upon contact with oral mucosa, which results in a cleansing and mild anti-inflammatory action.

Pharmacokinetics

Unknown.

Route	Onset	Peak	Duration
P.O.	Unknown	Unknown	Unknown
Otic	Unknown	Unknown	15-30 min

Contraindications and precautions

Contraindicated in patients with a perforated eardrum.

Interactions
None reported.

Effects on diagnostic tests
None reported.

Adverse reactions
GI: oral irritation or inflammation.

Overdose and treatment
Signs and symptoms of overdose include mild irritation to mucosal tissue or, if swallowed, irritation, inflammation, and burns in the mouth, throat, esophagus, or stomach. Gastric distention may result from liberation of oxygen. Accidental ocular exposure causes immediate pain and irritation, but severe injury is rare. Irrigate eyes with large amounts of warm water for at least 15 minutes. Accidental dermal exposure bleaches the exposed area. Wash exposed skin twice with soap and water. Treat oral exposure by immediate dilution with water. Spontaneous vomiting may occur.

Clinical considerations
- Don't use to treat swimmer's ear or itching of the ear canal.
- Don't use if patient has a perforated eardrum.
- Irrigation of ear may be necessary to aid removal of cerumen.
- Tip of dropper shouldn't touch ear or ear canal when using otic preparation.
- Remove cerumen remaining after instillation by using a soft rubber-bulb otic syringe to gently irrigate the ear canal with warm water.

Therapeutic monitoring
Patient should have regular checkup of his mouth and throat by doctor or dentist, to check for signs of inflammation or irritation.

Special populations
Pediatric patients. Oral preparations shouldn't be used in children under age 2; otic forms shouldn't be used by children under age 12.

Patient counseling
- Teach patient correct way to use product.
- Tell patient to report inflammation or persistent irritation.
- Warn patient not to use otic form for more than 4 consecutive days and to avoid contact with eyes.
- Instruct patient to keep otic solution in ear for at least 15 minutes by tilting head sideways or putting cotton in ear.
- Tell patient not to rinse mouth or drink for 5 minutes after use of oral preparation.

carboplatin
Paraplatin

Pharmacologic classification: alkylating agent (cell cycle–phase nonspecific)
Therapeutic classification: antineoplastic
Pregnancy risk category D

How supplied
Available by prescription only
Injection: 50-mg, 150-mg, 450-mg vials

Indications and dosages
Initial and secondary (palliative) treatment of ovarian carcinoma; ◇retinoblastoma; ◇advanced bladder cancer; ◇lung cancer; ◇head and neck cancer; ◇Wilms' tumor; ◇primary brain tumor; ◇testicular neoplasm; ◇cervical cancer
Adults: Initial recommended dose for single-agent therapy is 360 mg/m^2 I.V. on day 1. Dose is repeated q 4 weeks. In combination therapy (with cyclophosphamide), give 300 mg/m^2 I.V. on day 1 q 4 weeks for 6 cycles.
≡***Dosage adjustment.*** Dosage adjustments are based on the lowest post-treatment platelet or neutrophil value obtained in weekly blood counts.

Lowest platelet count (per mm^3)	Lowest neutrophil count (per mm^3)	Adjusted dose
> 100,000	> 2,000	125%
50,000 to 100,000	500 to 2,000	No adjustment
< 50,000	< 500	75%

In patients with impaired renal function, initial recommended dose is 250 mg/m^2 for creatinine clearance levels between 41 and 59 ml/minute; for creatinine clearance levels between 16 and 40 ml/minute, dose is 200 mg/m^2.

Pharmacodynamics
Antitumor action: Carboplatin causes cross-linking of DNA strands.

Pharmacokinetics
Absorption: Administered I.V.
Distribution: Volume of distribution is about equal to total body water. Drug isn't protein-bound but degraded to platinum-containing products, which are 87% protein-bound at 24 hours.
Metabolism: Hydrolyzed to form hydroxylated and aquated species. Half-life of drug is 2 to 3 hours; terminal half-life for platinum is 4 to 6 days.

Excretion: 65% is excreted by the kidneys within 12 hours, 71% within 24 hours. Enterohepatic recirculation may occur.

Route	Onset	Peak	Duration
I.V.	Unknown	Unknown	Unknown

Contraindications and precautions

Contraindicated in patients with history of hypersensitivity to cisplatin, platinum-containing compounds, or mannitol or in patients with severe bone marrow suppression or bleeding.

Interactions

Drug-drug. *Aspirin:* Increased risk of bleeding. Avoid use together.
Bone marrow suppressants (including radiation therapy): Increased hematologic toxicity. Monitor patient closely.
Myelosuppressive agents: Concurrent use can cause additive myelosuppression. Monitor patient.
Nephrotoxic agents: Produces additive nephrotoxicity of carboplatin. Use cautiously.

Effects on diagnostic tests

None reported.

Adverse reactions

CNS: dizziness, confusion, peripheral neuropathy, ototoxicity, central neurotoxicity, paresthesia, ***CVA***, asthenia.
CV: ***cardiac failure, embolism.***
EENT: visual disturbances, change in taste.
GI: constipation, diarrhea, *nausea, vomiting.*
GU: increased BUN, creatinine.
Hematologic: THROMBOCYTOPENIA, ***leukopenia***, NEUTROPENIA, ***anemia***, BONE MARROW SUPPRESSION.
Hepatic: increased AST or alkaline phosphatase levels.
Metabolic: decreased serum electrolyte levels.
Other: alopecia, ***hypersensitivity reactions***, pain, ***anaphylaxis.***

Overdose and treatment

Symptoms of overdose result from bone marrow suppression or hepatotoxicity. There is no known antidote for carboplatin overdose.

Clinical considerations

- Reconstitute with D_5W, normal saline solution, or sterile water for injection to make a concentration of 10 mg/ml.
- Drug can be further diluted to concentrations as low as 0.5 mg/ml using normal saline solution or D_5W. Infuse over at least 15 minutes.
- Store unopened vials at room temperature. Once reconstituted and diluted as directed, solution is stable at room temperature for 8 hours. Because drug doesn't contain antibacterial preservatives, discard unused drug after 8 hours.
- Needles or I.V. administration sets containing aluminum may precipitate drug and cause a loss of potency.
- Administration of carboplatin requires the supervision of a doctor experienced in the use of chemotherapeutic agents.

Therapeutic monitoring

- Although drug is promoted as causing less nausea and vomiting than cisplatin, it can cause severe emesis. Antiemetic therapy may be needed; monitor electrolyte levels regularly.

Special populations

Pregnant patients. May cause fetal harm. Carboplatin may be used during pregnancy if it's decided that the benefit outweighs the risk, or in life-threatening situations. Advise patient to avoid becoming pregnant while on carboplatin therapy.
Breast-feeding patients. It's unknown if carboplatin is distributed in breast milk; however, because of the potential for toxicity to the infant, discontinue breast-feeding.
Pediatric patients. Safety in children hasn't been established.
Geriatric patients. Patients over age 65 are at greater risk for neurotoxicity.

Patient counseling

- Stress importance of adequate fluid intake and increase in urine output, to facilitate uric acid excretion.
- Tell patient to report tinnitus immediately, to prevent permanent hearing loss. Patient should have audiometric testing before initial and subsequent course.
- Advise patient to avoid exposure to people with infections.
- Instruct patient to promptly report unusual bleeding or bruising.

carmustine (BCNU)

BiCNU, Gliadel

Pharmacologic classification: alkylating agent; nitrosourea (cell cycle–phase nonspecific)
Therapeutic classification: antineoplastic
Pregnancy risk category D

How supplied

Available by prescription only
Injection: 100-mg vial (lyophilized), with a 3-ml vial of absolute alcohol supplied as a diluent
Implant: 7.7 mg wafer

Indications and dosages

Dosage and indications may vary. Check current literature for recommended protocol.
◊***Brain;*** ◊***breast;*** ◊***GI tract;*** ◊***lung;*** ◊***hepatic cancer; Hodgkin's disease; ma-***

lignant lymphomas; ◇malignant melanomas; multiple myeloma
Adults: 75 to 100 mg/m^2 I.V. by slow infusion daily for 2 consecutive days, repeated q 6 weeks if platelet count is above 100,000/mm^3 and WBC count is above 4,000/mm^3.
≡ ***Dosage adjustment.*** Reduce dosage, p.r.n., using the following guidelines.

Nadir after prior dose		Percentage of prior dose to be given
Leukocytes/ mm^3	**Platelets/ mm^3**	
> 4,000	>100,000	100%
3,000-3,999	75,000-99,999	100%
2,000-2,999	25,000-74,999	70%
< 2,000	< 25,000	50%

Alternative therapy: 150 to 200 mg/m^2 I.V. slow infusion as a single dose, repeated q 6 to 8 weeks.
Recurrent glioblastoma and metastatic brain tumors (adjunct to surgery to prolong survival)
Adults: Implant 8 wafers in the resection cavity if allowed by size and shape of cavity.

Pharmacodynamics
Antineoplastic action: The cytotoxic action of carmustine is mediated through its metabolites, which inhibit several enzymes involved with DNA formation. This agent can also cause cross-linking of DNA. Cross-linking interferes with DNA, RNA, and protein synthesis. Cross-resistance between carmustine and lomustine has occurred.

Pharmacokinetics
Absorption: Not absorbed across the GI tract. Implant wafers are biodegradable in the human brain when implanted into the tumor resection cavity.
Distribution: Cleared rapidly from plasma. After I.V. administration, carmustine and its metabolites are distributed rapidly into CSF.
Metabolism: Metabolized extensively in the liver.
Excretion: About 60% to 70% of drug and its metabolites are excreted in urine within 96 hours, 6% to 10% is excreted as carbon dioxide by the lungs, and 1% is excreted in feces. Enterohepatic circulation and protein-binding can occur and may cause delayed hematologic toxicity.

Note: concerning implant wafer, the absorption, distribution, metabolism, and excretion of the copolymer in humans is unknown.

Route	Onset	Peak	Duration
I.V.	Unknown	Unknown	Unknown

Contraindications and precautions
Contraindicated in patients with hypersensitivity to drug.

Interactions
Drug-drug. *Anticoagulants, aspirin:* Increased risk of bleeding. Avoid use together.
Cimetidine: Increases the bone marrow toxicity of carmustine. Avoid use together.
Myelosuppressive agents: Concurrent use can cause additive myelosuppression. Monitor patient closely.

Effects on diagnostic tests
None reported.

Adverse reactions
CNS: ataxia, drowsiness.
EENT: ocular toxicities.
GI: *nausea beginning in 2 to 6 hours (can be severe), vomiting.*
GU: ***nephrotoxicity,*** azotemia, ***renal failure.***
Hematologic: ***cumulative bone marrow suppression*** (delayed 4 to 6 weeks, lasting 1 to 2 weeks); ***leukopenia; thrombocytopenia; acute leukemia, bone marrow dysplasia*** (after long-term use); anemia.
Hepatic: ***hepatotoxicity.***
Respiratory: ***pulmonary fibrosis.***
Skin: facial flushing, hyperpigmentation.
Other: *intense pain at infusion site from venous spasm;* possible hyperuricemia (in lymphoma patients when rapid cell lysis occurs).

Overdose and treatment
Signs and symptoms of overdose include leukopenia, thrombocytopenia, nausea, and vomiting. Treatment consists of supportive measures, including transfusion of blood components, antibiotics for infections that may develop, and antiemetics.

Clinical considerations
- Use double gloves and surgical instruments dedicated to the handling of implant wafers.
- Reconstitute 100-mg vial with the 3 ml of absolute alcohol provided by manufacturer, then dilute further with 27 ml sterile water for injection. Resultant solution contains 3.3 mg carmustine/ml in 10% ethanol. Dilute in normal saline or D_5W for I.V. infusion. Give at least 250 ml over 1 to 2 hours. Discard excess drug.
- Wear gloves to administer drug infusion and when changing I.V. tubing. Avoid contact with skin because carmustine causes a brown stain. If drug comes into contact with skin, wash off thoroughly.
- Solution is unstable in plastic I.V. bags. Administer only in glass containers.
- Carmustine may decompose at temperatures of more than 80° F (26.6° C).
- If powder liquefies or appears oily, discard it because it's a sign of decomposition.

■ Reconstituted solution may be stored in refrigerator for 24 hours (48 hours if reconstituted to 0.2 mg/ml in D_5W or normal saline solution).
■ Advise nurses not to mix with other drugs during administration.
■ To reduce pain on infusion, suggest further dilution or slow infusion rate.
■ Intense flushing of skin may occur during an I.V. infusion, but usually disappears within 2 to 4 hours.
■ Pulmonary toxicity is more likely in people who smoke.
■ At first sign of extravasation, discontinue infusion and infiltrate area with liberal injections of 0.5 mEq/ml sodium bicarbonate solution.
■ Drug has been applied topically in concentrations of 0.05% to 0.4% to treat mycosis fungoides.
■ Because drug crosses the blood-brain barrier, it may be used to treat primary brain tumors.

Therapeutic monitoring

■ Avoid I.M. injections when platelet count is less than 100,000/mm^3.
■ To reduce nausea, suggest giving antiemetic before administering.
■ Monitor patient's CBC.

Special populations

Pregnant patients. Advise women to avoid becoming pregnant and to report suspected pregnancy.
Breast-feeding patients. Active metabolites of drug have been found in breast milk. Therefore, it isn't advisable for women receiving drug to breast-feed their infants because of risk of serious adverse reactions, mutagenicity, and carcinogenicity in the infant.
Pediatric patients. Safety and effectiveness of carmustine in children haven't been established.

Patient counseling

■ Warn patient to watch for signs of infection and bone marrow toxicity (fever, sore throat, anemia, fatigue, easy bruising, nose or gum bleeds, melena). Patient should take temperature daily.
■ Remind patient to return for follow-up blood work weekly, or as needed, and to watch for signs and symptoms of infection.
■ Advise patient to avoid exposure to people with infections.
■ Tell patient to avoid OTC products containing aspirin because they may precipitate bleeding. Advise patient to report signs of bleeding promptly.

carteolol hydrochloride

Cartrol, Ocupress

Pharmacologic classification: beta blocker
Therapeutic classification: antihypertensive
Pregnancy risk category C

How supplied

Available by prescription only
Tablets: 2.5 mg, 5 mg
Ophthalmic solution: 1%

Indications and dosages

Hypertension
Adults: Initially, 2.5 mg P.O. as a single daily dose. Gradually increase the dose as required to 5 mg daily or 10 mg daily as a single dose.
◊***Angina***
Adults: 10 mg/day P.O.
≡ ***Dosage adjustment.*** Patients with substantial renal failure should receive the usual dose of carteolol scheduled at longer intervals as shown.

Creatinine clearance (ml/min)	Dosage interval (hr)
> 60	24
20 to 60	48
< 20	72

Open-angle glaucoma
Adults: 1 drop b.i.d. in eye.

Pharmacodynamics

Antihypertensive action: Drug is a nonselective beta-adrenergic blocking agent with intrinsic sympathomimetic activity (ISA). Its antihypertensive effects are probably caused by decreased sympathetic outflow from the brain and decreased cardiac output. Carteolol doesn't have a consistent effect on renin output.

Pharmacokinetics

Absorption: Absorbed rapidly. Bioavailability is about 85%.
Distribution: 20% to 30% bound to plasma proteins.
Metabolism: Only 30% to 50% is metabolized in the liver to 8-hydroxycarteolol, an active metabolite, and the inactive metabolite glucuronoside.
Excretion: Primarily renal. Plasma half-life is about 6 hours.

Route	Onset	Peak	Duration
P.O.	Unknown	1-3 hr	24 hr
Ophthalmic	Unknown	Unknown	Unknown

Contraindications and precautions

Contraindicated in patients hypersensitive to any component of drug and in those with bronchial asthma, severe COPD, sinus bradycardia, second- or third-degree AV block, overt cardiac failure, or cardiogenic shock.

Use cautiously in breast-feeding women and in patients with nonallergic bronchospastic disease, diabetes mellitus, hyperthyroidism, or decreased pulmonary function.

Interactions

Drug-drug. *Calcium channel blockers:* Increased risk of hypotension, left ventricular failure, and AV conduction disturbances. I.V. calcium antagonists should be used with caution.
Cardiac glycosides: May produce additive effects on slowing AV node conduction. Avoid use together.
Catecholamine-depleting drugs, such as reserpine, oral adrenergic blockers: May have an additive effect and contribute to the development of hypotension or bradycardia. Patients require close monitoring.
General anesthetics: Increased hypotensive effects. Careful observation for hypotension, bradycardia, or orthostatic hypotension is necessary.
Insulin and oral antidiabetic agents: May alter hypoglycemic response. Dose may need adjustment.
Drug-lifestyle. *Sun exposure:* Photophobia may occur with ophthalmic form of drug. Advise precautions.

Effects on diagnostic tests

None reported.

Adverse reactions

CNS: lassitude, fatigue, somnolence, *asthenia, paresthesia.*
CV: ***conduction disturbances.***
EENT: transient irritation, conjunctival hyperemia, *edema.*
GI: diarrhea, nausea, abdominal pain.
Musculoskeletal: *muscle cramps,* arthralgia.
Skin: rash.

Overdose and treatment

No information available. The likely symptoms are bradycardia, bronchospasm, heart failure, and hypotension.

Use atropine to treat symptomatic bradycardia. If no response is seen, cautiously use isoproterenol. Treat bronchospasm with a $beta_2$-agonist such as isoproterenol, or theophylline. Cardiac glycosides or diuretics may be useful in treating heart failure. Give vasopressors (epinephrine, dopamine, or norepinephrine) to combat hypotension.

Clinical considerations

Consider the recommendations relevant to all beta blockers as well as the following:

□ ***ALERT*** Discontinue drug at first sign of cardiac failure and notify doctor.
- Dosage of more than 10 mg/day doesn't produce a greater response; it may actually decrease response.
- Food may slow the rate, but not the extent, of carteolol absorption.
- Steady-state levels are reached rapidly (within 1 to 2 days) in patients with normal renal function.

Therapeutic monitoring

Monitor heart rate and blood pressure; slow heart rate must be reported to doctor.

Special populations

Breast-feeding patients. Drug may be excreted in breast milk. Use with caution in breast-feeding women.
Pediatric patients. Safety in children hasn't been established.
Geriatric patients. No specific age-related recommendations are available.

Patient counseling

- Advise patient to take drug exactly as prescribed and not to discontinue drug suddenly.
- Tell patient to report shortness of breath or difficulty breathing, unusually fast heartbeat, cough, or fatigue with exertion.
- Inform patient that transient stinging or discomfort may occur with ophthalmic use; if reaction is severe, he should call doctor immediately.
- Tell patient that if more than one topical ophthalmic drug is to be used, they should be administered at least 10 minutes apart.

carvedilol

Coreg

Pharmacologic classification: alpha-nonselective beta-adrenergic blocker
Therapeutic classification: antihypertensive, adjunct treatment for heart failure
Pregnancy risk category C

How supplied

Available by prescription only
Tablets: 3.125 mg, 6.25 mg, 12.5 mg, 25 mg

Indications and dosages

Hypertension
Adults: Dosage individualized. Initially, 6.25 mg P.O. b.i.d. with food; obtain standing systolic pressure 1 hour after initial dose. If tolerated, continue dosage for 7 to 14 days. Can increase to 12.5 mg P.O. b.i.d., repeating monitoring protocol as above. Maximum dose is 25 mg P.O. b.i.d. as tolerated.

Heart failure
Adults: Dosage individualized and adjusted carefully. Stabilize dosing of cardiac glycosides, diuretics, and ACE inhibitors before starting therapy. Initially, 3.125 mg P.O. b.i.d. with food for 2 weeks; if tolerated, possibly increasing to 6.25 mg P.O. b.i.d. for 2 weeks. Dose can be doubled q 2 weeks to highest level tolerated by patient. At initiation of new dose, observe patient for dizziness or light-headedness for 1 hour. Maximum dosing for patients weighing less than 187 lb (85 kg) is 25 mg P.O. b.i.d.; for those weighing more than 187 lb, give 50 mg P.O. b.i.d.

Pharmacodynamics
Antihypertensive action: Mechanism not established. Beta blockade reduces cardiac output and tachycardia. Alpha blockade is demonstrated by the attenuated pressor effects of phenylephrine, vasodilation, and decreases in peripheral vascular resistance.
Heart failure: Not fully established. Drug has been shown to decrease systemic blood pressure, pulmonary artery pressure, right atrial pressure, systemic vascular resistance, and heart rate while increasing stroke volume index.

Pharmacokinetics
Absorption: Rapidly and extensively metabolized following oral administration, with absolute bioavailability of 25% to 35% because of significant first-pass metabolism.
Distribution: Plasma levels are proportional to oral dose administered. Absorption is slowed when administered with food, as evidenced by a delay in the time to reach peak plasma levels with no significant difference in extent of bioavailability.
Metabolism: Extensively metabolized, primarily by aromatic ring oxidation and glucuronidation. The oxidative metabolites are further metabolized by conjugation via glucuronidation and sulfation. Demethylation and hydroxylation at the phenol ring produce three active metabolites with beta-blocking activity.
Excretion: Metabolites are primarily excreted via bile into the feces. Less than 2% of dose is excreted unchanged in urine.

Route	Onset	Peak	Duration
P.O.	Unknown	1-2 hr	7-10 hr

Contraindications and precautions
Contraindicated in patients with New York Heart Association (NYHA) class IV decompensated cardiac failure requiring I.V. inotropic therapy, bronchial asthma or related bronchospastic conditions, second- or third-degree AV block, sick sinus syndrome (unless a permanent pacemaker is in place), cardiogenic shock, severe bradycardia, or hypersensitivity to drug. Drug isn't recommended in patients with hepatic impairment.

Use cautiously in hypertensive patients with left ventricular failure, perioperative patients who receive anesthetics that depress myocardial function, such as ether, cyclopropane, trichloroethylene, or diabetic patients receiving insulin or oral antidiabetic agents, or in persons subject to spontaneous hypoglycemia. Also use with caution in patients with thyroid disease (may mask hyperthyroidism and drug withdrawal may precipitate thyroid storm or an exacerbation of hyperthyroidism), pheochromocytoma, Prinzmetal's variant angina, or peripheral vascular disease (may precipitate or aggravate symptoms of arterial insufficiency).

Interactions
Drug-drug. *Calcium channel blockers:* May cause isolated conduction disturbances; advise monitoring of ECG and blood pressure.
Catecholamine-depleting agents, such as reserpine, MAO inhibitors: May cause severe bradycardia or hypotension. Monitor patient closely.
Cimetidine: Increases bioavailability of carvedilol. Monitor vital signs closely.
Clonidine: May potentiate blood pressure and heart rate lowering effects. Monitor patient carefully.
Digoxin: Increased concentrations by about 15% while on concurrent therapy. Digoxin levels must be evaluated.
Insulin and oral antidiabetic agents: May enhance hypoglycemic properties; blood glucose levels must be checked.
Rifampin Reduces plasma levels of carvedilol by 70%. Vital signs must be monitored.
Drug-food. *Any food:* Delays rate of absorption of carvedilol but doesn't alter extent of bioavailability. Advise patient to take drug with food to minimize orthostatic effects.

Effects on diagnostic tests
None reported.

Adverse reactions
CNS: malaise, *dizziness, fatigue,* headache, hypesthesia, insomnia, pain, paresthesia, somnolence, vertigo.
CV: aggravated angina pectoris, ***AV block, bradycardia,*** chest pain, fluid overload, hypertension, hypotension, postural hypertension, syncope.
EENT: abnormal vision.
GI: abdominal pain, *diarrhea,* melena, nausea, periodontitis, vomiting.
GU: abnormal renal function, albuminuria, hematuria, impotence, urinary tract infection.
Hematologic: decreased PT, purpura, ***thrombocytopenia.***
Hepatic: increased ALT, AST.
Metabolic: dehydration, glycosuria, gout, hypercholesterolemia, *hyperglycemia,* hypertriglyceridemia, hypervolemia, hyperuricemia, hypoglycemia, hyponatremia, weight gain, in-

creased alkaline phosphatase, BUN, or nonprotein nitrogen.
Musculoskeletal: arthralgia, back pain, myalgia.
Respiratory: bronchitis, dyspnea, pharyngitis, rhinitis, sinusitis, *upper respiratory tract infection.*
Other: allergy, edema, fever, hypovolemia, peripheral edema, ***sudden death,*** viral infection.

Overdose and treatment

Overdose may cause severe hypotension, bradycardia, cardiac insufficiency, cardiogenic shock, and cardiac arrest. Respiratory effects, bronchospasm, vomiting, lapses of consciousness, and generalized seizures may also occur. Place patient in supine position. Gastric lavage or pharmacologically induced emesis may be effective shortly after ingestion. May use atropine 2 mg I.V. for bradycardia; glucagon 5 to 10 mg I.V. rapidly over 30 seconds, followed by continuous infusion at 5 mg/hour to support cardiovascular function; sympathomimetics (dobutamine, isoprenaline, adrenaline) at doses based on body weight and effect. If peripheral vasodilation dominates, administer epinephrine or norepinephrine, if necessary, and continuously monitor circulatory conditions. For therapy-resistant bradycardia, perform pacemaker therapy. For bronchospasm, give beta-sympathomimetics by aerosol or I.V. or aminophylline I.V. If seizures occur, slow I.V. injection of diazepam or clonazepam may be effective. If severe intoxication and symptoms of shock occur, continue treatment with antidotes for a sufficiently long period of time consistent with the drug's 7- to 10-hour half-life.

Clinical considerations

- Discontinue drug gradually over 1 to 2 weeks. Decrease dosage if heart rate is less than 55 beats/minute.
- Heart failure patients require monitoring for worsened condition, renal dysfunction, or fluid retention; diuretics may need to be increased; monitor diabetic patient for worsening of hyperglycemia.
- Patients on beta blocker therapy with history of severe anaphylactic reaction to several allergens may be more reactive to repeated challenge, either accidental, diagnostic, or therapeutic. They may be unresponsive to the usual doses of epinephrine used to treat allergic reactions.

Therapeutic monitoring

Mild hepatocellular injury may occur during therapy. At first sign of hepatic dysfunction, perform tests for hepatic injury or jaundice; if present, discontinue drug.

Special populations

Breast-feeding patients. It's unknown if drug is excreted in breast milk. Use cautiously.
Pediatric patients. Safety of drug in patients under age 18 hasn't been established.
Geriatric patients. Plasma levels must be monitored carefully; drug occurs about 50% higher in elderly compared with younger patients. No significant difference was found in adverse effects between older and younger patients; dizziness was slightly more common in the elderly.

Patient counseling

- Tell patient not to interrupt or discontinue drug without medical approval.
- Advise heart failure patient to call if weight gain or shortness of breath occurs.
- Inform patient that he may experience lowered blood pressure when standing. If dizziness occurs, advise him to sit or lie down. Fainting is rare.
- Caution patient against performing hazardous tasks during initiation of therapy. If dizziness or fatigue occur, tell him to call for an adjustment in dosage.
- Advise diabetic patient to report changes in serum glucose level promptly.
- Inform patients who wear contact lenses that decreased lacrimation may occur.

cascara sagrada

cascara sagrada aromatic fluidextract

Pharmacologic classification: anthraquinone glycoside mixture
Therapeutic classification: laxative
Pregnancy risk category C

How supplied

Available without a prescription
Tablets: 325 mg
Aromatic fluidextract: 1 g/ml with 19% alcohol

Indications and dosages

Acute constipation, preparation for bowel or rectal examination
Adults and children age 12 and older: 1 tablet P.O. h.s. or 2 to 6 ml of aromatic fluidextract P.O. once daily.
Children age 2 to 11: ½ of adult dose.
Children under age 2: ¼ of adult dose.

Pharmacodynamics

Laxative action: Cascara sagrada, obtained from the dried bark of the buckthorn tree *(Rhamnus purshiana),* contains cascarosides A and B (barbaloin glycosides) and cascarosides C and D (chrysaloin glycosides). Drug exerts a direct irritant action on the colon that promotes peristalsis and bowel motility. Cascara also enhances colonic fluid accumulation, thus increasing the laxative effect.

Pharmacokinetics
Absorption: Minimal drug absorption occurs in the small intestine. Although onset of action usually occurs in about 6 to 12 hours, onset may not occur for 3 or 4 days.
Distribution: May be distributed in the bile, saliva, and colonic mucosa.
Metabolism: Metabolized in the liver.
Excretion: Excreted in feces via biliary elimination, in urine, or in both.

Route	Onset	Peak	Duration
P.O.	6-10 hr	Variable	Variable

Contraindications and precautions
Contraindicated in patients with abdominal pain, nausea, vomiting, or other symptoms of appendicitis or acute surgical abdomen; acute surgical delirium; fecal impaction; and intestinal obstruction or perforation. Use cautiously in patients with rectal bleeding.

Interactions
None reported.

Effects on diagnostic tests
None reported.

Adverse reactions
GI: *nausea;* vomiting; diarrhea; loss of normal bowel function with excessive use; *abdominal cramps,* especially in severe constipation; malabsorption of nutrients; "cathartic colon" (syndrome resembling ulcerative colitis radiologically and pathologically) with chronic misuse; discoloration of rectal mucosa after long-term use.
Metabolic: hypokalemia, protein enteropathy, electrolyte imbalance (with excessive use).
Other: laxative dependence (with long-term or excessive use).

Overdose and treatment
No information available.

Clinical considerations
- Prescribe doses carefully; fluidextract preparation is five times as potent as aromatic fluid extract.
- Aromatic fluidextract tastes better than fluidextract.
- Cascara is a common ingredient in many so-called natural laxatives available without a prescription.

Therapeutic monitoring
Cascara turns alkaline urine pink to red, red to violet, or red to brown and turns acidic urine yellow to brown in the phenolsulfonphthalein excretion test.

Special populations
Pregnant patients. Bulk-forming or surfactant laxatives are preferred during pregnancy.
Breast-feeding patients. Cascara may be excreted in breast milk, which may result in increased incidence of diarrhea in infant.
Pediatric patients. Use with caution in children.
Geriatric patients. Because many elderly persons use laxatives, they're at particularly high risk for development of laxative dependence. Encourage them to use laxatives only for short periods.

Patient counseling
- Warn patient that drug may turn urine reddish pink or brown.
- Tell patient to take with a full glass of water.

castor oil
Emulsoil, Neoloid, Purge

Pharmacologic classification: glyceride, *Ricinus communis* derivative
Therapeutic classification: stimulant laxative
Pregnancy risk category X

How supplied
Available without a prescription
Liquid: 60 ml, 120 ml
Liquid (95%): 30 ml, 60 ml
Liquid emulsion: 60 ml (95%), 90 ml (67%)

Indications and dosages
Preparation for rectal or bowel examination or surgery; acute constipation (rarely)
Liquid
Adults: 15 to 60 ml (or 30 to 60 ml, 95%) P.O.
Children age 2 to 12: 5 to 15 ml P.O.
Liquid emulsion
Adults: 45 ml (67%) or 15 to 60 ml (95%) P.O. mixed with ½ to 1 glass liquid.
Children age 2 to 12: 15 ml (67%) or 5 to 15 ml (95%) P.O. mixed with ½ to 1 glass liquid.

Pharmacodynamics
Laxative action: Castor oil acts primarily in the small intestine, where it's metabolized to ricinoleic acid, which stimulates the intestine, promoting peristalsis and bowel motility.

Pharmacokinetics
Absorption: Unknown.
Distribution: Distributed locally, primarily in the small intestine.
Metabolism: Like other fatty acids, castor oil is metabolized by intestinal enzymes into its active form, ricinoleic acid.
Excretion: Excreted in feces.

Route	Onset	Peak	Duration
P.O.	2-6 hr	Variable	Variable

Contraindications and precautions
Contraindicated in patients with ulcerative bowel lesions; abdominal pain, nausea, vomiting, or other symptoms of appendicitis or acute surgical abdomen.

Also contraindicated in those with anal or rectal fissures, fecal impaction, or intestinal obstruction or perforation; and during menstruation or pregnancy. Use cautiously in patients with rectal bleeding.

Interactions
Drug-drug. *Intestinally absorbed drugs:* Castor oil may decrease absorption of these drugs. Monitor patient closely.
Drug-herb. *Male fern:* May increase absorption and increase risk of toxicity. Avoid use together.

Effects on diagnostic tests
None reported.

Adverse reactions
GI: *nausea;* vomiting; diarrhea; loss of normal bowel function with excessive use; *abdominal cramps,* especially in severe constipation; malabsorption of nutrients; "cathartic colon" (syndrome resembling ulcerative colitis radiologically and pathologically) with chronic misuse; laxative dependence with long-term or excessive use. May cause constipation after catharsis.
Other: hypokalemia, protein-losing enteropathy, other electrolyte imbalances (with excessive use).

Overdose and treatment
No information available.

Clinical considerations
- Failure to respond to drug may indicate acute condition requiring surgery.
- Castor oil isn't recommended for routine use in constipation; it's commonly used to evacuate the bowels before diagnostic or surgical procedures.
- Because of rapid onset of action, drug shouldn't be given at bedtime.
- Drug is most effective when taken on an empty stomach; shake well.
- Flavored preparations are available.

Therapeutic monitoring
Observe patient for signs and symptoms of dehydration.

Special populations
Pregnant patients. Drug shouldn't be used in pregnant women due to possibility of fetal abnormalities.
Breast-feeding patients. Breast-feeding women should seek medical approval before using castor oil.
Geriatric patients. With chronic use, geriatric patients may experience electrolyte depletion, resulting in weakness, incoordination, and orthostatic hypotension.

Patient counseling
- Advise pregnant women against use of castor oil.
- Recommend that drug be chilled or taken with juice or carbonated beverage for palatability.
- Instruct patient to shake emulsion well before taking it.
- Reassure patient that after response to drug he may not need to move bowels again for 1 or 2 days.

cefaclor
Ceclor, Ceclor CD

Pharmacologic classification: second-generation cephalosporin
Therapeutic classification: antibiotic
Pregnancy risk category B

How supplied
Available by prescription only
Tablets (extended-release): 375 mg, 500 mg
Capsules: 250 mg, 500 mg
Suspension: 125 mg/5 ml, 187 mg/5 ml, 250 mg/5 ml, 375 mg/5 ml

Indications and dosage
Infections of respiratory or urinary tract and skin; otitis media caused by susceptible organisms
Adults: 250 to 500 mg P.O. q 8 hours. Total daily dose shouldn't exceed 4 g. For extended-release tablets, 375 to 500 mg P.O. q 12 hours for 7 to 10 days.
Children: 20 mg/kg P.O. daily (40 mg/kg for severe infections and otitis media) in divided doses q 8 hours, not to exceed 1 g/day.
◇***Acute uncomplicated urinary tract infection***
Adults: 2 g P.O. as single dose.
≡***Dosage adjustment.*** Because cefaclor is dialyzable, patients receiving treatment with hemodialysis or peritoneal dialysis may require dosage adjustment.

Pharmacodynamics
Antibacterial action: Drug is primarily bactericidal; however, it may be bacteriostatic. Activity depends on the specific organism, extent of tissue penetration, drug dosage, and rate of organism multiplication. It acts by adhering to bacterial penicillin-binding proteins, thereby inhibiting cell-wall synthesis.

Cefaclor has the same bactericidal spectrum as other second-generation cephalosporins, except that it has increased activity against ampicillin- or amoxicillin-resistant *Haemophilus influenzae* and *Branhamella catarrhalis.*

Pharmacokinetics

Absorption: Well absorbed from the GI tract. Food will delay but not prevent complete GI tract absorption.
Distribution: Distributed widely into most body tissues and fluids; CSF penetration is poor. Cefaclor crosses the placenta; it's 25% protein-bound.
Metabolism: Not metabolized.
Excretion: Excreted primarily in urine by renal tubular secretion and glomerular filtration; small amounts of drug are excreted in breast milk. Elimination half-life is ½ to 1 hour in patients with normal renal function; end-stage renal disease prolongs half-life to 3 to 5½ hours. Hemodialysis removes cefaclor.

Route	Onset	Peak	Duration
P.O.	Unknown	½-1 hr	Unknown
P.O. (extended-release)	Unknown	½-2½ hr	Unknown

Contraindications and precautions

Contraindicated in patients with hypersensitivity to other cephalosporins. Use cautiously in patients with impaired renal function or penicillin allergy and in breast-feeding women.

Interactions

Drug-drug. *Antacids:* Absorption of extended release cefaclor is decreased if taken within 1 hour. Advise separate administration by 1 hour.
Chloramphenicol: Antagonistic effect. Don't use together.
Probenecid: Competitively inhibits renal tubular secretion of cephalosporins, resulting in higher, prolonged serum levels of these drugs. Patient must be monitored.
Nephrotoxic agents (vancomycin, colistin, polymyxin B, aminoglycosides) or loop diuretics: May increase the risk of nephrotoxicity. Patient must be monitored.

Effects on diagnostic tests

Cefaclor may cause false-positive Coombs' test results. Cefaclor also causes false-positive results in urine glucose tests using cupric sulfate (Benedict's reagent or Clinitest); use glucose oxidase tests (Chemstrip uG, Diastix, or glucose enzymatic test strip) instead.

Cefaclor causes false elevations in serum or urine creatinine levels in tests using Jaffé's reaction.

Adverse reactions

CNS: dizziness, headache, somnolence, malaise.
GI: *nausea,* vomiting, *diarrhea,* anorexia, dyspepsia, abdominal cramps, pseudomembranous colitis, oral candidiasis, transient increases in liver enzymes.
GU: vaginal moniliasis, vaginitis.
Hematologic: ***transient leukopenia,*** anemia, eosinophilia, ***thrombocytopenia,*** lymphocytosis.
Skin: *maculopapular rash,* dermatitis, pruritus.
Other: hypersensitivity reactions (serum sickness, ***anaphylaxis***), fever, ***Stevens-Johnson syndrome.***

Overdose and treatment

Clinical signs of overdose include neuromuscular hypersensitivity; seizure may follow high CNS concentrations. Remove cefaclor by hemodialysis or peritoneal dialysis.

Clinical considerations

Consider the recommendations relevant to all cephalosporins as well as the following:
- Total daily dose may be administered b.i.d. rather than t.i.d. with similar therapeutic effect.
- Stock oral suspension is stable for 14 days if refrigerated.

Therapeutic monitoring

To prevent toxic accumulation, reduced dosage may be required if patient's creatinine clearance is less than 40 ml/minute.

Special populations

Breast-feeding patients. Drug is distributed into breast milk; use with caution in breast-feeding women.
Pediatric patients. Drug can be used safely in children over age 1 month. Extended-release tablets should only be used in children age 16 and older.
Geriatric patients. No dosage adjustments appear to be needed.

Patient counseling

- Instruct patient to take extended-release tablets with food and not to cut, crush, or chew them.
- Tell patient to take the entire amount of medication exactly as prescribed, even if he feels better.

cefadroxil

Duricef

Pharmacologic classification: first-generation cephalosporin
Therapeutic classification: antibiotic
Pregnancy risk category B

How supplied

Available by prescription only
Tablets: 1 g
Capsules: 500 mg
Suspension: 125 mg/5 ml, 250 mg/5 ml, 500 mg/5 ml

Indications and dosages

Urinary tract, skin, and soft-tissue infections caused by susceptible organisms; pharyngitis; tonsillitis

Adults: 1 to 2 g P.O. daily, depending on the infection treated. Usually given once or twice daily.

Children: 30 mg/kg P.O. daily in two divided doses.

≡***Dosage adjustment.*** In patients with creatinine clearance less than 10 ml/minute, extend dosing interval to q 36 hours; if it ranges between 10 and 25 ml/minute, administer q 24 hours; and if it is between 25 and 50 ml/minute, give q 12 hours.

Because drug is dialyzable, patients receiving treatment with hemodialysis may require dosage adjustment.

Pharmacodynamics

Antibacterial action: Cefadroxil is primarily bactericidal; however, it may be bacteriostatic. Activity depends on the organism, tissue penetration, drug dosage, and rate of organism multiplication. It acts by adhering to bacterial penicillin-binding proteins, thereby inhibiting cell-wall synthesis.

Cefadroxil is active against many gram-positive cocci, including penicillinase-producing *Staphylococcus aureus* and *Staphylococcus epidermidis; Streptococcus pneumoniae,* group B streptococci, and group A beta-hemolytic streptococci; and susceptible gram-negative organisms, including *Klebsiella pneumoniae, Escherichia coli,* and *Proteus mirabilis.*

Pharmacokinetics

Absorption: Absorbed rapidly and completely from the GI tract after oral administration.

Distribution: Distributed widely into most body tissues and fluids, including the gallbladder, liver, kidneys, bone, bile, sputum, and pleural and synovial fluids; CSF penetration is poor. Drug crosses the placenta; it's 20% protein-bound.

Metabolism: Not metabolized.

Excretion: Excreted primarily unchanged in the urine by way of glomerular filtration and renal tubular secretion; small amounts may be excreted in breast milk. End-stage renal disease prolongs half-life to 25 hours. Drug can be removed by hemodialysis.

Route	Onset	Peak	Duration
P.O.	Unknown	1-2 hr	Unknown

Contraindications and precautions

Contraindicated in patients with hypersensitivity to drug or other cephalosporins. Use cautiously in patients with impaired renal function or penicillin allergy and in breast-feeding women.

Interactions

Drug-drug. *Probenecid*: Competitively inhibits renal tubular secretion of cephalosporins, resulting in higher, prolonged serum levels of these drugs. Use together cautiously.

Nephrotoxic agents (vancomycin, colistin, polymyxin B, aminoglycosides) or loop diuretics: May increase the risk of nephrotoxicity. Patients need close monitoring.

Bacteriostatic agents (chloramphenicol, erythromycin, tetracyclines): May interfere with bactericidal activity. Use with caution.

Effects on diagnostic tests

Cefadroxil causes false-positive results in urine glucose tests utilizing cupric sulfate (Benedict's reagent or Clinitest); use glucose oxidase test (Chemstrip uG, Diastix, or glucose enzymatic test strip) instead. Cefadroxil causes false elevations in serum or urine creatinine levels in tests using Jaffé's reaction.

Positive Coombs' test results occur in about 3% of patients taking cephalosporins.

Adverse reactions

CNS: ***seizures.***

GI: pseudomembranous colitis, *nausea,* vomiting, *diarrhea,* glossitis, abdominal cramps, oral candidiasis, transient increases in liver enzymes.

GU: genital pruritus, moniliasis, vaginitis, renal dysfunction.

Hematologic: ***transient neutropenia,*** eosinophilia, ***leukopenia,*** anemia, ***agranulocytosis, thrombocytopenia.***

Skin: *maculopapular and erythematous rashes,* urticaria.

Other: hypersensitivity reactions (serum sickness, ***anaphylaxis, angioedema***), dyspnea, fever.

Overdose and treatment

Clinical signs of overdose include neuromuscular hypersensitivity; seizure may follow high CNS concentrations. Remove cefadroxil by hemodialysis. Other treatment is supportive.

Clinical considerations

Consider the recommendations relevant to all cephalosporins; longer half-life of drug permits once- or twice-daily dosing.

Therapeutic monitoring

With large doses or prolonged therapy, monitor for superinfection, especially in high-risk patients.

Special populations

Breast-feeding patients. Drug is excreted in breast milk; use with caution in breast-feeding women.

Pediatric patients. Serum half-life is prolonged in neonates and infants under age 1.

Geriatric patients. Reduce dosage in geriatric patients with diminished renal function.

Patient counseling

- Inform patient of potential adverse reactions.
- Instruct patient to take medication with food to lessen GI discomfort.

cefamandole nafate

Mandol

Pharmacologic classification: second-generation cephalosporin
Therapeutic classification: antibiotic
Pregnancy risk category B

How supplied

Available by prescription only
For injection: 1 g, 2 g

Indications and dosages

Serious respiratory, GU, skin and soft-tissue, and bone and joint infections; septicemia; peritonitis from susceptible organisms

Adults: 500 mg to 1 g I.M. or I.V. q 4 to 8 hours. In life-threatening infections, up to 2 g q 4 hours may be needed.
Infants and children: 50 to 100 mg/kg I.M. or I.V. daily in equally divided doses q 4 to 8 hours. May be increased to total daily dose of 150 mg/kg (not to exceed maximum adult dose) for severe infections.

Total daily dose is same for I.M. or I.V. administration and depends on susceptibility of organism and severity of infection. Inject drug deep I.M. into a large muscle mass, such as the gluteus or the lateral aspect of the thigh.

≡ ***Dosage adjustment.*** In patients with impaired renal function, doses or frequency of administration must be modified according to degree of renal impairment, severity of infection, and susceptibility of organism. The following table gives appropriate doses for adults.

Creatinine clearance (ml/min/1.73 m²)	Severe infections	Life-threatening infections (maximum)
> 80	1 to 2 g q 6 hr	2 g q 4 hr
50 to 80	750 mg to 1.5 g q 6 hr	1.5 g q 4 hr; or 2 g q 6 hr
25 to 50	750 mg to 1.5 g q 8 hr	1.5 g q 6 hr; or 2 g q 8 hr
10 to 25	500 mg to 1 g q 8 hr	1 g q 6 hr; or 1.25 g q 8 hr
2 to 10	500 to 750 mg q 12 hr	670 mg q 8 hr; or 1 g q 12 hr
< 2	250 to 500 mg q 12 hr	500 mg q 8 hr; or 750 mg q 12 hr

Pharmacodynamics

Antibacterial action: Cefamandole is primarily bactericidal; however, it may be bacteriostatic. Activity depends on the organism, tissue penetration, drug dosage, and rate of organism multiplication. It acts by adhering to bacterial penicillin-binding proteins, thereby inhibiting cell-wall synthesis.

Cefamandole is active against *Escherichia coli* and other coliform bacteria, *Staphylococcus aureus* (penicillinase- and nonpenicillinase-producing), *Staphylococcus epidermidis,* group A beta-hemolytic streptococci, *Klebsiella, Haemophilus influenzae, Proteus mirabilis,* and *Enterobacter* as the second-generation drugs. *Bacteroides fragilis* and *Acinetobacter* are resistant.

Pharmacokinetics

Absorption: Not absorbed from the GI tract; must be given parenterally.
Distribution: Distributed widely into most body tissues and fluids, including the gallbladder, liver, kidneys, bone, sputum, bile, and pleural and synovial fluids; CSF penetration is poor. Cefamandole crosses the placenta; it's 65% to 75% protein-bound.
Metabolism: Not metabolized.
Excretion: Excreted primarily in urine by renal tubular secretion and glomerular filtration; small amounts of drug are excreted in breast milk. Elimination half-life is about ½ to 1 hour in patients with normal renal function; severe renal disease prolongs half-life to 12 to 18 hours.

Route	Onset	Peak	Duration
I.V., I.M.	Unknown	1½-2 hr	Unknown

Contraindications and precautions

Contraindicated in patients with hypersensitivity to drug or other cephalosporins. Use cautiously in patients with impaired renal function or penicillin allergy and in breast-feeding women.

Interactions

Drug-drug. *Anticoagulants*: May increase risk of bleeding. Avoid use together.
Probenecid: Competitively inhibits renal tubular secretion of cephalosporins, resulting in higher, prolonged serum levels of these drugs. Monitor patient closely.
Nephrotoxic agents (aminoglycosides, colistin, polymyxin B, vancomycin) or loop diuretics: May increase the risk of nephrotoxicity. Monitor patient closely.
Bacteriostatic agents (chloramphenicol, erythromycin, tetracyclines): May impair its bactericidal activity. Use with caution.
Drug-lifestyle. *Alcohol use:* May cause severe disulfiram-like reactions. Advise patient not to consume alcohol while on drug therapy.

Effects on diagnostic tests

Cefamandole causes false-positive results in urine glucose tests using cupric sulfate (Benedict's reagent or Clinitest); use glucose oxidase tests (Chemstrip uG, Diastix, or glucose enzymatic test strip) instead. Cefamandole also causes false elevations in serum or urine creatinine levels in tests using Jaffé's reaction. Drug may cause positive Coombs' test results and may elevate liver function test results or PT.

Adverse reactions

GI: pseudomembranous colitis, nausea, vomiting, *diarrhea,* oral candidiasis.
Hematologic: eosinophilia, coagulation abnormalities.
Skin: *maculopapular and erythematous rashes, urticaria.*
Other: hypersensitivity reactions (serum sickness, ***anaphylaxis***); transient increases in liver enzymes; *pain, induration, sterile abscesses,* temperature elevation, tissue sloughing (at injection site); *phlebitis, thrombophlebitis* (with I.V. injection).

Overdose and treatment

Signs of overdose include neuromuscular hypersensitivity. Seizure may follow high CNS concentrations. Hypoprothrombinemia and bleeding may occur; they may be treated with vitamin K or blood products. Some drug may be removed by hemodialysis.

Clinical considerations

- For most cephalosporin-sensitive organisms, cefamandole offers little advantage over other cephalosporins; it's less effective than cefoxitin against anaerobic infections. Some clinicians consider it inappropriate for pediatric use, especially for serious infections such as *Haemophilus influenzae.*
- For I.V. use, reconstitute 1 g with 10 ml of sterile water for injection, 5% dextrose injection, or normal saline injection. Administer slowly, over 3 to 5 minutes, or by intermittent infusion or continuous infusion in compatible solutions. Check package insert.
- Don't mix with I.V. infusions containing magnesium or calcium ions, which are chemically incompatible and may cause irreversible effects.
- For I.M. use, dilute 1 g of cefamandole in 3 ml of sterile water for injection, bacteriostatic water for injection, normal saline solution for injection, or 0.9% bacteriostatic saline for injection.
- Administer cefamandole deeply into large muscle mass to ensure maximum absorption. Rotate injection sites.
- I.M. cefamandole is less painful than cefoxitin injection; it doesn't require addition of lidocaine.
- After reconstitution, solution remains stable for 24 hours at room temperature or 96 hours under refrigeration. Solution should be light yellow to amber. Don't use solution if it's discolored or contains a precipitate.

Therapeutic monitoring

- PT requires monitoring for signs or symptoms of bleeding, with evaluation of PT and platelet level. Patient may require prophylactic use of vitamin K to prevent bleeding.
- Bleeding can be reversed by administering vitamin K or blood products.

Special populations

Breast-feeding patients. Drug is excreted in breast milk; use with caution in breast-feeding women. Safety hasn't been established.
Pediatric patients. Safety in infants under age 1 month hasn't been established.
Geriatric patients. Dosage reduction may be required in patients with diminished renal function. Hypoprothrombinemia and bleeding have been reported most frequently in geriatric, malnourished, and debilitated patients.

Patient counseling

Inform patient of potential adverse reactions.

cefazolin sodium

Ancef, Kefzol, Zolicef

Pharmacologic classification: first-generation cephalosporin
Therapeutic classification: antibiotic
Pregnancy risk category B

How supplied

Available by prescription only
Injection (parenteral): 500 mg, 1 g, 5g, 10 g, 20 g
Infusion: 500-mg or 1-g Redi Vials, Faspaks, or ADD-Vantage vials

Indications and dosages

Serious respiratory, GU, skin and soft-tissue, and bone and joint infections; biliary tract infections; septicemia, endocarditis from susceptible organisms; ◇perioperative prophylaxis; contaminated surgery
Adults: 250 mg I.M. or I.V. q 8 hours to 1 g q 8 hours. Maximum dose is 12 g/day in life-threatening situations.
Children over age 1 month: 25 to 100 mg/kg/day I.M. or I.V. in divided doses q 8 hours.

Total daily dose is same for I.M. or I.V. administration and depends on the susceptibility of organism and severity of infection. Inject cefazolin deep I.M. into a large muscle mass, such as the gluteus or the lateral aspect of the thigh.

≡ ***Dosage adjustment.*** Dose or frequency of administration must be modified according to the degree of renal impairment, severity of infection, susceptibility of organism, and serum levels of drug. Because drug can be removed by hemodialysis, patients undergoing hemodialysis may require dosage adjustment.

Creatinine clearance (ml/min/1.73 m²)	Adult dosage
≥ 55	Usual adult dose
35 to 54	Full dose q 8 hr or less frequently
11 to 34	½ usual dose q 12 hr
≤ 10	½ usual dose q 18 to 24 hr

Creatinine clearance (ml/min/1.73 m²)	Pediatric dosage
> 70	Usual pediatric dose
40 to 70	60% of normal daily dose q 12 hr
20 to 40	25% of normal daily dose q 12 hr
5 to 20	10% of normal daily dose q 24 hr

Pharmacodynamics

Antibacterial action: Cefazolin is primarily bactericidal; however, it may be bacteriostatic. Activity depends on the organism, tissue penetration, drug dosage, and rate of organism multiplication. It acts by adhering to bacterial penicillin-binding proteins, thereby inhibiting cell-wall synthesis.

Cefazolin is active against *Escherichia coli,* Enterobacteriaceae, *Haemophilus influenzae, Klebsiella, Proteus mirabilis, Staphylococcus aureus, Streptococcus pneumoniae,* and group A beta-hemolytic streptococci.

Pharmacokinetics

Absorption: Not well absorbed from the GI tract; must be given parenterally.

Distribution: Distributed widely into most body tissues and fluids, including the gallbladder, liver, kidneys, bone, sputum, bile, and pleural and synovial fluids; CSF penetration is poor. It crosses the placenta; it's 74% to 86% protein-bound.

Metabolism: Not metabolized.

Excretion: Excreted primarily unchanged in urine by renal tubular secretion and glomerular filtration; small amounts of drug are excreted in breast milk. Elimination half-life is about 1 to 2 hours in patients with normal renal function; end-stage renal disease prolongs half-life to 12 to 50 hours. Hemodialysis or peritoneal dialysis removes cefazolin.

Route	Onset	Peak	Duration
I.V.	Immediate	Immediate	Unknown
I.M.	Unknown	1-2 hr	Unknown

Contraindications and precautions

Contraindicated in patients with hypersensitivity to other cephalosporins. Use cautiously in patients with impaired renal function or penicillin allergy and in breast-feeding women.

Interactions

Drug-drug. *Probenecid*: Competitively inhibits renal tubular secretion of cephalosporins, resulting in higher, prolonged serum levels of these drugs. Patient requires close monitoring.
Nephrotoxic agents (aminoglycosides, colistin, polymyxin B, vancomycin) or loop diuretics: Concurrent use may increase the risk of nephrotoxicity. Patient requires close monitoring.
Bacteriostatic agents (chloramphenicol, erythromycin, tetracyclines): Concurrent use may interfere with bactericidal activity. Avoid use together.

Effects on diagnostic tests

Cephalosporins cause false-positive results in urine glucose tests utilizing cupric sulfate (Benedict's reagent or Clinitest); use glucose oxidase tests (Chemstrip uG, Diastix, or glucose enzymatic test strip) instead. Cefazolin causes false elevations in serum or urine creatinine levels in tests using Jaffé's reaction. Cefazolin also causes positive Coombs' test results.

Adverse reactions

GI: pseudomembranous colitis, nausea, anorexia, vomiting, *diarrhea,* glossitis, dyspepsia, abdominal cramps, anal pruritus, oral candidiasis.
GU: genital pruritus, candidiasis, vaginitis.
Hematologic: ***neutropenia, leukopenia,*** eosinophilia, ***thrombocytopenia.***
Hepatic: transient increases in liver enzymes.
Skin: *maculopapular and erythematous rashes, urticaria, pruritus,* ***Stevens-Johnson syndrome.***
Other: hypersensitivity reactions (serum sickness, ***anaphylaxis***); *pain, induration, sterile abscesses, tissue sloughing* (at injection site); *phlebitis, thrombophlebitis* (with I.V. injection).

Overdose and treatment

Clinical signs of overdose include neuromuscular hypersensitivity; seizure may follow high CNS concentrations. Cefazolin may be removed by hemodialysis.

Clinical considerations
Consider the recommendations relevant to all cephalosporins as well as the following:
- For I.M. use, reconstitute with sterile water, bacteriostatic water, or normal saline solution: 2 ml to a 500-mg vial, and 2.5 ml to a 1-g vial produces concentrations of 225 mg/ml, and 330 mg/ml respectively.
- Reconstituted solution is stable for 24 hours at room temperature and for 10 days if refrigerated.
- I.M. cefazolin injection is less painful than that of other cephalosporins.

Therapeutic monitoring
- For patients on sodium restrictions, note that cefazolin injection contains 2 mEq of sodium per gram of drug.
- Be sure to do electrolyte studies.

Special populations
Breast-feeding patients. Safety hasn't been established. Use drug with caution in breast-feeding women

Pediatric patients. Drug has been used in children. However, safety in infants under age 1 month hasn't been established.

Patient counseling
Inform patient of potential adverse reactions.

cefdinir
Omnicef

Pharmacologic classification: third-generation cephalosporin
Therapeutic classification: antibiotic
Pregnancy risk category B

How supplied
Available by prescription only
Capsules: 300 mg
Suspension: 125 mg/5 ml

Indications and dosages
Treatment of mild to moderate infections caused by susceptible strains of microorganisms for conditions of community-acquired pneumonia, acute exacerbations of chronic bronchitis, acute maxillary sinusitis, acute bacterial otitis media, and uncomplicated skin and skin structure infections

Adults and adolescents age 13 and older: 300 mg P.O. q 12 hours or 600 mg P.O. q 24 hours for 10 days. (Use q-12-hour doses for pneumonia and skin infections; treat acute otitis media for 5 to 10 days.)

Children age 6 months to 12 years: 7 mg/kg P.O. q 12 hours or 14 mg/kg P.O. q 24 hours for 10 days, up to maximum dose of 600 mg daily. (Use q-12-hour dosages for skin infections; treat acute otitis media for 5 to 10 days.)

Treatment of pharyngitis and tonsillitis

Adults and adolescents age 13 and older: 300 mg P.O. q 12 hours for 5 to 10 days or 600 mg P.O. q 24 hours for 10 days.

Children age 6 months to 12 years: 7 mg/kg P.O. q 12 hours for 5 to 10 days or 14 mg/kg P.O. q 24 hours for 10 days.

≡ ***Dosage adjustment.*** If creatinine clearance is less than 30 ml/minute, reduce dosage to 300 mg P.O. once daily for adults and 7 mg/kg P.O. (up to 300 mg) once daily for children.

In patients receiving chronic hemodialysis, 300 mg or 7 mg/kg P.O. at end of each dialysis session and subsequently every other day.

Pharmacodynamics
Antibiotic action: The bactericidal activity of cefdinir results from inhibition of cell wall synthesis. Drug is stable in the presence of some beta-lactamase enzymes, causing some microorganisms resistant to penicillins and cephalosporins to be susceptible to cefdinir. Excluding *Pseudomonas, Enterobacter, Enterococcus,* and methicillin-resistant *Staphylococcus* species, the spectrum of activity of cefdinir includes a broad range of gram-positive and gram-negative aerobic microorganisms.

Pharmacokinetics
Absorption: Estimated bioavailability of drug is 21% following administration of a 300-mg capsule dose, 16% following a 600-mg capsule dose, and 25% for the suspension.

Distribution: Mean volume of distribution for adults and children is 0.35 and 0.67 L/kg, respectively, and distribution to tonsil, sinus, lung, and middle ear tissue and fluid ranges from 15% to 35% of corresponding plasma levels. 60% to 70% bound to plasma proteins; binding is independent of concentration.

Metabolism: Not appreciably metabolized; its activity is due mainly to parent drug.

Excretion: Excreted principally by renal excretion; mean plasma elimination half-life is 1.7 hours. Drug clearance is reduced in patients with renal dysfunction.

Route	Onset	Peak	Duration
P.O.	Unknown	2-4 hr	Unknown

Contraindications and precautions
Contraindicated in patients with known allergy to cephalosporin class of antibiotics. Use cautiously in patients with known hypersensitivity to penicillin because of the possibility of cross-sensitivity with other beta-lactam antibiotics. Also use with caution in patients with history of colitis.

Interactions
Drug-drug. *Antacids (magnesium- and aluminum-containing) and iron supplements:* Decrease the rate of absorption and bioavailabil-

ity of cefdinir. These preparations should be given 2 hours before or after cefdinir dose.
Probenecid: Inhibits the renal secretion of cefdinir. Patient requires monitoring.
Drug-food. *Foods fortified with iron, such as infant formula:* Decrease the rate of absorption and bioavailability of cefdinir. Patient requires monitoring.

Effects on diagnostic tests
False-positive reactions for ketones (tests using nitroprusside only) and glucose (Clinitest, Benedict's solution, Fehling's solution) in the urine have been reported. Generally, cephalosporins can induce a positive direct Coombs' test.

Adverse reactions
CNS: headache.
GI: abdominal pain, *diarrhea,* nausea, vomiting.
GU: vaginal candidiasis, vaginitis.
Skin: rash.

Overdose and treatment
Information isn't available. Toxic signs of overdose with other beta-lactam antibiotics include nausea, vomiting, epigastric distress, diarrhea, and seizures. Drug removed by hemodialysis.

Clinical considerations
Pseudomembranous colitis has been reported with many antibiotics, including cefdinir, and should be considered in patients whose symptoms include diarrhea subsequent to antibiotic therapy or in those with history of colitis.

Therapeutic monitoring
As with many antibiotics, prolonged drug treatment may result in possible emergence and overgrowth of resistant organisms. Consider alternative therapy if superinfection occurs.

Special populations
Breast-feeding patients. Drug isn't detectable in breast milk following 600-mg doses.
Pediatric patients. Safety and efficacy in infants under age 6 months haven't been established. Pharmacokinetic data for the pediatric population are comparable to data for adults.
Geriatric patients. Cefdinir is well tolerated in all age groups. Safety and efficacy are comparable in geriatric patients and younger patients. Dosage adjustment isn't necessary unless patient has renal impairment.

Patient counseling
- Instruct patient to take antacids, iron supplements, and iron-fortified foods 2 hours before or after a cefdinir dose.
- Inform diabetic patient that each teaspoon of suspension contains 2.86 g of sucrose.
- Advise patient to report severe diarrhea or diarrhea accompanied by abdominal pain.

cefepime hydrochloride
Maxipime

Pharmacologic classification: semisynthetic third- or fourth-generation cephalosporin
Therapeutic classification: antibiotic
Pregnancy risk category B

How supplied
Available by prescription only
Injection: 500 mg/15 ml vial, 1 g/100 ml piggyback bottle, 1 g/ADD-Vantage vial, 1 g/15 ml vial, 2 g/100 ml piggyback bottle, 2 g/20 ml vial

Indications and dosages
Mild to moderate urinary tract infections caused by* Escherichia coli, Klebsiella pneumoniae, *or* Proteus mirabilis, *including cases associated with concurrent bacteremia with these microorganisms
Adults: 0.5 to 1 g I.M. (use I.M. route only for infections caused by *E. coli*), or I.V. infused over 30 minutes q 12 hours for 7 to 10 days.
***Severe urinary tract infections including pyelonephritis caused by* E. coli *or* K. pneumoniae**
Adults: 2 g I.V. infused over 30 minutes q 12 hours for 10 days.
Moderate to severe pneumonia caused by* Streptococcus pneumoniae, Pseudomonas aeruginosa, K. pneumoniae, *or* Enterobacter *species
Adults: 1 to 2 g I.V. infused over 30 minutes q 12 hours for 10 days.
***Moderate to severe uncomplicated skin and skin structure infections due to* Staphylococcus aureus *(methicillin-susceptible strains only) or* Streptococcus pyogenes**
Adults: 2 g I.V. infused over 30 minutes q 12 hours for 10 days.
Empiric therapy in febrile neutropenia
Adults: 2 g I.V. q 8 hours for 7 days or until neutropenia resolves.
Children weighing less than 88 lb (40 kg): 50 mg/kg I.V. q 8 hours.
Uncomplicated and complicated urinary tract infections, uncomplicated skin and skin structure infections, or pneumonia
Children weighing less than 88 lb (40 kg): 50 mg/kg I.V. q 12 hours.
◊ Alternatively, the American Academy of Pediatrics recommends for children older than 1 month a dosage of 1 to 2 g daily, divided b.i.d. for mild to moderate infections, or a dosage of 2 to 4 g daily divided b.i.d. for severe infections.

Pediatric dosages should not exceed the recommended adult dosages.

≡ *Dosage adjustment.* Adjust dosage in patients with impaired renal function. Consult manufacturer's recommendations. Patients receiving hemodialysis should receive a repeat dose at the end of dialysis. Patients undergoing continuous ambulatory peritoneal dialysis (CAPD) should receive the usual dose q 48 hours.

Pharmacodynamics
Antibiotic action: Cefepime exerts its bactericidal action by inhibition of cell-wall synthesis. It's usually active against gram-positive microorganisms such as *S. pneumoniae, S. aureus,* and *S. pyogenes* and gram-negative microorganisms such as *Enterobacter* species, *E. coli, K. pneumoniae, P. mirabilis,* and *P. aeruginosa.*

Pharmacokinetics
Absorption: Completely absorbed after I.M. administration.
Distribution: Widely distributed; about 20% bound to serum protein.
Metabolism: Metabolized rapidly.
Excretion: About 85% is excreted in urine as unchanged drug; less than 1% as the metabolite, 6.8% as the metabolite oxide, and 2.5% as an epimer of cefepime.

Route	Onset	Peak	Duration
I.V., I.M.	½ hr	1-2 hr	Unknown

Contraindications and precautions
Contraindicated in patients with hypersensitivity to drug, other cephalosporins, penicillins, or other beta-lactam antibiotics. Use cautiously in patients with history of GI disease (especially colitis), impaired renal function, or poor nutritional status and in those receiving a protracted course of antimicrobial therapy.

Interactions
Drug-drug. *Aminoglycosides:* May increase risk of nephrotoxicity and ototoxicity. Renal and hearing functions need close monitoring. *Potent diuretics such as furosemide:* May increase risk of nephrotoxicity. Renal function monitoring is necessary.

Effects on diagnostic tests
Cefepime may result in a false-positive reaction for glucose in the urine when using Clinitest tablets. Use glucose tests based on enzymatic glucose oxidase reactions (such as Chemstrip uG, Diastix, or glucose enzymatic test strip) instead. A positive direct Coombs' test may occur during treatment with drug.

Adverse reactions
CNS: headache.
GI: colitis, diarrhea, nausea, vomiting, oral moniliasis.
GU: vaginitis.
Skin: rash, pruritus, urticaria.
Other: phlebitis, pain, inflammation, fever.

Overdose and treatment
Overdose may result in the patient experiencing seizures, encephalopathy, and neuromuscular excitability. Patients who receive an overdose should be carefully observed and given supportive treatment. In the presence of renal insufficiency, hemodialysis, not peritoneal dialysis, is recommended to aid in the removal of cefepime from the body.

Clinical considerations
Consider the recommendations relevant to all cephalosporins as well as the following:
□ ***ALERT*** Names of some cephalosporins are similar. Use caution when dispensing.
- Do culture and sensitivity tests before giving first dose, if appropriate. Therapy may begin pending results.
- For I.V. administration, follow manufacturer guidelines closely when reconstituting drug. Variations occur in constituting drug for administration and depend on concentration of drug required and how drug is packaged (piggyback vial, ADD-Vantage vial, or regular vial). Type of diluent used for constitution varies, depending on product used. Use only solutions recommended by manufacturer. Administer the resulting solution over 30 minutes.
- Intermittent I.V. infusion with a Y-type administration set can be accomplished with compatible solutions. However, during infusion of a solution containing cefepime, discontinuing the other solution is recommended.
- For I.M. administration, constitute drug using sterile water for injection, normal saline solution, 5% dextrose injection, 5% or 1% lidocaine hydrochloride, or bacteriostatic water for injection with parabens or benzyl alcohol. Follow manufacturer guidelines for quantity of diluent to use.
- Inspect solution visually for particulate matter before administration. The powder and its solutions tend to darken depending on storage conditions. However, product potency isn't adversely affected when stored as recommended.

Therapeutic monitoring
Many cephalosporins may cause a decrease in prothrombin activity; patients at risk include those with renal or hepatic impairment or poor nutritional status and those receiving prolonged cefepime therapy. PT must be checked. Exogenous vitamin K can be given if necessary.

Special populations
Pregnant patients. Use drug only when clearly needed during pregnancy.
Breast-feeding patients. Drug is excreted in breast milk in very low concentrations; use cautiously.

Pediatric patients. Safety and effectiveness in children under age 2 months haven't been established.
Geriatric patients. Use caution when administering cefepime to geriatric patients. Dosage adjustment may be necessary in patients with impaired renal function.

Patient counseling

- Warn patient receiving drug I.M. that pain may occur at injection site.
- Instruct patient to report adverse reactions promptly.

cefixime

Suprax

Pharmacologic classification: third-generation cephalosporin
Therapeutic classification: antibiotic
Pregnancy risk category B

How supplied

Available by prescription only
Tablets: 200 mg, 400 mg
Powder for oral suspension: 100 mg/5 ml

Indications and dosages

Otitis media; acute bronchitis; acute exacerbations of chronic bronchitis, pharyngitis, tonsillitis; uncomplicated urinary tract infections caused by* Escherichia coli *and* Proteus mirabilis*; uncomplicated gonorrhea; ◇disseminated gonococcal infections
Adults and children weighing more than 110 lb (50 kg) or over age 12: 400 mg P.O. daily in one or two divided doses; for uncomplicated gonorrhea, 400 mg as a single dose.
Children over age 6 months weighing less than 110 lb (50 kg) or under age 12: 8 mg/kg P.O. daily in one or two divided doses.
≡ ***Dosage adjustment.*** In renally impaired patients, dosage must be adjusted based on degree of renal impairment, severity of infection, and susceptibility of organism. To prevent toxic accumulation in patients with creatinine clearance less than 60 ml/minute/1.73 m^2, reduced dosage may be needed.

Creatinine clearance (ml/min/1.73 m^2)	Adult dosage
> 60	Usual dose
20 to 60	75% of the usual dose
< 20 or patients receiving continuous ambulatory peritoneal dialysis	50% of the usual dose

Pharmacodynamics

Antibacterial action: Cefixime is primarily bactericidal; it acts by binding to penicillin-binding proteins in the bacterial cell wall, thereby inhibiting cell-wall synthesis.

It's used in the treatment of otitis media caused by *Haemophilus influenzae* (penicillinase- and nonpenicillinase-producing), *Moraxella (Branhamella) catarrhalis* (which is penicillinase-producing), and *Streptococcus pyogenes.* Substantial drug resistance has been noted. Cefixime is also active in the treatment of acute bronchitis and acute exacerbations of chronic bronchitis caused by *Streptococcus pneumoniae* and *H. influenzae* (penicillinase- and nonpenicillinase-producing), pharyngitis and tonsillitis caused by *S. pyogenes,* and uncomplicated urinary tract infections caused by *E. coli* and *P. mirabilis.*

Pharmacokinetics

Absorption: About 30% to 50% is absorbed following oral administration. The suspension form provides a higher serum level than the tablet form. Absorption is delayed by food, but the total amount absorbed is not affected.
Distribution: Widely distributed; about 65% is bound to plasma proteins.
Metabolism: About 50% is metabolized.
Excretion: Excreted primarily in the urine. In patients with end-stage renal disease, half-life may be prolonged to 11½ hours.

Route	Onset	Peak	Duration
P.O.	Unknown	3-4½ hr	Unknown

Contraindications and precautions

Contraindicated in patients with hypersensitivity to drug or other cephalosporins. Use cautiously in patients with impaired renal function.

Interactions

Drug-drug. *Carbamazepine:* Elevated carbamazepine levels reported when administered together. Avoid use together.
Probenecid: May inhibit excretion and increase blood levels of cefixime. Use together cautiously.
Salicylates: May increase serum level of cefixime. Use together cautiously.

Effects on diagnostic tests

Cefixime may cause false-positive results in urine glucose tests utilizing cupric sulfate (Benedict's reagent or Clinitest); use glucose oxidase tests (Chemstrip uG, Diastix, or glucose enzymatic test strip) instead. Cefixime may cause false-positive results in tests for urine ketones that utilize nitroprusside (but not nitroferricyanide).

False-positive direct Coombs' test results have been seen with other cephalosporins.

Adverse reactions

CNS: headache, dizziness.
GI: *diarrhea,* loose stools, abdominal pain, nausea, vomiting, dyspepsia, flatulence, pseudomembranous colitis.
GU: genital pruritus, vaginitis, genital candidiasis, transient increases in BUN and serum creatinine levels.
Hematologic: ***thrombocytopenia, leukopenia,*** eosinophilia.
Hepatic: transient increases in liver enzymes.
Skin: pruritus, rash, urticaria, erythema multiforme, ***Stevens-Johnson syndrome.***
Other: drug fever, hypersensitivity reactions (serum sickness, ***anaphylaxis***).

Overdose and treatment

No specific antidote available. Gastric lavage and supportive treatment are recommended. Peritoneal dialysis and hemodialysis will remove substantial quantities of drug.

Clinical considerations

Consider the recommendations relevant to all cephalosporins as well as the following:
□ ***ALERT.*** Names of some cephalosporins are similar. Use caution when dispensing.
- Cefixime is the first orally active, third-generation cephalosporin that's effective with once-daily dosage.
- The manufacturer suggests that tablets shouldn't be substituted for suspension when treating otitis media.

Therapeutic monitoring

- Evaluate patients with antibiotic-induced diarrhea for overgrowth of pseudomembranous colitis caused by *Clostridium difficile*. Mild cases usually respond to discontinuation of the drug; moderate to severe cases may require fluid, electrolyte, and protein supplementation. Oral vancomycin is the drug of choice for the treatment of antibiotic-associated *C. difficile* pseudomembranous colitis.
- Treat acute hypersensitivity reactions immediately. Emergency measures, such as airway management, pressor amines, epinephrine, oxygen, antihistamines, and corticosteroids, may be required.
- Some cephalosporins may cause seizures, especially in patients with renal failure who receive full therapeutic dosages. If seizures occur, discontinue drug and initiate anticonvulsant therapy.

Special populations

Pregnant patients. Use during pregnancy only when clearly needed.
Breast-feeding patients. Distribution of drug in breast milk is unknown. The manufacturer recommends discontinuation of breast-feeding during cefixime therapy.
Pediatric patients. The incidence of adverse GI effects in children receiving oral suspension is similar to those in adults receiving tablets.

Patient counseling

- Instruct patient to report rash, or symptoms of superinfection.
- Advise patient that oral suspension is stable for 14 days after reconstitution and doesn't require refrigeration.
- Tell patient to take all medication exactly as prescribed, even if he feels better.

cefoperazone sodium

Cefobid

Pharmacologic classification: third-generation cephalosporin
Therapeutic classification: antibiotic
Pregnancy risk category B

How supplied

Available by prescription only
Parenteral: 1 g, 2 g, 10 g
Infusion: 1 g, 2 g piggyback

Indications and dosages

Serious respiratory tract, intra-abdominal, gynecologic, skin and structure, urinary tract, and enterococcal infections; bacterial septicemia caused by susceptible organisms; perioperative prophylaxis
Adults: Usual dose is 1 to 2 g q 12 hours I.M. or I.V. In severe infections or infections caused by less sensitive organisms, the total daily dose or frequency may be increased up to 16 g/day in certain situations.
≡ ***Dosage adjustment.*** No dosage adjustment is usually necessary in patients with renal impairment. However, give doses of 4 g/day cautiously to patients with hepatic disease. Adults with combined hepatic and renal function impairment shouldn't receive more than 1 g (base) daily without serum determinations. In patients receiving hemodialysis treatments, schedule a dose to follow hemodialysis.

Pharmacodynamics

Antibacterial action: Cefoperazone is primarily bactericidal; however, it may be bacteriostatic. Activity depends on the organism, tissue penetration, drug dosage, and rate of organism multiplication. It acts by adhering to bacterial penicillin-binding proteins, thereby inhibiting cell-wall synthesis. Third-generation cephalosporins appear more active against some beta-lactamase-producing gram-negative organisms.

Cefoperazone is active against some gram-positive organisms and many enteric gram-negative bacilli, including *Streptococcus pneumoniae* and *Streptococcus pyogenes, Staphylococcus aureus* (penicillinase- and nonpenicillinase-producing), *Staphylococcus epidermidis, Escherichia coli, Klebsiella, Haemophilus influenzae, Enterobacter, Citrobacter, Proteus,* some *Pseudomonas* species (including *Pseudomonas aeruginosa),* and *Bacteroides fragilis. Acinetobacter* and *Listeria* usually are resistant. Cefoperazone is less effective than cefotaxime or ceftizoxime against Enterobacteriaceae but is slightly more active than those drugs against *Pseudomonas aeruginosa.*

Pharmacokinetics

Absorption: Not absorbed from the GI tract; must be given parenterally.
Distribution: Distributed widely into most body tissues and fluids, including the gallbladder, liver, kidneys, bone, sputum, bile, and pleural and synovial fluids; CSF penetration is achieved in patients with inflamed meninges. It crosses the placenta. Protein binding is dose-dependent and decreases as serum levels rise; average is 82% to 93%.
Metabolism: Not substantially metabolized.
Excretion: Excreted primarily in bile; some drug is excreted in urine by renal tubular secretion and glomerular filtration; and small amounts in breast milk. Elimination half-life is about 1½ to 2½ hours in patients with normal hepatorenal function; biliary obstruction or cirrhosis prolongs half-life to about 3½ to 7 hours. Hemodialysis removes cefoperazone.

Route	Onset	Peak	Duration
I.V.	Immediate	Immediate	Unknown
I.M.	Unknown	1-2 hr	Unknown

Contraindications and precautions

Contraindicated in patients with hypersensitivity to drug or other cephalosporins. Use cautiously in patients with impaired renal or hepatic function or penicillin allergy and in breast-feeding women.

Interactions

Drug-drug. *Aminoglycosides:* Concurrent use results in synergistic activity against *P. aeruginosa* and *Serratia marcescens;* such combined use slightly increases the risk of nephrotoxicity. Use together cautiously.
Anticoagulants: May increase risk of bleeding. Use together cautiously.
Clavulanic acid: Concurrent use results in synergistic activity against many Enterobacteriaceae, *B. fragilis, P. aeruginosa,* and *S. aureus.* Use together cautiously.
Probenecid: Competitively inhibits renal tubular secretions of cephalosporins, causing prolonged serum levels of these drugs. Use together cautiously.

Drug-lifestyle. *Alcohol use:* Can cause disulfiram-like reaction. Discourage use.

Effects on diagnostic tests

Cephalosporins cause false-positive results in urine glucose tests using cupric sulfate (Benedict's reagent or Clinitest); use glucose oxidase (Chemstrip uG, Diastix, or glucose enzymatic test strip) instead. Cefoperazone may cause positive Coombs' test results.

Adverse reactions

GI: pseudomembranous colitis, nausea, vomiting, *diarrhea.*
Hematologic: ***transient neutropenia,*** *eosinophilia,* anemia, hypoprothrombinemia, bleeding.
Hepatic: mildly elevated liver enzymes.
Skin: *maculopapular and erythematous rashes, urticaria.*
Other: hypersensitivity reactions (serum sickness, ***anaphylaxis***); *pain, induration, sterile abscesses, temperature elevation, tissue sloughing* (at injection site); *phlebitis, thrombophlebitis,* drug fever (with I.V. injection).

Overdose and treatment

Clinical signs of overdose include neuromuscular hypersensitivity. Seizure may follow high CNS concentrations. Hypoprothrombinemia and bleeding may occur and may require treatment with vitamin K or blood products. Hemodialysis removes cefoperazone.

Clinical considerations

Consider the recommendations relevant to all cephalosporins as well as the following:
- Diarrhea may be more common with drug than with other cephalosporins because of high degree of biliary excretion.
- Patients with biliary disease may need lower doses.
- For patients on sodium restriction, note that cefoperazone injection contains 1.5 mEq of sodium per gram of drug.
- To prepare I.M. injection, use the appropriate diluent, including sterile water for injection or bacteriostatic water for injection. Follow manufacturer's recommendations for mixing drug with sterile water for injection and lidocaine 2% injection. Final solution for I.M. injection will contain 0.5% lidocaine and will be less painful upon administration (recommended for concentrations of 250 mg/ml or greater). Inject cefoperazone deep I.M. into a large muscle mass, such as the gluteus or the lateral aspect of the thigh.
- Store drug in refrigerator and away from light before reconstituting.
- Allow solution to stand after reconstituting to allow foam to dissipate and solution to clear. Solution can be shaken vigorously to ensure complete drug dissolution.

- After reconstitution, solution is stable for 24 hours at a controlled room temperature or 3 days if refrigerated. Protecting drug from light is unnecessary.
- Because cefoperazone is dialyzable, patients undergoing treatment with hemodialysis may require dosage adjustment.

Therapeutic monitoring

Monitor INR regularly. Vitamin K promptly reverses bleeding if it occurs.

Special populations

Pregnant patients. Use during pregnancy only when clearly needed.
Breast-feeding patients. Drug is excreted in breast milk; use with caution in breast-feeding women.
Pediatric patients. Safety and effectiveness in children under age 12 haven't been established.
Geriatric patients. Hypoprothrombinemia and bleeding have been reported more frequently in geriatric patients. Use with caution, and monitor PT and check for signs of abnormal bleeding.

Patient counseling

- Inform patient of potential adverse reactions.
- Tell patient to report discomfort at I.V. site.

cefotaxime sodium

Claforan

Pharmacologic classification: third-generation cephalosporin
Therapeutic classification: antibiotic
Pregnancy risk category B

How supplied

Available by prescription only
Injection: 500 mg, 1 g, 2 g
Pharmacy bulk package: 10-g vial
Infusion: 1 g, 2 g

Indications and dosages

Serious lower respiratory, urinary, CNS, bone and joint, intra-abdominal, gynecologic, and skin infections; bacteremia; septicemia caused by susceptible organisms; ◇pelvic inflammatory disease
Adults and children weighing more than 110 lb (50 kg): Usual dose is 1 g I.V. or I.M. q 6 to 12 hours. Up to 12 g daily can be administered in life-threatening infections.
Children age 1 month to 12 years weighing less than 110 lb: 50 to 180 mg/kg/day I.V. in four or six equally divided doses. Higher doses are reserved for serious infections (such as meningitis).
Neonates age 1 to 4 weeks: 50 mg/kg I.V. q 8 hours.
Neonates up to age 1 week: 50 mg/kg I.V. q 12 hours.

Total daily dose is same for I.M. or I.V. administration and depends on susceptibility of organism and severity of infection. Inject cefotaxime deep I.M. into a large muscle mass, such as the gluteus or the lateral aspect of the thigh.

Uncomplicated gonorrhea
Adults and adolescents: 1 g I.M. as a single dose.
Perioperative prophylaxis
Adults: 1 g I.V. or I.M. 30 to 90 minutes before surgery.
◇Disseminated gonococcal infection
Adults: 1 g I.V. q 8 hours.
Neonates and infants: 25 to 50 mg/kg I.V. q 8 to 12 hours for 7 days or 50 to 100 mg/kg I.M. or I.V. q 12 hours for 7 days.
◇Gonococcal ophthalmia
Adults: 500 mg I.V. q.i.d.
Neonates: 100 mg I.V. or I.M. for one dose; may continue until ocular cultures are negative at 48 to 72 hours.
◇Gonorrheal meningitis or arthritis
Neonates and infants: 25 to 50 mg/kg I.V. q 8 to 12 hours for 10 to 14 days or 50 to 100 mg/kg I.M. or I.V. q 12 hours for 10 to 14 days.
≡***Dosage adjustment.*** In patients with impaired renal function, modify dose or frequency of administration based on degree of renal impairment, severity of infection, and susceptibility of organism. To prevent toxic accumulation, reduced dosage may be required in patients with creatinine clearance below 20 ml/minute.

Pharmacodynamics

Antibacterial action: Cefotaxime is primarily bactericidal; however, it may be bacteriostatic. Activity depends on the organism, tissue penetration, drug dosage, and rate of organism multiplication. It acts by adhering to bacterial penicillin-binding proteins, thereby inhibiting cell-wall synthesis.

Third-generation cephalosporins appear more active against some beta-lactamase-producing gram-negative organisms.

Cefotaxime is active against some gram-positive organisms and many enteric gram-negative bacilli, including streptococci (*Streptococcus pneumoniae* and *pyogenes*), *Staphylococcus aureus* (penicillinase- and nonpenicillinase-producing), *Staphylococcus epidermidis, Escherichia coli, Klebsiella* species, *Haemophilus influenzae, Enterobacter* species, *Proteus* species, *Peptostreptococcus* species, and some strains of *Pseudomonas aeruginosa. Listeria* and *Acinetobacter* are often resistant. The active metabolite of cefotaxime, desacetylcefotaxime, may act synergistically with the parent drug against some bacterial strains.

Pharmacokinetics

Absorption: Not absorbed from the GI tract; must be given parenterally.
Distribution: Distributed widely into most body tissues and fluids, including the gallbladder, liver, kidneys, bone, sputum, bile, and pleural and synovial fluids. Unlike most other cephalosporins, drug has adequate CSF penetration when meninges are inflamed; it crosses the placenta; 13% to 38% is protein-bound.
Metabolism: Metabolized partially to an active metabolite, desacetylcefotaxime.
Excretion: Excreted primarily in urine by renal tubular secretion; some drug may be excreted in breast milk. About 25% of cefotaxime is excreted in urine as the active metabolite; elimination half-life in normal adults is about 1 to 1½ hours for cefotaxime and about 1½ to 2 hours for desacetylcefotaxime; severe renal impairment prolongs the half-life of cefotaxime to 11½ hours and that of the metabolite to as much as 56 hours. Hemodialysis removes both drug and its metabolites.

Route	Onset	Peak	Duration
I.V.	Immediate	Immediate	Unknown
I.M.	Unknown	½ hr	Unknown

Contraindications and precautions

Contraindicated in patients with hypersensitivity to drug or other cephalosporins. Use cautiously in patients with impaired renal function or penicillin allergies and in breast-feeding women.

Interactions

Drug-drug. *Aminoglycoside:* Concurrent use results in apparent synergistic activity against Enterobacteriaceae and some strains of *P. aeruginosa* and *Serratia marcescens;* such combined use may increase risk of nephrotoxicity. Patient requires close monitoring.
Probenecid: May block renal tubular secretion of cefotaxime and prolong its half-life. Use together carefully.

Effects on diagnostic tests

Cephalosporins cause false-positive results in urine glucose tests using cupric sulfate (Benedict's reagent or Clinitest); use glucose oxidase (Chemstrip uG, Diastix, or glucose enzymatic test strip) instead. Cefotaxime also causes false elevations in urine creatinine levels in tests using Jaffé's reaction. Cefotaxime may cause positive Coombs' tests results.

Adverse reactions

CNS: headache.
GI: pseudomembranous colitis, nausea, vomiting, *diarrhea.*
GU: vaginitis, moniliasis, interstitial nephritis.
Hematologic: ***transient neutropenia,*** eosinophilia, hemolytic anemia, ***thrombocytopenia, agranulocytosis.***
Hepatic: transient increases in liver enzymes.
Skin: *maculopapular and erythematous rashes, urticaria.*
Other: hypersensitivity reactions (serum sickness, ***anaphylaxis***); elevated temperature; *pain, induration, sterile abscesses, temperature elevation, tissue sloughing* (at injection site); *phlebitis, thrombophlebitis* (with I.V. injection).

Overdose and treatment

Signs of overdose include neuromuscular hypersensitivity. Seizure may follow high CNS concentrations. Cefotaxime may be removed by hemodialysis.

Clinical considerations

Consider the recommendations relevant to all cephalosporins as well as the following:
◻ ***ALERT*** Names of some cephalosporins are similar. Use caution when dispensing.
- For patients on sodium restriction, note that cefotaxime contains 2.2 mEq of sodium per gram of drug.
- For I.M. injection, add 2 ml, 3 ml, or 5 ml of sterile or bacteriostatic water for injection to each 500-mg, 1-g, or 2-g vial. Shake well to dissolve drug completely. Check solution for particles and discoloration. Color ranges from light yellow to amber.
- Don't inject more than 1 g into a single I.M. site to prevent pain and tissue reaction.
- Don't mix with aminoglycosides or sodium bicarbonate or fluids with a pH above 7.5.
- For I.V. use, reconstitute all strengths of an I.V. dose with 10 ml of sterile water for injection. For infusion bottles, add 50 to 100 ml of normal saline solution injection or 5% dextrose injection. May be further reconstituted to 50 to 1,000 ml with fluids recommended by manufacturer.
- Give drug by direct intermittent I.V. infusion over 3 to 5 minutes. Cefotaxime also may be given more slowly into a flowing I.V. line of compatible solution.
- Solution is stable for 24 hours at room temperature or at least 10 days under refrigeration in the original container. Cefotaxime may be stored in disposable glass or plastic syringes for 24 hours at room temperature or 5 days in the refrigerator.

Therapeutic monitoring

With large doses or prolonged therapy, monitoring for superinfection is necessary, especially in high-risk patients.

Special populations

Breast-feeding patients. Drug is excreted in breast milk and should be used with caution in breast-feeding women.

Pediatric patients. Cefotaxime may be used in neonates, infants, and children.
Geriatric patients. Use with caution in geriatric patients with diminished renal function.

Patient counseling

- Inform patient of potential adverse reactions.
- Instruct patient to report discomfort at I.V. site.

cefotetan disodium

Cefotan

Pharmacologic classification: second-generation cephalosporin, cephamycin
Therapeutic classification: antibiotic
Pregnancy risk category B

How supplied

Available by prescription only
Injection: 1 g, 2 g
Injection: 10 g bulk package
Infusion: 1 g, 2 g piggyback vials; frozen, premixed solutions of 1 g, 2 g in 50 ml

Indications and dosages

Serious urinary, lower respiratory, gynecologic, skin, intra-abdominal, and bone and joint infections caused by susceptible organisms
Adults: 500 mg to 3 g I.V. or I.M. q 12 hours for 5 to 10 days. Up to 6 g daily in life-threatening infections.
◇ *Children:* 40 to 60 mg/kg daily I.V. divided in equally divided doses q 12 hours.
Preoperative prophylaxis; ◇ use in contaminated surgery
Adults: 1 to 2 g I.V. 30 to 60 minutes before surgery.
Postcesarean
Adults: 1 to 2 g I.V. as soon as umbilical cord is clamped.

Total daily dose is same for I.M. or I.V. administration and depends on the susceptibility of the organism and severity of infection. Inject cefotetan deep I.M. into a large muscle mass, such as the gluteus or the lateral aspect of the thigh.

≡ ***Dosage adjustment.*** In patients with impaired renal function, doses or frequency of administration must be modified based on degree of renal impairment, severity of infection, and susceptibility of organism. To prevent toxic accumulation, reduced dosage may be necessary in patients with creatinine clearance less than 30 ml/minute. Because drug is hemodialyzable, hemodialysis patients may require dosage adjustment.

Creatinine clearance (ml/min/1.73 m²)	Adult dosage
> 30	Usual adult dose
10 to 30	Usual adult dose q 24 hours; or one-half the usual adult dose q 12 hours
< 10	Usual adult dose q 48 hours; or one-fourth the usual adult dose q 12 hours
Hemodialysis patients	One-fourth the usual adult dose q 24 hours on the days between hemodialysis sessions; and one-half the usual adult dose on the day of hemodialysis

Pharmacodynamics

Antibacterial action: Cefotetan is primarily bactericidal; however, it may be bacteriostatic. Activity depends on the organism, tissue penetration, drug dosage, and rate of organism multiplication. It acts by adhering to bacterial penicillin-binding proteins, thereby inhibiting cell-wall synthesis.

Cefotetan is active against many gram-positive organisms and enteric gram-negative bacilli, including streptococci, *Staphylococcus aureus* (penicillinase- and nonpenicillinase-producing), *Staphylococcus epidermidis, Escherichia coli, Klebsiella* species, *Enterobacter* species, *Proteus* species, *Haemophilus influenzae, Neisseria gonorrhoeae,* and *Bacteroides* species (including some strains of *B. fragilis*); however, some *B. fragilis* strains, *Pseudomonas,* and *Acinetobacter* are resistant to cefotetan. Most Enterobacteriaceae are more susceptible to cefotetan than to other second-generation cephalosporins.

Pharmacokinetics

Absorption: Not absorbed from the GI tract; must be given parenterally.
Distribution: Distributed widely into most body tissues and fluids, including the gallbladder, liver, kidneys, bone, sputum, bile, and pleural and synovial fluids; CSF penetration is poor. Biliary concentration levels of cefotetan can be up to 20 times higher than serum levels in patients with good gallbladder function. Cefotetan crosses the placenta, and is 75% to 90% protein-bound.
Metabolism: Not metabolized.
Excretion: Excreted primarily in urine by glomerular filtration and some renal tubular secretion; 20% is excreted in the bile. Small amounts of drug are excreted in breast milk.

Elimination half-life is about 3 to 4½ hours in patients with normal renal function.

Route	Onset	Peak	Duration
I.V.	Immediate	Immediate	Unknown
I.M.	Unknown	1½-3 hr	Unknown

Contraindications and precautions
Contraindicated in patients with hypersensitivity to drug or other cephalosporins. Use cautiously in patients with impaired renal function or penicillin allergy and in breast-feeding women.

Interactions
Drug-drug. *Anticoagulants:* May increase risk of bleeding. Patient needs close monitoring.
Nephrotoxic agents (aminoglycosides, colistin, polymyxin B, vancomycin) or loop diuretics: May increase the risk of nephrotoxicity. Patient needs close monitoring.
Probenecid: May inhibit excretion and increase blood levels of cefotetan. Sometimes used for this effect. Patient needs close monitoring.
Drug-lifestyle. *Alcohol use:* May cause disulfiram-like reactions (flushing, sweating, tachycardia, headache, and abdominal cramping). Patient should avoid alcohol consumption while on therapy and shouldn't drink alcohol for several days after discontinuing cefotetan therapy.

Effects on diagnostic tests
Cefotetan also causes false-positive results in urine glucose tests using cupric sulfate (Benedict's reagent or Clinitest); use glucose oxidase tests (Chemstrip uG, Diastix, or glucose enzymatic test strip) instead. Cefotetan causes false elevations in serum or urine creatinine levels in tests using Jaffé's reaction. It may cause positive Coombs' test results.

Adverse reactions
GI: pseudomembranous colitis, transient increases in liver enzymes; nausea, *diarrhea.*
GU: ***nephrotoxicity.***
Hematologic: ***transient neutropenia,*** eosinophilia, hemolytic anemia, hypoprothrombinemia, bleeding, thrombocytosis, ***agranulocytosis, thrombocytopenia.***
Skin: *maculopapular and erythematous rashes, urticaria pain, induration, sterile abscesses, tissue sloughing* (at injection site); *phlebitis, thrombophlebitis* (with I.V. injection).
Other: hypersensitivity reactions (serum sickness, ***anaphylaxis***); elevated temperature.

Overdose and treatment
Clinical signs of overdose include neuromuscular hypersensitivity. Seizure may follow high CNS concentrations. Hypoprothrombinemia and bleeding may occur; they may be treated with vitamin K or blood products. Cefotetan may be removed by hemodialysis.

Clinical considerations
Consider the recommendations relevant to all cephalosporins as well as the following:
□ ***ALERT*** Names of some cephalosporins are similar. Use caution when dispensing.
- For I.V. use, reconstitute with sterile water for injection. Then it may be mixed with 50 to 100 ml D_5W or normal saline solution. Infuse intermittently over 30 to 60 minutes.
- For I.M. injection, cefotetan may be reconstituted with sterile water or bacteriostatic water for injection or with normal saline or 0.5% or 1% lidocaine hydrochloride. Shake to dissolve and let solution stand until clear.
- Reconstituted solution remains stable for 24 hours at room temperature or for 96 hours when refrigerated.

Therapeutic monitoring
- Assess for signs and symptoms of overt and occult bleeding. Monitor vital signs. Check CBC with differential, platelet levels, and PT for abnormalities.
- Bleeding can be reversed promptly by administering vitamin K.

Special populations
Pregnant patients. Use only when clearly needed.
Breast-feeding patients. Cephalosporins are excreted in breast milk; use with caution in breast-feeding women. Safety in breast-feeding women hasn't been established.
Pediatric patients. Safety in children hasn't been established.
Geriatric patients. Hypoprothrombinemia and bleeding have been reported more frequently in geriatric and debilitated patients.

Patient counseling
- Inform patient of potential adverse reactions.
- Tell patient to promptly report signs of bleeding and discomfort at I.V. site.

cefoxitin sodium
Mefoxin

Pharmacologic classification: second-generation cephalosporin, cephamycin
Therapeutic classification: antibiotic
Pregnancy risk category B

How supplied
Available by prescription only
Injection: 1 g, 2 g
Pharmacy bulk package: 10 g
Infusion: 1 g, 2 g in 50-ml containers

Indications and dosages
Serious respiratory, GU, gynecologic, skin, soft-tissue, bone and joint, blood,

and intra-abdominal infections caused by susceptible organisms
Adults: 1 to 2 g I.V. q 6 to 8 hours for uncomplicated forms of infection. Up to 12 g daily in life-threatening infections.
Children over age 3 months: 80 to 160 mg/kg I.V. daily given in four to six equally divided doses. Don't exceed 12 g/day.

Total daily dose is same for I.M. and I.V. administration and depends on susceptibility of organism and severity of infection. Inject cefoxitin deep I.M. into a large muscle mass, such as the gluteus or lateral aspect of the thigh.

Perioperative prophylaxis; ◇use in contaminated surgery
Adults: 2 g I.V. 30 to 60 minutes before surgery; then 2 g I.V. q 6 hours for 24 hours postoperatively.
Children over age 3 months: 30 to 40 mg/kg I.V. 30 to 60 minutes before surgery; then 30 mg/kg I.V. q 6 hours for 24 hours postoperatively. For contaminated surgery, 1 to 2 g I.V. q 6 hours with or without I.V. gentamicin (1.5 mg/kg q 8 hours) for 5 days.

Uncomplicated gonorrhea
Adults: Give 2 g I.M. as a single dose with 1 g probenecid P.O. at the same time or up to 30 minutes beforehand.

Pelvic inflammatory disease
Adults: 2 g I.V. q 6 hours. (If *Chlamydia trachomatis* is suspected, give additional antichlamydial coverage.)

≡***Dosage adjustment.*** In patients with impaired renal function, doses or frequency of administration must be modified based on degree of renal impairment, severity of infection, and susceptibility of organism. To prevent toxic accumulation, reduced dosage may be required in patients with creatinine clearance less than 50 ml/minute/1.73 m^2.

Creatinine clearance (ml/min/1.73 m^2)	Adult dosage
> 50	Usual adult dose
30 to 50	1 to 2 g q 8 to 12 hours
10 to 29	1 to 2 g q 12 to 24 hours
5 to 9	500 mg to 1 g q 12 to 24 hours
< 5	500 mg to 1 g q 24 to 48 hours

Pharmacodynamics
Antibacterial action: Cefoxitin is primarily bactericidal; however, it may be bacteriostatic. Activity depends on the organism, tissue penetration, drug dosage, and rate of organism multiplication. It acts by adhering to bacterial penicillin-binding proteins, thereby inhibiting cell-wall synthesis.

Cefoxitin is active against many gram-positive organisms and enteric gram-negative bacilli, including *Escherichia coli* and other coliform bacteria, *Staphylococcus aureus* (penicillinase- and nonpenicillinase-producing), *Staphylococcus epidermidis*, streptococci, *Klebsiella, Haemophilus influenzae,* and *Bacteroides* species (including *B. fragilis*). *Enterobacter, Pseudomonas,* and *Acinetobacter* are resistant to cefoxitin.

Pharmacokinetics
Absorption: Not absorbed from the GI tract; must be given parenterally.
Distribution: Distributed widely into most body tissues and fluids, including the gallbladder, liver, kidneys, bone, sputum, bile, and pleural and synovial fluids; CSF penetration is poor. Cefoxitin crosses the placenta, and is 50% to 80% protein-bound.
Metabolism: About 2% of a cefoxitin dose is metabolized.
Excretion: Excreted primarily in urine by renal tubular secretion and glomerular filtration; small amounts of drug are excreted in breast milk. Elimination half-life is about 0.7 to 1.1 hours in patients with normal renal function; half-life is prolonged in patients with severe renal dysfunction to 6.3 to 21.5 hours. Cefoxitin can be removed by hemodialysis but not by peritoneal dialysis.

Route	Onset	Peak	Duration
I.V.	Immediate	Immediate	Unknown
I.M.	Unknown	20-30 min	Unknown

Contraindications and precautions
Contraindicated in patients with hypersensitivity to drug or other cephalosporins. Use cautiously in patients with impaired renal function or penicillin allergy and in breast-feeding women.

Interactions
Drug-drug. *Bacteriostatic agents (tetracyclines, erythromycin, chloramphenicol):* May impair the bactericidal activity of cefoxitin. Avoid use together.
Nephrotoxic agents (vancomycin, colistin, polymyxin B, aminoglycosides) or loop diuretics: May increase the risk of nephrotoxicity. Patient must be monitored closely.
Probenecid: Competitively inhibits renal tubular secretion of cephalosporins, resulting in higher, prolonged serum levels of these drugs. Patient must be monitored closely.

Effects on diagnostic tests
Cefoxitin causes false-positive results in urine glucose tests using cupric sulfate (Benedict's reagent or Clinitest); use glucose oxidase tests (Chemstrip uG, Diastix, or glucose enzymatic test strip) instead. Cefoxitin also causes false elevations in serum or urine creatinine levels

in tests using Jaffé's reaction. May cause positive Coombs' test results.

Adverse reactions

CV: hypotension.
GI: pseudomembranous colitis, nausea, transient increases in liver enzymes, vomiting, *diarrhea.*
GU: ***acute renal failure.***
Hematologic: ***transient neutropenia,*** eosinophilia, ***hemolytic anemia,*** anemia, ***thrombocytopenia.***
Respiratory: dyspnea (with I.V. injection).
Skin: *maculopapular and erythematous rash, urticaria,* exfoliative dermatitis *pain, induration, sterile abscesses, tissue sloughing* (at injection site).
Other: hypersensitivity reactions (serum sickness, ***anaphylaxis***), elevated temperature; *phlebitis, thrombophlebitis.*

Overdose and treatment

Clinical signs of overdose include neuromuscular hypersensitivity. Seizure may follow high CNS concentrations. Cefoxitin may be removed by hemodialysis.

Clinical considerations

Consider the recommendations relevant to all cephalosporins as well as the following:
□ ***ALERT*** Names of some cephalosporins are similar. Use caution when dispensing.

- For I.V. use, reconstitute 1 g of cefoxitin with at least 10 ml of sterile water for injection, or 2 g of cefoxitin with 10 to 20 ml. Solutions of dextrose 5% and normal saline solution for injection can also be used.
- For I.M. injection, reconstitute with 0.5% to 1% lidocaine hydrochloride (without epinephrine) to minimize pain at injection site; or with sterile water for injection.
- Administer cefoxitin I.M. deep into a large muscle mass. Advise aspiration before injecting to prevent inadvertent injection into a blood vessel, and rotation of sites to prevent tissue damage.
- After reconstituting, shake vial and then let stand until clear to ensure complete drug dissolution. Solution is stable for 24 hours at room temperature, for 1 week if refrigerated, or 26 weeks if frozen.
- Solution may range from colorless to light amber and may darken during storage. Slight color change doesn't indicate loss of potency.
- Cefoxitin injection contains 2.3 mEq of sodium per gram of drug.

Therapeutic monitoring

Cefoxitin has been associated with thrombophlebitis. Frequent assessment of I.V. site for signs of infiltration or phlebitis is recommended.

Special populations

Pregnant patients. Use only when clearly needed.
Breast-feeding patients. Drug is excreted in breast milk; use with caution in breast-feeding women.
Pediatric patients. Dosage may need to be reduced in infants under age 3 months. Safety hasn't been established.
Geriatric patients. Dosage reduction may be necessary in patients with diminished renal function.

Patient counseling

Inform patient of potential adverse reactions.

cefpodoxime proxetil

Vantin

Pharmacologic classification: third-generation cephalosporin
Therapeutic classification: antibiotic
Pregnancy risk category B

How supplied

Available by prescription only
Tablets (film-coated): 100 mg, 200 mg
Oral suspension: 50 mg/5 ml, 100 mg/5 ml

Indications and dosages

***Acute, community-acquired pneumonia caused by non-beta-lactamase-producing strains of* Haemophilus influenzae *or* Streptococcus pneumoniae**
Adults: 200 mg P.O. q 12 hours for 14 days.
***Acute bacterial exacerbations of chronic bronchitis caused by non beta-lactamase-producing strains of* H. influenzae, S. pneumoniae, *or* Moraxella catarrhalis**
Adults: 200 mg P.O. q 12 hours for 10 days.
Uncomplicated gonorrhea in men and women; rectal gonococcal infections in women
Adults: 200 mg P.O. as a single dose. Follow with doxycycline 100 mg P.O. b.i.d. for 7 days.
***Uncomplicated skin and skin structure infections caused by* Staphylococcus aureus *or* Streptococcus pyogenes**
Adults: 400 mg P.O. q 12 hours for 7 to 14 days.
***Acute otitis media caused by* S. pneumoniae, H. influenzae, *or* M. catarrhalis**
Children age 2 months to 12 years: 5 mg/kg (not to exceed 200 mg) P.O. q 12 hours for 5 days.
***Pharyngitis or tonsillitis caused by* S. pyogenes**
Adults: 100 mg P.O. q 12 hours for 7 to 10 days.
Children age 2 months to 12 years: 5 mg/kg (not to exceed 100 mg) P.O. q 12 hours for 5 to 10 days.
***Uncomplicated urinary tract infections caused by* Escherichia coli, Klebsiella**

pneumoniae, Proteus mirabilis, *or* Staphylococcus saprophyticus
Adults: 100 mg P.O. q 12 hours for 7 days.
Acute maxillary sinusitis
Children age 2 months to 12 years: 5 mg/kg (up to 200 mg) q 12 hours for 10 days.
≡***Dosage adjustment.*** In patients with renal impairment when creatinine clearance is less than 30 ml/minute, increase dosage interval to q 24 hours. Patients receiving hemodialysis should get drug three times weekly, after dialysis.

Pharmacodynamics

Antibiotic action: A second-generation cephalosporin, cefpodoxime proxetil is a bactericidal agent that inhibits cell-wall synthesis. It's usually active against gram-positive aerobes, such as *Staphylococcus aureus* (including penicillinase-producing strains), *S. saprophyticus, S. pneumoniae,* and *S. pyogenes,* and gram-negative aerobes, such as *Escherichia coli, Haemophilus influenzae* (including beta-lactamase-producing strains), *Klebsiella pneumoniae, Branhamella catarrhalis, Neisseria gonorrhoeae* (including penicillinase-producing strains), and *Proteus mirabilis.*

Pharmacokinetics

Absorption: Absorbed via the GI tract. Absorption and mean peak plasma levels increase when drug is administered with food.
Distribution: Widely distributed to most tissues and fluids. Second-generation cephalosporins don't enter CSF even when the meninges are inflamed. Protein-binding ranges from 22% to 33% in serum and from 21% to 29% in plasma.
Metabolism: De-esterified to its active metabolite, cefpodoxime.
Excretion: Excreted primarily in urine.

Route	Onset	Peak	Duration
P.O.	Unknown	2-3 hr	Unknown

Contraindications and precautions

Contraindicated in patients with hypersensitivity to drug or other cephalosporins. Use cautiously in patients with impaired renal function or penicillin allergy and in breast-feeding women.

Interactions

Drug-drug. *Antacids* and *H_2 antagonists:* decrease absorption of cefpodoxime proxetil and shouldn't be administered together.
Probenecid: Decreases the excretion of cefpodoxime proxetil. Patient requires monitoring for cefpodoxime toxicity.
Drug-food. *Any food:* Increased absorption. Give drug with food.

Effects on diagnostic tests

Cefpodoxime proxetil may induce a positive direct Coombs' test.

Adverse reactions

CNS: headache.
GI: *diarrhea,* nausea, vomiting, abdominal pain.
GU: vaginal fungal infections.
Skin: rash.
Other: hypersensitivity reactions ***(anaphylaxis).***

Overdose and treatment

No information on drug overdose is available. Toxic symptoms after an overdose of beta-lactam antibiotics may include nausea, vomiting, epigastric distress, and diarrhea. In the event of serious toxic reaction from overdose, hemodialysis or peritoneal dialysis may aid in removing drug from the body, particularly if renal function is compromised.

Clinical considerations

□ ***ALERT*** Names of some cephalosporins are similar. Use caution when dispensing.
- Drug is highly stable in presence of beta-lactamase enzymes. As a result, many organisms resistant to penicillins and some cephalosporins, because of presence of beta-lactamases, may be susceptible to cefpodoxime proxetil.
- Cefpodoxime is inactive against most strains of *Pseudomonas, Enterobacter,* and *Enterococcus.*
- Specimens are obtained for culture and sensitivity tests before first dose. Therapy may begin pending test results.
- Store suspension in refrigerator (36° to 46° F [2° to 8° C]). Shake well before using. Discard unused portion after 14 days.

Therapeutic monitoring

- As with other antibiotics, prolonged use of cefpodoxime proxetil may result in overgrowth of nonsusceptible organisms. Repeated evaluation of the patient's condition is essential, and appropriate measures should be taken if superinfection occurs during therapy.

Special populations

Pregnant patients. Use only when clearly needed.
Breast-feeding patients. Drug is excreted in breast milk. Because of the potential for serious reactions in breast-fed infants, a decision must be made to discontinue breast-feeding or drug, taking into account the importance of drug to the woman.
Pediatric patients. Safety and efficacy in infants under age 6 months haven't been established.
Geriatric patients. No dose adjustment is necessary based on age. Any patient on dialysis,

especially the elderly, should receive the dose after dialysis treatment.

Patient counseling

- Tell patient to report rash or signs and symptoms of superinfection.
- Advise patient to continue taking drug for the prescribed course of therapy, even after feeling better.

cefprozil

Cefzil

Pharmacologic classification: second-generation cephalosporin
Therapeutic classification: antibiotic
Pregnancy risk category B

How supplied

Available by prescription only
Tablets: 250 mg, 500 mg
Oral suspension: 125 mg/5 ml, 250 mg/5 ml

Indications and dosages

***Pharyngitis or tonsillitis caused by* Streptococcus pyogenes**
Adults and children age 13 and older: 500 mg P.O. daily for at least 10 days.
Children age 2 to 12: 7.5 mg/kg P.O. q 12 hours for 10 days.
***Otitis media caused by* Streptococcus pneumoniae, Haemophilus influenzae, *and* Moraxella (Branhamella) catarrhalis**
Infants and children age 6 months to 12 years: 15 mg/kg P.O. q 12 hours for 10 days.
***Secondary bacterial infections of acute bronchitis and acute bacterial exacerbation of chronic bronchitis caused by* S. pneumoniae, H. influenzae, *and* M. (B.) catarrhalis**
Adults: 500 mg P.O. q 12 hours for 10 days.
***Uncomplicated skin and skin structure infections caused by* Staphylococcus aureus *and* S. pyogenes**
Adults and children age 13 and older: 250 mg P.O. b.i.d. or 500 mg daily to b.i.d. for 10 days.
Children age 2 to 12: 20 mg/kg P.O. q 24 hours for 10 days.
≡ ***Dosage adjustment.*** No adjustments are necessary for patients with creatinine clearance of more than 30 ml/minute. For patients with creatinine clearance of 30 ml/minute or less, dose should be reduced by 50%; however, dosing interval remains unchanged. Because drug is partially removed by hemodialysis, administer after the hemodialysis session.

Pharmacodynamics

Antibiotic action: Cefprozil interferes with bacterial cell-wall synthesis during cell replication, leading to osmotic instability and cell lysis. Action is bactericidal or bacteriostatic, depending on concentration.

Pharmacokinetics

Note: Pharmacokinetic data are derived from investigational studies that used an oral capsule formulation that isn't commercially available.
Absorption: About 95% absorbed from the GI tract.
Distribution: About 36% protein-bound.
Metabolism: Probably metabolized by the liver; plasma half-life increases only slightly in patients with impaired hepatic function.
Excretion: About 60% of a dose is recovered unchanged in the urine. Plasma half-life is 1⅓ hours in patients with normal renal function; 2 hours, impaired hepatic function; and 5¼ to 6 hours, end-stage renal disease. Drug is removed by hemodialysis.

Route	Onset	Peak	Duration
P.O.	Unknown	1½ hr	Unknown

Contraindications and precautions

Contraindicated in patients with hypersensitivity to drug or other cephalosporins. Use cautiously in patients with impaired renal function or penicillin allergy and in breast-feeding women.

Interactions

Drug-drug. *Aminoglycosides*: May increase the risk of nephrotoxicity of cephalosporins. Patient needs close monitoring.
Probenecid: May decrease excretion and increase blood levels of cefprozil. Use together cautiously.

Effects on diagnostic tests

Cephalosporins may produce a false-positive test for urine glucose with tests that use copper reduction method (Benedict's test, Fehling's solution, or Clinitest tablets). Instead, use enzymatic methods, such as glucose enzymatic test strip. A false-negative reaction may occur in the ferricyanide test for blood glucose.

Adverse reactions

CNS: dizziness, hyperactivity, headache, nervousness, insomnia, confusion, somnolence.
GI: *diarrhea, nausea,* vomiting, abdominal pain.
GU: elevated BUN level, elevated serum creatinine level, genital pruritus, vaginitis.
Hematologic: decreased leukocyte count, eosinophilia.
Hepatic: elevated liver enzymes, cholestatic jaundice (rare).
Skin: rash, urticaria, diaper rash.
Other: superinfection, hypersensitivity reactions (serum sickness, ***anaphylaxis***).

Overdose and treatment

Because drug is eliminated primarily by the kidneys, the manufacturer states that hemodialysis may aid in removal of drug in cases of extreme overdose, especially in patients with decreased renal function.

Clinical considerations

Consider the recommendations relevant to all cephalosporins as well as the following:

□ ***ALERT*** Names of some cephalosporins are similar. Use caution when dispensing.

- Obtain specimens for culture and sensitivity tests before first dose. Therapy may begin pending test results.
- Drug may cause overgrowth of nonsusceptible bacteria or fungi, so patient will be observed for signs and symptoms of superinfection.
- Advise patients with phenylketonuria that oral suspension contains 28 mg/5 ml phenylalanine.

Therapeutic monitoring

- Pseudomembranous colitis has been reported with nearly all antibacterial agents. It may occur in patients in whom diarrhea develops secondary to antibiotic therapy. Although most patients respond to withdrawal of drug therapy alone, it may be necessary to institute treatment with an antibacterial agent effective against *Clostridium difficile*, an organism linked to this disorder.

Special populations

Pregnant patients. Use during pregnancy or labor and delivery only when clearly needed.
Breast-feeding patients. It's unknown if drug is excreted in breast milk. Use with caution in breast-feeding women.
Pediatric patients. Oral suspensions contain drug in a bubble gum-flavored vehicle to improve palatability and compliance in children. Store reconstituted suspension in the refrigerator, and discard unused drug after 14 days. Shake suspension well before measuring dose.
Geriatric patients. Elderly volunteers (age 65 and older) exhibited a higher area under the plasma-concentration-versus-time curve and lower renal clearance compared with younger subjects.

Patient counseling

- Tell patient to take all of drug as prescribed, even if he feels better.
- Instruct patient to notify doctor if rash or symptoms of superinfection occur.

ceftazidime

Ceptaz, Fortaz, Tazicef, Tazidime

Pharmacologic classification: third-generation cephalosporin
Therapeutic classification: antibiotic
Pregnancy risk category B

How supplied

Available by prescription only
Injection: 500 mg, 1 g, 2 g
Injection: 6 g, 10 g bulk package
Infusion: 1 g, 2 g in 20-, 50-, and 100-ml vials and bags

Indications and dosages

Bacteremia, septicemia, and serious respiratory, urinary, gynecologic, bone and joint, intra-abdominal, CNS, and skin infections from susceptible organisms
Adults: 1 g I.V. or I.M. q 8 to 12 hours; up to 6 g daily in life-threatening infections.
Children age 1 month to 12 years: 30 to 50 mg/kg I.V. q 8 hours to a maximum of 6 g/day (Fortaz, Tazicef, and Tazidime only).
Neonates up to 4 weeks: 30 mg/kg I.V. q 12 hours (Fortaz, Tazicef, and Tazidime only).

Total daily dose is the same for I.M. or I.V. administration and depends on susceptibility of organism and severity of infection. Inject ceftazidime deep I.M. into a large muscle mass, such as the gluteus or lateral aspect of the thigh.

◇ ***Empiric therapy in febrile neutropenic patients***
Adults: 100 mg/kg I.V. daily in 3 divided doses; or 2 g I.V. q 8 hours either alone or in conjunction with an aminoglycoside such as amikacin.
Children age 2 years and older: 50 mg/kg (maximum 2 g) q 8 hours given I.V.

≡ ***Dosage adjustment.*** In patients with impaired renal function, doses or frequency of administration must be modified according to the degree of renal impairment, severity of infection, and susceptibility of organism. To prevent toxic accumulation, reduced dosage may be required in patients with creatinine clearance less than 50 ml/minute/1.73 m^2. In patients with creatinine clearance of 50 ml/minute or less, initially give 1 g loading dose then follow maintenance recommendations.

Creatinine clearance (ml/min/1.73 m^2)	Adult dosage
> 50	Usual adult dose
31 to 50	1 g q 12 hours
16 to 30	1 g q 24 hours
6 to 15	500 mg q 24 hours
≤ 5	500 mg q 48 hours
Hemodialysis patients	1 g after each hemodialysis period
Peritoneal dialysis patients	500 mg q 24 hours

Pharmacodynamics

Antibacterial action: Ceftazidime is primarily bactericidal; however, it may be bacteriostatic. Activity depends on the organism, tissue penetration, drug dosage, and rate of organism multiplication. It acts by adhering to bacterial penicillin-binding proteins, thereby inhibiting cell-wall synthesis. Third-generation cephalosporins appear more active against some beta-lactamase-producing gram-negative organisms.

Ceftazidime is active against some gram-positive organisms and many enteric gram-negative bacilli, as well as streptococci (*Streptococcus pneumoniae* and *S. pyogenes*); *Staphylococcus aureus* (penicillinase- and nonpenicillinase-producing); *Escherichia coli; Klebsiella* species; *Proteus* species; *Enterobacter* species; *Haemophilus influenzae; Pseudomonas* species; and some strains of *Bacteroides* species. It's more effective than any cephalosporin or penicillin derivative against *Pseudomonas*. Some other third-generation cephalosporins are more active against gram-positive organisms and anaerobes.

Pharmacokinetics

Absorption: Not absorbed from the GI tract; must be given parenterally.
Distribution: Distributed widely into most body tissues and fluids, including the gallbladder, liver, kidneys, bone, sputum, bile, and pleural and synovial fluids; unlike most other cephalosporins, ceftazidime has good CSF penetration; it crosses the placenta. Ceftazidime is 5% to 24% protein-bound.
Metabolism: Not metabolized.
Excretion: Excreted primarily in urine by glomerular filtration; small amounts of drug are excreted in breast milk. Elimination half-life is about 1½ to 2 hours in patients with normal renal function; up to 35 hours in patients with severe renal disease. Hemodialysis or peritoneal dialysis removes ceftazidime.

Route	Onset	Peak	Duration
I.V.	Immediate	Immediate	Unknown
I.M.	Unknown	1 hr	Unknown

Contraindications and precautions

Contraindicated in patients with hypersensitivity to drug or other cephalosporins. Use cautiously in breast-feeding women and in patients with poor renal function or penicillin allergy.

Interactions

Drug-drug. *Aminoglycosides:* Concurrent use results in synergistic activity against some strains of *Pseudomonas aeruginosa* and Enterobacteriaceae. Monitor for effects.
Chloramphenicol: Antagonistic effect. Avoid use together.
Probenicid: May inhibit excretion and increase levels. May be used as a therapeutic effect.
Quinolones: In vitro studies show synergistic effect against *Burkholderia cepacia.*

Effects on diagnostic tests

Ceftazidime causes false-positive results in urine glucose tests using cupric sulfate (Benedict's reagent or Clinitest); use glucose oxidase (Chemstrip uG, Diastix, or glucose enzymatic test strip) instead. Ceftazidime also causes false elevations in urine creatinine levels in tests using Jaffé's reaction. Ceftazidime may cause positive Coombs' test results.

Adverse reactions

CNS: headache, dizziness, paresthesia, ***seizures.***
GI: pseudomembranous colitis, nausea, vomiting, diarrhea, transient elevation in liver enzymes, candidiasis, abdominal cramps.
GU: vaginitis.
Hematologic: eosinophilia, thrombocytosis, ***leukopenia,*** hemolytic anemia, ***agranulocytosis, thrombocytopenia.***
Skin: *maculopapular and erythematous rash, urticaria, pain, induration, sterile abscesses, tissue sloughing* (at injection site).
Other: hypersensitivity reactions (serum sickness, ***anaphylaxis***), *phlebitis, thrombophlebitis* (with I.V. injection).

Overdose and treatment

Clinical signs of overdose include neuromuscular hypersensitivity. Seizure may follow high CNS concentrations. Drug may be removed by hemodialysis or peritoneal dialysis.

Clinical considerations

Consider the recommendations relevant to all cephalosporins as well as the following:

□ ***ALERT*** Names of some cephalosporins are similar. Use caution when dispensing.

- For patients on sodium restriction, note that ceftazidime contains 2.3 mEq of sodium per gram of drug.
- Ceftazidime powders (excluding Ceptaz) for injection contain 118 mg sodium carbonate per gram of drug; ceftazidime sodium is more water-soluble and is formed in situ upon reconstitution.
- Vials are supplied under reduced pressure. When antibiotic is dissolved, carbon dioxide is released and a positive pressure develops. Each brand of ceftazidime includes specific instructions for reconstitution. Read carefully.
- Because drug is hemodialyzable, patients undergoing treatments with hemodialysis or peritoneal dialysis may require dosage adjustment.
- Separate I.V. sites should be used for aminoglycosides and ceftazidime.

Therapeutic monitoring

With large doses or prolonged therapy, patients, especially high-risk patients, must be observed for superinfection.

Special populations

Pregnant patients. Use only when clearly needed.
Breast-feeding patients. Drug is excreted in breast milk; use with caution in breast-feeding women. Safety hasn't been established.

Pediatric patients. Only Fortaz, Tazicef, and Tazidime may be used in infants and children. Ceptaz shouldn't be used in children under age 12 because it contains arginine.
Geriatric patients. Reduced dosage may be necessary in geriatric patients with diminished renal function.

Patient counseling
- Advise patient to report discomfort at I.V. site.
- Tell patient to report rash or symptoms of superinfection.

ceftibuten
Cedax

Pharmacologic classification: third-generation cephalosporin
Therapeutic classification: antibiotic
Pregnancy risk category B

How supplied
Available by prescription only
Capsules: 400 mg
Oral suspension: 90 mg/5 ml, 180 mg/5 ml

Indications and dosages
***Acute bacterial exacerbations of chronic bronchitis due to* Haemophilus influenzae, Moraxella catarrhalis, *or* Streptococcus pneumoniae**
Adults and children age 12 and older: 400 mg P.O. daily for 10 days.
***Pharyngitis and tonsillitis due to* Streptococcus pyogenes; *acute bacterial otitis media due to* H. influenzae, M. catarrhalis, *or* S. pyogenes**
Adults and children age 12 and older: 400 mg P.O. daily for 10 days.
Children younger than 12: 9 mg/kg P.O. daily for 10 days. Children weighing more than 99 lb (45 kg) should receive the maximum daily dose of 400 mg.
≡ ***Dosage adjustment.*** No adjustments are necessary for patients with creatinine clearance of more than 50 ml/minute. Give 4.5 mg/kg (or 200 mg) daily to patients with creatinine clearance between 30 and 49 ml/minute and 2.25 mg/kg (or 100 mg) daily for those with creatinine clearance of 5 to 29 ml/minute. For patients undergoing hemodialysis two or three times weekly, give a single 400-mg dose (capsule form) or administer a single dose of 9 mg/kg (maximum dose, 400 mg) using oral suspension at the end of each hemodialysis session.

Pharmacodynamics
Antibiotic action: Ceftibuten exerts its bactericidal action by binding to essential target proteins of the bacterial cell wall. This binding leads to inhibition of cell-wall synthesis. It's usually active against gram-positive aerobes (*S. pneumoniae, S. pyogenes*) and gram-negative aerobes (*H. influenzae, M. catarrhalis*).

Pharmacokinetics
Absorption: Rapidly absorbed from GI tract. Food decreases the bioavailability of drug.
Distribution: 65% bound to plasma proteins.
Metabolism: Metabolized to its predominant component, cis-ceftibuten. About 10% of ceftibuten is converted to the transisomer.
Excretion: Excreted in urine and feces.

Route	Onset	Peak	Duration
P.O.	Unknown	2-4 hr	Unknown

Contraindications and precautions
Contraindicated in patients with hypersensitivity to the cephalosporin group of antibiotics. Use cautiously if administering to patients with history of hypersensitivity to penicillin because up to 10% of these patients will exhibit cross-sensitivity to a cephalosporin. Also use cautiously in patients with impaired renal function and GI disease (especially colitis).

Interactions
Drug-food. *Any food:* Decreased bioavailability of drug, which slows its absorption. Advise patient to take drug 2 hours before or 1 hour after a meal.

Effects on diagnostic tests
Although ceftibuten hasn't been known to affect the direct Coombs' test to date, other cephalosporins have caused a false-positive direct Coombs' test. Therefore, it should be recognized that a positive Coombs' test could be due to drug.

Adverse reactions
CNS: headache, dizziness, fatigue, paresthesia, somnolence, taste perversion, agitation, hyperkinesia, insomnia, irritability, rigors.
EENT: nasal congestion.
GI: nausea, dyspepsia, abdominal pain, vomiting, anorexia, constipation, dry mouth, eructation, flatulence, loose stools, melena.
GU: dysuria, hematuria, elevated BUN and serum creatinine level, vaginitis.
Hematologic: elevated amount of eosinophils, decreased hemoglobin level, altered platelet count, decreased leukocyte count.
Hepatic: elevated levels of liver enzymes, bilirubin, and alkaline phosphatase.
Respiratory: dyspnea.
Skin: rash, pruritus, diaper dermatitis, urticaria.
Other: candidiasis, dehydration, fever.

Overdose and treatment
Overdose of cephalosporins can cause cerebral irritation leading to seizures. Ceftibuten is readily dialyzable and significant quantities (65% of plasma levels) can be removed from the circulation by a single hemodialysis session. In-

formation with regarding the removal of ceftibuten by peritoneal dialysis doesn't exist.

Clinical considerations

Consider the recommendations relevant to all cephalosporins as well as the following:

- Pseudomembranous colitis has been reported with nearly all antibacterial agents; it may occur in patients in whom diarrhea develops secondary to antibiotic therapy. Although most patients respond to withdrawal of drug therapy alone, it may be necessary to institute treatment with an antibacterial agent effective against *Clostridium difficile*, an organism linked to this disorder.
- Obtain specimens for culture and sensitivity testing before first dose. Therapy may begin pending test results.
- When preparing oral suspension, first tap the bottle to loosen powder. Follow chart supplied by manufacturer for amount of water to add to powder when mixing oral suspension form. Add water in two portions, shaking well after each aliquot. After mixing, the suspension may be kept for 14 days and must be stored in the refrigerator.

Therapeutic monitoring

- Drug may cause overgrowth of nonsusceptible bacteria or fungi. Patient requires observation for signs and symptoms of superinfection.

Special populations

Breast-feeding patients. It isn't known if drug is excreted in breast milk. Use cautiously in breast-feeding women.
Pediatric patients. Safety and effectiveness in infants under age 6 months haven't been established.
Geriatric patients. Use with caution in geriatric patients. Dosage adjustment may be necessary if patient has impaired renal function.

Patient counseling

- Tell patient to take all of drug as prescribed, even if he's feeling better.
- Inform diabetic patient that oral suspension contains 1 g of sucrose per teaspoon of suspension.
- Instruct patient using oral suspension to shake bottle well before measuring dose.

ceftizoxime sodium

Cefizox

Pharmacologic classification: third-generation cephalosporin
Therapeutic classification: antibiotic
Pregnancy risk category B

How supplied

Available by prescription only
Injection: 500 mg, 1 g, 2 g, 10 g (bulk package)
Infusion: 1 g, 2 g in 100-ml vials

Indications and dosages

Bacteremia, septicemia, meningitis, pelvic inflammatory disease, and serious respiratory, urinary, gynecologic, intra-abdominal, bone and joint, and skin infections from susceptible organisms
Adults: Usual dosage is 500 mg to 2 g I.V. or I.M. q 8 to 12 hours. In life-threatening infections, 3 to 4 g I.V. q 8 hours.
Children age 6 months and older: 50 mg/kg I.V. or I.M. q 6 to 8 hours.

Total daily dose is same for I.M. or I.V. administration and depends on susceptibility of organism and severity of infection. Inject ceftizoxime deep I.M. into a large muscle mass, such as the gluteus or lateral aspect of the thigh.
Uncomplicated gonorrhea
Adults: 1 g I.M. given as a single dose.
≡***Dosage adjustment.*** In patients with impaired renal function, modify doses or frequency of administration according to degree of renal impairment, severity of infection, and susceptibility of organism. To prevent toxic accumulation, reduced dosage may be required in patients with creatinine clearance less than 80 ml/minute. The following table gives appropriate doses for adults.

Creatinine clearance (ml/min/1.73 m²)	Less severe infections	Life-threatening infections
> 80	Usual adult dose	Usual adult dose
50 to 79	500 mg q 8 hours	750 mg to 1.5 g q 8 hours
5 to 49	250 to 500 mg q 12 hours	500 mg to 1 g q 12 hours
0 to 4	500 mg q 48 hours; or 250 mg q 24 hours	500 mg to 1 g q 48 hours; or 500 mg q 24 hours

Pharmacodynamics

Antibacterial action: Ceftizoxime is primarily bactericidal; however, it may be bacteriostatic. Activity depends on the organism, tissue penetration, drug dosage, and rate of organism multiplication. It acts by adhering to bacterial penicillin-binding proteins, thereby inhibiting cell-wall synthesis. Third-generation cephalosporins appear more active against some beta-lactamase-producing gram-negative organisms.

Drug is active against some gram-positive organisms and many enteric gram-negative bacilli, as well as streptococci (*Streptococcus pneumoniae* and *pyogenes*); *Staphylococcus aureus* (penicillinase- and non-penicillinase-producing); *Staphylococcus epidermidis; Es-*

cherichia coli; Klebsiella species; Haemophilus influenzae; Enterobacter species; Proteus species; Bacteroides species (including Bacteroides fragilis); Peptostreptococcus species; some strains of Pseudomonas and Acinetobacter. Cefotaxime and moxalactam are slightly more active than ceftizoxime against gram-positive organisms but are less active against gram-negative organisms.

Pharmacokinetics

Absorption: Not absorbed from the GI tract; must be given parenterally.
Distribution: Distributed widely into most body tissues and fluids, including the gallbladder, liver, kidneys, bone, sputum, bile, and pleural and synovial fluids. Unlike most other cephalosporins, ceftizoxime has good CSF penetration and achieves adequate concentration in inflamed meninges; ceftizoxime crosses the placenta and is 30% protein-bound.
Metabolism: Not metabolized.
Excretion: Excreted primarily in urine by renal tubular secretion and glomerular filtration; small amounts of drug are excreted in breast milk. Elimination half-life is about 1½ to 2 hours in patients with normal renal function; severe renal disease prolongs half-life up to 30 hours. Hemodialysis or peritoneal dialysis removes minimal amounts of ceftizoxime.

Route	Onset	Peak	Duration
I.V.	Immediate	Immediate	Unknown
I.M.	Unknown	½-1½ hr	Unknown

Contraindications and precautions

Contraindicated in patients with hypersensitivity to ceftizoxime or other cephalosporins. Use cautiously in breast-feeding women and in patients with impaired renal function or penicillin allergy.

Interactions

Drug-drug. *Aminoglycosides:* May slightly increase the risk of nephrotoxicity. Avoid use. *Probenecid*: Competitively inhibits renal tubular secretion of cephalosporins, causing higher, prolonged serum levels. May be used for this effect.

Effects on diagnostic tests

Ceftizoxime causes false-positive results in urine glucose tests utilizing cupric sulfate (Benedict's reagent or Clinitest); use glucose oxidase (Chemstrip uG, Diastix, or glucose enzymatic test strip) instead. Ceftizoxime also causes false elevations in urine creatinine levels using Jaffé's reaction. Ceftizoxime may cause positive Coombs' test results.

Adverse reactions

GI: pseudomembranous colitis, nausea, anorexia, vomiting, *diarrhea*, transient elevation in liver enzymes (with I.V. injection).
GU: vaginitis.
Hematologic: ***transient neutropenia,*** eosinophilia, hemolytic anemia, thrombocytosis, anemia, ***thrombocytopenia.***
Respiratory: dyspnea.
Skin: *maculopapular and erythematous rash, urticaria pain, induration, sterile abscesses, tissue sloughing (at injected site).*
Other: hypersensitivity reactions (serum sickness, ***anaphylaxis***), elevated temperature, *phlebitis, thrombophlebitis.*

Overdose and treatment

Clinical signs of overdose include neuromuscular hypersensitivity. Seizure may follow high CNS concentrations. Ceftizoxime may be removed by hemodialysis.

Clinical considerations

Consider the recommendations relevant to all cephalosporins as well as the following:
☐ ***ALERT*** Names of some cephalosporins are similar. Use caution when dispensing.
- For patients on sodium restriction, note that ceftizoxime contains 2.6 mEq of sodium per gram of drug.
- Drug may be supplied as frozen, sterile solution in plastic containers. Thaw at room temperature. Thawed solution is stable for 24 hours at room temperature or for 21 days if refrigerated. Don't refreeze.
- For I.M. use, reconstitute with sterile water for injection. Shake vial well to ensure complete dissolution of drug. To administer a dose that exceeds 1 g, divide the dose and inject it into separate sites to prevent tissue injury.
- For I.V. use, reconstitute I.V. dose with sterile water for injection. Solution should clear after shaking well and range in color from yellow to amber. If particles are visible, discard solution. Reconstituted solution is stable for 24 hours at room temperature or 96 hours if refrigerated.
- Administer ceftizoxime I.V. as a direct injection slowly over 3 to 5 minutes directly or through tubing of compatible infusion fluid. If given as intermittent infusion, the reconstituted drug is diluted in 50 to 100 ml of compatible fluid. Check package insert.

Therapeutic monitoring

- If a severe hypersensitivity reaction occurs during therapy, discontinue drug and institute appropriate therapy (such as epinephrine, I.V. fluids, oxygen).

Special populations

Breast-feeding patients. Drug is excreted in breast milk; use with caution in breast-feeding women. Safety hasn't been established.
Pediatric patients. Safety and efficacy haven't been established in infants under age 6 months.
Geriatric patients. Reduced dosage may be necessary in geriatric patients with diminished renal function.

Patient counseling
- Inform patient of potential adverse reactions.
- Tell patient to report discomfort at I.V. site.

ceftriaxone sodium
Rocephin

Pharmacologic classification: third-generation cephalosporin
Therapeutic classification: antibiotic
Pregnancy risk category B

How supplied
Available by prescription only
Injection: 250 mg, 500 mg, 1 g, 2 g, 10-g bulk package
Infusion: 1 g, 2 g

Indications and dosages
Bacteremia, septicemia, and serious respiratory, bone, joint, urinary, gynecologic, intra-abdominal, and skin infections from susceptible organisms
Adults and children 12 and older: 1 to 2 g I.M. or I.V. once daily or in equally divided doses b.i.d. Total daily dose shouldn't exceed 4 g.
Children younger than 12: Total daily dose is 50 to 75 mg/kg I.M. or I.V., given in divided doses q 12 hours. Maximum daily dose is 2 g.
Gonococcal meningitis, endocarditis
Adults: 1 to 2 g I.V. q 12 hours for 10 to 14 days for meningitis and 3 to 4 weeks for endocarditis.
Children: 50 to 100 mg/kg (maximum daily dose, 4 g) I.M. or I.V. daily or divided q 12 hours for 7 to 14 days for meningitis and 28 days for endocarditis.

May give an initial dose of 100 mg/kg (not to exceed 4 g) I.M. or I.V. to initiate therapy. Total daily dose is same for I.M. or I.V. administration and depends on susceptibility of organism and severity of infection. Inject ceftriaxone deep I.M. into a large muscle mass, such as the gluteus or lateral aspect of the thigh.
Preoperative prophylaxis
Adults: 1 g I.M. or I.V. 30 minutes to 2 hours before surgery.
Uncomplicated gonorrhea
Adults: 125 to 250 mg I.M. given as a single dose; ◊ 1 to 2 g I.M. or I.V. daily until improvement occurs.
◊ **Haemophilus ducreyi *infection***
Adults: 250 mg I.M. as a single dose.
◊ Sexually transmitted epididymitis, pelvic inflammatory disease
Adults: 250 mg I.M. as a single dose; follow up with other antibiotics.
◊ Anti-infectives for sexual assault victims
Adults: 125 mg I.M. as a single dose in conjunction with other antibiotics.
◊ Lyme disease
Adults: 1 to 2 g I.M. or I.V. q 12 to 24 hours.
◊ Persisting or relapsing otitis media in pediatric patients
Children age 3 months and older: 50 mg/kg I.M. once daily for 3 days.
≡ ***Dosage adjustment.*** In patients with impaired hepatic and renal function, dose shouldn't exceed 2 g/day without monitoring serum drug levels.

Pharmacodynamics
Antibacterial action: Ceftriaxone is primarily bactericidal; however, it may be bacteriostatic. Activity depends on organism, tissue penetration, and drug dosage and on rate of organism multiplication. It acts by adhering to bacterial penicillin-binding proteins, thereby inhibiting cell-wall synthesis. Third-generation cephalosporins appear more active against some beta-lactamase-producing gram-negative organisms.

Ceftriaxone is active against some gram-positive organisms and many enteric gram-negative bacilli, as well as streptococci; *Streptococcus pneumoniae* and *pyogenes; Staphylococcus aureus* (penicillinase and non-penicillinase producing); *Staphylococcus epidermidis; Escherichia coli; Klebsiella* species; *Haemophilus influenzae, Enterobacter; Proteus;* some strains of *Pseudomonas* and *Peptostreptococcus* and spirochetes such as *Borrelia burgdorferi* (the causative organism of Lyme disease). Most strains of *Listeria, Pseudomonas,* and *Acinetobacter* are resistant. Generally, the activity of ceftriaxone is most like that of cefotaxime and ceftizoxime.

Pharmacokinetics
Absorption: Not absorbed from the GI tract and must be given parenterally.
Distribution: Distributed widely into most body tissues and fluids, including the gallbladder, liver, kidneys, bone, sputum, bile, and pleural and synovial fluids; unlike most other cephalosporins, ceftriaxone has good CSF penetration. Ceftriaxone crosses the placenta. Protein binding is dose-dependent and decreases as serum levels rise; average is 84% to 96%.
Metabolism: Partially metabolized.
Excretion: Excreted principally in urine; some drug is excreted in bile by biliary mechanisms, and small amounts are excreted in breast milk. Elimination half-life is 5½ to 11 hours in adults with normal renal function; severe renal disease prolongs half-life only moderately. Neither hemodialysis nor peritoneal dialysis will remove ceftriaxone.

Route	Onset	Peak	Duration
I.V.	Immediate	Immediate	Unknown
I.M.	Unknown	1½-4 hr	Unknown

Contraindications and precautions
Contraindicated in patients with hypersensitivity to ceftriaxone or other cephalosporins.

Use cautiously in breast-feeding women and in patients with penicillin allergy.

Interactions

Drug-drug. *Aminoglycosides:* Produces synergistic antimicrobial activity against *Pseudomonas aeruginosa* and some strains of Enterobacteriaceae. Monitor closely.
Probenecid: May increase clearance by blocking biliary secretion and displacement of ceftriaxone from plasma proteins. Avoid use together.
Quinolones: In vitro synergism against *S. pneumoniae.*

Effects on diagnostic tests

Ceftriaxone causes false-positive results in urine glucose tests utilizing cupric sulfate (Benedict's reagent or Clinitest); use glucose oxidase (Chemstrip uG, Diastix, or glucose enzymatic test strip) instead. Ceftriaxone also causes false elevations in urine creatinine levels in tests using Jaffé's reaction. Ceftriaxone may cause positive Coombs' test results.

Adverse reactions

CNS: headache, dizziness.
GI: pseudomembranous colitis, nausea, vomiting, diarrhea, urolithiasis, increased liver function tests, jaundice.
GU: genital pruritus, moniliasis, elevated BUN levels.
Hematologic: eosinophilia, thrombocytosis, ***leukopenia.***
Skin: pain, induration, tenderness (at injection site); phlebitis; *rash;* pruritus.
Other: hypersensitivity reactions (serum sickness, ***anaphylaxis***), elevated temperature, chills.

Overdose and treatment

Signs of overdose include neuromuscular hypersensitivity. Seizure may follow high CNS concentrations. Treatment is supportive.

Clinical considerations

Consider the recommendations relevant to all cephalosporins as well as the following:
□ ***ALERT*** Names of some cephalosporins are similar. Use caution when dispensing.
- For patients on sodium restriction, note that ceftriaxone injection contains 3.6 mEq of sodium per gram of drug.
- Dosage adjustment usually isn't necessary in patients with renal insufficiency because of partial biliary excretion.

Therapeutic monitoring

With large doses or prolonged therapy, monitor for superinfection in high-risk patients.

Special populations

Breast-feeding patients. Drug is distributed into breast milk. Use with caution in breast-feeding women.

Pediatric patients. Ceftriaxone may be used in neonates and children. Use cautiously in hyperbilirubinemic neonates due to the ability of the drug to displace bilirubin.

Patient counseling

- Inform patient of potential adverse reactions.
- Tell patient to report discomfort at I.V. site.

cefuroxime axetil

Ceftin

cefuroxime sodium

Kefurox, Zinacef

Pharmacologic classification: second-generation cephalosporin
Therapeutic classification: antibiotic
Pregnancy risk category B

How supplied

Available by prescription only
cefuroxime axetil
Tablets (film-coated): 125 mg, 250 mg, 500 mg
Suspension: 125 mg/5 ml, 250 mg/5 ml
cefuroxime sodium
Injection: 750 mg, 1.5 g, 7.5 g
Infusion: 750 mg, 1.5-g infusion packets

Indications and dosages

Serious lower respiratory, urinary tract, skin and skin-structure infections; septicemia; meningitis caused by susceptible organisms
Adults: Usual dosage is 750 mg to 1.5 g I.M. or I.V. q 8 hours, usually for 5 to 10 days. For life-threatening infections and infections caused by less susceptible organisms, 1.5 g I.M. or I.V. q 6 hours; for bacterial meningitis, up to 3 g I.V. q 8 hours.
Children and infants over age 3 months: 50 to 100 mg/kg/day I.M. or I.V. in divided doses q 6 to 8 hours. Some clinicians give 100 to 150 mg/kg/day. For meningitis, the usual starting dosage is 200 to 240 mg/kg/day I.V. in divided doses q 6 to 8 hours, reduced to 100 mg/kg/day when clinical improvement is seen. However, some clinicians prefer other agents for meningitis.

Total daily dose is same for I.M. and I.V. administration, and depends on susceptibility of organism and severity of infection. Inject cefuroxime deep I.M. into a large muscle mass, such as the gluteus or lateral aspect of the thigh.
Pharyngitis, tonsillitis, lower respiratory infection, urinary tract infection
Adults and children over age 12: 125 to 500 mg P.O. b.i.d. for 10 days.
Children under age 12 who can swallow pills: 125 to 250 mg P.O. b.i.d. (tablets) for 10 days.

Children age 3 months to 12 years: 20 mg/kg/day P.O. in divided doses b.i.d. (oral suspension) to maximum dose of 500 mg for 10 days.

Otitis media, impetigo

Children age 3 months to 12 years: 30 mg/kg/day P.O. oral suspension divided into two doses (maximum dose, 1 g) for 10 days.

Children who can swallow pills: 250 mg P.O. b.i.d. for 10 days.

Note: Compliance may be a problem when treating otitis media in children. Order suspension form if child is unable to swallow pills.

Perioperative prophylaxis

Adults: 1.5 g I.V. 30 to 60 minutes before surgery; then 750 mg I.M. or I.V. q 8 hours intraoperatively for a prolonged procedure. Open-heart surgery patients can receive 1.5 g I.V. at induction, then q 12 hours for 3 doses.

◇***Gonorrhea (urethral, endocervical, rectal)***

Adults: 1.5 g I.M. given as a single dose, alone or with other antibiotics.

***Lyme disease (erythema migrans) caused by* Borrelia burgdorferi**

Adults and children age 13 and older: 500 mg P.O. b.i.d. for 20 days.

≡***Dosage adjustment.*** Safety of drug in renal patients hasn't been established. In patients with impaired renal function, dose or frequency of administration must be modified based on degree of renal impairment, severity of infection, and susceptibility of organism. To prevent toxic accumulation, reduced I.M. or I.V. dosage may be required in patients with creatinine clearance of less than 20 ml/minute/1.73 m².

Creatinine clearance (ml/min/1.73 m²)	Adult dosage
>20	750 mg to 1.5 g q 8 hours
10 to 20	750 mg q 12 hours
<10	750 mg q 24 hours

Hemodialysis patients: 750 mg at end of each dialysis period in addition to regular dose.

Pharmacodynamics

Antibacterial action: Cefuroxime is primarily bactericidal; however, it may be bacteriostatic. Activity depends on the organism, tissue penetration, drug dosage, and rate of organism multiplication. It acts by adhering to bacterial penicillin-binding proteins, thereby inhibiting cell-wall synthesis.

Cefuroxime is active against many gram-positive organisms and enteric gram-negative bacilli, including *Streptococcus pneumoniae* and *S. pyogenes, Haemophilus influenzae, Klebsiella* species, *Staphylococcus aureus, Escherichia coli, Enterobacter,* and *Neisseria gonorrhoeae; Bacteroides fragilis, Pseudomonas,* and *Acinetobacter* are resistant to cefuroxime.

Pharmacokinetics

Absorption: Cefuroxime sodium isn't well absorbed from the GI tract and must be given parenterally. Cefuroxime axetil is better absorbed orally, with between 37% to 52% of an oral dose reaching the systemic circulation. Food appears to enhance absorption. Tablets and suspension aren't bioequivalent.

Distribution: Distributed widely into most body tissues and fluids, including the gallbladder, liver, kidneys, bone, bile, and pleural and synovial fluids; CSF penetration is greater than that of most first- and second-generation cephalosporins and achieves adequate therapeutic levels in inflamed meninges. Cefuroxime crosses the placenta, and is 33% to 50% protein-bound.

Metabolism: Not metabolized.

Excretion: Primarily excreted in urine by renal tubular secretion and glomerular filtration; elimination half-life is 1 to 2 hours in patients with normal renal function; end-stage renal disease prolongs half-life 15 to 22 hours. Some drug is excreted in breast milk. Hemodialysis removes cefuroxime.

Route	Onset	Peak	Duration
P.O.	Unknown	15-60 min	Unknown
I.V.	Immediate	Immediate	Unknown
I.M.	Unknown	2 hr	Unknown

Contraindications and precautions

Contraindicated in patients with hypersensitivity to cefuroxime or other cephalosporins. Use cautiously in breast-feeding women and in those with impaired renal function or penicillin allergy.

Interactions

Drug-drug. *Aminoglycosides:* Synergistic activity against some organisms; potential for increased nephrotoxicity. Monitor closely.

Diuretics: Increased risk of adverse effects. Patient requires close monitoring.

Probenecid: Competitively inhibits renal tubular secretion of cephalosporins, resulting in higher, prolonged serum levels of these drugs. Sometimes used for this effect.

Drug-food. *Any food:* Increased absorption. Advise patient to take drug with food.

Effects on diagnostic tests

Drug causes false-positive results in urine glucose tests using cupric sulfate (Benedict's reagent or Clinitest); use glucose oxidase tests (Chemstrip uG, Diastix, or glucose enzymatic test strip) instead. Cefuroxime also causes false elevations in serum or urine creatinine levels in tests using Jaffé's reaction. Cefuroxime may cause positive Coombs' test results.

Adverse reactions

GI: pseudomembranous colitis, nausea, anorexia, vomiting, *diarrhea.*
Hematologic: ***transient neutropenia,*** eosinophilia, ***hemolytic anemia, thrombocytopenia,*** decreased hemoglobin and hematocrit levels.
Hepatic: transient increases in liver enzymes.
Skin: *maculopapular and erythematous rash, urticaria, pain, induration, sterile abscesses, temperature elevation, tissue sloughing* (at injection site).
Other: hypersensitivity reactions (serum sickness, ***anaphylaxis***); *phlebitis, thrombophlebitis* (with I.V. injection).

Overdose and treatment

Clinical signs of overdose include neuromuscular hypersensitivity. Seizure may follow high CNS concentrations. Hemodialysis or peritoneal dialysis will remove cefuroxime.

Clinical considerations

Consider the recommendations relevant to all cephalosporins as well as the following:
☐ ***ALERT*** Names of some cephalosporins are similar. Use caution when dispensing.
- Tablets and suspension are not bioequivalent and cannot be substituted on a milligram per milligram basis.
- For patients on sodium restriction, note that cefuroxime sodium contains 2.4 mEq of sodium per gram of drug.
- Check solutions for particulate matter and discoloration. Solution may range in color from light yellow to amber without affecting potency.
- Advise shaking I.M. solution gently before administration to ensure complete drug dissolution, and giving deep I.M. in a large muscle mass, preferably the gluteus area. Advise aspiration before injecting to prevent inadvertent injection into a blood vessel. Rotate injection sites to prevent tissue damage. Ice to injection site may relieve pain.
- For direct intermittent I.V., inject solution slowly into vein over 3 to 5 minutes or slowly through tubing of free-running, compatible I.V. solution.
- Reconstituted solution retains potency for 24 hours at room temperature or for 48 hours if refrigerated.
- Because drug is hemodialyzable, patients undergoing treatment with hemodialysis or peritoneal dialysis may require dosage adjustments.
- Reconstituted suspension can be stored at room temperature or in refrigerator. Discard unused portion after 10 days. Shake well before each dose.

Therapeutic monitoring

With large doses or prolonged therapy, monitor for superinfection, especially in high-risk patients.

Special populations

Breast-feeding patients. Drug is excreted in breast milk; use with caution in breast-feeding women.
Pediatric patients. Safety in infants under age 3 months hasn't been established.
Geriatric patients. Use with caution in geriatric patients.

Patient counseling

- Inform patient of potential adverse reactions.
- Patient should report discomfort at I.V. site.

celecoxib

Celebrex

Pharmacologic classification: cyclooxygenase-2 (COX-2) inhibitor
Therapeutic classification: anti-inflammatory
Pregnancy risk category C

How supplied

Available by prescription only
Capsules: 100 mg, 200 mg

Indications and dosages

Relief of signs and symptoms of osteoarthritis
Adults: 200 mg P.O. daily as a single dose or divided equally twice daily.
For the relief of the signs and symptoms of rheumatoid arthritis
Adults: 100 to 200 mg P.O. twice daily.
≡ ***Dosage adjustment.*** In patients weighing less than 110 lb (50 kg), start at lowest recommended dosage. In patients with moderate hepatic impairment (Child-Pugh Class II), start therapy with reduced dosage.

Pharmacodynamics

Anti-inflammatory, analgesic, and antipyretic actions: Celecoxib is thought to act by selective inhibition of cyclooxygenase-2 (COX-2) resulting in decreased prostaglandin synthesis. Because celecoxib doesn't inhibit COX-1 at therapeutic concentrations, the reduction in symptoms of osteoarthritis and rheumatoid arthritis may be associated with a lower incidence of peripheral side effects.

Pharmacokinetics

***Absorption:*.** Steady-state plasma levels can be expected within 5 days if celecoxib is given in multiple dosages.
Distribution: Highly protein bound, primarily to albumin.
Metabolism: Primarily metabolized by cytochrome P-450-2C9.
Excretion: Eliminated primarily by hepatic metabolism; 27% is excreted into the urine.

Elimination half-life under fasting conditions is about 11 hours.

Route	Onset	Peak	Duration
P.O.	Unknown	3 hr	Unknown

Contraindications and precautions

Contraindicated in patients with severe hepatic impairment or hypersensitivity to celecoxib, sulfonamides, aspirin, or other NSAIDs and during the third trimester of pregnancy.

Use cautiously in patients with history of ulcers or GI bleeding, advanced renal disease, anemia, symptomatic liver disease, hypertension, edema, heart failure, or asthma. Also use cautiously in patients who smoke or use alcohol chronically, in those taking oral corticosteroids or anticoagulants, and in elderly or debilitated patients.

Interactions

Drug-drug. *Aluminum and magnesium antacids:* May decrease plasma levels of celecoxib. These agents must be given at least 1 hour apart.
Angiotensin-converting enzyme inhibitors: Diminish antihypertensive effects. Blood pressure monitoring is needed.
Aspirin: Increases risk of ulcers; low aspirin dosages can be used safely for prevention of cardiovascular events. Patient needs observation for signs and symptoms of gastrointestinal bleeding.
Fluconazole: Can increase concentration of celecoxib. May need adjustment of celecoxib to minimal effective dosage.
Furosemide: NSAIDs can reduce sodium excretion associated with diuretics, leading to sodium retention. Observe patient for swelling and increase in blood pressure.
Lithium: Increased concentration may occur. Lithium plasma levels require close monitoring.
Warfarin: A direct interaction hasn't been reported; however, observe patient for signs and symptoms of bleeding.
Drug-lifestyle. *Alcohol use:* May cause increased risk of gastrointestinal irritation or bleeding if being used long term. Discourage alcohol consumption. Observe patient for signs of bleeding.

Effects on diagnostic tests

None reported.

Adverse reactions

CNS: dizziness, *headache,* insomnia.
EENT: pharyngitis, rhinitis, sinusitis.
GI: abdominal pain, diarrhea, dyspepsia, flatulence, nausea.
GU: elevated blood urea nitrogen level.
Hepatic: elevated liver enzymes.
Metabolic: hyperchloremia, hypophosphatemia.
Respiratory: upper respiratory tract infection.
Skin: rash.
Other: *back pain, peripheral edema, accidental injury.*

Overdose and treatment

Common clinical signs of overdose include lethargy, drowsiness, nausea, vomiting, epigastric pain, and GI bleeding. Other possible symptoms include hypertension, acute renal failure, respiratory depression, and coma. Although there is no antidote for treatment of overdose, symptomatic and supportive care is usually sufficient. If a patient is seen within 4 hours of the overdose, emesis, activated charcoal, an osmotic cathartic, or a combination of these can be used. Because of the high protein binding, dialysis is unlikely to be effective.

Clinical considerations

- Patients may be allergic to celecoxib if they have an allergy to sulfonamides, aspirin, or other NSAIDs.
- Patient will need assessment for signs and symptoms of hepatic and renal toxicity, especially if the patient is dehydrated.
- Patients with a history of ulcers or GI bleeding are at higher risk for GI bleeding.

Therapeutic monitoring

- Aluminum and magnesium antacids may decrease the effect of celecoxib and should be administered at least an hour apart.

Special populations

Breast-feeding patients. It's unknown if celecoxib is excreted in human breast milk; however, it's been excreted in breast milk in animals. Risks and benefits must be determined before using celecoxib in breast-feeding women.
Pediatric patients. Drug hasn't been studied in patients under age 18.
Geriatric patients. Dosage adjustment isn't necessary unless the patient weighs less than 110 lb; however, geriatric patients experience more adverse effects overall.

Patient counseling

- Inform the patient that it may take several days before feeling consistent pain relief and to notify prescriber if no relief is experienced.
- Advise patient to immediately report any signs of swelling, excessive fatigue, yellowing of the skin, flu-like symptoms, any signs of bleeding or difficulty breathing.
- Instruct the patient to take drug with food if stomach upset occurs.

cephalexin hydrochloride
Keftab

cephalexin monohydrate
Biocef, Keflex, Novo-Lexin*

Pharmacologic classification: first-generation cephalosporin
Therapeutic classification: antibiotic
Pregnancy risk category B

How supplied
Available by prescription only
cephalexin hydrochloride
Tablets: 500 mg
cephalexin monohydrate
Tablets (film-coated): 250 mg, 500 mg
Capsules: 250 mg, 500 mg
Suspension: 125 mg/5 ml, 250 mg/5 ml

Indications and dosages
Respiratory, GU, skin and soft-tissue, or bone and joint infections caused by susceptible organisms
Adults: 250 mg to 1 g P.O. q 6 hours.
Children: 25 to 50 mg/kg/day P.O. divided into four doses. In patients over age 1 with streptococcal pharyngitis or skin and structure infections, dose may be administered q 12 hours.
Otitis media
Adults: 250 mg to 1 g P.O. q 6 hours.
Children: 75 to 100 mg/kg/day P.O. divided into four doses.
≡ ***Dosage adjustment.*** To prevent toxic accumulation in patients with impaired renal function and creatinine clearance less than 40 ml/minute, give reduced dosage. If creatinine clearance is less than 5 ml/minute, give 250 mg q 12 to 24 hours; if it ranges between 5 and 10 ml/minute, give 250 mg q 12 hours; and if it's 11 to 40 ml/minute, give 500 mg q 8 to 12 hours.

Pharmacodynamics
Antibacterial action: Cephalexin is primarily bactericidal; however, it may be bacteriostatic. Activity depends on the organism, tissue penetration, drug dosage, and rate of organism multiplication. It acts by adhering to bacterial penicillin-binding proteins, thereby inhibiting cell-wall synthesis.

Drug is active against many gram-positive organisms, including penicillinase-producing *Staphylococcus aureus* and *S. epidermidis, Streptococcus pneumoniae,* group B streptococci, and group A beta-hemolytic streptococci; susceptible gram-negative organisms include *Klebsiella pneumoniae, Escherichia coli, Proteus mirabilis,* and *Shigella.*

Pharmacokinetics
Absorption: Absorbed rapidly and completely from the GI tract after oral administration. The base monohydrate is probably converted to the hydrochloride in the stomach before absorption. Food delays but doesn't prevent complete absorption.
Distribution: Distributed widely into most body tissues and fluids, including the gallbladder, liver, kidneys, bone, sputum, bile, and pleural and synovial fluids; CSF penetration is poor. Cephalexin crosses the placenta, and is 6% to 15% protein-bound.
Metabolism: Not metabolized.
Excretion: Excreted primarily unchanged in urine by glomerular filtration and renal tubular secretion; small amounts of drug may be excreted in breast milk. Elimination half-life is about ½ to 1 hour in patients with normal renal function; 7½ to 14 hours in patients with severe renal impairment. Hemodialysis or peritoneal dialysis removes cephalexin.

Route	Onset	Peak	Duration
P.O.	Unknown	1 hr	Unknown

Contraindications and precautions
Contraindicated in patients with hypersensitivity to cephalosporins. Use cautiously in patients with impaired renal function or penicillin allergy and in breast-feeding women.

Interactions
Drug-drug. *Probenecid*: Competitively inhibits renal tubular secretion of cephalosporins, resulting in higher, prolonged serum levels of these drugs. May be used for this effect.
Nephrotoxic agents (aminoglycosides, colistin, polymyxin B, vancomycin), loop diuretics: May increase the risk of nephrotoxicity. Patient requires close monitoring.

Effects on diagnostic tests
Drug causes false-positive results in urine glucose tests utilizing cupric sulfate (Benedict's reagent or Clinitest); use glucose oxidase test (Chemstrip uG, Diastix, or glucose enzymatic test strip) instead. Cephalexin also causes false elevations in serum or urine creatinine levels in tests using Jaffé's reaction. Positive Coombs' test results occur in about 3% of patients taking cephalexin.

Adverse reactions
CNS: dizziness, headache, fatigue, agitation, confusion, hallucinations.
GI: pseudomembranous colitis, *nausea, anorexia,* vomiting, *diarrhea,* gastritis, transient increases in liver enzymes, glossitis, dyspepsia, abdominal pain, anal pruritus, tenesmus, oral candidiasis.
GU: genital pruritus and candidiasis, vaginitis, interstitial nephritis.

Hematologic: ***neutropenia,*** eosinophilia, anemia, ***thrombocytopenia.***
Musculoskeletal: arthritis, arthralgia, joint pain.
Skin: *maculopapular and erythematous rash, urticaria.*
Other: hypersensitivity reactions (serum sickness, ***anaphylaxis***).

Overdose and treatment
Clinical signs of overdose include neuromuscular hypersensitivity; seizure may follow high CNS concentrations. Remove cephalexin by hemodialysis or peritoneal dialysis. Other treatment is supportive.

Clinical considerations
Consider the recommendations relevant to all cephalosporins as well as the following:
- To prepare the oral suspension, add the required amount of water to the powder in two portions. Shake well after each addition. After mixing, store in refrigerator. Suspension is stable for 14 days without significant loss of potency. Store mixture in tightly closed container. Shake well before using.
- Because cephalexin is dialyzable, patients undergoing treatment with hemodialysis or peritoneal dialysis may require dosage adjustment.

Therapeutic monitoring
With large doses or prolonged therapy, patients need monitoring for superinfection, especially high-risk patients.

Special populations
Breast-feeding patients. Drug is distributed into breast milk; use with caution in breast-feeding women.
Pediatric patients. Serum half-life is prolonged in neonates and in infants under age 1. Safety and effectiveness in children haven't been established.
Geriatric patients. Reduce dosage in geriatric patients with diminished renal function.

Patient counseling
- Inform patient of potential adverse reactions.
- Instruct patient to take drug with food to avoid GI upset.

cephradine
Velosef

Pharmacologic classification: first-generation cephalosporin
Therapeutic classification: antibiotic
Pregnancy risk category B

How supplied
Available by prescription only
Capsules: 250 mg, 500 mg
Suspension: 125 mg/5 ml, 250 mg/5 ml

Indications and dosages
Serious respiratory, GU, skin and soft-tissue, bone and joint infections; septicemia; endocarditis; and otitis media
Adults: 250 to 500 mg P.O. q 6 hours. Severe or chronic infections may require larger or more frequent doses (up to 1 g P.O. q 6 hours).
Children over age 9 months: 25 to 100 mg/kg P.O. daily in equally divided doses q 6 to 12 hours.

Larger doses (up to 1 g q.i.d.) may be given for severe or chronic infections in all patients regardless of age and weight.
≡ ***Dosage adjustment.*** To prevent toxic accumulation, reduced dosage may be required in patients with creatinine clearance below 20 ml/minute.

Creatinine clearance (ml/min/1.73 m²)	Adult dosage
> 20	500 mg q 6 hours
5 to 20	250 mg q 6 hours
< 5	250 mg q 12 hours

For patients on chronic intermittent dialysis, give 250 mg initially; repeat in 12 hours and after 36 to 48 hours. Children may require dose modifications proportional to weight and severity of infection.

Pharmacodynamics
Antibacterial action: Primarily bactericidal; however, it may be bacteriostatic. Activity depends on the organism, tissue penetration, drug dosage, and rate of organism multiplication. It acts by adhering to bacterial penicillin-binding proteins, inhibiting cell-wall synthesis.

Like other first-generation cephalosporins, cephradine is active against many gram-positive organisms and some gram-negative organisms. Susceptible organisms include *Escherichia coli* and other coliform bacteria, group A beta-hemolytic streptococci, *Haemophilus influenzae, Klebsiella, Proteus mirabilis, Staphylococcus aureus, Streptococcus pneumoniae,* staphylococci, and *Streptococcus viridans.*

Pharmacokinetics
Absorption: Well absorbed from the GI tract.
Distribution: Distributed widely into most body tissues and fluids, including the gallbladder, liver, kidneys, bone, sputum, bile, and pleural and synovial fluids; CSF penetration is poor. Cephradine crosses the placenta, and is 6% to 20% protein-bound.
Metabolism: Not metabolized.
Excretion: Excreted primarily in urine by renal tubular and glomerular filtration; small amounts of drug are excreted in breast milk. Elimination half-life is about ½ to 2 hours in

normal renal function; end-stage renal disease prolongs half-life to 8 to 15 hours. Hemodialysis or peritoneal dialysis removes drug.

Route	Onset	Peak	Duration
P.O.	Unknown	1 hr	Unknown

Contraindications and precautions
Contraindicated in patients with hypersensitivity to drug and other cephalosporins. Use cautiously in patients with impaired renal function or penicillin allergy and in breast-feeding women.

Interactions
Drug-drug. *Probenecid:* Competitively inhibits renal tubular secretion of cephalosporins, resulting in higher, prolonged serum levels of these drugs. Sometimes used for this effect.
Nephrotoxic agents (aminoglycosides, colistin, polymyxin B, or vancomycin), loop diuretics: May increase the risk of nephrotoxicity. Patient requires close monitoring.
Bacteriostatic agents (chloramphenicol, erythromycin, or tetracyclines): May interfere with bactericidal activity. Avoid use together.

Effects on diagnostic tests
Drug causes false-positive results in urine glucose tests utilizing cupric sulfate (Benedict's reagent or Clinitest); use glucose oxidase tests (Chemstrip uG, Diastix, or glucose enzymatic test strip) instead. Cephradine also causes false elevations in serum or urine creatinine levels in tests using Jaffé's reaction. Cephradine may cause positive Coombs' test results.

Adverse reactions
CNS: dizziness, headache, malaise, paresthesia.
GI: pseudomembranous colitis, *nausea, anorexia,* vomiting, transient increases in liver enzymes, heartburn, abdominal cramps, *diarrhea,* oral candidiasis.
GU: genital pruritus and candidiasis, vaginitis.
Hematologic: ***transient neutropenia***, eosinophilia, ***thrombocytopenia.***
Skin: *maculopapular and erythematous rash, urticaria.*
Other: hypersensitivity reactions (serum sickness, ***anaphylaxis***).

Overdose and treatment
Clinical signs of overdose include neuromuscular hypersensitivity; seizure may follow high CNS concentrations. Remove cephradine by hemodialysis.

Clinical considerations
Consider the recommendations relevant to all cephalosporins as well as the following:
□ ***ALERT*** Names of some cephalosporins are similar. Use caution when dispensing.
■ Reconstituted oral suspension may be stored for 7 days at room temperature or for 14 days in the refrigerator.
■ Because drug is dialyzable, patients undergoing treatment with hemodialysis may require dosage adjustments.

Therapeutic monitoring
With large doses or prolonged therapy, monitor for superinfection, especially in high-risk patients.

Special populations
Breast-feeding patients. Drug is distributed into breast milk; use with caution in breast-feeding women. Safety hasn't been established.
Pediatric patients. Serum half-life is prolonged in neonates and infants under age 12 months. Safety hasn't been established.
Geriatric patients. Reduced dosage may be required in patients with reduced renal function. Use with caution.

Patient counseling
■ Inform patient of potential adverse reactions.
■ Inform patient to take drug with food to lessen GI upset.
■ Inform patient to take all medication as prescribed, even if he feels better.

cerivastatin sodium
Baycol

Pharmacologic classification: 3-hydroxy-3-methylglutaryl-coenzyme A (HMG-CoA) reductase inhibitor
Therapeutic classification: antilipemic
Pregnancy risk category X

How supplied
Available by prescription only
Tablets*:* 0.2 mg, 0.3 mg, 0.4 mg

Indications and dosages
Adjunct to diet for reducing elevated total and low-density lipoprotein (LDL) cholesterol, apo B, and triglyceride levels in patients with primary hypercholesterolemia and mixed dyslipidemia when diet and other nonpharmacologic measures have been inadequate
Adults: 0.4 mg, P.O., once daily in the evening.
≡ ***Dosage adjustment.*** In patients with significant renal impairment (creatinine clearance 60 ml/minute/1.73 m^2 or less), a starting dose of 0.2 mg or 0.3 mg daily is recommended.

Pharmacodynamics
Antilipemic action: Competitive inhibitor of HMG-CoA reductase that is responsible for conversion of HMG-CoA to mevalonate, a precursor of sterols including cholesterol. Reducing the level of cholesterol in hepatic cells

stimulates synthesis of LDL receptors, leading to an increase in uptake of LDL particles.

Pharmacokinetics

Absorption: Absorbed in the active form. Mean absolute bioavailability of 0.2-mg tablet is 60%, with peak levels occurring about 2½ hours after a dose. Absorption is similar if taken with an evening meal or 4 hours after an evening meal.
Distribution: Mean volume of distribution is 0.3 L/kg. More than 99% of circulating drug is bound to plasma proteins (80% bound to albumin).
Metabolism: Extensively metabolized to two active metabolites, M1 and M23. A demethylation reaction forms M1 and a hydroxylation reaction forms M23. The relative potencies of M1 and M23 are 50% and 80% of the active compound, respectively. Relative concentrations of these metabolites in comparison to the parent compound are significantly less. Therefore, cholesterol-lowering effect of cerivastatin is due primarily to parent compound.
Excretion: Doesn't occur in urine or feces; M1 and M23 are the major metabolites excreted by these routes. Following an oral dose of 0.4 mg ^{14}C-cerivastatin to healthy volunteers, excretion of radioactivity is about 24% in the urine and 70% in the feces. The parent compound, cerivastatin accounts for less than 2% of total radioactivity excreted.

Route	Onset	Peak	Duration
P.O.	1 wk	4 wk	Unknown

Contraindications and precautions

Contraindicated in patients with active liver disease, unexplained persistent elevations of serum transaminases, or known hypersensitivity to drug. Also contraindicated during pregnancy and in breast-feeding patients. Avoid use in women of childbearing age unless patient is highly unlikely to conceive because of potential for fetal harm. If patient becomes pregnant during therapy, discontinue drug. Use cautiously in patients with history of liver disease or chronic alcohol ingestion.

Interactions

Drug-drug. *Azole antifungals, cyclosporine, erythromycin, fibric acid derivatives, niacin:* May increase the risk of myopathy. Use together cautiously.
Cholestyramine: When given within 4 hours of drug, results in decreased absorption and decreased peak plasma levels of cerivastatin. Use together cautiously.
Drug-lifestyle. *Alcohol use:* May increase risk of liver toxicity. Don't use together.

Effects on diagnostic tests

None reported.

Adverse reactions

CNS: asthenia, dizziness, *headache*, insomnia.
CV: chest pain, peripheral edema.
EENT: *pharyngitis, rhinitis,* sinusitis.
GI: abdominal pain, constipation, diarrhea, dyspepsia, flatulence, nausea.
GU: urinary tract infection.
Hepatic: elevated transaminases, CK, alkaline phosphatase, gamma glutamyl transpeptidase, and bilirubin.
Musculoskeletal: arthralgia, back or leg pain, myalgia.
Respiratory: increased cough.
Skin: rash.
Other: flu syndrome.

Overdose and treatment

There are no specific recommendations regarding the treatment of overdose. If overdose occurs, treat symptomatically and provide supportive measures. Because of extensive drug binding to plasma proteins, hemodialysis may not enhance drug clearance.

Clinical considerations

- Withhold drug temporarily in patients with acute or serious conditions predisposing them to renal failure secondary to rhabdomyolysis; these include trauma; major surgery; severe metabolic, endocrine and electrolyte disorders; severe acute infection; hypotension; and uncontrolled seizures. Rare cases of rhabdomyolysis have been reported with other HMG-CoA reductase inhibitors.
- Therapy with lipid-lowering drugs should be a component of multiple risk factor intervention program and attempts should be made to control cholesterol with appropriate diet, exercise, and weight reduction before initiating therapy with lipid-lowering drugs.

Therapeutic monitoring

Before initiating treatment, exclude secondary causes for hypercholesterolemia and perform a baseline lipid profile. Periodic liver function tests and lipid levels should be done before starting treatment, at 6 and 12 weeks after initiation, or after an increase in dosage and periodically thereafter.

Special population

Pregnant patients. Drug should be given to women of childbearing age only if conception is highly unlikely and they've been warned of potential risks to fetus. Caution women that drug may cause fetal damage. Advise them to call doctor immediately if pregnancy occurs or is suspected.
Breast-feeding patients. Because of potential for adverse reactions in breast-fed infants, women taking cerivastatin shouldn't breast-feed.
Pediatric patients. Safety and efficacy in children haven't been established.

Geriatric patients. Plasma drug levels are similar in healthy elderly men over age 65 and in men under age 40.

Patient counseling

- Advise patient of importance of proper dietary management, weight control, and exercise.
- Explain importance of controlling elevated serum lipid levels.
- Tell patient to take drug in the evening with or without food.
- Tell patient to immediately report unexplained muscle pain, tenderness, or weakness, especially if accompanied by fever or malaise.

cetirizine hydrochloride

Zyrtec

Pharmacologic classification: selective H_1-receptor antagonist
Therapeutic classification: antihistamine
Pregnancy risk category B

How supplied

Available by prescription only
Tablets (film-coated): 5 mg, 10 mg
Syrup: 5 mg/ml

Indications and dosages

Seasonal allergic rhinitis, perennial allergic rhinitis, chronic urticaria
Adults and children age 6 and older: 5 or 10 mg P.O. daily.
≡***Dosage adjustment.*** In hemodialysis patients or those with hepatic impairment or creatinine clearance less than 31 ml/minute, 5 mg P.O. daily.

Pharmacodynamics

Antihistaminic action: Cetirizine's principal effects are mediated by way of selective inhibition of peripheral H_1 receptors.

Pharmacokinetics

Absorption: Rapidly absorbed.
Distribution: About 93% bound to plasma protein.
Metabolism: Metabolized to a very limited extent by oxidative O-dealkylation to a metabolite with negligible antihistaminic activity.
Excretion: Primarily excreted in urine with 50% as unchanged drug. A small amount is excreted in feces.

Route	Onset	Peak	Duration
P.O.	20-60 min	½-1½ hr	24 hr

Contraindications and precautions

Contraindicated in patients with hypersensitivity to drug or hydroxyzine. Use cautiously in patients with impaired renal function.

Interactions

Drug-drug. *Anticholinergics and CNS depressants:* May cause a possible additive effect. Avoid use together.
Theophylline: May cause decreased clearance of cetirizine. Patient requires close monitoring.
Drug-lifestyle. *Alcohol use:* May cause a possible additive effect. Avoid use together.

Effects on diagnostic tests

None reported.

Adverse reactions

CNS: somnolence, fatigue, dizziness.
EENT: pharyngitis.
GI: dry mouth.

Overdose and treatment

Overdose may result in somnolence. If overdose occurs, treatment should be symptomatic or supportive. There is no known specific antidote for cetirizine and the drug is not effectively removed by dialysis.

Clinical considerations

There is no information to indicate that abuse or dependency occurs with cetirizine use.

Therapeutic monitoring

Discontinue drug 4 days before performing diagnostic skin tests; it can prevent, reduce, or mask positive skin test response.

Special populations

Breast-feeding patients. Drug is reportedly excreted in breast milk. Avoid use of drug in breast-feeding women.
Pediatric patients. Safety and efficacy in children younger than age 6 haven't been established.
Geriatric patients. Half-life of the drug may be prolonged, as may be total body clearance. No dose adjustments are necessary, however.

Patient counseling

- Caution patient not to perform hazardous activities if somnolence occurs with drug use.
- Tell patient that coffee or tea may help reduce drowsiness.

chlorambucil

Leukeran

Pharmacologic classification: alkylating agent (cell cycle–phase nonspecific)
Therapeutic classification: antineoplastic
Pregnancy risk category D

How supplied

Available by prescription only
Tablets (sugar-coated): 2 mg

Indications and dosages

Dosage and indications may vary. Check current literature for recommended protocol.

Chronic lymphocytic leukemia, malignant lymphomas including lymphosarcoma, giant follicular lymphomas, Hodgkin's disease, ◇autoimmune hemolytic anemias, ◇nephrotic syndrome, ◇polycythemia vera, ◇macroglobulinemia, ◇ovarian neoplasms

Adults: 100 to 200 mcg/kg P.O. daily or 3 to 6 mg/m^2 P.O. daily as a single dose or in divided doses, for 3 to 6 weeks. Usual dose is 4 to 10 mg daily. Reduce dose if full course of radiation therapy is planned within 4 weeks.

◇Macroglobulinemia

Adults: 2 to 10 mg P.O. daily.

◇Metastatic trophoblastic neoplasia

Adults: 6 to 10 mg P.O. daily for 5 days; repeat q 1 to 2 weeks.

◇Idiopathic uveitis

Adults: 6 to 12 mg P.O. daily for 1 year.

◇Rheumatoid arthritis

Adults: 0.1 to 0.3 mg/kg P.O. daily.

Pharmacodynamics

Antineoplastic action: Drug exerts its cytotoxic activity by cross-linking strands of cellular DNA and RNA, disrupting normal nucleic acid function.

Pharmacokinetics

Absorption: Well absorbed from the GI tract.
Distribution: Not well understood. However, drug and its metabolites have been shown to be highly bound to plasma and tissue proteins.
Metabolism: Metabolized in the liver. Its primary metabolite, phenylacetic acid mustard, also possesses cytotoxic activity.
Excretion: Metabolites are excreted in urine. Half-life of parent compound is 2 hours; the phenylacetic acid metabolite, 2½ hours.

Route	Onset	Peak	Duration
P.O.	3-4 wk	1 hr	Unknown

Contraindications and precautions

Contraindicated in patients with hypersensitivity or resistance to previous therapy. Patients hypersensitive to other alkylating agents also may be hypersensitive to drug. Use cautiously in patients with history of head trauma or seizures and in those receiving other drugs that lower seizure threshold.

Interactions

Drug-drug. *Anticoagulants, aspirin:* Increased risk of bleeding. Avoid use together.
Myelosuppressive agents: Concurrent use can cause additive myelosuppression. Patient requires close monitoring.

Effects on diagnostic tests

None reported.

Adverse reactions

CNS: ***seizures,*** peripheral neuropathy, tremor, muscle twitching, confusion, agitation, ataxia, flaccid paresis.
GI: *nausea, vomiting, stomatitis,* diarrhea.
GU: *azoospermia, infertility.*
Hematologic: ***neutropenia,*** delayed up to 3 weeks, lasting up to 10 days after last dose; ***bone marrow suppression; thrombocytopenia;*** *anemia.*
Hepatic: ***hepatotoxicity.***
Respiratory: interstitial pneumonitis, ***pulmonary fibrosis*** (rare).
Skin: rash, hypersensitivity.
Other: allergic febrile reaction.

Overdose and treatment

Signs and symptoms of overdose include reversible pancytopenia in adults, and vomiting, ataxia, abdominal pain, muscle twitching, and major motor seizures in children.

Treatment is usually supportive with transfusion of blood components, if necessary, and appropriate anticonvulsant therapy if seizures occur. Induction of emesis, activated charcoal, and gastric lavage may be useful in removing unabsorbed drug. Drug is probably not dialyzable.

Clinical considerations

- Oral suspension can be prepared in the pharmacy by crushing tablets and mixing powder with a suspending agent and simple syrup.
- I.M. injections shouldn't be given when platelets are below 100,000/mm^3.
- Store tablets in a tightly closed, light-resistant container.

Therapeutic monitoring

- Drug-induced pancytopenia generally lasts 1 to 2 weeks but may persist for 3 to 4 weeks. It's reversible up to a cumulative dose of 6.5 mg/kg in a single course.
- To prevent hyperuricemia with resulting uric acid nephropathy, allopurinol may be used with adequate hydration.

Special populations

Pregnant patients. Drug should be used only in life-threatening cases, or when safer drugs can't be used or are ineffective. Inform patient of potential hazards to fetus.
Breast-feeding patients. It's unknown if drug is distributed into breast milk. Consider the risk of potential serious adverse reactions, mutagenicity, and carcinogenicity in breast-feeding infants and the woman's need for the medication in deciding whether to discontinue drug or breast-feed.
Pediatric patients. Safety and efficacy in children haven't been established. The potential benefits versus risks must be evaluated.

Patient counseling

- Emphasize importance of continuing medication despite nausea and vomiting, and of keeping appointments for periodic blood work.
- Advise patient to report if vomiting occurs shortly after taking dose or if symptoms of infection or bleeding are present.
- Tell patient to avoid exposure to people with infections.

chloramphenicol

Chloromycetin, Chloroptic, Econochlor, Fenicol*, Ophthochlor, Pentamycetin*

chloramphenicol sodium succinate

Chloromycetin Sodium Succinate, Pentamycetin*

Pharmacologic classification: dichloroacetic acid derivative
Therapeutic classification: antibiotic
Pregnancy risk category C

How supplied

Available by prescription only
Powder for solution: 25 mg/vial
Injection: 1-g vial
Ophthalmic solution: 0.5%
Ophthalmic ointment: 1%
Otic solution: 0.5%

Indications and dosages

Severe meningitis, brain abscesses, bacteremia, or other serious infections
Adults and children: 50 to 100 mg/kg I.V. daily, divided q 6 hours. Maximum dose, 100 mg/kg daily.
Premature infants and neonates weighing less than 4.4 lb (2 kg) or under age 7 days: 25 mg/kg I.V. daily.
Neonates weighing more than 4.4 lb and age 7 days or over: 25 mg/kg I.V. q 12 hours. I.V. route must be used to treat meningitis.
Superficial infections of the skin caused by susceptible bacteria
Adults and children: Rub into affected area b.i.d. or t.i.d.
External ear canal infection
Adults and children: Instill 2 to 3 drops into ear canal t.i.d or q.i.d.
Surface bacterial infection involving conjunctiva or cornea
Adults and children: Instill 2 drops of solution in eye q hour until condition improves, or instill q.i.d., depending on severity of infection. Apply small amount of ointment to lower conjunctival sac at bedtime as supplement to drops. To use ointment alone, apply small amount to lower conjunctival sac q 3 to 6 hours or more frequently, if necessary. Continue with treatment up to 48 hours after condition improves.

Pharmacodynamics

Antibacterial action: Chloramphenicol palmitate and chloramphenicol sodium succinate must be hydrolyzed to chloramphenicol before antimicrobial activity can take place. The active compound then inhibits bacterial protein synthesis by binding to the 50S subunit of the ribosome, thus inhibiting peptide bond formation.

Drug usually produces bacteriostatic effects on susceptible bacteria, including *Rickettsia, Chlamydia, Mycoplasma,* and certain *Salmonella* strains, as well as most gram-positive and gram-negative organisms. Chloramphenicol is used to treat *Haemophilus influenzae* infection, Rocky Mountain spotted fever, meningitis, lymphogranuloma, psittacosis, severe meningitis, and bacteremia.

Pharmacokinetics

Absorption: With I.V. administration, serum levels vary greatly, depending on patient's metabolism.
Distribution: Distributed widely to most body tissues and fluids, including CSF, liver, and kidneys; it readily crosses the placenta. About 50% to 60% of drug binds to plasma proteins.
Metabolism: Parent drug is metabolized primarily by hepatic glucuronyl transferase to inactive metabolites.
Excretion: About 8% to 12% of dose is excreted by the kidneys as unchanged drug; the remainder is excreted as inactive metabolites. (However, some drug may be excreted in breast milk.) Plasma half-life ranges from about 1½ to 4½ hours in adults with normal hepatic and renal function. Plasma half-life of parent drug is prolonged in patients with hepatic dysfunction. Peritoneal hemodialysis doesn't remove significant drug amounts. Plasma chloramphenicol levels may be elevated in patients with renal impairment after I.V. chloramphenicol administration.

Route	Onset	Peak	Duration
I.V.	Unknown	1-3 hr	Unknown
Ophthalmic	Unknown	Unknown	Unknown
Otic	Unknown	Unknown	Unknown

Contraindications and precautions

Contraindicated in patients with hypersensitivity to chloramphenicol. Use cautiously in patients with impaired renal or hepatic function, acute intermittent porphyria, or G6PD deficiency and in those taking drugs that suppress bone marrow function.

Interactions

Drug-drug. *Acetaminophen:* Causes an elevated serum chloramphenicol level (by an un-

known mechanism), possibly resulting in an enhanced pharmacologic effect. This may be useful.
Chlorpropamide, cyclophosphamide, dicumarol, phenobarbital, phenytoin, and tolbutamide: When used together, chloramphenicol inhibits hepatic metabolism (by inhibiting microsomal enzyme activity); that leads to prolonged plasma half-life of these drugs and possible toxicity from increased serum drug levels. Avoid use together.
Folic acid, iron salts, and *vitamin B_2:* Reduce the hematologic response to these substances. Patient requires close monitoring.
Penicillin: When used together, chloramphenicol may antagonize the bactericidal activity. If administering drug with penicillin, then penicillin should be given 1 hour or more before chloramphenicol to avoid reduction in the bactericidal activity of penicillin.

Effects on diagnostic tests
False elevation of urinary para-aminobenzoic acid (PABA) levels will result if chloramphenicol is administered during a bentiromide test for pancreatic function. Drug therapy will cause false-positive results on tests for urine glucose level using cupric sulfate (Clinitest).

Adverse reactions
CNS: headache, mild depression, confusion, delirium, peripheral neuropathy with prolonged therapy.
EENT: optic neuritis (in patients with cystic fibrosis), glossitis, decreased visual acuity, optic atrophy in children, stinging of eye after instillation, blurred vision (with ointment).
GI: nausea, vomiting, stomatitis, diarrhea, enterocolitis.
Hematologic: ***aplastic anemia, hypoplastic anemia, agranulocytosis, thrombocytopenia.***
Skin: possible contact sensitivity; burning, urticaria, pruritus, ***angioedema*** in hypersensitive patients.
Other: hypersensitivity reactions (fever, rash, urticaria, ***anaphylaxis***), hemoglobinuria, lactic acidosis, jaundice, ***gray syndrome in neonates (abdominal distention, gray cyanosis, vasomotor collapse, respiratory distress, death within a few hours of onset of symptoms).***

Overdose and treatment
Clinical effects of parenterally administered overdose include anemia and metabolic acidosis followed by hypotension, hypothermia, abdominal distention, and possible death.

Initial treatment is symptomatic and supportive. Drug may be removed by charcoal hemoperfusion.

Clinical considerations
- Culture and sensitivity tests may be done concurrently with first dose and repeated as needed.
- Use drug only when clearly indicated for severe infection. Because of drug's potential for severe toxicity, it should be reserved for potentially life-threatening infections.
- Refrigerate ophthalmic solution.
- For I.V. administration, reconstitute 1-g vial of powder for injection with 10 ml of sterile water for injection; concentration will be 100 mg/ml. Solution remains stable for 30 days at room temperature; however, refrigeration is recommended. Don't use cloudy solutions. Administer I.V. infusion slowly, over at least 1 minute. Check injection site daily for phlebitis and irritation.
- Therapeutic range is 10 to 20 mcg/ml for peak levels and 5 to 10 mcg/ml for trough levels.

Therapeutic monitoring
- CBC, platelet count, reticulocyte count, and serum iron level are necessary before therapy begins and every 2 days during therapy. Discontinue drug immediately if test results indicate anemia, reticulocytopenia, leukopenia, or thrombocytopenia.
- Observe patient for signs and symptoms of superinfection by nonsusceptible organisms.

Special populations
Breast-feeding patients. Drug is excreted in breast milk in low concentrations, posing risk of bone marrow depression and slight risk of gray syndrome. Alternative feeding method is recommended during treatment with chloramphenicol.
Pediatric patients. Use drug cautiously in children under age 2 because of risk of gray syndrome (although most cases occur in first 48 hours after birth). Drug has prolonged half-life in neonates, necessitating special dose.
Geriatric patients. Administer drug cautiously to geriatric patients with impaired liver function.

Patient counseling
- Instruct patient to report adverse reactions, especially nausea, vomiting, diarrhea, bleeding, fever, confusion, sore throat, or mouth sores.
- Tell patient to take drug for prescribed period and to take it exactly as directed, even after he feels better.
- Instruct patient to wash hands before and after applying topical ointment or solution.
- Warn patient using otic solution not to touch ear with dropper.
- Caution patient using topical cream to avoid sharing washcloths and towels with family members.
- Tell patient using ophthalmic drug to clean eye area of excess exudate before applying drug; show him how to instill drug in eye. Warn him not to touch applicator tip to eye or surrounding tissue. Instruct him to observe for signs and symptoms of sensitivity, such as itchy

eyelids or constant burning, and to discontinue drug and call immediately should any occur.

chlordiazepoxide

Libritabs

chlordiazepoxide hydrochloride

Librium, Mitran, Reposans-10

Pharmacologic classification: benzodiazepine
Therapeutic classification: antianxiety, anticonvulsant, sedative-hypnotic
Controlled substance schedule IV
Pregnancy risk category D

How supplied

Available by prescription only
Tablets: 5 mg, 10 mg, 25 mg
Capsules: 5 mg, 10 mg, 25 mg
Powder for injection: 100 mg/ampule

Indications and dosages

Mild to moderate anxiety and tension
Adults: 5 to 10 mg P.O. t.i.d. or q.i.d.
Children over age 6 and geriatric or debilitated patients: 5 mg P.O. b.i.d. to q.i.d. Maximum dose, 10 mg P.O. b.i.d. or t.i.d.
Severe anxiety and tension
Adults: 20 to 25 mg P.O. t.i.d. or q.i.d.
Withdrawal symptoms of acute alcoholism
Adults: 50 to 100 mg P.O., I.M., or I.V. Maximum dose, 300 mg/day.
Preoperative apprehension and anxiety
Adults: 5 to 10 mg P.O. t.i.d. or q.i.d. on day before surgery; or 50 to 100 mg I.M. 1 hour before surgery.

Note: Parenteral form isn't recommended in children under age 12.

Pharmacodynamics

Anxiolytic action: Chlordiazepoxide depresses the CNS at the limbic and subcortical levels of the brain. It produces an antianxiety effect by influencing the effect of the neurotransmitter gamma-aminobutyric acid (GABA) on its receptor in the ascending reticular activating system, which increases inhibition and blocks both cortical and limbic arousal after stimulation of the reticular formation.
Anticonvulsant action: Drug suppresses the spread of seizure activity produced by the epileptogenic foci in the cortex, thalamus, and limbic structures by enhancing presynaptic inhibition.

Pharmacokinetics

Absorption: When given orally, is absorbed well through the GI tract. I.M. administration results in erratic absorption.
Distribution: Distributed widely throughout the body; 90% to 98% is protein-bound.
Metabolism: Metabolized in the liver to several active metabolites.
Excretion: Most metabolites are excreted in urine as glucuronide conjugates. Half-life of drug is 5 to 30 hours.

Route	Onset	Peak	Duration
P.O.	Unknown	½-4 hr	Unknown
I.V.	1-5 min	Unknown	15-60 min
I.M.	15-30 min	Unknown	Unknown

Contraindications and precautions

Contraindicated in patients hypersensitive to drug. Use cautiously in patients with impaired renal or hepatic function, mental depression, or porphyria.

Interactions

Drug-drug. *Antacids:* May delay the absorption of chlordiazepoxide. Monitor closely.
Cimetidine and possibly disulfiram: Diminishes hepatic metabolism of chlordiazepoxide, which increases its plasma levels. Patient requires careful monitoring.
Haloperidol: May decrease serum levels. Avoid use together.
Levodopa: May decrease the therapeutic effects of levodopa. Avoid use together.
Oral contraceptives: May impair the metabolism of chlordiazepoxide. Avoid use together.
Phenothiazines, narcotics, barbiturates, antihistamines, MAO inhibitors, general anesthetics, and antidepressants: Chlordiazepoxide potentiates the CNS depressant effects. Avoid use together.
Phenytoin and digoxin: Levels may be increased. Avoid use together.
Drug-lifestyle. *Alcohol use:* Potentiates the CNS depressant effects. Discourage use together.
Heavy smoking: Accelerates chlordiazepoxide's metabolism, thus lowering clinical effectiveness. Discourage use together.

Effects on diagnostic tests

Minor changes in EEG patterns, usually low-voltage, fast activity, may occur during and after chlordiazepoxide therapy.

Chlordiazepoxide may cause a false-positive pregnancy test, depending on method used. It may also alter urinary 17-ketosteroids (Zimmerman reaction), urine alkaloid determination (Frings thin layer chromatography method), and urinary glucose determinations (with Chemstrip uG and Diastix, but not glucose enzymatic test strip).

Adverse reactions

CNS: *drowsiness, lethargy,* ataxia, confusion, extrapyramidal symptoms, EEG changes.
GI: nausea, constipation.

GU: increased or decreased libido, menstrual irregularities.
Hematologic: ***agranulocytosis.***
Hepatic: jaundice.
Skin: *swelling, pain at injection site,* skin eruptions, edema.

Overdose and treatment
Signs and symptoms of overdose include somnolence, confusion, coma, hypoactive reflexes, dyspnea, labored breathing, hypotension, bradycardia, slurred speech, and unsteady gait or impaired coordination.

Support blood pressure and respiration until drug effects subside; monitor vital signs. Flumazenil, a specific benzodiazepine antagonist, may be useful. Mechanical ventilatory assistance via endotracheal tube may be required to maintain a patent airway and support adequate oxygenation. Use I.V. fluids and vasopressors, such as dopamine and phenylephrine, to treat hypotension as needed. Use gastric lavage if ingestion was recent, but only if an endotracheal tube is in place to prevent aspiration. Induce emesis if the patient is conscious. After emesis or lavage, administer activated charcoal with a cathartic as a single dose. Don't administer barbiturates if excitation occurs. Dialysis is of limited value.

Clinical considerations
Consider the recommendations relevant to all benzodiazepines as well as the following:
- I.M. administration isn't recommended because of erratic and slow absorption. However, if I.M. route is used, reconstitute with special diluent only. Don't use diluent if hazy. Discard unused portion. Inject I.M. deep into large muscle mass.
- For I.V. administration, reconstitute drug with sterile water or normal saline solution and infuse slowly, directly into a large vein, at a rate not exceeding 50 mg/minute for adults. Don't infuse chlordiazepoxide into small veins. Avoid extravasation into subcutaneous tissue. Observe infusion site for phlebitis. Keep resuscitation equipment nearby in case of an emergency.
- Prepare solutions for I.V. or I.M. use immediately before administration. Discard unused portions.
- Lower doses are effective in patients with renal or hepatic dysfunction. Closely monitor renal and hepatic studies for signs of dysfunction.

Therapeutic monitoring
- Patients should remain in bed under observation for at least 3 hours after parenteral administration of chlordiazepoxide.

Special populations
Breast-feeding patients. The breast-fed infant of a woman who uses chlordiazepoxide may become sedated, have feeding difficulties, or lose weight. Drug shouldn't be given to breast-feeding women.
Pediatric patients. Safety of oral form hasn't been established in children under age 6. Safety of parenteral form hasn't been established in children under age 12.
Geriatric patients. Geriatric patients demonstrate a greater sensitivity to the CNS depressant effects of drug. Some may require supervision with ambulation and activities of daily living during initiation of therapy or after an increase in dose. Lower doses are usually effective in geriatric patients because of decreased elimination. Parenteral administration of drug is more likely to cause apnea, hypotension, and bradycardia in geriatric patients.

Patient counseling
- Warn patient that sudden changes in position may cause dizziness. Advise patient to dangle legs a few minutes before getting out of bed to prevent falls and injury.
- Warn patient not to abruptly stop using drug because withdrawal symptoms may occur.

chloroquine hydrochloride
Aralen Hydrochloride

chloroquine phosphate
Aralen Phosphate

Pharmacologic classification: 4-aminoquinoline
Therapeutic classification: antimalarial, amebicide, anti-inflammatory
Pregnancy risk category C

How supplied
Available by prescription only
chloroquine hydrochloride
Injection: 50 mg/ml (40 mg/ml base)
chloroquine phosphate
Tablets: 500 mg (300-mg base)

Indications and dosages
Suppressive prophylaxis
Adults: Give 500 mg (300-mg base) P.O. on same day once weekly beginning 2 weeks before exposure.
Children: 5 mg (base)/kg P.O. on same day once weekly (not to exceed adult dosage) beginning 2 weeks before exposure.
Treatment of acute attacks of malaria
Adults: 1 g (600-mg base) P.O. followed by 500 mg (300-mg base) P.O. after 6 to 8 hours; then a single dose of 500 mg (300-mg base) P.O. for next 2 days or 4 to 5 ml (160- to 200-mg base) I.M. and repeated in 6 hours if needed; change to P.O. as soon as possible.
Children: Initial dose is 10 mg (base)/kg P.O.; then 5 mg (base)/kg after 6 hours. Third dose

is 5 mg (base)/kg 18 hours after second dose; fourth dose is 5 mg (base)/kg 24 hours after third dose; or 5 mg (base)/kg I.M. May repeat in 6 hours and change to P.O. as soon as possible.

Extraintestinal amebiasis

Adults: 1 g (600-mg base) daily for 2 days, then 500 mg (300-mg base) daily for 2 to 3 weeks or 4 to 5 ml (160- to 200-mg base) I.M. for 10 to 12 days; change to P.O. as soon as possible. Administer in conjunction with an intestinal amebicide.

◇ ***Rheumatoid arthritis***

Adults: 250 mg P.O. daily (chloroquine phosphate) with evening meal.

◇ ***Lupus erythematosus***

Adults: 250 mg P.O. daily (chloroquine phosphate) with evening meal; reduce dosage gradually over several months when lesions regress.

Pharmacodynamics

Antimalarial action: Chloroquine binds to DNA, interfering with protein synthesis. It also inhibits both DNA and RNA polymerases.

Amebicidal action: Mechanism of action is unknown.

Anti-inflammatory action: Mechanism of action is unknown. Drug may antagonize histamine and serotonin and inhibit prostaglandin effects by inhibiting conversion of arachidonic acid to prostaglandin F_2; it also may inhibit chemotaxis of polymorphonuclear leukocytes, macrophages, and eosinophils.

Chloroquine's spectrum of activity includes the asexual erythrocytic forms of *Plasmodium malariae, P. ovale, P. vivax,* many strains of *P. falciparum,* and *Entamoeba histolytica.*

Pharmacokinetics

Absorption: Absorbed readily and almost completely.

Distribution: 55% bound to plasma proteins. It concentrates in erythrocytes, liver, spleen, kidneys, heart, and brain and is strongly bound in melanin-containing cells.

Metabolism: About 30% of an administered dose is metabolized by the liver to monodesethylchloroquine and bidesethylchloroquine.

Excretion: About 70% of an administered dose is excreted unchanged in urine; unabsorbed drug is excreted in feces. Small amounts of the drug may be present in urine for months after the drug is discontinued. Renal excretion is enhanced by urinary acidification. Drug is excreted in breast milk.

Route	Onset	Peak	Duration
P.O.	Unknown	1-3 hr	Unknown
I.M.	Unknown	½ hr	Unknown

Contraindications and precautions

Contraindicated in patients with hypersensitivity to drug and in those with retinal or visual field changes or porphyria. Use cautiously in patients with GI, neurologic, or blood disorders.

Interactions

Drug-drug. *Cimetidine:* May reduce oral clearance and metabolism. Patient must be monitored for toxicity.

Kaolin, magnesium and aluminum salts: May decrease absorption of chloroquine. Advise separate administration times.

Intradermal human diploid cell rabies vaccine: May interfere with antibody response. Use together cautiously.

Drug-lifestyle. *Sun exposure:* May exacerbate drug-induced dermatoses. Advise patient to avoid excessive sun exposure.

Effects on diagnostic tests

May cause inversion or depression of the T wave or widening of the QRS complex on ECG.

Adverse reactions

CNS: mild and transient headache, psychic stimulation, ***seizures,*** dizziness, neuropathy.

CV: hypotension, ECG changes, AV block, cardiomyopathy.

EENT: visual disturbances (blurred vision; difficulty in focusing; reversible corneal changes; typically irreversible, sometimes progressive or delayed retinal changes, such as narrowing of arterioles; macular lesions; pallor of optic disk; optic atrophy; patchy retinal pigmentation, typically leading to blindness); ototoxicity (nerve deafness, vertigo, tinnitus).

GI: anorexia, abdominal cramps, diarrhea, nausea, vomiting, stomatitis.

Hematologic: ***agranulocytosis, aplastic anemia,*** hemolytic anemia, ***thrombocytopenia.***

Skin: pruritus, lichen planus eruptions, skin and mucosal pigmentary changes, pleomorphic skin eruptions.

Overdose and treatment

Symptoms of drug overdose may appear within 30 minutes after ingestion and may include headache, drowsiness, visual changes, CV collapse, and seizures followed by respiratory and cardiac arrest. Treatment is symptomatic. Empty stomach by emesis or lavage. After lavage, activated charcoal in an amount at least five times the estimated amount of drug ingested may be helpful if given within 30 minutes of ingestion.

Ultra-short-acting barbiturates may help control seizures. Intubation may become necessary. Peritoneal dialysis and exchange transfusions also may be useful. Forced fluids and acidification of the urine are helpful after the acute phase.

Clinical considerations

□ ***ALERT*** Drug dosage may be discussed in milligrams or milligrams base. Be aware of the difference.

- Resistance of *P. falciparum* to chloroquine has spread to most areas with malaria except the Dominican Republic, Haiti, Central America west of the Panama Canal, and Egypt.
- It may also be advisable for traveler to take sulfadoxine and pyrimethamine (Fansidar) with him on his travels. Instruct patient to take drug if a febrile illness occurs and professional medical care isn't available. Emphasize that such self-treatment is a temporary measure and that he must seek medical care as soon as possible. He should continue prophylaxis after the treatment dose of Fansidar.

Therapeutic monitoring

- Baseline and periodic ophthalmologic examinations are necessary in prolonged or high-dosage therapy.
- Assist patient in obtaining audiometric examinations before, during, and after therapy, especially if therapy is long-term.

Special populations

Breast-feeding patients. Safety hasn't been established. Use with caution in breast-feeding women.
Pediatric patients. Children are extremely susceptible to toxicity; monitor closely for adverse effects.

Patient counseling

- Tell patient to report blurred vision, increased sensitivity to light, hearing loss, pronounced GI disturbances, or muscle weakness promptly.
- Advise patient to take drug immediately before or after meals on the same day each week to minimize gastric distress. Patients who can't tolerate drug because of GI distress may tolerate hydroxychloroquine.

chlorpheniramine maleate

Aller-Chlor, Chlo-Amine, Chlor-100, Chlor-Pro, Chlorspan-12, Chlortab-4, Chlortab-8, Chlor-Trimeton, Chlor-Tripolon*, Novo-Pheniram*, Pfeiffer's Allergy, Phenetron, Teldrin

Pharmacologic classification: propylamine-derivative antihistamine
Therapeutic classification: antihistamine (H_1-receptor antagonist)
Pregnancy risk category B

How supplied

Available with or without a prescription
Tablets: 4 mg
Tablets (chewable): 2 mg
Tablets (extended-release): 8 mg, 12 mg
Capsules (extended-release): 8 mg, 12 mg
Syrup: 2 mg/5 ml
Injection: 10 mg/ml

Indications and dosages

Rhinitis, allergy symptoms
Adults and children age 12 and older: 4 mg of tablets or syrup P.O. q 4 to 6 hours; or 8 to 12 mg of extended-release tablets b.i.d. or t.i.d. Maximum dose, 24 mg/day; 10 to 20 mg S.C., I.V., or I.M. also may be used.
Children age 6 to 11: 2 mg of tablets or syrup P.O. q 4 to 6 hours; or one 8-mg extended-release tablet in 24 hours. Maximum dose, 12 mg/day.
Children age 2 to 5: 1 mg of syrup P.O. q 4 to 6 hours. Maximum dose, 6 mg/day. Safety and efficacy of extended release preparations for children under age 6 haven't been established.

Pharmacodynamics

Antihistamine action: Antihistamines compete with histamine for H_1-receptor sites on smooth muscle of the bronchi, GI tract, uterus, and large blood vessels; they bind to cellular receptors, preventing access of histamine, thereby suppressing histamine-induced allergic symptoms. They don't directly alter histamine or its release.

Pharmacokinetics

Absorption: Well absorbed from the GI tract. Food in the stomach delays absorption but doesn't affect bioavailability.
Distribution: Distributed extensively into the body; drug is about 72% protein-bound.
Metabolism: Metabolized largely in GI mucosal cells and liver (first-pass effect).
Excretion: Half-life is 12 to 43 hours in adults and 10 to 13 hours in children; drug and metabolites are excreted in urine.

Route	Onset	Peak	Duration
P.O.	15-60 min	2-6 hr	24 hr
I.V.	15-60 min	Immediate	24 hr
I.M., S.C.	15-60 min	Unknown	24 hr

Contraindications and precautions

Contraindicated in patients having acute asthmatic attacks. Antihistamines aren't recommended for breast-feeding women because small amounts of drug are excreted in breast milk.

Use cautiously in the elderly and in patients with increased intraocular pressure, hyperthyroidism, CV or renal disease, hypertension, bronchial asthma, urine retention, prostatic hyperplasia, bladder neck obstruction, or stenosing peptic ulcers.

Interactions

Drug-drug. *CNS depressants:* Increased sedation. Use together cautiously.
MAO inhibitors: Increased anticholinergic effects.
Epinephrine: Chlorpheniramine enhances the effects. Patient requires monitoring.

Sulfonylureas: May diminish the effects. Advise patient to report effectiveness of treatment.
Heparin: Chlorpheniramine may partially counteract the anticoagulant action. Avoid using together.
Drug-lifestyle. *Alcohol use:* Additive sedation may occur when antihistamines are given with chlorpheniramine. Discourage use together.

Effects on diagnostic tests

Discontinue drug 4 days before diagnostic skin tests; antihistamines can prevent, reduce, or mask positive skin test response.

Adverse reactions

CNS: *stimulation,* sedation, *drowsiness,* excitability (in children).
CV: hypotension, palpitations, weak pulse.
GI: epigastric distress, *dry mouth.*
GU: urine retention.
Respiratory: thick bronchial secretions.
Skin: rash, urticaria, local stinging, burning sensation (after parenteral administration), pallor.

Overdose and treatment

Signs and symptoms of overdose may include either CNS depression (sedation, reduced mental alertness, apnea, and CV collapse) or CNS stimulation (insomnia, hallucinations, tremors, and seizures). Atropine-like symptoms, such as dry mouth, flushed skin, fixed and dilated pupils, and GI symptoms, are common, especially in children.

Treat overdose by inducing emesis with ipecac syrup (in conscious patient), followed by activated charcoal to reduce further drug absorption. Use gastric lavage if patient is unconscious or ipecac fails. Treat hypotension with vasopressors, and control seizures with diazepam or phenytoin. Don't give stimulants. Administering ammonium chloride or vitamin C to acidify urine promotes drug excretion.

Clinical considerations

Consider the recommendations relevant to all antihistamines as well as the following:

- Don't use parenteral solutions intradermally.
- Administer I.V. solution slowly, over 1 minute.

Therapeutic monitoring

If symptoms occur during or after parenteral dose, discontinue drug and inform doctor.

Special populations

Breast-feeding patients. Antihistamines such as chlorpheniramine shouldn't be used during breast-feeding. Many of these drugs are secreted in breast milk, exposing the infant to risks of unusual excitability; premature infants are at particular risk for seizures.
Pediatric patients. Drug isn't indicated for use in premature or newborn infants. Children, especially those under age 6, may experience paradoxical hyperexcitability.
Geriatric patients. Geriatric patients are usually more sensitive to adverse effects of antihistamines and are especially likely to experience a greater degree of dizziness, sedation, hyperexcitability, dry mouth, and urine retention than younger patients. Symptoms usually respond to a decrease in medication dosage.

Patient counseling

- Instruct patient to swallow extended-release tablets whole; they shouldn't be crushed or chewed.
- Inform patient to store syrup and parenteral solution away from light.

chlorpromazine hydrochloride

Chlorpromanyl-5*, Chlorpromanyl-20*, Largactil*, Novo-Chlorpromazine*, Ormazine, Thorazine, Thor-Prom

Pharmacologic classification: aliphatic phenothiazine
Therapeutic classification: antipsychotic, antiemetic
Pregnancy risk category C

How supplied

Available by prescription only
Tablets: 10 mg, 25 mg, 50 mg, 100 mg, 200 mg
Capsules (sustained-release): 30 mg, 75 mg, 150 mg
Syrup: 10 mg/5 ml
Oral concentrate: 30 mg/ml, 100 mg/ml
Suppositories: 25 mg, 100 mg
Injection: 25 mg/ml

Indications and dosages

Psychosis
Adults: 30 to 75 mg P.O. daily in two to four divided doses. Dosage may be increased twice weekly by 20 to 50 mg until symptoms are controlled. Most patients respond to 200 mg daily, but doses up to 800 mg may be necessary. 25 to 50 mg may be given I.M., and may be repeated in 1 hour, if needed. Gradually increase subsequent I.M. doses over several days to a maximum of 400 mg q 4 to 6 hours. Switch to oral therapy as soon as possible.
Children age 6 months and older: 0.55 mg/kg P.O. q 4 to 6 hours; or I.M. q 6 to 8 hours; or 1.1 mg/kg P.R. q 6 to 8 hours. Maximum I.M. dose is 40 mg in children under age 5 or weighing less than 50 lb (22.7 kg), and 75 mg in children age 5 to 12 or weighing 50 to 100 lb (22.7 to 45.5 kg).
Nausea, vomiting
Adults: 10 to 25 mg P.O. q 4 to 6 hours, p.r.n.; or 50 to 100 mg P.R. q 6 to 8 hours, p.r.n.; or 25 mg I.M. initially. If no hypotension occurs,

25 to 50 mg I.M. q 3 to 4 hours may be given, p.r.n., until vomiting stops.
Children 6 months and older: 0.55 mg/kg P.O. q 4 to 6 hours, p.r.n.; or I.M. q 6 to 8 hours, p.r.n.; or 1.1 mg/kg P.R. q 6 to 8 hours, p.r.n. Maximum I.M. dose in children younger than 5 or weighing less than 50 lb (22.7 kg) is 40 mg. Maximum I.M. dose in children age 5 to 12 or weighing 50 to 100 lb (22.7 to 45.5 kg) is 75 mg.

Intractable hiccups; acute intermittent porphyria
Adults: 25 to 50 mg P.O. or I.M. t.i.d. or q.i.d. For hiccups, if symptoms persist, 25 to 50 mg diluted in 500 to 1,000 ml of normal saline solution and infuse I.V. slowly with patient in supine position.

Tetanus
Adults: 25 mg to 50 mg I.M. or I.V. t.i.d. or q.i.d.
Children age 6 months and older: 0.55 mg/kg I.M. or I.V. q 6 to 8 hours. Maximum parenteral dose in children weighing less than 50 lb (22.7 kg) is 40 mg daily; for children weighing 50 to 100 lb (22.7 to 45.5 kg), maximum parenteral dose is 75 mg daily, except in severe cases.

Surgery
Adults: Preoperatively, 25 to 50 mg P.O. 2 to 3 hours before surgery or 12.5 to 25 mg I.M. 1 to 2 hours before surgery; during surgery, 12.5 mg I.M., repeated in 30 minutes, if needed, or fractional 2 mg doses I.V. at 2-minute intervals up to maximum of 25 mg; postoperatively, 10 to 25 mg P.O. q 4 to 6 hours or 12.5 to 25 mg I.M., repeated in 1 hour, if needed.
Children age 6 months and older: Preoperatively, 0.55 mg/kg P.O. 2 to 3 hours before surgery or I.M. 1 to 2 hours before surgery; during surgery, 0.275 mg/kg I.M., repeated in 30 minutes, if needed, or fractional 1 mg doses I.V. at 2-minute intervals, up to maximum of 0.275 mg/kg; postoperatively, 0.55 mg/kg P.O. or I.M., oral dose repeated q 4 to 6 hours or I.M. dose repeated in 1 hour, if needed, and if hypotension doesn't occur.

Pharmacodynamics

Antipsychotic action: Drug is thought to exert its antipsychotic effects by postsynaptic blockade of CNS dopamine receptors, thereby inhibiting dopamine-mediated effects; antiemetic effects are attributed to dopamine receptor blockade in the medullary chemoreceptor trigger zone (CTZ). Drug has many other central and peripheral effects; it produces both alpha and ganglionic blockade and counteracts histamine- and serotonin-mediated activity. Its most prominent adverse reactions are antimuscarinic and sedative.

Pharmacokinetics

Absorption: Rate and extent of absorption vary with route of administration. Oral tablet absorption is erratic; sustained-release preparations have similar absorption. Oral concentrates and syrups are much more predictable; I.M. drug is absorbed rapidly.
Distribution: Distributed widely into the body, including breast milk; concentration is usually higher in CNS than in plasma. Steady-state serum level is achieved within 4 to 7 days. Drug is 91% to 99% protein-bound.
Metabolism: Metabolized extensively by the liver and forms 10 to 12 metabolites; some are pharmacologically active.
Excretion: Mostly excreted as metabolites in urine; some is excreted in feces via the biliary tract. It may undergo enterohepatic circulation.

Route	Onset	Peak	Duration
P.O.	½-1 hr	Unknown	4-6 hr
P.O. (extended)	½-1 hr	Unknown	10-12 hr
I.V., I.M.	Unknown	Unknown	Unknown
P.R.	>1 hr	Unknown	3-4 hr

Contraindications and precautions

Contraindicated in patients with hypersensitivity to drug or in patients experiencing CNS depression, bone marrow suppression, subcortical damage, and coma.

Use cautiously in acutely ill or dehydrated children; geriatric or debilitated patients; and in patients with impaired renal or hepatic function, severe CV disease, glaucoma, prostatic hyperplasia, respiratory or seizure disorders, hypocalcemia, reaction to insulin or electroconvulsive therapy, or exposure to heat, cold, or organophosphate insecticides.

Interactions

Drug-drug. *Antiarrhythmic agents, quinidine, disopyramide, and procainamide:* Increased incidence of arrhythmias and conduction defects. Avoid use together.
Anticholinergic drugs: Increased anticholinergic activity, aggravated parkinsonian symptoms. Use with caution.
Beta blockers: May inhibit chlorpromazine metabolism, increasing plasma levels and toxicity. Patient requires close monitoring.
CNS depressants, parenteral magnesium sulfate: Additive effects are likely. Avoid use together.
Centrally acting antihypertensive drugs: Chlorpromazine may decrease blood pressure. Patient requires close monitoring.
Epinephrine: Chlorpromazine may cause epinephrine reversal. Avoid use together.
Lithium: May cause severe neurologic toxicity, and a decreased therapeutic response to chlorpromazine. Avoid use together.
Propylthiouracil: Concurrent use increases risk of agranulocytosis. Avoid use together.
Sympathomimetics: Concurrent use may decrease their stimulatory and pressor effects. Avoid use together.

Warfarin: Decreased effect of oral anticoagulants. Monitor INR and PT.
Drug-food. *Caffeine:* Pharmacokinetic alterations and subsequent decreased therapeutic response. Avoid caffeinated foods and beverages.
Drug-lifestyle. *Heavy smoking:* May reduce therapeutic response to chlorpromazine. Discourage use.
Alcohol use: Additive effects are likely after use. Discourage use.
Sun exposure: Photosensitivity reactions may result. Take precautions.

Effects on diagnostic tests

Drug causes false-positive test results for urinary porphyrins, urobilinogen, amylase, and 5-hydroxyindoleacetic acid because of darkening of urine by metabolites; it also causes false-positive results in urine pregnancy tests using human chorionic gonadotropin.

Adverse reactions

CNS: extrapyramidal reactions, drowsiness, sedation, ***seizures,*** tardive dyskinesia, pseudoparkinsonism, dizziness, ***neuroleptic malignant syndrome.***
CV: *orthostatic hypotension,* tachycardia, ECG changes.
EENT: ocular changes, blurred vision, nasal congestion.
GI: *dry mouth, constipation,* nausea.
GU: *urine retention,* menstrual irregularities, gynecomastia, inhibited ejaculation, priapism.
Hematologic: ***leukopenia, agranulocytosis,*** eosinophilia, hemolytic anemia, ***aplastic anemia, thrombocytopenia.***
Hepatic: jaundice, abnormal liver function test results.
Skin: *mild photosensitivity,* allergic reactions, *pain at I.M. injection site,* sterile abscess, skin pigmentation.
After abrupt withdrawal of long-term therapy: gastritis, nausea, vomiting, dizziness, tremor.

Overdose and treatment

CNS depression is characterized by deep, unarousable sleep and possible coma, hypotension, or hypertension, extrapyramidal symptoms, abnormal involuntary muscle movements, agitation, seizures, arrhythmias, ECG changes, hypothermia or hyperthermia, and autonomic nervous system dysfunction.

Treatment is symptomatic and supportive, including maintaining vital signs, airway, stable body temperature, and fluid and electrolyte balance.

Don't induce vomiting: drug inhibits cough reflex, and aspiration may occur. Use gastric lavage, then activated charcoal and sodium chloride cathartics; dialysis doesn't help. Regulate body temperature as needed. Treat hypotension with I.V. fluids: don't give epinephrine. Treat seizures with parenteral diazepam or barbiturates; arrhythmias with parenteral phenytoin (1 mg/kg with rate adjusted to blood pressure); extrapyramidal reactions with benztropine 1 to 2 mg or parenteral diphenhydramine 10 to 50 mg.

Clinical considerations

Consider the recommendations relevant to all phenothiazines as well as the following:
□ ***ALERT*** I.V. form should be used only during surgery or for severe hiccups. Dilute injection to 1 mg/ml with normal saline solution and administer at a rate of 1 mg/2 minutes for children and 1 mg/minute for adults.
- Sustained-release preparations shouldn't be crushed or opened, but swallowed whole.
- Oral formulations may cause stomach upset and may be administered with food or fluid.
- Dilute concentrate in 2 to 4 oz of liquid, preferably water, carbonated drinks, fruit juice, tomato juice, milk, pudding, or applesauce.
- Store suppository form in a cool place.
- Give I.M. injection deep in the upper outer quadrant of the buttocks. Injection is usually painful; massaging the area after administration may prevent abscess formation.
- Liquid and injectable forms may cause a rash if skin contact occurs.
- Solution for injection may be slightly discolored. Don't use if drug is excessively discolored or if a precipitate is evident. Monitor blood pressure before and after parenteral administration.

Therapeutic monitoring

If tissue irritation occurs, chlorpromazine injection may be diluted with normal saline solution or 2% procaine.

Special populations

Breast-feeding patients. Drug is excreted in breast milk. Potential benefits to the woman should outweigh potential harm to the infant.
Pediatric patients. Drug isn't recommended for patients under age 6 months. Sudden infant death syndrome has been reported to occur in children younger than age 1 receiving drug. Extrapyramidal effects may be more common in children.
Geriatric patients. Older patients tend to require lower doses, adjusted individually. Adverse reactions, especially tardive dyskinesia and other extrapyramidal effects, are more likely to develop in geriatric patients.

Patient counseling

- Explain risks of dystonic reactions and tardive dyskinesia, and tell patient to report abnormal involuntary body movements or painful muscle contractions.
- Warn patient to avoid extremely hot or cold baths or exposure to temperature extremes,

sunlamps, or tanning beds. Drug may cause thermoregulatory changes.
- Tell patient not to spill the liquid preparation on the skin because rash and irritation may result.
- Instruct patient to take drug exactly as prescribed and not to double dose to compensate for missed ones.
- Explain that many drug interactions are possible. Patient should seek medical approval before taking any self-prescribed medications.
- Tell patient not to stop taking drug suddenly.
- Encourage patient to report difficulty urinating, sore throat, dizziness, fever, or fainting.
- Advise patient to avoid hazardous activities that require alertness until the effect of the drug is established. Excessive sedative effects tend to subside after several weeks.
- Explain what fluids are appropriate for diluting the concentrate and the dropper technique for measuring dose. Teach patient how to use suppository form.
- Inform patient that sugarless chewing gum or hard candy, ice chips, or artificial saliva may help to alleviate dry mouth.

chlorpropamide

Diabinese, Novo-Propamide*

Pharmacologic classification: sulfonylurea
Therapeutic classification: antidiabetic
Pregnancy risk category C

How supplied

Available by prescription only
Tablets: 100 mg, 250 mg

Indications and dosages

Adjunct to diet to lower blood glucose levels in patients with non-insulin-dependent diabetes mellitus (type 2)
Adults: 250 mg P.O. daily with breakfast or in divided doses if GI disturbances occur. First dosage increase may be made after 5 to 7 days because of extended duration of action, then dosage may be increased q 3 to 5 days by 50 to 125 mg, if needed, to a maximum of 750 mg daily.
≡ ***Dosage adjustment.*** In adults over age 65, initial dose should be 100 to 125 mg daily.
To change from insulin to oral therapy
Adults: If insulin dosage is less than 40 U daily, insulin may be stopped and oral therapy started as above. If insulin dosage is 40 U or more daily, start oral therapy as above, with insulin dose reduced 50% the first few days. Further insulin reductions should be made based on patient response.

Pharmacodynamics

Antidiabetic action: Chlorpropamide lowers blood glucose levels by stimulating insulin release from beta cells in the pancreas. After prolonged administration, it produces hypoglycemic effects through extrapancreatic mechanisms, including reduced basal hepatic glucose production and enhanced peripheral sensitivity to insulin; the latter may result either from an increased number of insulin receptors or from changes in events that follow insulin binding.
Antidiuretic action: Drug appears to potentiate the effects of minimal levels of antidiuretic hormone.

Pharmacokinetics

Absorption: Absorbed readily from the GI tract. Maximum decrease in serum glucose levels at 3 to 6 hours.
Distribution: Distribution isn't fully understood, but is probably similar to that of the other sulfonylureas. It's highly protein-bound.
Metabolism: About 80% of drug is metabolized by the liver. Whether the metabolites have hypoglycemic activity is unknown.
Excretion: Excreted in urine. Rate of excretion depends on urinary pH; it increases in alkaline urine and decreases in acidic urine. Duration of action is up to 60 hours; half-life is 36 hours.

Route	Onset	Peak	Duration
P.O.	1 hr	2-4 hr	24 hr

Contraindications and precautions

Contraindicated for treating type 1 diabetes (insulin-dependent) or diabetes that can be adequately controlled by diet. Also contraindicated in patients with type 2 diabetes complicated by ketosis, acidosis, diabetic coma, major surgery, severe infections, or severe trauma, or during pregnancy or breast-feeding as well as in those with hypersensitivity to drug.

Use cautiously in geriatric, debilitated, or malnourished patients and in those with porphyria or impaired renal or hepatic function.

Interactions

Drug-drug. *Anticoagulants:* May increase plasma levels of both drugs and, after continued therapy, may reduce plasma levels and anticoagulant effects. Monitor patient closely.
Beta blockers: May increase the risk of hypoglycemia. Monitor patient closely.
Chloramphenicol, guanethidine, insulin, MAO inhibitors, probenecid, salicylates, or sulfonamides: May enhance hypoglycemic effects by displacing chlorpropamide from its protein-binding sites. Avoid use together.
Drug-lifestyle. *Alcohol use:* May produce a disulfiram-like reaction. Discourage use together.
Smoking: Increases corticosteroid release. May require higher dosages of chlorpropamide.

Effects on diagnostic tests
None reported.

Adverse reactions
CNS: paresthesia, fatigue, dizziness, vertigo, malaise, headache.
EENT: tinnitus.
GI: nausea, heartburn, epigastric distress.
GU: tea-colored urine.
Hematologic: ***leukopenia, thrombocytopenia, aplastic anemia, agranulocytosis,*** hemolytic anemia.
Metabolic: ***prolonged hypoglycemia, dilutional hyponatremia,*** alterations in cholesterol, alkaline phosphatase, bilirubin, urine phenyl ketone, porphyrins, protein levels, and cephalin flocculation.
Skin: rash, pruritus, erythema, urticaria.
Other: ***hypersensitivity reactions.***

Overdose and treatment
Signs and symptoms of overdose include low blood glucose levels, tingling of lips and tongue, hunger, nausea, decreased cerebral function (lethargy, yawning, confusion, agitation, and nervousness), increased sympathetic activity (tachycardia, sweating, and tremor), and ultimately seizures, stupor, and coma.

Mild hypoglycemia (without loss of consciousness or neurologic findings) can be treated with oral glucose and dosage adjustments. If patient loses consciousness or experiences neurologic symptoms, he should receive rapid injection of dextrose 50%, followed by a continuous infusion of dextrose 10% at a rate to maintain blood glucose levels greater than 100 mg/dl. Because of chlorpropamide's long half-life, monitor patient for 3 to 5 days.

Clinical considerations
Consider the recommendations relevant to all sulfonylureas as well as the following:
- To avoid GI intolerance in those patients who require dosages of 250 mg/day or more and to improve control of hyperglycemia, divided doses are recommended. These are given before the morning and evening meals.
- Geriatric, debilitated, or malnourished patients and those with impaired renal or hepatic function usually require a lower initial dosage.
- Patients switching from chlorpropamide to another sulfonylurea should be monitored closely for 1 week because of chlorpropamide's prolonged retention in the body.
- Because of the long duration of action of the drug, adverse reactions, especially hypoglycemia, may be more frequent or severe than with some other sulfonylureas.
- Patients with severe diabetes who don't respond to 500 mg usually won't respond to higher doses.
- Oral hypoglycemic agents have been associated with an increased risk of CV mortality compared with diet or diet and insulin treatments.

Therapeutic monitoring
- Drug may accumulate in patients with renal insufficiency. Observe patient for signs such as dysuria, anuria, and hematuria.
- Chlorpropamide may potentiate antidiuretic effects of vasopressin. Monitor patient for drowsiness, muscle cramps, seizures, unconsciousness, water retention, and weakness.

Special populations
Breast-feeding patients. Drug is excreted in breast milk and shouldn't be used in breast-feeding women.
Pediatric patients. Drug is ineffective in insulin-dependent (type 1, juvenile-onset) diabetes.
Geriatric patients. Geriatric patients may be more sensitive to the effects of drug because of reduced metabolism and elimination. They're more likely to develop neurologic symptoms of hypoglycemia. Avoid drug in geriatric patients because of its longer duration of action. Geriatric patients usually require a lower initial dosage.

Patient counseling
- Emphasize importance of following prescribed diet, as well as the exercise and medical regimen.
- Instruct patient to take medication at the same time each day. If a dose is missed, it should be taken immediately, unless it's almost time for the next dose. Patient should never double the dose.
- Encourage patient to wear a medical identification bracelet or necklace.
- Instruct patient to take drug with food if it causes GI upset.
- Teach patient how to monitor blood glucose, urine glucose, and ketone levels, as needed.
- Teach patient to recognize the signs and symptoms of hypoglycemia and hyperglycemia and what to do if they occur.

chlorzoxazone
Paraflex, Parafon Forte DSC, Remular-S

Pharmacologic classification: benzoxazole derivative
Therapeutic classification: skeletal muscle relaxant
Pregnancy risk category C

How supplied
Available by prescription only
Tablets: 250 mg, 500 mg
Tablets (film-coated): 250 mg

Indications and dosages

Adjunct in acute, painful musculoskeletal conditions

Adults: 250, 500, or 750 mg P.O. t.i.d. or q.i.d. Reduce to lowest effective dose after response is obtained.
Children: 20 mg/kg or 600 mg/m² P.O. daily divided t.i.d. or q.i.d., or 125 to 500 mg t.i.d. or q.i.d., depending on age and weight.

Pharmacodynamics

Skeletal muscle relaxant action: Chlorzoxazone doesn't relax skeletal muscle directly, but apparently it does so through its sedative effects. However, exact mechanism of action is unknown. Animal studies suggest that drug modifies central perception of pain without eliminating peripheral pain reflexes.

Pharmacokinetics

Absorption: Rapidly and completely absorbed from the GI tract.
Distribution: Widely distributed in the body.
Metabolism: Metabolized in the liver to inactive metabolites. The half-life of chlorzoxazone is 66 minutes.
Excretion: Excreted in urine as glucuronide metabolite.

Route	Onset	Peak	Duration
P.O.	1 hr	1-2 hr	3-4 hr

Contraindications and precautions

Contraindicated in patients with hypersensitivity to drug or impaired hepatic function.

Interactions

Drug-drug. *CNS depressants:* Produce further CNS depression. Avoid use together.
MAO inhibitors or tricyclic antidepressants: May result in increased CNS depression, respiratory depression, and hypotensive effects. Reduce dosage of one or both agents.
Drug-lifestyle. *Alcohol use:* Produces further CNS depression. Discourage alcohol use.

Effects on diagnostic tests

None reported.

Adverse reactions

CNS: *drowsiness, dizziness, light-headedness,* malaise, headache, overstimulation, tremor.
GI: anorexia, nausea, vomiting, heartburn, abdominal distress, constipation, diarrhea.
GU: urine discoloration (orange or purple-red).
Hepatic: hepatic dysfunction.
Skin: urticaria, redness, pruritus, petechiae, bruising, ***angioneurotic edema, anaphylaxis.***

Overdose and treatment

Signs and symptoms of overdose include nausea, vomiting, diarrhea, drowsiness, dizziness, light-headedness, headache, malaise, or sluggishness, followed by loss of muscle tone, decreased or absent deep tendon reflexes, respiratory depression, and hypotension.

To treat overdose, induce emesis or perform gastric lavage followed by activated charcoal. Closely monitor vital signs and neurologic status. Provide general supportive measures, including maintenance of adequate airway and assisted ventilation. Use caution if administering pressor agents.

Clinical considerations

- Drug may cause drowsiness.
- Urine may turn orange or reddish purple.

Therapeutic monitoring

Monitor liver function tests in patients receiving long-term therapy. Watch for early signs of hepatic dysfunction or abnormal liver enzymes.

Special populations

Pregnant patients. Use only when benefits outweigh the risks. Safety hasn't been established.
Breast-feeding patients. It's unknown if drug is excreted in breast milk. No clinical problems have been reported.
Pediatric patients. Tablets may be crushed and mixed with food, milk, or fruit juice to aid dosing in children.
Geriatric patients. Geriatric patients may be more sensitive to the effects of the drug.

Patient counseling

- Caution patient to avoid hazardous activities that require alertness or physical coordination until CNS depression is determined.
- Advise patient to store drug away from direct heat or light (not in bathroom medicine cabinet, where heat and humidity cause deterioration of drug).
- Tell patient to take missed dose only if remembered within 1 hour of scheduled time. If beyond 1 hour, patient should skip dose and go back to regular schedule. Patient shouldn't double the dose.
- Inform patient not to stop taking drug without calling for specific instructions.
- Warn athletic patient that skeletal muscle relaxants are banned in competition sponsored by the U.S. Olympics Committee and the National Collegiate Athletic Association. Use can lead to disqualification.

cholestyramine

Questran, Questran Light

Pharmacologic classification: anion exchange resin
Therapeutic classification: antilipemic, bile acid sequestrant
Pregnancy risk category C

How supplied

Available by prescription only

Powder: 378-g cans, 9-g single-dose packets (Questran). 5-g single dose packets (Questran Light). Each scoop of powder or single-dose packet contains 4 g of cholestyramine resin.

Indications and dosages

Primary hyperlipidemia and hypercholesterolemia unresponsive to dietary measures alone; to reduce the risks of atherosclerotic coronary artery disease and MI; to relieve pruritus associated with partial biliary obstruction; ◇cardiac glycoside toxicity

Adults: 4 g P.O. before meals and h.s. not to exceed 32 g daily. Can be given in one to six divided doses.

Children age 6 to 12: 80 mg/kg or 2.35 g/m^2 P.O. t.i.d.

Pharmacodynamics

Antilipemic action: Bile is normally excreted into the intestine to facilitate absorption of fat and other lipid materials. Cholestyramine binds with bile acid, forming an insoluble compound that's excreted in feces. With less bile available in the digestive system, less fat and lipid materials in food are absorbed, more cholesterol is used by the liver to replace its supply of bile acids, and the serum cholesterol level decreases. In partial biliary obstruction, excess bile acids accumulate in dermal tissue, resulting in pruritus; by reducing levels of dermal bile acids, cholestyramine combats pruritus.

Drug can also act as an antidiarrheal in postoperative diarrhea caused by bile acids in the colon.

Pharmacokinetics

Absorption: Not absorbed. Cholesterol levels may begin to decrease 24 to 48 hours after the start of therapy and may continue to fall for up to 12 months. In some patients, the initial decrease is followed by a return to or above baseline cholesterol levels on continued therapy. Relief of pruritus associated with cholestasis occurs 1 to 3 weeks after initiation of therapy. Diarrhea associated with bile acids may cease in 24 hours.

Distribution: None.

Metabolism: None.

Excretion: Insoluble cholestyramine with bile acid complex is excreted in feces.

Route	Onset	Peak	Duration
P.O.	Unknown	Unknown	2-4 wk

Contraindications and precautions

Contraindicated in patients with hypersensitivity to bile-acid sequestering resins and in those with complete biliary obstruction. Use cautiously in patients with coronary artery disease or a predisposition to constipation.

Interactions

Drug-drug. *Acetaminophen, corticosteroids, thiazide diuretics, thyroid preparations, cardiac glycosides:* May reduce absorption of these medications. Administer other drugs 1 hour before or 4 to 6 hours after cholestyramine. Readjustment must also be made when cholestyramine is withdrawn, to prevent high-dose toxicity.

Warfarin: May decrease anticoagulant effects. Avoid use together. Careful monitoring of PT and INR is mandatory.

Effects on diagnostic tests

Cholecystography using iopanoic acid will yield abnormal results because iopanoic acid is also bound by cholestyramine.

Adverse reactions

CNS: headache, anxiety, vertigo, dizziness, insomnia, fatigue, syncope, tinnitus.

GI: *constipation, **fecal impaction,*** hemorrhoids, *abdominal discomfort,* flatulence, *nausea,* vomiting, steatorrhea, GI bleeding, diarrhea, anorexia.

GU: hematuria, dysuria.

Hematologic: anemia; ecchymoses; bleeding tendencies.

Hepatic: alters serum concentrations of ALT, AST.

Metabolic: alters serum concentrations of chloride, phosphorus, potassium, calcium, and sodium; hyperchloremic acidosis (with long-term use or very high doses).

Musculoskeletal: backache; muscle and joint pain; osteoporosis.

Skin: *rash;* irritation of skin, tongue, and perianal area.

Other: *vitamin A, D, E, and K deficiencies from decreased absorption.*

Overdose and treatment

Drug overdose hasn't been reported. Chief potential risk is intestinal obstruction; treatment would depend on location and degree of obstruction and on amount of gut motility.

Clinical considerations

- To mix, sprinkle powder on surface of preferred beverage or wet food, let stand a few minutes and stir to obtain uniform suspension; avoid excess foaming by using large glass and mixing slowly. Use at least 90 ml of water or other fluid, soup, milk, or pulpy fruit; rinse container and have patient drink this liquid to be sure he ingests entire dose.
- Drug has been used to treat cardiac glycoside overdose because it binds these agents and prevents enterohepatic recycling. When used as an adjunct to hyperlipidemia, monitor levels of cardiac glycosides and other drugs to ensure appropriate dosage during and after therapy with cholestyramine.

- Questran Light contains aspartame and provides 1.6 calories per packet or scoop.

Therapeutic monitoring
- Monitor serum cholesterol level frequently during first few months of therapy and periodically thereafter.
- Monitor bowel function. Treat constipation promptly by decreasing dosage, adding a stool softener, or discontinuing drug.
- Observation of patient for signs of vitamin A, D, or K deficiency is necessary.

Special populations
Pregnant patients. Use dietary management.
Breast-feeding patients. Safety in breast-feeding women hasn't been established.
Pediatric patients. Children may be at greater risk of hyperchloremic acidosis during cholestyramine therapy. Safe dosage hasn't been established for children under age 6.
Geriatric patients. Patients over age 60 are more likely to experience adverse GI effects as well as adverse nutritional effects.

Patient counseling
- Encourage patient to comply with continued blood testing and special diet; although therapy isn't curative, it helps control serum cholesterol level.
- Encourage patient to control weight and to stop smoking as part of attempt to increase awareness of other cardiac risk factors.
- Tell patient not to take the powder in dry form; teach him to mix drug with fluids or pulpy fruits.

choline magnesium trisalicylates
Tricosal, Trilisate

choline salicylate
Arthropan

Pharmacologic classification: salicylate
Therapeutic classification: nonnarcotic analgesic, antipyretic, anti-inflammatory
Pregnancy risk category C

How supplied
Available by prescription only
Tablets: 500 mg, 750 mg, 1,000 mg of salicylate (as choline and magnesium salicylate)
Solution: 500 mg of salicylate/5 ml (as choline and magnesium salicylate); 870 mg/5 ml (as choline salicylate)

Indications and dosages
Rheumatoid arthritis, osteoarthritis
Adults: 1,500 mg P.O. b.i.d. or 3,000 mg h.s.
≡***Dosage adjustment.*** In geriatric patients, give 750 mg t.i.d.
Arthritis, mild; antipyresis
Adults: 2,000 to 3,000 mg P.O. daily in divided doses b.i.d.
Mild-to-moderate pain and fever
Children: Based on weight, and the doses should be divided b.i.d.
Children weighing 26 to 28.5 lb (12 to 13 kg): 500 mg P.O. daily.
Children weighing 30 to 37.5 lb (14 to 17 kg): 750 mg P.O. daily.
Children weighing 39 to 48.5 lb (18 to 22 kg): 1,000 mg P.O. daily.
Children weighing 50 to 59.5 lb (23 to 27 kg): 1,250 mg P.O. daily.
Children weighing 61 to 70.5 lb (28 to 32 kg): 1,500 mg P.O. daily.
Children weighing 73 to 81.5 lb (33 to 37 kg): 1,750 mg P.O. daily.

Pharmacodynamics
Analgesic action: Choline salicylates produce analgesia by an ill-defined effect on the hypothalamus (central action) and by blocking generation of pain impulses (peripheral action). The peripheral action may involve inhibition of prostaglandin synthesis.
Anti-inflammatory action: These drugs exert their anti-inflammatory effect by inhibiting prostaglandin synthesis; they may also inhibit the synthesis or action of other inflammation mediators.
Antipyretic action: Choline salicylates relieve fever by acting on the hypothalamic heat-regulating center to produce peripheral vasodilation. This increases peripheral blood supply and promotes sweating, which leads to loss of heat and to cooling by evaporation. These drugs don't affect platelet aggregation and shouldn't be used to prevent thrombosis.

Pharmacokinetics
Absorption: Absorbed rapidly and completely from the GI tract.
Distribution: Protein binding depends on concentration and ranges from 75% to 90%, decreasing as serum level increases. Severe toxic effects may occur at serum levels greater than 400 mcg/ml.
Metabolism: Hydrolyzed to salicylate in the liver.
Excretion: Metabolites are excreted in urine.

Route	Onset	Peak	Duration
P.O.	Unknown	1-2 hr	Unknown

Contraindications and precautions
Contraindicated in patients hypersensitive to drug. Also contraindicated in patients with hemophilia, bleeding ulcers, hemorrhagic states,

and for patients who consume three or more alcoholic beverages per day. Use cautiously in patients with impaired renal or hepatic function, peptic ulcer disease, or gastritis. Don't give to children or teenagers with chickenpox or influenza-like illnesses.

Interactions

Drug-drug. *Ammonium chloride, urine acidifiers:* Increase choline salicylate blood levels; monitor for choline salicylate blood levels and thus toxicity.
Antacids: Delay and decrease absorption of choline salicylates. Patient requires close monitoring.
Corticosteroids: Enhance salicylate elimination; observe for decreased effect.
Corticosteroids, antibiotics, NSAIDs: Enhanced risk of adverse GI effects. Use together with caution.
Lithium carbonate: Choline salicylates decrease renal clearance, increasing serum lithium levels and the risk of adverse effects. Monitor patient closely.
Methotrexate: Concurrent use may cause displacement of bound methotrexate and inhibition of renal excretion. Avoid using together.
Phenytoin, sulfonylureas, warfarin: Concurrent use may cause displacement of either drug, and adverse effects. Monitor therapy closely for both drugs.
Warfarin: Salicylates enhance the hypoprothrombinemic effects. Avoid using together.
Drug-food. *Food:* Delays and decreases absorption of choline salicylates. Give on an empty stomach.
Drug-lifestyle. *Alcohol use:* Enhanced risk of adverse GI effects. Avoid use together.

Effects on diagnostic tests

Choline salicylates may interfere with urinary glucose analysis performed via Chemstrip uG, Diastix, glucose enzymatic test strip, Clinitest, and Benedict's solution. These drugs also interfere with urinary 5-hydroxyindole acetic acid and vanillylmandelic acid.

Adverse reactions

EENT: tinnitus, hearing loss.
GI: GI distress, nausea, vomiting.
GU: ***acute tubular necrosis with renal failure.***
Skin: rash.
Other: elevated free T_4 levels, hypersensitivity reactions ***(anaphylaxis), Reye's syndrome.***

Overdose and treatment

Signs and symptoms of overdose include metabolic acidosis with respiratory alkalosis, hyperpnea, and tachypnea from increased carbon dioxide production and direct stimulation of the respiratory center.

To treat overdose of choline salicylates, empty stomach immediately by inducing emesis with ipecac syrup, if patient is conscious, or by gastric lavage. Administer activated charcoal via nasogastric tube. Provide symptomatic and supportive measures (respiratory support and correction of fluid and electrolyte imbalances). Monitor laboratory parameters and vital signs closely. Hemodialysis is effective in removing choline salicylates but is used only in severe poisoning. Forced diuresis with alkalinizing agent accelerates salicylate excretion.

Clinical considerations

Consider the recommendations relevant to all salicylates as well as the following:
- Choline salicylates shouldn't be mixed with antacids.
- Administer oral solution of choline salicylate mixed with fruit juice. Follow with a full 8-oz (240 ml) glass of water to ensure passage into stomach.

Therapeutic monitoring

Monitor serum magnesium levels to prevent possible magnesium toxicity.

Special populations

Pregnant patients. Avoid use of choline salicylates in the third trimester of pregnancy.
Breast-feeding patients. Salicylates are distributed into breast milk. Avoid use in breast-feeding women.
Pediatric patients. Safety of long-term drug use in children under age 14 hasn't been established. Because of epidemiologic association with Reye's syndrome, the Centers for Disease Control and Prevention recommend that children with chickenpox or flulike symptoms not be given salicylates. Toxicity can develop rapidly in febrile, dehydrated children. Usually, they shouldn't receive more than five doses in 24 hours.
Geriatric patients. Patients over age 60 may be more susceptible to the toxic effects of these drugs.

Patient counseling

Warn patient not to take drug longer than prescribed or to increase dosage without consulting a doctor.

cidofovir

Vistide

Pharmacologic classification: nucleotide analogue
Therapeutic classification: antiviral
Pregnancy risk category C

How supplied

Available by prescription only
Injection: 75 mg/ml

Indications and dosages

Cytomegalovirus (CMV) retinitis in patients with AIDS; ◇acyclovir-resistant herpes simplex infections in immunocompromised patients

Adults: Give 5 mg/kg I.V. infused over 1 hour once weekly for 2 consecutive weeks followed by a maintenance dosage of 5 mg/kg I.V. infused over 1 hour once q 2 weeks. Probenecid must be administered concomitantly.

≡***Dosage adjustment.*** For patients with creatinine clearance of 41 to 55 ml/minute, reduce induction and maintenance dosages to 2 mg/kg; if creatinine clearance is 30 to 40 ml/minute, reduce induction and maintenance dosages to 1.5 mg/kg; if creatinine clearance is 20 to 29 ml/minute, reduce induction and maintenance dosages to 1 mg/kg; and if creatinine clearance is 19 ml/minute or less, reduce induction and maintenance doses to 0.5 mg/kg.

Pharmacodynamics

Antiviral action: Cidofovir suppresses CMV replication by selective inhibition of viral DNA synthesis.

Pharmacokinetics

Absorption: Administered only I.V.
Distribution: Unknown.
Metabolism: Not metabolized.
Excretion: 80% to 100% is excreted unchanged in urine.

Route	Onset	Peak	Duration
I.V.	Unknown	Unknown	Unknown

Contraindications and precautions

Contraindicated in patients with hypersensitivity to drug or history of clinically severe hypersensitivity to probenecid or other sulfa-containing medications. Do not administer as a direct intraocular injection (direct injection may be associated with significant decreases in intraocular pressure and vision impairment). Use cautiously in patients with impaired renal function.

Interactions

Drug-drug. *Nephrotoxic drugs (such as amphotericin B, aminoglycosides, foscarnet, and I.V. pentamidine):* May increase nephrotoxicity. Avoid use together.
Ganciclovir ocular implants: May result in profound hypotony. Cidofovir shouldn't be given within one month before or after placement of implant.

Effects on diagnostic tests

None reported.

Adverse reactions

CNS: malaise; *asthenia, headache,* amnesia, anxiety, confusion, ***seizure,*** depression, dizziness, abnormal gait, hallucinations, insomnia, neuropathy, paresthesia, somnolence, vasodilation.
CV: hypotension, postural hypotension, pallor, syncope, tachycardia.
EENT: amblyopia, conjunctivitis, eye disorders, ocular hypotony, iritis, retinal detachment, taste perversion, uveitis, abnormal vision, pharyngitis, rhinitis, sinusitis.
GI: *nausea, vomiting, diarrhea, anorexia, abdominal pain,* dry mouth, colitis, constipation, tongue discoloration, dyspepsia, dysphagia, flatulence, gastritis, melena, oral candidiasis, rectal disorders, stomatitis, aphthous stomatitis, mouth ulceration.
GU: *elevated creatinine levels,* ***nephrotoxicity,*** *proteinuria,* decreased creatinine clearance levels, glycosuria, hematuria, urinary incontinence, urinary tract infection.
Hematologic: NEUTROPENIA, *anemia,* ***thrombocytopenia.***
Hepatic: hepatomegaly, abnormal liver function tests, increased alkaline phosphatase levels.
Metabolic: fluid imbalances, hyperglycemia, hyperlipemia, hypocalcemia, hypokalemia, weight loss.
Musculoskeletal: arthralgia, myasthenia, myalgia.
Respiratory: asthma, bronchitis, coughing, dyspnea, hiccups, increased sputum, lung disorders, pneumonia.
Skin: *rash, alopecia,* acne, skin discoloration, dry skin, herpes simplex, pruritus, sweating, urticaria.
Other: *fever; infections; chills;* allergic reactions; facial edema; pain in back, chest, or neck; *sarcoma,* ***sepsis.***

Overdose and treatment

No information on drug overdose is available. However, hemodialysis and hydration may reduce drug plasma concentrations in patients who receive an overdose of the drug. Probenecid may reduce the potential for nephrotoxicity in patients who receive a drug overdose through reduction of active tubular secretion.

Clinical considerations

- Renal impairment is the major toxicity of cidofovir. To minimize possible nephrotoxicity, use I.V. prehydration with normal saline and administer probenecid with each cidofovir infusion.
- Administer normal saline solution, 1 L, over a 1- to 2-hour period immediately before each cidofovir infusion. Administer a second liter in patients who can tolerate the additional fluid load. If the second liter is given, administer it either at the start of the cidofovir infusion or immediately afterward; infuse it over a 1- to 3-hour period.
- Give probenecid, 2 g, P.O. 3 hours before the cidofovir dose and 1 g at 2 hours, and again at

8 hours after completion of the 1-hour infusion (total 4 g).

- To prepare infusion, extract the appropriate amount of cidofovir from the vial with a syringe and transfer the dose to an infusion bag containing 100 ml normal saline solution. The entire volume is infused I.V. at a constant rate over a 1-hour period. Use a standard infusion pump for administration.
- Because of the mutagenic properties of cidofovir, prepare drug in a class II laminar flow biological safety cabinet. Personnel preparing drug should wear surgical gloves and a closed front surgical-type gown with knit cuffs.
- If drug contacts the skin, wash membranes and flush thoroughly with water. Place excess drug and all other materials used in the admixture preparation and administration in a leak-proof, puncture-proof container. The recommended method of disposal is high temperature incineration.
- Administer cidofovir infusion admixtures within 24 hours of preparation; refrigerator or freezer storage shouldn't be used to extend this 24-hour period. If admixtures aren't to be used immediately, they may be refrigerated at 36 to 46° F (2 to 8° C) for no more than 24 hours. Allow refrigerated admixtures to equilibrate to room temperature before use.
- No other drug and supplements should be added to the cidofovir admixture for concurrent administration. Compatibility with Ringer's solution, lactated Ringer's solution, or bacteriostatic infusion fluids hasn't been evaluated.
- Drug is indicated only for the treatment of CMV retinitis in patients with AIDS. Safety and efficacy of drug haven't been established for treating other CMV infections, congenital or neonatal CMV disease, and CMV disease in patients not infected with HIV.
- In animal studies, cidofovir was carcinogenic and teratogenic and caused hypospermia.
- Fanconi's syndrome and decreased serum bicarbonate levels associated with evidence of renal tubular damage have been reported in patients receiving cidofovir. Monitor patient closely.
- Discontinue zidovudine therapy or reduce dosage by 50% in patients receiving zidovudine on the days cidofovir is administered because probenecid reduces metabolic clearance of zidovudine.

Therapeutic monitoring

- WBC counts with differential should be monitored before each dose.
- Monitor renal function (serum creatinine and urine protein) before each dose of the drug and modify the dosage for changes in renal function.
- Granulocytopenia has been observed in association with cidofovir treatment; monitor neutrophil counts during therapy.
- Intraocular pressure, visual acuity, and ocular symptoms should be monitored periodically.
- Drug shouldn't be initiated in patients with baseline serum creatinine exceeding 1.5 mg/dl or calculated creatinine clearances of 55 ml/minute or less unless the potential benefits exceed the potential risks.

Special populations

Pregnant patients. Instruct women of childbearing potential to use effective contraception during and for 1 month after treatment with cidofovir. Tell men to practice barrier contraceptive methods during and for 3 months after drug treatment.

Breast-feeding patients. It isn't known if drug is excreted in breast milk. Drug shouldn't be given to breast-feeding women.

Pediatric patients. Safety and effectiveness in children haven't been established.

Geriatric patients. Use with caution when administering cidofovir to geriatric patients. Dosage adjustment will be necessary if patient is renally impaired.

Patient counseling

- Inform patient that drug isn't a cure for CMV retinitis and that regular ophthalmologic follow-up examinations are necessary.
- Alert patients on zidovudine therapy that they'll need to obtain dosage guidelines on days that cidofovir is administered.
- Tell patient that close monitoring of renal function will be needed during cidofovir therapy and that an abnormality may require a change in cidofovir therapy.
- Stress importance of completing a full course of probenecid with each cidofovir dose. Tell patient to take probenecid after a meal to decrease nausea.
- Advise patient that cidofovir is considered a potential carcinogen in humans.

cilostazol

Pletal

Pharmacologic classification: quinolinone phosphodiesterase inhibitor
Therapeutic classification: antiplatelet agent
Pregnancy risk category C

How supplied

Available by prescription only
Tablets: 50 mg, 100 mg

Indications and dosages

Intermittent claudication

Adults: 100 mg P.O. b.i.d., taken ½ hour before or 2 hours after breakfast and dinner.

Pharmacodynamics

Antiplatelet action: Mechanism of action not fully understood. Believed to be due to inhibition of the enzyme phosphodiesterase (type III), causing an increase of cAMP in platelets and blood vessels, resulting in inhibition of platelet aggregation and vasodilation. Cilostazol reversibly inhibits platelet aggregation induced by various stimuli, such as thrombin, adenosine diphosphate, collagen, arachidonic acid, epinephrine, and stress.

Pharmacokinetics

Absorption: Absorbed following oral administration. A high fat meal increases peak serum levels about 90% and bioavailability by 25%. Absolute bioavailability isn't known.
Distribution: 95% to 98% protein-bound, primarily to albumin.
Metabolism: Extensively metabolized by hepatic cytochrome P-450 enzyme system, primarily CYP3A4.
Excretion: Excreted primarily in urine, mostly of metabolites (about 74%). Remaining drug is eliminated in the feces (about 20%). Half life of cilostazol and active metabolites is about 11 to 13 hours.

Route	Onset	Peak	Duration
P.O.	Unknown	Unknown	Unknown

Contraindications and precautions

Contraindicated in patients with heart failure of any severity. It's also contraindicated in patients with known or suspected hypersensitivity to any of its components. Use cautiously in patients with severe underlying heart disease and in combination with other drugs having antiplatelet activity.

Interactions

Drug-drug. *Erythromycin and other macrolides, omeprazole, diltiazem, strong inhibitors of CYP3A4, such as ketoconazole, itraconazole, fluconazole, miconazole, fluvoxamine, fluoxetine, nefazodone, and sertraline:* Increase peak serum levels of cilostazol or one of its metabolites. Avoid use together.
Drug-food. *Grapefruit juice:* May increase cilostazol levels. Discourage use together.
Drug-lifestyle. *Smoking:* Decreases drug exposure by about 20%. Discourage smoking.

Effects on diagnostic tests

None reported.

Adverse reactions

CNS: *headache, dizziness,* vertigo.
CV: *palpitation,* tachycardia.
EENT: *pharyngitis, rhinitis.*
GI: *abnormal stools, diarrhea,* dyspepsia, abdominal pain, flatulence, nausea.
Musculoskeletal: back pain, myalgia.
Respiratory: cough aggravation.
Other: *infection,* peripheral edema.

Overdose and treatment

Clinical signs of overdose include severe headache, diarrhea, hypotension, tachycardia, and, possibly, cardiac arrhythmias. Observe patient carefully and give supportive treatment. Because drug is highly protein-bound, it may not be efficiently removed by hemodialysis.

Clinical considerations

- A thorough medication history must be obtained before initiating therapy.
- Several drugs that inhibit the enzyme phosphodiesterase have caused decreased survival in patients with class III-IV heart failure. Therefore, cilostazol is contraindicated in patients with congestive heart failure.

Therapeutic monitoring

There's uncertainty concerning cardiovascular risk in long-term use or in patients with severe underlying heart disease.

Special populations

Breast-feeding patients. Because drug is excreted in breast milk, a decision should be made to discontinue nursing or discontinue drug.
Pediatric patients. Safety and effectiveness haven't been established in pediatric patients.
Geriatric patients. No overall differences in safety, efficacy, or pharmacokinetics have been observed between geriatric and younger patients.

Patient counseling

- Instruct patient that cilostazol should be taken at least ½ hour before or 2 hours after breakfast and dinner.
- Tell patient that a beneficial effect won't be noticed before 2 to 4 weeks, and that it may take as long as 12 weeks before a beneficial effect is experienced.
- To chart effects of drug therapy, advise patient to keep a log of how far he's able to walk without pain.

cimetidine

Tagamet, Tagamet HB

Pharmacologic classification: H_2-receptor antagonist
Therapeutic classification: antiulcer
Pregnancy risk category B

How supplied

Available by prescription only
Tablets: 200 mg, 300 mg, 400 mg, 800 mg
Injection: 300 mg/2 ml, 300 mg/50 ml normal saline (premixed)
Liquid: 300 mg/5 ml
Available without a prescription
Tablets: 200 mg

Indications and dosages

Duodenal ulcer (short-term treatment)
Adults: 800 mg P.O. h.s. for maximum of 8 weeks. Alternatively, give 400 mg P.O. b.i.d. or 300 mg P.O. q.i.d. with meals and h.s. When healing occurs, stop treatment or give h.s. dose only to control nocturnal hypersecretion.
Parenteral: 300 mg diluted to 20 ml with normal saline solution or other compatible I.V. solution by I.V. push over 5 minutes q 6 hours. Or 300 mg diluted in 50 ml dextrose 5% solution or other compatible I.V. solution by I.V. infusion over 15 to 20 minutes q 6 to 8 hours. Or 300 mg I.M. q 6 to 8 hours (no dilution necessary). To increase dose, give more frequently to maximum daily dose of 2,400 mg.
Duodenal ulcer prophylaxis
Adults: 400 mg P.O. h.s.
Active benign gastric ulcer
Adults: 800 mg P.O. h.s., or 300 mg P.O. q.i.d. with meals and h.s. for up to 8 weeks.
Pathologic hypersecretory conditions (such as Zollinger-Ellison syndrome, systemic mastocytosis, and multiple endocrine adenomas); ◇short-bowel syndrome
Adults: 300 mg P.O. q.i.d. with meals and h.s.; adjust to patient needs. Maximum daily dose, 2,400 mg.
Parenteral: 300 mg diluted to 20 ml with normal saline solution or other compatible I.V. solution by I.V. push over 5 minutes q 6 to 8 hours. Or 300 mg diluted in 50 ml dextrose 5% solution or other compatible I.V. solution by I.V. infusion over 15 to 20 minutes q 6 to 8 hours. To increase dosage, give 300 mg doses more frequently to maximum daily dose of 2,400 mg.
Symptomatic relief of gastroesophageal reflux
Adults: 800 mg P.O. b.i.d. or 400 mg q.i.d., before meals and h.s.
◇Active upper GI bleeding, peptic esophagitis, stress ulcer
Adults: 1 to 2 g I.V. or P.O. daily, in four divided doses.
Continuous infusion for patients unable to tolerate oral medication
Adults: 37.5 mg/hour (900 mg/day) by continuous I.V. infusion. Use an infusion pump if total volume is below 250 ml/day.
Heartburn, acid indigestion, sour stomach
Adults: 200 mg P.O. up to a maximum of b.i.d. (400 mg).
≡***Dosage adjustment.*** In patients with renal failure, recommended dosage is 300 mg P.O. or I.V. q 8 to 12 hours at end of dialysis. Dosage may be decreased further if hepatic failure is also present.

Pharmacodynamics

Antiulcer action: Cimetidine competitively inhibits histamine's action at H_2 receptors in gastric parietal cells, inhibiting basal and nocturnal gastric acid secretion (such as from stimulation by food, caffeine, insulin, histamine, betazole, or pentagastrin). Cimetidine may also enhance gastromucosal defense and healing.

A 300-mg oral or parenteral dose inhibits about 80% of gastric acid secretion for 4 to 5 hours.

Pharmacokinetics

Absorption: About 60% to 75% of oral dose is absorbed. Absorption rate (but not extent) may be affected by food.
Distribution: Distributed to many body tissues. About 15% to 20% of drug is protein-bound. Cimetidine apparently crosses the placenta and is distributed in breast milk.
Metabolism: About 30% to 40% of dose is metabolized in the liver. Drug has a half-life of 2 hours in patients with normal renal function; half-life increases with decreasing renal function.
Excretion: Excreted primarily in urine (48% of oral dose, 75% of parenteral dose); 10% of oral dose is excreted in feces. Some drug is excreted in breast milk.

Route	Onset	Peak	Duration
P.O.	Unknown	45-90 min	4-5 hr
I.V.	Unknown	Immediate	Unknown
I.M.	Unknown	Unknown	Unknown

Contraindications and precautions

Contraindicated in patients hypersensitive to drug. Use with caution in elderly or debilitated patients.

Interactions

Drug-drug. *Beta blockers (such as propranolol), phenytoin, lidocaine, procainamide, quinidine, benzodiazepines, disulfiram, metronidazole, xanthines, tricyclic antidepressants, oral contraceptives, isoniazid, warfarin, carmustine, and triamterene:* Cimetidine decreases the metabolism of these drugs, increasing potential toxicity and possibly necessitating dosage reduction. Monitor patient closely.
Digoxin: Serum digoxin levels may be reduced. Patient requires close monitoring.
Ferrous salts, ketoconazole, indomethacin, and tetracyclines: May affect the absorption of these drugs altering gastric pH. Avoid use together.
Flecainide: Serum levels of flecainide may be increased. Avoid use together.
Drug-herb. *Guarana:* May increase caffeine serum levels or prolong serum caffeine half-life. Patient requires close monitoring.
Pennyroyal: May change the rate of formation of toxic metabolites of pennyroyal. Avoid use together.
Yerba maté: May decrease clearance of yerba maté methylxanthines and cause toxicity. Use together cautiously.

Drug-lifestyle. *Smoking:* May increase gastric acid secretion and worsen disease. Discourage use together.

Effects on diagnostic tests
Cimetidine may antagonize pentagastrin's effect during gastric acid secretion tests; it may cause false-negative results in skin tests using allergen extracts.

Adverse reactions
CNS: confusion, dizziness, headache, peripheral neuropathy, somnolence, hallucinations.
GI: *mild and transient diarrhea.*
GU: transient elevations in serum creatinine levels, impotence, mild gynecomastia if used for over 1 month.
Hematologic: ***agranulocytosis*** (rare), ***neutropenia, thrombocytopenia*** (rare), ***aplastic anemia*** (rare).
Hepatic: jaundice (rare); increases prolactin levels, serum alkaline phosphatase levels, and serum creatinine levels.
Musculoskeletal: muscle pain, arthralgia.
Other: hypersensitivity reactions.

Overdose and treatment
Clinical effects of overdose include respiratory failure and tachycardia. Overdose is rare; intake of up to 10 g has caused no untoward effects.

Support respiration and maintain a patent airway. Induce emesis or use gastric lavage; follow with activated charcoal to prevent further absorption. Treat tachycardia with propranolol if necessary. Hemodialysis removes drug.

Clinical considerations
Consider the recommendations relevant to all H_2-receptor antagonists as well as the following:

☐ ***ALERT*** For I.V. use, cimetidine must be diluted before administration. Don't dilute drug with sterile water for injection; use normal saline solution or D_5W to a total volume of 20 ml. FD and C blue dye #2 used in Tagamet tablets may impair interpretation of Hemoccult and Gastroccult tests on gastric content aspirate. Be sure to wait at least 15 minutes after tablet administration before drawing the sample, and follow test manufacturer's instructions closely.

- For I.M. administration, drug may be given undiluted. Injection may be painful.
- After administration of the liquid via nasogastric tube, flush tube to clear it and ensure passage of drug to stomach.
- Since hemodialysis removes drug, schedule dose after dialysis session.

Therapeutic monitoring
Assess for abdominal pain. Note any blood in emesis, stool, or gastric aspirate.

Special populations
Breast-feeding patients. Drug is excreted in breast milk. Avoid use in breast-feeding women.
Geriatric patients. Use caution when administering cimetidine to geriatric patients because of the potential for adverse reactions affecting the CNS.

Patient counseling
- Instruct patient to take drug as directed and to continue taking it even after pain subsides, to allow for adequate healing.
- Urge patient to avoid smoking, because it may increase gastric acid secretion and worsen disease.

ciprofloxacin (systemic)
Cipro

Pharmacologic classification: fluoroquinolone antibiotic
Therapeutic classification: antibiotic
Pregnancy risk category C

How supplied
Available by prescription only
Tablets (film-coated): 100 mg, 250 mg, 500 mg, 750 mg
Injection for infusion: 200 mg/20-ml vial; 400 mg/40-ml vial; 200 mg in 100 ml D_5W; 400 mg in 200 ml D_5W
Oral suspension: 250 mg/5 ml, 500 mg/5 ml

Indications and dosages
Mild to moderate urinary tract infection caused by susceptible bacteria
Adults: 250 mg P.O. or 200 mg I.V. q 12 hours.
Infectious diarrhea, mild to moderate respiratory tract infections, bone and joint infections, severe or complicated urinary tract infections
Adults: 500 mg P.O. q 12 hours or 400 mg I.V. q 12 hours.
Severe or complicated infections of the respiratory tract, bones, joints, skin, or skin structures; ◇mycobacterial infections
Adults: 750 mg P.O. q 12 hours or 400 mg I.V. q 12 hours.
Typhoid fever
Adults: 500 mg P.O. q 12 hours.
Intra-abdominal infections (in combination with metronidazole)
Adults: 500 mg P.O. q 12 hours
***Treatment of mild to moderate acute sinusitis caused by* Haemophilus influenzae, Streptococcus pneumoniae, *or* Moraxella catarrhalis; *mild to moderate chronic bacterial prostatitis caused by* Escherichia coli *or* Proteus mirabilis**
Adults: 400 mg I.V. infusion given over 60 minutes every 12 hours.
◇Uncomplicated gonorrhea
Adults: 250 mg P.O. as a single dose.

◊**Neisseria meningitidis** ***in nasal passages***
Adults: 500 to 750 mg P.O. as a single dose, or 250 mg P.O. b.i.d. for 2 days, or 500 mg P.O. b.i.d. for 5 days.
≡***Dosage adjustment.*** For patients with renal failure, refer to the following tables.

Oral Ciprofloxacin

Creatinine clearance (ml/min)	Adult dosage
> 50	No adjustment
30 to 50	250 to 500 mg q 12 hr
5 to 29	250 to 500 mg q 18 hr

I.V. Ciprofloxacin

Creatinine clearance (ml/min)	Adult dosage
> 30	No adjustment
5 to 29	200 to 400 mg. I.V. q 18 to 24 hr

Hemodialysis patients: 200 to 400 mg q 24 hours after dialysis period.

Pharmacodynamics

Antibiotic action: Ciprofloxacin inhibits DNA gyrase, preventing bacterial DNA replication. The following organisms have been reported to be susceptible (in-vitro) to ciprofloxacin: *Campylobacter jejuni, Citrobacter diversus, Citrobacter freundii, Enterobacter cloacae, Escherichia coli* (including enterotoxigenic strains), *Haemophilus parainfluenzae, Klebsiella pneumoniae, Morganella morganii, Proteus mirabilis, Proteus vulgaris, Providencia stuartii, Providencia rettgeri, Pseudomonas aeruginosa, Serratia marcescens, Shigella flexneri, Shigella sonnei, Staphylococcus aureus* (penicillinase- and non-penicillinase-producing strains), *Staphylococcus epidermidis, Streptococcus faecalis,* and *Streptococcus pyogenes.*

Pharmacokinetics

Absorption: About 70% is absorbed after oral tablet administration. Food delays rate of absorption but not extent.
Distribution: Peak serum levels occur within 1 to 2 hours after oral tablet dosing. Drug is 20% to 40% protein-bound; CSF levels are only about 10% of plasma levels.
Metabolism: Metabolism is probably hepatic. Four metabolites have been identified; each has less antimicrobial activity than the parent compound.
Excretion: Excretion is primarily renal. Serum half-life is about 4 hours in adults with normal renal function.

Route	Onset	Peak	Duration
P.O. (Tab)	Unknown	½-2⅓ hr	Unknown
P.O. (Susp)	Unknown	Unknown	Unknown
I.V.	Unknown	Immediate	Unknown

Contraindications and precautions

Contraindicated in patients sensitive to fluoroquinolone antibiotics. Use cautiously in patients with CNS disorders or those at risk for seizures.

Interactions

Drug-drug. *Aluminum-, calcium-,* and *magnesium-containing antacid supplements:* May interfere with ciprofloxacin absorption. Antacids may be safely administered 2 hours before or 6 hours after ciprofloxacin.
Beta-lactams and aminoglycosides: Synergistic effects have occurred with concurrent use. Avoid use together.
Probenecid: Concurrent use interferes with renal tubular secretion and results in higher plasma levels of ciprofloxacin. Avoid use together.
Sucralfate: Reduces absorption of ciprofloxacin by 50%. Avoid use together.
Theophylline: Increased risk of theophylline toxicity. Closer monitoring of theophylline levels may be necessary.
Warfarin: PT has increased with use of ciprofloxacin and warfarin. Avoid use together.
Drug-herb. *Yerba maté methylxanthines:* May decrease clearance of yerba maté methylxanthines and cause toxicity; use together cautiously.
Drug-lifestyle. *Sun exposure:* Photosensitivity reaction may occur from sun exposure. Advise patient to take precautions.
Drug-food. *Caffeine:* Ciprofloxacin also prolongs elimination half-life of caffeine.
Vitamins, minerals, and iron: May interfere with absorption of ciprofloxacin. Avoid use together.

Effects on diagnostic tests

None reported.

Adverse reactions

CNS: headache, restlessness, tremor, dizziness, fatigue, drowsiness, insomnia, depression, light-headedness, confusion, hallucinations, ***seizures,*** paresthesia.
GI: *nausea, diarrhea,* vomiting, abdominal pain or discomfort, oral candidiasis, elevated liver enzymes, pseudomembranous colitis, dyspepsia, flatulence, constipation.
GU: crystalluria, increased serum creatinine and BUN levels, interstitial nephritis.
Musculoskeletal: arthralgia, joint or back pain, joint inflammation, joint stiffness, aching, neck or chest pain.

Skin: *rash,* photosensitivity, toxic epidermal necrolysis, exfoliative dermatitis.
Other: photosensitivity, ***Stevens-Johnson syndrome,*** hypersensitivity; thrombophlebitis, burning, pruritus, erythema, edema (with I.V. administration).

Overdose and treatment

To treat drug overdose, empty the stomach by induced vomiting or lavage. Provide general supportive measures and maintain hydration. Peritoneal dialysis or hemodialysis may be helpful, particularly if patient's renal function is compromised.

Clinical considerations

Duration of therapy depends on type and severity of infection. Therapy should continue for 2 days after symptoms have abated. Most infections are well controlled in 1 to 2 weeks, but bone or joint infections may require therapy for 4 weeks or longer.

Therapeutic monitoring

Patient's intake and output require monitoring, as well as observation for signs of crystalluria.

Special populations

Breast-feeding patients. Drug may be secreted in breast milk. Consider discontinuing breast-feeding or drug therapy to avoid serious toxicity in the infant.
Pediatric patients. Avoid use in children.

Patient counseling

- Tell patient that drug may be taken without regard to meals. The preferred time is 2 hours after a meal.
- Advise patient to avoid taking drug with antacids, iron, or calcium and to drink plenty of fluids during therapy.
- Inform patient that because dizziness, lightheadedness, or drowsiness may occur, he should avoid hazardous activities that require mental alertness until CNS effects of drug are determined.

ciprofloxacin hydrochloride (ophthalmic)

Ciloxan

Pharmacologic classification: fluoroquinolone
Therapeutic classification: antibacterial
Pregnancy risk category C

How supplied

Available by prescription only
Ophthalmic solution: 0.3% in 2.5- and 5-ml containers

Indications and dosages

***Corneal ulcers caused by* Pseudomonas aeruginosa, Staphylococcus aureus, Staphylococcus epidermidis, Streptococcus pneumoniae, *and possibly* Serratia marcescens *and* Streptococcus viridans**
Adults and children over age 12: Instill 2 drops in the affected eye q 15 minutes for first 6 hours, then 2 drops q 30 minutes for remainder of first day. On day 2, instill 2 drops hourly. On days 3 to 14, instill 2 drops q 4 hours.
***Bacterial conjunctivitis caused by* S. aureus *and* S. epidermidis *and possibly* S. pneumoniae**
Adults and children over age 12: Instill 1 or 2 drops into the conjunctival sac of affected eye q 2 hours while awake, for first 2 days. Then 1 or 2 drops q 4 hours while awake, for next 5 days.

Pharmacodynamics

Antibacterial action: Inhibits bacterial DNA gyrase, an enzyme necessary for bacterial replication. Bacteriostatic or bactericidal, depending on concentration.

Pharmacokinetics

Absorption: Systemic absorption is limited. The maximum plasma concentration is less than 5 ng/ml, and the mean plasma concentration is usually below 2.5 ng/ml.
Distribution: Unknown.
Metabolism: Unknown.
Excretion: Unknown.

Route	Onset	Peak	Duration
Ophthalmic	Unknown	Unknown	Unknown

Contraindications and precautions

Contraindicated in patients with history of hypersensitivity to drug or other fluoroquinolone antibiotics. Use with caution in breast-feeding women.

Interactions

None reported.

Effects on diagnostic tests

None reported.

Adverse reactions

EENT: *local burning or discomfort, white crystalline* precipitate (in the superficial portion of the corneal defect in patients with corneal ulcers), *margin crusting, crystals or scales, foreign body sensation, itching, conjunctival hyperemia,* bad or bitter taste in mouth, corneal staining, allergic reactions, keratopathy, lid edema, tearing, photophobia, decreased vision.
GI: nausea.

Overdose and treatment

A topical overdose of drug may be flushed from the eye with warm tap water.

Clinical considerations

If corneal epithelium is still compromised after 14 days of treatment, continue therapy.

Therapeutic monitoring

Drug must be discontinued at first sign of hypersensitivity reactions, such as rash, itching eyelids, redness or swelling, and the doctor must be notified.

Special populations

Breast-feeding patients. It's unknown if drug is excreted in breast milk after application to the eye; however, systemically administered ciprofloxacin has been detected in breast milk. Use with caution.
Pediatric patients. Safety and efficacy in children under age 12 haven't been established.

Patient counseling

- Teach patient how to instill drug correctly. Remind him not to touch the tip of the bottle with his hands and to avoid contact of the tip with the eye or surrounding tissue.
- Remind patient not to share washcloths or towels with other family members to avoid spreading infection.
- Advise patient to wash hands before and after instilling solution.

cisapride

Propulsid

Pharmacologic classification: serotonin-4 receptor agonist
Therapeutic classification: GI prokinetic
Pregnancy risk category C

How supplied

Available by prescription only
Tablets: 10 mg, 20 mg
Suspension: 1 mg/1 ml

Indications and dosages

Symptomatic treatment of nocturnal heartburn due to gastroesophageal reflux disease that doesn't respond adequately to lifestyle modifications, antacids, and gastric acid-reducing agents
Adults: 10 mg P.O. q.i.d. at least 15 minutes before meals and h.s. Dose may be increased to 20 mg q.i.d., if needed.

Pharmacodynamics

GI prokinetic action: Cisapride is thought to enhance release of acetylcholine at the myenteric plexus, increasing GI motility. Cisapride doesn't induce muscarinic or nicotinic receptor stimulation, nor does it inhibit acetylcholinesterase activity. It also doesn't increase or decrease basal- or pentagastrin-induced gastric acid secretion, or block dopamine receptors.

Pharmacokinetics

Absorption: Rapidly absorbed.
Distribution: Extensively distributed (the volume of distribution is about 180 L). About 97.5% to 98% binds to plasma proteins, mainly to albumin.
Metabolism: Extensively metabolized in the liver. Norcisapride, formed by N-dealkylation, is the principal metabolite in plasma, feces, and urine.
Excretion: Excreted in urine and feces. Unchanged drug accounts for less than 10% of urinary and fecal recovery after oral administration. The mean terminal half-life ranges from 6 to 12 hours.

Route	Onset	Peak	Duration
P.O.	30-60 min	1-2 hr	Unknown

Contraindications and precautions

Contraindicated in patients hypersensitive to drug. Also contraindicated in patients in whom increased GI motility may be harmful, such as those with mechanical obstruction, hemorrhage, or perforation of the GI tract.

Use of drug with macrolides, antifungals, protease inhibitors, nefazodone, and grapefruit juice is contraindicated. Also contraindicated in patients with history of prolonged QT intervals, ventricular arrhythmias, ischemic heart disease, uncorrected electrolyte disorders (such as hypokalemia, hypomagnesemia), and heart, renal, or respiratory failure. Use cautiously in breast-feeding women.

Interactions

Drug-drug. *Anticholinergic agents:* May decrease cisapride's therapeutic effects. Patient requires close monitoring.
Anticoagulant: Administration of cisapride during anticoagulant therapy has led to increased coagulation times. It's advisable to check coagulation time 1 week after the start and discontinuation of cisapride therapy, with an appropriate adjustment of the anticoagulant dose, if necessary.
Cimetidine: Coadministration leads to an increased peak plasma level of cisapride. GI absorption of cimetidine and ranitidine is accelerated when they are coadministered with cisapride. Monitor closely.
Digoxin: May increase the absorption of digoxin. Avoid use together.
Clarithromycin, erythromycin, fluconazole, indinavir, itraconazole, ketoconazole, miconazole, nefazodone, ritonavir, troleandomycin, and agents that inhibit cytochrome P-450 IIIA4: Concurrent use is contraindicated because of the increased risk of prolonged QT intervals and arrhythmias.
Drug-food. *Grapefruit juice:* Increased cisapride availability. Avoid use together.
Drug-lifestyle. *Alcohol use:* Enhanced sedation. Avoid use together.

Effects on diagnostic tests
None reported.

Adverse reactions
CNS: *headache,* insomnia, anxiety, nervousness.
EENT: abnormal vision.
GI: *diarrhea, abdominal pain,* nausea, constipation, flatulence, dyspepsia.
GU: urinary frequency, urinary tract infection, vaginitis.
Respiratory: rhinitis, sinusitis, cough, upper respiratory tract infections.
Skin: rash, pruritus.
Other: pain, fever, viral infections, arthralgia.

Overdose and treatment
Symptoms of overdose may include retching, borborygmi, flatulence, and increased stool and urinary frequency. Treatment should include gastric lavage or activated charcoal, close observation, and general supportive measures.

Clinical considerations
- Cisapride may affect the absorption of other drugs by accelerating gastric emptying. Closely monitor patient receiving narrow therapeutic ratio drugs or other drugs that require careful adjustment and reassess plasma levels.
- Protect 20-g tablets from light; protect all products from moisture.

Therapeutic monitoring
Cases of serious arrhythmias have been reported in patients receiving cisapride. Monitor ECG closely.

Special populations
Pregnant patients: Give only when potential benefits outweigh risk to fetus.
Breast-feeding patients. Drug is excreted in breast milk at concentrations about 1/20 of those observed in plasma. Use caution when administering cisapride to breast-feeding patients.
Pediatric patients. Safety and effectiveness in children haven't been established.
Geriatric patients. Steady-state plasma levels of cisapride are generally higher in older patients because of a moderately prolonged elimination half-life. Therapeutic doses, however, are similar to those used in younger adults. Monitor closely for adverse effects.

Patient counseling
- Instruct patient to take cisapride at least 15 minutes before meals and at bedtime.
- Warn patient that drug may accelerate the sedative effects of benzodiazepines and alcohol.

cisatracurium besylate
Nimbex

Pharmacologic classification: nondepolarizing neuromuscular blocker
Therapeutic classification: skeletal muscle relaxant
Pregnancy risk category B

How supplied
Available by prescription only
Injection: 2 mg/ml, 10 mg/ml

Indications and dosages
Adjunct to general anesthesia, to facilitate tracheal intubation, and to provide skeletal muscle relaxation during surgery or mechanical ventilation in the intensive care unit
Adults and children age 12 and older: Initially, 0.15 or 0.20 mg/kg I.V.; then 0.03 mg/kg I.V. q 40 to 50 minutes after an initial dose of 0.15 mg/kg and q 50 to 60 minutes following an initial dose of 0.20 mg/kg for maintenance in prolonged surgical procedures. Alternatively, administer 3 mcg/kg/minute maintenance infusion after initial dose and then decrease to 1 to 2 mcg/kg/minute, p.r.n.
Children age 2 to 12: 0.1 mg/kg I.V. over 5 to 10 seconds. Administer 3 mcg/kg/minute maintenance I.V. infusion after initial dose and then decrease to 1 to 2 mcg/kg/minute, p.r.n., in prolonged surgical procedures.
Maintenance of neuromuscular blockade in intensive care unit
Adults: 3 mcg/kg/minute I.V. infusion.

Note: Dosage requirements among patients vary widely. Also, dosages may increase or decrease over time.

Pharmacodynamics
Skeletal muscle relaxation action: Cisatracurium binds competitively to cholinergic receptors on the motor end-plate to antagonize the action of acetylcholine, resulting in blockage of neuromuscular transmission.

Pharmacokinetics
Absorption: Only administered I.V.
Distribution: Volume of distribution is limited by its large molecular weight and high polarity. Drug binding to plasma proteins hasn't been successfully studied because of its rapid degradation at physiologic pH.
Metabolism: The degradation of cisatracurium is largely independent of liver metabolism. It's believed drug undergoes Hofmann elimination (a pH- and temperature-dependent chemical process) to form laudanosine and the monoquaternary acrylate metabolite.

Excretion: The metabolites of cisatracurium are excreted primarily in urine and feces. Elimination half-life is between 22 and 29 minutes.

Route	Onset	Peak	Duration
I.V.	1-3 min	2-5 min	25-44 min

Contraindications and precautions

Contraindicated in patients with hypersensitivity to drug, other bis-benzylisoquinolinium agents, or benzyl alcohol. Use cautiously in pregnant patients.

Interactions

Drug-drug. *Aminoglycosides, bacitracin, clindamycin, colistin, lincomycin, lithium, local anesthetics, magnesium salts, polymyxins, procainamide, quinidine, tetracyclines, and colistimethate sodium:* May enhance the neuromuscular blocking action of cisatracurium. Use together cautiously.
Carbamazepine, phenytoin: May cause slightly shorter duration of neuromuscular blockage requiring higher infusion rate requirements. Monitor patient closely.
Isoflurane, enflurane administered with nitrous oxide or oxygen: May prolong the clinically effective duration of action of initial and maintenance dosages of cisatracurium. In long surgical procedures, less frequent maintenance dosing, lower maintenance dosages, or reduced infusion rates of cisatracurium may be needed.
Succinylcholine: Shorter time to onset of maximum neuromuscular block. Close monitoring of patient is necessary.

Effects on diagnostic tests

None reported.

Adverse reactions

CV: bradycardia, hypotension.
Respiratory: ***bronchospasm.***
Skin: flushing, rash.

Overdose and treatment

Overdose with neuromuscular blocking agents may result in neuromuscular block beyond the time needed for surgery and anesthesia. The primary treatment is maintenance of a patent airway and controlled ventilation until recovery of normal neuromuscular function is assured. Once recovery from neuromuscular block begins, further recovery may be facilitated by administration of an anticholinesterase agent (neostigmine, edrophonium) and an appropriate anticholinergic agent.

Clinical considerations

□ ***ALERT*** For I.V. use, 20-ml vial is intended for use in the intensive care unit only. Drug isn't compatible with propofol injection or ketorolac injection for Y-site administration. Drug is acidic and may also not be compatible with an alkaline solution having a pH greater than 8.5, such as barbiturate solutions for Y-site administration. Drug shouldn't be diluted in lactated Ringer's injection USP because of chemical instability.

- Drug isn't recommended for rapid sequence endotracheal intubation because of its intermediate onset of action.
- Cisatracurium has no known effect on consciousness, pain threshold, or cerebration. To avoid patient distress, neuromuscular block shouldn't be induced before patient is unconscious.
- Drug is a colorless to slightly yellow or greenish-yellow solution. Inspect vial visually for particulate matter and discoloration before administration. Solutions that aren't clear or contain visible particulates shouldn't be used.
- To avoid inaccurate dosing, perform neuromuscular monitoring on a nonparetic limb in patients with hemiparesis or paraparesis.
- In patients with neuromuscular disease (myasthenia gravis and myasthenic syndrome), prolonged neuromuscular block may occur. The use of a peripheral nerve stimulator and a dose not exceeding 0.02 mg/kg is recommended to assess the level of neuromuscular block and to monitor dosage requirements.
- Because patients with burns have been shown to develop resistance to nondepolarizing neuromuscular blocking agents, these patients may require increased dosing requirements and exhibit shortened duration of action. Monitor closely.

Therapeutic monitoring

- Monitor neuromuscular function during drug administration with a nerve stimulator. Additional doses of drug shouldn't be given before there is a definite response to nerve stimulation. If no response occurs, discontinue infusion until a response returns.
- Monitor patient's acid-base balance and electrolyte levels. Acid-base or serum electrolyte abnormalities may potentiate or antagonize the action of cisatracurium.
- Monitor patient for malignant hyperthermia.

Special populations

Breast-feeding patients. Use caution when administering cisatracurium to breast-feeding women because it isn't known if drug is excreted in breast milk.
Pediatric patients. Safety and effectiveness in children under age 2 haven't been established.
Geriatric patients. Use with caution when administering cisatracurium to geriatric patients. The time to maximum block is about 1 minute slower in geriatric patients.

Patient counseling

- Reassure patient and family that patient will be monitored continuously throughout drug use; explain reason for its use.

■ All procedures and events must be explained to the patient since the drug doesn't interfere with patient's ability to hear.

cisplatin (cis-platinum)

Platinol, Platinol AQ

Pharmacologic classification: alkylating agent (cell cycle–phase nonspecific)
Therapeutic classification: antineoplastic
Pregnancy risk category D

How supplied

Available by prescription only
Injection: 1 mg/ml (50-mg, or 100-mg vials)

Indications and dosages

Indications and dosages may vary. Check current literature for recommended protocol.
Adjunctive therapy in metastatic testicular cancer
Adults: 20 mg/m^2 I.V. daily for 5 days. Repeat q 3 weeks for three cycles or more. Usually used in therapeutic regimen with bleomycin and vinblastine.
Adjunctive therapy in metastatic ovarian cancer
Adults: 75 to 100 mg/m^2 I.V. Repeat q 4 weeks or 50 mg/m^2 I.V. q 3 weeks with concurrent doxorubicin hydrochloride therapy.
Treatment of advanced bladder cancer
Adults: 50 to 70 mg/m^2 I.V. once q 3 to 4 weeks. Patients who have received other antineoplastics or radiation therapy should receive 50 mg/m^2 q 4 weeks.
◊ ***Head and neck cancer***
Adults: 80 to 120 mg/m^2 I.V. once q 3 weeks.
◊ ***Cervical cancer***
Adults: 50 mg/m^2 I.V. once q 3 weeks.
◊ ***Non-small-cell lung cancer***
Adults: 70 to 120 mg/m^2 I.V. once q 3 to 6 weeks.
◊ ***Brain tumor***
Children: 60 mg/m^2 I.V. for 2 days q 3 to 4 weeks.
◊ ***Osteogenic sarcoma or neuroblastoma***
Children: 90 mg/m^2 I.V. q 3 weeks.

Note: Prehydration and mannitol diuresis may significantly reduce renal toxicity and ototoxicity.

Pharmacodynamics

Antineoplastic action: Cisplatin exerts its cytotoxic effects by binding with DNA and inhibiting DNA synthesis and, to a lesser extent, by inhibition of protein and RNA synthesis. Cisplatin also acts as a bifunctional alkylating agent, causing intrastrand and interstrand cross-links of DNA. Interstrand cross-linking appears to correlate well with the cytotoxicity of drug.

Pharmacokinetics

Absorption: Not administered orally or intramuscularly.
Distribution: Distributed widely into tissues, with the highest concentrations found in the kidneys, liver, and prostate. Drug can accumulate in body tissues, with drug being detected up to 6 months after the last dose. Cisplatin doesn't readily cross the blood-brain barrier. Drug is extensively and irreversibly bound to plasma proteins and tissue proteins.
Metabolism: Metabolic fate of cisplatin is unclear.
Excretion: Excreted primarily unchanged in urine. In patients with normal renal function, the half-life of the initial elimination phase is 25 to 79 minutes and the terminal phase 58 to 78 hours. The terminal half-life of total cisplatin is up to 10 days.

Route	Onset	Peak	Duration
I.V.	Unknown	Unknown	Several days

Contraindications and precautions

Contraindicated in patients with hypersensitivity to drug or to other platinum-containing compounds and in those with severe renal disease, hearing impairment, or myelosuppression.

Interactions

Drug-drug. *Aminoglycosides:* Concurrent use potentiates the cumulative nephrotoxicity caused by cisplatin. Therefore, aminoglycosides shouldn't be used within 2 weeks of cisplatin therapy, and renal function studies should be monitored carefully.
Aspirin: Increased risk of bleeding. Avoid use together.
Loop diuretics: Concurrent use increases the risk of ototoxicity; closely monitor patient's audiologic status.
Phenytoin: May decrease serum level of phenytoin. Monitor phenytoin level.

Effects on diagnostic tests

None reported.

Adverse reactions

CNS: *peripheral neuritis,* loss of taste, ***seizures,*** neuropathy.
EENT: *tinnitus, hearing loss, ototoxicity,* vestibular toxicity.
GI: *nausea, vomiting* (beginning 1 to 4 hours after dose and lasting 24 hours).
GU: more prolonged and SEVERE RENAL TOXICITY with repeated courses of therapy.
Hematologic: MYELOSUPPRESSION; ***leukopenia, thrombocytopenia; anemia;*** nadirs in circulating platelet and WBC counts on days 18 to 23, with recovery by day 39.
Metabolism: *hypomagnesemia,* hypokalemia, hypocalcemia, hyponatremia, hypophosphatemia, hyperuricemia.
Other: ***anaphylactoid reaction.***

Overdose and treatment

Signs and symptoms of overdose include leukopenia, thrombocytopenia, nausea, and vomiting.

Treatment is generally supportive and includes transfusion of blood components, antibiotics for possible infections, and antiemetics. Cisplatin can be removed by dialysis, but only within 3 hours after administration.

Clinical considerations

- Review hematologic status and creatinine clearance before therapy.
- Reconstitute 10-mg vial with 10 ml and 50-mg vial with 50 ml of sterile water for injection to yield a concentration of 1 mg/ml. The drug may be diluted further in a sodium chloride-containing solution for I.V. infusion.
- Don't use aluminum needles for reconstitution or administration of cisplatin; a black precipitate may form. Use stainless steel needles.
- Drug is stable for 24 hours in normal saline solution at room temperature. Don't refrigerate because precipitation may occur. Discard solution containing precipitate.
- Infusions are most stable in chloride-containing solutions, such as normal saline, 0.45% saline, or 0.225% saline.
- Mannitol may be given as a 12.5-g I.V. bolus before starting cisplatin infusion. Follow by infusion of mannitol at rate of up to 10 g/hour, as necessary, to maintain urine output during cisplatin infusion and for 6 to 24 hours after infusion.
- I.V. sodium thiosulfate may be administered with cisplatin infusion to decrease risk of nephrotoxicity.
- Hydrate patient, with P.O. fluids if possible, or with normal saline solution before giving drug. Maintain urine output of 100 ml/hour for 4 consecutive hours before and 24 hours after infusion.
- Nausea and vomiting may be severe and protracted (up to 24 hours). Antiemetics can be started 24 hours before therapy. Monitor fluid intake and output. Continue I.V. hydration until patient can tolerate adequate oral intake.
- High-dose metoclopramide (2 mg/kg I.V.) has been used to prevent and treat nausea and vomiting. Dexamethasone 10 to 20 mg has been administered I.V. with metoclopramide to help alleviate nausea and vomiting. Many patients respond favorably to treatment with ondansetron (Zofran). Pretreatment with this 5-HT_3 antagonist should begin 30 minutes before cisplatin therapy is started.
- Treat extravasation with local injections of a 1/6 M sodium thiosulfate solution (prepared by mixing 4 ml of sodium thiosulfate 10% and 6 ml of sterile water for injection).
- Anaphylactoid reaction usually responds to immediate treatment with epinephrine, corticosteroids, or antihistamines.
- Avoid contact with skin. If contact occurs, wash drug off immediately with soap and water.

Therapeutic monitoring

- Monitor CBC, platelet count, and renal function studies before initial and subsequent doses. Don't repeat dose unless platelet count is more than 100,000/mm^3, WBC count is more than 4,000/mm^3, serum creatinine level is less than 1.5 mg/dl, or BUN level is less than 25 mg/dl.
- Renal toxicity becomes more severe with repeated doses. Renal function must return to normal before next dose can be given.
- Monitor electrolytes extensively; aggressive supplementation is often required after a course of therapy.

Special populations

Pregnant patients. Caution women of childbearing age not to become pregnant during therapy. Also recommend consulting with doctor before becoming pregnant.

Breast-feeding patients. It's unknown if cisplatin is distributed into breast milk. However, because of risk to infant of serious adverse reactions, mutagenicity, and carcinogenicity, breast-feeding isn't recommended during therapy.

Pediatric patients. Pediatric dosages of cisplatin haven't been fully established. Unlabeled uses of cisplatin include osteogenic sarcoma and neuroblastoma. Ototoxicity appears to be more severe in children.

Patient counseling

- Stress importance of adequate fluid intake and increase in urine output, to facilitate uric acid excretion.
- Tell patient to report tinnitus immediately, to prevent permanent hearing loss. Patient should have audiometric tests before initial and subsequent courses.
- Advise patient to avoid exposure to people with infections.
- Inform patient to promptly report unusual bleeding or bruising.

citalopram hydrobromide

Celexa

Pharmacologic classification: selective serotonin reuptake inhibitor
Therapeutic classification: antidepressant
Pregnancy risk category C

How supplied

Available by prescription only
Tablets: 20 mg, 40 mg

Indications and dosages

Depression
Adults: Initially, 20 mg P.O. once daily, increasing to 40 mg daily after no less than 1 week. Maximum recommended dose is 40 mg daily.
Elderly: 20 mg/day P.O. with titration to 40 mg/day for nonresponding patients.
≡***Dosage adjustment.*** For patients with hepatic impairment, use 20 mg/day P.O. with titration to 40 mg/day only for nonresponding patients.

Pharmacodynamics

Antidepressant action: A selective serotonin reuptake inhibitor (SSRI) whose action is presumed to be linked to potentiation of serotonergic activity in the central nervous system resulting from inhibition of neuronal reuptake of serotonin.

Pharmacokinetics

Absorption: Absolute bioavailability is 80% following oral administration.
Distribution: Highly bound to plasma proteins (80%).
Metabolism: Extensively metabolized primarily by cytochrome P-4503A4 and cytochrome P-4502C19 to inactive metabolites.
Excretion: About 20% of drug is excreted in urine. Elimination half-life is about 35 hours. In geriatric patients over age 60, the half-life is increased up to 30%.

Route	Onset	Peak	Duration
P.O.	Unknown	4 hr	Unknown

Contraindications and precautions

Contraindicated in patients also taking MAO inhibitors or within 14 days of MAO inhibitor therapy and in those with hypersensitivity to drug or its inactive ingredients.

Interactions

Drug-drug. *Carbamazepine:* May increase citalopram clearance; monitor for effects.
CNS drugs: Have additive effects; use together cautiously.
Drugs that inhibit cytochrome P-450 isoenzymes 3A4 and 2C19: Decreased clearance of citalopram; monitor patient closely.
Imipramine, other tricyclic antidepressants: Concentration of imipramine metabolite desipramine increased by about 50%; use together cautiously.
Lithium: May enhance serotonergic effect of citalopram; use with caution, and monitor lithium level.
MAO inhibitors: Serious, sometimes fatal, reactions may occur; don't use drug within 14 days of MAO inhibitor use.
Warfarin: Prothrombin time is increased by 5%; patient needs careful monitoring.
Drug-lifestyle. *Alcohol use:* May increase CNS effects. Avoid use together.

Adverse reactions

CNS: tremor, *somnolence, insomnia,* anxiety, agitation, dizziness, paresthesia, migraine, impaired concentration, amnesia, depression, apathy, *suicide attempt,* confusion, fatigue.
CV: tachycardia, orthostatic hypotension, hypotension.
EENT: rhinitis, sinusitis, abnormal accommodation.
GI: *dry mouth, nausea,* diarrhea, anorexia, dyspepsia, vomiting, abdominal pain, taste perversion, increased saliva, flatulence, decreased and increased weight, increased appetite.
GU: dysmenorrhea, amenorrhea, ejaculation disorder, impotence, polyuria.
Musculoskeletal: arthralgia, myalgia.
Respiratory: upper respiratory tract infection, coughing.
Skin: rash, pruritus.
Other: *increased sweating,* fever, yawning, decreased libido, SIADH, hyponatremia.

Clinical considerations

- Use cautiously in patients with history of mania, seizures, suicidal ideation, or hepatic or renal impairment.
- Be aware that, although drug hasn't been shown to impair psychomotor performance, any psychoactive drug has the potential to impair judgment, thinking, or motor skills.

Therapeutic monitoring

The possibility of a suicide attempt is inherent in depression and may persist until significant remission occurs. Closely observe high-risk patients at the start of drug therapy. Reduce risk of overdose by limiting the amount of drug available per refill.

Special populations

Breast-feeding patients. Drug is excreted in breast milk with subsequent effects in the infant; therefore, a decision to discontinue drug or breast-feeding should be made during drug therapy
Pediatric patients. Safety and effectiveness haven't been established.
Geriatric patients. Use cautiously in the elderly since greater sensitivity to drug hasn't been ruled out.

Patient counseling

- Inform patient that although improvement may occur within 1 to 4 weeks, he should continue therapy as prescribed.
- Instruct patient to exercise caution when operating hazardous machinery, including automobiles, because of the potential of psychoactive drugs to impair judgment, thinking, and motor skills.

■ Advise patient to consult doctor before taking other prescription or OTC medications.
■ Tell patient that drug may be taken in the morning or evening without regard to meals.

cladribine

Leustatin

Pharmacologic classification: purine nucleoside analogue
Therapeutic classification: antineoplastic
Pregnancy risk category D

How supplied

Available by prescription only
Injection: 1 mg/ml

Indications and dosages

Active hairy cell leukemia
Adults: 0.09 mg/kg daily by continuous I.V. infusion for 7 days.
◇***Advanced cutaneous T-cell lymphomas, chronic lymphocytic leukemia, malignant lymphomas, acute myeloid leukemias, autoimmune hemolytic anemia, mycosis fungoides, or Sézary syndrome***
Adults: Usually 0.1 mg/kg/day by continuous I.V. infusion for 7 days.

Pharmacodynamics

Antineoplastic action: Cladribine enters tumor cells, where it's phosphorylated by deoxycytidine kinase and subsequently converted into an active triphosphate deoxynucleotide. This metabolite impairs synthesis of new DNA, inhibits repair of existing DNA, and disrupts cellular metabolism.

Pharmacokinetics

Absorption: Not administered P.O. or I.M.
Distribution: About 20% of cladribine is bound to plasma proteins.
Metabolism: Information not available.
Excretion: For patients with normal renal function, the mean terminal half-life of cladribine is 5½ hours.

Route	Onset	Peak	Duration
I.V.	4 mo	Unknown	> 8 mo

Contraindications and precautions

Contraindicated in patients hypersensitive to drug. Use cautiously in patients with impaired renal or hepatic function.

Interactions

Drug-drug. *Amphotericin B:* May increase the risk of nephrotoxicity, hypotension and bronchospasm. Patient requires close monitoring.

Effects on diagnostic tests

None reported.

Adverse reactions

CNS: *malaise, headache, fatigue,* dizziness, insomnia, asthenia.
CV: tachycardia, edema.
EENT: epistaxis.
GI: *nausea, decreased appetite, vomiting, diarrhea,* constipation, abdominal pain.
GU: acute renal insufficiency.
Hematologic: NEUTROPENIA, ***anemia, thrombocytopenia.***
Musculoskeletal: *trunk pain, myalgia, arthralgia.*
Respiratory: *abnormal breath or chest sounds, cough,* shortness of breath.
Skin: *rash, pruritus, erythema, purpura,* petechiae, *local reaction at the injection site.*
Other: *fever,* INFECTION, *chills, diaphoresis,* hyperuricemia.

Overdose and treatment

High doses of cladribine have been associated with irreversible neurologic toxicity (paraparesis/quadriparesis), acute nephrotoxicity, and severe bone marrow suppression that results in neutropenia, anemia, and thrombocytopenia. No antidote specific to cladribine overdose is known. Besides discontinuation of cladribine, treatment consists of careful observation and appropriate supportive measures. It isn't known if drug can be removed from the circulation by dialysis or hemofiltration.

Clinical considerations

■ Fever is commonly observed during the first month of therapy and frequently requires antibiotic therapy.
■ Because of risk of hyperuricemia from tumor lysis, administer allopurinol during therapy.
■ For a 24-hour infusion, add the calculated dose to a 500-ml infusion bag of normal saline solution injection. Once diluted, administer promptly or store in the refrigerator for no more than 8 hours before administration. Don't use solutions that contain dextrose because studies have shown increased degradation of drug. Because the product doesn't contain bacteriostatic agents, use strict aseptic technique to prepare the admixture. Solutions containing cladribine shouldn't be mixed with other I.V. drugs or infused simultaneously via a common I.V. line.
■ Alternatively, prepare a 7-day infusion solution, using bacteriostatic sodium chloride injection, which contains 0.9% benzyl alcohol. First, pass the calculated amount of drug through a disposable 0.22-micron hydrophilic syringe filter into a sterile infusion reservoir. Next, add sufficient bacteriostatic sodium chloride injection to bring the total volume to 100 ml. Clamp off the line; then disconnect and discard the filter. If necessary, aseptically aspirate air bubbles from the reservoir, using a new filter or sterile vent filter assembly.

- Physical and chemical stability are acceptable using Pharmacia Deltec medication cassettes.
- Refrigerate unopened vials at 36° to 46° F (2° to 8° C), and protect from light. Although freezing doesn't adversely affect the drug, a precipitate may form; this will disappear if the drug is allowed to warm to room temperature gradually and the vial is vigorously shaken. Don't heat, microwave, or refreeze.

Therapeutic monitoring

- Cladribine is a toxic drug, and some toxicity is expected during treatment. Monitor hematologic function closely, especially during the first 4 to 8 weeks of therapy. Severe bone marrow suppression, including neutropenia, anemia, and thrombocytopenia, has commonly been observed in patients treated with drug; many patients also have preexisting hematologic impairment from their disease.

Special populations

Pediatric patients. Safety and effectiveness in children haven't been established.
Breast-feeding patients. It isn't known if drug is excreted in breast milk. A decision should be made whether to discontinue breast-feeding or drug, taking into account the importance of drug to the woman.
Pregnant patients. Women of childbearing age should avoid pregnancy during drug therapy because of risk of fetal malformations.

Patient counseling

- Teach patient to watch for signs of infection and bleeding (easy bruising, nosebleeds).
- Tell patient to take his temperature daily.

clarithromycin

Biaxin

Pharmacologic classification: macrolide
Therapeutic classification: antibiotic
Pregnancy risk category C

How supplied

Available by prescription only
Tablets: 250 mg, 500 mg
Suspension: 125 mg/5 ml, 250 mg/5 ml

Indications and dosages

***Pharyngitis or tonsillitis caused by* Streptococcus pyogenes**
Adults: 250 mg P.O. q 12 hours for 10 days.
Children: 15 mg/kg/day P.O. divided q 12 hours for 10 days.
***Acute maxillary sinusitis caused by* Streptococcus pneumoniae, Haemophilus influenzae, *or* Moraxella catarrhalis**
Adults: 500 mg P.O. q 12 hours for 14 days.
Children: 15 mg/kg/day P.O. divided q 12 hours for 10 days.
***Acute exacerbations of chronic bronchitis caused by* M. (Branhamella) catarrhalis *or* S. pneumoniae; *pneumonia caused by* S. pneumoniae *or* Mycoplasma pneumoniae**
Adults: 250 mg P.O. q 12 hours for 7 to 14 days.
***Acute exacerbations of chronic bronchitis caused by* H. influenzae**
Adults: 500 mg P.O. q 12 hours for 7 to 14 days.
***Uncomplicated skin and skin structure infections caused by* Staphylococcus aureus *or* S. pyogenes**
Adults: 250 mg P.O. q 12 hours for 7 to 14 days.
Prophylaxis and treatment of disseminated infection due to* Mycobacterium avium *complex
Adults: 500 mg P.O. b.i.d.
Children: 7.5 mg/kg P.O. b.i.d. up to 500 mg b.i.d.
***Acute otitis media caused by* H. influenzae, M. catarrhalis, *or* S. pneumoniae**
Children: 7.5 mg/kg P.O. b.i.d. up to 500 mg b.i.d.
H. pylori *eradication to reduce risk of duodenal ulcer recurrence*
Adult: 500 mg Biaxin in combination with 30 mg lansoprazole and 1 g amoxicilin, all given q 12 hours for 10 to 14 days. Alternatively, dual therapy with 500 mg Biaxin q 8 hours and 40 mg omeprazole once daily for 14 days.
≡ ***Dosage adjustment.*** In patients with creatinine clearance of less than 30 ml/minute, cut dose in half or double frequency interval.

Pharmacodynamics

Antibiotic action: Clarithromycin, a macrolide antibiotic, binds to the 50S subunit of bacterial ribosomes, blocking protein synthesis. It is bacteriostatic or bactericidal, depending on the concentration.

Pharmacokinetics

Absorption: Rapidly absorbed from the GI tract; absolute bioavailability is about 50%. Although food slightly delays onset of absorption, clarithromycin may be taken without regard to meals because food doesn't alter the total amount of drug absorbed.
Distribution: Widely distributed; because it readily penetrates cells, tissue concentrations are higher than plasma levels. Plasma half-life is dose-dependent; half-life is 3 to 4 hours at doses of 250 mg q 12 hours and increases to 5 to 7 hours at doses of 500 mg q 12 hours.
Metabolism: Clarithromycin's major metabolite, 14-hydroxy clarithromycin, has significant antimicrobial activity. It's about twice as active against *H. influenzae* as the parent drug.
Excretion: In patients taking 250 mg q 12 hours, about 20% is eliminated in the urine unchanged; this increases to 30% in patients taking 500 mg q 12 hours. The major metabo-

lite accounts for about 15% of drug in the urine. Elimination half-life of the active metabolite is dose-dependent: 5 to 6 hours with 250 mg q 12 hours; 7 hours with 500 mg q 12 hours.

Route	Onset	Peak	Duration
P.O.	Unknown	2-4 hr	Unknown

Contraindications and precautions
Contraindicated in patients with hypersensitivity to erythromycin or other macrolides who have preexisting cardiac abnormalities or electrolyte disturbances. Use cautiously in patients with impaired renal or hepatic function.

Interactions
Drug-drug. *Cyclosporine, triazolam, phenytoin:* Decreased metabolism of these drugs. Close monitoring of patient is needed.
Digoxin: Increased levels. Monitor patient for signs of digoxin toxicity.
Ergotamine, dihydroergotamine: Acute ergot toxicity. Avoid use together.
Theophylline, carbamazepine: May increase serum levels. Monitor plasma levels of these agents carefully.
Warfarin: Increased INR with other macrolides, and possibly with clarithromycin. Monitor patient closely.

Effects on diagnostic tests
None reported.

Adverse reactions
CNS: headache.
GI: *diarrhea, nausea, abnormal taste,* dyspepsia, abdominal pain or discomfort.
GU: elevated BUN and creatinine.
Hematologic: increased PT; decreased WBCs.
Hepatic: elevated liver function tests.

Overdose and treatment
No information available.

Clinical considerations
- Obtain specimen for culture and sensitivity tests before giving first dose. Therapy may begin pending test results.
- Reconstituted suspension shouldn't be refrigerated; discard any unused portion after 14 days.

Therapeutic monitoring
Drug may cause overgrowth of nonsusceptible bacteria or fungi. Monitor for signs and symptoms of superinfection.

Special populations
Breast-feeding patients. It's unknown if drug is excreted in breast milk; however, other macrolides have been found in breast milk. Use with caution.

Pediatric patients. Safety and efficacy in children under age 12 haven't been established.

Patient counseling
- Tell patient to take all of drug as prescribed, even if he feels better.
- Inform patient that he may take drug without regard to meals.
- Instruct patient to shake suspension well before use; don't refrigerate. Discard unused portion after 10 days.

clemastine fumarate
Tavist, Tavist Allergy

Pharmacologic classification: ethanolamine-derivative antihistamine
Therapeutic classification: antihistamine (H_1-receptor antagonist)
Pregnancy risk category C

How supplied
Available without a prescription
Tablets: 1.34 mg (Tavist Allergy), 2.68 mg (Tavist)
Syrup: 0.5 mg /5 ml

Indications and dosages
Rhinitis, allergy symptoms
Adults and children age 12 or over: 1.34 to 2.68 mg P.O. b.i.d. or t.i.d. Maximum recommended daily dose: 8.04 mg.
Children age 6 to 11: 0.67 mg P.O. b.i.d.; not to exceed 4.02 mg/day.
Allergic skin manifestation of urticaria and angioedema
Adults and children age 12 or over: 2.68 mg P.O. up to t.i.d. maximum.
Children age 6 to 11: 1.34 mg P.O. b.i.d.; not to exceed 4.02 mg/day.

Pharmacodynamics
Antihistamine action: Antihistamines compete with histamine for histamine H_1-receptor sites on the smooth muscle of the bronchi, GI tract, uterus, and large blood vessels; by binding to cellular receptors, they prevent access of histamine and suppress histamine-induced allergic symptoms, even though they don't prevent its release.

Pharmacokinetics
Absorption: Absorbed readily from the GI tract.
Distribution: Unknown.
Metabolism: Extensively metabolized.
Excretion: Excreted in urine

Route	Onset	Peak	Duration
P.O.	15-60 min	5-7 hr	12 hr

Contraindications and precautions
Contraindicated in patients with hypersensitivity to drug or other antihistamines of simi-

lar chemical structure; in those with acute asthma; in neonates or premature infants; and in breast-feeding patients.

Use cautiously in the elderly and in patients with increased intraocular pressure, glaucoma, hyperthyroidism, CV or renal disease, hypertension, bronchial asthma, pyloroduodenal obstruction, prostatic hyperplasia, bladder neck obstruction, and stenosing peptic ulcers.

Interactions

Drug-drug. *MAO inhibitors:* Prolong and intensify the central depressant and anticholinergic effects. Don't use together.
CNS depressants: Increased sedation. Use together cautiously.
Sulfonylureas: May diminish the effects. Patient requires close monitoring.
Heparin: May partially counteract the anticoagulant effect. Monitor patient closely.
Drug-lifestyle. *Alcohol use*: Additive CNS depression may occur. Discourage use together.
Sun exposure: Photosensitivity reactions may occur. Advise patient to take precautions.

Effects on diagnostic tests

Discontinue clemastine 4 days before diagnostic skin tests; antihistamines can prevent, reduce, or mask positive skin test response.

Adverse reactions

CNS: *sedation, drowsiness,* ***seizures,*** nervousness, tremor, confusion, restlessness, vertigo, headache, *sleepiness, dizziness, incoordination,* fatigue.
CV: hypotension, palpitations, tachycardia.
GI: *epigastric distress,* anorexia, diarrhea, nausea, vomiting, constipation, *dry mouth.*
GU: urine retention, urinary frequency.
Hematologic: hemolytic anemia, ***thrombocytopenia, agranulocytosis.***
Respiratory: *thick bronchial secretions.*
Skin: rash, urticaria, photosensitivity, diaphoresis.
Other: ***anaphylactic shock.***

Overdose and treatment

Signs and symptoms of overdose may include either CNS depression (sedation, reduced mental alertness, apnea, and CV collapse) or CNS stimulation (insomnia, hallucinations, tremors, or seizures). Anticholinergic symptoms, such as dry mouth, flushed skin, fixed and dilated pupils, and GI symptoms, are common, especially in children.

Treat overdose by inducing emesis with ipecac syrup (in conscious patient), followed by activated charcoal to reduce further drug absorption. Use gastric lavage if patient is unconscious or if ipecac fails. Treat hypotension with vasopressors, and control seizures with diazepam or phenytoin. Don't give stimulants.

Clinical considerations

Consider the recommendations relevant to all antihistamines; drug is indicated for treatment of urticaria only at dosages of 2.68 mg up to t.i.d.

Therapeutic monitoring

Monitor blood counts during long-term therapy; observe for signs of blood dyscrasias.

Special populations

Breast-feeding patients. Drug shouldn't be used during breast-feeding because it's secreted in breast milk, exposing infant to risks of unusual excitability; premature infants are at particular risk for seizures.
Pediatric patients. Drug isn't indicated for use in premature infants or neonates. Children, especially those under age 6, may experience paradoxical hyperexcitability.
Geriatric patients. Geriatric patients are more susceptible to the sedative effect of drug and may experience dizziness or hypotension more readily than younger people. Instruct older patient to change positions slowly and gradually.

Patient counseling

- Inform patient of potential adverse reactions.
- Tell patient to report if tolerance develops because a different antihistamine may need to be prescribed.

clindamycin hydrochloride

Cleocin

clindamycin palmitate hydrochloride

Cleocin Pediatric

clindamycin phosphate

Cleocin Phosphate, Cleocin T

Pharmacologic classification: lincomycin derivative
Therapeutic classification: antibiotic
Pregnancy risk category NR (B, vaginal and topical creams)

How supplied

Available by prescription only
Capsules: 75 mg, 150 mg, 300 mg
Solution (granules): 75 mg/5 ml
Injection: 150 mg/ml
Infusion for I.V. use: 150 mg/ml (300 mg, 600 mg, 900 mg)
Gel, lotion, topical solution, pledgets: 1%
Vaginal cream: 2%

Indications and dosages

Infections caused by sensitive organisms
Adults: 150 to 450 mg P.O. q 6 hours; or 600 to 2,700 mg/day I.M. or I.V. divided into two to four equal doses.
Children over age 1 month: 8 to 20 mg/kg/day P.O. or 20 to 40 mg/kg/day I.V. divided into three or four equal doses.
Children under age 1 month: 15 to 20 mg/kg/day I.V. divided into three or four equal doses.
Bacterial vaginosis
Adults: 100 mg (1 applicatorful of clindamycin phosphate) intravaginally h.s. for 7 days.
Acne vulgaris
Adults: Apply thin film of topical solution, gel, or lotion to affected areas b.i.d.
◇ ***Toxoplasmosis (cerebral or ocular) in immunocompromised patients***
Adults and adolescents: 300 to 450 mg P.O. q 6 to 8 hours with pyrimethamine (25 to 75 mg once daily) and leucovorin (10 to 25 mg once daily).
Infants and children: 20 to 30 mg/kg daily P.O. in 4 divided doses with oral pyrimethamine (1 mg/kg daily) and oral leucovorin (5 mg once every 3 days).
◇ **Pneumocystis carinii *pneumonia***
Adults: 600 mg I.V. q 6 hours or 300 to 450 mg P.O. q.i.d. With primaquine, give 15 to 30 mg P.O. daily.

Pharmacodynamics

Antibacterial action: Drug inhibits bacterial protein synthesis by binding to ribosome's 50S subunit. Clindamycin may produce bacteriostatic or bactericidal effects on susceptible bacteria, including most aerobic gram-positive cocci and anaerobic gram-negative and gram-positive organisms. It's considered a first-line drug in the treatment of *Bacteroides fragilis* and most other gram-positive and gram-negative anaerobes. It's also effective against *Mycoplasma pneumoniae, Leptotrichia buccalis,* and some gram-positive cocci and bacilli.

Pharmacokinetics

Absorption: When administered orally, drug is absorbed rapidly and almost completely from the GI tract, regardless of formulation. Drug may also be given I.M. with good absorption. With 300-mg dose, peak levels are about 6 mcg/ml; with 600-mg dose, about 10 mcg/ml.
Distribution: Distributed widely to most body tissues and fluids (except CSF) and crosses the placenta. About 93% of drug is bound to plasma proteins.
Metabolism: Metabolized partially to inactive metabolites.
Excretion: About 10% of dose is excreted unchanged in urine; rest is excreted as inactive metabolites (with some drug excreted in breast milk). Plasma half-life is 2½ to 3 hours in patients with normal renal function; 3½ to 5 hours in anephric patients; and 7 to 14 hours in patients with hepatic disease. Peritoneal dialysis and hemodialysis don't remove drug.

Route	Onset	Peak	Duration
P.O.	Unknown	45-60 min	Unknown
I.V.	Unknown	Immediate	Unknown
I.M.	Unknown	3 hr	Unknown
Topical, intravaginal	Unknown	Unknown	Unknown

Contraindications and precautions

Contraindicated in patients with hypersensitivity to the antibiotic congener lincomycin; in those with a history of ulcerative colitis, regional enteritis, or antibiotic-associated colitis; and in those with a history of atopic reactions.

Use cautiously in patients with asthma, impaired renal or hepatic function, or history of GI diseases or significant allergies.

Interactions

Drug-drug. *Acne preparations:* Topical clindamycin may cause a cumulative irritant or drying effect. Monitor patient carefully.
Diphenoxylate, opiates: May prolong or worsen clindamycin-induced diarrhea. Patient requires close monitoring.
Erythromycin: May block clindamycin from reaching its site of action. Avoid use together.
Kaolin: May reduce GI absorption of clindamycin. Separate administration times.
Neuromuscular blocking agents: May potentiate the neuromuscular blockade. Patient requires close monitoring.
Drug-food. *Diet foods with sodium cyclamate:* Decreased serum concentration of drug. Don't use together.

Effects on diagnostic tests

None reported.

Adverse reactions

GI: *nausea,* vomiting, abnormal liver function test results, abdominal pain, ***diarrhea, pseudomembranous colitis.***
GU: *cervicitis, vaginitis, Candida albicans* overgrowth, *vulvar irritation.*
Hematologic: ***transient leukopenia,*** eosinophilia, ***thrombocytopenia.***
Hepatic: jaundice.
Skin: maculopapular rash, urticaria, dryness, *redness,* pruritus, swelling, irritation, contact dermatitis, burning.
Other: ***anaphylaxis.***

Overdose and treatment

No information available.

Clinical considerations

- Take culture and sensitivity tests before treatment starts; repeat as needed.
- Don't refrigerate reconstituted oral solution because it will thicken. Drug remains stable for 2 weeks at room temperature.
- I.M. preparation should be given deep I.M. Rotate sites. Doses exceeding 600 mg aren't recommended.
- I.M. injection may increase creatine kinase levels because of muscle irritation.
- For I.V. infusion, dilute each 300 mg in 50 ml of D_5W, normal saline, or lactated Ringer's solution and give no faster than 30 mg/minute. Don't administer more than 1.2 g/hour.
- Topical form may produce adverse systemic effects.

Therapeutic monitoring

Monitor renal, hepatic, and hematopoietic functions during prolonged therapy.

Special populations

Breast-feeding patients. Drug is excreted in breast milk. Advise breast-feeding women to use alternative feeding method during clindamycin therapy.
Pediatric patients. Administer drug cautiously, if at all, to neonates and infants. Monitor closely, especially for diarrhea.
Geriatric patients. Geriatric patients may tolerate drug-induced diarrhea poorly. Monitor closely for change in bowel frequency and dehydration.

Patient counseling

- Warn patient that I.M. injection may be painful.
- Instruct patient to report adverse effects, especially diarrhea. Warn patient not to self-treat diarrhea.
- Advise patient to take capsules with 8 oz (240 ml) of water to prevent dysphagia.
- Instruct patient using topical solution to wash, rinse, and dry affected areas before application. Warn patient not to use topical solution near eyes, nose, mouth, or other mucous membranes, and caution about sharing washcloths and towels with family members.

clobetasol propionate

Dermovate*, Temovate

Pharmacologic classification: topical adrenocorticoid
Therapeutic classification: anti-inflammatory
Pregnancy risk category C

How supplied

Available by prescription only
Cream: 0.05%
Gel: 0.05%
Ointment: 0.05%
Solution: 0.05%

Indications and dosages

Inflammation of corticosteroid-responsive dermatoses
Adults: Apply a thin layer to affected skin areas b.i.d., once in the morning and once at night. Limit treatment to 14 days, with no more than 50 g of the cream or ointment or 50 ml of lotion (25 mg total) weekly.

Pharmacodynamics

Anti-inflammatory action: Drug is effective because of anti-inflammatory, antipruritic, and vasoconstrictive actions; however, the exact mechanism of its actions is unknown. Clobetasol is a high-potency group I fluorinated corticosteroid that's usually reserved for the management of severe dermatoses that haven't responded satisfactorily to a less potent formulation.

Pharmacokinetics

Absorption: Amount absorbed depends on the potency of the preparation, the amount applied, and the nature of the skin at the application site. It ranges from about 1% in areas with a thick stratum corneum (such as the palms, soles, elbows, and knees) to as high as 36% in areas with a thin stratum corneum (face, eyelids, and genitals). Absorption increases in areas of skin damage, inflammation, or occlusion. Some systemic absorption of topical steroids occurs, especially through the oral mucosa.
Distribution: After topical application, clobetasol is distributed throughout the local skin. Any drug absorbed into the circulation is rapidly removed from the blood and distributed into muscle, liver, skin, intestines, and kidneys.
Metabolism: After topical administration, drug is metabolized primarily in the skin. The small amount absorbed into systemic circulation is metabolized primarily in the liver to inactive compounds.
Excretion: Inactive metabolites are excreted by the kidneys, primarily as glucuronides and sulfates, but also as unconjugated products. Small amounts of the metabolites are also excreted in feces.

Route	Onset	Peak	Duration
Topical	Unknown	Unknown	Unknown

Contraindications and precautions

Contraindicated in patients hypersensitive to corticosteroids.

Interactions

None reported.

Effects on diagnostic tests

None reported.

Adverse reactions
Skin: burning, pruritus, irritation, dryness, erythema, folliculitis, perioral dermatitis, allergic contact dermatitis, hypopigmentation, hypertrichosis, acneiform eruptions.
Other: ***hypothalamic-pituitary-adrenal (HPA) axis suppression,*** Cushing's syndrome, hyperglycemia, glucosuria.

Overdose and treatment
No information available.

Clinical considerations
Consider the recommendations relevant to all topical adrenocorticoids as well as the following:
- Don't use occlusive dressings or bandages. Don't cover or wrap treated area unless instructed by doctor.
- Apply sparingly in light film.
- "Pulse" therapy is sometimes used with topical steroids of this potency, that is, b.i.d. for 3 days, then none for 3 days. Intermittent use prevents cumulative effects. Drug suppresses HPA axis at doses as low as 2 g/day.

Therapeutic monitoring
Discontinue drug and notify doctor if skin infection, striae, or atrophy occurs.

Special populations
Pregnant patients. There's possibility of teratogenic effects; avoid use in pregnancy.
Pediatric patients. Drug treatment isn't recommended in patients under age 12.

Patient counseling
- Inform patient of potential adverse reactions.
- Advise patient to avoid contact with eyes.
- Warn patient not to use drug for longer than 14 days.

clofibrate
Atromid-S

Pharmacologic classification: fibric acid derivative
Therapeutic classification: antilipemic
Pregnancy risk category C

How supplied
Available by prescription only
Capsules: 500 mg

Indications and dosages
Hyperlipidemia and xanthoma tuberosum; type III hyperlipidemia that doesn't respond adequately to diet
Adults: 2 g P.O. daily in two to four divided doses. Some patients may respond to lower doses as assessed by serum lipid monitoring.
◇***Diabetes insipidus***
Adults: 1.5 to 2 g P.O. daily in divided doses.
≡***Dosage adjustment.*** Decreased renal function may require reduced dosage frequency (q 12 to 18 hours).

Pharmacodynamics
Antilipemic action: Clofibrate may lower serum triglyceride levels by accelerating catabolism of very low-density lipoproteins; drug lowers serum cholesterol levels (to a lesser degree) by inhibiting cholesterol biosynthesis. Both mechanisms are unknown. Drug is closely related to gemfibrozil.

Pharmacokinetics
Absorption: Absorbed slowly but completely from GI tract. Serum triglyceride levels decrease in 2 to 5 days, with peak clinical effect at 21 days.
Distribution: Distributed into extracellular space as its active form, clofibric acid, which is up to 98% protein-bound. Animal studies suggest that fetal concentration levels may exceed maternal concentration levels.
Metabolism: Hydrolyzed by serum enzymes to clofibric acid, which is metabolized by the liver.
Excretion: 20% is excreted unchanged in urine; 70% is eliminated in urine as conjugated metabolite. Plasma half-life after a single dose ranges from 6 to 25 hours; in patients with renal impairment and cirrhosis, half-life can be as long as 113 hours.

Route	Onset	Peak	Duration
P.O.	Unknown	2-6 hr	Unknown

Contraindications and precautions
Contraindicated in patients with significant hepatic or renal dysfunction, primary biliary cirrhosis, or hypersensitivity to drug and in pregnant or breast-feeding women. Use cautiously in patients with peptic ulcer or history of gallbladder disease.

Interactions
Drug-drug. *Oral anticoagulants*: Clofibrate potentiates the effects; if such a combination is necessary, reduce oral anticoagulant dosage by 50%, and evaluate PT and INR frequently.
Cholestyramine: Concurrent use reduces absorption rate of clofibrate. Avoid use together.
Furosemide: Concurrent use may cause increased diuresis; use cautiously.
Sulfonylureas: Clofibrate may enhance the effects of sulfonylureas, causing hypoglycemia; a dosage adjustment may be needed.

Effects on diagnostic tests
None reported.

Adverse reactions
CNS: fatigue, weakness, drowsiness, dizziness, headache.
CV: ***arrhythmias,*** angina, ***thromboembolic events,*** intermittent claudication.
GI: *nausea, diarrhea, vomiting,* stomatitis, *dyspepsia,* flatulence, ***cholelithiasis, cholecystitis.***
GU: impotence and decreased libido, renal dysfunction (dysuria, hematuria, proteinuria, decreased urine output).
Hematologic: ***leukopenia,*** anemia, eosinophilia.
Hepatic: gallstones, *transient and reversible elevations of liver function test results,* hepatomegaly.
Musculoskeletal: myalgia and arthralgia.
Skin: rash, urticaria, pruritus, dry skin and hair.
Other: *weight gain; polyphagia.*

Overdose and treatment
No information available.

Clinical considerations
- Clofibrate shouldn't be used indiscriminately; it may pose an increased risk of gallstones, heart disease, and cancer.
- Clofibrate may increase risk of death from cancer, postcholecystectomy complications, and pancreatitis.

Therapeutic monitoring
- Monitor serum cholesterol and triglyceride levels regularly during clofibrate therapy.
- Observe patient for following serious adverse reactions: thrombophlebitis, pulmonary embolism, angina, and dysrhythmias; monitor renal and hepatic function, blood counts, and serum electrolyte and blood glucose levels.

Special populations
Breast-feeding patients. Clofibrate may enter breast milk; alternative feeding method is recommended during therapy.
Pediatric patients. Safety and efficacy haven't been established in children under age 14.

Patient counseling
- Warn patient to report flulike symptoms immediately.
- Stress importance of close medical supervision and of reporting adverse reactions; encourage compliance with prescribed regimen and diet.
- Warn patient not to exceed prescribed dose.
- Advise patient to take drug with food to minimize GI discomfort.
- Emphasize that drug therapy won't replace diet, exercise, and weight reduction for the control of hyperlipidemia.

clomiphene citrate
Clomid, Milophene, Serophene

Pharmacologic classification: chlorotrianisene derivative
Therapeutic classification: ovulation stimulant
Pregnancy risk category X

How supplied
Available by prescription only
Tablets: 50 mg

Indications and dosages
To induce ovulation
Adults: 50 mg P.O. daily for 5 days, starting any time in women who have had no recent uterine bleeding; or 50 mg P.O. daily starting on day 5 of menstrual cycle (first day of menstrual flow is day 1). Dose may be increased to 100 mg if ovulation doesn't occur. Repeat the 5-day course each ovulatory cycle until conception occurs or until 3 courses of therapy are completed.
◇***Male infertility***
Adults: 50 to 400 mg P.O. daily for 2 to 12 months.

Pharmacodynamics
Ovulation stimulant action: Mechanism of action for inducing ovulation in anovulatory females is unknown. Drug may stimulate release of pituitary gonadotropin, follicle-stimulating hormone (FSH), and luteinizing hormone (LH), which results in development and maturation of the ovarian follicle, ovulation, and subsequent development and function of corpus luteum.

Pharmacokinetics
Absorption: Absorbed readily from the GI tract.
Distribution: May undergo enterohepatic recirculation or may be stored in body fat.
Metabolism: Metabolized by the liver.
Excretion: Half-life is about 5 days. Drug is excreted principally in feces via biliary elimination.

Route	Onset	Peak	Duration
P.O.	Unknown	Unknown	Unknown

Contraindications and precautions
Contraindicated during pregnancy and in patients with undiagnosed abnormal genital bleeding, ovarian cyst not due to polycystic ovarian syndrome, hepatic disease or dysfunction, uncontrolled thyroid or adrenal dysfunction, or presence of organic intracranial lesion (such as a pituitary tumor).

Interactions
None reported.

Effects on diagnostic tests
None reported.

Adverse reactions
CNS: headache, restlessness, insomnia, dizziness, light-headedness, depression, fatigue, aggressive behavior.
EENT: blurred vision, diplopia, scotoma, photophobia.
GI: nausea, vomiting, bloating, distention, weight gain.
GU: urinary frequency and polyuria; abnormal uterine bleeding; *ovarian enlargement* and cyst formation, which regress spontaneously when drug is stopped.
Hematologic: ***thrombocytopenia, leukopenia,*** anemia.
Respiratory: pharyngitis, rhinitis, sinusitis, coughing, epistaxis, dyspnea.
Skin: alopecia, urticaria, rash, dermatitis.
Other: *hot flashes,* reversible *breast discomfort;* increased levels of serum thyronine, thyroxine-binding globulin, sex hormone-binding globulin, sulfobromophthalein retention and FSH and LH secretion.

Overdose and treatment
No information available.

Clinical considerations
- Advise patient to stop drug and notify doctor immediately if abdominal symptoms or pain occur; these may indicate ovarian enlargement or ovarian cyst. Also, immediately report visual disturbances.
- Human chorionic gonadotropin (5,000 to 10,000 U) may be administered 5 to 7 days after the last dose of drug to stimulate ovulation.

Therapeutic monitoring
Patient must be monitored closely because of risk of serious adverse effects.

Special populations
Pregnant patients. Contraindicated during pregnancy because of teratogenic possibilities. Advise patient to discontinue drug and contact her doctor if she suspects she's pregnant.

Patient counseling
- Advise patient of possibility of multiple births, which increases with higher doses.
- Patient should take basal body temperature every morning (starting on day 1 of menstrual period) and chart on a graph to detect ovulation.
- Instruct patient on importance of properly timed coitus.
- Warn patient to avoid hazardous tasks until response to drug is known because dizziness or visual disturbances may occur.

clomipramine hydrochloride
Anafranil

Pharmacologic classification: tricyclic antidepressant (TCA)
Therapeutic classification: antiobsessional
Pregnancy risk category C

How supplied
Available by prescription only
Capsules: 25 mg, 50 mg, 75 mg

Indications and dosages
Treatment of obsessive-compulsive disorder (OCD)
Adults: Initially, 25 mg P.O. daily, gradually increasing to 100 mg P.O. daily (in divided doses, with meals) during the first 2 weeks. Maximum dosage, 250 mg daily. After titration, entire daily dose may be given h.s.
Children and adolescents: Initially, 25 mg P.O. daily, gradually increased to a maximum of 3 mg/kg or 100 mg P.O. daily, whichever is smaller (in divided doses, with meals) over the first 2 weeks. Maximum daily dose is 3 mg/kg or 200 mg, whichever is smaller. After titration, entire daily dose may be given h.s.

Pharmacodynamics
Antiobsessional action: A selective inhibitor of serotonin (5-HT) reuptake into neurons within the CNS. It may also have some blocking activity at postsynaptic dopamine receptors. The exact mechanism by which clomipramine treats OCD is unknown.

Pharmacokinetics
Absorption: Well absorbed from GI tract, but extensive first-pass metabolism limits bioavailablity to about 50%.
Distribution: Distributed well into lipophilic tissues; the volume of distribution is about 12 L/kg; 98% is bound to plasma proteins.
Metabolism: Metabolism is primarily hepatic. Several metabolites have been identified; desmethylclomipramine is the primary active metabolite.
Excretion: About 66% is excreted in the urine and the remainder in the feces. Mean elimination half-life of the parent compound is about 36 hours; the elimination half-life of desmethylclomipramine has a mean of 69 hours. After multiple dosing, the half-life may increase.

Route	Onset	Peak	Duration
P.O.	≥ 2 wk	2-6 hr	Unknown

Contraindications and precautions
Contraindicated in patients with hypersensitivity to drug or other TCAs; in those who have taken MAO inhibitors within the previous 14

days; and in patients during acute recovery period after MI.

Use cautiously in patients with urine retention, suicidal tendencies, glaucoma, increased intraocular pressure, brain damage, or seizure disorders and in those taking medications that may lower the seizure threshold. Also use cautiously in patients with impaired renal or hepatic function, hyperthyroidism, or tumors of the adrenal medulla and in those undergoing elective surgery or receiving thyroid medication or electroconvulsive treatment.

Interactions

Drug-drug. *MAO inhibitors:* May cause hyperpyretic crisis, seizures, coma, and death. Don't use together.
Barbiturates: Decrease TCA blood levels. Monitor patient for decreased effectiveness.
Barbiturates, CNS depressants: May cause an exaggerated depressant effect when used concomitantly with TCAs. Avoid use together.
Methylphenidate: May increase TCA blood levels. Patient needs close monitoring.
Epinephrine, norepinephrine: May produce an increased hypertensive effect in patients taking TCAs. Avoid use together.
Drug-lifestyle. *Alcohol use:* Exaggerated depressant effect when used with TCAs. Discourage use together.
Smoking: Lower levels of clomipramine have been noted. Advise patient to avoid smoking.
Sun exposure: Increased risk of photosensitivity. Advise patient to take precautions.

Effects on diagnostic tests

None reported.

Adverse reactions

CNS: *somnolence, tremor, dizziness, headache, insomnia, nervousness, myoclonus, fatigue,* EEG changes, ***seizures.***
CV: postural hypotension, palpitations, tachycardia.
EENT: *pharyngitis, rhinitis, visual changes.*
GI: *dry mouth, constipation, nausea, dyspepsia, increased appetite,* diarrhea, *anorexia, abdominal pain.*
GU: *urinary hesitancy,* urinary tract infection, *dysmenorrhea, ejaculation failure, impotence.*
Hematologic: purpura, anemia.
Skin: *diaphoresis,* rash, pruritus, dry skin.
Other: *myalgia, weight gain, altered libido.*

Overdose and treatment

Signs and symptoms of clomipramine overdose are similar to those of other TCAs and have included sinus tachycardia, intraventricular block, hypotension, irritability, fixed and dilated pupils, drowsiness, delirium, stupor, hyperreflexia, and hyperpyrexia.

Treatment should include gastric lavage with large quantities of fluid. Continue lavage for 12 hours because the anticholinergic effects of the drug slow gastric emptying. Hemodialysis, peritoneal dialysis, and forced diuresis are ineffective because of the high degree of plasma protein binding. Support respirations and monitor cardiac function. Treat shock with plasma expanders or corticosteroids; treat seizures with diazepam.

Clinical considerations

□ ***ALERT*** To minimize risk of overdose, dispense drug in small quantities.
- Don't withdraw drug abruptly.
- Activation of mania or hypomania may occur with clomipramine therapy.

Therapeutic monitoring

Patient needs observation for urinary retention and constipation. Suggest stool softener or high-fiber diet, as needed, and encourage adequate fluid intake.

Special populations

Breast-feeding patients. It isn't known if drug is excreted in breast milk. Use with caution in breast-feeding women.

Patient counseling

- Warn patient to avoid hazardous activities that require alertness or good psychomotor coordination until adverse CNS effects are known. This is especially important during initial titration period when daytime sedation and dizziness may occur.
- Suggest that dry mouth may be relieved with saliva substitutes or sugarless candy or gum.
- Tell patient adverse GI effects can be minimized by taking drug with meals during the titration period. Later, the entire daily dose may be taken at bedtime to limit daytime drowsiness.
- Inform patient to avoid using OTC medications, particularly antihistamines and decongestants, unless recommended by doctor or pharmacist.
- Encourage patient to continue therapy, even if adverse reactions are troublesome. Advise patient not to stop taking it without notifying caregiver.

clonazepam

Klonopin, Rivotril*

Pharmacologic classification: benzodiazepine
Therapeutic classification: anticonvulsant
Controlled substance schedule IV
Pregnancy risk category C

How supplied

Available by prescription only
Tablets: 0.5 mg, 1 mg, 2 mg

Indications and dosages

Absence and atypical absence seizures; akinetic and myoclonic seizures; ◇generalized tonic-clonic seizures

Adults: Initial dosage shouldn't exceed 1.5 mg P.O. daily, divided into three doses. May be increased by 0.5 to 1 mg q 3 days until seizures are controlled. Maximum recommended daily dose, 20 mg.

Children up to age 10 or weighing 66 lb (30 kg) or less: 0.01 to 0.03 mg/kg P.O. daily (not to exceed 0.05 mg/kg daily), divided q 8 hours. Increase dosage by 0.25 to 0.5 mg q third day to a maximum maintenance dosage of 0.1 to 0.2 mg/kg daily.

◇Leg movements during sleep; ◇adjunct treatment in schizophrenia

Adults: 0.5 to 2 mg P.O. h.s.

◇Parkinsonian dysarthria

Adults: 0.25 to 0.5 mg P.O. daily.

◇Acute manic episodes

Adults: 0.75 to 16 mg P.O. daily.

◇Multifocal tic disorders

Adults: 1.5 to 12 mg P.O. daily.

◇Neuralgia

Adults: 2 to 4 mg P.O. daily.

Pharmacodynamics

Anticonvulsant action: Mechanism of anticonvulsant activity is unknown; drug appears to act in the limbic system, thalamus, and hypothalamus. Drug is used to treat myoclonic, atonic, and absence seizures resistant to other anticonvulsants and to suppress or eliminate attacks of sleep-related nocturnal myoclonus (restless legs syndrome).

Pharmacokinetics

Absorption: Well absorbed from the GI tract.
Distribution: Distributed widely throughout the body; about 85% protein-bound.
Metabolism: Metabolized by the liver to several metabolites. The half-life of drug is 18 to 39 hours.
Excretion: Excreted in urine.

Route	Onset	Peak	Duration
P.O.	20-60 min	1-2 hr	6-12 hr

Contraindications and precautions

Contraindicated in patients with significant hepatic disease; in those with sensitivity to benzodiazepines; and in patients with acute angle-closure glaucoma. Use cautiously in children and in patients with mixed-type seizures, respiratory disease, or glaucoma.

Interactions

Drug-drug. *CNS depressants, anticonvulsants:* Additive CNS depressant effects. Avoid use together.
Valproic acid: May induce absence seizures. Don't use together.
Ritonavir: May significantly increase levels of clonazepam. Patient requires close monitoring.
Drug-lifestyle. *Alcohol use:* Additive CNS depressant effects. Don't use together.

Effects on diagnostic tests

None reported.

Adverse reactions

CNS: *drowsiness, ataxia, behavioral disturbances* (especially in children), slurred speech, tremor, confusion, psychosis, agitation.
CV: palpitations.
EENT: nystagmus, abnormal eye movements, sore gums.
GI: constipation, gastritis, change in appetite, nausea, anorexia, increased liver function tests, diarrhea.
GU: dysuria, enuresis, nocturia, urine retention.
Hematologic: ***leukopenia, thrombocytopenia,*** eosinophilia.
Respiratory: ***respiratory depression,*** chest congestion, shortness of breath.
Skin: rash.

Overdose and treatment

Symptoms of overdose may include ataxia, confusion, coma, decreased reflexes, and hypotension. Treat overdose with gastric lavage and supportive therapy. Flumazenil, a specific benzodiazepine antagonist, may be useful. Vasopressors should be used to treat hypotension. Carefully monitor vital signs, ECG, and fluid and electrolyte balance. Clonazepam isn't dialyzable.

Clinical considerations

- Abrupt withdrawal may precipitate status epilepticus; after long-term use, lower dosage gradually.
- Monitor for oversedation, especially in geriatric patients.

Therapeutic monitoring

Monitor CBC and liver function tests periodically.

Special populations

Breast-feeding patients. Alternative feeding method is recommended during clonazepam therapy.
Pediatric patients. Long-term safety in children hasn't been established.
Geriatric patients. Geriatric patients may require lower doses because of diminished renal function; such patients also are at greater risk for oversedation from CNS depressants.

Patient counseling

- Explain rationale for therapy and risks and benefits that may be anticipated.

- Teach patient signs and symptoms of adverse reactions and need to report them promptly.
- Warn patient not to discontinue drug or change dosage unless prescribed.
- Advise patient to avoid tasks that require mental alertness until degree of sedative effect is determined.

clonidine hydrochloride

Catapres, Catapres-TTS, Dixarit*

Pharmacologic classification: centrally acting alpha-adrenergic agonist
Therapeutic classification: antihypertensive
Pregnancy risk category C

How supplied

Available by prescription only
Tablets: 0.1 mg, 0.2 mg, 0.3 mg
Transdermal: TTS-1 (releases 0.1 mg/24 hours); TTS-2 (releases 0.2 mg/24 hours); TTS-3 (releases 0.3 mg/24 hours)

Indications and dosages

Hypertension
Adults: Initially, 0.1 mg P.O. b.i.d.; then increased by 0.1 to 0.2 mg daily or every few days until desired response is achieved. Usual dose range is 0.2 to 0.6 mg daily in divided doses. Maximum effective dose is 2.4 mg/day. If transdermal patch is used, apply to area of hairless intact skin once q 7 days.
Children: No dosing recommendations for children.
◇***Adjunctive therapy in nicotine withdrawal***
Adults: Initially, 0.15 mg P.O. daily, gradually increased to 0.4 mg P.O. daily as tolerated. Alternatively, apply transdermal patch (0.2 mg/24 hours) and replace weekly for the first 2 or 3 weeks after smoking cessation.
◇***Prophylaxis for vascular headache***
Adults: 0.025 mg P.O. b.i.d. to q.i.d. up to 0.15 mg P.O. daily in divided doses.
◇***Adjunctive treatment of menopausal symptoms***
Adults: 0.025 to 0.075 mg P.O. b.i.d.
◇***Adjunctive therapy in opiate withdrawal***
Adults: 5 to 17 mcg/kg P.O. daily in divided doses for up to 10 days. Adjust dosage to avoid hypotension and excessive sedation, and slowly withdraw drug.
◇***Ulcerative colitis***
Adults: 0.3 mg P.O. t.i.d.
◇***Neuralgia***
Adults: 0.2 mg P.O. daily.
◇***Tourette syndrome***
Adults: 0.15 to 0.2 mg P.O. daily.
◇***Diabetic diarrhea***
Adults: 0.15 to 1.2 mg/day P.O. or 1 to 2 patches/week (0.3 mg/24 hours).
◇***Growth delay in children***
Children: 0.0375 to 0.15 mg/m^2 P.O. daily.
◇***To diagnose pheochromocytoma***
Adults: 0.3 mg given once.

Pharmacodynamics

Antihypertensive action: Clonidine decreases peripheral vascular resistance by stimulating central alpha-adrenergic receptors, thus decreasing cerebral sympathetic outflow; drug may also inhibit renin release. Initially, clonidine may stimulate peripheral alpha-adrenergic receptors, producing transient vasoconstriction.

Pharmacokinetics

Absorption: Absorbed well from the GI tract when administered orally; absorbed well percutaneously after transdermal topical administration.
Distribution: Distributed widely into the body.
Metabolism: Metabolized in the liver, where nearly 50% is transformed to inactive metabolites.
Excretion: About 65% of a given dose is excreted in urine; 20% is excreted in feces. Half-life of clonidine ranges from 6 to 20 hours in patients with normal renal function. After oral administration, the antihypertensive effect lasts up to 8 hours; after transdermal application, the antihypertensive effect persists for up to 7 days.

Route	Onset	Peak	Duration
P.O.	½-1 hr	2-4 hr	12-24 hr
Transdermal	2-3 days	2-3 days	7-8 days

Contraindications and precautions

Contraindicated in patients with hypersensitivity to drug. Transdermal form is contraindicated in patients with hypersensitivity to any component of the adhesive layer of the transdermal system. Use cautiously in patients with severe coronary disease, recent MI, cerebrovascular disease, and impaired hepatic or renal function.

Interactions

Drug-drug. *Barbiturates:* Clonidine may increase CNS depressant effects. Avoid using together.
Tricyclic antidepressants, MAO inhibitors, tolazoline: May inhibit the antihypertensive effects of clonidine. Avoid use together.
Propranolol or other beta blockers: May have an additive effect, producing bradycardia. Avoid use together.
Drug-herb. *Capsicum:* May reduce antihypertensive effectiveness. Avoid use together.
Drug-lifestyle. *Alcohol use:* Increases CNS depressant effects. Discourage alcohol use.

Effects on diagnostic tests
Clonidine may decrease urinary excretion of vanillylmandelic acid and catecholamines; and may cause a weakly positive Coombs' test.

Adverse reactions
CNS: *drowsiness, dizziness,* fatigue, *sedation, weakness,* malaise, agitation, depression.
CV: orthostatic hypotension, bradycardia, *severe rebound hypertension.*
GI: *constipation, dry mouth,* nausea, vomiting, anorexia.
GU: urine retention, impotence, loss of libido.
Metabolic: possible slight increase in serum glucose levels.
Skin: *pruritus, dermatitis* (with transdermal patch), rash.
Other: weight gain.

Overdose and treatment
Clinical signs of overdose include bradycardia, CNS depression, respiratory depression, hypothermia, apnea, seizures, lethargy, agitation, irritability, diarrhea, and hypotension; hypertension has also been reported.

After overdose with oral clonidine, don't induce emesis because rapid onset of CNS depression can lead to aspiration. After adequate airway is assured, empty stomach by gastric lavage followed by administration of activated charcoal. If overdose occurs in patients receiving transdermal therapy, remove transdermal patch. Further treatment is usually symptomatic and supportive.

Clinical considerations
□ ***ALERT*** Remove transdermal systems when attempting defibrillation or synchronized cardioversion because of electrical conductivity.
- Clonidine may be used to lower blood pressure quickly in some hypertensive emergencies.
- Don't discontinue abruptly; reduce dosage gradually over 2 to 4 days to prevent severe rebound hypertension.
- Patients with renal impairment may respond to smaller doses of drug.
- Give drug 4 to 6 hours before scheduled surgery.
- Patient may need oral antihypertensive therapy during the initiation of transdermal therapy.

Therapeutic monitoring
- Nursing staff should monitor pulse and blood pressure frequently; dosage is usually adjusted to patient's response and tolerance.
- Daily weight must be recorded during initiation of therapy to monitor fluid retention.

Special populations
Breast-feeding patients. Clonidine is distributed into breast milk. An alternate feeding method is recommended during treatment.
Pediatric patients. Efficacy and safety in children haven't been established; use drug only if potential benefit outweighs risk.
Geriatric patients. Geriatric patients may require lower doses because they may be more sensitive to the hypotensive effects of clonidine. Monitor renal function closely.

Patient counseling
- Explain disease and rationale for therapy; emphasize importance of follow-up visits in establishing therapeutic regimen.
- Teach patient signs and symptoms of adverse effects and need to report them; patient should also report excessive weight gain (more than 5 lb [2.27 kg] weekly).
- Warn patient to avoid hazardous activities that require mental alertness until tolerance develops to CNS effects.
- Advise patient to avoid sudden position changes to minimize orthostatic hypotension.
- Inform patient that ice chips, hard candy, or gum will relieve dry mouth.
- Warn patient to call for specific instructions before taking OTC cold preparations.
- Advise taking last dose at bedtime to ensure night-time blood pressure control.
- Tell patient not to discontinue drug suddenly; rebound hypertension may develop.
- Teach patient to rotate transdermal patch site weekly.

clopidogrel bisulfate
Plavix

Pharmacologic classification: inhibitor of ADP-induced platelet aggregation
Therapeutic classification: antiplatelet agent
Pregnancy risk category B

How supplied
Available by prescription only
Tablets: 75 mg

Indications and dosages
To reduce atherosclerotic events (MI, CVA, vascular death) in patients with atherosclerosis documented by recent CVA, MI, or peripheral arterial disease
Adults: 75 mg P.O. once daily with or without food.

Pharmacodynamics
Antiplatelet action: Inhibits the binding of adenosine diphosphate (ADP) to its platelet receptor and the subsequent ADP-mediated activation of glycoprotein IIb/IIIa complex, thereby inhibiting platelet aggregation. Because clopidogrel acts by irreversibly modifying the platelet ADP receptor, platelets exposed to the drug are affected for their life span.

Pharmacokinetics

Absorption: After repeated oral doses, plasma levels of parent compound, which has no platelet-inhibiting effect, are very low and generally below quantification limit. Pharmacokinetic evaluations are generally stated in terms of the main circulating metabolite. Rapidly absorbed after oral dosing. Following oral administration, about 50% of dose is absorbed.
Distribution: Clopidogrel and main circulating metabolite binds reversibly to human plasma proteins (98% and 94%, respectively).
Metabolism: Extensively metabolized by the liver. Main circulating metabolite is the carboxylic acid derivative that has no effect on platelet aggregation. It represents about 85% of circulating drug. Elimination half-life of main circulating metabolite is 8 hours after single and repeated doses.
Excretion: Following oral administration, about 50% is excreted in the urine and 46% in feces.

Route	Onset	Peak	Duration
P.O.	2 hr	Unknown	5 days

Contraindications and precautions

Contraindicated in patients with pathologic bleeding, such as peptic ulcer or intracranial hemorrhage, and in those with known hypersensitivity to drug or its components.

Use with caution in patients at risk for increased bleeding from trauma, surgery, or other pathologic conditions and in those with hepatic impairment or severe hepatic disease.

Interactions

Drug-drug. *Aspirin, NSAIDs:* May increase risk for GI bleeding; Use together cautiously. *Heparin, warfarin:* Safety hasn't been established. Use together cautiously.
Drug-herb. *Red clover:* May cause increased bleeding if taken with drug. Use together cautiously.

Effects on diagnostic tests

None reported.

Adverse reactions

CNS: asthenia, depression, dizziness, fatigue, headache, paresthesia, syncope.
CV: chest pain, edema, hypertension, palpitation.
EENT: epistaxis, rhinitis.
GI: abdominal pain, constipation, diarrhea, dyspepsia, gastritis, hemorrhage, nausea, vomiting.
GU: urinary tract infection.
Hematologic: purpura.
Respiratory: bronchitis, coughing, dyspnea, upper respiratory infection.
Skin: rash, pruritus.
Other: arthralgia, flu symptoms, pain.

Overdose and treatment

No adverse effects were reported after single oral administration of 600 mg (equivalent to eight standard 75-mg tablets). The bleeding time was prolonged by a factor of 1.7, which is similar to that observed with the therapeutic dosage of 75 mg daily.

Based on biological plausibility, platelet transfusion may be appropriate to reverse the pharmacologic effects of clopidogrel if quick reversal is required.

Clinical considerations

- Drug is usually used in patients who are hypersensitive or intolerant to aspirin.
- If patient is to undergo surgery and an antiplatelet effect isn't desired, drug should be stopped 7 days before surgery.

Therapeutic monitoring

Instruct patient to report unusual bleeding or bruising.

Special populations

Breast-feeding patients. It isn't known if drug or its metabolites are distributed in breast milk. Assess risks and benefits before continuing drug in breast-feeding women.
Pediatric patients. Safety and efficacy in children haven't been established.

Patient counseling

- Inform patient it may take longer than usual to stop bleeding; therefore, advise him to refrain from activities in which trauma and bleeding may occur. Encourage use of seat belts.
- Tell patient to inform doctor or dentist of clopidogrel use before scheduling surgery or taking new drugs.
- Inform patient that drug may be taken without regard to meals.

clorazepate dipotassium

Novo-Clopate*, Tranxene*, Tranxene-SD, Tranxene-SD Half Strength

Pharmacologic classification: benzodiazepine
Therapeutic classification: antianxiety agent, anticonvulsant, sedative-hypnotic
Controlled substance schedule IV
Pregnancy risk category NR

How supplied

Available by prescription only
Tablets: 3.75 mg, 7.5 mg, 11.25 mg, 15 mg, 22.5 mg
Capsules: 3.75 mg, 7.5 mg, 15 mg

Indications and dosages

Acute alcohol withdrawal
Adults: Day 1—initially, 30 mg P.O., followed by 30 to 60 mg P.O. in divided doses; day 2—

45 to 90 mg P.O. in divided doses; day 3—22.5 to 45 mg P.O. in divided doses; day 4—15 to 30 mg P.O. in divided doses; gradually reduce daily dose to 7.5 to 15 mg.

Anxiety

Adults: 15 to 60 mg P.O. daily.

As an adjunct in treatment of partial seizures

Adults and children over age 12: Maximum recommended initial dose is 7.5 mg P.O. t.i.d. Dosage increases shouldn't exceed 7.5 mg/week. Maximum daily dose shouldn't exceed 90 mg.

Children age 9 to 12: Maximum recommended initial dose is 7.5 mg P.O. b.i.d. Dosage increases shouldn't exceed 7.5 mg/week. Maximum daily dose shouldn't exceed 60 mg.

Pharmacodynamics

Anxiolytic and sedative actions: Clorazepate depresses the CNS at the limbic and subcortical levels of the brain. It produces an antianxiety effect by enhancing the effect of the neurotransmitter gamma-aminobutyric acid (GABA) on its receptor in the ascending reticular activating system, which increases inhibition and blocks both cortical and limbic arousal.

Anticonvulsant action: Drug suppresses spread of seizure activity produced by epileptogenic foci in the cortex, thalamus, and limbic structures by enhancing presynaptic inhibition.

Pharmacokinetics

Absorption: After oral administration, clorazepate is hydrolyzed in the stomach to desmethyldiazepam, which is absorbed completely and rapidly.

Distribution: Distributed widely throughout the body. About 80% to 95% of an administered dose is bound to plasma protein.

Metabolism: Metabolized in the liver to conjugated oxazepam.

Excretion: Inactive glucuronide metabolites are excreted in urine. The half-life of desmethyldiazepam ranges from 30 to 100 hours.

Route	Onset	Peak	Duration
P.O.	Unknown	½-2 hr	Unknown

Contraindications and precautions

Contraindicated in patients with hypersensitivity to drug or other benzodiazepines and acute angle-closure glaucoma. Avoid use in pregnant patients, especially during the first trimester.

Use cautiously in patients with impaired renal or hepatic function, suicidal tendencies, or history of drug abuse.

Interactions

Drug-drug. *Phenothiazines, narcotics, barbiturates, antihistamines, MAO inhibitors, general anesthetics, antidepressants:* Potentiate the CNS depressant effects. Avoid use together.

Cimetidine, disulfiram: Increase plasma concentration. Avoid use together.

Haloperidol: Reduces serum levels. Patient requires close monitoring.

Levodopa: Decreases therapeutic effectiveness. Avoid use together.

Drug-lifestyle. *Alcohol use:* Potentiates CNS depressant effects. Discourage alcohol use.

Heavy smoking: Accelerates clorazepate's metabolism, thus lowering clinical effectiveness. Discourage smoking.

Effects on diagnostic tests

None reported.

Adverse reactions

CNS: *drowsiness,* dizziness, nervousness, confusion, headache, insomnia, depression, irritability, tremor.

CV: hypotension, minor changes in EEG patterns.

EENT: blurred vision, diplopia.

GI: nausea, vomiting, abdominal discomfort, dry mouth, elevated liver function test.

GU: urine retention, incontinence.

Skin: rash.

Overdose and treatment

Signs and symptoms of overdose include somnolence, confusion, coma, hypoactive reflexes, dyspnea, labored breathing, hypotension, bradycardia, slurred speech, and unsteady gait or impaired coordination.

Support blood pressure and respiration until drug effects subside; monitor vital signs. Flumazenil, a specific benzodiazepine antagonist, may be useful. Mechanical ventilatory assistance via endotracheal tube may be required to maintain a patent airway and support adequate oxygenation. Treat hypotension with I.V. fluids and vasopressors such as dopamine and phenylephrine, as needed. Induce emesis if patient is conscious. Use gastric lavage if ingestion was recent, but only if an endotracheal tube is present to prevent aspiration. After emesis or lavage, administer activated charcoal with a cathartic as a single dose. Dialysis is of limited value. Don't use barbiturates because they may worsen CNS adverse effects.

Clinical considerations

Consider the recommendations relevant to all benzodiazepines as well as the following:

- Lower doses are effective in geriatric patients and patients with renal or hepatic dysfunction.
- Store in a cool, dry place away from direct light.

Therapeutic monitoring

Monitor liver, renal, and hematopoietic function studies periodically in patients receiving repeated or prolonged therapy.

Special populations

Breast-feeding patients. The breast-fed infant of a woman who uses clorazepate may become sedated, have feeding difficulties, or lose weight. Avoid use in breast-feeding women.

Pediatric patients. Safety hasn't been established in children under age 9.

Geriatric patients. Lower doses are usually effective in geriatric patients because of decreased elimination. Use with caution. Geriatric patients who receive this drug require supervision with ambulation and activities of daily living during initiation of therapy or after an increase in dose.

Patient counseling

- Advise patient of potential for physical and psychological dependence with chronic use of clorazepate.
- Instruct patient not to alter drug regimen without medical approval.
- Warn patient that sudden position changes may cause dizziness. Advise patient to dangle legs for a few minutes before getting out of bed to prevent falls and injury.
- Advise patient to take antacids 1 hour before or after clorazepate.
- Inform patient not to suddenly stop taking drug.

clotrimazole

FemCare, Gyne-Lotrimin, Lotrimin, Lotrimin AF, Mycelex, Mycelex-G, Mycelex OTC, Mycelex-7

Pharmacologic classification: synthetic imidazole derivative
Therapeutic classification: topical antifungal
Pregnancy risk category B (C, oral form)

How supplied

Available by prescription only
Vaginal tablets: 100 mg, 200 mg, 500 mg
Topical cream: 1%
Topical lotion: 1%
Topical solution: 1%
Oral lozenges: 10 mg
Available without a prescription
Vaginal tablets: 100 mg
Vaginal cream: 1%
Combination pack: Vaginal tablets 500 mg/topical cream 1% 7 g

Indications and dosages

Tinea pedis, tinea cruris, tinea versicolor, tinea corporis, cutaneous candidiasis
Adults and children: Apply thinly and massage into cleansed affected and surrounding area, morning and evening, for prescribed period (usually 1 to 4 weeks; however, therapy may take up to 8 weeks).

Vulvovaginal candidiasis
Adults: Insert one tablet intravaginally h.s. for 7 consecutive days. If vaginal cream is used, insert one applicatorful intravaginally, h.s. for 7 to 14 consecutive days.

Treatment of oropharyngeal candidiasis
Adults and children: Usual dosage is one lozenge P.O. five times daily for 14 consecutive days.

Prophylaxis of oropharyngeal candidiasis in immunocompromised patients
Adults: 1 lozenge t.i.d. for duration of chemotherapy.

◇***Keratitis***
Adults: 1% ointment in sterile peanut oil q 2 to 4 hours for up to 6 weeks.

Pharmacodynamics

Antifungal action: Clotrimazole alters cell membrane permeability by binding with phospholipids in the fungal cell membrane. Clotrimazole inhibits or kills many fungi, including yeast and dermatophytes, and also is active against various species of gram-positive bacteria.

Pharmacokinetics

Absorption: Absorption is limited with topical administration. Absorption following dissolution of a lozenge in the mouth not determined.
Distribution: Distributed minimally with local application.
Metabolism: Unknown.
Excretion: Unknown.

Route	Onset	Peak	Duration
P.O.	Unknown	Unknown	3 hr
Topical, intravaginal	Unknown	Unknown	Unknown

Contraindications and precautions

Contraindicated in patients hypersensitive to drug. Also contraindicated for ophthalmic use.

Interactions

None reported.

Effects on diagnostic tests

None reported.

Adverse reactions

GI: nausea, vomiting, unpleasant mouth sensation (with lozenges); lower abdominal cramps, abnormal liver function test.
GU: *mild vaginal burning or irritation* (with vaginal use), cramping, urinary frequency.
Skin: blistering, *erythema,* edema, pruritus, burning, stinging, peeling, urticaria, skin fissures, general irritation.

Overdose and treatment

Discontinue therapy.

Clinical considerations
Improvement is usually demonstrated within 1 week; if no improvement occurs in 4 weeks, review diagnosis.

Therapeutic monitoring
Patients given clotrimazole oral lozenges, especially those who have preexisting liver dysfunction, should have periodic liver function tests.

Special populations
Pregnant patients. Use lozenges only when potential benefits outweigh the risks.
Breast-feeding patients. It's unknown if drug is excreted in breast milk. Use drug with caution in breast-feeding women.
Pediatric patients. Drug isn't recommended for use in children under age 3.

Patient counseling
- Advise patient that lozenges must dissolve slowly (15 to 30 minutes) in the mouth to achieve maximum effect. Tell patient not to chew lozenges.
- Instruct patients using intravaginal application to insert drug high into the vagina and to refrain from sexual contact during treatment period to avoid reinfection. Also tell patient to use a sanitary napkin to prevent staining of clothing and to absorb discharge.
- Tell patient to complete the full course of therapy. Improvement usually will be noted within 1 week. Patient should call if no improvement occurs in 4 weeks or if condition worsens.
- Advise patient to watch for and report irritation or sensitivity and, if this occurs, to discontinue use.

cloxacillin sodium
Tegopen

Pharmacologic classification: penicillinase-resistant penicillin
Therapeutic classification: antibiotic
Pregnancy risk category B

How supplied
Available by prescription only
Capsules: 250 mg, 500 mg
Oral solution: 125 mg/5 ml (after reconstitution)

Indications and dosages
Systemic infections caused by penicillinase-producing staphylococci organisms
Adults: 250 to 500 mg P.O. q 6 hours.
Children: 50 to 100 mg/kg P.O. daily, divided into doses given q 6 hours.

Pharmacodynamics
Antibiotic action: Cloxacillin is bactericidal; it adheres to bacterial penicillin-binding proteins, thereby inhibiting bacterial cell-wall synthesis.

Cloxacillin resists the effects of penicillinases—enzymes that inactivate penicillin—and therefore is active against many strains of penicillinase-producing bacteria; this activity is most pronounced against penicillinase-producing staphylococci; some strains may remain resistant. Cloxacillin is also active against gram-positive aerobic and anaerobic bacilli but has no significant effect on gram-negative bacilli.

Pharmacokinetics
Absorption: Absorbed rapidly but incompletely (37% to 60%) from the GI tract; it's relatively acid stable. Food may decrease both rate and extent of absorption.
Distribution: Distributed widely. CSF penetration is poor but enhanced in meningeal inflammation. Cloxacillin crosses the placenta, and is 90% to 96% protein-bound.
Metabolism: Only partially metabolized.
Excretion: Excreted in urine by renal tubular secretion and glomerular filtration; also excreted in breast milk. Elimination half-life in adults is ½ to 1 hour, extended minimally to 2½ hours in patients with renal impairment.

Route	Onset	Peak	Duration
P.O.	Unknown	2 hr	6 hr

Contraindications and precautions
Contraindicated in patients with hypersensitivity to drug or other penicillins.

Interactions
Drug-drug. *Aminoglycosides:* Produce synergistic bactericidal effects against *Staphylococcus aureus.* However, the drugs are physically and chemically incompatible and are inactivated when mixed or given together.
Probenecid: Increases serum levels of cloxacillin. Probenecid may be used for this purpose.
Drug-food. *Foods:* Decrease drug absorption. Advise taking drug on an empty stomach.
Fruit juices and carbonated beverages: May inactivate drug. Don't give together.

Effects on diagnostic tests
Cloxacillin alters test results for urine and serum proteins; it produces false-positive or elevated results in turbidimetric urine and serum protein tests using sulfosalicylic acid or trichloroacetic acid; it also reportedly produces false results on the Bradshaw screening test for Bence Jones protein.

Cloxacillin may falsely decrease serum aminoglycoside levels.

Adverse reactions
CNS: lethargy, hallucinations, ***seizures,*** anxiety, confusion, agitation, depression, dizziness, fatigue.
GI: *nausea,* vomiting, *epigastric distress, diarrhea,* enterocolitis, pseudomembranous colitis, black "hairy" tongue, transient elevations in liver function study results, abdominal pain.
GU: interstitial nephritis, nephropathy.
Hematologic: eosinophilia, anemia, ***thrombocytopenia, leukopenia,*** hemolytic anemia, ***agranulocytosis.***
Hepatic: intrahepatic cholestasis.
Other: hypersensitivity reactions (rash, urticaria, chills, fever, sneezing, wheezing, ***anaphylaxis***), overgrowth of nonsusceptible organisms.

Overdose and treatment
Signs of overdose include neuromuscular irritability or seizures. No specific recommendation is available. Treatment is symptomatic. After recent ingestion (within 4 hours), empty the stomach by induced emesis or gastric lavage; follow with activated charcoal to reduce absorption. Cloxacillin isn't appreciably removed by hemodialysis or peritoneal dialysis.

Clinical considerations
Consider the recommendations relevant to all penicillins as well as the following:
- Give dose on empty stomach with water only.
- Refrigerate oral suspension and discard any unused medication after 14 days. Unrefrigerated suspension is stable for 3 days.

Therapeutic monitoring
Periodically assess renal, hepatic, and hematopoietic function in patients receiving long-term therapy.

Special populations
Breast-feeding patients. Drug is excreted in breast milk; use cautiously in breast-feeding women.
Pediatric patients. Elimination of cloxacillin is reduced in neonates; safety of drug in neonates hasn't been established.

Patient counseling
- Inform patient of potential adverse reactions (such as fever, chills, or rash); advise him to report adverse reactions promptly.
- Instruct patient to take drug on an empty stomach and take with water only.
- Tell patient to refrigerate oral suspension and to discard any unused suspension after the course of treatment.

clozapine
Clozaril

Pharmacologic classification: tricyclic dibenzodiazepine derivative
Therapeutic classification: antipsychotic
Pregnancy risk category B

How supplied
Available by prescription only
Tablets: 25 mg, 100 mg

Indications and dosages
Treatment of schizophrenia in severely ill patients unresponsive to other therapies
Adults: Initially, 12.5 mg P.O. once or twice daily, adjusted upward at 25 to 50 mg daily (if tolerated) to a daily dose of 300 to 450 mg by end of 2 weeks. Individual dosage is based on clinical response, patient tolerance, and adverse reactions. Subsequent increases of dosage should occur no more than once or twice weekly and shouldn't exceed 100 mg. Many patients respond to doses of 300 to 600 mg daily, but some patients require as much as 900 mg daily. Don't exceed 900 mg/day.

Pharmacodynamics
Antipsychotic action: Clozapine binds to dopamine receptors (D-1, D-2, D-3, D-4, and D-5) within the limbic system of the CNS. It also may interfere with adrenergic, cholinergic, histaminergic, and serotoninergic receptors.

Pharmacokinetics
Absorption: Food doesn't appear to interfere with bioavailability. Only 27% to 50% of the dose reaches systemic circulation.
Distribution: About 95% bound to serum proteins.
Metabolism: Metabolism is nearly complete; very little unchanged drug appears in the urine.
Excretion: About 50% appears in the urine and 30% in the feces, mostly as metabolites. Elimination half-life appears proportional to dose and may range from 4 to 66 hours.

Route	Onset	Peak	Duration
P.O.	Unknown	2½ hr	4-12 hr

Contraindications and precautions
Contraindicated in patients with uncontrolled epilepsy or history of clozapine-induced agranulocytosis; in patients with a WBC count below 3,500/mm³; in patients with severe CNS depression or coma; in patients taking other drugs that suppress bone marrow function; and in those with myelosuppressive disorders.

Use cautiously in patients with renal, hepatic, or cardiac disease, prostatic hyperplasia, or angle-closure glaucoma and in those receiving general anesthesia.

Use cautiously with other drugs metabolized by cytochrome P-450 2D6, including antidepressants, phenothiazines, carbamazepine, and type IC antiarrhythmics (propafenone, flecainide, encainide) or drugs that inhibit this enzyme, such as quinidine.

Interactions

Drug-drug. *Antihypertensives:* May potentiate the hypotensive effects. Check blood pressure frequently.
Anticholinergics: May potentiate the anticholinergic effects of clozapine. Avoid use together.
Benzodiazepines: Concurrent use may pose a risk of respiratory arrest and severe hypotension. Avoid use together.
Bone marrow suppressants: Increased bone marrow toxicity. Use together cautiously.
CNS-active drugs: Potential for additive effects. Use together cautiously.
Phenytoin: Clozapine may decrease levels. May lower the seizure threshold; avoid use together.
Warfarin, digoxin, highly protein-bound drugs: Increased serum levels. Monitor closely for adverse reactions.
Drug-herb. *Nutmeg:* May reduce effectiveness of drug. Avoid use together.
Drug-food. *Caffeine-containing beverages:* May inhibit antipsychotic effects of clozapine. Patient requires close monitoring.
Drug-lifestyle. *Alcohol use:* Increased CNS depression. Advise patient to avoid alcohol.
Smoking: May reduce plasma clozapine concentrations. Discourage smoking.

Effects on diagnostic tests

None reported.

Adverse reactions

CNS: *drowsiness, sedation, **seizures,*** dizziness, syncope, vertigo, headache, tremor, disturbed sleep or nightmares, restlessness, hypokinesia or akinesia, agitation, rigidity, akathisia, confusion, fatigue, insomnia, hyperkinesia, weakness, lethargy, ataxia, slurred speech, depression, myoclonus, anxiety, neuroleptic malignant syndrome.
CV: *tachycardia, hypotension,* hypertension, chest pain, ECG changes, orthostatic hypotension.
GI: *dry mouth, constipation,* nausea, vomiting, *excessive salivation,* heartburn, constipation, diarrhea.
GU: urinary abnormalities (urinary frequency or urgency, urine retention), incontinence, abnormal ejaculation.
Hematologic: ***leukopenia, agranulocytosis.***
Musculoskeletal: muscle pain or spasm, muscle weakness.
Skin: rash.
Other: fever, weight gain, visual disturbances, diaphoresis.

After abrupt withdrawal of long-term therapy: Possible abrupt recurrence of psychotic symptoms. Monitor patient closely.

Overdose and treatment

Fatalities have occurred at doses exceeding 2.5 g. Symptoms include drowsiness, delirium, coma, hypotension, hypersalivation, tachycardia, respiratory depression, and, rarely, seizures.

Treat symptomatically. Establish an airway and ensure adequate ventilation. Gastric lavage with activated charcoal and sorbitol may be effective. Monitor vital signs. Avoid epinephrine (and derivatives), quinidine, and procainamide when treating hypotension and arrhythmias.

Clinical considerations

- When discontinuing clozapine therapy, drug must be withdrawn gradually (over a 1- to 2-week period). However, changes in the patient's clinical status (including the development of leukopenia) may require abrupt discontinuation of the drug. If so, monitor closely for recurrence of psychotic symptoms.
- To reinstate therapy in patients withdrawn from drug, follow usual guidelines for dosage buildup. However, re-exposure of the patient may increase the risk and severity of adverse reactions. If therapy was terminated for WBC counts of less than 2,000/mm^3 or granulocyte counts of less than 1,000/mm^3, drug shouldn't be reinstated.
- Some patients experience transient fevers (temperature of more than 100.4° F [38° C]), especially in the first 3 weeks of therapy. Monitor patient closely.

Therapeutic monitoring

- For the first 6 months, clozapine therapy must be given with a monitoring program that ensures weekly testing of WBC counts. Blood tests must be performed weekly, and no more than a 1-week supply of drug can be distributed. Blood testing then can be done every other week.
- Patient needs periodic assessment for abnormal body movement.

Special populations

Breast-feeding patients. Animal studies have shown that drug is excreted in breast milk. Women taking clozapine shouldn't breast-feed.
Pediatric patients. Safety in children hasn't been established.
Geriatric patients. Geriatric patients may require reduced dosages, because they may be more sensitive to adverse reactions, especially orthostatic hypotension, dry mouth, and constipation. Monitor closely.

Patient counseling

- Warn patient about risk of developing agranulocytosis. Safe use of drug requires blood tests weekly for the first 6 months, then every other week to monitor for agranulocytosis.

- Advise patient to promptly report flulike symptoms, fever, sore throat, lethargy, malaise, or other signs of infection.
- Advise patient to call before taking OTC drugs or alcohol.
- Tell patient that ice chips or sugarless candy or gum may help to relieve dry mouth.
- Warn patient to rise slowly to upright position to avoid orthostatic hypotension.

codeine phosphate
codeine sulfate

Pharmacologic classification: opioid
Therapeutic classification: analgesic, antitussive
Controlled substance schedule II
Pregnancy risk category C

How supplied
Available by prescription only
Tablets: 15 mg, 30 mg, 60 mg; 30 mg, 60 mg (soluble)
Oral solution: 15 mg/5 ml codeine phosphate
Injection: 15 mg/ml, 30 mg/ml, 60 mg/ml codeine phosphate

Indications and dosages
Mild to moderate pain
Adults: 15 to 60 mg P.O. or 15 to 60 mg (phosphate) S.C. or I.M. q 4 to 6 hours, p.r.n., or around-the-clock.
Children: 0.5 mg/kg (or 15 mg/m^2) P.O. q 4 to 6 hours, or 0.5 mg/kg (or 15 mg/m^2) (phosphate) S.C. or I.M.
Nonproductive cough
Adults and children age 12 and older: 10 to 20 mg P.O. q 4 to 6 hours. Maximum dose is 120 mg/24 hours.
Children age 6 to 11: 5 to 10 mg P.O. q 4 to 6 hours, not to exceed 60 mg daily.
Children age 2 to 6: 1 mg/kg P.O. daily divided into four equal doses, administered q 4 to 6 hours, not to exceed 30 mg in 24 hours.

Pharmacodynamics
Analgesic action: Codeine (methylmorphine) has analgesic properties that result from its agonist activity at the opiate receptors.
Antitussive action: Codeine has a direct suppressant action on the cough reflex center.

Pharmacokinetics
Absorption: Well absorbed after oral or parenteral administration. It's about two-thirds as potent orally as parenterally.
Distribution: Distributed widely throughout the body; it crosses the placenta and enters breast milk.
Metabolism: Metabolized mainly in the liver, by demethylation or by conjugation with glucuronic acid.
Excretion: Excreted mainly in the urine as norcodeine and free and conjugated morphine.

Route	Onset	Peak	Duration
P.O.	30-45 min	1-2 hr	4-6 hr
I.V.	Immediate	Immediate	4-6 hr
I.M.	10-30 min	½-1 hr	4-6 hr
S.C.	10-30 min	Unknown	4-6 hr

Contraindications and precautions
Contraindicated in patients with hypersensitivity to drug. Use cautiously in patients with impaired renal or hepatic function, head injuries, increased intracranial pressure, increased CSF pressure, hypothyroidism, Addison's disease, acute alcoholism, CNS depression, bronchial asthma, COPD, respiratory depression, or shock, and in geriatric or debilitated patients.

Interactions
Drug-drug. *Anticholinergics:* Concurrent use may cause paralytic ileus. Monitor closely.
CNS depressants, narcotic analgesics, general anesthetics, antihistamines, phenothiazines, barbiturates, benzodiazepines, sedative-hypnotics, tricyclic antidepressants, MAO inhibitors, muscle relaxants: Potentiate drug's respiratory and CNS depression, sedation, and hypotensive effects. Use together with extreme caution.
Cimetidine: Increases respiratory and CNS depression. Avoid using together.
Digitoxin, phenytoin, rifampin: Drug accumulation and enhanced effects may result. Patient requires close monitoring.
Drug-lifestyle. *Alcohol use:* Potentiates respiratory and CNS depression, sedation, and hypotensive effects of drug. Discourage alcohol use.

Effects on diagnostic tests
Drug may increase plasma amylase and lipase levels, delay gastric emptying, increase biliary tract pressure resulting from contraction of the sphincter of Oddi, and may interfere with hepatobiliary imaging studies.

Adverse reactions
CNS: *sedation, clouded sensorium, euphoria, dizziness, light-headedness.*
CV: *hypotension,* bradycardia.
GI: *nausea, vomiting, constipation, dry mouth,* ileus.
GU: *urine retention.*
Respiratory: ***respiratory depression.***
Skin: pruritus, flushing, *diaphoresis.*
Other: physical dependence.

Overdose and treatment
The most common signs and symptoms of overdose are CNS depression, respiratory depression, and miosis (pinpoint pupils). Other acute toxic effects include hypotension, bradycardia, hypothermia, shock, apnea, cardiopulmonary arrest, circulatory collapse, pulmonary edema, and seizures.

To treat acute overdose, first establish adequate respiratory exchange via a patent airway and ventilation as needed; administer narcotic antagonist (naloxone) to reverse respiratory depression. (Because the duration of action of codeine is longer than that of naloxone, repeated naloxone dosing is necessary.) Naloxone shouldn't be given unless the patient has clinically significant respiratory or CV depression. Monitor vital signs closely.

If patient shows signs and symptoms within 2 hours of ingestion of an oral overdose, empty the stomach immediately by inducing emesis (ipecac syrup) or using gastric lavage. Use caution to avoid risk of aspiration. Administer activated charcoal via nasogastric tube for further removal of drug in an oral overdose.

Provide symptomatic and supportive treatment (continued respiratory support, correction of fluid or electrolyte imbalance). Monitor laboratory parameters, vital signs, and neurologic status closely.

Clinical considerations
Consider the recommendations relevant to all opioids as well as the following:

☐ ***ALERT*** Don't mix with other solutions because codeine phosphate is incompatible with many drugs.
- Codeine and aspirin have additive analgesic effects. Give together for maximum pain relief.
- Codeine has much less abuse potential than morphine.
- Patients who become physically dependent on drug may experience acute withdrawal syndrome if given a narcotic antagonist.

Therapeutic monitoring
- Monitor cough type and frequency.
- Monitor respiratory and circulatory status.

Special populations
Breast-feeding patients. Drug is excreted in breast milk; assess risk to benefit ratio before administering.

Pediatric patients. Administer cautiously to children. Codeine-containing cough preparations may be hazardous in young children. Use a calibrated measuring device and don't exceed the recommended daily dose.

Geriatric patients. Lower doses are usually indicated for geriatric patients, who may be more sensitive to the therapeutic and adverse effects of drug.

Patient counseling
- Inform patient that codeine may cause drowsiness, dizziness, or blurring of vision; tell him to use caution while driving or performing tasks that require mental alertness.
- Instruct patient to ask for or to take drug before pain is intense.
- Advise patient that GI distress from oral medication can be lessened when drug is taken with milk.

colchicine

Pharmacologic classification: Colchicum autumnale alkaloid
Therapeutic classification: antigout
Pregnancy risk category C (oral), D (parenteral)

How supplied
Available by prescription only
Injection: 0.5 mg/ml
Tablets: 0.5 mg , 0.6 mg

Indications and dosages
To prevent acute attacks of gout as prophylactic or maintenance therapy
Adults: 0.5 or 0.6 mg P.O. one to four times weekly.
To prevent attacks of gout in patients undergoing surgery
Adults: 0.5 to 0.6 mg P.O. t.i.d. 3 days before and 3 days after surgery.
Acute gout, acute gouty arthritis
Adults: Initially, 0.5 to 1.2 mg P.O., followed by 0.5 to 1.2 mg P.O. q 1 to 2 hours; total daily dose is usually 4 to 8 mg P.O.; give until pain is relieved or until nausea, vomiting, or diarrhea ensues. Or 2 mg I.V. followed by 0.5 mg I.V. q 6 hours if necessary. Total I.V. dose over 24 hours (one course of treatment) not to exceed 4 mg.
◊ ***Familial Mediterranean fever***
Colchicine has been used effectively to treat familial Mediterranean fever (hereditary disorder characterized by acute episodes of fever, peritonitis, and pleuritis).
Adults: 1 to 2 mg/day P.O. in divided doses.
◊ ***Amyloidosis suppressant***
Adults: 500 to 600 mcg P.O. once daily to b.i.d.
◊ ***Dermatitis herpetiformis suppressant***
Adults: 600 mcg P.O. b.i.d. or t.i.d.
◊ ***Hepatic cirrhosis***
Adults: 1 mg P.O. 5 days weekly.
◊ ***Primary biliary cirrhosis***
Adults: 0.6 mg b.i.d.

Pharmacodynamics
Antigout action: Colchicine's exact mechanism of action is unknown, but it's involved in leukocyte migration inhibition; reduction of lactic acid production by leukocytes, resulting

in decreased deposits of uric acid; and interference with kinin formation.
Anti-inflammatory action: Colchicine reduces the inflammatory response to deposited uric acid crystals and diminishes phagocytosis.

Pharmacokinetics

Absorption: When administered P.O., rapidly absorbed from the GI tract. Unchanged drug may be reabsorbed from the intestine by biliary processes.
Distribution: Distributed rapidly into various tissues after reabsorption from the intestine. It's concentrated in leukocytes and distributed into the kidneys, liver, spleen, and intestinal tract, but is absent in the heart, skeletal muscle, and brain.
Metabolism: Metabolized partially in the liver and also slowly metabolized in other tissues.
Excretion: Excreted primarily in the feces, with lesser amounts excreted in urine.

Route	Onset	Peak	Duration
P.O.	< 12 hr	½-2 hr	Unknown
I.V.	6-12 hr	Unknown	Unknown

Contraindications and precautions

Contraindicated in patients with hypersensitivity to drug; blood dyscrasias; or serious CV, renal, or GI disease. Use cautiously in geriatric or debilitated patients and in those with early signs of CV, renal, or GI disease.

Interactions

Drug-drug. *Cyclosporine:* Increased GI toxicity with concurrent use. Dose may require adjustment.
Erythromycin: Increased serum colchicine levels. May need to reduce colchicine dosage.
Loop diuretics: May decrease efficacy of colchicine prophylaxis. Avoid use together.
Phenylbutazone: May increase risk of leukopenia or thrombocytopenia. Avoid use together.
Vitamin B: Impaired absorption. Avoid use together.
Drug-lifestyle. *Alcohol use:* May inhibit drug action. Discourage alcohol use.

Effects on diagnostic tests

Colchicine may cause false-positive results of urine tests for RBCs or hemoglobin.

Adverse reactions

CNS: peripheral neuritis.
GI: *nausea, vomiting, abdominal pain, diarrhea.*
GU: reversible azoospermia.
Hematologic: ***aplastic anemia, thrombocytopenia, and agranulocytosis*** (with long-term use); nonthrombocytopenic purpura.
Hepatic: increased alkaline phosphatase, AST, and ALT levels.
Skin: alopecia, urticaria, dermatitis, hypersensitivity reactions.
Other: severe local irritation if extravasation occurs, myopathy.

Overdose and treatment

Signs and symptoms of overdose include nausea, vomiting, abdominal pain, and diarrhea. Diarrhea may be severe and bloody from hemorrhagic gastroenteritis. Burning sensations in the throat, stomach, and skin also may occur. Extensive vascular damage may result in shock, hematuria, and oliguria, indicating kidney damage. Patient develops severe dehydration, hypotension, and muscle weakness with an ascending paralysis of the CNS. Patient usually remains conscious, but delirium and convulsions may occur. Death may result from respiratory depression.

There is no known specific antidote. Treatment begins with gastric lavage and preventive measures for shock. Recent studies support the use of hemodialysis and peritoneal dialysis; atropine and morphine may relieve abdominal pain; paregoric usually is administered to control diarrhea and cramps. Respiratory assistance may be needed.

Clinical considerations

- To avoid cumulative toxicity, a course of oral colchicine shouldn't be repeated for at least 3 days; a course of I.V. colchicine shouldn't be repeated for several weeks.
- Advise nurse not to administer I.M. or S.C.; severe local irritation occurs.
- Give colchicine by slow I.V. push over 2 to 5 minutes by direct I.V. injection or into tubing of a free-flowing I.V. with compatible I.V. fluid. Avoid extravasation. Don't dilute colchicine injection with bacteriostatic normal saline solution, dextrose 5% injection, or any other fluid that might change pH of colchicine solution. If lower concentration of colchicine injection is needed, dilute with sterile water or normal saline solution. However, if diluted solution becomes turbid, don't inject.
- Drug must be discontinued if weakness, anorexia, nausea, vomiting, or diarrhea appears. First sign of acute overdose may be GI symptoms, followed by vascular damage, muscle weakness, and ascending paralysis. Delirium and convulsions may occur without loss of consciousness.
- Store drug in a tightly closed, light-resistant container, away from moisture and high temperatures.

Therapeutic monitoring

Obtain baseline laboratory studies, including CBC, before initiating therapy and periodically thereafter.

Special populations

Breast-feeding patients. Safety hasn't been established in breast-feeding women. It isn't known if drug is excreted in breast milk.

Pediatric patients. Safety and efficacy in children haven't been established.
Geriatric patients. Administer with caution to geriatric or debilitated patients, especially those with renal, GI, or heart disease or hematologic disorders. Reduce dosage if weakness, anorexia, nausea, vomiting, or diarrhea appears.

Patient counseling

- Advise patient to report rash, sore throat, fever, unusual bleeding, bruising, tiredness, weakness, numbness, or tingling.
- Tell patient to discontinue drug as soon as gout pain is relieved or at the first sign of nausea, vomiting, stomach pain, or diarrhea, and to report persistent symptoms.

colestipol hydrochloride

Colestid

Pharmacologic classification: anion exchange resin
Therapeutic classification: antilipemic
Pregnancy risk category C

How supplied

Available by prescription only
Tablets: 1 g
Granules for oral suspension: 5 g/packet, 300 g and 500 g multidose with calibrated scoop.

Indications and dosages

Primary hypercholesterolemia and xanthomas
Adults: Tablets: Initially, 2 g P.O. once daily or b.i.d., then increase in 2-g increments at 1- to 2-month intervals. Usual dosage is 2 to 16 g P.O. daily given as a single dose or in divided doses.
Granules: Initially, 5 g P.O. once daily or b.i.d., then increase in 5-g increments at 1- to 2-month intervals. Usual dosage is 5 to 30 g P.O. daily given as a single dose or in divided doses.
◊ *Children:* 10 to 20 g or 500 mg/kg P.O. daily in two to four divided doses (lower doses of 125 to 250 mg/kg used when serum cholesterol levels were 15% to 20% above normal after only dietary management).
◊ ***Digitoxin overdose***
Adults: Initially, 10 g P.O. followed by 5 g P.O. q 6 to 8 hours.

Pharmacodynamics

Antilipemic action: Bile is normally excreted into the intestine to facilitate absorption of fat and other lipid materials. Colestipol binds with bile acid, forming an insoluble compound that is excreted in feces. With less bile available in the digestive system, less fat and lipid materials in food are absorbed, more cholesterol is used by the liver to replace its supply of bile acids, and the serum cholesterol level decreases.

Pharmacokinetics

Absorption: Not absorbed. Cholesterol levels may decrease in 24 to 48 hours, with peak effect occurring at 1 month. In some patients, the initial decrease is followed by a return to or above baseline cholesterol levels on continued therapy.
Distribution: None.
Metabolism: None.
Excretion: Excreted in feces; cholesterol levels return to baseline within 1 month after therapy stops.

Route	Onset	Peak	Duration
P.O.	1 mo	Unknown	1 mo

Contraindications and precautions

Contraindicated in patients with hypersensitivity reactions to bile-acid sequestering resins. Use cautiously in patients prone to constipation and in those with conditions aggravated by constipation, such as symptomatic coronary artery disease.

Interactions

Drug-drug. *Cardiac glycosides, digoxin, digitoxin, tetracycline, penicillin G, chenodiol, thiazide diuretics:* Colestipol impairs absorption, thus decreasing their therapeutic effect. Other drugs should be given 1 hour before or 4 hours after colestipol.
Any oral drug: May require adjustment to compensate for possible binding with colestipol; readjustment must also be made when colestipol is withdrawn to prevent high-dose toxicity.

Effects on diagnostic tests

None reported.

Adverse reactions

CNS: headache, dizziness, anxiety, vertigo, insomnia, fatigue, syncope, tinnitus.
GI: *constipation,* ***fecal impaction,*** hemorrhoids, abdominal discomfort, flatulence, nausea, vomiting, steatorrhea, ***GI bleeding,*** diarrhea, anorexia, difficulty swallowing, transient espohageal obstruction.
GU: dysuria, hematuria.
Hematologic: anemia, ecchymoses, bleeding tendencies.
Musculoskeletal: backache, muscle and joint pain, osteoporosis.
Skin: rash, irritation of tongue and perianal area.
Other: vitamin A, D, E, and K deficiencies from decreased absorption; hyperchloremic acidosis with long-term use or high dosage; alterations in serum levels of alkaline phosphatase, ALT, AST, chloride, phosphorus, potassium, and sodium.

Overdose and treatment

Overdose of colestipol hasn't been reported. Chief potential risk is intestinal obstruction; treatment would depend on location and degree of obstruction and on amount of gut motility.

Clinical considerations

- To mix, sprinkle granules on surface of preferred beverage or wet food, let stand a few minutes, and stir to obtain uniform suspension; avoid excess foaming by using large glass and mixing slowly. Use at least 90 ml of water or other fluid, soups, milk, or pulpy fruit; rinse container and have patient drink this to be sure he ingests entire dose. Tablets should be swallowed whole.
- Drug effects are most successful if used together with a diet and exercise program.
- Bowel habits must be monitored; and constipation treated promptly by decreasing dosage, increasing fluid intake, adding a stool softener, or discontinuing drug.

Therapeutic monitoring

- Monitor levels of cardiac glycosides and other drugs to ensure appropriate dosage during and after therapy with colestipol.
- Serum cholesterol levels must be checked frequently during first few months of therapy and periodically thereafter.
- Patient needs observation for signs of vitamin A, D, or K deficiency.

Special populations

Breast-feeding patients. Safety in breast-feeding women hasn't been established.
Pediatric patients. Safety in children hasn't been established. Drug isn't usually recommended; however, it's been used in a limited number of children with hypercholesteremia.
Geriatric patients. Geriatric patients are more likely to experience adverse GI effects, as well as adverse nutritional effects.

Patient counseling

- Explain disease process and rationale for therapy and encourage patient to comply with continued blood testing and special diet; although therapy isn't curative, it helps control serum cholesterol levels.
- Teach patient how to administer drug. To enhance palatability, tell patient to mix and refrigerate the next daily dose the previous evening.

corticotropin (adrenocorticotropic hormone, ACTH)

ACTH, Acthar, Cortrophin-Zinc, H.P. Acthar Gel

Pharmacologic classification: anterior pituitary hormone
Therapeutic classification: diagnostic aid, replacement hormone, multiple sclerosis, and nonsuppurative thyroiditis treatment
Pregnancy risk category C

How supplied

Available by prescription only
Injection: 25 U/vial, 40 U/vial
Repository injection: 40 U/ml, 80 U/ml

Indications and dosages

Diagnostic test of adrenocortical function
Adults: Up to 80 U I.M. or S.C. in divided doses; or a single dose of repository form; or 10 to 25 U (aqueous form) in 500 ml of D_5W I.V. over 8 hours, between blood samplings.

Individual dosages vary with adrenal glands' sensitivity to stimulation and with the specific disease. Infants and younger children require larger doses per kilogram than do older children and adults.
Replacement hormone
Adults*:* 20 U S.C. or I.M. q.i.d.
Exacerbations of multiple sclerosis
Adults*:* 80 to 120 U I.M. daily for 2 to 3 weeks.
Severe allergic reactions, collagen disorders, dermatologic disorders, inflammation
Adults: 40 to 80 U/day I.M. or S.C. Adjust dosage based upon patient response.
Infantile spasms
Infants: 20 to 40 U I.M. (of repository injection) daily or 80 U I.M. every other day for 3 months or 1 month after spasm ceases.

Pharmacodynamics

Diagnostic action: Corticotropin is used to test adrenocortical function. Corticotropin binds with a specific receptor in the adrenal cell plasma membrane, stimulating the synthesis of the entire spectrum of adrenal steroids, one of which is cortisol. The effect of corticotropin is measured by analyzing plasma cortisol before and after drug administration. In patients with primary adrenocortical insufficiency, corticotropin doesn't increase plasma cortisol levels significantly.
Anti-inflammatory action: In nonsuppurative thyroiditis and acute exacerbations of multiple sclerosis, corticotropin stimulates release of adrenal cortex hormones, which combat tissue responses to inflammatory processes.

Pharmacokinetics

Absorption: Absorbed rapidly after I.M. administration.
Distribution: Exact distribution of corticotropin is unknown, but it's removed rapidly from plasma by many tissues.
Metabolism: Unknown.
Excretion: Probably excreted by the kidneys. Half-life is about 15 minutes.

Route	Onset	Peak	Duration
I.V., I.M.	Rapid	1 hr	2-4 hr
I.M. (repository)	Unknown	Unknown	3 days
S.C.	Unknown	Unknown	Unknown

Contraindications and precautions

Contraindicated in patients with peptic ulcer, scleroderma, osteoporosis, systemic fungal infections, ocular herpes simplex, peptic ulceration, heart failure, hypertension, sensitivity to pork and pork products, adrenocortical hyperfunction or primary insufficiency, or Cushing's syndrome. Also contraindicated in those who have had surgery recently.

Use cautiously in pregnant patients and in women of childbearing age. Also use cautiously in patients being immunized and in those with latent tuberculosis, hypothyroidism, cirrhosis, acute gouty arthritis, psychotic tendencies, renal insufficiency, diverticulitis, ulcerative colitis, thromboembolic disorders, seizures, uncontrolled hypertension, or myasthenia gravis.

Use with caution if surgery or emergency treatment is required.

Interactions

Drug-drug. *Cardiac glycosides:* May increase the risk of arrhythmias or digitalis toxicity associated with hypokalemia; close monitoring is necessary.
Cortisone, hydrocortisone, or estrogens: May elevate plasma cortisol levels abnormally. Use with caution.
Diuretics, amphotericin B, carbonic anhydrase inhibitors: Accentuate the electrolyte loss associated with diuretic therapy. Monitor serum blood levels, especially potassium.
Hepatic enzyme-inducing agents: May increase corticotropin metabolism. Patient requires close monitoring.
Insulin or oral antidiabetic agents: May require increased dosage of the antidiabetic agent; monitor blood glucose levels closely.
Salicylates, NSAIDs, and indomethacin: Increased risk of GI bleeding. Avoid use together.

Effects on diagnostic tests

Corticotropin therapy alters protein-bound iodine levels; radioactive iodine (^{131}I) uptake and T_3 uptake; total protein values; serum amylase, urine amino acid, serotonin, uric acid and 17-ketosteroid levels; and leukocyte counts.

Adverse reactions

CNS: ***seizures,*** *dizziness,* vertigo, ***increased intracranial pressure with papilledema,*** pseudotumor cerebri.
CV: hypertension, ***heart failure,*** necrotizing vasculitis, ***shock.***
EENT: cataracts, glaucoma.
GI: ***peptic ulceration with perforation and hemorrhage,*** pancreatitis, abdominal distention, ulcerative esophagitis, nausea, vomiting.
GU: menstrual irregularities.
Metabolic: activation of latent diabetes mellitus, *sodium and fluid retention,* calcium and potassium loss, hypokalemic alkalosis, negative nitrogen balance.
Musculoskeletal: muscle weakness, steroid myopathy, loss of muscle mass, osteoporosis, suppression of growth in children, vertebral compression fractures.
Respiratory: pneumonia.
Skin: impaired wound healing; thin, fragile skin; petechiae; ecchymoses; facial erythema; diaphoresis; acne; hyperpigmentation; allergic reactions; hirsutism.
Other: abscess and septic infection, cushingoid symptoms, progressive increase in antibodies, loss of corticotropin stimulatory effect, hypersensitivity reactions (rash, ***bronchospasm***).

Overdose and treatment

Specific information unavailable. Treatment is supportive, as appropriate.

Clinical considerations

- Cosyntropin is less antigenic and less likely to cause allergic reactions than corticotropin. However, allergic reactions occur rarely with corticotropin.
- In patient with suspected sensitivity to porcine proteins, perform skin testing. To decrease the risk of anaphylactic reaction in patient with limited adrenal reserves, 1 mg of dexamethasone may be given at midnight before the corticotropin test and 0.5 mg at start of test.
- Observe neonates of corticotropin-treated women for signs of hypoadrenalism.
- Counteract edema by low-sodium, high-potassium intake; nitrogen loss by high-protein diet; and psychotic symptoms by reducing corticotropin dosage or administering sedatives.
- Drug may mask signs of chronic disease and decrease host resistance and ability to localize infection.
- Refrigerate reconstituted product and use within 24 hours.
- If administering gel, it must be warmed to room temperature, drawn into a large needle, and given slowly, deep I.M. with a 22G needle.
- Don't discontinue drug abruptly, especially after prolonged therapy. An addisonian crisis may occur.

Therapeutic monitoring
Monitor weight, fluid exchange, and resting blood pressure levels until minimal effective dosage is achieved.

Special populations
Breast-feeding patients. Safety hasn't been established. Because the potential for severe adverse reactions exists, benefits and risks must be weighed.
Pediatric patients. Use with caution because prolonged use of drug inhibits skeletal growth. Intermittent administration is recommended.

Patient counseling
- Warn patient that injection is painful.
- Tell patient to report marked fluid retention, muscle weakness, abdominal pain, seizures, or headache.
- Instruct patient not to be vaccinated during corticotropin therapy.
- Teach patient how to monitor for edema, and tell him about the need for fluid and salt restriction as appropriate.
- Warn patient not to stop drug except as prescribed. Tell him that abrupt discontinuation may provoke severe adverse reactions.

cortisone acetate
Cortone

Pharmacologic classification: glucocorticoid, mineralocorticoid
Therapeutic classification: anti-inflammatory, replacement therapy
Pregnancy risk category NR

How supplied
Available by prescription only
Tablets: 5 mg, 10 mg, 25 mg
Injection (I.M. use): 50 mg/ml suspension

Indications and dosages
Adrenal insufficiency, allergy, inflammation
Adults: 25 to 300 mg P.O. or 20 to 300 mg I.M. daily or on alternate days. Dosage highly individualized, depending on severity of disease.
Children: 20 to 300 mg/m^2 P.O. daily in four divided doses or 7 to 37.5 mg/m^2 I.M. once or twice daily. Dosage must be highly individualized.

Pharmacodynamics
Adrenocorticoid replacement: Cortisone acetate is an adrenocorticoid with both glucocorticoid and mineralocorticoid properties. A weak anti-inflammatory agent, drug has only about 80% of the anti-inflammatory activity of an equal weight of hydrocortisone. It's a potent mineralocorticoid, however, having twice the potency of prednisone. Cortisone (or hydrocortisone) is usually the drug of choice for replacement therapy in patients with adrenal insufficiency. It's usually not used for inflammatory or immunosuppressant activity because of the extremely large doses that must be used and because of the unwanted mineralocorticoid effects. Injectable form has a slow onset but a long duration of action. It's usually used only when the oral dosage form can't be used.

Pharmacokinetics
Absorption: Absorbed readily after oral administration.
Distribution: Distributed rapidly to muscle, liver, skin, intestines, and kidneys. Cortisone is extensively bound to plasma proteins (transcortin and albumin). Only the unbound portion is active. Cortisone is distributed into breast milk and through the placenta.
Metabolism: Metabolized in the liver to the active metabolite hydrocortisone, which in turn is metabolized to inactive glucuronide and sulfate metabolites. Duration of hypothalamic-pituitary-adrenal (HPA) axis suppression is 1¼ to 1½ days.
Excretion: Inactive metabolites and small amounts of unmetabolized drug are excreted by the kidneys. Insignificant quantities of the drug are also excreted in feces. Biological half-life of cortisone is 8 to 12 hours.

Route	Onset	Peak	Duration
P.O.	Variable	1-2 hr	Variable
I.M.	24-48 hr	Variable	Variable

Contraindications and precautions
Contraindicated in patients with hypersensitivity to drug or its ingredients or systemic fungal infections. Use cautiously in patients with renal disease, recent MI, GI ulcer, hypertension, osteoporosis, diabetes mellitus, hypothyroidism, cirrhosis, diverticulitis, ulcerative colitis, recent intestinal anastomosis, thromboembolic disorders, seizures, myasthenia gravis, heart failure, tuberculosis, ocular herpes, emotional instability, or psychotic tendencies.

Interactions
Drug-drug. *Oral anticoagulants:* When used together, cortisone may decrease the effects. PT must be checked.
Barbiturates, phenytoin, or rifampin: Decreased corticosteroid effects. Monitor closely.
Cardiac glycosides: Hypokalemia may increase the risk of toxicity in patients concurrently receiving cardiac glycosides. Avoid use together.
Cholestyramine, colestipol, or antacids: Decrease cortisone's effect by adsorbing the corticosteroid, decreasing the amount absorbed. Patient needs careful monitoring.
Diuretic or amphotericin B therapy: Cortisone may enhance hypokalemia associated with diuretic or amphotericin B therapy. Monitor serum blood levels closely, especially potassium.

Estrogens: May reduce the metabolism of cortisone. The half-life of cortisone is then prolonged. Avoid use together.
Insulin or oral antidiabetic agents: Cause hyperglycemia, which may require dosage adjustment.
Isoniazid and salicylates: When used together, cortisone increases the metabolism of isoniazid and salicylates. Use together cautiously.
NSAIDs: May increase the risk of GI ulceration. Avoid use together.
Toxoids or inactivated vaccines: Cortisone may have a diminished response to toxoids or inactivated vaccines. Avoid use together.
Drug-lifestyle. *Alcohol use:* Increased risk of gastric irritation and GI ulceration. Advise patient to avoid alcohol.

Effects on diagnostic tests
Drug therapy suppresses reactions to skin tests; causes false-negative results in the nitroblue tetrazolium test for systemic bacterial infections; and decreases ^{131}I uptake and protein-bound iodine concentrations in thyroid function tests.

Adverse reactions
Most adverse reactions to corticosteroids are dose- or duration-dependent.
CNS: euphoria, insomnia, psychotic behavior, pseudotumor cerebri, vertigo, headache, paresthesia, ***seizures.***
CV: ***heart failure,*** hypertension, edema, ***arrhythmias,*** thrombophlebitis, ***thromboembolism.***
EENT: cataracts, glaucoma.
Endocrine: menstrual irregularities, cushingoid symptoms (moonface, buffalo hump, central obesity).
GI: *peptic ulcer,* GI irritation, increased appetite, pancreatitis, nausea, vomiting.
Musculoskeletal: muscle weakness, osteoporosis.
Skin: delayed wound healing, acne, various skin eruptions, atrophy at I.M. injection sites.
Other: hirsutism, susceptibility to infections; possible hypokalemia, hyperglycemia, and carbohydrate intolerance; growth suppression in children; ***acute adrenal insufficiency may follow increased stress (infection, surgery, trauma) or abrupt withdrawal after long-term therapy.*** Increased glucose and cholesterol levels; decreased serum potassium, calcium, thyroxine, and triiodothyronine levels; and increased urine glucose and calcium levels.
After abrupt withdrawal: rebound inflammation, fatigue, weakness, arthralgia, fever, dizziness, lethargy, depression, fainting, orthostatic hypotension, dyspnea, anorexia, hypoglycemia. After prolonged use, sudden withdrawal may be fatal.

Overdose and treatment
Acute ingestion, even in massive doses, is rarely a clinical problem. Toxic signs and symptoms rarely occur if the drug is used for less than 3 weeks, even at large dosage ranges. However, chronic use causes adverse physiologic effects.

Clinical considerations
□ ***ALERT*** Check for sensitivity to any other corticosteroid medication. Drug isn't for I.V. use. For better results and less toxicity, give a once-daily dose in the morning.

Therapeutic monitoring
- Monitor serum electrolyte and blood glucose levels.
- Monitor for fluid and electrolyte imbalance.

Special populations
Pediatric patients. Chronic use of cortisone in children and adolescents may delay growth and maturation.
Geriatric patients. Use with caution in geriatric patients in whom osteoporosis is more likely to develop.

Patient counseling
- Inform patient of potential adverse reactions.
- Tell patient not to discontinue drug abruptly or without doctor's consent.
- Advise patient to avoid exposure to infections (such as measles and chicken pox) and to notify doctor if such exposure occurs.
- Instruct patient to carry a card indicating his need for supplemental glucocorticoids during stress. This card should contain doctor's name, medication, and dose taken.

cosyntropin
Cortrosyn

Pharmacologic classification: anterior pituitary hormone
Therapeutic classification: diagnostic
Pregnancy risk category C

How supplied
Available by prescription only
Injection: 0.25 mg

Indications and dosages
Diagnostic test of adrenocortical function
Adults and children age 2 and older: 0.25 to 0.75 mg I.M. or I.V. (unless label prohibits I.V. administration) between blood samplings. To administer as I.V. infusion, dilute 0.25 mg in D_5W or normal saline solution, and infuse over 6 hours (40 mcg/hour).
Children under age 2: 0.125 mg I.M. or I.V.

Pharmacodynamics
Diagnostic action: Cosyntropin is used to test adrenal function. Drug binds with a specific

receptor in the adrenal cell plasma membrane to initiate synthesis of its entire spectrum of hormones, one of which is cortisol. In patients with primary adrenocortical insufficiency, cosyntropin doesn't increase plasma cortisol levels significantly.

Pharmacokinetics

Absorption: Inactivated by the proteolytic enzymes in the GI tract. After I.M. administration, cosyntropin is absorbed rapidly. After rapid I.V. administration in patients with normal adrenocortical function, plasma cortisol levels begin to increase within 5 minutes and double within 15 to 30 minutes. Peak levels begin to decrease in 2 to 4 hours.
Distribution: Not fully understood, but drug is removed rapidly from plasma by many tissues.
Metabolism: Unknown.
Excretion: Probably excreted by the kidneys.

Route	Onset	Peak	Duration
I.V.	Rapid	45-60 min	Unknown
I.M., S.C.	Unknown	45-60 min	Unknown

Contraindications and precautions

Contraindicated in patients with hypersensitivity to drug.

Interactions

Drug-drug. *Blood, plasma products:* Inactivate cosyntropin. Avoid administration together. *Cortisone, hydrocortisone, or estrogens:* May cause abnormally elevated plasma cortisol levels. Avoid use together.

Effects on diagnostic tests

None reported.

Adverse reactions

CNS: ***seizures,*** dizziness, vertigo, ***increased intracranial pressure with papilledema,*** pseudotumor cerebri.
EENT: cataracts, glaucoma.
GI: peptic ulcer, ***pancreatitis,*** abdominal distension, ulcerative esophagitis, nausea, vomiting.
Musculoskeletal: fractures, muscle weakness, steroid myopathy, loss of muscle mass, osteoporosis, vertebral compression.
Skin: pruritus; impaired wound healing; thin, fragile skin; petechiae; ecchymoses; facial erythema; diaphoresis; acne; hyperpigmentation; hirsutism.
Other: flushing, hypersensitivity reactions, cushingoid symptoms, menstrual irregularities, alterations in blood glucose levels.

Overdose and treatment

Acute overdose requires no therapy other than symptomatic treatment and supportive care, as appropriate.

Clinical considerations

- High plasma cortisol levels may be reported erroneously in patients receiving spironolactone, cortisone, or hydrocortisone when fluorometric analysis is used. This doesn't occur with the radioimmunoassay or competitive protein-binding method. However, therapy can be maintained with prednisone, dexamethasone, or betamethasone because these aren't detectable by the fluorometric method.
- More cortisol is secreted if dosage is given slowly, not rapidly I.V.
- Cosyntropin is less antigenic than corticotropin and less likely to produce allergic reactions.
- For rapid screening, plasma cortisol levels are determined before and 30 minutes after administration of 0.25 mg I.M. or I.V. injection over 2 minutes. Some clinicians prefer plasma cortisol concentration determinations at 60 minutes after injection of cosyntropin.
- Reconstitute powder by adding 1 ml of normal saline solution to 0.25-mg vial to yield a solution containing 0.25 mg/ml.
- Reconstituted solution remains stable at room temperature for 24 hours or for 21 days at 36° to 46° F (2° to 8° C).

Therapeutic monitoring

A normal response to cosyntropin includes: The control plasma cortisol level should exceed 5 mcg/100 ml plasma; 30 minutes after the injection, cortisol levels increase by 7 mcg/100 ml above control; 30-minute cortisol levels exceed 18 mcg/100 ml.

Patient counseling

- Inform patient taking spironolactone, cortisone, hydrocortisone, or estrogen that these medications may interfere with test results.
- Tell patient to report adverse effects immediately.

co-trimoxazole (trimethoprim-sulfamethoxazole)

Apo-Sulfatrim*, Bactrim, Bactrim DS, Bactrim I.V., Cotrim, Cotrim D.S., Novo-Trimel*, Roubac*, Septra, Septra DS, Septra I.V., SMZ-TMP, Sulfatrim

Pharmacologic classification: sulfonamide and folate antagonist
Therapeutic classification: antibiotic
Pregnancy risk category C

How supplied

Available by prescription only
Tablets: trimethoprim 80 mg and sulfamethoxazole 400 mg; trimethoprim 160 mg and sulfamethoxazole 800 mg

Suspension: trimethoprim 40 mg and sulfamethoxazole 200 mg/5 ml
Injectable: trimethoprim 16 mg/ml and sulfamethoxazole 80 mg/ ml

Indications and dosages

Urinary tract infections and shigellosis
Adults: 1 double-strength or 2 regular-strength tablets P.O. q 12 hours for 10 to 14 days or 5 days for shigellosis. Or, 8 to 10 mg/kg (based on trimethoprim) I.V. daily given in 2 to 4 equally divided doses for up to 14 days (5 days for shigellosis). Maximum daily dose, 960 mg.
Children over age 2 months: 8 mg/kg trimethoprim and 40 mg/kg sulfamethoxazole P.O. daily in two divided doses q 12 hours (10 days for urinary tract infections; 5 days for shigellosis).
Primary prophylaxis against toxoplasmosis in HIV-infected patients
Adults and adolescents: 160 mg (based on trimethoprim) daily P.O.
Children: 150 mg/m^2 (based on trimethoprim) P.O. daily in 2 divided doses.
Otitis media
Children over age 2 months: 8 mg/kg trimethoprim and 40 mg/kg sulfamethoxazole P.O. daily, in two divided doses q 12 hours for 10 days.
Pneumocystis carinii *pneumonitis*
Adults and children over age 2 months: 15 to 20 mg/kg trimethoprim and 75 to 100 mg/kg sulfamethoxazole P.O. daily, in equally divided doses, q 6 to 8 hours for 14 to 21 days.
Prophylaxis of* P. carinii *pneumonia
Adults: 160 mg (based on trimethoprim) daily.
Children: 150 mg/m^2 (based on trimethoprim) per day in 2 divided doses for 3 consecutive days each week.
Chronic bronchitis
Adults: 1 double-strength or 2 regular-strength tablets P.O. q 12 hours for 14 days.
Traveler's diarrhea
Adults: 1 double-strength or 2 regular-strength tablets P.O. q 12 hours for 5 days.

Note: For the following unlabeled uses, dosages refer to oral trimethoprim (as co-trimoxazole).

◇ ***Septic agranulocytosis***
Adults: 2.5 mg/kg I.V. q.i.d.; for prophylaxis, 80 to 160 mg b.i.d.
◇ ***Nocardia infection***
Adults: 640 mg P.O. daily for 7 months.
◇ ***Pharyngeal gonococcal infections***
Adults: 720 mg P.O. daily for 5 days.
◇ ***Chancroid***
Adults: 160 mg P.O. b.i.d for 7 days.
◇ ***Pertussis***
Adults: 320 mg P.O. daily in two divided doses.
Children: 40 mg/kg/day P.O. in two divided doses.
◇ ***Cholera***
Adults: 160 mg P.O. b.i.d for 3 days.
Children: 5 mg/kg P.O. b.i.d for 3 days.
◇ ***Isosporiasis***
Adults: 160 mg P.O. q.i.d. for 10 days, followed by 160 mg b.i.d. for 3 weeks.
≡ ***Dosage adjustment.*** In patients with impaired renal function, adjust dose or frequency of administration of parenteral form according to degree of renal impairment, severity of infection, and susceptibility of organism.

Pharmacodynamics

Antibacterial action: Co-trimoxazole is generally bactericidal; it acts by sequential blockade of folic acid enzymes in the synthesis pathway. The sulfamethoxazole component inhibits formation of dihydrofolic acid from para-aminobenzoic (PABA), whereas trimethoprim inhibits dihydrofolate reductase. Both drugs block folic acid synthesis, preventing bacterial cell synthesis of essential nucleic acids.

Co-trimoxazole is effective against *E. coli, Klebsiella, Enterobacter, P. mirabilis, H. influenzae, S. pneumoniae, S. aureus, Acinetobacter, Salmonella, Shigella,* and *P. carinii.*

Pharmacokinetics

Absorption: Well absorbed from the GI tract after oral administration.
Distribution: Distributed widely into body tissues and fluids, including middle ear fluid, prostatic fluid, bile, aqueous humor, and CSF. Protein binding is 44% for trimethoprim, 70% for sulfamethoxazole. Drug crosses the placenta.
Metabolism: Metabolized by the liver.
Excretion: Both components of co-trimoxazole are excreted primarily in urine by glomerular filtration and renal tubular secretion; some is excreted in breast milk. Trimethoprim's plasma half-life in patients with normal renal function is 8 to 11 hours, extended to 26 hours in severe renal dysfunction; sulfamethoxazole's plasma half-life is normally 10 to 13 hours, extended to 30 to 40 hours in severe renal dysfunction. Hemodialysis removes some co-trimoxazole.

Route	Onset	Peak	Duration
P.O.	Unknown	1-4 hr	Unknown
I.V.	Immediate	Immediate	Unknown

Contraindications and precautions

Contraindicated in patients with hypersensitivity to trimethoprim or sulfonamides, severe renal impairment (creatinine clearance of less than 15 ml/minute), or porphyria; in those with megaloblastic anemia caused by folate deficiency; in pregnant women at term; in breast-feeding women; and in children under age 2 months.

Use cautiously in patients with impaired renal or hepatic function, severe allergies, severe bronchial asthma, G6PD deficiency, or blood dyscrasia.

Interactions

Drug-drug. *Oral anticoagulants:* Co-trimoxazole may inhibit hepatic metabolism, en-

hancing anticoagulant effects. Observe patient for signs of bleeding.
PABA: Concurrent use antagonizes sulfonamide effects. Monitor patient closely.
Oral sulfonylureas: Concurrent use enhances their hypoglycemic effects. Monitor blood glucose levels.
Phenytoin: Co-trimoxazole may inhibit metabolism of phenytoin. Dosage adjustment may be necessary.
Tricyclic antidepressants: May decrease antidepressant effect. Monitor patient closely.
Indomethacin: May increase plasma levels of sulfamethoxazole. Dosage adjustment may be necessary.
Digoxin: Increase serum digoxin levels. Monitor serum levels closely.
Pyrimethamine: May cause megaloblastic anemia in pyrimethamine doses greater than 25 mg weekly. Avoid use together.
Methotrexate: Concurrent use can increase levels. Use together cautiously.
Zidovudine: Serum levels of zidovudine may be increased. Monitor patient carefully.
Cyclosporine: Decreased therapeutic effect and an increased risk of nephrotoxicity. Avoid use together.
Drug-lifestyle. *Sun exposure:* Photosensitivity reaction may occur. Advise precautions.

Effects on diagnostic tests
Trimethoprim can interfere with serum methotrexate assay as determined by the competitive binding protein technique. No interference occurs if radioimmunoassay is used.

Adverse reactions
CNS: headache, mental depression, aseptic meningitis, tinnitus, apathy, ***seizures,*** hallucinations, ataxia, nervousness, fatigue, muscle weakness, vertigo, insomnia.
GI: *nausea, vomiting, diarrhea,* abdominal pain, anorexia, stomatitis, ***pancreatitis,*** pseudomembranous colitis.
GU: *toxic nephrosis with oliguria and anuria,* crystalluria, hematuria, interstitial nephritis.
Hematologic: ***agranulocytosis, aplastic anemia,*** megaloblastic anemia, ***thrombocytopenia, leukopenia, hemolytic anemia, pancytopenia.***
Hepatic: jaundice, ***hepatic necrosis.***
Respiratory: pulmonary infiltrates.
Skin: ***erythema multiforme (Stevens-Johnson syndrome),*** generalized skin eruptions, epidermal necrolysis, exfoliative dermatitis, photosensitivity, urticaria, pruritus.
Other: hypersensitivity reactions (*serum sickness, drug fever,* ***anaphylaxis***), thrombophlebitis, arthralgia, myalgia, rhabdomyolysis.

Overdose and treatment
Clinical signs of overdose include mental depression, drowsiness, anorexia, jaundice, confusion, headache, nausea, vomiting, diarrhea, facial swelling, slight elevations in liver function test results, and bone marrow depression.

Treat by emesis or gastric lavage, followed by supportive care (correction of acidosis, forced oral fluid, and I.V. fluids). Treatment of renal failure may be required; transfuse appropriate blood products in severe hematologic toxicity; use folinic acid to rescue bone marrow. Hemodialysis has limited ability to remove co-trimoxazole. Peritoneal dialysis isn't effective.

Clinical considerations
Consider the recommendations relevant to all sulfonamides as well as the following:
□ ***ALERT*** Note that DS means double-strength.
□ ***ALERT*** Occasionally, dosage is written as trimethoprim component; check it carefully.
□ ***ALERT*** Drug isn't for I.M. use.
- Co-trimoxazole has been used effectively to treat chronic bacterial prostatitis and as prophylaxis against recurrent urinary tract infection in women and traveler's diarrhea.
- For I.V. use, dilute infusion in D_5W. Don't mix with other drugs. Don't administer by rapid infusion or bolus injection. Infuse slowly over 60 to 90 minutes.
- I.V. infusion must be diluted before use. Each 5 ml should be added to 125 ml D_5W. Don't refrigerate solution; diluted solutions must be used within 6 hours. A dilution of 5 ml per 75 ml D_5W may be prepared for patients requiring fluid restriction, but these solutions should be used within 2 hours.
- Check solution carefully for precipitate before starting infusion. Don't use solution containing a precipitate.
- Assess I.V. site for signs of phlebitis or infiltration.
- Shake oral suspension thoroughly before administering.

Therapeutic monitoring
Monitor renal and liver function tests.

Special populations
Pregnant patients. Use only when extremely necessary in pregnant women.
Breast-feeding patients. Drug isn't recommended in breast-feeding women.
Pediatric patients. Drug isn't recommended for infants under age 2 months.
Geriatric patients. In geriatric patients, diminished renal function may prolong half-life. Such patients also have an increased risk of adverse reactions.

Patient counseling
- Inform patient of potential adverse reactions.
- Tell patient to take drug as prescribed, even if he feels better.
- Instruct patient to take oral dose with 8 oz. (240 ml) of water on an empty stomach.

cromolyn sodium

Gastrocrom, Intal Aerosol Spray, Intal Nebulizer Solution, Nasalcrom, Opticrom

Pharmacologic classification: chromone derivative
Therapeutic classification: mast cell stabilizer, antiasthmatic
Pregnancy risk category B

How supplied

Available by prescription only
Aerosol: 800 mcg/metered spray
Solution: 20 mg/2 ml for nebulization
Ophthalmic solution: 4%
Oral concentrate: 100 mg/5ml
Available without a prescription
Nasal solution: 5.2 mg/metered spray (40 mg/ml)

Indications and dosages

Adjunct in treatment of severe perennial bronchial asthma
Adults and children over age 5: 2 inhalations q.i.d. at regular intervals; aqueous solution administered through a nebulizer, 1 ampule q.i.d.
Prevention and treatment of allergic rhinitis
Adults and children age 6 and older: 1 spray (5.2 mg) of nasal solution in each nostril t.i.d. or q.i.d. May give up to six times daily.
Prevention of exercise-induced bronchospasm
Adults and children over age 5: 2 metered sprays using inhaler no more than 1 hour before anticipated exercise.

Inhalation of 20 mg of oral inhalation solution may be used in adults or children age 2 and older. Repeat inhalation as required for protection during long exercise.
Allergic ocular disorders (giant papillary conjunctivitis, vernal keratoconjunctivitis, vernal keratitis, allergic keratoconjunctivitis)
Adults and children over age 4: Instill 1 to 2 drops in each eye 4 to 6 times daily at regular intervals. One drop contains about 1.6 mg cromolyn sodium.
Systemic mastocytosis
Adults: 200 mg P.O. q.i.d.
Children age 2 to 12: 100 mg P.O. q.i.d.
Children under age 2: 20 mg/kg daily P.O. divided in four equal doses.
◊ ***Food allergy, inflammatory bowel disease***
Adults: 200 mg P.O. q.i.d. 15 to 20 minutes before meals.

Pharmacodynamics

Antiasthmatic action: Cromolyn prevents release of mediators of type I allergic reactions, including histamine and slow-reacting substance of anaphylaxis (SRS-A), from sensitized mast cells after the antigen-antibody union has taken place. Cromolyn doesn't inhibit binding of IgE to mast cells nor the interaction between cell-bound IgE and the specific antigen. It does inhibit the release of substances (such as histamine and SRS-A) in response to IgE binding to mast cells. Main site of action occurs locally on the lung mucosa, nasal mucosa, and eyes.
Bronchodilating action: Besides mast cell stabilization, recent evidence suggests that drug may have a bronchodilating effect by an unknown mechanism. Comparative studies have shown cromolyn and theophylline to be equally efficacious but less effective than orally inhaled $beta_2$-adrenergic agonists in preventing this bronchospasm.
Ocular antiallergy action: Cromolyn inhibits degranulation of sensitized mast cells that occurs after exposure to specific antigens, preventing release of histamine and SRS-A.

Cromolyn has no direct anti-inflammatory, vasoconstrictor, antihistamine, antiserotonin, or corticosteroid-like properties.

Cromolyn dissolved in water and given orally has been found to be effective in managing food allergy, inflammatory bowel disease (Crohn's disease, ulcerative colitis), and systemic mastocytosis.

Pharmacokinetics

Absorption: Only 0.5% to 2% of an oral dose is absorbed. The amount reaching the lungs depends on patient's ability to use inhaler correctly, amount of bronchoconstriction, and size or presence of mucus plugs. The degree of absorption depends on method of administration; most absorption occurs with the aerosol via metered-dose inhaler, and least occurs with the administration of the solution via power-operated nebulizer. Less than 7% of an intranasal dose of cromolyn as a solution is absorbed systemically. Only minimal absorption (0.03%) of an ophthalmic dose occurs after instillation into the eye. Absorption half-life from the lung is 1 hour. A plasma concentration of 9 ng/ml can be achieved 15 minutes following a 20-mg dose.
Distribution: Cromolyn doesn't cross most biological membranes because it's ionized and lipid-insoluble at the body's pH. Less than 0.1% of a dose crosses to the placenta; it isn't known if drug is distributed into breast milk.
Metabolism: None significant.
Excretion: Excreted unchanged in urine (50%) and bile (about 50%). Small amounts may be excreted in the feces or exhaled. Elimination half-life is 81 minutes.

Route	Onset	Peak	Duration
P.O., inhalation, intranasal, ophthalmic	Unknown	Unknown	Unknown

Contraindications and precautions
Contraindicated in patients experiencing acute asthma attacks or status asthmaticus and in patients with hypersensitivity to drug. Use inhalation form cautiously in patients with cardiac disease or arrhythmias.

Interactions
None reported.

Effects on diagnostic tests
None reported.

Adverse reactions
CNS: dizziness, headache.
EENT: *irritated throat and trachea,* nasal congestion, pharyngeal irritation, *sneezing,* nasal burning and irritation, epistaxis, lacrimation, swollen parotid gland, bad taste in mouth.
GI: nausea, esophagitis, abdominal pain.
GU: dysuria, urinary frequency.
Musculoskeletal: joint swelling and pain.
Respiratory: ***bronchospasm*** (after inhalation of dry powder), *cough,* wheezing, *eosinophilic pneumonia.*
Skin: rash, urticaria.
Other: ***angioedema.***

Overdose and treatment
No information available.

Clinical considerations
- Bronchospasm or cough occasionally occur after inhalation and may require stopping therapy. Prior bronchodilation may help but it may still be necessary to stop the cromolyn therapy.
- Asthma symptoms may recur if cromolyn dosage is reduced below the recommended dosage.
- Use reduced dosage in patients with impaired renal or hepatic function.
- Eosinophilic pneumonia or pulmonary infiltrates with eosinophilia requires stopping drug.
- Nasal solution may cause nasal stinging or sneezing immediately after instillation of drug but this reaction rarely requires discontinuation of drug.
- Watch for recurrence of asthmatic symptoms when corticosteroids are also used. Use only when acute episode has been controlled, airway is cleared, and patient is able to inhale.
- Protect oral solution and ophthalmic solution from direct sunlight.
- Therapeutic effects may not be seen for 2 to 4 weeks after initiating therapy.

Therapeutic monitoring
- Pulmonary status must be monitored before and immediately after therapy.
- Pulmonary function tests are needed to confirm significant bronchodilator-reversible component of airway obstruction in patients considered for cromolyn therapy.

Special populations
Pregnant patients. Animal studies have shown adverse fetal effects when cromolyn sodium is administered parenterally in high doses with high-dose isoproterenol.
Pediatric patients. Cromolyn use in children under age 5 is limited to the inhalation route of administration. The safety of the nebulizer solution in children under age 2 hasn't been established. Safety of nasal solution in children under age 6 hasn't been established.

Patient counseling
- Teach correct use of metered-dose inhaler: exhale completely before placing mouthpiece between lips, then inhale deeply and slowly with steady, even breath; remove inhaler from mouth, hold breath for 5 to 10 seconds, and exhale.
- Urge patient to call doctor if drug causes wheezing or coughing.
- Instruct patient with asthma or seasonal or perennial allergic rhinitis to administer drug at regular intervals to ensure clinical effectiveness.
- Advise patient that gargling and rinsing mouth after administration can help reduce mouth dryness.
- Tell patient taking prescribed adrenocorticoids to continue taking them during therapy, if appropriate.
- Instruct patient who uses a bronchodilator inhaler to administer dose about 5 minutes before taking cromolyn (unless otherwise indicated); explain that this step helps reduce adverse reactions.

cyanocobalamin (vitamin B_{12})
Bedoz,* Cobex, Crystamine, Cyanoject, Cyomin, Rubesol-1000, Rubramin PC, Vibal

hydroxocobalamin (vitamin B_{12})
Hydrobexan, Hydro-Cobex, LA-12

Pharmacologic classification: water-soluble vitamin
Therapeutic classification: vitamin, nutrition supplement
Pregnancy risk category C (parenteral)

How supplied
Available by prescription only
Injection: 100 mcg/ml, 1,000 mcg/ml
Tablets: 25 mcg, 50 mcg, 100 mcg, 250 mcg, 500 mcg, 1,000 mcg

Indications and dosages
RDA for vitamin B_{12}
Neonates and infants up to age 6 months: 0.4 mcg

Infants age 6 months to 1 year: 0.5 mcg
Children age 1 to 3 years: 0.9 mcg
Children age 4 to 8 years: 1.2 mcg
Children age 9 to 13 years: 1.8 mcg
Adults and children age 14 and older: 2.4 mcg
Pregnant women: 2.6 mcg
Breast-feeding women: 2.8 mcg

Vitamin B_{12} deficiency from any cause except malabsorption related to pernicious anemia or other GI disease

Adults: 30 mcg S.C. or I.M. daily for 5 to 10 days, depending on severity of deficiency. Maintenance dosage is 100 to 200 mcg I.M. once monthly. For subsequent prophylaxis, advise adequate nutrition and daily RDA vitamin B_{12} supplements.
Children: 1 to 5 mg given in single doses of 100 mcg I.M. or S.C. over the course of 2 or more weeks. Maintenance dosage is 60 mcg/month I.M. or S.C.

Schilling test flushing dose

Adults and children: 1,000 mcg I.M. in a single dose.

Pharmacodynamics

Nutritional action: Vitamin B_{12} can be converted to coenzyme B_{12} in tissues and, as such, is essential for conversion of methyl-malonate to succinate and synthesis of methionine from homocystine, a reaction that also requires folate. Without coenzyme B_{12} folate deficiency occurs. Vitamin B_{12} is also associated with fat and carbohydrate metabolism and protein synthesis. Cells characterized by rapid division (epithelial cells, bone marrow, and myeloid cells) appear to have the greatest requirement for vitamin B_{12}.

Vitamin B_{12} deficiency may cause megaloblastic anemia, GI lesions, and neurologic damage; it begins with an inability to produce myelin followed by gradual degeneration of the axon and nerve. Parenteral administration of vitamin B_{12} completely reverses the megaloblastic anemia and GI symptoms of vitamin B_{12} deficiency.

Pharmacokinetics

Absorption: After oral administration, vitamin B_{12} is absorbed irregularly from the distal small intestine. Vitamin B_{12} is protein-bound, and this bond must be split by proteolysis and gastric acid before absorption. Absorption depends on sufficient intrinsic factor and calcium. Vitamin B_{12} is inadequate in malabsorptive states and in pernicious anemia. After oral administration of doses of less than 3 mcg, peak plasma levels aren't reached for 8 to 12 hours.
Distribution: Distributed into the liver, bone marrow, and other tissues, including the placenta. At birth, the vitamin B_{12} concentration in neonates is three to five times that in the mother. Vitamin B_{12} is distributed into breast milk in concentrations about equal to the maternal vitamin B_{12} concentration. Unlike cyanocobalamin, hydroxocobalamin is absorbed more slowly parenterally and may be taken up by the liver in larger quantities; it also produces a greater increase in serum cobalamin levels and less urinary excretion.
Metabolism: Cyanocobalamin and hydroxocobalamin are metabolized in the liver.
Excretion: In healthy persons receiving only dietary vitamin B_{12}, about 3 to 8 mcg of the vitamin is secreted into the GI tract daily, mainly from bile, and all but about 1 mcg is reabsorbed; less than 0.25 mcg is usually excreted in the urine daily. When vitamin B_{12} is administered in amounts that exceed the binding capacity of plasma, the liver, and other tissues, it's free in the blood for urinary excretion.

Route	Onset	Peak	Duration
P.O.	Unknown	8-12 hr	Unknown
I.M., S.C.	Unknown	1 hr	Unknown

Contraindications and precautions

Contraindicated in patients hypersensitive to vitamin B_{12} or cobalt and in patients with early Leber's disease. Use cautiously in anemic patients with coexisting cardiac, pulmonary, or hypertensive disease and in those with severe vitamin B_{12}-dependent deficiencies.

Interactions

Drug-drug. *Aminoglycosides, colchicine, extended-release potassium preparations, aminosalicylic acid and its salts, anticonvulsants, cobalt irradiation of the small bowel:* Concurrent use decreases vitamin B_{12} absorption from the GI tract. Don't use together.
Colchicine: Concurrent administration may increase neomycin-induced malabsorption of vitamin B_{12}. Don't use together.
Ascorbic acid: May destroy vitamin B_{12}; shouldn't be administered within 1 hour of taking vitamin B_{12}.
Chloramphenicol: Antagonized hematopoietic response. Don't give together.
Drug-lifestyle. *Alcohol use:* Decreases vitamin B_{12} absorption from the GI tract. Advise patient to avoid alcohol use.
Smoking: Tell patient to avoid smoking, which appears to increase requirement for vitamin B_{12}.

Effects on diagnostic tests

Vitamin B_{12} therapy may cause false-positive results for intrinsic factor antibodies, which are present in the blood of half of all patients with pernicious anemia.

Methotrexate, pyrimethamine, and most anti-infectives invalidate diagnostic blood assays for vitamin B_{12}.

Adverse reactions

CV: peripheral vascular thrombosis, pulmonary edema, heart failure.
GI: transient diarrhea.

Skin: itching, transitory exanthema, urticaria.
Other: ***anaphylaxis, anaphylactoid reactions*** (with parenteral administration); pain, burning (at S.C. or I.M. injection sites).

Overdose and treatment
Not applicable. Even in large doses, vitamin B_{12} isn't usually toxic.

Clinical considerations
- Recommended RDA for vitamin B_{12} is 0.3 mcg in infants to 2 mcg in adults, as follows:
  Infants up to age 6 months: 0.3 mcg
  Children age 6 months to 1 year: 0.5 mcg
  Children age 1 to 3: 0.7 mcg
  Children age 4 to 6: 1 mcg
  Children age 7 to 10: 1.4 mcg
  Children age 11 to adult: 2 mcg
  Pregnant women: 2.2 mcg
  Breast-feeding women: 2.6 mcg
- Determine patient's diet and drug history, including patterns of alcohol use, to identify poor nutritional habits.
- Administer oral solution promptly after mixing with fruit juice. Ascorbic acid causes instability of vitamin B_{12}. Protect oral solution from light.
- Administer oral vitamin B_{12} with meals to increase absorption.
- Monitor bowel function because regularity is essential for consistent absorption of oral preparations.
- Don't mix the parenteral form with dextrose solutions, alkaline or strongly acidic solutions, or oxidizing and reducing agents, because anaphylactic reactions may occur with I.V. use.
- Parenteral therapy is preferred for patients with pernicious anemia because oral administration may be unreliable. In patients with neurologic complications, prolonged inadequate oral therapy may lead to permanent spinal cord damage. Oral therapy is appropriate for mild conditions without neurologic signs and for those patients who refuse or are sensitive to the parenteral form.
- Patients with a history of sensitivities and those suspected of being sensitive to vitamin B_{12} should receive an intradermal test dose before therapy begins. Sensitization to vitamin B_{12} may develop after as many as 8 years of treatment.
- Expect therapeutic response to occur within 48 hours; it's measured by laboratory values and effect on fatigue, GI symptoms, anorexia, pallid or yellow complexion, glossitis, distaste for meat, dyspnea on exertion, palpitation, neurologic degeneration (paresthesia, loss of vibratory and position sense and deep reflexes, incoordination), psychotic behavior, anosmia, and visual disturbances.
- Therapeutic response to vitamin B_{12} may be impaired by concurrent infection, uremia, folic acid or iron deficiency, or drugs having bone marrow suppressant effects. Large doses of vitamin B_{12} may improve folate-deficient megaloblastic anemia.
- Patients with mild peripheral neurologic defects may respond to concomitant physical therapy. Usually, neurologic damage that doesn't improve after 12 to 18 months of therapy is considered irreversible. Severe vitamin B_{12} deficiency that persists for 3 months or longer may cause permanent spinal cord degeneration.

Therapeutic monitoring
- Monitor vital signs in patients with cardiac disease and those receiving parenteral vitamin B_{12}. Watch for symptoms of pulmonary edema, which tend to develop early in therapy.
- Expect reticulocyte level to rise in 3 to 4 days, peak in 5 to 8 days, and then gradually decline as erythrocyte count and hemoglobin rise to normal levels (in 4 to 6 weeks).
- Monitor potassium levels during the first 48 hours, especially in patients with pernicious anemia or megaloblastic anemia. Potassium supplements may be required. Conversion to normal erythropoiesis increases erythrocyte potassium requirement and can result in fatal hypokalemia in these patients.
- Continue periodic hematologic evaluations throughout patient's lifetime.

Special populations
Breast-feeding patients. Vitamin B_{12} is excreted in breast milk in levels that approximate the maternal vitamin B_{12} level. The Food and Nutrition Board of the National Academy of Sciences-National Research Council recommends that breast-feeding women consume 2.6 mcg/day of vitamin B_{12}.
Pediatric patients. Safety and efficacy of vitamin B_{12} for use in children haven't been established. Intake for children should be 0.5 to 2 mcg daily, as recommended by the Food and Nutrition Board of the National Academy of Sciences-National Research Council.

Some of these products contain benzyl alcohol, which has been associated with a fatal "gasping syndrome" in premature infants.

Patient counseling
- Emphasize importance of a well-balanced diet. To prevent progression of subacute combined degeneration, don't use folic acid instead of vitamin B_{12} to prevent anemia.
- Instruct patient to report infection or disease in case his condition requires increased dosage of vitamin B_{12}.
- Tell patient with pernicious anemia that he must have lifelong treatment with vitamin B_{12} to prevent recurring symptoms and the risk of incapacitating and irreversible spinal cord damage.
- Instruct patient to store tablets in a tightly closed container at room temperature.

cyclobenzaprine hydrochloride

Flexeril

Pharmacologic classification: tricyclic antidepressant derivative
Therapeutic classification: skeletal muscle relaxant
Pregnancy risk category B

How supplied

Available by prescription only
Tablets: 10 mg

Indications and dosages

Adjunct in acute, painful musculoskeletal conditions
Adults: 20 to 40 mg P.O. divided b.i.d. to q.i.d.; maximum dose, 60 mg daily. Drug shouldn't be administered for more than 2 weeks.
◇ ***Fibrositis***
Adults: 10 to 40 mg P.O. daily.

Pharmacodynamics

Skeletal muscle relaxant action: Cyclobenzaprine relaxes skeletal muscles through an unknown mechanism of action. Cyclobenzaprine is a CNS depressant.

Drug also potentiates the effects of norepinephrine and exhibits anticholinergic effects similar to those of tricyclic antidepressants, including central and peripheral antimuscarinic actions, sedation, and an increase in heart rate.

Pharmacokinetics

Absorption: Almost completely absorbed during first pass through GI tract.
Distribution: About 93% is plasma protein-bound.
Metabolism: During first pass through GI tract and liver, drug and metabolites undergo enterohepatic recycling. The half-life of cyclobenzaprine is 1 to 3 days.
Excretion: Excreted primarily in urine as conjugated metabolites; also in feces via bile as unchanged drug.

Route	Onset	Peak	Duration
P.O.	1 hr	3-8 hr	12-24 hr

Contraindications and precautions

Contraindicated in patients who have received MAO inhibitors within 14 days; during acute recovery phase of MI; and in patients with hyperthyroidism, hypersensitivity to drug, heart block, arrhythmias, conduction disturbances, or heart failure. Use cautiously in geriatric or debilitated patients and in those with increased intraocular pressure, glaucoma, or urine retention.

Interactions

Drug-drug. *CNS depressants:* May potentiate the CNS depression. Avoid use together.
Antidyskinetics or antimuscarinics: Antimuscarinic effects may be potentiated when used together. Use together cautiously.
Guanadrel or guanethidine: Cyclobenzaprine may decrease or block the antihypertensive effects. Avoid use together.
MAO inhibitors: Hyperpyretic crisis, seizures and death have occurred with concomitant administration of MAO inhibitors and tricyclics; the potential for this interaction with cyclobenzaprine also exists. Allow 14 days to elapse after discontinuance of MAO inhibitor therapy before starting cyclobenzaprine, and allow 5 to 7 days after discontinuance of cyclobenzaprine therapy and start of MAO inhibitor.
Drug-lifestyle. *Alcohol use:* May potentiate CNS depressant effects when used together. Advise patient to avoid alcohol use.

Effects on diagnostic tests

None reported.

Adverse reactions

CNS: *drowsiness,* headache, insomnia, fatigue, asthenia, nervousness, confusion, paresthesia, *dizziness,* depression, visual disturbances, ***seizures.***
CV: tachycardia, syncope, ***arrhythmias,*** palpitations, hypotension, vasodilation.
EENT: blurred vision, *dry mouth.*
GI: dyspepsia, abnormal taste, constipation, nausea.
GU: urine retention, urinary frequency.
Skin: rash, urticaria, pruritus.
Other: with high doses, watch for adverse reactions similar to those of other tricyclic antidepressants.

Overdose and treatment

Signs and symptoms of overdose include severe drowsiness, troubled breathing, syncope, seizures, tachycardia, arrhythmias, hallucinations, increase or decrease in body temperature, and vomiting.

To treat overdose, induce emesis or perform gastric lavage. As ordered, give 20 to 30 g activated charcoal every 4 to 6 hours for 24 to 48 hours. Take ECG and monitor cardiac functions for arrhythmias. Monitor vital signs, especially body temperature and ECG. Maintain adequate airway and fluid intake. If needed, 1 to 3 mg I.V. physostigmine may be given to combat severe life-threatening antimuscarinic effects. Provide supportive therapy for arrhythmias, cardiac failure, circulatory shock, seizures, and metabolic acidosis as necessary.

Clinical considerations

- Drug may cause effects and adverse reactions similar to those of other tricyclic antidepressants.

■ Note that the antimuscarinic effect of the drug may inhibit salivary flow, resulting in development of dental caries, periodontal disease, oral candidiasis, and mouth discomfort.
■ Drug is intended for short-term (2 or 3 weeks) treatment, because risk-benefit ratio associated with prolonged use isn't known. Additionally, muscle spasm accompanying acute musculoskeletal conditions is usually transient.
■ Spasmolytic effect usually begins within 1 or 2 days and may be manifested by lessening of pain and tenderness and an increase in range of motion and ability to perform activities of daily living.

Therapeutic monitoring
■ Monitor patient for GI problems.
■ Be alert for nausea, headache, and malaise, which may occur if drug is stopped abruptly after long-term therapy.

Special populations
Pediatric patients. Drug isn't recommended for children under age 15.
Geriatric patients. Geriatric patients are more sensitive to the effects of the drug.

Patient counseling
■ Warn patient about possible drowsiness and dizziness. Tell him to avoid hazardous activities that require alertness until reaction to drug is known.
■ Advise patient to relieve dry mouth (anticholinergic effect) with frequent clear water rinses, extra fluid intake, or with sugarless gum or candy.
■ Tell patient to report discomfort immediately.
■ Advise patient to use cough and cold preparations cautiously because some products contain alcohol.
■ Instruct patient to check with dentist to minimize risk of dental disease (tooth decay, fungal infections, or gum disease) if treatment lasts longer than 2 weeks.

cyclopentolate hydrochloride

AK-Pentolate, Cyclogyl, Minims Cyclopentolate*, Pentolair

Pharmacologic classification: anticholinergic
Therapeutic classification: cycloplegic, mydriatic
Pregnancy risk category C

How supplied
Available by prescription only
Ophthalmic solution: 0.5%, 1%, 2%

Indications and dosages
Diagnostic procedures requiring mydriasis and cycloplegia
Adults: Instill 1 drop of 1% solution in eye, followed by another drop in 5 minutes, 40 to 50 minutes before procedure. Use 2% solution in heavily pigmented irises.
Children: Instill 1 drop of 0.5%, 1%, or 2% solution in each eye, followed by 1 drop of 0.5% or 1% solution in 5 minutes, if necessary, 40 to 50 minutes before procedure.

Pharmacodynamics
Cycloplegic and mydriatic action: Anticholinergic action prevents the sphincter muscle of the iris and the muscle of the ciliary body from responding to cholinergic stimulation. This results in unopposed adrenergic influence, producing pupillary dilation (mydriasis) and paralysis of accommodation (cycloplegia).

Pharmacokinetics
Absorption: Rapid onset of action and shorter duration of action than atropine or homatropine.
Distribution: Unknown.
Metabolism: Unknown.
Excretion: Recovery from mydriasis usually occurs in about 24 hours; recovery from cycloplegia may occur in 6 to 24 hours.

Route	Onset	Peak	Duration
Ophthalmic	Rapid	½-1¼ hr	¼-1 day

Contraindications and precautions
Contraindicated in patients with glaucoma, hypersensitivity to drug or belladonna alkaloids, or adhesions between the iris and lens. Use cautiously in children, the elderly, and in patients with increased intraocular pressure.

Interactions
Drug-drug. *Carbachol, cholinesterase inhibitors, or pilocarpine:* Cyclopentolate may interfere with the antiglaucoma action of these drugs. Avoid use together.
Drug-lifestyle. *Sun exposure:* Photophobia may occur. Advise patient to take precautions.

Effects on diagnostic tests
None reported.

Adverse reactions
CNS: irritability, confusion, somnolence, hallucinations, ataxia, ***seizures,*** behavioral disturbances in children.
CV: tachycardia.
EENT: eye burning on instillation, blurred vision, eye dryness, *photophobia,* ocular congestion, contact dermatitis in eye, conjunctivitis, increased intraocular pressure, tran-

sient stinging and burning, irritation, hyperemia.
GU: urine retention.
Skin: dryness.

Overdose and treatment

Signs and symptoms of overdose include flushing, warm dry skin, dry mouth, dilated pupils, delirium, hallucinations, tachycardia, bladder distention, ataxia, hypotension, respiratory depression, coma, and death. Induce emesis or give activated charcoal. Use physostigmine to antagonize cyclopentolate's anticholinergic activity, and in severe toxicity; propranolol may be used to treat symptomatic tachyarrhythmias unresponsive to physostigmine.

Clinical considerations

- Superior to homatropine hydrobromide, cyclopentolate has a shorter duration of action.
- Recovery usually occurs within 24 hours; however, 1 to 2 drops of a 1% or 2% pilocarpine solution instilled into the eye may reduce recovery time to 3 to 6 hours.
- To minimize systemic absorption, doctor should apply light finger-pressure to lacrimal sac during and for 1 to 2 minutes following topical instillation especially in children and when the 2% solution is used.

Therapeutic monitoring

Assess patient's CNS status.

Special populations

Breast-feeding patients. No data are available; however, use drug with extreme caution in breast-feeding women because of potential for CNS and cardiopulmonary effects in infants.
Pediatric patients. Avoid getting preparation in child's mouth while administering. Infants and young children may experience an increased sensitivity to the cardiopulmonary and CNS effects of drug. Young infants shouldn't be given solution more concentrated than 0.5%.
Geriatric patients. Use drug with caution in geriatric patients because undiagnosed narrow-angle glaucoma may be present.

Patient counseling

- Warn patient that drug will cause burning sensation when instilled.
- Advise patient to protect eyes from bright illumination; dark glasses may reduce sensitivity.
- Teach patient to instill drug. Warn him not to touch tip of dropper to eye or surrounding tissue.

cyclophosphamide

Cytoxan, Neosar

Pharmacologic classification: alkylating agent (cell cycle–phase nonspecific)
Therapeutic classification: antineoplastic
Pregnancy risk category D

How supplied

Available by prescription only
Tablets: 25 mg, 50 mg
Injection: 100-mg, 200-mg, 500-mg, 1-g, 2-g vials

Indications and dosages

Dosage and indications may vary. Check literature for recommended protocols.
Breast, head, neck, lung, and ovarian carcinoma; Hodgkin's disease; chronic lymphocytic or myelocytic and acute lymphoblastic leukemia; neuroblastoma; retinoblastoma; malignant lymphomas; multiple myeloma; mycosis fungoides; sarcomas; severe rheumatoid disorders; glomerular and nephrotic syndrome (in children); immunosuppression after transplants
Adults: 40 to 50 mg/kg I.V. in divided doses over 2 to 5 days. Oral dosing for initial and maintenance dosage is 1 to 5 mg/kg P.O. daily.
◇***Polymyositis***
Adults: 1 to 2 mg/kg P.O. daily.
◇***Rheumatoid arthritis***
Adults: 1.5 to 3 mg/kg P.O. daily.
◇***Wegener's granulomatosis***
Adults: 1 to 2 mg/kg P.O. daily (usually administered with prednisone).
◇***Nephrotic syndrome in children***
Children: 2.5 to 3 mg/kg P.O. daily for 60 to 90 days.
≡***Dosage adjustment.*** Adjust dosage of cyclophosphamide in patients with renal impairment.

Pharmacodynamics

Antineoplastic action: Cytotoxic action of cyclophosphamide is mediated by its two active metabolites. These metabolites function as alkylating agents, preventing cell division by cross-linking DNA strands. This results in an imbalance of growth within the cell, leading to cell death. Cyclophosphamide also has significant immunosuppressive activity.

Pharmacokinetics

Absorption: Almost completely absorbed from the GI tract at doses of 100 mg or less. Higher doses (300 mg) are about 75% absorbed.
Distribution: Distributed throughout the body, although only minimal amounts have been found in saliva, sweat, and synovial fluid. The concentration in the CSF is too low for treat-

ment of meningeal leukemia. The active metabolites are about 50% bound to plasma proteins.
Metabolism: Metabolized to its active form by hepatic microsomal enzymes. The activity of these metabolites is terminated by metabolism to inactive forms.
Excretion: Eliminated primarily in urine, with 15% to 30% excreted as unchanged drug. The elimination half-life ranges from 3 to 12 hours.

Route	Onset	Peak	Duration
P.O., I.V.	Unknown	Unknown	Unknown

Contraindications and precautions
Contraindicated in patients with hypersensitivity to drug or with severe bone marrow suppression. Use cautiously in patients with impaired renal or hepatic function, leukopenia, thrombocytopenia, or malignant cell infiltration of bone marrow and in those who have recently undergone radiation therapy or chemotherapy.

Interactions
Drug-drug. *Barbiturates, phenytoin, chloral hydrate*: Increases rate of cyclophosphamide metabolism. Use cautiously.
Corticosteroids: Inhibit cyclophosphamide metabolism, reducing its effect. Eventual reduction of dose or discontinuation of steroids may increase cyclophosphamide metabolism to a toxic level. Use with extreme caution.
Allopurinol, chloramphenicol, chloroquine, imipramine, phenothiazines, potassium iodide, and vitamin A: May inhibit cyclophosphamide metabolism. Monitor patient closely.
Succinylcholine: Prolonged respiratory distress and apnea. Use succinylcholine with caution or not at all.
Doxorubicin: Use of cyclophosphamide may potentiate the cardiotoxic effects. Avoid use together.

Effects on diagnostic tests
Drug may suppress positive reaction to *Candida,* mumps, trichophytin, and tuberculin TB skin tests. A false-positive result for the Papanicolaou test may occur.

Adverse reactions
CV: *cardiotoxicity* (with very high doses and with doxorubicin).
GI: anorexia, *nausea, vomiting* (within 6 hours); abdominal pain; stomatitis; mucositis, ***hepatotoxicity.***
GU: HEMORRHAGIC CYSTITIS, fertility impairment.
Hematologic: ***leukopenia,*** nadir between days 8 to 15, recovery in 17 to 28 days; ***thrombocytopenia; anemia.***
Respiratory: ***pulmonary fibrosis*** (with high doses).
Other: *reversible alopecia,* ***secondary malignant disease, anaphylaxis,*** hypersensitivity reactions; increased serum uric acid levels and decreased serum pseudocholinesterase levels.

Overdose and treatment
Signs and symptoms of overdose include myelosuppression, alopecia, nausea, vomiting, and anorexia.

Treatment is generally supportive and includes transfusion of blood components and antiemetics. Drug is dialyzable.

Clinical considerations
- Follow institutional guidelines for safe preparation, administration, and disposal of chemotherapeutic drugs.
- Reconstitute vials with appropriate volume of bacteriostatic or sterile water for injection to give a concentration of 20 mg/ml.
- Reconstituted solution is stable 6 days if refrigerated or 24 hours at room temperature.
- Drug can be given by direct I.V. push into a running I.V. line or by infusion in normal saline solution or D_5W.
- I.M. injections shouldn't be given when platelet counts are low.
- Oral medication should be taken with or after a meal. Higher oral doses (400 mg) may be tolerated better if divided into smaller doses.
- Administration with cold foods such as ice cream may improve toleration of oral dose.
- Push fluid (3 L daily) to prevent hemorrhagic cystitis. Some clinicians use uroprotectant agents such as mesna. Drug shouldn't be given at bedtime, because voiding afterward is too infrequent to avoid cystitis. If hemorrhagic cystitis occurs, discontinue drug. Cystitis can occur months after therapy has been discontinued.
- Reduced drug dosage is warranted if patient is also receiving corticosteroid therapy and develops viral or bacterial infections.
- Monitor for cyclophosphamide toxicity if patient's corticosteroid therapy is discontinued.
- Nausea and vomiting are most common with high doses of I.V. cyclophosphamide.
- Drug has been used successfully to treat many nonmalignant conditions, for example, multiple sclerosis, because of its immunosuppressive activity.

Therapeutic monitoring
- Monitor uric acid, CBC, and renal and hepatic functions.
- Observe for hematuria and dysuria.

Special populations
Pregnant patients. Advise both male and female patients to practice contraception while taking drug and for 4 months after because drug has teratogenic properties.

Breast-feeding patients. Drug is excreted into breast milk; therefore, discontinue breast-feeding because of risk of serious adverse reactions, mutagenicity, and carcinogenicity in the infant.

Patient counseling

- Emphasize importance of continuing medication despite nausea and vomiting.
- Advise patient to report to doctor vomiting that occurs shortly after an oral dose.
- Warn patient that alopecia is likely to occur, but that it's reversible.
- Encourage adequate fluid intake to prevent hemorrhagic cystitis and to facilitate uric acid excretion.
- Tell patient to promptly report unusual bleeding or bruising.
- Advise patient to avoid individuals with infections and to call immediately if fever, chills, or signs of infection occur.

cycloserine

Seromycin

Pharmacologic classification: isoxizolidone, d-alanine analogue
Therapeutic classification: antitubercular
Pregnancy risk category C

How supplied

Available by prescription only
Capsules: 250 mg

Indications and dosages

Adjunctive treatment in pulmonary or extrapulmonary tuberculosis
Adults: Initially, 250 mg P.O. q 12 hours for 2 weeks; then, if blood levels are below 25 to 30 mcg/ml and there are no clinical signs of toxicity, dosage is increased to 250 mg P.O. q 8 hours for 2 weeks. If optimum blood levels are still not achieved, and there are no signs of clinical toxicity, then dosage is increased to 250 mg P.O. q 6 hours. Maximum dose is 1 g/day. If CNS toxicity occurs, drug is discontinued for 1 week, then resumed at 250 mg/ day for 2 weeks. If no serious toxic effects occur, dosage is increased by 250-mg increments q 10 days until blood levels reach 25 to 30 mcg/ml.
◇ *Children:* 10 to 20 mg/kg (maximum, 750 to 1,000 mg) P.O. daily administered in two equally divided doses.
Urinary tract infections
Adults: 250 mg P.O. q 12 hours for 2 weeks.

Pharmacodynamics

Antibiotic action: Cycloserine inhibits bacterial cell utilization of amino acids, thereby inhibiting cell-wall synthesis. Its action is bacteriostatic or bactericidal, depending on organism susceptibility and drug concentration at infection site. Cycloserine is active against *Mycobacterium tuberculosis, M. bovis,* and some strains of *M. kansasii, M. marinum, M. ulcerans, M. avium, M. smegmatis,* and *M. intracellulare.* It's also active against some gram-negative and gram-positive bacteria, including *Staphylococcus aureus, Enterobacter,* and *Escherichia coli.* Cycloserine is considered adjunctive therapy in tuberculosis and is combined with other antitubercular agents to prevent or delay development of drug resistance by *M. tuberculosis.*

Pharmacokinetics

Absorption: About 80% of oral dose is absorbed from the GI tract.
Distribution: Distributed widely into body tissues and fluids, including CSF. Drug crosses the placenta; it doesn't bind to plasma proteins.
Metabolism: May be metabolized partially.
Excretion: Excreted primarily in urine by glomerular filtration. Small amounts of drug are excreted in feces and breast milk. Elimination plasma half-life in adults is 10 hours. Drug is hemodialyzable.

Route	Onset	Peak	Duration
P.O.	Unknown	4-8 hr	Unknown

Contraindications and precautions

Contraindicated in patients with hypersensitivity to drug and in those with seizure disorders, depression or severe anxiety, psychosis, severe renal insufficiency, or excessive concurrent use of alcohol. Use cautiously in patients with impaired renal function.

Interactions

Drug-drug. *Isoniazid, ethionamide:* Increase hazard of CNS toxicity, drowsiness, and dizziness. Use with extreme caution.
Phenytoin: Cycloserine may inhibit metabolism of phenytoin, producing toxic blood levels. Dosage adjustment may be required.
Drug-lifestyle. *Alcohol use:* May increase incidence of seizures. Discourage alcohol use.

Effects on diagnostic tests

None reported.

Adverse reactions

CNS: ***seizures,*** drowsiness, somnolence, headache, tremor, dysarthria, vertigo, confusion, loss of memory, ***possible suicidal tendencies,*** psychosis, hyper-irritability, character changes, aggression, paresthesia, paresis, hyperreflexia, ***coma.***
CV: ***sudden-onset heart failure.***
Other: hypersensitivity reactions (allergic dermatitis), skin rash, elevated transaminase level.

Overdose and treatment

Signs of overdose include CNS depression accompanied by dizziness, hyperreflexia, confusion, or seizures.

Treat with gastric lavage and supportive care, including oxygen, I.V. fluids, pressor agents (for circulatory shock), and body temperature stabilization. Treat seizures with anticonvulsants and pyridoxine.

Clinical considerations

- Drug should be taken after meals to avoid gastric irritation.
- Specimens for culture and sensitivity testing will be done before first dose, but therapy can begin pending test results; repeat periodically to detect drug resistance.
- Pyridoxine (200 to 300 mg daily) may be used to treat or prevent neurotoxic effects.
- Anticonvulsants, tranquilizers, or sedatives may be prescribed to relieve adverse reactions.

Therapeutic monitoring

- Monitor hematologic, renal, and liver function studies before and periodically during therapy to minimize toxicity; toxic reactions may occur at blood levels in excess of 30 mcg/ml.
- Assess level of consciousness and neurologic function; monitor for personality changes and other early signs of CNS toxicity.

Special populations

Breast-feeding patients. Drug is excreted in breast milk; use cautiously in breast-feeding women.
Geriatric patients. Because geriatric patients commonly have renal impairment, which decreases excretion of drugs, use drug with caution.

Patient counseling

- Explain rationale for long-term therapy.
- Teach signs and symptoms of hypersensitivity and other adverse reactions, and emphasize need to report any unusual effects and rash promptly.
- Warn patient to avoid hazardous tasks that require mental alertness because drug may cause patient to become drowsy or dizzy.
- Advise patient to take drug after meals to avoid gastric irritation.
- Urge patient to complete entire prescribed regimen, to comply with instructions for around-the-clock dosage, and not to discontinue drug without medical approval.
- Explain importance of follow-up appointments.

cyclosporine

Neoral, Sandimmune

Pharmacologic classification: polypeptide antibiotic
Therapeutic classification: immunosuppressant
Pregnancy risk category C

How supplied

Available by prescription only
Capsules: 25 mg, 50 mg, 100 mg
Oral solution: 100 mg/ml
Emulsion solution: 100 mg
Injection: 50 mg/ml
Capsules for microemulsion: 25 mg, 100 mg

Indications and dosages

Prophylaxis of organ rejection in kidney, liver, heart, bone marrow, ◇pancreas, ◇cornea transplants

Adults and children: 15 mg/kg P.O. daily 4 to 12 hours before transplantation. Continue daily dose postoperatively for 1 to 2 weeks. Then, gradually reduce dosage by 5% weekly to maintenance level of 5 to 10 mg/kg/day. Alternatively, administer an I.V. concentrate of 5 to 6 mg/kg 4 to 12 hours before transplantation.

Postoperatively, administer 5 to 6 mg/kg daily as an I.V. dilute solution infusion (50 mg per 20 to 100 ml infused over 2 to 6 hours) until patient can tolerate oral forms.

Note: Sandimmune and Neoral aren't bioequivalent and can't be used interchangeably without doctor supervision. When converting to Neoral from Sandimmune, start with same daily dose (1:1) and follow serum trough levels frequently.

Pharmacodynamics

Immunosuppressant action: Exact mechanism is unknown; purportedly, its action is related to the inhibition of induction of interleukin-2, which plays a role in both cellular and humoral immune responses.

Pharmacokinetics

Absorption: Absorption after oral administration varies widely between patients and in the same individual. Only 30% of an oral dose reaches systemic circulation. Neoral has a greater bioavailability than Sandimmune.
Distribution: Distributed widely outside the blood volume. About 33% to 47% is found in plasma; 4% to 9%, in leukocytes; 5% to 12%, in granulocytes; and 41% to 58%, in erythrocytes. In plasma, about 90% is bound to proteins, primarily lipoproteins. Cyclosporine crosses the placenta; cord blood levels are about 60% those of maternal blood. Cyclosporine enters breast milk.

Metabolism: Metabolized extensively in the liver.
Excretion: Primarily excreted in the feces (biliary excretion) with only 6% of drug found in urine.

Route	Onset	Peak	Duration
P.O.	Unknown	3½ hr	Unknown
I.V.	Unknown	Unknown	Unknown

Contraindications and precautions
Contraindicated in patients hypersensitive to drug or to polyoxyethylated castor oil (found in injectable form).

Interactions
Drug-drug. *Amphotericin B or aminoglycosides:* Increase nephrotoxicity and amphotericin may increase cyclosporine blood levels. Avoid use together.
Immunosuppressive agents (except corticosteroids): Increased risk of malignancy (lymphoma) and susceptibility to infection. Avoid use together.
Erythromycin, ketoconazole, diltiazem, verapamil, fluconazole, itraconazole, and possibly corticosteroids: Increase plasma cyclosporine levels; reduced dosage of cyclosporine may be necessary.
Phenytoin, rifampin, phenobarbital, and co-trimoxazole: Lower plasma levels of cyclosporine. Monitor patient closely.
Drug-food. *Grapefruit juice:* Can increase trough concentrations. Avoid use together.
Drug-herb. *Pill-bearing spurge:* May inhibit CYPSA enzyme effecting drug metabolism; use together cautiously.

Effects on diagnostic tests
None reported.

Adverse reactions
CNS: *tremor, headache,* ***seizures,*** confusion, paresthesia.
CV: hypertension.
EENT: *gum hyperplasia,* oral candidiasis, sinusitis.
GI: *nausea, vomiting,* diarrhea, abdominal discomfort.
GU: ***nephrotoxicity.***
Hematologic: anemia, ***leukopenia, thrombocytopenia,*** hemolytic anemia.
Hepatic: ***hepatotoxicity.***
Skin: acne, flushing.
Other: increased low-density lipoprotein levels, *infections,* hirsutism, ***anaphylaxis,*** gynecomastia.

Overdose and treatment
Signs and symptoms of overdose include extensions of common adverse effects. Hepatotoxicity and nephrotoxicity often accompany nausea and vomiting; tremor and seizures may occur. Up to 2 hours after ingestion, empty stomach by induced emesis or lavage; thereafter, treat supportively. Monitor vital signs and fluid and electrolyte levels closely. Drug isn't removed by hemodialysis or charcoal hemoperfusion.

Clinical considerations
- Cyclosporine usually is prescribed with corticosteroids.
- Consider possible kidney rejection before discontinuation of drug for suspected nephrotoxicity.
- Give dose at the same time each day. Measure oral solution carefully in oral syringe and mix with plain or chocolate milk or fruit juice to increase palatability; serve in a glass to minimize drug adherence to container walls. Drug can be taken with food to minimize nausea.
- Neoral capsules and oral solution are bioequivalent. Sandimmune capsules and oral solution have decreased bioavailability compared with Neoral.

Therapeutic monitoring
Monitor hepatic and renal function tests routinely; hepatotoxicity may occur in first month after transplantation, but renal toxicity may be delayed for 2 to 3 months.

Special populations
Breast-feeding patients. Safety hasn't been established; avoid use in breast-feeding women.
Pediatric patients. Safety and efficacy haven't been established; however, drug has been used in children as young as age 6 months. Use with caution.

Patient counseling
- Teach patient about rationale for therapy; explain possible adverse effects and importance of reporting them, especially fever, sore throat, mouth sores, abdominal pain, unusual bleeding or bruising, pale stools, or dark urine.
- Encourage compliance with therapy and follow-up visits.
- Teach patient how and when to take medication for optimal benefit and minimal discomfort; caution against discontinuing drug without medical approval.
- Advise patient to make oral solution more palatable by diluting with room temperature milk, chocolate milk, or orange juice. Don't use grapefruit juice or food when taking Neoral.
- Tell patient not to rinse syringe with water.

cyproheptadine hydrochloride
Periactin

Pharmacologic classification: piperidine-derivative antihistamine
Therapeutic classification: antihistamine (H_1-receptor antagonist), antipruritic
Pregnancy risk category B

How supplied
Available by prescription only
Tablets: 4 mg
Syrup: 2 mg/5 ml

Indications and dosages
Allergy symptoms, pruritus, cold urticaria, allergic conjunctivitis, appetite stimulant, vascular cluster headaches
Adults: 4 mg P.O. t.i.d. or q.i.d. Maximum dose, 0.5 mg/kg daily.
Children age 7 to 14: 4 mg P.O. b.i.d. or t.i.d. Maximum dose, 16 mg daily.
Children age 2 to 6: 2 mg P.O. b.i.d. or t.i.d. Maximum dose, 12 mg daily.
◇ ***Cushing's syndrome***
Adults: 8 to 24 mg P.O. daily in divided doses.

Pharmacodynamics
Antihistamine action: Antihistamines compete with histamine for H_1-receptor sites on smooth muscle of the bronchi, GI tract, uterus, and large blood vessels; they bind to cellular receptors, preventing access of histamine, thereby suppressing histamine-induced allergic symptoms. They don't directly alter histamine or its release.

Drug also displays significant anticholinergic and antiserotonin activity.

Pharmacokinetics
Absorption: Well absorbed from the GI tract.
Distribution: Unknown.
Metabolism: Appears to be almost completely metabolized in the liver.
Excretion: Drug's metabolites are excreted primarily in urine; unchanged drug isn't excreted in urine. Small amounts of unchanged cyproheptadine and metabolites are excreted in feces.

Route	Onset	Peak	Duration
P.O.	15-60 min	6-9 hr	Unknown

Contraindications and precautions
Contraindicated in patients with hypersensitivity to drug or other drugs of similar chemical structure; in those with acute asthma, angle-closure glaucoma, stenosing peptic ulcer, symptomatic prostatic hyperplasia, bladder neck obstruction, and pyloroduodenal obstruction; in concurrent therapy with MAO inhibitors; in neonates or premature infants; in geriatric or debilitated patients, and in breast-feeding patients.

Use cautiously in patients with increased intraocular pressure, hyperthyroidism, CV disease, hypertension, or bronchial asthma.

Interactions
Drug-drug. *MAO inhibitors:* Prolong and intensify their central depressant and anticholinergic effects. Avoid use together.
CNS depressants: Additive sedative effects result when cyproheptadine is used. Avoid use together.
Thyrotropin-releasing hormone: Serum amylase and prolactin levels may be increased. Monitor patient closely.
Drug-lifestyle. *Alcohol use:* Additive sedative effects result when cyproheptadine is used with alcohol. Discourage alcohol use.
Sun exposure: Photosensitivity reactions may occur. Advise patient to take precautions.

Effects on diagnostic tests
Discontinue drug 4 days before diagnostic skin tests. Antihistamines can prevent, reduce, or mask positive skin test response.

Adverse reactions
CNS: *drowsiness,* dizziness, headache, fatigue, sedation, sleepiness, incoordination, confusion, restlessness, insomnia, nervousness, tremor, ***seizures,*** toxic psychosis.
CV: hypotension, palpitations, tachycardia.
GI: nausea, vomiting, epigastric distress, *dry mouth,* diarrhea, constipation.
GU: urine retention, urinary frequency.
Hematologic: hemolytic anemia, ***leukopenia, agranulocytosis, thrombocytopenia.***
Skin: rash, urticaria, photosensitivity.
Other: weight gain, ***anaphylactic shock.***

Overdose and treatment
Signs and symptoms of overdose may include either CNS depression (sedation, reduced mental alertness, apnea, and CV collapse) or CNS stimulation (insomnia, hallucinations, tremors, or seizures). Anticholinergic symptoms, such as dry mouth, flushed skin, fixed and dilated pupils, and GI symptoms, are common, especially in children.

Treat overdose by inducing emesis with ipecac syrup (in conscious patient), followed by activated charcoal to reduce further drug absorption. Use gastric lavage if patient is unconscious or ipecac fails. Treat hypotension with vasopressors, and control seizures with diazepam or phenytoin. Don't give stimulants.

Clinical considerations
Consider the recommendations relevant to all antihistamines as well as the following:
- Drug can cause weight gain. Monitor weight.

■ Drug also has been used experimentally to stimulate appetite and increase weight gain in children.
■ In some patients, sedative effect disappears within 3 or 4 days.

Therapeutic monitoring
Assess patient's CNS status.

Special populations
Breast-feeding patients. Antihistamines such as cyproheptadine shouldn't be used during breast-feeding. Many of these drugs are secreted in breast milk, exposing the infant to risks of unusual excitability; premature infants are at particular risk for seizures.
Pediatric patients. CNS stimulation (agitation, confusion, tremors, hallucinations) is more common in children and may require dosage reduction. Drug isn't indicated for use in newborn or premature infants.
Geriatric patients. Geriatric patients are more susceptible to the sedative effect of drug. Instruct patient to change positions slowly and gradually. Geriatric patients may experience dizziness or hypotension more readily than younger patients.

Patient counseling
■ Inform patient about potential adverse reactions.
■ Tell patient that GI distress can be reduced by taking drug with food or milk.
■ Instruct patient to report to doctor if tolerance to drug develops, because a different antihistamine may need to be prescribed.

cytarabine (ara-C, cytosine arabinoside)
Cytosar-U

Pharmacologic classification: antimetabolite (cell cycle–phase specific, S phase)
Therapeutic classification: antineoplastic
Pregnancy risk category D

How supplied
Available by prescription only
Injection: 100-mg, 500-mg, 1-g, 2-g vials
Injection: 20 mg/ml (100 mg); 20 mg/ml pharmacy bulk package (1g)

Indications and dosages
Dosage and indications may vary. Check literature for recommended protocols.
Acute myelocytic and other acute leukemias
Adults and children: 200 mg/m² I.V. daily by continuous I.V. infusion for 5 days at approximately 2-week intervals for remission induction; or 30 mg/m² intrathecally (range, 5 to 75 mg/m²) q 4 days until CSF findings are normal, then followed by one additional dose.
◊Dosages up to 3 g/m² q 12 hours for up to 12 doses have been given by continuous infusion for refractory acute leukemias.

Pharmacodynamics
Antineoplastic action: Cytarabine requires conversion to its active metabolite within the cell. This metabolite acts as a competitive inhibitor of the enzyme DNA polymerase, disrupting the normal synthesis of DNA.

Pharmacokinetics
Absorption: Poorly absorbed (less than 20%) across the GI tract because of rapid deactivation in the gut lumen. After I.M. or subcutaneous administration, peak plasma levels are less than after I.V. administration.
Distribution: Rapidly distributed widely through the body. About 13% of the drug is bound to plasma proteins. Drug penetrates the blood-brain barrier only slightly after a rapid I.V. dose; however, when administered by continuous I.V. infusion, CSF levels achieve a concentration 40% to 60% of that of plasma levels.
Metabolism: Metabolized primarily in the liver but also in the kidneys, GI mucosa, and granulocytes.
Excretion: Biphasic elimination of drug, with an initial half-life of 8 minutes and a terminal phase half-life of 1 to 3 hours. Cytarabine and its metabolites are excreted in urine. Less than 10% of a dose is excreted as unchanged drug in urine.

Route	Onset	Peak	Duration
I.V., intrathecal	Unknown	Unknown	Unknown
S.C.	Unknown	20-60 min	Unknown

Contraindications and precautions
Contraindicated in patients hypersensitive to drug. Use cautiously in patients with impaired hepatic function.

Interactions
Drug-drug. *Methotrexate*: When used together, cytarabine decreases the cellular uptake of methotrexate, reducing its effectiveness. Avoid use together.
Gentamicin: Cytarabine may antagonize the activity of gentamicin. Use cautiously.
Digoxin: Combination chemotherapy (including cytarabine) may decrease digoxin absorption even several days after stopping chemotherapy. Digoxin capsules and digitoxin don't appear to be affected. Patient effect and serum digoxin levels must be evaluated.

Effects on diagnostic tests
None reported.

Adverse reactions
CNS: neurotoxicity, malaise, dizziness, headache.
EENT: conjunctivitis.
GI: *nausea; vomiting;* diarrhea; anorexia; anal ulcer; abdominal pain; oral ulcers in 5 to 10 days; high dose given rapidly I.V. may cause projectile vomiting.
GU: renal dysfunction.
Hematologic: ***leukopenia,*** with initial WBC count nadir 7 to 9 days after drug is stopped and a second (more severe) nadir 15 to 24 days after drug is stopped; anemia; reticulocytopenia; ***thrombocytopenia,*** with platelet count nadir occurring between days 12 to 15; *megaloblastosis.*
Hepatic: hepatotoxicity (usually mild and reversible), jaundice.
Musculoskeletal: myalgia, bone pain.
Skin: rash, pruritus.
Other: flulike syndrome, hyperuricemia, infection, fever, thrombophlebitis, ***anaphylaxis,*** edema.

Overdose and treatment
Signs and symptoms of overdose include myelosuppression, nausea, vomiting, and megaloblastosis. Treatment is usually supportive and includes transfusion of blood components and antiemetics.

Clinical considerations
- To reconstitute the 100-mg vial for I.V. administration use 5 ml bacteriostatic water for injection (20 mg/ml) and for the 500-mg vial with 10 ml bacteriostatic water for injection (50 mg/ml).
- Drug may be further diluted with D_5W or normal saline solution for continuous I.V. infusion.
- For intrathecal injection, dilute drug in 5 to 15 ml of lactated Ringer's solution, Elliot's B solution, or normal saline solution with no preservative, and administer after withdrawing an equivalent volume of CSF.
- Don't reconstitute drug with bacteriostatic diluent for intrathecal administration because the preservative, benzyl alcohol, has been associated with a higher incidence of neurologic toxicity.
- Reconstituted solutions are stable for 48 hours at room temperature. Infusion solutions up to a concentration of 5 mg/ml are stable for 7 days at room temperature. Discard cloudy reconstituted solution.
- Dose modification may be required in thrombocytopenia, leukopenia, renal or hepatic disease, and after other chemotherapy or radiation therapy.
- Excellent mouth care can help prevent adverse oral reactions.
- Nausea and vomiting are more frequent when large doses are administered rapidly by I.V. push. These reactions are less frequent with infusion. To reduce nausea, give antiemetic before administering.
- Steroid eyedrops (dexamethasone) may be prescribed to prevent drug-induced keratitis.
- Avoid I.M. injections of any drugs in patient with severely depressed platelet count (thrombocytopenia) to prevent bleeding.
- Pyridoxine supplements may be administered to prevent neuropathies; reportedly, however, prophylactic use of pyridoxine doesn't prevent cytarabine neurotoxicity.

Therapeutic monitoring
- Watch for signs of infection (cough, fever, sore throat). Monitor CBC.
- Monitor intake and output carefully. Maintain high fluid intake and give allopurinol, if ordered, to avoid urate nephropathy in leukemia induction therapy. Monitor uric acid and plasma digoxin levels.
- Monitor hepatic function.
- Monitor patients receiving high doses for cerebellar dysfunction.

Special populations
Breast-feeding patients. It isn't known if drug is excreted in breast milk. However, because of the risk of serious adverse reactions, mutagenicity, and carcinogenicity in the infant, breast-feeding isn't recommended.
Pregnant patients. Caution women of childbearing age to avoid becoming pregnant during therapy. Also, recommend consulting with doctor before becoming pregnant. Drug may harm fetus.

Patient counseling
- Encourage adequate fluid intake to increase urine output and facilitate excretion of uric acid.
- Advise patient to avoid exposure to people with infections. Tell him to call doctor immediately if signs of infection or unusual bleeding occur.

D

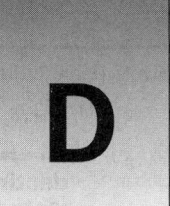

dacarbazine (DTIC)

DTIC-Dome

Pharmacologic classification: alkylating agent (cell cycle-phase nonspecific)
Therapeutic classification: antineoplastic
Pregnancy risk category C

How supplied

Available by prescription only
Injection: 100 mg, 200 mg

Indications and dosages

Dosage and indications may vary. Check current literature for recommended protocols.

Metastatic malignant melanoma

Adults: 2 to 4.5 mg/kg I.V. daily for 10 days, then repeat q 4 weeks as tolerated; or 250 mg/m^2 I.V. daily for 5 days, repeated at 3-week intervals.

Hodgkin's disease

Adults: 150 mg/m^2 I.V. (in combination with other agents) for 5 days, repeat q 4 weeks; or 375 mg/m^2 on day 1 of a combination regimen, repeated q 15 days.

≡ ***Dosage adjustment.*** Reduce dosage when giving repeated doses to patients with severely impaired renal function. Use lower dose if renal function or bone marrow is impaired.

Pharmacodynamics

Antineoplastic action: Three mechanisms have been proposed to explain the cytotoxicity of dacarbazine: alkylation, in which DNA and RNA synthesis are inhibited; antimetabolite activity as a false precursor for purine synthesis; and binding with protein sulfhydryl groups.

Pharmacokinetics

Absorption: Because of poor absorption from the GI tract, dacarbazine isn't administered orally.

Distribution: Believed to localize in body tissues, especially the liver. It crosses the blood-brain barrier to a limited extent and is minimally bound to plasma proteins.

Metabolism: Rapidly metabolized in the liver to several compounds, some of which may be active.

Excretion: Eliminated in a biphasic manner, with an initial phase half-life of 19 minutes and terminal phase of 5 hours in patients with normal renal and hepatic function. About 30% to 45% of a dose is excreted unchanged in urine.

Route	Onset	Peak	Duration
I.V.	Unknown	Unknown	Unknown

Contraindications and precautions

Contraindicated in patients hypersensitive to drug. Use cautiously in patients with impaired bone marrow function.

Interactions

Drug-drug. *Anticoagulants, aspirin:* Increased risk of bleeding. Avoid use together.
Bone marrow suppressants: Additive toxicity. Patient requires careful monitoring.
Amphotericin B: Increased risk of nephrotoxicity. Patient requires careful monitoring.
Phenobarbitol, phenytoin: Increased risk of toxicity. Patient requires careful monitoring.
Drug-lifestyle. *Sun exposure:* Photosensitivity reactions may occur, especially during the first 2 days of therapy. Advise patient to take precautions.

Effects on diagnostic tests

None reported.

Adverse reactions

CNS: facial paresthesia.
GI: *severe nausea and vomiting, anorexia,* diarrhea (rare).
GU: increased serum BUN.
Hematologic: ***leukopenia, thrombocytopenia.***
Hepatic: transient increase in liver enzyme levels, ***hepatotoxicity*** (rare).
Skin: phototoxicity, rash, facial flushing.
Other: *flulike syndrome* (fever, malaise; myalgia, beginning 7 days after treatment ends and lasting possibly 7 to 21 days), alopecia, ***anaphylaxis;*** severe pain (if I.V. solution infiltrates or if solution is too concentrated); tissue damage.

Overdose and treatment

Signs and symptoms of overdose include myelosuppression and diarrhea. Treatment is supportive and includes transfusion of blood components and monitoring of hematologic parameters.

Clinical considerations

- Follow all procedures for safe handling, administration, and disposal of chemotherapeutic drugs.
- To reconstitute drug for I.V. administration, use a volume of sterile water for injection that gives a concentration of 10 mg/ml (9.9 ml for 100-mg vial, 19.7 ml for 200-mg vial).
- Drug may be diluted further with D_5W or normal saline solution to a volume of 100 to 200 ml for I.V. infusion over 30 minutes. Increase volume or slow the rate of infusion to decrease pain at infusion site.
- Drug may be administered by I.V. push over 1 to 2 minutes.
- A change in solution color from ivory to pink indicates some drug degradation. During infusion, protect solution from light to avoid possible drug breakdown.
- Treatment of extravasation with application of hot packs may relieve burning sensation, local pain, and irritation.
- Discard refrigerated solution after 72 hours; room temperature solution after 8 hours.
- Nausea and vomiting may be minimized by administering dacarbazine by I.V. infusion and by hydrating patient 4 to 6 hours before therapy.
- Avoid all I.M. injections when platelet count is less than $100,000/mm^3$.

Therapeutic monitoring

- Monitor uric acid levels.
- Stop drug if WBC count goes to $3,000/mm^3$ or platelet count goes to $100,000/mm^3$. Monitor CBC.
- Monitor daily temperature. Observe for signs of infection.

Special populations

Pregnant patients. Counsel patient to avoid pregnancy. Advise her to inform doctor immediately if she suspects she's pregnant.
Breast-feeding patients. It isn't known if drug is excreted in breast milk. However, because of risk of serious adverse reactions, mutagenicity, and carcinogenicity in the infant, breast-feeding isn't recommended during therapy.

Patient counseling

- Instruct patient to avoid contact with people who have infections and to report signs of infection or unusual bleeding immediately.
- Reassure patient that growth of hair should return 4 to 8 weeks after treatment has ended, but hair is usually of a different texture and its color will be lost as therapy continues.
- Reassure patient that flulike syndrome may be treated with mild antipyretics such as acetaminophen.
- Teach the patient the signs and symptoms of bleeding, and instruct him to report them promptly.

dactinomycin (actinomycin D)

Cosmegen

Pharmacologic classification: antibiotic antineoplastic (cell cycle–phase nonspecific)
Therapeutic classification: antineoplastic
Pregnancy risk category C

How supplied

Available by prescription only
Injectable: 500-mcg vial

Indications and dosages

Dosage and indications may vary. Check current literature for recommended protocols.
Uterine cancer, testicular cancer, Wilms' tumor, rhabdomyosarcoma, Ewing's sarcoma, sarcoma botryoides, ◇Kaposi's sarcoma, ◇acute organ (kidney or heart) rejection, ◇malignant melanoma, ◇acute lymphocytic leukemia, ◇advanced tumors of breast or ovary, ◇Paget's disease of bone
Adults: 500 mcg (0.5 mg) I.V. daily for a maximum of 5 days. Maximum dose is 15 mcg/kg/day or 400 to 600 $mcg/m^2/day$ for 5 days. After bone marrow recovery, course may be repeated.
Children: 15 mcg/kg (0.015 mg/kg) I.V. daily for a maximum of 5 days. Alternatively, give a total dosage of 2,500 mcg/m^2 I.V. over a 1-week period. Maximum dose is 15 mcg/kg/day or 400 to 600 $mcg/m^2/day$. After bone marrow recovery, course may be repeated.

For isolation-perfusion, use 50 mcg/kg for lower extremity or pelvis; 35 mcg/kg for upper extremity.

Dose should be based on body surface area in obese or edematous patients.

Pharmacodynamics

Antineoplastic action: Dactinomycin exerts its cytotoxic activity by intercalating between DNA base pairs and uncoiling the DNA helix. The result is inhibition of DNA synthesis and DNA-dependent RNA synthesis.

Pharmacokinetics

Absorption: Because of its vesicant properties, dactinomycin must be administered I.V.
Distribution: Widely distributed into body tissues, with highest levels found in the bone marrow and nucleated cells. Drug doesn't cross the blood-brain barrier to a significant extent.

Metabolism: Only minimally metabolized in the liver.
Excretion: Excreted in the urine and bile. Plasma elimination half-life of drug is 36 hours.

Route	Onset	Peak	Duration
I.V.	Unknown	Unknown	Unknown

Contraindications and precautions
Contraindicated in patients with chickenpox or herpes zoster.

Interactions
Drug-drug. *Bone marrow suppressants*: May cause additive toxicity. Patient requires close monitoring.
Vitamin K derivatives: Decrease effectiveness of drug. Patient requires close monitoring.

Effects on diagnostic tests
None reported.

Adverse reactions
CNS: malaise, fatigue, lethargy.
GI: *anorexia, nausea, vomiting,* abdominal pain, diarrhea, *stomatitis,* ulceration, proctitis.
Hematologic: ***anemia, leukopenia, thrombocytopenia, pancytopenia, aplastic anemia, agranulocytosis.***
Hepatic: ***hepatotoxicity.***
Metabolic: increased blood and urine levels of uric acid, hypocalcemia.
Musculoskeletal: myalgia.
Skin: *erythema;* desquamation; *hyperpigmentation of skin, especially in previously irradiated areas; acnelike eruptions* (reversible).
Other: phlebitis and severe damage to soft tissue at injection site, reversible alopecia, fever, ***death.***

Overdose and treatment
Signs and symptoms of overdose include myelosuppression, nausea, vomiting, glossitis, and oral ulceration.

Treatment is generally supportive and includes antiemetics and transfusion of blood components.

Clinical considerations
- To reconstitute for I.V. administration, add 1.1 ml of preservative-free sterile water for injection to drug to give a concentration of 0.5 mg/ml. Don't use a preserved diluent, because precipitation may occur.
- Use gloves when preparing and administering this drug.
- Drug may be diluted further with D_5W or normal saline solution for administration by I.V. infusion.
- Discard unused solution because it doesn't contain preservatives.
- Drug may be administered by I.V. push injection into the tubing of a freely flowing I.V. infusion. Don't administer through an in-line I.V. filter.
- Use body surface area calculation in obese or edematous patients.
- Treatment of extravasation includes topical administration of dimethyl sulfoxide and cold compresses.
- To reduce nausea, give an antiemetic before administering. Nausea usually occurs within 30 minutes of a dose.
- Patients who have received other cytotoxic drugs or radiation within 6 weeks of dactinomycin may exhibit erythema, followed by hyperpigmentation or edema, or both; desquamation; vesiculation; and, rarely, necrosis.

Therapeutic monitoring
- Monitor CBC daily and platelet counts every third day. Leukocyte and platelet nadirs usually occur 14 to 21 days after completion of course of therapy. Observe for signs of bleeding.
- Monitor renal and hepatic functions.

Special populations
Breast-feeding patients. Distribution of drug in breast milk is unknown. However, because of risks of serious adverse reactions, mutagenicity, and carcinogenicity in infants, breast-feeding isn't recommended.
Pediatric patients. Restrict use of drug in infants age 6 months or over; adverse reactions are more frequent in infants under age 6 months.

Patient counseling
- Advise patient to avoid exposure to people with infections.
- Warn patient that alopecia may occur but is usually reversible.
- Tell patient to report sore throat, fever, or signs of bleeding promptly.

dalteparin sodium
Fragmin

Pharmacologic classification: low-molecular-weight heparin derivative
Therapeutic classification: anticoagulant
Pregnancy risk category B

How supplied
Available by prescription only
Injection: 2,500 anti-factor Xa IU/0.2 ml, 5,000 anti-factor Xa IU/0.2 ml

Indications and dosages
Prophylaxis against deep vein thrombosis (DVT) in patients undergoing abdominal surgery who are at risk for thromboembolic complications (including those who are over age 40, obese, undergoing general anesthesia lasting longer than 30 minutes,

and with history of DVT or pulmonary embolism)
Adults: 2,500 IU S.C. daily, starting 1 to 2 hours before surgery and repeated once daily for 5 to 10 days postoperatively. In abdominal surgery patients at high risk for thromboembolic complications (such as those with malignant disease), 5,000 IU S.C. daily starting on the evening before surgery and repeated once daily for 5 to 10 days postoperatively. Alternatively, 2500 IU S.C. within 1 to 2 hours before surgery, followed 12 hours later by a second dose of 2,500 IU S.C. , then 5,000 IU S.C. once daily for 5 to 10 days postoperatively.
Prophylaxis against deep vein thrombosis in patients undergoing hip replacement surgery
Adults: 2,500 IU S.C. within 2 hours before surgery and second dose 2,500 IU S.C. in the evening of surgery (at least 6 hours after first dose). If surgery is performed in the evening, omit second dose on day of surgery. Starting on first postoperative day, administer 5,000 IU S.C. once daily for 5 to 10 days. Alternatively, 5,000 IU S.C. on the evening before surgery, followed by 5,000 IU S.C. once daily starting in the evening of surgery for 5 to 10 days postoperatively.

Pharmacodynamics
Anticoagulant action: Drug acts by enhancing the inhibition of factor Xa and thrombin by antithrombin.

Pharmacokinetics
Absorption: Absolute bioavailability measured in anti-factor Xa activity is about 87%.
Distribution: Volume of distribution for dalteparin anti-factor Xa activity is 40 to 60 ml/kg.
Metabolism: Unknown.
Excretion: Unknown.

Route	Onset	Peak	Duration
S.C.	Unknown	4 hr	Unknown

Contraindications and precautions
Contraindicated in patients with hypersensitivity to drug, heparin, or pork products; active major bleeding; or thrombocytopenia associated with positive in vitro tests for antiplatelet antibody in the presence of drug.

Use with extreme caution in patients with history of heparin-induced thrombocytopenia or in those with increased risk of hemorrhage, such as those with severe uncontrolled hypertension, bacterial endocarditis, congenital or acquired bleeding disorders, active ulceration and angiodysplastic GI disease, hemorrhagic stroke; or shortly after brain, spinal, or ophthalmic surgery. Use cautiously in patients with bleeding diathesis, thrombocytopenia, or platelet defects; severe liver or kidney insufficiency; hypertensive or diabetic retinopathy; and recent GI bleeding.

Interactions
Drug-drug. *Oral anticoagulants, platelet inhibitors:* May increase risk of bleeding. Use together with caution.

Effects on diagnostic tests
None reported.

Adverse reactions
Hematologic: ***thrombocytopenia,*** hemorrhage, ecchymoses, bleeding complications.
Hepatic: elevated AST and ALT levels.
Skin: pruritus, rash, *hematoma,* pain or skin necrosis (rare) (at injection site).
Other: fever, ***anaphylactoid reactions*** (rare).

Overdose and treatment
Overdose may cause hemorrhagic complications. These may generally be stopped by the slow I.V. injection of protamine sulfate (1% solution), at a dose of 1 mg protamine for every 100 anti-factor Xa IU of dalteparin given. A second infusion of 0.5 mg protamine sulfate per 100 anti-factor Xa IU of dalteparin may be administered if the activated partial thromboplastin time (APTT) measured 2 to 4 hours after the first infusion remains prolonged. Even with these additional doses of protamine sulfate, the APTT may remain more prolonged than would usually be found following administration of conventional heparin.

Clinical considerations
□ ***ALERT*** Dalteparin should never be administered I.M.
□ ***ALERT*** Drug isn't interchangeable (unit for unit) with unfractionated heparin or other low-molecular-weight heparins.
- Patients receiving dalteparin who require neuraxial anesthesia or spinal puncture may be at increased risk for development of an epidural or spinal hematoma, which can result in long-term or permanent paralysis.
- Patient should assume a sitting or lying down position when drug is administered. Inject dalteparin S.C. deeply. Injection sites include a U-shaped area around the navel, the upper outer side of the thigh, or the upper outer quadrangle of the buttock. Rotate sites daily. When the area around the navel or the thigh is used, use the thumb and forefinger to lift up a fold of skin while the injection is being given. Insert the entire length of the needle at a 45- to 90-degree angle.
- Don't mix drug with other injections or infusions unless specific compatibility data are available that support such mixing.

Therapeutic monitoring
- Periodic routine CBC, including platelet count, and stool occult blood tests are recommended in patients receiving treatment with dalteparin. Patients don't require regular monitoring of PT, INR, or APTT.

- Monitor patient closely for thrombocytopenia.
- Discontinue drug if a thromboembolic event occurs despite dalteparin prophylaxis.

Special populations

Breast-feeding patients. It isn't known if drug is excreted in breast milk; use with caution in breast-feeding women.
Pediatric patients. Safety and effectiveness in children haven't been established.

Patient counseling

- Instruct patient and his family to watch for signs of bleeding and report them to his doctor immediately.
- Tell patient to avoid OTC medications containing aspirin or other salicylates.

danaparoid sodium

Orgaran

Pharmacologic classification: glycosaminoglycan
Therapeutic classification: antithrombotic
Pregnancy risk category B

How supplied

Available by prescription only
Ampule: 750 anti-Xa units/0.6 ml
Syringe: 750 anti-Xa units/0.6 ml

Indications and dosages

Prophylaxis against postoperative deep vein thrombosis (DVT), which may lead to pulmonary embolism in patients undergoing elective hip replacement surgery
Adults: 750 anti-Xa units S.C. b.i.d. beginning 1 to 4 hours preoperatively; then no sooner than 2 hours after surgery. Continue treatment for 7 to 10 days postoperatively or until risk of DVT has diminished.

Pharmacodynamics

Antithrombotic action: Prevents fibrin formation by inhibiting generation of thrombin by anti-Xa and anti-IIa. Because of its predominant anti-Xa activity, danaparoid injection has little effect on clotting assays such as PT, INR, and partial thromboplastin time (PTT). Drug has only minor effect on platelet function and platelet aggregability.

Pharmacokinetics

Drug pharmacokinetics have been described by monitoring its biologic activity (plasma anti-Xa activity) because no specific chemical assay methods are currently available.
Absorption: S.C. administration is about 100% bioavailable, compared with same dose administered I.V. Onset and duration are unknown.
Distribution: Not reported.
Metabolism: Not reported.
Excretion: Mainly eliminated through the kidneys. Mean value for the terminal half-life is about 24 hours. In patients with severely impaired renal function, elimination half-life of plasma anti-Xa activity may be prolonged.

Route	Onset	Peak	Duration
S.C.	Unknown	2-5 hr	Unknown

Contraindications and precautions

Contraindicated in patients with hypersensitivity to drug or to pork products, severe hemorrhagic diathesis (such as hemophilia or idiopathic thrombocytopenic purpura), active major bleeding (including hemorrhagic stroke in the acute phase), or type II thrombocytopenia associated with positive in vitro tests for antiplatelet antibody in the presence of the drug.

Use with extreme caution in patients at increased risk of hemorrhage, such as in severe uncontrolled hypertension, acute bacterial endocarditis, congenital or acquired bleeding disorders, active ulcerative and angiodysplastic GI disease, nonhemorrhagic stroke, postoperative use of indwelling epidural catheter; or shortly after brain, spinal, or ophthalmic surgery.

Use cautiously in patients with impaired renal function and in those receiving oral anticoagulants or platelet inhibitors.

Interactions

Drug-drug. *Oral anticoagulants, platelet inhibitors:* May increase the risk of bleeding; use together cautiously.

Effects on diagnostic tests

Monitoring of anticoagulant activity of oral anticoagulants by PT and Thrombotest is unreliable within 5 hours after danaparoid administration.

Adverse reactions

CNS: insomnia, headache, asthenia, dizziness.
CV: peripheral edema, ***hemorrhage.***
GI: *nausea, constipation,* vomiting.
GU: urinary tract infection, urine retention.
Hematologic: anemia.
Musculoskeletal: joint disorder, pain.
Skin: rash, pruritus.
Other: *fever,* pain at injection site, infection.

Overdose and treatment

Overdose of danaparoid injection may lead to bleeding complications. The effects of danaparoid on anti-Xa activity can't be currently antagonized with other known agents. Although protamine sulfate partially neutralizes the anti-Xa activity of danaparoid and can be safely coadministered, there's no evidence that protamine sulfate is capable of reducing severe nonsurgical bleeding during treatment with danaparoid. If serious bleeding occurs, stop drug and administer blood or blood products as needed.

Symptoms of acute toxicity after I.V. dosing were respiratory depression, prostration, and twitching.

Clinical considerations

□ ***ALERT*** Drug isn't interchangeable (unit for unit) with heparin or low-molecular-weight heparin.

□ ***ALERT*** Don't give drug I.M.

- Drug contains sodium sulfite, which may cause allergic-type reactions, including anaphylactic symptoms and life-threatening or less severe asthmatic episodes in certain patients. The overall prevalence of sulfite allergy in the general population is unknown and probably low. Sulfite sensitivity is seen more frequently in asthmatic than in nonasthmatic patients.
- Risks and benefits of danaparoid injection should be carefully considered before use in patients with severely impaired renal function or hemorrhagic disorders.
- To administer drug, have patient lie down. Give S.C. injection deeply, using a 25G to 26G needle. Alternate injection sites between the left and right anterolateral and posterolateral abdominal wall. Gently pull up a skin fold with thumb and forefinger and insert entire length of the needle into tissue. Don't rub or pinch afterward.

Therapeutic monitoring

- Periodic, routine CBCs (including platelet count) and fecal occult blood tests are recommended during therapy. Patients don't require regular monitoring of PT, INR, or PTT.
- Drug has little effect on PT, INR, PTT, fibrinolytic activity, and bleeding time.
- Monitor patient's hematocrit and blood pressure closely; a decrease in either may signal hemorrhage. If serious bleeding occurs, stop drug and transfuse blood products if needed.

Special populations

Breast-feeding patients. It isn't known if drug is excreted in breast milk; use cautiously in breast-feeding women.

Pediatric patients. Safety and effectiveness in children haven't been established.

Patient counseling

- Instruct patient and family to watch for and report signs of bleeding.
- Tell patient to avoid OTC drugs containing aspirin or other salicylates.

danazol

Cyclomen*, Danocrine

Pharmacologic classification: androgen
Therapeutic classification: antiestrogen, androgen
Pregnancy risk category X

How supplied

Available by prescription only
Capsules: 50 mg, 100 mg, 200 mg

Indications and dosages

Mild endometriosis
Adults: initially, 100 to 200 mg P.O. b.i.d. uninterrupted for 3 to 6 months; may continue for 9 months. Subsequent dosage based on patient response.

Moderate to severe endometriosis
Adults: 400 mg P.O. b.i.d. uninterrupted for 3 to 6 months; may continue for 9 months.

Fibrocystic breast disease
Adults: 100 to 400 mg P.O. daily in two divided doses uninterrupted for 2 to 6 months.

Prevention of hereditary angioedema
Adults: 200 mg P.O. b.i.d. or t.i.d., continued until favorable response is achieved. Then, decrease dosage by half at 1- to 3-month intervals.

Pharmacodynamics

Antiestrogenic action: The antiestrogenic actions of danazol cause regression and atrophy of normal and ectopic endometrial tissue. Drug also decreases the rate of growth and nodularity of abnormal breast tissue in fibrocystic breast disease.

Androgenic action: The androgenic effects of danazol increase levels of the C1 and C4 components of complement, which reduces the frequency and severity of attacks associated with hereditary angioedema.

Pharmacokinetics

Absorption: Amount absorbed by the body isn't proportional to the administered dose; doubling drug dose produces an increase of only 35% to 40% in drug absorption.

Distribution: Unknown.

Metabolism: Metabolized to 2-hydroxymethylethisterone.

Excretion: Unknown.

Route	Onset	Peak	Duration
P.O.	1 mo	6-8 wk	Variable

Contraindications and precautions

Contraindicated in patients with undiagnosed abnormal genital bleeding; porphyria; or impaired renal, cardiac, or hepatic function; during pregnancy; and in breast-feeding patients.

Use cautiously in patients with seizure disorders or migraine headaches.

Interactions

Drug-drug. *Cyclosporine:* Can increase cyclosporine levels and increase chance of nephrotoxicity. Patient requires close monitoring.
Warfarin-type anticoagulants: Prolonged PT and INR. Monitor PT and INR.
Carbamazepine: May increase the plasma levels of carbamazepine in patients taking both drugs. Patient requires careful reevaluation.

Effects on diagnostic tests

Glucose tolerance test results may be abnormal. Total serum T_4 may be decreased; T_3 may be increased.

Adverse reactions

CNS: dizziness, headache, sleep disorders, fatigue, tremor, irritability, excitation, lethargy, mental depression, chills, paresthesia.
CV: elevated blood pressure.
EENT: visual disturbances.
GI: gastric irritation, nausea, vomiting, diarrhea, constipation, change in appetite.
GU: hematuria, *hypoestrogenic effects (flushing, diaphoresis, vaginitis—including itching, dryness,* and *burning— vaginal bleeding, nervousness, emotional lability, menstrual irregularities).*
Hematologic: prolonged PT and INR (especially in patients on anticoagulant therapy).
Hepatic: reversible jaundice, elevated liver enzyme levels, hepatic dysfunction.
Musculoskeletal: muscle cramps or spasms.
Other: androgenic effects in women *(weight gain, hirsutism,* hoarseness, clitoral enlargement, *decreased breast size,* acne, edema, changes in libido, *oily skin or hair,* voice deepening).

Overdose and treatment

No information available. Empty stomach by induced emesis or gastric lavage; follow with activated charcoal to reduce absorption. Treatment is supportive.

Clinical considerations

Consider the recommendations relevant to all androgens as well as the following:

- To treat endometriosis and fibrocystic breast disease, begin danazol therapy during menstruation.
- Danazol provides alternative therapy for patients who can't tolerate or fail to respond to other means of therapy. (It isn't indicated in cases in which surgery is the best choice.)

Therapeutic monitoring

- Because drug may cause hepatic dysfunction, perform periodic liver function studies.
- Advise patient taking danazol for fibrocystic disease to examine breasts regularly. Tell patient to immediately report if breast nodule enlarges during treatment.

Special populations

Breast-feeding patients. Because of the potential for serious adverse reactions in the infant, a decision should be made to discontinue breast-feeding or the drug, depending on the importance of drug to patient.
Pediatric patients. Use with caution because of possible androgenic effects. Use danazol with extreme caution in children to avoid precocious puberty and premature closure of the epiphyses. Conduct X-ray examinations every 6 months to assess skeletal maturation.
Geriatric patients. Use with caution. Observe geriatric male patients for the development of prostatic hypertrophy; symptomatic prostatic hypertrophy or prostatic carcinoma mandates discontinuation of danazol.

Patient counseling

- Tell patient desiring birth control to use a nonhormonal contraceptive; during danazol treatment, ovulation may not be suppressed by hormonal contraceptives.
- Advise patient to report voice changes or other signs of virilization promptly. Some androgenic effects such as deepening of the voice may not be reversible on discontinuation of drug.
- Instruct patient to immediately report nausea, vomiting, headache, and visual disturbances, which may suggest pseudotumor cerebri.
- Advise women that amenorrhea usually occurs after 6 to 8 weeks of therapy.
- Advise men that periodic evaluation of semen may be indicated.

dantrolene sodium

Dantrium

Pharmacologic classification: hydantoin derivative
Therapeutic classification: skeletal muscle relaxant
Pregnancy risk category C

How supplied

Available by prescription only
Capsules: 25 mg, 50 mg, 100 mg
Injection: 20 mg parenteral (contains 3 g mannitol)

Indications and dosages

Spasticity resulting from upper motor neuron disorders
Adults: 25 mg P.O. daily, increased gradually in increments of 25 mg at 4- to 7-day intervals, up to 100 mg b.i.d. to q.i.d., to maximum of 400 mg daily.
Children over age 5: 0.5 mg/kg P.O. b.i.d., increased to t.i.d., then q.i.d. Increase dosage

further, p.r.n., by 0.5 mg/kg up to 3 mg/kg b.i.d. to q.i.d. Maximum dose is 100 mg q.i.d.
Prevention of malignant hyperthermia in susceptible patients who require surgery
Adults: 4 to 8 mg/kg/day P.O. given in three to four divided doses for 1 to 2 days before procedure; administer last dose 3 to 4 hours before procedure. Alternatively, give 2.5 mg/kg I.V. over 1 hour about 75 minutes before anesthesia.
Management of malignant hyperthermia crisis
Adults and children: Initially, 1 mg/kg I.V.; then continue until symptoms subside or maximum cumulative dose of 10 mg/kg has been reached.
Prevention of recurrence of malignant hyperthermia after crisis
Adults: 4 to 8 mg/kg/day P.O. given in four divided doses for up to 3 days after crisis. Alternatively, give 1 mg/kg or more I.V. based on clinical situation.
◊ ***To reduce succinylcholine-induced muscle fasciculations and postoperative muscle pain***
Adults weighing less than 99 lb (45 kg): 100 mg P.O. 2 hours before succinylcholine.
Adults weighing more than 99 lb: 150 mg P.O. 2 hours before succinylcholine.

Pharmacodynamics
Skeletal muscle relaxant action: A hydantoin derivative, dantrolene is chemically and pharmacologically unrelated to other skeletal muscle relaxants. It directly affects skeletal muscle, reducing muscle tension. It interferes with the release of calcium ions from the sarcoplasmic reticulum, resulting in decreased muscle contraction. This mechanism is of particular importance in malignant hyperthermia when increased myoplasmic calcium ion concentrations activate acute catabolism in the skeletal muscle cell. Dantrolene prevents or reduces the increase in myoplasmic calcium levels associated with malignant hyperthermia crises.

Pharmacokinetics
Absorption: 35% of oral dose is absorbed through GI tract, with serum half-life reached within 8 to 9 hours after oral administration. Therapeutic effect in patients with upper motor neuron disorders may take 1 week or more.
Distribution: Substantially plasma protein-bound, mainly to albumin.
Metabolism: Metabolized in the liver to its less active 5-hydroxy derivatives, and to its amino derivative by reductive pathways.
Excretion: Excreted in urine as metabolites.

Route	Onset	Peak	Duration
P.O.	Unknown	5 hr	Unknown
I.V.	Unknown	Unknown	3 hr after infusion ends

Contraindications and precautions
Contraindicated in patients when spasticity is used to maintain motor function in those with upper motor neuron disorders, for spasms in rheumatic disorders, in patients with active hepatic disease, and in breast-feeding women. Contraindicated in combination with verapamil in management of malignant hyperthermia. Use cautiously in women (especially those taking estrogen), in patients over age 35, and in patients with severely impaired cardiac or pulmonary function or preexisting hepatic disease.

Interactions
Drug-drug. *CNS depressant drugs:* Increase CNS depression. Avoid use together.
Estrogen: increased risk of hepatotoxicity. Use together cautiously.
Verapamil: Has resulted in cardiac collapse. Don't use together.
Drug-lifestyle. *Alcohol use*: Increases CNS depression. Advise patient to avoid alcohol.

Effects on diagnostic tests
None reported.

Adverse reactions
CNS: *muscle weakness, drowsiness, dizziness, light-headedness, malaise, fatigue, headache, confusion, nervousness, insomnia,* ***seizures.***
CV: tachycardia, blood pressure changes.
EENT: excessive lacrimation, speech disturbance, altered taste, diplopia, visual disturbances.
GI: anorexia, constipation, cramping, dysphagia, metallic taste, severe diarrhea, GI bleeding.
GU: urinary frequency, hematuria, incontinence, nocturia, dysuria, crystalluria, difficult erection, urine retention.
Hepatic: altered liver function test results; ***hepatitis.***
Musculoskeletal: myalgia, back pain.
Respiratory: pleural effusion with pericarditis.
Skin: eczematous eruption, pruritus, urticaria.
Other: abnormal hair growth, diaphoresis, chills, fever.

Overdose and treatment
Signs and symptoms of overdose include exaggeration of adverse reactions, particularly CNS depression, and nausea and vomiting.

Treatment includes supportive measures, gastric lavage, and observation of symptoms. Maintain adequate airway, have emergency ventilation equipment on hand, monitor ECG, and administer large quantities of I.V. solutions to prevent crystalluria. Monitor vital signs closely. The benefit of dialysis isn't known.

Clinical considerations
- To prepare suspension for single oral dose, dissolve contents of appropriate number of capsules in fruit juice or other suitable liquid.

■ Before therapy begins, patient's baseline neuromuscular functions—posture, gait, coordination, range of motion, muscle strength and tone, presence of abnormal muscle movements, and reflexes—should be checked and documented for later comparisons.
■ Drug may cause muscle weakness and impaired walking ability. Use with caution and carefully supervise patients receiving drug for prophylactic treatment for malignant hyperthermia.
■ Because of the risk of hepatic injury, discontinue drug if improvement isn't evident within 45 days.
■ Risk of hepatotoxicity may be greater in women, patients over age 35, and in those taking other medications (especially estrogen) or high dantrolene doses (400 mg or more daily) for prolonged periods.
■ Clinical signs of malignant hyperthermia include skeletal muscle rigidity (often the first sign), sudden tachycardia, cardiac arrhythmias, cyanosis, tachypnea, severe hypercarbia, unstable blood pressure, rapidly rising temperature, acidosis, and shock.
■ In malignant hyperthermia crisis, give drug by rapid I.V. injection as soon as reaction is recognized.
■ To reconstitute, add 60 ml sterile water for injection to 20-mg vial. Don't use bacteriostatic water, D_5W, or normal saline for injection. Store reconstituted solution away from direct sunlight at room temperature, and discard after 6 hours.

Therapeutic monitoring
Perform baseline and regularly scheduled liver function tests (alkaline phosphatase, ALT, AST, and total bilirubin), blood cell counts, and renal function tests.

Special populations
Breast-feeding patients. Contraindicated for use in breast-feeding women.
Pediatric patients. Drug isn't recommended for long-term use in children under age 5.
Geriatric patients. Use drug with extreme caution in geriatric patients.

Patient counseling
■ Instruct patient to report promptly the onset of jaundice: yellow skin or sclerae, dark urine, clay-colored stools, itching, and abdominal discomfort. Hepatotoxicity occurs more frequently between the third and twelfth month of therapy.
■ Advise patient susceptible to malignant hyperthermia to wear medical identification (e.g., Medic Alert) indicating diagnosis, doctor's name and telephone number, drug causing reaction, and treatment used.
■ Advise patient to avoid excessive or unnecessary exposure to sunlight and to use protective clothing and a sunscreen agent because photosensitivity reactions may occur.
■ Warn patient to avoid hazardous activities that require alertness until CNS depressant effects are determined. Drug may cause drowsiness.
■ Advise patient to report adverse reactions immediately.
■ Tell patient to store drug away from heat and direct light (not in bathroom medicine cabinet). Keep out of reach of children.
■ If patient misses a dose, tell him to take it within 1 hour; otherwise, he should omit the dose and return to regular dosing schedule. Tell him not to double the dose.

dapsone
Avlosulfon*

Pharmacologic classification: synthetic sulfone
Therapeutic classification: antileprotic, antimalarial
Pregnancy risk category C

How supplied
Available by prescription only
Tablets: 25 mg, 100 mg

Indications and dosages
Treatment of multibacillary leprosy
Adults: 100 mg P.O. daily plus rifampin and clofazimine given for 12 months.
Children age 10 to 14 years: 50 mg daily P.O. plus rifampin and clofazimine given for 12 months.
Children under 10 years: Give appropriately adjusted dosage plus rifampin and clofazimine for 12 months.
Treatment of paucibacillary leprosy
Adults: 100 mg P.O. daily plus rifampin given for 6 months.
Children age 10 to 14 years: 50 mg daily P.O. plus rifampin given for 6 months.
Children under 10 years: Give appropriately adjusted dosage plus rifampin for 6 months.
Prophylaxis for leprosy patient's close contacts
Adults and children age 12 and older: 50 mg P.O. daily.
Children age 6 to 12: 25 mg P.O. daily.
Children age 2 to 5: 25 mg P.O. three times weekly.
Infants age 6 to 23 months: 12 mg P.O. three times weekly.
Infants under age 6 months: 6 mg P.O. three times weekly.
Dermatitis herpetiformis
Adults: Initially, 50 mg P.O. daily; may increase dose, p.r.n., to obtain full control.
≡ ***Dosage adjustment.*** Dapsone levels are influenced by acetylation rates. Patients with high acetylation rates may require dose adjustments.

◊ ***Malaria suppression or prophylaxis***
Adults: 100 mg P.O. weekly, with pyrimethamine 12.5 mg P.O. weekly.
Children: 2 mg/kg P.O. weekly, with pyrimethamine 0.25 mg/kg weekly.

Continue prophylaxis throughout exposure and 6 months after exposure.

◊ ***Treatment of* Pneumocystis carinii *pneumonia***
Adults: 100 mg P.O. daily. Usually administered with trimethoprim, 20 mg/kg daily, for 21 days.

◊ ***Prophylaxis of* P. carinii *pneumonia***
Adults: 50 mg b.i.d or 100 mg daily P.O.

◊ ***Prophylaxis against toxoplasmosis in HIV-infected patients***
Adults and adolescents: 50 mg daily with pyrimethamine 50 mg once weekly and leucovorin 25 mg once weekly, P.O.
Children age 1 month or older: 2 mg/kg or 15 mg/m^2 (maximum 25 mg) P.O. once daily plus pyrimethamine and leucovorin.

Pharmacodynamics
Antibiotic action: Drug is bacteriostatic and bactericidal; like sulfonamides, it's thought to act principally by inhibition of folic acid. It acts against *Mycobacterium leprae* and *Mycobacterium tuberculosis* and has some activity against *P. carinii* and *Plasmodium.*

Pharmacokinetics
Absorption: When given orally, drug is rapidly and almost completely absorbed.
Distribution: Distributed widely into most body tissues and fluids; 50% to 90% is protein-bound.
Metabolism: Undergoes acetylation by liver enzymes; rate varies and is genetically determined. Almost 50% of blacks and whites are slow acetylators, and more than 80% of Chinese, Japanese, and Inuits are fast acetylators.
Excretion: Excreted primarily in urine; small amounts of drug are excreted in feces; and substantial amounts in breast milk. Dapsone undergoes enterohepatic circulation; half-life in adults ranges between 10 and 50 hours (average 28 hours). Orally administered charcoal may enhance excretion. Dapsone is dialyzable.

Route	Onset	Peak	Duration
P.O.	Unknown	4-8 hr	Unknown

Contraindications and precautions
Contraindicated in patients with hypersensitivity to drug. Use cautiously in patients with impaired renal, hepatic, or CV disease; refractory types of anemia; and G6PD deficiency.

Interactions
Drug-drug. *Activated charcoal*: Decreases GI absorption of dapsone. Monitor carefully.
Didanosine: May produce a possible therapeutic failure of dapsone, leading to an increase in infection. Avoid use together.
Folic acid antagonists such as methotrexate: Increased risk of adverse hematologic reactions. Avoid use together.
PABA: May antagonize the effect of dapsone by interfering with the primary mechanism of action. Monitor for lack of efficacy.
Probenecid: Reduces urinary excretion of dapsone metabolites, increasing plasma levels. Monitor patient closely.
Rifampin: Increased hepatic metabolism of dapsone. Monitor for lack of efficacy.
Trimethoprim: Increased serum levels of both drugs may occur, possibly increasing the pharmacologic and toxic effects of each drug. Patient requires careful monitoring.
Drug-lifestyle. *Sun exposure:* Photosensitivity reactions may occur. Tell patient to take precautions.

Effects on diagnostic tests
None reported.

Adverse reactions
CNS: insomnia, psychosis, headache, paresthesia, peripheral neuropathy, vertigo.
CV: tachycardia.
EENT: tinnitus, blurred vision.
GI: anorexia, abdominal pain, nausea, vomiting, ***pancreatitis.***
GU: albuminuria, nephrotic syndrome, renal papillary necrosis, male infertility.
Hematologic: ***hemolytic anemia*** (dose-related), ***agranulocytosis, aplastic anemia.***
Respiratory: pulmonary eosinophilia.
Skin: lupus erythematosus, phototoxicity, ***exfoliative dermatitis, toxic erythema, erythema multiforme, toxic epidermal necrolysis, morbilliform and scarlatiniform reactions, urticaria, erythema nodosum.***
Other: fever, tachycardia, ***pancreatitis,*** infectious mononucleosis-like syndrome, ***sulfone syndrome (fever, malaise, jaundice [with hepatic necrosis], exfoliative dermatitis, lymphadenopathy, methemoglobinemia, hemolytic anemia).***

Leprosy reactional states
During therapy for leprosy, two types of reactions related to the effectiveness of dapsone therapy may occur.

Type I, reversal reaction, includes erythema, followed by swelling of skin and nerve lesions in tuberculoid patients; skin lesions may ulcerate and multiply, and acute neuritis may cause neural dysfunction. Severe cases require hospitalization, analgesics, corticosteroids, and nerve trunk decompression while dapsone therapy is continued.

Type II, erythema nodosum leprosum, occurs primarily in lepromatous leprosy, with an incidence of about 50% during the first year of therapy. Signs and symptoms include tender erythematous skin nodules, fever, malaise, orchitis, neuritis, albuminuria, iritis, joint swelling, epistaxis, and depression; skin lesions may ulcerate. Treatment includes one or more of the following drugs while dapsone is continued: corticosteroids, analgesics, and thalidomide.

Additional treatment guidelines are available from National Hansen's Disease Center at the U.S. Public Health Service at Carville, LA, 1-800-642-2477.

Overdose and treatment

Signs of overdose include nausea, vomiting, and hyperexcitability, occurring within minutes or up to 24 hours after ingestion; methemoglobin-induced depression, cyanosis, and seizures may occur. Hemolysis is a late complication (up to 14 days after ingestion).

Treatment is by gastric lavage, followed by activated charcoal; dapsone-induced methemoglobinemia (in patients without G6PD deficiency) can be given methylene blue. Hemodialysis may also be used to enhance elimination.

Clinical considerations

- Give drug with or after meals to avoid gastric irritation. Ensure adequate fluid intake.
- Specimens for culture and sensitivity testing should be done before first dose, but therapy may begin before test results are complete; repeat periodically to detect drug resistance.
- Isolation of patient with inactive leprosy isn't required; however, be sure to disinfect surfaces in contact with discharge from nose or skin lesions.
- Therapeutic effect on leprosy may not be evident until 3 to 6 months after start of therapy.
- Because drug is dialyzable, patients undergoing hemodialysis may require dosage adjustments.

Therapeutic monitoring

- Monitor dapsone serum levels periodically to maintain effective levels. Levels of 0.1 to 7 mcg/ml (average 2.3 mcg/ml) are usually effective and safe.
- Monitor vital signs frequently during early weeks of drug therapy. Frequent or high fever may require reduced dosage or discontinuation of drug.
- Patient requires observation for adverse effects and monitoring of hematologic and liver function studies to minimize toxicity.
- Watch skin and mucous membranes for early signs of allergic reactions or leprosy reactional states.

Special populations

Breast-feeding patients. Dapsone is excreted in breast milk and is tumorigenic in animals. An alternative feeding method is recommended during therapy with dapsone.

Pediatric patients. Use drug with caution in children.

Geriatric patients. Geriatric patients often have decreased renal function, which decreases drug excretion. Use with caution in geriatric patients.

Patient counseling

- Explain disease process and rationale for long-term therapy to patient and family; emphasize that improvement may not occur for 3 to 6 months and that treatment must continue for at least 1 to 2 years.
- Teach signs and symptoms of hypersensitivity and other adverse reactions, and emphasize need to report these promptly; explain possibility of cumulative effects; urge patient to report any unusual effects or reactions and to report loss of appetite, nausea, or vomiting promptly.
- Teach patient how to take drug and of the need to comply with prescribed regimen. Encourage patient to report no improvement or worsening of symptoms after 3 months of drug treatment. Urge patient not to discontinue drug without medical approval.
- Explain importance of follow-up visits and need to monitor close contacts at 6- to 12-month intervals for 10 years.
- Teach sanitary disposal of secretions from nose or skin lesions.
- Assure patient and family that inactive leprosy is no barrier to employment or school attendance.
- New mothers need not be separated from infant during therapy; teach signs of cyanosis and methemoglobinemia.

daunorubicin citrate liposomal

DaunoXome

Pharmacologic classification: anthracycline
Therapeutic classification: antineoplastic
Pregnancy risk category D

How supplied

Available by prescription only
Injection: 2 mg/ml (equivalent to 50 mg daunorubicin base)

Indications and dosages

First-line cytotoxic therapy for advanced HIV-associated Kaposi's sarcoma
Adults: 40 mg/ m^2 I.V. over 60 minutes once every 2 weeks. Continue treatment until there is evidence of progressive disease or until other complications of HIV preclude continuation of therapy.

≡***Dosage adjustment.*** In patients with impaired hepatic and renal function, reduce dosage as follows: If serum bilirubin is 1.2 to 3 mg/dl, give three-fourths the normal dose; if serum bilirubin or creatinine is greater than 3 mg/dl, give one-half the normal dose.

Pharmacodynamics

Antineoplastic action: Daunorubicin exerts its cytotoxic activity by intercalating between DNA base pairs and uncoiling the DNA helix. This results in the inhibition of DNA synthesis and DNA-dependent RNA synthesis. The drug may also inhibit polymerase activity. The liposomal preparation of daunorubicin maximizes the selectivity of daunorubicin for solid tumors in situ. After penetrating the tumor, daunorubicin is released over time to exert its antineoplastic activity.

Pharmacokinetics

Absorption: Must be administered I.V. because of its vesicant nature.
Distribution: Thought to be distributed primarily in the vascular fluid volume.
Metabolism: Metabolized by the liver into active metabolites.
Excretion: Apparent elimination half-life is 4½ hours.

Route	Onset	Peak	Duration
I.V.	Unknown	Unknown	Unknown

Contraindications and precautions

Contraindicated in patients who have experienced a severe hypersensitivity reaction to daunorubicin citrate liposomal or any constituents of this product. Use cautiously in patients with myelosuppression, preexisting cardiac disease, previous radiotherapy encompassing the heart, prior anthracycline use (doxorubicin more than 300 mg/m² or equivalent), hepatic or renal dysfunction.

Interactions

None reported.

Effects on diagnostic tests

None reported.

Adverse reactions

CNS: *headache, neuropathy,* depression, dizziness, insomnia, amnesia, anxiety, ataxia, confusion, ***seizures,*** hallucination, tremor, hypertonia, meningitis, *fatigue,* malaise, emotional lability, abnormal gait, hyperkinesia, somnolence, abnormal thinking.
CV: ***cardiomyopathy (dose related),*** chest pain, hypertension, palpitation, syncope, ***arrhythmias, pericardial effusion, pericardial tamponade, cardiac arrest,*** angina pectoris, ***pulmonary hypertension,*** flushing, edema, tachycardia, ***MI.***
EENT: *rhinitis,* stomatitis, sinusitis, abnormal vision, conjunctivitis, tinnitus, eye pain, deafness, taste disturbances, earache, gingival bleeding, tooth caries, dry mouth.
GI: *nausea, diarrhea, abdominal pain, vomiting, anorexia,* constipation, ***GI hemorrhage,*** gastritis, dysphagia, stomatitis, increased appetite, melena, hemorrhoids, tenesmus.
GU: dysuria, nocturia, polyuria.
Hematologic: **NEUTROPENIA.**
Hepatic: hepatomegaly.
Musculoskeletal: *rigors, back pain,* arthralgia, myalgia.
Respiratory: *cough, dyspnea,* hemoptysis, hiccups, pulmonary infiltration, increased sputum.
Skin: alopecia, pruritus, *increased sweating,* dry skin, seborrhea, folliculitis.
Other: *fever,* splenomegaly, lymphadenopathy, *opportunistic infections, allergic reactions,* influenza-like symptoms, dehydration, thirst, injection site inflammation.

Overdose and treatment

The symptoms of acute overdose are an increased severity of adverse effects such as myelosuppression, fatigue, nausea and vomiting. Treatment is usually supportive.

Clinical considerations

- Administer only under the supervision of clinicians specializing in cancer chemotherapy.

☐ ***ALERT*** Daunorubicin citrate liposomal exhibits unique pharmacokinetic properties compared to conventional daunorubicin hydrochloride and shouldn't be substituted on a milligram per milligram basis.

- Dilute drug with D_5W before administration. Withdraw the calculated volume of drug from the vial and transfer it into an equivalent amount of D_5W. The recommended concentration after dilution should be 1 mg/ml.
- Don't mix daunorubicin citrate liposomal with other drugs, saline, bacteriostatic agents, or any other solution.
- After dilution, immediately administer I.V. over 60 minutes. If unable to use immediately, refrigerate at 36° to 46° F (2° to 8° C) for a maximum of 6 hours.
- Don't use in-line filters for the I.V. infusion.
- A triad of back pain, flushing and chest tightness may occur within the first 5 minutes of the infusion. This triad subsides after stopping the infusion and generally doesn't recur when the infusion is administered at a slower rate.
- Because local tissue necrosis is possible, monitor I.V. site closely to avoid extravasation.
- Follow procedures for proper handling and disposal of antineoplastics.

Therapeutic monitoring

- Monitor and assess cardiac function regularly before administering each dose because of the potential risk for cardiac toxicity and heart failure. Perform determination of left ventricular ejection fraction at total cumulative doses of 320 mg/m^2 and every 160 mg/m^2 thereafter.

- Careful hematologic monitoring is required because severe myelosuppression may occur. Repeat blood counts before each dose. Withhold treatment if absolute granulocyte count is less than 750 $cells/mm^3$.
- Monitor patient closely for signs of opportunistic infections especially because patients with HIV infection are immunocompromised.

Special populations

Pregnant patients. Drug causes severe maternal toxicity and embryolethality; advise patient to avoid becoming pregnant during treatment.
Breast-feeding patients. Safety during breast-feeding hasn't been established. Because of the potential for serious adverse effects occurring in the nursing infant, avoid breast-feeding.
Pediatric patients. Safety and efficacy haven't been established in pediatric patients.
Geriatric patients. Safety and efficacy haven't been established in geriatric patients.

Patient counseling

- Inform patient that alopecia may occur, but is usually reversible.
- Instruct patient to report sore throat, fever, or any other signs of infection; tell patient to avoid exposure to people with infections.
- Advise patient to report suspected or confirmed pregnancy while receiving the drug.
- Tell patient to report back pain, flushing, and chest tightness during the infusion.

daunorubicin hydrochloride

Cerubidine

Pharmacologic classification: antibiotic antineoplastic (cell cycle–phase nonspecific)
Therapeutic classification: antineoplastic
Pregnancy risk category D

How supplied

Available by prescription only
Injection: 20-mg vials (with 100 mg of mannitol)

Indications and dosages

Dosage and indications may vary. Check current literature for recommended protocols.
Remission induction in acute nonlymphocytic leukemia (myelogenous, monocytic, erythroid)
Adults under age 60: 45 mg/m^2 I.V. daily on days 1 to 3 of first course and on days 1 and 2 of subsequent courses. Give all courses in combination with cytosine arabinoside infusions.
Adults age 60 and older: 30 mg/m^2 I.V. daily on days 1 to 3 of first course and on days 1 and 2 of subsequent courses. Give all courses in combination with cytosine arabinoside infusions.
Remission induction in acute lymphocytic leukemia
Adults: 45 mg/m^2/day I.V. on days 1 to 3; give in combination with vincristine, prednisone, and l-asparaginase.
Children age 2 and older: 25 mg/m^2 I.V. on day 1 weekly for up to 6 weeks, if needed; give in combination with vincristine and prednisone.
Children under age 2 or with a body surface area of less than 0.5 m^2: Calculate dose based on body weight (1 mg/kg), rather than body surface area.
≡ ***Dosage adjustment.*** Use reduced dosage if patient has hepatic or renal impairment. In patients with serum bilirubin of 1.2 to 3 mg/dl, reduce dose by 25%; with serum bilirubin or creatinine levels of more than 3 mg/dl, reduce dose by 50%.

Pharmacodynamics

Antineoplastic action: Drug exerts its cytotoxic activity by intercalating between DNA base pairs and uncoiling the DNA helix. The result is inhibition of DNA synthesis and DNA-dependent RNA synthesis. Drug may also inhibit polymerase activity.

Pharmacokinetics

Absorption: Owing to its vesicant nature, drug must be given I.V.
Distribution: Widely distributed into body tissues, with the highest levels being found in the spleen, kidneys, liver, lungs, and heart. It doesn't cross the blood-brain barrier.
Metabolism: Extensively metabolized in the liver by microsomal enzymes. One of the metabolites has cytotoxic activity.
Excretion: Primarily excreted in bile, with a small portion excreted in urine. Plasma elimination has been described as biphasic, with an initial phase half-life of 45 minutes and a terminal phase half-life of 18½ hours.

Route	Onset	Peak	Duration
I.V.	Unknown	Unknown	Unknown

Contraindications and precautions

No known contraindications. Use cautiously in patients with myelosuppression or impaired cardiac, renal, or hepatic function.

Interactions

Drug-drug. *Heparin sodium, dexamethasone phosphate:* Admixture of these agents results in the formation of a precipitate. Don't mix daunorubicin with either heparin sodium or dexamethasone phosphate.
Doxorubicin: Additive cardiotoxicity. Patient requires close monitoring.
Hepatotoxic drugs: Increase the risk of hepatotoxicity. Patient requires close monitoring.

Effects on diagnostic tests
None reported.

Adverse reactions
CV: ***irreversible cardiomyopathy*** (dose-related), ECG changes.
GI: *nausea, vomiting,* diarrhea, *mucositis* (may occur 3 to 7 days after administration).
GU: red urine (transient).
Hematologic: ***bone marrow suppression*** (lowest blood counts 10 to 14 days after administration).
Hepatic: ***hepatotoxicity.***
Metabolic: hyperuricemia.
Skin: rash.
Other: *severe cellulitis, tissue sloughing* (if drug extravasates); *alopecia,* fever, chills.

Overdose and treatment
Signs and symptoms of overdose include myelosuppression, nausea, vomiting, and stomatitis. Treatment is usually supportive and includes transfusion of blood components and antiemetics.

Clinical considerations
□ *ALERT* Reddish color of drug looks similar to that of doxorubicin (Adriamycin). Don't confuse the two drugs.
- Erythematous streaking along the vein or flushing in the face indicates that the drug is being administered too rapidly.
- To reconstitute drug for I.V. administration, add 4 ml of sterile water for injection to a 20-mg vial to give a concentration of 5 mg/ml.
- Drug may be diluted further into 100 ml of D_5W or normal saline solution and infused over 30 to 45 minutes.
- For I.V. push administration, reconstituted drug is withdrawn into a syringe containing 10 to 15 ml of normal saline or D_5W and injected over 2 to 3 minutes into the tubing of a freely flowing I.V. infusion. Reconstituted solution is stable for 24 hours at room temperature and 48 hours in refrigeration.
- Extravasation may be treated with topical application of dimethyl sulfoxide and ice packs to the site.
- Antiemetics may be used to prevent or treat nausea and vomiting.
- Darkening or redness of the skin may occur in prior radiation fields.
- ECG monitoring or monitoring of systolic injection fraction may help to identify early changes associated with drug-induced cardiomyopathy. An ECG or determination of systolic injection fraction should be performed before each course of therapy.
- To prevent cardiomyopathy, limit cumulative dose in adults to 500 to 600 mg/m^2 (400 to 450 mg/m^2 when patient has been receiving other cardiotoxic agents, such as cyclophosphamide, or radiation therapy that encompasses the heart).

Therapeutic monitoring
- Monitor CBC and hepatic function.
- A high resting pulse rate must be reported to doctor (a sign of cardiac adverse reactions).
- Don't use a scalp tourniquet or apply ice to prevent alopecia, because doing so may compromise effectiveness of drug.

Special populations
Breast-feeding patients. It isn't known if drug is excreted in breast milk. However, because of potential for serious adverse reactions, mutagenicity, and carcinogenicity in the infant, breast-feeding isn't recommended.
Pediatric patients. Children have an increased incidence of drug-induced cardiotoxicity, which may occur at lower doses. Total lifetime dosage for children over age 2 is 300 mg/m^2; for children under age 2, 10 mg/kg.
Geriatric patients. Geriatric patients have an increased incidence of drug-induced cardiotoxicity. Monitor for hematologic toxicity because some geriatric patients have poor bone marrow reserve.

Patient counseling
- Warn patient that urine may be red for 1 to 2 days and that this is a drug effect, not bleeding.
- Advise patient that alopecia may occur, but that it's usually reversible.
- Tell patient to avoid exposure to people with infections.
- Encourage adequate fluid intake to increase urine output and facilitate excretion of uric acid.
- Warn patient that nausea and vomiting may be severe and may last for 24 to 48 hours.
- Instruct patient to call if a sore throat, fever, or signs of bleeding occurs.

deferoxamine mesylate
Desferal

Pharmacologic classification: chelating agent
Therapeutic classification: heavy metal antagonist
Pregnancy risk category C

How supplied
Available by prescription only
Injectable powder for injection: 500-mg vial

Indications and dosages
Acute iron intoxication
Adults and children: 1 g I.M. or I.V. (I.M. injection is preferred route for all patients in shock), followed by 500 mg I.M. or I.V. q 4 hours for two doses; then 500 mg I.M. or I.V. q 4 to 12 hours, if needed. I.V. infusion rate shouldn't exceed 15 mg/kg/hour for the first 1 g. Subsequently, rate shouldn't exceed

125 mg/hour. Don't exceed 6 g in 24 hours. (reserve I.V. infusion for patients in CV collapse.)
Chronic iron overload resulting from multiple transfusions
Adults and children: 500 mg to 1 g I.M. daily and 2 g slow I.V. infusion in separate solution along with each unit of blood transfused. I.V. infusion rate shouldn't exceed 15 mg/kg/hour. Alternatively, give 1 to 2 g via an S.C. infusion pump over 8 to 24 hours.

Pharmacodynamics
Chelating action: Deferoxamine chelates iron by binding ferric ions to the 3 hydroxamic groups of the molecule, preventing it from entering into further chemical reactions. It also chelates aluminum to a lesser extent.

Pharmacokinetics
Absorption: Absorbed poorly after oral administration; however, absorption may occur in patients with acute iron toxicity.
Distribution: Distributed widely into the body after parenteral administration.
Metabolism: Small amounts are metabolized by plasma enzymes.
Excretion: Excreted in urine as unchanged drug or as ferrioxamine, the deferoxamine-iron complex.

Route	Onset	Peak	Duration
I.V., I.M., S.C.	Unknown	Unknown	Unknown

Contraindications and precautions
Contraindicated in patients with severe renal disease or anuria. Use cautiously in patients with impaired renal function.

Interactions
Ascorbic acid: Increases availability of iron for chelation. Administer together except for patients with cardiac failure.

Effects on diagnostic tests
None reported.

Adverse reactions
CV: tachycardia (with long-term use).
EENT: blurred vision, cataracts, hearing loss, visual field defects.
GI: diarrhea, abdominal discomfort (with long-term use), nausea, vomiting.
GU: dysuria (with long-term use).
Musculoskeletal: leg cramps.
Other: hypersensitivity reactions (cutaneous wheal formation, pruritus, rash, ***anaphylaxis***); pain and induration at injection site; fever; *erythema, urticaria, hypotension,* ***shock*** (after too-rapid I.V. administration), susceptibility to infection.

Overdose and treatment
Acute intoxication is anticipated to include extension and exacerbation of adverse reactions. Treat symptomatically. Drug can be removed by hemodialysis.

Clinical considerations
□ ***ALERT*** Observe closely and be prepared to treat hypersensitivity reactions; have epinephrine 1:1,000 available.
- Use I.M. route for acute iron intoxication if patient isn't in shock. If patient is in shock, administer I.V. slowly; avoid S.C. route.
- Drug has been used to treat iron overload from congenital anemias and in the diagnosis and treatment of primary hemochromatosis. It's been applied topically to remove corneal rust rings and has been used I.V. or intraperitoneally to promote aluminum excretion or removal.
- Drug has also been used experimentally as a chelator to reduce aluminum levels in bones of patients with renal failure and in patients presenting with dialysis-induced encephalopathy. It also slows cognitive deterioration by 50%.

Therapeutic monitoring
- Monitor fluid intake and output carefully.
- Monitor renal, vision, and hearing function throughout therapy.

Special populations
Pregnant patients. Drug can cause fetal anomalies. Don't administer to pregnant patient unless the benefits outweigh the risks.
Pediatric patients. Drug is safe and effective in children over age 3. Monitor child's growth.
Geriatric patients. Use drug with caution because geriatric patients are more likely to have visual or hearing impairment and renal dysfunction than younger patients.

Patient counseling
- Advise patient that ophthalmic and, possibly, audiometric examinations are needed every 3 to 6 months during continuous therapy; stress importance of reporting changes in vision or hearing.
- Explain that drug may turn urine red.

delavirdine mesylate
Rescriptor

Pharmacologic classification: nonnucleoside reverse-transcriptase inhibitor of HIV-1
Therapeutic classification: antiviral
Pregnancy risk category C

How supplied
Available by prescription only
Tablets: 100 mg, 200 mg

Indications and dosages

HIV infection

Adults: 400 mg P.O. t.i.d.; use with other antiretroviral agents as appropriate.

Pharmacodynamics

Antiviral action: Delavirdine is a non-nucleoside reverse transcriptase (RT) inhibitor of HIV-1. It binds directly to RT and blocks RNA- and DNA-dependent DNA polymerase activities.

Pharmacokinetics

Absorption: Rapidly absorbed following oral administration.

Distribution: 98% bound to plasma proteins, primarily albumin. Distribution into CSF, saliva, and semen is about 0.4%, 6%, and 2%, respectively, of the corresponding plasma levels.

Metabolism: Converted to several inactive metabolites; primarily metabolized in liver by cytochrome P-450 3A (CYP3A) enzyme system; however, CYP2D6 may also be involved. Delavirdine can reduce CYP3A activity and can inhibit its own metabolism; this is usually reversed within 1 week after discontinuation of the drug. CYP2C9 and CYP2C19 activity may also be reduced by delavirdine.

Excretion: After many doses, 44% of the dose was recovered in feces and 51% was excreted in urine. Less than 5% of the dose was recovered unchanged in urine. Mean elimination half-life was 5¾ hours.

Route	Onset	Peak	Duration
P.O.	Unknown	1 hr	Unknown

Contraindications and precautions

Contraindicated in patients with hypersensitivity to formulation of drug. Use caution when administering to patients with impaired hepatic function. Nonnucleoside RT inhibitors, when used alone or in combination, may confer cross-resistance to other drugs in that class.

Interactions

Drug-drug. *Phenobarbital:* Use drugs together cautiously.

Nonsedating antihistamines, indinavir, saquinavir, clarithromycin, dapsone, rifabutin, benzodiazepines, sedative hypnotics, quinidine, warfarin, calcium channel blockers, ergot alkaloid preparations, amphetamines, and cisapride: Increase or prolong both therapeutic and adverse effects. Avoid use together; however, reduced doses of indinavir with delavirdine may be used.

Ketoconazole, clarithromycin, and fluoxetine: Cause a 50% increase in delavirdine bioavailability. Patient requires monitoring.

Carbamazepine, phenobarbital, phenytoin, rifabutin, rifampin: Decrease plasma delavirdine levels; use with caution.

Antacids: Reduced absorption of delavirdine. Separate doses by at least 1 hour.

H_2-receptor antagonists: Increased gastric pH reduces absorption of delavirdine. Long-term use of these drugs with delavirdine isn't recommended.

Didanosine: Coadministration with delavirdine results in 20% decrease in absorption of both drugs. Separate doses by at least 1 hour.

Indinavir: Increased plasma levels. Consider a lower dose of indinavir when given with delavirdine.

Saquinavir: Five-fold increase in bioavailability. Monitor AST and ALT levels frequently when used together.

Effects on diagnostic tests

None reported.

Adverse reactions

CNS: asthenia, *fatigue,* headache, abnormal coordination, agitation, amnesia, anxiety, change in dreams, lethargy, malaise, cognitive impairment, confusion, depression, disorientation, emotional lability, hallucinations, hyperesthesia, hyperreflexia, hypesthesia, impaired concentration, insomnia, manic symptoms, muscle cramps, nervousness, neuropathy, nightmares, nystagmus, paralysis, paranoid symptoms, paresthesia, restlessness, somnolence, tingling, tremor, vertigo, weakness, pallor.

CV: ***bradycardia,*** palpitation, orthostatic hypotension, syncope, tachycardia, vasodilation, chest pain.

EENT: blepharitis, conjunctivitis, diplopia, dry eyes, ear pain, photophobia, taste perversion, tinnitus.

GI: *nausea,* vomiting, diarrhea, anorexia, aphthous stomatitis, bloody stools, colitis, constipation, decreased appetite, diverticulitis, duodenitis, dry mouth, dyspepsia, dysphagia, enteritis, esophagitis, fecal incontinence, flatulence, gagging, gastritis, gastroesophageal reflux, ***GI bleeding,*** gingivitis, gum hemorrhage, increased thirst and appetite, increased saliva, mouth ulcer, nonspecific ***hepatitis, pancreatitis,*** sialadenitis, stomatitis, tongue edema or ulceration, abdominal cramps, distention, pain (generalized or localized).

GU: breast enlargement, renal calculi, epididymitis, hematuria, hemospermia, impotence, renal pain, metrorrhagia, nocturia, polyuria, proteinuria, vaginal moniliasis, decreased libido.

Hematologic: bruises, ***anemia,*** ecchymosis, eosinophilia, ***granulocytosis, neutropenia, pancytopenia,*** petechia, prolonged PTT, purpura, spleen disorder, ***thrombocytopenia.***

Hepatic: *increased ALT and AST levels.*

Metabolic: alcohol intolerance; bilirubinemia; hyperkalemia; hyperuricemia; hypocalcemia; hyponatremia; hypophosphatemia; increased gamma-glutamyltransferase, lipase, serum alkaline phosphatase, serum amylase, and serum CK; peripheral edema; weight gain or loss.

Musculoskeletal: flank pain, back pain, pain (generalized or localized), neck rigidity, arthralgia or arthritis of single and many joints, bone pain, leg cramps, muscular weakness, myalgia, tendon disorder, tenosynovitis, tetany.
Respiratory: upper respiratory infection, bronchitis, chest congestion, cough, dyspnea, epistaxis, laryngismus, pharyngitis, rhinitis, sinusitis.
Skin: epidermal cyst, *rash, pruritus,* ***angioedema,*** dermal leukocytoblastic vasculitis, dermatitis, desquamation, diaphoresis, dry skin, erythema multiforme, folliculitis, fungal dermatitis, alopecia, nail disorder, petechial rash, seborrhea, skin nodule, ***Stevens-Johnson syndrome,*** urticaria.
Other: ***allergic reaction,*** chills, edema (generalized or localized), fever, flu syndrome, lip edema, sebaceous cyst, trauma.

Overdose and treatment

Although no information is available, provide supportive treatment. Remove drug by gastric lavage or emesis, if needed. Dialysis is unlikely to be effective because drug is highly protein-bound.

Clinical considerations

- Rash is more common in patients with lower CD4+ cell counts and usually occurs within the first 3 weeks of treatment. Severe rash has occurred in 3.6% of patients. In most cases, rash lasted less than 2 weeks and didn't require dose reduction or drug discontinuation. Most patients were able to resume therapy after treatment interruption caused by rash.
- Rash occurs mainly on the upper body and proximal arms, with decreasing lesion intensity on the neck and face and less on the rest of the trunk and limbs. Erythema multiforme and Stevens-Johnson syndrome are rarely seen, and have resolved after drug was stopped. Occurrence of drug-related rash after 1 month of therapy is uncommon unless prolonged interruption of drug treatment occurs.
- Symptomatic relief may be obtained by using diphenhydramine, hydroxyzine, or topical corticosteroids.

Therapeutic monitoring

- Neutropenia (absolute neutrophil count less than 750/mm³), anemia (hemoglobin less than 7 g/dl), thrombocytopenia (platelet count less than 50,000/mm³), ALT and AST (more than five times upper limit of normal), bilirubin (more than 2½ times upper limit of normal) and amylase (more than twice upper limit of normal) may occur while on delavirdine. Monitor patient carefully.
- Monitor patients with hepatic or renal impairment because effect of drug hasn't been studied.

Special populations

Breast-feeding patients. Women infected with HIV are advised not to breast-feed.
Pediatric patients. Safety and effectiveness haven't been studied in patients under age 16.
Geriatric patients. Safety and effectiveness haven't been studied in patients over age 65.

Patient counseling

- Instruct patient to discontinue drug and call doctor if severe rash or symptoms such as fever, blistering, oral lesions, conjunctivitis, swelling, or muscle or joint aches occur.
- Tell patient that drug isn't a cure for HIV-1 infection. He may continue to acquire illnesses associated with HIV-1 infection, including opportunistic infections. Therapy doesn't reduce the incidence or frequency of such illnesses.
- Advise patient to remain under medical supervision when taking drug because long-term effects aren't known.
- Inform patient to take drug as prescribed and not to alter doses without medical approval. If a dose is missed, tell him to take the next dose as soon as possible; he shouldn't double the next dose.
- Inform patient that drug may be dispersed in water before ingestion. Add tablets to at least 3 oz (90 ml) of water, allow to stand for a few minutes, and stir until a uniform dispersion occurs. Tell patient to drink dispersion promptly, rinse glass, and swallow the rinse to ensure that entire dose is consumed.
- Advise patient with achlorhydria to take drug with an acidic beverage such as orange or cranberry juice.
- Advise patient to report the use of other prescription or OTC medications to doctor.

demeclocycline hydrochloride

Declomycin

Pharmacologic classification: tetracycline antibiotic
Therapeutic classification: antibiotic
Pregnancy risk category D

How supplied

Available by prescription only
Tablets (film-coated): 150 mg, 300 mg

Indications and dosages

Infections caused by susceptible organisms
Adults: 150 mg P.O. q 6 hours, or 300 mg P.O. q 12 hours.
Children over age 8: 6.6 to 13.2 mg/kg P.O. daily, divided q 6 to 12 hours.

Gonorrhea
Adults: 600 mg P.O. initially, then 300 mg P.O. q 12 hours for 4 days (total, 3 g).
◇ ***SIADH secretion (a hypo-osmolar state)***
Adults: 600 to 1,200 mg P.O. daily in three or four divided doses.

Pharmacodynamics

Antibacterial action: Demeclocycline is bacteriostatic. Tetracyclines bind reversibly to ribosomal subunits, thereby inhibiting bacterial protein synthesis. Demeclocycline is active against many gram-negative and gram-positive organisms, *Mycoplasma, Rickettsia, Chlamydia,* and spirochetes.

Pharmacokinetics

Absorption: About 60% to 80% is absorbed from the GI tract after oral administration; peak serum levels occur at 3 to 4 hours. Food or milk reduces absorption by 50%; antacids chelate with tetracyclines and further reduce absorption. Drug has the greatest affinity of all tetracyclines for calcium ions.
Distribution: Distributed widely into body tissues and fluids, including synovial, pleural, prostatic, and seminal fluids; bronchial secretions; saliva; and aqueous humor; CSF penetration is poor. Drug crosses the placenta; about 36% to 91% is protein-bound.
Metabolism: Not metabolized.
Excretion: Excreted primarily unchanged in urine by glomerular filtration; some drug may be excreted in breast milk. Plasma half-life is 10 to 17 hours in adults with normal renal function. Hemodialysis and peritoneal dialysis remove only minimal amounts of demeclocycline.

Route	Onset	Peak	Duration
P.O.	Unknown	3-4 hr	Unknown

Contraindications and precautions

Contraindicated in patients with hypersensitivity to drug or other tetracyclines. Use cautiously in women during second half of pregnancy, in children under age 8, and in patients with impaired renal or hepatic function.

Interactions

Drug-drug. *Antacids containing aluminum, calcium, or magnesium or laxatives containing aluminum, magnesium, calcium and antidiarrheals, iron products, zinc, and sodium bicarbonate:* Oral absorption of tetracyclines is impaired by concurrent use. Avoid using together.
Penicillin: May interfere with bactericidal action of penicillin; administer penicillin 2 to 3 hours before tetracycline.
Methoxyflurane: Increases the risk of nephrotoxicity. Avoid use together.
Oral anticoagulants: Increased anticoagulant effect. Monitor INR and PT, dose may require adjustment.
Digoxin: Lowered dosages of digoxin because of increased bioavailability. Monitor serum digoxin levels.
Oral contraceptives: May render oral contraceptives less effective. Breakthrough bleeding has been reported. Recommend a nonhormonal birth control method.
Drug-food. *Food, milk, other dairy products:* May impair absorption of tetracyclines. Antibiotic must be given 1 hour before or 2 hours after these food products.
Drug-lifestyle. *Sun exposure:* May potentiate photosensitivity reactions. Advise patient to take precautions.

Effects on diagnostic tests

Drug causes false-negative results in urine tests using glucose oxidase reagent (Diastix, Chemstrip uG, or glucose enzymatic test strip). It also causes false elevations in fluorometric tests for urinary catecholamines.

Adverse reactions

CNS: ***intracranial hypertension (pseudotumor cerebri),*** dizziness.
CV: pericarditis.
EENT: dysphagia, glossitis, tinnitus, visual disturbances.
GI: anorexia, *nausea, vomiting, diarrhea,* enterocolitis, anogenital inflammation, ***pancreatitis.***
GU: *increased BUN level.*
Hematologic: ***neutropenia,*** eosinophilia, ***thrombocytopenia, hemolytic anemia.***
Hepatic: elevated liver enzymes.
Skin: *maculopapular and erythematous rash, photosensitivity, increased pigmentation, urticaria.*
Other: hypersensitivity reactions ***(anaphylaxis),*** diabetes insipidus syndrome (polyuria, polydipsia, weakness), permanent tooth discoloration or bone growth retardation if used in children under age 8.

Overdose and treatment

Clinical signs of overdose are usually limited to the GI tract. Treatment may include antacids or gastric lavage if ingestion occurred within the preceding 4 hours.

Clinical considerations

Consider the recommendations relevant to all tetracyclines as well as the following:
◘ ***ALERT*** Check expiration date. Outdated or deteriorated tetracyclines have been associated with reversible nephrotoxicity (Fanconi's syndrome).
▪ As an anti-infective, drug is usually reserved for patients intolerant of other antibiotics.

Therapeutic monitoring
- A reversible diabetes insipidus syndrome has been reported with long-term use of demeclocycline; monitor patient for this disorder (weakness, polyuria, polydipsia).
- Monitor renal and liver function tests.
- Monitor fluid balance and daily weights in patients with impaired renal or liver function.

Special populations
Pregnant patients. Advise women taking oral contraceptives to use barrier contraceptives for duration of drug treatment.
Breast-feeding patients. Avoid use of drug in breast-feeding women.
Pediatric patients. Don't use drug in children under age 8.

Patient counseling
- Instruct patient to take entire amount of medication exactly as prescribed, even if he feels better.
- Tell patient to report signs and symptoms of superinfection.
- Advise patient not to expose drug to light or heat; store in tightly capped container.
- Stress good oral hygiene.

desipramine hydrochloride
Norpramin

Pharmacologic classification: dibenzazepine tricyclic antidepressant
Therapeutic classification: antidepressant
Pregnancy risk category NR

How supplied
Available by prescription only
Tablets: 10 mg, 25 mg, 50 mg, 75 mg, 100 mg, 150 mg
Tablets (film-coated): 10 mg, 25 mg, 50 mg, 75 mg, 100 mg, 150 mg

Indications and dosages
Depression
Adults: 100 to 200 mg P.O. daily in divided doses, increasing to maximum of 300 mg daily. Alternatively, the entire dose can be given once daily, usually h.s.
Geriatric patients and adolescents: 25 to 100 mg P.O. daily, increasing gradually to a maximum of 100 mg daily (maximum 150 mg/daily only for the severely ill in these age groups).

Pharmacodynamics
Antidepressant action: Drug is thought to exert its antidepressant effects by inhibiting reuptake of norepinephrine and serotonin in CNS nerve terminals (presynaptic neurons), which results in increased concentrations and enhanced activity of these neurotransmitters in the synaptic cleft. Desipramine more strongly inhibits reuptake of norepinephrine than serotonin; it has a lesser incidence of sedative effects and less anticholinergic and hypotensive activity than its parent compound, imipramine.

Pharmacokinetics
Absorption: Absorbed rapidly from the GI tract after oral administration.
Distribution: Distributed widely into the body, including the CNS and breast milk. Drug is 90% protein-bound. Proposed therapeutic plasma levels (parent drug and metabolite) range from 125 to 300 ng/ml.
Metabolism: Metabolized by the liver; a significant first-pass effect may explain variability of serum levels in different patients taking the same dosage.
Excretion: Excreted primarily in urine.

Route	Onset	Peak	Duration
P.O.	Unknown	4-6 hr	2-4 wk

Contraindications and precautions
Contraindicated in patients with hypersensitivity to drug, in those who have taken MAO inhibitors within the previous 14 days, and in patients during acute recovery phase of MI.

Use with extreme caution in patients with history of seizure disorders or urine retention, CV or thyroid disease, or glaucoma, and in those taking thyroid medication.

Interactions
Drug-drug. *Cimetidine, fluoxetine, fluvoxamine, paroxetine, sertraline:* May increase serum desipramine levels. Patient requires careful monitoring.
MAO inhibitors: May cause severe excitation, hyperpyrexia, or seizures, usually with high dosage. Avoid use together.
Clonidine, ephedrine, epinephrine, norepinephrine, phenylephrine, phenylpropanolamine: May increase blood pressure; use with caution.
Warfarin: May increase PT and cause bleeding. Monitor PT and INR.
Thyroid medication, pimozide, antiarrhythmic agents: May increase incidence of cardiac arrhythmias and conduction defects. Avoid use together.
Clonidine, guanabenz, guanadrel, guanethidine, methyldopa, reserpine: Desipramine may decrease hypotensive effects. Avoid use together.
Disulfiram, ethchlorvynol: May cause delirium and tachycardia. Avoid use together.
CNS depressants: Additive effects. Avoid use together.
Barbiturates: Induce desipramine metabolism and decrease therapeutic efficacy. Patient requires careful monitoring.
Phenothiazines, haloperidol: Decrease its metabolism, decreasing therapeutic efficacy. Patient requires careful monitoring.

Cimetidine, methylphenidate, oral contraceptives, propoxyphene, beta blockers: May inhibit desipramine metabolism, increasing plasma levels and toxicity. Avoid use together.
Selective serotonin-uptake inhibiting agents: Patient may become toxic to tricyclic antidepressant at much lower dosages. Dosage reduction may be needed.
Drug-lifestyle. *Alcohol use:* May enhance CNS depression. Encourage patient to avoid alcohol use.
Heavy smoking: May lower plasma levels of desipramine. Discourage smoking.
Sun exposure: May increase risk of photosensitivity. Advise patient to take precautions.

Effects on diagnostic tests
None reported.

Adverse reactions
CNS: *drowsiness, dizziness,* excitation, tremor, weakness, confusion, anxiety, restlessness, agitation, headache, nervousness, EEG changes, ***seizures,*** extrapyramidal reactions.
CV: orthostatic hypotension, *tachycardia, ECG changes,* hypertension.
EENT: *blurred vision,* tinnitus, mydriasis.
GI: *dry mouth, constipation,* nausea, vomiting, anorexia, paralytic ileus.
GU: *urine retention.*
Hematologic: decreased WBC counts.
Hepatic: elevated liver function tests.
Metabolic: hyperglycemia, hypoglycemia.
Skin: rash, urticaria, photosensitivity.
Other: *diaphoresis,* ***hypersensitivity reaction, sudden death*** (in children).
After abrupt withdrawal of long-term therapy: nausea, headache, malaise (doesn't indicate addiction).

Overdose and treatment
The first 12 hours after acute ingestion are a stimulatory phase characterized by excessive anticholinergic activity (agitation, irritation, confusion, hallucinations, parkinsonian symptoms, hyperthermia, seizures, urine retention, dry mucous membranes, pupillary dilatation, constipation, and ileus). This is followed by CNS depressant effects, including hypothermia, decreased or absent reflexes, sedation, hypotension, cyanosis; and cardiac irregularities, including tachycardia, conduction disturbances, and quinidine-like effects on the ECG.

Severity of overdose is best indicated by widening of the QRS complex, which usually represents a serum level in excess of 1,000 ng/ml; serum levels are generally not helpful. Metabolic acidosis may follow hypotension, hypoventilation, and seizures.

Treatment is symptomatic and supportive, including maintaining airway, stable body temperature, and fluid and electrolyte balance. Induce emesis with ipecac if patient is conscious; follow with gastric lavage and activated charcoal to prevent further absorption. Dialysis is of little use. Physostigmine may be used with caution to reverse CV abnormalities or coma; too rapid administration may cause seizures. Treat seizures with parenteral diazepam or phenytoin; arrhythmias, with parenteral phenytoin or lidocaine; and acidosis, with sodium bicarbonate. Don't give barbiturates; these may enhance CNS and respiratory depressant effects.

Clinical considerations
Consider the recommendations relevant to all tricyclic antidepressants as well as the following:
- Dispense drug in the smallest possible quantities to depressed outpatients, as suicide has been accomplished with drug.
- Drug has a lesser incidence of sedative effects and fewer anticholinergic and hypotensive effects than its parent compound imipramine.
- Tolerance usually develops to the sedative effects of the drug during initial weeks of therapy.
- Drug shouldn't be withdrawn abruptly; rather, it should be tapered gradually over 3 to 6 weeks.
- Discontinue drug at least 48 hours before surgical procedures.
- Drug therapy in patients with bipolar illness may induce a hypomanic state.

Therapeutic monitoring
Recommend that standing and sitting blood pressure be checked to assess orthostasis before administration of desipramine.

Special populations
Breast-feeding patients. Drug is excreted in breast milk in levels equal to those in maternal serum. The potential benefit to the woman should outweigh the possible adverse reactions in the infant.
Pediatric patients. Drug isn't recommended for patients under age 12. Sudden death has been reported in children using drug.
Geriatric patients. Geriatric patients may be more susceptible to adverse cardiovascular and anticholinergic effects.

Patient counseling
- Tell patient to take the full dose at bedtime to alleviate daytime sedation.
- Explain that full effects of drug may not become apparent for 4 weeks or more after initiation of therapy.
- Tell patient to take the medication exactly as prescribed and not to double the dose for missed ones.
- To prevent dizziness, advise patient to lie down for about 30 minutes after each dose at start of therapy and to avoid sudden orthostatic changes, especially when rising to upright position.

- Warn patient not to stop taking drug suddenly.
- Encourage patient to report unusual or troublesome effects, especially confusion, movement disorders, rapid heartbeat, dizziness, fainting, or difficulty urinating.
- Tell patient sugarless chewing gum or hard candy or ice may alleviate dry mouth.
- Stress importance of regular dental hygiene to avoid caries.

desmopressin acetate

DDAVP, Stimate

Pharmacologic classification: posterior pituitary hormone
Therapeutic classification: antidiuretic, hemostatic
Pregnancy risk category B

How supplied

Available by prescription only
Tablets: 0.1 mg
Nasal solution: 0.1 mg/ml, 1.5 mg/ml
Injection: 4 mcg/ml in 1-ml single-dose ampules and 10-ml multiple-dose vials

Indications and dosages

Central cranial diabetes insipidus, temporary polyuria, polydipsia associated with pituitary trauma
Adults: 0.1 to 0.4 ml (10 to 40 mcg) intranasally in one to three divided doses daily. Adjust morning and evening doses separately for adequate diurnal rhythm of water turnover. Use the lowest effective dosage.

Alternatively, 0.05 mg P.O. b.i.d. initially. Adjust individual dosage in increments of 0.1 mg to 1.2 mg daily, divided into two or three doses. Optimal dosage range is 0.1 to 0.8 mg daily in divided doses. Or give 0.5 ml (2 mcg) to 1 ml (4 mcg) I.V. or S.C. daily, usually in two divided doses.
Children age 3 months to 12 years: 0.05 to 0.3 ml (5 to 30 mcg) intranasally daily in one or two doses.
Hemophilia A, von Willebrand's disease
Adults and children: 0.3 mcg/kg diluted in normal saline solution and infused I.V. slowly over 15 to 30 minutes. May repeat dosage, if necessary, as indicated by laboratory response and patient's condition. Alternatively, give one spray per nostril.
Primary nocturnal enuresis
Children age 6 and older: 20 mcg (two to four metered sprays), intranasally h.s. Dosage adjusted according to response. Maximum recommended dose is 40 mcg daily.

Pharmacodynamics

Antidiuretic action: Drug is used to control or prevent signs and complications of neurogenic diabetes insipidus. The site of action is primarily at the renal tubular level. Desmopressin increases water permeability at the renal tubule and collecting duct, resulting in increased urine osmolality and decreased urinary flow rate.
Hemostatic action: Desmopressin increases factor VIII activity by releasing endogenous factor VIII from plasma storage sites.

Pharmacokinetics

Absorption: Destroyed in the GI tract. After intranasal administration, 10% to 20% of dose is absorbed through nasal mucosa.
Distribution: Not fully understood.
Metabolism: Unknown.
Excretion: Plasma levels decline in two phases: the half-life of the fast phase is about 8 minutes; the slow phase, 75 minutes. Duration of action after intranasal administration is 8 to 20 hours; after I.V. administration, 12 to 24 hours for mild hemophilia and about 3 hours for von Willebrand's disease.

Route	Onset	Peak	Duration
P.O.	1 hr	1-1½ hr	8-12 hr
I.V.	15-30 min	Unknown	4-12 hr
Nasal	1 hr	1-5 hr	8-12 hr

Contraindications and precautions

Contraindicated in patients hypersensitive to drug and in patients with type IIB von Willebrand's disease. Use cautiously in patients with coronary artery insufficiency or hypertensive CV disease, or in those with conditions associated with fluid and electrolyte imbalances, such as cystic fibrosis, because these patients are susceptible to hyponatremia.

Interactions

Drug-drug. *Carbamazepine, chlorpropamide, clofibrate:* May potentiate the antidiuretic action of desmopressin action. Avoid use together.
Demeclocycline, epinephrine, heparin, lithium, norepinephrine: May decrease the antidiuretic effect. Use together cautiously.
Drug-lifestyle. *Alcohol use:* May increase risk of adverse effects. Avoid use together.

Effects on diagnostic tests

None reported.

Adverse reactions

CNS: headache.
CV: slight rise in blood pressure (at high dosage).
EENT: rhinitis, epistaxis, sore throat, cough.
GI: nausea, abdominal cramps.
GU: vulval pain.
Other: flushing, local erythema, swelling, burning (after injection).

Overdose and treatment

Signs and symptoms of overdose include drowsiness, listlessness, headache, confusion, anuria, and weight gain (water intoxication). Treatment requires water restriction and temporary withdrawal of desmopressin until polyuria occurs. Severe water intoxication may require osmotic diuresis with mannitol, hypertonic dextrose, or urea—alone or with furosemide.

Clinical considerations

Consider the recommendations relevant to all posterior pituitary hormones as well as the following:

- Desmopressin may be administered intranasally through a flexible catheter called a rhinyle. A measured quantity is drawn up into the catheter, one end is inserted into patient's nose, and patient blows on the other end to deposit drug into nasal cavity. Alternatively, drug is newly available in nasal spray, which may be easier for some patients.
- Patients may be switched from intranasal to S.C. desmopressin (such as during episodes of rhinorrhea). They should receive 1/10 of their usual dosage parenterally.
- Desmopressin isn't indicated for hemophilia A patients with factor VIII levels up to 5% or in patients with severe von Willebrand's disease.
- Drug therapy may enable some patients to avoid the hazards of contaminated blood products.

Therapeutic monitoring

- Monitor for early signs of water intoxication—drowsiness, listlessness, headache, confusion, anuria, and weight gain—to prevent seizures, coma, and death.
- Patient's fluid intake requires adjustment to reduce risk of water intoxication and of sodium depletion, especially in young or elderly patients.
- Weigh patient daily and observe for edema.

Special populations

Pediatric patients. Drug isn't recommended in infants under age 3 months because of their increased tendency to develop fluid imbalance. Use with caution in infants because of risk of hyponatremia and water intoxication. Safety and efficacy of parenteral desmopressin haven't been established for management of diabetes insipidus in children under age 12.
Geriatric patients. Geriatric patients have an increased risk of hyponatremia and water intoxication; therefore, restriction of their fluid intake is recommended. Because geriatric patients are more sensitive to effects of drug, they may need a lower dosage.

Patient counseling

- Teach patient correct administration technique, then evaluate his proficiency at drug administration and accurate measurement on return visits; some may have difficulty measuring and inhaling drug into nostrils.
- Emphasize that patient shouldn't increase or decrease dosage unless it's prescribed.
- Assist patient in planning a schedule for fluid intake if oral fluids must be reduced to decrease the possibility of water intoxication and hyponatremia. A diuretic may be administered if excessive fluid retention occurs.
- Tell patient to store drug away from heat and direct light, not in bathroom, where heat and moisture can cause drug to deteriorate.

desonide

DesOwen, Tridesilon

Pharmacologic classification: topical adrenocorticoid
Therapeutic classification: anti-inflammatory
Pregnancy risk category C

How supplied

Available by prescription only
Cream, lotion, ointment: 0.05%

Indications and dosages

Adjunctive therapy for inflammation in acute and chronic corticosteroid-responsive dermatoses
Adults and children: Apply sparingly to affected area b.i.d. to q.i.d.

Pharmacodynamics

Anti-inflammatory action: Desonide stimulates the synthesis of enzymes needed to decrease the inflammatory response. Desonide is a group I.V. nonfluorinated glucocorticoid with a potency similar to that of alclometasone dipropionate 0.05% and fluocinolone acetonide 0.01%.

Pharmacokinetics

Absorption: Amount absorbed depends on the amount applied and on the nature of the skin at the application site. It ranges from about 1% in areas with a thick stratum corneum (such as the palms, soles, elbows, and knees) to as much as 36% in areas of the thinnest stratum corneum (face, eyelids, and genitals). Absorption increases in areas of skin damage, inflammation, or occlusion. Some systemic absorption of topical steroids occurs, especially through the oral mucosa.
Distribution: After topical application, desonide is distributed throughout the local skin layer. Any drug that's absorbed into circulation is removed rapidly from the blood and distributed into muscle, liver, skin, intestines, and kidneys.
Metabolism: After topical administration, drug is metabolized primarily in the skin. The small amount that's absorbed into systemic circula-

tion is metabolized primarily in the liver to inactive compounds.
Excretion: Inactive metabolites are excreted by the kidneys, primarily as glucuronides and sulfates, but also as unconjugated products. Small amounts of the metabolites are also excreted in feces.

Route	Onset	Peak	Duration
Topical	Unknown	Unknown	Unknown

Contraindications and precautions
Contraindicated in patients hypersensitive to drug.

Interactions
None significant.

Effects on diagnostic tests
None reported.

Adverse reactions
Metabolic: hyperglycemia, glucosuria.
Skin: burning, pruritus, irritation, dryness, erythema, folliculitis, perioral dermatitis, allergic contact dermatitis, hypertrichosis, hypopigmentation, acneiform eruptions; *maceration of skin, secondary infection, atrophy, striae, miliaria* (with occlusive dressings).
Other: ***hypothalamic-pituitary-adrenal axis suppression,*** Cushing's syndrome.

Overdose and treatment
No information available.

Clinical considerations
- Gently wash skin before applying. Rub medication in gently, leaving a thin coat. When treating hairy sites, part hair and apply directly to lesions.
- Avoid using plastic pants or tight-fitting diapers on treated area in young child.

Therapeutic monitoring
Monitor for skin infection, striae, or atrophy; if these develop, stop drug and notify doctor.

Special populations
Pediatric patients. Children may be more susceptible to systemic absorption leading to hypothalamic-pituitary-adrenal axis suppression.

Patient counseling
- Teach patient to apply drug.
- If occlusive dressing is ordered, advise patient not to leave dressing in place longer than 12 hours each day, or as ordered, and not to use occlusive dressings on infected or exudative lesions.
- Tell patient to report adverse effects immediately.

dexamethasone (ophthalmic suspension)
Maxidex

dexamethasone sodium phosphate
AK-Dex, Decadron, Dexair, I-Methasone, Ocu-Dex

Pharmacologic classification: corticosteroid
Therapeutic classification: ophthalmic anti-inflammatory
Pregnancy risk category C

How supplied
Available by prescription only
dexamethasone
Ophthalmic suspension: 0.1%
dexamethasone sodium phosphate
Ophthalmic ointment: 0.05%
Ophthalmic solution: 0.1%

Indications and dosages
Uveitis; iridocyclitis; inflammation of eyelids, conjunctiva, cornea, anterior segment of globe; corneal injury from burns or penetration by foreign bodies; allergic conjunctivitis; suppression of graft rejection after keratoplasty
Adults and children: Instill 1 to 2 drops of suspension or solution or apply 1.25 to 2.5 cm of ointment into conjunctival sac. For initial therapy of severe cases, instill the solution or suspension into the conjunctival sac every hour, gradually discontinue dose as patient's condition improves. In mild condition, use drops up to four to six times daily or apply ointment t.i.d. or q.i.d. As patient's condition improves, taper dose to b.i.d. then once daily. Treatment may extend from a few days to several weeks.

Pharmacodynamics
Anti-inflammatory action: Corticosteroids stimulate the synthesis of enzymes needed to decrease the inflammatory response. Dexamethasone, a long-acting fluorinated synthetic adrenocorticoid with strong anti-inflammatory activity and minimal mineralocorticoid activity, is 25 to 30 times more potent than an equal weight of hydrocortisone.

Drug is poorly soluble and therefore has a slower onset of action but a longer duration of action when applied in a liquid suspension. The sodium phosphate salt is highly soluble and has a rapid onset but short duration of action.

Pharmacokinetics
Absorption: After ophthalmic administration, drug is absorbed through the aqueous humor. Because only low doses are administered, little if any systemic absorption occurs.

Distribution: Distributed throughout the local tissue layers. Drug absorbed into circulation is rapidly removed from the blood and distributed into muscle, liver, skin, intestines, and kidneys.
Metabolism: Primarily metabolized locally. The small amount absorbed into systemic circulation is metabolized primarily in the liver to inactive compounds.
Excretion: Inactive metabolites are excreted by the kidneys, primarily as glucuronides and sulfates, but also as unconjugated products. Small amounts of the metabolites are also excreted in feces.

Route	Onset	Peak	Duration
Ophthalmic	Unknown	Unknown	Unknown

Contraindications and precautions
Contraindicated in patients with acute superficial herpes simplex (dendritic keratitis), vaccinia, varicella, or other fungal or viral diseases of cornea and conjunctiva; ocular tuberculosis; or acute, purulent, untreated infections of the eye.

Use cautiously in patients with corneal abrasions that may be infected (especially with herpes). Also use cautiously in patients with glaucoma because intraocular pressure may increase. Glaucoma medications may need to be increased to compensate.

Interactions
None reported.

Effects on diagnostic tests
None reported.

Adverse reactions
EENT: increased intraocular pressure; thinning of cornea, interference with corneal wound healing, increased susceptibility to viral or fungal corneal infection, corneal ulceration; glaucoma exacerbation, cataracts, defects in visual acuity and visual field, optic nerve damage; mild blurred vision; burning, stinging, or redness of eyes; watery eyes, discharge, discomfort, ocular pain, foreign body sensation (with excessive or long-term use).
Other: systemic effects and adrenal suppression (with excessive or long-term use).

Overdose and treatment
None reported.

Clinical considerations
□ ***ALERT*** Warn patient to call immediately and stop drug if visual acuity changes or visual field diminishes.
- Shake suspension well before use.
- Drug isn't recommended for long-term use.

Therapeutic monitoring
Monitor for signs of corneal ulceration; may require stopping drug.

Patient counseling
- Teach patient how to instill eye drops or ointment. Advise him to wash hands before and after administering, and warn him not to touch tip of dropper to eye or surrounding tissue.
- Tell patient to apply light finger pressure on lacrimal sac for 1 minute after installation.
- Warn patient not to share medication.

dexamethasone (systemic)
Decadron, Deronil*, Dexasone*, Dexone, Hexadrol

dexamethasone acetate
Dalalone D.P., Decadron-LA, Decaject-L.A., Dexasone-L.A., Dexone L.A., Solurex LA

dexamethasone sodium phosphate
AK-Dex, Dalalone, Decadrol, Decadron, Decaject, Dexameth, Dexasone, Dexone, Hexadrol Phosphate, Oradexon*, Solurex

Pharmacologic classification: glucocorticoid
Therapeutic classification: anti-inflammatory, immunosuppressant
Pregnancy risk category NR

How supplied
Available by prescription only
dexamethasone
Tablets: 0.25 mg, 0.5 mg, 0.75 mg, 1 mg, 1.5 mg, 2 mg, 4 mg, 6 mg
Elixir: 0.5 mg/5 ml
Oral solution: 0.5 mg/0.5 ml, 0.5 mg/5 ml
dexamethasone acetate
Injection: 8 mg/ml, 16 mg/ml suspension
dexamethasone sodium phosphate
Injection: 4 mg/ml, 10 mg/ml
Injection (I.V. use only): 24 mg/ml

Indications and dosages
Cerebral edema
dexamethasone sodium phosphate
Adults: Initially, 10 mg I.V., then 4 mg I.M. q 6 hours for 2 to 4 days, then taper over 5 to 7 days.
Inflammatory conditions, allergic reactions, neoplasias
Adults: 0.75 to 9 mg P.O. daily divided b.i.d., t.i.d., or q.i.d.
Children: 0.024 to 0.34 mg/kg P.O. daily in four divided doses.
dexamethasone acetate
Adults: 4 to 16 mg intra-articularly or into soft tissue q 1 to 3 weeks; 0.8 to 1.6 mg into lesions q 1 to 3 weeks; or 8 to 16 mg I.M. q 1 to 3 weeks, p.r.n.

dexamethasone sodium phosphate
Adults: 0.2 to 6 mg intra-articularly, intralesionally, or into soft tissue; or 0.5 to 9 mg I.M.
Shock (other than adrenal crisis)
dexamethasone sodium phosphate
Adults: 1 to 6 mg/kg I.V. daily as a single dose; or 40 mg I.V. q 2 to 6 hours, p.r.n.
Dexamethasone suppression test
Adults: 0.5 mg P.O. q 6 hours for 48 hours.
Adrenal insufficiency
Adults: 0.75 to 9 mg P.O. daily in divided doses.
Children: 0.024 to 0.34 mg/kg P.O. daily in four divided doses.
dexamethasone sodium phosphate
Adults: 0.5 to 9 mg I.M. or I.V. daily.
Children: 0.235 to 1.25 mg/m^2 I.M. or I.V. once daily or b.i.d.
Tuberculous meningitis
Adults: 8 to 12 mg daily tapered over 6 to 8 weeks.
◊ ***Prevention of hyaline membrane disease in premature infants***
Adults: 5 mg (phosphate) I.M. t.i.d. to mother for 2 days before delivery.
◊ ***Prevention of cancer chemotherapy-induced nausea and vomiting***
Adults: 10 to 20 mg I.V. before administration of chemotherapy. Additional doses (individualized for each patient and usually lower than initial dose) may be administered I.V. or P.O. for 24 to 72 hours following cancer chemotherapy, if needed.

Pharmacodynamics

Anti-inflammatory action: Dexamethasone stimulates the synthesis of enzymes needed to decrease the inflammatory response. It causes suppression of the immune system by reducing activity and volume of the lymphatic system, producing lymphocytopenia (primarily T-lymphocytes), decreasing passage of immune complexes through basement membranes, and possibly by depressing reactivity of tissue to antigen-antibody interactions.

Drug is a long-acting synthetic adrenocorticoid with strong anti-inflammatory activity and minimal mineralocorticoid properties. It's 25 to 30 times more potent than an equal weight of hydrocortisone.

The acetate salt is a suspension and shouldn't be used I.V. It's particularly useful as an anti-inflammatory agent in intra-articular, intradermal, and intralesional injections.

The sodium phosphate salt is highly soluble and has a more rapid onset and a shorter duration of action than does the acetate salt. It's most commonly used for cerebral edema and unresponsive shock. It can also be used in intra-articular, intralesional, or soft tissue inflammation. Other uses for dexamethasone are symptomatic treatment of bronchial asthma, chemotherapy-induced nausea, and as a diagnostic test for Cushing's syndrome.

Pharmacokinetics

Absorption: After oral administration, drug is absorbed readily. The suspension for injection has a variable onset and duration of action, depending on whether it's injected into an intra-articular space, a muscle, or the blood supply to the muscle. After I.V. injection, dexamethosone is rapidly and completely absorbed into the tissues.
Distribution: Removed rapidly from the blood and distributed to muscle, liver, skin, intestines, and kidneys. Dexamethasone is bound weakly to plasma proteins (transcortin and albumin). Only the unbound portion is active. Adrenocorticoids are distributed into breast milk and through the placenta.
Metabolism: Metabolized in the liver to inactive glucuronide and sulfate metabolites.
Excretion: Inactive metabolites and small amounts of unmetabolized drug are excreted by the kidneys. Insignificant quantities of drug are also excreted in feces; biologic half-life is 36 to 54 hours.

Route	Onset	Peak	Duration
P.O.	1-2 hr	1-2 hr	2½ days
I.V.	1 hr	1 hr	Variable
I.M.	1 hr	1 hr	6 days
I.M. (acetate)	1 hr	8 hr	Unknown

Contraindications and precautions

Contraindicated in patients hypersensitive to any component of drug and in those with systemic fungal infections.

Use cautiously in patients with recent MI, GI ulcer, renal disease, hypertension, osteoporosis, diabetes mellitus, hypothyroidism, cirrhosis, diverticulitis, nonspecific ulcerative colitis, recent intestinal anastomoses, thromboembolic disorders, seizures, myasthenia gravis, heart failure, tuberculosis, ocular herpes simplex, emotional instability, and psychotic tendencies. Because some formulations contain sulfite preservatives, also use cautiously in patients sensitive to sulfites.

Interactions

Drug-drug. *Insulin or oral antidiabetic agents:* Cause hyperglycemia. May require dosage adjustment.
Oral anticoagulants: Decrease the effects. Monitor PT and INR closely.
Isoniazid and salicylates: Dexamethasone increases the metabolism of isoniazid and salicylates. Patient requires careful monitoring.
Diuretic or amphotericin B therapy: Hypokalemia. Monitor serum potassium levels.
Cardiac glycosides: Hypokalemia may increase the risk of toxicity. May need dose adjustment.
Barbiturates, phenytoin, rifampin: May cause decreased corticosteroid effects. Dose adjustment may be necessary.

Cholestyramine, colestipol, antacids: Decrease the corticosteroid effect. Monitor patient closely; patient may need dosage adjustment.
Estrogens: May reduce the metabolism of dexamethasone by increasing the concentration of transcortin. Patient requires careful monitoring.
Aspirin, NSAIDs: May increase the risk of GI ulceration. Use together cautiously.
Skin-test antigens: Decrease response. Defer skin testing until therapy is completed.
Toxoids and vaccines: Decrease antibody response and increase risk of neurologic complications. Avoid use together.
Drug-lifestyle: *Alcohol use:* Increases risk of gastric irritation and GI ulceration. Advise patient to avoid alcohol.

Effects on diagnostic tests

Dexamethasone causes false-negative results in the nitroblue tetrazolium test for systemic bacterial infections and decreases ^{131}I uptake and protein-bound iodine levels in thyroid function tests.

Adverse reactions

Most adverse reactions to corticosteroids are dose dependent or duration dependent.
CNS: *euphoria, insomnia,* psychotic behavior, pseudotumor cerebri, vertigo, headache, paresthesia, ***seizures.***
CV: ***heart failure,*** hypertension, edema, ***arrhythmias,*** thrombophlebitis, ***thromboembolism.***
EENT: cataracts, glaucoma.
Endocrine: menstrual irregularities, cushingoid state (moonface, buffalo hump, central obesity).
GI: *peptic ulceration,* GI irritation, increased appetite, ***pancreatitis,*** nausea, vomiting.
Metabolic: hypokalemia, hypocalcemia, hyperglycemia, carbohydrate intolerance, decreased levels of thyroxine, and triiodothyronine, and increased urine glucose and calcium levels.
Musculoskeletal: muscle weakness, osteoporosis, growth suppression in children.
Skin: delayed wound healing, acne, various skin eruptions; atrophy (at I.M. injection sites).
Other: hirsutism, susceptibility to infections; ***acute adrenal insufficiency may follow increased stress (infection, surgery, or trauma) or abrupt withdrawal after long-term therapy.***
After abrupt withdrawal: rebound inflammation, fatigue, weakness, arthralgia, fever, dizziness, lethargy, depression, fainting, orthostatic hypotension, dyspnea, anorexia, hypoglycemia. ***After prolonged use, sudden withdrawal may be fatal.***

Overdose and treatment

Acute ingestion, even in massive doses, rarely poses a clinical problem. Toxic signs and symptoms rarely occur if drug is used for less than 3 weeks, even at large dosage ranges. However, long-term use causes adverse physiologic effects, including suppression of the hypothalamic-pituitary-adrenal axis, cushingoid appearance, muscle weakness, and osteoporosis.

Clinical considerations

- Determine whether patient is sensitive to other corticosteroid medications.
- For better results and less toxicity, a once-daily dose in the morning is recommended.
- Give drug by I.M. injection deep into gluteal muscle. Rotate sites. Avoid S.C. injection.
- Drug is being used investigationally to prevent hyaline membrane disease (respiratory distress syndrome) in premature infants. The suspension (phosphate salt) is administered I.M. to the mother two or three times daily for 2 days before delivery.

Therapeutic monitoring

- Patient's weight, blood pressure, and serum electrolyte levels must be checked frequently.
- Monitor for depression or psychotic episodes.

Special populations

Pediatric patients. Chronic use of drug in children and adolescents may delay growth and maturation.

Patient counseling

- Tell patient not to discontinue drug abruptly or without doctor's consent.
- Instruct patient to take medication with food or milk.
- Teach patient signs of early adrenal insufficiency: fatigue, muscular weakness, joint pain, fever, anorexia, nausea, dyspnea, dizziness, and fainting.

dexamethasone sodium phosphate

Decadron Phosphate

Pharmacologic classification: corticosteroid
Therapeutic classification: anti-inflammatory
Pregnancy risk category C

How supplied

Available by prescription only
dexamethasone
Aerosol: 0.01%, 0.04%

Indications and dosages

Inflammation of corticosteroid-responsive dermatoses
Adults and children: Apply sparingly t.i.d. or q.i.d. For aerosol use on scalp, shake can well and apply to dry scalp after shampooing. Hold

can upright. Slide applicator tube under hair so that it touches scalp. Spray while moving tube to all affected areas, keeping tube under hair and in contact with scalp throughout spraying, which should take about 2 seconds. Inadequately covered areas may be spot sprayed. Slide applicator tube through hair to touch scalp, press and immediately release spray button. Don't massage medication into scalp or spray forehead or eyes.

Pharmacodynamics

Anti-inflammatory action: Dexamethasone is a synthetic fluorinated corticosteroid. It's usually classed as a group VII potency anti-inflammatory agent. Occlusive dressings may be used in severe cases. The aerosol spray is usually used for dermatologic conditions of the scalp.

Pharmacokinetics

Absorption: Absorption depends on the potency of the preparation, the amount applied, the vehicle used, and the nature of the skin at the application site. It ranges from about 1% in areas with a thick stratum corneum (such as the palms, soles, elbows, and knees) to 25% in areas of the thinnest stratum corneum (face, eyelids, and genitals). Inflamed or damaged skin may absorb more than 33%. Absorption increases in areas of skin damage, inflammation, or occlusion. Some systemic absorption occurs, especially through the oral mucosa.
Distribution: After topical administration, dexamethasone is distributed throughout the local skin layer, If absorbed into circulation, drug is distributed rapidly into muscle, liver, skin, intestines, and kidneys.
Metabolism: After topical administration, dexamethasone is metabolized primarily in the skin. The small amount that's absorbed into systemic circulation is primarily metabolized in the liver to inactive compounds.
Excretion: Inactive metabolites are excreted by the kidneys, primarily as glucuronides and sulfates, but also as unconjugated products. Small amounts of the metabolites are also excreted in feces.

Route	Onset	Peak	Duration
Topical	Unknown	Unknown	Unknown

Contraindications and precautions

Contraindicated in patients hypersensitive to drug.

Interactions

None significant.

Effects on diagnostic tests

None reported.

Adverse reactions

Metabolic: hyperglycemia, glucosuria.
Skin: burning, pruritus, irritation, dryness, erythema, folliculitis, hypertrichosis, acneiform eruptions, perioral dermatitis, hypopigmentation, allergic contact dermatitis; *maceration, secondary infection, atrophy, striae, miliaria* (with occlusive dressings).
Other: ***hypothalamic-pituitary-adrenal axis suppression,*** Cushing's syndrome.

Overdose and treatment

Topical corticosteroids can be absorbed in sufficient amounts to produce systemic effects.

Clinical considerations

- Gently wash skin before applying.
- To prevent skin damage, rub cream in gently, leaving a thin coat.
- When treating hairy sites, part hair and apply directly to lesions.
- Continue treatment for a few days after lesions clear, as ordered.

Therapeutic monitoring

Stop drug and contact doctor if skin infection, striae, or atrophy occurs.

Special populations

The same considerations apply to all patients.

Patient counseling

- Teach patient and family how to apply drug.
- Inform patient that if occlusive dressings are ordered and a fever develops, he should notify doctor and remove dressing.
- Advise patient not to leave occlusive dressing on more than 12 hours each day.
- Tell patient not to use occlusive dressing on infected or exudative lesions.

dexrazoxane

Zinecard

Pharmacologic classification: intracellular chelating agent
Therapeutic classification: cardioprotective
Pregnancy risk category C

How supplied

Available by prescription only
Injection: 250 mg, 500 mg in single-dose vials

Indications and dosages

Reduction of incidence and severity of doxorubicin-induced cardiomyopathy in women with metastatic breast cancer who have received a cumulative doxorubicin dose of 300 mg/m² but would benefit from continued therapy with doxorubicin
Adults: Dosage ratio of dexrazoxane to doxorubicin must be 10:1, such as 500 mg/m^2 dexrazoxane:50 mg/m^2 doxorubicin. After reconstitution, administer dexrazoxane by slow

I.V. push or rapid drip I.V. infusion. After completion of dexrazoxane administration and before a total elapsed time of 30 minutes from the beginning of the dexrazoxane administration, give the I.V. injection of the doxorubicin dose.

Pharmacodynamics
Cardioprotective action: The specific mechanism of action of dexrazoxane is unknown. Drug is a cyclic derivative of EDTA that readily penetrates cell membranes. Studies suggest that drug is converted intracellularly to a ring-opened chelating agent that interferes with iron-mediated free radical generation believed to be responsible, in part, for anthracycline-induced cardiomyopathy.

Pharmacokinetics
Absorption: Given I.V.
Distribution: Unknown. Drug isn't bound to plasma proteins.
Metabolism: Not believed to be metabolized.
Excretion: Primarily excreted in urine.

Route	Onset	Peak	Duration
I.V.	Unknown	Unknown	Unknown

Contraindications and precautions
Contraindicated in patients who aren't receiving doxorubicin as part of the chemotherapy regimen. Use cautiously in all patients because additive effects of immunosuppression may occur from concomitant administration of cytotoxic drugs.

Interactions
None significant.

Effects on diagnostic tests
None reported.

Adverse reactions
The following reactions (except for pain on injection) may be attributed to the FAC regimen (fluorouracil, doxorubicin, cyclophosphamide) given shortly after dexrazoxane.
CNS: *fatigue, malaise, **neurotoxicity.***
GI: *nausea, vomiting, anorexia, stomatitis, diarrhea,* esophagitis, dysphagia.
Hematologic: ***hemorrhage.***
Skin: urticaria.
Other: *alopecia, fever, infection, pain on injection, **sepsis,*** streaking at I.V. insertion site, erythema, phlebitis, extravasation.

Overdose and treatment
There are no known reports of overdose, although myelosuppression is most likely to occur. Because dexrazoxane isn't bound to plasma protein, peritoneal dialysis or hemodialysis may be effective in removing drug from body. Manage suspected overdose with good supportive care until resolution of myelosuppression and related conditions is complete. Management of overdose should include treatment of infections, fluid regulation, and maintenance of nutritional requirements.

Clinical considerations
☐ ***ALERT*** Doxorubicin shouldn't be given before dexrazoxane. Also, dexrazoxane isn't recommended for use with the initiation of doxorubicin therapy but only after a cumulative dosage of doxorubicin of 300 mg/m^2 has been reached and continuation of doxorubicin is desired.
- Drug must be diluted with the diluent supplied with drug (0.167 M sodium lactate injection) to give a concentration of 10 mg dexrazoxane for each milliliter of sodium lactate. Give reconstituted solution by slow I.V. push or rapid drip I.V. infusion from a bag.
- Reconstituted solution, when transferred to an empty infusion bag, is stable for 6 hours from the time of reconstitution when stored at controlled room temperature (36° to 46° F [2° to 8° C]) or under refrigeration. Discard unused solution.
- Reconstituted drug may be diluted with either normal saline solution or D_5W injection to a concentration range of 1.3 to 5.0 mg/ml in I.V. infusion bags. The resultant solution is also stable for 6 hours under the same storage conditions as the diluted drug.
- Dexrazoxane shouldn't be mixed with other drugs because of possible incompatibility.
- Use caution when handling and preparing the reconstituted solution; follow same precautions as handling antineoplastic agents. Be sure to use gloves. If drug powder or solution contacts the skin or mucosa, immediately wash thoroughly with soap and water.

Therapeutic monitoring
- Monitor CBC closely because drug is always used with other cytotoxic drugs and it may add to the myelosuppressive effects of cytotoxic drugs itself.
- The administration of Zinecard with doxorubicin doesn't eliminate the possibility of cardiac toxicity. Carefully monitor cardiac function.

Special populations
Breast-feeding patients. Because of the potential for serious adverse effects in breast-fed infants, breast-feeding isn't recommended.
Pediatric patients. Safety and effectiveness in children haven't been established.

Patient counseling
- Inform patient of need for drug during continued doxorubicin therapy.
- Warn patient to watch for signs of infection (fever, sore throat, fatigue) and bleeding (easy bruising, nose bleeds, bleeding gums, melena). Tell patient to take temperature daily and

teach him infection control and bleeding precautions.
- Inform patient that alopecia may occur but that it's usually reversible.

dextroamphetamine sulfate
Dexedrine, Ferndex

Pharmacologic classification: amphetamine
Therapeutic classification: CNS stimulant, short-term adjunctive anorexigenic agent, sympathomimetic amine
Controlled substance schedule II
Pregnancy risk category C

How supplied
Available by prescription only
Tablets: 5 mg, 10 mg
Capsules (sustained-release): 5 mg, 10 mg, 15 mg

Indications and dosages
Narcolepsy
Adults: 5 to 60 mg P.O. daily in divided doses. Long-acting dosage forms allow once-daily dosing.
Children over age 12: 10 mg P.O. daily, with 10-mg increments weekly, as indicated.
Children age 6 to 12: 5 mg P.O. daily, with 5-mg increments weekly, as indicated.
◇ ***Short-term adjunct in exogenous obesity***
Adults: 5 to 30 mg P.O. daily 30 to 60 minutes before meals in divided doses of 5 to 10 mg. Alternatively, give one 10- or 15-mg sustained-release capsule daily as a single dose in the morning.
Attention deficit hyperactivity disorder
Children age 6 and older: 5 mg P.O. once daily or b.i.d., with 5-mg increments weekly, p.r.n. Total daily dose should rarely exceed 40 mg.
Children age 3 to 5: 2.5 mg P.O. daily, with 2.5-mg increments weekly, as necessary; not recommended for children under age 3.

Pharmacodynamics
CNS stimulant action: Amphetamines are sympathomimetic amines with CNS stimulant activity; in hyperactive children, they have a paradoxical calming effect.
Anorexigenic action: Anorexigenic effects are thought to occur in the hypothalamus, where decreased smell and taste acuity decreases appetite. They may be tried for short-term control of refractory obesity, with caloric restriction and behavior modification.

The cerebral cortex and reticular activating system appear to be the primary sites of activity; amphetamines release nerve terminal stores of norepinephrine, promoting nerve impulse transmission. At high dosages, effects are mediated by dopamine.

Amphetamines are used to treat narcolepsy and as adjuncts to psychosocial measures in attention deficit disorder in children. Their precise mechanism of action in these conditions is unknown.

Pharmacokinetics
Absorption: Rapidly absorbed from the GI tract.
Distribution: Distributed widely throughout the body.
Metabolism: Unknown.
Excretion: Excreted in urine.

Route	Onset	Peak	Duration
P.O.	Unknown	2 hr	Unknown
P.O. (extended)	Unknown	8-10 hr	Unknown

Contraindications and precautions
Contraindicated in patients with hypersensitivity or idiosyncrasy to the sympathomimetic amines, within 14 days of MAO inhibitor therapy, and in those with hyperthyroidism, moderate to severe hypertension, symptomatic CV disease, glaucoma, advanced arteriosclerosis, and history of drug abuse. Use cautiously in patients with motor and phonic tics, Tourette syndrome, and agitated states.

Interactions
Drug-drug. *MAO inhibitors:* May cause hypertensive crisis. Don't use together or within 14 days after MAO inhibitor has been discontinued.
Antihypertensives: May antagonize antihypertensive effects. Avoid use together.
Alkalizing agents, antacids, sodium bicarbonate, acetazolamide: Enhance renal reabsorption. Patient requires monitoring for enhanced amphetamine effects.
Ascorbic acid, acidifying agents, ammonium chloride: Enhance dextroamphetamine excretion and shorten duration of action. Monitor for decreased amphetamine effects.
Adrenergic blockers: Inhibited by amphetamines. Avoid use together.
Chlorpromazine: Inhibits the central stimulant effects of amphetamines. Can be used to treat amphetamine poisoning.
CNS stimulants, theophylline, phenothiazines, haloperidol, tricyclic antidepressants: Increase CNS effects. Avoid use together.
Barbiturates: Antagonize dextroamphetamine by CNS depression. Avoid use together.
Insulin and oral antidiabetic: Dextroamphetamine may alter requirements. Monitor blood glucose levels.
Lithium carbonate: May inhibit antiobesity and stimulating effects of amphetamines. Monitor patient closely.
Meperidine: Amphetamines potentiate the analgesic effect. Use together cautiously.

Methenamine therapy: Increases urinary excretion of amphetamines and reduces efficacy. Monitor patient closely.
Norepinephrine: Amphetamines enhance the adrenergic effect. Monitor patient closely.
Phenobarbitol, phenytoin: May produce a synergistic anticonvulsant action. Monitor patient closely.
Drug-food. *Caffeine:* May increase amphetamine and related amine effects. Use cautiously.

Effects on diagnostic tests
None reported.

Adverse reactions
CNS: *restlessness,* tremor, *insomnia,* dizziness, headache, chills, overstimulation, dysphoria, euphoria.
CV: *tachycardia, palpitations,* hypertension, ***arrhythmias.***
GI: dry mouth, unpleasant taste, diarrhea, constipation, anorexia, weight loss, other GI disturbances.
GU: impotence, altered libido.
Skin: urticaria.

Overdose and treatment
Individual responses to overdose vary widely. Toxic symptoms may occur at 15 and 30 mg and can cause severe reactions; however, doses of 400 mg or more have not always proved fatal.

Symptoms of overdose include restlessness, tremor, hyperreflexia, tachypnea, confusion, aggressiveness, hallucinations, and panic; fatigue and depression usually follow excitement stage. Other symptoms may include arrhythmias, shock, alterations in blood pressure, nausea, vomiting, diarrhea, and abdominal cramps; death is usually preceded by seizures and coma.

Treat overdose symptomatically and supportively: if ingestion is recent (within 4 hours), use gastric lavage or emesis and sedate with a barbiturate; monitor vital signs and fluid and electrolyte balance. Urinary acidification may enhance excretion. Saline catharsis (magnesium citrate) may hasten GI evacuation of unabsorbed sustained-release drug.

Clinical considerations
Consider the recommendations relevant to all amphetamines as well as the following:
- Drug may elevate plasma corticosteroid levels and may interfere with urinary steroid determinations.
- Give dextroamphetamine 30 to 60 minutes before meals when using as an anorexigenic agent. To minimize insomnia, avoid giving within 6 hours of bedtime.
- For narcolepsy, patient should take first dose on awakening.

Therapeutic monitoring
- Take vital signs regularly, and observe patient for signs of excessive stimulation.
- When tolerance to anorexigenic effect develops, dosage should be discontinued, not increased.
- Monitor blood and urine glucose levels. Drug may alter daily insulin requirement in patients with diabetes.

Special populations
Breast-feeding patients. Safety hasn't been established. Alternative feeding method is recommended during therapy with dextroamphetamine sulfate.
Pediatric patients. Drug isn't recommended for treatment of obesity in children under age 12.
Geriatric patients. Use lower doses in geriatric patients. Avoid using drug in geriatric patients with cardiovascular, CNS, or GI disturbances.

Patient counseling
- Teach parents to provide drug-free periods for children with attention deficit disorder, especially during periods of reduced stress.
- Warn patient to avoid hazardous activities that require alertness until CNS response is determined.
- Instruct patient to take drug early in the day to minimize insomnia.
- Tell patient not to crush sustained-release forms or to increase dosage.

dextromethorphan hydrobromide
Balminil D.M.*, Benylin DM Cough, Broncho-Grippol-DM*, Delsym, DM Syrup*, Hold, Koffex*, Mediquell, Neo-DM*, Robidex*, Sedatuss*, St. Joseph Cough Suppressant for Children, Sucrets Cough Control Formula, Suppress, Trocal, Vicks Formula 44

Pharmacologic classification: levorphanol derivative (dextrorotatory methyl ether)
Therapeutic classification: antitussive (nonnarcotic)
Pregnancy risk category C

How supplied
Available without a prescription
Syrup: 10 mg/5 ml, 15 mg/15 ml
Solution: 3.5 mg/5 ml, 5 mg/5 ml, 7.5 mg/5 ml, 10 mg/5 ml, 12.5 mg/5 ml, 15 mg/5 ml
Lozenges: 5 mg, 7.5 mg, 15 mg
Tablets: 200 mg
Capsules (liquid-filled): 30 mg

Indications and dosages

Nonproductive cough (chronic)

Adults and children age 12 and older: 10 to 20 mg P.O. q 4 hours; or 30 mg q 6 to 8 hours; or controlled-release liquid b.i.d. (60 mg b.i.d.). Maximum dose is 120 mg daily.
Children age 6 to 12: 5 to 10 mg P.O. q 4 hours; or 15 mg q 6 to 8 hours; or controlled-release liquid b.i.d. (30 mg b.i.d.). Maximum dose is 60 mg daily.
Children age 2 to 6: 2.5 to 5 mg P.O. q 4 hours; or 7.5 mg q 6 to 8 hours; or sustained-action liquid 15 mg b.i.d. Maximum dose is 30 mg daily.

Pharmacodynamics

Antitussive action: Dextromethorphan suppresses the cough reflex by direct action on the cough center in the medulla. Dextromethorphan is almost equal in antitussive potency to codeine but causes no analgesia or addiction and little or no CNS depression and has no expectorant action; it also produces fewer subjective and GI adverse effects than codeine. Treatment is intended to relieve cough frequency without abolishing protective cough reflex. In therapeutic doses, drug doesn't inhibit ciliary activity.

Pharmacokinetics

Absorption: Absorbed readily from the GI tract.
Distribution: Unknown.
Metabolism: Metabolized extensively by the liver. Plasma half-life is about 11 hours.
Excretion: Little is excreted unchanged. Metabolites are excreted primarily in urine; about 7% to 10% is excreted in feces.

Route	Onset	Peak	Duration
P.O.	< ½ hr	Unknown	3-6 hr

Contraindications and precautions

Contraindicated in patients currently taking MAO inhibitors or within 2 weeks of discontinuing MAO inhibitors. Use cautiously in atopic children, sedated or debilitated patients, and those patients confined to the supine position. Also use cautiously in patients with a sensitivity to aspirin.

Interactions

Drug-drug. *MAO inhibitors:* May cause nausea, hypotension, excitation, hyperpyrexia, and coma; dextromethorphan shouldn't be given to patients at any interval less than 2 weeks after MAO inhibitors are discontinued.
Selegiline: May cause confusion, coma, or hyperpyrexia. Avoid use together.
Drug-herb. *Parsley*: May promote or produce serotonin syndrome. Avoid use together.

Effects on diagnostic tests

None reported.

Adverse reactions

CNS: drowsiness, dizziness.
GI: nausea, vomiting, stomach pain.

Overdose and treatment

Signs and symptoms of overdose may include nausea, vomiting, drowsiness, dizziness, blurred vision, nystagmus, shallow respirations, urine retention, toxic psychosis, stupor, and coma.

Treatment of overdose involves administering activated charcoal to reduce drug absorption and I.V. naloxone to support respiration. Other symptoms are treated supportively.

Clinical considerations

- Treatment is intended to relieve cough intensity and frequency, without completely abolishing the protective cough reflex.
- May be used with percussion and chest vibration.

Therapeutic monitoring

Note nature and frequency of coughing.

Special populations

Breast-feeding patients. Safety hasn't been established.
Pediatric patients. Don't use syrup, tablets, or lozenges in children under age 2. Sustained-action liquid may be used in children under age 2, but dosage must be individualized.

Patient counseling

- Tell patient to report persistent cough of more than 7 days.
- Instruct patient to use sugarless throat lozenges for throat irritation and resulting cough.
- Recommend a humidifier to filter out dust, smoke, and air pollutants.

diazepam

Apo-Diazepam*, Dizac, Novodipam*, Valium, Vivol*, Diastat, Zetran

Pharmacologic classification: benzodiazepine
Therapeutic classification: antianxiety; skeletal muscle relaxant; amnesic; anticonvulsant; sedative-hypnotic
Controlled substance schedule IV
Pregnancy risk category D

How supplied

Available by prescription only
Tablets: 2 mg, 5 mg, 10 mg
Capsules (extended-release): 15 mg
Oral solution: 5 mg/ml; 5 mg/5 ml, 10 mg/10 ml
Injection: 5 mg/ml in ampules, vials, and disposable syringes
Rectal gel: 2.5 mg, 5 mg, 10 mg, 15 mg, 20 mg twin packs

Indications and dosages

Anxiety
Adults: Depending on severity, 2 to 10 mg P.O. b.i.d. to q.i.d. or 15 to 30 mg extended-release capsules P.O. once daily. Alternatively, 2 to 10 mg I.M. or I.V. q 3 to 4 hours, p.r.n.
Children age 6 months and older: 1 to 2.5 mg P.O. t.i.d. or q.i.d.; increase dose gradually, as needed and tolerated.
Acute alcohol withdrawal
Adults: 10 mg P.O. t.i.d. or q.i.d. for the first 24 hours; reduce to 5 mg t.i.d. or q.i.d., p.r.n.; or 10 mg I.M. or I.V. initially, followed by 5 to 10 mg q 3 to 4 hours, p.r.n.
Muscle spasm
Adults: 2 to 10 mg P.O. b.i.d. to q.i.d.; or 15 to 30 mg extended-release capsules once daily. Alternatively, 5 to 10 mg I.M. or I.V. q 3 to 4 hours, p.r.n.
Tetanus
Infants over age 30 days to children age 5: 1 to 2 mg I.M. or I.V. slowly, repeated q 3 to 4 hours.
Children age 5 and older: 5 to 10 mg I.M. or I.V. slowly q 3 to 4 hours, p.r.n.
Adjunct to convulsive disorders
Adults: 2 to 10 mg P.O. b.i.d. to q.i.d.
Children age 6 months and older: Initially, 1 to 2.5 mg P.O. t.i.d. or q.i.d.; increase dose as tolerated and needed.
Adjunct to anesthesia, endoscopic procedures
Adults: 5 to 10 mg I.M. before surgery; or administer I.V. slowly just before procedure, titrating dose to effect. Usually, less than 10 mg is used, but up to 20 mg may be given.
Cardioversion
Adults: Administer 5 to 15 mg I.V. 5 to 10 minutes before procedure.
Status epilepticus
Adults: 5 to 10 mg I.V. (preferred) or I.M. initially, repeated at 10- to 15-minute intervals up to a maximum dose of 30 mg. Repeat q 2 to 4 hours, p.r.n.
Children age 5 and older: 1 mg I.V. q 2 to 5 minutes up to a maximum dose of 10 mg; repeat in 2 to 4 hours, p.r.n.
Infants over age 30 days to children age 5: 0.2 to 0.5 mg I.V. q 2 to 5 minutes up to a maximum dose of 5 mg.
Control of acute repetitive seizure activity in patients already taking antiepileptic drugs
Children age 12 and older: 0.2 mg/kg P.R. using applicator. A second dose may be given 4 to 12 hours after the first dose, if needed.
Children age 6 to 11: 0.3 mg/kg P.R. using applicator. A second dose may be given 4 to 12 hours after the first dose, if needed.
Children age 2 to 5 years: 0.5 mg/kg P.R. using applicator. A second dose may be given 4 to 12 hours after the first dose, if needed.

Pharmacodynamics

Anxiolytic and sedative-hypnotic actions: Diazepam depresses the CNS at the limbic and subcortical levels of the brain. It produces an antianxiety effect by influencing the effect of the neurotransmitter gamma-aminobutyric acid on its receptor in the ascending reticular activating system, which increases inhibition and blocks cortical and limbic arousal.
Anticonvulsant action: Diazepam suppresses the spread of seizure activity produced by epileptogenic foci in the cortex, thalamus, and limbic structures by enhancing presynaptic inhibition.
Amnesic action: The exact mechanism of action is unknown.
Skeletal muscle relaxant action: The exact mechanism is unknown, but it's believed to involve inhibiting polysynaptic afferent pathways.

Pharmacokinetics

Absorption: When administered orally, drug is absorbed through the GI tract. I.M. administration results in erratic absorption of the drug; Drug is well absorbed rectally and reaches peak plasma levels in 1½ hours.
Distribution: Distributed widely throughout the body. About 85% to 95% of an administered dose is bound to plasma protein.
Metabolism: Metabolized in the liver to the active metabolite desmethyldiazepam.
Excretion: Most metabolites of diazepam are excreted in urine, with only small amounts excreted in feces. Half-life of desmethyldiazepam is 30 to 200 hours. Duration of sedative effect is 3 hours; this may be prolonged up to 90 hours in elderly patients and in patients with hepatic or renal dysfunction. Anticonvulsant effect is 30 to 60 minutes after I.V. administration.

Route	Onset	Peak	Duration
P.O.	½ hr	2 hr	3-8 hr
I.V.	1-5 min	Immediate	15-60 min
I.M.	Unknown	2 hr	Unknown
P.R.	Unknown	1-5 hr	Unknown

Contraindications and precautions

Contraindicated in patients with hypersensitivity or narrow angle glaucoma; in patients experiencing shock, coma, or acute alcohol intoxication (parenteral form); and in children under age 6 months (oral form). Use cautiously in the elderly, in debilitated patients, and in those with impaired hepatic or renal function, depression, or chronic open-angle glaucoma. Avoid use in pregnant women, especially during the first trimester.

Interactions

Drug-drug. *Antidepressants, antihistamines, barbiturates, general anesthetics, MAO inhibitors, narcotics, phenothiazines:* Diazepam

potentiates the CNS depressant effects. Avoid use together.
Cimetidine and possibly disulfiram: Diminished hepatic metabolism of diazepam, which increases its plasma concentration. Patient requires close monitoring.
Antacids: Decrease the rate of absorption of diazepam. Avoid use together.
Haloperidol: May change the seizure patterns; benzodiazepines also may reduce the serum levels of *haloperidol.* Avoid use together.
Digoxin: Diazepam reportedly can decrease digoxin clearance; monitor patients for digoxin toxicity.
Nondepolarizing neuromuscular blocking agents, such as pancuronium and succinylcholine: Intensified and prolonged respiratory depression. Don't use together.
Oral contraceptives: May impair the metabolism of diazepam. Patient requires close monitoring.
Levodopa: Diazepam may inhibit the therapeutic effect of levodopa. Monitor patient carefully.
Drug-lifestyle. *Alcohol use:* Diazepam potentiates the CNS depressant effects of alcohol. Advise patient to avoid use together.
Heavy smoking: Accelerates metabolism of diazepam, lowering clinical effectiveness. Advise patient to avoid use together.

Effects on diagnostic tests
None reported.

Adverse reactions
CNS: *drowsiness,* slurred speech, tremor, transient amnesia, fatigue, ataxia, headache, insomnia, paradoxical anxiety, hallucinations, changes in EEG patterns.
CV: hypotension, ***CV collapse,*** *bradycardia.*
EENT: diplopia, blurred vision, nystagmus.
GI: nausea, constipation.
GU: incontinence, urine retention, altered libido.
Hematologic: ***neutropenia.***
Hepatic: elevated liver function tests, *jaundice.*
Musculoskeletal: *dysarthria.*
Respiratory: ***respiratory depression.***
Skin: rash.
Other: physical or psychological dependence, ***acute withdrawal syndrome*** after sudden discontinuation in physically dependent persons, *pain, phlebitis* (at injection site).

Overdose and treatment
Signs and symptoms of overdose include somnolence, confusion, coma, hypoactive reflexes, dyspnea, labored breathing, hypotension, bradycardia, slurred speech, and unsteady gait or impaired coordination.

Support blood pressure and respiration until drug effects subside; monitor vital signs. Mechanical ventilatory assistance via endotracheal tube may be required to maintain a patent airway and support adequate oxygenation. Flumazenil, a specific benzodiazepine antagonist, may be useful, but shouldn't be administered during status epilepticus. Use I.V. fluids and vasopressors such as dopamine and phenylephrine to treat hypotension as needed. If the patient is conscious, induce emesis; use gastric lavage if ingestion was recent, but only if an endotracheal tube is present to prevent aspiration. After emesis or lavage, administer activated charcoal with a cathartic as a single dose. Dialysis is of limited value.

Clinical considerations
Consider the recommendations relevant to all benzodiazepines as well as the following:
- Don't discontinue drug suddenly; decrease dosage slowly over 8 to 12 weeks after long-term therapy.
- To enhance taste, oral solution can be mixed with liquids or semisolid foods, such as applesauce or pudding, immediately before administration.
- Extended-release capsule should be swallowed whole; don't let patient crush or chew it.
- Shake oral suspension well before administering.
- When prescribing with opiates for endoscopic procedures, reduce opiate dose by at least one-third.
- Parenteral forms of diazepam may be diluted in normal saline solution; a slight precipitate may form, but the solution can still be used.
- Diazepam interacts with plastic. Don't store diazepam in plastic syringes or administer it in plastic administration sets, which decreases availability of the infused drug.
- I.V. route is preferred because of rapid and more uniform absorption.
- For I.V. administration, infuse drug slowly, directly into a large vein, at a rate not exceeding 5 mg/minute for adults or 0.25 mg/kg of body weight over 3 minutes for children. Don't inject diazepam into small veins to avoid extravasation into subcutaneous tissue. Observe infusion site for phlebitis. If direct I.V. administration isn't possible, inject diazepam directly into I.V. tubing at point closest to vein insertion site to prevent extravasation.
- Administration by continuous I.V. infusion isn't recommended.
- Inject I.M. dose deep into deltoid muscle. Aspirate for backflow to prevent inadvertent intra-arterial administration. Use I.M. route only if I.V. or oral routes are unavailable.
- Patient should remain in bed under observation for at least 3 hours after parenteral administration of diazepam to prevent potential hazards; keep resuscitation equipment nearby.
- Lower doses are effective in patients with renal or hepatic dysfunction.

■ Anticipate possible transient increase in frequency or severity of seizures when diazepam is used as adjunctive treatment of convulsive disorders. Impose seizure precautions.
■ Don't mix diazepam with other drugs in a syringe or infusion container.
■ Use Diastat rectal gel to treat no more than five episodes per month and no more than one episode every 5 days.

Therapeutic monitoring

■ During prolonged therapy, periodically monitor blood counts and liver function studies.
■ Assess gag reflex postendoscopy and before resuming oral intake to prevent aspiration.

Special populations

Pregnant patients. Warn female patient to call her doctor immediately if she becomes pregnant.
Breast-feeding patients. Diazepam is excreted in breast milk. The breast-fed infant of a woman who uses diazepam may become sedated, have feeding difficulties, or lose weight. Avoid use of drug in breast-feeding women.
Pediatric patients. Safe use of oral diazepam in infants under age 6 months hasn't been established. Safe use of parenteral diazepam in infants under age 30 days hasn't been established. Closely observe neonates whose mothers took diazepam for a prolonged period during pregnancy; the infants may show withdrawal symptoms. Use of rectal diazepam during labor may cause neonatal flaccidity. Safety and efficacy of rectal diazepam haven't been established in children under age 2.
Geriatric patients. Geriatric patients are more sensitive to the CNS depressant effects of diazepam. Use with caution. Lower doses are usually effective in geriatric patients because of decreased elimination. Geriatric patients who receive this drug require assistance with walking and activities of daily living during initiation of therapy or after an increase in dose. Parenteral administration of this drug is more likely to cause apnea, hypotension, and bradycardia in geriatric patients.

Patient counseling

■ Advise patient of the potential for physical and psychological dependence with long-term use.
■ Warn patient that sudden changes of position can cause dizziness. Advise patient to dangle legs for a few minutes before getting out of bed to prevent falls and injury.
■ Caution patient to avoid alcohol while taking diazepam.
■ Advise patient not to suddenly discontinue drug.
■ Teach patient's caregiver when to use rectal gel (to control bouts of increased seizure activity) and how to monitor and record patient's clinical response.
■ Teach patient's caregiver how to administer rectal gel.

diazoxide

Hyperstat IV, Proglycem

Pharmacologic classification: peripheral vasodilator
Therapeutic classification: antihypertensive, antihypoglycemic
Pregnancy risk category C

How supplied

Available by prescription only
Capsules: 50 mg
Oral suspension: 50 mg/ml in 30-ml bottle
Injection: 15 mg/ml in 20-ml ampule

Indications and dosages

Hypertensive crisis
Adults and children: 1 to 3 mg/kg I.V. (up to a maximum of 150 mg) q 5 to 15 minutes until an adequate reduction in blood pressure is achieved.

Note: The use of 300-mg I.V. bolus push is no longer recommended. Switch to therapy with oral antihypertensives as soon as possible.

Hypoglycemia from hyperinsulinism
Adults and children: Usual daily dose is 3 to 8 mg/kg/day P.O. divided in two or three equal doses.
Infants and newborns: Usual daily dose is 8 to 15 mg/kg/day P.O. divided in two or three equal doses.

Pharmacodynamics

Antihypertensive action: Diazoxide directly relaxes arteriolar smooth muscle, causing vasodilation and reducing peripheral vascular resistance, thus reducing blood pressure.
Antihypoglycemic action: Diazoxide increases blood glucose levels by inhibiting pancreatic secretion of insulin, by stimulating catecholamine release, or by increasing hepatic release of glucose.

Diazoxide is a nondiuretic congener of thiazide diuretics.

Pharmacokinetics

Absorption: After I.V. administration, blood pressure should decrease promptly, with maximum decrease in under 5 minutes. After oral administration, hyperglycemic effect begins in 1 hour.
Distribution: Distributed throughout the body; highest level is found in kidneys, liver, and adrenal glands; diazoxide crosses placenta and blood-brain barrier. Drug is about 90% protein-bound.
Metabolism: Metabolized partially in the liver.
Excretion: Excreted slowly by the kidneys. Duration of antihypertensive effect varies wide-

ly, ranging from 30 minutes to 72 hours (average 3 to 12 hours) after I.V. administration; after oral administration, antihypoglycemic effect persists for about 8 hours. Antihypertensive and antihypoglycemic effects may be prolonged in patients with renal dysfunction.

Route	Onset	Peak	Duration
P.O.	Unknown	Unknown	Unknown
I.V.	1 min	2-5 min	2-12 hr

Contraindications and precautions

Parenteral form is contraindicated in patients with hypersensitivity to drug, other thiazides, or sulfonamide-derived drugs, and in the treatment of compensatory hypertension (such as that associated with coarctation of the aorta or arteriovenous shunt). Oral form is contraindicated in patients with functional hypoglycemia.

Use cautiously in patients with uremia or impaired cerebral or cardiac function.

Interactions

Drug-drug. *Antihypertensives:* Diazoxide may potentiate antihypertensive effects; especially if I.V. diazoxide is administered within 6 hours after patient has received another antihypertensive agent. Use together cautiously.
Phenytoin: May increase metabolism and decrease the plasma protein binding of phenytoin. Monitor patient closely.
Diuretics: May potentiate antihypoglycemic, hyperuricemic, or antihypertensive effects of diazoxide. Monitor patient closely.
Warfarin: Diazoxide may displace warfarin, bilirubin, or other highly protein-bound substances from protein-binding sites. Avoid use together.
Thiazides: May enhance effects of diazoxide. Use together cautiously.
Insulin and oral antidiabetics: Diazoxide may alter insulin and oral antidiabetic requirements in previously stable diabetic patients. Monitor blood glucose levels.

Effects on diagnostic tests

Diazoxide inhibits glucose-stimulated insulin release and may cause false-negative insulin response to glucagon.

Adverse reactions

CNS: dizziness, weakness; headache, malaise, anxiety, insomnia, paresthesia (with oral form); headache, ***seizures, paralysis, cerebral ischemia,*** light-headedness, euphoria (with parenteral form).
CV: ***arrhythmias,*** tachycardia, hypotension, hypertension (with oral form); *sodium and water retention, orthostatic hypotension,* diaphoresis, flushing, warmth, angina, myocardial ischemia, ECG changes, ***shock, MI*** (with parenteral form).
EENT: diplopia, transient cataracts, blurred vision, lacrimation (with oral administration), optic nerve infarction (with parenteral form).
GI: abdominal discomfort, diarrhea; nausea, vomiting, anorexia, taste alteration (with oral form); *nausea, vomiting,* dry mouth, constipation (with parenteral form).
GU: azotemia, reversible nephrotic syndrome, decreased urine output, hematuria, albuminuria (with oral administration).
Hematologic: ***leukopenia, thrombocytopenia,*** anemia, eosinophilia, excessive bleeding (with oral administration).
Metabolic: *sodium and fluid retention, ketoacidosis and hyperosmolar nonketotic syndrome, hyperuricemia, hyperglycemia.*
Skin: rash, pruritus (with oral administration).
Other: hirsutism; fever (with oral administration); inflammation and pain resulting from extravasation.

Overdose and treatment

Overdose is manifested primarily by hyperglycemia; ketoacidosis and hypotension may occur.

Treat acute overdose supportively and symptomatically. If hyperglycemia develops, give insulin and replace fluid and electrolyte losses; use vasopressors if hypotension fails to respond to conservative treatment. Prolonged monitoring may be necessary because of the long half-life of diazoxide.

Clinical considerations

- Diazoxide is used to treat only hypoglycemia resulting from hyperinsulinism; it isn't used to treat functional hypoglycemia. It may be used temporarily to control preoperative or postoperative hypoglycemia in patients with hyperinsulinism.
- I.V. use of diazoxide is seldom necessary for more than 4 or 5 days.
- Significant hypotension doesn't occur after oral administration in doses used to treat hypoglycemia.
- Drug may be given by constant I.V. infusion (7.5 to 30 mg/minute) until adequate blood pressure reduction occurs.

Therapeutic monitoring

- Monitor blood pressure and ECG continuously. Keep norepinephrine available.
- After I.V. injection, monitor blood pressure every 5 minutes for 15 to 30 minutes, then hourly when patient is stable. Discontinue if severe hypotension develops or if blood pressure continues to decrease 30 minutes after drug infusion; keep patient recumbent during this time and have norepinephrine available. Monitor I.V. site for infiltration or extravasation.
- Intake and output must be monitored carefully. If fluid or sodium retention develops, diuretics may be given 30 to 60 minutes after di-

azoxide. Patient must be recumbent for 8 to 10 hours after diuretic administration.

- Monitor daily blood glucose and electrolyte levels, watching diabetic patients closely for severe hyperglycemia or hyperglycemic hyperosmolar nonketotic coma; also monitor daily urine glucose and ketone levels, intake and output, and weight. Check serum uric acid levels frequently.

Special populations
Breast-feeding patients. It isn't known if drug is excreted in breast milk; an alternative feeding method is recommended during therapy.
Pediatric patients. Use with caution in children.
Geriatric patients. Geriatric patients may have a more pronounced hypotensive response.

Patient counseling
- Explain that orthostatic hypotension can be minimized by rising slowly and avoiding sudden position changes.
- Tell patient to report adverse effects immediately, including pain and redness at injection site, which may indicate infiltration.
- Instruct patient to check weight daily and report gains of more than 5 lb/week; diazoxide causes sodium and water retention.
- Reassure patient that excessive hair growth is a common reaction that subsides when drug treatment is completed.

dibucaine
Nupercainal

Pharmacologic classification: local anesthetic (amine)
Therapeutic classification: local amide anesthetic
Pregnancy risk category B

How supplied
Available without a prescription
Ointment (rectal or topical): 1%
Cream (topical): 0.5%

Indications and dosages
Temporary relief of pain and itching associated with abrasions, sunburn, minor burns, insect bites, and other minor skin conditions
Adults and children: Apply to affected areas, p.r.n. Maximum daily dose of 1% ointment is 30 g for adults and 7.5 g for children.
Temporary relief of pain, itching, and burning caused by hemorrhoids
Adults: Instill 1% ointment into rectum using a rectal applicator each morning and evening and after each bowel movement, p.r.n. Apply additional ointment topically to anal tissues. Maximum daily dose is 30 g.

Pharmacodynamics
Anesthetic action: Dibucaine inhibits conduction of nerve impulses and decreases cell membrane permeability to ions, anesthetizing local nerve endings.

Pharmacokinetics
Absorption: Dibucaine has limited absorption.
Distribution: None.
Metabolism: None.
Excretion: None.

Route	Onset	Peak	Duration
Topical, P.R.	Unknown	Unknown	Unknown

Contraindications and precautions
Contraindicated in patients with known hypersensitivity to drug, sulfites, or other amide-type local anesthetics and for use on large skin areas, on broken skin or mucous membranes, and in eyes.

Interactions
None reported.

Effects on diagnostic tests
None reported.

Adverse reactions
Skin: irritation, inflammation, contact dermatitis, cutaneous lesions.
Other: ***hypersensitivity reactions*** (urticaria, edema, burning, stinging, tenderness).

Note: Discontinue drug if sensitization occurs or if condition worsens.

Overdose and treatment
Clean area thoroughly with mild soap and water.

Clinical considerations
- Use dibucaine topically only for short periods.
- Don't use in or near the eye.

Therapeutic monitoring
If rectal bleeding, rash, pain, swelling, or other symptoms develop, notify doctor immediately and discontinue use of medication.

Special populations
Breast-feeding patients. Drug shouldn't be used in breast-feeding women.
Pediatric patients. Adjust dosage to patient's age, size, and physical condition.
Geriatric patients. Adjust dosage to patient's age, size, and physical condition.

Patient counseling
- Advise patient to call if condition worsens or if symptoms persist for more than 7 days after use.
- Explain correct use of drug.

- Emphasize need to wash hands thoroughly after use.
- Caution patient to apply drug sparingly to minimize untoward effects.
- Tell patient to keep drug out of reach of children.

diclofenac potassium

Cataflam

diclofenac sodium

Voltaren, Voltaren-XR

Pharmacologic classification: NSAID
Therapeutic classification: antiarthritic, anti-inflammatory
Pregnancy risk category B

How supplied

Available by prescription only
diclofenac potassium
Tablets: 50 mg
diclofenac sodium
Tablets (delayed-release): 25 mg, 50 mg, 75 mg
Tablets (extended-release): 100 mg
Ophthalmic drops: 0.1%

Indications and dosages

Osteoarthritis
Adults: 50 mg P.O. b.i.d. or t.i.d., or 75 mg P.O. b.i.d. (diclofenac sodium only).
Ankylosing spondylitis
Adults: 25 mg P.O. q.i.d. An additional 25 mg dose may be needed h.s.
Rheumatoid arthritis
Adults: 50 mg P.O. t.i.d. or q.i.d. Alternatively, 75 mg P.O. b.i.d. (diclofenac sodium only).
Analgesia and primary dysmenorrhea
Adults: 50 mg (diclofenac potassium only) P.O. t.i.d. Alternatively, 100 mg (diclofenac potassium only) P.O. initially, followed by 50 mg doses, up to a maximum dose of 200 mg in first 24 hours; subsequent dosing should follow 50 mg t.i.d. regimen.

Pharmacodynamics

Anti-inflammatory action: Diclofenac exerts its anti-inflammatory and antipyretic actions through an unknown mechanism that may involve inhibition of prostaglandin synthesis.

Pharmacokinetics

Absorption: After oral administration, diclofenac is rapidly and almost completely absorbed. Absorption is delayed by food.
Distribution: Highly (nearly 100%) protein-bound.
Metabolism: Undergoes first-pass metabolism, with 60% of unchanged drug reaching systemic circulation. The principal active metabolite, 48-hydroxydiclofenac, has about 3% of the activity of the parent compound. Mean terminal half-life is about 1¼ to 1¾ hours after an oral dose.
Excretion: About 40% to 60% is excreted in the urine; the balance is excreted in the bile. The 4'-hydroxy metabolite accounts for 20% to 30% of the dose excreted in the urine; the other metabolites account for 10% to 20%; 5% to 10% is excreted unchanged in the urine. More than 90% is excreted within 72 hours. Moderate renal impairment doesn't alter the elimination rate of unchanged diclofenac but may reduce the elimination rate of the metabolites. Hepatic impairment doesn't appear to affect the pharmacokinetics of diclofenac.

Route	Onset	Peak	Duration
P.O.	10 min	1 hr	8 hr
P.O. (enteric)	30 min	2-3 hr	8 hr
P.O. (extended-release)	Unknown	Unknown	Unknown

Contraindications and precautions

Oral form is contraindicated in patients with hypersensitivity to drug and in those with hepatic porphyria or a history of asthma, urticaria, or other allergic reactions after taking aspirin or other NSAIDs. Avoid use during late pregnancy or while breast-feeding. Ophthalmic solution is contraindicated in patients with hypersensitivity to any component of the drug and in those wearing soft contact lenses; also avoid use during late pregnancy.

Use oral form cautiously in patients with history of peptic ulcer disease, hepatic or renal dysfunction, cardiac disease, hypertension, or conditions associated with fluid retention.

Use ophthalmic solution cautiously in patients with hypersensitivity to aspirin, phenylacetic acid derivatives, and other NSAIDs and in surgical patients with known bleeding tendencies or in those receiving medications that may prolong bleeding time.

Interactions

Drug-drug. *Aspirin:* Lowers plasma levels of diclofenac. Concurrent use isn't recommended.
Warfarin: Affects platelet function. Requires close monitoring of anticoagulant dosage.
Cyclosporine, digoxin, methotrexate: Increases the toxicity of these drugs. Monitor patient and serum levels closely.
Lithium: Decreases renal clearance of lithium and increases plasma levels; may lead to lithium toxicity. Monitor serum levels closely.
Insulin or oral antidiabetic agents: May alter the patient's response to these agents. Monitor blood glucose levels closely.
Diuretics: Concurrent use of diclofenac may inhibit the action of diuretics. Monitor patient closely.

Potassium-sparing diuretics: May increase serum potassium levels. Monitor serum potassium levels closely.
Beta blockers: May blunt antihypertensive effects. Don't use together.
Phenytoin: May increase serum levels. Monitor for toxicity.
Drug-lifestyle. *Sun exposure:* May cause photosensitivity reactions. Advise patient to take precautions.

Effects on diagnostic tests
None reported.

Adverse reactions
Unless otherwise noted, the following adverse reactions refer to oral administration of drug:
CNS: anxiety, depression, dizziness, drowsiness, insomnia, irritability, headache.
CV: ***heart failure,*** hypertension, edema.
EENT: *tinnitus,* laryngeal edema, swelling of the lips and tongue, blurred vision, eye pain, night blindness, epistaxis, taste disorder, reversible hearing loss; *transient stinging and burning, increased intraocular pressure, keratitis,* anterior chamber reaction, ocular allergy (with ophthalmic solution).
GI: *abdominal pain or cramps, constipation, diarrhea, indigestion, nausea,* vomiting, abdominal distention, flatulence, peptic ulceration, ***bleeding,*** melena, bloody diarrhea, appetite change, colitis.
GU: proteinuria, ***acute renal failure***, oliguria, interstitial nephritis, papillary necrosis ***nephrotic syndrome,*** fluid retention.
Hematologic: increased platelet aggregation time.
Hepatic: elevated liver enzymes, jaundice, *hepatitis,* ***hepatotoxicity.***
Metabolic: hypoglycemia; hyperglycemia.
Musculoskeletal: back, leg, or joint pain.
Respiratory: asthma.
Skin: rash, pruritus, urticaria, eczema, dermatitis, alopecia, photosensitivity, bullous eruption, ***Stevens-Johnson syndrome*** (rare), allergic purpura.
Other: ***anaphylaxis; anaphylactoid reactions; angioedema;*** viral infection (with ophthalmic solution).

Overdose and treatment
No information available. There is no special antidote. Supportive and symptomatic treatment may include induction of vomiting or gastric lavage. Treatment with activated charcoal or dialysis may also be appropriate.

Clinical considerations
- Administration with other drugs, such as glucocorticoids, that produce adverse GI effects may aggravate such effects.
- Because the anti-inflammatory, antipyretic, and analgesic effects of diclofenac may mask the usual signs of infection, monitor carefully for infection.

Therapeutic monitoring
- Monitor renal function during treatment. Use with caution and at reduced dosage in patients with renal impairment.
- Periodic ophthalmologic examinations are recommended during prolonged therapy.
- Monitor liver function during therapy. Abnormal liver function test results and severe hepatic reactions may occur.
- Periodic evaluation of hematopoietic function is recommended because bone marrow abnormalities have occurred. Regular check of hemoglobin level is important to detect toxic effects on the GI tract.

Special populations
Breast-feeding patients. Low levels of diclofenac have been measured in breast milk. Risk-to-benefit ratio must be considered.
Pediatric patients. Drug isn't recommended for use in children.
Geriatric patients. Use with caution in geriatric patients; they may be more susceptible to adverse reactions, especially GI toxicity and nephrotoxicity. Reduce dosage to lowest level that controls symptoms.

Patient counseling
- Advise patient to take drug with meals or milk to avoid GI upset.
- Teach patient to restrict salt intake, as diclofenac may cause edema, especially if patient is hypertensive.
- Instruct patient to report symptoms that may be related to GI ulceration, such as epigastric pain and black or tarry stools, as well as other unusual symptoms such as skin rash, pruritus or significant edema or weight gain.

dicloxacillin sodium
Dycill, Dynapen, Pathocil

Pharmacologic classification: penicillinase-resistant penicillin
Therapeutic classification: antibiotic
Pregnancy risk category NR

How supplied
Available by prescription only
Capsules: 125 mg, 250 mg, 500 mg
Oral suspension: 62.5 mg/5 ml (after reconstitution)

Indications and dosages
Systemic infections caused by penicillinase-producing staphylococci
Adults and children weighing 88 lb (40 kg) or more: 125 to 250 mg P.O. q 6 hours.
Infants and children over age 1 month weighing less than 88 lb (40 kg): 12.5 to 50 mg/kg

P.O. daily, divided into doses given q 6 hours. Serious infection may require higher dosage (75 to 100 mg/kg/day in divided doses q 6 hours).

Pharmacodynamics

Antibiotic action: Dicloxacillin is bactericidal; it adheres to bacterial penicillin-binding proteins, thus inhibiting bacterial cell wall synthesis. Dicloxacillin resists the effects of penicillinases—enzymes that inactivate penicillin—and is thus active against many strains of penicillinase-producing bacteria; this activity is most important against penicillinase-producing staphylococci; some strains may remain resistant. Dicloxacillin is also active against a few gram-positive aerobic and anaerobic bacilli but has no significant effect on gram-negative bacilli.

Pharmacokinetics

Absorption: Absorbed rapidly but incompletely (35% to 76%) from the GI tract; it's relatively acid stable. Food may decrease both rate and extent of absorption.
Distribution: Distributed widely into bone, bile, and pleural and synovial fluids. CSF penetration is poor but is enhanced by meningeal inflammation. Drug crosses the placenta, and is 95% to 99% protein-bound.
Metabolism: Metabolized only partially.
Excretion: Excreted in urine by renal tubular secretion and glomerular filtration; also excreted in breast milk. Elimination half-life in adults is ½ to 1 hour, extended minimally to 2¼ hours in patients with renal impairment.

Route	Onset	Peak	Duration
P.O.	Unknown	2 hr	6 hr

Contraindications and precautions

Contraindicated in patients with hypersensitivity to drug or other penicillins. Use cautiously in patients with other drug allergies, especially to cephalosporins, or in those with mononucleosis.

Interactions

Drug-drug. *Aminoglycosides:* Dicloxacillin may falsely decrease serum aminoglycoside levels. Monitor patient carefully.
Probenecid: Blocks renal tubular secretion of dicloxacillin, raising its serum levels. Probenecid may be used for this purpose.
Oral contraceptives: May decrease their efficacy. Recommend additional form of contraceptive during penicillin therapy.

Effects on diagnostic tests

Dicloxacillin alters test results for urine and serum proteins; it produces false-positive or elevated results in turbidimetric urine and serum protein tests using sulfosalicylic acid or trichloroacetic acid; it also reportedly produces false results on the Bradshaw screening test for Bence Jones protein.

Adverse reactions

CNS: neuromuscular irritability, ***seizures,*** lethargy, hallucinations, anxiety, confusion, agitation, depression, dizziness, fatigue.
GI: *nausea,* vomiting, *epigastric distress,* flatulence, *diarrhea,* enterocolitis, pseudomembranous colitis, black "hairy" tongue, abdominal pain.
GU: interstitial nephritis, nephropathy.
Hematologic: eosinophilia, anemia, ***thrombocytopenia, leukopenia,*** hemolytic anemia, ***agranulocytosis.***
Hepatic: transient elevations in liver function study results, cholestasis, ***hepatitis.***
Other: hypersensitivity reactions (pruritus, urticaria, rash, ***anaphylaxis***), overgrowth of nonsusceptible organisms.

Overdose and treatment

Clinical signs of overdose include neuromuscular irritability or seizures. No specific recommendations. Treatment is supportive. After recent ingestion (4 hours or less), empty the stomach by induced emesis or gastric lavage; follow with activated charcoal to reduce absorption. Drug isn't appreciably dialyzable.

Clinical considerations

Consider the recommendations relevant to all penicillins as well as the following:
- Aminoglycosides produce synergistic bactericidal effects against *Staphylococcus aureus.* However, the drugs are physically and chemically incompatible and are inactivated when mixed or given together. Dicloxacillin may falsely decrease serum aminoglycoside levels.
- Give drug with water only; acid in fruit juice or carbonated beverage may inactivate drug.
- Give dose on empty stomach; food decreases absorption.

Therapeutic monitoring

Regularly assess renal, hepatic, and hematopoietic function during prolonged therapy.

Special populations

Breast-feeding patients. Dicloxacillin is excreted into breast milk; use drug with caution in breast-feeding women.
Pediatric patients. Elimination of dicloxacillin is reduced in neonates; safety in neonates hasn't been established.
Geriatric patients. Half-life may be prolonged in geriatric patients because of impaired renal function.

Patient counseling

- Tell patient to report severe diarrhea promptly. He should also report rash or itching.
- Instruct patient to complete full course of therapy as prescribed, even if he feels better.

dicyclomine hydrochloride

Antispas, A-Spas, Bentyl, Bentylol*, Byclomine, Dibent, Formulex*, Lomine*, Neoquess, Or-Tyl, Spasmoban*, Spasmoject

Pharmacologic classification: anticholinergic
Therapeutic classification: antimuscarinic, GI antispasmodic
Pregnancy risk category B

How supplied

Available by prescription only
Tablets: 20 mg
Capsules: 10 mg
Syrup: 10 mg/5 ml
Injection: 10 mg/ml in 2-ml vials, 10-ml vials, 2-ml ampules

Indications and dosages

Irritable bowel syndrome and other functional GI disorders
Adults: Initially, 20 mg P.O. q.i.d., then increase to 40 mg P.O. q.i.d. during first week of therapy unless precluded by adverse reactions. Alternatively, give 20 mg I.M. q 4 to 6 hours.
Children age 2 and older: 10 mg P.O. t.i.d. or q.i.d.
Infants age 6 to 23 months: 5 to 10 mg P.O. t.i.d. or q.i.d.
◊***Infant colic***
Infants age 6 months and older: 5 to 10 mg P.O. t.i.d. or q.i.d. Adjust dosage according to patient's needs and response.

Note: High environmental temperatures may induce heatstroke during drug use. If symptoms occur, the discontinue drug.

Pharmacodynamics

Antispasmodic action: Dicyclomine exerts a nonspecific, direct spasmolytic action on smooth muscle. It also has some local anesthetic properties that may contribute to spasmolysis in the GI and biliary tracts.

Pharmacokinetics

Absorption: About 67% of an oral dose is absorbed from the GI tract.
Distribution: Largely unknown.
Metabolism: Unknown.
Excretion: After oral administration, 80% of a dose is excreted in urine and 10% in feces.

Route	Onset	Peak	Duration
P.O., I.M.	Unknown	1-1½ hr	Unknown

Contraindications and precautions

Contraindicated in patients with obstructive uropathy, obstructive disease of the GI tract, reflux esophagitis, severe ulcerative colitis, myasthenia gravis, hypersensitivity to anticholinergics, unstable CV status in acute hemorrhage, or glaucoma. Also contraindicated in breast-feeding patients and in children under age 6 months.

Use cautiously in patients with autonomic neuropathy, hyperthyroidism, coronary artery disease, arrhythmias, heart failure, hypertension, hiatal hernia, hepatic or renal disease, prostatic hyperplasia, and ulcerative colitis.

Interactions

Drug-drug. *Antacids:* Decrease oral absorption of anticholinergics. Dicyclomine should be given at least 1 hour before antacids.
Amantadine, antihistamines, antiparkinsonian agents, dysopyramide, glutethimide, meperidine, phenothiazines, procainamide, quinidine, tricyclic antidepressants: May cause additive adverse effects. Avoid use together.
Levodopa and ketoconazole: Decreased GI absorption. Avoid use together.
Digoxin (slowly dissolving tablets): Higher serum digoxin levels when administered with anticholinergics. Monitor digoxin levels closely.
Oral potassium supplements (especially wax-matrix formulations): Potassium-induced GI ulcerations may be increased. Use together cautiously.
Methotrimeprazine: May enhance risk of extrapyramidal reactions. Avoid use together.

Effects on diagnostic tests

None reported.

Adverse reactions

CNS: *headache; dizziness;* insomnia; lightheadedness; drowsiness; nervousness, confusion, excitement (in elderly patients).
CV: *palpitations,* tachycardia.
EENT: blurred vision, increased intraocular pressure, mydriasis.
GI: nausea, vomiting, *constipation, dry mouth,* abdominal distention, heartburn, paralytic ileus.
GU: *urinary hesitancy, urine retention,* impotence.
Skin: urticaria, decreased sweating or possible anhidrosis, other dermal manifestations, local irritation.
Other: fever, allergic reactions, dependence.

Dicyclomine is a synthetic tertiary derivative that may have atropine-like adverse reactions.

Overdose and treatment

Clinical signs of overdose include curare-like symptoms of CNS stimulation followed by depression, and such psychotic symptoms as disorientation, confusion, hallucinations, delusions, anxiety, agitation, and restlessness. Peripheral effects may include dilated, nonreactive pupils; hot, flushed, dry skin; tachycardia; hypertension; and increased respiration.

Treatment is primarily symptomatic and supportive, as necessary. Maintain patent airway. If patient is alert, induce emesis (or use gastric lavage) and follow with a saline cathartic and activated charcoal to prevent further drug absorption. In severe cases, physostigmine may be administered to block the antimuscarinic effects of dicyclomine. Give fluids, as needed, to treat shock; diazepam to control psychotic symptoms; and pilocarpine (instilled into the eyes) to relieve mydriasis. If urine retention occurs, catheterization may be necessary.

Clinical considerations

Consider the recommendations relevant to all anticholinergics as well as the following:
☐ ***ALERT*** Never give dicyclomine I.V. or S.C.
- Be prepared to adjust dose, based on patient's needs and response.

Therapeutic monitoring

Monitor vital signs and urine output carefully.

Special populations

Breast-feeding patients. Dicyclomine may be excreted in breast milk; it may also decrease milk production. Breast-feeding women should avoid use of drug.
Pediatric patients. Safety and effectiveness in children haven't been established. Administer cautiously to infants age 6 months or over; seizures have been reported. Drug is contraindicated in infants under age 6 months.
Geriatric patients. Administer drug cautiously to geriatric patients. Lower doses are indicated.

Patient counseling

- Tell patient that syrup formulation may be diluted with water.
- Warn patient that high environmental temperatures may induce heatstroke while drug is being used; tell patient to avoid exposure to such temperatures.
- Advise patient to avoid driving and other hazardous activities if drowsiness or blurred vision occurs; and report rash or other skin eruption.

didanosine (ddI)

Videx

Pharmacologic classification: purine analogue
Therapeutic classification: antiviral
Pregnancy risk category B

How supplied

Available by prescription only
Tablets (chewable): 25 mg, 50 mg, 100 mg, 150 mg
Powder for oral solution (buffered): 100 mg/packet, 167 mg/packet, 250 mg/packet
Powder for oral solution (pediatric): 2 g and 4 g in 4- and 8-ounce bottles, respectively

Indications and dosages

Treatment of HIV infection when antiretroviral therapy is warranted
Adults weighing 132 lb (60 kg) or more: 200 mg (tablets) P.O. b.i.d., or 400 mg once daily, or 250 mg buffered powder P.O. b.i.d.
Adults weighing less than 132 lb: 125 mg (tablets) P.O. b.i.d. or 250 mg once daily, or 167 mg buffered powder P.O. b.i.d.
Children: 120 mg/m^2 P.O. b.i.d. To prevent gastric acid degradation, children over age 1 should receive a 2-tablet dose, and children under age 1 should receive a 1-tablet dose.
≡ ***Dosage adjustment.*** Patients with renal or hepatic impairment may need their dosage adjusted.

Pharmacodynamics

Antiviral actions: Didanosine is a synthetic purine analogue of deoxyadenosine. After didanosine enters the cell, it's converted to its active form dideoxyadenosine triphosphate (ddATP), which inhibits replication of HIV by preventing DNA replication. In addition, ddATP inhibits the enzyme HIV-RNA dependent DNA polymerase (reverse transcriptase).

Pharmacokinetics

Absorption: Degrades rapidly in gastric acid. Commercially available preparations contain buffers to raise stomach pH. Bioavailability averages about 33%; tablets may exhibit better bioavailability than buffered powder for oral solution. Food can decrease absorption by 50%.
Distribution: Widely distributed; drug penetration into the CNS varies, but CSF levels average 46% of concurrent plasma levels.
Metabolism: Metabolism isn't fully understood, but is probably similar to that of endogenous purines.
Excretion: Excreted in urine as allantoin, hypoxanthine, xanthine, and uric acid. Serum half-life averages 0.8 hours.

Route	Onset	Peak	Duration
P.O.	Unknown	½-1 hr	Unknown

Contraindications and precautions

Contraindicated in patients with history of hypersensitivity to any component of the formulation. Use very cautiously in patients with history of pancreatitis. Also use cautiously in patients with peripheral neuropathy, impaired renal or hepatic function, or hyperuricemia.

Interactions

Drug-drug. *Ketoconazole, dapsone, drugs that require gastric acid for adequate absorption:* Decreased buffering action of didanosine. Administer such drugs 2 hours before didanosine.
Tetracyclines, fluoroquinolones: Decreased absorption from buffering agents in didanosine tablets or antacids in pediatric suspension. Avoid use together.

Antacids containing magnesium or aluminum hydroxides: May produce enhanced adverse effects, such as diarrhea or constipation. Avoid use together.
Itraconazole: May decrease serum levels of itraconazole. Avoid use together.
Drug-food. *Any food:* Decreased rate of absorption. Give drug on an empty stomach at least 30 minutes before a meal.

Effects on diagnostic tests

None reported.

Adverse reactions

CNS: *headache,* ***seizures,*** confusion, anxiety, nervousness, asthenia, abnormal thinking, twitching, depression, *peripheral neuropathy.*
GI: *diarrhea, nausea, vomiting, abdominal pain,* ***pancreatitis,*** dry mouth, anorexia.
Hematologic: ***leukopenia,*** granulocytosis, ***thrombocytopenia,*** anemia.
Hepatic: ***hepatic failure,*** elevated liver enzymes, hepatomegaly.
Metabolic: increased serum uric acid levels. lactic acidosis.
Musculoskeletal: myopathy.
Respiratory: pneumonia, dyspnea.
Skin: rash, pruritus, sarcoma.
Other: pain, infection, ***allergic reactions,*** *chills, fever.*

Overdose and treatment

No specific information exists regarding the treatment of overdose; however, possible effects of overdose include diarrhea, pancreatitis, peripheral neuropathy, hyperuricemia, and hepatic dysfunction. Treatment is supportive. No specific antidote is known, and it's unknown if drug is dialyzable.

Clinical considerations

☐ ***ALERT*** Didansene shouldn't be used as monotherapy.
☐ ***ALERT*** Pediatric powder for oral solution must be prepared by the pharmacist before dispensing. It must be constituted with water, then diluted with antacid (manufacturer recommends either Mylanta Double Strength Liquid or Maalox TC) to a final concentration of 10 mg/ml. The admixture is stable for 30 days if refrigerated at 36° to 46° F (2° to 8° C). Be sure to shake well before measuring the dose.
☐ ***ALERT*** Don't confuse drug with other antivirals that use abbreviations for identification.

- Most patients over age 1 should receive two tablets per dose. Tablets contain buffers that raise stomach pH to levels that prevent degradation of the active drug. Tablets should be thoroughly chewed before swallowing, and the patient should drink at least 1 oz of water with each dose. If tablets are manually crushed, mix drug in 1 oz (30 ml) water; stir to disperse uniformly, then have patient drink it immediately. Single-dose packets containing buffered powder for oral solution are available.
- To administer buffered powder for oral solution, carefully open the packet and pour the contents into 4 oz (120 ml) water. Don't use fruit juice or other acidic beverages. Stir for 2 or 3 minutes until the powder dissolves completely. Administer immediately.
- Consider substituting the chewable tablets if diarrhea occurs.
- When preparing powder or crushing tablets, avoid excessive dispersal of drug particles into the air.

Therapeutic monitoring

- The major toxicity of drug use is pancreatitis, which has been fatal in some cases. It must be considered when abdominal pain, nausea, and vomiting develop or biochemical markers are elevated. Discontinue use of drug until pancreatitis is excluded. If pancreatitis is confirmed, don't use the drug again.

Special populations

Breast-feeding patients. It's unknown if drug is excreted in breast milk. Because of risk of serious adverse effects in the infant, breast-feeding isn't recommended
Pediatric patients. Retinal depigmentation has occurred in some children receiving drug. Children should receive dilated retinal examinations at least every 6 months or if a change in vision occurs.

Patient counseling

- Tell patient to take drug on an empty stomach to ensure adequate absorption, to chew tablets thoroughly before swallowing, and to drink at least 1 oz (30 ml) water with each dose.
- Remind patient using buffered powder for oral solution not to use fruit juice or other acidic beverages, to allow 3 minutes for powder to dissolve completely, and to take immediately. Be sure he understands how to mix the solution.

diflunisal

Dolobid

Pharmacologic classification: NSAID, salicylic acid derivative
Therapeutic classification: nonnarcotic analgesic, antipyretic, anti-inflammatory
Pregnancy risk category C

How supplied

Available by prescription only
Tablets (film-coated): 250 mg, 500 mg

Indications and dosages

Mild to moderate pain

Adults: Initiate therapy with 1 g, then 500 mg P.O. daily in two or three divided doses, usually q 8 to 12 hours. Maximum dose is 1,500 mg daily.

≡ ***Dosage adjustment.*** In adults over age 65, start with one half the usual adult dose.

Rheumatoid arthritis and osteoarthritis

Adults: 500 to 1,000 mg P.O. daily in two divided doses, usually q 12 hours. Maximum dose is 1,500 mg daily.

≡ ***Dosage adjustment.*** In adults over age 65, start with one half the usual dose.

Pharmacodynamics

Analgesic, antipyretic, and anti-inflammatory actions: Mechanisms of action are unknown, but are probably related to inhibition of prostaglandin synthesis. Diflunisal is a salicylic acid derivative, but isn't hydrolyzed to free salicylate in vivo.

Pharmacokinetics

Absorption: Absorbed rapidly and completely via the GI tract.

Distribution: Highly protein-bound.

Metabolism: Metabolized in the liver; it isn't metabolized to salicylic acid.

Excretion: Excreted in urine. Half-life is 8 to 12 hours.

Route	Onset	Peak	Duration
P.O.	1 hr	2-3 hr	8-12 hr

Contraindications and precautions

Contraindicated in patients with hypersensitivity to the drug or for whom acute asthmatic attacks, urticaria, or rhinitis are precipitated by aspirin or other NSAIDs. Use cautiously in patients with GI bleeding, history of peptic ulcer disease, renal impairment, and compromised cardiac function, hypertension, or other conditions predisposing patient to fluid retention.

Because of the epidemiologic association with Reye's syndrome, the Center for Disease Control and Prevention recommends not giving salicylates to children and teenagers with chickenpox or influenza-like illness.

Interactions

Drug-drug. *Anticoagulants, thrombolytic drugs:* Potentiate their anticoagulant effects. Use together cautiously.

Highly protein-bound drugs, such as phenytoin, sulfonylureas, and warfarin: May cause displacement of either drug and adverse effects. Monitor patient closely for both drugs.

Steroids, antibiotics, NSAIDs: May potentiate the adverse GI effects of diflunisal; use together with caution.

Aspirin, antacids: Delay and decrease the absorption of diflunisal. Monitor for decreased therapeutic effect.

Hydrochlorothiazide: Increases the plasma concentration of hydrochlorothiazide; decreases its hyperuricemic, diuretic, antihypertensive, and natriuretic effects. Avoid use together.

Furosemide: Decreases the hyperuricemic effect of furosemide. Monitor patient carefully.

Antihypertensives: Decrease their effect on blood pressure; blood pressure must be monitored closely.

Cyclosporine, diuretics, gold compounds: May increase nephrotoxic potential. Avoid use together.

Indomethacin: Decreased renal clearance of indomethacin. Fatal GI hemorrhage has also been reported. Avoid use together.

Acetaminophen: May increase serum acetaminophen levels by as much as 50%, leading to potential hepatotoxicity. This interaction may also be nephrotoxic. Avoid use together.

Lithium: May result in increased lithium serum levels. Monitor lithium levels closely.

Methotrexate, verapamil, nifedipine: Diflunisal may decrease the renal excretion of these drugs. Monitor patient carefully.

Probenecid: May decrease renal clearance of diflunisal. Monitor patient closely.

Sulindac: Diflunisal decreases blood levels of sulindac's active metabolite. Monitor patient carefully for reduced effect.

Drug-lifestyle. *Alcohol use:* May potentiate the adverse GI effects of diflunisal. Advise patient to avoid alcohol consumption.

Effects on diagnostic tests

None reported.

Adverse reactions

CNS: *dizziness,* somnolence, insomnia, *headache,* fatigue.

EENT: *tinnitus, visual disturbances* (rare).

GI: *nausea, dyspepsia, GI pain, diarrhea,* vomiting, constipation, flatulence.

GU: increased serum BUN and creatinine, renal impairment, hematuria, interstitial nephritis.

Hematologic: prolonged bleeding time.

Hepatic: increased liver function tests.

Metabolic: hyperkalemia, hypouricemia.

Skin: *rash,* pruritus, sweating, stomatitis, ***erythema multiforme, Stevens-Johnson syndrome.***

Overdose and treatment

Signs and symptoms of overdose include drowsiness, nausea, vomiting, hyperventilation, tachycardia, sweating, tinnitus, disorientation, stupor, and coma.

To treat overdose of diflunisal, empty stomach immediately by inducing emesis with ipecac syrup if patient is conscious, or by gastric lavage. Administer activated charcoal via nasogastric tube. Provide symptomatic and supportive measures (respiratory support and correction of fluid and electrolyte imbalances). Monitor laboratory parameters and vital signs closely. Hemodialysis has little effect.

Clinical considerations

Consider the recommendations relevant to all NSAIDs as well as the following:

◻ ***ALERT*** Don't give salicylates to children and teenagers with chickenpox or flulike symptoms because of the epidemiologic association with Reye's syndrome.

- Diflunisal is recommended for twice-daily dosing for added patient convenience and compliance.
- Don't break, crush, or allow patient to chew diflunisal. Patient should swallow medication whole.
- Administer diflunisal with water, milk, or meals to minimize GI upset.
- Don't administer with aspirin or acetaminophen.
- Evaluate patient's response to diflunisal therapy as evidenced by a reduction in pain or inflammation. Monitor vital signs frequently, especially temperature.
- Institute safety measures to prevent injury if patient experiences CNS effects.

Therapeutic monitoring

- Monitor results of laboratory tests, especially renal and liver function studies. Assess presence and amount of peripheral edema. Monitor weight frequently.
- Assess patient for signs and symptoms of potential hemorrhage, such as bruising, petechiae, coffee ground emesis, and black, tarry stools.

Special populations

Breast-feeding patients. Because drug is excreted in breast milk, breast-feeding isn't recommended.

Pediatric patients. Don't use long-term diflunisal therapy in children under age 14; safety hasn't been established.

Geriatric patients. Patients over age 60 may be more susceptible to the toxic effects (particularly GI toxicity) of this drug. The effects of this drug on renal prostaglandins may cause fluid retention and edema, a significant drawback for geriatric patients, especially those with heart failure or hypertension.

Patient counseling

- Instruct patient in diflunisal regimen and need for compliance. Advise him to report adverse reactions.
- Tell patient to take diflunisal with foods to minimize GI upset and to swallow capsule whole.
- Caution patient to avoid activities requiring alertness or concentration, such as driving, until CNS effects are known.
- Instruct patient in safety measures to prevent injury.

digoxin

Lanoxicaps, Lanoxin, Novodigoxin*

Pharmacologic classification: cardiac glycoside
Therapeutic classification: antiarrhythmic, inotropic
Pregnancy risk category C

How supplied

Available by prescription only
Tablets: 0.125 mg, 0.25 mg
Capsules: 0.05 mg, 0.10 mg, 0.20 mg
Elixir: 0.05 mg/ml
Injection: 0.1 mg/ml (pediatric), 0.25 mg/ml, 0.5 mg/2 ml

Indications and dosages

Heart failure, atrial fibrillation and flutter, paroxysmal atrial tachycardia

Tablets, elixir

Adults: For rapid digitalization, give 0.75 to 1.25 mg P.O. over 24 hours in two or more divided doses q 6 to 8 hours. For slow digitalization, give 0.125 to 0.5 mg daily for 5 to 7 days. Maintenance dosage is 0.125 to 0.5 mg daily.

Children age 10 and older: 10 to 15 mcg/kg P.O. over 24 hours in two or more divided doses q 6 to 8 hours. Maintenance dosage is 25% to 35% of total digitalizing dose.

Children age 5 to 10: 20 to 35 mcg/kg P.O. over 24 hours in two or more divided doses q 6 to 8 hours. Maintenance dosage is 25% to 35% of total digitalizing dose.

Children age 2 to 5: 30 to 40 mcg/kg P.O. over 24 hours in two or more divided doses q 6 to 8 hours. Maintenance dosage is 25% to 35% of total digitalizing dose.

Infants age 1 month to 2 years: 35 to 60 mcg/kg P.O. over 24 hours in two or more divided doses q 6 to 8 hours. Maintenance dosage is 25% to 35% of total digitalizing dose.

Neonates: 25 to 35 mcg/kg P.O. over 24 hours in two or more divided doses q 6 to 8 hours. Maintenance dosage is 25% to 35% of total digitalizing dose.

Premature infants: 20 to 30 mcg/kg P.O. over 24 hours in two or more divided doses q 6 to 8 hours. Maintenance dosage is 20% to 30% of total digitalizing dose.

Capsules

Adults: For rapid digitalization, give 0.4 to 0.6 mg P.O. initially, followed by 0.1 to 0.3 mg q 6 to 8 hours, as needed and tolerated, for 24 hours. For slow digitalization, give 0.05 to 0.35 mg daily in two divided doses for 7 to 22 days, as needed, until therapeutic serum levels are

reached. Maintenance dosage is 0.05 to 0.35 mg daily in one or two divided doses.
Children: Digitalizing dose is based on child's age and is administered in three or more divided doses over the first 24 hours. Initial dose should be 50% of the total dose; subsequent doses are given q 4 to 8 hours as needed and tolerated.
Children age 10 and older: For rapid digitalization, give 8 to 12 mcg/kg P.O. over 24 hours, divided as above. Maintenance dosage is 25% to 35% of total digitalizing dose, given daily as a single dose.
Children age 5 to 10: For rapid digitalization, give 15 to 30 mcg/kg P.O. over 24 hours, divided as above. Maintenance dosage is 25% to 35% of total digitalizing dose, divided and given in two or three equal portions daily.
Children age 2 to 5: For rapid digitalization, give 25 to 35 mcg/kg P.O. over 24 hours, divided as above. Maintenance dosage is 25% to 35% of total digitalizing dose, divided and given in two or three equal portions daily.

Injection

Adults: For rapid digitalization, give 0.4 to 0.6 mg I.V. initially, followed by 0.1 to 0.3 mg I.V. q 4 to 8 hours, as needed and tolerated, for 24 hours. For slow digitalization, give appropriate daily maintenance dosage for 7 to 22 days as needed until therapeutic serum levels are reached. Maintenance dosage is 0.125 to 0.5 mg I.V. daily in one or two divided doses.
Children: Digitalizing dose is based on child's age and is administered in three or more divided doses over the first 24 hours. Initial dose should be 50% of total dose; subsequent doses are given q 4 to 8 hours as needed and tolerated.
Children age 10 and older: For rapid digitalization, give 8 to 12 mcg/kg I.V. over 24 hours, divided as above. Maintenance dosage is 25% to 35% of total digitalizing dose, given daily as a single dose.
Children age 5 to 10: For rapid digitalization, give 15 to 30 mcg/kg I.V. over 24 hours, divided as above. Maintenance dosage is 25% to 35% of total digitalizing dose, divided and given in two or three equal portions daily.
Children age 2 to 5: For rapid digitalization, give 25 to 35 mcg/kg I.V. over 24 hours, divided as above. Maintenance dosage is 25% to 35% of total digitalizing dose, divided and given in two or three equal portions daily.
Infants age 1 month to 2 years: For rapid digitalization, give 30 to 50 mcg/kg I.V. over 24 hours, divided as above. Maintenance dosage is 25% to 35% of total digitalizing dose, divided and given in two or three equal portions daily.
Neonates: For rapid digitalization, give 20 to 30 mcg/kg I.V. over 24 hours, divided as above. Maintenance dosage is 25% to 35% of the total digitalizing dose, divided and given in two or three equal portions daily.
Premature infants: For rapid digitalization, give 15 to 25 mcg/kg I.V. over 24 hours, divided as above. Maintenance dosage is 20% to 30% of the total digitalizing dose, divided and given in two or three equal portions daily.
≡ ***Dosage adjustment.*** Reduce dosage in patients with impaired renal function. Hypothyroid patients are highly sensitive to glycosides; hyperthyroid patients may need larger doses.

Pharmacodynamics

Digoxin is the most widely used cardiac glycoside. Many oral forms and a parenteral form are available, facilitating use of the drug in both acute and long-term clinical settings.
Inotropic action: The effect of digoxin on the myocardium is dose related and involves both direct and indirect mechanisms. It directly increases the force and velocity of myocardial contraction, AV node refractory period, and total peripheral resistance; at higher doses, it also increases sympathetic outflow. It indirectly depresses the SA node and prolongs conduction to the AV node. In patients with heart failure, increased contractile force boosts cardiac output, improves systolic emptying, and decreases diastolic heart size. It also reduces ventricular end-diastolic pressure and, consequently, pulmonary and systemic venous pressures. Increased myocardial contractility and cardiac output reflexively reduce sympathetic tone in patients with heart failure. This compensates for the direct vasoconstrictive action of the drug, thereby reducing total peripheral resistance. It also slows increased heart rate and causes diuresis in edematous patients.
Antiarrhythmic action: Digoxin-induced heart-rate slowing in patients without heart failure is negligible and stems mainly from vagal (cholinergic) and sympatholytic effects on the SA node; however, with toxic doses, heart-rate slowing results from direct depression of SA node automaticity. Therapeutic doses produce little effect on the action potential, but toxic doses increase the automaticity (spontaneous diastolic depolarization) of all cardiac regions except the SA node.

Pharmacokinetics

Absorption: With tablet or elixir administration, 60% to 85% of dose is absorbed. With capsule form, bioavailability increases. About 90% to 100% of a dose is absorbed. With I.M. administration, about 80% of dose is absorbed.
Distribution: Distributed widely in body tissues; highest levels occur in the heart, kidneys, intestine, stomach, liver, and skeletal muscle; lowest levels are in the plasma and brain. Digoxin crosses both the blood-brain barrier and the placenta; fetal and maternal digoxin levels are equivalent at birth. About 20% to 30% of drug is bound to plasma proteins. Usual therapeutic range for steady-state serum levels is 0.5 to 2 ng/ml. In treatment of atrial tachyarrhyth-

mias, higher serum levels (such as 2 to 4 ng/ml) may be needed. Because of long half-life of drug, achievement of steady-state levels may take 7 days or longer, depending on patient's renal function. Toxic symptoms may appear within the usual therapeutic range; however, these are more frequent and serious with levels above 2.5 ng/ml.
Metabolism: In most patients, a small amount of digoxin apparently is metabolized in the liver and gut by bacteria. This metabolism varies and may be substantial in some patients. Drug undergoes some enterohepatic recirculation (also variable). Metabolites have minimal cardiac activity.
Excretion: Most of dose is excreted by the kidneys as unchanged drug. Some patients excrete a substantial amount of metabolized or reduced drug. In patients with renal failure, biliary excretion is a more important excretion route. In healthy patients, terminal half-life is 30 to 40 hours. In patients lacking functioning kidneys, half-life increases to at least 4 days.

Route	Onset	Peak	Duration
P.O.	1½-2 hr	2-6 hr	3-4 days
I.M.	30 min	4-6 hr	Unknown
I.V.	5-30 min	1-4 hr	3-4 days

Contraindications and precautions

Contraindicated in patients with hypersensitivity to drug, digitalis-induced toxicity, ventricular fibrillation, or ventricular tachycardia unless caused by heart failure.

Use very cautiously in the elderly and in patients with acute MI, incomplete AV block, sinus bradycardia, PVCs, chronic constrictive pericarditis, hypertrophic cardiomyopathy, renal insufficiency, severe pulmonary disease, or hypothyroidism.

Interactions

Drug-drug. *Amiloride:* Inhibits digoxin effect and increases digoxin excretion. Monitor for altered digoxin effect.
Antacids, magnesium trisilicate, kaolin-pectin, aminosalicylic acid, sulfasalazine: Decrease absorption of orally administered digoxin. Monitor for altered digoxin effect. Separate administration times as far as possible from each other.
Anticholinergics: May increase digoxin absorption of oral digoxin tablets. Monitor blood levels and observe for toxicity.
Cholestyramine, colestipol, metoclopramide: Impair absorption. Monitor digoxin levels closely. Space doses by giving digoxin 1½ hours before or 2 hours after other drugs.
Cytotoxic agents, radiation therapy: Decrease digoxin absorption if the intestinal mucosa is damaged. Use of digoxin elixir or capsules is recommended in this situation.
Amiodarone, diltiazem, nifedipine, verapamil, quinidine: Increased serum digoxin levels, predisposing the patient to toxicity. Avoid use together.
Procainamide, propranolol, verapamil: Additive cardiac effects. Avoid use together.
Sympathomimetics, such as ephedrine, epinephrine, and isoproterenol, or rauwolfia alkaloids: May increase the risk of arrhythmias. Avoid use together.
Antibiotics: Increase in digoxin bioavailability and, consequently, increased serum digoxin levels. Monitor digoxin levels closely; separate administration times.
I.V. calcium: Synergistic effects that precipitate arrhythmias. Avoid use together.
Diuretics, such as ethacrynic acid, furosemide, and bumetanide: May cause hypokalemia and hypomagnesemia; Monitor blood levels closely.
Thiazides and parenteral calcium: May cause hypercalcemia. Monitor serum calcium levels.
Amphotericin B, carbenicillin, ticarcillin, corticosteroids, corticotropin, edetate disodium, laxatives, and sodium polystyrene sulfonate: Possible digoxin toxicity. Monitor digoxin levels closely.
Glucagon, large dextrose doses, and dextrose-insulin infusions: Digitalis toxicity. Avoid use together.
Succinylcholine: May precipitate cardiac arrhythmias by potentiating effects of digoxin. Avoid use together.
Drug-herb. *Betel palm, fumitory, goldenseal, lily-of-the-valley, motherwort, rue, shepherd's purse:* Enhance cardiac effects. Monitor patient closely.
Siberian ginseng, licorice, oleander, squill: May enhance toxicity. Avoid use together.

Effects on diagnostic tests

None reported.

Adverse reactions

The following signs of toxicity may occur with all cardiac glycosides:
CNS: *fatigue, generalized muscle weakness, agitation, hallucinations,* headache, malaise, dizziness, vertigo, stupor, paresthesia.
CV: ***arrhythmias*** (most commonly, conduction disturbances with or without AV block, PVCs, and supraventricular arrhythmias) that may lead to increased severity of ***heart failure*** and hypotension. ***Toxic effects on the heart may be life-threatening and require immediate attention.***
EENT: *yellow-green halos around visual images, blurred vision,* light flashes, photophobia, diplopia.
GI: *anorexia, nausea,* vomiting, diarrhea.

Overdose and treatment

Clinical effects of overdose are primarily GI, CNS, and cardiac reactions.

Severe intoxication may cause hyperkalemia, which may develop rapidly and result in life-threatening cardiac manifestations. Cardiac signs of digoxin toxicity may occur with or without other toxicity signs and commonly precede other toxic effects. Because toxic cardiac effects also can occur as manifestations of heart disease, determining whether these effects result from underlying heart disease or digoxin toxicity may be difficult. Digoxin has caused almost every kind of arrhythmia; various combinations of arrhythmias may occur in the same patient. Patients with chronic digoxin toxicity commonly have ventricular arrhythmias or AV conduction disturbances. Patients with digoxin-induced ventricular tachycardia have a high mortality because ventricular fibrillation or asystole may result.

If toxicity is suspected, discontinue drug and obtain serum drug level measurements. Usually, drug takes at least 6 hours to distribute between plasma and tissue and reach equilibrium; plasma levels drawn earlier may show higher digoxin levels than those present after drug is distributed into the tissues.

Other treatment measures include immediate emesis induction, gastric lavage, and administration of activated charcoal to reduce absorption of drug remaining in the gut. Repeated doses of activated charcoal (such as 50 g q 6 hours) may help reduce further absorption, especially of any drug undergoing enterohepatic recirculation. Some clinicians advocate cholestyramine administration if digoxin was recently ingested; however, it may not be useful if the ingestion is life threatening. Interacting drugs probably should be discontinued. Ventricular arrhythmias may be treated with I.V. potassium (replacement dose; but not in patients with significant AV block), I.V. phenytoin, I.V. lidocaine, or I.V. propranolol. Refractory ventricular tachyarrhythmias may be controlled with overdrive pacing. Procainamide may be used for ventricular arrhythmias that don't respond to the above treatments. In severe AV block, asystole, and hemodynamically significant sinus bradycardia, atropine restores a normal rate.

Administration of digoxin-specific antibody fragments (digoxin immune Fab, or Digibind) is a treatment for life-threatening digoxin toxicity. Each 40 mg of digoxin immune Fab binds about 0.6 mg of digoxin in the bloodstream. The complex is then excreted in the urine, rapidly decreasing serum levels and therefore cardiac drug levels.

Clinical considerations

□ ***ALERT*** Beware of sound-alikes: digoxin and doxepin, cesoxyn, or digitoxin.

□ ***ALERT*** Excessive slowing of heart rate (60 beats/minute or less) may be a sign of digitalis toxicity. Withhold drug and notify doctor.

- Obtain baseline heart rate and rhythm, blood pressure, and serum electrolyte levels before giving first dose.
- Monitor clinical status. Take apical-radial pulse for a full minute. Watch for significant changes (sudden rate increase or decrease, pulse deficit, irregular beats, and especially regularization of a previously irregular rhythm). Check blood pressure and obtain 12-lead ECG if these changes occur.
- Question patient about use of cardiac glycosides within the previous 2 to 3 weeks before administering a loading dose. Always divide loading dose over first 24 hours unless clinical situation indicates otherwise.
- GI absorption may be reduced in patients with heart failure, especially right heart failure.
- Because digoxin may predispose patients to postcardioversion asystole, most clinicians withhold digoxin 1 or 2 days before elective cardioversion in patients with atrial fibrillation. (However, consider consequences of increased ventricular response to atrial fibrillation if drug is withheld.)
- Calcium must not be given rapidly I.V. to patient receiving digoxin. Calcium affects cardiac contractility and excitability in much the same way that digoxin does and may lead to serious arrhythmias.
- Digoxin solution is enclosed in newly available soft capsule (Lanoxicaps). Because these capsules are better absorbed than tablets, dose is usually slightly less.

Therapeutic monitoring

- Dose is adjusted to patient's clinical condition and renal function; monitor ECG and serum levels of digoxin, calcium, potassium, and magnesium as well as serum creatinine. Therapeutic serum digoxin levels range from 0.5 to 2 ng/ml. Take corrective action before hypokalemia occurs.

Special populations

Pediatric patients. Pediatric patients have a poorly defined range of serum levels; however, toxicity apparently doesn't occur at same levels considered toxic in adults. Divided daily dosing is recommended for infants and children under age 10; older children require adult doses proportional to body weight.

Geriatric patients. Use digoxin with caution in geriatric patients (especially if renally compromised); adjust dosage to prevent systemic accumulation.

Patient counseling

- Inform patient and responsible family member about drug action, medication regimen, how to take pulse, reportable signs, and follow-up plans. Patient must understand importance of follow-up laboratory tests and have access to outpatient laboratory facilities.

- Instruct patient not to take an extra dose of digoxin if dose is missed.
- Tell patient to call doctor if severe nausea, vomiting, or diarrhea occurs because these conditions may make patient more susceptible to toxicity.
- Advise patient to use the same brand consistently.
- Tell patient to call doctor before using OTC preparations, especially those high in sodium.

digoxin immune Fab (ovine)

Digibind

Pharmacologic classification: antibody fragment
Therapeutic classification: cardiac glycoside antidote
Pregnancy risk category C

How supplied

Available by prescription only
Injection: 38-mg vial

Indications and dosages

Potentially life-threatening digoxin or digitoxin intoxication
Adults and children: Administered I.V. over 30 minutes or as a bolus if cardiac arrest is imminent. Dosage varies based on amount of drug to be neutralized; average dose for adults is 6 vials (228 mg). However, if toxicity resulted from acute digoxin ingestion and neither a serum digoxin level nor an estimated ingestion amount is known, 10 to 20 vials (380 to 760 mg) should be administered. See package insert for complete, specific dosage instructions.

Pharmacodynamics

Cardiac glycoside antidote: Specific antigen-binding fragments bind to free digoxin in extracellular fluid and intravascularly to prevent and reverse pharmacologic and toxic effects of the cardiac glycoside. This binding is preferential for digoxin and digitoxin; preliminary evidence suggests some binding to other digoxin derivatives and cardioactive metabolites.

Once free digoxin is bound and removed from serum, tissue-bound digoxin is released into the serum to maintain efflux-influx balance. As digoxin is released, it's bound and removed by digoxin immune Fab, resulting in a reduction of serum and tissue digoxin. Cardiac glycoside toxicity begins to subside within 30 minutes after completion of a 15- to 30-minute I.V. infusion of digoxin immune Fab. The onset of action and response is variable and appears to depend on rate of infusion, dose administered relative to body load of glycoside, and possibly other, as yet unidentified, factors. Reversal of toxicity, including hyperkalemia, is usually complete within 2 to 6 hours after administration of digoxin immune Fab.

Pharmacokinetics

Absorption: Peak serum levels occur at the completion of I.V. infusion. Digoxin immune Fab has a serum half-life of 15 to 20 hours. The association reaction between Fab fragments and glycoside molecules appears to occur rapidly; data are limited.
Distribution: Distribution isn't fully characterized. After I.V. administration, drug appears to be distributed rapidly throughout extracellular space, into both plasma and interstitial fluid. It isn't known whether digoxin immune Fab crosses the placental barrier or is distributed into breast milk.
Metabolism: Unknown.
Excretion: Excreted in urine via glomerular filtration.

Route	Onset	Peak	Duration
I.V.	30 min	End of infusion	15-20 hr

Contraindications and precautions

No known contraindications. Use cautiously in patients known to be allergic to ovine proteins. In these high-risk patients, skin testing is recommended because drug is derived from digoxin-specific antibody fragments obtained from immunized sheep.

Interactions

Drug-drug. *Cardiac glycosides, including digoxin, digitoxin, and lanatoside C:* When used together, digoxin immune Fab binds cardiac glycosides. This also occurs if redigitalization is attempted before elimination of digoxin immune Fab is complete (several days with normal renal function; 1 week or longer with renal impairment). Drug is used for this effect.

Effects on diagnostic tests

Digoxin immune Fab therapy alters standard cardiac glycoside determinations by radioimmunoassay procedures. Results may be falsely increased or decreased, depending on separation method used. Serum potassium levels may decrease rapidly.

Adverse reactions

CV: ***heart failure,*** rapid ventricular rate (both caused by reversal of cardiac glycoside's therapeutic effects).
Metabolic: hypokalemia.
Other: hypersensitivity reactions ***(anaphylaxis).***

Overdose and treatment

Limited information is available; however, administration of doses larger than needed for neutralizing the cardiac glycoside may subject the patient to increased risk of allergic or febrile reaction or delayed serum sickness. Large doses may also prolong the time span required before redigitalization.

Clinical considerations

- Measure serum digoxin or digitoxin levels before giving antidote because serum levels may be difficult to interpret after therapy with antidote.
- Give I.V. using a 0.22-micron filter needle over 30 minutes or as a bolus injection when cardiac arrest is imminent. Dose depends on amount of digoxin to be neutralized. Each 38-mg vial binds about 0.5 mg of digoxin or digitoxin. Reconstitute vial with 4 ml of sterile water for injection, mix gently, and use immediately. May be stored in refrigerator up to 4 hours.
- To determine appropriate dose, divide the total digitalis body load by 0.5; the resultant number estimates the number of vials required for appropriate dose. Alternatively, in cases of acute ingestion of known quantity of digitalis, multiply the amount of digitalis ingested in milligrams by 0.80 (to account for incomplete absorption).
- Skin testing may be appropriate for high-risk patients. One of two methods may be used: *Intradermal test*—dilute 0.1 ml of reconstituted solution in 9.9 ml of sterile saline for injection; then withdraw and inject 0.1 ml of this solution intradermally. Inspect site after 20 minutes for signs of erythema or urticaria. *Scratch test*—dilute as for intradermal test. Place one drop of diluted solution on skin and make a ¼" scratch through the drop with a sterile needle. Inspect site after 20 minutes for signs of erythema or urticaria. If results are positive, avoid use of digoxin immune Fab unless necessary. If systemic reaction occurs, treat symptomatically.
- Pretreat patients with sensitivity or allergy to sheep or ovine products, or when skin test results are positive, with an antihistamine such as diphenhydramine and a corticosteroid before administering digoxin immune Fab.
- Keep medications and equipment for cardiopulmonary resuscitation readily available during administration of digoxin immune Fab for patients who respond poorly to withdrawal of inotropic effects of digoxin. Dopamine or dobutamine, or other cardiac load-reducing agents, may be used. Catecholamines may aggravate arrhythmias induced by digitalis toxicity; use with caution.

Therapeutic monitoring

- Closely monitor temperature, blood pressure, ECG, and potassium level before, during, and after administration of antidote.
- Potassium levels must be checked repeatedly because severe digitalis intoxication can cause life-threatening hyperkalemia, and reversal by digoxin immune Fab may lead to rapid hypokalemia.

Special populations

Breast-feeding patients. It's unknown if digoxin immune Fab is excreted in breast milk; use cautiously in breast-feeding women.

Pediatric patients. Consider the risk-to-benefit ratio. Adverse effects haven't occurred in infants and small children. Monitor for volume overload in small children. Very small doses may require diluting reconstituted solution with 36 ml of sterile saline for injection to produce a 1 mg/ml solution.

Infants may require smaller doses; manufacturer recommends reconstituting as directed and administering with a tuberculin syringe.

Patient counseling

- Explain use and administration to patient and family.
- Instruct patient to report adverse effects immediately.

dihydrotachysterol

DHT, DHT Intensol, Hytakerol

Pharmacologic classification: vitamin D analogue
Therapeutic classification: antihypocalcemic
Pregnancy risk category C

How supplied

Available by prescription only
Tablets: 0.125 mg, 0.2 mg, 0.4 mg
Capsules: 0.125 mg
Solution: 0.2 mg/ml (Intensol)

Indications and dosages

Hypocalcemia associated with hypoparathyroidism and pseudohypoparathyroidism
Adults: Initially, 0.8 to 2.4 mg P.O. daily for several days. Maintenance dosage is 0.2 to 1 mg daily, as required for normal serum calcium levels. Average dose is 0.6 mg daily.
Children: Initially, 1 to 5 mg P.O. daily for 4 days, then continue dosage or reduce to one fourth the initial amount. Usual maintenance dosage is 0.5 to 1.5 mg daily, as required for normal serum calcium levels.

Prevention of thyroidectomy-induced hypocalcemia
Adults: 0.25 mg P.O. daily given with calcium supplements until danger of hypocalcemic tetany has passed.

◇ ***Familial hypophosphatemia***
Adults and children: 0.5 to 2 mg P.O. daily (until healing of bones occurs). Maintenance dosage is 0.2 to 1.5 mg daily.

◇ ***Renal osteodystrophy in chronic uremia***
Adults: 0.1 to 0.6 mg P.O. daily.
Children: 0.1 to 0.5 mg P.O. daily.

◇ ***Osteoporosis***
Adults: 0.6 mg P.O. daily given with calcium and fluoride.

Pharmacodynamics

Antihypocalcemic action: Once activated to its 25-hydroxy form, drug works with parathyroid hormone to regulate levels of calcium. It appears to have little activity as the parent compound.

Pharmacokinetics

Absorption: Absorbed readily from the small intestine.
Distribution: Distributed widely; it is largely protein-bound.
Metabolism: Metabolized in the liver, and has a duration of action up to 9 weeks.
Excretion: Excreted in urine and bile.

Route	Onset	Peak	Duration
P.O.	Several hours	1-2 wk	9 wk

Contraindications and precautions

Contraindicated in patients with hypercalcemia or vitamin D toxicity. Use cautiously in those with a history of renal calculi. Drug isn't recommended in breast-feeding women.

Interactions

Drug-drug. *Magnesium-containing antacids:* May alter absorption of dihydrotachysterol. Avoid use together.
Barbiturates, phenytoin, primidone: May increase metabolism and therefore reduce activity of dihydrotachysterol. Avoid use together.
Mineral oil, orlistat: May interfere with intestinal absorption of vitamin D analogues. Avoid use together.
Cholestyramine, colestipol: Decreased absorption of vitamin D analogues. Avoid use together.
Cardiac glycosides: Increased risk of arrhythmias. Avoid use together.
Corticosteroids: Counteract vitamin D analogue effects. Don't use together.
Other vitamin D analogues: Increase toxicity. Avoid use together.
Thiazide diuretics: May cause hypercalcemia. Use together cautiously.

Effects on diagnostic tests

None reported.

Adverse reactions

CNS: headache, somnolence, irritability, psychosis (rare).
CV: hypertension, ***arrhythmias.***
EENT: conjunctivitis, photophobia, rhinorrhea.
GI: nausea, vomiting, constipation, polydipsia, pancreatitis, metallic taste, dry mouth, anorexia, diarrhea.
GU: polyuria, nocturia, decreased libido, nephrocalcinosis.
Hepatic: altered serum alkaline phosphatase.
Metabolic: weight loss; alterations in cholesterol levels and electrolytes, such as magnesium, phosphate, and calcium, in serum and urine.
Musculoskeletal: weakness, bone and muscle pain.
Other: thirst, hyperthermia.

Overdose and treatment

Hypercalcemia is the only sign of overdose. Treatment involves discontinuing therapy, instituting a low-calcium diet, increasing fluid intake, and providing supportive measures. In severe cases, death from cardiac and renal failure has occurred. Calcitonin administration may help reverse hypercalcemia.

Clinical considerations

- Adequate dietary calcium intake is necessary; usually supplemented with 10 to 15 g oral calcium lactate or gluconate daily.
- 1 mg of dihydrotachysterol is equivalent to 120,000 units ergocalciferol (vitamin D_2).
- Store in tightly closed, light-resistant container. Don't refrigerate.

Therapeutic monitoring

- Monitor serum and urine calcium levels. Observe patient for signs and symptoms of hypercalcemia.
- There is some evidence that monitoring urine calcium and urine creatinine is helpful in screening for hypercalciuria. The ratio of urine calcium to urine creatinine should be less than or equal to 0.18. A value of more than 0.2 suggests hypercalciuria, and the dose should be decreased regardless of serum calcium level.

Special populations

Breast-feeding patients. Don't use in breast-feeding women.
Pediatric patients. Some infants may be hyperreactive to drug.

Patient counseling

- Explain importance of a calcium-rich diet.
- Tell patient to report early signs of hypercalcemia; thirst, headache, vertigo, tinnitus, or anorexia promptly.

diltiazem hydrochloride

Cardizem, Cardizem CD, Cardizem SR, Dilacor XR, Tiazac

Pharmacologic classification: calcium channel blocker
Therapeutic classification: antianginal
Pregnancy risk category C

How supplied

Available by prescription only
Tablets: 30 mg, 60 mg, 90 mg, 120 mg
Capsules (extended-release): 60 mg, 90 mg, 120 mg, 180 mg, 240 mg, 300 mg, 360 mg

Capsules, extended-release, (containing multiple 60-mg beads): 120 mg, 180 mg, 240 mg
Injection: 5 mg/ml (25 mg and 50 mg)
Injection: 25 mg
Injection (for I.V. infusion only): 100 mg

Indications and dosages

Management of Prinzmetal's or variant angina or chronic stable angina pectoris
Adults: 30 mg P.O. q.i.d. before meals and h.s. Increase dose gradually to maximum of 360 mg/day divided into three to four doses, as indicated. Alternatively, give 120 or 180 mg (extended-release) P.O. once daily. Adjust over a 7- to 14-day period as needed and tolerated up to a maximum dose of 480 mg daily.
Hypertension
Adults: 60 to 120 mg P.O. b.i.d. (sustained-release). Adjust up to maximum recommended dose of 360 mg/day, as necessary. Alternatively, give 180 to 240 mg (extended-release) P.O. once daily. Adjust dose based on patient response to a maximum dose of 480 mg/day.
Atrial fibrillation or flutter; paroxysmal supraventricular tachycardia
Adults: 0.25 mg/kg I.V. as a bolus injection over 2 minutes. Repeat after 15 minutes if response isn't adequate with a dose of 0.35 mg/kg I.V. over 2 minutes. Follow bolus with continuous I.V. infusion at 5 to 15 mg/hour (for up to 24 hours).

Pharmacodynamics

Antianginal or antihypertensive action: By dilating systemic arteries, diltiazem decreases total peripheral resistance and afterload, slightly reduces blood pressure, and increases cardiac index when given in high doses (more than 200 mg). Afterload reduction, which occurs at rest and with exercise, and the resulting decrease in myocardial oxygen consumption account for the effectiveness of diltiazem in controlling chronic stable angina.

Diltiazem also decreases myocardial oxygen demand and cardiac work by reducing heart rate, relieving coronary artery spasm (through coronary artery vasodilation), and dilating peripheral vessels. These effects relieve ischemia and pain. In patients with Prinzmetal's angina, diltiazem inhibits coronary artery spasm, increasing myocardial oxygen delivery.
Antiarrhythmic action: By impeding the slow inward influx of calcium at the AV node, diltiazem decreases conduction velocity and increases refractory period, thereby decreasing the impulses transmitted to the ventricles in atrial fibrillation or flutter. The end result is a decreased ventricular rate.

Pharmacokinetics

Absorption: About 80% of a dose is absorbed rapidly from the GI tract. However, only about 40% of drug enters systemic circulation because of a significant first-pass effect in the liver.
Distribution: About 70% to 85% of circulating drug is bound to plasma proteins.
Metabolism: Metabolized in the liver.
Excretion: About 35% is excreted in the urine and about 65% in the bile as unchanged drug and inactive and active metabolites. Elimination half-life is 3 to 9 hours. Half-life may increase in geriatric patients; however, renal dysfunction doesn't appear to affect half-life.

Route	Onset	Peak	Duration
P.O.	½-1 hr	2-3 hr	6-8 hr
P.O. (extended)	2-3 hr	10-14 hr	12-24 hr
I.V.	3 min	Immediate	1-10 hr

Contraindications and precautions

Contraindicated in patients with sick sinus syndrome or second- or third-degree AV block in the absence of an artificial pacemaker; in supraventricular tachycardias associated with a bypass tract such as in Wolfe-Parkinson-White syndrome or Lown-Ganong-Levine syndrome; and in patients with left ventricular failure, hypotension (systolic blood pressure less than 90 mm Hg), hypersensitivity to the drug, acute MI, and pulmonary congestion (documented by X-ray). Use cautiously in the elderly and in patients with heart failure or impaired hepatic or renal function.

Interactions

Drug-drug. *Anesthetics:* Effects may be potentiated. Monitor patient.
Beta blockers: Combined effects that result in heart failure, conduction disturbances, arrhythmias, and hypotension. Use together cautiously.
Cyclosporine: Increased serum cyclosporine levels and subsequent cyclosporine-induced nephrotoxicity. If used together, monitor cyclosporine levels.
Cimetidine: May increase plasma level of diltiazem. Carefully monitor patient.
Digoxin: Diltiazem may increase serum levels of digoxin. Monitor for toxicity.
Furosemide: Forms a precipitate when mixed with diltiazem injection. Drug needs to be administered through separate I.V. lines.

Effects on diagnostic tests

None reported.

Adverse reactions

CNS: *headache,* dizziness, asthenia, somnolence.
CV: *edema,* ***arrhythmias,*** flushing, bradycardia, hypotension, conduction abnormalities, ***heart failure,*** AV block, abnormal ECG.
GI: *nausea, constipation,* abdominal discomfort.
Hepatic: acute hepatic injury.
Skin: *rash.*

Overdose and treatment

Clinical effects of overdose primarily are extensions of adverse reactions of drug. Heart block, asystole, and hypotension are the most serious effects and require immediate attention.

Treatment may involve I.V. isoproterenol, norepinephrine, epinephrine, atropine, or calcium gluconate administered in usual doses. Adequate hydration must be ensured. Inotropic agents, including dobutamine and dopamine, may be used, if necessary. If severe conduction disturbances (such as heart block and asystole) with hypotension that doesn't respond to drug therapy develops, initiate cardiac pacing immediately with cardiopulmonary resuscitation measures, as indicated.

Clinical considerations

Consider the recommendations relevant to all calcium channel blockers as well as the following:

- Sublingual nitroglycerin may be administered concomitantly, as needed, if patient has acute angina symptoms.
- Diltiazem has been used investigationally to prevent reinfarction after non Q-wave MI; as an adjunct in the treatment of peripheral vascular disorders; and in the treatment of several spastic smooth muscle disorders, including esophageal spasm.

Therapeutic monitoring

- Monitor blood pressure and heart rate during initiation of therapy and dosage adjustments.
- If systolic blood pressure is less than 90 mm Hg or heart rate is less than 60 beats/minute, withhold dose and notify doctor.

Special populations

Breast-feeding patients. Drug is excreted in breast milk; therefore, patients should discontinue breast-feeding during diltiazem therapy.
Geriatric patients. Use drug with caution in geriatric patients because the half-life may be prolonged.

Patient counseling

- Tell patient that nitrate therapy prescribed during titration of diltiazem dosage may cause dizziness. Urge patient to continue compliance.
- Inform patient of proper use, dose, and adverse effects associated with diltiazem use.
- Instruct patient to continue taking drug even when feeling better.
- Tell patient to report feelings of lightheadedness or dizziness and to avoid sudden position changes.

dimenhydrinate

Apo-Dimenhydrinate*, Calm-X, Dimetabs, Dinate, Dommanate, Dramamine, Dramocen, Dramoject, Dymenate, Gravol*, Hydrate, PMS-Dimenhydrinate*, Wehamine

Pharmacologic classification: ethanol-amine-derivative antihistamine
Therapeutic classification: antihistamine (H_1-receptor antagonist), antiemetic, antivertigo
Pregnancy risk category B

How supplied

Available with or without a prescription
Tablets: 50 mg
Tablets (chewable): 50 mg
Tablets (film-coated): 50 mg
Solution: 12.5 mg/5 ml
Injection: 50 mg/ml

Indications and dosages

Prophylaxis and treatment of nausea, vomiting, dizziness associated with motion sickness
Adults and children age 12 and older: 50 to 100 mg q 4 to 6 hours P.O., I.V., or I.M. For I.V. administration, dilute each 50-mg dose in 10 ml of normal saline solution and inject slowly over 2 minutes.
Children: 1.25 mg/kg/day or 37.5 mg/m²/day P.O. or I.M. q.i.d. not to exceed 300 mg/day, or according to the following schedule:
Children age 6 to 12: 25 to 50 mg P.O. q 6 to 8 hours; maximum dose is 150 mg/day.
Children age 2 to 6: 12.5 to 25 mg P.O. q 6 to 8 hours; maximum dose is 75 mg/day.
◊***Meniere's disease***
Adults: 50 mg I.M. for acute attack; maintenance dosage is 25 to 50 mg P.O. t.i.d.

Pharmacodynamics

Antiemetic and antivertigo action: Dimenhydrinate probably inhibits nausea and vomiting by centrally depressing sensitivity of the labyrinth apparatus that relays stimuli to the chemoreceptor trigger zone and stimulates the vomiting center in the brain.

Pharmacokinetics

Absorption: Well absorbed.
Distribution: Well distributed throughout the body and crosses the placenta.
Metabolism: Metabolized in the liver.
Excretion: Metabolites are excreted in urine.

Route	Onset	Peak	Duration
P.O.	15-30 min	Unknown	3-6 hr
I.V.	Immediate	Unknown	3-6 hr
I.M.	20-30 min	Unknown	3-6 hr

Contraindications and precautions
Contraindicated in patients hypersensitive to drug or its components. I.V. product contains benzyl alcohol, which has been associated with a fatal "gasping syndrome" in premature infants and low birth weight infants.

Use cautiously in patients with seizures, acute angle-closure glaucoma, or enlarged prostate gland and in those receiving ototoxic drugs.

Interactions
Drug-drug. *Other CNS depressants, such as antianxiety agents, barbiturates, sleeping agents, and tranquilizers:* Additive CNS sedation and depression. Avoid use together.
Aminoglycosides, cisplatin, loop diuretics, salicylates, vancomycin: Dimenhydrinate may mask the signs of ototoxicity, which can be caused by these drugs. Monitor patient closely.
Drug-lifestyle. *Alcohol use:* May cause additive CNS depression. Advise patient to avoid alcohol use.

Effects on diagnostic tests
Dimenhydrinate may alter or confuse test results for xanthines (caffeine, aminophylline) because of its 8-chlorotheophylline content; discontinue dimenhydrinate 4 days before diagnostic skin tests to avoid preventing, reducing, or masking test response.

Adverse reactions
CNS: *drowsiness,* headache, dizziness, confusion, nervousness, insomnia (especially in children), vertigo, tingling and weakness of hands, lassitude, excitation.
CV: palpitations, hypotension, tachycardia, tightness of chest.
EENT: blurred vision, dry respiratory passages, diplopia, nasal congestion.
GI: dry mouth, nausea, vomiting, diarrhea, epigastric distress, constipation, anorexia.
Respiratory: wheezing, thickened bronchial secretions.
Skin: photosensitivity, urticaria, rash.
Other: ***anaphylaxis.***

Overdose and treatment
Signs and symptoms of overdose may include either CNS depression (sedation, reduced mental alertness, apnea, and CV collapse) or CNS stimulation (insomnia, hallucinations, tremors, or seizures). Anticholinergic symptoms, such as dry mouth, flushed skin, fixed and dilated pupils, and GI symptoms, are likely to occur, especially in children.

Use gastric lavage to empty stomach contents; emetics may be ineffective. Diazepam or phenytoin may be used to control seizures. Provide supportive treatment.

Clinical considerations
Consider the recommendations relevant to all antihistamines as well as the following:
- ☐ ***ALERT*** Most I.V. products contain benzyl alcohol, which has been associated with a fatal "gasping syndrome" in premature infants and low-birth-weight infants.
- Incorrectly administered or undiluted I.V. solution is irritating to veins and may cause sclerosis.
- Parenteral solution is incompatible with many drugs; don't mix other drugs in the same syringe.
- To prevent motion sickness, patient should take medication 30 minutes before traveling and again before meals and at bedtime.
- Antiemetic effect may diminish with prolonged use.

Therapeutic monitoring
- Advise safety measures for all patients; dimenhydrinate has a high incidence of drowsiness. Tolerance to CNS depressant effects usually develops within a few days.

Special populations
Breast-feeding patients. Avoid use of antihistamines during breast-feeding. Many of these drugs, including dimenhydrinate, are excreted in breast milk, exposing the infant to risks of unusual excitability; premature infants are at particular risk for seizures.
Pediatric patients. Safety in neonates hasn't been established. Infants and children under age 6 may experience paradoxical hyperexcitability. I.V. dosage for children hasn't been established.
Geriatric patients. Geriatric patients are usually more sensitive to adverse effects of antihistamines than younger patients and are especially likely to experience a greater degree of dizziness, sedation, hyperexcitability, dry mouth, and urine retention.

Patient counseling
- Tell patient to avoid hazardous activities, such as driving or operating heavy machinery, until adverse CNS effects of drug are known.
- Tell patient to take drug for motion sickness 30 minutes before exposure.

dimercaprol
BAL in Oil

Pharmacologic classification: chelating agent
Therapeutic classification: heavy metal antagonist
Pregnancy risk category NR

How supplied
Available by prescription only
Injection: 100 mg/ml

Indications and dosages

Severe arsenic or gold poisoning
Adults and children: 3 mg/kg deep I.M. q 4 hours for 2 days, then q.i.d. on day 3; then b.i.d. for 10 days.
Mild arsenic or gold poisoning
Adults and children: 2.5 mg/kg deep I.M. q.i.d. for 2 days, then b.i.d. on day 3; then once daily for 10 days.
Severe gold dermatitis
Adults and children: 2.5 mg/kg deep I.M. q 4 hours for 2 days, then b.i.d. for 7 days.
Gold-induced thrombocytopenia
Adults and children: 100 mg deep I.M. b.i.d. for 15 days.
Mercury poisoning
Adults and children: Initially, 5 mg/kg deep I.M., then 2.5 mg/kg daily or b.i.d. for 10 days.
Acute lead encephalopathy or blood lead level greater than 100 mcg/dl
Adults and children: 4 mg/kg (or 75 to 83 mg/m^2) deep I.M. injection, then give simultaneously with edetate calcium disodium (250 mg/m^2) q 4 hours for 3 to 5 days. Use separate injection sites.

Pharmacodynamics

Chelating action: The sulfhydryl groups of dimercaprol form heterocyclic ring complexes with heavy metals, particularly arsenic, mercury, and gold, preventing or reversing their binding to body ligands.

Pharmacokinetics

Absorption: Absorbed slowly through the skin.
Distribution: Distributed to all tissues, mainly the intracellular space, with the highest levels of dimercaprol occurring in the liver and kidneys.
Metabolism: Uncomplexed dimercaprol is metabolized rapidly to inactive products.
Excretion: Most dimercaprol-metal complexes and inactive metabolites are excreted in urine and feces.

Route	Onset	Peak	Duration
I.M.	Unknown	30-60 min	4 hr

Contraindications and precautions

Contraindicated in patients with hepatic dysfunction (except postarsenical jaundice). Use cautiously in patients with hypertension or oliguria. Avoid use in pregnant women unless required to treat a life-threatening acute poisoning.

Interactions

Drug-drug. *Cadmium, iron, selenium, uranium:* Form toxic complexes with dimercaprol. Delay iron therapy for 24 hours after stopping dimercaprol.

Effects on diagnostic tests

Dimercaprol therapy blocks thyroid uptake of ^{131}I, causing decreased values.

Adverse reactions

CNS: pain or tightness in throat, chest, or hands; headache; paresthesia; muscle pain or weakness, anxiety.
CV: *transient increase in blood pressure* (returns to normal in 2 hours), *tachycardia.*
EENT: blepharospasm, conjunctivitis, lacrimation, rhinorrhea, excessive salivation.
GI: *nausea; vomiting; burning sensation in lips, mouth, and throat; abdominal pain.*
Other: *fever* (especially in children).

Overdose and treatment

Clinical signs of overdose include vomiting, seizures, stupor, coma, hypertension, and tachycardia; effects subside in 1 to 6 hours. Support CV and respiratory status; control seizures with diazepam.

Clinical considerations

□ ***ALERT*** Administer drug by deep I.M. injection only.

- Treat patient as soon as possible after poisoning for optimal therapeutic effect.
- Adverse effects of dimercaprol are usually mild and transitory and occur in about one half of patients who receive an I.M. dose of 5 mg/kg. In patients who receive doses in excess of 5 mg/kg, adverse effects usually occur within 30 minutes after injection and subside in 1 to 6 hours.
- Drug has strong garlic odor.

Therapeutic monitoring

Monitor vital signs and intake and output during therapy, and keep urine alkaline to prevent renal failure.

Special populations

Pregnant patients. Safety in pregnancy hasn't been established, and drug shouldn't be used unless judged by a doctor to be necessary to treat a life-threatening acute poisoning.
Pediatric patients. Fever is common, usually appearing after the second or third dose, and may persist throughout therapy. Acrodynia in infants and children has been treated with 3 mg/kg of dimercaprol I.M. every 4 hours for 2 days, then every 6 hours for 1 day, followed by every 12 hours for 7 to 8 days.
Geriatric patients. Use drug with caution.

Patient counseling

- Advise patient that drug may cause a bad taste in the mouth or bad breath. It also may cause a burning sensation of the lips, mouth, throat, eyes, and penis, and pain in the teeth.

diphenhydramine hydrochloride

Benadryl, Benadryl Allergy, Benylin, Compoz, Diphen AF, Diphen Cough, Diphenadryl, Hydramine, Nervine Nighttime Sleep-Aid, Nytol, QuickCaps, Sleep-Eze 3, Sominex, Tusstat, Twilite

Pharmacologic classification: ethanolamine-derivative antihistamine
Therapeutic classification: antihistamine (H_1-receptor antagonist), antiemetic, antivertigo, antitussive, sedative-hypnotic, topical anesthetic, antidyskinetic (anticholinergic)
Pregnancy risk category B

How supplied

Available with or without a prescription
Tablets: 25 mg, 50 mg
Tablets (film-coated): 25 mg, 50 mg
Tablets (chewable): 12.5 mg
Capsules: 25 mg, 50 mg
Capsules (liquid-filled): 25 mg, 50 mg
Elixir: 12.5 mg/5 ml
Solution: 12.5 mg/5 ml
Injection: 10 mg/ml, 50 mg/ml
Cream (topical): 1%, 2%
Gel (topical): 1%, 2%
Solution (topical): 1%, 2%
Spray: 1%, 2%
Stick (Topical): 2%

Indications and dosages

Rhinitis, allergy symptoms, motion sickness, Parkinson's disease
Adults and children age 12 and older: 25 to 50 mg P.O. t.i.d. or q.i.d.; or 10 to 50 mg I.V. or deep I.M. Maximum I.M. or I.V. dose is 400 mg daily.
Children under age 12: 5 mg/kg daily P.O., deep I.M., or I.V. in divided doses q.i.d. Maximum dose is 300 mg daily.
Nonproductive cough
Adults and children age 12 and older: 25 mg P.O. q 4 to 6 hours. Maximum dose is 150 mg daily.
Children age 6 to 12: 12.5 mg P.O. q 4 to 6 hours. Maximum dose is 75 mg daily.
Children age 2 to 6: 6.25 mg P.O. q 4 to 6 hours. Maximum dose is 25 mg daily.
Insomnia
Adults: 50 mg P.O. h.s.
Sedation
Adults: 25 to 50 mg P.O., or deep I.M., p.r.n.

Pharmacodynamics

Antihistamine action: Antihistamines compete for H_1 receptor sites on the smooth muscle of the bronchi, GI tract, uterus, and large blood vessels; by binding to cellular receptors, they prevent access of histamine and suppress histamine-induced allergic symptoms, even though they don't prevent its release.
Antivertigo, antiemetic, and antidyskinetic actions: Central antimuscarinic actions of antihistamines probably are responsible for these effects of diphenhydramine.
Antitussive action: Drug suppresses the cough reflex by a direct effect on the cough center.
Sedative action: Mechanism of the CNS depressant effects of diphenhydramine is unknown.
Anesthetic action: Drug is structurally related to local anesthetics, which prevent initiation and transmission of nerve impulses; this is the probable source of its topical and local anesthetic effects.

Pharmacokinetics

Absorption: Well absorbed from the GI tract.
Distribution: Distributed widely throughout the body, including the CNS; drug crosses the placenta and is excreted in breast milk. Drug is about 82% protein-bound.
Metabolism: About 50% to 60% of an oral dose of diphenhydramine is metabolized by the liver before reaching the systemic circulation (first-pass effect); virtually all available drug is metabolized by the liver within 24 to 48 hours.
Excretion: Plasma elimination half-life of drug is about 2½ to 9 hours; drug and metabolites are excreted primarily in urine.

Route	Onset	Peak	Duration
P.O.	15 min	1-4 hr	6-8 hr
I.V.	Immediate	1-4 hr	6-8 hr
I.M.	Unknown	1-4 hr	6-8 hr
Topical	Unknown	Unknown	Unknown

Contraindications and precautions

Contraindicated in patients with hypersensitivity to drug, during acute asthmatic attacks, and in neonates, premature neonates, and breast-feeding patients.

Use with extreme caution in patients with angle-closure glaucoma, prostatic hyperplasia, pyloroduodenal and bladder neck obstruction, asthma or COPD, increased intraocular pressure, hyperthyroidism, CV disease, hypertension, and stenosing peptic ulcer.

Interactions

Drug-drug. *MAO inhibitors:* Increased anticholinergic effects. Don't use together.
CNS depressants, such as barbiturates, tranquilizers, and sleeping aids, antianxiety agents: Additive CNS depression. Use together cautiously.
Sulfonylureas: Diphenhydramine may diminish the effects of sulfonylureas. Monitor patient closely.

Epinephrine: Enhanced effects. Monitor patient closely.
Heparin: Partially counteracts the anticoagulant effects of heparin. Monitor PT and INR.
Drug-lifestyle. *Alcohol use:* May cause additive CNS depression. Use cautiously.
Sun exposure: May cause photosensitivity reactions. Advise patient to take precautions.

Effects on diagnostic tests
Discontinue drug 4 days before diagnostic skin tests; antihistamines can prevent, reduce, or mask positive skin test response.

Adverse reactions
CNS: *drowsiness,* confusion, insomnia, headache, vertigo, *sedation, sleepiness, dizziness, incoordination,* fatigue, restlessness, tremor, nervousness, ***seizures.***
CV: palpitations, hypotension, tachycardia.
EENT: diplopia, blurred vision, tinnitus.
GI: *nausea,* vomiting, diarrhea, *dry mouth,* constipation, *epigastric distress,* anorexia.
GU: dysuria, urine retention, urinary frequency.
Hematologic: hemolytic anemia, ***thrombocytopenia, agranulocytosis.***
Respiratory: nasal congestion, *thickening of bronchial secretions.*
Skin: urticaria, photosensitivity, rash.
Other: ***anaphylactic shock.***

Overdose and treatment
Drowsiness is the usual symptom of overdose. Seizures, coma, and respiratory depression may occur with profound overdose. Anticholinergic symptoms, such as dry mouth, flushed skin, fixed and dilated pupils, and GI symptoms, are common, especially in children.

Treat overdose by inducing emesis with ipecac syrup (in conscious patient), followed by activated charcoal to reduce further drug absorption. Use gastric lavage if patient is unconscious or ipecac fails. Treat hypotension with vasopressors and control seizures with diazepam or phenytoin. Don't give stimulants.

Clinical considerations
Consider the recommendations relevant to all antihistamines as well as the following:
- Diphenhydramine injection is compatible with most I.V. solutions but is incompatible with some drugs; check compatibility before mixing in the same I.V. line.
- Alternate injection sites to prevent irritation. Administer deep I.M. into large muscle.
- Drowsiness is the most common adverse effect during initial therapy but usually disappears with continued use of drug.
- Injectable and elixir solutions are light-sensitive; protect them from light.

Therapeutic monitoring
Be sure the I.V. site is patent. Drug given perivascularly causes tissue irritation.

Special populations
Breast-feeding patients. Avoid use of antihistamines during breast-feeding. Many of these drugs are secreted in breast milk, exposing the infant to risks of unusual excitability; premature infants are at particular risk for seizures.
Pediatric patients. Drug shouldn't be used in premature infants or neonates. Infants and children, especially those under age 6, may experience paradoxical hyperexcitability.
Geriatric patients. Geriatric patients are usually more sensitive to adverse effects of antihistamines than younger patients and are especially likely to experience a greater degree of dizziness, sedation, hyperexcitability, dry mouth, and urine retention. Symptoms usually respond to a decrease in medication dosage.

Patient counseling
- Advise patient that drowsiness is very common initially, but may be reduced with continued use of drug.
- Advise patient undergoing skin testing for allergies to notify doctor of current drug therapy.

diphenoxylate hydrochloride and atropine sulfate
Lofene, Logen, Lomanate, Lomotil, Lonox

Pharmacologic classification: opiate
Therapeutic classification: antidiarrheal
Controlled substance schedule V
Pregnancy risk category C

How supplied
Available by prescription only
Tablets: 2.5 mg diphenoxylate hydrochloride and 0.025 mg atropine sulfate per tablet
Liquid: 2.5 mg diphenoxylate hydrochloride and 0.025 mg atropine sulfate/5 ml

Indications and dosages
Acute, nonspecific diarrhea
Adults: 5 mg diphenoxylate component P.O. q.i.d., then adjust, p.r.n.
Children age 2 and older: 0.3 to 0.4 mg/kg diphenoxylate component P.O. daily in four divided doses using the liquid form; or administer according to diphenoxylate component, as follows:
Children age 8 to 12: 2 mg P.O. five times daily.
Children age 5 to 8: 2 mg P.O. q.i.d.
Children age 2 to 5: 2 mg P.O. t.i.d.

Pharmacodynamics
Antidiarrheal action: Diphenoxylate is a meperidine analogue that inhibits GI motility locally and centrally. In high doses, it may produce an opiate effect. Atropine is added in subtherapeutic doses to prevent abuse by deliberate overdose.

Pharmacokinetics
Absorption: About 90% of an oral dose is absorbed.
Distribution: Distributed in breast milk.
Metabolism: Metabolized extensively by the liver.
Excretion: Metabolites are excreted mainly in feces via the biliary tract, with lesser amounts excreted in urine.

Route	Onset	Peak	Duration
P.O.	45-60 min	3 hr	3-4 hr

Contraindications and precautions
Contraindicated in patients with hypersensitivity to diphenoxylate or atropine, acute diarrhea resulting from poison until toxic material is eliminated from GI tract, acute diarrhea caused by organisms that penetrate intestinal mucosa, or diarrhea resulting from antibiotic-induced pseudomembranous enterocolitis or enterotoxin-producing bacteria; also contraindicated in patients with obstructive jaundice and in children under age 2.

Use cautiously in children age 2 and older; in patients with hepatic disease, narcotic dependence, or acute ulcerative colitis; and in pregnant women. Stop therapy immediately if abdominal distention or other signs of toxic megacolon develop.

Interactions
Drug-drug. *MAO inhibitors*: may precipitate hypertensive crisis. Avoid use together.
CNS depressants such as barbiturates, narcotic agents, tranquilizers: May result in an increased depressant effect. Avoid use together.
Drug-lifestyle. *Alcohol use*: May enhance CNS depression. Avoid use together.

Effects on diagnostic tests
Diphenoxylate may decrease urinary excretion of phenolsulfonphthalein (PSP) during the PSP excretion test.

Adverse reactions
CNS: *sedation, dizziness,* headache, drowsiness, lethargy, restlessness, depression, euphoria, malaise, confusion, numbness in extremities.
CV: tachycardia.
EENT: mydriasis.
GI: *dry mouth,* nausea, vomiting, abdominal discomfort or distention, ***paralytic ileus,*** anorexia, fluid retention in bowel or megacolon (may mask depletion of extracellular fluid and electrolytes, especially in young children treated for acute gastroenteritis), increased serum amylase, ***pancreatitis,*** swollen gums, possible physical dependence with long-term use.
GU: urine retention.
Respiratory: ***respiratory depression.***
Skin: pruritus, rash, dry skin.
Other: ***angioedema, anaphylaxis.***

Overdose and treatment
Clinical effects of overdose include drowsiness, low blood pressure, marked seizures, apnea, blurred vision, miosis, flushing, dry mouth and mucous membranes, and psychotic episodes.

Treatment is supportive; maintain airway and support vital functions. A narcotic antagonist, such as naloxone, may be given. Gastric lavage may be performed. Monitor patient for 48 to 72 hours.

Clinical considerations
- Drug is usually ineffective in treating antibiotic-induced diarrhea.
- Reduce dosage as soon as symptoms are controlled.

Therapeutic monitoring
- Monitor vital signs and intake and output; observe patient for adverse reactions, especially CNS reactions.
- Monitor bowel function.

Special populations
Geriatric patients. Geriatric patients may be more susceptible to respiratory depression and to exacerbation of preexisting glaucoma.
Pediatric patients. Drug is contraindicated in children under age 2; some children may experience respiratory depression. Children, especially those with Down syndrome, appear to be particularly sensitive to atropine content of drug.
Breast-feeding patients. Drug is excreted in breast milk; drug effects have been reported in breast-fed infants of women taking drug.

Patient counseling
- Warn patient to take drug exactly as ordered and not to exceed recommended dose.
- Advise patient to maintain adequate fluid intake during course of diarrhea and teach him about diet and fluid replacement.
- Caution patient to avoid driving during drug therapy because drowsiness and dizziness may occur.
- Advise patient to call doctor if drug isn't effective within 48 hours.
- Warn patient that prolonged use may result in tolerance and that use of larger-than-recommended doses may result in drug dependence.

diphtheria and tetanus toxoids, adsorbed

Pharmacologic classification: toxoid
Therapeutic classification: diphtheria and tetanus prophylaxis
Pregnancy risk category C

How supplied

Available by prescription only
Available in pediatric (DT) and adult (Td) strengths
Injection (for pediatric use): 6.6 limit flocculation (Lf) units of diphtheria toxoid and 5 Lf units of tetanus toxoid per 0.5 ml, in 5-ml vials; 7.5 Lf units of diphtheria toxoid and 7.5 Lf units of tetanus toxoid per 0.5 ml, in multidose vials; 10 Lf units of diphtheria toxoid and 5 Lf units of tetanus toxoid per 0.5 ml in single-dose and 5-ml vials; 12.5 Lf units of diphtheria toxoid and 5 Lf units of tetanus toxoid per 0.5 ml, in 5-ml vials
Injection (for adult use): 2 Lf units of diphtheria toxoid and 2 Lf units of tetanus toxoid per 0.5 ml in multidose vials; 2 Lf units of diphtheria toxoid and 5 Lf units of tetanus toxoid per 0.5 ml in single-dose and multidose vials

Indications and dosages

Primary immunization
Adults and children age 7 and older: Use adult strength. Give 0.5 ml I.M. 4 to 8 weeks apart for two doses and a third dose 6 to 12 months later. Booster dose is 0.5 ml I.M. q 10 years.
Children age 1 to 7: Use pediatric strength. Give two 0.5-ml doses I.M. 4 to 8 weeks apart. Give a third dose 6 to 12 months after the second injection. If final immunizing dose is given after the 7th birthday, use the adult strength.
Infants age 6 weeks to 1 year: Use pediatric strength. Give three 0.5-ml doses I.M. 4 to 8 weeks apart. Give a fourth dose 6 to 12 months after third injection.

Pharmacodynamics

Diphtheria and tetanus prophylaxis: Diphtheria and tetanus toxoids promote active immunization to diphtheria and tetanus by inducing production of antitoxins.

Pharmacokinetics

No information available.

Route	Onset	Peak	Duration
I.M.	Unknown	Unknown	10 yr

Contraindications and precautions

Contraindicated in immunosuppressed patients and in those receiving radiation or corticosteroid therapy. Defer vaccination in patients with respiratory illness and during polio outbreaks; also defer in those with acute illness except during emergency. When polio is a risk, a single antigen is used. In children under age 6, use only when diphtheria, tetanus, and pertussis combination is contraindicated because of pertussis component. DT shouldn't be used in children age 7 or older because of an increased incidence of adverse reactions. Drug is also contraindicated in patients with history of adverse reactions to constituents of drug.

Interactions

Drug-drug. *Corticosteroids, immunosuppressants:* May impair the immune response to diphtheria and tetanus toxoids. Avoid elective immunization under these circumstances.

Effects on diagnostic tests

None reported.

Adverse reactions

CNS: malaise, headache.
CV: flushing, tachycardia, hypotension.
Skin: *pain, stinging, edema, erythema, induration at injection site,* urticaria, pruritus.
Other: ***anaphylaxis,*** chills, fever, ***shock.***

Overdose and treatment

No information available.

Clinical considerations

- Obtain a thorough history of allergies and reactions to immunizations.
- Epinephrine solution 1:1,000 should be available to treat allergic reactions.
- Diphtheria and tetanus toxoids are used primarily when pertussis vaccine is contraindicated or used separately.
- These toxoids aren't used to treat active tetanus or diphtheria infections.
- To prevent sciatic nerve damage, avoid administration in gluteal muscle. During primary immunization, don't inject same site more than once.

Therapeutic monitoring

Document manufacturer, lot number, date of injection, and name and title of person administering injection on permanent record or log.

Special populations

Pregnant patients. Teratogenicity hasn't been reported. Immunization during pregnancy is recommended when needed.
Pediatric patients. Children age 7 and older have an increased risk of development of adverse reactions when preparations containing more than 7 Lf units of diphtheria toxoid are administered; therefore, children age 7 and older should receive Td (adult) preparations, not the pediatric (DT) preparation.

Patient counseling

- Inform patient that he may experience discomfort at the injection site and that a nodule

may develop there and persist for several weeks after immunization. Fever, headache, upset stomach, general malaise, or body aches and pains may also develop. Tell patient to relieve such effects with acetaminophen.
- Tell patient to report distressing adverse reactions.

diphtheria and tetanus toxoids and pertussis vaccine, adsorbed (DTP)

Acel-Imune, diphtheria and tetanus toxoids and acellular pertussis vaccine adsorbed (DTaP), DTwP, Tri-Immunol, Tripedia

Pharmacologic classification: combination toxoid and vaccine
Therapeutic classification: diphtheria, tetanus, and pertussis prophylaxis
Pregnancy risk category C

How supplied

Available by prescription only
Whole-cell vaccine
Injection: 6.7 limit flocculation (Lf) units inactivated diphtheria, 5 Lf units inactivated tetanus, and 4 protective units pertussis per 0.5 ml in 2.5-, 5-, and 7.5-ml vials
Acellular vaccine
Injection: 6.7 Lf units inactivated diphtheria, 5 Lf units inactivated tetanus, and 46.8 mcg acellular pertussis antigens per 0.5 ml in single-dose and 7.5-ml vials; 7.5 Lf units inactivated diphtheria, 5 Lf units inactivated tetanus, and 40 mcg acellular pertussis antigen per 0.5 ml in 5-ml vials; 15 Lf units of inactivated diphtheria, 6 Lf units inactivated tetanus, and 40 mcg acellualr pertussis antigens per 0.5 ml in 7.5-ml vials; 25 Lf units of inactivated diphtheria, 10 Lf units inactivated tetanus, and 58 mcg acellular pertussis vaccine per 0.5 ml in 0.5-ml vials

Indications and dosages

Primary immunization
Children age 6 weeks to 7 years: Give 0.5 ml I.M. 4 to 8 weeks apart for three doses and a fourth dose 6 to 12 months after the third dose.
Booster immunization
Booster dosage is 0.5 ml I.M. when starting school at age 4 to 6 unless fourth dose in series was administered after child's 4th birthday; then, a booster isn't necessary at time of school entrance. Not advised for adults or for children age 7 or older.

Note: The acellular vaccine may be used only for the fourth or fifth dose in children age 15 months (Tripedia) or 17 months (Acel-Imune) to 7 years who have been immunized with three or four doses of the whole-cell vaccine.

Pharmacodynamics

Diphtheria, tetanus, and pertussis (whooping cough) prophylaxis: Vaccine promotes active immunity to diphtheria, tetanus, and pertussis by inducing production of antitoxin and antibodies.

Pharmacokinetics

No information available.

Route	Onset	Peak	Duration
I.M.	2 wk after last dose	Unknown	4-6 yr

Contraindications and precautions

Contraindicated in immunosuppressed patients and in those on corticosteroid therapy or with history of seizures. Defer vaccination in patients with acute febrile illness. Children with preexisting neurologic disorders shouldn't receive pertussis component. Also, children who exhibit neurologic signs after injection shouldn't receive pertussis component in any succeeding injections. Give diphtheria and tetanus toxoids (called DT) instead.

Interactions

Drug-drug. *Corticosteroids, immunosuppressants:* May impair the immune response to the toxoids and vaccine. Patient shouldn't have elective immunization under these circumstances.

Effects on diagnostic tests

None reported.

Adverse reactions

CNS: ***encephalopathy, seizures,*** peripheral neuropathy.
Hematologic: thrombocytopenic purpura.
Skin: soreness, redness, expected nodule remaining several weeks at injection site, urticaria.
Other: ***anaphylaxis,*** *fever,* ***hypersensitivity reactions, shock.***

Overdose and treatment

No information available.

Clinical considerations

□ ***ALERT*** Vaccine isn't routinely given to individuals age 7 and older; it may be used only in special circumstances.
- Obtain history of allergies and reactions to immunizations, especially to pertussis vaccine.
- Epinephrine solution 1:1,000 should be available to treat allergic reactions.
- Vaccine may be given at same time as trivalent oral polio vaccine and, if indicated, when the patient receives vaccines against *Haemophilus influenzae* type b, measles, mumps, and rubella.
- Don't use to treat active tetanus, diphtheria, or pertussis infections.

Therapeutic monitoring
Acellular vaccine may be associated with a lower incidence of local pain and fever.

Patient counseling
- Explain to parents that child may experience discomfort at the injection site after immunization and that a nodule may develop there and persist for several weeks. Fever, upset stomach, or general malaise may also develop. Recommend acetaminophen liquid to relieve such discomfort.
- Tell parents to report worrisome or intolerable reactions promptly.
- Stress importance of keeping scheduled appointments for subsequent doses. Full immunization requires a series of injections.

dipivefrin hydrochloride
Propine

Pharmacologic classification: sympathomimetic
Therapeutic classification: antiglaucoma
Pregnancy risk category B

How supplied
Available by prescription only
Ophthalmic solution: 0.1%

Indications and dosages
To reduce intraocular pressure in chronic open-angle glaucoma
Adults: For initial glaucoma therapy, 1 drop in eye q 12 hours; then adjust dose based on patient response as determined by tonometric readings.

Pharmacodynamics
Antiglaucoma action: Dipivefrin is a prodrug converted to epinephrine in the eye. It decreases aqueous humor production and enhances outflow. It's often used with a miotic agent.

Pharmacokinetics
Absorption: Absorbed quickly.
Distribution: Unknown.
Metabolism: Unknown.
Excretion: Unknown.

Route	Onset	Peak	Duration
Ophthalmic	½ hr	1 hr	> 12 hr

Contraindications and precautions
Contraindicated in patients with angle-closure glaucoma or hypersensitivity to drug. Use cautiously in patients with asthma, hypersensitivity to epinephrine, and aphakia or CV disease.

Interactions
Drug-drug. *Ophthalmic beta blockers, osmotic agents, carbonic anhydrase inhibitors:* Dipivefrin may enhance the lowering of intraocular pressure. Use together cautiously.
Sympathomimetics: Possible additive effects if significant systemic absorption occurs. Patient requires close monitoring.
Digoxin, anesthetics, tricyclic antidepressants: Increased risk of cardiac arrhythmias. Patient requires close monitoring.

Effects on diagnostic tests
None reported.

Adverse reactions
CV: tachycardia, hypertension, ***arrhythmias.***
EENT: eye burning or stinging, conjunctival injection, conjunctivitis, mydriasis, allergic reaction, photophobia.

Overdose and treatment
Overdose is rare with ophthalmic use but may cause the following effects after accidental ingestion: hypertension with tachycardia or bradycardia, arrhythmias, precordial pain, anxiety, nervousness, insomnia, muscle tremor, cerebral hemorrhage, seizures, altered mental status, anorexia, nausea and vomiting, and acute renal failure. To treat oral overdose, dilute immediately then initiate emesis followed by activated charcoal and a cathartic, unless patient is comatose or obtunded. Monitor urinary output. As ordered, treat seizures with I.V. diazepam and hypertension with nitroprusside; treat arrhythmias appropriately, depending on the type of arrhythmia. Preparations containing sulfites may cause GI or cardiac toxicities and hypotension.

Clinical considerations
- Drug may cause fewer adverse reactions than with conventional epinephrine therapy; it's often used with other antiglaucoma agents.
- Store away from heat and light.

Therapeutic monitoring
Monitor patient for hypertension.

Special populations
Geriatric patients. Use drug with caution in geriatric patients to avoid precipitating narrow-angle glaucoma.

Patient counseling
- Teach patient the correct way to instill drops and warn him not to touch eye with dropper.
- Teach patient that if also using other eye drops, he should instill dipivefrin first, then wait at least 5 minutes before using the other drops.
- Instruct patient not to blink more than usual and not to close his eyes tightly after instillation.
- Tell patient instillation of drug may cause transient burning or stinging.

dipyridamole

Persantine

Pharmacologic classification: pyrimidine analogue
Therapeutic classification: coronary vasodilator, platelet aggregation inhibitor
Pregnancy risk category B

How supplied

Available by prescription only
Tablets: 25 mg, 50 mg, 75 mg
Injection: 10 mg/2 ml

Indications and dosages

Alternative to exercise in thallium myocardial perfusion imaging
Adults: 0.142 mg/kg/minute I.V. infused over 4 minutes (0.57 mg/kg total).
Inhibition of platelet adhesion in patients with prosthetic heart valves, in combination with warfarin or aspirin
Adults: 75 to 100 mg P.O. q.i.d.
◇ ***Chronic angina pectoris***
Adults: 50 mg P.O. t.i.d. at least 1 hour before meals; 2 to 3 months of therapy may be required to achieve a clinical response.
◇ ***Prevention of thromboembolic complications in patients with various thromboembolic disorders other than prosthetic heart valves***
Adults: 150 to 400 mg P.O. daily (in combination with warfarin or aspirin).

Pharmacodynamics

Coronary vasodilating action: Dipyridamole increases coronary blood flow by selectively dilating the coronary arteries. Coronary vasodilator effect follows inhibition of serum adenosine deaminase, which allows accumulation of adenosine, a potent vasodilator. Dipyridamole inhibits platelet adhesion by increasing effects of prostacyclin or by inhibiting phosphodiesterase.

Pharmacokinetics

Absorption: Absorption is variable and slow; bioavailability ranges from 27% to 59%.
Distribution: Animal studies indicate wide distribution in body tissues; small amounts cross the placenta. Protein binding ranges from 91% to 97%.
Metabolism: Metabolized by the liver.
Excretion: Elimination occurs via biliary excretion of glucuronide conjugates. Some dipyridamole and conjugates may undergo enterohepatic circulation and fecal excretion; a small amount is excreted in urine. Half-life varies from 1 to 12 hours.

Route	Onset	Peak	Duration
P.O.	Unknown	75 min	Unknown

Contraindications and precautions

No known contraindications. Use cautiously in patients with hypotension.

Interactions

Drug-drug. *Aminophylline:* Inhibits the action of dipyridamole. Avoid use together.
Oral anticoagulants and heparin: Can enhance the effects of oral anticoagulants and heparin. Monitor closely.

Effects on diagnostic tests

None reported.

Adverse reactions

CNS: *headache, dizziness.*
CV: flushing, fainting, *hypotension;* angina, chest pain, *blood pressure lability, hypertension* (with I.V. infusion).
GI: *nausea,* vomiting, diarrhea, abdominal distress.
Hematologic: increased bleeding time.
Skin: rash, irritation (with undiluted injection), pruritus.

Overdose and treatment

Clinical signs of overdose include peripheral vasodilation and hypotension. Maintain blood pressure and treat symptomatically.

Clinical considerations

- Give drug at least 1 hour before meals.
- When used as a pharmacologic "stress test," total doses beyond 60 mg appear to be unnecessary.
- Dilute I.V. form to at least a 1:2 ratio with 0.45% saline injection, normal saline injection, or D_5W to a total volume of 20 to 50 ml. Inject thallium within 5 minutes of dipyridamole.

Therapeutic monitoring

- Monitor blood pressure.
- Be alert for adverse reactions, including signs of bleeding and prolonged bleeding time, especially at high doses and during long-term therapy.

Special populations

Breast-feeding patients. Safety in breast-feeding women hasn't been established.
Pediatric patients. Dosage hasn't been established in children.

Patient counseling

- Explain that clinical response may require 2 to 3 months of continuous therapy; encourage patient compliance.
- Discuss adverse reactions and how to manage therapy.

dirithromycin

Dynabac

Pharmacologic classification: macrolide
Therapeutic classification: antibiotic
Pregnancy risk category C

How supplied

Available by prescription only
Tablets: 250 mg

Indications and dosages

Acute bacterial exacerbations of chronic bronchitis due to* Moraxella catarrhalis *or* Streptococcus pneumoniae; *secondary bacterial infection of acute bronchitis due to* M. catarrhalis *or* S. pneumoniae; *uncomplicated skin and skin structure infections due to* Staphylococcus aureus *(methicillin susceptible)
Adults and children age 12 and older: 500 mg P.O. daily with food for 7 days.
***Community-acquired pneumonia due to* Legionella pneumophila, Mycoplasma pneumoniae, *or* S. pneumoniae**
Adults and children age 12 and older: 500 mg P.O. daily with food for 14 days.
***Pharyngitis or tonsillitis due to* Streptococcus pyogenes**
Adults and children age 12 and older: 500 mg P.O. daily with food for 10 days.

Pharmacodynamics

Antibiotic action: Dirithromycin inhibits bacterial RNA-dependent protein synthesis by binding to the 50S subunit of the ribosome. Its spectrum of activity includes gram-positive aerobes such as *S. aureus* (methicillin-susceptible strains only), *S. pneumoniae, S. pyogenes;* gram-negative aerobes such as *L. pneumophila* and *M. catarrhalis;* and other bacteria such as *M. pneumoniae.*

Pharmacokinetics

Absorption: Rapidly absorbed from GI tract and converted by nonenzymatic hydrolysis to the microbiologically active compound erythromycylamine. Food slightly increases bioavailability of drug.
Distribution: Widely distributed throughout the body. The protein binding of erythromycylamine ranges from 15% to 30%.
Metabolism: Undergoes little to no hepatic metabolism.
Excretion: Primarily eliminated in bile or feces with a small amount in urine. Mean half-life of erythromycylamine is about 8 hours.

Route	Onset	Peak	Duration
P.O.	Unknown	4 hr	Unknown

Contraindications and precautions

Contraindicated in patients with hypersensitivity to dirithromycin, erythromycin, or other macrolide antibiotics.

Use cautiously in patients with hepatic insufficiency and in pregnant women.

Interactions

Drug-drug. *Antacids and H_2 antagonists:* Absorption may be slightly enhanced when dirithromycin is administered immediately after these drugs.
Theophylline: Dirithromycin may alter steady-state plasma level of theophylline. Monitor theophylline plasma levels. Dosage adjustments may be needed.
Alfentanil, anticoagulants, bromocriptine, carbamazepine, cyclosporine, digoxin, disopyramide, ergotamine, hexobarbital, lovastatin, phenytoin, triazolam, valproate: These drugs interact with erythromycin products; it isn't known if these same drug interactions occur with dirithromycin. Use caution during coadministration.
Drug-food. *Any food:* Increases absorption; administer drug with food.

Effects on diagnostic tests

None reported.

Adverse reactions

CNS: headache, dizziness, vertigo, insomnia, asthenia.
GI: abdominal pain, nausea, diarrhea, vomiting, dyspepsia, GI disorder, flatulence.
Hematologic: increased platelet, eosinophil, and neutrophil counts.
Metabolic: hyperkalemia, decreased bicarbonate levels, increased CK levels.
Respiratory: increased cough, dyspnea.
Skin: rash, pruritus, urticaria.
Other: pain (nonspecific).

Overdose and treatment

The symptoms of a macrolide antibiotic overdose may include nausea, vomiting, epigastric distress, and diarrhea. Treatment should be supportive because forced diuresis, dialysis, and hemoperfusion haven't been established to be helpful for an overdose of dirithromycin.

Clinical considerations

- Obtain culture and sensitivity tests before initiating drug treatment. Therapy may begin pending results.
- Don't use drug in patients with known, suspected, or potential bacteremias because serum levels are inadequate to provide antibacterial coverage of the bloodstream.

Therapeutic monitoring

Monitor patient for superinfection. Drug may cause overgrowth of nonsusceptible bacteria or fungi.

Special populations

Breast-feeding patients. It isn't known if dirithromycin is excreted in breast milk; administer cautiously to breast-feeding women.
Pediatric patients. Safety and effectiveness in children under age 12 haven't been established.

Patient counseling

- Tell patient to take all of drug as prescribed, even after he feels better.
- Instruct patient to take drug with food or within 1 hour of having eaten. Tell him not to cut, chew, or crush the tablet.

disopyramide phosphate

Norpace, Norpace CR, Rythmodan*, Rythmodan-LA*

Pharmacologic classification: pyridine derivative antiarrhythmic, group IA antiarrhythmic
Therapeutic classification: ventricular antiarrhythmic, supraventricular antiarrhythmic, atrial antitachyarrhythmic
Pregnancy risk category C

How supplied

Available by prescription only
Capsules: 100 mg, 150 mg
Capsules (extended-release): 100 mg, 150 mg

Indications and dosages

PVCs (unifocal, multifocal, or coupled); ventricular tachycardia; ◇conversion of atrial fibrillation, atrial flutter, and paroxysmal atrial tachycardia to normal sinus rhythm
Adults: Initially, 200 to 300 mg loading dose. Usual maintenance dosage is 150 mg P.O. q 6 hours or 300 mg (extended-release) P.O. q 12 hours; for patients weighing less than 110 lb (50 kg), give 100 mg P.O. q 6 hours or 200 mg (extended-release) P.O. q 12 hours; and for patients with cardiomyopathy or possible cardiac decompensation, give 100 mg P.O. q 6 to 8 hours initially and then adjust as indicated.
Children age 12 to 18: 6 to 15 mg/kg/day P.O.
Children age 4 to 12: 10 to 15 mg/kg/day P.O.
Children age 1 to 4: 10 to 20 mg/kg/day P.O.
Children younger than 1: 10 to 30 mg/kg/day P.O.

All children's doses should be divided equally and given q 6 hours. Extended-release capsules not recommended for use in children.
≡ ***Dosage adjustment.*** Geriatric patients may need dosage reduction. Adults with hepatic insufficiency or moderately impaired renal function should receive 100 mg P.O. q 6 hours or 200 mg (extended-release) q 12 hours. Patients with severely impaired renal function should receive only 100 mg (regular-release) at the following intervals.

Creatinine clearance (ml/minute)	Dosage interval
30 to 40	q 8 hr
15 to 30	q 12 hr
< 15	q 24 hr

Pharmacodynamics

Antiarrhythmic action: A class IA antiarrhythmic agent, disopyramide depresses phase O of the action potential. It's considered a myocardial depressant because it decreases myocardial excitability and conduction velocity and may depress myocardial contractility. It also possesses anticholinergic activity that may modify the direct myocardial effects of the drug. In therapeutic doses, disopyramide reduces conduction velocity in the atria, ventricles, and His-Purkinje system. By prolonging the effective refractory period (ERP), it helps control atrial tachyarrhythmias (however, this indication is unapproved in the United States). Its anticholinergic action, which is much greater than quinidine's, may increase AV node conductivity.

Disopyramide also has a greater myocardial depressant (negative inotropic) effect than quinidine. It helps manage premature ventricular beats by suppressing automaticity in the His-Purkinje system and ectopic pacemakers. At therapeutic doses, it usually doesn't prolong the QRS segment duration and PR interval but may prolong the QT interval.

Pharmacokinetics

Absorption: Rapidly and well absorbed from the GI tract; about 60% to 80% of drug reaches systemic circulation.
Distribution: Well distributed throughout extracellular fluid but isn't extensively bound to tissues. Plasma protein binding varies, depending on drug levels, but generally ranges from about 50% to 65%. Usual therapeutic serum level ranges from 2 to 4 mcg/ml, although some patients may require up to 7 mcg/ml. Levels above 9 mcg/ml generally are considered toxic.
Metabolism: Metabolized in the liver to one major metabolite that possesses little antiarrhythmic activity but greater anticholinergic activity than the parent compound.
Excretion: About 90% of an orally administered dose is excreted in the urine as unchanged drug and metabolites; 40% to 60% is excreted as unchanged drug. Usual elimination half-life is about 7 hours but lengthens in patients with renal or hepatic insufficiency. Duration of effect is usually 6 to 7 hours.

Route	Onset	Peak	Duration
P.O.	½-3½ hr	2-2½ hr	1½-8½ hr

Contraindications and precautions
Contraindicated in patients with hypersensitivity to drug, cardiogenic shock, or second- or third-degree heart block in the absence of an artificial pacemaker.

Use very cautiously and, if possible, avoid in patients with heart failure. Use cautiously in patients with underlying conduction abnormalities, urinary tract diseases (especially prostatic hyperplasia), hepatic or renal impairment, myasthenia gravis, or acute angle-closure glaucoma.

Interactions
Drug-drug. *Antiarrhythmic agents:* May cause additive or antagonistic cardiac effects and additive toxicity. Monitor closely.
Rifampin: May impair antiarrhythmic activity of disopyramide. Monitor patient closely.
Anticholinergic agents: May cause additive anticholinergic effects. Monitor patient closely.
Warfarin: May potentiate anticoagulant effects. Monitor PT and INR closely.
Oral antidiabetic agents, insulin: Additive hypoglycemia. Monitor blood glucose levels.
Erythromycin: Increases disopyramide levels causing arrhythmias and increased QT intervals. Avoid use together.
Drug-herb. *Jimson weed:* May adversely affect the function of the cardiovascular system. Avoid use together.

Effects on diagnostic tests
None reported.

Adverse reactions
CNS: dizziness, agitation, depression, fatigue, muscle weakness, syncope.
CV: *hypotension, **heart failure, heart block,*** edema, ***arrhythmias,*** shortness of breath, chest pain.
EENT: *blurred vision, dry eyes or nose.*
GI: nausea, vomiting, anorexia, bloating, abdominal pain, diarrhea.
Hepatic: cholestatic jaundice.
Metabolic: hypoglycemia (rare), weight gain.
Musculoskeletal: aches, pain, muscle weakness.
Skin: rash, pruritus, dermatosis.

Overdose and treatment
Signs and symptoms of overdose include anticholinergic effects, severe hypotension, widening of QRS complex and QT interval, ventricular arrhythmias, cardiac conduction disturbances, bradycardia, heart failure, asystole, loss of consciousness, seizures, apnea episodes, and respiratory arrest.

Treatment involves general supportive measures (including respiratory and CV support) and hemodynamic and ECG monitoring. If ingestion was recent, gastric lavage, emesis induction, and administration of activated charcoal may decrease absorption. Isoproterenol or dopamine may be administered to correct hypotension after adequate hydration has been ensured. Digoxin and diuretics may be administered to treat heart failure. Hemodialysis and charcoal hemoperfusion may effectively remove disopyramide. Some patients may require intra-aortic balloon counterpulsation, mechanically assisted respiration, or endocardial pacing.

Clinical considerations
□ ***ALERT*** Patients with atrial flutter or fibrillation should be digitalized before disopyramide administration to ensure that enhanced AV conduction doesn't lead to ventricular tachycardia.
- Correct underlying electrolyte abnormalities, especially hypokalemia, before administering drug because disopyramide may be ineffective in patients with these problems.
- Don't give sustained-release capsules for rapid control of ventricular arrhythmias if therapeutic blood drug levels must be attained rapidly, or if patient has cardiomyopathy, possible cardiac decompensation, or severe renal impairment.
- If drug causes constipation, administer laxatives and ensure proper diet.
- Drug is commonly prescribed for patients who can't tolerate quinidine or procainamide.
- Pharmacist may prepare disopyramide suspension; 100-mg capsules are used with cherry syrup to prepare suspension (this may be best form for young children).
- Drug is removed by hemodialysis. Dosage adjustments may be necessary in patients undergoing dialysis.

Therapeutic monitoring
Patient must be monitored for signs of developing heart block, such as QRS complex widening by more than 25% or QT interval lengthening by more than 25% above baseline.

Special populations
Breast-feeding patients. Drug is excreted in breast milk; recommend alternative infant feeding methods during drug therapy.
Pediatric patients. Although safety and effectiveness of drug in children haven't been established, current recommendations call for total daily dose given in equally divided doses every 6 hours or at intervals based on individual requirements. Monitor pediatric patients during initial adjustment period; dose adjustment should begin at lower end of recommended ranges. Monitor serum drug levels and therapeutic response carefully.
Geriatric patients. Monitor closely for toxicity signs; also monitor serum electrolyte and drug levels.

Patient counseling

- When changing from immediate-release to sustained-release capsules, advise patient to begin taking sustained-release capsule 6 hours after last immediate-release capsule.
- Teach patient importance of taking drug on time, exactly as prescribed. To do this, he may have to use an alarm clock for night doses.
- Advise patient to use sugarless gum or hard candy to relieve dry mouth.

disulfiram

Antabuse

Pharmacologic classification: aldehyde dehydrogenase inhibitor
Therapeutic classification: alcoholic deterrent
Pregnancy risk category C

How supplied

Available by prescription only
Tablets: 250 mg, 500 mg

Indications and dosages

Adjunct in management of chronic alcoholism
Adults: Give maximum dose of 500 mg P.O. as a single dose in the morning for 1 to 2 weeks. Can be taken in evening if drowsiness occurs. Maintenance dosage is 125 to 500 mg daily (average dose 250 mg) until permanent self-control is established. Treatment may continue for months or years.

Pharmacodynamics

Antialcoholic action: Disulfiram irreversibly inhibits aldehyde dehydrogenase, which prevents the oxidation of alcohol after the acetaldehyde stage. It interacts with ingested alcohol to produce acetaldehyde levels five to ten times higher than are produced by normal alcohol metabolism. Excess acetaldehyde produces a highly unpleasant reaction (nausea and vomiting) to even a small quantity of alcohol. Tolerance to disulfiram doesn't occur; rather, sensitivity to alcohol increases with longer duration of therapy.

Pharmacokinetics

Absorption: Absorbed completely after oral administration, but 3 to 12 hours may be required before effects occur.
Distribution: Highly lipid-soluble and initially localized in adipose tissue.
Metabolism: Mostly oxidized in the liver and excreted in urine as free drug and metabolites (for example, diethyldithiocarbamate, diethylamine, and carbon disulfide).
Excretion: 5% to 20% is unabsorbed and is eliminated in feces. A small amount is eliminated through the lungs, but most is excreted in the urine. Several days may be required for total elimination of drug.

Route	Onset	Peak	Duration
P.O.	1-2 hr	Unknown	14 days

Contraindications and precautions

Contraindicated in patients intoxicated by alcohol and within 12 hours of alcohol ingestion; in those with psychoses, myocardial disease, coronary occlusion, or hypersensitivity to disulfiram or to other thiuram derivatives used in pesticides and rubber vulcanization; and in patients receiving metronidazole, paraldehyde, alcohol, or alcohol-containing preparations.

Use with extreme caution in patients with diabetes mellitus, hypothyroidism, seizure disorder, cerebral damage, or nephritis or hepatic cirrhosis or insufficiency and with concurrent phenytoin therapy. Drug shouldn't be administered during pregnancy.

Interactions

Drug-drug. *Alfentanil:* May prolong duration of effect. Closely monitor patient.
Bacampicillin: May precipitate disulfiram reaction. Don't use together.
Diazepam, midazolam, chlordiazepoxide, barbiturates, CNS depressants, coumarin anticoagulants, paraldehyde, phenytoin: Disulfiram may increase the blood level of these drugs. Use together cautiously.
Tricyclic antidepressants, especially amitriptyline: May cause transient delirium. Closely monitor patient.
Metronidazole: Psychosis or confusion. Avoid use together.
Isoniazid: Ataxia, unsteady gait, or marked behavioral changes. Don't use together.
Drug-herb. *Passion flower, pill-bearing spurge, squaw vine, squill, sundew, sweet flag, tormentil, valerian, yarrow, pokeweed:* Disulfiram reaction if herbal form contains alcohol. Don't use together.
Drug-food. *Caffeine:* Exaggerated or prolonged effects of caffeine may occur. Advise patient to avoid caffeine.
Drug-lifestyle. *Alcohol use (all sources including cough syrups, liniments, shaving lotions, back-rub preparations):* May precipitate disulfiram reaction. Alcohol reaction may occur as long as 2 weeks after single disulfiram dose; the longer patient remains on drug, the more sensitive he becomes to alcohol. Advise patient to be alert for and avoid use of these products.
Marijuana: Disulfiram produces a synergistic CNS stimulation when used with marijuana. Advise patient to avoid use.

Effects on diagnostic tests

Disulfiram may decrease urinary vanillylmandelic acid excretion and increase urinary concentrations of homovanillic acid. Decrease of ^{131}I; uptake or protein-bound iodine levels may occur rarely.

Adverse reactions

CNS: drowsiness, headache, fatigue, delirium, depression, neuritis, peripheral neuritis, polyneuritis, restlessness, psychotic reactions.
EENT: optic neuritis.
GI: metallic or garlic aftertaste.
GU: impotence.
Metabolic: elevated serum cholesterol.
Skin: acneiform or allergic dermatitis, occasional eruptions.
Other: disulfiram reaction (precipitated by ethanol use), which may include flushing, throbbing headache, dyspnea, nausea, copious vomiting, diaphoresis, thirst, chest pain, palpitations, hyperventilation, hypotension, syncope, anxiety, weakness, blurred vision, confusion, arthropathy.

In severe reactions: respiratory depression, CV collapse, arrhythmias, MI, acute heart failure, seizures, unconsciousness, or death.

Overdose and treatment

Overdose symptoms include GI upset and vomiting, abnormal EEG findings, drowsiness, altered consciousness, hallucinations, speech impairment, incoordination, and coma. Treat overdose by gastric aspiration or lavage along with supportive therapy.

Treatment of alcohol-induced disulfiram reaction is supportive and symptomatic. These reactions aren't usually life-threatening. Emergency equipment and drugs should be available because arrhythmias and severe hypotension may occur. Treat severe reactions like shock by administering plasma or electrolyte solutions, as needed. Large I.V. doses of ascorbic acid, iron, and antihistamines have been used but are of questionable value. Hypokalemia has been reported; it requires careful monitoring and potassium supplements.

Clinical considerations

□ ***ALERT*** Caution patient's family that disulfiram should never be given to the patient without his knowledge; severe reaction or death could result if patient ingests alcohol.
- Disulfiram shouldn't be administered for at least 12 hours after the last alcohol ingestion.
- Drug use requires close medical supervision. Patients should clearly understand consequences of disulfiram therapy and give informed consent before use.
- Use drug only in patients who are cooperative and well motivated, and who are receiving supportive psychiatric therapy.

Therapeutic monitoring

Complete physical examination and laboratory studies (CBC, electrolytes, transaminases) should precede therapy and be repeated regularly.

Special populations

Pregnant patients. Drug shouldn't be administered during pregnancy.

Patient counseling

- Explain that although disulfiram can help discourage use of alcohol, it isn't a cure for alcoholism.
- Warn patient to avoid all sources of alcohol: sauces or soups made with sherry or other wines or alcohol (even "cooking alcohol"), some herbal preparations, and cough syrups. External applications of after-shave lotion, liniments, or other topical preparations may cause disulfiram reaction (because of the products' alcohol content).
- Warn patient that drug may cause drowsiness.
- Instruct patient to carry identification card stating that disulfiram is being used and including the telephone number of the doctor or clinic to contact if a reaction occurs.

dobutamine hydrochloride

Dobutrex

Pharmacologic classification: adrenergic, $beta_1$ agonist
Therapeutic classification: inotropic
Pregnancy risk category B

How supplied

Available by prescription only
Injection: 12.5 mg/ml in 20-ml vials (parenteral)
Premixed: 0.5 mg/ml (125 or 250 mg) in 5% dextrose; 1 mg/ml (250 or 500 mg) in 5% dextrose; 2 mg/ml (500 mg) in 5% dextrose; 4 mg/ml (1,000 mg) in 5% dextrose

Indications and dosages

To increase cardiac output in short-term treatment of cardiac decompensation caused by depressed contractility
Adults: 2 to 20 mcg/kg/minute as an I.V. infusion. Rarely, infusion rates up to 40 mcg/kg/minute may be needed. Adjust dosage carefully to patient response.
≡ ***Dosage adjustment.*** Geriatric patients require lower doses because they may be more sensitive to the effects of the drug.

Pharmacodynamics

Inotropic action: Dobutamine selectively stimulates $beta_1$-adrenergic receptors to increase myocardial contractility and stroke volume, resulting in increased cardiac output (a positive inotropic effect in patients with normal hearts or in heart failure). At therapeutic doses, dobutamine decreases peripheral resistance (afterload), reduces ventricular filling pressure (preload), and may facilitate AV node conduction. Systolic blood pressure and pulse pressure may remain unchanged or increased from increased cardiac output. Increased myocardial contractility results in increased coronary blood flow and myocardial oxygen consumption. Heart rate usually remains unchanged; however, excessive doses do have chronotropic effects. Dobutamine doesn't appear to affect dopaminergic receptors, nor does it cause renal or mesenteric vasodilation; however, urine flow may increase because of increased cardiac output.

Pharmacokinetics

Absorption: After I.V. administration, onset of action occurs quickly.
Distribution: Widely distributed throughout the body.
Metabolism: Metabolized by the liver and by conjugation to inactive metabolites.
Excretion: Excreted mainly in urine, with minor amounts in feces, as its metabolites and conjugates.

Route	Onset	Peak	Duration
I.V.	1-2 min	10 min	< 5 min after infusion ends

Contraindications and precautions

Contraindicated in patients with hypersensitivity to drug or its formulation and in those with idiopathic hypertrophic subaortic stenosis. Use cautiously in patients with a history of hypertension or after recent myocardial infarction. Drug may precipitate an exaggerated pressor response.

Interactions

Drug-drug. *Inhalation hydrocarbon anesthetics:* May trigger ventricular arrhythmias. Patient requires careful ECG monitoring.
Beta blockers: May antagonize the cardiac effects of dobutamine. Don't use together.
Bretylium: May potentiate actions of vasopressors on adrenergic receptors. Monitor closely for arrhythmias.
Guanadrel, guanethidine: May potentiate the pressor effects of dobutamine, possibly resulting in hypertension and cardiac arrhythmias. Monitor patient closely.
Nitroprusside: May cause higher cardiac output and lower pulmonary wedge pressure. Monitor patient closely.
Rauwolfia alkaloids: May prolong the actions of dobutamine (a denervation supersensitivity response). Monitor patient closely.
Tricyclic antidepressants: May potentiate pressor response. Use with caution.
Drug-herb. *Rue:* May increase inotropic potential. Use cautiously.

Effects on diagnostic tests

None reported.

Adverse reactions

CNS: headache.
CV: *increased heart rate,* ***hypertension, PVCs,*** angina, nonspecific chest pain, palpitations, hypotension.
GI: nausea, vomiting.
Respiratory: shortness of breath, ***asthmatic episodes.***
Other: phlebitis, hypersensitivity reactions ***(anaphylaxis).***

Overdose and treatment

Signs and symptoms of overdose include nervousness and fatigue. No treatment is necessary beyond dosage reduction or withdrawal of drug.

Clinical considerations

Consider the recommendations relevant to all adrenergics as well as the following:
□ ***ALERT*** Dobutamine is incompatible with alkaline solution (sodium bicarbonate). Also, don't mix with or give through same I.V. line as heparin, hydrocortisone, cefazolin, or penicillin.
- Before administration of dobutamine, correct hypovolemia with appropriate plasma volume expanders.
- Before giving dobutamine, administer a cardiac glycoside if patient has atrial fibrillation (dobutamine increases AV conduction).
- Adjust dose to meet individual needs and achieve desired clinical response. Drug must be administered by I.V. infusion using an infusion pump or other device to control flow rate.
- Concentration of infusion solution shouldn't exceed 5,000 mcg/ml; use the solution within 24 hours. Rate and duration of infusion depend on patient response.

Therapeutic monitoring

- Monitor ECG, blood pressure, cardiac output, and pulmonary wedge pressure. Monitor serum electrolytes, especially potassium.
- Most patients experience an increase of 10 to 20 mm Hg in systolic blood pressure; some show an increase of 50 mm Hg or more. Most also experience an increase in heart rate of 5 to 15 beats/minute; some show increases of 30 or more beats/minute. Premature ventricular arrhythmias may also occur in about 5% of patients. Dosage reduction may be necessary when these occur.

Special populations

Breast-feeding patients. It's unknown if dobutamine is excreted in breast milk. Administer cautiously to breast-feeding women.
Pediatric patients. Increases cardiac output and systemic pressure in children. Use with caution in pediatric patients.
Geriatric patients. Use with caution in geriatric patients.

Patient counseling

- Advise patient to report adverse reactions, especially dyspnea and drug-induced headache.
- Instruct patient to report pain at I.V. site.

docetaxel

Taxotere

Pharmacologic classification: taxoid
Therapeutic classification: antineoplastic
Pregnancy risk category D

How supplied

Available by prescription only
Injection: 20 mg, 80 mg

Indications and dosages

Treatment of patients with locally advanced or metastatic breast cancer who have progressed during anthracycline-based therapy or have relapsed during anthracycline-based adjuvant therapy
Adults: 60 to 100 mg/m^2 I.V. over 1 hour q 3 weeks.
◊ ***Non-small-cell lung carcinoma***
Monotherapy
Adults: 100 mg/m^2 I.V. over 1 hour q 3 weeks.
In combination with other agents
Adults: 75 to 100 mg/m^2 I.V. over 1 hour q 3 weeks.

Pharmacodynamics

Antineoplastic action: Docetaxel acts by disrupting the microtubular network in cells that's essential for mitotic and interphase cellular functions.

Pharmacokinetics

Absorption: Administered I.V.
Distribution: About 94% protein-bound.
Metabolism: Undergoes oxidative metabolism.
Excretion: Eliminated primarily in feces with a small amount being eliminated in urine.

Route	Onset	Peak	Duration
I.V.	Rapid	Unknown	Unknown

Contraindications and precautions

Contraindicated in patients with history of severe hypersensitivity to drug or other drugs formulated with polysorbate 80. Docetaxel shouldn't be used in patients with neutrophil counts of less than 1,500 cells/mm^3.

Interactions

Drug-drug. *Compounds that induce, inhibit, or are metabolized by cytochrome P-450 3A4, such as cyclosporine, ketoconazole, erythromycin, and troleandomycin:* Metabolism of docetaxel may be modified by concomitant administration. Use together cautiously.

Effects on diagnostic tests

None reported.

Adverse reactions

CNS: paresthesia, dysesthesia, pain (including burning sensation), weakness.
CV: fluid retention, hypotension, chest tightness.
GI: *stomatitis,* nausea, vomiting, diarrhea.
Hematologic: *anemia,* **NEUTROPENIA, FEBRILE NEUTROPENIA,** ***myelosuppression*** (dose-limiting), **LEUKOPENIA, THROMBOCYTOPENIA.**
Hepatic: *increased liver function tests.*
Musculoskeletal: *myalgia,* arthralgia, back pain.
Respiratory: dyspnea.
Skin: *alopecia,* maculopapular eruptions, desquamation, nail pigmentation alteration, onycholysis, nail pain, flushing, rash.
Other: **HYPERSENSITIVITY REACTIONS,** *infections,* drug fever, chills.

Overdose and treatment

Signs and symptoms of overdose may include bone marrow suppression, peripheral neurotoxicity, and mucositis. There's no known antidote for docetaxel. Closely monitor patient's vital functions.

Clinical considerations

- Patients with bilirubin values greater than the upper limits of normal (ULN) should generally not receive docetaxel. Also, patients with ALT or AST that exceeds 1.5 times ULN concomitant with alkaline phosphatase greater than 2.5 times ULN should generally not receive drug.
- Premedicate patient with oral corticosteroids such as dexamethasone 16 mg daily for 5 days starting 1 day before docetaxel administration, to reduce the incidence and severity of fluid retention and hypersensitivity reactions.
- Docetaxel requires dilution before administration using the diluent supplied with drug. Allow drug and diluent to stand at room temperature for about 5 minutes before mixing. After adding the entire contents of diluent to the vial of docetaxel, gently rotate the vial for about 15 seconds. Then allow solution to stand for a few minutes to allow any foam to dissipate.
- To prepare the docetaxel infusion solution, aseptically withdraw the required amount of premix solution from the vial and inject into a 250-ml infusion bag or bottle of normal saline solution or D_5W solution to produce a final concentration of 0.3 to 0.9 mg/ml. Doses exceeding 240 mg require a larger volume of infusion solution so a concentration of 0.9 mg/ml of docetaxel isn't exceeded. Thoroughly mix the infusion by manual rotation.
- Use caution during preparation and administration of docetaxel. Use of gloves is recom-

mended. If solution contacts skin, wash skin immediately and thoroughly with soap and water. If docetaxel contacts mucous membranes, flush membranes thoroughly with water. Mark all waste materials with CHEMOTHERAPY HAZARD labels.

- Contact of the undiluted concentrate with plasticized polyvinyl chloride equipment or devices used to prepare solutions for infusion isn't recommended. Prepare and store infusion solutions in bottles (glass, polypropylene) or plastic bags (polypropylene, polyolefin) and administer through polyethylene-lined administration sets.

Therapeutic monitoring

- Monitor patient closely for hypersensitivity reactions, especially during the first and second infusions. If minor reactions such as flushing or localized skin reactions occur, interruption of therapy isn't required. More severe reactions require the immediate discontinuation of docetaxel and aggressive treatment.
- Bone marrow toxicity is the most frequent and dose-limiting toxicity. Frequent blood count monitoring is necessary during therapy.
- Patients who are dosed initially at 100 mg/m^2 and who experience either febrile neutropenia, a neutrophil count less than 500 cells/mm^3 for more than 1 week, severe or cumulative cutaneous reactions, or severe peripheral neuropathy during docetaxel therapy should have dosage adjusted from 100 to 75 mg/m^2. If the patient continues to experience these reactions, dosage should either be decreased from 75 to 55 mg/m^2 or the treatment discontinued.
- Patients who are dosed initially at 60 mg/m^2 and who don't experience febrile neutropenia, a neutrophil count less than 500 cells/mm^3 for more than 1 week, severe or cumulative cutaneous reactions, or severe peripheral neuropathy during docetaxel therapy may tolerate higher doses.

Special populations

Pregnant patients. Advise patient of childbearing age to avoid becoming pregnant during therapy with docetaxel because of the potential harm to the fetus.
Breast-feeding patients. Because of potential for serious adverse reactions in breast-fed infants, it's recommended that breast-feeding be discontinued during docetaxel therapy.
Pediatric patients. Safety and effectiveness in children under age 16 haven't been established.

Patient counseling

- Warn patient that alopecia occurs in almost 80% of all patients.
- Tell patient to promptly report a sore throat, fever, unusual bruising, or bleeding.

docusate calcium

Pro-Cal-Sof, Surfak

docusate potassium

Dialose, Diocto-K, Kasof

docusate sodium

Colace, Diocto, Dioeze, Diosuccin, Disonate, DOK, DOS, Doxinate, D-S-S, Duosol, Modane Soft, Pro-Sof, Regulax SS, Regulex*, Regutol

Pharmacologic classification: surfactant
Therapeutic classification: emollient laxative
Pregnancy risk category C

How supplied

Available without a prescription
Tablets: 100 mg
Capsules: 50 mg, 100 mg, 240 mg, 250 mg
Syrup: 16.7 mg/5 ml, 20 mg/5 ml
Solution: 10 mg/ml

Indications and dosages

Stool softener
docusate sodium
Adults and children age 12 and older: 50 to 200 mg P.O. daily until bowel movements are normal. Alternatively, add 50 to 100 mg to saline or oil retention enema to treat fecal impaction.
Children age 6 to 12: 40 to 120 mg P.O. daily.
Children age 3 to 6: 20 to 60 mg P.O. daily.
Children under age 3: 10 to 40 mg P.O. daily.
docusate calcium or potassium
Adults: 240 mg (calcium) or 100 to 300 mg (potassium) P.O. daily until bowel movements are normal. Higher doses are for initial therapy. Adjust dose to individual response.
Children age 6 and older: 50 to 150 mg (calcium) or 100 mg (potassium) P.O. daily.

Pharmacodynamics

Laxative action: Docusate salts act as detergents in the intestine, reducing surface tension of interfacing liquids; this promotes incorporation of fat and additional liquid, softening the stool.

Pharmacokinetics

Absorption: Absorbed minimally in the duodenum and jejunum.
Distribution: Distributed primarily locally, in the gut.
Metabolism: None.
Excretion: Excreted in feces.

Route	Onset	Peak	Duration
P.O.	24-72 hr	24-72 hr	24-72 hr

Contraindications and precautions
Contraindicated in patients hypersensitive to drug and in those with intestinal obstruction, undiagnosed abdominal pain, vomiting or other signs of appendicitis, fecal impaction, or acute surgical abdomen.

Interactions
Drug-drug. *Mineral oil:* Docusate salts may increase absorption of mineral oil and cause toxicity. Separate administration times.

Effects on diagnostic tests
None reported.

Adverse reactions
GI: bitter taste, mild abdominal cramping, diarrhea, laxative dependence (with long-term or excessive use).

Overdose and treatment
No information available.

Clinical considerations
- Liquid or syrup must be given in 6 to 8 oz (180 to 240 ml) of milk or fruit juice or in infant's formula to prevent throat irritation.
- Avoid using docusate sodium in sodium-restricted patients.
- Docusate salts are available in combination with casanthranol (Peri-Colace), senna (Senokot, Gentlax), and phenolphthalein (Ex-Lax, Feen-a-Mint, Correctol).
- Docusate salts are the preferred laxative for most patients who must avoid straining at stool, such as those recovering from MI or rectal surgery. They also are used commonly to treat patients with postpartum constipation.

Therapeutic monitoring
- Before giving for constipation, determine whether patient has adequate fluid intake, exercise, and diet.
- Discontinue drug if severe cramping occurs; notify doctor.

Special populations
Breast-feeding patients. Because absorption of docusate salts is minimal, they presumably pose no risk to breast-feeding infants.
Geriatric patients. Docusate salts are good choices for geriatric patients because they rarely cause laxative dependence, cause fewer adverse effects, and are gentler than some other laxatives.

Patient counseling
- Docusate salts lose their effectiveness over time; advise patient to report failure of medication.
- Teach patient about dietary sources of bulk, which include bran and other cereals, fresh fruit, and vegetables.

dolasetron mesylate
Anzemet

Pharmacologic classification: selective serotonin 5-HT_3 receptor antagonist
Therapeutic classification: antinauseant, antiemetic
Pregnancy risk category B

How supplied
Available by prescription only
Tablets: 50 mg, 100 mg
Injection: 20 mg/ml as 12.5 mg/0.625 ml ampules or 100 mg/5 ml vials

Indications and dosages
Prevention of nausea and vomiting associated with cancer chemotherapy
Adults: 100 mg P.O. given as a single dose 1 hour before chemotherapy; or 1.8 mg/kg as a single I.V. dose given 30 minutes before chemotherapy; or a fixed dose of 100 mg I.V. given 30 minutes before chemotherapy.
Children age 2 to 16: 1.8 mg/kg P.O. given 1 hour before chemotherapy; or 1.8 mg/kg as a single I.V. dose given 30 minutes before chemotherapy. Injectable form can be mixed with apple or apple-grape juice and administered P.O. 1 hour before chemotherapy. Maximum daily dose of 100 mg.
Prevention of postoperative nausea and vomiting
Adults: 100 mg P.O. within 2 hours before surgery; 12.5 mg as a single I.V. dose about 15 minutes before cessation of anesthesia.
Children age 2 to 16: 1.2 mg/kg P.O. given within 2 hours before surgery, up to maximum of 100 mg; or 0.35 mg/kg (up to 12.5 mg) given as a single I.V. dose about 15 minutes before the cessation of anesthesia. Injectable form (1.2 mg/kg up to 100-mg dose) can be mixed with apple or apple-grape juice and administered P.O. 2 hours before surgery.
Treatment of postoperative nausea and vomiting (I.V. form only)
Adults: 12.5 mg as a single I.V. dose as soon as nausea or vomiting occurs.
Children age 2 to 16: 0.35 mg/kg, up to a maximum dose of 12.5 mg, given as a single I.V. dose as soon as nausea or vomiting occurs.

Pharmacodynamics
Antinauseant and antiemetic actions: A selective serotonin 5-HT_3 receptor antagonist that blocks the action of serotonin. 5-HT_3 receptors are located on the nerve terminals of the vagus nerve in the periphery and in the central chemoreceptor trigger zone. Blocking the activity of the serotonin receptors prevents serotonin from stimulating the vomiting reflex.

Pharmacokinetics

Absorption: Orally administered dolasetron, injection, the I.V. solution, and tablets are bioequivalent. Oral dolasetron is well absorbed, although parent drug is rarely detected in plasma due to rapid and complete metabolism to the most clinically relevant metabolite, hydrodolasetron.
Distribution: Widely distributed in the body, with a mean apparent volume of distribution of 5.8 L/kg; 69% to 77% of hydrodolasetron is bound to plasma protein.
Metabolism: A ubiquitous enzyme, carbonyl reductase, mediates the reduction of dolasetron to hydrodolasetron. CYP2D6 and CYP3A are responsible for subsequent hydroxylation and N-oxidation of hydrodolasetron, respectively.
Excretion: Two-thirds of dose is excreted in the urine and one-third in the feces. Mean elimination half-life of hydrodolasetron is 8 hours.

Route	Onset	Peak	Duration
P.O.	Rapid	1 hr	8 hr
I.V.	Rapid	36 min	7 hr

Contraindications and precautions

Contraindicated in patients hypersensitive to drug.

Use drug cautiously in patients with or at risk for development of prolonged cardiac conduction intervals, particularly QTc. These include patients taking antiarrhythmic drugs or other drugs that lead to QT interval prolongation; hypokalemia or hypomagnesemia; patients with a potential for electrolyte abnormalities, including those receiving diuretics; patients with congenital prolonged QT interval syndrome; and those who have received cumulative high-dose anthracycline therapy.

Interactions

Drug-drug. *Drugs that prolong ECG intervals, such as antiarrhythmic drugs:* Can increase the risk of arrhythmias. Monitor patient closely.
Drugs that inhibit the P-450 enzymes, such as cimetidine: Can increase hydrodolasetron levels. Monitor patient for adverse effects.
Drugs that induce the P-450 enzyme, such as rifampin: May decrease hydrodolasetron levels. Monitor patient for decreased efficacy of antiemetic.

Effects on diagnostic tests

None reported.

Adverse reactions

CNS: *headache*, dizziness, drowsiness, fatigue.
CV: ***arrhythmias,*** ECG changes, hypotension, hypertension, tachycardia, bradycardia.
GI: *diarrhea*, dyspepsia, abdominal pain, constipation, anorexia.
GU: oliguria, urinary retention.
Hepatic: elevation of liver function tests.
Skin: pruritus, rash.
Other: fever, chills, pain at injection site.

Overdose and treatment

There is no specific antidote for dolasetron overdose; provide supportive care. It isn't known whether drug is removed by hemodialysis or peritoneal dialysis.

Clinical considerations

□ ***ALERT*** Safety and efficacy of several drug doses haven't been evaluated. Efficacy studies have all been conducted with single doses of drug.
- Injection can be infused as rapidly as 100 mg/30 seconds or diluted in 50 ml compatible solution and infused over 15 minutes.
- Injection for oral administration is stable in apple or apple-grape juice for 2 hours at room temperature.

Therapeutic monitoring

Monitor ECG and blood pressure carefully.

Special populations

Breast-feeding patients. It isn't known if drug is excreted in breast milk. Use caution when administering drug to breast-feeding women.
Pediatric patients. There's no experience in pediatric patients under age 2. Efficacy in pediatric patients age 2 to 17 receiving cancer chemotherapy is consistent with that in adults. No efficacy information has been collected in pediatric postoperative nausea and vomiting studies.
Geriatric patients. Dosage adjustment isn't needed in patients over age 65. Effectiveness in prevention of nausea and vomiting in geriatric patients is no different from that in younger age groups.

Patient counseling

- Inform patient that oral doses of drug must be taken 1 to 2 hours before surgery or 1 hour before chemotherapy to be effective.
- Instruct patient not to mix injection in juice for oral administration until just before dosing.
- Tell patient to report if nausea or vomiting occurs.

donepezil hydrochloride

Aricept

Pharmacologic classification: acetylcholinesterase inhibitor
Therapeutic classification: cholinomimetic
Pregnancy risk category C

How supplied

Available by prescription only
Tablets: 5 mg, 10 mg

Indications and dosages

Mild to moderate dementia of the Alzheimer's type

Adults: Initially, 5 mg P.O. daily h.s. After 4 to 6 weeks, dosage may be increased to 10 mg daily.

Pharmacodynamics

Anticholinesterase action: Drug is believed to inhibit the enzyme acetylcholinesterase in the CNS, increasing the concentration of acetylcholine and temporarily improving cognitive function in patients with Alzheimer's disease. Drug doesn't alter the course of the underlying disease process.

Pharmacokinetics

Absorption: Well absorbed with a relative bioavailability of 100%. Steady state is reached within 15 days.

Distribution: Steady-state volume of distribution is 12 L/kg. Donepezil is about 96% bound to plasma proteins, mainly to albumins (about 75%) and alpha$_1$-acid glycoprotein (about 21%) over the concentration range of 2 to 1,000 ng/ml.

Metabolism: Extensively metabolized to four major metabolites (two are known to be active) and several minor metabolites (not all have been identified). Donepezil is metabolized by CYP 450 isoenzymes 2D6 and 3A4 and undergoes glucuronidation.

Excretion: Both excreted in the urine intact and extensively metabolized by the liver. Elimination half-life is about 70 hours and mean apparent plasma clearance is 0.13 L/hour/kg. About 17% of drug is eliminated by the kidneys as unchanged drug.

Route	Onset	Peak	Duration
P.O.	Unknown	3-4 hr	Unknown

Contraindications and precautions

Contraindicated in patients with known hypersensitivity to drug or to piperidine derivatives. Use very cautiously in patients with "sick sinus syndrome" or other supraventricular cardiac conduction conditions because drug may cause bradycardia. Use cautiously in patients with CV disease, asthma, or history of ulcer disease and in those taking NSAIDs.

Interactions

Drug-drug. *Anticholinergics:* May interfere with anticholinergic activity. Monitor patient.

Carbamazepine, dexamethasone, phenobarbital, phenytoin, rifampin: May increase rate of elimination of donepezil. Monitor patient.

Cholinomimetics, cholinesterase inhibitors: May produce synergistic effect. Monitor patient closely.

Bethanechol, succinylcholine: May produce additive effects. Monitor patient closely.

Drug-herb. *Jaborandi tree, pill-bearing spurge:* Additive effect may occur when used concomitantly and the risk of toxicity may be increased. Use together cautiously.

Effects on diagnostic tests

None reported.

Adverse reactions

CNS: abnormal dreams or crying, aggression, aphasia, ataxia, dizziness, fatigue, depression, *headache, insomnia,* irritability, nervousness, paresthesia, restlessness, somnolence, ***seizures,*** tremor, vertigo.

CV: ***atrial fibrillation,*** chest pain, hypertension, vasodilation, hypotension, syncope.

EENT: blurred vision, cataract, eye irritation, sore throat.

GI: anorexia, bloating, *diarrhea,* epigastric pain, fecal incontinence, GI bleeding, *nausea,* vomiting.

GU: frequent urination, hot flashes, nocturia, increased libido.

Hematologic: ecchymosis.

Metabolic: dehydration, weight loss.

Musculoskeletal: arthritis, bone fracture, muscle cramps, toothache.

Respiratory: bronchitis, dyspnea.

Skin: diaphoresis, pruritus, urticaria.

Other: influenza, pain.

Overdose and treatment

Overdose can result in cholinergic crisis characterized by severe nausea, vomiting, salivation, sweating, bradycardia, hypotension, respiratory depression, collapse, and seizures. Increasing muscle weakness may also occur and may result in death if respiratory muscles are involved. Tertiary anticholinergics such as atropine may be used as an antidote for drug overdose. I.V. atropine sulfate titrated to effect is recommended; give an initial dose of 1 to 2 mg I.V. and base subsequent doses on response. Atypical responses in blood pressure and heart rate have been reported with other cholinomimetics when coadministered with quaternary anticholinergics such as glycopyrrolate. It isn't known whether donepezil or its metabolites can be removed by dialysis.

Clinical considerations

- Diarrhea, nausea, and vomiting occur more frequently with the 10-mg dose than with the 5-mg dose. These effects are mostly mild and transient, sometimes lasting 1 to 3 weeks, and resolve during continued drug therapy.
- Although not observed in clinical trials, drug may cause bladder outflow obstruction.
- Cholinomimetics have potential to cause generalized seizures. However, seizure activity also may be due to Alzheimer's disease.

Therapeutic monitoring
- Drug may increase gastric acid secretion. Closely monitor patients at increased risk for development of ulcers for symptoms of active or occult GI bleeding.

Special populations
Breast-feeding patients. It isn't known if donepezil is excreted in breast milk. Avoid use of donepezil in breast-feeding women.
Pediatric patients. Safety and efficacy in children haven't been established.
Geriatric patients. Mean plasma drug levels of geriatric patients with Alzheimer's disease are comparable with those observed in young healthy volunteers.

Patient counseling
- Explain to patient and caregiver that drug doesn't alter disease but can stabilize or alleviate symptoms. Effects of therapy depend on drug administration at regular intervals.
- Tell caregiver to give drug in the evening, just before bedtime.
- Advise patient and caregiver to immediately report significant adverse effects or changes in overall health status.
- Tell patient to inform his doctor that he's using this drug before he receives anesthesia.

dopamine hydrochloride
Intropin

Pharmacologic classification: adrenergic
Therapeutic classification: inotropic, vasopressor
Pregnancy risk category C

How supplied
Available by prescription only
Injection: 40 mg/ml, 80 mg/ml, and 160 mg/ml parenteral concentrate for injection for I.V. infusion; 0.8 mg/ml (200 or 400 mg) in D_5W, 1.6 mg/ml (400 or 800 mg) in D_5W, and 3.2 mg/ml (800 mg) in D_5W parenteral injection for I.V. infusion

Indications and dosages
Adjunct in shock to increase cardiac output, blood pressure, and urine flow
Adults and children: 2 to 5 mcg/kg/minute I.V. infusion, up to 20 to 50 mcg/kg/minute. Infusion rate may be increased by 1 to 4 mcg/kg/minute at 10- to 30-minute intervals until optimum response is achieved. In severely ill patient, infusion may begin at 5 mcg/kg/minute and gradually increased by increments of 5 to 10 mcg/kg/minute until optimum response is achieved, up to 20-50 mcg/kg/minute.
Short-term treatment of severe, refractory, chronic heart failure
Adults: Initially, 0.5 to 2 mcg/kg/minute I.V. infusion. Dosage may be increased until desired renal response occurs. Average dosage, 1 to 3 mcg/kg/minute.

Pharmacodynamics
Vasopressor action: An immediate precursor of norepinephrine, dopamine stimulates dopaminergic, beta-adrenergic, and alpha-adrenergic receptors of the sympathetic nervous system. The main effects produced are dose dependent. It has a direct stimulating effect on $beta_1$ receptors (in I.V. doses of 2 to 10 mcg/kg/minute) and little or no effect on $beta_2$ receptors. In I.V. doses of 0.5 to 2 mcg/kg/minute it acts on dopaminergic receptors, causing vasodilation in the renal, mesenteric, coronary, and intracerebral vascular beds; in I.V. doses of more than 10 mcg/kg/minute, it stimulates alpha receptors.

Low to moderate doses result in cardiac stimulation (positive inotropic effects) and renal and mesenteric vasodilation (dopaminergic response). High doses result in increased peripheral resistance and renal vasoconstriction.

Pharmacokinetics
Absorption: Rapid onset of action, with a short duration.
Distribution: Widely distributed throughout the body; however, it doesn't cross the blood-brain barrier.
Metabolism: Metabolized to inactive compounds in the liver, kidneys, and plasma by MAO and catechol-O-methyltransferase. About 25% is metabolized to norepinephrine within adrenergic nerve terminals.
Excretion: Excreted in urine, mainly as its metabolites.

Route	Onset	Peak	Duration
I.V.	5 min	Unknown	< 10 min after infusion ends

Contraindications and precautions
Contraindicated in patients with uncorrected tachyarrhythmias, pheochromocytoma, or ventricular fibrillation.

Use cautiously in patients with occlusive vascular disease, cold injuries, diabetic endarteritis, and arterial embolism; in those taking MAO inhibitors; and in pregnant women.

Interactions
Drug-drug. *MAO inhibitors:* May prolong and intensify the effects of dopamine. Avoid use together.
Beta blockers: Antagonize the cardiac effects of dopamine. Don't use together.

Alpha blockers: Antagonize the peripheral vasoconstriction caused by high doses of dopamine. Don't use together.
Ergot alkaloids: Extreme elevations in blood pressure. Don't use together.
General anesthetics, especially halothane and other halogenated hydrocarbons: Ventricular arrhythmias and hypertension. Don't use together.
Phenytoin: Hypotension and bradycardia. Monitor blood pressure and heart rate closely.
Diuretics: Increases diuretic effects of both agents. Don't use together.
Oxytocics: Advanced vasoconstriction. Dosage adjustments may be needed.

Effects on diagnostic tests
Dopamine may cause elevated urinary catecholamine levels.

Adverse reactions
CNS: headache.
CV: ectopic beats, tachycardia, anginal pain, palpitations, *hypotension; **bradycardia**,* conduction disturbances, hypertension, vasoconstriction, widening of QRS complex (less frequently).
Endocrine: decreased TSH, growth hormone, and prolactin.
GI: nausea, vomiting.
GU: azotemia.
Metabolic: hyperglycemia.
Respiratory: dyspnea, ***asthmatic episodes.***
Other: necrosis and tissue sloughing with extravasation, piloerection, ***anaphylactic reactions.***

Overdose and treatment
Signs and symptoms of overdose include excessive, severe hypertension. No treatment is necessary beyond dosage reduction or withdrawal of drug. If that fails to lower blood pressure, a short-acting alpha blocking agent may be helpful.

Clinical considerations
Consider the recommendations relevant to all adrenergics as well as the following.
☐ ***ALERT*** Severe hypotension may result with abrupt withdrawal of infusion; therefore, reduce dose gradually. Expand blood volume with I.V. fluids, if necessary.
- Correct hypovolemia with plasma volume expanders before administration of dopamine.
- Dopamine is administered by I.V. infusion using an infusion device to control rate of flow.
- Don't mix other drugs in dopamine solutions. Discard solutions after 24 hours.
- Give drug into a large vein to prevent the possibility of extravasation. If necessary to administer in hand or ankle veins, change injection site to larger vein as soon as possible. Monitor continuously for free flow. Central venous access is recommended.
- Dose may require adjustment to meet individual needs of patient and to achieve desired clinical response. If dose required to obtain desired systolic blood pressure exceeds optimum rate of renal response, reduce dose as soon as hemodynamic condition is stabilized.
- If extravasation occurs, stop infusion and infiltrate site promptly with 10 to 15 ml saline injection containing 5 to 10 mg of phentolamine. Use syringe with a fine needle, and infiltrate area liberally with phentolamine solution. In children, 0.1 to 0.2 mg/kg up to 10 mg per dose is recommended.

Therapeutic monitoring
During infusion monitor ECG, blood pressure, cardiac output, central venous pressure, pulmonary artery wedge pressure, pulse rate, urine output, and color and temperature of extremities.

Special populations
Pregnant patients. Use only when potential benefits outweigh the risks to the fetus.
Breast-feeding patients. It isn't known if drug is excreted into breast milk; use drug with caution in breast-feeding women.
Pediatric patients. No increase in adverse effects has been noted in children.
Geriatric patients. Lower doses are indicated because geriatric patients may be more sensitive to effects of the drug.

Patient counseling
- Advise patient to report adverse reactions.
- Inform patient of need for frequent monitoring of his vital signs and condition.

dorzolamide hydrochloride
Trusopt

Pharmacologic classification: sulfonamide
Therapeutic classification: antiglaucoma
Pregnancy risk category C

How supplied
Available by prescription only
Ophthalmic solution: 2%

Indications and dosages
Treatment of increased intraocular pressure in patients with ocular hypertension or open-angle glaucoma
Adults: Instill 1 drop in the conjunctival sac of affected eye t.i.d.

Pharmacodynamics
Antiglaucoma action: Dorzolamide inhibits carbonic anhydrase in the ciliary processes of the eye, which decreases aqueous humor secretion, presumably by slowing the formation

of bicarbonate ions with subsequent reduction in sodium and fluid transport. The result is a reduction in intraocular pressure.

Pharmacokinetics

Absorption: Reaches the systemic circulation when applied topically.
Distribution: Accumulates in RBCs during chronic dosing as a result of binding to carbonic anhydrase II.
Metabolism: Unknown.
Excretion: Primarily excreted unchanged in urine.

Route	Onset	Peak	Duration
Ophthalmic	Unknown	Unknown	Unknown

Contraindications and precautions

Contraindicated in patients with hypersensitivity to any component of drug or in those with impaired renal function. Use cautiously in patients with impaired hepatic function.

Interactions

Drug-drug. *Oral carbonic anhydrase inhibitors*: May cause additive effects. Don't administer together.

Effects on diagnostic tests

None reported.

Adverse reactions

CNS: asthenia, headache, fatigue.
EENT: *ocular burning, stinging, discomfort; superficial punctate keratitis; ocular allergic reactions; blurred vision; lacrimation; dryness; photophobia;* iridocyclitis, redness, eyelid crusting, ocular pain.
GI: *bitter taste,* nausea.
GU: urolithiasis.
Skin: rash.

Overdose and treatment

Overdose may result in electrolyte imbalance, acidosis, and possible CNS effects. Monitor serum electrolyte levels (especially potassium) and blood pH levels. Treatment is supportive.

Clinical considerations

- Because dorzolamide is a sulfonamide and is absorbed systemically, the same types of adverse reactions that are attributable to sulfonamides may occur with topical administration of dorzolamide.
- If more than one topical ophthalmic drug is being used, administer drugs at least 10 minutes apart.

Therapeutic monitoring

Inform patient to report ocular reactions, particularly conjunctivitis and lid reactions, and discontinue drug.

Special populations

Breast-feeding patients. It isn't known if drug is excreted in breast milk. Because of the risk for serious adverse reactions to the breast-fed infant, use in breast-feeding women isn't recommended.
Pediatric patients. Safety and effectiveness in children haven't been established.
Geriatric patients. Use with caution because greater sensitivity to drug may occur in older adults.

Patient counseling

- Teach patient how to instill drops. Advise him to wash hands before and after instilling solution, and warn him not to touch dropper or tip to eye or surrounding tissue.
- Advise patient to apply light finger pressure on lacrimal sac for 1 minute after instillation to minimize systemic absorption of drug.
- Tell patient not to wear soft contact lenses while using drug.
- Stress importance of compliance with recommended therapy.

doxacurium chloride

Nuromax

Pharmacologic classification: nondepolarizing neuromuscular blocker
Therapeutic classification: skeletal muscle relaxant
Pregnancy risk category C

How supplied

Available by prescription only
Injection: 1 mg/ml

Indications and dosages

To provide skeletal muscle relaxation for endotracheal intubation and during surgery as an adjunct to general anesthesia
Adults: Dosage is highly individualized; 0.05 mg/kg rapid I.V. produces adequate conditions for endotracheal intubation in 5 minutes in about 90% of patients when used as part of a thiopental-narcotic induction technique. Lower doses may require longer delay before intubation is possible. Neuromuscular blockade at this dose lasts an average of 100 minutes.
Children over age 2: Dosage is highly individualized; an initial dose of 0.03 mg/kg I.V. administered during halothane anesthesia produces effective blockade in 7 minutes and has a duration of 30 minutes. Under the same conditions, 0.05 mg/kg produces a blockade in 4 minutes and lasts 45 minutes.
Maintenance of neuromuscular blockade during long procedures
Adults and children over age 2: After initial dose of 0.05 mg/kg I.V., maintenance dosages of 0.005 and 0.01 mg/kg prolong neuromus-

cular blockade for an average of 30 minutes and 45 minutes, respectively. Children usually require more frequent administration of maintenance dosages.

≡ ***Dosage adjustment.*** Adjust dosage to ideal body weight in obese patients (patients whose weight is 30% or more above their ideal weight) to avoid prolonged neuromuscular blockade.

Pharmacodynamics

Skeletal muscle relaxant action: Doxacurium binds competitively to cholinergic receptors on the motor end-plate to antagonize the action of acetylcholine, resulting in a block of neuromuscular transmission.

Pharmacokinetics

Absorption: Effects are rapid after I.V. administration.
Distribution: Plasma protein binding of drug is about 30% in human plasma.
Metabolism: Not metabolized.
Excretion: Primarily eliminated as unchanged drug in urine and bile.

Route	Onset	Peak	Duration
I.V.	2 min	3-6 min	Variable

Contraindications and precautions

Contraindicated in patients with hypersensitivity to drug and in neonates. Drug contains benzyl ethanol, which has been associated with death in newborns.

Use cautiously, perhaps at a reduced dose, in debilitated patients; in patients with metastatic cancer, severe electrolyte disturbances, or neuromuscular diseases; and in those in whom potentiation or difficulty in reversal of neuromuscular blockade is anticipated. Patients with myasthenia gravis or myasthenic syndrome (Eaton-Lambert syndrome) are particularly sensitive to the effects of nondepolarizing relaxants. Shorter-acting agents are recommended for use in such patients.

Interactions

Drug-drug. *Alkaline solutions:* Drug is physically incompatible with alkaline solutions; precipitate may form. These drugs shouldn't be administered through the same I.V. line.
Isoflurane, enflurane, halothane: Decrease the effective dose required to produce a 50% suppression of the response to ulnar nerve stimulation of doxacurium by 30% to 45%. May also prolong the clinically effective duration of action of doxacurium by up to 25%. Don't use together.
Antibiotics (aminoglycosides, such as gentamycin, kanamycin, neomycin, and streptomycin, tetracyclines, bacitracin, polymyxins, lincomycin, clindamycin, colistin, and colistimethate sodium), magnesium salts, lithium, local anesthetics, procainamide, and quinidine: Neuromuscular blocking action of doxacurium may be enhanced. Use together cautiously. Monitor for excessive weakness.
Carbamazepine, phenytoin: Delay onset of neuromuscular blockade induced by doxacurium and shorten its duration. Monitor patient.

Effects on diagnostic tests

None reported.

Adverse reactions

Respiratory: dyspnea, ***respiratory depression, respiratory insufficiency or apnea.***
Musculoskeletal: prolonged muscle weakness.

Overdose and treatment

Overdose with neuromuscular blocking agents such as doxacurium may result in neuromuscular block beyond the time needed for surgery and anesthesia. The primary treatment is maintenance of a patent airway and controlled ventilation until recovery of normal neuromuscular function is assured. Once initial evidence of recovery is observed, further recovery may be facilitated by administration of an anticholinesterase agent (such as neostigmine or edrophonium) in conjunction with an appropriate anticholinergic agent.

Clinical considerations

- All times of onset and duration of neuromuscular blockade are averages; considerable individual variation in dosages is normal.
- As with other nondepolarizing neuromuscular blocking agents, a reduction in dosage of doxacurium must be considered in cachectic or debilitated patients; in patients with neuromuscular diseases, severe electrolyte abnormalities, or carcinomatosis; and in other patients in whom potentiation of neuromuscular block or difficulty with reversal is anticipated. Increased doses of doxacurium may be required in burn patients.
- Drug has no effect on consciousness or pain threshold. To avoid distress to the patient, it shouldn't be administered until patient's consciousness is obtunded by general anesthetic.
- Drug may prolong neuromuscular block in patients undergoing renal transplantation, and onset and duration of the block may vary with patients undergoing liver transplantation.
- Use drug only under direct medical supervision by caregivers familiar with use of neuromuscular blocking agents and in airway management. Don't use unless facilities and equipment for mechanical ventilation, oxygen therapy, and intubation and an antagonist are within reach.
- Use of a peripheral nerve stimulator will permit the most advantageous use of doxacurium, minimize the possibility of overdose or underdose, and assist in the evaluation of recovery.

- Doxacurium is acidic (pH 3.9 to 5.0) and may not be compatible with alkaline solutions having a pH above 8.5 (such as barbiturate solutions).
- Doxacurium diluted up to 1:10 in D_5W injection, USP or normal saline injection, USP, is physically and chemically stable when stored in polypropylene syringes at 41° to 77° F (5° to 25° C) for up to 24 hours. Because dilution reduces preservative effectiveness of benzyl alcohol, use aseptic technique to prepare diluted product. Use diluted product immediately; discard any unused portion after 8 hours.

Therapeutic monitoring

- Monitor ECG, especially for bradycardia.
- Monitor respirations until patient is fully recovered from neuromuscular blockade, as evidenced by tests of muscle strength (such as hand grips, head lift, and ability to cough).

Special populations

Breast-feeding patients. It isn't known if drug is excreted in breast milk. Use cautiously when administrating to breast-feeding women.
Pediatric patients. Drug use hasn't been studied in children under age 2.
Geriatric patients. Geriatric patients may be more sensitive to the effects of the drug. They may experience a slower onset of the blockade and a longer duration.

Patient counseling

Reassure patient and family that he will be monitored at all times.

doxapram hydrochloride

Dopram

Pharmacologic classification: analeptic
Therapeutic classification: CNS and respiratory stimulant
Pregnancy risk category B

How supplied

Available by prescription only
Injection: 20 mg/ml (benzyl alcohol 0.9%)

Indications and dosages

Postanesthesia respiratory stimulation
Adults: 0.5 to 1 mg/kg of body weight as a single I.V. injection (not to exceed 1.5 mg/kg) or as several injections q 5 minutes, not to exceed 2 mg/kg total dosage. Alternatively, 250 mg in 250 ml of normal saline solution or D_5W infused at an initial rate of 5 mg/minute I.V. until a satisfactory response is achieved. Maintain at 1 to 3 mg/minute. Recommended total dose for infusion shouldn't exceed 4 mg/kg.
Drug-induced CNS depression
Adults: For injection, priming dose of 2 mg/kg I.V. repeated in 5 minutes and again q 1 to 2 hours until patient awakens (and if relapse occurs). Maximum daily dose is 3 g.

For infusion, priming dose of 2 mg/kg I.V., repeated in 5 minutes and again in 1 to 2 hours if needed. If response occurs, give I.V. infusion (1 mg/ml) at 1 to 3 mg/minute until patient awakens. Don't infuse for longer than 2 hours or administer more than 3 g/day. May resume I.V. infusion after a rest period of 30 minutes to 2 hours, if needed.
Chronic pulmonary disease associated with acute hypercapnia
Adults: Infusion of 1 to 2 mg/minute (using 2 mg/ml solution). Maximum dose is 3 mg/minute for a maximum duration of 2 hours. Don't use drug with mechanical ventilation. Use infusion pump to regulate rate.

Pharmacodynamics

Respiratory stimulant action: Doxapram increases respiratory rate by direct stimulation of the medullary respiratory center and possibly by indirect action on chemoreceptors in the carotid artery and aortic arch. Doxapram causes increased release of catecholamines.

Pharmacokinetics

Absorption: After I.V. administration, effects are rapid.
Distribution: Distributed throughout the body.
Metabolism: 99% metabolized by the liver.
Excretion: Metabolites are excreted in urine.

Route	Onset	Peak	Duration
I.V.	20-40 sec	1-2 min	5-12 min

Contraindications and precautions

Contraindicated in patients with seizure disorders; head injury; CV disorders; frank, uncompensated heart failure; severe hypertension; CVA; respiratory failure or incompetence secondary to neuromuscular disorders; muscle paresis; flail chest; obstructed airway; pulmonary embolism; pneumothorax; restrictive respiratory disease; acute bronchial asthma or extreme dyspnea; or hypoxia not associated with hypercapnia. Drug also contraindicated in neonates because product contains benzyl alcohol.

Use cautiously in patients with bronchial asthma, severe tachycardia or arrhythmias, cerebral edema or increased CSF pressure, hyperthyroidism, pheochromocytoma, or metabolic disorders.

Interactions

Drug-drug. *MAO inhibitors, sympathomimetic drugs*: Added pressor effects. Use together cautiously.
Anesthetics such as cyclopropane enflurane, and halothane: Sensitize the myocardium to catecholamines. Discontinue at least 10 minutes before giving doxapram.

Neuromuscular blockers: Doxapram temporarily may mask residual effects of neuromuscular blockers used after anesthesia. Monitor patient closely.

Effects on diagnostic tests
None reported.

Adverse reactions
CNS: ***seizures,*** *headache,* dizziness, apprehension, disorientation, hyperactivity, bilateral Babinski's signs, paresthesia.
CV: *chest pain and tightness, variations in heart rate, hypertension,* lowered T waves, ***arrhythmias.***
EENT: sneezing, ***laryngospasm.***
GI: nausea, vomiting, diarrhea.
GU: urine retention, bladder stimulation with incontinence, increased BUN levels, albuminuria.
Hematologic: decreased erythrocyte and leukocyte counts, reduced hemoglobin and hematocrit levels.
Musculoskeletal: muscle spasms.
Respiratory: cough, ***bronchospasm,*** dyspnea, rebound hypoventilation.
Skin: pruritus.
Other: hiccups, diaphoresis, flushing.

Overdose and treatment
Signs of overdose include hypertension, tachycardia, arrhythmias, skeletal muscle hyperactivity, and dyspnea.

Treatment is supportive. Keep oxygen and resuscitative equipment available, but use oxygen with caution because rapid increase in partial pressure of oxygen can suppress carotid chemoreceptor activity. Keep I.V. anticonvulsants available to treat seizures.

Clinical considerations
- Use of doxapram as an analeptic is strongly discouraged; use only in surgery or emergency room.
- Establish adequate airway before administering drug; prevent aspiration of vomitus by placing patient on his side.
- For I.V. infusion, dilute to 1 mg/ml. Doxapram shouldn't be infused faster than recommended rate because hemolysis may occur. Use only on an intermittent basis; maximum infusion period is 2 hours.
- Avoid repeated injections in the site for long periods because of risk of thrombophlebitis or local skin irritation.
- Don't combine doxapram, which is acidic, with alkaline solutions, such as thiopental sodium; solution is compatible with D_5W or $D_{10}W$ and normal saline solution.
- Give oxygen cautiously to patients with COPD who are narcotized or those who have just undergone surgery; doxapram-stimulated respiration increases oxygen demand.

Therapeutic monitoring
Monitor blood pressure, heart rate, deep tendon reflexes, and arterial blood gas (ABG) levels before giving drug and every 30 minutes afterward. Discontinue drug if ABG levels deteriorate or mechanical ventilation is started.

Special populations
Breast-feeding patients. Safety in breast-feeding women hasn't been established. Distribution into breast milk is unknown.
Pediatric patients. Safety in children under age 12 hasn't been established.
Geriatric patients. No specific recommendations exist for use in geriatric patients. However, geriatric patients may be predisposed to one of several illnesses that preclude its use.

Patient counseling
Inform patient, if alert, and family of need for drug; answer questions and address concerns.

doxazosin mesylate
Cardura

Pharmacologic classification: alpha blocker
Therapeutic classification: antihypertensive
Pregnancy risk category C

How supplied
Available by prescription only
Tablets: 1 mg, 2 mg, 4 mg, 8 mg

Indications and dosages
Essential hypertension
Adult: Dosage must be individualized. Initially, administer 1 mg P.O. daily and determine effect on standing and supine blood pressure at 2 to 6 hours and 24 hours after dosing. If necessary, increase dose to 2 mg daily. To minimize adverse reactions, adjust dose slowly (dosage typically increased only q 2 weeks). If necessary, increase dose to 4 mg daily, then 8 mg. Maximum daily dose is 16 mg, but doses exceeding 4 mg daily are associated with a greater incidence of adverse reactions.
Benign prostatic hyperplasia
Adults: Initially, 1 mg P.O. once daily in the morning or evening; increase to 2 mg and, thereafter, to 4 mg and 8 mg once daily. Recommended adjustment interval is 1 to 2 weeks.

Pharmacodynamics
Hypotensive action: Doxazosin selectively blocks postsynaptic $alpha_1$-adrenergic receptors, dilating both resistance (arterioles) and capacitance (veins) vessels. It lowers both supine and standing blood pressure, producing more pronounced effects on diastolic pressure. Maximum reductions occur 2 to 6 hours after dosing and are associated with a small in-

crease in standing heart rate. Doxazosin has a greater effect on blood pressure and heart rate in the standing position.
Benign prostatic hyperplasia: Doxazosin improves urine flow related to relaxation of smooth muscles produced by blockade of alpha adrenoreceptors in the bladder neck and prostate.

Pharmacokinetics
Absorption: Readily absorbed from the GI tract after oral administration.
Distribution: 98% protein-bound. It's distributed in breast milk in levels about 20 times greater than in maternal plasma.
Metabolism: Extensively metabolized in the liver by *O*-demethylation or hydroxylation. Secondary peaking of plasma levels suggests enterohepatic recycling.
Excretion: 63% is excreted in bile and feces (4.8% as unchanged drug); 9% is excreted in urine.

Route	Onset	Peak	Duration
P.O.	1-2 hr	2-3 hr	24 hr

Contraindications and precautions
Contraindicated in patients with hypersensitivity to drug and quinazoline derivatives (including prazosin and terazosin). Use cautiously in patients with impaired hepatic function.

Interactions
Drug-drug. *Clonidine:* Antihypertensive effects of clonidine may be decreased. Monitor patient closely.
Drug-herb. *Butcher's broom:* Possibly reduce effects of doxazosin; avoid use together.

Effects on diagnostic tests
None reported.

Adverse reactions
CNS: *dizziness,* vertigo, somnolence, drowsiness, *asthenia, headache.*
CV: *orthostatic hypotension,* hypotension, edema, palpitations, ***arrhythmias,*** tachycardia.
EENT: rhinitis, pharyngitis, abnormal vision.
GI: nausea, vomiting, diarrhea, constipation.
Hematologic: mean WBC and neutrophil counts may be decreased.
Musculoskeletal: arthralgia, myalgia, pain.
Respiratory: dyspnea.
Skin: rash, pruritus.

Overdose and treatment
Keep patient supine to restore blood pressure and heart rate. If necessary, treat shock with volume expanders. Administer vasopressors and monitor and support renal function.

Clinical considerations
- Tolerance to antihypertensive effects of doxazosin hasn't been observed.
- No apparent differences exist in the hypotensive response of whites and blacks or of geriatric patients.
- First-dose effect (orthostatic hypotension) occurs with doxazosin but is less pronounced than with prazosin or terazosin.

Therapeutic monitoring
Orthostatic effects are most likely to occur 2 to 6 hours after dose. Monitor blood pressure during this time after the first dose and after subsequent increases in dosage. Daily doses above 4 mg increase the potential of excessive orthostatic effects.

Special populations
Breast-feeding patients. Drug accumulates in breast milk at levels about 20 times greater than in maternal plasma.
Pediatric patients. Safety and efficacy in children haven't been established.
Geriatric patients. Use drug with caution in geriatric patients with underlying autonomic dysfunction or arrhythmias.

Patient counseling
- Tell patient that orthostatic hypotension and syncope may occur, especially after first few doses and with dosage changes. Patient should rise slowly to prevent orthostatic hypotension.
- Caution patient that drug may cause drowsiness and somnolence. Patient should avoid driving and other hazardous tasks that require alertness for 12 to 24 hours after first dose, after dosage increases, and after resumption of interrupted therapy.
- Tell patient to report bothersome palpitations or dizziness.
- Inform patient drug may be taken with food if nausea occurs. Tell patient that nausea should improve as therapy continues.

doxepin hydrochloride
Adapin, Sinequan, Triadapin*

Pharmacologic classification: tricyclic antidepressant
Therapeutic classification: antidepressant
Pregnancy risk category NR

How supplied
Available by prescription only
Capsules: 10 mg, 25 mg, 50 mg, 75 mg, 100 mg, 150 mg
Oral concentrate: 10 mg/ml

Indications and dosages
Depression or anxiety
Adults: Initially, 25 to 75 mg P.O. daily in divided doses, to a maximum of 300 mg daily. Alternatively, give entire maintenance dosage

once daily with a maximum dose of 150 mg P.O.
≡ ***Dosage adjustment.*** Reduce dosage in geriatric, debilitated, or adolescent patients and in those receiving other medications (especially anticholinergics).

Pharmacodynamics
Antidepressant action: Doxepin is thought to exert its antidepressant effects by inhibiting reuptake of norepinephrine and serotonin in CNS nerve terminals (presynaptic neurons), which results in increased levels and enhanced activity of these neurotransmitters in the synaptic cleft. Doxepin more actively inhibits reuptake of serotonin than norepinephrine. Anxiolytic effects of this drug usually precede antidepressant effects. Doxepin also may be used as an anxiolytic. Doxepin has the greatest sedative effect of all tricyclic antidepressants; tolerance to this effect usually develops in a few weeks.

Pharmacokinetics
Absorption: Absorbed rapidly from the GI tract after oral administration.
Distribution: Distributed widely into the body, including the CNS and breast milk. Drug is 90% protein-bound. Steady-state is achieved within 7 days. Therapeutic levels (parent drug and metabolite) are thought to range from 150 to 250 ng/ml.
Metabolism: Metabolized by the liver to the active metabolite desmethyldoxepin. A significant first-pass effect may explain variability of serum levels in different patients taking the same dosage.
Excretion: Mostly excreted in urine.

Route	Onset	Peak	Duration
P.O.	Unknown	2 hr	Unknown

Contraindications and precautions
Contraindicated in patients with hypersensitivity to drug, glaucoma, or tendency to retain urine.

Interactions
Drug-drug. *Sympathomimetics, such as ephedrine, epinephrine, norepinephrine, phenylephrine, and phenylpropanolamine:* May increase blood pressure. Use with caution.
Warfarin: May increase PT and INR and cause bleeding. Monitor PT and INR.
Clonidine: Increases hypertensive effect. Monitor blood pressure closely.
Thyroid medication; pimozide; antiarrhythmic agents such as disopyramide, procainamide and quinidine: May increase incidence of cardiac arrhythmias and conduction defects. Monitor ECG closely.
Centrally acting antihypertensive drugs: Doxepin may decrease hypotensive effects. Monitor blood pressure closely.
Disulfiram, ethchlorvynol: Cause delirium and tachycardia. Monitor patient closely.
CNS depressants: Additive effects are likely after use of doxepin. Avoid use together.
Atropine, other anticholinergic drugs: Oversedation, paralytic ileus, visual changes, and severe constipation. Monitor patient closely.
Metrizamide: Increased risk of seizures. Avoid use together.
MAO inhibitors: May cause severe excitation, hyperpyrexia, or seizures, usually with high dose. Monitor patient closely.
Barbiturates: Induce doxepin metabolism and decrease therapeutic efficacy. Monitor patient closely; dosage adjustment may be necessary.
Phenothiazines, haloperidol: Decrease its metabolism, decreasing therapeutic efficacy. Avoid use together.
Methylphenidate, cimetidine, fluoxetine, sertraline, oral contraceptives, propoxyphene, beta blockers: May inhibit doxepin metabolism, increasing plasma levels and toxicity. Monitor serum level closely.
Drug-food. *Carbonated beverages or grape juice:* Incompatible; don't give together.
Drug-lifestyle. *Alcohol use:* Enhanced CNS depression. Advise patient to avoid use together.
Heavy smoking: Induces doxepin metabolism and decreases therapeutic efficacy. Advise patient to avoid use together.
Sun exposure: Increases risk of photosensitivity reactions. Advise patient to take precautions.

Effects on diagnostic tests
None reported.

Adverse reactions
CNS: *drowsiness, dizziness,* confusion, numbness, hallucinations, paresthesia, ataxia, weakness, headache, ***seizures,*** extrapyramidal reactions.
CV: *orthostatic hypotension, tachycardia,* ECG changes.
EENT: *blurred vision,* tinnitus.
GI: *dry mouth, constipation,* nausea, vomiting, anorexia.
GU: urine retention.
Hematologic: ***eosinophilia, bone marrow depression.***
Hepatic: elevated liver function tests.
Metabolic: hyperglycemia, hypoglycemia.
Skin: *diaphoresis,* rash, urticaria, photosensitivity.
Other: *hypersensitivity reaction.*
After abrupt withdrawal of long-term therapy: nausea, headache, malaise (doesn't indicate addiction).

Overdose and treatment
The first 12 hours after acute ingestion are a stimulatory phase characterized by excessive anticholinergic activity (agitation, irritation, confusion, hallucinations, hyperthermia, parkin-

sonian symptoms, seizures, urine retention, dry mucous membranes, pupillary dilatation, constipation, and ileus). This is followed by CNS depressant effects, including hypothermia, decreased or absent reflexes, sedation, hypotension, cyanosis, and cardiac irregularities, including tachycardia, conduction disturbances, and quinidine-like effects on the ECG.

Severity of overdose is best indicated by widening of QRS complex. Usually, this represents a serum level in excess of 1,000 ng/ml. Serum levels are usually not helpful. Metabolic acidosis may follow hypotension, hypoventilation, and seizures.

Treatment is symptomatic and supportive, including maintaining airway, stable body temperature, and fluid and electrolyte balance. Induce emesis with ipecac if patient is conscious; follow with gastric lavage and activated charcoal to prevent further absorption. Dialysis is of little use. Physostigmine may be cautiously used to reverse central anticholinergic effects. Treat seizures with parenteral diazepam or phenytoin; arrhythmias with parenteral phenytoin or lidocaine; and acidosis with sodium bicarbonate. Don't give barbiturates: these may enhance CNS and respiratory depressant effects.

Clinical considerations

□ ***ALERT*** Because hypertensive episodes have occurred during surgery in patients receiving TCAs, be aware that drug should be gradually discontinued several days before surgery.

- Recommendations for administration of doxepin, care of patients during therapy, and use in pediatric patients are the same as those for all tricyclic antidepressants.

Therapeutic monitoring

- If signs of psychosis occur or increase, expect dosage to be reduced.
- Record mood changes. Monitor patient for suicidal tendencies, and allow only a minimum supply of the drug.

Special populations

Breast-feeding patients. Drug is excreted in breast milk. Avoid use of drug in breast-feeding women, especially if high doses are used.
Pediatric patients. Doxepin is rarely used for the treatment of anxiety in pediatric patients.
Geriatric patients. Adverse CNS reactions, orthostatic hypotension, and GI and GU disturbances are more likely to develop in geriatric patients.

Patient counseling

- Teach patient to dilute oral concentrate with 4 oz (120 ml) of water, milk, or juice (grapefruit, orange, pineapple, prune, or tomato). Drug is incompatible with carbonated beverages.
- Tell patient to use ice chips, sugarless gum or hard candy, or saliva substitutes to treat dry mouth.
- Warn patient to avoid taking other drugs while taking doxepin unless they've been prescribed.
- Instruct patient to take full dose at bedtime.

doxercalciferol

Hectorol

Pharmacologic classification: synthetic vitamin D analogue
Therapeutic classification: parathyroid hormone antagonist
Pregnancy risk category B

How supplied

Available by prescription only
Capsules: 2.5 mcg

Indication, route, and dosage

Reduction of elevated intact parathyroid hormone (PTH) levels in the management of secondary hyperparathyroidism in patients undergoing long-term renal dialysis
Adults: Initially, 10 mcg P.O. three times weekly at dialysis. Dosage adjusted as needed to lower intact PTH levels to 150 to 300 pg/ml. Dosage may be increased by 2.5 mcg at 8-week intervals if the intact PTH level isn't decreased by 50% and fails to reach target range. Maximum dose is 20 mcg P.O. three times weekly. If intact PTH levels go below 100 pg/ml, suspend drug for 1 week, then resume at a dose that's at least 2.5 mcg lower than the last administered dose.

Pharmacodynamics

PTH antagonist action: Once activated, doxercalciferol and other biologically active vitamin D metabolites regulate blood calcium levels required for essential body functions. Doxercalciferol acts directly on the parathyroid glands to suppress PTH synthesis and secretion.

Pharmacokinetics

Absorption: Absorbed from the GI tract.
Distribution: No information available.
Metabolism: Metabolized to its active forms in the liver.
Excretion: The major metabolite of doxercalciferol attains peak blood levels at 11 to 12 hours after repeated oral doses. Elimination half-life is 32 to 37 hours, with a range of up to 96 hours.

Route	Onset	Peak	Duration
P.O.	Unknown	11-12 hr	Unknown

Contraindications and precautions

Contraindicated in patients with a recent history of hypercalcemia, hyperphosphatemia, or vitamin D toxicity. Use cautiously in patients with hepatic insufficiency and frequently monitor calcium, phosphorus, and intact PTH levels in these patients.

Interactions

Drug-drug. *Cholestyramine, mineral oil:* Reduce intestinal absorption of doxercalciferol. Avoid use together.
Glutethimide, phenobarbital, and other enzyme inducers; phenytoin and other enzyme inhibitors: May affect the metabolism of doxercalciferol. Adjust dosage as appropriate.
Magnesium-containing antacids: May cause hypermagnesemia. Avoid use together.
Calcium-containing or nonaluminum-containing phosphate binders: May cause hypercalcemia or hyperphosphatemia and decrease effectiveness of doxercalciferol. Use cautiously together and adjust dose of phosphate binders as appropriate.
Vitamin D supplements: May cause additive effects and hypercalcemia. Avoid use together.
Orlistat: May interfere with intestinal absorption of vitamin D analogues. Avoid use together.

Adverse reactions

CNS: *dizziness, headache, malaise,* sleep disorder.
CV: bradycardia, *edema.*
GI: anorexia, dyspepsia, *nausea, vomiting,* constipation.
Metabolic: weight gain.
Musculoskeletal: arthralgia.
Respiratory: *dyspnea.*
Skin: pruritus.
Other: abscess.

Effects on diagnostic tests

None reported.

Overdose and treatment

Excessive doses of doxercalciferol can cause hypercalcemia, hypercalciuria, hyperphosphatemia, and oversuppression of PTH secretion. For hypercalcemia of greater than 1 mg/dl above the upper limit of normal, suspend doxercalciferol therapy immediately, institute a low-calcium diet, and withdraw calcium supplements. Check serum calcium levels weekly until levels return to normal, usually in 2 to 7 days. Dialysis, using a low-calcium or calcium-free dialysate, may correct persistently or markedly elevated serum calcium levels. When serum calcium levels have returned to within normal limits, drug can be restarted at a dose that's at least 2.5 mcg lower than prior therapy.

For acute overdose, treatment should consist of general supportive measures. Within 10 minutes of ingestion, induce vomiting or perform gastric lavage to prevent further absorption. If postingestion time is more than 10 minutes, administer mineral oil to promote fecal elimination. Monitor serum calcium levels, the rate of urinary calcium excretion, and ECG findings. If serum calcium levels are persistently and markedly elevated, consider drugs, such as corticosteroids or phosphates, or therapeutic measures, such as dialysis or forced diuresis.

Clinical considerations

- Management of secondary hyperparathyroidism may prevent bone disease in patients with renal failure.
- Doxercalciferol is administered with dialysis (approximately every other day). Dosing must be individualized and based on intact PTH levels, with monitoring of serum calcium and phosphorus levels before doxercalciferol therapy and weekly thereafter.
- Calcium-based or nonaluminum-containing phosphate binders and a low-phosphate diet are used to control serum phosphorus levels in dialysis patients. Expect adjustments in doses of doxercalciferol and therapies such as dietary phosphate binders in order to sustain PTH suppression and maintain serum calcium and phosphorus levels within acceptable ranges.
- Progressive hypercalcemia secondary to vitamin D overdose may require emergency attention. Acute hypercalcemia may exacerbate arrhythmias and seizures and affect the action of digoxin. Chronic hypercalcemia can lead to vascular and soft-tissue calcification.

Therapeutic monitoring

If hypercalcemia, hyperphosphatemia, or a product of serum calcium times serum phosphorus (Ca × P) that's greater than 70 is noted, administration of doxercalciferol must be stopped, as ordered, until these parameters are lowered.

Special populations

Breast-feeding patients. It's unknown if doxercalciferol is excreted in human milk, but other vitamin D derivatives are and the potential for serious adverse reactions in nursing infants exists. Based on importance of drug to the woman, it should be decided whether breast-feeding or drug should be discontinued.
Pediatric patients. Safety and efficacy in pediatric patients haven't been established.

Patient counseling

- Inform patient that dose must be adjusted over several months to achieve satisfactory PTH suppression.
- Instruct patient to adhere to a low-phosphorus diet and to follow instructions regarding calcium supplementation.
- Tell patient to obtain his health care provider's approval before using OTC drugs, including antacids and vitamin preparations containing calcium or vitamin D.
- Inform patient that early signs and symptoms of hypercalcemia include weakness, headache, somnolence, nausea, vomiting, dry mouth, constipation, muscle pain, bone pain, and metallic taste. Late signs and symptoms include polyuria, polydipsia, anorexia, weight loss, nocturia, conjunctivitis, pancreatitis, photophobia.

doxorubicin hydrochloride

Adriamycin PFS, Adriamycin RDF, Rubex

Pharmacologic classification: antineoplastic antibiotic (cell cycle–phase nonspecific)
Therapeutic classification: antineoplastic
Pregnancy risk category D

How supplied

Available by prescription only
Injection: 10 mg, 20 mg, 50 mg, 100 mg, 150 mg vials
Injection (preservative-free): 2 mg/ml (10 mg, 20 mg, 50 mg, 75 mg, and 200 mg)

Indications and dosages

Dosage and indications may vary. Check current literature for recommended protocol or for information on liposomal doxorubicin.

Bladder, breast, lung, ovarian, stomach, and thyroid cancers; Hodgkin's disease; acute lymphoblastic and myeloblastic leukemia; Wilms' tumor; neuroblastoma; lymphoma; sarcoma
Adults: 60 to 75 mg/m² I.V. as a single dose q 21 days; or 25 to 30 mg/m² I.V. as a single daily dose on days 1 to 3 of 4-week cycle. Alternatively, 20 mg/m² I.V. once weekly. Maximum cumulative dosage is 550 mg/m² (450 mg/m² in patients who have received chest irradiation).

Pharmacodynamics

Antineoplastic action: Doxorubicin exerts its cytotoxic activity by intercalating between DNA base pairs and uncoiling the DNA helix. The result is inhibition of DNA synthesis and DNA-dependent RNA synthesis. Doxorubicin also inhibits protein synthesis.

Pharmacokinetics

Absorption: Because of its vesicant effects, doxorubicin must be administered I.V.
Distribution: Distributed widely into body tissues, with the highest levels found in the liver, heart, and kidneys. It doesn't cross the blood-brain barrier.
Metabolism: Extensively metabolized by hepatic microsomal enzymes to several metabolites, one of which possesses cytotoxic activity.
Excretion: Excreted primarily in bile. A minute amount is eliminated in urine. The plasma elimination of doxorubicin is described as biphasic with a half-life of about 15 to 30 minutes in the initial phase and 16½ hours in the terminal phase.

Route	Onset	Peak	Duration
I.V.	Unknown	Unknown	Unknown

Contraindications and precautions

Contraindicated in patients with marked myelosuppression induced by previous treatment with other antitumor agents or by radiotherapy and in those who have received lifetime cumulative dosage of 550 mg/m².

Interactions

Drug-drug. *Streptozocin:* Increases the plasma half-life of doxorubicin, increasing the activity of doxorubicin. Dosage may have to be adjusted.
Cyclophosphamide, daunorubicin: Potentiate the cardiotoxicity of doxorubicin through additive effects on the heart. Avoid use together.
Heparin sodium, fluorouracil, aminophylline, cephalosporins, dexamethasone phosphate, hydrocortisone sodium phosphate: Result in a precipitate when mixed with doxorubicin. Administer through separate I.V. lines.
Digoxin: Levels may be decreased if used with doxorubicin. Monitor serum digoxin levels closely.
Cyclophosphamide: Doxorubicin may worsen induced hemorrhagic cystitis. Monitor patient closely.
Mercaptopurine: Hepatotoxicity. Don't use together.
Drug-herb. *Green tea:* May enhance the antitumor activity of doxorubicin. Monitor patient closely.

Effects on diagnostic tests

None reported.

Adverse reactions

CV: cardiac depression, seen in such ECG changes as sinus tachycardia, T-wave flattening, ST-segment depression, voltage reduction; ***arrhythmias; acute left ventricular failure; irreversible cardiomyopathy.***
EENT: conjunctivitis.
GI: *nausea, vomiting,* diarrhea, *stomatitis,* esophagitis, anorexia.
GU: red urine (transient).
Hematologic: *leukopenia during days 10 to 15 with recovery by day 21;* ***thrombocytopenia;*** **MYELOSUPPRESSION.**
Metabolic: hyperuricemia.
Skin: urticaria, facial flushing.
Other: *severe cellulitis or tissue sloughing* (if drug extravasates); *complete alopecia within 3 to 4 weeks* (hair may regrow 2 to 5 months after drug is stopped); fever; chills; ***anaphylaxis.***

Overdose and treatment

Signs and symptoms of overdose include myelosuppression, nausea, vomiting, mucositis, and irreversible myocardial toxicity.

Treatment is usually supportive and includes transfusion of blood components, antiemetics, antibiotics for infections which may develop, symptomatic treatment of mucositis, and cardiac glycoside preparations.

Clinical considerations

ALERT Reddish color is similar to that of daunorubicin. Don't confuse the two drugs.
- If signs of heart failure occur, stop drug and notify doctor.
- The alternative dosage schedule (once-weekly dosing) has been found to cause a lower incidence of cardiomyopathy.
- To reconstitute, add 5 ml of normal saline injection, USP, to the 10-mg vial, 10 ml to the 20-mg vial, and 25 ml to the 50-mg vial, to yield a concentration of 2 mg/ml.
- Drug may be further diluted with normal saline solution or D_5W and administered by I.V. infusion.
- Drug may be administered by I.V. push injection over 5 to 10 minutes into the tubing of a freely flowing I.V. infusion.
- If cumulative dose exceeds 550 mg/m^2 body surface area, cardiac adverse reactions, which begin 2 weeks to 6 months after stopping drug, develop in 30% of patients. With high doses of doxorubicin, consider concomitant dosing with the cardioprotective agent dexrazoxane.
- The occurrence of streaking along a vein or facial flushing indicates that drug is being administered too rapidly.
- Applying a scalp tourniquet or ice may decrease alopecia. However, don't use these if treating leukemias or other neoplasms in which stem cells may be present in scalp.
- Discontinue drug or slow rate of infusion if tachycardia develops. Treat extravasation with topical application of dimethyl sulfoxide and ice packs.
- Esophagitis is very common in patients who have also received radiation therapy.

Therapeutic monitoring
- Monitor CBC and hepatic function.
- Decrease dosage as follows if serum bilirubin level increases: 50% of dose when bilirubin level is 1.2 to 3 mg/100 ml; 25% of dose when bilirubin level exceeds 3 mg/100 ml.

Special populations
Breast-feeding patients. It isn't known if doxorubicin is excreted in breast milk. However, because of the risk of serious adverse reactions, mutagenicity, and carcinogenicity in the infant, breast-feeding isn't recommended.
Pediatric patients. Children under age 2 have a higher incidence of drug-induced cardiotoxicity.
Geriatric patients. Patients over age 70 have an increased incidence of drug-induced cardiotoxicity. Take caution in geriatric patients with low bone marrow reserve to prevent serious hematologic toxicity.

Patient counseling
- Encourage adequate fluid intake to increase urine output and facilitate excretion of uric acid.
- Advise patient to avoid exposure to people with infections.
- Warn patient that alopecia will occur. Explain that hair growth should resume 2 to 5 months after drug is stopped.
- Advise patient that urine will appear red for 1 to 2 days after the dose and doesn't indicate bleeding. The urine may stain clothes.
- Instruct patient not to receive immunizations during therapy and for several weeks after. Other members of the patient's household should also not receive immunizations during the same period.
- Tell patient to call doctor if unusual bruising or bleeding or signs of an infection occur.

doxorubicin hydrochloride liposomal
Doxil

Pharmacologic classification: anthracycline
Therapeutic classification: antineoplastic
Pregnancy risk category D

How supplied
Available by prescription only
Injection: 2 mg/ml

Indication, route, and dosage
Metastatic carcinoma of the ovary in patients with disease that is refractory to both paclitaxel- and platinum-based chemotherapy regimens.
Adults: 50 mg/m^2 (doxorubicin hydrochloride equivalent) I.V. at an initial infusion rate of 1 mg/minute once every 4 weeks for a minimum of 4 courses. Continue treatment as long as the patient doesn't progress, shows no evidence of cardiotoxicity, and continues to tolerate treatment. If no infusion-related adverse events are observed, increase infusion rate to complete administration over 1 hour.
AIDS-related Kaposi's sarcoma in patients with disease that has progressed on prior combination chemotherapy or in patients who are intolerant to such therapy
Adults: 20 mg/m^2 (doxorubicin hydrochloride equivalent) I.V. over 30 minutes, once every 3 weeks, for as long as patients respond satisfactorily and tolerate treatment.
≡***Dosage adjustment.*** For patients with impaired hepatic function, reduce dosage as follows: If serum bilirubin is 1.2 to 3 mg/dl give ½ normal dose; if serum bilirubin is over 3 mg/dl give ¼ normal dose.

The dose modifications shown in the tables on the next page are recommended for managing palmar-plantar erythrodysesthesia, hematologic toxicity, and stomatitis.

PALMAR-PLANTAR ERYTHRODYSESTHESIA

Grade	Symptoms	Dosage adjustment
1	Mild erythema, swelling, or desquamation not interfering with daily activities	Redose unless patient has experienced a previous grade 3 or 4 skin toxicity If so, delay up to 2 weeks and decrease dose by 25%. Return to original dose interval.
2	Erythema, desquamation, or swelling interfering with, but not precluding, normal physical activities; small blisters or ulcerations less than 2 cm in diameter	Delay dosing up to 2 weeks or until resolved to grade 0-1. If after 2 weeks there's no resolution, discontinue drug.
3	Blistering, ulceration, or swelling interfering with walking or normal daily activities; can't wear regular clothing	Delay dosing up to 2 weeks or until resolved to grade 0-1. Decrease dose by 25% and return to original dose interval. If after 2 weeks there's no resolution, discontinue drug.
4	Diffuse or local process causing infectious complications, or a bedridden state or hospitalization	Delay dosing up to 2 weeks or until resolved to grade 0-1. Decrease dose by 25% and return to original dose interval. If after 2 weeks there's no resolution, discontinue drug.

HEMATOLOGIC TOXICITY

Grade	ANC (cells/mm³)	Platelets (cells/mm³)	Dosage adjustment
1	1500 - 1900	75,000 - 150,000	Resume treatment with no dose reduction.
2	1000 - < 1500	50,000 - < 75,000	Wait until ANC > 1,500 and platelets > 75,000; redose with no dose reduction.
3	500 - 999	25,000 - < 50,000	Wait until ANC ≥ 1,500 and platelets ≥ 75,000; redose with no dose reduction.
4	< 500	< 25,000	Wait until ANC ≥ 1,500 and platelets ≥ 75,000; redose at 25% dose reduction or continue full dose with cytokine support.

STOMATITIS

Grade	Symptoms	Dosage adjustment
1	Painless ulcers, erythema, or mild soreness	Redose unless patient has experienced previous grade 3 or 4 toxicity. If so, delay up to 2 weeks and decrease dose by 25%. Return to original dose interval.
2	Painful erythema, edema, or ulcers, but can eat	Delay dosing up to 2 weeks or until resolved to grade 0-1. If after 2 weeks there's no resolution, discontinue drug.
3	Painful erythema, edema, or ulcers, and can't eat	Delay dosing up to 2 weeks or until resolved to grade 0-1. Decrease dose by 25% and return to original dose interval. If after 2 weeks there's no resolution, discontinue drug.
4	Requires parenteral or enteral support	Delay dosing up to 2 weeks or until resolved to grade 0-1. Decrease dose by 25% and return to original dose interval. If after 2 weeks there's no resolution, discontinue drug.

Pharmacodynamics

Antineoplastic action: Doxorubicin hydrochloride liposomal is doxorubicin hydrochloride encapsulated in liposomes which, due to their small size and persistence in the circulation, are able to penetrate the altered vasculature of tumors. The mechanism of action of doxorubicin hydrochloride is thought to be related to its ability to bind DNA and inhibit nucleic acid synthesis.

The mechanism of action of the drug, which consists of doxorubicin hydrochloride encapsulated in liposomes, is thought to be related to its ability to bind DNA and inhibit nucleic acid synthesis.

Pharmacokinetics

Absorption: Unknown.
Distribution: Distributed mostly to vascular fluid. Plasma protein binding hasn't been determined; however, the plasma protein binding of doxorubicin is about 70%.
Metabolism: Doxorubicinol, the major metabolite of doxorubicin, is detected at very low levels in the plasma.
Excretion: Plasma elimination is slow and is described as biphasic, with a half-life of about 5 hours in the first phase and 55 hours in the second phase at doses of 10 to 20 mg/m^2.

Route	Onset	Peak	Duration
I.V.	Unknown	Unknown	Unknown

Contraindications and precautions

Contraindicated in patients with a history of hypersensitivity reactions to the conventional formulation of doxorubicin hydrochloride or any component in the liposomal formulation. Also, contraindicated in patients with marked myelosuppression or those who have received a lifetime cumulative dosage of 550 mg/m^2 or 400 mg/m^2 who have received radiotherapy to the mediastinal area or concomitant therapy with other cardiotoxic agents, such as cyclophosphamide. Use in patients with a history of cardiovascular disease only when the benefit of the drug outweighs the risk to the patient.

Use cautiously in patients who have received other anthracyclines. The total dose of doxorubicin hydrochloride administered to the individual patient should also take into account any previous or concomitant therapy with related compounds such as daunorubicin. Heart failure and cardiomyopathy may be encountered after discontinuation of therapy.

Interactions

None reported; however, doxorubicin hydrochloride liposomal may interact with drugs known to interact with the conventional formulation of doxorubicin hydrochloride.

Effects on diagnostic tests

None reported.

Adverse reactions

CNS: *asthenia*, paresthesia, headache, somnolence, dizziness, depression, insomnia, anxiety, malaise, emotional lability, fatigue.
CV: chest pain, hypotension, tachycardia, peripheral edema, cardiomyopathy, ***heart failure, arrhythmias,*** pericardial effusion.
EENT: *mucous membrane disorder,* mouth ulceration, pharyngitis, rhinitis, conjunctivitis, retinitis, optic neuritis.
GI: *nausea, vomiting, constipation, anorexia, diarrhea,* abdominal pain, dyspepsia, oral moniliasis, enlarged abdomen, esophagitis, dysphagia, *stomatitis,* taste perversion, glossitis.
GU: albuminuria.
Hematologic: LEUKOPENIA, NEUTROPENIA, THROMBOCYTOPENIA, *anemia,* increased PT.
Hepatic: hyperbilirubinemia.
Metabolic: dehydration, weight loss, hypocalcemia, hyperglycemia.
Musculoskeletal: myalgia, back pain.
Respiratory: dyspnea, increased cough, pneumonia.
Skin: *rash, alopecia,* dry skin, pruritus, skin discoloration, skin disorder, exfoliative dermatitis, herpes zoster, sweating, *palmar-plantar erythrodysesthesia,* alopecia.
Other: fever, allergic reaction, chills, infection, infusion-related reactions.

Overdose and treatment

Acute overdose with doxorubicin hydrochloride causes increases in mucositis, leukopenia and thrombocytopenia. Treatment of acute overdose consists of treatment of the severely myelosuppressed patient with hospitalization, antibiotics, platelet and granulocyte transfusions, and symptomatic treatment of mucositis.

Clinical considerations

- Patient's hepatic function must be evaluated before therapy, and dosage adjusted accordingly.

☐ ***ALERT*** Doxorubicin hydrochloride liposomal exhibits unique pharmacokinetic properties compared to conventional doxorubicin hydrochloride and shouldn't be substituted on a mg per mg basis.

- Follow procedures for proper handling and disposal of antineoplastic drugs.
- Dilute appropriate dose (up to a maximum of 90 mg) in 250 ml of D_5W using aseptic technique. Refrigerate diluted solution at 36° to 46° F (2° to 8° C) and administer within 24 hours.

☐ ***ALERT*** Carefully check the label on the I.V. bag before administering. Accidental substitution of doxorubicin hydrochloride liposomal for conventional doxorubicin hydrochloride has resulted in severe side effects.

- Don't use with in-line filters.
- Infuse drug I.V. over 30 to 60 minutes depending on the dose; carefully monitor the patient during infusion. Acute infusion-associated reactions (flushing, shortness of breath, facial swelling, headache, chills, back pain, tightness in the chest or throat, or hypotension) may occur. These reactions resolve over several hours to a day once the infusion is stopped. The reaction may resolve by slowing the infusion rate.

■ Don't give I.M. or S.C. Avoid extravasation. If signs or symptoms of extravasation occur, stop the I.V. infusion immediately and restart in another vein. The application of ice over the site of extravasation for about 30 minutes may be helpful in alleviating the local reaction.

Therapeutic monitoring

■ Drug may potentiate the toxicity of other antineoplastic therapies.
■ Monitor cardiac function closely by endomyocardial biopsy, echocardiography, or gated radionuclide scans. If results indicate possible cardiac injury, the benefit of continued therapy must be weighed against the risk of myocardial injury.
■ Monitor CBC, including platelets, before each dose and frequently throughout therapy. Leukopenia is usually transient. Hematologic toxicity may require dose reduction or suspension or delay of therapy. Persistent severe myelosuppression may result in superinfection or hemorrhage. Patient may require G-CSF (or GM-CSF) to support blood counts.

Special populations

Breast-feeding patients. It isn't known if drug is excreted in breast milk. Because many drugs are excreted in breast milk and because of the potential for serious adverse reactions in nursing infants, women should discontinue nursing before taking this drug.
Pediatric patients. Safety and effectiveness in pediatric patients haven't been established.
Geriatric patients. No overall differences were observed between elderly and younger subjects, but greater sensitivity in some older individuals can't be ruled out.

Patient counseling

■ Tell patient to notify his health care provider if he experiences symptoms of hand-foot syndrome such as tingling or burning, redness, flaking, bothersome swelling, small blisters, or small sores on the palms of hands or soles of feet.
■ Advise patient to report symptoms of stomatitis such as painful redness, swelling, or sores in the mouth.
■ Advise patient to avoid exposure to people with infections. Tell patient to report temperature of 100.5° F (38° C) or higher.
■ Inform patient to report nausea, vomiting, tiredness, weakness, rash, or mild hair loss.
■ Advise women of childbearing age to avoid pregnancy during therapy.

doxycycline
Vibramycin

doxycycline calcium
Vibramycin

doxycycline hyclate
Doryx, Doxy-100, Doxy-200, Doxy-Caps, Vibramycin, Vibra-Tabs

doxycycline monohydrate
Monodox, Vibramycin

Pharmacologic classification: tetracycline
Therapeutic classification: antibiotic
Pregnancy risk category D

How supplied

Available by prescription only
doxycycline calcium
Oral suspension: 50 mg/5 ml
doxycycline hyclate
Tablets (film-coated): 100 mg
Capsules: 50 mg
Capsules (delayed-release): 100 mg
Injection: 100 mg, 200 mg
doxycycline monohydrate
Capsules: 50 mg, 100 mg
Oral suspension: 25 mg/5 ml

Indications and dosages

Infections caused by sensitive organisms
Adults and children weighing 99 lb (45 kg) and over: 100 mg P.O. q 12 hours on day 1, then 100 mg P.O. daily; or 200 mg I.V. on day 1 in one or two infusions, then 100 to 200 mg I.V. daily.
Children over age 8 weighing less than 99 lb (45 kg): 4.4 mg/kg P.O. or I.V. daily, divided q 12 hours day 1, then 2.2 to 4.4 mg/kg daily.
Give I.V. infusion slowly (minimum 1 hour). Infusion must be completed within 12 hours (within 6 hours in lactated Ringer's solution or D_5W in lactated Ringer's solution).
Gonorrhea in patients allergic to penicillin
Adults: 100 mg P.O. b.i.d. for 7 days; or 300 mg P.O. initially and repeat dose in 1 hour.
◇***Syphilis in patients allergic to penicillin***
Adults: 100 mg P.O. b.i.d. for 2 weeks (early detection) or 4 weeks (if more than 1 year's duration).
Chlamydia trachomatis, ***nongonococcal urethritis, and uncomplicated urethral, endocervical, or rectal infections***
Adults: 100 mg P.O. b.i.d. for at least 7 days.
Acute pelvic inflammatory disease (PID)
Adults: 250 mg I.M. ceftriaxone, followed by 100 mg doxycycline P.O. b.i.d. for 10 to 14 days.

***Acute epididymoorchitis caused by* C. trachomatis *or* Neisseria gonorrhoeae**
Adults: 100 mg P.O. b.i.d for at least 10 days.
◇ ***Prevention of traveler's diarrhea commonly caused by enterotoxigenic* E. coli**
Adults: 100 mg P.O. daily for up to 3 days.
◇ ***Prophylaxis for rape victims***
Adults and adolescents: 100 mg P.O. b.i.d. for 7 days after a single 2-g oral dose of metronidazole is given in conjunction with a single 125-mg I.M. dose of ceftriaxone.
Chemoprophylaxis for malaria in travelers to areas where chloroquine-resistant* Plasmodium falciparum *is endemic and mefloquine is contraindicated
Adults: 100 mg P.O. once daily. Begin prophylaxis 1 to 2 days before travel to malarious areas; continue daily while in affected area, and continue for 4 weeks after return from malarious area.
Children over age 8: Give 2 mg/kg P.O. daily as a single dose; don't exceed 100 mg daily. Use the same dosage schedule as for adults.
◇ ***Lyme disease***
Adults and children age 9 and older: 100 mg P.O. b.i.d. or t.i.d. for 10 to 30 days.
◇ ***Pleural effusions associated with cancer***
Adults: 500 mg of doxycycline diluted in 250 ml of normal saline and instilled into pleural space via a chest tube.
Trachoma
Adults: 2.5 to 4 mg/kg P.O. once daily for 36 to 40 days.

Pharmacodynamics
Antibacterial action: Doxycycline is bacteriostatic; it binds reversibly to ribosomal units, thereby inhibiting bacterial protein synthesis.

Spectrum of activity of the drug includes many gram-negative and gram-positive organisms, *Mycoplasma, Rickettsia, Chlamydia,* and spirochetes.

Pharmacokinetics
Absorption: About 90% to 100% is absorbed after oral administration. Doxycycline has the least affinity for calcium of all tetracyclines; its absorption is insignificantly altered by milk or other dairy products.
Distribution: Distributed widely into body tissues and fluids, including synovial, pleural, prostatic, and seminal fluids; bronchial secretions; saliva; and aqueous humor. CSF penetration is poor. Doxycycline readily crosses the placenta, and is 25% to 93% protein-bound.
Metabolism: Insignificantly metabolized; some hepatic degradation occurs.
Excretion: Excreted primarily unchanged in urine by glomerular filtration; some may be excreted in breast milk. Plasma half-life is 22 to 24 hours after multiple dosing in adults with normal renal function; 20 to 30 hours in patients with severe renal impairment. Some drug is excreted in feces.

Route	Onset	Peak	Duration
P.O.	Unknown	1½-4 hr	Unknown
I.V.	Immediate	Unknown	Unknown

Contraindications and precautions
Contraindicated in patients with hypersensitivity to drug or other tetracyclines. Use cautiously in patients with impaired renal or hepatic function. Use during last half of pregnancy and in children under age 8 may cause permanent discoloration of teeth, enamel defects, and bone growth retardation.

Interactions
Drug-drug. *Antacids containing aluminum, calcium, or magnesium or laxatives containing magnesium; oral iron products, sodium bicarbonate, zinc:* Decrease oral absorption of doxycycline. Give antibiotic 1 hour before or 2 hours after any of these medications.
Carbamazepine , phenobarbital: May cause decreased antibiotic effect. Avoid use together.
Digoxin: Increased bioavailability. Monitor serum digoxin levels. Lowered dosages of digoxin may be needed.
Methoxyflurane: Causes nephrotoxicity with tetracyclines. Monitor serum levels carefully.
Oral anticoagulants: Increased anticoagulant effect. Monitor PT and INR and adjust dose as needed.
Oral contraceptives: Decrease contraceptive effectiveness and increase risk of breakthrough bleeding. Use a nonhormonal form of birth control.
Penicillin: May antagonize bactericidal effects. Administer penicillin 2 to 3 hours before tetracycline.
Drug-lifestyle. *Alcohol use:* May decrease antibiotic effect. Avoid use together.
Sun exposure: May cause photosensitivity reactions. Patient should take precautions.

Effects on diagnostic tests
Doxycycline causes false-negative results in urine tests using glucose oxidase reagent (Diastix, Chemstrip uG, or glucose enzymatic test strip); parenteral dosage form may cause false-negative Clinitest results.

Doxycycline also causes false elevations in fluorometric tests for urinary catecholamines.

Adverse reactions
CNS: ***intracranial hypertension (pseudotumor cerebri).***
CV: pericarditis.
EENT: glossitis, dysphagia.
GI: anorexia, *epigastric distress, nausea,* vomiting, *diarrhea,* oral candidiasis, enterocolitis, anogenital inflammation.

Hematologic: ***neutropenia,*** eosinophilia, ***thrombocytopenia,*** hemolytic anemia.
Hepatic: elevated liver enzymes.
Skin: *maculopapular and erythematous rashes, photosensitivity, increased pigmentation, urticaria.*
Other: hypersensitivity reactions ***(anaphylaxis);*** permanent discoloration of teeth, enamel defects, bone growth retardation if used in children under age 8; superinfection; thrombophlebitis.

Overdose and treatment

Signs of overdose are usually limited to the GI tract; give antacids or empty stomach by gastric lavage if ingestion occurred within the preceding 4 hours.

Clinical considerations

Consider the recommendations relevant to all tetracyclines as well as the following:
☐ ***ALERT*** Don't confuse sound-alike drugs: doxycycline and doxylamine and dicyclomine.
☐ ***ALERT*** Check expiration date. Outdated or deteriorated tetracyclines have been associated with reversible nephrotoxicity (Fanconi's syndrome).

- Reconstitute powder for injection with sterile water for injection. Use 10 ml in a 100-mg vial and 20 ml in a 200-mg vial. Dilute solution to 100 to 1,000 ml for I.V. infusion. Don't infuse solutions more concentrated than 1 mg/ml.
- Reconstituted solution is stable for 72 hours if refrigerated and protected from light.
- Drug may not be given S.C. or I.M.
- Drug may be used in patients with impaired renal function; it doesn't accumulate or cause a significant rise in BUN levels.

Therapeutic monitoring

- With larger doses or prolonged therapy, monitor for superinfection, especially in high-risk patients.
- Tell patient to check tongue for fungal infection. Stress good oral hygiene.

Special populations

Breast-feeding patients. Avoid use in breast-feeding women.
Pediatric patients. Avoid use of drug in children under age 8 unless other drugs prove ineffective or are contraindicated.

Patient counseling

- Instruct patient to take entire amount of medication as prescribed, even if he feels better.
- Tell patient to take oral form of medication with food or milk if GI upset occurs.

droperidol

Inapsine

Pharmacologic classification: butyrophenone derivative
Therapeutic classification: tranquilizer
Pregnancy risk category C

How supplied

Available by prescription only
Injection: 2.5 mg/ml

Indications and dosages

Delirium
Adults: 5 mg I.M., p.r.n. It's given for its quick onset and sedative quality.
Anesthetic premedication
Adults: 2.5 to 10 mg I.M. 30 to 60 minutes before induction of general anesthesia.
Children age 2 to 12: 0.088 to 0.165 mg/kg I.V. or I.M.
Adjunct for induction of general anesthesia
Adults: 0.22 to 0.275 mg/kg I.V. (preferably) or I.M. with an analgesic or general anesthetic.
Children: 0.088 to 0.165 mg/kg I.V. or I.M.
Adjunct for maintenance of general anesthesia
Adults: 1.25 to 2.5 mg I.V.
For use without a general anesthetic during diagnostic procedures
Adults: 2.5 to 10 mg I.M. 30 to 60 minutes before the procedure. Additional doses of 1.25 to 2.5 mg I.V. are given, p.r.n.
Adjunct to regional anesthesia
Adults: 2.5 to 5 mg I.M. or slow I.V. injection.
◇***Antiemetic in conjunction with cancer chemotherapy***
Adults: 6.25 mg I.M. or by slow I.V. injection.

Pharmacodynamics

Tranquilizer action: Droperidol produces marked sedation by directly blocking subcortical receptors. Droperidol also blocks CNS receptors at the chemoreceptor trigger zone, producing an antiemetic effect.

Pharmacokinetics

Absorption: Well absorbed after I.M. injection. Some alteration of consciousness may persist for 12 hours.
Distribution: Not well understood; drug crosses the blood-brain barrier and is distributed in the CSF. It also crosses the placenta.
Metabolism: Metabolized by the liver to *p*-fluoro-phenylacetic acid and *p*-hydroxypiperidine.
Excretion: Excreted in urine and feces.

Route	Onset	Peak	Duration
I.V., I.M.	3-10 min	½ hr	2-4 hr

Contraindications and precautions

Contraindicated in patients with known hypersensitivity or intolerance to drug. Use cautiously in patients with hypotension and other CV disease because of its vasodilatory effects, in patients with hepatic or renal disease in whom drug clearance may be impaired, and in patients taking other CNS depressants, including alcohol, opiates, and sedatives, because droperidol may potentiate the effects of these drugs.

Interactions

Drug-drug. *Opiates, other analgesics, other CNS depressants, such as barbiturates, tranquilizers, and sedative-hypnotics:* Additive CNS depression. When used together, reduce dosage of both drugs.
Fentanyl citrate: May cause hypertension and respiratory depression. Avoid use together if possible.
Drug-lifestyle. *Alcohol use:* Drug potentiates CNS depressant effects. Advise patient to avoid alcohol.

Effects on diagnostic tests

None reported.

Adverse reactions

CNS: *sedation,* altered consciousness, postoperative hallucinations, extrapyramidal reactions (dystonia [extended tongue, stiff rotated neck, upward rotation of eyes], akathisia [restlessness], fine tremors of limbs), temporarily altered EEG pattern.
CV: *hypotension* with rebound tachycardia, ***bradycardia*** (occasional), hypertension when combined with fentanyl or other parenteral analgesics (rare), decreased pulmonary artery pressure.
Respiratory: ***Respiratory depression.***

Note: Discontinue drug if patient shows signs of ***hypersensitivity, severe persistent hypotension, respiratory depression, paradoxical hypertension, or dystonia.***

Overdose and treatment

Signs of overdose include extension of the pharmacologic actions of the drug. Treat overdose symptomatically and supportively.

Clinical considerations

☐ ***ALERT*** Have fluids and other measures to manage hypotension readily available.

- Droperidol has been used for its antiemetic effects in preventing or treating chemotherapy-induced nausea and vomiting, especially that produced by cisplatin.

Therapeutic monitoring

- Vital signs must be monitored and patient observed for extrapyramidal reactions. Droperidol is related to haloperidol and is more likely than other antipsychotics to cause extrapyramidal symptoms.
- Observe patient for postoperative hallucinations or emergence delirium and drowsiness.

Special populations

Breast-feeding patients. It's unknown if droperidol is excreted in breast milk.
Pediatric patients. Safety and efficacy in children under age 2 haven't been established.
Geriatric patients. Use drug with caution. Geriatric patients are more prone to extrapyramidal reactions, CNS disturbances, and CV side effects.

Patient counseling

- Advise patient of possible postoperative effects.
- Warn patient to rise slowly to prevent orthostatic hypotension.

E

econazole nitrate

Spectazole

Pharmacologic classification: synthetic imidazole derivative
Therapeutic classification: antifungal
Pregnancy risk category C

How supplied
Available by prescription only
Cream: 1% (water-soluble base)

Indications and dosages
Cutaneous candidiasis
Adults and children: Gently rub sufficient quantity into affected areas b.i.d. in the morning and evening.
Tinea pedis, tinea cruris, tinea corporis, and tinea versicolor
Adults and children: Gently rub into affected area once daily.

Pharmacodynamics
Antifungal action: Although exact mechanism of action is unknown, drug is thought to exert its effects by altering cellular membranes and interfering with intracellular enzymes. Econazole is active against many fungi, including dermatophytes and yeasts, as well as some gram-positive bacteria.

Pharmacokinetics
Absorption: Minimal but rapid percutaneous absorption.
Distribution: Minimal.
Metabolism: Unknown.
Excretion: Unknown.

Route	Onset	Peak	Duration
Topical	Unknown	Unknown	Unknown

Contraindications and precautions
Contraindicated in patients hypersensitive to drug.

Interactions
Drug-drug. *Corticosteroids:* Can inhibit the antifungal activity of econazole nitrate, in a concentration-dependent manner, in the treatment of *Saccharomyces cerevisiae* and *Candida albicans*. Avoid use together.

Effects on diagnostic tests
None reported.

Adverse reactions
Skin: burning, pruritus, stinging, erythema.

Overdose and treatment
No overdose information available. If a reaction suggesting sensitivity or chemical irritation occurs, discontinue therapy.

Clinical considerations
Wash affected area with soap and water, and dry thoroughly before applying drug.

Therapeutic monitoring
Relief of symptoms usually occurs within 1 to 2 weeks of therapy.

Special populations
Breast-feeding patients. It's unknown if drug is excreted in breast milk. Use with caution in breast-feeding women.

Patient counseling
- Tell patient to wash hands well after application
- Caution patient to use medication as directed for the entire period of treatment, even though symptoms may lessen.
- Instruct patient with tinea pedis (athlete's foot) to wear well-fitting, well-ventilated shoes, and to change all-cotton socks daily.

edrophonium chloride

Enlon, Reversol, Tensilon

Pharmacologic classification: cholinesterase inhibitor
Therapeutic classification: cholinergic agonist, diagnostic
Pregnancy risk category NR

How supplied
Available by prescription only
Injection: 10 mg/ml in 1-ml ampule, 10-ml vial, 15-ml vial

Indications and dosages
Curare antagonist (to reverse neuromuscular blocking action)
Adults: 10 mg I.V. given over 30 to 45 seconds, repeated, p.r.n., to 40 mg maximum dose. Larg-

er doses may potentiate rather than antagonize effect of curare.

Diagnostic aid in myasthenia gravis

Adults: 2 mg I.V. within 15 to 30 seconds, then 8 mg if no response (increase in muscular strength) occurs. Alternatively, 10 mg I.M. If cholinergic reaction occurs, 2 mg I.M. 30 minutes later to rule out false-negative response.

Children weighing over 75 lb (34 kg): 2 mg I.V. If no response within 45 seconds, give 1 mg q 45 seconds to maximum dose of 10 mg; alternatively, 5 mg I.M.

Children weighing 75 lb or less: 1 mg I.V. If no response within 45 seconds, give 1 mg q 45 seconds to maximum dose of 5 mg; alternatively, 2 mg I.M.

Infants: 0.5 mg I.V.

To differentiate myasthenic crisis from cholinergic crisis

Adults: 1 mg I.V. If no response occurs in 1 minute, repeat dose once. Increased muscular strength confirms myasthenic crisis; no increase or exaggerated weakness confirms cholinergic crisis.

Tensilon test for evaluating treatment requirements in myasthenia gravis

Adults: 1 to 2 mg I.V. administered 1 hour after oral intake of drug being used in treatment. Response will be myasthenic in the undertreated patient, adequate in the controlled patient, and cholinergic in the overtreated patient.

◇ ***To terminate paroxysmal atrial tachycardia or as an aid in diagnosing supraventricular tachyarrhythmias and evaluating the function of demand pacemakers***

Adults: 10 mg I.V. over 5 minutes.

≡ ***Dosage adjustment.*** In elderly or digitalized adults, 5 to 7 mg I.V. over 5 minutes.

To slow supraventricular tachyarrhythmias unresponsive to a cardiac glycoside

Adults: 2 mg/minute I.V. test dose, followed by 2 mg q minute until a total dose of 10 mg is given. If heart rate decreases in response to this dose, infusion of 0.25 mg/minute may be started; rate of infusion may be increased to 2 mg/minute if necessary.

Pharmacodynamics

Cholinergic action: Edrophonium blocks hydrolysis of acetylcholine by cholinesterase, resulting in acetylcholine accumulation at cholinergic synapses. This leads to increased cholinergic receptor stimulation at the neuromuscular junction and vagal sites. Edrophonium is a short-acting agent, which makes it particularly useful for the diagnosis of myasthenia gravis.

Pharmacokinetics

Absorption: No information available.

Distribution: Not clearly identified.

Metabolism: Exact metabolic fate is unknown; drug isn't hydrolyzed by cholinesterases.

Excretion: Exact excretion mode is unknown.

Route	Onset	Peak	Duration
I.V.	< 1 min	Unknown	5-20 min
I.M.	2-10 min	Unknown	10-30 min

Contraindications and precautions

Contraindicated in patients with hypersensitivity to anticholinesterase agents and in those with mechanical obstruction of the intestine or urinary tract. Use cautiously in patients with bronchial asthma or arrhythmias.

Interactions

Drug-drug. *Aminoglycosides and anesthetics:* May potentiate prolonged or enhanced muscle weakness. Use together cautiously.

Cardiac glycosides: May increase the heart's sensitivity to edrophonium. Use together cautiously.

Cholinergic drugs: May lead to additive toxicity. Avoid use together.

Corticosteroids: May decrease the cholinergic effects of edrophonium; when corticosteroids are stopped, however, cholinergic effects may increase, possibly affecting muscle strength. Observe for lack of drug effect.

Ganglionic blockers, such as mecamylamine: May lead to a critical blood pressure decrease. Avoid use together.

Magnesium: Administration has a direct depressant effect on skeletal muscle. Avoid use together.

Procainamide and quinidine: May reverse the cholinergic effect of edrophonium on muscle. Use together cautiously.

Succinylcholine: May cause prolonged respiratory depression from plasma esterase inhibition. Avoid use together.

Drug-herb. *Jaborandi tree and pill-bearing spurge:* May cause an additive effect and increased risk of toxicity. Use with caution.

Effects on diagnostic tests

None reported.

Adverse reactions

CNS: *seizures,* weakness.

CV: hypotension, bradycardia, **AV block,** ***cardiac arrest.***

EENT: excessive lacrimation, diplopia, miosis, conjunctival hyperemia.

GI: nausea, vomiting, *diarrhea, abdominal cramps,* dysphagia, excessive salivation.

GU: urinary frequency, incontinence.

Musculoskeletal: dysarthria, muscle cramps, muscle fasciculation.

Respiratory: ***paralysis of muscles of respiration, central respiratory paralysis, bron-***

chospasm, laryngospasm, increased bronchial secretions.
Skin: diaphoresis.

Overdose and treatment

Signs and symptoms of overdose include muscle weakness, nausea, vomiting, diarrhea, blurred vision, miosis, excessive tearing, bronchospasm, increased bronchial secretions, hypotension, incoordination, excessive sweating, cramps, fasciculations, paralysis, bradycardia or tachycardia, excessive salivation, and restlessness or agitation. Muscles first weakened by overdose include neck, jaw, and pharyngeal muscles, followed by muscle weakening of the shoulder, upper extremities, pelvis, outer eye, and legs.

Discontinue drug immediately. Support respiration; bronchial suctioning may be performed. Atropine may be given to block the muscarinic effects of edrophonium but won't counter the paralytic effects of the drug on skeletal muscle. Avoid atropine overdose, because it may lead to bronchial plug formation.

Clinical considerations

- When giving edrophonium to differentiate myasthenic crisis from cholinergic crisis, evaluate patient's muscle strength closely.
- For easier administration, use a tuberculin syringe with an I.V. needle.
- Atropine sulfate injection should always be readily available as an antagonist for the muscarinic effects of edrophonium.

Therapeutic monitoring

Monitor for adverse reactions and for therapeutic effects.

Special populations

Pregnant patients. Drug may cause uterine irritability and induce premature labor when given I.V. to patients near term.
Breast-feeding patients. Safety hasn't been established. Breast-feeding women should avoid edrophonium.
Pediatric patients. Children may require I.M. administration; with this route, drug effects may be delayed for 2 to 10 minutes.
Geriatric patients. Geriatric patients may be more sensitive to effects of this drug. Use with caution.

Patient counseling

Tell patient that the adverse effects of the drug will be transient because of its short duration of effect.

efavirenz

Sustiva

Pharmacologic classification: nonnucleoside, reverse transcriptase inhibitor (NNRTI)
Therapeutic classification: antiretroviral
Pregnancy risk category C

How supplied

Available by prescription only
Capsules: 50 mg, 100 mg, 200 mg

Indications and dosages

Treatment of HIV-1 infection
Adults: 600 mg P.O. once daily in combination with a protease inhibitor or nucleoside analogue reverse transcriptase inhibitors.
Children 3 years and older weighing 88 lb (40 kg) or more: 600 mg P.O. once daily in combination with a protease inhibitor or nucleoside analogue reverse transcriptase inhibitors.
Children 3 years and older weighing 22 to under 88 lb (10 to under 40 kg): Give the following doses in combination with a protease inhibitor or nucleoside analogue reverse transcriptase inhibitors.
Children weighing 22 to under 33 lb (10 to under 15 kg): 200 mg P.O. once daily.
Children weighing 33 to under 44 lb (15 to under 20 kg): 250 mg P.O. once daily.
Children weighing 44 to under 55 lb (20 to under 25 kg): 300 mg P.O. once daily.
Children weighing 55 to under 72 lb (25 to under 32.5 kg): 350 mg P.O. once daily.
Children weighing 72 to under 88 lb (32.5 to under 40 kg): 400 mg P.O. once daily.

Pharmacodynamics

Antiretroviral action: Efavirenz inhibits the transcription of HIV-1 RNA to DNA, a critical step in the viral replication process. Therefore, drug lowers the amount of HIV in the blood (the viral load) and increases CD4 lymphocytes.

Pharmacokinetics

Absorption: Relative bioavailability increased by about 50% when taken with a high-fat meal.
Distribution: Highly bound to plasma proteins (about 99.5% to 99.75%); also distributed into the cerebrospinal fluid.
Metabolism: Metabolized primarily by cytochrome P-450 3A4 and cytochrome P-450 2B6 to hydroxylated inactive metabolites.
Excretion: 14% to 34% is excreted in urine (less than 1% is excreted unchanged), and 16% to 61% is excreted in feces. Terminal elimination half-life is 52 to 76 hours.

Route	Onset	Peak	Duration
P.O.	Unknown	3-5 hr	Unknown

Contraindications and precautions

Contraindicated in patients with hypersensitivity to efavirenz or its components. Use cautiously in patients with hepatic impairment or in those concurrently receiving hepatotoxic medications.

Interactions

Drug-drug. *Cisapride, ergot derivatives, midazolam, and triazolam:* Competition for cytochrome P-450 enzyme system may result in inhibition of the metabolism of these drugs and cause serious or life-threatening adverse events (such as arrhythmias, prolonged sedation, or respiratory depression). Avoid use together.
Clarithromycin and indinavir: May decrease plasma levels. Consider alternative therapy or dosage adjustment.
Drugs that induce the cytochrome P-450 enzyme system (such as phenobarbital, rifampin, and rifabutin): Increase clearance of efavirenz, resulting in lower plasma levels. Avoid use together.
Estrogens and ritonavir: Increase plasma levels. Monitor patient.
Oral contraceptives: Potential interaction of efavirenz with oral contraceptives hasn't been determined. Advise use of a reliable method of barrier contraception in addition to use of oral contraceptives.
Psychoactive drugs: May cause additive CNS effects. Avoid use together.
Saquinavir: Plasma levels of saquinavir decrease significantly. Don't use with saquinavir as sole protease inhibitor. Use of saquinavir also decreases AUC of efavirenz by 12% to 13%.
Warfarin: Plasma levels and effects of warfarin are potentially increased or decreased. Recommend monitoring INR.
Drug-food. *High-fat meals:* May increase absorption of drug. Instruct patient to maintain a proper low-fat diet.
Drug-lifestyle. *Alcohol use:* Enhances CNS effects. Advise patient to avoid alcohol use.

Effects on diagnostic tests

Drug therapy may cause false-positive urine cannabinoid test results.

Adverse reactions

CNS: abnormal dreams or thinking, agitation, amnesia, confusion, depersonalization, depression, *dizziness*, euphoria, fatigue, hallucinations, headache, hypoesthesia, impaired concentration, insomnia, somnolence, nervousness.
GI: abdominal pain, anorexia, *diarrhea*, dyspepsia, flatulence, *nausea*, vomiting, pancreatitis.
GU: hematuria, kidney stones.
Hepatic: increased AST, ALT, and total cholesterol.
Skin: increased sweating, ***erythema multiforme, Stevens-Johnson syndrome, toxic epidermal necrolysis,*** *rash,* pruritus.
Other: fever.

Overdose and treatment

Overdose has resulted in symptoms of the nervous system and involuntary muscle contractions. Treatment should involve supportive care, including frequent monitoring of vital signs and observation of clinical status. Activated charcoal may be given to aid in the removal of unabsorbed drug. Efavirenz is unlikely to be removed by hemodialysis.

Clinical considerations

- Use drug in combination with other antiretroviral agents because resistant viruses emerge rapidly when used alone. Drug shouldn't be used as monotherapy, or added on as a single agent to a failing regimen.
- Combination with ritonavir is associated with a higher frequency of adverse effects (such as dizziness, nausea, paresthesia) and laboratory abnormalities (elevated liver enzymes).

Therapeutic monitoring

- Recommend monitoring liver function and cholesterol levels.
- Monitor patient for adverse reactions.

Special populations

Pregnant patients. Pregnancy must be ruled out before starting therapy in women of childbearing age.
Breast-feeding patients. HIV-infected women shouldn't breast-feed their infants to avoid risking transmitting the disease. The drug is excreted in breast milk of animals. Instruct women not to nurse their infants.
Pediatric patients. Children may be more prone to adverse reactions, especially diarrhea, nausea, vomiting, and rash.
Geriatric patients. Geriatric patients may be more susceptible to the CNS effects of the drug.

Patient counseling

- Instruct patient to take drug with water, juice, milk, or soda. It may be taken without regard to meals.
- Inform patient that drug isn't a cure for HIV infection and that it won't affect the development of opportunistic infections and other complications associated with HIV disease or transmission of HIV to others through sexual contact or blood contamination.
- Instruct patient to take drug at the same time daily and always in combination with other antiretroviral drugs.
- Tell patient to take drug exactly as prescribed and not to discontinue it without medical approval.
- Instruct patient to report adverse reactions.

- Inform patient that rash in the most common adverse effect. If this occurs, tell patient to report it immediately, because it may be serious in rare cases.
- Advise patient that dizziness, difficulty sleeping or concentrating, drowsiness, or unusual dreams may occur the first few days of therapy. Reasure him that these symptoms generally resolve after 2 to 4 weeks and may be less problematic if drug is taken at bedtime.
- Tell patient to avoid alcoholic beverages, driving, or operating machinery until the effects of the drug are known.

enalaprilat

Vasotec I.V.

enalapril maleate

Vasotec

Pharmacologic classification: ACE inhibitor
Therapeutic classification: antihypertensive
Pregnancy risk category C (D, in second and third trimesters)

How supplied

Available by prescription only
Tablets: 2.5 mg, 5 mg, 10 mg, 20 mg
Injection: 1.25 mg/ml in 2-ml vials

Indications and dosages

Hypertension
Adults: For patient not receiving diuretics, initially 5 mg P.O. once daily, then adjusted according to response. Usual dosage range is 10 to 40 mg daily as a single dose or two divided doses. Alternatively, 1.25 mg I.V. infusion q 6 hours over 5 minutes. For patient on diuretics, initially 2.5 mg P.O. once daily. Alternatively, administer 0.625 mg I.V. over 5 minutes; repeat in 1 hour, if needed, then follow with 1.25 mg I.V. q 6 hours.
To convert from I.V. therapy to oral therapy
Adults: If patient wasn't given diuretics and was receiving 1.25 mg I.V. q 6 hours, then initially, 5 mg P.O. once daily. If patient was being given diuretics and was receiving 0.625 mg I.V. q 6 hours, then 2.5 mg P.O. once daily. Adjust dose according to response.
To convert from oral therapy to I.V. therapy
Adults: 1.25 mg I.V. over 5 minutes q 6 hours.
≡ ***Dosage adjustment.*** In hypertensive patients with renal failure who have a creatinine clearance less than 30 ml/minute, begin therapy at 2.5 mg/day. Gradually adjust dosage according to response. Patients undergoing hemodialysis should receive a supplemental dose of 2.5 mg on days of dialysis.
Heart failure
Adults: Initially, 2.5 mg P.O. once or twice daily. Usual maintenance dose is 5 to 20 mg P.O. daily, given in two divided doses. Maximum daily dose is 40 mg P.O. in two divided doses.
Asymptomatic left ventricular dysfunction
Adults: Initially, 2.5 mg P.O. b.i.d.; adjust to targeted daily dose of 20 mg (in divided doses) as tolerated.
≡ ***Dosage adjustment.*** In patients with heart failure and renal impairment or hyponatremia (serum sodium less than 130 mEq/L or serum creatinine of more than 1.6 mg/dl), begin therapy with 2.5 mg P.O. daily. Increase dosage to 2.5 mg b.i.d., then 5 mg b.i.d. and higher as indicated, usually at intervals of 4 days or more.

Pharmacodynamics

Antihypertensive action: Enalapril inhibits ACE, preventing conversion of angiotensin I to angiotensin II, a potent vasoconstrictor. Reduced angiotensin II levels decrease peripheral arterial resistance, thus lowering blood pressure, and decrease aldosterone secretion, thus reducing sodium and water retention.

Pharmacokinetics

Absorption: About 60% of a given dose is absorbed from the GI tract.
Distribution: Full distribution pattern is unknown; drug doesn't appear to cross the blood-brain barrier.
Metabolism: Metabolized extensively to the active metabolite enalaprilat.
Excretion: About 94% of a dose is excreted in urine and feces as enalaprilat and enalapril.

Route	Onset	Peak	Duration
P.O.	1 hr	4-6 hr	24 hr
I.V.	15 min	1-4 hr	6 hr

Contraindications and precautions

Contraindicated in patients with hypersensitivity to drug or history of angioedema related to previous treatment with an ACE inhibitor. Use cautiously in patients with impaired renal function. Avoid use in patients at high risk for cardiogenic shock.

Interactions

Drug-drug. *Diuretics, phenothiazines, or other antihypertensive drugs:* Increase antihypertensive effects. Use together cautiously.
Insulin, oral antidiabetic agents: Increased risk of hypoglycemia, especially at the initiation of enalapril therapy. Recommend close monitoring of glucose level.
Lithium: Decreased renal clearance of lithium. Recommend monitoring lithium level.
NSAIDs and aspirin: May decrease the antihypertensive effect of enalapril. Use together cautiously.

Potassium-sparing diuretics and potassium supplements: Enhanced diuretic effects and possibly hyperkalemia. Use together cautiously.
Rifampin: Decreased pharmacologic effects of rifampin. Closely monitor patient.
Drug-food. *Salt substitutes:* May enhance effects, thereby causing hyperkalemia.

Effects on diagnostic tests
None reported.

Adverse reactions
CNS: *headache, dizziness, fatigue,* vertigo, asthenia, syncope.
CV: *hypotension,* chest pain, bradycardia.
GI: diarrhea, nausea, abdominal pain, vomiting.
GU: elevated BUN and serum creatinine levels, decreased renal function (in patients with bilateral renal artery stenosis or heart failure).
Hematologic: ***neutropenia, thrombocytopenia, agranulocytosis.***
Hepatic: increased liver enzyme and bilirubin levels.
Respiratory: *dry, persistent, tickling, nonproductive cough;* dyspnea.
Skin: rash.
Other: ***angioedema.***

Overdose and treatment
The most likely clinical sign is hypotension. After acute ingestion, empty stomach by induced emesis or gastric lavage. Follow with activated charcoal to reduce absorption. Consider hemodialysis in severe cases. Subsequent treatment is usually symptomatic and supportive.

Clinical considerations
- Discontinue diuretic therapy 2 to 3 days before beginning enalapril therapy to reduce risk of hypotension; if drug doesn't adequately control blood pressure, reinstate diuretics.
- Give drug without regard to meals; food doesn't appear to affect absorption.

Therapeutic monitoring
- Proteinuria and nephrotic syndrome may occur in patients on enalapril therapy.
- WBC and differential counts should be done before treatment, every 2 weeks for 3 months, and periodically thereafter.

Special populations
Pregnant patients. Neonatal and fetal death may occur when drug is administered during second and third trimesters.
Breast-feeding patients. It's unknown if drug is excreted in breast milk; an alternative feeding method is recommended during therapy.
Pediatric patients. Safety and efficacy of enalapril in children haven't been established; use only if potential benefit outweighs risk.
Geriatric patients. Geriatric patients may need lower doses because of impaired drug clearance.

Patient counseling
- Tell patient to report light-headedness, especially in first few days, so dosage can be adjusted; signs of infection, such as sore throat and fever, because drug may decrease WBC count; facial swelling or difficulty breathing, because drug may cause angioedema; and loss of taste, which may necessitate discontinuing drug.
- Advise patient not to change position suddenly to minimize orthostatic hypotension.
- Warn patient to seek medical approval before taking OTC cold preparations, particularly cough medications.

enoxaparin sodium
Lovenox

Pharmacologic classification: low-molecular-weight heparin
Therapeutic classification: anticoagulant
Pregnancy risk category B

How supplied
Available by prescription only
Ampules: 30 mg/0.3 ml
Syringes (prefilled): 30 mg/0.3 ml, 40 mg/0.4 ml
Syringes (graduated prefilled): 60 mg/0.6 ml, 80 mg/0.8 ml, 100 mg/1 ml

Indications and dosages
Prevention of deep vein thrombosis (DVT), which may lead to pulmonary embolism, following hip or knee replacement surgery
Adults: 30 mg S.C. q 12 hours for 7 to 10 days. Give initial dose between 12 and 24 hours postoperatively provided hemostasis has been established.
Prevention of DVT, which may lead to pulmonary embolism, following abdominal surgery
Adults: 40 mg S.C. once daily for 7 to 10 days. Give initial dose 2 hours before surgery.
Prevention of ischemic complications of unstable angina and non-Q-wave MI, when concurrently administered with aspirin
Adults: 1 mg/kg S.C. q 12 hours for 2 to 8 days in conjunction with oral aspirin therapy (100 to 325 mg once daily).

Note: To minimize risk of bleeding following vascular instrumentation during the treatment of unstable angina, adhere precisely to the intervals recommended between enoxaparin doses.
Inpatient treatment of acute DVT with and without pulmonary embolism when ad-

ministered in conjunction with warfarin sodium
Adults: 1 mg/kg S.C. every 12 hours; alternatively, 1.5 mg/kg S.C. once daily (at the same time every day) for 5 to 7 days until therapeutic oral anticoagulant effect (INR 2 to 3) has been achieved. Warfarin sodium therapy is usually initiated within 72 hours of enoxaparin injection.
Outpatient treatment of acute DVT without pulmonary embolism when administered in conjunction with warfarin sodium
Adults: 1 mg/kg S.C. every 12 hours for 5 to 7 days until therapeutic oral anticoagulant effect (INR 2 to 3) has been achieved. Warfarin sodium therapy is usually initiated within 72 hours of enoxaparin injection.

Pharmacodynamics
Anticoagulant action: Enoxaparin is a low-molecular-weight heparin that accelerates formation of antithrombin III-thrombin complex and deactivates thrombin, preventing conversion of fibrinogen to fibrin. It has a higher anti-factor Xa to anti-factor IIa activity than unfractionated heparin.

Pharmacokinetics
Absorption: Bioavailability is 92%
Distribution: Volume of distribution of anti-factor Xa activity is about 6 L.
Metabolism: Information not available.
Excretion: Elimination half-life based on anti-factor Xa activity is about 4½ hours after S.C. administration.

Route	Onset	Peak	Duration
S.C.	Unknown	3-5 hr	24 hr

Contraindications and precautions
Contraindicated in patients with hypersensitivity to drug or heparin or pork products; in patients with active, major bleeding or thrombocytopenia; and in those who demonstrate antiplatelet antibodies in the presence of drug.

Use with extreme caution in patients with history of heparin-induced thrombocytopenia. Use cautiously in patients with conditions that put them at increased risk for hemorrhage, such as bacterial endocarditis; congenital or acquired bleeding disorders; ulcer disease; angiodysplastic GI disease; hemorrhagic stroke; or recent spinal, eye, or brain surgery; or in those treated concomitantly with NSAIDs, platelet inhibitors, or other anticoagulants that affect hemostasis.

Use with extreme caution in patients with postoperative indwelling epidural catheters. Cases of epidural or spinal hematomas have been reported with the use of enoxaparin and spinal or epidural anesthesia or spinal puncture, resulting in long-term or permanent paralysis.

Also use cautiously in patients with a bleeding diathesis, uncontrolled arterial hypertension, or history of recent GI ulceration, diabetic retinopathy, and hemorrhage.

Use with care in the elderly and patients with renal insufficiency who may show delayed elimination of enoxaparin.

Interactions
Drug-drug. *Other anticoagulants, antiplatelet agents, and NSAIDs:* Increased risk of bleeding. May also lead to spinal or epidural hematomas in patients with spinal punctures or epidural or spinal anesthesia. Patient requires careful monitoring.
Plicamycin and valproic acid: May cause hypoprothrombinemia and inhibit platelet aggregation. Monitor patient closely.

Effects on diagnostic tests
Enoxaparin may decrease patient's platelet count and may increase AST and ALT levels.

Adverse reactions
CNS: confusion, ***neurologic injury*** when used with spinal or epidural puncture.
CV: edema, peripheral edema, CV toxicity (chest pain, dizziness, irregular heartbeat).
GI: nausea.
Hematologic: hypochromic anemia, ***thrombocytopenia, hemorrhage,*** ecchymoses, bleeding complications.
Hepatic: elevated liver enzymes.
Skin: *rash, hives.*
Other: irritation, pain, hematoma, erythema (at injection site); fever; pain; ***angioedema.***

Overdose and treatment
Accidental overdose after drug administration may lead to hemorrhagic complications. This may be largely neutralized by the slow I.V. injection of protamine sulfate (1%) solution. The dose of protamine sulfate should be equal to the dose of enoxaparin injection (1 mg of protamine neutralizes 1 mg of enoxaparin).

Clinical considerations
- Enoxaparin isn't intended for I.M. administration.
- Drug can't be used interchangeably (unit for unit) with unfractionated heparin or other low-molecular-weight heparins.
- Don't mix drug with other injections or infusions.
- Screen all patients before prophylactic administration of enoxaparin to rule out a bleeding disorder.
- Don't expel air bubble from syringe before injecting drug because drug may be lost.

Therapeutic monitoring
Monitor for adverse reactions including angioedema.

Special populations

Breast-feeding patients. It isn't known if drug is excreted in breast milk. Use cautiously when administering to breast-feeding women.
Pediatric patients. Safety and efficacy of enoxaparin in children haven't been established.

Patient counseling

- Explain risk of adverse reactions.
- Instruct patient to watch for signs of bleeding.
- Caution patient against use of aspirin or other salicylates.

ephedrine

ephedrine hydrochloride

ephedrine sulfate

Pretz-D

Pharmacologic classification: adrenergic
Therapeutic classification: bronchodilator, vasopressor (parenteral form), nasal decongestant
Pregnancy risk category C

How supplied

Available with and without a prescription
Capsules: 25 mg, 50 mg
Nasal spray: 0.25%
Injection: 25 mg/ml, 50 mg/ml (parenteral)

Indications and dosages

To correct hypotensive states
Adults: 25 to 50 mg I.M. or S.C., or 10 to 25 mg via slow I.V. bolus. If necessary, a second I.M. dose of 50 mg or I.V. dose of 25 mg may be administered. Additional I.V. doses may be given in 5 to 10 minutes. Maximum dose is 150 mg daily.
Children: 3 mg/kg or 100 mg/m^2 S.C. or I.V. daily, divided into four to six doses.
Orthostatic hypotension
Adults: 25 mg P.O. once daily to q.i.d.
Children: 3 mg/kg P.O. daily, divided into four to six doses.
Bronchodilator or nasal decongestant
Adults and children older than 12: 12.5 to 50 mg P.O. q 3 to 4 hours, p.r.n., not to exceed 150 mg in 24 hours.

As nasal decongestant: 2 to 3 sprays in each nostril not more often than q 4 hours.
Children age 6 to 12: 6.25 to 12.5 mg P.O. q 4 hours, not to exceed 75 mg in 24 hours.

As nasal decongestant: 1 to 2 sprays in each nostril, not more often than q 4 hours. *Alternatively, children age 2 and older:* 2 to 3 mg/kg or 100 mg/m^2 P.O. daily in four to six divided doses.
Severe, acute bronchospasm
Adults: 12.5 to 25 mg I.M., S.C., or I.V.
Enuresis
Adults: 25 to 50 mg P.O. h.s.
Myasthenia gravis
Adults: 25 mg P.O. t.i.d. or q.i.d.

Pharmacodynamics

Direct- and indirect-acting sympathomimetic action: Ephedrine stimulates both alpha- and beta-adrenergic receptors. Release of norepinephrine from its storage sites is one of its indirect effects. In therapeutic doses, ephedrine relaxes bronchial smooth muscle and produces cardiac stimulation with increased systolic and diastolic blood pressure when norepinephrine stores aren't depleted.
Bronchodilator action: Ephedrine relaxes bronchial smooth muscle by stimulating beta$_2$-adrenergic receptors, resulting in increased vital capacity, relief of mild bronchospasm, improved air exchange, and decreased residual volume.
Vasopressor action: Drug produces positive inotropic effects with low doses by action on beta$_1$-receptors in the heart. Vasodilation results from its effect on beta$_2$-adrenergic receptors; vasoconstriction results from its alpha-adrenergic effects. Pressor effects may result from vasoconstriction or cardiac stimulation; however, when peripheral vascular resistance is decreased, blood pressure elevation results from increased cardiac output.
Nasal decongestant action: Ephedrine stimulates alpha-adrenergic receptors in blood vessels of nasal mucosa, producing vasoconstriction and nasal decongestion.

Pharmacokinetics

Absorption: Rapidly and completely absorbed after oral, S.C., or I.M. administration.
Distribution: Widely distributed throughout the body.
Metabolism: Slowly metabolized in the liver by oxidative deamination, demethylation, aromatic hydroxylation, and conjugation.
Excretion: Dose is mostly excreted unchanged in urine; rate of excretion depends on urine pH.

Route	Onset	Peak	Duration
P.O.	15-60 min	Unknown	3-5 hr
I.V.	5 min	Unknown	1 hr
I.M., S.C.	10-20 min	Unknown	½-1 hr
Nasal spray	Unknown	Unknown	Unknown

Contraindications and precautions

Contraindicated in patients with hypersensitivity to drug and other sympathomimetics; in those with porphyria, severe coronary artery disease, arrhythmias, angle-closure glaucoma, psychoneurosis, angina pectoris, substantial organic heart disease, CV disease; and in those taking MAO inhibitors.

Nasal solution is contraindicated in patients with angle-closure glaucoma, psychoneurosis, angina pectoris, substantial organic heart disease, CV disease, and hypersensitivity to drug or other sympathomimetics.

Use with extreme caution in elderly men and in those with hypertension, hyperthyroidism, nervous or excitable states, diabetes, and prostatic hyperplasia. Use nasal solution cautiously in patients with hyperthyroidism, hypertension, diabetes mellitus, or prostatic hyperplasia.

Interactions

Drug-drug. *Acetazolamide:* May increase serum ephedrine levels. Monitor patient for toxicity.
Alpha blockers: Unopposed beta-adrenergic effects, resulting in hypotension. Avoid use together.
Antihypertensives: Decreased effects of antihypertensives. Blood pressure must be monitored.
Atropine: Blocks reflex bradycardia and enhances pressor effects. Monitor patient carefully.
Beta blockers: Unopposed alpha-adrenergic effects, resulting in hypertension. Blood pressure must be monitored.
Ergot alkaloids: May enhance vasoconstrictor activity. Monitor patient cautiously.
General anesthetics (especially cyclopropane, halothane) and cardiac glycosides: May sensitize myocardium to effects of ephedrine, causing arrhythmias. Monitor patient closely.
Guanadrel, guanethidine: Enhanced pressor effects of ephedrine. Monitor patient and blood pressure closely.
Levodopa: Enhanced risk of ventricular arrhythmias. Monitor patient closely.
MAO inhibitors and tricyclic antidepressants: Enhanced pressor effects; may cause hypertensive crisis. Allow 14 days to lapse after withdrawal of MAO inhibitor before using ephedrine.
Reserpine, methyldopa, diuretics: Decrease pressor effects of ephedrine. Monitor patient carefully.
Sympathomimetic agents: Increased effects and toxicity. Avoid use together.
Theophylline: Causes more adverse reactions than either drug when used alone. Use together cautiously.

Effects on diagnostic tests

None reported.

Adverse reactions

CNS: *insomnia, nervousness,* dizziness, headache, euphoria, confusion, delirium; nervousness, excitation (with nasal solution).
CV: *palpitations,* tachycardia, hypertension, precordial pain; *tachycardia* (with nasal solution), ***arrhythmias.***
EENT: dry nose and throat; rebound nasal congestion with long-term or excessive use, mucosal irritation (with nasal solution).
GI: nausea, vomiting, anorexia.
GU: urine retention, painful urination due to visceral sphincter spasm.
Musculoskeletal: muscle weakness.
Skin: diaphoresis.

Overdose and treatment

Signs and symptoms of overdose include exaggeration of common adverse reactions, especially arrhythmias, extreme tremor or seizures, nausea and vomiting, fever, and CNS and respiratory depression.

Treatment requires supportive and symptomatic measures. If patient is conscious, induce emesis with ipecac followed by activated charcoal. If patient is depressed or hyperactive, perform gastric lavage. Maintain airway and blood pressure. Don't administer vasopressors. Monitor vital signs closely.

A beta blocker (such as propranolol) may be used to treat arrhythmias. A cardioselective beta blocker is recommended in asthmatic patients. Phentolamine may be used for hypertension, paraldehyde or diazepam for seizures, and dexamethasone for pyrexia.

Clinical considerations

Consider the recommendations relevant to all adrenergics. As a pressor agent, ephedrine isn't a substitute for blood, plasma, fluids, or electrolytes. Correct fluid volume depletion before administration.

Therapeutic monitoring

- Tolerance may develop after prolonged or excessive use; increased dose may be needed. Also, if drug is discontinued for a few days and readministered, effectiveness may be restored.
- With parenteral dosing, monitor vital signs closely during infusion. Tachycardia is common.

Special populations

Pregnant patients. It isn't known if drug is safe for use during pregnancy. Use drug during pregnancy only when clearly indicated.
Breast-feeding patients. Avoid use in breast-feeding women.
Pediatric patients. Use cautiously in children.
Geriatric patients. Administer cautiously because geriatric patients may be more sensitive to effects of the drug. Lower doses may be recommended.

Patient counseling

- Instruct patient to clear nose before instilling nasal solutions.
- Tell patient using OTC product to follow directions on label, to take last dose a few hours before bedtime to reduce possibility of in-

somnia, to take only as directed, and not to increase dose or frequency.
- Advise patient to store drug away from heat and light (not in bathroom medicine cabinet) and to keep out of reach of children.
- Instruct patient who misses a dose to take it as soon as remembered if within 1 hour. If beyond 1 hour, patient should skip dose and return to regular schedule.
- Teach patient to be aware of palpitations and significant pulse rate changes.

epinephrine
Bronkaid Mist, Bronkaid Mistometer*, EpiPen, EpiPen Jr., Primatene Mist, Sus-Phrine

epinephrine bitartrate
AsthmaHaler

epinephrine hydrochloride
Adrenalin Chloride, AsthmaNefrin, Epifrin, Glaucon, microNefrin, Vaponefrin

epinephryl borate
Epinal

Pharmacologic classification: adrenergic
Therapeutic classification: bronchodilator, vasopressor, cardiac stimulant, local anesthetic (adjunct), topical antihemorrhagic, antiglaucoma
Pregnancy risk category C

How supplied
Available by prescription only
Injection: 0.01 mg/ml (1:100,000), 0.1 mg/ml (1:10,000), 0.5 mg/ml (1:2,000), 1 mg/ml (1:1,000) parenteral; 5 mg/ml (1:200) parenteral suspension
Ophthalmic: 0.1%, 0.25%, 0.5%, 1%, 2% solution
Available without a prescription
Nebulizer inhaler: 1% (1:100), 1.25%, 2.25%
Aerosol inhaler: 160 mcg, 200 mcg, 250 mcg/metered spray
Nasal solution: 0.1%

Indications and dosages
Bronchospasm, hypersensitivity reactions, anaphylaxis
Adults: Initially, 0.1 to 0.5 mg (0.1 to 0.5 ml of a 1:1,000 solution) S.C. or I.M.; may be repeated at 10- to 15-minute intervals, p.r.n. Alternatively, 0.1 to 0.25 mg (1 to 2.5 ml of a 1:10,000 solution) I.V. slowly over 5 to 10 minutes. May be repeated q 5 to 15 minutes if needed or followed by a 1 to 4 mcg/minute I.V. infusion.
Children: 0.01 mg/kg (0.01 ml/kg of a 1:1,000 solution) or 0.3 mg/m^2 (0.3 ml/ m^2 of a 1:1,000 solution) S.C. Dose not to exceed 0.5 mg. May be repeated at 20-minute to 4-hour intervals, p.r.n. Alternatively, 0.02 to 0.025 mg/kg (0.004 to 0.005 ml/kg) or 0.625 mg/ m^2 (0.125 ml/ m^2) of a 1:200 solution. May be repeated but not more often than q 6 hours. Alternatively, 0.1 mg (10 ml of a 1:100,000 dilution) I.V. slowly over 5 to 10 minutes followed by a 0.1 to 1.5 mcg/kg/minute I.V. infusion.
Bronchodilator
Adults and children: 1 inhalation via metered aerosol, repeated once if needed after 1 minute; subsequent doses shouldn't be repeated for at least 3 hours. Alternatively, 1 or 2 deep inhalations via hand-bulb nebulizer of a 1% (1:100) solution; may be repeated at 1- to 2-minute intervals. Alternatively, 0.03 ml (0.3 mg) of a 1% solution via intermittent positive pressure breathing.
To restore cardiac rhythm in cardiac arrest
Adults: Initially, 0.5 to 1 mg (range, 0.1 to 1 mg to 10 ml of a 1:10,000 solution) I.V. bolus; may be repeated q 3 to 5 minutes, p.r.n. Alternatively, initial dose followed by 0.3 mg S.C. or 1 to 4 mcg/minute I.V. infusion. Alternatively, 1 mg (10 ml of a 1:10,000 solution) intratracheally, or 0.1 to 1 mg (1 to 10 ml of a 1:10,000 solution) by intracardiac injection.
Children: Initially, 0.01 mg/kg (0.1 ml/kg of a 1:10,000 solution) I.V. bolus or intratracheally; may be repeated q 5 minutes, p.r.n.

Alternatively, initially, 0.1 mcg/kg/minute; may increase in increments of 0.1 mcg/kg/minute to a maximum of 1 mcg/kg/minute. Alternatively, 0.005 to 0.01 mg/kg (0.05 to 0.1 ml/kg of a 1:10,000 solution) by intracardiac injection.
Infants: Initially, 0.01 to 0.03 mg/kg (0.1 to 0.3 ml/kg of a 1:10,000 solution) I.V. bolus or by intratracheal injection. May be repeated q 5 minutes, p.r.n.
Hemostatic use
Adults: 1:50,000 to 1:1,000, applied topically.
To prolong local anesthetic effect
Adults and children: 1:500,000 to 1:50,000 mixed with local anesthetic.
Open-angle glaucoma
Adults: 1 or 2 drops of 1% to 2% solution instilled daily or b.i.d.
Nasal congestion, local superficial bleeding
Adults and children: Instill 1 or 2 drops of solution.

Pharmacodynamics
Epinephrine acts directly by stimulating alpha- and beta-adrenergic receptors in the sympathetic nervous system. Its main therapeutic effects include relaxation of bronchial smooth muscle, cardiac stimulation, and dilation of skeletal muscle vasculature.

Bronchodilator action: Epinephrine relaxes bronchial smooth muscle by stimulating $beta_2$-adrenergic receptors. Epinephrine constricts bronchial arterioles by stimulating alpha-adrenergic receptors, resulting in relief of bronchospasm, reduced congestion and edema, and increased tidal volume and vital capacity. By inhibiting histamine release, it may reverse bronchiolar constriction, vasodilation, and edema.
CV and vasopressor actions: As a cardiac stimulant, epinephrine produces positive chronotropic and inotropic effects by action on $beta_1$-receptors in the heart, increasing cardiac output, myocardial oxygen consumption, and force of contraction and decreasing cardiac efficiency. Vasodilation results from its effect on $beta_2$-receptors; vasoconstriction results from alpha-adrenergic effects.
Local anesthetic (adjunct) action: Epinephrine acts on alpha receptors in skin, mucous membranes, and viscera; it produces vasoconstriction, which reduces absorption of local anesthetic, thus prolonging its duration of action, localizing anesthesia, and decreasing risk of anesthetic's toxicity.
Local vasoconstriction action: Epinephrine's effect results from action on alpha receptors in skin, mucous membranes, and viscera, which produces vasoconstriction and hemostasis in small vessels.
Antiglaucoma action: Epinephrine's exact mechanism of lowering intraocular pressure is unknown. When applied topically to the conjunctiva or injected into the interior chamber of the eye, epinephrine constricts conjunctival blood vessels, contracts the dilator muscle of the pupil, and may dilate the pupil.

Pharmacokinetics

Absorption: Well absorbed after S.C. or I.M. injection; epinephrine has a rapid onset of action and short duration of action.
Distribution: Distributed widely throughout the body.
Metabolism: Metabolized at sympathetic nerve endings, liver, and other tissues to inactive metabolites.
Excretion: Excreted in urine, mainly as its metabolites and conjugates.

Route	Onset	Peak	Duration
I.V.	Immediate	5 min	Short
I.M.	Variable	Unknown	1-4 hr
S.C.	5-15 min	½ hr	1-4 hr
Inhalation	1-5 min	Unknown	1-3 hr

Contraindications and precautions

Contraindicated in patients with angle-closure glaucoma, shock (other than anaphylactic shock), organic brain damage, cardiac dilation, arrhythmias, coronary insufficiency, or cerebral arteriosclerosis. Also contraindicated in patients during general anesthesia with halogenated hydrocarbons or cyclopropane and in patients in labor (may delay second stage).

Some commercial products contain sulfites; contraindicated in patients with sulfite allergies except when epinephrine is being used for treatment of serious allergic reactions or other emergencies.

In conjunction with local anesthetics, epinephrine is contraindicated for use on fingers, toes, ears, nose, and genitalia.

Ophthalmic preparation is contraindicated in patients with angle-closure glaucoma or when nature of the glaucoma hasn't been established and in patients with hypersensitivity to the drug, organic mental syndrome, or cardiac dilation and coronary insufficiency. Nasal solution is contraindicated in patients with hypersensitivity to drug.

Use with extreme caution in patients with longstanding bronchial asthma and emphysema in whom degenerative heart disease has developed. Also use cautiously in geriatric patients and in those with hyperthyroidism, CV disease, hypertension, psychoneurosis, and diabetes.

Use ophthalmic preparation cautiously in the elderly and in patients with diabetes, hypertension, Parkinson's disease, hyperthyroidism, aphakia (eye without lens), cardiac disease, cerebral arteriosclerosis, or bronchial asthma.

Interactions

Drug-drug. *Other sympathomimetics:* Additive effects and toxicity. Avoid use together.
Alpha blockers: Antagonize vasoconstriction and hypertension. Avoid use together.
Antidiabetic agents: May decrease blood sugar effects. Dosage adjustments may be necessary.
Beta blockers such as propranolol: Antagonize cardiac and bronchodilating effects of epinephrine. Monitor patient carefully.
Doxapram, mazindol, and methylphenidate: May enhance CNS stimulation or pressor effects. Monitor patient closely.
General anesthetics (especially cyclopropane, halothane) and cardiac glycosides: May sensitize the myocardium to effects of epinephrine, causing arrhythmias. Patient requires ECG monitoring.
Guanadrel and guanethidine: Decreased hypotensive effects while potentiating effects of epinephrine, resulting in hypertension and arrhythmias. Patient and blood pressure require close monitoring.
Levodopa: Enhances risk of cardiac arrhythmias. Monitor patient carefully.
MAO inhibitors: Increased risk of hypertensive crisis. Recommend monitoring blood pressure closely.
Miotics: Reduce the ciliary spasm, mydriasis, blurred vision, and increased intraocular pres-

sure that may occur with miotics or epinephrine alone. May be used for this reason concomitantly.
Oxytocics or ergot alkaloids: May cause severe hypertension. Avoid use together.
Phenothiazines: Reversal of pressor effects. Avoid use together.
Topical miotics, topical beta blockers, osmotic agents, and carbonic anhydrase inhibitors: May cause additive lowering of intraocular pressure. Avoid use together.
Tricyclic antidepressants, antihistamines, and thyroid hormones: May potentiate adverse cardiac effects of epinephrine. Avoid use together.

Effects on diagnostic tests
Epinephrine interferes with tests for urinary catecholamines.

Adverse reactions
CNS: *nervousness, tremor,* vertigo, *headache,* disorientation, agitation, *drowsiness,* fear, pallor, dizziness, weakness, ***cerebral hemorrhage, CVA.*** In patients with Parkinson's disease, drug increases rigidity, tremor; brow ache, headache, light-headedness (with ophthalmic preparation); nervousness, excitation (with nasal solution).
CV: *palpitations;* widened pulse pressure; *hypertension; tachycardia;* ***ventricular fibrillation; shock;*** anginal pain; ECG changes, including a decreased T-wave amplitude; palpitations, tachycardia, ***arrhythmias,*** hypertension (with ophthalmic preparation); *tachycardia (with nasal solution).*
EENT: corneal or conjunctival pigmentation or corneal edema in long-term use; follicular hypertrophy; chemosis; conjunctivitis; iritis; hyperemic conjunctiva; maculopapular rash; eye pain; allergic lid reaction; ocular irritation; eye stinging, burning, and tearing on instillation (with ophthalmic preparation); rebound nasal congestion; slight sting upon application (with nasal solution).
GI: *nausea, vomiting.*
GU: increased BUN levels.
Metabolic: increased blood glucose and serum lactic acid levels.
Respiratory: dyspnea.
Skin: urticaria, pain, hemorrhage (at injection site).

Overdose and treatment
Signs and symptoms of overdose may include a sharp increase in systolic and diastolic blood pressure, increase in venous pressure, severe anxiety, irregular heartbeat, severe nausea or vomiting, severe respiratory distress, unusually large pupils, unusual paleness and coldness of skin, pulmonary edema, renal failure, and metabolic acidosis.

Treatment includes symptomatic and supportive measures, because epinephrine is rapidly inactivated in the body. Monitor vital signs closely. Phentolamine may be needed for hypotension; beta blockers (such as propranolol) may be needed for arrhythmias.

Clinical considerations
Consider the recommendations relevant to all adrenergics as well as the following:
- After S.C. or I.M. injection, massaging the site may hasten absorption.
- Epinephrine is destroyed by oxidizing agents, alkalis (including sodium bicarbonate), halogens, permanganates, chromates, nitrates, and salts of easily reducible metals such as iron, copper, and zinc.
- Avoid I.M. injection into buttocks. Epinephrine-induced vasoconstriction favors growth of the anaerobe *Clostridium perfringens.*
- Intracardiac administration requires external cardiac massage to move drug into coronary circulation.
- Breathing treatment should start with first symptoms of bronchospasm. Patient should use the fewest number of inhalations that provide relief. To prevent excessive dosage, at least 1 or 2 minutes should elapse before taking additional inhalations of epinephrine. Dosage requirements vary.
- Ophthalmic preparation may cause mydriasis with blurred vision and sensitivity to light in some patients being treated for glaucoma. Drug is usually administered at bedtime or after prescribed miotic to minimize these symptoms.
- When using separate solutions of epinephrine and a topical miotic, instill the miotic 2 to 10 minutes before epinephrine.

Therapeutic monitoring
- Blood pressure, pulse, respirations, and urine output must be monitored, and the patient observed closely. Epinephrine may widen pulse pressure. If arrhythmias occur, discontinue epinephrine immediately. Watch for changes in intake and output ratio.
- Patients, especially geriatric patients, should have regular tonometer readings during continuous therapy.

Special populations
Pregnant patients. Drug inhibits spontaneous or oxytocin-induced labor. With dose sufficient to reduce uterine contractions, drug may cause a prolonged period of uterine atony with hemorrhage. Drug should be used during pregnancy only if the potential benefits justify the possible risks to the fetus.
Breast-feeding patients. Drug is excreted in breast milk. Patient should avoid breast-feeding during therapy with epinephrine.
Pediatric patients. Safety and efficacy of ophthalmic epinephrine in children haven't been established. Use with caution.

Geriatric patients. Geriatric patients may be more sensitive to effects of epinephrine; lower doses are indicated.

Patient counseling

- Urge patient to report diminishing effect. Repeated or prolonged use of epinephrine can cause tolerance to effects of drug. Continuing to take epinephrine despite tolerance can be hazardous. Interrupting drug therapy for 12 hours to several days may restore responsiveness to drug.

Inhalation therapy

- Instruct patient in correct use of inhaler.
- Warn patient that overuse or too-frequent use can cause severe adverse reactions.
- Tell patient to save applicator; refills may be available.
- Advise patient to contact prescriber immediately if he receives no relief within 20 minutes or if condition worsens.

Nasal therapy

- Tell patient to contact prescriber if symptoms aren't relieved in 20 minutes or if they become worse, and to report bronchial irritation, nervousness, or sleeplessness, which require dosage reduction.
- Warn patient that intranasal applications may sting slightly and cause rebound congestion or drug-induced rhinitis after prolonged use. Nose drops should be used for 3 or 4 days only. Encourage patient to use drug exactly as prescribed.
- Tell patient to rinse nose dropper or spray tip with hot water after each use to avoid contaminating the solution.
- Instruct patient to gently press finger against nasolacrimal duct for at least 1 or 2 minutes immediately after drug instillation to avoid excessive systemic absorption.

Ophthalmic therapy

- To minimize systemic absorption, tell patient to press finger to lacrimal sac during and for 1 to 2 minutes after instillation of eye drops.
- To prevent contamination, tell patient not to touch applicator tip to any surface and to keep container tightly closed.
- Tell patient not to use epinephrine solution if it's discolored or contains a precipitate.
- Advise patient to remove soft contact lenses before instilling eye drops to avoid staining or damaging them.
- Tell patient to apply a missed dose as soon as possible. If it's close to time for next dose, the patient should wait and apply at regularly scheduled time.
- Tell patient to store drug away from heat and light (not in bathroom medicine cabinet where heat and moisture can cause drug to deteriorate) and out of reach of children.

epirubicin hydrochloride

Ellence

Pharmacologic classification: anthracycline
Therapeutic classification: antineoplastic
Pregnancy risk category D

How supplied

Available by prescription only
Injection: 2 mg/ml

Indications and dosages

Adjuvant therapy in patients with evidence of axillary node tumor involvement following resection of primary breast cancer

Adults: 100 to120 mg/m^2 I.V. infusion over 3 to 5 minutes via a free-flowing I.V. solution on day 1 of each cycle q 3 to 4 weeks, or divided equally in two doses on days 1 and 8 of each cycle. Maximum cumulative (lifetime) dose is 900 mg/m^2.

Dosage modification after the first cycle is based on toxicity. For patients experiencing platelet counts less than 50,000/mm^3, absolute neutrophil count (ANC) less than 250/mm^3, neutropenic fever, or grade 3 or 4 nonhematologic toxicity, reduce the day-1 dose in subsequent cycles to 75% of the day-1 dose given in the current cycle. Delay day-1 therapy in subsequent cycles until platelets are at least 100,000/mm^3, ANC is at least 1,500/mm^3, and nonhematologic toxicities recover to grade 1.

For patients receiving divided doses (days 1 and 8), the day-8 dose should be 75% of the day-1 dose if platelet counts are 75,000 to 100,000/mm^3 and ANC is 1,000 to 1,499/mm^3. If day-8 platelet counts are less than 75,000 /mm^3, ANC is less than 1000/mm^3, or grade 3 or 4 nonhematologic toxicity has occurred, the day-8 dose should be omitted.

≡ ***Dosage adjustment.*** In patients with bone marrow dysfunction (heavily pretreated patients, patients with bone marrow depression, or those with neoplastic bone marrow infiltration), start at lower doses of 75 to 90 mg/m^2. In hepatic dysfunction, if bilirubin is 1.2 to 3 mg/dl or AST is two to four times upper limit of normal, give one half the recommended starting dose. If bilirubin is greater than 3 mg/dl or AST is greater than four times upper limit of normal, then give one fourth the recommended starting dose. Effects in patients with severe hepatic impairment haven't been evaluated, so epirubicin shouldn't be used in these patients. In patients with severe renal dysfunction (serum creatinine over 5 mg/dl), consider lower dosages.

Pharmacodynamics

Antineoplastic action: The precise mechanisms of cytotoxic effects of epirubicin aren't completely known. Epirubicin is thought to form a complex with DNA by intercalation between nucleotide base pairs; thereby inhibiting DNA, RNA, and protein synthesis; DNA cleavage occurs, resulting in cytocidal activity. The drug may also generate cytotoxic free radicals as well as interfere with replication and transcription of DNA.

Pharmacokinetics

Absorption: Drug is a vesicant and must be given I.V.
Distribution: Rapidly and widely distributed into tissues. It binds to plasma proteins, predominantly albumin, and appears to concentrate in red blood cells.
Metabolism: Extensively and rapidly metabolized by the liver. Several metabolites form with little to no cytotoxic activity.
Excretion: Eliminated mostly by biliary excretion and, to a lesser extent, urinary excretion.

Route	Onset	Peak	Duration
I.V.	Unknown	Unknown	Unknown

Contraindications and precautions

Contraindicated in patients with hypersensitivity to this drug, other anthracyclines, or anthracenediones. Also contraindicated in patients with baseline neutrophil counts of less than 1,500 cells/mm^3, in patients with severe myocardial insufficiency or recent myocardial infarction, in patients whose previous treatment with anthracyclines reached total cumulative doses, and in patients with severe hepatic dysfunction.

Use cautiously in patients with active or dormant cardiac disease, patients with prior or concomitant radiotherapy to the mediastinal and pericardial area, previous therapy with other anthracyclines or anthracenediones, or with other cardiotoxic drugs.

Interactions

Drug-drug. *Calcium channel blockers, other cardioactive compounds:* May increase risk of heart failure. Recommend monitoring cardiac function closely.
Cimetidine: Increases concentrations of epirubicin by 50%. Avoid use together.
Cytotoxic drugs: Additive toxicities (especially hematologic and gastrointestinal) may occur; monitor patient closely.
Radiation therapy: Effects may be enhanced. Monitor patient carefully.

Effects on diagnostic tests

None reported.

Adverse reactions

CNS: lethargy.
CV: cardiomyopathy, ***heart failure, cardiotoxicity,*** sinus tachycardia, ECG changes, ***AV block, ventricular tachycardia.***
EENT: conjunctivitis, keratitis.
GI: nausea, vomiting, diarrhea, anorexia, mucositis.
GU: *amenorrhea.*
Hematologic: LEUKOPENIA, NEUTROPENIA, ***febrile neutropenia,*** *anemia,* THROMBOCYTOPENIA.
Skin: alopecia, rash, itch, skin changes, urticaria.
Other: infection, fever, hot flashes, local toxicity, photosensitivity, ***anaphylaxis.***

Overdose and treatment

Signs and symptoms of overdose are similar to known toxicities of drug. Provide supportive treatment as needed until recovery of toxicities. Monitor for signs of heart failure, which may occur months after therapy, and provide supportive therapy as appropriate.

Clinical considerations

- Don't give drug I.M. or S.C.
- Patients receiving 120 mg/m^2 of epirubicin should also receive prophylactic antibiotic therapy with co-trimoxazole or a fluoroquinolone.
- Use of antiemetics before epirubicin may be necessary to reduce nausea and vomiting.
- Anthracycline-induced leukemia may occur.
- Administration of drug after previous radiation therapy may induce an inflammatory cell reaction at the site of irradiation.
- Administer epirubicin under the supervision of a doctor who is experienced in the use of cancer chemotherapy.
- Pregnant health care providers shouldn't handle this drug.
- Contraceptive methods should be used by both male and female patients.

Therapeutic monitoring

- Monitor left ventricular ejection fraction (LVEF) regularly during therapy; discontinue drug at the first sign of impaired cardiac function. Early signs of cardiac toxicity may include sinus tachycardia, ECG abnormalities, tachyarrhythmias, bradycardia, AV block, and bundle branch block.
- Obtain baseline total bilirubin, AST, creatinine, and CBC including ANC, and evaluate cardiac function by measuring LVEF before therapy.
- Obtain total and differential WBC, RBC, and platelet counts before and during each cycle of therapy.
- WBC nadir is usually reached 10 to14 days after drug administration, and returns to normal by day 21.
- Recommend monitoring serum uric acid, potassium, calcium phosphate, and creatinine immediately after initial chemotherapy administration in patients susceptible to tumor lysis syndrome. Hydration, urine alkalinization, and prophylaxis with allopurinol may prevent hyperuricemia and minimize potential complications of tumor lysis syndrome.

■ Delayed cardiac toxicity may occur 2 to 3 months after completion of treatment and is dependent upon the cumulative dose of epirubicin. Don't exceed a cumulative dose of 900 mg/m^2.

Special populations
Breast-feeding patients. It isn't known if drug is excreted in breast milk. Because many drugs, including anthracyclines, are excreted in human milk and because of the potential for serious adverse reactions in nursing infants from epirubicin, women should discontinue nursing before taking this drug.
Pediatric patients. Safety and efficacy haven't been established in pediatric patients. They may be at greater risk for anthracycline-induced cardiotoxicity and heart failure.
Geriatric patients. Plasma clearance is decreased in elderly women. Monitor closely for toxicity in geriatric patients, especially women over age 70.

Patient counseling
■ Advise patient to report nausea, vomiting, stomatitis, dehydration, fever, evidence of infection, or symptoms of heart failure (tachycardia, dyspnea, edema).
■ Inform patient of the risk of cardiac damage and treatment-related leukemia with use of drug.
■ Advise men to use effective contraception during treatment.
■ Advise women that irreversible amenorrhea or premature menopause may occur.
■ Tell patient that hair regrowth usually occurs within 2 to 3 months after therapy is discontinued.

epoetin alfa (erythropoietin)
Epogen, Procrit

Pharmacologic classification: glycoprotein
Therapeutic classification: antianemic
Pregnancy risk category C

How supplied
Available by prescription only
Injection: 2,000 units, 3,000 units, 4,000 units, 10,000 units, 20,000 units, 40,000 units

Indications and dosages
Anemia associated with chronic renal failure
Adults: Initiate therapy at 50 to 100 units/kg I.V. or S.C. three times weekly. Patients receiving dialysis should receive drug I.V.; patients with chronic renal failure who aren't on dialysis may receive drug S.C. or I.V.

Reduce dosage when target hematocrit is reached or if hematocrit increases more than 4 points within a 2-week period. Increase dosage if hematocrit doesn't increase by 5 to 6 points after 8 weeks of therapy and hematocrit is below target range. Maintenance dosage is highly individualized.

Anemia related to zidovudine therapy in patients infected with HIV
Adults: Before therapy, determine endogenous serum epoetin alfa levels. Patients with levels of 500 milliunits/ml or more are unlikely to respond to therapy.

Initial dose for patients with levels of less than 500 milliunits/ml who are receiving 4,200 mg weekly or less of zidovudine is 100 units/kg I.V. or S.C. three times weekly for 8 weeks. If response is inadequate after 8 weeks, increase dose by increments of 50 to 100 units/kg three times weekly and reevaluate response q 4 to 8 weeks. Individualize maintenance dosage to maintain response, which may be influenced by zidovudine dose or infection or inflammation.

Anemia secondary to cancer chemotherapy
Adults: 150 units/kg S.C. three times weekly for 8 weeks or until target hemoglobin level is reached. If response isn't satisfactory after 8 weeks, increase dose up to 300 units/kg S.C. three times weekly.

Reduction of need for allogeneic blood transfusion in anemic patients scheduled to undergo elective, noncardiac, nonvascular surgery
Adults: 300 units/kg/day S.C. daily for 10 days before surgery, on day of surgery, and for 4 days after surgery. Alternatively, 600 units/kg S.C. in once-weekly doses (21, 14, and 7 days before surgery), plus a fourth dose on day of surgery. Before initiating treatment, establish that hemoglobin level is above 10 g/dl and less than or equal to 13 g/dl.

Pharmacodynamics
Antianemic action: Epoetin alfa is a glycoprotein consisting of 165 amino acids synthesized using recombinant DNA technology. It mimics naturally occurring erythropoietin, which is produced by the kidneys. It stimulates the division and differentiation of cells within bone marrow to produce RBCs.

Pharmacokinetics
Absorption: May be given S.C. or I.V.
Distribution: Unknown.
Metabolism: Unknown.
Excretion: Unknown.

Route	Onset	Peak	Duration
I.V.	Unknown	Immediate	Unknown
S.C.	Unknown	5-24 hr	Unknown

Contraindications and precautions
Contraindicated in patients with uncontrolled hypertension and hypersensitivity to mammalian cell-derived products or albumin (human).

Interactions
None reported.

Effects on diagnostic tests
None reported.

Adverse reactions
CNS: *headache, **seizures**, paresthesia, fatigue, asthenia,* dizziness.
CV: *hypertension, edema.*
GI: *nausea, vomiting, diarrhea.*
GU: increased BUN and creatinine.
Metabolic: increased uric acid, phosphorus, and potassium levels.
Musculoskeletal: *arthralgia.*
Respiratory: *cough, shortness of breath.*
Skin: *rash,* urticaria.
Other: increased clotting of arteriovenous grafts, *pyrexia, injection site reactions.*

Overdose and treatment
Maximum safe dose hasn't been established. Doses up to 1,500 units/kg have been administered three times weekly for 3 weeks without direct toxic effects.

The drug can cause polycythemia; phlebotomy may be used to bring hematocrit within appropriate levels.

Clinical considerations
- For HIV-infected patients treated with zidovudine, measure hematocrit once weekly until stabilized and then periodically.
- Most patients eventually require supplemental iron therapy. Before and during therapy, monitor patient's iron stores, including serum ferritin and transferrin saturation.

Therapeutic monitoring
- Routine monitoring of CBC with differential and platelet counts is recommended.
- Recommend measuring hematocrit twice weekly until it has stabilized and during adjustment to a maintenance dosage in patients with chronic renal failure. An interval of 2 to 6 weeks may elapse before a dosage change is reflected in the hematocrit level.
- Recommend monitoring hematocrit at least twice weekly during initiation of therapy and during any dosage adjustment. Close monitoring of blood pressure is also recommended.
- If a patient fails to respond to epoetin alfa therapy, consider the following possible causes: vitamin deficiency, iron deficiency, underlying infection, occult blood loss, underlying hematologic disease, hemolysis, aluminum intoxication, osteitis fibrosa cystica, or increased dosage of zidovudine.

Special populations
Pregnant patients. Use drug during pregnancy only when benefits outweigh risks to fetus.
Breast-feeding patients. It's unknown if drug is excreted in breast milk. Use with caution in breast-feeding women.
Pediatric patients. Safety and efficacy in children haven't been established.

Patient counseling
- Explain importance of regularly monitoring blood pressure in light of potential drug effects.
- Advise patient to adhere to dietary restrictions during therapy. Make sure he understands that drug won't influence disease process.

epoprostenol sodium
Flolan

Pharmacologic classification: naturally occurring prostaglandin
Therapeutic classification: vasodilator, antiplatelet aggregator
Pregnancy risk category B

How supplied
Available by prescription only
Injection: 0.5 mg/17-ml vial, 1.5 mg/17-ml vial

Indications and dosages
Long-term I.V. treatment of primary pulmonary hypertension in New York Heart Association (NYHA) class III and class IV patients
Adults: Initially for acute dose ranging, 2 ng/kg/minute as an I.V. infusion; increase in increments of 2 ng/kg/minute q 15 minutes or longer until dose-limiting pharmacologic effects are elicited. Begin maintenance (chronic) dosing with 4 ng/kg/minute less than the maximum tolerated infusion rate as determined during acute dose ranging. If the maximum tolerated infusion rate is less than 5 ng/kg/minute, begin maintenance infusion at one-half the maximum tolerated infusion rate. Base subsequent dosage adjustments on persistence, recurrence, or worsening of patient's symptoms of primary pulmonary hypertension and the occurrence of adverse events because of excessive doses of drug. Increases in dose from the initial maintenance dosage can generally be expected and are done in increments of 1 to 2 ng/kg/minute at intervals of at least 15 minutes.

Pharmacodynamics
Vasodilator and antiplatelet actions: Epoprostenol causes direct vasodilation of pulmonary and systemic arterial vascular beds and inhibits platelet aggregation.

Pharmacokinetics
Absorption: Administered I.V.
Distribution: Unknown.
Metabolism: Extensively metabolized.
Excretion: Excreted primarily in urine with a small amount excreted in feces.

Route	Onset	Peak	Duration
I.V.	Unknown	Unknown	Unknown

Contraindications and precautions
Contraindicated in patients with hypersensitivity to drug or structurally related compounds. Long-term use of drug is also contraindicated in patients with heart failure because of severe left ventricular systolic dysfunction or in those in whom pulmonary edema develops during initial dose ranging.

Interactions
Drug-drug. *Anticoagulants, antiplatelet agents:* May increase risk of bleeding. Monitor closely for bleeding.
Antihypertensive agents, diuretics, or other vasodilators: May cause additional reduction in blood pressure. Recommend monitoring blood pressure closely.

Effects on diagnostic tests
None reported.

Adverse reactions
CNS: *headache, anxiety, nervousness, agitation, dizziness, hyperesthesia, paresthesia.*
CV: *tachycardia; hypotension, chest pain,* bradycardia (during initial dose ranging).
GI: *nausea, vomiting;* abdominal pain, dyspepsia (during initial dose ranging); *diarrhea* (during maintenance dosing).
Hematologic: ***thrombocytopenia.***
Musculoskeletal: musculoskeletal pain, back pain, *jaw pain, myalgia, nonspecific musculoskeletal pain* (during maintenance dosing).
Respiratory: dyspnea.
Skin: *flushing.* sweating (during initial dose ranging).
Other: *flulike symptoms, chills, fever,* ***sepsis.***

Overdose and treatment
Overdose may result in flushing, headache, hypotension, tachycardia, nausea, vomiting, and diarrhea. Treatment usually requires dose reduction of epoprostenol.

Clinical considerations
- Drug should be used only by staff experienced in the diagnosis and treatment of primary pulmonary hypertension. Determining the appropriate dose for the patient must be done in a setting with adequate personnel and equipment for physiologic monitoring and emergency care.
- Before use, protect reconstituted solutions of the drug from light and refrigerate at 36° to 46° F (2° to 8° C) if not used immediately. Don't freeze reconstituted solutions of drug. Discard reconstituted solution that's been frozen. Discard reconstituted solution if it's been refrigerated for more than 48 hours.
- Avoid abrupt withdrawal or sudden large reductions in infusion rates.
- Administer anticoagulant therapy during long-term use of drug, unless contraindicated. Monitor PT and INR closely.

Therapeutic monitoring
- During maintenance infusion, the occurrence of dose-related pharmacologic events similar to those observed during initial dosing may necessitate a decrease in infusion rate, but the adverse event may occasionally resolve without dosage adjustment.
- Monitor for adverse reactions.

Special populations
Breast-feeding patients. It isn't known if drug is excreted in breast milk. Use cautiously in breast-feeding women.
Pediatric patients. Safety and efficacy in children haven't been established.
Geriatric patients. In general, dose selection for a geriatric patient should be cautious, reflecting the greater frequency of decreased hepatic, renal, or cardiac function and of concomitant disease or other drug therapy.

Patient counseling
- Ensure that patient and family understand before therapy is begun that there's a high likelihood that I.V. therapy with epoprostenol will be needed for prolonged periods, possibly years, and that the patient or family has the ability to accept and care for a permanent I.V. catheter and infusion pump.
- Instruct patient and family how to reconstitute drug and administer drug via infusion pump using sterile technique. Explain how to use infusion pump. Stress importance of maintaining continuous drug therapy. Provide patient and family with instructions on how to switch to a new infusion pump in the event of pump failure. Also instruct patient and family on how to store drug.
- Instruct patient to report adverse reactions regarding drug therapy immediately because dosage adjustments may be necessary.
- Provide patient with telephone number to obtain assistance for 24-hour support.

eptifibatide
Integrilin

Pharmacologic classification: glycoprotein IIb/IIIa (GP IIb/IIIa) inhibitor
Therapeutic classification: antiplatelet agent
Pregnancy risk category B

How supplied
Available by prescription only
Injection: 2 mg /ml, 10-ml vial, 0.75 mg/ml, 100-ml vials

Indications and dosages

Acute coronary syndrome (unstable angina or non-Q-wave MI) in patients being managed medically and in those undergoing percutaneous coronary intervention

Adults: 180 mcg/kg (up to maximum dose of 22.6 mg) I.V. bolus as soon as possible following diagnosis, followed by a continuous I.V. infusion of 2 mcg/kg/minute (up to maximum infusion rate of 15 mg/hour) for up to 72 hours. Infusion rate may be decreased to 0.5 mcg/kg/minute during percutaneous coronary intervention. Infusion should then be continued for an additional 20 to 24 hours after the procedure for up to 96 hours of therapy.

Treatment in patients without signs and symptoms of acute coronary syndrome who are undergoing percutaneous coronary intervention

Adults: I.V. bolus of 135 mcg/kg administered immediately before procedure, followed by a continuous infusion of 0.5 mcg/kg/minute for 20 to 24 hours.

Pharmacodynamics

Antiplatelet action: Reversibly inhibits platelet aggregation by preventing the binding of fibrinogen, von Willebrand factor, and other adhesion molecules to the GP IIb/IIIa receptor on human platelets.

Pharmacokinetics

Absorption: Not applicable with I.V. administration.

Distribution: 25% bound to plasma proteins.

Metabolism: Not reported. No major metabolites have been detected in human plasma.

Excretion: Elimination half-life is 2½ hours. Most of drug is excreted in urine.

Route	Onset	Peak	Duration
I.V.	Immediate	Immediate	4-6 hr after end of infusion

Contraindications and precautions

Contraindicated in patients with known hypersensitivity to drug or its ingredients.

Contraindicated in patients with a history of bleeding diathesis or evidence of active abnormal bleeding within previous 30 days; severe hypertension (systolic blood pressure exceeding 200 mm Hg or diastolic blood pressure of more than 110 mm Hg) not adequately controlled on antihypertensive therapy; major surgery within previous 6 weeks; history of stroke within 30 days; history of hemorrhagic stroke; current or planned use of another parenteral GP IIb/IIIa inhibitor; or a platelet count of less than 100,000/mm^3.

Contraindicated in patients whose serum creatinine is 2 mg/dl or higher (for the 180 mcg/kg bolus and 2 mcg/kg/minute infusion) or 4 mg/dl or higher (for the 135 mcg/kg bolus and 0.5 mcg/kg/minute infusion); or in patients who are dependent on renal dialysis.

Use cautiously in patients at increased risk of bleeding and patients weighing more than 315 lb (143 kg).

Interactions

Drug-drug. *Clopidogrel, dipyridamole, NSAIDs, oral anticoagulants (warfarin), thrombolytics, and ticlopidine:* Increased risk of bleeding. Monitor patient closely.

Other inhibitors of platelet receptor GP IIb/IIIa: May potentiate serious bleeding. Don't administer together.

Effects on diagnostic tests

None reported.

Adverse reactions

CV: hypotension.

GU: hematuria.

Hematologic: ***bleeding, thrombocytopenia.***

Other: bleeding at femoral artery access site.

Overdose and treatment

Limited data exist. Few patients received doses greater than or equal to two times the recommended dose.

Clinical considerations

- Recommend performing baseline laboratory tests before start of drug therapy: hematocrit, hemoglobin, and platelet count, serum creatinine level, PT, INR, and PTT.
- Drug may be administered in same I.V. line as alteplase, atropine, dobutamine, heparin, lidocaine, meperidine, metoprolol, midazolam, morphine, nitroglycerin, or verapamil.
- Drug may be administered in same I.V. line with normal saline or normal saline solution and 5% dextrose, and solution may contain up to 60 mEq/L of potassium chloride.
- Don't administer drug in same I.V. line as furosemide.
- Use drug in conjunction with heparin and aspirin.
- Discontinue eptifibatide and heparin and achieve sheath hemostasis by standard compressive techniques at least 4 hours before hospital discharge. The arterial access site is the most common site of bleeding.
- If patient is to undergo coronary artery bypass graft surgery, stop infusion before surgery.
- Minimize use of arterial and venous punctures, I.M. injections, and use of urinary catheters, nasotracheal tubes, and nasogastric tubes.

Therapeutic monitoring

- Monitor patient for bleeding.
- If patient's platelet count is less than 100,000/mm^3, discontinue eptifibatide and heparin.

Special populations

Breast-feeding patients. It isn't known if drug is excreted in breast milk. Administer cautiously to breast-feeding women.
Pediatric patients. Safety in children hasn't been established.
Geriatric patients. Drug has been used in patients as old as age 94. No significant difference shown compared to younger population.

Patient counseling

- Advise patient of potential adverse reactions.
- Instruct patient to report chest discomfort or other adverse events immediately.
- Caution patient to avoid activities that might cause bleeding or bruising.

ergocalciferol (vitamin D_2)

Calciferol, Drisdol, Vitamin D

Pharmacologic classification: vitamin
Therapeutic classification: antihypocalcemic
Pregnancy risk category C

How supplied

Available by prescription only
Capsules: 1.25 mg (50,000 units)
Injection: 12.5 mg (500,000 units)/ml
Available without a prescription
Liquid: 8,000 units/ml in 60-ml dropper bottle

Indications and dosages

Nutritional rickets or osteomalacia
Adults: 25 to 125 mcg P.O. daily if patient has normal GI absorption. With severe malabsorption, 250 mcg to 7.5 mg P.O. or 250 mcg I.M. daily.
Children: 25 to 125 mcg P.O. daily if patient has normal GI absorption. With malabsorption, 250 to 625 mcg P.O. daily.
Familial hypophosphatemia
Adults: 250 mcg to 1.5 mg P.O. daily with phosphate supplements.
Children: 1 to 2 mg P.O. daily with phosphate supplements. Increase daily dose in 250- to 500-mcg increments at 3- to 4-month intervals until adequate response is obtained.
Vitamin D-dependent rickets
Adults: 250 mcg to 1.5 mg P.O. daily.
Children: 75 to 125 mcg P.O. daily.
Anticonvulsant-induced rickets and osteomalacia
Adults: 50 mcg to 1.25 mg P.O. daily.
Hypoparathyroidism and pseudohypoparathyroidism
Adults: 625 mcg to 5 mg P.O. daily with calcium supplements.
Children: 1.25 to 5 mg P.O. daily with calcium supplements.
◇ ***Fanconi's syndrome***
Adults: 1.25 to 5 mg. P.O. daily.
Children: 625 mcg to 1.25 mg P.O. daily.
◇ ***Osteoporosis***
Adults: 25 to 250 mcg P.O. daily or 1.25 mg P.O. weekly with calcium and fluoride supplements.

Pharmacodynamics

Antihypocalcemic action: Once activated, ergocalciferol acts to regulate the serum levels of calcium by regulating absorption from the GI tract and resorption from bone.

Pharmacokinetics

Absorption: Absorbed readily from the small intestine.
Distribution: Distributed widely and bound to proteins stored in the liver.
Metabolism: Metabolized in the liver and kidneys. It has an average half-life of 24 hours and a duration of up to 6 months.
Excretion: Bile (feces) is the primary excretion route. A small percentage is excreted in urine.

Route	Onset	Peak	Duration
P.O., I.M.	2-24 hr	4-12 hr	2 days-6 mo

Contraindications and precautions

Contraindicated in patients with hypercalcemia, hypervitaminosis A, or renal osteodystrophy with hyperphosphatemia. Use with extreme caution, if at all, in patients with impaired renal function, heart disease, renal stones, or arteriosclerosis.

Interactions

Drug-drug. *Cardiac glycosides:* May result in arrhythmias. Patient requires close monitoring.
Cholestyramine, colestipol, and excessive use of mineral oil: Interfere with absorption of ergocalciferol. Avoid use together.
Corticosteroids: Counteract effects of drug. Monitor patient carefully.
Magnesium-containing antacids: May lead to hypermagnesemia. Monitor magnesium level.
Orlistat: May decrease absorption of vitamin D analogues. Separate drugs by 2 hours.
Phenobarbital or phenytoin: May increase metabolism of drug to inactive metabolites. Use together cautiously.
Thiazide diuretics: May cause hypercalcemia in patients with hypoparathyroidism. Monitor patient closely.
Verapamil: Atrial fibrillation may occur when supplemental calcium and calciferol have induced hypercalcemia. Patient requires careful monitoring.

Effects on diagnostic tests

None reported.

Adverse reactions
Adverse reactions listed usually occur only in vitamin D toxicity.
CNS: headache, weakness, somnolence, decreased libido, overt psychosis, irritability.
CV: *calcifications of soft tissues, including the heart,* hypertension, ***arrhythmias.***
EENT: rhinorrhea, conjunctivitis (calcific), photophobia.
GI: anorexia, nausea, vomiting, constipation, dry mouth, metallic taste, polydipsia.
GU: polyuria, albuminuria, hypercalciuria, nocturia, ***impaired renal function,*** reversible azotemia.
Hepatic: elevated liver enzymes (falsely or actually).
Metabolic: ***hypercalcemia,*** hyperthermia, increased serum cholesterol levels, weight loss.
Musculoskeletal: bone and muscle pain, bone demineralization.
Skin: pruritus.

Overdose and treatment
Signs and symptoms of overdose include hypercalcemia, hypercalciuria, and hyperphosphatemia, which may be treated by stopping therapy, starting a low-calcium diet, and increasing fluid intake. A loop diuretic, such as furosemide, may be given with saline I.V. infusion to increase calcium excretion. Provide supportive measures. In severe cases, death from cardiac or renal failure may occur. Calcitonin may decrease hypercalcemia.

Clinical considerations
- I.M. injection of ergocalciferol dispersed in oil is preferable in patients who are unable to absorb the oral form.
- Patients with hyperphosphatemia require dietary phosphate restrictions and binding agents to avoid metastatic calcifications and renal calculi.
- Doses of 60,000 IU daily can cause hypercalcemia.

Therapeutic monitoring
- Monitor eating and bowel habits; dry mouth, nausea, vomiting, metallic taste, and constipation can be early signs of toxicity.
- When high therapeutic doses are used, frequent serum and urine calcium, potassium, and urea determinations should be made.
- Malabsorption caused by inadequate bile or hepatic dysfunction may require addition of exogenous bile salts.

Special populations
Breast-feeding patients. Very little drug is excreted in breast milk; however, effect on infants of amounts exceeding RDA levels of vitamin D isn't known.
Pediatric patients. Some infants may be hyperreactive to drug.

Patient counseling
- Caution patient not to increase daily dose.
- Tell patient to avoid magnesium-containing antacids and mineral oil.
- Instruct patient to swallow tablets whole without crushing or chewing.

ergonovine maleate
Ergotrate Maleate

Pharmacologic classification: ergot alkaloid
Therapeutic classification: oxytocic
Pregnancy risk category NR

How supplied
Available by prescription only
Injection: 0.2-mg/ml ampules

Indications and dosages
Prevent or treat postpartum and postabortion hemorrhage due to uterine atony or subinvolution
Adults: 0.2 mg I.M. q 2 to 4 hours, maximum five doses; or 0.2 mg I.V. (only for severe uterine bleeding or other life-threatening emergency) over 1 minute while blood pressure and uterine contractions are monitored. I.V. dose may be diluted to 5 ml with normal saline injection.
◊ ***To diagnose coronary artery spasm (Prinzmetal's angina)***
Adults: 0.1 to 0.4 mg I.V. for one dose.

Pharmacodynamics
Oxytocic action: Ergonovine maleate stimulates contractions of uterine and vascular smooth muscle. This produces intense uterine contractions, followed by periods of relaxation. The drug produces vasoconstriction of primarily capacitance blood vessels, causing an increased CVP and elevated blood pressure.

The clinical effect is secondary to contraction of the uterine wall around bleeding vessels, producing hemostasis.

Pharmacokinetics
Absorption: Absorption is rapid following I.M. administration.
Distribution: Unknown.
Metabolism: Metabolized in the liver.
Excretion: Primarily nonrenal elimination in feces has been suggested.

Route	Onset	Peak	Duration
I.V.	Immediate	Unknown	Unknown
I.M.	2-5 min	Unknown	Unknown

Contraindications and precautions
Contraindicated in patients sensitive to ergot preparations; in threatened spontaneous abortion, induction of labor, or before delivery of placenta because captivation of placenta may

occur; and in those with history of allergic or idiosyncratic reactions to drug.

Because of the potential for adverse CV effects, use cautiously in patients with hypertension, toxemia, sepsis, occlusive vascular disease, and hepatic, renal, and cardiac disease.

Interactions

Drug-drug. *Cardiac glycosides:* Enhanced vasoconstriction. Avoid use together.
Local anesthetics with vasoconstrictors (lidocaine with epinephrine): Enhanced vasoconstriction. Use cautiously.
Other ergot alkaloids and sympathomimetic amines: Enhanced vasoconstrictor potential. Monitor patient carefully.
Drug-lifestyle. *Smoking:* Enhances vasoconstriction. Advise patient not to smoke.

Effects on diagnostic tests

None reported.

Adverse reactions

CNS: headache, confusion, dizziness, ringing in ears.
CV: chest pain, weakness in legs (peripheral vasospasm), hypertension, thrombophlebitis.
GI: nausea, vomiting, diarrhea, cramping.
Metabolic: decreased serum prolactin.
Musculoskeletal: pain in arms, legs, or lower back.
Respiratory: shortness of breath.
Other: itching; sweating; ***hypersensitivity reactions, signs of shock.***

Note: Discontinue drug if hypertension or allergic reactions occur.

Overdose and treatment

Signs and symptoms of overdose include seizures, with nausea, vomiting, diarrhea, dizziness, fluctuations in blood pressure, weak pulse, chest pain, tingling, and numbness and coldness in the extremities. Rarely, gangrene has occurred. Treat seizures with anticonvulsants and hypercoagulability with heparin; give vasodilators to improve blood flow. Gangrene may require amputation.

Clinical considerations

- Contractions begin immediately after I.V. injection. May continue for 45 minutes after I.V. injection.
- Hypocalcemia may decrease patient response; I.V. administration of calcium salts is necessary.
- High doses during delivery may cause uterine tetany and possible infant hypoxia or intracranial hemorrhage.
- Drug has been used as a diagnostic agent for angina pectoris.

Therapeutic monitoring

Monitor blood pressure, pulse rate, uterine response, and character and amount of vaginal bleeding. Watch for sudden changes in vital signs and frequent periods of uterine relaxation.

Special populations

Pregnant patients. High doses during delivery may cause uterine tetany and possible infant hypoxia or intracranial hemorrhage.
Breast-feeding patients. Ergot alkaloids inhibit lactation. Drug is excreted in breast milk, and ergotism has been reported in breast-fed infants of women given other ergot alkaloids. Use with caution.

Patient counseling

- Tell patient not to smoke while taking drug.
- Advise patient of possible adverse reactions.

ergotamine tartrate

Cafergot, Ergomar, Ergostat, Gynergen, Medihaler Ergotamine, Wigraine

Pharmacologic classification: ergot alkaloid
Therapeutic classification: vasoconstrictor
Pregnancy risk category X

How supplied

Available by prescription only
Tablets (S.L.): 2 mg
Tablets: 1 mg* (with or without caffeine 100 mg)
Aerosol inhaler: 360 mcg/metered spray
Suppositories: 2 mg (with caffeine 100 mg)

Indications and dosages

To prevent or abort vascular headache, including migraine and cluster headaches
Adults: Initially, 2 mg S.L. or P.O., then 1 to 2 mg S.L. or P.O. q 30 minutes, to maximum 6 mg per attack or in 24 hours, and 10 mg weekly. Alternatively, initially 1 inhalation; if not relieved in 5 minutes, repeat 1 inhalation. May repeat inhalations at least 5 minutes apart up to maximum of 6 inhalations per 24 hours or 15 inhalations weekly. Patient may also use rectal suppositories. Initially, 2 mg P.R. at onset of attack; repeat in 1 hour, p.r.n. Maximum dose is 2 suppositories per attack or 5 suppositories weekly.
◇ *Children:* 1 mg S.L. in older children and adolescents; if no improvement, additional 1-mg dose may be given in 30 minutes.

Pharmacodynamics

Vasoconstricting action: By stimulating alpha-adrenergic receptors, ergotamine in therapeutic doses causes peripheral vasoconstriction (if vascular tone is low); however, if vascular tone is high, it produces vasodilation. In high doses, it's a competitive alpha blocker. In therapeutic doses, it inhibits the reuptake of norepinephrine, which increases the vasoconstricting activity of ergotamine. A weaker serotonin antagonist, it reduces the increased rate of platelet aggregation caused by serotonin.

In the treatment of vascular headaches, ergotamine probably causes direct vasoconstriction of dilated carotid artery beds while decreasing the amplitude of pulsations. Its serotoninergic and catecholamine effects also seem to be involved.

Pharmacokinetics

Absorption: Rapidly absorbed after inhalation and variably absorbed after oral administration. Peak levels occur in ½ to 3 hours. Caffeine may increase rate and extent of absorption. Drug undergoes first-pass metabolism after oral administration.
Distribution: Widely distributed throughout the body.
Metabolism: Extensively metabolized in the liver.
Excretion: Part of dose (4%) is excreted in urine within 96 hours; remainder is presumed to be excreted in feces. Ergotamine is dialyzable. Onset of action depends on how promptly drug is given after onset of headache.

Route	Onset	Peak	Duration
P.O.	Variable	½-3 hr	Variable
S.L., Inhalation	Variable	Unknown	Variable
P.R.	Unknown	Unknown	Unknown

Contraindications and precautions

Contraindicated in patients with peripheral and occlusive vascular diseases, coronary artery disease, hypertension, hepatic or renal dysfunction, severe pruritus, sepsis, or hypersensitivity to ergot alkaloids and during pregnancy.

Interactions

Drug-drug. *Erythromycin and other macrolides:* May cause symptoms of ergot toxicity. Vasodilators (nifedipine, nitroprusside, or prazosin) may be ordered to treat ergot toxicity.
Propranolol or other beta blockers: Increased vasoconstrictor effects. Monitor patient carefully.
Drug-food. *Caffeine:* May increase rate and extent of absorption. Advise patient to avoid caffeine.
Drug-lifestyle. *Alcohol use:* May worsen headache. Advise patient to avoid alcohol use.
Smoking: May increase adverse effects. Caution patient to avoid smoking.

Effects on diagnostic tests

None reported.

Adverse reactions

CNS: numbness and tingling in fingers and toes.
CV: transient tachycardia or bradycardia, precordial distress and pain, increased arterial pressure, angina, peripheral vasoconstriction.
GI: nausea, vomiting.
Musculoskeletal: weakness in legs, muscle pain in extremities.
Skin: pruritus, localized edema.

Overdose and treatment

Signs and symptoms of overdose include adverse vasospastic effects, nausea, vomiting, lassitude, impaired mental function, delirium, severe dyspnea, hypotension or hypertension, rapid pulse, weak pulse, unconsciousness, spasms of the limbs, seizures, and shock.

Treatment is supportive and symptomatic, with prolonged and careful monitoring. If patient is conscious and ingestion is recent, empty stomach by emesis or gastric lavage; if comatose, perform gastric lavage after placement of endotracheal tube with cuff inflated. Activated charcoal and a saline (magnesium sulfate) cathartic may be used. Provide respiratory support. Apply warmth (not direct heat) to ischemic extremities if vasospasm occurs. As needed, administer vasodilators (nitroprusside, prazosin, or tolazoline) and, if necessary, I.V. diazepam to treat convulsions. Dialysis may be helpful.

Clinical considerations

Consider the recommendations relevant to all alpha blockers as well as the following:
- Drug is most effective when used in prodromal stage of headache or as soon as possible after onset. Provide quiet, low-light environment to relax patient after dose is administered.
- Sublingual tablet is preferred during early stage of attack because of its rapid absorption.
- Drug isn't effective for muscle contraction headaches.

Therapeutic monitoring

- Rebound headache or increased duration or frequency of headache may occur when drug is stopped.
- If patient experiences severe vasoconstriction with tissue necrosis, administer I.V. sodium nitroprusside or intra-arterial tolazoline. I.V. heparin and 10% dextran 40 in D_5W injection also may be administered to prevent vascular stasis and thrombosis.

Special populations

Pregnant patients. Drug is contraindicated in women who are or may become pregnant.
Breast-feeding patients. Drug is excreted in breast milk; therefore, use with caution in breast-feeding women. Excessive drug use may inhibit lactation.
Pediatric patients. Safety and efficacy of ergotamine in children haven't been established.
Geriatric patients. Administer cautiously to geriatric patients.

Patient counseling

- Instruct patient in correct use of drug.
- Urge patient to immediately report to prescriber feelings of numbness or tingling in fingers or toes or red or violet blisters on hands or feet.
- Caution patient to avoid alcoholic beverages and smoking.
- Warn patient to avoid prolonged exposure to very cold temperatures, which may increase adverse effects of drug.
- Advise patient who uses an inhaler to call prescriber promptly if mouth, throat, or lung infection occurs or if condition worsens. Cough, hoarseness, or throat irritation may occur. Patient should gargle and rinse mouth after each dose to help prevent hoarseness and irritation.
- Advise patient not to exceed recommended dosage.

erythromycin base

E-Base, E-Mycin, ERYC, ERYC Sprinkle*, Ery-Tab, Erythromycin Base/Filmtabs, Ilotycin, PCE, Robimycin

erythromycin estolate

erythromycin ethylsuccinate

E.E.S., EryPed, Pediazole

erythromycin gluceptate

Ilotycin Gluceptate

erythromycin lactobionate

Erythrocin Lactobionate

erythromycin stearate

Apo-Erythro-S*, Erythrocin Stearate Filmtab, Novo-Rythro*

erythromycin (topical)

Akne-Mycin, A/T/S, Del-Mycin, Erycette, EryDerm, Erymax, Ery-Sol, Erythra-Derm, Staticin, Theramycin Z, T-Stat

erythromycin (ophthalmic)

Ilotycin

Pharmacologic classification: erythromycin
Therapeutic classification: antibiotic
Pregnancy risk category B

How supplied

Available by prescription only
erythromycin base
Tablets (enteric-coated): 250 mg, 333 mg, 500 mg
Pellets (enteric-coated): 250 mg
erythromycin estolate
Capsules: 250 mg
Suspension: 125 mg/5 ml, 250 mg/5 ml
erythromycin ethylsuccinate
Tablets (chewable): 200 mg
Tablets: 400 mg
Oral suspension: 200 mg/5 ml, 400 mg/5 ml
Powder for oral suspension: 100 mg/2.5 ml, 200 mg/5 ml, 400 mg/5 ml (after reconstitution)
Granules for oral suspension: 200 mg/5 ml (after reconstitution)
erythromycin gluceptate
Injection: 500-mg, 1-g vials
erythromycin lactobionate
Injection: 500-mg, 1-g vials
erythromycin stearate
Tablets (film-coated): 250 mg, 500 mg
erythromycin (topical)
Topical gel: 2%
Topical ointment: 2%
Topical solution: 1.5%, 2%
erythromycin (ophthalmic)
Ointment: 5 mg/g

Indications and dosages

***Acute pelvic inflammatory disease caused by* Neisseria gonorrhoeae**
Adults: 500 mg I.V. (gluceptate, lactobionate) q 6 hours for 3 days, then 250 mg (base, estolate, stearate) or 400 mg (ethylsuccinate) P.O. q 6 hours for 7 days.
Endocarditis prophylaxis for dental procedures in patients allergic to penicillin
Adults: Initially, 800 mg (ethylsuccinate) or 1 g (stearate) P.O. 2 hours before procedure; then 400 mg (ethylsuccinate) or 500 mg (stearate) P.O. 6 hours later.
Children: Initially, 20 mg/kg (ethylsuccinate or stearate) P.O. 2 hours before procedure, then 10 mg/kg 6 hours later.
Intestinal amebiasis in patients who can't receive metronidazole
Adults: 250 mg (base, estolate, stearate) or 400 mg (ethylsuccinate) P.O. q 6 hours for 10 to 14 days.
Children: 30 to 50 mg/kg (base, estolate, ethylsuccinate, stearate) P.O. daily, divided q 6 hours for 10 to 14 days.

Note: Base and stearate forms not available in liquid form.

Mild to moderately severe respiratory tract, skin, and soft-tissue infections caused by susceptible organisms
Adults: 250 to 500 mg (base, estolate, stearate) P.O. q 6 hours; or 400 to 800 mg (ethylsuccinate) P.O. q 6 hours; or 15 to 20 mg/kg (gluceptate, lactobionate) I.V. daily, in divided doses q 6 hours.
Children: 30 mg/kg to 50 mg/kg (oral erythromycin salts) P.O. daily, in divided doses q 6 hours; or 15 to 20 mg/kg I.V. daily, in divided doses q 4 to 6 hours.

Syphilis
Adults: 500 mg (base, estolate, stearate) P.O. q.i.d. for 14 days.
Legionnaire's disease
Adults: 500 mg to 1 g I.V. or P.O. (base, estolate, stearate) or 800 mg to 1,600 mg (ethylsuccinate) P.O. q 6 hours for 21 days.
Uncomplicated urethral, endocervical, or rectal infections when tetracyclines are contraindicated
Adults: 500 mg (base, estolate, stearate) or 800 mg (ethylsuccinate) P.O. q.i.d. for at least 7 days.
Urogenital* Chlamydia trachomatis *infections during pregnancy
Adults: 500 mg (base, estolate, stearate) P.O. q.i.d. for at least 7 days or 250 mg (base, estolate, stearate) or 400 mg (ethylsuccinate) P.O. q.i.d. for at least 14 days.
Conjunctivitis caused by* C. trachomatis *in neonates
Neonates: 50 mg/kg/day P.O. in four divided doses for at least 2 weeks.
***Pneumonia of infancy caused by* C. trachomatis**
Infants: 50 mg/kg/day P.O. in four divided doses for at least 3 weeks.
Topical treatment of acne vulgaris
Adults and children: Apply to the affected area b.i.d.
Prophylaxis of ophthalmia neonatorum
Neonates: Apply 1-cm long ribbon ointment in the lower conjunctival sac of each eye no later than 1 hour after birth. Use new tube for each infant and don't flush after instillation.
Acute and chronic conjunctivitis, trachoma, other eye infections
Adults and children: Apply 1-cm long ribbon ointment directly into infected eye up to six times daily, depending on severity of infection.

Pharmacodynamics

Antibacterial action: Erythromycin inhibits bacterial protein synthesis by binding to the ribosomal 50S subunit. It's used in the treatment of infection with *Haemophilus influenzae, Entamoeba histolytica, Mycoplasma pneumoniae, Corynebacterium diphtheriae, Corynebacterium minutissimum, Legionella pneumophila,* and *Bordetella pertussis.* It may be used as an alternative to penicillins or tetracycline in the treatment of infection with *Streptococcus pneumoniae, Streptococcus viridans, Listeria monocytogenes, Staphylococcus aureus, C. trachomatis, N. gonorrhoeae,* and *Treponema pallidum.*

Pharmacokinetics

Absorption: Because base salt is acid-sensitive, it must be buffered or have enteric coating to prevent destruction by gastric acids. Acid salts and esters (estolate, ethylsuccinate, and stearate) aren't affected by gastric acidity and therefore are well absorbed. Give base and stearate preparations on an empty stomach. Absorption of estolate and ethylsuccinate preparations is unaffected or possibly even enhanced by presence of food. When administered topically, drug is absorbed minimally.
Distribution: Distributed widely to most body tissues and fluids except CSF, where it's distributed only in low levels. Drug crosses the placenta. About 80% of base and 96% of erythromycin estolate are protein-bound.
Metabolism: Metabolized partially in the liver to inactive metabolites.
Excretion: Excreted mainly unchanged in bile. Only small drug amounts (less than 5%) are excreted in urine; some drug is excreted in breast milk. In patients with normal renal function, plasma half-life is about 1½ hours. Drug isn't dialyzable.

Route	Onset	Peak	Duration
P.O.	Unknown	1-4 hr	Unknown
I.V.	Unknown	Immediate	Unknown
Topical	Unknown	Unknown	Unknown

Contraindications and precautions

Contraindicated in patients with hypersensitivity to drug or other macrolides. Erythromycin estolate is contraindicated in patients with hepatic disease. Use erythromycin salts cautiously in patients with impaired hepatic function.

Interactions

Drug-drug. *Carbamazepine:* Increased carbemazepine blood levels and increased risk of toxicity. Monitor patient and carbemazepine levels closely.
Cisapride: Increased cisapride levels leading to toxicity. Patient requires close monitoring.
Clindamycin and lincomycin: May be antagonistic. Avoid use together.
Cyclosporine: Increased serum cyclosporine levels and possible nephrotoxicity. Patient requires close monitoring.
Digoxin: Increased serum digoxin levels. Monitor for digitalis toxicity.
Disopyramide: Increased disopyramide plasma levels resulting in some cases in arrhythmias and increased QT intervals. Patient requires ECG monitoring.
Isotretinoin: May cause cumulative dryness, resulting in excessive skin irritation. Monitor patient carefully.
Midazolam and triazolam: Increased effects of these drugs. Use together cautiously.
Oral anticoagulants: Excessive anticoagulant effect. Monitor PT and INR closely.
Theophylline: Increased serum theophylline levels and decreased erythromycin blood level. Use together cautiously.
Drug-herb. *Pill-bearing spurge:* Inhibition of CYP3A enzymes affecting drug metabolism. Avoid use together.

Drug-lifestyle. *Abrasive or medicated soaps or cleansers; acne preparations or other preparations containing peeling agents (benzoyl peroxide, resorcinol, salicylic acid, sulfur, tretinoin); alcohol-containing products (after-shave, perfumed toiletries, cosmetics, shaving creams or lotions); astringent soaps or cosmetics; medicated cosmetics or cover-ups:* May cause cumulative dryness, resulting in excessive dryness. Use together cautiously.

Effects on diagnostic tests
Erythromycin may interfere with fluorometric determination of urinary catecholamines. False elevation of liver function tests using colorimetric assays may occur (rare).

Adverse reactions
CV: ***ventricular arrhythmias.***
EENT: bilateral reversible hearing loss (with high systemic or oral doses in patients with renal or hepatic insufficiency); slowed corneal wound healing, blurred vision (with ophthalmic administration).
GI: *abdominal pain, cramping, nausea, vomiting, diarrhea* (with oral or systemic administration).
Hepatic: cholestatic jaundice (with estolate).
Skin: urticaria, rash, eczema (with oral or systemic administration); urticaria, dermatitis (with ophthalmic administration); sensitivity reactions, erythema, burning, *dryness, pruritus,* irritation, peeling, oily skin (with topical application).
Other: overgrowth of nonsusceptible bacteria or fungi; ***anaphylaxis;*** fever (with oral or systemic administration); *venous irritation, thrombophlebitis* (after I.V. injection); overgrowth of nonsusceptible organisms (with long-term use); ***hypersensitivity reactions,*** including itching and burning eyes (with ophthalmic administration).

Overdose and treatment
No information available.

Clinical considerations
- Absorption of estolate and ethylsuccinate preparations is unaffected or possibly even enhanced by presence of food.
- Erythromycin estolate may cause serious hepatotoxicity (reversible cholestatic jaundice) in adults.
- Don't administer erythromycin lactobionate with other drugs because of chemical instability. Reconstituted solutions are acidic and should be completely administered within 8 hours of preparation.
- Drug may cause overgrowth of nonsusceptible bacteria or fungi.
- Although drug is bacteriostatic, it may be bactericidal in high levels or against highly susceptible organisms.

Therapeutic monitoring
- Perform culture and sensitivity tests before treatment starts and then as needed.
- Recommend monitoring liver function tests for increased serum bilirubin, AST, and alkaline phosphatase levels. Other erythromycin salts can cause less severe hepatotoxicity. (Patients in whom hepatotoxicity develops from erythromycin estolate may react in a similar fashion to any erythromycin preparation.)

Special populations
Pregnant patients. Use drug during pregnancy only when clearly indicated.
Breast-feeding patients. Although drug is excreted in breast milk, no adverse reactions have been reported. Administer cautiously to breast-feeding women.

Patient counseling
- Instruct patient to take oral form with full glass of water 1 hour before or 2 hours after meals; enteric-coated tablets may be taken with meals.
- Advise patient not to take drug with fruit juice. If patient takes chewable tablets, tell him not to swallow them whole.
- If patient uses topical solution, instruct patient to wash, rinse, and dry affected areas before applying it. Warn patient not to apply solution near eyes, nose, mouth, or other mucous membranes.
- Instruct patient to wash hands before and after applying ophthalmic ointment. Instruct him to cleanse eye area of excess exudate before applying ointment. Warn him not to allow tube to touch the eye or surrounding tissue. Instruct him to promptly report signs of sensitivity, such as itching eyelids and constant burning.
- Tell patient to take drug exactly as directed and to continue taking it for prescribed period, even after he feels better.
- Instruct patient to report adverse reactions promptly.

esmolol hydrochloride
Brevibloc

Pharmacologic classification: beta blocker
Therapeutic classification: antiarrhythmic
Pregnancy risk category C

How supplied
Available by prescription only
Injection: 10 mg/ml in 10-ml vials; 250 mg/ml in 10-ml ampules

Indications and dosages
Supraventricular tachycardia
Adults: Dosage range is 50 to 200 mcg/kg/minute; average dose is 100 mcg/kg/minute.

Individual dosage adjustment requires stepwise titration in which each step consists of a loading dose followed by a maintenance infusion.

To begin treatment, administer a loading infusion of 500 mcg/kg/minute for 1 minute followed by a 4-minute maintenance infusion of 50 mcg/kg/minute. If tachycardia doesn't subside within 5 minutes, repeat loading dose and follow with maintenance infusion increased to 100 mcg/kg/minute. Continue titration, repeating loading infusion and increasing each maintenance infusion by 50 mcg/kg/minute. As patient's heart rate or blood pressure reaches a safety endpoint, omit loading infusion and reduce the increase in maintenance infusion from 50 to 25 mcg/kg/minute or less; also, increase the interval between titration steps from 5 to 10 minutes.

Intraoperative and postoperative tachycardia and hypertension
Adults: For immediate control, 80 mg (about 1 mg/kg) I.V. bolus dose over 30 seconds followed by a 150-mcg/kg/minute infusion, if necessary; for gradual control, a loading I.V. infusion of 500 mcg/kg/minute for 1 minute, followed by a 4-minute maintenance infusion of 50 mcg/kg/minute. If an adequate therapeutic effect isn't observed within 5 minutes, repeat the same loading dose and follow with a maintenance infusion increased to 100 mcg/kg/minute (see supraventricular tachycardia, above).

Pharmacodynamics

Antiarrhythmic action: Esmolol, a beta blocker with rapid onset and very short duration of action, decreases blood pressure and heart rate in a dose-related, titratable manner. Its hemodynamic effects are similar to those of propranolol, but it doesn't increase vascular resistance.

Pharmacokinetics

Absorption: Absorption is immediate after I.V. infusion.
Distribution: Distributed rapidly throughout the plasma. Distribution half-life is about 2 minutes. Esmolol is 55% protein-bound.
Metabolism: Hydrolyzed rapidly by plasma esterases.
Excretion: Excreted by the kidneys as metabolites. Elimination half-life is about 9 minutes.

Route	Onset	Peak	Duration
I.V.	Immediate	30 min	30 min after infusion

Contraindications and precautions

Contraindicated in patients with sinus bradycardia, heart block greater than first-degree, cardiogenic shock, or overt heart failure. Use cautiously in patients with impaired renal function, diabetes, or bronchospasm.

Interactions

Drug-drug. *Insulin or oral antidiabetic agents:* May mask symptoms of developing hypoglycemia. Patient requires close observation.
Antihypertensives: May potentiate their hypotensive effects. Dosage adjustments may be necessary.
I.V. digoxin: Increased digoxin blood levels 10% to 20%. Dosage adjustment may be required.
I.V. morphine: Increases esmolol steady-state levels by 46%. Patient requires careful monitoring.
Nondepolarizing neuromuscular blocking agents, such as succinylcholine, gallamine, metocurine, pancuronium, or tubocurarine: May potentiate and prolong their action; careful postoperative monitoring of patient is necessary after concurrent or sequential use, especially if there's a possibility of incomplete reversal of neuromuscular blockade.
I.V. phenytoin: Additive cardiac depressant effects. Patient requires close monitoring.
Reserpine and other catecholamine-depleting drugs: Additive and possibly excessive beta-adrenergic blockade with bradycardia and hypotension. Close observation is recommended.
Sympathomimetic amines having beta-adrenergic stimulant activity: Mutual but transient inhibition of therapeutic effects. Use together cautiously.
Xanthines, especially aminophylline or theophylline: Mutual inhibition of therapeutic effects and (except for dyphylline) may decrease theophylline clearance, especially in patients with increased theophylline clearance induced by smoking; concurrent use requires careful monitoring to prevent toxic accumulation of theophylline.

Effects on diagnostic tests

None reported.

Adverse reactions

CNS: dizziness, somnolence, headache, agitation, fatigue, confusion.
CV: HYPOTENSION (sometimes with diaphoresis), peripheral ischemia.
GI: *nausea,* vomiting.
Respiratory: ***bronchospasm,*** wheezing, dyspnea, nasal congestion.
Other: inflammation, induration (at infusion site).

Overdose and treatment

Limited information is available. Hypotension would be the most likely symptom.

Symptoms of esmolol overdose usually disappear quickly after esmolol is withdrawn. In addition to immediate discontinuation of esmolol infusion, treatment is supportive and symptomatic.

Glucagon has been reported to effectively combat the CV effects (bradycardia, hypotension) of overdose with beta blockers. An I.V. dose of 2 to 3 mg is administered over 30 seconds and repeated if necessary, followed by infusion at 5 mg/hour until patient's condition has stabilized.

Clinical considerations

- I.V. infusion concentrations exceeding 10 mg of esmolol hydrochloride per ml may produce irritation.
- Drug isn't compatible with 5% sodium bicarbonate injection USP.
- Diluted solutions of esmolol hydrochloride are stable for at least 24 hours at room temperature.
- To convert to other antiarrhythmic therapy after control has been achieved with esmolol, reduce infusion rate of esmolol by 50% 30 minutes after administration of first dose of the alternative agent. If after the second dose of the alternative agent a satisfactory response is maintained for 1 hour, then discontinue esmolol.

Therapeutic monitoring

Monitor patient's pulse and blood pressure.

Special populations

Pregnant patients. Use in third trimester may cause fetal bradycardia. Use drug during pregnancy only when benefits to patient outweigh potential risk to fetus.
Breast-feeding patients. It isn't known if drug is excreted in breast milk; however, no problems associated with breast-feeding women have been reported.
Pediatric patients. Adequate and well-controlled studies haven't been done. Safety and efficacy in children haven't been established.
Geriatric patients. Geriatric patients may be less sensitive to some effects of beta blockers. However, reduced metabolic and excretory capabilities in many geriatric patients may lead to increased myocardial depression and require dosage reduction of beta blockers. Base dosage adjustment on clinical response.

Patient counseling

Advise patient to report adverse events including pain at I.V. site.

estazolam

ProSom

Pharmacologic classification: benzodiazepine
Therapeutic classification: hypnotic
Controlled substance schedule IV
Pregnancy risk category X

How supplied

Available by prescription only
Tablets: 1 mg, 2 mg

Indications and dosages

Short-term management of insomnia characterized by difficulty in falling asleep, frequent nocturnal awakenings, or early-morning awakenings
Adults: Initially, 1 mg P.O. h.s.; may increase to 2 mg as needed and tolerated.
≡ ***Dosage adjustment.*** In small or debilitated older adults, initially, 0.5 mg P.O. h.s.; may increase with care to 1 mg if needed.

Pharmacodynamics

Hypnotic action: Estazolam depresses the CNS at the limbic and subcortical levels of the brain. It produces a sedative-hypnotic effect by potentiating the effect of the neurotransmitter gamma-aminobutyric acid on its receptor in the ascending reticular activating system, which increases inhibition and blocks both cortical and limbic arousal.

Pharmacokinetics

Absorption: Rapidly and completely absorbed through the GI tract.
Distribution: 93% protein-bound.
Metabolism: Extensively metabolized in the liver.
Excretion: Metabolites are excreted primarily in the urine. Less than 5% is excreted in urine as unchanged drug; 4% of a 2-mg dose is excreted in feces. Elimination half-life ranges from 10 to 24 hours; clearance is accelerated in smokers.

Route	Onset	Peak	Duration
P.O.	Unknown	1-3 hr	Unknown

Contraindications and precautions

Contraindicated in pregnant women or patients with hypersensitivity to drug. Use cautiously in patients with depression, suicidal tendencies, and hepatic, renal, or pulmonary disease.

Interactions

Drug-drug. *Cimetidine, disulfiram, oral contraceptives, and isoniazid:* May diminish hepatic metabolism, resulting in increased plasma levels of estazolam. Monitor patient for increased CNS depressant effects.
Phenothiazines, narcotics, antihistamines, MAO inhibitors, barbiturates, general anesthetics, and tricyclic antidepressants: Increased CNS effects. Avoid use together.
Phenytoin and digoxin: Increased level of these drugs, with possible toxicity. Monitor patient closely.
Probenecid: Increased benzodiazepine effect. Monitor patient carefully.
Rifampin: Increases clearance and decreases half-life of estazolam. Monitor for decrease in drug effect.
Theophylline: Antagonizes pharmacologic effects of estazolam. Monitor patient for drug effectiveness.

Drug-lifestyle. *Alcohol use:* May cause excessive respiratory and CNS depression. Advise patient to avoid alcohol.
Heavy smoking: Accelerates metabolism of estazolam, resulting in diminished clinical efficacy. Advise patient to avoid smoking.
Caffeine: May enhance CNS effects. Discourage use.

Effects on diagnostic tests
None reported.

Adverse reactions
CNS: fatigue, dizziness, *daytime drowsiness, somnolence, asthenia, hypokinesia, abnormal thinking.*
GI: dyspepsia, abdominal pain.
Hepatic: AST levels may be increased.
Musculoskeletal: back pain, stiffness.

Overdose and treatment
Somnolence, confusion with reduced or absent reflexes, respiratory depression, apnea, hypotension, impaired coordination, slurred speech, seizures, or coma can occur from benzodiazepine overdose. If excitation occurs, don't use barbiturates. Several agents may have been ingested. Perform gastric evacuation and lavage immediately. Monitor respiration, pulse rate, and blood pressure. Use symptomatic and supportive measures. Maintain airway and administer fluids. Flumazenil, a specific benzodiazepine antagonist, may be useful.

Clinical considerations
Consider the recommendations relevant to all benzodiazepines; withdraw drug slowly after prolonged use.

Therapeutic monitoring
Recommend regularly performing blood counts, urinalysis, and blood chemistry analyses.

Special populations
Pregnant patients. Drug can cause harm to fetus when administered during pregnancy. Safety during labor and delivery hasn't been established.
Breast-feeding patients. It isn't known if drug is excreted in breast milk. Avoid use in breast-feeding women.
Pediatric patients. Safety and efficacy in children haven't been established.
Geriatric patients. Geriatric patients may be more susceptible to CNS depressant effects of estazolam. Use with caution. Lower dosage may be required. To prevent injury from dizziness and falls, recommend supervising geriatric patients during daily living activities, especially at the start of treatment and after an increase in dosage.

Patient counseling
- Advise the patient to avoid caffeine or other stimulants.
- Tell patient to avoid alcohol and other CNS depressants.
- Advise patient to immediately report if she suspects pregnancy or plans to become pregnant during therapy.
- Warn patient that drug may cause drowsiness. Advise special caution and avoidance of driving or operating hazardous machinery until adverse CNS effects of the drug are known.
- Caution patient not to discontinue drug abruptly after taking it daily for prolonged period and not to vary dosage or increase dosage unless prescribed. Drug should be taken until sleep pattern is established and then slowly tapered as prescribed.
- Inform patient that nocturnal sleep may be disturbed for 1 or 2 nights after drug is stopped.

esterified estrogens
Estratab, Menest

Pharmacologic classification: estrogen
Therapeutic classification: estrogen replacement, antineoplastic
Pregnancy risk category X

How supplied
Available by prescription only
Tablets: 0.3 mg, 0.625 mg, 1.25 mg, 2.5 mg

Indications and dosages
Palliative treatment of advanced inoperable prostatic cancer
Adults: 1.25 to 2.5 mg P.O. t.i.d.
Breast cancer
Men and postmenopausal women: 10 mg P.O. t.i.d. for 3 or more months.
Female hypogonadism
Adults: 2.5 mg P.O. daily to t.i.d. in cycles of 20 days on, 10 days off.
Castration, primary ovarian failure
Adults: 2.5 mg P.O. daily to t.i.d. in cycles of 3 weeks on, 1 week off.
Vasomotor menopausal symptoms
Adults: 0.3 to 1.25 mg P.O. daily in cycles of 3 weeks on, 1 week off; dosage may be increased to 2.5 or 3.75 mg P.O. daily, if necessary.
Atrophic vaginitis and atrophic urethritis
Adults: 0.3 to 1.25 mg P.O. daily in cycles of 3 weeks on, 1 week off.

Pharmacodynamics
Estrogenic action: Esterified estrogen mimics the action of endogenous estrogen in treating female hypogonadism, menopausal symptoms, and atrophic vaginitis. It inhibits growth of hormone-sensitive tissue in advanced, inoperable prostatic cancer and in certain carefully

selected cases of breast cancer in men and postmenopausal women.

Pharmacokinetics
Absorption: After oral administration, esterified estrogens are well absorbed from the GI tract.
Distribution: About 50% to 80% plasma protein-bound, particularly the estradiol-binding globulin. Distribution occurs throughout the body with highest levels appearing in fat.
Metabolism: Metabolized primarily in the liver, where estrogens are conjugated with sulfate and glucuronide.
Excretion: Eliminated through the kidneys in the form of sulfate or glucuronide conjugates.

Route	Onset	Peak	Duration
P.O.	Unknown	Unknown	Unknown

Contraindications and precautions
Contraindicated in patients with breast cancer (except metastatic disease), estrogen-dependent neoplasia, active thrombophlebitis or thromboembolic disorders, undiagnosed abnormal genital bleeding, hypersensitivity to drug, history of thromboembolic disease, during pregnancy or breast-feeding.

Use cautiously in patients with history of hypertension, mental depression, liver impairment, or cardiac or renal dysfunction and in those with bone diseases, migraine, seizures, or diabetes mellitus.

Interactions
Drug-drug. *Drugs that induce hepatic metabolism, such as rifampin, barbiturates, primidone, carbamazepine, and phenytoin:* Decreased estrogenic effects. Use together cautiously.
Anticoagulants: Decreased effects of warfarin-type anticoagulants. Monitor patient closely.
Corticosteroids: Enhanced effects. Monitor patient's fluid and electrolyte status.
Cyclosporine: Increased risk of toxicity. Monitor patient closely.
Dantrolene and other hepatotoxic medications: Increased risk of hepatotoxicity. Monitor patient carefully.
Estrogens: Decreased effectiveness of tamoxifen. Monitor patient for drug effects.
Insulin or oral antidiabetic agents: May require adjustment because estradiol may increase blood glucose levels.
Drug-food. *Caffeine:* Increased serum caffeine levels. Advise patient to avoid caffeine.
Drug-lifestyle. *Smoking:* Increased risk of adverse CV effects. Advise patient to avoid smoking.

Effects on diagnostic tests
None reported.

Adverse reactions
CNS: headache, dizziness, chorea, depression, ***seizures.***
CV: thrombophlebitis; *thromboembolism;* hypertension; edema; ***increased risk of CVA, pulmonary embolism, MI.***
EENT: worsening of myopia or astigmatism, intolerance of contact lenses.
GI: *nausea,* vomiting, abdominal cramps, bloating, anorexia, increased appetite, weight changes, ***pancreatitis,*** gallbladder disease.
GU: in women, breakthrough bleeding, altered menstrual flow, dysmenorrhea, amenorrhea, ***increased risk of endometrial cancer, possibility of increased risk of breast cancer,*** cervical erosion, altered cervical secretions, enlargement of uterine fibromas, vaginal candidiasis; breast changes (tenderness, enlargement, secretion); in men, gynecomastia, testicular atrophy, impotence.
Hematologic: increased PT and INR and clotting factors VII to X and norepinephrine-induced platelet aggregability.
Hepatic: cholestatic jaundice, ***hepatic adenoma.***
Metabolic: decreased serum folate, pyridoxine, and antithrombin III levels; increased triglyceride, glucose, and phospholipid levels; hypercalcemia.
Skin: melasma, rash, hirsutism or hair loss, erythema nodosum, dermatitis.

Overdose and treatment
Serious toxicity after overdose of these drugs hasn't been reported. Nausea may occur. Provide appropriate supportive care.

Clinical considerations
Clinical considerations are the same as for all estrogens.

Therapeutic monitoring
Therapeutic monitoring is the same as for all estrogens.

Special populations
Pregnant patients. Drug is contraindicated during pregnancy.
Breast-feeding patients. Esterified estrogens are contraindicated in breast-feeding women.

Patient counseling
Patient counseling is the same as for all estrogens.

estradiol

Climara, Estrace, Estrace Vaginal Cream, Estraderm, Vivelle

estradiol cypionate

depGynogen, Depo-Estradiol Cypionate, Depogen, Estro-Cyp, Estrofem

estradiol valerate

Delestrogen*, Dioval 40, Dioval XX, Estra-L 40, Gynogen L.A. 10, Gynogen L.A. 20, Valergen-20

polyestradiol phosphate

Estradurin

Pharmacologic classification: estrogen
Therapeutic classification: estrogen replacement, antineoplastic
Pregnancy risk category X

How supplied

Available by prescription only
estradiol
Tablets: 0.5 mg, 1 mg, 2 mg
Vaginal: 0.1 mg/g cream (in nonliquefying base)
Transdermal: 4 mg/10 cm^2 (delivers 0.05 mg/24 hours); 8 mg/20 cm^2 (delivers 0.1 mg/24 hours)
estradiol cypionate
Injection: 5 mg/ml (in oil)
estradiol valerate
Injection: 10 mg/ml, 20 mg/ml, 40 mg/ml (in oil)
polyestradiol phosphate
Injection: 40 mg/2 ml

Indications and dosages

Atrophic vaginitis, atrophic dystrophy of the vulva, vasomotor menopausal symptoms, hypogonadism, female castration, primary ovarian failure
estradiol (tablets)
Adults: 1 to 2 mg P.O. daily, in cycles of 21 days on and 7 days off or cycles of 5 days on and 2 days off; or 0.2 to 1 mg I.M. weekly.
estradiol valerate
Adults: 10 to 20 mg I.M. once a month.
estradiol (transdermal)
Adults: Place one Estraderm transdermal patch on trunk of the body, preferably the abdomen, twice weekly. Administer on an intermittent cyclic schedule (3 weeks on and 1 week off).
Atrophic vaginitis
estradiol (vaginal cream)
Adults: 2 to 4 g daily for 1 to 2 weeks. When vaginal mucosa is restored, begin maintenance dosage of 1 g one to three times weekly.
Female hypogonadism
estradiol cypionate
Adults: 1.5 to 2 mg I.M. at monthly intervals.
Inoperable breast cancer
estradiol (tablets)
Adults: 10 mg P.O. t.i.d. for 3 months.
Inoperable prostatic cancer
estradiol valerate
Adults: 30 mg I.M. q 1 to 2 weeks.
estradiol (tablets)
Adults: 1 to 2 mg P.O. t.i.d.
polyestradiol phosphate
Adults: 40 mg I.M. q 2 to 4 weeks.

Pharmacodynamics

Estrogenic action: Estradiol mimics the action of endogenous estrogen in treating female hypogonadism, menopausal symptoms, and atrophic vaginitis. It inhibits growth of hormone-sensitive tissue in advanced, inoperable prostatic cancer and in certain carefully selected cases of breast cancer in men and postmenopausal women.

Pharmacokinetics

Absorption: After oral administration, estradiol and other natural unconjugated estrogens are well absorbed but substantially inactivated by the liver. Therefore, unconjugated estrogens are usually administered parenterally.

After I.M. administration, absorption begins rapidly and continues for days. The cypionate and valerate esters administered in oil have prolonged durations of action because of their slow absorption characteristics.

Topically applied estradiol is absorbed readily into the systemic circulation.

Distribution: Estradiol and other natural estrogens are about 50% to 80% plasma protein-bound, particularly the estradiol-binding globulin. Distribution occurs throughout the body, with highest levels appearing in fat.

Metabolism: Steroidal estrogens, including estradiol, are metabolized primarily in the liver, where they are conjugated with sulfate and glucuronide. Because of the rapid rate of metabolism, nonesterified forms of estrogen, including estradiol, must usually be administered daily.

Excretion: The majority of estrogen elimination occurs through the kidneys in the form of sulfate or glucuronide conjugates.

Route	Onset	Peak	Duration
P.O., I.M., Transdermal, Intravaginal	Unknown	Unknown	Unknown

Contraindications and precautions

Contraindicated in patients with thrombophlebitis or thromboembolic disorders, estrogen-dependent neoplasia, breast or reproductive organ cancer (except for palliative treatment), or undiagnosed abnormal genital bleeding and during pregnancy. Also contraindicated in patients with history of thrombophlebitis or thromboembolic disorders associated with previous estrogen use (except for palliative treatment of breast and prostate cancer).

Use cautiously in patients with cerebrovascular or coronary artery disease, asthma, bone diseases, migraine, seizures, or cardiac, hepatic, or renal dysfunction and in women with a strong family history of breast cancer or who have breast nodules, fibrocystic disease, or abnormal mammographic findings.

Interactions

Drug-drug. *Drugs that induce hepatic metabolism, such as rifampin, barbiturates, primidone, carbamazepine, and phenytoin:* Decreased estrogenic effects from a given dose. These drugs are known to accelerate the rate of metabolism of certain other agents. Monitor patient closely.
Insulin or oral antidiabetic agents: May require adjustment because drug affects blood glucose.
Warfarin-type anticoagulants: Decreased anticoagulant effect. May necessitate dosage adjustment.
Corticosteroids: May cause enhanced effects. Monitor patient closely.
Cyclosporine: May increase risk of toxicity. Monitor patient and cyclosprine levels frequently.
Dantrolene, other hepatotoxic medications: May increase risk of hepatotoxicity. Monitor patient closely.
Tamoxifen: Decreased effects of tamoxifen. Monitor patient closely.
Drug-food. *Caffeine:* May increase serum caffeine levels. Advise patient to avoid caffeine.
Drug-lifestyle. *Smoking:* Increases risk of adverse CV effects. Advise patient to avoid smoking.

Effects on diagnostic tests

None reported.

Adverse reactions

CNS: headache, dizziness, chorea, depression, ***seizures.***
CV: thrombophlebitis; ***thromboembolism;*** hypertension; edema; ***increased risk of CVA, pulmonary embolism, MI.***
EENT: worsening of myopia or astigmatism, intolerance of contact lenses.
GI: *nausea,* vomiting, abdominal cramps, bloating, anorexia, increased appetite, weight changes, ***pancreatitis,*** gallbladder disease.
GU: in women, breakthrough bleeding, altered menstrual flow, dysmenorrhea, amenorrhea, ***increased risk of endometrial cancer, possibility of increased risk of breast cancer,*** cervical erosion, altered cervical secretions, enlargement of uterine fibromas, vaginal candidiasis; breast changes (tenderness, enlargement, secretion); in men, gynecomastia, testicular atrophy, impotence.
Hematologic: increased PT and INR and clotting factors VII to X and norepinephrine-induced platelet aggregability.
Hepatic: cholestatic jaundice, ***hepatic adenoma.***
Metabolic: decreased serum folate, pyridoxine, and antithrombin III levels; increased triglyceride, glucose, and phospholipid levels; hypercalcemia.
Skin: melasma, rash, hirsutism or hair loss, erythema nodosum, dermatitis.

Overdose and treatment

Serious toxicity after overdose of drug hasn't been reported. Nausea may occur. Provide appropriate supportive care.

Clinical considerations

Clinical considerations are the same as for all other estrogen products.

Therapeutic monitoring

Consider the recommendations for all estrogen products; monitor patch site for skin reactions when using transdermal form of drug administration.

Special populations

Pregnant patients. Drug is contraindicated in pregnant women.
Breast-feeding patients. Drug is contraindicated in breast-feeding women.
Geriatric patients. Frequent physical examinations are recommended in postmenopausal women taking estrogen.

Patient counseling

- Tell patient not to apply patch to breast area.
- Remind patient not to use the same skin site for at least 1 week after removal of the transdermal system.

estradiol/norethindrone acetate transdermal system

CombiPatch

Pharmacologic classification: estrogen/progestin
Therapeutic classification: postmenopausal agent
Pregnancy risk category X

How supplied

Available by prescription only
Transdermal: 9 cm^2 system (0.05 mg estradiol and 0.14 mg norethindrone); 16 cm^2 system (0.05 mg estradiol and 0.25 mg norethindrone)

Indications and dosages

Moderate-to-severe vasomotor symptoms associated with menopause, vulvar and vaginal atrophy, and hypoestrogenemia due to hypogonadism, castration, or pri-

mary ovarian failure in women with an intact uterus
Adults: Continuous combined regimen—9 cm^2 patch worn continuously on the lower abdomen. Remove old system and apply new system twice weekly during a 28-day cycle. May increase to 16 cm^2 patch if more progestin is desired.
Continuous sequential regimen—patch can be applied as a sequential regimen in combination with an estradiol-only transdermal system (such as Alora, Esclim, Estraderm, Vivelle). A 0.05-mg estradiol-only transdermal patch is worn for first 14 days of a 28-day cycle; replace system twice weekly according to product directions. For remainder of 28-day cycle, apply the 9 cm^2 patch system to the lower abdomen and replace twice weekly. May increase to 16 cm^2 patch if more progestin is desired.

Women not currently receiving continuous estrogen or estrogen/progestin therapy may start therapy at any time.

Women currently receiving continuous hormone replacement therapy should complete the current cycle of therapy before initiating therapy. Women often experience withdrawal bleeding at the completion of the cycle; first day of withdrawal bleeding would be an appropriate time to initiate therapy.

Pharmacodynamics
Hormone action: Estrogen replacement therapy can reduce the frequency of menopausal symptoms by replacing the naturally declining levels that occur in postmenopausal women.

Pharmacokinetics
Absorption: Estradiol and norethindrone are well absorbed transdermally.
Distribution: Estradiol is primarily bound to sex hormone binding protein (SHBG) and norethindrone is primarily bound to albumin and SHBG.
Metabolism: Estradiol is minimally metabolized. Norethindrone is metabolized primarily by the liver.
Excretion: Elimination half-life of estradiol is 2 to 3 hours; of norethindrone, 6 to 8 hours.

Route	Onset	Peak	Duration
Transdermal	12-24 hr	Unknown	Unknown

Contraindications and precautions
Contraindicated in women who may be pregnant, have known or suspected breast cancer, known or suspected estrogen-dependent neoplasia, undiagnosed abnormal genital bleeding, active thrombophlebitis, thromboembolic disorders or stroke, or known hypersensitivity to estrogen, progestin, or any component of the patch. Use cautiously in patients with impaired liver function, asthma, epilepsy, migraine, and cardiac or renal dysfunction.

Interactions
None reported.

Effects on diagnostic tests
Drug may cause a reduced response to the metyrapone test and sulfobromophthalein retention. Increased thyroid-binding globulin may lead to increased total T_3 and T_4 levels and decreased T_3 resin uptake. Free T_4 and T_3 levels are unaffected.

Adverse reactions
CNS: *asthenia,* depression, insomnia, nervousness, dizziness, *headache.*
CV: INR, activated partial thromboplastin time, and platelet aggregation times may be altered; platelet count and fibrinogen activity may increase.
EENT: tooth disorder, *pharyngitis, rhinitis, sinusitis.*
GI: *abdominal pain, diarrhea,* dyspepsia, flatulence, *nausea,* constipation.
GU: *dysmenorrhea, leukorrhea, menstrual disorder,* suspicious Papanicolaou smear, *vaginitis,* menorrhagia, vaginal hemorrhage.
Musculoskeletal: arthralgia, *back pain.*
Respiratory: *respiratory disorder,* bronchitis.
Skin: application site reactions, acne.
Other: *accidental injury, flu syndrome, pain, breast pain,* peripheral edema, breast enlargement, infection.

Overdose and treatment
Nausea and withdrawal bleeding are the most common consequences of overdose. Treatment should involve discontinuation or removal of the patch. Medical treatment may be initiated.

Clinical considerations
- Combination estrogen/progestin regimens are indicated for women with an intact uterus.
- Progestins taken with estrogen drugs significantly reduce, but don't eliminate, the risk of endometrial cancer associated with the use of estrogen.
- Store norethindrone patches in refrigerator before dispensing. Once dispensed, system may be stored at a temperature under 77° F (25° C) for up to 3 months.

Therapeutic monitoring
- Reevaluate hormonal therapy every 3 to 6 months.
- Blood pressure increases have been associated with estrogen use. Monitor patient's blood pressure regularly.

Special populations
Pregnant patients. Contraindicated during pregnancy.
Breast-feeding patients. Estrogen and progestin are excreted in breast milk. The patch shouldn't be used during breast-feeding.

Patient counseling
- Instruct patient to apply patch system to a smooth (fold-free), clean, dry, nonirritated area

of skin on the lower abdomen, avoiding the waistline. Application sites should be rotated, with an interval of at least 1 week between applications to the same site.
- Don't apply patch on or near the breasts.
- Advise patient of potential for adverse events.
- Tell patient she may store patches at room temperature for up to 3 months.

estramustine phosphate sodium
Emcyt

Pharmacologic classification: estrogen, alkylating agent
Therapeutic classification: antineoplastic
Pregnancy risk category NR

How supplied
Available by prescription only
Capsules: 140 mg

Indications and dosages
Dosage and indications may vary. Check literature for recommended protocols.
Palliative treatment of metastatic or progressive cancer of the prostate
Adults: 10 to 16 mg/kg P.O. in three or four divided doses. Usual dose is 14 mg/kg daily. Therapy should continue for up to 3 months and, if successful, be maintained as long as patient responds.

Pharmacodynamics
Antineoplastic action: Exact mechanism of action is unclear. However, the estrogenic portion of the molecule may act as a carrier of the drug to facilitate selective uptake by tumor cells with estradiol hormone receptors, such as those in the prostate gland. At that point, the nitrogen mustard portion of the drug acts as an alkylating agent.

Pharmacokinetics
Absorption: After oral administration, about 75% of a dose is absorbed across the GI tract.
Distribution: Estramustine is distributed widely into body tissues.
Metabolism: Extensively metabolized in the liver.
Excretion: Drug and its metabolites are eliminated primarily in feces, with a small amount excreted in urine. Terminal phase of plasma elimination has a half-life of 20 hours.

Route	Onset	Peak	Duration
P.O.	Unknown	Unknown	Unknown

Contraindications and precautions
Contraindicated in patients hypersensitive to estradiol and nitrogen mustard and in those with active thrombophlebitis or thromboembolic disorders, except when the actual tumor mass is the cause of the thromboembolic phenomenon. Contraindicated in pregnant and breast-feeding women.

Use cautiously in patients with history of thrombophlebitis or thromboembolic disorders and cerebrovascular or coronary artery disease.

Interactions
Drug-drug. *Calcium-containing drugs, such as antacids:* Impaired absorption of estramustine. They shouldn't be taken together.
Anticoagulants: Decreased anticoagulant effect. May require increased dosage of anticoagulants.
Drug-food. *Calcium-rich foods, such as milk and dairy products:* May impair absorption of estramustine. Drug shouldn't be taken with these foods.

Effects on diagnostic tests
Estramustine therapy may cause a reduced response to the metyrapone test. Glucose tolerance may be decreased.

Adverse reactions
CNS: lethargy, insomnia, headache, anxiety.
CV: chest pain, ***MI,*** sodium and fluid retention, thrombophlebitis, ***heart failure, stroke.***
GI: *nausea, vomiting,* diarrhea, anorexia, flatulence, GI bleeding, thirst.
GU: *painful gynecomastia and breast tenderness.*
Hematologic: ***leukopenia, thrombocytopenia,*** increased norepinephrine-induced platelet aggregability.
Hepatic: elevated liver enzymes.
Metabolic: decreased serum folate, pyridoxine, phosphate, and pregnanediol levels; increased ceruloplasmin, cortisol, prolactin PT, sodium, triglyceride, and phospholipid levels.
Musculoskeletal: leg cramps.
Respiratory: ***edema, pulmonary embolism,*** dyspnea.
Skin: rash, pruritus, dry skin, flushing.
Other: thinning of hair.

Overdose and treatment
Signs and symptoms of overdose include headache, nausea, vomiting, and myelosuppression.

Treatment is usually supportive and includes induction of emesis, gastric lavage, transfusion of blood components, and appropriate symptomatic therapy. Hematologic monitoring should continue for at least 6 weeks after the ingestion.

Clinical considerations
Consider the recommendations relevant to all alkylating agents as well as the following:
- Store capsules in refrigerator.
- Phenothiazines can be used to treat nausea and vomiting.

- Estramustine may cause hypertension.
- Drug may exaggerate preexisting peripheral edema or heart failure.

Therapeutic monitoring

- Recommend monitoring blood pressure at baseline and routinely during therapy.
- Recommend monitoring glucose tolerance periodically during therapy.
- Patients may continue estramustine as long as they're responding favorably. Some patients have taken drug for more than 3 years.
- Recommend monitoring weight gain regularly in these patients.

Special populations

Pregnant patients. Drug is contraindicated during pregnancy.
Breast-feeding patients. Drug is contraindicated in breast-feeding women.
Geriatric patients. Use with caution in geriatric patients, who are more likely to have vascular disorders, because the use of estrogen is associated with vascular complications.

Patient counseling

- Emphasize importance of continuing medication despite nausea and vomiting.
- Advise patient to call immediately if vomiting occurs shortly after a dose is taken.
- Because of possibility of mutagenic effects, advise patients of childbearing age to use contraceptive measures.

estrogen and progestin

Alesse-28, Brevicon, Demulen 1/35, Demulen 1/35-28, Enovid, Loestrin 21 1/20, Loestrin 21 1.5/30, Loestrin Fe 1/20, Loestrin Fe 1.5/30, Lo/Ovral, Lo/Ovral-28, Modicon 21, Modicon 28, Nordette-21, Nordette-28, Norinyl 1+35 21-Day, Norinyl 1+35 28-Day, Norinyl 1+50 21-Day, Norinyl 1+50 28-Day, Norinyl 1+80 28-Day, Ortho-Novum 1/35 21, Ortho-Novum 1/35 28, Ortho-Novum 1/50 21, Ortho-Novum 1/50 28, Ortho-Novum 7/7/7-21, Ortho-Novum 7/7/7-28, Ortho-Novum 10/11-21, Ortho-Novum 10/11-28, Ovcon-35, Ovcon-50, Ovral, Ovral-28, Tri-Norinyl-21, Tri-Norinyl-28, Triphasil-21, Triphasil-28

Pharmacologic classification: estrogen with progestin
Therapeutic classification: contraceptive (hormonal)
Pregnancy risk category X

How supplied

Available by prescription only
Tablets—monophasic type
Mestranol 0.1 mg and norethynodrel 2.5 mg
Mestranol 0.1 mg and norethindrone 2 mg
Mestranol 0.1 mg and ethynodiol diacetate 1 mg
Mestranol 0.08 mg and norethindrone 1 mg
Mestranol 0.05 mg and norethindrone 1 mg
Ethinyl estradiol 0.02 mg and levonorgestrel 0.1 mg
Ethinyl estradiol 0.05 mg and norethindrone 1 mg
Ethinyl estradiol 0.05 mg and norethindrone acetate 1 mg
Ethinyl estradiol 0.05 mg and ethynodiol diacetate 1 mg
Ethinyl estradiol 0.05 mg and norethindrone acetate 2.5 mg
Ethinyl estradiol 0.05 mg and norgestrel 0.5 mg
Ethinyl estradiol 0.035 mg and norethindrone 1 mg
Ethinyl estradiol 0.035 mg and norethindrone 0.5 mg
Ethinyl estradiol 0.035 mg and norethindrone 0.4 mg
Ethinyl estradiol 0.035 mg and ethynodiol diacetate 1 mg
Ethinyl estradiol 0.03 mg and norethindrone acetate 1.5 mg
Ethinyl estradiol 0.03 mg and norgestrel 0.3 mg
Ethinyl estradiol 0.03 mg and levonorgestrel 0.15 mg
Ethinyl estradiol 0.02 mg and norethindrone 1 mg
Tablets—biphasic type
10 tablets ethinyl estradiol 0.035 mg and norethindrone 0.5 mg; 11 tablets ethinyl estradiol 0.035 mg and norethindrone 1 mg
Tablets—triphasic type
7 tablets ethinyl estradiol 0.035 mg and norethindrone 0.5 mg; 9 tablets ethinyl estradiol 0.035 mg and norethindrone 1 mg; 5 tablets ethinyl estradiol 0.035 mg and norethindrone 0.5 mg
7 tablets ethinyl estradiol 0.035 mg and norethindrone 0.5 mg; 7 tablets ethinyl estradiol 0.035 mg and norethindrone 0.75 mg; 7 tablets ethinyl estradiol 0.035 mg and norethindrone 1 mg
6 tablets ethinyl estradiol 0.03 and levonorgestrel 0.05 mg; 5 tablets ethinyl estradiol 0.04 mg and levonorgestrel 0.075 mg; 10 tablets ethinyl estradiol 0.03 mg and levonorgestrel 0.125 mg

Indications and dosages

Contraception
Monophasic
Adults: One tablet P.O. daily, beginning on day 5 of menstrual cycle (first day of menstrual flow is day 1), or on the first Sunday after onset of menstruation, or on day 1 of menstrual cycle depending on specific contraceptive. With 20- and 21-tablet packages, new dosing cycle begins 7 days after last tablet taken. With 28-tablet packages, dosage is one tablet daily without interruption; extra tablets are placebos or

contain iron. If next menstrual period doesn't begin on schedule, rule out pregnancy before starting new dosing cycle. If menstrual period begins, start new dosing cycle 7 days after last tablet was taken. If all doses have been taken on schedule and one menstrual period is missed, continue dosing cycle. If two consecutive menstrual periods are missed, pregnancy test is required before new dosing cycle is started.

Biphasic

Adults: One color tablet P.O. daily (Ortho-Novum 10/11) for 10 days, then next color tablet for 11 days.

Triphasic

Adults: One tablet P.O. daily (Ortho-Novum 7/7/7, Tri-Norinyl, Triphasil) in the sequence specified by the manufacturer.

Hypermenorrhea

Adults: Use high-dose combinations only. Dosage is same as for contraception.

Endometriosis

Adults: Cyclic therapy: One 10-mg tablet P.O. daily (Ortho-Novum) for 20 days from day 5 to day 24 of menstrual cycle. Suppressive therapy: One 5- or 10-mg tablet P.O. daily (Enovid) for 2 weeks, starting on day 5 of menstrual cycle. Continue without interruption for 6 to 9 months, increasing dose by 5 to 10 mg q 2 weeks, up to 20 mg daily. Up to 40 mg daily may be needed if breakthrough bleeding occurs.

Pharmacodynamics

Contraceptive action: Estrogen components of oral contraceptives inhibit the release of follicle-stimulating hormone, thereby stopping follicular development and suppressing ovulation.

Progestin components of oral contraceptives inhibit the release of luteinizing hormone, preventing ovulation even in the event of incomplete suppression of follicular development. Progestins also change the endometrial environment to inhibit nidation (implantation of the fertilized egg into the endometrium) and cause thickening of the cervical mucus, blocking the upward migration of sperm.

Pharmacokinetics

Absorption: Most components of oral contraceptives are absorbed relatively well from the GI tract. Bioavailabilities range from 40% to 70%; considerable individual variation exists in extent of absorption.

Distribution: Protein binding of the various drugs used in oral contraceptives is high, ranging from 80% to 98%. These agents are distributed extensively into virtually all body tissues.

Metabolism: These drugs undergo metabolic transformation before excretion; their rates of metabolism may thus be affected by agents that induce or inhibit metabolism.

Excretion: Very little, if any, is excreted unchanged in urine or feces. They appear primarily as sulfate and glucuronide conjugates.

Route	Onset	Peak	Duration
P.O.	Unknown	1-2 hr	Unknown

Contraindications and precautions

Oral contraceptives are contraindicated in patients with thromboembolic disorders, cerebrovascular or coronary artery disease, or MI because of their association with thromboembolic disease; in patients with known or suspected cancer of the breast or reproductive organs or with benign or malignant liver tumors because of their association with tumorigenesis; in patients with undiagnosed abnormal vaginal bleeding; in women known or believed to be pregnant or breast-feeding; in adolescents with incomplete epiphyseal closure; and in women smokers over age 35.

Use oral contraceptives cautiously in patients with systemic lupus erythematosus, hypertension, mental depression, migraine, epilepsy, asthma, diabetes mellitus, amenorrhea, scanty or irregular periods, fibrocystic breast disease, family history (mother, grandmother, sister) of breast or genital tract cancer, or renal or gallbladder disease. Advise patient to report development or worsening of any of these conditions. Prolonged therapy may be inadvisable in women who plan to become pregnant.

Interactions

Drug-drug. *Aminoglutethimide, ampicillin, antihistamines, barbiturates, carbamazepine, chloramphenicol, griseofulvin, isoniazid, neomycin, nitrofurantoin, phenylbutazone, phenytoin, primidone, penicillin V, rifampin, sulfonamides, and tetracycline:* Increased metabolism of oral contraceptives, resulting in reduced efficacy, breakthrough bleeding, and occasionally contraceptive failure. Monitor patient for drug effects.

Insulin or oral antidiabetic agents: Serum glucose may be affected; dose adjustment may be required.

Oral warfarin-type anticoagulants and anticonvulsants, antihypertensives, and tricyclic antidepressants: Countereffects may occur. Avoid use together.

Drug-food. *Caffeine:* May increase serum caffeine levels. Advise patient to avoid caffeine.

Drug-lifestyle. *Smoking:* Increases risk of CV effects. Advise patient not to smoke.

Effects on diagnostic tests

None reported.

Adverse reactions

CNS: headache, dizziness, depression, lethargy, migraine.

CV: ***thromboembolism,*** hypertension, edema, increase in varicosities.
EENT: worsening of myopia or astigmatism, intolerance of contact lenses, unexplained loss of vision, optic neuritis, diplopia, retinal thrombosis, papilledema.
GI: *nausea, vomiting,* abdominal cramps, bloating, diarrhea, constipation, changes in appetite, weight gain, bowel ischemia.
GU: breakthrough bleeding, granulomatous colitis, dysmenorrhea, amenorrhea, cervical erosion or abnormal secretions, enlargement of uterine fibromas, vaginal candidiasis, urinary tract infections, breast tenderness, enlargement, or secretion.
Hematologic: increased prothrombin and clotting factors VII to X, plasminogen, norepinephrine-induced platelet aggregation, fibrinogen; decreased antithrombin III.
Hepatic: gallbladder disease, cholestatic jaundice, ***liver tumors.***
Metabolic: hyperglycemia, hypercalcemia, folic acid deficiency; increased sulfobromophthalein retention, thyroid-binding globulin, triglycerides, phospholipids, transcortin and corticosteroids, transferrin, prolactin, renin, and vitamin A; decreased metyrapone, pregnanediol excretion, free T_3 resin uptake, glucose tolerance, zinc, and vitamin B_{12}.
Skin: rash, acne, seborrhea, oily skin, erythema multiforme, hyperpigmentation.
Other: libido changes, possible increased risk of congenital anomalies.

Note: Adverse effects may be more serious, frequent, and rapid in onset with high-dose than with low-dose combinations.

Overdose and treatment

Serious toxicity after drug overdose hasn't been reported. Nausea and vomiting, as well as withdrawal bleeding, may occur.

Clinical consideration

Consider the recommendations relevant to all estrogens and progestins as well as the following:

- Astigmatic error and myopic refractive error may be increased twofold to threefold, usually after 6 months of oral contraceptive therapy.
- If patient becomes hypersensitive, discontinue the drug.
- Changes in ocular contour and lubricant quality of tears may necessitate change in size and shape of contact lenses.

Therapeutic monitoring

- Therapeutic monitoring considerations are the same as those relevant to all estrogens and progestins.
- Breakthrough bleeding in patients taking high-dose estrogen-progestin combinations for menstrual disorders may necessitate dosage adjustment.

Special populations

Pregnant patients. Drug is contraindicated during pregnancy.
Breast-feeding patients. Oral contraceptives are contraindicated in breast-feeding women.
Pediatric patients. To avoid later fertility and menstrual problems, hormonal contraception isn't advised for the adolescent until after at least 2 years of well-established menstrual cycles and completion of physiologic maturation. An estrogen-dominant agent is the best choice for the adolescent with scanty menses, moderate or severe acne, or candidiasis. A progestin-dominant agent is the best choice for the adolescent with dysmenorrhea, hypermenorrhea, fibrocystic breast disease, or cyclic premenstrual weight gain.

Patient counseling

- Advise patient of potential adverse reactions and inform her that these should diminish after 3 to 6 dosing cycles (months).
- Advise patient to use an additional method of birth control for the first week of administration in the initial cycle (unless using day-1 start).
- Instruct patient to take drug at the same time each day at 24-hour intervals for efficacy of medication, to keep tablets in original container, and to take them in correct (color-coded) sequence.
- Tell patient that night-time dosing may reduce incidence of nausea and headaches.
- Suggest taking drug with or immediately after food to reduce nausea.
- Stress importance of annual Papanicolaou smears and gynecologic examinations while taking estrogen-progestin combinations.
- Advise patient of increased risks associated with simultaneous use of cigarettes and oral contraceptives, especially the risk of serious cardiovascular side effects. Strongly advise women who use oral contraceptives not to smoke.
- Instruct patient as follows regarding missed doses.

Monophasic or biphasic cycles

For 20-, 21-, or 24-day dosing schedule:

- If one regular dose is missed, take tablet as soon as possible; if remembered on the next day, take two tablets, then continue regular dosing schedule.
- If two consecutive days are missed, take two tablets a day for next 2 days, then resume regular dosing schedule.
- If 3 consecutive days are missed, discontinue drug and substitute other contraceptive method until period begins or pregnancy is ruled out. Then start new cycle of tablets.

For 28-day dosing schedule:

- Follow instructions for 21-day dosing schedule; if one of the last seven tablets is missed, be sure to take first tablet of next month's cycle on regularly scheduled day.

Triphasic cycle
For 21-day dosing schedule:
- If 1 day is missed, take dose as soon as possible; if remembered on the next day, take two tablets, then continue regular dosing schedule while using additional method of contraception for remainder of cycle.
- If 2 consecutive days are missed, take two tablets daily for next 2 days, then continue regular schedule while using additional contraceptive method for remainder of cycle.
- If 3 consecutive days are missed, discontinue drug and use other contraceptive method until period begins or pregnancy is ruled out. Then start new cycle of tablets.

For 28-day dosing schedule:
- Follow instructions for 21-day dosing schedule; if one of the last seven tablets was missed, be sure to take first tablet of next month's cycle on regularly scheduled day.

estrogenic substances, conjugated
Premarin

Pharmacologic classification: estrogen
Therapeutic classification: estrogen replacement, antineoplastic, antiosteoporotic
Pregnancy risk category X

How supplied
Available by prescription only
Tablets: 0.3 mg, 0.625 mg, 0.9 mg, 1.25 mg, 2.5 mg
Injection: 25 mg/5 ml
Vaginal cream: 0.0625%

Indications and dosages
Abnormal uterine bleeding (hormonal imbalance)
Adults: 25 mg I.V. or I.M. Repeat dose in 6 to 12 hours, if necessary.
Castration and primary ovarian failure
Adults: Initially, 1.25 mg P.O. daily in cycles of 3 weeks on, 1 week off. Adjust dose p.r.n.
Prevention of osteoporosis
Adults: 0.625 mg P.O. daily given continuously, or cyclically, 25 days on, 5 days off.
Female hypogonadism
Adults: 0.3 to 0.625 mg P.O. daily, given cyclically 3 weeks on, 1 week off.
Vasomotor menopausal symptoms
Adults: 0.625 mg P.O. daily, or cyclically 25 days on, 5 days off.
Atrophic vaginitis or kraurosis vulvae
Adults: 0.3 to 1.25 mg or more P.O. daily. Alternatively, 0.5 to 2 g intravaginally or topically once daily in cycles of 3 weeks on, 1 week off.
Palliative treatment of inoperable prostatic cancer
Adults: 1.25 to 2.5 mg P.O. t.i.d.
Palliative treatment of breast cancer
Adults: 10 mg P.O. t.i.d. for 3 months or more.

Pharmacodynamics
Estrogenic action: Conjugated estrogenic substances mimic the action of endogenous estrogen in treating female hypogonadism, menopausal symptoms, and atrophic vaginitis. They inhibit growth of hormone-sensitive tissue in advanced, inoperable prostatic cancer and in certain carefully selected cases of breast cancer in men and postmenopausal women; they also retard progression of osteoporosis by enhancing calcium and phosphate retention and limiting bone decalcification.

Pharmacokinetics
Absorption: Not well characterized. After I.M. administration, absorption begins rapidly and continues for days.
Distribution: Conjugated estrogens are about 50% to 80% plasma protein-bound and distributed throughout the body, with highest levels appearing in fat.
Metabolism: Conjugated estrogens are metabolized primarily in the liver, where they are conjugated with sulfate and glucuronide. Because of the rapid rate of metabolism, nonesterified forms of estrogen, including estradiol, must usually be administered daily.
Excretion: The majority of estrogen elimination occurs through the kidneys, in the form of sulfate or glucuronide conjugates, or both.

Route	Onset	Peak	Duration
P.O., I.V., I.M., Intravaginal	Unknown	Unknown	Unknown

Contraindications and precautions
Contraindicated in patients with thrombophlebitis or thromboembolic disorders, estrogen-dependent neoplasia, breast or reproductive organ cancer (except for palliative treatment), or undiagnosed abnormal genital bleeding and during pregnancy.

Use cautiously in patients with cerebrovascular or coronary artery disease, asthma, bone disease, migraine, seizures, or cardiac, hepatic, or renal dysfunction or in women with family history (mother, grandmother, sister) of breast or genital tract cancer or who have breast nodules, fibrocystic disease, or abnormal mammographic findings.

Interactions
Drug-drug. *Drugs that induce hepatic metabolism (such as barbiturates, carbamazepine, phenytoin, primidone, and rifampin):* May result in decreased estrogenic effects from a given dose. These drugs are known to accelerate

the rate of metabolism of certain other agents. Use together cautiously.
Insulin or oral antidiabetic agents: May require dosage adjustment as a result of effects of blood glucose level.
Warfarin-type anticoagulants: Decreased anticoagulant effect. Dosage adjustment may be necessary.
Corticosteroids: Enhanced effects. Use together cautiously.
Cyclosporine: Increased risk of toxicity. Monitor patient carefully.
Dantrolene, other hepatotoxic medications: May increase risk of hepatotoxicity.
Tamoxifen: Decreased effects of tamoxifen. Monitor patient closely.
Drug-food. *Caffeine:* May increase serum caffeine levels. Advise patient to avoid caffeine.
Drug-lifestyle. *Smoking:* Increases risk of adverse CV effects. Advise patient to avoid smoking.

Effects on diagnostic tests
Therapy with estrogens increases sulfobromophthalein retention. Increases in the thyroid-binding globulin concentration may occur, resulting in increased total thyroid levels (measured by protein-bound iodine or total T_4) and decreased uptake of free T_3 resin. Glucose tolerance may be impaired. Pregnanediol excretion may decrease.

Adverse reactions
CNS: headache, dizziness, chorea, depression, ***seizures.***
CV: thrombophlebitis; ***thromboembolism;*** hypertension; edema; ***increased risk of CVA, pulmonary embolism, MI.***
EENT: worsening of myopia or astigmatism, intolerance of contact lenses.
GI: *nausea,* vomiting, abdominal cramps, bloating, anorexia, increased appetite, ***pancreatitis,*** gallbladder disease.
GU: in women, breakthrough bleeding, altered menstrual flow, dysmenorrhea, amenorrhea, ***increased risk of endometrial cancer, possibility of increased risk of breast cancer,*** cervical erosion, altered cervical secretions, enlargement of uterine fibromas, vaginal candidiasis; breast changes (tenderness, enlargement, secretion); in men, gynecomastia, testicular atrophy, impotence.
Hematologic: increased PT and INR and clotting factors VII to X and norepinephrine-induced platelet aggregability.
Hepatic: cholestatic jaundice, ***hepatic adenoma.***
Metabolic: decreased serum folate, pyridoxine, and antithrombin III levels; increased triglyceride, glucose, and phospholipid levels; hypercalcemia, weight changes.
Skin: melasma, urticaria, flushing (with rapid I.V. administration), hirsutism or hair loss, erythema nodosum, dermatitis.

Overdose and treatment
Serious toxicity after drug overdose hasn't been reported. Nausea may occur. Provide appropriate supportive care.

Clinical considerations
Consider the recommendations relevant to all estrogens as well as the following:
- For the rapid treatment of dysfunctional uterine bleeding or reduction of surgical bleeding, parenteral administration is preferred.
- Refrigerate before reconstitution. Reconstituted drug may be safely stored in refrigeration for up to 60 days.

Therapeutic monitoring
Therapeutic monitoring is the same as for all other estrogens.

Special populations
Pregnant patients. Drug is contraindicated during pregnancy.
Breast-feeding patients. Estrogens are contraindicated in breast-feeding women.
Geriatric patients. Chronic use for menopausal symptoms may be associated with increased risk of certain types of cancer. Frequent physical examinations are recommended.

Patient counseling
Advise patient to report adverse experiences.

estropipate
Ogen, Ortho-Est

Pharmacologic classification: estrogen
Therapeutic classification: estrogen replacement
Pregnancy risk category X

How supplied
Estropipate is available as estrone sodium sulfate. Available by prescription only.
Tablets: 0.625 mg, 1.25 mg, 2.5 mg

Indications and dosages
Atrophic vaginitis, kraurosis vulvae, and vasomotor menopausal symptoms
Adults: 0.625 to 5 mg P.O. daily for 21 days, followed by 7 days off therapy.
Female hypogonadism, primary ovarian failure, or after castration
Adults: 1.25 to 7.5 mg P.O. daily for 3 weeks, followed by 8 to 10 days off therapy. Cycle may be repeated if no withdrawal bleeding occurs within 10 days of discontinuing therapy.
Prevention of osteoporosis
Adults: 0.625 mg P.O. daily for 25 days of a 31-day cycle.

Pharmacodynamics
Estrogenic action: Estropipate mimics the action of endogenous estrogen in treating female

hypogonadism, menopausal symptoms, and atrophic vaginitis.

Pharmacokinetics

Absorption: After oral administration, estropipate (and other synthetic derivatives of the natural estrogens) are rapidly absorbed after oral administration.
Distribution: About 50% to 80% plasma protein-bound. Distribution occurs throughout the body, with highest levels appearing in fat.
Metabolism: Steroidal estrogens are metabolized primarily in the liver, where they are conjugated with sulfate and glucuronide. Usually, because of the rapid rate of metabolism, many forms of estrogen must be administered daily.
Excretion: Mostly eliminated through the kidneys in the form of sulfate or glucuronide conjugates.

Route	Onset	Peak	Duration
P.O.	Unknown	Unknown	Unknown

Contraindications and precautions

Contraindicated in patients with thrombophlebitis or thromboembolic disorders, estrogen-dependent neoplasia, breast or reproductive organ cancer (except for palliative treatment), or undiagnosed abnormal genital bleeding and during pregnancy.

Use cautiously in patients with cerebrovascular or coronary artery disease, asthma, bone diseases, mental depression, migraine, seizures, or cardiac, hepatic, or renal dysfunction or in women with family history (mother, grandmother, sister) of breast or genital tract cancer or who have breast nodules, fibrocystic disease, or abnormal mammographic findings.

Interactions

Drug-drug. *Drugs that induce hepatic metabolism, such as rifampin, barbiturates, primidone, carbamazepine, phenytoin:* May result in decreased estrogenic effects from a given dose. These drugs are known to accelerate the rate of metabolism of certain other agents. Use together cautiously.
Insulin or oral antidiabetic agents: May require dosage adjustment because of effects of blood glucose level.
Warfarin-type anticoagulants: Decreased anticoagulant effect. Dosage adjustment may be necessary.
Cyclosporine: Increased risk of toxicity. Monitor cyclosporine levels.
Dantrolene, other hepatotoxic medications: May increase risk of hepatotoxicity.
Tamoxifen: Decreased effects of tamoxifen. Monitor patient closely.
Drug-food. *Caffeine:* May increase serum caffeine levels. Advise patient to avoid caffeine.
Drug-lifestyle. *Smoking:* Increases risk of adverse CV effects. Advise patient to avoid smoking.

Effects on diagnostic tests

Therapy with estrogens increases sulfobromophthalein retention. Increases in the thyroid-binding globulin concentration may occur, resulting in increased total thyroid levels (measured by protein-bound iodine or total T_4) and decreased uptake of free T_3 resin. Glucose tolerance may be impaired. Pregnanediol excretion may decrease.

Adverse reactions

CNS: headache, dizziness, depression, migraine, ***seizures.***
CV: ***increased risk of CVA, pulmonary embolism, MI, thromboembolism,*** thrombophlebitis, edema.
EENT: worsening of myopia or astigmatism, intolerance of contact lenses.
GI: vomiting, abdominal cramps, bloating, gallbladder disease.
GU: in women, breakthrough bleeding, increased size of uterine fibromas, dysmenorrhea, amenorrhea, vaginal candidiasis, ***increased risk of endometrial cancer, possibility of increased risk of breast cancer,*** altered menstrual flow, cervical erosion, altered cervical secretions, breast changes (tenderness, enlargement, secretion); in men, gynecomastia, testicular atrophy; cystitis-like syndrome, condition resembling premenstrual syndrome; libido changes.
Hematologic: increased PT and clotting factors VII to X and norepinephrine-induced platelet aggregability.
Hepatic: cholestatic jaundice, ***hepatic adenoma.***
Metabolic: decreased serum folate, pyridoxine, and antithrombin III levels; increased triglyceride, glucose, and phospholipid levels; hypercalcemia, weight changes.
Skin: ***erythema multiforme,*** erythema nodosum, hair loss, hemorrhagic eruption, hirsutism, melasma.
Other: aggravation of porphyria.

Overdose and treatment

Serious toxicity after overdose of this drug hasn't been reported. Nausea may occur. Provide appropriate supportive care.

Clinical considerations

Consider the recommendations relevant to all estrogens as well as the following:
- When used for progressive, inoperable prostate cancer, remission should be apparent within 3 weeks of therapy.
- When submitting specimens to pathologist for evaluation, be sure to note that patient is taking estrogens.

Therapeutic monitoring
Therapeutic monitoring is the same as for all estrogens.

Special populations
Pregnant patients. Drug is contraindicated during pregnancy.
Breast-feeding patients. Drug is contraindicated in breast-feeding women.
Geriatric patients. Frequent physical examinations are recommended for postmenopausal women taking estrogens.

Patient counseling
Patient counseling is the same as for all estrogens.

etanercept
Enbrel

Pharmacologic classification: tumor necrosis factor (TNF) blocker
Therapeutic classification: antirheumatic
Pregnancy risk category B

How supplied
Available by prescription only
Injection: 25 mg single-use vial

Indications and dosages
Reduction in signs and symptoms of moderately to severely active rheumatoid arthritis in patients with demonstrated inadequate response to one or more disease-modifying antirheumatic drugs; or in combination with methotrexate in patients who don't respond adequately to methotrexate alone
Adults: 25 mg S.C. twice weekly.
Children age 4 to 17 years: 0.4 mg/kg (maximum dose 25 mg) S.C. twice weekly for 3 months.

Pharmacodynamics
Antirheumatic action: Binds specifically to tumor necrosis factor (TNF) and blocks its action with cell-surface TNF receptors, reducing inflammatory and immune responses found in rheumatoid arthritis.

Pharmacokinetics
Absorption: Not reported.
Distribution: Not reported.
Metabolism: Not reported.
Excretion: Elimination half-life is 115 hours.

Route	Onset	Peak	Duration
S.C.	Unknown	72 hr	Unknown

Contraindications and precautions
Contraindicated in patients with sepsis and hypersensitivity to etanercept or any of its components.

Live vaccines are contraindicated during drug therapy.

Use cautiously in patients with underlying diseases that predispose them to infection, such as diabetes, heart failure, or history of active or chronic infections.

Interactions
None reported.

Effects on diagnostic tests
None reported.

Adverse reactions
CNS: asthenia, *headache,* dizziness.
EENT: *rhinitis,* pharyngitis, sinusitis.
GI: abdominal pain, dyspepsia.
Respiratory: *upper respiratory tract infections,* cough, respiratory disorder.
Skin: *injection site reaction,* rash.
Other: *infections,* malignancies.

Clinical considerations
- Anti-TNF therapies, including etanercept, may affect defenses against infection.
- Live vaccines shouldn't be given concurrently during drug therapy.
- Juvenile rheumatoid arthritis patients should, if possible, be brought up-to-date with all immunizations in compliance with current immunization guidelines before initiating treatment.
- Don't add other medications or diluents to reconstituted solution.
- Injection sites should be at least 1" apart; areas where skin is tender, bruised, red, or hard should never be used. Recommended sites include the thigh, abdomen, or upper arm. Rotate sites regularly.

Therapeutic monitoring
- Positive antinuclear antibodies (ANA) or positive anti-double-stranded DNA antibodies may developed as measured by radioimmunoassay and *Crithidia lucilae* assay.
- Monitor for infections.

Special populations
Breast-feeding patients. Advise breast-feeding women to discontinue nursing during drug therapy.
Pediatric patients. Safety and efficacy haven't been studied in children under age 4. Children with juvenile rheumatoid arthritis are more susceptible to the adverse effects of abdominal pain and vomiting than adults with rheumatoid arthritis.
Geriatric patients. No overall differences in safety and efficacy have been noted between geriatric and younger adults; however, greater

sensitivity to drug effects by geriatric patients can't be ruled out.

Patient counseling

- Instruct patient who will be self-administering drug about mixing and injection techniques, including rotation of injection sites.
- Tell patient that injection site reactions generally occur within first month of therapy and decrease thereafter.
- Inform patient of importance of avoiding live vaccine administration while receiving drug. Stress importance of alerting health care providers of drug use.
- Instruct patient to promptly report signs and symptoms of infection.

ethacrynate sodium

ethacrynic acid

Edecrin

Pharmacologic classification: loop diuretic
Therapeutic classification: diuretic
Pregnancy risk category B

How supplied

Available by prescription only
Tablets: 25 mg, 50 mg
Injectable: 50 mg (with 62.5 mg of mannitol and 0.1 mg of thimerosal)

Indications and dosages

Acute pulmonary edema
Adults: 50 mg or 0.5 to 1 mg/kg I.V. to a maximum dose of 100 mg of ethacrynate sodium I.V. slowly over several minutes.
Edema
Adults: 50 to 200 mg P.O. daily. Refractory cases may require up to 200 mg b.i.d.
Children: Initially, 25 mg P.O., given cautiously and increased in 25-mg increments daily until desired effect is achieved.
◇***Hypertension***
Adults: Initially, 25 mg P.O. daily. Adjust dose, as necessary. Maximum maintenance dosage is 200 mg P.O. daily in two divided doses.

Pharmacodynamics

Diuretic action: Ethacrynic acid inhibits sodium and chloride reabsorption in the proximal part of the ascending loop of Henle, promoting the excretion of sodium, water, chloride, and potassium.

Pharmacokinetics

Absorption: Absorbed rapidly from the GI tract.
Distribution: Ethacrynic acid accumulates in the liver of animals. Ethacrynic acid doesn't enter the CSF, and its distribution into breast milk or the placenta is unknown.
Metabolism: Metabolized by the liver to a potentially active metabolite.
Excretion: 30% to 65% is excreted in urine and 35% to 40% is excreted in bile as the metabolite. Duration of action is 6 to 8 hours after oral administration and about 2 hours after I.V. administration.

Route	Onset	Peak	Duration
P.O.	30 min	2 hr	6-8 hr
I.V.	5 min	15-30 min	2 hr

Contraindications and precautions

Contraindicated in infants and in patients with anuria or hypersensitivity to drug. Use cautiously in patients with electrolyte abnormalities or impaired hepatic function.

Interactions

Drug-drug. *Aminoglycosides, some cephalosporins, or other ototoxic drugs, such as cisplatin:* May increase the incidence of deafness; avoid use of such combinations.
Antihypertensive agents: Increased antihypertensive effect. Patients may require dosage reduction.
Cardiac glycosides: Increased risk of digitalis toxicity from ethacrynate-induced hypokalemia. Recommend monitoring digitalis and potassium levels.
Diuretics, such as metolazone: May enhance the diuretic effect of the other drugs; reduce dosage when adding ethacrynic acid to a diuretic regimen.
Insulin or oral antidiabetic agents: Elevated blood glucose; dosages may need to be increased.
Lithium: Reduced renal clearance of lithium; monitor lithium levels. Dosage adjustment may be necessary.
NSAIDs: Decreased diuretic effectiveness; possible risk of renal failure. Use together cautiously.
Potassium-sparing diuretics, such as spironolactone, triamterene, and amiloride: Decreased potassium loss induced by ethacrynic acid. May be used as a therapeutic advantage.
Other potassium-depleting drugs, such as steroids and amphotericin B: Severe potassium loss may occur. Monitor patient closely.
Warfarin: May potentiate anticoagulant effects. Use together cautiously.

Effects on diagnostic tests

None reported.

Adverse reactions

CNS: confusion, fatigue, vertigo, headache, malaise.
CV: volume depletion and dehydration, orthostatic hypotension.
EENT: transient deafness (with too-rapid I.V. injection), blurred vision, tinnitus, hearing loss.

GI: diarrhea, anorexia, nausea, vomiting, GI bleeding, ***pancreatitis.***
GU: oliguria, hematuria, nocturia, polyuria, frequent urination, azotemia.
Hematologic: ***agranulocytosis,*** *neutropenia,* ***thrombocytopenia.***
Metabolic: hypokalemia; hypochloremic alkalosis; asymptomatic hyperuricemia; fluid and electrolyte imbalances, including dilutional hyponatremia, hypocalcemia, hypomagnesemia; hyperglycemia; impaired glucose tolerance.
Other: fever, chills.

Overdose and treatment
Signs and symptoms of overdose include profound electrolyte and volume depletion, which may precipitate circulatory collapse.

Treatment of ethacrynic acid overdose is primarily supportive; empty stomach by inducing emesis or gastric lavage. Replace fluid and electrolytes as needed.

Clinical considerations
Consider the recommendations relevant to all loop diuretics as well as the following:
- Administer drug slowly over 20 to 30 minutes, by I.V. infusion or by direct I.V. injection over a period of several minutes; rapid injection may cause hypotension.
- Drug shouldn't be administered simultaneously with whole blood or blood products; hemolysis may occur.
- I.V. ethacrynate sodium has been used to treat hypercalcemia and to manage ethylene glycol poisoning and bromide intoxication.

Therapeutic monitoring
- Periodically assess hearing function in patients receiving high-dose therapy. Ethacrynic acid may potentiate ototoxicity of other medications.

Special populations
Pregnant patients. Use drug during pregnancy only when clearly indicated.
Breast-feeding patients. Don't use drug in breast-feeding women.
Pediatric patients. Ethacrynate sodium and ethacrynic acid shouldn't be administered to infants. Safety in children hasn't been established.
Geriatric patients. Geriatric and debilitated patients require close observation because they're more susceptible to drug-induced diuresis. Excessive diuresis promotes rapid dehydration, leading to hypovolemia, hypokalemia, hyponatremia, and circulatory collapse. Reduced dosages may be indicated.

Patient counseling
- Advise patient receiving I.V. form of drug to report pain or irritation at I.V. site immediately.
- Notify diabetic patient that antidiabetic dosage may need to be increased.

ethambutol hydrochloride
Myambutol

Pharmacologic classification: semisynthetic antitubercular
Therapeutic classification: antitubercular
Pregnancy risk category NR

How supplied
Available by prescription only
Tablets: 100 mg, 400 mg

Indications and dosages
Adjunctive treatment in pulmonary tuberculosis
Adults and children age 13 and older: Initial treatment for patients who haven't received previous antitubercular therapy, 15 mg/kg P.O. daily single dose. Retreatment: 25 mg/kg P.O. daily single dose for 60 days with at least one other antitubercular drug; then decrease to 15 mg/kg P.O. daily single dose.

Pharmacodynamics
Antitubercular action: Ethambutol is bacteriostatic; it interferes with mycolic acid incorporation into the mycobacterial cell wall. Ethambutol is active against *Mycobacterium tuberculosis, M. bovis,* and *M. marinum,* some strains of *M. kansasii, M. avium, M. fortuitum,* and *M. intracellulare,* and the combined strain of *M. avium* and *M. intracellulare* (MAC). Ethambutol is considered adjunctive therapy in tuberculosis and is combined with other antitubercular agents to prevent or delay development of drug resistance by *M. tuberculosis.*

Pharmacokinetics
Absorption: Absorbed rapidly from the GI tract.
Distribution: Distributed widely into body tissues and fluids, especially into lungs, erythrocytes, saliva, and kidneys; lesser amounts distribute into brain, ascitic, pleural, and cerebrospinal fluids. Ethambutol is 8% to 22% protein-bound.
Metabolism: Undergoes partial hepatic metabolism.
Excretion: After 24 hours, about 50% of unchanged ethambutol and 8% to 15% of its metabolites are excreted in urine; 20% to 25% is excreted in feces. Small amounts of drug may be excreted in breast milk. Plasma half-life in adults is about 3¼ hours; half-life is prolonged in decreased renal or hepatic function. Ethambutol can be removed by peritoneal dialysis and, to a lesser extent, by hemodialysis.

Route	Onset	Peak	Duration
P.O.	Unknown	2-4 hr	Unknown

Contraindications and precautions
Contraindicated in children under age 13 and in patients with optic neuritis or hypersensitivity to drug. Use cautiously in patients with impaired renal function, cataracts, recurrent eye inflammations, gout, and diabetic retinopathy.

Interactions
Drug-drug. *Agents that produce neurotoxicity:* Increased neurotoxic effects. Avoid use together.
Aluminum salts: May delay and reduce the absorption of ethambutol. Separate administration times by several hours.

Effects on diagnostic tests
None reported.

Adverse reactions
CNS: headache, malaise, dizziness, mental confusion, possible hallucinations, peripheral neuritis (numbness and tingling of extremities).
EENT: optic neuritis (related to dose and duration of treatment).
GI: anorexia, nausea, vomiting, abdominal pain, GI upset.
Hematologic: ***thrombocytopenia.***
Hepatic: abnormal liver function tests.
Metabolic: elevated uric acid level.
Musculoskeletal: joint pain, precipitation of acute gout.
Respiratory: bloody sputum.
Skin: dermatitis, pruritus, toxic epidermal necrolysis.
Other: ***anaphylactoid reactions,*** fever.

Overdose and treatment
No specific recommendation is available. Treatment is supportive. After recent ingestion (4 hours or less), empty stomach by induced emesis or gastric lavage. Follow with activated charcoal to decrease absorption.

Clinical considerations
- Drug can be given with food if necessary to prevent gastric irritation; food doesn't interfere with absorption.
- Specimens for culture and sensitivity testing should be collected before first dose, but therapy can begin before test results are complete; repeat periodically to detect drug resistance.

Therapeutic monitoring
- Assess visual status before therapy; test visual acuity and color discrimination monthly in patients taking more than 15 mg/kg/day. Visual disturbances are dose-related and reversible if detected in time.
- Recommend monitoring blood (including serum uric acid), renal, and liver function studies before and periodically during therapy to minimize toxicity.
- Monitor for change in renal function. Dosage reduction may be necessary.

Special populations
Pregnant patients. Use drug during pregnancy only when benefits justify risk to the fetus.
Breast-feeding patients. Drug is excreted in breast milk. Use cautiously in breast-feeding women.
Pediatric patients. Drug isn't recommended for use in children under age 13.

Patient counseling
- Inform patient of the potential for hypersensitivity and other adverse reactions, and emphasize need to report these reactions. Urge patient to report any unusual effects, especially blurred vision, red-green color blindness, or changes in urine elimination.
- Assure patient that visual alterations will disappear within several weeks or months after drug is discontinued.
- Urge patient to complete the prescribed regimen, to comply with instructions for daily dosage, to avoid missing doses, and not to discontinue drug without medical approval. Explain importance of keeping follow-up appointments.

ethinyl estradiol
Estinyl

Pharmacologic classification: estrogen
Therapeutic classification: estrogen replacement, antineoplastic
Pregnancy risk category X

How supplied
Available by prescription only
Tablets: 0.02 mg, 0.05 mg

Indications and dosages
Palliative treatment of metastatic breast cancer (at least 5 years after menopause)
Adults: 1 mg P.O. t.i.d. for at least 3 months.
Female hypogonadism
Adults: 0.05 mg P.O. daily to t.i.d. for 2 weeks monthly, followed by 2 weeks progesterone therapy; continue for three to six monthly dosing cycles, followed by 2 months off.
Vasomotor menopausal symptoms
Adults: 0.02 to 0.05 mg P.O. daily for cycles of 3 weeks on, 1 week off.
Palliative treatment of metastatic inoperable prostatic cancer
Adults: 0.15 to 2 mg P.O. daily.

Pharmacodynamics
Estrogenic action: Ethinyl estradiol mimics the action of endogenous estrogen in treating female hypogonadism and menopausal symptoms. It inhibits growth of hormone-sensitive tissue in advanced, inoperable prostatic can-

cer and in certain carefully selected cases of breast cancer in men and postmenopausal women.

Pharmacokinetics

Absorption: After oral administration, estradiol is well absorbed but substantially inactivated by the liver.
Distribution: About 50% to 80% plasma protein-bound, particularly estradiol-binding globulin. Distribution occurs throughout the body, with highest levels appearing in fat.
Metabolism: Steroidal estrogens, including estradiol, are metabolized primarily in the liver, where they are conjugated with sulfate and glucuronide. Because of the rapid rate of metabolism, nonesterified forms of estrogen, including estradiol, must usually be administered daily.
Excretion: The majority of estrogen elimination occurs through the kidneys in the form of sulfate or glucuronide conjugates.

Route	Onset	Peak	Duration
P.O.	Unknown	Unknown	Unknown

Contraindications and precautions

Contraindicated in patients with thrombophlebitis or thromboembolic disorders, estrogen-dependent neoplasia, breast or reproductive organ cancer (except for palliative treatment), and undiagnosed abnormal genital bleeding and during pregnancy.

Use cautiously in patients with cerebrovascular or coronary artery disease, asthma, mental depression, bone disease, or cardiac, hepatic, or renal dysfunction and in women with a family history (mother, grandmother, sister) of breast or genital tract cancer or who have breast nodules, fibrocystic disease, or abnormal mammographic findings.

Interactions

Drug-drug. *Drugs that induce hepatic metabolism (such as barbiturates, carbamazepine, primidone, and rifampin):* May result in decreased estrogenic effects from a given dose. These drugs are known to accelerate the rate of metabolism of certain other agents. Use together cautiously.
Insulin or oral antidiabetic agents: May require dosage adjustment as a result of effects of blood glucose level.
Warfarin-type anticoagulants: Decreased anticoagulant effect. Dosage adjustment may be necessary.
Cyclosporine: Increased risk of toxicity. Recommend monitoring cyclosporine levels.
Dantrolene, other hepatotoxic medications: May increase risk of hepatotoxicity.
Tamoxifen: Decreased effects of tamoxifen. Monitor patient closely.
Drug-food. *Caffeine:* May increase serum caffeine levels. Advise patient to avoid caffeine.
Drug-lifestyle. *Smoking:* Increases risk of adverse CV effects. Advise patient to avoid smoking.

Effects on diagnostic tests

None reported.

Adverse reactions

CNS: headache, dizziness, chorea, depression, *seizures.*
CV: thrombophlebitis; ***thromboembolism;*** hypertension; edema; ***increased risk of CVA, pulmonary embolism, MI.***
EENT: worsening of myopia or astigmatism, intolerance of contact lenses.
GI: *nausea,* vomiting, abdominal cramps, bloating, anorexia, increased appetite, gallbladder disease.
GU: in women, breakthrough bleeding, altered menstrual flow, dysmenorrhea, amenorrhea, ***increased risk of endometrial cancer, possibility of increased risk of breast cancer,*** cervical erosion, altered cervical secretions, enlargement of uterine fibromas, vaginal candidiasis, breast changes (tenderness, enlargement, secretion); in men, gynecomastia, testicular atrophy, impotence.
Hematologic: increased PT and INR and clotting factors VII to X, and norepinephrine-induced platelet aggregability.
Hepatic: cholestatic jaundice, ***hepatic adenoma.***
Metabolic: decreased serum folate, pyridoxine, and antithrombin III levels; increased triglyceride, glucose, and phospholipid levels; hypercalcemia, weight changes.
Skin: melasma, urticaria, flushing (with rapid I.V. administration), hirsutism or hair loss, erythema nodosum, dermatitis.

Overdose and treatment

Serious toxicity after overdose of this drug hasn't been reported. Nausea may occur. Provide appropriate supportive care.

Clinical considerations

Consider the recommendations relevant to all other estrogens. Because of risk of thromboembolism, discontinue drug therapy at least 1 month before procedures associated with prolonged immobilization or thromboembolism.

Therapeutic monitoring

- Monitor patient for adverse reactions.
- Recommend periodically monitoring serum lipid levels, blood pressure, body weight, and hepatic function as ordered.

Special populations

Pregnant patients. Drug is contraindicated for use during pregnancy.
Breast-feeding patients. Drug is contraindicated in breast-feeding women.

Geriatric patients. Use with caution in patients whose condition may be aggravated by fluid retention.

Patient counseling

- Provide patient with a package insert describing adverse reactions of estrogen as well as a verbal explanation.
- Emphasize importance of regular physical examinations.
- Warn patient to immediately report abdominal pain; pain, numbness, or stiffness in legs or buttocks; pressure or pain in chest; shortness of breath; severe headaches; visual disturbances such as blind spots, flashing lights, or blurriness; vaginal bleeding or discharge; breast lumps; swelling of hands or feet; yellow skin or sclera; dark urine; or light-colored stools.
- Tell diabetic patient to report elevated blood glucose test results; antidiabetic medication dosage may be adjusted.

ethosuximide

Zarontin

Pharmacologic classification: succinimide derivative
Therapeutic classification: anticonvulsant
Pregnancy risk category C

How supplied

Available by prescription only
Capsules: 250 mg
Syrup: 250 mg/5 ml

Indications and dosages

Absence seizures
Adults and children age 6 and older: Initially, 250 mg P.O. b.i.d. May increase by 250 mg q 4 to 7 days up to 1.5 g daily.
Children age 3 to 6: 250 mg P.O. daily. Optimal dose is 20 mg/kg/day.

Pharmacodynamics

Anticonvulsant action: Ethosuximide raises the seizure threshold; it suppresses characteristic spike-and-wave pattern by depressing neuronal transmission in the motor cortex and basal ganglia. It's indicated for absence seizures refractory to other drugs.

Pharmacokinetics

Absorption: Absorbed from the GI tract; steady-state plasma levels occur in 4 to 7 days.
Distribution: Distributed widely throughout the body; protein binding is minimal.
Metabolism: Metabolized extensively in the liver to several inactive metabolites.
Excretion: Excreted in urine, with small amounts in bile and feces. Plasma half-life is about 60 hours in adults and about 30 hours in children.

Route	Onset	Peak	Duration
P.O.	Unknown	3-7 hr	Unknown

Contraindications and precautions

Contraindicated in patients with hypersensitivity to succinimide derivatives. Use with extreme caution in patients with hepatic or renal disease.

Interactions

Drug-drug. *Other CNS depressants (anxiolytics, antidepressants, antipsychotics, other anticonvulsants, narcotics):* Additive CNS depression and sedation. Monitor patient closely.
Phenytoin: Increased serum phenytoin levels. Monitor patient carefully.
Valproic acid: Increased or decreased serum levels of ethosuximide. Monitor patient closely.
Drug-lifestyle. *Alcohol use:* Additive CNS depression and sedation. Advise patient to avoid alcohol.

Effects on diagnostic tests

Ethosuximide may cause false-positive Coombs' test results. May also cause abnormal results of renal function tests.

Adverse reactions

CNS: *drowsiness, headache, fatigue, dizziness, ataxia, irritability, hiccups, euphoria, lethargy, depression, psychosis.*
EENT: myopia, tongue swelling, gingival hyperplasia.
GI: *nausea, vomiting, diarrhea, weight loss, cramps, anorexia, epigastric and abdominal pain.*
GU: vaginal bleeding, urinary frequency, abnormal renal function tests.
Hematologic: *leukopenia,* eosinophilia, ***agranulocytosis,*** pancytopenia.
Hepatic: elevated liver enzyme levels.
Skin: urticaria, pruritic and erythematous rash, hirsutism, ***Stevens-Johnson syndrome.***

Overdose and treatment

Symptoms of ethosuximide overdose, when used alone or with other anticonvulsants, include CNS depression, ataxia, stupor, and coma. Treatment is symptomatic and supportive. Carefully monitor vital signs and fluid and electrolyte balance.

Clinical considerations

- Administer ethosuximide with food to minimize GI distress.
- Abrupt discontinuation of drug may precipitate petit mal seizures.

Therapeutic monitoring

- Observe patient for dermatologic reactions, joint pain, unexplained fever, or unusual bruis-

ing or bleeding (which may signal hematologic or other severe adverse reactions).
- Recommend performing CBC, liver function tests, and urinalysis periodically.
- Therapeutic plasma levels range from 40 to 100 mcg/ml.

Special populations

Pregnant patients. Safety hasn't been established.
Breast-feeding patients. Safety hasn't been established. Advise nursing women to use alternative feeding method during therapy with ethosuximide.
Pediatric patients. Don't use drug in children under age 3.
Geriatric patients. Use with caution in geriatric patients.

Patient counseling

- Advise patient to take drug with food or milk to prevent GI distress, to avoid use with alcoholic beverages, and to avoid hazardous tasks that require alertness if drug causes drowsiness, dizziness, or blurred vision.
- Inform patient that drug may color urine pink to reddish-brown.
- Tell patient to report to prescriber the following effects: rash, joint pain, fever, sore throat, or unusual bleeding or bruising.
- Advise patient to contact prescriber immediately if pregnancy is suspected.

etidronate disodium

Didronel

Pharmacologic classification: pyrophosphate analogue
Therapeutic classification: antihypercalcemic
Pregnancy risk category C

How supplied

Available by prescription only
Tablets: 200 mg, 400 mg
Injection: 50 mg/ml (300-mg ampule)

Indications and dosages

Symptomatic Paget's disease
Adults: 5 mg/kg P.O. daily as a single dose 2 hours before a meal with water or juice. Patient shouldn't eat, consume milk or milk products, or take antacids or vitamins with mineral supplements for 2 hours after dose. May give up to 10 mg/kg/day in severe cases, not to exceed 6 months. Maximum dose is 20 mg/kg/day, not to exceed 3 months.
Heterotopic ossification in spinal cord injuries
Adults: 20 mg/kg/day P.O. for 2 weeks, then 10 mg/kg/day for 10 weeks. Total treatment period is 12 weeks.
Heterotopic ossification after total hip replacement
Adults: 20 mg/kg/day P.O. for 1 month before total hip replacement and for 3 months afterward.
Hypercalcemia associated with malignancy
Adults: 7.5 mg/kg I.V. daily for 3 days. May repeat up to 7 days. Then wait 7 days before beginning a second course of treatment.

Pharmacodynamics

Bone-metabolism inhibitor action: Although the exact mechanism isn't known, etidronate acts on bone by adsorbing to hydroxyapatite crystals in the bone, thereby inhibiting their growth and dissolution. It also decreases the number of osteoclasts in bone, thereby slowing excessive remodeling of pagetic or heterotopic bone.

Pharmacokinetics

Absorption: Absorption following an oral dose is variable and is decreased in the presence of food. Absorption may also be dose-related.
Distribution: About half of the dose is distributed to bone.
Metabolism: Not metabolized.
Excretion: About 50% of drug is excreted within 24 hours in urine.

Route	Onset	Peak	Duration
P.O.	1 mo (in Paget's)	Unknown	Unknown
I.V.	24 hr	After 3rd infusion	Unknown

Contraindications and precautions

Contraindicated in patients with known hypersensitivity to drug or in those with clinically overt osteomalacia. Use cautiously in patients with impaired renal function.

Interactions

Drug-drug. *Antacids containing calcium, magnesium, or aluminum; mineral supplements containing calcium, iron, magnesium, or aluminum:* Can inhibit absorption. Avoid use within 2 hours of dose.
Drug-food. *Foods containing large amounts of calcium, such as milk and dairy products:* Can prevent oral absorption. Avoid use within 2 hours of dose.

Effects on diagnostic tests

None reported.

Adverse reactions

CNS: ***seizures.***
GI: reactions occur most frequently at dosage of 20 mg/kg daily—diarrhea, increased frequency of bowel movements, nausea, constipation, stomatitis.
Hepatic: abnormal hepatic function.
Metabolic: *elevated serum phosphate level.*

Musculoskeletal: increased or recurrent bone pain, pain at previously asymptomatic sites, increased risk of fracture.
Respiratory: dyspnea.
Other: fever, fluid overload, *hypersensitivity reactions.*

Overdose and treatment
Signs and symptoms of overdose include diarrhea, nausea, and hypocalcemia. Treat with gastric lavage and emesis. Administer calcium if required.

Clinical considerations
Drug should be taken in a single dose. However, if nausea occurs, dosage may be divided.

Therapeutic monitoring
Monitor drug effect by serum alkaline phosphate and urinary hydroxyproline excretion; both are lowered by effective therapy.

Special populations
Pregnant patients. Use drug during pregnancy only when clearly indicated.
Breast-feeding patients. Use drug with caution in breast-feeding women.
Pediatric patients. Safety and efficacy for use in children haven't been established.

Patient counseling
- Instruct patient to take drug on an empty stomach with water or juice and to avoid food, milk or milk products, antacids, and vitamins with mineral supplements for 2 hours.
- Remind patient that improvement may take at least 3 months and may continue even after the drug is stopped.

etodolac
Lodine, Lodine XL

Pharmacologic classification: NSAID
Therapeutic classification: antiarthritic
Pregnancy risk category C

How supplied
Available by prescription only
Capsules: 200 mg, 300 mg
Tablets: 400 mg
Tablets (extended-release): 400 mg, 500 mg, 600 mg

Indications and dosages
Acute and chronic management of osteoarthritis, rheumatoid arthritis, and pain
Adults: For acute pain, give 200 to 400 mg P.O. q 6 to 8 hours, p.r.n., not to exceed 1,200 mg daily. For patients weighing 132 lb (60 kg) or less, total daily dose shouldn't exceed 20 mg/kg.

For osteoarthritis or rheumatoid arthritis, give 800 to 1,200 mg P.O. daily in divided doses initially, followed by adjustments of 600 to 1,200 mg in divided doses: 200 mg P.O. t.i.d. or q.i.d.; 300 mg P.O. b.i.d., t.i.d., or q.i.d.; 400 mg P.O. b.i.d. or t.i.d. Total daily dose shouldn't exceed 1,200 mg. For patients weighing 132 lb or less, total daily dose shouldn't exceed 20 mg/kg, or 400 to 1,000 mg P.O. daily (extended-release form). Adjust dosage to lowest effective dose based on patient response. Don't exceed maximum dose of 1,000 mg daily.

Pharmacodynamics
Antiarthritic action: Mechanism of action is unknown but is presumed to be associated with inhibition of prostaglandin biosynthesis.

Pharmacokinetics
Absorption: Well-absorbed from GI tract. Antacids don't appear to affect absorption of etodolac; however, they can decrease peak levels reached by 15% to 20% but have no effect when peak levels are reached.
Distribution: Found in liver, lungs, heart, and kidneys.
Metabolism: Extensively metabolized in the liver.
Excretion: Excreted in urine primarily as metabolites; 16% is excreted in feces.

Route	Onset	Peak	Duration
P.O.	30 min	1-2 hr	4-12 hr
P.O. (extended)	Unknown	3-12 hr	6-12 hr

Contraindications and precautions
Contraindicated in patients with hypersensitivity to drug and in those with history of aspirin- or NSAID-induced asthma, rhinitis, urticaria, or other allergic reactions.

Use cautiously in patients with impaired renal or hepatic function, history of peptic ulcer disease, cardiac disease, hypertension, or conditions associated with fluid retention.

Interactions
Drug-drug. *Antacids:* Decreased peak levels of the drug. Monitor patient for decreased effects of etodolac.
Aspirin: Reduces protein-binding of etodolac without altering its clearance and may increase GI toxicity. Avoid use together.
Cyclosporine: Impaired elimination and increased risk of nephrotoxicity. Avoid use together.
Digoxin, lithium, and methotrexate: Increased levels of these drugs. Monitor drug levels.
Diuretics and beta blockers: May blunt effects of drug. Monitor patient carefully.
Phenytoin: Increased serum levels of phenytoin. Monitor patient for signs of toxicity.
Warfarin: Decreased protein-binding of warfarin but doesn't change its clearance. No dosage adjustment is necessary, but monitor INR and watch for bleeding.

Drug-lifestyle. *Alcohol use:* Increases risk of adverse effects. Advise patient to avoid alcohol.
Sun exposure: Photosensitivity reactions may result from sun exposure. Advise patient to take precautions.

Effects on diagnostic tests
A false-positive test for urinary bilirubin may be caused by phenolic metabolites.

Adverse reactions
CNS: *asthenia, malaise, dizziness,* depression, drowsiness, nervousness, insomnia.
CV: hypertension, ***heart failure,*** syncope, flushing, palpitations, edema, fluid retention.
EENT: blurred vision, tinnitus, photophobia, dry mouth.
GI: *dyspepsia, flatulence, abdominal pain, diarrhea, nausea,* constipation, gastritis, melena, vomiting, anorexia, peptic ulceration with or without *GI bleeding* or perforation, ulcerative stomatitis, thirst.
GU: dysuria, urinary frequency, ***renal failure.***
Hematologic: anemia (rare), ***leukopenia, thrombocytopenia,*** hemolytic anemia, ***agranulocytosis.***
Hepatic: elevated liver function tests, ***hepatitis.***
Metabolic: decreased serum uric acid levels, weight gain.
Respiratory: asthma.
Skin: pruritus, rash, ***Stevens-Johnson syndrome.***
Other: chills, fever.

Overdose and treatment
Signs of overdose include lethargy, drowsiness, nausea, vomiting, and epigastric pain. Rare symptoms include GI bleeding, coma, renal failure, hypertension, and anaphylaxis. Treatment is symptomatic and supportive, including stomach decontamination.

Clinical considerations
- Use caution with concurrent use of diuretics in patients with cardiac, renal, or hepatic failure.
- Etodolac 1,200 mg was shown to cause less GI bleeding than ibuprofen 2,400 mg daily, indomethacin 200 mg daily, naproxen 750 mg daily, or piroxicam 20 mg daily.

Therapeutic monitoring
- Monitor for signs and symptoms of GI ulceration and bleeding.
- In chronic conditions, a therapeutic response to therapy is most often seen within 2 weeks.

Special populations
Pregnant patients. Avoid drug during third trimester.
Breast-feeding patients. It's unknown if drug is excreted in breast milk. Use cautiously.
Pediatric patients. Safety and efficacy haven't been established in children under age 18.
Geriatric patients. Drug is well tolerated in older and younger adults and generally doesn't require age-related dosage adjustments. No age-related differences have been reported.

Patient counseling
- Advise patient of the potential for adverse events and instruct him to report to prescriber any GI effects of drug.
- Tell patient that drug may be taken with food.

etoposide
Toposar, VePesid

Pharmacologic classification: podophyllotoxin (cell cycle-phase specific, G2 and late S phases)
Therapeutic classification: antineoplastic
Pregnancy risk category D

How supplied
Available by prescription only
Capsules: 50 mg
Injection: 20 mg/ml multiple-dose vials

Indications and dosages
Dosage and indications may vary. Check literature for current protocol.
Small-cell carcinoma of the lung
Adults: 70 mg/m^2/day P.O. (rounded to the nearest 50 mg) for 4 days; or 100 mg/m^2 P.O. (rounded to the nearest 50 mg) daily for 5 days. Repeat q 3 to 4 weeks. Alternatively, 35 mg/m^2 I.V. daily for 4 days or 50 mg/m^2 I.V. daily for 5 days. Repeat q 3 to 4 weeks.
Testicular carcinoma
Adults: 50 to 100 mg/m^2 I.V. daily on days 1 to 5; or 100 mg/m^2/day on days 1, 3, and 5 of a regimen repeated q 3 or 4 weeks.
◇***AIDS-related Kaposi's sarcoma***
Adults: 150 mg/m^2 daily I.V. for 3 consecutive days every 4 weeks. Repeat cycles as necessary.
≡***Dosage adjustment.*** Dosage reduction may be required in patients with impaired renal function.

Pharmacodynamics
Antineoplastic action: Etoposide exerts its cytotoxic action by arresting cells in the metaphase portion of cell division. Drug also inhibits cells from entering mitosis and depresses DNA and RNA synthesis.

Pharmacokinetics
Absorption: Only moderately absorbed across the GI tract after oral administration. Etoposide's bioavailability ranges from 25% to 75%, with an average of 50% of the dose being absorbed.

Distribution: Distributed widely into body tissues; the highest levels are found in the liver, spleen, kidneys, healthy brain tissue, and brain tumor tissue. It crosses the blood-brain barrier to a limited and variable extent. Etoposide is about 94% bound to serum albumin.
Metabolism: Only a small portion of a dose of etoposide is metabolized. Metabolism occurs in the liver.
Excretion: Excreted primarily in the urine as unchanged drug. A smaller portion of a dose is excreted in the feces. The plasma elimination of etoposide is described as biphasic, with an initial phase half-life of about ½ to 2 hours and a terminal phase of about 5¼ to 11 hours.

Route	Onset	Peak	Duration
P.O., I.V.	Unknown	Unknown	Unknown

Contraindications and precautions
Contraindicated in patients hypersensitive to drug. Use cautiously in patients who have had cytotoxic or radiation therapy.

Interactions
Drug-drug. *Cisplatin:* Etoposide increases cytotoxicity of cisplatin against certain tumors. May be used for this purpose.
Warfarin: Concurrent administration may cause elongation of PT and INR. Monitor patient closely.

Effects on diagnostic tests
None reported.

Adverse reactions
CNS: peripheral neuropathy.
CV: hypotension (from too-rapid infusion).
GI: *nausea and vomiting, anorexia, diarrhea,* abdominal pain, *stomatitis.*
Hematologic: *anemia,* ***myelosuppression*** (dose-limiting), **LEUKOPENIA, THROMBOCYTOPENIA.**
Other: *reversible alopecia,* ***anaphylaxis*** (rare), phlebitis at injection site (infrequent).

Overdose and treatment
Signs and symptoms of overdose include myelosuppression, nausea, and vomiting. Treatment is usually supportive and includes transfusion of blood components, antiemetics, and appropriate symptomatic therapy.

Clinical considerations
- Pretreatment with antiemetics may reduce frequency and duration of nausea and vomiting.
- At doses below 200 mg, extent of absorption after oral administration isn't affected by food.
- Have diphenhydramine, hydrocortisone, epinephrine, and airway available in case of an anaphylactic reaction.
- Etoposide has produced complete remissions in small-cell lung cancer and testicular cancer.

Therapeutic monitoring
- Monitor blood pressure before infusion and at 30-minute intervals during infusion. If systolic blood pressure goes below 90 mm Hg, stop infusion.
- Monitor CBC. Drug shouldn't be given if platelet count is less than 50,000/mm^3 or absolute neutrophil count is less than 500/mm^3.
- GI toxicity occurs more frequently after oral administration.

Special populations
Pregnant patients. High risk for fetal harm. During pregnancy, use drug only for life-threatening conditions or severe disease when much safer drugs aren't available or are ineffective.
Breast-feeding patients. Because drug is excreted into breast milk, its use in breast-feeding women isn't recommended.
Pediatric patients. Safety and effectiveness in children haven't been established.
Geriatric patients. Geriatric patients may be particularly susceptible to the hypotensive effects of etoposide.

Patient counseling
- Advise patient of potential adverse reactions and instruct to contact prescriber immediately if vomiting occurs shortly after dose.
- Advise patient to report to prescriber sore throat, fever, or unusual bruising or bleeding.
- Advise patient to avoid exposure to people with infections.
- Tell patient not to receive immunizations during therapy with etoposide and that other family members also shouldn't receive immunizations during duration of therapy.
- Advise patient to use contraceptive measures during therapy.

etoposide phosphate
Etopophos

Pharmacologic classification: semisynthetic derivative of podophyllotoxin
Therapeutic classification: antineoplastic
Pregnancy risk category D

How supplied
Available by prescription only
Capsules: 50 mg
Injection: Vials containing etoposide phosphate equivalent to 100 mg etoposide/5 ml

Indications and dosages
Adjunct treatment of refractory testicular cancer
Adults: Etoposide phosphate doses equivalent to 50 to 100 mg/m^2/day of etoposide I.V. on

days 1 through 5 of each cycle and given in conjunction with other approved chemotherapeutic agents. Cycle is repeated when adequate recovery from drug toxicity has occurred (usually at 3- to 4-week intervals). Alternatively, etoposide phosphate doses equivalent to 100 mg/m²/day of etoposide I.V. on days 1, 3, and 5 of each cycle and given in conjunction with other approved chemotherapeutic agents. Cycle is repeated at 3- to 4-week intervals if adequate recovery from drug toxicity has occurred. Infusion rate may range from 5 minutes to 210 minutes, or VePesid may be given P.O. Recommended dose is two times the I.V. dose rounded to the nearest 50 mg.

Adjunct treatment of small-cell lung cancer
Adults: Dosage is individualized but may range from etoposide phosphate doses equivalent to 35 mg/m²/day etoposide I.V. for 4 days to etoposide phosphate doses equivalent to 50 mg/m²/day etoposide I.V. for 5 days and given in conjunction with other approved chemotherapeutic agents. Cycle is repeated when adequate recovery from drug toxicity has occurred (usually at 3- to 4-week intervals). Infusion rate may range from 5 minutes to 210 minutes.

◊***AIDS-related Kaposi's sarcoma***
Adults: 150 mg/m² daily I.V. for 3 consecutive days every 4 weeks. Repeat cycles as necessary.

≡***Dosage adjustment.*** In patients with renal failure with creatinine clearance above 50 ml/minute, give usual dosage; for creatinine clearance between 15 and 50 ml/minute, give 75% of usual dosage.

Pharmacodynamics

Antineoplastic action: Although action of drug is unknown, it's believed to exert cytotoxicity by arresting cells in the metaphase portion of cell division. Drug may also inhibit cells from entering mitosis and depressing DNA and RNA synthesis.

Pharmacokinetics

Absorption: Only administered as an I.V. infusion.
Distribution: Distribution is believed to be similar to etoposide. Etoposide crosses the blood-brain barrier to a limited and variable extent and is about 97% bound to serum albumin.
Metabolism: Rapidly and completely converted to etoposide in plasma.
Excretion: After etoposide phosphate is converted to etoposide, etoposide is excreted primarily in the urine as unchanged drug. A smaller portion of a dose is excreted in the feces. The plasma elimination of etoposide is described as biphasic, with an initial phase half-life of about ½ to 2 hours and a terminal phase of about 5¼ to 11 hours.

Route	Onset	Peak	Duration
P.O., I.V.	Unknown	Unknown	Unknown

Contraindications and precautions

Contraindicated in patients with history of hypersensitivity to etoposide phosphate, etoposide, or other components of the formulation.

Interactions

Drug-drug. *High-dose cyclosporine:* May increase the toxic effects of etoposide phosphate because of delayed excretion of the drug. Monitor patient closely for drug effects.
Levamisole hydrochloride: Known to inhibit phosphatase activities. Avoid using any drug known to inhibit phosphatase activities.
Warfarin: Prolonged PT and INR. Monitor patient carefully.

Effects on diagnostic tests

None reported.

Adverse reactions

CNS: *asthenia, malaise,* dizziness, peripheral neurotoxicity.
CV: hypertension, hypotension.
GI: *nausea, vomiting, anorexia, mucositis,* constipation, abdominal pain, diarrhea, taste alteration.
Hematologic: *anemia,* ***myelosuppression*** (dose-limiting), **LEUKOPENIA, THROMBOCYTOPENIA, NEUTROPENIA.**
Skin: facial flushing, rash.
Other: *reversible alopecia, chills, fever,* phlebitis, ***anaphylaxis.***

Overdose and treatment

Because etoposide phosphate is rapidly converted to etoposide, signs and symptoms of overdose would be expected to be similar. Signs of overdose of etoposide include myelosuppression, nausea, and vomiting. Treatment is usually supportive and includes transfusion of blood components, antiemetics, and appropriate symptomatic therapy.

Clinical considerations

- Use of gloves is recommended when handling etoposide phosphate. If etoposide phosphate solution comes into contact with the skin or mucosa, immediately and thoroughly wash the skin with soap and water and flush the mucosa with water.
- After reconstitution, solution may be administered without further dilution or it can be further diluted to levels as low as 0.1 mg/ml etoposide with either D_5W injection or normal saline solution.
- Patients with low serum albumin may be at an increased risk for etoposide-associated toxicities.

Therapeutic monitoring

- Monitor CBC. Observe patient for signs of bone marrow depression. Withhold drug if platelet count is less than 50,000/mm^3 or absolute neutrophil count is less than 500/mm^3 until the blood counts have sufficiently recovered.
- Advise prescriber if an anaphylactic reaction occurs, terminate infusion immediately and administer pressor agents, corticosteroids, antihistamines, or volume expanders, as needed.

Special populations

Pregnant patients. High risk for fetal harm. During pregnancy, use drug only for life-threatening conditions or severe disease when much safer drugs aren't available or are ineffective.
Breast-feeding patients. Drug isn't contraindicated in breast-feeding women.
Pediatric patients. Safety and efficacy in children haven't been established. Anaphylactic reactions have been reported in pediatric patients who received etoposide.
Geriatric patients. Geriatric patients may be particularly susceptible to the hypotensive effects of etoposide.

Patient counseling

- Advise patient to avoid exposure to people with infections.
- Tell patient to promptly report a sore throat, fever, unusual bruising, or bleeding.
- Reassure patient that hair should grow back after treatment has ended.
- Tell patient to store capsules in refrigerator.

F

famciclovir

Famvir

Pharmacologic classification: synthetic acyclic guanine derivative
Therapeutic classification: antiviral
Pregnancy risk category B

How supplied

Available by prescription only
Tablets: 125 mg, 250 mg, 500 mg

Indications and dosages

Management of acute herpes zoster in immunocompromised patients
Adults: 500 mg P.O. q 8 hours for 7 days.
≡ ***Dosage adjustment.*** In adults with reduced renal function, adjust dosage using this table.

Creatinine clearance (ml/min)	Dosage
≥ 60	500 mg q 8 hr
40 to 59	500 mg q 12 hr
20 to 39	500 mg q 24 hr
< 20	250 mg q 48 hr

Recurrent genital herpes in immunocompromised patients
Adults: 125 mg P.O. b.i.d. for 5 days.
≡ ***Dosage adjustment.*** In adults with reduced renal function, adjust dosage using this table.

Creatinine clearance (ml/min)	Dosage
≥ 40	125 mg q 12 hr
20 to 39	125 mg q 24 hr
< 20	125 mg q 48 hr

◊ ***Chronic suppression or maintenance prophylaxis of HSV infection in HIV-infected patients***
Adults: 500 mg P.O. b.i.d.

Pharmacodynamics

Antiviral action: Famciclovir, a prodrug, changes to an active antiviral compound, penciclovir. It enters viral cells (herpes simplex types 1 and 2, varicella zoster), where it inhibits DNA polymerase, viral DNA synthesis, and, thus, viral replication.

Pharmacokinetics

Absorption: Absolute bioavailability of famciclovir is 77%. Because bioavailability isn't affected by food intake, the drug can be taken without regard to meals.
Distribution: Less than 20% protein-bound.
Metabolism: Extensively metabolized in the liver to the active drug penciclovir (98.5%) and other inactive metabolites.
Excretion: Primarily eliminated in the urine.

Route	Onset	Peak	Duration
P.O.	Unknown	1 hr	Unknown

Contraindications and precautions

Contraindicated in patients with hypersensitivity to drug. Use cautiously in patients with impaired renal or hepatic function.

Interactions

Drug-drug. *Probenecid or other drugs significantly eliminated by active renal tubular secretion:* May result in increased plasma levels of penciclovir. Monitor patient for increased adverse effects.

Effects on diagnostic tests

May interfere with cross-matching studies or hematologic studies.

Adverse reactions

CNS: headache, fatigue, dizziness, paresthesia, somnolence.
EENT: pharyngitis, sinusitis.
GI: diarrhea, nausea, vomiting, constipation, anorexia, abdominal pain.
Musculoskeletal: back pain, arthralgia.
Skin: pruritus; zoster-related signs, symptoms, and complications.
Other: fever, injury, pain, rigors.

Overdose and treatment

No acute overdose reported. Give symptomatic and supportive therapy. It isn't known if hemodialysis removes famciclovir from the blood. However, hemodialysis enhances elimination of acyclovir, a related nucleoside analogue.

Clinical considerations

Drug may be given without regard to meals.

Therapeutic monitoring
Recommend monitoring renal and liver function tests.

Special populations
Pregnant patients. Use drug during pregnancy only when clearly indicated.
Breast-feeding patients. It isn't known if drug is excreted in breast milk. Use drug with caution in breast-feeding women.
Pediatric patients. Safety and effectiveness haven't been established in children under age 18.

Patient counseling
- Explain that treatment is more effective when started within 48 hours of rash onset.
- Inform patient that drug isn't a cure for genital herpes but can decrease the duration and severity of symptoms.
- Advise patient of potential adverse reactions.

famotidine
Pepcid, Pepcid AC

Pharmacologic classification: H_2-receptor antagonist
Therapeutic classification: antiulcer
Pregnancy risk category B

How supplied
Available by prescription only
Tablets: 20 mg, 40 mg
Injection: 10 mg/ml
Injection, premixed: 20 mg/50 ml normal saline solution
Suspension: 40 mg/5 ml
Available without a prescription (Pepcid AC)
Tablets: 10 mg

Indications and dosages
Duodenal and gastric ulcer
Adults: For acute therapy, 40 mg P.O. h.s. for 4 to 8 weeks; for maintenance therapy, 20 mg P.O. h.s.
Pathologic hypersecretory conditions (such as Zollinger-Ellison syndrome)
Adults: 20 mg P.O. q 6 hours. As much as 160 mg q 6 hours may be administered.
Short-term treatment of gastroesophageal reflux disease (GERD)
Adults: 20 to 40 mg P.O. b.i.d. for up to 12 weeks.
◇ ***Hospitalized patients with intractable ulcers or hypersecretory conditions or patients who can't take oral medication, patients with GI bleeding; to control gastric pH in critically ill patients***
Adults: 20 mg I.V. q 12 hours.
Prevention or treatment of heartburn
Pepcid AC
Adults: 10 mg P.O. when symptoms occur; or 10 mg P.O. 1 hour before meals for prevention of symptoms. Drug can be used b.i.d. if necessary.
≡ ***Dosage adjustment.*** In patients with severe renal insufficiency (creatinine clearance less than 10 ml/minute), dosage may be reduced to 20 mg h.s., or the dosing interval may be prolonged to 36 to 48 hours to avoid excess accumulation of drug.

Pharmacodynamics
Antiulcer action: Famotidine competitively inhibits action of histamine at H_2-receptors in gastric parietal cells. This inhibits basal and nocturnal gastric acid secretion from stimulation by such factors as caffeine, food, and pentagastrin.

Pharmacokinetics
Absorption: When administered orally, about 40% to 45% of dose is absorbed.
Distribution: Distributed widely to many body tissues.
Metabolism: About 30% to 35% of an administered dose is metabolized by the liver.
Excretion: Most is excreted unchanged in urine. Famotidine has a longer duration of effect than its 2½- to 4-hour half-life suggests.

Route	Onset	Peak	Duration
P.O.	1 hr	1-3 hr	12 hr
I.V.	Unknown	30 min	12 hr

Contraindications and precautions
Contraindicated in patients hypersensitive to drug.

Interactions
Drug-drug. *Enteric-coated drugs:* Enteric coatings may dissolve too rapidly because of increased gastric pH. Use together cautiously.
Ketoconazole: Decreased absorption of ketoconazole. Increased dose of ketoconazole may be necessary.

Effects on diagnostic tests
Drug may antagonize pentagastrin during gastric acid secretion tests. In skin tests using allergen extracts, drug may cause false-negative results.

Adverse reactions
CNS: *headache,* dizziness, vertigo, malaise, paresthesia.
EENT: tinnitus, taste disorder, orbital edema.
GI: diarrhea, constipation, anorexia, dry mouth.
GU: increased BUN and creatinine levels.
Hepatic: elevated liver enzymes.
Musculoskeletal: musculoskeletal pain.
Skin: acne, dry skin, flushing.
Other: transient irritation (at I.V. site), palpitations, fever.

Overdose and treatment
Overdose hasn't been reported. Treatment should include gastric lavage or induced eme-

sis, followed by activated charcoal to prevent further absorption and supportive and symptomatic therapy. Hemodialysis doesn't remove famotidine.

Clinical considerations
Consider the recommendations relevant to all H_2-receptor antagonists as well as the following:
- Drug isn't recommended for use longer than 8 weeks in patients with uncomplicated duodenal ulcer.
- After administration via nasogastric tube, flush tube to clear it and ensure passage of drug to stomach.
- Antacids may be administered concurrently.
- Drug appears to cause fewer adverse reactions and drug interactions than cimetidine.

◻ ***ALERT*** Don't confuse drug with drugs of similar names, such as felodipine.

Therapeutic monitoring
Therapeutic monitoring is as for all H_2-receptor antagonists.

Special populations
Pregnant patients. Use drug during pregnancy only when clearly indicated.
Breast-feeding patients. Drug may be excreted in breast milk. Use with caution in breast-feeding women.
Geriatric patients. Use drug cautiously in geriatric patients because of increased risk of adverse reactions, particularly those affecting the CNS.

Patient counseling
- Caution patient to take drug only as directed and to continue taking doses, even after pain subsides, to ensure adequate healing.
- Instruct patient to take dose at bedtime.

felodipine
Plendil

Pharmacologic classification: calcium channel blocker
Therapeutic classification: antihypertensive
Pregnancy risk category C

How supplied
Available by prescription only
Tablets (extended-release): 2.5 mg, 5 mg, 10 mg

Indications and dosages
Hypertension
Adults: 5 mg P.O. daily. Adjust dosage based on patient response, generally at intervals not less than 2 weeks. Usual dose is 2.5 to 10 mg P.O. daily; doses exceeding 10 mg daily increase rate of peripheral edema and vasodilatory adverse effects.

≡***Dosage adjustment.*** Geriatric patients or patients with impaired hepatic function should receive a starting dose of 2.5 mg daily. Doses of more than 10 mg shouldn't be considered.

Pharmacodynamics
Antihypertensive action: A dihydropyridine-derivative calcium channel blocker, felodipine blocks the entry of calcium ions into vascular smooth muscle and cardiac cells. This type of calcium channel blocker shows some selectivity for smooth muscle as compared with cardiac muscle. Effects on vascular smooth muscle are relaxation and vasodilation.

Pharmacokinetics
Absorption: Almost completely absorbed, but extensive first-pass metabolism reduces absolute bioavailability to about 20%.
Distribution: Over 99% bound to plasma proteins.
Metabolism: Metabolism probably hepatic; at least 6 inactive metabolites known.
Excretion: Over 70% of a dose appears in urine, and 10% appears in feces as metabolites.

Route	Onset	Peak	Duration
P.O.	2-5 hr	2½-5 hr	24 hr

Contraindications and precautions
Contraindicated in patients hypersensitive to drug. Use cautiously in patients with impaired hepatic function or heart failure, especially those receiving beta blockers.

Interactions
Drug-drug. *Anticonvulsants:* May decrease plasma level of felodipine.
Cimetidine: Decreases the clearance of felodipine. Use lower doses of felodipine.
Digoxin: Decreased peak serum levels of digoxin, but total absorbed drug is unchanged. Clinical significance is unknown.
Metoprolol: Concurrent use may alter the pharmacokinetics of metoprolol. No dosage adjustment appears necessary; however, monitor for adverse effects.
Theophylline: May slightly decrease theophylline levels. Monitor patient for drug effects.
Drug-food. *Grapefruit juice:* May increase bioavailability and effect of drug when taken together. Avoid use together.

Effects on diagnostic tests
None reported.

Adverse reactions
CNS: *headache,* dizziness, paresthesia, asthenia.
CV: *flushing, peripheral edema,* chest pain, palpitations.
EENT: rhinorrhea, pharyngitis, gingival hyperplasia.

GI: abdominal pain, nausea, constipation, diarrhea.
Musculoskeletal: muscle cramps, back pain.
Respiratory: upper respiratory infection, cough.
Skin: rash.

Overdose and treatment
Expected symptoms include peripheral vasodilation, bradycardia, and hypotension. Provide supportive care. I.V. fluids or sympathomimetics may be useful in treating hypotension, and atropine (0.5 to 1 mg I.V.) may treat bradycardia. It isn't known if drug may be removed by dialysis.

Clinical considerations
Consider the recommendations relevant to all calcium channel blockers as well as the following:
- Peripheral edema appears to be both dose- and age-dependent. It's more common in patients taking higher doses, especially those age 60 and older.
- Drug may be administered without regard to meals. However, a small study reported a more than twofold increase of bioavailability when drug was taken with doubly concentrated grapefruit juice compared with water or orange juice.

Therapeutic monitoring
Monitor as for all calcium channel blockers.

Special populations
Pregnant patients. Use drug in pregnancy only when benefits justify risk to fetus.
Breast-feeding patients. It's unknown if drug is excreted in breast milk. Because of risk of serious adverse effects to the infant, breast-feeding isn't recommended.
Pediatric patients. Safety and efficacy in children haven't been established.
Geriatric patients. Higher blood levels of drug are seen in geriatric patients. Mean clearance of drug from geriatric hypertensive patients (average age 74) was less than half of that observed in young patients (average age 26). Check blood pressure closely during dosage adjustment. Maximum daily dose is 10 mg.

Patient counseling
- Tell patient to observe good oral hygiene and to see a dentist regularly because drug has been associated with mild gingival hyperplasia.
- Remind patient to swallow tablet whole and not to crush or chew it.
- Inform patient that he should continue taking drug, even when feeling better. He should watch his diet and call before taking other medications, including OTC drugs.

fenofibrate (micronized)
Tricor

Pharmacologic classification: fibric acid derivative
Therapeutic classification: antihyperlipidemic
Pregnancy risk category C

How supplied
Available by prescription only
Capsules: 67 mg

Indications and dosages
Adjunct to diet for treatment of patients with very high serum triglyceride levels (type IV and V hyperlipidemia) who are at high risk of pancreatitis and who don't respond adequately to diet alone
Adults: Initiate therapy with one (67-mg) capsule P.O. once daily. Based on response, increase dose if necessary following repeat triglyceride levels at 4- to 8-week intervals to maximum dose of three capsules daily (201 mg).
≡ ***Dosage adjustment.*** Minimize dose in renally impaired patients. Initiate therapy at dose of 67 mg/day and increase only after effects on renal function and triglyceride levels have been evaluated at this dose.

Pharmacodynamics
Antihyperlipidemic action: Exact mechanism of action isn't known; drug is thought to lower triglyceride levels by inhibiting triglyceride synthesis, resulting in a decrease in the amount of very-low-density lipoprotein released into the circulation. Fenofibrate may stimulate the breakdown of triglyceride-rich protein.

Pharmacokinetics
Absorption: Well absorbed. Food increases the absorption of drug by 35%.
Distribution: Steady-state plasma levels are achieved within 5 days after initiation of therapy. Drug is almost entirely bound to plasma protein.
Metabolism: Rapidly hydrolyzed by esterases to fenofibric acid, an active metabolite. Fenofibric acid is primarily conjugated with glucuronic acid and excreted in urine.
Excretion: Primarily excreted in the urine; 25% is excreted in the feces; elimination half-life is 20 hours.

Route	Onset	Peak	Duration
P.O.	Unknown	6-8 hr	Unknown

Contraindications and precautions
Contraindicated in patients with preexisting gallbladder disease, hepatic dysfunction (including primary biliary cirrhosis), severe renal dysfunction, unexplained persistent liver function abnormalities, or hypersensitivity to drug.

Interactions

Drug-drug. *Coumarin-type anticoagulants:* Protein binding displacement of the anticoagulant and potentiation of its effects. Use extreme caution; reduce dose of anticoagulant to maintain PT and INR within desired range.
HMG-CoA inhibitors (statins): No data are available on use of statins with fenofibrate; however, because of risk of myopathy, rhabdomyolysis, and acute renal failure reported with the combination use of statins with gemfibrozil (another fibrate derivative), these drugs shouldn't be given together.
Bile acid resins: May bind and inhibit absorption of fenofibrate. Fenofibrate should be taken 1 hour before or 4 to 6 hours after taking these agents.
Cyclosporine: Cyclosporine-induced renal dysfunction may compromise the elimination of fenofibrate. Use cyclosporine and fenofibrate together cautiously.

Effect on diagnostic tests

None reported.

Adverse reactions

CNS: dizziness, miscellaneous pain, asthenia, fatigue, paresthesia, insomnia, headache.
CV: ***arrhythmias.***
EENT: eye irritation, eye floaters, earache, conjunctivitis, blurred vision, rhinitis, sinusitis.
GI: dyspepsia, eructation, flatulence, increased appetite, nausea, vomiting, abdominal pain, constipation, diarrhea.
GU: polyuria, vaginitis, increased creatinine and BUN levels.
Hematologic: decreased hemoglobin.
Hepatic: elevated liver enzymes.
Metabolic: decreased uric acid levels.
Musculoskeletal: arthralgia.
Respiratory: cough.
Skin: urticaria, pruritis, rash.
Other: *infections,* decreased libido, flu syndrome.

Overdose and treatment

No cases of overdose have been reported. If overdose does occur, initiate supportive measures. Because drug is highly protein-bound, hemodialysis is unlikely to be of value.

Clinical considerations

- Fenofibrate lowers serum uric acid levels in normal patients as well as hyperuricemic patients by increasing uric acid excretion.
- Drug shouldn't be used for primary or secondary prevention of coronary artery disease.
- If possible, change or discontinue the use of beta blocking agents, estrogens, and thiazide diuretics because they may increase plasma triglyceride levels.
- Pancreatitis may occur in patients receiving fenofibrate; myositis and rhabdomyolysis may occur in those with renal failure. Assess creatine kinase levels in patients with myalgia, muscle tenderness, or weakness.

Therapeutic monitoring

- Advise prescriber to withdraw therapy in patients who don't achieve an adequate response after 2 months of treatment with the maximum daily dose.
- Drug may cause excretion of cholesterol into the bile leading to cholelithiasis. If suspected, perform appropriate tests and discontinue drug.
- Mild to moderate decreases in hemoglobin, hematocrit, and WBC count may occur on initiation of therapy but stabilize on long-term administration.

Special populations

Breast-feeding patients. Don't use drug in breast-feeding patients; either the drug or breast-feeding should be discontinued.
Pediatric patients. Drug isn't indicated for use in children. Safety and efficacy haven't been established.
Geriatric patients. Drug acts similarly in the elderly (ages 77 to 87) as in young adults; similar dosing regimens can be used.

Patient counseling

- Advise patient to promptly report symptoms of unexplained muscle weakness, pain, or tenderness, especially if it's accompanied by malaise or fever.
- Instruct patient to take drug with meals to optimize drug absorption.

fenoldopam mesylate

Corlopam

Pharmacologic classification:
dopamine D_1-like receptor agonist
Therapeutic classification: antihypertensive
Pregnancy risk category B

How supplied

Available by prescription only
Ampules: 10 mg/ml in single-dose 1-ml, 2-ml, 5-ml ampules

Indications and dosages

Short-term (up to 48 hours) in-hospital management of severe hypertension when rapid but quickly reversible reduction of blood pressure is indicated, including malignant hypertension with deteriorating end-organ function
Adults: Administer by continuous I.V. infusion. Infusion rate is initiated at 0.025 to 0.3 mcg/kg/minute and titrated upward or downward at a frequency not exceeding q 15 minutes to achieve desired blood pressure. Recommended increments for titration are 0.05 to 0.1 mcg/kg/minute.

Pharmacodynamics
Antihypertensive action: Rapid-acting vasodilator. Fenoldopam is an agonist for D_1-like dopamine receptors and binds with moderate affinity to $alpha_2$-adrenoreceptors. No significant affinity for D_2-like receptors, $alpha_1$ or beta adrenoreceptors, 5HT, $5HT_2$, or muscarinic receptors has been noted. In addition, fenoldopam has no effect on ACE activity, although it may increase norepinephrine plasma levels.

Pharmacokinetics
Absorption: Not reported. Drug is given by I.V. infusion only.
Distribution: Not reported. Steady-state plasma levels of 3.2 to 4 ng/ml were reported with infusion rates of 0.1 mcg/kg/minute.
Metabolism: Principle routes of conjugation are methylation, glucuronidation, and sulfation.
Excretion: Elimination is largely by conjugation, without participation of cytochrome P-450 enzymes. Elimination half-life is reported to be about 5 minutes. Following I.V. administration, 90% of drug is excreted in urine and 10% in the feces. Only 4% of drug is excreted unchanged.

Route	Onset	Peak	Duration
I.V.	15 min	20 min	Unknown

Contraindications and precautions
No contraindications are known. Use cautiously because drug is a rapid-acting, potent vasodilator that may precipitate severe hypotension.

Use with caution in patients with glaucoma or ocular hypertension because dose-dependent increases in intraocular pressure may occur. Drug may cause symptomatic hypotension; use particular caution when administering to patients who have sustained an acute cerebral infarction or hemorrhage.

Fenoldopam contains sodium metabisulfite, which may cause allergic-type reactions (including anaphylactic symptoms and severe asthmatic episodes in certain susceptible individuals). Sulfite sensitivity is more frequent in asthmatic than in nonasthmatic people.

Interactions
Drug-drug. *Beta blockers:* Unexpected hypotension could result from beta-blocker inhibition of the reflex response to fenoldopam. Avoid use together.

Effects on diagnostic tests
None reported.

Adverse reactions
CNS: dizziness, headache, insomnia.
CV: hypotension, orthostatic hypotension, palpitations, *bradycardia*, tachycardia, angina, ***MI, heart failure,*** T-wave inversion, flushing.
EENT: nasal congestion.
GI: nausea, vomiting, abdominal pain, constipation, diarrhea.
GU: oliguria, urinary tract infection.
Hematologic: leukocytosis, bleeding.
Metabolic: increased BUN and creatinine, serum glucose, LD, transaminases; hypokalemia.
Musculoskeletal: limb cramp, back pain.
Respiratory: dyspnea.
Other: pyrexia, nonspecific chest pain, injection site reaction.

Overdose and treatment
Intentional overdose hasn't been reported. The most likely reaction would be excessive hypotension, which should be treated with drug discontinuation and appropriate supportive measures.

Clinical considerations
- Drug causes a dose-related tachycardia, which diminishes over time but remains substantial at higher doses.
- Diluted solution is stable at room temperature for at least 24 hours.
- Drug may be abruptly discontinued or infusion gradually tapered. Oral antihypertensive agents can be added once blood pressure is stable during infusion or after its discontinuation.

Therapeutic monitoring
- Monitor blood pressure frequently during infusions; monitor blood pressure and heart rate every 15 minutes until patient is stable.
- Monitor serum electrolytes and watch for hypokalemia.

Special populations
Pregnant patients. Use during pregnancy only if clearly needed.
Breast-feeding patients. Drug may be excreted in breast milk; use caution in administering to breast-feeding women.
Pediatric patients. Safety and efficacy in children haven't been established.

Patient counseling
- Advise patient that drug causes dose-related decreases in blood pressure and increases in heart rate.
- Encourage patient to report adverse reactions promptly.

fenoprofen calcium
Nalfon

Pharmacologic classification: NSAID
Therapeutic classification: nonnarcotic analgesic, antipyretic, anti-inflammatory
Pregnancy risk category NR

How supplied
Available by prescription only
Tablets: 600 mg
Capsules: 200 mg, 300 mg

Indications and dosages

Rheumatoid arthritis and osteoarthritis
Adults: 300 to 600 mg P.O. t.i.d. or q.i.d. Maximum dose is 3.2 g daily.
Mild to moderate pain
Adults: 200 mg P.O. q 4 to 6 hours, p.r.n.
◊ ***Fever***
Adults: Single oral doses up to 400 mg P.O.
◊ ***Acute gouty arthritis***
Adults: 800 mg P.O. q 6 hours; decrease dose based on patient response.

Pharmacodynamics

Analgesic, anti-inflammatory, and antipyretic actions: Mechanisms of action unknown, but drug is thought to inhibit prostaglandin synthesis. Fenoprofen decreases platelet aggregation and may prolong bleeding time.

Pharmacokinetics

Absorption: Absorbed rapidly and completely from the GI tract.
Distribution: About 99% is protein-bound.
Metabolism: Metabolized in the liver.
Excretion: Excreted chiefly in urine with a serum half-life of 2½ to 3 hours. A small amount is excreted in feces.

Route	Onset	Peak	Duration
P.O.	15-30 min	2 hr	4-6 hr

Contraindications and precautions

Contraindicated during pregnancy and in patients with hypersensitivity to drug, significantly impaired renal function, or history of aspirin- or NSAID-induced asthma, rhinitis, or urticaria.

Use cautiously in the elderly and in patients with history of GI events, peptic ulcer disease, compromised cardiac function, or hypertension.

Interactions

Drug-drug. *Anticoagulants and thrombolytic drugs (coumarin derivatives, heparin, streptokinase, urokinase):* May potentiate anticoagulant effects. Use together cautiously.
Antihypertensives or diuretics: Decreased effectiveness. Monitor patient for effects.
Aspirin: May decrease the bioavailability of fenoprofen. Avoid use together.
Coumarin derivatives, phenytoin, verapamil, or nifedipine: Toxicity may occur. Use together cautiously.
Diuretics: Increased nephrotoxic potential. Use together with caution.
Drugs that inhibit platelet aggregation (such as dextran, dipyridamole, mezlocillin, piperacillin, sulfinpyrazone, ticarcillin, valproic acid) or with cefamandole, cefoperazone, plicamycin, aspirin, salicylates, or other anti-inflammatory agents: Bleeding problems may occur. Avoid use together.
Gold compounds, other anti-inflammatory agents, or acetaminophen: Increased nephrotoxicity may occur. Use together cautiously.
Insulin or oral antidiabetic agents: Increased hypoglycemic effects. Dosage may require adjustment.
Methotrexate and lithium: May decrease the renal clearance of fenoprofen.
Salicylates, anti-inflammatory agents, corticotropin, or corticosteroids: May cause increased GI adverse reactions, including ulceration and hemorrhage. Avoid use together.
Drug-lifestyle. *Alcohol use:* May increase risk of adverse GI reactions. Avoid use together.

Effects on diagnostic tests

Drug may cause false elevations in both free and total serum T_3, but thyroid-stimulating hormone and T_4 are unaffected.

Adverse reactions

CNS: *headache,* dizziness, *somnolence,* fatigue, nervousness, asthenia, tremor, confusion.
CV: peripheral edema, palpitations.
EENT: tinnitus, blurred vision, decreased hearing.
GI: *epigastric distress, nausea,* ***GI bleeding,*** vomiting, occult blood loss, peptic ulceration, constipation, anorexia, *dyspepsia,* flatulence.
GU: oliguria, interstitial nephritis, proteinuria, reversible ***renal failure,*** papillary necrosis, cystitis, hematuria, increased BUN and creatinine.
Hematologic: prolonged bleeding time, anemia, ***aplastic anemia, agranulocytosis, thrombocytopenia, hemorrhage,*** bruising, hemolytic anemia.
Hepatic: elevated enzymes, ***hepatitis.***
Metabolic: hyperkalemia.
Respiratory: dyspnea, upper respiratory tract infections, nasopharyngitis.
Skin: *pruritus,* rash, urticaria, increased diaphoresis.
Other: ***anaphylaxis, angioedema.***

Overdose and treatment

Little is known about the acute toxicity of fenoprofen. Nonoliguric renal failure, tachycardia, and hypotension have been observed. Other symptoms include drowsiness, dizziness, confusion and lethargy, nausea, vomiting, headache, tinnitus, and blurred vision. Elevations in serum creatinine and BUN levels have been reported. To treat an overdose of fenoprofen, empty stomach immediately by inducing emesis with ipecac syrup or by gastric lavage. Administer activated charcoal via nasogastric tube. Provide symptomatic and supportive measures (respiratory support and correction of fluid and electrolyte imbalances). Monitor laboratory parameters and vital signs closely. Dialysis is of little value.

Clinical considerations
Consider the recommendations relevant to all NSAIDs. Fenoprofen has been used to treat fever, acute gouty arthritis, and juvenile arthritis.

Therapeutic monitoring
- Monitor for potential CNS effects. Institute safety measures to prevent injury.
- Monitor renal, hepatic, and auditory function in patients on long-term therapy. Stop drug if abnormalities occur.

Special populations
Breast-feeding patients. Because drug is excreted in breast milk, avoid use in breast-feeding women.
Pediatric patients. Safe use of fenoprofen in children hasn't been established. Drug isn't recommended for use in children under age 14.
Geriatric patients. Patients over age 60 may be more susceptible to the toxic effects of fenoprofen, especially adverse GI reactions. Use with caution. The effects of drug on renal prostaglandins may cause fluid retention and edema, a significant drawback for geriatric patients and those with heart failure.

Patient counseling
- Tell patient to avoid activities that require alertness or concentration until CNS effects of drug are known.
- Advise patient to call prescriber for specific instruction before taking OTC analgesics.

fentanyl citrate
Sublimaze

fentanyl transdermal system
Duragesic-25, Duragesic-50, Duragesic-75, Duragesic-100

fentanyl transmucosal
Fentanyl Oralet

Pharmacologic classification: opioid agonist
Therapeutic classification: analgesic, adjunct to anesthesia, anesthetic
Controlled substance schedule II
Pregnancy risk category C

How supplied
Available by prescription only
Injection: 50 mcg/ml
Transdermal system: Patches designed to release 25 mcg, 50 mcg, 75 mcg, or 100 mcg of fentanyl/hour.
Transmucosal: 100 mcg, 200 mcg, 300 mcg, 400 mcg

Indications and dosages
Preoperatively
Adults: 50 to 100 mcg I.M. 30 to 60 minutes before surgery.
Children and adults under 33 lb (15 kg): 5 mcg/kg as lozenge P.O. for patient to suck until dissolved, 20 to 40 minutes before surgery.
Adjunct to general anesthetic
Low-dose regimen for minor procedures
Adults: 2 mcg/kg I.V.
Moderate-dose regimen for major procedures
Adults: Initial dose is 2 to 20 mcg/kg I.V.; may give additional doses of 25 to 100 mcg I.V. or I.M., p.r.n.
High-dose regimen for complicated procedures
Adults: Initial dose is 20 to 50 mcg/kg I.V.; additional doses of 25 mcg to one-half the initial dose may be administered, p.r.n.
Adjunct to anesthesia (lozenge)
Adults and children older than 2 years: 5 mcg/kg lozenge P.O.
Adjunct to regional anesthesia
Adults: 50 to 100 mcg I.M. or slow I.V. over 1 to 2 minutes.
Induction and maintenance of anesthesia
Children age 2 to 12: Reduced dose as low as 1.7 to 3.3 mcg/kg.
Postoperative analgesic
Adults: 50 to 100 mcg I.M. q 1 to 2 hours, p.r.n.
Management of chronic pain in patients who can't be managed by lesser means
Adults: Apply one transdermal system to a portion of the upper torso on an area of skin that isn't irritated and hasn't been irradiated. Initiate therapy with the 25-mcg/hour system; adjust dosage as needed and tolerated. Each system may be worn for 72 hours.
≡ ***Dosage adjustment.*** Lower doses are usually indicated for geriatric patients who may be more sensitive to the therapeutic and adverse effects of drug.

Pharmacodynamics
Analgesic action: Fentanyl binds to the opiate receptors as an agonist to alter the patient's perception of painful stimuli, thus providing analgesia for moderate to severe pain. Its CNS and respiratory depressant effects are similar to those of morphine. Drug has little hypnotic activity and rarely causes histamine release.

Pharmacokinetics
Absorption: Onset of action after I.V. administration is immediate.
Distribution: Redistribution has been suggested as the main cause of the brief analgesic effect of fentanyl.
Metabolism: Metabolized in the liver.
Excretion: Excreted in the urine as metabolites and unchanged drug. Elimination half-life is about 7 hours after parenteral use, 5 to 15

hours after transmucosal use, and 18 hours after transdermal use.

Route	Onset	Peak	Duration
I.V.	1-2 min	3-5 min	½-1 hr
I.M.	7-15 min	20-30 min	1-2 hr
Transdermal	12-24 hr	1-3 days	Variable
Transmucosal	5-15 min	20-50 min	Unknown

Contraindications and precautions

Contraindicated in patients with known intolerance of drug. Use cautiously in geriatric or debilitated patients and in those with head injuries, increased CSF pressure, COPD, decreased respiratory reserve, compromised respirations, arrhythmias, or hepatic, renal, or cardiac disease.

Interactions

Drug-drug. *Anticholinergics:* Avoid use together.
Cimetidine: May increase respiratory and CNS depression; such use requires that dosage of fentanyl be reduced by one-quarter to one-third.
CNS depressants (narcotic analgesics, general anesthetics, antihistamines, phenothiazines, barbiturates, benzodiazepines, sedative-hypnotics, tricyclic antidepressants, muscle relaxants): Potentiates respiratory and CNS depression, sedation, and hypotensive effects of drug. Use together cautiously.
Droperidol: Hypotension and a decrease in pulmonary artery pressure. Use together cautiously.
Drugs that are extensively metabolized in the liver (rifampin, phenytoin, digitoxin): Drug accumulation and enhanced effects may result from use together. Use together cautiously.
General anesthetics; diazepam: Severe CV depression may result. Avoid use together.
MAO inhibitors: Increased CNS effects. The manufacturer warns that fentanyl shouldn't be given to a patient who has received an MAO inhibitor within the past 14 days.
Narcotic antagonists: May cause acute withdrawal syndrome. Use with caution.
Spinal anesthesia and some peridural anesthetics: When used together, fentanyl can alter respiration by blocking intercostal nerves. Avoid use together.
Drug-lifestyle. *Alcohol use:* May cause additive effects. Advise patient to avoid alcohol use.

Effects on diagnostic tests

None reported.

Adverse reactions

CNS: *sedation, somnolence, clouded sensorium, euphoria,* dizziness, headache, *confusion, asthenia,* nervousness, hallucinations, anxiety, depression.
CV: *hypotension,* hypertension, ***arrhythmias,*** chest pain.
GI: *nausea, vomiting, constipation,* ileus, abdominal pain, *dry mouth,* anorexia, diarrhea, dyspepsia, increased plasma amylase and lipase levels.
GU: *urine retention.*
Respiratory: ***respiratory depression,*** hypoventilation, dyspnea, ***apnea.***
Skin: reaction at application site (erythema, papules, edema), *pruritus, diaphoresis.*
Other: physical dependence.

Overdose and treatment

The most common signs and symptoms are extensions of its actions. They include CNS depression, respiratory depression, and miosis. Other acute toxic effects include hypotension, bradycardia, hypothermia, shock, apnea, cardiopulmonary arrest, circulatory collapse, pulmonary edema, and seizures.

To treat acute overdose, first establish adequate respiratory exchange via a patent airway and ventilation as needed; administer a narcotic antagonist (naloxone) to reverse respiratory depression. (Because the duration of action of fentanyl is longer than that of naloxone, repeated dosing may be necessary.) Naloxone shouldn't be given unless the patient has clinically significant respiratory or CV depression. Monitor vital signs closely.

Provide symptomatic and supportive treatment. Monitor laboratory values, vital signs, and neurologic status closely.

Clinical considerations

Consider the recommendations relevant to all opioid (narcotic) agonists as well as the following:

- The high lipid solubility of fentanyl may contribute to this potential adverse effect.
- Fentanyl may cause bradycardia. Pretreatment with an anticholinergic (such as atropine or glycopyrrolate) may minimize this effect.
- High doses can produce muscle rigidity. This effect can be reversed by naloxone.
- Many anesthesiologists use epidural and intrathecal fentanyl as a potent adjunct to epidural anesthesia.

Transdermal form

- Transdermal fentanyl isn't recommended for postoperative pain.
- Dosage adjustments in patients using the transdermal system should be made gradually. Reaching steady-state levels of a new dose may take up to 6 days; delay dose adjustment until after at least two applications.
- Most patients experience good control of pain for 3 days while wearing the transdermal system, although a few may need a new application after 48 hours. Because serum fentanyl level increases for the first 24 hours after application, analgesic effect can't be evaluated for the first day.
- When reducing opiate therapy or switching to a different analgesic, withdraw the transder-

mal system gradually. Because the serum level of fentanyl decreases very gradually after removal, give half of the equianalgesic dose of the new analgesic 12 to 18 hours after removal.

Therapeutic monitoring

- Observe patient for delayed onset of respiratory depression.
- Monitor patient's heart rate.
- Monitor patient for at least 12 hours for adverse reactions to the transdermal system. Serum levels of fentanyl decrease very gradually and may take as long as 17 hours to decline by 50%.

Special populations

Pregnant patients. Drug use is contraindicated during pregnancy unless benefits outweigh risks to fetus.
Breast-feeding patients. Drug is excreted in breast milk; don't administer to breast-feeding women.
Pediatric patients. Safe use in children under age 2 hasn't been established for parenteral or transmucosal (buccal) use. Safe use in children under age 12 for transdermal system hasn't been established. Transdermal system also should not be used in children under age 18 weighing less than 110 lb (50 kg), and the buccal form should not be used in any child weighing less than 33 lb (15 kg).
Geriatric patients. Use with caution in geriatric patients.

Patient counseling

- Advise patient of proper application of the transdermal patch.
- Tell patient to apply to a new site if another patch is needed after 72 hours.
- Warn patient to keep lozenges out of reach of children.
- Advise patient on proper disposal of lozenges.

ferrous fumarate

Femiron, Feostat, Fumasorb, Fumerin, Hemocyte, Ircon, Ircon-FA, Neo-Fer*, Nephro-Fer, Novofumar*, Palafer*, Span-FF

Pharmacologic classification: oral iron supplement
Therapeutic classification: hematinic
Pregnancy risk category A

How supplied

Available without a prescription. Ferrous fumarate is 33% elemental iron.
Tablets: 63 mg, 195 mg, 200 mg, 324 mg, 325 mg, 350 mg
Tablets (chewable): 100 mg
Capsules (extended-release): 325 mg
Suspension: 100 mg/5 ml
Drops: 45 mg/0.6 ml

Indications and dosages

Iron-deficiency states
Adults: 50 to 100 mg P.O. of elemental iron, t.i.d. Adjust dose gradually, as needed and as tolerated.
Children: 4 to 6 mg/kg P.O. daily divided into three doses.
≡ ***Dosage adjustment.*** Geriatric patients may need higher doses because reduced gastric secretions and achlorhydria may lower capacity for iron absorption.

Pharmacodynamics

Hematinic action: Ferrous fumarate replaces iron, an essential component in the formation of hemoglobin.

Pharmacokinetics

Absorption: Absorbed from the entire length of the GI tract, but primary absorption sites are the duodenum and proximal jejunum. Up to 10% of iron is absorbed by healthy individuals; patients with iron-deficiency anemia may absorb up to 60%. Enteric coating and some extended-release formulas have decreased absorption because they're designed to release iron past the points of highest absorption; food may decrease absorption by 33% to 50%.
Distribution: Transported through GI mucosal cells directly into the blood, where it's immediately bound to a carrier protein, transferrin, and transported to the bone marrow for incorporation into hemoglobin. Iron is highly protein-bound.
Metabolism: Liberated by the destruction of hemoglobin, but is conserved and reused by the body.
Excretion: Healthy individuals lose only small amounts of iron daily. Men and postmenopausal women lose about 1 mg/day, and premenopausal women about 1.5 mg/day. The loss usually occurs in nails, hair, feces, and urine; trace amounts are lost in bile and sweat.

Route	Onset	Peak	Duration
P.O.	4 days	7-10 days	2-4 mo

Contraindications and precautions

Contraindicated in patients with primary hemochromatosis or hemosiderosis, hemolytic anemia unless iron-deficiency anemia is also present, peptic ulcer disease, regional enteritis, or ulcerative colitis and in those receiving repeated blood transfusions. Use cautiously on long-term basis.

Interactions

Drug-drug. *Antacids, aluminum-containing phosphate binders, cholestyramine, cimetidine, and vitamin E:* Decrease ferrous fumarate absorption. Separate doses by 1- to 2-hour intervals.
Chloramphenicol: Delays response to iron therapy. Monitor patient carefully.

Doxycycline: May interfere with ferrous fumarate absorption even when doses are separated. Avoid use together.
L-thyroxine: May decrease L-thyroxine absorption. Separate doses by at least 2 hours. Monitor thyroid function.
Levodopa and methyldopa: May decrease absorption of these drugs. Monitor patient carefully.
Penicillamine: Decreased penicillamine absorption; separate doses by at least 2 hours.
Quinolones: Drug may decrease absorption of quinolones. Monitor patient closely.
Tetracycline: Inhibits absorption of both drugs; give tetracycline 3 hours after or 2 hours before iron supplement.
Vitamin C: Increases iron absorption. May be used as a beneficial drug interaction.
Drug-food. *Yogurt, cheese, eggs, milk, whole-grain breads, cereals, tea, coffee:* May impair oral iron absorption. Don't use together.

Effects on diagnostic tests

Ferrous fumarate blackens feces and may interfere with tests for occult blood in the stool; the guaiac test and orthotoluidine test may yield false-positive results, but the benzidine test is usually not affected.

Iron overload may decrease uptake of technetium 99m and thus interfere with skeletal imaging.

Adverse reactions

GI: *nausea,* epigastric pain, vomiting, *constipation,* diarrhea, black stools, anorexia.
Other: temporary staining of teeth (with suspension and drops).

Overdose and treatment

The lethal dose of iron is between 200 and 250 mg/kg; fatalities have occurred with lower doses. Symptoms may follow ingestion of 20 to 60 mg/kg. Clinical signs of acute overdose may occur as follows:

Between 30 minutes and 8 hours after ingestion, patient may experience lethargy, nausea and vomiting, green then tarry stools, weak and rapid pulse, hypotension, dehydration, acidosis, and coma. If death doesn't immediately ensue, symptoms may clear for about 24 hours.

At 12 to 48 hours, symptoms may return, accompanied by diffuse vascular congestion, pulmonary edema, shock, seizures, anuria, and hyperthermia. Death may follow.

Treatment requires immediate support of airway, respiration, and circulation. In conscious patient with intact gag reflex, induce emesis with ipecac; if not, empty stomach by gastric lavage. Follow emesis with lavage, using a 1% sodium bicarbonate solution, to convert iron to the less irritating, poorly absorbed form (phosphate solutions have been used, but carry hazard of other adverse effects). X-ray abdomen to determine continued presence of excess iron; if serum iron levels exceed 350 mg/dl, deferoxamine may be used for systemic chelation.

Survivors are likely to sustain organ damage, including pyloric or antral stenosis, hepatic cirrhosis, CNS damage, and intestinal obstruction.

Clinical considerations

- Drug may cause dark-colored stools.
- Drug may stain teeth.

Therapeutic monitoring

Monitor for adverse reactions and for evidence of therapeutic results.

Special populations

Breast-feeding patients. Iron supplements are often recommended for breast-feeding women; no adverse effects of such use have been documented.
Pediatric patients. Iron overdose may be fatal in children; treat immediately.
Geriatric patients. Because iron-induced constipation is common in geriatric patients, stress proper diet to these patients.

Patient counseling

- Instruct patient to take tablets with orange juice or water, but not with milk or antacids.
- Tell patient to take suspension with straw and place drops at back of throat.

ferrous gluconate

Apo-Ferrous Gluconate*, Fergon, Ferralet, Fertinic*, Novoferrogluc*, Simron

Pharmacologic classification: oral iron supplement
Therapeutic classification: hematinic
Pregnancy risk category A

How supplied

Available without a prescription. Ferrous gluconate is 11.6% elemental iron.
Tablets: 300 mg (contains 35 mg Fe^+), 320 mg, 325 mg (320-mg tablet contains 37 mg Fe^+)
Capsules: 86 mg (contains 10 mg Fe^+), 325 mg (contains 38 mg Fe^+)
Elixir: 300 mg/5 ml (contains 35 mg Fe^+)

Indications and dosages

Iron deficiency

Adults: 325 mg P.O. q.i.d., dosage increased as needed and tolerated, up to 650 mg q.i.d.
Children age 2 to 12: 3 mg/kg/day P.O. in three or four divided doses.
Children age 6 months to 2 years: Up to 6 mg/kg/day P.O. in three or four divided doses.
Infants: 10 to 25 mg/day P.O. divided into three or four doses.
≡ ***Dosage adjustment.*** Geriatric patients may need higher doses because reduced gastric se-

cretions and achlorhydria may lower capacity for iron absorption.

Pharmacodynamics

Hematinic action: Ferrous gluconate replaces iron, an essential component in the formation of hemoglobin.

Pharmacokinetics

Absorption: Absorbed from the entire length of the GI tract, but primary absorption sites are the duodenum and proximal jejunum. Up to 10% of iron is absorbed by healthy individuals; patients with iron-deficiency anemia may absorb up to 60%. Food may decrease absorption by 33% to 50%.
Distribution: Transported through GI mucosal cells directly into the blood, where it's immediately bound to a carrier protein, transferrin, and transported to the bone marrow for incorporation into hemoglobin. Iron is highly protein-bound.
Metabolism: Liberated by the destruction of hemoglobin, but is conserved and reused by the body.
Excretion: Healthy individuals lose only small amounts of iron daily. Men and postmenopausal women lose about 1 mg/day, premenopausal women about 1.5 mg/day. Loss usually occurs in nails, hair, feces, and urine; trace amounts are lost in bile and sweat.

Route	Onset	Peak	Duration
P.O.	4 days	7-10 days	2-4 mo

Contraindications and precautions

Contraindicated in patients with peptic ulceration, regional enteritis, ulcerative colitis, hemosiderosis, primary hemochromatosis, or hemolytic anemia unless iron deficiency anemia is also present and in those receiving repeated blood transfusions. Use cautiously on long-term basis.

Interactions

Drug-drug. *Antacids, aluminum-containing phosphate binders, cholestyramine, cimetidine, vitamin E:* Decrease ferrous fumarate absorption. Separate doses by 1- to 2-hour intervals.
Chloramphenicol: Delays response to iron therapy. Monitor patient carefully.
Doxycycline: May interfere with ferrous fumarate absorption even when doses are separated. Avoid use together.
L-thyroxine: May decrease L-thyroxine absorption. Separate doses by at least 2 hours. Monitor thyroid function.
Levodopa and methyldopa: May decrease absorption of these drugs. Monitor patient carefully.
Penicillamine: Decreased penicillamine absorption; separate doses by at least 2 hours.
Quinolones: May decrease absorption of quinolones. Monitor patient closely.
Tetracycline: Inhibits absorption of both drugs; give tetracycline 3 hours after or 2 hours before iron supplement.
Vitamin C: Increased iron absorption. May be used as a beneficial drug interaction.
Drug-food. *Yogurt, cheese, eggs, milk, whole-grain breads, cereals, tea, coffee:* May impair oral iron absorption. Avoid use together.

Effects on diagnostic tests

Ferrous gluconate blackens feces and may interfere with test for occult blood in the stools; the guaiac test and orthotoluidine test may yield false-positive results, but the benzidine test is usually not affected.

Iron overload may decrease uptake of technetium 99m and thus interfere with skeletal imaging.

Adverse reactions

GI: *nausea,* epigastric pain, vomiting, *constipation,* diarrhea, *black stools,* anorexia.
Other: temporary staining of teeth (with elixir).

Overdose and treatment

The lethal dose of iron is between 200 to 250 mg/kg; fatalities have occurred with lower doses. Symptoms may follow ingestion of 20 to 60 mg/kg. Clinical signs of acute overdose may occur as follows:

Between 30 minutes and 8 hours after ingestion, patient may experience lethargy, nausea and vomiting, green then tarry stools, weak and rapid pulse, hypotension, dehydration, acidosis, and coma. If death doesn't immediately ensue, symptoms may clear for about 24 hours.

At 12 to 48 hours, symptoms may return, accompanied by diffuse vascular congestion, pulmonary edema, shock, seizures, anuria, and hyperthermia. Death may follow.

Treatment requires immediate support of airway, respiration, and circulation. In conscious patient with intact gag reflex, induce emesis with ipecac; if not, empty stomach by gastric lavage. Follow emesis with lavage, using a 1% sodium bicarbonate solution, to convert iron to less irritating, poorly absorbed form (phosphate solutions have been used, but carry hazard of other adverse effects). Take abdominal X-ray to determine continued presence of excess iron; if serum iron levels exceed 350 mg/dl, deferoxamine may be used for systemic chelation.

Survivors are likely to sustain organ damage, including pyloric or antral stenosis, hepatic cirrhosis, CNS damage, and intestinal obstruction.

Clinical considerations

Drug can be given between meals or with some food, but absorption may be decreased.

Therapeutic monitoring

Monitor for adverse reactions and for evidence of therapeutic effect.

Special populations

Breast-feeding patients. Iron supplements are often recommended for breast-feeding women; no adverse effects of such use have been documented.
Pediatric patients. Overdose may be fatal in children; treat immediately.
Geriatric patients. Iron-induced constipation is common in geriatric patients; stress proper diet to these patients.

ferrous sulfate

Apo-Ferrous Sulfate*, Feosol, Feratab, Fer-In-Sol, Fer-Iron, Fero-Grad-500*, Fero-Gradumet, Ferospace, Ferralyn Lanacaps, Ferra-TD, Mol-Iron, Novoferrosulfa*, PMS Ferrous Sulfate*, Slow FE

Pharmacologic classification: oral iron supplement
Therapeutic classification: hematinic
Pregnancy risk category A

How supplied

Available without a prescription. Ferrous sulfate is 20% elemental iron; dried and powdered (exsiccated), it is about 32% elemental iron.
Tablets: 195 mg, 300 mg, 324 mg, 325 mg; 200 mg (exsiccated); 160 mg (exsiccated, extended-release); 525 mg (timed-release)
Capsules: 150 mg, 190 mg, 250 mg
Capsules (extended-release): 150 mg, 159 mg, 250 mg
Syrup: 90 mg/5 ml
Elixir: 220 mg/5 ml
Liquid: 75 mg/0.6 ml, 125 mg/ml

Indications and dosages

Iron deficiency
Adults: 300 mg P.O. b.i.d.; dosage gradually increased to 300 mg q.i.d. as needed and tolerated. For extended-release capsule, 150 to 250 mg P.O. once or twice daily; for extended-release tablets, 160 to 525 mg once or twice daily.
Children age 2 to 12: 3 mg/kg/day P.O. in three or four divided doses.
Children age 6 months to 2 years: up to 6 mg/kg/day P.O. in three or four divided doses.
Infants: 10 to 25 mg/day P.O. in three or four divided doses.
≡ ***Dosage adjustment.*** Geriatric patients may need higher doses because reduced gastric secretions and achlorhydria may lower capacity for iron absorption.

Pharmacodynamics

Hematinic action: Ferrous sulfate replaces iron, an essential component in the formation of hemoglobin.

Pharmacokinetics

Absorption: Absorbed from the entire length of the GI tract, but primary absorption sites are the duodenum and proximal jejunum. Up to 10% of iron is absorbed by healthy individuals; patients with iron-deficiency anemia may absorb up to 60%. Enteric coating and some extended-release formulas have decreased absorption because they're designed to release iron past the points of highest absorption; food may decrease absorption by 33% to 50%.
Distribution: Transported through GI mucosal cells directly into the blood, where it's immediately bound to a carrier protein, transferrin, and transported to the bone marrow for incorporation into hemoglobin. Iron is highly protein-bound.
Metabolism: Liberated by the destruction of hemoglobin, but is conserved and reused by the body.
Excretion: Healthy individuals lose very little iron each day. Men and postmenopausal women lose about 1 mg/day, and premenopausal women about 1.5 mg/day. The loss usually occurs in nails, hair, feces, and urine; trace amounts are lost in bile and sweat.

Route	Onset	Peak	Duration
P.O.	4 days	7-10 days	2-4 mo

Contraindications and precautions

Contraindicated in patients with hemosiderosis, primary hemochromatosis, hemolytic anemia unless iron deficiency anemia is also present, peptic ulceration, ulcerative colitis, or regional enteritis and in those receiving repeated blood transfusions. Use cautiously on long-term basis.

Interactions

Drug-drug. *Antacids, aluminum-containing phosphate binders, cholestyramine, cimetidine, and vitamin E:* Decrease ferrous fumarate absorption. Separate doses by 1- to 2-hour intervals.
Chloramphenicol: Delays response to iron therapy. Monitor patient carefully.
Doxycycline: May interfere with ferrous fumarate absorption even when doses are separated. Avoid use together.
L-thyroxine: May decrease L-thyroxine absorption. Separate doses by at least 2 hours. Monitor thyroid function.
Levodopa and methyldopa: May decrease absorption of these drugs. Monitor carefully.
Penicillamine: Decreased penicillamine absorption; separate doses by at least 2 hours.
Quinolones: Drug may decrease absorption of quinolones. Monitor patient closely.
Tetracycline: Inhibits absorption of both drugs; give tetracycline 3 hours after or 2 hours before iron supplement.
Vitamin C: Increases iron absorption. May be used as a beneficial drug interaction.

Drug-food. *Yogurt, cheese, eggs, milk, whole-grain breads, cereals, tea, coffee:* May impair oral iron absorption. Avoid use together.

Effects on diagnostic tests
Ferrous sulfate blackens feces and may interfere with tests for occult blood in the stool; the guaiac test and orthotoluidine test may yield false-positive results, but the benzidine test is usually not affected.

Iron overload may decrease uptake of technetium 99m and thus interfere with skeletal imaging.

Adverse reactions
GI: *nausea,* epigastric pain, vomiting, *constipation, black stools,* diarrhea, anorexia.
Other: temporary staining of teeth (with liquid forms).

Overdose and treatment
The lethal dose of iron is 200 to 250 mg/kg; fatalities have occurred with lower doses. Symptoms may follow ingestion of 20 to 60 mg/kg. Clinical signs of acute overdose may occur as follows:

Between 30 minutes and 8 hours after ingestion, patient may experience lethargy, nausea and vomiting, green then tarry stools, weak and rapid pulse, hypotension, dehydration, acidosis, and coma. If death doesn't immediately ensue, symptoms may clear for about 24 hours.

At 12 to 48 hours, symptoms may return, accompanied by diffuse vascular congestion, pulmonary edema, shock, seizures, anuria, and hyperthermia. Death may follow.

Treatment requires immediate support of airway, respiration, and circulation. In conscious patient with intact gag reflex, induce emesis with ipecac; if not, empty stomach by gastric lavage. Follow emesis with lavage, using a 1% sodium bicarbonate solution, to convert iron to less irritating, poorly absorbed form (phosphate solutions have been used, but carry hazard of other adverse effects). Take abdominal X-ray to determine continued presence of excess iron; if serum iron levels exceed 350 mg/dl, deferoxamine may be used for systemic chelation.

Survivors are likely to sustain organ damage, including pyloric or antral stenosis, hepatic cirrhosis, CNS damage, and intestinal obstruction.

Clinical considerations
- Drug may be taken with meals to minimize GI effects; maximum absorption will occur if drug is taken between meals.
- Drug may cause dark-colored stools.
- Drug may stain teeth.

Therapeutic monitoring
Monitor for adverse reactions and for evidence of therapeutic effects.

Special populations
Breast-feeding patients. Iron supplements often are recommended for breast-feeding women; no adverse effects have been documented.
Pediatric patients. Extended-release iron capsules or tablets are usually not recommended for children. Overdose may be fatal; treat immediately.
Geriatric patients. Iron-induced constipation is common in geriatric patients; stress proper diet to minimize this adverse effect.

Patient counseling
- Instruct patient not to crush or chew extended-release forms.
- Inform parents that three or four tablets can cause serious iron poisoning in children.

fexofenadine hydrochloride
Allegra

Pharmacologic classification: H_1-receptor antagonist
Therapeutic classification: antihistaminic
Pregnancy risk category C

How supplied
Available by prescription only
Capsules: 60 mg

Indications and dosages
Seasonal allergic rhinitis
Adults and children age 12 and older: 60 mg P.O. b.i.d.
≡ ***Dosage adjustment.*** In patients with impaired renal function, 60 mg P.O. once daily.

Pharmacodynamics
Antihistaminic action: Principal effects of fexofenadine are mediated through a selective inhibition of peripheral H_1 receptors.

Pharmacokinetics
Absorption: Rapidly absorbed.
Distribution: 60% to 70% bound to plasma protein.
Metabolism: About 5% of drug is metabolized.
Excretion: Mainly excreted in feces; less so in urine. Mean elimination half-life of drug is 14½ hours.

Route	Onset	Peak	Duration
P.O.	Unknown	3 hr	14 hr

Contraindications and precautions
Contraindicated in patients with hypersensitivity to drug or its components. Use cautiously in patients with impaired renal function.

Interactions
None reported.

Effects on diagnostic tests
Possible interference with antigen skin-testing procedures. Discontinue drug 24 to 48 hours before test.

Adverse reactions
CNS: fatigue, drowsiness.
GI: nausea, dyspepsia.
GU: dysmenorrhea.
Other: viral infection.

Overdose and treatment
Overdose of up to 800 mg did not result in significant clinical adverse reactions. If overdose occurs, treatment should be symptomatic or supportive. Fexofenadine isn't effectively removed by hemodialysis.

Clinical considerations
No information indicates that abuse or dependency occurs with fexofenadine use.

Therapeutic monitoring
Monitor for adverse reactions.

Special populations
Pregnant patients. Use drug only during pregnancy when potential benefit outweighs risk to fetus.
Breast-feeding patients. It isn't known if drug is excreted in breast milk. Caution is recommended when administering fexofenadine to breast-feeding women.
Pediatric patients. Safety and efficacy in children under age 12 haven't been established.

Patient counseling
- Caution patient not to perform hazardous activities if drowsiness is experienced with drug use.
- Instruct patient not to exceed prescribed dosage and to take drug only when needed.

filgrastim (granulocyte colony-stimulating factor, G-CSF)
Neupogen

Pharmacologic classification: biologic response modifier
Therapeutic classification: colony-stimulating factor
Pregnancy risk category C

How supplied
Available by prescription only
Injection: 300 mcg/ml in 1-ml and 1.6-ml single-dose vials

Indications and dosages
To decrease incidence of infection after cancer chemotherapy for nonmyeloid malignancies, chronic severe neutropenia, after bone marrow transplantation in cancer patients; to treat ◇agranulocytosis, ◇pancytopenia with colchicine overdose, ◇acute leukemia ◇myelodysplastic syndrome, ◇hematologic toxicity with zidovudine antiviral therapy
Adults: Initially, 5 mcg/kg S.C. or I.V. as a single daily dose; may increase dose incrementally by 5 mcg/kg for each course of chemotherapy according to duration and severity of absolute neutrophil count (ANC) nadir.

Don't administer earlier than 24 hours after or within 24 hours before chemotherapy.

Give filgrastim daily for up to 2 weeks until ANC nadir reaches 10,000/mm^3 after the anticipated chemoinduced ANC nadir. Duration of treatment depends on the myelosuppressive potential of the chemotherapy used. Discontinue if ANC nadir surpasses 10,000/mm^3.
Acquired immune deficiency syndrome (AIDS)
Adults: 0.3 to 3.6 mcg/kg/day S.C. or I.V.
Aplastic anemia
Adults: 800 to 1,200 mcg/m^2/day S.C. or I.V.
Hairy cell leukemia, myelodysplasia
Adults: 15 to 500 mcg/m^2/day S.C. or I.V.

Pharmacodynamics
Immunostimulant action: Filgrastim is a naturally occurring cytokine glycoprotein that stimulates proliferation, differentiation, and functional activity of neutrophils, causing a rapid increase in WBC counts within 2 to 3 days in patients with normal bone marrow function or 7 to 14 days in patients with bone marrow suppression. Blood counts return to pretreatment levels, usually within 1 week after therapy ends.

Pharmacokinetics
Absorption: After S.C. bolus dose, blood levels suggest rapid absorption.
Distribution: Unknown.
Metabolism: Unknown.
Excretion: Elimination half-life is about 3½ hours.

Route	Onset	Peak	Duration
I.V.	5-60 min	24 hr	1-7 days
S.C.	5-60 min	2-8 hr	1-7 days

Contraindications and precautions
Contraindicated in patients hypersensitive to proteins derived from *Escherichia coli* or to drug or its components.

Interactions
Drug-drug. *Chemotherapeutic agents:* Cause rapidly dividing myeloid cells to be potentially sensitive to cytotoxic agents. Don't use within 24 hours before or after a dose of one of these agents.

Lithium: Use with caution in patients taking lithium.

Effects on diagnostic tests
None reported.

Adverse reactions
CNS: headache, weakness, *fatigue.*
CV: ***MI, arrhythmias,*** chest pain, transient hypotension.
GI: *nausea, vomiting, diarrhea, mucositis,* stomatitis, constipation.
GU: increased serum creatinine.
Hematologic: ***thrombocytopenia,*** leukocytosis, transient increases in neutrophils.
Hepatic: elevated liver enzymes.
Metabolic: elevations in uric acid.
Musculoskeletal: *skeletal pain.*
Respiratory: dyspnea, cough.
Skin: *alopecia,* rash, cutaneous vasculitis.
Other: *fever,* ***hypersensitivity reactions.***

Overdose and treatment
Maximum tolerated dose hasn't been determined. There have been no reports of overdose.

Clinical considerations
- Store drug in refrigerator; don't freeze.
- Filgrastim isn't compatible with normal saline solution.

Therapeutic monitoring
- Obtain CBC and platelet counts before and twice weekly during therapy.
- Regular monitoring of hematocrit and platelet counts is recommended.
- Adult respiratory distress syndrome may occur in septic patients because of the influx of neutrophils at the site of inflammation.
- MI and arrhythmias have occurred; closely monitor patients with preexisting cardiac conditions.
- Bone pain is the most frequent adverse reaction and may be controlled with nonnarcotic analgesics if mild to moderate or may require narcotic analgesics if severe.

Special populations
Breast-feeding patients. It's unknown if drug is excreted in breast milk. Risk-to-benefit ratio must be assessed.
Pediatric patients. Efficacy hasn't been established, but there's no evidence of greater toxicity in children than in adults.
Geriatric patients. No age-related problems have been reported.

Patient counseling
- Review "Information for Patients" section of package insert with patient. Thorough instruction is essential if home use is prescribed.
- Manufacturer has hotline to answer questions about insurance reimbursement procedures. Hotline operates from Monday through Friday 9 a.m. to 5 p.m. Eastern Standard Time: 1-800-272-9376; in Washington, D.C., 1-202-637-6698.

finasteride
Propecia, Proscar

Pharmacologic classification: steroid (synthetic 4-azasteroid) derivative
Therapeutic classification: androgen synthesis inhibitor
Pregnancy risk category X

How supplied
Available by prescription only
Tablets: 1 mg, 5 mg

Indications and dosages
Symptomatic BPH, ◇adjuvant therapy after radical prostatectomy, ◇first-stage prostate cancer, ◇acne, ◇hirsutism
Adult (men only): 5 mg P.O. daily, usually for 6 to 12 months.
◇Male pattern baldness (androgenetic alopecia)
Adults: 1 mg P.O. daily, usually for 3 months or more. Continued use is recommended to sustain benefit. Withdrawal of treatment leads to reversal of effect within 12 months.

Pharmacodynamics
Androgen synthesis inhibition action: Finasteride competitively inhibits steroid 5μ, an enzyme responsible for formation of the potent androgen 5μ-dihydrotestosterone (DHT) from testosterone. Because DHT influences development of the prostate gland, decreasing levels of this hormone in adult men should relieve the symptoms associated with BPH. In men with male pattern baldness, the balding scalp contains miniaturized hair follicles and increased amounts of DHT. Finasteride decreases scalp and serum DHT levels in these men.

Pharmacokinetics
Absorption: Average bioavailability of drug was 63% in one study.
Distribution: About 90% bound to plasma proteins. Drug crosses the blood-brain barrier.
Metabolism: Extensively metabolized by the liver; at least 2 metabolites have been identified. Metabolites are responsible for less than 20% of total activity of the drug.
Excretion: Part of oral dose (39%) is excreted in urine as metabolites; 57% is excreted in feces. No unchanged drug is found in urine.

Route	Onset	Peak	Duration
P.O.	Unknown	1-2 hr	24 hr

Contraindications and precautions
Contraindicated in patients hypersensitive to drug. Although drug isn't used in women, man-

ufacturer indicates pregnancy as a contraindication.

Interactions

Drug-drug. *Theophylline:* Clinically insignificant increases in theophylline clearance and decreased half-life (10%) have been observed. Use together with caution.

Effects on diagnostic tests

None reported.

Adverse reactions

GU: impotence, decreased volume of ejaculate, decreased libido.
CV: Nonbeneficial decreased prostate-specific antigen serum levels (PSA).

Overdose and treatment

Experience with overdose is limited. Patients have received single doses of 400 mg and doses of up to 80 mg daily for 3 months without adverse effects.

Clinical considerations

- Closely evaluate patient for conditions that might mimic BPH before therapy, including hypotonic bladder, prostate cancer, infection, stricture, or other neurologic conditions.

◻ *ALERT* All women of childbearing age should avoid exposure to drug and semen of patient receiving this drug. Exposure to broken or crushed tablet or with semen of patient during pregnancy presents hazard to male fetus.

- Because it's not possible to identify prospectively which patients will respond to finasteride, a minimum of 6 months of therapy may be necessary.
- Long-term effects of drug on the complications of BPH, including acute urinary obstruction, or the incidence of surgery aren't known.
- Current investigations aim to determine effectiveness of drug as adjuvant therapy after radical prostatectomy; as adjunctive treatment of prostate cancer; acne, and hirsutism.

Therapeutic monitoring

- Carefully monitor patients who have large residual urine volumes or severely diminished urine flows. Not all patients respond to drug, and these patients may not be candidates for finasteride therapy.
- Recommend carefully evaluating sustained increases in serum PSA. In patients receiving finasteride therapy, this could indicate noncompliance to therapy.

Special populations

Pregnant patients. Not indicated for use in women; potential hazard to male fetus when pregnant women come in contact with broken or crushed tablet or semen of male patient receiving drug.
Breast-feeding patients. It's unknown if drug is excreted in breast milk; however, it isn't indicated for use in women.
Pediatric patients. Drug isn't indicated for use in children.
Geriatric patients. Although elimination rate of drug is decreased in geriatric patients, dosage adjustments aren't necessary.

Patient counseling

- Advise patient that anyone who is or may become pregnant must not handle crushed tablets or have contact with patient's semen because of risk of adverse effects on a male fetus.
- Explain that drug may decrease the volume of ejaculate but doesn't appear to impair normal sexual function. However, impotence and decreased libido have occurred in less than 4% of patients treated with drug.

flecainide acetate

Tambocor

Pharmacologic classification: benzamide derivative local anesthetic (amide)
Therapeutic classification: ventricular antiarrhythmic
Pregnancy risk category C

How supplied

Available by prescription only
Tablets: 50 mg, 100 mg, 150 mg

Indications and dosages

Life-threatening ventricular tachycardia and PVCs
Adults: 100 mg P.O. q 12 hours; may increase in increments of 50 mg b.i.d. q 4 days until efficacy is achieved. Maximum dose is 400 mg daily.
Paroxysmal supraventricular tachycardia, paroxysmal atrial fibrillation or flutter in patients without structural heart disease
Adults: 50 mg P.O. q 12 hours; may increase in increments of 50 mg b.i.d. q 4 days until efficacy is achieved. Maximum dose is 300 mg/day.
≡ ***Dosage adjustment.*** Reduce dosage in patients with renal impairment (creatinine clearance of less than 35 ml/minute/1.73 m^2) beginning at 100 mg/day (50 mg b.i.d.); increase dosage cautiously at intervals longer than 4 days. For patients with less severe renal failure, initial dose is 100 mg q 12 hours, increasing cautiously at intervals longer than 4 days.

Pharmacodynamics

Antiarrhythmic action: A class IC antiarrhythmic agent, flecainide suppresses SA node automaticity and prolongs conduction in the atria, AV node, ventricles, accessory pathways, and His-Purkinje system. It has the most pronounced effect on the His-Purkinje system, as shown by QRS complex widening; this leads to a prolonged QT interval. The drug has relatively little effect on action potential duration except in Purkinje's fibers, where it shortens it. A proarrhythmic (arrhythmogenic) effect may result from the potent effects of the drug on the conduction system. Effects on the sinus node are strongest in patients with sinus node disease (sick sinus syndrome). Flecainide also exerts a moderate negative inotropic effect.

Pharmacokinetics

Absorption: Rapidly and almost completely absorbed from the GI tract; bioavailability of commercially available tablets is 85% to 90%.
Distribution: Apparently well distributed throughout the body. Only about 40% binds to plasma proteins. Trough serum levels ranging from 0.2 to 1 mcg/ml provide the greatest therapeutic benefit. Trough serum levels higher than 0.7 mcg/ml have been associated with increased adverse effects.
Metabolism: Metabolized in the liver to inactive metabolites. About 30% of an orally administered dose escapes metabolism and is excreted in the urine unchanged.
Excretion: Elimination half-life averages about 20 hours. Plasma half-life may be prolonged in patients with heart failure and renal disease.

Route	Onset	Peak	Duration
P.O.	Immediate	2-3 hr	Unknown

Contraindications and precautions

Contraindicated in patients with hypersensitivity to drug or cardiogenic shock and in those with preexisting second- or third-degree AV block or right bundle branch block when associated with a left hemiblock (in the absence of an artificial pacemaker).

Use cautiously in patients with heart failure, cardiomyopathy, severe renal or hepatic disease, prolonged QT interval, sick sinus syndrome, or blood dyscrasia.

Tambocor has demonstrated proarrythmic effects in patients with atrial fibrillation or flutter; therefore it isn't recommended for use in these patients.

Interactions

Drug-drug. *Acidifying and alkalizing agents:* Alkalization decreases renal flecainide excretion, and acidification increases it. Monitor patient carefully.
Beta blockers: May cause additive negative inotropic effects. Monitor patient carefully.
Digoxin: May cause increased serum digoxin levels. Monitor digoxin levels.
Cimetidine: May decrease both the renal and nonrenal clearance of flecainide. Monitor patient carefully.
High-dose antacids, carbonic anhydrase inhibitors, sodium bicarbonate: Marked effect on urine acidity; monitor for possible subtherapeutic or toxic levels and effects.
Other antiarrhythmic drugs: May cause additive, synergistic, or antagonistic cardiac effects and may cause additive adverse effects. Use together cautiously and monitor patient.
Drug-lifestyle. *Smoking:* May lower flecainide serum levels.

Adverse reactions

CNS: *dizziness, headache,* fatigue, tremor, anxiety, insomnia, depression, malaise, paresthesia, ataxia, vertigo, *light-headedness, syncope,* asthenia.
CV: *new or worsened* ***arrhythmias,*** chest pain, flushing, edema, ***heart failure, cardiac arrest,*** palpitations.
EENT: *blurred vision and other visual disturbances.*
GI: nausea, constipation, abdominal pain, dyspepsia, vomiting, diarrhea, anorexia.
Respiratory: *dyspnea.*
Skin: rash.
Other: fever.

Overdose and treatment

Clinical effects of overdose include increased PR and QT intervals, increased QRS complex duration, decreased myocardial contractility, conduction disturbances, and hypotension.

Treatment generally involves symptomatic and supportive measures along with ECG, blood pressure, and respiratory monitoring. Inotropic agents, including dopamine and dobutamine, may be used. Hemodynamic support, including use of an intra-aortic balloon pump and transvenous pacing, may be needed. Because of long half-life of drug, supportive measures may need to be continued for extended periods. Hemodialysis is ineffective in reducing serum drug levels.

Clinical considerations

□ ***ALERT*** Tambocor has been associated with excessive mortality or nonfatal cardiac arrest rate in national multicenter trials. Its use should be restricted to those patients in whom the benefits outweigh the risks.
- Tambocor is a strong negative inotrope and may cause or worsen heart failure, especially in those with cardiomyopathy, preexisting heart failure, or low ejection fraction.
- Hypokalemia or hyperkalemia may alter drug effects and should be corrected before drug therapy begins.
- Initiation of therapy should be done in the hospital with careful monitoring of patient with symptomatic heart failure, sinus node dysfunction, sustained ventricular tachycardia, or underlying structural heart disease and in patient changing from another antiarrhythmic in whom discontinuation of current antiarrhythmic is likely to cause life-threatening arrhythmias.
- Loading doses may exacerbate arrhythmias and therefore aren't recommended. Dosage ad-

justments should be made at intervals of at least 4 days because of long half-life of drug.
- Most patients can be adequately maintained on an every-12-hour dosage schedule, but some need to receive drug every 8 hours.
- Twice-daily dosing improves patient compliance.
- Full therapeutic effect of drug may take 3 to 5 days. I.V. lidocaine may be administered while awaiting full effect.
- Flecainide is a first class IC antiarrhythmic. Incidence of adverse effects increases when trough serum drug levels exceed 0.7 mcg/ml. Recommend periodically monitoring blood levels, especially in patients with renal failure or heart failure. Therapeutic levels range from 0.2 to 1.0 mcg/ml.
- Drug may increase acute and chronic endocardial pacing thresholds and may suppress ventricular escape rhythms. Determine pacing threshold before drug is administered, after 1 week of therapy, and regularly thereafter. It shouldn't be given to patients with preexisting poor thresholds or nonprogrammable artificial pacemakers unless pacing rescue is available.
- In heart failure and myocardial dysfunction, initial dose shouldn't exceed 100 mg every 12 hours; common initial dose is 50 mg every 12 hours.
- Use in hepatic impairment hasn't been fully evaluated; however, because flecainide is metabolized extensively (probably in the liver), use in patients with significant hepatic impairment only when benefits clearly outweigh risks. Dosage reduction may be necessary; monitor patient carefully for signs of toxicity. Serum levels also must be monitored.

Therapeutic monitoring
- Monitor for signs of toxicity.
- Monitor cardiac status.
- Monitor drug compliance.

Special populations
Breast-feeding patients. Limited data indicate that drug is excreted in breast milk. Breast-feeding isn't recommended during flecainide therapy because of the risk of adverse effects on the infant.
Pediatric patients. Safety and efficacy haven't been established in children under age 18. Limited data suggest usefulness in management of paroxysmal reentrant supraventricular tachycardia.
Geriatric patients. Geriatric patients are more susceptible to adverse effects. Monitor patient carefully.

Patient counseling
- Advise patient to closely follow administration instruction.
- Warn patient of potential adverse drug effects.

floxuridine
FUDR

Pharmacologic classification: antimetabolite (cell cycle-phase specific, S phase)
Therapeutic classification: antineoplastic
Pregnancy risk category D

How supplied
Available by prescription only
Injection: 500-mg vials

Indications and dosages
Dosage and indications may vary. Check current literature for recommended protocol.
Palliative management of GI adenocarcinoma metastatic to the liver; brain, head, neck, gallbladder, bile duct cancer
Adults: 0.1 to 0.6 mg/kg daily by intra-arterial infusion; or 0.4 to 0.6 mg/kg daily into hepatic artery.
◇ ***Solid tumors***
Adults: 0.5 to 1 mg/kg daily by I.V. infusion for 6 to 15 days or until toxicity occurs; or 30 mg/kg daily by single injection for 5 days, then 15 mg/kg every other day for up to 11 days or until toxicity occurs.

Pharmacodynamics
Antineoplastic action: Floxuridine exerts its cytotoxic activity after conversion to its active form, by competitively inhibiting the enzyme thymidylate synthetase; this halts DNA synthesis and leads to cell death.

Pharmacokinetics
Absorption: Not administered orally.
Distribution: Crosses the blood-brain barrier to a limited extent.
Metabolism: Metabolized to fluorouracil in the liver after intra-arterial infusions and rapid I.V. injections.
Excretion: About 60% of a dose is excreted through the lungs as carbon dioxide. A small amount is excreted by the kidneys as unchanged drug and metabolites.

Route	Onset	Peak	Duration
Intra-arterial	Unknown	Unknown	Unknown

Contraindications and precautions
Contraindicated in patients with poor nutritional state, bone marrow suppression, or serious infection. Use in pregnancy only if the potential benefits justify the potential risk to tbe fetus.

Use cautiously in patients following high-dose pelvic radiation therapy or use of alkylating agents and in those with impaired renal or hepatic function.

Interactions
Drug-lifestyle. *Sun exposure:* May increase skin reaction. Advise patient to take precautions.

Effects on diagnostic tests
None reported.

Adverse reactions
CNS: cerebellar ataxia, malaise, weakness, headache, lethargy, disorientation, confusion, euphoria.
CV: myocardial ischemia, angina.
EENT: blurred vision, nystagmus, photophobia, epistaxis.
GI: *anorexia, stomatitis, nausea, vomiting, diarrhea, bleeding, enteritis,* GI ulceration.
Hematologic: ***leukopenia, anemia, thrombocytopenia, agranulocytosis.***
Hepatic: elevated liver enzymes, increased bilirubin, ***drug-induced hepatotoxicity.***
Skin: *erythema,* dermatitis, pruritus, rash, alopecia, photosensitivity.
Other: thrombophlebitis, ***anaphylaxis,*** fever.

Overdose and treatment
Signs and symptoms of overdose include myelosuppression, diarrhea, alopecia, dermatitis, and hyperpigmentation.

Treatment is usually supportive and includes transfusion of blood components and antidiarrheal agents.

Clinical considerations
- Reconstituted drug solutions are stable for 14 days when refrigerated.
- Drug is often administered via hepatic arterial infusion in treating hepatic metastases.

Therapeutic monitoring
- Instruct prescriber to discontinue drug if severe skin and GI adverse reactions occur.
- Monitor patient's intake and output, CBC, and renal and hepatic function.
- Therapeutic effect may be delayed 1 to 6 weeks.

Special populations
Pregnant patients. Women of childbearing age should avoid this drug to avoid toxicity to fetus. Use only when potential benefits to pregnant woman justify risks to fetus.
Breast-feeding patients. It isn't known if drug is excreted in breast milk. However, because of risk of serious adverse reactions, mutagenicity, and carcinogenicity in the infant, breast-feeding isn't recommended.

Patient counseling
Advise patient to report nausea, vomiting, stomach pain, signs of infection, or unusual bruising or bleeding.

fluconazole
Diflucan

Pharmacologic classification: bis-triazole derivative
Therapeutic classification: antifungal
Pregnancy risk category C

How supplied
Available by prescription only
Tablets: 50 mg, 100 mg, 150 mg, 200 mg
Injection: 200 mg/100 ml, 400 mg/200 ml
Suspension: 350 mg/35 ml, 1,400 mg/35 ml

Indications and dosages
Oropharyngeal and esophageal candidiasis
Adults: 200 mg P.O. or I.V. on day 1 followed by 100 mg P.O. or I.V. once daily. As much as 400 mg daily has been used for esophageal disease. Treatment should continue for at least 2 weeks after resolution of symptoms.
Children: 6 mg/kg on day 1, followed by 3 mg/kg for at least 2 weeks.
Systemic candidiasis
Adults: Up to 400 mg P.O. or I.V. once daily. Treatment should be continued for at least 2 weeks after resolution of symptoms.
Cryptococcal meningitis
Adults: 400 mg I.V. or P.O. on day 1, followed by 200 mg once daily. Continue treatment for 10 to 12 weeks after CSF culture becomes negative. For suppression of relapse in patients with AIDS, give 200 mg once daily.
Vaginal candidiasis
Adults: 150 mg P.O. as a single dose.
Urinary tract infection or peritonitis
Adults: 50 to 200 mg P.O. or I.V. daily.
Prophylaxis in patients undergoing bone marrow transplantation
Adults: 400 mg P.O. or I.V. daily for several days before transplantation and 7 days after neutrophil count rises above 1,000 cells/ mm³.
◇ ***Candidal infection, long-term suppression in patients with HIV infection***
Adults: 100 to 200 mg P.O. or I.V. daily.
◇ ***Prophylaxis against mucocutaneous candidiasis, cryptococcosis, coccidioidomycosis, or histoplasmosis in patients with HIV infection***
Adults: 200 to 400 mg P.O. or I.V. daily.
Children and infants: 2 to 8 mg/kg P.O. daily.
≡ ***Dosage adjustment.*** Patients with renal impairment should have their dosages adjusted based on this table:

Creatinine clearance (ml/min)	Percentage of usual adult dosage
> 50	100
21 to 49	50
11 to 20	25

Patients receiving hemodialysis should receive one full dose after each session.

Pharmacodynamics

Antifungal action: Fluconazole exerts its fungistatic effects by inhibiting fungal cytochrome P-450. The spectrum of activity includes *Cryptococcus neoformans, Candida* (including systemic *C. albicans), Aspergillus flavus, Aspergillus fumigatus, Coccidioides immitis,* and *Histoplasma capsulatum.*

Pharmacokinetics

Absorption: After oral administration, absorption is rapid and complete.
Distribution: Well distributed to various sites, including CNS, saliva, sputum, blister fluid, urine, normal skin, nails, and blister skin. CNS levels approach 50% to 90% of that of serum. Fluconazole is 12% protein-bound.
Metabolism: Partially metabolized.
Elimination: Primarily excreted via the kidneys. More than 80% of an administered dose is excreted unchanged in the urine. Excretion rate diminishes as renal function decreases.

Route	Onset	Peak	Duration
P.O.	Unknown	1-2 hr	30 hr
I.V.	Immediate	Unknown	Unknown

Contraindications and precautions

Contraindicated in patients with hypersensitivity to drug and other drugs in same class.

Interactions

Drug-drug. *Cimetidine:* May reduce serum levels of fluconazole. Monitor patient carefully.
Cisapride: Concurrent use may cause prolongation of the QT interval, resulting in arrhythmias and serious CV effects. Don't use together.
Cyclosporine: Increased cyclosporine levels. Monitor cyclosporine levels.
Hydrochlorothiazide: Decreased fluconazole clearance, elevating serum levels of the drug. Use together cautiously.
Phenytoin: May significantly increase phenytoin serum levels. Monitor phenytoin levels.
Rifampin: Can lower fluconazole levels. Monitor patient for drug effects.
Rifampin, isoniazid, sulfonylureas, phenytoin, valproic acid: Elevated hepatic transaminase levels. Monitor patient carefully.
Sulfonylureas, tolbutamide, glyburide, and glipizide: Concurrent use increases hypoglycemic effects. Use together cautiously and monitor blood glucose.
*Tacrolimus:*Increased concentration of tacrolimus. Monitor patient carefully.
Theophylline: Increased theophylline levels. Monitor theophylline levels.
Warfarin: Enhanced hypoprothrombinemic effects. Monitor PT and INR closely.
Zidovudine: Increased activity of zidovine may occur. Monitor patient carefully.
Drug-food. *Caffeine:* May increase plasma caffeine levels. Advise avoiding caffeine.

Effects on diagnostic tests

None reported.

Adverse reactions

CNS: headache.
GI: *nausea,* vomiting, abdominal pain, diarrhea.
Hepatic: ***hepatotoxicity*** (rare), elevated liver enzymes.
Skin: rash, ***Stevens-Johnson syndrome*** (rare), alopecia.
Other: ***anaphylaxis.***

Overdose and treatment

Treatment is largely supportive.

Clinical considerations

- Adjust dose in those with renal dysfunction.
- Fluconazole isn't compatible with other I.V. medications.
- Bioavailability of oral drug is comparable to I.V. dosing.
- Adverse reactions (including transaminase elevations) are more frequent and more severe in patients with severe underlying illness (including AIDS and malignancies).

Therapeutic monitoring

Monitor for anaphylaxis and other adverse reactions.

Special populations

Pregnant patients. Fluconazole shouldn't be given to pregnant HIV-infected women and should be discontinued if pregnancy occurs. Use in pregnancy only if potential benefits outweigh the risk to the fetus.
Breast-feeding patients. Drug is excreted in breast milk at levels similar to those of plasma. Therefore, use in breast-feeding women isn't recommended.
Pediatric patients. Safety and efficacy in children under age 6 months aren't established.

Patient counseling

Warn patient of potential adverse reactions and advise to promptly report any adverse drug events to prescriber.

flucytosine (5-FC)

Ancobon

Pharmacologic classification: fluorinated pyrimidine
Therapeutic classification: antifungal
Pregnancy risk category C

How supplied

Available by prescription only
Capsules: 250 mg, 500 mg

Indications and dosages

***Severe fungal infections caused by susceptible strains of* Candida *and* Cryptococcus**
Adults : 50 to 150 mg/kg/day P.O., administered in divided doses q 6 hours.
◇ ***Chromomycosis***
Adults: 150 mg/kg P.O. daily.
≡ ***Dosage adjustment.*** In patients with renal failure who have a creatinine clearance of 50 ml/minute or less, reduce dosage by 20% to 80%. Alternatively, in patients with creatinine clearance of 20 to 40 ml/minute, increase dosage interval to q 12 hours; creatinine clearance of 10 to 20 ml/minute, increase dosage interval to q 24 hours; and for those with creatinine clearance of less than 10 ml/minute, increase dosage interval to q 24 to 48 hours. Monitor serum levels. Flucytosine is removed by hemodialysis and peritoneal dialysis.

Dosage of 20 to 50 mg/kg P.O. immediately after hemodialysis q 2 to 3 days ensures therapeutic blood levels.

Pharmacodynamics

Antifungal action: Flucytosine penetrates fungal cells, where it's converted to fluorouracil, which interferes with pyrimidine metabolism; it also may be converted to fluorodeoxyuredylic acid, which interferes with DNA synthesis. Because human cells lack the enzymes needed to convert drug to these toxic metabolites, flucytosine is selectively toxic to fungal, not host cells. It's active against some strains of *Cryptococcus* and *Candida.*

Pharmacokinetics

Absorption: About 75% to 90% of an oral dose is absorbed. Food decreases rate of absorption.
Distribution: Distributed widely into the liver, kidneys, spleen, heart, bronchial secretions, joints, peritoneal fluid, and aqueous humor. CSF levels vary from 60% to 100% of serum levels. It's 2% to 4% bound to plasma proteins.
Metabolism: Only small amounts are metabolized.
Excretion: About 75% to 95% of a dose is excreted unchanged in urine; less than 10% is excreted unchanged in feces. Serum half-life is 2½ to 6 hours with normal renal function; as long as 1,160 hours with creatinine clearance less than 2 ml/minute.

Route	Onset	Peak	Duration
P.O.	Unknown	2-6 hr	Unknown

Contraindications and precautions

Contraindicated in patients with hypersensitivity to drug. Use cautiously in patients with impaired renal or hepatic function and bone marrow suppression.

Interactions

Drug-drug. *Amphotericin B:* Synergistic effects and possible enhanced toxicity. Monitor patient carefully.

Effects on diagnostic tests

Flucytosine causes falsely elevated creatinine values on iminohydrolase enzymatic assay.

Adverse reactions

CNS: headache, vertigo, sedation, fatigue, weakness, confusion, hallucinations, psychosis, ataxia, hearing loss, paresthesia, parkinsonism, peripheral neuropathy.
CV: ***cardiac arrest, myocardial toxicity, ventricular dysfunction.***
GI: nausea, vomiting, diarrhea, abdominal pain, emesis, dry mouth, duodenal ulcer, ***hemorrhage,*** ulcerative colitis.
GU: azotemia, elevated creatinine and BUN levels, crystalluria, ***renal failure.***
Hematologic: anemia, ***leukopenia, bone marrow suppression, thrombocytopenia,*** **eosinophilia,** ***agranulocytosis, aplastic anemia.***
Hepatic: elevated liver enzymes, elevated serum alkaline phosphatase, jaundice.
Metabolic: hypoglycemia, hypokalemia.
Respiratory: ***respiratory arrest,*** chest pain, dyspnea.
Skin: occasional rash, pruritus, urticaria, photosensitivity, allergic reactions, ***toxic epidermal necrolysis.***

Overdose and treatment

Flucytosine overdose may affect CV and pulmonary function. Treatment is largely supportive. Induced emesis or lavage may be useful within 4 hours after ingestion. Activated charcoal and osmotic cathartics also may be helpful. Flucytosine is readily removed by either hemodialysis or peritoneal dialysis.

Clinical considerations

- Hematologic studies and renal and hepatic function studies should precede therapy and should be repeated frequently thereafter.
- Giving capsules over 15-minute period helps reduce nausea, vomiting, and GI distress.

Therapeutic monitoring

- Monitor intake and output to ensure adequate renal function.
- Prolonged serum levels in excess of 100 mcg/ml may be associated with toxicity; recommend monitoring serum levels, especially in patients with renal insufficiency.

Special populations

Pregnant patients. Use drug only when potential benefits justify risk to fetus.
Breast-feeding patients. Safety hasn't been established in breast-feeding women.
Pediatric patients. Safety and efficacy in children haven't been established.

Patient counseling

- Advise patient of adverse reactions and the need to report them.
- Tell patient to call prescriber promptly if urine output decreases or signs of bleeding or bruising occur.
- Explain that adequate response may require several weeks or months of therapy.
- Advise patient to adhere to medical regimen and to return as instructed for follow-up visits.

fludarabine phosphate

Fludara

Pharmacologic classification: antimetabolite
Therapeutic classification: antineoplastic
Pregnancy risk category D

How supplied

Available by prescription only
Injection: 50 mg as lyophilized powder

Indications and dosages

Treatment of B-cell chronic lymphocytic leukemia (CLL) in patients who haven't responded or responded inadequately to at least one standard alkylating agent regimen, ◊ mycosis fungoides, ◊ hairy-cell leukemia, ◊ Hodgkin's and malignant lymphoma

Adults: Usually, 25 mg/m² I.V. over 30 minutes (◊ rapid I.V. injection or continuous I.V. infusion) for 5 consecutive days q 28 days. Therapy based on patient response and tolerance.

◊ Chronic lymphocytic leukemia

Adults: Usually, 18 to 30 mg/m² I.V. over 30 minutes (◊ rapid I.V. injection or continuous I.V. infusion) for 5 consecutive days q 28 days. Therapy based on patient response and tolerance.

Pharmacodynamics

Antineoplastic action: After rapid conversion of fludarabine to its active metabolite, the metabolite appears to inhibit DNA synthesis by inhibiting DNA polymerase alpha, ribonucleotide reductase, and DNA primase. The exact mechanism of action isn't fully established.

Pharmacokinetics

Absorption: Administered I.V.
Distribution: Widely distributed with a volume of distribution of 96 to 98 L/m² at steady state.
Metabolism: Rapidly dephosphorylated and then phosphorylated intracellularly to its active metabolite.
Excretion: 23% is excreted in urine as unchanged active metabolite. Half-life is about 10 hours.

Route	Onset	Peak	Duration
I.V.	7-12 wk	Unknown	Unknown

Contraindications and precautions

Contraindicated in patients hypersensitive to drug or its components. Use cautiously in patients with renal insufficiency.

Interactions

Drug-drug. *Other myelosuppressive agents:* Concurrent use may cause additive toxicity. Don't use with other myelosuppresive agents. *Pentostatin:* Increases risk of pulmonary toxicity. Avoid use together.

Effects on diagnostic tests

None reported.

Adverse reactions

CNS: *fatigue, malaise, weakness, paresthesia,* peripheral neuropathy, headache, sleep disorder, depression, cerebellar syndrome, ***CVA,*** agitation, ***confusion, coma.***
CV: *edema,* angina, transient ischemic attack, phlebitis, ***arrhythmias, heart failure,*** supraventricular tachycardia, deep venous thrombosis, ***aneurysm, hemorrhage.***
EENT: *visual disturbances,* hearing loss, delayed blindness (with high doses), sinusitis, pharyngitis, epistaxis.
GI: *nausea, vomiting, diarrhea,* constipation, *anorexia,* stomatitis, ***GI bleeding,*** esophagitis, mucositis.
GU: dysuria, *urinary infection* or hesitancy, proteinuria, hematuria, ***renal failure.***
Hematologic: ***hemolytic anemia,*** **MYELOSUPPRESSION.**
Hepatic: ***liver failure,*** cholelithiasis.
Metabolic: hypocalcemia, hyperkalemia, hyperglycemia, dehydration, hyperuricemia, hyperphosphatemia.
Musculoskeletal: *myalgia.*
Respiratory: *cough, pneumonia, dyspnea, upper respiratory tract infection,* allergic pneumonitis, hemoptysis, hypoxia, bronchitis.
Skin: alopecia, diaphoresis, *rash,* pruritus, seborrhea.
Other: *fever, chills, infection, pain,* tumor lysis syndrome, ***anaphylaxis, death*** (with very high doses).

Overdose and treatment

Irreversible CNS toxicity characterized by delayed blindness, coma, and death is associated with high doses. Severe thrombocytopenia and neutropenia secondary to bone marrow suppression also occur. There's no specific antidote, and treatment consists of discontinuing therapy and taking supportive measures.

Clinical considerations

- Drug has been used investigationally in the treatment of malignant lymphoma, macroglobulinemic lymphoma, prolymphocytic leukemia or prolymphocytoid variant of CLL, mycosis fungoides, hairy cell leukemia, and Hodgkin's disease.
- Administer drug under the direct supervision of a doctor experienced in antineoplastic therapy.
- Tumor lysis syndrome (hyperuricemia, hyperphosphatemia, hypocalcemia, metabolic acidosis, hyperkalemia, hematuria, urate crystalluria, and renal failure) has occurred in CLL patients with large tumors.
- Severe neurologic effects, including blindness, are seen when high doses are used to treat acute leukemia.
- Advanced age, renal insufficiency, and bone marrow impairment may predispose patient to severe toxicity; toxic effects are dose-dependent.
- Optimal duration of therapy hasn't been established; three additional cycles after achieving maximal response are recommended before discontinuing drug.

Therapeutic monitoring

Careful hematologic monitoring is required, especially of neutrophil and platelet counts.

Special populations

Breast-feeding patients. It's unknown if drug is excreted in breast milk. Risk-benefit ratio must be determined.
Pediatric patients. Safety and efficacy in children haven't been established.
Geriatric patients. Advanced age may increase toxicity potential.

Patient counseling

Tell patient to avoid contact with infected persons and report signs of infection or unusual bleeding immediately.

fludrocortisone acetate

Florinef

Pharmacologic classification: mineralocorticoid, glucocorticoid
Therapeutic classification: mineralocorticoid replacement therapy
Pregnancy risk category C

How supplied

Available by prescription only
Tablets: 0.1 mg

Indications and dosages

Adrenal insufficiency (partial replacement), salt-losing adrenogenital syndrome
Adults: 0.1 to 0.2 mg P.O. daily.
Children: 0.05 to 0.1 mg P.O. daily.
Postural hypotension in diabetic patients, ◇orthostatic hypotension
Adults: 0.1 to 0.4 mg P.O. daily.
Postural hypotension due to levodopa therapy
Adults: 0.05 to 0.2 mg P.O. daily.

Pharmacodynamics

Adrenal hormone replacement: Fludrocortisone, a synthetic glucocorticoid with potent mineralocorticoid activity, is used for partial replacement of steroid hormones in adrenocortical insufficiency and in salt-losing forms of congenital adrenogenital syndrome. In treating adrenocortical insufficiency, an exogenous glucocorticoid must also be administered for adequate control. (Cortisone or hydrocortisone are usually the drugs of choice for replacement because they produce both mineralocorticoid and glucocorticoid activity.) Fludrocortisone is administered on a variable schedule ranging from three times weekly to twice daily, depending on individual requirements.

Pharmacokinetics

Absorption: Absorbed readily from the GI tract.
Distribution: Removed rapidly from blood and distributed to muscle, liver, skin, intestines, and kidneys. It has a plasma half-life of about 30 minutes. It's extensively bound to plasma proteins (transcortin and albumin). Only the unbound portion is active. Adrenocorticoids are distributed into breast milk and through the placenta.
Metabolism: Metabolized in the liver to inactive glucuronide and sulfate metabolites.
Excretion: Inactive metabolites and small amounts of unmetabolized drug are excreted by the kidneys. Insignificant quantities of drug are also excreted in feces. Biologic half-life is 18 to 36 hours; plasma half-life is 3½ hours or more.

Route	Onset	Peak	Duration
P.O.	Variable	2 hr	1-2 days

Contraindications and precautions

Contraindicated in patients with systemic fungal infections or hypersensitivity to drug.

Use cautiously in patients with hypothyroidism, cirrhosis, ocular herpes simplex, emotional instability, psychotic tendencies, nonspecific ulcerative colitis, diverticulitis, fresh intestinal anastamoses, peptic ulcer, renal insufficiency, hypertension, osteoporosis, and myasthenia gravis.

Interactions

Drug-drug. *Barbiturates, phenytoin, rifampin:* May cause decreased corticosteroid effects. Monitor patient carefully.
Cardiac glycosides: If hypokalemia occurs, there's increased risk of toxicity. Monitor patient closely.

Isoniazid and salicylates: Increased metabolism of these drugs. Monitor patient for drug effects.
Thiazide diuretics or amphotericin B: Concurrent use may enhance hypokalemia. Monitor electrolytes.
Drug-food. *Sodium-containing medications or foods:* May increase blood pressure. Sodium intake may need to be adjusted.

Effects on diagnostic tests

Recommend performing glucose tolerance tests only if necessary, because severe hypoglycemia tends to develop in addisonian patients within 3 hours of the test.

Adverse reactions

CV: *sodium and water retention,* hypertension, cardiac hypertrophy, edema, ***heart failure.***
Metabolic: increased serum sodium levels, hypokalemia.
Skin: bruising, diaphoresis, urticaria, allergic rash.

Overdose and treatment

Acute toxicity is manifested as an extension of the therapeutic effect, such as disturbances in fluid and electrolyte balance, hypokalemia, edema, hypertension, and cardiac insufficiency. In acute toxicity, administer symptomatic treatment and correct fluid and electrolyte imbalance.

Clinical considerations

Consider the recommendations relevant to all systemic adrenocorticoids as well as the following:
- Use only with other supplemental measures, such as glucocorticoids, control of electrolytes, and control of infection.
- Supplemental dosages may be required in times of physiologic stress from serious illness, trauma, or surgery.

Therapeutic monitoring

Monitor for significant patient weight gain, edema, hypertension, or severe headaches.

Special populations

Pediatric patients. Long-term use in children and adolescents may delay growth and maturation.

Patient counseling

- Teach patient to recognize signs of electrolyte imbalance: muscle weakness, paresthesia, numbness, fatigue, anorexia, nausea, altered mental status, increased urination, altered heart rhythm, severe or continuing headaches, unusual weight gain, or swelling of the feet.
- Tell patient to take missed doses as soon as possible, unless it's almost time for the next dose, and not to double the dose.

flumazenil

Romazicon

Pharmacologic classification: benzodiazepine antagonist
Therapeutic classification: antidote
Pregnancy risk category C

How supplied

Available by prescription only
Injection: 0.1 mg/ml in 5-ml and 10-ml multiple-dose vials

Indications and dosages

Complete or partial reversal of sedative effects of benzodiazepines after anesthesia or short diagnostic procedures (conscious sedation)
Adults: Initially, 0.2 mg I.V. over 15 seconds. If patient doesn't reach desired level of consciousness after 45 seconds, repeat dose. Repeat at 1-minute intervals until a cumulative dose of 1 mg has been given (initial dose plus four additional doses). Most patients respond after 0.6 to 1 mg of drug. If resedation occurs, dose may be repeated after 20 minutes, but no more than 1 mg should be given at one time, and patient shouldn't receive more than 3 mg/hour.
Management of suspected benzodiazepine overdose
Adults: Initially, 0.2 mg I.V. over 30 seconds. If patient doesn't reach desired level of consciousness after 30 seconds, administer 0.3 mg over 30 seconds. If patient still doesn't respond adequately, give 0.5 mg over 30 seconds, then repeat 0.5-mg doses at 1-minute intervals until a cumulative dose of 3 mg has been given. Most patients with benzodiazepine overdose respond to cumulative doses between 1 and 3 mg; rarely, patients who respond partially after 3 mg may require additional doses. Don't give more than 5 mg over 5 minutes initially; sedation that persists after this dose is unlikely to be caused by benzodiazepines. If resedation occurs, dose may be repeated after 20 minutes, but no more than 1 mg should be given at one time, and patient shouldn't receive more than 3 mg/hour.

Pharmacodynamics

Antidote action: Flumazenil competitively inhibits the actions of benzodiazepines on the gamma-aminobutyric acid—benzodiazepine receptor complex.

Pharmacokinetics

Absorption: No information available.
Distribution: After administration, drug redistributes rapidly (initial distribution half-life is 7 to 15 minutes). It's about 50% bound to plasma proteins.

Metabolism: Rapidly extracted from the blood and metabolized by the liver. Metabolites that have been identified are inactive. Ingestion of food during an I.V. infusion enhances extraction of drug from plasma, probably by increasing hepatic blood flow.
Excretion: About 90% to 95% is excreted in the urine as metabolites; the remainder is excreted in feces. Plasma half-life is about 54 minutes.

Route	Onset	Peak	Duration
I.V.	1-2 min	6-10 min	Variable

Contraindications and precautions
Contraindicated in patients hypersensitive to drug or benzodiazepines; in patients who show evidence of serious tricyclic antidepressant overdose; and in those who received a benzodiazepine to treat a potentially life-threatening condition such as status epilepticus.

Use cautiously in alcohol-dependent or psychiatric patients, in those at high risk for seizures, or in those with head injuries, signs of seizures, or recent high intake of benzodiazepines, such as patients in the intensive care unit.

Interactions
Drug-drug. *Antidepressants and drugs that can cause seizures or arrhythmias:* May cause seizures or arrhythmias after flumazenil removes the effects of the benzodiazepine overdose. Flumazenil shouldn't be used in mixed overdose, especially when seizures (from any cause) are likely to occur.

Effects on diagnostic tests
None reported.

Adverse reactions
CNS: *dizziness, abnormal or blurred vision, headache, seizures,* agitation, emotional lability, tremor, insomnia.
CV: ***arrhythmias,*** cutaneous vasodilation, palpitations.
GI: nausea, vomiting.
Respiratory: dyspnea, hyperventilation.
Skin: *diaphoresis.*
Other: *pain* (at injection site).

Overdose and treatment
In clinical trials, large doses of flumazenil were administered I.V. to volunteers in the absence of a benzodiazepine agonist. No serious adverse reactions, clinical signs or symptoms, or altered laboratory tests were noted.

In patients with benzodiazepine overdose, large doses of flumazenil may produce agitation or anxiety, hyperesthesia, increased muscle tone, or seizures. Seizures may be treated with barbiturates, phenytoin, or benzodiazepines.

Clinical considerations
- Because duration of action of flumazenil is shorter than that of benzodiazepines, advise prescriber to monitor patient carefully and administer additional drug as needed. Duration and degree of effect depend on plasma levels of the sedating benzodiazepine and the dose of flumazenil.
- Resedation may occur after reversal of benzodiazepine effect.
- Flumazenil can be administered by direct injection or diluted with a compatible solution.

Therapeutic monitoring
Monitor patient for resedation according to duration of drug being reversed. Usually, serious resedation is unlikely in patient who fails to show signs of resedation 2 hours after a 1-mg dose of flumazenil.

Special populations
Breast-feeding patients. It's unknown if drug is excreted in breast milk. Use cautiously in breast-feeding women.
Pediatric patients. Because no clinical data exist regarding risks, benefits, or dosage range in children, manufacturer doesn't recommend its use.

Patient counseling
Because of risk of resedation, advise patient to avoid hazardous activities (such as driving a car), alcohol, CNS depressants, and OTC drugs within 24 hours of the procedure.

flunisolide
Nasal inhalant
Nasalide

Oral inhalant
AeroBid, AeroBid-M

Pharmacologic classification: glucocorticoid
Therapeutic classification: anti-inflammatory, antiasthmatic
Pregnancy risk category C

How supplied
Available by prescription only
Nasal inhalant: 25 mcg/metered spray; 200 doses/bottle
Oral inhalant: 250 mcg/metered spray; at least 100 doses/inhaler

Indications and dosages
Corticosteroid-dependent asthma
Adults: Two inhalations b.i.d. for a total daily dose of 1 mg. Don't exceed 8 inhalations (2 mg)/day.
Children age 6 and older: Two inhalations b.i.d. Don't exceed 4 inhalations daily.

Seasonal or perennial rhinitis
Adults: 2 sprays (50 mcg) in each nostril b.i.d. (total dose 200 mcg/day). If needed, increase to 2 sprays in each nostril t.i.d. (total dose 300 mcg/day).
Children age 6 to 14: 1 spray (25 mcg) in each nostril t.i.d. or 2 sprays (50 mcg) in each nostril b.i.d. (total dose 150 to 200 mcg/day).

Pharmacodynamics
Anti-inflammatory action: Flunisolide stimulates the synthesis of enzymes needed to decrease the inflammatory response. The anti-inflammatory and vasoconstrictor potency of topically applied flunisolide is several hundred times greater than that of hydrocortisone and about equal to that of an equal weight of triamcinolone; the metabolite, 6-beta-hydroxy-flunisolide, has about three times the activity of hydrocortisone.
Antiasthmatic action: The nasal inhalant form is used in the symptomatic treatment of seasonal or perennial rhinitis. In patients who require corticosteroids to control symptoms, the oral inhalant form is used to treat bronchial asthma.

Pharmacokinetics
Absorption: About 50% of a nasally inhaled dose is absorbed systemically. After oral inhalation, about 40% of dose is absorbed from the lungs and GI tract; only about 20% of an orally inhaled dose reaches systemic circulation unmetabolized because of extensive metabolism in the liver. Onset of action usually occurs in a few days but may take as long as 4 weeks.
Distribution: Distribution following intranasal administration or oral inhalation hasn't been described. No evidence exists of tissue storage of flunisolide or its metabolites.
Metabolism: When swallowed, undergoes rapid metabolism in the liver or GI tract to several metabolites, one of which has glucocorticoid activity. Flunisolide and its 6-beta-hydroxy metabolite are eventually conjugated in the liver, by glucuronic acid or surface sulfate, to inactive metabolites.
Excretion: Excretion pathway is unknown when drug is given as inhalant; however, when it's given systemically, metabolites are excreted in roughly equal portions in feces and urine. Biologic half-life of drug averages about 2 hours.

Route	Onset	Peak	Duration
Inhalation	Variable	10-30 min	Unknown

Contraindications and precautions
Contraindicated in patients hypersensitive to drug. Use of nasal inhalant is contraindicated in the presence of untreated localized infection involving nasal mucosa; oral inhalant shouldn't be used in patients with status asthmaticus or respiratory infections.

Use nasal inhalant cautiously in patients with tuberculosis; untreated fungal, bacterial, or systemic viral or ocular herpes simplex infections; or septal ulcers, trauma, surgery in the nasal region. Oral inhalant isn't recommended for patients with asthma controlled by bronchodilators or other noncorticosteroids alone or those patients with nonasthma bronchial diseases.

Interactions
None reported.

Effects on diagnostic tests
None reported.

Adverse reactions
CNS: headache (with nasal inhalant); dizziness, irritability, nervousness (with oral inhalant).
CV: chest pain, edema (with oral inhalant).
EENT: nasopharyngeal fungal infection; *mild, transient nasal burning and stinging,* stinging, dryness, sneezing, epistaxis, watery eyes (with nasal inhalant).
GI: nausea, vomiting (with nasal inhalant); dry mouth, abdominal pain, decreased appetite, *nausea, vomiting, diarrhea, upset stomach* (with oral inhalant).
Respiratory: *upper respiratory tract infection* (with oral inhalant).
Skin: rash, pruritus (with oral inhalant).
Other: *cold symptoms, flu,* fever (with oral inhalant).

Overdose and treatment
No information available.

Clinical considerations
Recommendations for use of flunisolide and for care and teaching of the patient during therapy are the same as those for all inhalant adrenocorticoids.

Therapeutic monitoring
- Monitor for adverse reactions
- Monitor for development of oral fungal infections.

Special populations
Pregnant patients. Use drug during pregnancy only when potential benefits justify risk to fetus.
Breast-feeding patients. Use drug with caution in breast-feeding patients.
Pediatric patients. Safety and efficacy haven't been established in children under age 6 months.

Patient counseling
- Inform patient that drug doesn't relieve emergency asthma attacks.
- Advise patient of proper administration method.

fluocinonide

Lidemol*, Lidex, Lidex-E, Lyderm*

Pharmacologic classification: topical adrenocorticoid
Therapeutic classification: anti-inflammatory
Pregnancy risk category C

How supplied

Available by prescription only
Cream, gel, ointment, solution: 0.05%

Indications and dosages

Inflammation of corticosteroid-responsive dermatoses
Adults and children: Apply sparingly b.i.d. or t.i.d. Occlusive dressings may be used for severe or resistant dermatoses.

Pharmacodynamics

Anti-inflammatory action: Fluocinonide stimulates the synthesis of enzymes needed to decrease the inflammatory response. Fluocinonide is a high-potency fluorinated glucocorticoid categorized as a group II topical corticosteroid.

Pharmacokinetics

Absorption: Amount absorbed depends on amount applied and on nature of skin at application site. It ranges from about 1% in areas of thick stratum corneum (such as the palms, soles, elbows, and knees) to as high as 36% in areas of thin stratum corneum (face, eyelids, and genitals). Absorption increases in areas of skin damage, inflammation, or occlusion. Some systemic absorption of corticosteroids occurs, especially through the oral mucosa.
Distribution: After topical application, is distributed throughout the local skin. Any drug absorbed into circulation is removed rapidly from the blood and distributed into muscle, liver, skin, intestines, and kidneys.
Metabolism: After topical administration, is metabolized primarily in the skin. The small amount absorbed into systemic circulation is metabolized primarily in the liver to inactive compounds.
Excretion: Inactive metabolites are excreted by the kidneys, primarily as glucuronides and sulfates, but also as unconjugated products. Small amounts of metabolites are excreted in feces.

Route	Onset	Peak	Duration
Topical	Unknown	Unknown	Unknown

Contraindications and precautions

Contraindicated in patients hypersensitive to drug.

Interactions

None significant.

Effects on diagnostic tests

None reported.

Adverse reactions

Metabolic: hyperglycemia, glucosuria.
Skin: burning, pruritus, irritation, dryness, erythema, folliculitis, hypertrichosis, hypopigmentation, acneiform eruptions, perioral dermatitis, allergic contact dermatitis; *maceration, secondary infection, atrophy, striae, miliaria* (with occlusive dressings).
Other: ***hypothalamic-pituitary-adrenal axis suppression***, Cushing's syndrome.

Overdose and treatment

No information available.

Clinical considerations

Clinical considerations are the same as for all topical adrenocorticoids.

Therapeutic monitoring

Therapeutic monitoring is the same as for all topical adrenocorticoids.

Special populations

Drug use recommendations in pregnant and breast-feeding women and pediatric and geriatric patients is the same as for all topical adrenocorticoids.

fluorouracil (5-FU)

Adrucil, Efudex, Fluoroplex

Pharmacologic classification: antimetabolite (cell cycle-phase specific, S phase)
Therapeutic classification: antineoplastic
Pregnancy risk category D (injection), X (cream)

How supplied

Available by prescription only
Injection: 50 mg/ml in 10-ml, 20-ml, 50-ml, 100-ml vials
Cream: 1%, 5%
Topical solution: 1%, 2%, 5%

Indications and dosages

Dosage and indications may vary. Check current literature for recommended protocol.
Palliative management of colon, rectal, breast, ◇ovarian, ◇cervical, gastric, ◇bladder, ◇liver, pancreatic cancers
Adults and children: 12 mg/kg I.V. for 4 days, then if no toxicity occurs, give 6 mg/kg I.V. on days 6, 8, 10, and 12. Maintenance therapy is a repeated course q 30 days. Don't exceed 800 mg/day (400 mg/day in severely ill patients).

Actinic or solar keratoses
Adults: Sufficient cream or lotion to cover lesions b.i.d. for 2 to 4 weeks. Usually, 1% preparations are used on head, neck, and chest, 2% and 5% on hands.
Superficial basal cell carcinomas
Adults: 5% solution or cream in a sufficient amount to cover lesion b.i.d. for 3 to 6 weeks, up to 12 weeks.

Pharmacodynamics
Antineoplastic action: Fluorouracil exerts its cytotoxic activity by acting as an antimetabolite, competing for the enzyme that's important in the synthesis of thymidine, an essential substrate for DNA synthesis. Therefore, DNA synthesis is inhibited. Drug also inhibits RNA synthesis to a lesser extent.

Pharmacokinetics
Absorption: Given parenterally because it's absorbed poorly after oral administration.
Distribution: Distributes widely into all areas of body water and tissues, including tumors, bone marrow, liver, and intestinal mucosa. Fluorouracil crosses the blood-brain barrier to a significant extent.
Metabolism: A small amount is converted in the tissues to the active metabolite, with most of drug degraded in the liver.
Excretion: Metabolites are primarily excreted through the lungs as carbon dioxide. A small portion of a dose is excreted in urine as unchanged drug.

Route	Onset	Peak	Duration
I.V., Topical	Unknown	Unknown	Unknown

Contraindications and precautions
Contraindicated in patients hypersensitive to drug; patients who are in a poor nutritional state; patients with bone marrow suppression (WBC counts of 5,000/mm^3 or less or platelet counts of 100,000/ mm^3 or less); patients with potentially serious infections; and in those who have had major surgery within the previous month.

Use cautiously in patients after high-dose pelvic radiation therapy or use of alkylating agents. Also use with caution in patients with widespread neoplastic infiltration of bone marrow and impaired renal or hepatic function.

Interactions
Drug-drug. *Leucovorin calcium and prior treatment with alkylating agents:* May enhance toxicity. Use with extreme caution.
Drug-lifestyle. *Sun exposure:* May cause photosensitivity reactions. Advise patient to take precautions.

Effects on diagnostic tests
None reported.

Adverse reactions
CNS: acute cerebellar syndrome, confusion, disorientation, euphoria, ataxia, headache, *weakness, malaise.*
CV: ***myocardial ischemia,*** angina.
EENT: nystagmus.
GI: *stomatitis, GI ulcer* (may precede leukopenia), *nausea, vomiting, diarrhea, anorexia,* GI bleeding.
Hematologic: ***leukopenia, thrombocytopenia, agranulocytosis,*** anemia; WBC count nadir 9 to 14 days after first dose; platelet count nadir in 7 to 14 days.
Metabolic: hypoalbuminemia because of drug-induced protein malabsorption.
Skin: *reversible alopecia; dermatitis; erythema; scaling; pruritus;* nail changes; pigmented palmar creases; erythematous, contact dermatitis; desquamative rash of hands and feet with long-term use ("hand-foot syndrome").
Other: *pain, burning,* soreness, suppuration, swelling (with topical use), ***anaphylaxis,*** thrombophlebitis.

Overdose and treatment
Signs and symptoms of overdose include myelosuppression, diarrhea, alopecia, dermatitis, hyperpigmentation, nausea, and vomiting. Treatment is usually supportive and includes transfusion of blood components, antiemetics, and antidiarrheals.

Clinical considerations
- Drug may be administered I.V. push over 1 to 2 minutes.
- Drug may be further diluted in D_5W or normal saline solution for infusions up to 24 hours in duration.
- Solution is more stable in plastic I.V. bags than in glass bottles.
- Don't refrigerate fluorouracil.
- Drug can be diluted in 120 ml of water and administered orally; however, this isn't an FDA-approved method of administration, and absorption is erratic.
- Topical application to larger ulcerated areas may cause systemic toxicity.

Therapeutic monitoring
- General photosensitivity occurs for 2 to 3 months after a dose.
- Recommend monitoring intake and output, CBC, and renal and hepatic function.

Special populations
Pregnant patients. During pregnancy, use drug only for life-threatening or serious situations when no other safe alternatives are available.
Breast-feeding patients. It isn't known if drug is excreted in breast milk. However, because of potential for serious adverse reactions, mutagenicity, and carcinogenicity in the infant, breast-feeding isn't recommended.

Pediatric patients. Safety and efficacy for use in children haven't been established.

Patient counseling

- Warn patient to avoid strong sunlight or ultraviolet light because it will intensify the skin reaction. Encourage use of sunscreens.
- Tell patient to avoid exposure to people with infections. Advise patient to promptly report signs of infection or unusual bleeding.
- Reassure patient that hair should grow back after treatment is discontinued.
- Advise patient to apply topical fluorouracil with gloves and wash hands thoroughly after application.
- Warn patient that treated area may be unsightly during therapy and for several weeks after therapy is stopped. Complete healing may not occur until 1 or 2 months after treatment is stopped.

fluoxetine

Prozac, Prozac Pulvules

Pharmacologic classification: selective serotonin reuptake inhibitor (SSRI)
Therapeutic classification: antidepressant
Pregnancy risk category C

How supplied

Available by prescription only
Tablets: 10 mg
Capsules: 10 mg, 20 mg
Oral solution: 20 mg/5 ml

Indications and dosages

Depression, ◇panic disorder; ◇bipolar disorder; ◇alcohol dependence; ◇cataplexy; ◇myoclonus
Adults: 20 mg P.O. daily in the morning. Increase dosage, p.r.n., after several weeks to 40 mg daily with a dose in the morning and midday. Don't exceed 80 mg daily.
Obsessive-compulsive disorder
Adults: Initially, 20 mg P.O. daily. Gradually increase dosage as needed and tolerated to 60 to 80 mg daily.
◇Obesity
Adults: 20 to 60 mg P.O. daily.
◇Eating disorders
Adults: 60 to 80 mg P.O. daily.

Pharmacodynamics

Antidepressant action: The antidepressant action of fluoxetine is purportedly related to its inhibition of CNS neuronal uptake of serotonin. Fluoxetine blocks uptake of serotonin, but not of norepinephrine, into human platelets. Animal studies suggest that it's a much more potent uptake inhibitor of serotonin than of norepinephrine.

Pharmacokinetics

Absorption: Well absorbed after oral administration. Absorption isn't altered by food.
Distribution: Apparently highly protein-bound (about 95%).
Metabolism: Metabolized primarily in the liver to active metabolites.
Excretion: Excreted by the kidneys. Elimination half-life is 2 to 3 days. Norfluoxetine (the primary active metabolite) has an elimination half-life of 7 to 9 days.

Route	Onset	Peak	Duration
P.O.	Unknown	Unknown	Unknown

Contraindications and precautions

Contraindicated in patients hypersensitive to drug and in patients taking MAO inhibitors within 14 days of starting therapy. Use cautiously in patients at high risk of suicide or in those with a history of seizures, diabetes mellitus, or renal, hepatic, or CV disease.

Interactions

Drug-drug. *Cyproheptadine:* May reverse or decrease pharmacologic effect. Monitor patient closely.
Flecainide, carbamazepine, and vinblastine: Increased serum levels of these drugs. Monitor serum levels and the patient for adverse effects.
Insulin, oral antidiabetic agents: Altered blood glucose levels. May alter requirements for antidiabetic medication.
Lithium and tricyclic antidepressants: Increased adverse CNS effects. Avoid use together.
Phenytoin: Increased plasma phenytoin levels and risk of toxicity. Serum phenytoin level must be monitored; dosage adjustment may be needed.
Tryptophan: Increased adverse CNS effects (agitation, restlessness) and GI distress. Use with caution.
Warfarin and other highly protein-bound drugs: Increased plasma levels of fluoxetine or other highly protein-bound drugs. Monitor patient closely.
Drug-lifestyle. *Alcohol use:* May increase CNS depression. Advise patient to avoid alcohol.

Effects on diagnostic tests

None reported.

Adverse reactions

CNS: *nervousness, anxiety, insomnia, headache, drowsiness, tremor, dizziness, asthenia,* fatigue.
CV: palpitations, hot flashes.
EENT: nasal congestion, pharyngitis, cough, sinusitis.
GI: *nausea, diarrhea, dry mouth, anorexia, dyspepsia,* constipation, abdominal pain, vomiting, flatulence, increased appetite.
GU: sexual dysfunction.

Musculoskeletal: muscle pain.
Respiratory: upper respiratory infection, respiratory distress.
Skin: *rash, pruritus,* diaphoresis.
Other: flulike syndrome, *weight loss,* fever.

Overdose and treatment

Symptoms of overdose include agitation, restlessness, hypomania, and other signs of CNS excitation; and, in patients who took higher doses of fluoxetine, nausea and vomiting.

To treat fluoxetine overdose, establish and maintain an airway; ensure adequate oxygenation and ventilation. Activated charcoal, which may be used with sorbitol, may be as effective as emesis or lavage.

Monitor cardiac and vital signs, and provide usual supportive measures. Fluoxetine-induced seizures that don't subside spontaneously may respond to diazepam. Forced diuresis, dialysis, hemoperfusion, and exchange transfusion are unlikely to be of benefit.

Clinical considerations

- Advise prescriber to consider the inherent risk of suicide until significant improvement of depressive state occurs. High-risk patients should have close supervision during initial drug therapy. To reduce risk of suicidal overdose, use the smallest quantity of pulvules consistent with good management.
- Full antidepressant effect may be delayed until 4 weeks of treatment or longer.
- Treatment of acute depression usually requires at least several months of continuous drug therapy; optimal duration of therapy hasn't been established.
- Because of its long elimination half-life, changes in fluoxetine dosage won't be reflected in plasma for several weeks, affecting titration to final dose and withdrawal from treatment.
- Fluoxetine therapy may activate mania or hypomania.
- Prescribe lower or less frequent dosages in patients with renal or hepatic impairment. Consider lower or less frequent dosages in elderly patients and others with concurrent disease or multiple drug therapy.

Therapeutic monitoring

Patient must be closely monitored for improvement of depressive state and inherent risk of suicide.

Special populations

Pregnant patients. Avoid using drug during pregnancy. Because of the long half-life of the drug, patient planning to become pregnant should consult prescriber to ascertain when risk to fetus has passed.
Breast-feeding patients. Drug is excreted in milk and shouldn't be used by breast-feeding patients.
Pediatric patients. Safety and efficacy in children haven't been established.
Geriatric patients. No overall differences in safety and efficacy in geriatric patients were observed; however, the elderly may exhibit increased sensitivity to the drug.

Patient counseling

- Inform patient drug may cause dizziness or drowsiness. Advise patient to avoid hazardous tasks that require alertness until CNS response to drug is established.
- Caution patient to avoid ingestion of alcohol and to seek medical approval before taking other drugs.
- Tell patient to promptly report rash or hives, anxiety, nervousness, anorexia (especially in underweight patients), suspicion of pregnancy, or intent to become pregnant.

fluphenazine decanoate
Modecate*, Prolixin Decanoate

fluphenazine enanthate
Moditen Enanthate*, Prolixin Enanthate

fluphenazine hydrochloride
Permitil, Prolixin

Pharmacologic classification: phenothiazine (piperazine derivative)
Therapeutic classification: antipsychotic
Pregnancy risk category NR

How supplied

Available by prescription only
fluphenazine decanoate
Depot injection: 25 mg/ml
fluphenazine enanthate
Depot injection: 25 mg/ml
fluphenazine hydrochloride
Tablets: 1 mg, 2.5 mg, 5 mg, 10 mg
Oral concentrate: 5 mg/ml (Prolixin contains 14% alcohol and Permitil contains 1% alcohol)
Elixir: 2.5 mg/5 ml (with 14% alcohol)
I.M. injection: 2.5 mg/ml

Indications and dosages

Psychotic disorders
Adults: Initially, 0.5 to 10 mg fluphenazine hydrochloride P.O. daily in divided doses q 6 to 8 hours; may increase cautiously to 20 mg. Maintenance dosage is 1 to 5 mg P.O. daily. I.M. doses are one-third to one-half that of oral doses (starting dose is 1.25 mg I.M.).
≡ ***Dosage adjustment.*** Use lower doses for geriatric patients (1 to 2.5 mg daily).

Pharmacodynamics

Antipsychotic action: Fluphenazine is thought to exert its antipsychotic effects by postsynaptic blockade of CNS dopamine receptors, thereby inhibiting dopamine-mediated effects.

Fluphenazine has many other central and peripheral effects; it produces both alpha and ganglionic blockade and counteracts histamine- and serotonin-mediated activity. Its most prominent adverse reactions are extrapyramidal.

Pharmacokinetics

Absorption: Rate and extent of absorption vary with route of administration; oral tablet absorption is erratic and variable.
Distribution: Distributed widely into the body, including breast milk. CNS levels are usually higher than those in plasma. Drug is 91% to 99% protein-bound.
Metabolism: Metabolized extensively by the liver, but no active metabolites are formed; duration of action is about 6 to 8 hours after oral administration; 1 to 6 weeks (average, 2 weeks) after I.M. depot administration.
Excretion: Mostly excreted in urine via the kidneys; some is excreted in feces via the biliary tract.

Route	Onset	Peak	Duration
P.O.	< 1 hr	½ hr	6-8 hr
I.M. (HCl)	< 1hr	1½-2 hr	6-8 hr
I.M.	24-72 hr	Unknown	1-6 wk
S.C.	Unknown	Unknown	Unknown

Contraindications and precautions

Contraindicated in patients with hypersensitivity or in patients experiencing coma, CNS depression, bone marrow suppression or other blood dyscrasia, subcortical damage, or liver damage.

Use cautiously in geriatric or debilitated patients and in those with pheochromocytoma, severe CV disease, peptic ulcer disease, exposure to extreme hot or cold (including antipyretic therapy), exposure to phosphorus insecticides, respiratory or seizure disorders, hypocalcemia, severe reaction to insulin or electroconvulsive therapy, mitral insufficiency, glaucoma, or prostatic hyperplasia. Use parenteral form cautiously in patients with asthma and those allergic to sulfites.

Interactions

Drug-drug. *Aluminum- and magnesium-containing antacids and antidiarrheals:* Decreased absorption. Monitor patient.
Antiarrhythmic agents, quinidine, disopyramide, and procainamide: Increased incidence of arrhythmias and conduction defects. Avoid use together.
Atropine or other anticholinergic drugs, including antidepressants, MAO inhibitors, phenothiazines, antihistamines, meperidine, and antiparkinsonian agents: Oversedation, paralytic ileus, visual changes, and severe constipation. Avoid use together.
Beta blockers: Increased plasma levels and toxicity. Monitor patient closely.
Bromocriptine: Antagonized therapeutic effect of bromocriptine on prolactin secretion. Monitor patient for drug effect.
Centrally acting antihypertensive drugs such as guanethidine, guanabenz, guanadrel, clonidine, methyldopa, and reserpine: Inhibition of blood pressure response; patient requires close monitoring.
CNS depressants, including analgesics, barbiturates, narcotics, tranquilizers, and general, spinal, or epidural anesthetics, or parenteral magnesium sulfate: Additive effects of oversedation, respiratory depression, and hypotension are likely. Avoid use together.
Dopamine: Decreased vasoconstricting effects. Monitor patient carefully.
Levodopa: Decreased effectiveness and increased toxicity of levodopa. Monitor patient carefully.
Lithium: May result in severe neurologic toxicity with an encephalitis-like syndrome and a decreased therapeutic response to fluphenazine. Monitor patient closely.
Metrizamide: Increased risk of seizures. Patient requires close observation.
Nitrates: May result in hypotension. Check blood pressure frequently.
Phenobarbital: Enhanced renal excretion. Monitor patient closely.
Phenytoin and tricyclic antidepressants: Inhibited metabolism and increased toxicity of these drugs. Monitor patient closely.
Propylthiouracil: Increased risk of agranulocytosis. Monitor patient carefully.
Sympathomimetics including epinephrine, phenylephrine, phenylpropanolamine, and ephedrine (often found in nasal sprays) and appetite suppressants: May decrease their stimulatory and pressor effects. Use with caution.
Drug-food. *Caffeine:* May increase metabolism of fluphenazine. Advise patient to avoid caffeine.
Drug-lifestyle. *Alcohol use:* May increase CNS depression. Advise patient not to drink alcohol.
Smoking: Increased metabolism of fluphenazine. Advise patient to avoid smoking.
Sun exposure: May increase risk of photosensitivity. Advise patient to take precautions.

Effects on diagnostic tests

Fluphenazine causes false-positive test results for urinary porphyrins, urobilinogen, amylase, and 5-hydroxyindoleacetic acid, because of darkening of urine by metabolites; it also causes false-positive urine pregnancy test results using human chorionic gonadotropin.

Fluphenazine elevates test results for liver enzymes and causes quinidine-like ECG effects.

Adverse reactions

CNS: *extrapyramidal reactions, tardive dyskinesia, sedation, pseudoparkinsonism, EEG changes, drowsiness, seizures,* dizziness.
CV: *orthostatic hypotension,* tachycardia, ECG changes.
EENT: ocular changes, *blurred vision,* nasal congestion.
GI: *dry mouth, constipation.*
GU: *urine retention,* dark urine, menstrual irregularities, gynecomastia, inhibited ejaculation.
Hematologic: ***leukopenia, agranulocytosis,*** eosinophilia, hemolytic anemia, ***aplastic anemia, thrombocytopenia.***
Hepatic: cholestatic jaundice, abnormal liver function test results.
Metabolic: elevated protein-bound iodine, weight gain, increased appetite.
Skin: mild photosensitivity, allergic reactions.
Other: rarely, ***neuroleptic malignant syndrome.***
After abrupt withdrawal of long-term therapy: gastritis, nausea, vomiting, dizziness, tremor, feeling of warmth or cold, diaphoresis, tachycardia, headache, insomnia.

Overdose and treatment

CNS depression is characterized by deep, unarousable sleep and possible coma, hypotension or hypertension, extrapyramidal symptoms, dystonia, abnormal involuntary muscle movements, agitation, seizures, arrhythmias, ECG changes, hypothermia or hyperthermia, and autonomic nervous system dysfunction.

Treatment is symptomatic and supportive, including maintaining vital signs, airway, stable body temperature, and fluid and electrolyte balance.

Don't induce vomiting: drug inhibits cough reflex, and aspiration may occur. Use gastric lavage, then activated charcoal and saline cathartics; dialysis doesn't help. Regulate body temperature as needed. Treat hypotension with I.V. fluids: don't give epinephrine. Treat seizures with parenteral diazepam or barbiturates; arrhythmias with parenteral phenytoin (1 mg/kg with rate titrated to blood pressure); extrapyramidal reactions with benztropine 1 to 2 mg or parenteral diphenhydramine at 10 to 50 mg.

Clinical considerations

Consider the recommendations relevant to all phenothiazines as well as the following:

- Note that depot injection (25 mg/ml) and I.M. injection (2.5 mg/ml) aren't interchangeable.
- Depot injection isn't recommended for patients who aren't stabilized on a phenothiazine. This form has a prolonged elimination; its action couldn't be terminated in case of adverse reactions.

Therapeutic monitoring

Recommendations are the same as for all phenothiazines.

Special populations

Pregnant patients. Recommendations are the same as for all phenothiazines.
Breast-feeding patients. Drug is excreted in breast milk. Use with caution; potential benefits to the woman should outweigh the potential harm to the infant.
Pediatric patients. Safety and efficacy in children under age 12 haven't been established.
Geriatric patients. Recommendations are the same as for all phenothiazines.

Patient counseling

- Inform patient that drug may cause dizziness or drowsiness. Advise patient to avoid hazardous tasks that require alertness until CNS response to drug is established.
- Tell patient to avoid ingestion of alcohol and to seek medical approval before taking other drugs.
- Instruct patient to promptly report rash or hives, anxiety, nervousness, anorexia (especially in underweight patients), suspicion of pregnancy, or intent to become pregnant.

flurazepam hydrochloride

Apo-Flurazepam*, Dalmane, Novoflupam*

Pharmacologic classification: benzodiazepine
Therapeutic classification: sedative-hypnotic
Controlled substance schedule IV
Pregnancy risk category X

How supplied

Available by prescription only
Capsules: 15 mg, 30 mg

Indications and dosages

Insomnia
Adults: 15 to 30 mg P.O. h.s.
≡ ***Dosage adjustment.*** In patients over age 65, 15 mg P.O. h.s.

Pharmacodynamics

Sedative action: Flurazepam depresses the CNS at the limbic and subcortical levels of the brain. It produces a sedative effect by potentiating the effect of the neurotransmitter gamma-aminobutyric acid on its receptor in the ascending reticular activating system, which increases inhibition and blocks both cortical and limbic arousal.

Pharmacokinetics

Absorption: When administered orally, flurazepam is absorbed rapidly through the GI tract.
Distribution: Distributed widely throughout the body. About 97% of administered dose is bound to plasma protein.
Metabolism: Metabolized in the liver to the active metabolite desalkylflurazepam.
Excretion: Desalkylflurazepam is excreted in urine; half-life is 50 to 100 hours.

Route	Onset	Peak	Duration
P.O.	< 20 min	1-2 hr	7-10 hr

Contraindications and precautions

Contraindicated in patients with hypersensitivity to drug and during pregnancy.

Use cautiously in patients with impaired renal or hepatic function, chronic pulmonary insufficiency, mental depression, suicidal tendencies, or history of drug abuse.

Interactions

Drug-drug. *Phenothiazines, narcotics, barbiturates, antihistamines, MAO inhibitors, general anesthetics, and antidepressants:* Increased CNS depressant effects of these drugs. Use together cautiously.
Digoxin: Serum levels may increase resulting in toxicity. Monitor patient closely.
Disulfiram, isoniazid, oral contraceptives, cimetidine, and ritonavir: May decrease metabolism of benzodiazepines, leading to toxicity. Monitor patient carefully.
Levodopa: Decreased therapeutic effect of levodopa. Monitor patient for drug effects.
Phenytoin: Increased phenytoin levels. Recommend monitoring serum levels of phenytoin.
Rifampin: Enhanced metabolism of benzodiazepines. Monitor patient closely.
Theophylline: May act as an antagonist with flurazepam. Monitor patient closely.
Drug-lifestyle. *Alcohol use:* Excessive CNS and respiratory depression. Advise patient to avoid alcohol.
Heavy smoking: Accelerates metabolism of flurazepam. Monitor patient for drug effect.

Effects on diagnostic tests

None reported.

Adverse reactions

CNS: *daytime sedation, dizziness, drowsiness, disturbed coordination,* lethargy, confusion, *headache,* light-headedness, nervousness, hallucinations, staggering, ataxia, disorientation, changes in EEG patterns, *coma.*
GI: nausea, vomiting, heartburn, diarrhea, abdominal pain.
Hepatic: elevated liver enzymes.
Other: physical or psychological dependence.

Overdose and treatment

Signs and symptoms of overdose include somnolence, confusion, hypoactive reflexes, dyspnea, labored breathing, hypotension, bradycardia, slurred speech, unsteady gait or impaired coordination, and, eventually, coma.

Support blood pressure and respiration until drug effects subside; monitor vital signs. Mechanical ventilatory assistance via endotracheal (ET) tube may be required to maintain a patent airway and support adequate oxygenation. Use I.V. fluids to promote diuresis and vasopressors such as dopamine and phenylephrine to treat hypotension, as needed. Flumazenil, a specific benzodiazepine antagonist, may be useful as an adjunct to supportive therapy.

If patient is conscious, induce emesis. Use gastric lavage if ingestion was recent, but only if an ET tube is present to prevent aspiration. After emesis or lavage, administer activated charcoal with a cathartic as a single dose. Dialysis is of limited value. Don't use barbiturates if excitation occurs to avoid exacerbation of excitatory state or potentiation of CNS depressant effects.

Clinical considerations

Consider the recommendations relevant to all benzodiazepines as well as the following:

- Studies have demonstrated a "carryover effect." Drug is most effective after 3 or 4 nights of use because of long half-life. Don't increase dose more frequently than every 5 days.
- Recommend monitoring hepatic function and AST, ALT, bilirubin, and alkaline phosphatase levels for changes.
- Drug is useful for patients who have trouble falling asleep and who awaken frequently at night and early in the morning.
- Although prolonged use isn't recommended, this drug has proven effective for up to 4 weeks of continuous use.
- Rapid withdrawal after prolonged use can cause withdrawal symptoms.
- Lower doses are effective in patients with renal or hepatic dysfunction.

Therapeutic monitoring

Recommendations are the same as for all benzodiazepines.

Special populations

Pregnant patients. Drug is contraindicated during pregnancy.
Breast-feeding patients. Drug is excreted in breast milk. A breast-fed infant may become sedated, have feeding difficulties, or lose weight. Avoid use in breast-feeding women.
Pediatric patients. Closely observe a neonate for withdrawal symptoms if the mother took

flurazepam during pregnancy. Use of flurazepam during labor may cause neonatal flaccidity. Drug isn't for use in children under age 15. Neonates are more sensitive to flurazepam because of slower metabolism. The possibility of toxicity is greatly increased.
Geriatric patients. Geriatric patients are more susceptible to CNS depressant effects of flurazepam. They may require assistance and supervision with walking and daily activities during initiation of therapy or after an increase in dose. Lower doses usually are effective in geriatric patients because of decreased elimination.

Patient counseling
- Warn patient to avoid alcohol while taking drug.
- Emphasize the potential for excessive CNS depression if drug is taken with alcohol, even if it's taken the evening before ingestion of alcohol.
- Advise patient that rebound insomnia may occur after stopping drug, not to discontinue medication abruptly after prolonged therapy, and not to exceed prescribed dosage.

flurbiprofen
Ansaid

Pharmacologic classification: NSAID, phenylalkanoic acid derivative
Therapeutic classification: antiarthritic
Pregnancy risk category B

How supplied
Available by prescription only
Tablets: 50 mg, 100 mg

Indications and dosages
Rheumatoid arthritis and osteoarthritis
Adults: 200 to 300 mg P.O. daily, divided b.i.d., t.i.d., or q.i.d.
≡ ***Dosage adjustment.*** Patients with end-stage renal disease may accumulate flurbiprofen metabolites, but half-life of parent compound is unchanged. Monitor patient closely and adjust dosage accordingly.

Pharmacodynamics
Anti-inflammatory action: An NSAID, flurbiprofen interferes with the synthesis of prostaglandins.

Pharmacokinetics
Absorption: Well absorbed after oral administration. Administering with food alters rate, but not extent, of absorption.
Distribution: Highly bound (more than 99%) to plasma proteins.
Metabolism: Metabolized primarily in the liver. The major metabolite shows little anti-inflammatory activity.
Excretion: Excreted primarily in urine. Average elimination half-life is 6 to 10 hours.

Route	Onset	Peak	Duration
P.O.	Unknown	1½ hr	Unknown

Contraindications and precautions
Contraindicated in patients with hypersensitivity to drug, or history of aspirin- or NSAID-induced asthma, urticaria, or other allergic-type reactions.

Use cautiously in geriatric or debilitated patients and those with history of peptic ulcer disease, herpes simplex keratitis, impaired renal or hepatic function, cardiac disease, or conditions associated with fluid retention.

Interactions
Drug-drug. *Oral anticoagulants:* Increased bleeding tendencies. Avoid use together.
Aspirin: May decrease flurbiprofen levels and increase GI toxicity. Avoid use together.
Beta blockers: Antihypertensive effect of beta blockers may be impaired. Monitor patient carefully.
Cyclosporine: Increased risk of nephrotoxicity. Use together with extreme caution.
Diuretics: Decreased diuretic effect. Monitor patient carefully.
Lithium: Lithium levels may be increased. Recommend monitoring serum levels.
Methotrexate: May cause increased risk of methotrexate toxicity. Avoid use together.
Drug-lifestyle. *Alcohol use:* Increased risk of adverse GI reactions. Advise patient to avoid alcohol.
Sun exposure: May potentiate photosensitivity reactions. Advise patient to take precautions.

Effects on diagnostic tests
None reported.

Adverse reactions
CNS: *headache,* anxiety, insomnia, dizziness, increased reflexes, tremors, amnesia, asthenia, drowsiness, malaise, depression.
CV: *edema,* ***heart failure,*** hypertension, vasodilation.
EENT: rhinitis, tinnitus, visual changes, epistaxis.
GI: *dyspepsia, diarrhea, abdominal pain, nausea,* constipation, *bleeding,* flatulence, vomiting.
GU: *symptoms suggesting urinary tract infection,* hematuria, interstitial nephritis, ***renal failure.***
Hematologic: ***thrombocytopenia,*** *neutropenia,* anemia, ***aplastic anemia.***
Hepatic: *elevated liver enzymes, jaundice.*
Metabolic: weight changes.
Respiratory: asthma.
Skin: rash, photosensitivity, urticaria, ***angioedema.***

Overdose and treatment
Overdose has resulted in lethargy, coma, respiratory depression, epigastric pain, and distress.

Treatment should be supportive. Emptying the stomach by emesis or lavage would be of little use if the ingestion took place more than an hour before treatment, but is still recommended.

Clinical considerations
Consider the recommendations relevant to all NSAIDs. Advise prescriber to closely monitor patient with impaired hepatic or renal function and geriatric or debilitated patients; they may need lower doses. These patients may be at risk for renal toxicity. Recommend periodically monitoring renal function.

Therapeutic monitoring
Patients receiving long-term therapy should have periodic liver function studies, ophthalmologic and auditory examinations, and hematocrit determinations.

Special populations
Pregnant patients. Recommendations are the same as for all NSAIDs.
Breast-feeding patients. A breast-feeding woman taking 200 mg of flurbiprofen daily could deliver as much as 0.1 mg to the infant daily. Breast-feeding isn't recommended while using the drug.
Pediatric patients. Safety in children hasn't been established.

Patient counseling
- Advise patient to discontinue the drug and contact prescriber promptly if GI bleeding occurs.
- Tell patient to take drug with food, milk, or antacid to minimize GI upset.
- Advise patient to avoid hazardous activities that require alertness until the adverse CNS effects of the drug are known.
- Tell patient to immediately report to prescriber edema, substantial weight gain, black stools, rash, itching, or visual disturbances.

flutamide
Eulexin

Pharmacologic classification: nonsteroidal antiandrogen
Therapeutic classification: antineoplastic
Pregnancy risk category D

How supplied
Available by prescription only
Capsules: 125 mg

Indications and dosages
Treatment of metastatic prostatic carcinoma (stage D2) in combination with luteinizing hormone-releasing hormone analogues, such as leuprolide acetate
Adults (men only): 250 mg P.O. q 8 hours.

Pharmacodynamics
Antitumor action: Flutamide inhibits androgen uptake or prevents binding of androgens in nucleus of cells within target tissues. Prostatic carcinoma is known to be androgen-sensitive.

Pharmacokinetics
Absorption: Rapidly and completely absorbed after oral administration.
Distribution: Concentrates in the prostate in animals. Drug and its active metabolite are about 95% protein-bound.
Metabolism: Metabolism is rapid, with at least six metabolites identified. More than 97% of drug is metabolized within 1 hour of administration.
Excretion: More than 95% is excreted in urine.

Route	Onset	Peak	Duration
P.O.	Unknown	2 hr	Unknown

Contraindications and precautions
Contraindicated in patients hypersensitive to drug and in patients with severe hepataic impairment.

Interactions
None reported.

Effects on diagnostic tests
Elevation of plasma testosterone and estradiol levels has been reported. Serum ALT, AST, bilirubin, and creatinine levels may be increased.

Adverse reactions
CNS: *drowsiness, confusion, depression, anxiety, nervousness.*
CV: *peripheral edema, hypertension.*
GI: *diarrhea, nausea, vomiting.*
GU: *impotence, loss of libido.*
Hematologic: anemia, ***leukopenia, thrombocytopenia,*** hemolytic anemia.
Hepatic: elevated liver enzyme levels, ***hepatitis.***
Skin: rash, photosensitivity.
Other: *hot flashes,* gynecomastia.

Overdose and treatment
No experience with overdose in humans has been reported. Dosage as high as 1,500 mg daily for 36 weeks has been reported without serious adverse effects.

Clinical considerations
Flutamide must be taken continuously with the agent used for medical castration (such as

leuprolide acetate) to produce full benefit of therapy. Leuprolide suppresses testosterone production, while flutamide inhibits testosterone action at the cellular level. Together they can impair the growth of androgen-responsive tumors.

Therapeutic monitoring

- Monitor patient for adverse reactions.
- Recommend monitoring liver function tests and CBC.

Special populations

Pediatric patients. Safety in children hasn't been established.

Patient counseling

- Tell patient not to discontinue either leuprolide or flutamide without medical approval.
- Explain that some symptoms may worsen initially before they improve.

fluticasone propionate

Cutivate, Flonase, Flovent

Pharmacologic classification: corticosteroid
Therapeutic classification: topical/inhalation anti-inflammatory
Pregnancy risk category C

How supplied

Available by prescription only
Cream: 0.05%
Ointment: 0.005%
Metered nasal spray: 50 mcg/actuation
Inhalation aerosol: 44 mcg/actuation, 110 mcg/actuation, 220 mcg/actuation
Inhalation powder: 50-mcg, 100-mcg, 250-mcg rotadisk

Indications and dosages

Relief of inflammation and pruritus of corticosteroid-responsive dermatoses
Adults: Apply sparingly to affected area b.i.d. and rub in gently and completely.
Allergic rhinitis
Adults: 2 sprays in each nostril once daily or 1 spray b.i.d.
Management of nasal symptoms of seasonal and perennial allergic rhinitis in children
Adolescents and children age 4 and older: Initially, 1 spray (50 mcg) in each nostril once daily. If patient doesn't respond or symptoms are severe, increase to 2 sprays in each nostril daily. Once adequate control is achieved, decrease dose to 1 spray in each nostril daily. Maximum dose is 2 sprays in each nostril daily.
Maintenance treatment of asthma as prophylactic therapy
Adults and children 12 and older: 88 to 220 mcg inhalation aerosol b.i.d., adjusting to maximum 440 mcg inhalation aerosol b.i.d.
Adults and adolescents: 100 mcg inhalation powder b.i.d., adjusting to maximum 500 mcg inhalation powder b.i.d.
Children age 4 to 11: 50 mcg inhalation powder b.i.d., adjusting to maximum 100 mcg inhalation powder b.i.d.

See also package insert for dosing considerations in combination with oral corticosteroids.

Pharmacodynamics

Anti-inflammatory action: Fluticasone stimulates synthesis of enzymes needed to decrease inflammation.

Pharmacokinetics

Absorption: Amount absorbed depends on the amount applied, application site, vehicle used, use of occlusive dressing, and integrity of epidermal barrier. Some systemic absorption does occur.
Distribution: Distributed throughout the local skin.
Metabolism: Metabolized primarily by the skin. Absorbed drug is extensively metabolized by the liver.
Excretion: Less than 5% is excreted in urine as metabolites; rest is excreted in feces as parent drug and metabolites.

Route	Onset	Peak	Duration
Topical, Inhalation	Unknown	Unknown	Unknown

Contraindications and precautions

Contraindicated in patients hypersensitive to drug or its components and in patients with viral, fungal, herpetic, or tubercular skin lesions.

Flovent inhalation aerosol and powder are contraindicated as the primary treatment in status asthmaticus or other acute episodes of asthma where intensive measures are required.

Use care when transferring patients from systemically active corticosteroids to Flovent inhalation aerosol or powder; deaths have occurred in asthmatic patients during and after transfer from systemic corticosteroids to less systemically available inhalation corticosteroids. During periods of stress or severe asthma attack, instruct patients who have been withdrawn from systemic corticosteroids to resume oral corticosteroids in large doses immediately and contact their doctors for further assistance.

Interactions

Drug-drug. *Ketoconazole:* May result in increased mean fluticasone levels. Exercise care when fluticasone is coadministered with long-term ketoconazole and other known cytochrome P-450 3A4 inhibitors.

Effects on diagnostic tests
None reported.

Adverse reactions
CNS: dizziness, giddiness.
GU: dysmenorrhea.
Metabolic: hyperglycemia, glucosuria.
Musculoskeletal: pain in joints, sprain or strain aches and pains, pain in limbs.
Respiratory: bronchitis, chest congestion.
Skin: stinging, burning, pruritus, irritation, dryness, erythema, folliculitis, skin atrophy, leukoderma, vesicles, numbness of fingers, rash, hypertrichosis, acneiform eruptions, hypopigmentation, perioral dermatitis, allergic contact dermatitis, secondary infection, striae, miliaria.
Other: ***hypothalamic-pituitary-adrenal axis suppression,*** Cushing's syndrome, fever.

Clinical considerations
- Not used for treatment of rosacea, perioral dermatitis, or acne.
- Mixing with other bases or vehicles may affect potency far beyond expectations.
- Flovent inhalation aerosol and powder aren't indicated for the relief of acute bronchospasm.

Therapeutic monitoring
- During withdrawal from oral corticosteroids, some patients may experience symptoms of systemically active corticosteroid withdrawal, such as joint or musculoskeletal pain, malaise, and depression, despite maintenance or improvement of respiratory function.
- Because of the possibility of systemic absorption of inhalation corticosteroids, carefully observe patients treated with these drugs for any evidence of systemic corticosteroid effects. Take special care during periods of stress or postoperatively for adrenal insufficiency.

Special populations
Pregnant patients. Use drug during pregnancy only when potential benefits justify risks to fetus.
Breast-feeding patients. Use with caution in breast-feeding women because it's unknown if topical or inhalation corticosteroids undergo sufficient absorption to produce systemic effects in the infant.
Pediatric patients. Safety and efficacy of topical form haven't been established in children. Safety and efficacy of nasal form haven't been established in children under age 12; use of drug isn't recommended in these patients. A reduction of growth velocity in children or teenagers may occur as a result of the use of corticosteroids for treatment or from inadequate control of chronic disease such as asthma. The benefits of asthma control from corticosteroid therapy must be weighed against the possibility of growth suppression in these patients.

Patient counseling
- Advise patient that proper application includes washing area prior to application and applying agent sparingly and rubbing it in lightly.
- Instruct patient to report burning, irritation, or persistent or worsened condition.
- Tell patient to avoid prolonged use, contact with eyes, or use around genital area, rectal area, on face, and in skin creases.
- Inform patient to rinse mouth well after corticosteroid inhalation.
- Inform patient on inhalation corticosteroids to avoid exposure and to consult doctor immediately if he has been exposed to chicken pox or measles.
- Instruct patient on proper administration using the nasal spray pump, including the need to prime the pump.

fluvastatin sodium
Lescol

Pharmacologic classification: hydroxymethylglutaryl-coenzyme A (HMG-CoA) reductase inhibitor
Therapeutic classification: cholesterol-lowering antilipemic
Pregnancy risk category X

How supplied
Available by prescription only
Capsules: 20 mg, 40 mg

Indications and dosages
Reduction of low-density lipoprotein and total cholesterol levels in patients with primary hypercholesterolemia (types IIa and IIb) when response to diet and other nonpharmacologic measures has been inadequate
Adults: Initially, 20 mg P.O. h.s. Increase dose as necessary to a maximum of 40 mg daily.
≡ ***Dosage adjustment.*** With a persistent increase in ALT or AST levels of at least three times the upper limit of normal, withdrawal of fluvastatin is recommended. Because fluvastatin is cleared hepatically, with less than 5% of the dose excreted into urine, dosage adjustments for mild to moderate renal impairment aren't necessary. Exercise caution with severe impairment.

Pharmacodynamics
Antilipemic action: Fluvastatin is a competitive inhibitor of HMG-CoA reductase, which is responsible for the conversion of HMG-CoA to mevalonate, a precursor of sterols, including cholesterol. This enzyme is an early (and rate-limiting) step in the synthetic pathway of

cholesterol. Fluvastatin increases high-density lipoproteins and decreases low-density lipoproteins, very-low-density lipoproteins, and plasma triglycerides.

Pharmacokinetics

Absorption: Absorbed rapidly and virtually completely (98%) after oral administration on an empty stomach.
Distribution: Over 98% of circulating drug is bound to plasma proteins.
Metabolism: Completely metabolized in the liver. It has no active metabolites.
Excretion: About 5% is excreted in urine and 90% in feces.

Route	Onset	Peak	Duration
P.O.	Unknown	1 hr	Unknown

Contraindications and precautions

Contraindicated in patients with hypersensitivity to drug; in those with active liver disease or conditions associated with unexplained persistent elevations of serum transaminase levels; in pregnant and breast-feeding women; and in women of childbearing age unless there's no risk of pregnancy.

Use cautiously in patients with impaired renal function and history of hepatic disease or heavy alcohol consumption.

Interactions

Drug-drug. *Cholestyramine or colestipol:* May bind fluvastatin in the GI tract and decrease absorption. Administer fluvastatin at bedtime, at least 2 hours after the resin, to avoid significant interaction from the drug binding to the resin.
Cimetidine, omeprazole, and ranitidine: Decreased fluvastatin metabolism. Monitor patient closely.
Cyclosporine and other immunosuppressants, erythromycin, gemfibrozil, and niacin: Increased risk of polymyositis and rhabdomyolysis when administered with fluvastatin. Avoid use together.
Digoxin: Altered pharmacokinetics of digoxin. Recommend monitoring patient's serum digoxin levels carefully.
Rifampin: Enhanced fluvastatin metabolism and decreases plasma levels. Monitor patient closely for lack of effect.
Warfarin: Increased anticoagulant effect with bleeding. Monitor patient closely.
Drug-lifestyle. *Alcohol use:* Increased risk of hepatotoxicity. Monitor patient carefully.

Effects on diagnostic tests

None reported.

Adverse reactions

CNS: headache, fatigue, dizziness, insomnia.
GI: dyspepsia, diarrhea, nausea, vomiting, abdominal pain, constipation, flatulence, tooth disorder.
Hepatic: increased liver enzyme levels, increased bilirubin levels.
Hematologic: ***thrombocytopenia, leukopenia, hemolytic anemia.***
Metabolic: Thyroid function test abnormalities can occur.
Musculoskeletal: arthropathy, muscle pain.
Respiratory: sinusitis, *upper respiratory infection,* rhinitis, cough, pharyngitis, bronchitis.
Other: *hypersensitivity reactions* (rash, pruritus).

Overdose and treatment

No specific information on overdose is available. If an accidental overdose occurs, treat symptomatically and institute supportive measures as required. The dialyzability of fluvastatin and its metabolites in humans is unknown.

Clinical considerations

- Initiate fluvastatin therapy only after diet and other nonpharmacologic therapies have proven ineffective.
- Drug may be taken without regard to meals; however, efficacy is enhanced if drug is taken in the evening.

Therapeutic monitoring

- Monitor patient closely for signs of myositis.
- Liver function tests should be performed at the start of therapy, every 4 to 6 weeks during the first 3 months of therapy, every 6 to 12 weeks during the next 12 months, and at 6-month intervals thereafter.

Special populations

Pregnant patients. Drug shouldn't be used during pregnancy.
Breast-feeding patients. Preclinical data suggest that drug is excreted in breast milk in a 2:1 ratio (milk:plasma). The potential for serious adverse reactions in nursing infants indicates that breast-feeding women shouldn't take fluvastatin.
Pediatric patients. Safety and efficacy in patients under age 18 haven't been established. Use in pediatric patients isn't recommended.

Patient counseling

- Instruct patient to take fluvastatin at bedtime to enhance effectiveness.
- Warn patient to restrict alcohol intake because of potentially serious adverse effects.
- Tell patient to report to prescriber adverse reactions, particularly muscle aches and pains.

fluvoxamine maleate

Luvox

Pharmacologic classification: selective serotonin reuptake inhibitor (SSRI)
Therapeutic classification: anticompulsive
Pregnancy risk category C

How supplied

Available by prescription only
Tablets: 25 mg, 50 mg, 100 mg

Indications and dosages

Obsessive-compulsive disorder
Adults: Initially, 50 mg P.O. daily h.s. Increase in 50-mg increments q 4 to 7 days until maximum benefit is achieved. Maximum daily dose is 300 mg. Give total daily doses exceeding 100 mg in two divided doses.
≡ ***Dosage adjustment.*** Because the elderly and patients with hepatic impairment have been observed to have decreased clearance of fluvoxamine maleate, dosage adjustment may be appropriate.

Pharmacodynamics

Anticompulsive action: The exact mechanism of action is unknown. Fluvoxamine is a potent selective inhibitor of the neuronal uptake of serotonin, which is thought to improve obsessive-compulsive behavior.

Pharmacokinetics

Absorption: Absolute bioavailability of drug is 53%.
Distribution: Mean apparent volume of distribution is about 25 L/kg. About 80% of drug is bound to plasma protein (mostly albumin).
Metabolism: Extensively metabolized in the liver mostly by oxidative demethylation and deamination.
Excretion: Metabolites are primarily excreted in urine.

Route	Onset	Peak	Duration
P.O.	Unknown	3-8 hr	Unknown

Contraindications and precautions

Contraindicated in patients with hypersensitivity to drug or to other phenylpiperazine antidepressants and within 14 days of MAO inhibitor therapy. Use cautiously in patients with hepatic dysfunction, concomitant conditions that may affect hemodynamic responses or metabolism, or history of mania or seizures.

Interactions

Drug-drug. *Benzodiazepines, theophylline, and warfarin:* Reduced clearance of these drugs. Use together cautiously. However, diazepam shouldn't be coadministered with fluvoxamine. An adjustment in diazepam dosage may be necessary.
Carbamazepine, clozapine, methadone, metoprolol, propranolol, and tricyclic antidepressants: Elevated serum levels of fluvoxamine. Use together with caution and monitor patient closely for adverse reactions. Dosage adjustments may be necessary.
Diltiazem: May cause bradycardia; therefore, monitor patient's heart rate.
Lithium and tryptophan: May enhance effects of fluvoxamine; use together cautiously.
MAO inhibitors: May cause severe excitation, hyperpyrexia, myoclonus, delirium, and coma. Avoid use together.
Drug-lifestyle. *Smoking:* May decrease effectiveness of drug. Advise patient to avoid smoking.

Effects on diagnostic tests

None reported.

Adverse reactions

CNS: headache, asthenia, somnolence, insomnia, nervousness, dizziness, tremor, anxiety, hypertonia, agitation, depression, CNS stimulation, taste perversion.
CV: palpitations, vasodilation.
EENT: amblyopia.
GI: *nausea, diarrhea, constipation, dyspepsia,* anorexia, *vomiting,* flatulence, tooth disorder, dysphagia, *dry mouth.*
GU: decreased libido, abnormal ejaculation, urinary frequency, impotence, anorgasmia, urine retention.
Respiratory: upper respiratory infection, dyspnea, yawning.
Skin: sweating.
Other: flulike syndrome, chills.

Overdose and treatment

Common signs and symptoms of fluvoxamine overdose include drowsiness, vomiting, diarrhea, and dizziness; coma, tachycardia, bradycardia, hypotension, ECG abnormalities, liver function abnormalities, and seizures may also occur. Symptoms such as aspiration pneumonitis, respiratory difficulties, or hypokalemia may occur because of loss of consciousness or vomiting.

Treatment is supportive. Besides maintaining an open airway and monitoring vital signs and ECG, administration of activated charcoal may be as effective as emesis or lavage. Because absorption with overdose may be delayed, measures to minimize absorption may be necessary for up to 24 hours after ingestion. Dialysis isn't believed to be beneficial.

Clinical considerations

- Allow at least 14 days after stopping fluvoxamine before starting patient on an MAO inhibitor.
- Allow at least 14 days after MAO inhibitor therapy has been discontinued before starting patient on fluvoxamine.

Therapeutic monitoring

Monitor patient for suicidal tendencies, and allow a minimum supply of drug.

Special populations

Pregnant patients. Drug shouldn't be used during pregnancy.
Breast-feeding patients. Drug is excreted in breast milk and shouldn't be given to breast-feeding women.
Pediatric patients. Safety and efficacy in children under age 18 haven't been established.
Geriatric patients. Drug clearance is decreased by about 50% in geriatric patients compared with younger patients. Administer drug cautiously in this age group and adjust dosage slowly during initiation of therapy.

Patient counseling

- Warn patient not to engage in hazardous activity until CNS effects are known and to avoid alcoholic beverages.
- Alert patient that smoking may decrease the effectiveness of drug.
- Inform patient that several weeks of therapy may be required to obtain the full antidepressant effect. Once improvement is seen, advise patient not to discontinue the drug until directed by doctor.
- Advise patient to contact prescriber before taking OTC drugs because of possible drug interactions.

folic acid

Folvite

Pharmacologic classification: folic acid derivative
Therapeutic classification: vitamin supplement
Pregnancy risk category A

How supplied

Available by prescription only
Tablets: 1 mg
Injection: 10-ml vials (folic acid 5 mg/ml contains 1.5% benzyl alcohol and EDTA; Folvite 5 mg/ml contains 1.5% benzyl alcohol)
Available without a prescription
Tablets: 0.4 mg, 0.8 mg

Indications and dosages

Megaloblastic or macrocytic anemia secondary to folic acid deficiency, hepatic disease, alcoholism, intestinal obstruction, excessive hemolysis
Pregnant and breast-feeding patients: 0.8 mg P.O., S.C., or I.M. daily.
Adults and children age 4 and older: 0.4 mg P.O., S.C., or I.M. daily for 4 to 5 days. After anemia secondary to folic acid deficiency is corrected, proper diet and RDA supplements are necessary to prevent recurrence.
Children under age 4: Up to 0.3 mg P.O., S.C., or I.M. daily.
Prevention of megaloblastic anemia of pregnancy and fetal damage
Adults: 1 mg P.O., S.C., or I.M. daily during pregnancy.
Nutritional supplement
Adults: Give 0.15 to 0.2 mg P.O., S.C., or I.M. daily for men; give 0.15 to 0.18 mg P.O., S.C., or I.M. daily for women.
Children: 0.05 mg P.O. daily.
Tropical sprue
Adults: 3 to 15 mg P.O. daily.

Pharmacodynamics

Nutritional action: Exogenous folate is required to maintain normal erythropoiesis and to perform nucleoprotein synthesis. Folic acid stimulates production of RBCs, WBCs, and platelets in certain megaloblastic anemias.

Dietary folic acid is present in foods, primarily as reduced folate polyglutamate. This vitamin may be absorbed only after hydrolysis, reduction, and methylation occur in the GI tract. Conversion to active tetrahydrofolate may require vitamin B_{12}.

Oral synthetic form of folic acid is a monoglutamate and is absorbed completely after administration, even in malabsorption syndromes.

Pharmacokinetics

Absorption: Absorbed rapidly from the GI tract, mainly from the proximal part of the small intestine. Normal serum folate levels range from 0.005 to 0.015 mcg/ml. Usually, serum levels less than 0.005 mcg/ml indicate folate deficiency; those less than 0.002 mcg/ml usually result in megaloblastic anemia.
Distribution: The active tetrahydrofolic acid and its derivatives are distributed into all body tissues; the liver contains about half of the total body folate stores. Folate is actively concentrated in the CSF. Folic acid is distributed into breast milk.
Metabolism: Metabolized in the liver to *N*-methyltetrahydrofolic acid, the main form of folate storage and transport.
Excretion: A single 0.1-mg to 0.2-mg dose usually results in only a trace amount of drug in urine. After administering large doses, excessive folate is excreted unchanged in urine. Small amounts of folic acid have been recovered in feces. About 0.05 mg/day of normal body folate stores is lost by a combination of

urinary and fecal excretion and oxidative cleavage of the molecule.

Route	Onset	Peak	Duration
P.O.	20-30 min	2-3 hr	3-6 hr
I.V.	5 min	10 min	3-6 min
I.M.	10-20 min	<1 hr	3-6 hr

Contraindications and precautions
Contraindicated in patients with undiagnosed anemia because it may mask pernicious anemia, and in those with pernicious anemia and other megaloblastic anemias where vitamin B_{12} is deficient.

Interactions
Drug-drug. *Aminosalicylic acid, chloramphenicol, methotrexate, oral contraceptives, sulfasalazine, pyrimethamine, trimethoprim, triamterene:* May act as antagonists to folic acid. Monitor patient for decreased drug effect.
Anticonvulsants such as phenobarbital and phenytoin: Increased anticonvulsant metabolism and decreased blood levels of the anticonvulsants. Recommend monitoring serum blood levels.
Phenytoin and primidone: Decreased serum folate levels; symptoms of folic acid deficiency in long-term therapy. Monitor patient closely.
Pyrimethamine: Interference with antimicrobial actions of pyrimethamine against toxoplasmosis. Avoid use together.

Effects on diagnostic tests
Falsely low serum and erythrocyte folate levels may occur with the *Lactobacillus casei* assay in patients receiving anti-infectives, such as tetracycline, which suppress the growth of this organism.

Adverse reactions
CNS: general malaise.
Respiratory: ***bronchospasm.***
Skin: allergic reactions (rash, pruritus, erythema).

Overdose and treatment
Folic acid is relatively nontoxic. Adverse GI and CNS effects have been reported rarely in patients receiving 15 mg of folic acid daily for 1 month.

Clinical considerations
- The RDA for folic acid is 25 to 200 mcg in children and 180 to 200 mcg in adults; 100 mcg/day is considered an adequate oral supplement. Pregnant women require 400 mcg daily. During the first 6 months of breast-feeding, women require 280 mcg daily; during the second 6 months, this requirement decreases to 260 mcg daily.
- The preferred route of administration for folic acid is P.O. The manufacturer recommends deep I.M., S.C., or I.V. only when P.O. treatment isn't feasible or when malabsorption is suspected.
- Patients undergoing renal dialysis are at risk for folate deficiency.
- Protect folic acid injections from light.

Therapeutic monitoring
Recommend monitoring CBC to measure effectiveness of drug treatment.

Special populations
Pregnant patients. Prepregnancy initiation of drug therapy may reduce risk of fetal neural tube defects.
Breast-feeding patients. Folic acid is excreted in breast milk. Daily doses of 0.8 mg are sufficient to maintain a normoblastic bone marrow after clinical symptoms have subsided and blood components have returned to normal.

Patient counseling
Advise patient of potential adverse reactions.

fomivirsen sodium
Vitravene

Pharmacologic classification: phosphorothioate oligonucleotide
Therapeutic classification: antiviral
Pregnancy risk category C

How supplied
Available by prescription only
Intravitreal injection: Preservative-free, single-use vials containing 0.25 ml, 6.6 mg/ml

Indications and dosages
Local treatment of CMV retinitis in patients with AIDS, who are intolerant of or have a contraindication to other treatments or who were insufficiently responsive to previous treatments
Adults: Induction dose is 330 mcg (0.05 ml) by intravitreal injection every other week for two doses. Subsequent maintenance dosage is 330 mcg (0.05 ml) by intravitreal injection once every 4 weeks after induction.

Pharmacodynamics
Antiviral action: Drug inhibits human CMV replication by binding to the target mRNA and subsequently inhibiting virus replication.

Pharmacokinetics
No information available.

Route	Onset	Peak	Duration
Intravitreal	Unknown	Unknown	Unknown

Contraindications and precautions
Contraindicated in patients with hypersensitivity to drug or its components or in those who have been treated within 2 to 4 weeks with either I.V. or intravitreal cidofovir because of an increased risk of exaggerated ocular inflammation.

Interactions
None reported.

Effects on diagnostic tests
None reported.

Adverse reactions
CNS: asthenia, headache, abnormal thinking, depression, dizziness, neuropathy, pain.
CV: chest pain.
EENT: abnormal or blurred vision, anterior chamber inflammation, cataract, conjunctival hemorrhage, decreased visual acuity, desaturation of color vision, eye pain, floaters, increased intraocular pressure, *ocular inflammation, iritis,* photophobia, retinal detachment, retinal edema, retinal hemorrhage, retinal pigment changes, *uveitis, vitritis,* application site reaction, conjunctival hyperemia, conjunctivitis, corneal edema, decreased peripheral vision, eye irritation, hypotony, keratic precipitates, optic neuritis, photopsia, retinal vascular disease, visual field defect, vitreous hemorrhage, vitreous opacity, sinusitis.
GI: abdominal pain, anorexia, diarrhea, nausea, vomiting, oral candidiasis, *pancreatitis.*
GU: catheter infection, ***kidney failure.***
Hematologic: anemia, lymphoma-like reaction, ***neutropenia, thrombocytopenia.***
Hepatic: abnormal liver function, increased GGT.
Metabolic: decreased weight, dehydration.
Musculoskeletal: back pain.
Respiratory: bronchitis, dyspnea, increased cough, pneumonia.
Skin: rash, sweating.
Other: allergic reactions, cachexia, fever, flu-like syndrome, infection, ***sepsis,*** systemic CMV.

Overdose and treatment
None reported.

Clinical considerations
□ ***ALERT*** Drug is for ophthalmic use by intravitreal injection only.
■ Drug provides localized therapy limited to the treated eye and doesn't provide treatment for systemic CMV disease.
■ Ocular inflammation (uveitis) is most common during induction dosing.

Therapeutic monitoring
■ Monitor light perception and optic nerve head perfusion postinjection.
■ Monitor for increased intraocular pressure. This is usually transient and returns to normal without treatment or with temporary use of topical medications.
■ Monitor patient for extraocular CMV disease or disease in the contralateral eye.

Special populations
Pregnant patients. Safety and efficacy in pregnant women haven't been reported.
Breast-feeding patients. It's unknown if drug is excreted in breast milk. Discontinue drug or nursing.
Pediatric patients. Safety and efficacy in children haven't been established.
Geriatric patients. Safety and efficacy in patients over age 65 haven't been established.

Patient counseling
■ Inform patient that drug isn't a cure for CMV retinitis and that some patients continue to experience progression of retinitis during and following treatment.
■ Tell patient that drug treats only the eye in which it has been injected and that CMV may also exist in the body. Stress importance of follow-up visits to monitor progress and to check for additional infections.
■ Advise HIV-infected patient to continue taking antiretroviral therapy as indicated.

foscarnet sodium (phosphonoformic acid)
Foscavir

Pharmacologic classification: pyrophosphate analogue
Therapeutic classification: antiviral
Pregnancy risk category C

How supplied
Available by prescription only
Injection: 24 mg/ml in 250-ml and 500-ml vials

Indications and dosages
Cytomegalovirus (CMV) retinitis in patients with AIDS
Adults: Initially, 60 mg/kg I.V. as an induction treatment in patients with normal renal function. Administer as an I.V. infusion over 1 hour q 8 hours for 2 or 3 weeks, depending on response. Follow with a maintenance infusion of 90 mg/kg daily administered over 2 hours; increase as needed and tolerated to 120 mg/kg daily if disease shows signs of progression.
Mucocutaneous acyclovir-resistant herpes simplex virus (HSV) infection
Adults: 40 mg/kg I.V. Administer as an I.V. infusion over 1 hour q 8 to 12 hours for 2 or 3 weeks, depending on response.
◊ ***Varicella zoster infection***
Adults: 40 mg/kg I.V. q 8 hours for 10 to 21 days.

HSV INFECTION

Induction dose		
Creatinine clearance (ml/min/kg)	*Equivalent to 80 mg/kg/day (40 mg/kg q 12 hr)*	*Equivalent to 120 mg/kg/day (40 mg/kg q 8 hr)*
> 1.4	40 q 12 hr	40 q 8 hr
> 1.0 – 1.4	30 q 12 hr	30 q 8 hr
> 0.8 – 1.0	20 q 12 hr	35 q 12 hr
> 0.6 – 0.8	35 q 24 hr	25 q 12 hr
> 0.5 – 0.6	25 q 24 hr	40 q 24 hr
≥ 0.4 – 0.5	20 q 24 hr	35 q 24 hr
< 0.4	Not recommended	Not recommended

CMV INFECTION

Induction dose		
Creatinine clearance (ml/min/kg)	*Equivalent to 180 mg/kg/day (60 mg/kg q 8 hr)*	*Equivalent to 180 mg/kg/day (90 mg/kg q 12 hr)*
> 1.4	60 q 8 hr	90 q 12 hr
> 1.0 – 1.4	45 q 8 hr	70 q 12 hr
> 0.8 – 1.0	50 q 12 hr	50 q 12 hr
> 0.6 – 0.8	40 q 12 hr	80 q 24 hr
> 0.5 – 0.6	60 q 24 hr	60 q 24 hr
≥ 0.4 – 0.5	50 q 24 hr	50 q 24 hr
< 0.4	Not recommended	Not recommended
Maintenance dose		
Creatinine clearance (ml/min/kg)	*Equivalent to 90 mg/kg/day (Once daily)*	*Equivalent to 120 mg/kg/day (Once daily)*
> 1.4	90 q 24 hr	120 q 24 hr
> 1.0 – 1.4	70 q 24 hr	90 q 24 hr
> 0.8 – 1.0	50 q 24 hr	65 q 24 hr
> 0.6 – 0.8	80 q 48 hr	105 q 48 hr
> 0.5 – 0.6	60 q 48 hr	80 q 48 hr
≥ 0.4 – 0.5	50 q 48 hr	65 q 48 hr
< 0.4	Not recommended	Not recommended

≡ ***Dosage adjustment.*** For adult patients with renal failure, calculate weight-adjusted creatinine clearance (ml/minute/kg):
For men:

$$\text{creatinine clearance (per kg)} = \frac{(140 - \text{age})}{(\text{serum creatinine} \times 72)};$$

For women: Multiply the above value by 0.85.
Administer the drug according to the above tables.

Pharmacodynamics

Antiviral action: An analogue of pyrophosphate (important in enzymatic reactions), drug inhibits known herpes viruses in vitro by blocking the pyrophosphate binding site on DNA polymerases and reverse transcriptases.

Pharmacokinetics

Absorption: Unknown.
Distribution: About 14% to 17% bound to plasma proteins; drug is deposited in bone.
Metabolism: Unknown.
Excretion: About 80% to 90% appears in urine unchanged. Drug clearance is dependent on

renal function. Plasma half-life is about 3 hours.

Route	Onset	Peak	Duration
I.V.	Unknown	Immediate	Unknown

Contraindications and precautions
Contraindicated in patients with hypersensitivity to drug. Use with extreme caution in patients with impaired renal function.

Interactions
Drug-drug. *Nephrotoxic drugs, such as amphotericin B and aminoglycosides:* Increased risk of nephrotoxicity. Avoid use together.
Pentamidine: Increased risk of nephrotoxicity; severe hypocalcemia has also been reported. Don't use together.
Zidovudine: Increased incidence or severity of anemia. Recommend monitoring blood counts.

Effects on diagnostic tests
None reported.

Adverse reactions
CNS: *headache,* ***seizures,*** fatigue, malaise, asthenia, paresthesia, dizziness, hypoesthesia, neuropathy, tremor, ataxia, generalized spasms, dementia, stupor, sensory disturbances, meningitis, aphasia, abnormal coordination, EEG abnormalities, depression, confusion, anxiety, insomnia, somnolence, nervousness, amnesia, agitation, aggressive reaction, hallucinations.
CV: *hypertension, palpitations, ECG abnormalities, sinus tachycardia,* cerebrovascular disorder, *first-degree AV block, hypotension, flushing,* edema.
EENT: visual disturbances, taste perversion, eye pain, conjunctivitis.
GI: *nausea, diarrhea, vomiting, abdominal pain, anorexia,* constipation, dysphagia, rectal hemorrhage, dry mouth, dyspepsia, melena, flatulence, ulcerative stomatitis, *pancreatitis.*
GU: *abnormal renal function, decreased creatinine clearance and increased serum creatinine levels, albuminuria, dysuria, polyuria, urethral disorder, urine retention, urinary tract infections, acute renal failure,* moniliasis.
Hematologic: *anemia,* ***granulocytopenia, leukopenia, bone marrow suppression, thrombocytopenia,*** platelet abnormalities, thrombocytosis, WBC count abnormalities.
Hepatic: abnormal hepatic function, increased liver enzymes.
Metabolic: hypokalemia, hypomagnesemia, hypophosphatemia or hyperphosphatemia, hypocalcemia.
Musculoskeletal: leg cramps, back or chest pain, arthralgia, myalgia.
Respiratory: *cough, dyspnea,* pneumonitis, sinusitis, pharyngitis, rhinitis, respiratory insufficiency, pulmonary infiltration, stridor, pneumothorax, ***bronchospasm,*** hemoptysis, flulike symptoms.
Skin: *rash, increased sweating,* pruritus, skin ulceration, erythematous rash, seborrhea, skin discoloration, facial edema.
Other: *fever,* lymphadenopathy, pain, infection, sepsis, rigors, inflammation and pain at infusion site, lymphoma-like disorder, sarcoma, bacterial or fungal infections, abscess, ***death.***

Clinical considerations
- Anemia is common (up to 33% of patients treated with drug) and may be severe enough to require transfusions.
- Don't exceed the recommended dosage, infusion rate, or frequency of administration. All doses must be individualized according to patient's renal function.
- An infusion pump must be used to administer foscarnet.
- Foscarnet may be active against certain CMV strains resistant to ganciclovir.

Therapeutic monitoring
Recommend monitoring renal function and for anemia.

Special populations
Breast-feeding patients. It's unknown if drug is excreted in breast milk; however, animal studies indicate that drug may concentrate in breast milk when administered at high doses. Use with caution.
Pediatric patients. Safety and efficacy in children haven't been established. In animals, up to 40% of a dose is deposited in the teeth and bones; similar deposition may be seen in growing children.
Geriatric patients. It's unknown if age alters drug response. However, geriatric patients are likely to have preexisting renal function impairment, which requires alterations in dosage.

Patient counseling
- Warn patient of the high frequency of adverse reactions and the need for ongoing laboratory studies.
- Advise patient to report to prescriber perioral tingling, numbness in the extremities, and paresthesia.

fosinopril sodium
Monopril

Pharmacologic classification: ACE inhibitor
Therapeutic classification: antihypertensive
Pregnancy risk category C (D, second and third trimesters)

How supplied
Available by prescription only
Tablets: 10 mg, 20 mg, 40 mg

Indications and dosages

Treatment of hypertension

Adults: Initially, 10 mg P.O. daily; adjust dose based on blood pressure response at peak and trough levels. Usual dose: 20 to 40 mg daily; maximum up to 80 mg daily. Dose may be divided.

Treatment of heart failure

Adults: Initially, 10 mg P.O. daily; maximum dose up to 40 mg daily. Doses may be divided.

Pharmacodynamics

Antihypertensive action: Fosinopril is believed to lower blood pressure primarily by suppressing the renin-angiotensin-aldosterone system, although it's also been effective in patients with low-renin hypertension.

Pharmacokinetics

Absorption: Absorbed slowly through GI tract, primarily via proximal small intestine.
Distribution: More than 95% is protein-bound.
Metabolism: Hydrolyzed primarily in the liver and gut wall by esterases.
Excretion: Part of drug (50%) is excreted in urine, the remainder in feces.

Route	Onset	Peak	Duration
P.O.	1 hr	3 hr	24 hr

Contraindications and precautions

Contraindicated in patients with hypersensitivity to drug or other ACE inhibitors and in breast-feeding women. Use cautiously in those patients with impaired renal or hepatic function.

Interactions

Drug-drug. *Antacids:* May impair absorption of fosinopril; separate administration by at least 2 hours.
Diuretics and other antihypertensives: Excessive hypotension may occur. Effect may be minimized by stopping diuretic.
Lithium: Increased serum lithium levels and lithium toxicity may occur. Recommend monitoring lithium levels frequently.
Potassium supplements or potassium-sparing diuretics: Concurrent use may result in hyperkalemia. Recommend monitoring potassium levels.
Drug-food. *Salt substitutes containing potassium:* Risk of hyperkalemia. Advise patient to avoid use of potassium salt substitutes.

Effects on diagnostic tests

False low measurements of digoxin levels may result with the DIGI TAB radioimmunoassay kit for digoxin; other kits may be used.

Adverse reactions

CNS: headache, dizziness, fatigue, syncope, paresthesia, sleep disturbance, ***CVA.***
CV: chest pain, angina, ***MI, hypertensive crisis,*** rhythm disturbances, palpitations, hypotension, orthostatic hypotension.
EENT: tinnitus, sinusitis.
GI: nausea, vomiting, diarrhea, *pancreatitis,* dry mouth, abdominal distention, abdominal pain, constipation.
GU: sexual dysfunction, elevations of BUN and serum creatinine, renal insufficiency.
Hematologic: decreased hematocrit or hemoglobin may occur.
Hepatic: elevated liver function tests, *hepatitis.*
Metabolic: hyperkalemia.
Musculoskeletal: arthralgia, musculoskeletal pain, myalgia, gout.
Respiratory: *dry, persistent, tickling, nonproductive cough; bronchospasm.*
Skin: urticaria, rash, photosensitivity, pruritus.
Other: decreased libido, *angioedema.*

Overdose and treatment

Overdose has never been reported; however, the most common sign of overdose is likely to be hypotension. Treat with infusion of normal saline. Hemodialysis and peritoneal dialysis aren't effective in removing the drug.

Clinical considerations

- Diuretic therapy is usually discontinued 2 to 3 days before start of ACE inhibitor therapy to reduce risk of hypotension. If fosinopril doesn't adequately control blood pressure, diuretic may be reinstituted with care.
- Incidence of orthostatic hypotension is low.
- Blood pressure is lowered within 1 hour of a single dose of 10 to 40 mg.

Therapeutic monitoring

- Recommend monitoring potassium levels.
- Recommend performing CBC with differential counts before therapy, then every 2 weeks for 3 months and periodically thereafter.

Special populations

Pregnant patients. Drug is Category D in second and third trimesters of pregnancy.
Breast-feeding patients. Avoid use of drug; significant levels have been detected in breast milk.
Pediatric patients. Safety and efficacy in children haven't been established.
Geriatric patients. No age-related differences have been observed.

Patient counseling

- Tell patient to take dose 1 hour before or 2 hours after food or antacids.
- Advise patient to report to prescriber lightheadedness in the first few days of therapy and signs of infection such as fever or sore throat. He should also contact his prescriber and discontinue drug immediately if the following oc-

cur: swelling of tongue, lips, face, mucous membranes, eyes, lips, or extremities; difficulty swallowing or breathing; or hoarseness.
- Advise patient to maintain the same salt intake as before therapy, because salt restriction can lead to precipitous decrease in blood pressure with initial doses of this drug. Large reductions in blood pressure may also occur with excessive perspiration and dehydration.
- Warn patient to avoid sudden position changes until effect of drug is known; however, orthostatic hypotension is infrequent.

fosphenytoin sodium

Cerebyx

Pharmacologic classification: hydantoin derivative
Therapeutic classification: anticonvulsant
Pregnancy risk category D

How supplied

Available by prescription only
Injection: 2 ml (150 mg fosphenytoin sodium equivalent to 100 mg phenytoin sodium), 10 ml (750 mg fosphenytoin sodium equivalent to 500 mg phenytoin sodium)

Indications and dosages

Status epilepticus
Adults: Give 15 to 20 mg phenytoin sodium equivalent (PE)/kg I.V. at 100 to 150 PE/minute as a loading dose and then, 4 to 6 mg PE/kg/day I.V. as a maintenance dosage. (Phenytoin may be used instead of fosphenytoin as maintenance using the appropriate dose.)
Prevention and treatment of seizures during neurosurgery
Adults: Administer 10 to 20 mg PE/kg I.M. or I.V. at an I.V. infusion rate not exceeding 150 mg PE/minute as a loading dose. Maintenance dosage is 4 to 6 mg PE/kg/day I.V.
Short-term substitution for oral phenytoin therapy
Adults: Same total daily dose as oral phenytoin sodium therapy given as a single daily dose I.M. or I.V. at an I.V. infusion rate not exceeding 150 mg PE/minute. (Some patients may require more frequent dosing.)

Pharmacodynamics

Anticonvulsant action: Because fosphenytoin is a prodrug of phenytoin, its anticonvulsant action is that of phenytoin. Phenytoin stabilizes neuronal membranes and limits seizure activity by modulating voltage-dependent sodium channels of neurons, inhibiting calcium flux across neuronal membranes, modulating voltage-dependent calcium channels of neurons, and enhancing sodium-potassium adenosine triphosphatase activity of neurons and glial cells.

Pharmacokinetics

Absorption: No information available.
Distribution: About 95% to 99% is bound to plasma proteins, primarily albumin. Volume of distribution increases with dose and rate and ranges from 4.3 to 10.8 L.
Metabolism: Conversion half-life of fosphenytoin to phenytoin is about 15 minutes. Phosphatases are believed to play a major role in the conversion.
Excretion: Unknown, although it isn't excreted in urine.

Route	Onset	Peak	Duration
I.V.	Unknown	End of infusion	Unknown
I.M.	Unknown	30 min	Unknown

Contraindications and precautions

Contraindicated in patients with hypersensitivity to the drug or its components, phenytoin, or other hydantoins. Also contraindicated in patients with sinus bradycardia, SA block, second- and third-degree AV block, and Adams-Stokes syndrome because of the effect of parenteral phenytoin on ventricular automaticity.

Use cautiously in patients with hypotension, severe myocardial insufficiency, impaired renal or hepatic function, hypoalbuminemia, porphyria, diabetes mellitus, and history of hypersensitivity to similarly structured drugs, such as barbiturates and succinimides.

Interactions

Drug-drug. *Drugs that may increase plasma phenytoin levels (and thus its therapeutic effects), such as amiodarone, chloramphenicol, chlordiazepoxide, cimetidine, diazepam, dicumarol, disulfiram, estrogens, ethosuximide, fluoxetine, H_2-antagonists, halothane, isoniazid, methylphenidate, phenothiazines, phenylbutazone, salicylates, succinimides, sulfonamides, tolbutamide, and trazodone:* Increased plasma phenytoin levels. Monitor patient carefully.
Carbamazepine or reserpine: Plasma phenytoin levels may be decreased. Use together cautiously.
Coumarin, digitoxin, doxycycline, estrogens, furosemide, oral contraceptives, rifampin, quinidine, theophylline, and vitamin D: Efficacy may be decreased by phenytoin due to increased hepatic metabolism.
Phenobarbital, valproic acid, sodium valproate: May increase or decrease plasma phenytoin levels. Monitor patient closely.
Tricyclic antidepressants: Lower seizure threshold and may require adjustments in phenytoin dosage.
Drug-lifestyle. *Acute alcohol use:* Increased plasma phenytoin concentration.
Long-term alcohol use: Decreased plasma phenytoin levels. Advise patient to avoid alcohol.

Effects on diagnostic tests
Fosphenytoin may produce artificially low results in dexamethasone or metyrapone tests.

Adverse reactions
CNS: increased or decreased reflexes, speech disorders, dysarthria, asthenia, ***intracranial hypertension, cerebral hemorrhage,*** thinking abnormalities, nervousness, hypesthesia, extrapyramidal syndrome, brain edema, headache, *nystagmus, dizziness, somnolence, ataxia,* stupor, incoordination, stupor, paresthesia, agitation, tremor, vertigo.
CV: hypertension, ***cardiac arrest,*** palpitation, sinus bradycardia, atrial flutter, ***bundle branch block,*** cardiomegaly, orthostatic hypotension, ***pulmonary embolus,*** QT interval prolongation, thrombophlebitis, ventricular extrasystoles, ***heart failure,*** vasodilation, tachycardia, hypotension.
EENT: taste perversion, deafness, visual field defect, eye pain, conjunctivitis, photophobia, hyperacusis, mydriasis, parosmia, ear pain, taste loss, tinnitus, diplopia, amblyopia.
GI: constipation, dyspepsia, diarrhea, anorexia, GI hemorrhage, increased salivation, tenesmus, tongue edema, dysphagia, flatulence, gastritis, ileus, nausea, dry mouth, vomiting.
GU: urine retention, oliguria, dysuria, vaginitis, albuminuria, genital edema, kidney failure, polyuria, urethral pain, urinary incontinence, vaginal moniliasis.
Hematologic: ***thrombocytopenia,*** anemia, leukocytosis, hypochromic anemia, ***leukopenia, agranulocytosis, granulocytopenia, pancytopenia,*** ecchymosis.
Hepatic: elevated liver enzymes.
Metabolic: diabetes insipidus, hypokalemia, hyperglycemia, hypophosphatemia, alkalosis, acidosis, dehydration, hyperkalemia, ketosis, decreased serum levels of T_4.
Musculoskeletal: myasthenia, myopathy, leg cramps, arthralgia, myalgia, pelvic pain, back pain.
Respiratory: cyanosis, pneumonia, pharyngitis, sinusitis, hyperventilation, rhinitis, ***apnea,*** aspiration pneumonia, asthma, dyspnea, atelectasis, increased cough, increased sputum, epistaxis, hypoxia, pneumothorax, hemoptysis, bronchitis.
Skin: petechia, rash, maculopapular rash, urticaria, sweating, skin discoloration, contact dermatitis, pustular rash, skin nodule, *pruritus.*
Other: lymphadenopathy.

Overdose and treatment
There have been no reports of fosphenytoin overdose. However, because it's a prodrug of phenytoin, overdose may be similar. Early signs of phenytoin overdose may include drowsiness, nausea, vomiting, nystagmus, ataxia, dysarthria, tremor, and slurred speech; hypotension, respiratory depression, and coma may follow. Death is caused by respiratory and circulatory depression. Estimated lethal dose of phenytoin in adults is 2 to 5 g.

Formate and phosphate are metabolites of fosphenytoin and, therefore, may contribute to signs of toxicity following overdose. Signs of formate toxicity are similar to those of methanol toxicity and are associated with severe anion-gap metabolic acidosis. Large amounts of phosphate, delivered rapidly, could potentially cause hypocalcemia with paresthesia, muscle spasms, and seizures. Ionized free calcium levels can be measured and, if low, used to guide treatment.

Treatment is with gastric lavage or emesis and followed by supportive treatment. Monitor vital signs and fluid and electrolyte balance. Forced diuresis is of little or no value. Hemodialysis or peritoneal dialysis may be helpful.

Clinical considerations
- Always prescribe and dispense fosphenytoin in phenytoin sodium equivalent units (PE). Don't make adjustments in the recommended doses when substituting fosphenytoin for phenytoin and vice versa.
- Administer dose of I.V. fosphenytoin used to treat status epilepticus at a maximum rate of 150 mg PE/minute. The typical infusion of drug administered to a 110-lb (50-kg) patient takes 5 to 7 minutes, whereas that of an identical molar dose of phenytoin can't be accomplished in less than 15 to 20 minutes because of the untoward CV effects that accompany the direct I.V. administration of phenytoin at rates of more than 50 mg/minute. Don't use I.M. fosphenytoin because therapeutic phenytoin levels may not be reached as rapidly as with I.V. administration.
- If rapid phenytoin loading is a primary goal, I.V. administration of fosphenytoin is preferred because the time to achieve therapeutic plasma phenytoin levels is greater following I.M. than that following I.V. administration.
- Patients receiving fosphenytoin at doses of 20 mg PE/kg at 150 mg PE/minute are expected to experience some sensory discomfort, with the groin being the most common location. The occurrence and intensity of the discomfort can be lessened by slowing or temporarily stopping the infusion.
- The phosphate load provided by fosphenytoin (0.0037 mmol phosphate/mg PE fosphenytoin) must be taken into consideration when treating patients who require phosphate restriction, such as those with severe renal impairment.
- Discontinue drug in patients with acute hepatotoxicity and don't readminister to these patients.
- I.M. drug administration generates systemic phenytoin levels similar enough to oral pheny-

toin sodium to allow essentially interchangeable use.

- A dose of 15 to 20 mg PE/kg of fosphenytoin infused I.V. at 100 to 150 mg PE/minute yields plasma-free phenytoin levels over time that approximate those achieved when an equivalent dose of phenytoin sodium (such as parenteral dilantin) is administered at 50 mg/minute I.V.
- Interpretation of total phenytoin plasma levels should be made cautiously in patients with renal or hepatic disease or hypoalbuminemia due to an increased fraction in unbound phenytoin. Unbound phenytoin levels may be more useful in these patients. Also, these patients are at increased risk for both the frequency and severity of adverse reactions when fosphenytoin is administered I.V.

Therapeutic monitoring

- Recommend monitoring patient's ECG, blood pressure, and respiration continuously throughout the period where maximal serum phenytoin levels occur, about 10 to 20 minutes after the end of fosphenytoin infusions. Severe CV complications are most commonly encountered in geriatric or gravely ill patients. Reduction in rate of administration or discontinuation of dosing may be needed.
- Discontinue drug if rash appears. If rash is exfoliative, purpuric, or bullous or if lupus erythematosus, Stevens-Johnson syndrome, or toxic epidermal necrolysis is suspected, don't resume use of drug; seek alternative therapy. If rash is mild (measles-like or scarlatiniform), therapy may be resumed after it has completely disappeared. If rash recurs on reinstitution of therapy, further fosphenytoin or phenytoin administration is contraindicated.
- Following drug administration, it's recommended that phenytoin levels not be monitored until conversion to phenytoin is essentially complete; about 2 hours after the end of an I.V. infusion or 4 hours after I.M. administration.

Special populations

Breast-feeding patients. Because it's unknown if fosphenytoin is excreted in breast milk, breast-feeding isn't recommended.
Pediatric patients. Safety and efficacy in children haven't been established.
Geriatric patients. Geriatric patients metabolize and excrete phenytoin slowly; therefore, administer fosphenytoin cautiously to older adults.

Patient counseling

- Warn patient that sensory disturbances may occur with I.V. drug administration.
- Tell patient to report adverse reactions, especially rash, immediately.

furosemide

Apo-Furosemide*, Lasix, Lasix Special*, Novosemide*, Uritol*

Pharmacologic classification: loop diuretic
Therapeutic classification: diuretic, antihypertensive
Pregnancy risk category C

How supplied

Available by prescription only
Tablets: 20 mg, 40 mg, 80 mg
Solution: 10 mg/ml, 40 mg/5 ml
Injection: 10 mg/ml

Indications and dosages

Acute pulmonary edema
Adults: 40 mg I.V. injected slowly; then 80 mg I.V. within 1 hour, p.r.n.
Infants and children: 1 mg/kg I.M. or I.V. q 2 hours until response is achieved; maximum dose is 6 mg/kg/day.
Edema
Adults: 20 to 80 mg P.O. daily in morning, with second dose given in 6 to 8 hours, carefully adjusted up to 600 mg daily, p.r.n.; or 20 to 40 mg I.M. or I.V. Increase by 20 mg q 2 hours until desired response is achieved. I.V. dosage should be given slowly over 1 to 2 minutes.
Infants and children: 2 mg/kg/day P.O., increased by 1 to 2 mg/kg in 6 to 8 hours, p.r.n., carefully adjusted not to exceed 6 mg/kg/day.
Hypertension
Adults: 40 mg P.O. b.i.d. Adjust dosage according to response.
◊ ***Hypercalcemia***
Adults: 80 to 100 mg I.V. q 1 to 2 hours; or 120 mg P.O. daily.
≡ ***Dosage adjustment.*** Reduced dosages may be indicated in geriatric patients.

Pharmacodynamics

Diuretic action: Loop diuretics inhibit sodium and chloride reabsorption in the proximal part of the ascending loop of Henle, promoting the excretion of sodium, water, chloride, and potassium.
Antihypertensive action: This drug effect may be the result of renal and peripheral vasodilatation and a temporary increase in glomerular filtration rate and a decrease in peripheral vascular resistance.

Pharmacokinetics

Absorption: About 60% of a given furosemide dose is absorbed from the GI tract after oral administration. Food delays oral absorption but doesn't alter diuretic response. Diuresis begins in 30 to 60 minutes; peak diuresis occurs 1 to 2 hours after oral administration. Diuresis follows I.V. administration within 5 minutes and peaks in 20 to 60 minutes.

Distribution: About 95% is plasma protein-bound. It crosses the placenta and distributes into breast milk.
Metabolism: Metabolized minimally by the liver.
Excretion: About 50% to 80% of a dose is excreted in urine; plasma half-life is about 30 minutes. Duration of action is 6 to 8 hours after oral administration and about 2 hours after I.V. administration.

Route	Onset	Peak	Duration
P.O.	20-30 min	1-2 hr	6-8 hr
I.V.	5 min	½ hr	2 hr

Contraindications and precautions
Contraindicated in patients with anuria or history of hypersensitivity to drug. Use cautiously in hepatic cirrhosis and during pregnancy.

Interactions
Drug-drug. *Ethacrynic acid, aminoglycoside antibiotics, and cisplatin:* Can potentiate ototoxicity. Don't use together.
Antidiabetic agents: Decreased hypoglycemic effects. Recommend monitoring glucose levels.
Other antihypertensives: Increased risk of hypotension. Recommend checking blood pressure frequently.
Cardiac glycosides, neuromuscular blockers, and lithium: Increased risk of toxicity. Recommend monitoring potassium levels.
Corticosteroids, corticotropin, amphotericin B, metolazone: Increased risk of hypokalemia. Recommend monitoring potassium levels.
NSAIDs: May inhibit diuretic response. Use together cautiously.
Salicylates: May cause salicylate toxicity. Use together cautiously.
Sucralfate: May reduce diuretic and antihypertensive effect. Separate administration by 2 hours.
Drug-herb. *Aloe:* May increase drug effects. Use together cautiously.
Drug-lifestyle. *Sun exposure:* Potentiates photosensitivity reactions. Advise patient to take precautions.

Effects on diagnostic tests
None reported.

Adverse reactions
CNS: vertigo, headache, dizziness, paresthesia, restlessness.
CV: volume depletion and dehydration, orthostatic hypotension.
EENT: transient deafness with too rapid I.V. injection, blurred vision.
GI: abdominal discomfort and pain, diarrhea, anorexia, nausea, vomiting, constipation, *pancreatitis.*
GU: nocturia, polyuria, frequent urination, altered renal function tests, oliguria.
Hematologic: ***agranulocytosis, leukopenia, thrombocytopenia,*** azotemia, anemia, ***aplastic anemia.***
Hepatic: altered liver function test results.
Metabolic: hypokalemia; hypochloremic alkalosis; asymptomatic hyperuricemia; fluid and electrolyte imbalances, including dilutional hyponatremia, hypocalcemia, hypomagnesemia; hyperglycemia and impaired glucose tolerance.
Musculoskeletal: muscle spasm; weakness.
Skin: dermatitis, purpura.
Other: fever; transient pain (at I.M. injection site); thrombophlebitis (with I.V. administration).

Overdose and treatment
Signs and symptoms of overdose include profound electrolyte and volume depletion, which may precipitate circulatory collapse. Treatment is chiefly supportive; replace fluids and electrolytes.

Clinical considerations
Consider the recommendations relevant to all loop diuretics. Give I.V. furosemide slowly, over 1 to 2 minutes; for I.V. infusion, dilute furosemide in D_5W, normal saline solution, or lactated Ringer's solution, and use within 24 hours. If high-dose furosemide therapy is needed, administer as a controlled infusion not exceeding 4 mg/minute.

Therapeutic monitoring
Recommendations are the same as for all loop diuretics.

Special populations
Pregnant patients. Use cautiously during pregnancy.
Breast-feeding patients. Drug shouldn't be used by breast-feeding women.
Pediatric patients. Use drug with caution in neonates. The usual pediatric dosage can be used, but extend dosing intervals. Sorbitol content of oral preparations may cause diarrhea, especially at high doses.
Geriatric patients. Geriatric and debilitated patients require close observation because they're more susceptible to drug-induced diuresis. Excessive diuresis promotes rapid dehydration, leading to hypovolemia, hypokalemia, hyponatremia, and circulatory collapse.

Patient counseling
Warn patient that photosensitivity reaction may occur. Explain that reaction is a photoallergy in which ultraviolet radiation alters drug structure, causing allergic reactions in some individuals.

G

gabapentin
Neurontin

Pharmacologic classification: 1-amino-methyl cyclohexoneacetic acid
Therapeutic classification: anticonvulsant
Pregnancy risk category C

How supplied
Available by prescription only
Capsules: 100 mg, 300 mg, 400 mg

Indications and dosages
Adjunctive treatment of partial seizures with and without secondary generalization
Adults: 300 mg P.O. on day 1, 300 mg P.O. b.i.d. on day 2, and 300 mg P.O. t.i.d. on day 3. Increase dosage as needed and tolerated to 1,800 mg daily, in three divided doses. Usual dose is 300 to 600 mg P.O. t.i.d., although doses up to 3,600 mg/day have been well tolerated.
≡ ***Dosage adjustment.*** In adult patients with renal failure, if creatinine clearance is more than 60 ml/minute, give 400 mg P.O. t.i.d.; if creatinine clearance is between 30 and 60 ml/minute, give 300 mg P.O. b.i.d.; if creatinine clearance is between 15 and 30 ml/minute, give 300 mg P.O. daily; and if creatinine clearance is less than 15 ml/minute, give 300 mg P.O. every other day. Patients on hemodialysis should receive a loading dose of 300 to 400 mg P.O.; then 200 mg to 300 mg P.O. q 4 hours after hemodialysis.

Pharmacodynamics
Anticonvulsant action: The mechanism of action of gabapentin is unknown. Although it's structurally related to gamma-aminobutyric acid (GABA), it doesn't interact with GABA receptors, isn't converted metabolically into GABA or a GABA agonist, and doesn't inhibit GABA uptake or degradation. Gabapentin doesn't exhibit affinity for other common receptor sites.

Pharmacokinetics
Absorption: Drug bioavailability isn't dose proportional. A 400-mg dose, for example, is about 25% less bioavailable than a 100-mg dose. Over the recommended dose range of 300 to 600 mg t.i.d., however, differences in bioavailability aren't large and bioavailability is about 60%. Food has no effect on the rate or extent of absorption.
Distribution: Circulates largely unbound (less than 3%) to plasma protein. Drug crosses the blood-brain barrier with about 20% of the corresponding plasma levels found in CSF.
Metabolism: Not appreciably metabolized in humans.
Excretion: Eliminated from the systemic circulation by renal excretion as unchanged drug. Its elimination half-life is 5 to 7 hours. Drug can be removed from plasma by hemodialysis.

Route	Onset	Peak	Duration
P.O.	Unknown	Unknown	Unknown

Contraindications and precautions
Contraindicated in patients hypersensitive to drug.

Interactions
Drug-drug. *Antacids:* Decrease absorption of gabapentin. Separate administration of the two drugs by at least 2 hours.

Effects on diagnostic tests
Gabapentin causes false-positive results with the Ames N-Multistix SG dipstick test for urinary protein when added to other antiepileptic drugs. The more specific sulfosalicylic acid precipitation procedure is recommended to determine the presence of urine protein.

Adverse reactions
CNS: *fatigue, somnolence, dizziness, ataxia, nystagmus, tremor,* nervousness, dysarthria, amnesia, depression, abnormal thinking, twitching, incoordination.
CV: peripheral edema, vasodilation.
EENT: *diplopia, rhinitis,* pharyngitis, dry throat, coughing, dental abnormalities, *amblyopia.*
GI: nausea, vomiting, dyspepsia, dry mouth, constipation.
GU: impotence.
Hematologic: ***leukopenia,*** decreased WBC count.
Metabolic: increased appetite, weight gain.
Musculoskeletal: back pain, myalgia, fractures.
Skin: pruritus, abrasion.

Overdose and treatment

Acute overdose of gabapentin may cause double vision, slurred speech, drowsiness, lethargy, and diarrhea. Supportive care is recommended. Gabapentin can be removed by hemodialysis and may be indicated by the patient's clinical state or in patients with significant renal impairment.

Clinical considerations

- Don't suddenly withdraw other anticonvulsant drugs in patients starting gabapentin therapy. Discontinue drug therapy or substitute alternative medication gradually over at least 1 week to minimize risk of precipitating seizures.
- Drug can be taken without regard to meals.

Therapeutic monitoring

- Routine monitoring of plasma drug levels isn't necessary. Drug doesn't appear to alter plasma levels of other anticonvulsants.
- Sulfosalicylic acid precipitation procedure is recommended to determine the presence of urine protein. Don't use Ames N-Multistix SG dipstick to test for urine protein; false-positive results can occur.

Special populations

Pregnant patients. Data concerning use during pregnancy is inadequate; however, gabapentin has shown to be tetragenic in mice and rats.

Breast-feeding patients. It's unknown if drug is excreted in breast milk. Discontinue breast-feeding if gabapentin therapy is initiated because of potential for serious adverse reactions.

Pediatric patients. Safety and efficacy in children under age 12 haven't been established.

Patient counseling

- Instruct patient to take first dose at bedtime to minimize drowsiness, dizziness, fatigue, and ataxia.
- Warn patient to avoid driving or operating heavy machinery until adverse CNS effects of drug are known.
- Inform patient that drug can be taken without regard to meals.

ganciclovir (DHPG)

Cytovene

Pharmacologic classification: synthetic nucleoside

Therapeutic classification: antiviral

Pregnancy risk category C

How supplied

Available by prescription only

Injection: 500-mg vial

Capsules: 250 mg, 500 mg

Indications and dosages

Treatment of cytomegalovirus (CMV) retinitis

Adults: Initially, 5 mg/kg I.V. (given at a constant rate over 1 hour) q 12 hours for 14 to 21 days; followed by a maintenance dosage of 5 mg/kg I.V. once daily for 7 days weekly; or 6 mg/kg I.V. once daily for 5 days weekly. These I.V. infusions should be given at a constant rate over 1 hour. Alternately, a maintenance dosage of 1,000 mg P.O. t.i.d. or 500 mg P.O. q 3 hours while awake (six times daily) may be used.

Prevention of CMV in transplant recipients

Adults: 5 mg/kg I.V. over 1 hour q 12 hours for 7 to 14 days, followed by a maintenance dosage of 5 mg/kg once daily for 7 days weekly or 6 mg/kg once daily for 5 days weekly.

◇***Other CMV infections***

Adults: 5 mg/kg I.V. over 1 hour q 12 hours for 14 to 21 days; or 2.5 mg/kg I.V. q 8 hours for 14 to 21 days.

≡***Dosage adjustment.*** Adjust dosage in patients with renal failure. Consider a dosage reduction for patients with neutropenia, anemia, or thrombocytopenia.

Pharmacodynamics

Antiviral action: Ganciclovir is a synthetic nucleoside analogue of 2′-deoxyguanosine. It competitively inhibits viral DNA polymerase, and may be incorporated within viral DNA to cause early termination of DNA replication. It has shown activity against CMV, herpes simplex virus type 1 and type 2 (HSV-1 and HSV-2), varicella zoster virus, Epstein-Barr virus, and hepatitis B virus.

Pharmacokinetics

Absorption: Less than 7% is absorbed after oral administration.

Distribution: Only 2% to 3% protein-bound. It preferentially concentrates within CMV-infected cells because of action of cellular kinases that convert it to ganciclovir triphosphate.

Metabolism: Most (over 90%) is excreted unchanged.

Excretion: Elimination half-life is about 3 hours in patients with normal renal function; it can be as long as 30 hours in patients with severe renal failure. The primary route of excretion is through the kidneys by glomerular filtration and some renal tubular secretion.

Route	Onset	Peak	Duration
P.O.	Unknown	1¾-3 hr	Unknown
I.V.	Unknown	Immediate	Unknown

Contraindications and precautions

Contraindicated in patients with hypersensitivity to drug and with an absolute neutrophil count less than 500 mm^3 or a platelet count below 25,000 mm³. Use cautiously in patients with impaired renal function.

Interactions

Drug-drug. *Cytotoxic drugs:* Additive toxicity (bone marrow depression, stomatitis, alopecia). Monitor patient closely.
Imipenem-cilastatin: Increased risk of seizures. Monitor patient closely.
Immunosuppressants, such as azathioprine, cyclosporine, corticosteroids: Enhanced immune and bone marrow suppression. Use together cautiously.
Probenecid: Decreased renal clearance of ganciclovir. Monitor patient closely.
Zidovudine: Higher incidence of neutropenia. Monitor patient closely.

Effects on diagnostic tests

None reported.

Adverse reactions

CNS: altered dreams, confusion, ataxia, headache, ***seizures, coma,*** dizziness, somnolence, tremor, abnormal thinking, agitation, amnesia, anxiety, neuropathy, paresthesia, asthenia.
EENT: retinal detachment (in CMV retinitis patients).
GI: *nausea, vomiting, diarrhea, anorexia, abdominal pain,* flatulence, dyspepsia, dry mouth.
GU: increased serum creatinine levels.
Hematologic: ***granulocytopenia, thrombocytopenia, leukopenia,*** *anemia.*
Hepatic: abnormal liver function tests.
Respiratory: pneumonia.
Skin: *rash; sweating;* pruritus, inflammation, pain (at injection site).
Other: phlebitis, chills, ***sepsis,*** *fever,* infection.

Overdose and treatment

Overdose may result in emesis, neutropenia, or GI disturbances. Treatment should be symptomatic and supportive. Hemodialysis may be useful. Hydrate the patient to reduce plasma levels.

Clinical considerations

- Drug has a high potential for toxicity; use only when the potential for benefit outweighs risk.
- Reconstitute with sterile water for injection. Don't reconstitute with bacteriostatic water for injection because this may lead to the formation of a precipitate. Reconstituted solutions are stable for 12 hours. Don't refrigerate.

☐ *ALERT* Don't administer S.C., I.M., or as a rapid I.V. bolus.

- Administer drug over 1 hour because of its high potential for toxicity.

Therapeutic monitoring

- Recommend monitoring CBC to detect neutropenia, which may occur in as many as 40% of patients. It usually appears after about 10 days of therapy, and may be associated with a higher dosage (15 mg/kg/day). Neutropenia is reversible, but may necessitate discontinuation of therapy. Patient may resume drug therapy when blood counts return to normal.
- Adverse reactions occur frequently, can be reduced with reduction of dose, and generally resolve when drug therapy is discontinued.

Special populations

Breast-feeding patients. Don't use drug in breast-feeding women. Instruct women to discontinue breast-feeding until at least 72 hours after last treatment.
Pediatric patients. Little data are available on drug use in children under age 12. Use with extreme caution, keeping in mind the potential for carcinogenic and reproductive toxicity.
Geriatric patients. Use cautiously in geriatric patients with compromised renal function.

Patient counseling

- Inform patient that maintenance infusions are necessary to prevent recurrence of disease.
- Instruct patient to have regular eye examinations to monitor retinitis.
- Advise patient to immediately report signs or symptoms of infection (fever, sore throat) or easy bruising or bleeding.
- Instruct patient to take oral dose with food.

ganirelix acetate

Antagon

Pharmacologic classification: gonadotropin-releasing hormone (GnRH) antagonist
Therapeutic classification: fertility agent
Pregnancy risk category X

How supplied

Available by prescription only
Injection: 250 mcg/0.5 ml in prefilled syringes

Indications and dosages

Inhibition of premature luteinizing hormone (LH) surges in women undergoing medically supervised, controlled ovarian hyperstimulation
Adults: 250 mcg S.C. once daily during early to midfollicular phase of menstrual cycle. Continue daily until enough follicles of sufficient size are confirmed by ultrasound; human chorionic gonadotropin is then administered to induce final maturation of follicles.

Pharmacodynamics

LH suppression action: GnRH, secreted by the pituitary gland, stimulates the synthesis and secretion of gonadotropins, LH, and follicle-stimulating hormone (FSH). In midcycle, a large increase in GnRH leads to a large surge in LH secretion, causing ovulation, an increase in progesterone levels, and a decrease in estradiol levels. Ganirelix blocks pituitary GnRH receptors and suppresses LH and, to a smaller degree, FSH secretions. By suppressing LH and FSH secretions in the early to mid menstrual cycle, ganirelix stops premature gonadotropin surges that could interfere with a trial of medically supervised, controlled ovarian hyperstimulation.

Pharmacokinetics

Absorption: Rapidly absorbed after S.C. injection with an average of 91.1% absorbed.
Distribution: Most (81.9%) is bound to plasma proteins.
Metabolism: Unmetabolized drug is found in urine up to 24 hours after dose. Two metabolites have been detected in feces.
Excretion: Primary excretion route is fecal; metabolites can be detected nearly 8 days after a dose.

Route	Onset	Peak	Duration
S.C.	Unknown	Unknown	Unknown

Contraindications and precautions

Contraindicated in patients with known hypersensitivity to ganirelix or its components or to GnRH or GnRH analogue. Also contraindicated in pregnant women. Use with caution in patients with potential hypersensitivity to GnRH and in those with latex allergies because the product packaging contains natural rubber latex.

Interactions

None reported.

Effects on diagnostic tests

None reported.

Adverse reactions

CNS: headache.
GI: abdominal pain, nausea.
GU: vaginal bleeding, gynecologic abdominal pain, ovarian hyperstimulation syndrome.
Skin: injection site reaction.
Other: ***fetal death.***

Overdose and treatment

No information available.

Clinical considerations

- Only health care providers experienced in infertility treatments should prescribe this drug.
- Before starting treatment, ensure that patient isn't pregnant.
- The natural rubber latex packaging of this product may cause allergic reactions in hypersensitive patients.

Therapeutic monitoring

- After first injection, patients who report previous or potential hypersensitivity to GnRH must be monitored closely.
- Increased WBC count and decreased bilirubin levels and hematocrit have occurred in patients receiving ganirelix injections.

Special populations

Pregnant patients. Drug may cause fetal death; don't use in pregnancy.
Breast-feeding patients. The amount of drug excreted in human milk is unknown; drug shouldn't be used by breast-feeding women.
Pediatric patients. Ganirelix use hasn't been studied in pediatric patients.
Geriatric patients. Ganirelix use hasn't been sufficiently studied in patients age 65 and older.

Patient counseling

- Tell patient that the correct use of ganirelix injection is extremely important to the success of the infertility treatments.
- Provide patient with information on proper technique for S.C. administration of drug.
- Advise patient to store drug at room temperature, away from heat and light, and out of children's reach.
- Instruct patient to discontinue drug and contact prescriber as soon as pregnancy is suspected.

gemcitabine hydrochloride

Gemzar

Pharmacologic classification: nucleoside analogue
Therapeutic classification: antitumor
Pregnancy risk category D

How supplied

Available by prescription only
Powder for injection: 200-mg/10 ml, 1-g/50 ml vials

Indications and dosages

Locally advanced (nonresectable stage II or stage III) or metastatic pancreatic adenocarcinoma (stage IV) and in patients previously treated with fluorouracil
Adults: 1,000 mg/m^2 I.V. over 30 minutes once weekly for up to 7 weeks or until toxicity necessitates reducing or holding a dose. Treatment course of 7 weeks is followed by 1 week rest. Subsequent dosage cycles consist of one infusion weekly for 3 out of 4 consecutive weeks.
≡ ***Dosage adjustment.*** Adjust dosage if bone marrow suppression is detected. Give full dose if absolute granulocyte count (AGC) is 1,000/mm^3 or more and platelet count is 100,000/mm^3 or more. If AGC is 500/mm^3 to

999/mm³, or if platelet count is 50,000/mm³ to 99,000/mm³, give 75% of dose. Hold dose if AGC is less than 500/mm³ or platelet count is less than 50,000/mm³. Adjust dosage for subsequent cycles based on AGC and platelet count nadirs and degree of nonhematologic toxicity.

Advanced non-small cell lung cancer
Adults: 1,000 mg/m² I.V. over 30 minutes once weekly for up to 7 weeks or until toxicity necessitates reducing or holding a dose. Treatment course of 7 weeks is followed by 1 week rest. Subsequent dosage cycles consist of one infusion weekly for 3 out of 4 consecutive weeks.

Inoperable, locally advanced (stage IIIA or IIIB) or metastatic (stage IV) non-small cell lung carcinoma as initial treatment in combination with cisplatin
4-week schedule
Adults: 1,000 mg/m² I.V. over 30 minutes on days 1, 8, and 15 of each 28-day cycle. Cisplatin is administered on day 1 after gemcitabine administration is completed.
3-week schedule
Adults: 1,250 mg/m² I.V. over 30 minutes on days 1 and 8 of each 21-day cycle. Cisplatin is administered on day 1 after gemcitabine administration is completed.
≡ ***Dosage adjustment.*** When used in combination with cisplatin, reduce dosage by 50% in the occurrence of severe nonhematologic toxicity.

◇ ***Advanced or metastatic bladder cancer***
Adults: 1,200 mg/m to 1,250 mg/m² I.V. over 30 minutes, once a week for 3 weeks of a 4 week cycle.

Pharmacodynamics
Cytotoxic action: Drug is cell-phase specific; it inhibits DNA synthesis and blocks progression of cells through G1/S-phase boundary.

Pharmacokinetics
Absorption: Not reported.
Distribution: Volume of distribution (V_d) increases with increased infusion time. Following an infusion lasting under 70 minutes, V_d was 50 L/m², suggesting that drug isn't extensively distributed. The V_d increased to 370 L/m² for longer infusions, reflecting slow equilibration of gemcitabine with the tissue compartment. Plasma protein-binding is negligible. Longer infusion time results in longer drug half-life.
Metabolism: Metabolized to an inactive uracil metabolite.
Excretion: Drug clearance decreases with increasing age; it's also less in women than men. This results in an increased half-life with increased age and in women. A total of 92% to 98% of drug has been recovered almost entirely in urine.

Route	Onset	Peak	Duration
I.V.	Unknown	Unknown	Unknown

Contraindications and precautions
Contraindicated in patients with hypersensitivity to drug.

Interactions
None reported.

Effects on diagnostic tests
None reported.

Adverse reactions
CNS: *paresthesia, somnolence.*
CV: *edema, peripheral edema.*
GI: *constipation, diarrhea, nausea, stomatitis, vomiting.*
GU: *elevated BUN* and creatinine, *hematuria, proteinuria.*
Hematologic: *anemia,* LEUKOPENIA, NEUTROPENIA, THROMBOCYTOPENIA, HEMORRHAGE.
Hepatic: *elevated liver enzymes.*
Respiratory: bronchospasm, *dyspnea.*
Skin: *alopecia, rash.*
Other: *fever, flulike symptoms,* INFECTION, *pain.*

Overdose and treatment
There's no known antidote for drug overdose. If overdose is suspected, monitor patient with appropriate blood counts and provide supportive therapy.

Clinical considerations
☐ ***ALERT*** Preparation and administration of parenteral form of drug is associated with mutagenic, teratogenic, and carcinogenic risks for personnel.
- Prolongation of infusion time beyond 60 minutes and more frequently than weekly dosing have been shown to increase drug toxicity.
- Age, gender, and renal impairment may predispose patient to toxicity.
- Exercise caution when drug is used for patients with renal and hepatic impairment.

Therapeutic monitoring
- Monitor renal and hepatic function tests before treatment and periodically thereafter.
- Recommend monitoring CBC, differential, and platelet count before giving each dose. Drug can suppress bone marrow function as manifested by leukopenia, thrombocytopenia, and anemia.
- When drug is used in combination with cisplatin, recommend monitoring serum concentrations of creatinine, potassium, calcium, and magnesium.

Special populations

Breast-feeding patients. It's unknown if drug is excreted in breast milk. Avoid use in breast-feeding women.
Pediatric patients. Drug hasn't been studied in pediatric patients.
Geriatric patients. Drug clearance is affected by age; however, dosage adjustment isn't indicated.

Patient counseling

- Advise patient to take temperature daily and to watch for signs of infection (fever, sore throat, fatigue) and bleeding (easy bruising, nosebleeds, bleeding gums, melena).

gemfibrozil

Lopid

Pharmacologic classification: fibric acid derivative
Therapeutic classification: antilipemic
Pregnancy risk category C

How supplied

Available by prescription only
Tablets: 600 mg

Indications and dosages

Type IV hyperlipidemia (hypertriglyceridemia) and severe hypercholesterolemia unresponsive to diet and other drugs; reducing risk of cardiac disease, only in type IIb patients without history of disease
Adults: 1,200 mg P.O. administered in two divided doses 30 minutes before morning and evening meals.

Pharmacodynamics

Antilipemic action: Gemfibrozil decreases serum triglyceride levels and very-low-density lipoprotein (VLDL) cholesterol while increasing serum high-density lipoprotein cholesterol, inhibits lipolysis in adipose tissue, and reduces hepatic triglyceride synthesis. Drug is closely related to clofibrate pharmacologically.

Pharmacokinetics

Absorption: Well absorbed from GI tract. Plasma levels of VLDL decrease in 2 to 5 days with decreases in plasma VLDL levels occurring over several months.
Distribution: 95% protein-bound.
Metabolism: Metabolized by the liver.
Excretion: Eliminated mostly in urine but some is excreted in feces. After a single dose, half-life is 1½ hours; after multiple doses, half-life decreases to about 1¼ hours.

Route	Onset	Peak	Duration
P.O.	2-5 days	4 wk	Unknown

Contraindications and precautions

Contraindicated in patients with hypersensitivity to drug, hepatic or severe renal dysfunction (including primary biliary cirrhosis), and preexisting gallbladder disease.

Interactions

Drug-drug. *Oral anticoagulants:* Enhanced effect of oral anticoagulants, increasing risk of hemorrhage. Adjust anticoagulant dose to maintain the desired PT and INR, and monitor frequently.
Lovastatin, simvastatin, pravastatin: Myopathy with rhabdomyolysis can occur. Avoid use together.

Effects on diagnostic tests

None reported.

Adverse reactions

CNS: headache, fatigue, vertigo.
CV: atrial fibrillation.
GI: abdominal and epigastric pain, diarrhea, nausea, vomiting, *dyspepsia,* constipation, acute appendicitis.
Hematologic: anemia, ***leukopenia,*** eosinophilia, ***thrombocytopenia.***
Hepatic: bile duct obstruction, elevated liver enzymes.
Metabolic: hypokalemia.
Skin: rash, dermatitis, pruritus, eczema.

Overdose and treatment

In overdose, immediately induce emesis or initiate gastric lavage.

Clinical considerations

- Because drug is pharmacologically related to clofibrate, adverse reactions associated with clofibrate may also occur with gemfibrozil. Some studies suggest clofibrate increases risk of death from cancer, postcholecystectomy complications, and pancreatitis. These hazards haven't been studied in gemfibrozil, however.
- Before initiating gemifibrozil therapy, aggressively attempt treatment through behavioral changes (diet and exercise) as well as identification and treatment of possible underlying causes of hyperlipoproteinemia.

Therapeutic monitoring

Recommend monitoring serum lipoprotein concentrations regularly; discontinue drug if a substantial lipid response isn't obtained.

Special populations

Breast-feeding patients. Safety in breast-feeding women hasn't been established.
Pediatric patients. Safety and efficacy in children under age 18 haven't been established.

Patient counseling

- Instruct patient to report adverse reactions promptly; and to comply with prescribed regimen, diet, and exercise.
- Warn patient not to exceed prescribed dose.

gentamicin sulfate

Cidomycin*, Garamycin, Genoptic, Genoptic S.O.P., Gentacidin, Gentak, Gentafair, Gentasol, Jenamicin

Pharmacologic classification: aminoglycoside
Therapeutic classification: antibiotic
Pregnancy risk category NR

How supplied

Available by prescription only
Injection: 40 mg/ml (adult), 10 mg/ml (pediatric), 2 mg/ml (intrathecal)
Ophthalmic ointment: 3 mg/g
Ophthalmic solution: 3 mg/ml
Topical cream or ointment: 0.1%

Indications and dosages

Serious infections caused by susceptible organisms
Adults with normal renal function: 3 mg/kg/day I.M. or I.V. infusion (in 50 to 100 ml of normal saline solution or D_5W infused over 30 minutes to 2 hours) daily in divided doses q 8 hours. May be given by direct I.V. push if necessary. For life-threatening infections, patient may receive up to 5 mg/kg/day in three to four divided doses.
Children with normal renal function: 2 to 2.5 mg/kg I.M. or I.V. infusion q 8 hours.
Infants and neonates over age 1 week with normal renal function: 2.5 mg/kg I.M. or I.V. infusion q 8 hours.
Neonates under age 1 week: 2.5 mg/kg I.M. or I.V. infusion q 12 hours. For I.V. infusion, dilute in normal saline solution or D_5W and infuse over 30 minutes to 2 hours.
Meningitis
Adults: Systemic therapy as above; may also use 4 to 8 mg intrathecally daily.
Children: Systemic therapy as above; may also use 1 to 2 mg intrathecally daily.
Endocarditis prophylaxis for GI or GU procedure or surgery
Adults: 1.5 mg/kg I.M. or I.V. 30 to 60 minutes before procedure or surgery and q 8 hours after, for two doses. Give separately with aqueous penicillin G or ampicillin.
Children: 2 mg/kg I.M. or I.V. 30 to 60 minutes before procedure or surgery and q 8 hours after, for two doses. Give separately with aqueous penicillin G or ampicillin.
External ocular infections caused by susceptible organisms
Adults and children: Instill 1 to 2 drops in eye q 4 hours. In severe infections, may use up to 2 drops q hour. Apply ointment to lower conjunctival sac b.i.d. or t.i.d.
Primary and secondary bacterial infections; superficial burns; skin ulcers; and infected lacerations, abrasions, insect bites, or minor surgical wounds
Adults and children over age 1: Rub in small amount gently t.i.d. or q.i.d., with or without gauze dressing.
Pelvic inflammatory disease
Adults: Initially, 2 mg/kg I.M. or I.V.; then 1.5 mg/kg q 8 hours.
≡***Dosage adjustment.*** In patients with renal failure, initial dose is same as for those with normal renal function. Subsequent doses and frequency determined by renal function studies and blood levels; keep peak serum levels between 4 and 10 mcg/ml and trough serum levels between 1 and 2 mcg/ml. One method is to administer 1-mg/kg doses and adjust the dosing interval based on steady-state serum creatinine, using the following formula:

$$\frac{\text{Creatinine}}{(\text{mg/100 ml})} \times 8 = \frac{\text{dosing interval}}{(\text{hours})}$$

Posthemodialysis to maintain therapeutic blood levels
Adults: 1 to 1.7 mg/kg I.M. or I.V. infusion after each dialysis.
Children: 2 to 2.5 mg/kg I.M. or I.V. infusion after each dialysis.

Pharmacodynamics

Antibiotic action: Gentamicin is bactericidal; it binds directly to the 30S ribosomal subunit, thus inhibiting bacterial protein synthesis. Its spectrum of activity includes many aerobic gram-negative organisms (including most strains of *Pseudomonas aeruginosa*) and some aerobic gram-positive organisms. Gentamicin may act against some bacterial strains resistant to other aminoglycosides; bacterial strains resistant to gentamicin may be susceptible to tobramycin, netilmicin, or amikacin.

Pharmacokinetics

Absorption: Absorbed poorly after oral administration.
Distribution: Distributed widely after parenteral administration; intraocular penetration is poor. CSF penetration is low even in patients with inflamed meninges. Intraventricular administration produces high levels throughout the CNS. Protein-binding is minimal. Gentamicin crosses the placenta.
Metabolism: Not metabolized.
Excretion: Excreted primarily in urine by glomerular filtration; small amounts may be excreted in bile and breast milk. Drug's elimination half-life in adults is 2 to 3 hours. In pa-

tients with severe renal damage, half-life may extend to 24 to 60 hours.

Route	Onset	Peak	Duration
I.V.	Immediate	30-90 min	Unknown
I.M.	Unknown	30-90 min	Unknown
Intrathecal	Unknown	Unknown	Unknown
Topical	Unknown	Unknown	Unknown
Ophthalmic	Unknown	Unknown	Unknown

Contraindications and precautions

Contraindicated in patients hypersensitive to drug or in those who may exhibit cross-sensitivity with other aminoglycosides such as neomycin.

Use systemic treatment cautiously in neonates, infants, the elderly, or in patients with renal or neuromuscular disorders.

Interactions

Drug-drug. *Dimenhydrinate, other antiemetic and antivertigo drugs:* May mask gentamicin-induced ototoxicity. Use with caution.
Ethacrynic acid, furosemide, bumetanide, urea, mannitol: Increased hazard of ototoxicity. Use cautiously.
General anesthetics or neuromuscular blocking agents, such as succinylcholine and tubocurarine): Increased neuromuscular blockade. Monitor patient closely.
Indomethacin: Increased serum peak and trough levels of gentamicin. Recommend monitoring serum gentamicin levels closely.
Methoxyflurane, polymyxin B, vancomycin, capreomycin, cisplatin, cephalosporins, amphotericin B, acyclovir, other aminoglycosides: May increase the hazard of nephrotoxicity, ototoxicity, or neurotoxicity. Use together cautiously.
Penicillin: Results in synergistic bactericidal effect against *P. aeruginosa, Escherichia coli, Klebsiella, Citrobacter, Enterobacter, Serratia,* and *Proteus mirabilis*; however, the drugs are physically and chemically incompatible and are inactivated when mixed or given together. Don't mix drugs together.

Effects on diagnostic tests

None reported.

Adverse reactions

CNS: headache, lethargy, encephalopathy, confusion, dizziness, ***seizures,*** numbness, peripheral neuropathy (with injected form).
CV: hypotension (with injected form).
EENT: *ototoxicity,* blurred vision (with injected form); burning, stinging, blurred vision (with ophthalmic ointment), transient irritation (with ophthalmic solution), conjunctival hyperemia (with ophthalmic form).
GI: vomiting, nausea (with injected form).
GU: *nephrotoxicity* (with injected form).
Hematologic: anemia, eosinophilia, ***leukopenia, thrombocytopenia, granulocytopenia*** (with injected form).
Musculoskeletal: muscle twitching, myasthenia gravis-like syndrome.
Respiratory: *apnea* (with injected form).
Skin: rash, urticaria, pruritus, tingling (with injected form); minor skin irritation, possible photosensitivity, allergic contact dermatitis (with topical administration).
Other: fever, ***anaphylaxis,*** pain at injection site (with injected form); ***hypersensitivity reactions,*** overgrowth of nonsusceptible organisms (with ophthalmic form and long-term use).

Note: Systemic absorption from excessive use may cause systemic toxicities.

Overdose and treatment

Signs of overdose include ototoxicity, nephrotoxicity, and neuromuscular toxicity. Drug can be removed by hemodialysis or peritoneal dialysis. Treatment with calcium salts or anticholinesterases reverses neuromuscular blockade.

Clinical considerations

Consider the recommendations relevant to all aminoglycosides as well as the following:

☐ ***ALERT*** Use preservative-free formulations when intrathecal route is ordered.

- Because drug is dialyzable, patients undergoing hemodialysis may need dosage adjustments.

Therapeutic monitoring

Increased risk of toxicity is associated with prolonged peak serum level of more than 10 mcg/ml and trough serum level of more than 2 mcg/ml.

Patient counseling

- Inform patient of the proper administration technique.
- Instruct patient to promptly report to prescriber if lesions worsen or skin irritation occurs.

glimepiride

Amaryl

Pharmacologic classification: sulfonylurea
Therapeutic classification: antidiabetic
Pregnancy risk category C

How supplied

Available by prescription only
Tablets: 1 mg, 2 mg, 4 mg

Indications and dosages

Adjunct to diet and exercise to lower blood glucose level in patients with non-insulin-dependent diabetes mellitus whose hyper-

glycemia can't be managed by diet and exercise alone
Adults: Initially, 1 to 2 mg P.O. once daily with first main meal of the day; usual maintenance dosage is 1 to 4 mg P.O. once daily. Maximum recommended dose is 8 mg once daily. After dose of 2 mg is reached, increase dosage in increments not exceeding 2 mg at 1- to 2-week intervals based on patient's blood glucose response.
Adjunct to insulin therapy in patients with non-insulin-dependent diabetes mellitus whose hyperglycemia can't be managed by diet and exercise in conjunction with an oral hypoglycemic agent
Adults: 8 mg P.O. once daily with first main meal of the day in combination with low-dose insulin. Upward adjustments of insulin should be done weekly as needed and guided by patient's blood glucose response.
Adjunct to metformin therapy in patients with type 2 (non-insulin-dependent) diabetes mellitus whose hyperglycemia can't be managed by diet, exercise, and glimepiride or metformin alone
Adults: 8 mg P.O. once daily with first main meal of the day, in combination with metformin if patient doesn't respond adequately to glimepiride monotherapy. Adjust dosages based on patient's blood glucose response to determine minimum effective dosage of each drug.
≡ ***Dosage adjustment.*** Patients with renal impairment require cautious dosing. Give 1 mg P.O. once daily with first main meal of the day, followed by appropriate dosage adjustment as necessary.

Pharmacodynamics
Antidiabetic action: Exact mechanism of glimepiride to lower blood glucose level appears to depend on stimulating the release of insulin from functioning pancreatic beta cells. Also, drug can lead to increased sensitivity of peripheral tissues to insulin.

Pharmacokinetics
Absorption: Completely absorbed from the GI tract.
Distribution: Protein binding is greater than 99.5%.
Metabolism: Completely metabolized by oxidative biotransformation.
Excretion: Metabolites are excreted in urine (about 60%) and feces (about 40%).

Route	Onset	Peak	Duration
P.O.	Unknown	2-3 hr	> 24 hr

Contraindications and precautions
Contraindicated in patients with hypersensitivity to drug and in those with diabetic ketoacidosis (with or without coma) because this condition should be treated with insulin. Use cautiously in debilitated or malnourished patients and in those with adrenal, pituitary, hepatic, or renal insufficiency because these patients are more susceptible to the hypoglycemic action of glucose-lowering drugs.

Interactions
Drug-drug. *Beta blockers:* May mask symptoms of hypoglycemia. Monitor patient carefully.
Insulin: Increased potential for hypoglycemia. May require dosage adjustment.
NSAIDs and other drugs that are highly protein-bound, such as salicylates, sulfonamides, chloramphenicol, coumarins, probenecid, MAO inhibitors and beta blockers: May potentiate the hypoglycemic action of sulfonylureas such as glimepiride. May require dosage adjustment.
Thiazides and other diuretics, estrogens, oral contraceptives, corticosteroids, phenothiazines, thyroid products, phenytoin, nicotinic acid, sympathomimetics, and isoniazid: Tend to produce hyperglycemia. May require dosage adjustment.
Drug-lifestyle. *Alcohol use:* Alters glycemic control, most commonly hypoglycemia. May also cause disulfiram-like reaction. Advise patient to avoid alcohol.

Effects on diagnostic tests
None reported.

Adverse reactions
CNS: dizziness, asthenia, headache.
EENT: changes in accommodation, blurred vision.
GI: vomiting, abdominal pain, nausea, diarrhea.
Hematologic: ***leukopenia,*** hemolytic anemia, ***agranulocytosis, thrombocytopenia, aplastic anemia, pancytopenia.***
Hepatic: cholestatic jaundice, elevated transaminase levels.
Metabolic: hypoglycemia.
Skin: allergic skin reactions (pruritus, erythema, urticaria, morbilliform or maculopapular eruptions).

Overdose and treatment
Overdose of sulfonylureas can produce hypoglycemia. Mild hypoglycemic symptoms without loss of consciousness or neurologic findings should be treated aggressively with oral glucose and adjustments in drug dosage and meal patterns. Monitor patient closely until he's out of danger. Severe hypoglycemic reactions with coma, seizure, or other neurologic impairment occur infrequently but constitute medical emergencies requiring immediate hospitalization. If hypoglycemic coma occurs or is suspected, give a rapid I.V. injection of concentrated (50%) glucose solution followed by continuous infusion of a more dilute (10%) glucose solution at a rate that will maintain the blood glucose at a level of

more than 100 mg/dl. Monitor patient closely for at least 24 to 48 hours because hypoglycemia may recur after apparent clinical recovery.

Clinical considerations

Consider the recommendations relevant to all sulfonylureas as well as the following:

- In geriatric, debilitated, or malnourished patients or in patients with renal or hepatic insufficiency, the initial dosing, dose increments, and maintenance dosage should be conservative to avoid hypoglycemic reactions.
- Oral hypoglycemic agents have been associated with an increased risk of CV mortality compared with diet or diet and insulin therapy.

Therapeutic monitoring

- Recommend monitoring fasting blood glucose level periodically to determine therapeutic response. Also recommend monitoring glycosylated hemoglobin, usually every 3 to 6 months, to more precisely assess long-term glycemic control.
- During maintenance therapy, discontinue glimepiride if satisfactory lowering of blood glucose level is no longer achieved. Secondary failures to glimepiride monotherapy can be treated with glimepiride-insulin combination therapy.

Special populations

Breast-feeding patients. It's unknown if drug is excreted in breast milk. Because of the potential for hypoglycemia in nursing infants, avoid giving drug to breast-feeding women.
Pediatric patients. Safety and efficacy in children haven't been established.
Geriatric patients. Geriatric patients may be more sensitive to the effects of drug because of reduced metabolism and elimination.

Patient counseling

- Instruct patient to take drug with first meal of the day.
- Make sure patient understands that therapy relieves symptoms but doesn't cure disease.
- Stress importance of adhering to specific diet, weight reduction, exercise, and personal hygiene programs. Explain how and when to perform self-monitoring of blood glucose level.
- Teach patient how to recognize and manage signs and symptoms of hyperglycemia and hypoglycemia.
- Advise patient to carry medical identification regarding diabetic status.

glipizide

Glucotrol, Glucotrol XL

Pharmacologic classification: sulfonylurea
Therapeutic classification: antidiabetic
Pregnancy risk category C

How supplied

Available by prescription only
Tablets: 5 mg, 10 mg
Tablets (extended-release): 5 mg, 10 mg

Indications and dosages

Adjunct to diet to lower blood glucose levels in patients with non-insulin-dependent diabetes mellitus
Adults: Initially, 5 mg P.O. daily 30 minutes before breakfast; adjust dose in increments of 2.5 to 5 mg. Usual maintenance dosage is 10 to 15 mg daily. Maximum recommended daily dose is 40 mg. Divide total daily doses of more than 15 mg except when using extended-release tablets.
≡***Dosage adjustment.*** Initial dosage in geriatric patients or those with hepatic disease may be 2.5 mg.
Extended-release tablets
Adults: Initially, 5 mg P.O. daily. May increase to 10 mg after 3 months based on glycosylated hemoglobin measurement. Subsequent dose adjustments should be based on glycosylated hemoglobin measurements at 3-month intervals. If no response after 3 months on higher dose, previous dose should be resumed. Maximum daily dose is 20 mg.
To replace insulin therapy
Adults: If insulin dose is more than 20 units daily, patient may be started at usual dose of glipizide plus 50% of insulin dosage. If insulin dose is less than 20 units, insulin may be discontinued.

Pharmacodynamics

Antidiabetic action: Glipizide decreases blood glucose levels by stimulating insulin release from functioning beta cells in the pancreas. After prolonged administration, the hypoglycemic effects of the drug appear to reflect extrapancreatic effects, possibly including reduction of basal hepatic glucose production and enhanced peripheral sensitivity to insulin.

Pharmacokinetics

Absorption: Absorbed rapidly and completely from the GI tract.
Distribution: Probably distributed within the extracellular fluid. It's about 92% to 99% protein-bound.
Metabolism: Metabolized almost completely by the liver to inactive metabolites.
Excretion: Excreted primarily in urine; small amounts are excreted in feces. Renal clearance

of unchanged glipizide increases with increasing urinary pH. Duration of action is 10 to 24 hours; half-life is 2 to 4 hours.

Route	Onset	Peak	Duration
P.O.	15-30 min	1-3 hr	4 hr
P.O. (extended-release)	2-3 hr	6-12 hr	24 hr

Contraindications and precautions

Contraindicated in patients with hypersensitivity to drug, diabetic ketoacidosis with or without coma, and during pregnancy or breast-feeding.

Use cautiously in patients with impaired renal or hepatic function and in geriatric, malnourished, or debilitated patients.

Interactions

Drug-drug. *Adrenocorticoids, glucocorticoids, amphetamines, baclofen, corticotropin, epinephrine, estrogens, ethacrynic acid, furosemide, oral contraceptives, phenytoin, thiazide diuretics, triamterene, thyroid hormones:* May increase glucose levels. Dosage adjustments may be required.
Anabolic steroids, chloramphenicol, clofibrate, guanethidine, insulin, MAO inhibitors, probenecid, salicylates, sulfonamides: Enhanced hypoglycemic effect by displacing glipizide from protein-binding sites. Monitor patient.
Anticoagulants: Increased plasma levels of both drugs and, after continued therapy, may reduce plasma levels and effectiveness of the anticoagulant. Monitor patient carefully.
Antifungal antibiotics such as miconazole, fluconazole: Increased plasma levels of glipizide and hypoglycemia. Monitor patient.
Beta blockers, including ophthalmics: May mask symptoms of hypoglycemia. Monitor and observe patient closely.
Cimetidine: Potentiates hypoglycemic effects by preventing hepatic metabolism. Monitor patient closely.
Corticosteroids, glucagon, rifampin, thiazide diuretics: May decrease hypoglycemic response. Monitor patient closely.
Hydantoins: Increased blood levels of hydantoins. Monitor blood levels.
Drug-lifestyle. *Alcohol use:* Altered glycemic control. May also cause a disulfiram-like reaction. Advise patient to avoid alcohol.
Smoking: Increased corticosteroid release, requiring higher dosages. Discourage smoking.

Effects on diagnostic tests

None reported.

Adverse reactions

CNS: *asthenia,* dizziness, drowsiness, headache, pain, tremor, nervousness, insomnia, anxiety, depression, hypesthesia, paresthesia.
GI: nausea, constipation, diarrhea, flatulence, dyspepsia, vomiting.
GU: altered BUN level.
Hematologic: ***leukopenia,*** hemolytic anemia, ***agranulocytosis, thrombocytopenia, aplastic anemia.***
Hepatic: cholestatic jaundice, altered liver enzymes.
Metabolic: altered cholesterol, ***hypoglycemia.***
Skin: rash, pruritus.

Overdose and treatment

Signs and symptoms include low blood glucose levels, tingling of lips and tongue, hunger, nausea, decreased cerebral function, increased sympathetic activity, and, ultimately, seizures, stupor, and coma.

Mild hypoglycemia responds to treatment with oral glucose and dosage adjustments. If patient loses consciousness or experiences other neurologic changes, he should receive a rapid injection of dextrose 50%, followed by continuous infusion of dextrose 10% at a rate to maintain blood glucose levels more than 100 mg/dl. Monitor for 24 to 48 hours.

Clinical considerations

Consider the recommendations relevant to all sulfonylureas as well as the following:

- To improve glucose control in patients who receive 15 mg/day or more, doses can be divided and given 30 minutes before the morning and evening meals.
- Some patients taking glipizide can be controlled on a once-daily regimen; others show better response with divided dosing.
- Drug has a mild diuretic effect that may be useful in patients with heart failure or cirrhosis.
- Patients who may be more sensitive to drug, such as elderly, debilitated, or malnourished individuals, should begin therapy with lower doses (2.5 mg once daily).
- Oral antidiabetic agents have been associated with an increased risk of CV mortality as compared with diet or diet and insulin therapy.

Therapeutic monitoring

- When substituting glipizide for chlorpropamide, monitor patient carefully during the first week because of the prolonged retention of chlorpropamide.
- Recommend monitoring blood glucose, urine glucose, ketone levels, and glycosylated hemoglobin.

Special populations

Pregnant patients. Use in pregnancy is usually not recommended. If glipizide must be used, manufacturer recommends that drug be discontinued at least 1 month before expected delivery to prevent neonatal hypoglycemia.
Pediatric patients. Safety and efficacy in children haven't been established.

Geriatric patients. Geriatric patients may be more sensitive to the effects of drug. Hypoglycemia causes more neurologic symptoms in geriatric patients.

Patient counseling

- Emphasize importance of following prescribed diet, exercise, and medical regimen.
- Tell patient that, if a dose is missed, it should be taken immediately, unless it's almost time to take the next dose. Patient shouldn't double the dose.
- Advise patient to avoid alcohol and products containing alcohol when taking glipizide.
- Suggest that drug be taken with food if glipizide causes GI upset.
- Provide patient with instruction on how to monitor blood glucose, urine glucose, and ketone levels, as prescribed.
- Teach patient how to recognize and manage the signs and symptoms of hyperglycemia and hypoglycemia.

glucagon

Pharmacologic classification: antihypoglycemic
Therapeutic classification: antihypoglycemic, diagnostic
Pregnancy risk category B

How supplied

Available by prescription only
Powder for injection: 1 mg (1 unit)/vial, 10 mg (10 units)/vial

Indications and dosages

Severe hypoglycemia
Adults and children weighing more than 44 lb (20 kg): 1 mg S.C., I.M., or I.V. May repeat dose after 15 minutes if patient fails to respond. When patient responds, give supplemental carbohydrates.
Children weighing less than 44 lb: 0.5 mg S.C., I.M., or I.V. Alternatively, 20 to 30 mcg/kg. May repeat dose after 15 minutes if patient fails to respond. When patient responds, give supplemental carbohydrates.
Diagnostic aid for radiographic examination of stomach, duodenum, and small intestine
Adults: 1 or 2 mg I.M. or 0.25 to 2 mg I.V. For relaxation of the stomach, use 0.5. mg I.V. or 2 mg I.M.

Pharmacodynamics

Antihypoglycemic action: Glucagon increases plasma glucose levels and causes smooth muscle relaxation and an inotropic myocardial effect because of the stimulation of adenylate cyclase to produce cAMP. cAMP initiates a series of reactions that leads to the degradation of glycogen to glucose. Hepatic stores of glycogen are necessary for glucagon to exert an antihypoglycemic effect.
Diagnostic action: The mechanism by which glucagon relaxes the smooth muscles of the GI tract hasn't been fully defined.

Pharmacokinetics

Absorption: Glucagon is destroyed in the GI tract; therefore, it must be given parenterally. Administration to comatose hypoglycemic patients (with normal liver glycogen stores) usually produces a return to consciousness within 20 minutes.
Distribution: Not fully understood.
Metabolism: Degraded extensively by the liver, in the kidneys and plasma, and at its tissue receptor sites in plasma membranes.
Excretion: Metabolic products are excreted by the kidneys. Half-life is about 3 to 10 minutes.

Route	Onset	Peak	Duration
I.V.	Immediate	½ hr	60-90 min
I.M., S.C.	Unknown	Unknown	Unknown

Contraindications and precautions

Contraindicated in patients with pheochromocytoma or hypersensitivity to drug. Use cautiously in patients with insulinoma.

Interactions

Drug-drug. *Epinephrine:* Increases and prolongs the hyperglycemic effect. Recommend monitoring blood glucose levels.
Phenytoin: Appears to inhibit glucagon-induced insulin release. Use with caution as a diagnostic agent in patients with diabetes mellitus.

Effects on diagnostic tests

None reported.

Adverse reactions

CV: hypotension.
GI: nausea, vomiting.
Metabolic: hypokalemia.
Respiratory: respiratory distress.
Other: ***hypersensitivity reactions*** (***bronchospasm,*** rash, dizziness, light-headedness).

Overdose and treatment

Signs and symptoms of overdose include nausea, vomiting, and hypokalemia. Treat symptomatically.

Clinical considerations

- Glucagon should be used only under direct medical supervision.
- For I.V. drip infusion, glucagon is compatible with dextrose solution but forms a precipitate in chloride solutions.
- Glucagon has a positive inotropic and chronotropic action on the heart and may be used to treat overdose of beta blockers.

- Mixed solutions with diluent are stable for 48 hours when stored at 41° F (5° C). Following reconstitution with sterile water, use immediately. Discard unused portion.

Therapeutic monitoring
If patient experiences nausea and vomiting from glucagon administration and can't retain some form of sugar for 1 hour, consider administration of I.V. dextrose.

Special populations
Breast-feeding patients. It's unknown if drug is excreted in breast milk.
Pediatric patients. Glucagon has been used safely and effectively for the treatment of hypoglycemia in children. Safety and efficacy in diagnostic procedures haven't been established.

Patient counseling
- Provide patient with instructions on how to mix and inject medication properly.
- Tell patient to expect response usually within 20 minutes after injection.

glyburide
DiaBeta, Glynase PresTab, Micronase

Pharmacologic classification: sulfonylurea
Therapeutic classification: antidiabetic
Pregnancy risk category C

How supplied
Available by prescription only
Tablets: 1.25 mg, 2.5 mg, 5 mg
Tablets (micronized): 1.5 mg, 3 mg, 6 mg

Indications and dosages
Adjunct to diet to lower blood glucose levels in patients with non-insulin-dependent diabetes mellitus
Adults: Initially, 2.5 to 5 mg P.O. daily with breakfast. Start patients who are more sensitive to hypoglycemic drugs at 1.25 mg daily. Usual maintenance dosage is 1.25 to 20 mg daily, either as a single dose or in divided doses.

For micronized tablets, initially give 1.5 to 3 mg P.O. with breakfast. Usual maintenance dosage is 0.75 to 12 mg P.O. daily.
≡ ***Dosage adjustment.*** In geriatric, debilitated, or malnourished patients or those with renal or liver dysfunction, start therapy with 1.25 mg once daily.
To replace insulin therapy
Adults: If insulin dose is more than 40 units/day, patient may be started on 5 mg of glyburide daily plus 50% of the insulin dose. Patients maintained on less than 20 units/day should receive 2.5 to 5 mg/day; those maintained on 20 to 40 units/day should receive 5 mg/day. In all patients, glyburide is substituted and insulin discontinued abruptly.

For micronized tablets, if insulin dose is more than 40 units/day, give 3 mg P.O. with a 50% reduction in insulin. Patients maintained on 20 to 40 units/day should receive 3 mg P.O. as a single daily dose; those maintained on less than 20 units/day should receive 1.5 to 3 mg/day as a single dose.

Pharmacodynamics
Antidiabetic action: Glyburide decreases blood glucose levels by stimulating insulin release from functioning beta cells in the pancreas. After prolonged administration, the hypoglycemic effects of the drug appear to be related to extrapancreatic effects, possibly including reduction of basal hepatic glucose production and enhanced peripheral sensitivity to insulin. The latter may result either from an increase in the number of insulin receptors or from changes in events subsequent to insulin binding.

Pharmacokinetics
Absorption: Almost completely absorbed from GI tract. A micronized tablet results in significant absorption; a 3-mg micronized tablet provides blood levels similar to a 5-mg conventional tablet.
Distribution: 99% protein-bound. Its distribution isn't fully understood.
Metabolism: Metabolized completely by the liver to inactive metabolites.
Excretion: Excreted as metabolites in urine and feces in equal proportions. Its duration of action is 24 hours; its half-life is 10 hours.

Route	Onset	Peak	Duration
P.O.	1-4 hr	4 hr	24 hr

Contraindications and precautions
Contraindicated in patients with hypersensitivity to drug or diabetic ketoacidosis with or without coma, and during pregnancy or breastfeeding. Use cautiously in patients with impaired renal or hepatic function and in geriatric, malnourished, or debilitated patients.

Interactions
Drug-drug. *Adrenocorticoids, diazoxide, glucocorticoids, amphetamines, baclofen, corticotropin, epinephrine, ethacrynic acid, furosemide, glucagon, phenytoin, rifampin, thiazide diuretics, triamterene, thyroid hormones:* Increased blood glucose levels. Dosage adjustments may be required.
Anabolic steroids, chloramphenicol, clofibrate, guanethidine, insulin, MAO inhibitors, probenecid, salicylates, sulfonamides: Enhanced hypoglycemic effect by displacing glyburide from its protein-binding sites. Recommend monitoring glucose levels; monitor patient carefully.

Anticoagulants: May increase plasma levels of both drugs and, after continued therapy, may reduce plasma levels and anticoagulant effect. Recommend monitoring blood glucose and PT.
Beta blockers, including ophthalmics: Increased risk of hypoglycemia. Use together cautiously.
Hydantoins: May increase blood levels of hydantoins. Recommend monitoring blood levels.
Drug-lifestyle. *Alcohol use:* Altered glycemic control, most commonly hypoglycemia. May also cause a disulfiram-like reaction consisting of nausea, vomiting, abdominal cramps, and headaches. Discourage use together.
Smoking: May increase corticosteroid release; patients who smoke may require higher dosages of glipizide. Advise patient to stop smoking.

Effects on diagnostic tests

Glyburide therapy alters cholesterol, alkaline phosphatase, and BUN levels.

Adverse reactions

EENT: changes in accommodation or blurred vision.
GI: nausea, epigastric fullness, heartburn.
GU: altered BUN levels.
Hematologic: ***leukopenia,*** hemolytic anemia, ***agranulocytosis, thrombocytopenia, aplastic anemia.***
Hepatic: cholestatic jaundice, ***hepatitis,*** abnormal liver function.
Metabolic: altered cholesterol level, ***hypoglycemia.***
Musculoskeletal: arthralgia, myalgia.
Skin: rash, pruritus, other allergic reactions.
Other: ***angioedema.***

Overdose and treatment

Signs and symptoms of overdose include low blood glucose levels, tingling of lips and tongue, hunger, nausea, decreased cerebral function (lethargy, yawning, confusion, agitation, and nervousness), increased sympathetic activity (tachycardia, sweating, and tremor) and, ultimately, seizures, stupor, and coma.

Mild hypoglycemia, without loss of consciousness or neurologic findings, responds to treatment with oral glucose and dosage adjustments. Patient with severe hypoglycemia should be hospitalized immediately. If hypoglycemic coma is suspected, the patient should receive rapid injection of dextrose 50%, followed by a continuous infusion of dextrose 10% at a rate to maintain blood glucose levels greater than 100 mg/dl. Monitor for 24 to 48 hours.

Clinical considerations

Consider the recommendations relevant to all sulfonylureas as well as the following:

- To improve control in patients receiving 10 mg/day or more, divided doses, usually given before the morning and evening meals, are recommended.
- Some patients taking glyburide may be controlled effectively on a once-daily regimen, whereas others show better response with divided dosing.
- Glyburide is a second-generation sulfonylurea oral antidiabetic agent. It appears to cause fewer adverse reactions than first-generation drugs.
- Drug has a mild diuretic effect that may be useful in patients with chronic heart failure or cirrhosis.
- Oral antidiabetic agents have been associated with an increased risk of CV mortality compared with diet or diet and insulin therapy.

Therapeutic monitoring

- When substituting glyburide for chlorpropamide, monitor patient closely during the first week because of the prolonged retention of chlorpropamide in the body.
- Recommend monitoring blood glucose, urine glucose, and ketone levels.

Special populations

Pediatric patients. Glyburide is ineffective in insulin-dependent (type 1, juvenile-onset) diabetes. Safety and efficacy in children haven't been established.
Geriatric patients. Geriatric patients may be more sensitive to effects of drug because of reduced metabolism and elimination. Hypoglycemia causes more neurologic symptoms in geriatric patients.

Patient counseling

- Emphasize importance of following prescribed diet, exercise, and medical regimen.
- Advise patient to avoid alcohol and alcohol-containing products while taking glyburide.
- Suggest drug be taken with food if GI upset occurs.
- Provide patient with instruction on how to monitor blood glucose, urine glucose, and ketone levels.
- Inform patient of the signs and symptoms of hyperglycemia and hypoglycemia and what to do if they occur.

glycopyrrolate

Robinul, Robinul Forte

Pharmacologic classification: anticholinergic
Therapeutic classification: antimuscarinic, GI antispasmodic
Pregnancy risk category B

How supplied

Available by prescription only
Tablets: 1 mg, 2 mg
Injection: 0.2 mg/ml in 1-ml, 2-ml, 5-ml, 20-ml vials

Indications and dosages

Blockade of cholinergic effects of anticholinesterase drugs used to reverse neuromuscular blockade
Adults and children: 0.2 mg I.V. for each 1 mg neostigmine or 5 mg of pyridostigmine. May be given I.V. without dilution or may be added to dextrose injection and infused.
Preoperatively to diminish secretions and block cardiac vagal reflexes
Adults and children over age 2: 0.0044 mg/kg of body weight given I.M. 30 to 60 minutes before anesthesia.
Adjunctive therapy in peptic ulcers and other GI disorders
Adults: 1 to 2 mg P.O. t.i.d. or 0.1 mg I.M. t.i.d. or q.i.d. Dosage should be individualized.

Pharmacodynamics

Anticholinergic action: Glycopyrrolate inhibits muscarinic actions of acetylcholine on autonomic effectors innervated by postganglionic cholinergic nerves. That action blocks adverse muscarinic effects associated with anticholinesterase agents used to reverse curariform-induced neuromuscular blockade. Glycopyrrolate decreases secretions and GI motility by the same mechanism. Glycopyrrolate blocks cardiac vagal reflexes by blocking vagal inhibition of the SA node.

Pharmacokinetics

Absorption: Poorly absorbed from GI tract (10% to 25%) after oral administration.
Distribution: Rapidly distributed. Because it's a quaternary amine, it doesn't cross the blood-brain barrier or enter the CNS.
Metabolism: Exact metabolic fate is unknown.
Excretion: Small amount of drug is eliminated in the urine as unchanged drug and metabolites. Drug is mostly excreted unchanged in feces or bile.

Route	Onset	Peak	Duration
P.O.	Unknown	Unknown	8-12 hr
I.V.	1 min	Unknown	3-7 hr
I.M., S.C.	15-30 min	30-45 min	3-7 hr

Contraindications and precautions

Contraindicated in patients with hypersensitivity to drug and in those with glaucoma, obstructive uropathy, obstructive disease of the GI tract, myasthenia gravis, paralytic ileus, intestinal atony, unstable CV status in acute hemorrhage, severe ulcerative colitis, or toxic megacolon.

Use cautiously in patients with autonomic neuropathy, hyperthyroidism, coronary artery disease, arrhythmias, heart failure, hypertension, hiatal hernia, hepatic or renal disease, and ulcerative colitis. Also use with caution in hot or humid conditions where drug-induced heatstroke may occur.

Interactions

Drug-drug. *Amantadine, antihistamines, antiparkinsonian agents, disopyramide, glutethimide, meperidine, phenothiazines, procainamide, quinidine, tricyclic antidepressants:* Additive adverse effects. Avoid use together.
Antacids: Decrease oral absorption of anticholinergics. Give glycopyrrolate at least 1 hour before antacids.
Slowly dissolving digoxin tablets: May yield higher serum digoxin levels when administered with anticholinergics. Use cautiously; dose adjustment may be needed.
Levodopa, ketoconazole: Decreased GI absorption. Separate administration times by 2 to 3 hours.
Oral potassium supplements, especially wax-matrix formulations: Increased incidence of potassium-induced GI ulcerations. Use cautiously.

Effects on diagnostic tests

None reported.

Adverse reactions

CNS: weakness, nervousness, insomnia, drowsiness, dizziness, headache, confusion or excitement (in elderly patients).
CV: palpitations, tachycardia.
EENT: *dilated pupils, blurred vision,* photophobia, increased intraocular pressure.
GI: *constipation, dry mouth,* nausea, loss of taste, abdominal distension, vomiting, epigastric distress.
GU: *urinary hesitancy, urine retention,* impotence.
Skin: urticaria, decreased sweating or anhidrosis, other dermal manifestations.
Other: allergic reactions ***(anaphylaxis),*** fever.

Overdose and treatment

Clinical effects of overdose include such peripheral effects as dilated, nonreactive pupils; blurred vision; flushed, hot, dry skin; dryness of mucous membranes; dysphagia; decreased or absent bowel sounds; urine retention; hyperthermia; tachycardia; hypertension; and increased respiration.

Treatment is primarily symptomatic and supportive, as needed. If patient is alert, induce emesis (or use gastric lavage) and follow with a saline cathartic and activated charcoal to prevent further drug absorption. In severe life-threatening cases, physostigmine may be administered to block antimuscarinic effects of glycopyrrolate. Give fluids, as needed, to treat shock. If urine retention occurs, catheterization may be necessary.

Clinical considerations

Consider the recommendations relevant to all anticholinergics as well as the following:

- Even slight overdose can lead to toxicity.
- For immediate treatment of bradycardia, some clinicians prefer atropine over glycopyrrolate.
- Don't mix glycopyrrolate with I.V. solutions containing sodium chloride or bicarbonate.
- Drug may be administered with neostigmine or physostigmine in same syringe.
- Drug is incompatible with thiopental, methohexital, secobarbital, pentobarbital, chloramphenicol, dimenhydrinate, and diazepam.

Therapeutic monitoring

- Monitor patient closely for toxicity.
- Monitor patient for CNS effects and for urinary hesitancy or urine retention.

Special populations

Breast-feeding patients. Drug may be excreted in breast milk, possibly resulting in infant toxicity. Breast-feeding women should avoid this drug, which may decrease milk production.
Pediatric patients. Drug not recommended for peptic ulcer in children under age 12. Manufacturer recommends that drug not be used in neonates under age 1 month because glycopyrrolate injection contains benzyl alcohol.
Geriatric patients. Administer glycopyrrolate cautiously to geriatric patients. However, glycopyrrolate may be the preferred anticholinergic in geriatric patients.

Patient counseling

- Instruct patient to take oral drug 30 to 60 minutes before meals.
- Warn patient to avoid activities that require alertness until CNS effects of drug are known.
- Advise patient to contact prescriber to report signs of urinary hesitancy or urine retention.

gold sodium thiomalate

Aurolate

Pharmacologic classification: gold salt
Therapeutic classification: antiarthritic
Pregnancy risk category C

How supplied

Available by prescription only
Injection: 50 mg/ml with benzyl alcohol

Indications and dosages

Rheumatoid arthritis, ◇psoriatic arthritis, ◇Felty's syndrome
Adults: Initially, 10 mg I.M.; then 25 mg in second week and continue for a third dose the following week. Continue until 1 g (cumulative) has been given, unless toxicity occurs. If improvement occurs without toxicity before initial 1-g dose, a maintenance dosage of 25 to 50 mg every other week for 2 to 20 weeks may be started. Then continue to every third then every fourth week indefinitely. Weekly injections may be restarted anytime, if necessary. If patient doesn't respond after reaching initial 1-g dose, then discontinue therapy, or give 25 to 50 mg I.M. for an additional 10 weeks, or increase dose by 10 mg q 1 to 4 weeks (maximum dose per injection is 100 mg).
Children: Initiate therapy with 10-mg test dose, then give 1 mg/kg weekly. Continue dosage and administration as listed for adults. Maximum single dose for children under age 12 is 50 mg.
◇Palindromic rheumatism
Adults: Initially, 10 to 15 mg I.M. weekly until dose of 1 g is reached.
◇Pemphigus
Adults: Initially, 10 mg I.M.; then 25 mg I.M. for second week, then 50 mg I.M. weekly. When patient is off corticosteroid therapy, maintenance dosage of 25 to 50 mg I.M. q 2 weeks may be administered.

Pharmacodynamics

Antiarthritic action: Gold sodium thiomalate is thought to be effective against rheumatoid arthritis by altering the immune system to reduce inflammation. Although the exact mechanism of action remains unknown, these compounds have reduced serum levels of immunoglobulins and rheumatoid factors in patients with arthritis.

Pharmacokinetics

Absorption: Absorption is rapid.
Distribution: Higher tissue levels occur with parenteral gold salts, with a mean steady-state plasma level of 1 to 5 mcg/ml. Drug is distributed widely throughout the body in lymph nodes, bone marrow, kidneys, liver, spleen, and tissues. About 85% to 90% is protein-bound.
Metabolism: Not broken down into its elemental form. The half-life with cumulative dosing is 14 to 40 days.
Excretion: About 70% is excreted in the urine, 30% in feces.

Route	Onset	Peak	Duration
I.M.	Unknown	3-6 hr	Unknown

Contraindications and precautions

Contraindicated in patients with hypersensitivity to drug; in those with history of severe toxicity from previous exposure to gold or heavy metals, hepatitis, or exfoliative dermatitis; and in patients with severe uncontrollable diabetes, renal disease, hepatic dysfunction, uncontrolled heart failure, systemic lupus erythematosus, colitis, or Sjögren's syndrome. Also contraindicated in patients with urticaria, eczema, hemorrhagic conditions, or severe hematologic disorders and in those who have recently received radiation therapy.

Use with extreme caution in patients with rash, marked hypertension, compromised cerebral or CV function, or history of renal or hepatic disease, drug allergies, or blood dyscrasias.

Interactions

Drug-drug. *Other drugs known to cause blood dyscrasias:* Additive risk of hematologic toxicity. Avoid use together.
Drug-lifestyle. *Sun or ultraviolet light exposure:* May cause photosensitivity reactions. Advise patient to use precautions.

Effects on diagnostic tests

Serum protein-bound iodine test, especially when done by the chloric acid digestion method, gives false readings during and for several weeks after gold therapy.

Adverse reactions

Adverse reactions to gold are considered severe and potentially life-threatening.
CNS: confusion, hallucinations, ***seizures.***
CV: *bradycardia*, hypotension.
EENT: corneal gold deposition, corneal ulcers.
GI: *metallic taste, stomatitis, diarrhea,* anorexia, abdominal cramps, nausea, vomiting, ulcerative enterocolitis.
GU: albuminuria, proteinuria, *nephrotic syndrome,* nephritis, acute tubular necrosis, hematuria, ***acute renal failure.***
Hematologic: ***thrombocytopenia*** (with or without purpura), ***aplastic anemia, agranulocytosis, leukopenia,*** eosinophilia, anemia.
Hepatic: ***hepatitis,*** jaundice, elevated liver function tests.
Skin: diaphoresis, photosensitivity, *rash, dermatitis,* erythema, exfoliative dermatitis.
Other: ***anaphylaxis, angioedema.***

Overdose and treatment

When severe reactions to gold occur, corticosteroids, dimercaprol (a chelating agent), or penicillamine may be given to aid in the recovery. Prednisone 40 to 100 mg/day in divided doses is recommended to manage severe renal, hematologic, pulmonary, or enterocolitic reactions to gold. Dimercaprol may be used together with corticosteroids to facilitate the removal of the gold when the corticosteroid treatment alone is ineffective.

Clinical considerations

- Administer all gold salts I.M., preferably intragluteally. Normal color of drug is pale yellow; don't use if it darkens.
- Patient should remain recumbent for 10 to 20 minutes and remain under medical observation for 30 minutes after administration because of possible anaphylactic reaction.
- Vasomotor adverse effects are more common with gold sodium thiomalate than with other gold salts.

Therapeutic monitoring

- Obtain patient's urine for analysis for protein and sediment changes before each injection.
- Recommend monitoring patient's CBC and platelet count monthly or before every other injection. Stop drug if platelet count decreases to less than 100,000/mm^3.
- Most adverse reactions are readily reversible if drug is discontinued immediately.
- If adverse reactions are mild, some rheumatologists order resumption of gold therapy after 2 to 3 weeks' rest.

Special populations

Breast-feeding patients. Drug isn't recommended for use in breast-feeding women.
Pediatric patients. Use in children under age 6 isn't recommended.
Geriatric patients. Administer usual adult dose. Use cautiously in patients with decreased renal function.

Patient counseling

- Inform patient that beneficial drug effect may be delayed for 3 months.
- Explain that vasomotor adverse reactions—faintness, weakness, dizziness, flushing, nausea, vomiting, diaphoresis—may occur immediately after injection. Advise patient to lie down until symptoms subside.
- Tell patient that stomatitis is often preceded by a metallic taste; this symptom must be reported to prescriber immediately.
- Advise patient to report rash or other skin problems to prescriber immediately.

gonadorelin acetate

Lutrepulse

Pharmacologic classification: gonadotropin-releasing hormone (GnRH)
Therapeutic classification: fertility
Pregnancy risk category B

How supplied

Available by prescription only
Injection: 0.8 mg/10 ml, 3.2 mg/10 ml, in 10-ml vials
Supplied as a kit with I.V. supplies and portable infusion pump

Indications and dosages

To induce ovulation in women with primary hypothalamic amenorrhea

Adults: 5 mcg I.V. q 90 minutes (using a Lutrepulse pump, 0.8 mg solution at 50 microliters/pulse) for 21 days. If no response after three treatment intervals, dosage may be increased. Usual dose is 1 to 20 mcg.

Pharmacodynamics

Ovulation-stimulating action: Mimics the action of GnRH, which results in the synthesis and release of luteinizing hormone (LH) from the anterior pituitary. LH subsequently acts on the reproductive organs to regulate hormone synthesis.

Pharmacokinetics

Absorption: Administered I.V. using a portable pump designed to administer the drug in a pulsatile fashion to mimic the endogenous hormone.

Distribution: Low plasma volume of distribution (10 to 15 L) and high rate of clearance from plasma.

Metabolism: Rapidly metabolized. Several biologically inactive peptide fragments have been identified.

Excretion: Excreted primarily in urine. The high initial clearance rate (half-life of 2 to 10 minutes) is followed by a somewhat slower terminal half-life of 10 to 40 minutes.

Route	Onset	Peak	Duration
I.V.	Unknown	Unknown	10-40 min

Contraindications and precautions

Contraindicated in patients hypersensitive to drug, in women with conditions that could be complicated by pregnancy (such as prolactinoma), in those who are anovulatory from any cause other than a hypothalamic disorder, and in those with ovarian cysts.

Interactions

Drug-drug. *Ovary-stimulating drugs:* Risk of ovarian hyperstimulation. Avoid use together.

Effects on diagnostic tests

None reported.

Adverse reactions

GU: multiple pregnancy, ovarian hyperstimulation.

Skin: hematoma, local infection, inflammation, mild phlebitis.

Overdose and treatment

No harmful effects are expected if the pump were to malfunction and deliver the entire contents of the highest concentration vial (3.2 mg). Bolus doses of up to 3,000 mcg haven't proven harmful in clinical trials; however, continuous exposure (nonpulsatile administration) to gonadorelin may temporarily reduce pituitary responsiveness.

Clinical considerations

To mimic the action of the naturally occurring hormone, gonadorelin requires a pulsatile administration with a special portable infusion pump. The pulse period is set at 1 minute (drug is infused over 1 minute); pulse interval is set at 90 minutes.

Therapeutic monitoring

- Close monitoring of dosage and ultrasonography of the ovaries are necessary to monitor drug response. Patients usually require pelvic ultrasound on days 7 and 14 after establishment of a baseline scan, although the interval between scans may be shortened.
- Regular pelvic examinations and midluteal phase serum progesterone determinations are necessary.
- Similar drugs have caused anaphylaxis; monitor patients for signs and symptoms of anaphylaxis.

Special populations

Breast-feeding patients. It's unknown if drug is excreted in breast milk; however, there's no reason to administer drug to a breast-feeding woman.

Pediatric patients. Safety and efficacy in patients under age 18 haven't been established.

Patient counseling

- Inform patient of the signs and symptoms of hypersensitivity reactions (hives, wheezing, difficulty breathing) and instruct her to report them immediately.
- Stress that a multiple pregnancy is possible (incidence about 12%).

goserelin acetate

Zoladex, Zoladex 3-month

Pharmacologic classification: synthetic decapeptide
Therapeutic classification: luteinizing hormone-releasing hormone (LHRH; GnRH) analogue
Pregnancy risk category X (10.8-mg implant); D (3.6-mg implant)

How supplied

Available by prescription only
Implant: 3.6 mg, 10.8 mg

Indications and dosages

Palliative treatment of advanced carcinoma of the prostate, endometriosis, advanced breast carcinoma

Adults: 1 (3.6 mg) implant S.C. q 28 days into the upper abdominal wall for 6 months. Treat-

ment of endometriosis shouldn't exceed 6 months.
Palliative treatment of advanced carcinoma of the prostate
Men: 1 (10.8 mg) implant S.C. q 12 weeks into the upper abdominal wall.

Pharmacodynamics
Hormonal action: Chronic administration of goserelin, an LHRH, acts on the pituitary to decrease the release of follicle-stimulating hormone (FSH) and luteinizing hormone. In men, the result is dramatically decreased serum levels of testosterone.

Pharmacokinetics
Absorption: Slowly absorbed from implant site.
Distribution: Administration of the implant results in measurable levels of drug in serum throughout the dosing period.
Metabolism: Clearance of goserelin following S.C. administration of the drug is rapid and occurs via a combination of hepatic metabolism and urinary excretion.
Excretion: Elimination half-life is about 4¼ hours in patients with normal renal function. Substantial renal impairment prolongs half-life, but this doesn't appear to increase the incidence of adverse effects.

Route	Onset	Peak	Duration
S.C.	Unknown	12-15 days	Unknown

Contraindications and precautions
Contraindicated in patients with hypersensitivity to LHRH, LHRH agonist analogues, or goserelin acetate. Also contraindicated during pregnancy or in breast-feeding women. The 10.8-mg implant is contraindicated for use in women.

Use cautiously in patients at risk for osteoporosis, chronic alcohol or tobacco abuse, or use of anticonvulsants or corticosteroids.

Interactions
None reported.

Effects on diagnostic tests
None reported.

Adverse reactions
CNS: lethargy, pain (worsened in the first 30 days), dizziness, *insomnia, asthenia,* anxiety, *depression, headache,* chills, *emotional lability.*
CV: edema, ***heart failure, arrhythmias,*** *peripheral edema,* ***CVA,*** hypertension, ***MI,*** peripheral vascular disorder, chest pain.
GI: nausea, vomiting, diarrhea, constipation, ulcer, anorexia, abdominal pain.
GU: *impotence, sexual dysfunction, lower urinary tract symptoms,* renal insufficiency, urinary obstruction, *vaginitis,* urinary tract infection, amenorrhea, increased serum testosterone levels during the first week of therapy.
Hematologic: anemia.
Metabolic: increased serum acid phosphatase initially (will decrease by week 4), hyperglycemia, weight increase.
Musculoskeletal: gout, back pain.
Respiratory: COPD, upper respiratory infection.
Skin: rash, *diaphoresis, acne, seborrhea,* hirsutism.
Other: *changes in libido, hot flashes, infection,* breast swelling and tenderness, *changes in breast size,* breast pain.

Overdose and treatment
No information is available regarding accidental or intentional overdose. In animal studies, doses up to 1 mg/kg/day didn't produce non-endocrine-related symptoms.

Clinical considerations
- Give drug every 28 days for the 3.6-mg implant and every 12 weeks for the 10.8-mg implant, always under direct medical supervision. Local anesthesia may be used before injection.
- In the unlikely event of the need to surgically remove goserelin, it may be localized by ultrasound.

Therapeutic monitoring
- Monitor for adverse reactions.
- Recommend monitoring drug serum levels.

Special populations
Breast-feeding patients. It's unknown if drug is excreted in breast milk.
Pediatric patients. Safety and efficacy in children under age 18 haven't been established.

Patient counseling
- Advise patient to report on time for each new implant.
- Advise patient to immediately report to prescriber any implant-site reactions or other adverse reactions.

granisetron hydrochloride
Kytril

Pharmacologic classification: selective 5-hydroxytryptamine (5-HT_3) receptor antagonist
Therapeutic classification: antiemetic, antinausea
Pregnancy risk category B

How supplied
Available by prescription only
Tablets: 1 mg
Injection: 1 mg/ml

Indications and dosages
Prevention of nausea and vomiting associated with emetogenic cancer chemotherapy
Adults and children age 2 to 16: 10 mcg/kg I.V. infused over 5 minutes. Begin infusion within 30 minutes before administration of chemotherapy.
Oral form
Adults: 1 mg P.O. b.i.d. Give the first 1-mg tablet 1 hour before chemotherapy administration and the second tablet 12 hours after the first. Give only on days when chemotherapy is given. Continued treatment while not on chemotherapy hasn't been found to be useful.

Pharmacodynamics
Antiemetic action: Granisetron as a selective 5-hydroxytryptamine (5-HT_3) receptor antagonist is thought to bind to serotonin receptors of the 5-HT_3 type located peripherally on vagal nerve terminals and centrally in the chemoreceptor trigger zone of the area postrema. This binding blocks serotonin stimulation and subsequent vomiting after emetogenic stimuli, such as cisplatin.

Pharmacokinetics
Absorption: Not determined.
Distribution: Distributed freely between plasma and RBCs. Plasma protein-binding is about 65%.
Metabolism: Metabolized by the liver, possibly mediated by the cytochrome P-450 3A subfamily.
Excretion: About 12% is eliminated unchanged in the urine in 48 hours; the remainder is excreted as metabolites: 48% in the urine and 38% in the feces.

Route	Onset	Peak	Duration
P.O., I.V.	Unknown	Unknown	Unknown

Contraindications and precautions
Contraindicated in patients hypersensitive to drug.

Interactions
Drug-herb. *Horehound:* Enhanced serotonergic effects. Avoid use together.

Effects on diagnostic tests
None reported.

Adverse reactions
CNS: *headache, asthenia,* somnolence, dizziness, anxiety.
CV: hypertension.
GI: diarrhea, *constipation,* abdominal pain, *nausea,* vomiting, decreased appetite.
Hematologic: *leukopenia,* anemia, ***thrombocytopenia.***
Hepatic: elevated liver function tests.
Skin: alopecia.
Other: fever.

Overdose and treatment
No antidote for overdose exists. Give symptomatic treatment. Overdose of up to 38.5 mg of granisetron has been reported without symptoms or only the occurrence of a slight headache.

Clinical considerations
- Don't mix with other drugs; information about compatibility is limited.
- Diluted solutions are stable for 24 hours at room temperature.
- No dosage adjustment is recommended for patients with renal impairment or hepatic disease.

Therapeutic monitoring
Monitor for decreased symptoms and for any increase in nausea or abdominal pain.

Special populations
Breast-feeding patients. It's unknown if drug is excreted in breast milk.
Pediatric patients. Safety and efficacy in children under age 2 haven't been established. Safety and efficacy in children haven't been established for the oral form.

Patient counseling
Tell patient to watch for signs of an anaphylactoid reaction—local or generalized hives, chest tightness, wheezing, and dizziness or weakness—and to report them immediately.

griseofulvin microsize
Fulvicin-U/F, Grifulvin V, Grisactin

griseofulvin ultramicrosize
Fulvicin P/G, Grisactin Ultra, Gris-PEG

Pharmacologic classification: penicillium antibiotic
Therapeutic classification: antifungal
Pregnancy risk category C

How supplied
Available by prescription only
Microsize
Capsules: 250 mg
Tablets: 250 mg, 500 mg
Oral suspension: 125 mg/5 ml
Ultramicrosize
Tablets: 125 mg, 165 mg, 250 mg, 330 mg
Tablets (film-coated): 125 mg, 250 mg

Indications and dosages
Tinea corporis, tinea capitis, tinea barbae, or tinea cruris infections
Adults: 330 mg ultramicrosize P.O. daily, or 500 mg microsize P.O. daily.

Children weighing 30 to 50 lb (14 to 23 kg): 82.5 to 165 mg ultramicrosize P.O. daily, or 125 to 250 mg microsize P.O. daily.
Children weighing more than 50 lb: 165 to 330 mg ultramicrosize P.O. daily, or 250 to 500 mg microsize P.O. daily.
Tinea pedis or tinea unguium infections
Adults: 660 mg ultramicrosize P.O. daily or 1 g microsize P.O. daily.
Children weighing 30 to 50 lb (14 to 23 kg): 82.5 to 165 mg ultramicrosize P.O. daily, or 125 to 250 mg microsize P.O. daily.
Children weighing more than 50 lb: 165 to 330 mg ultramicrosize P.O. daily, or 250 to 500 mg microsize P.O. daily.

Pharmacodynamics
Antifungal action: Griseofulvin disrupts fungal cell's mitotic spindle, interfering with cell division; it also may inhibit DNA replication. Drug also enters keratin precursor cells, slowing fungal growth. Active against *Trichophyton, Microsporum,* and *Epidermophyton.*

Pharmacokinetics
Absorption: Absorbed primarily in the duodenum and varies among individuals. Ultramicrosize preparations are absorbed almost completely; microsize absorption ranges from 25% to 70% and may be increased by giving with a high-fat meal.
Distribution: Concentrates in skin, hair, nails, fat, liver, and skeletal muscle; it's tightly bound to new keratin.
Metabolism: Oxidatively demethylated and conjugated with glucuronic acid to inactive metabolites in the liver.
Excretion: About 50% of drug and its metabolites is excreted in urine and 33% in feces within 5 days. Less than 1% of a dose appears unchanged in urine. Drug is also excreted in perspiration. Elimination half-life is 9 to 24 hours.

Route	Onset	Peak	Duration
P.O.	Unknown	4-8 hr	Unknown

Contraindications and precautions
Contraindicated in those with hypersensitivity to drug and in those with porphyria or hepatocellular failure. Also contraindicated in pregnant women or women who intend to become pregnant during therapy. Use cautiously in penicillin-sensitive patients.

Interactions
Drug-drug. *Barbiturates:* Impaired absorption of griseofulvin. Dosage may need to be increased.
Oral contraceptives: Decrease efficacy of contraceptives. Suggest alternative method of contraception.
Phenobarbital: Decreases griseofulvin blood levels as a result of decreased absorption or increased metabolism. Avoid use together.
Warfarin: Decreased PT and INR. Dosage adjustment may be needed.
Drug-food. *High-fat meals:* Increased absorption. May be given together.
Drug-lifestyle. *Alcohol use:* Increased in alcohol effect, producing tachycardia, diaphoresis, and flushing. Advise patient to avoid alcohol.

Effects on diagnostic tests
None reported.

Adverse reactions
CNS: headache (in early stages of treatment), transient decrease in hearing, fatigue with large doses, occasional mental confusion, impaired performance of routine activities, psychotic symptoms, dizziness, insomnia, paresthesia of the hands and feet after extended therapy.
EENT: oral thrush.
GI: nausea, vomiting, flatulence, diarrhea, epigastric distress, ***bleeding.***
GU: proteinuria, menstrual irregularities.
Hematologic: *leukopenia,* ***granulocytopenia*** (requires discontinuation of drug), porphyria.
Hepatic: ***hepatotoxicity.***
Skin: *rash, urticaria,* photosensitivity, angioneurotic edema.
Other: *hypersensitivity reactions* (rash), lupus erythematosus.

Overdose and treatment
Symptoms of overdose include headache, lethargy, confusion, vertigo, blurred vision, nausea, vomiting, and diarrhea. Treatment is supportive. After recent ingestion (within 4 hours), empty stomach by induced emesis or gastric lavage. Follow with activated charcoal to decrease absorption. A cathartic may also be helpful.

Clinical considerations
- Confirm identification of organism before therapy begins.
- Give drug with or after meals, consisting of a high-fat content (if allowed), to minimize GI distress.
- Treatment of tinea pedis may require combined oral and topical therapy.

□ ***ALERT*** Because griseofulvin ultramicrosize is dispersed in polyethylene glycol, it's absorbed more rapidly and completely than microsize and is effective at one-half to two-thirds the usual griselfulvin dose. Don't interchange preparations.

Therapeutic monitoring
- Assess nutrition and monitor food intake; drug may alter taste sensation, suppressing appetite.
- Check CBCs regularly for possible adverse effects; monitor renal and liver function studies periodically.

Special populations
Pregnant patients. Contraindicated in pregnant women or women who intend to become pregnant during therapy.
Breast-feeding patients. Safety hasn't been established in breast-feeding women.
Pediatric patients. Microsize griseofulvin has been used in children as young as 3 months. Manufacturer states that dosage of ultramicrosize griseofulvin has not been established in children age 2 years and younger.

Patient counseling
- Encourage patient to maintain adequate nutritional intake.
- Stress importance of completing prescribed regimen to prevent relapse even though symptoms may abate quickly.
- Tell patient to report adverse reactions to prescriber immediately.
- Advise patient to avoid exposure to intense indoor light and sunlight to reduce the risk of photosensitivity reactions.
- Explain that drug may potentiate alcohol effects, and advise patient to avoid alcohol during therapy.

guaifenesin
Amonidrin, Anti-Tuss, Balminil Expectorant*, Breonesin, Fenesin, Gee-Gee, Genatuss, GG-Cen, Glyate, Glycotuss, Glytuss, Guiatuss, Humibid L.A., Humibid Sprinkle, Hytuss, Hytuss 2X, Malotuss, Mytussin, Naldecon Senior EX, Organidin NR, Resyl*, Robitussin, Scot-Tussin

Pharmacologic classification: propanediol derivative
Therapeutic classification: expectorant
Pregnancy risk category C

How supplied
Available by prescription only
Capsules: 300 mg
Tablets: 600 mg
Available without a prescription
Tablets: 100 mg, 200 mg
Tablets (extended-release): 600 mg
Capsules: 200 mg
Capsules (extended-release): 300 mg
Syrup: 100 mg/5 ml, 200 mg/5 ml

Indications and dosages
Expectorant
Adults and children age 12 and older: 100 to 400 mg P.O. q 4 hours; maximum dose is 2.4 g/day.
Children age 6 to 11: 100 to 200 mg P.O. q 4 hours; maximum dose is 1.2 g/day.
Children age 2 to 5: 50 to 100 mg P.O. q 4 hours; maximum dose is 600 mg/day.
Children under age 2: Individualize dosage.
Extended-release
Adults and children over age 12: 600 to 1,200 mg P.O. q 12 hours, not to exceed 2,400 mg in 24 hours.
Children age 6 to 12: 600 mg P.O. q 12 hours, not to exceed 1,200 mg in 24 hours.
Children age 2 to 6: 300 mg P.O. q 12 hours, not to exceed 600 mg in 24 hours.

Pharmacodynamics
Expectorant action: Guaifenesin increases respiratory tract fluid by reducing adhesiveness and surface tension, decreasing viscosity of the secretions and thereby facilitating their removal.

Pharmacokinetics
Unknown.

Route	Onset	Peak	Duration
P.O.	Unknown	Unknown	Unknown

Contraindications and precautions
Contraindicated in patients hypersensitive to drug.

Interactions
None significant.

Effects on diagnostic tests
Drug may cause color interference with tests for 5-hydroxyindoleacetic acid and vanillylmandelic acid.

Adverse reactions
CNS: dizziness, headache.
GI: vomiting and nausea (with large doses).
Skin: rash.

Overdose and treatment
No information available.

Clinical considerations
Efficacy of guaifenesin as an expectorant hasn't been clearly established because of conflicting results of clinical studies.

Therapeutic monitoring
Patient should be re-evaluated if symptoms persist for more than 1 week, if cough recurs, or if cough is accompanied by fever, rash, or persistent headache.

Special populations
Breast-feeding patients. It's unknown if drug is distributed in breast milk. Safety in breast-feeding women hasn't been established.
Pediatric patients. Individualize dosage for children under age 2.
Geriatric patients. No specific recommendations are available. Most liquid preparations contain alcohol (3.5% to 10%).

Patient counseling
- Advise patient to take drug with a glass of water to help loosen mucus in lungs.
- Advise patient to use sugarless throat lozenges to decrease throat irritation and associated cough and to report cough that persists longer than 7 days.

guanabenz acetate
Wytensin

Pharmacologic classification: centrally acting antiadrenergic
Therapeutic classification: antihypertensive
Pregnancy risk category C

How supplied
Available by prescription only
Tablets: 4 mg, 8 mg

Indications and dosages
Hypertension (generally considered a step 2 agent)
Adults: Initially, 2 to 4 mg P.O. b.i.d. Dosage may be increased in increments of 4 to 8 mg/day q 1 to 2 weeks. The usual maintenance dosage ranges from 8 to 16 mg daily. Maximum dose is 32 mg b.i.d.
Children age 12 and older: Initially, 0.5 to 4 mg P.O. daily; maintenance dosage ranges from 4 to 24 mg daily, administered in two divided doses.
◇***Management of opiate withdrawal***
Adults: 4 mg P.O. b.i.d. to q.i.d.

Pharmacodynamics
Antihypertensive action: Guanabenz decreases blood pressure by stimulating central $alpha_2$-adrenergic receptors, decreasing cerebral sympathetic outflow and thus decreasing peripheral vascular resistance. Guanabenz may also antagonize antidiuretic hormone (ADH) secretion and ADH activity in the kidney.

Pharmacokinetics
Absorption: After oral administration, 70% to 80% is absorbed from the GI tract.
Distribution: Appears to be distributed widely into the body, and is about 90% protein-bound.
Metabolism: Metabolized extensively in the liver; several metabolites are formed.
Excretion: Guanabenz and its metabolites are excreted primarily in urine; remaining drug is excreted in feces.

Route	Onset	Peak	Duration
P.O.	1 hr	2-5 hr	6-12 hr

Contraindications and precautions
Contraindicated in patients with hypersensitivity to drug. Use cautiously in the elderly and in patients with impaired renal or hepatic function, severe coronary insufficiency, recent MI, and cerebrovascular disease.

Interactions
Drug-drug. *Diuretics and other antihypertensive agents:* Increased risk of excessive hypotension. Recommend monitoring blood pressure frequently.
Phenothiazines, benzodiazepines, barbiturates, other sedatives: Increased CNS depressant effects. Use together cautiously.
Tricyclic antidepressants, MAO inhibitors: Inhibit antihypertensive effects of guanabenz. Recommend monitoring blood pressure frequently.
Drug-lifestyle. *Alcohol use:* Increased CNS depressant effects. Advise patient to avoid alcohol.

Effects on diagnostic tests
None reported.

Adverse reactions
CNS: *drowsiness, sedation, dizziness, weakness,* headache.
CV: *rebound hypertension.*
GI: *dry mouth.*
Hepatic: elevations in liver enzyme levels.
Metabolic: may reduce serum cholesterol and total triglyceride levels slightly.

Overdose and treatment
Clinical signs of overdose include bradycardia, CNS depression, respiratory depression, hypothermia, apnea, seizures, lethargy, agitation, irritability, diarrhea, and hypotension.

Don't induce emesis; CNS depression occurs rapidly. After adequate respiration is assured, empty stomach by gastric lavage; then give activated charcoal and a saline cathartic to decrease absorption. Follow with symptomatic and supportive care.

Clinical considerations
- Abrupt discontinuation of guanabenz causes severe rebound hypertension; reduce dosage gradually over 2 to 4 days.
- Reduced dosages may be required in patients with hepatic impairment.

Therapeutic monitoring
- Monitor for adverse reactions, including CNS effects.
- Recommend monitoring liver enzyme level and serum triglyceride levels.

Special populations
Breast-feeding patients. It's unknown if guanabenz is distributed into breast milk; an alternative feeding method is recommended during therapy.
Pediatric patients. Drug has been used to treat hypertension in a limited number of children

over age 12; safety and efficacy in younger children haven't been established.
Geriatric patients. Geriatric patients may be more sensitive to antihypertensive and sedative effects of guanabenz.

Patient counseling
- Explain signs and symptoms of adverse effects and importance of reporting them.
- Warn patient to avoid hazardous activities that require mental alertness and to avoid alcohol and other CNS depressants.
- Suggest taking drug at bedtime until tolerance develops to sedation, drowsiness, and other CNS effects.
- Warn patient to seek medical approval before taking OTC cold preparations.
- Advise patient not to discontinue drug suddenly; severe rebound hypertension may occur.

guanadrel sulfate
Hylorel

Pharmacologic classification: adrenergic neuron blocker
Therapeutic classification: antihypertensive
Pregnancy risk category B

How supplied
Available by prescription only
Tablets: 10 mg, 25 mg

Indications and dosages
Hypertension
Adults: Initially, 5 mg P.O. b.i.d.; adjust dosage until blood pressure is controlled. Most patients require 20 to 75 mg daily, usually given b.i.d. (400 mg daily is rarely used).
≡ ***Dosage adjustment.*** In patient with renal impairment, if creatinine clearance is 30 to 60 ml/minute, reduce dose to 5 mg q 24 hours; if creatinine clearance is less than 30 ml/minute, increase dosing interval to q 48 hours.

Pharmacodynamics
Antihypertensive action: Guanadrel reduces blood pressure by peripheral inhibition of norepinephrine release in adrenergic nerve endings, thus decreasing arteriolar vasoconstriction.

Pharmacokinetics
Absorption: Absorbed rapidly and almost completely from the GI tract.
Distribution: Distributed widely into the body; and is about 20% protein-bound. It doesn't enter the CNS.
Metabolism: About 40% to 50% of a given dose is metabolized by the liver.
Excretion: Drug and its metabolites are eliminated primarily in urine. Plasma half-life is about 10 hours but varies considerably with each individual.

Route	Onset	Peak	Duration
P.O.	2 hr	4-6 hr	4-14 hr

Contraindications and precautions
Contraindicated in patients with hypersensitivity to drug, known or suspected pheochromocytoma, or frank heart failure. Also contraindicated in patients receiving MAO inhibitors or within 1 week of discontinuing MAO inhibitor therapy.

Use cautiously in patients with regional vascular disease, bronchial asthma, or peptic ulcer disease.

Interactions
Drug-drug. *Other antihypertensive agents, diuretics:* Enhanced antihypertensive effects. Monitor blood pressure closely.
MAO inhibitors, ephedrine, norepinephrine, methylphenidate, tricyclic antidepressants, phenothiazines, or amphetamines: May antagonize antihypertensive effects of guanadrel. Dosage adjustment may be needed.
Drug-lifestyle. *Alcohol use:* Increased risk of guanadrel-induced orthostatic hypotension. Monitor blood pressure frequently.

Effects on diagnostic tests
None reported.

Adverse reactions
CNS: *fatigue, drowsiness, faintness, headache, confusion, paresthesia.*
CV: *palpitations, chest pain, peripheral edema, orthostatic hypotension.*
EENT: *glossitis, visual disturbances.*
GI: *diarrhea,* dry mouth, *indigestion,* constipation, anorexia, nausea, vomiting, abdominal pain.
GU: impotence, *ejaculation disturbances, nocturia, urination frequency.*
Metabolic: *weight gain.*
Musculoskeletal: *aching limbs, leg cramps.*
Respiratory: *shortness of breath, cough.*

Overdose and treatment
Signs of overdose include hypotension, dizziness, blurred vision, and syncope.

After acute ingestion, empty stomach by induced emesis or gastric lavage. The effect of activated charcoal in absorbing guanadrel hasn't been determined. Further treatment is usually symptomatic and supportive.

Clinical considerations
- Separate use of guanadrel and MAO inhibitors by at least 1 week.
- Discontinue guanadrel 48 to 72 hours before surgery, to minimize risk of vascular collapse during anesthesia.

Therapeutic monitoring
- Monitor supine and standing blood pressure, especially during periods of dosage adjustment.
- Assess for signs and symptoms of edema.

Special populations
Breast-feeding patients. It's unknown if drug is excreted in breast milk. An alternative feeding method is recommended during therapy.
Pediatric patients. Safety and efficacy in children haven't been established; use drug only if potential benefit outweighs risk.
Geriatric patients. Geriatric patients may be more sensitive to orthostatic hypotension.

Patient counseling
- Instruct patient to report excessive weight gain (more than 5 lb [2.25 kg] weekly).
- Explain that orthostatic hypotension can be minimized by rising slowly from a supine position and avoiding sudden position changes; it may be aggravated by fever, hot weather, hot showers, prolonged standing, exercise, and alcohol.
- Warn patient to avoid hazardous activities that require mental alertness and to take drug at bedtime until tolerance develops to sedation, drowsiness, and other CNS effects.
- Warn patient to seek medical approval before taking OTC cold preparations.

guanethidine monosulfate
Ismelin

Pharmacologic classification: adrenergic neuron blocker
Therapeutic classification: antihypertensive
Pregnancy risk category C

How supplied
Available by prescription only
Tablets: 10 mg, 25 mg

Indications and dosages
Moderate to severe hypertension, ◊signs and symptoms of thyrotoxicosis
Adults: Initially, 10 mg P.O. once daily; increase by 10 mg at weekly to monthly intervals, as necessary. Usual dose is 25 to 50 mg once daily; some patients may require up to 300 mg.

Pharmacodynamics
Antihypertensive action: Guanethidine acts peripherally; it decreases arteriolar vasoconstriction and reduces blood pressure by inhibiting norepinephrine release and depleting norepinephrine stores in adrenergic nerve endings.

Pharmacokinetics
Absorption: Absorbed incompletely from the GI tract. Maximal antihypertensive effects usually aren't evident for 1 to 3 weeks.
Distribution: Distributed throughout the body; it's not protein-bound but demonstrates extensive tissue binding.
Metabolism: Undergoes partial hepatic metabolism to pharmacologically less active metabolites.
Excretion: Drug and metabolites are excreted primarily in urine; small amounts are excreted in feces. Elimination half-life after chronic administration is biphasic.

Route	Onset	Peak	Duration
P.O.	Unknown	8 hr	3-4 days

Contraindications and precautions
Contraindicated in patients with pheochromocytoma, frank heart failure, or hypersensitivity to drug and in those receiving MAO inhibitors. Use cautiously in patients with severe cardiac disease, recent MI, cerebrovascular disease, peptic ulcer, impaired renal function, or bronchial asthma, and in those taking other antihypertensive agents.

Interactions
Drug-drug. *Amphetamines, ephedrine, MAO inhibitors, methylphenidate, norepinephrine, phenothiazines, tricyclic antidepressants, or oral contraceptives:* May antagonize the antihypertensive effect of guanethidine. Discontinue MAO inhibitor therapy 1 week before starting guanethidine. Dosage may need adjustment.
Cardiac glycosides: May result in additive bradycardia.
Diuretics, other antihypertensive agents, levodopa: May potentiate antihypertensive effect of guanethidine. Use together cautiously.
Norepinephrine, metaraminol, oral sympathomimetic nasal decongestants: Guanethidine potentiates pressor effects of such agents. Monitor blood pressure closely.
Rauwolfia alkaloids (reserpine): May cause excessive orthostatic hypotension, bradycardia, and mental depression.
Drug-lifestyle. *Alcohol use:* Increased hypotensive effect of guanethidine. Advise patient to avoid alcohol.

Effects on diagnostic tests
None reported.

Adverse reactions
CNS: *syncope, fatigue, headache, drowsiness, paresthesia, confusion.*
CV: *palpitations, chest pain, orthostatic hypotension, peripheral edema, bradycardia,* ***heart failure.***
EENT: *visual disturbances,* glossitis.

GI: *diarrhea, indigestion, constipation, anorexia,* nausea, vomiting.
GU: *nocturia, urination frequency, ejaculation disturbances,* impotence.
Metabolic: *weight gain.*
Musculoskeletal: *aching limbs, leg cramps.*
Respiratory: shortness of breath, cough.

Overdose and treatment
Signs of overdose include hypotension, blurred vision, syncope, bradycardia, and severe diarrhea.

After acute ingestion, empty stomach by induced emesis or gastric lavage and give activated charcoal to reduce absorption. Further treatment is usually symptomatic and supportive.

Clinical considerations
- When drug is replacing MAO inhibitors, wait at least 1 week before initiating guanethidine; if replacing ganglionic blocking agents, withdraw them slowly to prevent a spiking blood pressure response during the transfer period.
- Dosage requirements may be reduced in the presence of fever.
- Discontinue drug 2 to 3 weeks before elective surgery to reduce risk of CV collapse during anesthesia.

Therapeutic monitoring
- If diarrhea develops, atropine or paregoric may be prescribed.
- Monitor patient for adverse reactions.

Special populations
Breast-feeding patients. Small amounts of drug are excreted in breast milk; recommend alternative feeding method during therapy.
Pediatric patients. Safety and efficacy in children haven't been established.
Geriatric patients. Geriatric patients may be more sensitive to drug's antihypertensive effects.

Patient counseling
- Tell patient to report persistent diarrhea and excessive weight gain (5 lb [2.25 kg] weekly). Advise patient not to discontinue the drug but to call prescriber for further instructions.
- Warn patient to avoid hazardous activities that require mental alertness and to take drug at bedtime until tolerance develops to sedation, drowsiness, and other CNS effects.
- Advise patient to avoid sudden position changes, strenuous exercise, heat, and hot showers, to minimize orthostatic hypotension; and to relieve dry mouth with ice chips, hard candy, or gum.
- Tell patient if a dose is missed not to double the next scheduled dose but to take only the next scheduled dose.
- Advise patient to seek medical approval before taking OTC cold preparations.

H

Haemophilus b vaccines

Haemophilus b conjugate vaccine, diphtheria CRM protein conjugate (HbOC)
HibTITER

Haemophilus b conjugate vaccine, diphtheria toxoid conjugate (PRP-D)
ProHIBiT

Haemophilus b conjugate vaccine, meningococcal protein conjugate (PRP-OMP)
PedvaxHIB

Haemophilus b polysaccharide conjugate vaccine, tetanus toxoid (PRP-T)
ActHIB, OmniHIB

Pharmacologic classification: vaccine
Therapeutic classification: bacterial vaccine
Pregnancy risk category C

How supplied
Available by prescription only
Conjugate vaccine, diphtheria CRM_{197}
Injection: 10 mcg of purified *Haemophilus* b saccharide and about 25 mcg CRM_{197} protein per 0.5 ml
Conjugate vaccine, diphtheria toxoid conjugate
Injection: 25 mcg of *Haemophilus influenzae* type b (Hib) capsular polysaccharide and 18 mcg of diphtheria toxoid protein per 0.5 ml
Conjugate vaccine, meningococcal protein conjugate
Injection: 7.5 mcg *Haemophilus* b capsular polysaccharide, 125 mcg *Neisseria meningitidis* OMPC per 0.5 ml.
Conjugate vaccine, tetanus toxoid
Powder for injection: 10 mcg *Haemophilus* b purified capsular polysaccharide, 24 mcg of tetanus toxoid, and 8.5% sucrose

Indications and dosages
Routine immunization
***Haemophilus* b conjugate vaccine, diphtheria CRM_{197} protein conjugate**
Children age 2 to 6 months: 0.5 ml I.M.; repeat in 2 months and again in 4 months (for total of three doses). A booster dose is required at age 15 months.
Previously unvaccinated children age 7 to 11 months: 0.5 ml I.M.; repeat in 2 months (for total of two doses before age 15 months). A booster dose is required at age 15 months (but no sooner than 2 months after last vaccination).
Previously unvaccinated children age 12 to 14 months: 0.5 ml I.M. A booster dose is required at age 15 months (but no sooner than 2 months after last vaccination).
Previously unvaccinated children age 15 to 60 months: 0.5 ml I.M.
***Haemophilus* b conjugate vaccine, diphtheria toxoid conjugate**
Children age 15 to 60 months: 0.5 ml I.M.
***Haemophilus* b conjugate vaccine, meningococcal protein conjugate**
Previously unvaccinated infants age 2 to 10 months: 0.5 ml I.M. ideally at 2 months. Repeat 2 months later (or as soon as possible thereafter). Administer a booster dose of 0.5 ml I.M. at 12 to 15 months (but no sooner than 2 months after last vaccination).
Previously unvaccinated children age 11 to 14 months: 0.5 ml I.M.; repeat in 2 months.
Previously unvaccinated children age 15 to 71 months: 0.5 ml I.M.
***Haemophilus* b polysaccharide conjugate vaccine, tetanus toxoid**
Previously unvaccinated children age 2 to 6 months: Three 0.5-ml I.M. doses, at 8-week intervals followed by a booster dose at age 15 to 18 months.
Previously unvaccinated children age 7 to 11 months: Two 0.5-ml I.M. doses at 8-week intervals, followed by a booster dose at age 15 to 18 months.
Previously unvaccinated children age 12 to 14 months: 0.5 ml I.M., followed by a booster dose at age 15 to 18 months. Administer no earlier than 2 months after previous dose.
Previously unvaccinated children age 15 to 60 months: 0.5 ml I.M.

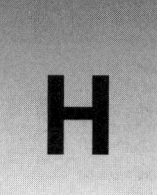

Pharmacodynamics
Prophylactic action: Vaccine promotes active immunity to *H. influenzae* type b.

Pharmacokinetics
Absorption: After I.M. or S.C. administration, increases in *H. influenzae* type b capsular antibody levels in serum are detectable in about 2 weeks and peak within 3 weeks.
Distribution: Limited data indicate that antibodies to *H. influenzae* type b can be detected in fetal blood and in breast milk after administration of the vaccine to pregnant and breast-feeding patients women.
Metabolism: No information available.
Excretion: The vaccine polysaccharide has been detected in urine for up to 11 days after administration to children.

Route	Onset	Peak	Duration
I.M.	2 wk after last dose	Unknown	Several yr

Contraindications and precautions
Contraindicated in patients with acute illness or hypersensitivity to any component of vaccine, including thimerosal. Don't administer to patients less than 10 days before or during treatment with immunosuppressive drugs or irradiation.

Interactions
Drug-drug. *Corticosteroids or immunosuppressants:* May impair immune response to the vaccine. Avoid vaccination under these circumstances.

Effects on diagnostic tests
For days or weeks after administration, *Haemophilus* b (Hib) may interfere with antigen detection tests.

Adverse reactions
CNS: irritability.
GI: diarrhea, vomiting.
Skin: *erythema, pain at injection site.*
Other: ***anaphylaxis,*** fever.

Overdose and treatment
No information available.

Clinical considerations
- Epinephrine solution 1:1,000 should be available to treat allergic reactions.

□ ***ALERT*** Vaccine types are age specific. Check labeling as well as current U.S. Health Service Advisory Committee on Immunization Practices (ACIP) and American Academy of Pediatrics (AAP) recommendations.

- Vaccine may be given simultaneously with diphtheria, tetanus, and pertussis (DTP) vaccine; measles, mumps, and rubella (MMR) vaccine; poliovirus vaccine, inactivated (IPV); meningococcal vaccine; or pneumococcal vaccine, but should be administered at different sites.
- Administer same vaccine throughout the vaccination series; no data are available to support the interchangeability of the vaccines.
- Children under age 24 months in whom invasive *H. influenzae* type b disease develops should be vaccinated because natural immunity may not develop.
- Vaccination shouldn't be used to prevent invasive disease associated with *H. influenzae* type b disease because of the time required to develop immunity. Instead, use chemoprophylaxis (with drugs such as rifampin) in both vaccinated and unvaccinated individuals because children with immunity may carry and transmit the organism. However, if every child in a household or day-care group has been fully vaccinated, chemoprophylaxis isn't necessary.
- A conjugate vaccine containing meningococcal proteins won't prevent meningococcal disease; one containing diphtheria proteins won't produce immunity against diphtheria; and one containing the tetanus toxoid conjugate won't produce immunity against tetanus toxoid. Administer DTP vaccine according to the recommended schedule.
- Some vaccine products may contain thimerosal.

Therapeutic monitoring
- Adverse reactions generally occur within the first 24 hours.
- Monitor for anaphylaxis, injection site reactions, and fever.

Special populations
Pregnant patients. Generally not recommended for use in pregnant women.
Pediatric patients. Safety and efficacy of PRP-D haven't been established for patients under age 1. Safety and efficacy of PRP-OMP haven't been established for patients under age 2 months. Safety and efficacy of PRP-T haven't been established for patients under age 6 weeks.

Patient counseling
- *H. influenzae* type b is a cause of meningitis in infants and preschool children. Explain to parents that this vaccine will protect children only against meningitis caused by this organism.
- Tell parents that child may experience swelling and inflammation at injection site and fever. Recommend acetaminophen liquid for fever.
- Tell parents to report worrisome or persistent adverse reactions promptly.

haloperidol

Apo-Haloperidol*, Haldol, Novo-Peridol*, Peridol*

haloperidol decanoate

Haldol Decanoate, Haldol Decanoate 100, Haldol LA*

haloperidol lactate

Haldol, Haldol Concentrate, Haloperidol Intensol

Pharmacologic classification: butyrophenone
Therapeutic classification: antipsychotic
Pregnancy risk category C

How supplied

Available by prescription only
haloperidol
Tablets: 0.5 mg, 1 mg, 2 mg, 5 mg, 10 mg, 20 mg
haloperidol decanoate
Injection: 50 mg/ml, 100 mg/ml
haloperidol lactate
Oral concentrate: 2 mg/ml
Injection: 5 mg/ml

Indications and dosages

Psychotic disorders, ◇alcohol dependence
Adults: Dosage varies for each patient and symptoms. Initial dosage range is 0.5 to 5 mg P.O. b.i.d. or t.i.d.; or 2 to 5 mg I.M. q 4 to 8 hours, increased rapidly if necessary for prompt control. Maximum dose is 100 mg P.O. daily. Doses of more than 100 mg have been used to treat patients who have severely resistant conditions.
Psychotic patients who require prolonged therapy
Adults: 100 mg I.M. of haloperidol decanoate q 4 weeks. Experience with doses of more than 450 mg monthly is limited.
Control of tics, vocal utterances in Tourette syndrome
Adults: 0.5 to 5 mg P.O. b.i.d. or t.i.d., increased, p.r.n.
Children age 3 to 12: 0.05 to 0.075 mg/kg/day given b.i.d. or t.i.d.
◇Delirium
Adults: 1 to 2 mg I.V. every 2 to 4 hours.

Pharmacodynamics

Antipsychotic action: Haloperidol is thought to exert its antipsychotic effects by strong postsynaptic blockade of CNS dopamine receptors, thereby inhibiting dopamine-mediated effects; its pharmacologic effects are most similar to those of piperazine antipsychotics. Its mechanism of action in Tourette syndrome is unknown.

Haloperidol has many other central and peripheral effects; it has weak peripheral anticholinergic effects and antiemetic effects, produces both alpha and ganglionic blockade, and counteracts histamine- and serotonin-mediated activity. Its most prominent adverse reactions are extrapyramidal.

Pharmacokinetics

Absorption: Rate and extent of absorption vary with route of administration.
Distribution: Distributed widely into the body, with high levels in adipose tissue. Drug is 90% to 92% protein-bound.
Metabolism: Metabolized extensively by the liver; there may be only one active metabolite that's less active than parent drug.
Excretion: About 40% of a given dose is excreted in urine within 5 days; about 15% is excreted in feces via the biliary tract.

Route	Onset	Peak	Duration
P.O.	Unknown	3-6 hr	Unknown
I.M. (decanoate)	Unknown	3-9 days	Unknown
I.M. (lactate)	Unknown	10-20 min	Unknown

Contraindications and precautions

Contraindicated in patients with hypersensitivity or in those experiencing parkinsonism, coma, or CNS depression.

Use haloperidol cautiously in geriatric or debilitated patients; in patients with history of seizures, EEG abnormalities, CV disorders, allergies, narrow angle glaucoma, or urine retention; and in those receiving anticoagulant, anticonvulsant, antiparkinsonian, or lithium medications.

Interactions

Drug-drug. *Aluminum- and magnesium-containing antacids and antidiarrheals*: Separate administration times by 2 hours.
Antiarrhythmic agents, disopyramide, procainamide, quinidine: Increased incidence of arrhythmias and conduction defects. Avoid use together.
Atropine or other anticholinergic drugs, including antidepressants, antihistamines, MAO inhibitors, meperidine, phenothiazines, and antiparkinsonian agents: Oversedation, paralytic ileus, visual changes, and severe constipation. Use with caution.
Beta blockers: May inhibit haloperidol metabolism, increasing plasma levels and toxicity. Use with caution.
Bromocriptine: Haloperidol antagonizes the therapeutic effect of bromocriptine on prolactin secretion.
Centrally acting antihypertensive drugs (such as clonidine, guanabenz, guanadrel, guanethidine, methyldopa, reserpine): Inhibited blood

pressure response. Monitor blood pressure carefully.
CNS depressants, including analgesics, barbiturates, narcotics, tranquilizers, and general, spinal, or epidural anesthetics, or with parenteral magnesium sulfate: Increased CNS depression. Avoid use together.
Dopamine: Decreased vasoconstricting effects.
Levodopa: Decreased effectiveness and increased toxicity of levodopa. Avoid use together.
Lithium: May result in severe neurologic toxicity with an encephalitis-like syndrome, and a decreased therapeutic response to haloperidol. Use with caution; monitor patient.
Metrizamide: Increased risk of seizures. Avoid use together.
Nitrates: Hypotension. Monitor blood pressure frequently.
Phenobarbital: Enhanced renal excretion. Monitor patient closely.
Phenytoin: Inhibited metabolism and increased toxicity of phenytoin. Avoid use together.
Propylthiouracil: Increases risk of agranulocytosis. Avoid use together.
Rifampin: Decreased haloperidol concentrations; decreased efficacy. Monitor carefully.
Sympathomimetics, including epinephrine, phenylephrine, phenylpropanolamine, and ephedrine (often found in nasal sprays), and appetite suppressants: May decrease stimulatory and pressor effects of these drugs. Monitor patient carefully.
Drug-herb. *Nutmeg*: Loss of symptom control; interference with existing therapy for psychiatric illnesses. Avoid use together.
Drug-lifestyle. *Heavy smoking:* Increased metabolism of haloperidol. Discourage smoking.

Effects on diagnostic tests
None reported.

Adverse reactions
CNS: *severe extrapyramidal reactions, tardive dyskinesia,* sedation, drowsiness, lethargy, headache, insomnia, confusion, vertigo, ***seizures.***
CV: tachycardia, hypotension, hypertension, ECG changes.
EENT: *blurred vision.*
GI: dry mouth, anorexia, constipation, diarrhea, nausea, vomiting, dyspepsia.
GU: urine retention, menstrual irregularities, gynecomastia, priapism.
Hematologic: ***leukopenia,*** leukocytosis.
Hepatic: altered liver function tests, jaundice.
Skin: rash, other skin reactions, diaphoresis.
Other: ***neuroleptic malignant syndrome*** (rare).

Overdose and treatment
Overdose is manifested as greater acuity of adverse reactions and can include deep, unarousable sleep, coma, hypotension, hypertension, extrapyramidal symptoms, dystonia, abnormal involuntary muscle movements, agitation, seizures, arrhythmias, ECG changes (may show QT interval prolongation and torsades de pointes), hypothermia, hyperthermia, and autonomic nervous system dysfunction. Overdose with long-acting decanoate requires prolonged recovery time.

Treatment is symptomatic and supportive, including maintaining vital signs, airway, stable body temperature, and fluid and electrolyte balance. Ipecac may be used to induce vomiting, with due regard for antiemetic properties of haloperidol and hazard of aspiration. Gastric lavage also may be used, followed by activated charcoal and saline cathartics; dialysis doesn't help.

Regulate body temperature as needed. Treat hypotension with I.V. fluids; don't give epinephrine. Treat seizures with parenteral diazepam or barbiturates; arrhythmias, with parenteral phenytoin (1 mg/kg I.V. with rate titrated to blood pressure not to exceed 50 mg/minute with ECG monitoring; may repeat every 5 minutes up to 10 mg/kg); extrapyramidal reactions with benztropine at 1 to 2 mg or parenteral diphenhydramine at 10 to 50 mg.

Clinical considerations
- Drug has few CV adverse effects and may be preferred in patients with cardiac disease.
- Dose of 2 mg is therapeutic equivalent of 100 mg chlorpromazine.
- When changing from tablets to decanoate injection, patient should initially receive 10 to 20 times the oral dose once monthly (not more than 100 mg).

Therapeutic monitoring
- Assess patient periodically for extrapyramidal reactions and tardive dyskinesia.
- Don't withdraw drug abruptly except when required because abrupt withdrawal may cause severe adverse reaction.

Special populations
Pediatric patients. Safety and efficacy of drug injection in children haven't been established and oral drug isn't recommended for children under age 3.
Geriatric patients. Drug is especially useful for agitation associated with senile dementia. Tardive dyskinesia may occur more often, especially in elderly women. Geriatric patients usually require lower initial doses and a more gradual dosage titration.

Patient counseling
- Warn patient against activities that require alertness and good psychomotor coordination until CNS response to drug is determined. Drowsiness and dizziness usually subside after a few weeks.
- Tell patient to report adverse effects to prescriber.

■ Instruct patient to avoid combining with alcohol or other depressants.

heparin sodium

Heparin Lock Flush, Hep-Lock, Hep-Lock U/P, Liquaemin

Pharmacologic classification: anticoagulant
Therapeutic classification: anticoagulant
Pregnancy risk category C

How supplied

Available products are derived from bovine lung or porcine intestinal mucosa. All are injectable and available by prescription only.

heparin sodium
Vials: 1,000 units/ml, 5,000 units/ml, 10,000 units/ml, 20,000 units/ml, 40,000 units/ml
Unit-dose ampules: 1,000 units/ml, 5,000 units/ml, 10,000 units/ml
Disposable syringes: 1,000 units/ml, 2,500 units/ml, 5,000 units/ml, 7,500 units/ml, 10,000 units/ml, 20,000 units/ml
Carpuject: 5,000 units/ml
Premixed I.V. solutions: 1,000 units in 500 ml normal saline solution; 2,000 units in 1,000 ml normal saline solution; 12,500 units in 250 ml 0.45% saline solution; 25,000 units in 250 ml 0.45% saline solution; 25,000 units in 500 ml 0.45% saline solution; 10,000 units in 100 ml D_5W; 12,500 units in 250 ml D_5W; 25,000 units in 250 ml D_5W; 25,000 units in 500 ml D_5W

heparin sodium flush
Vials: 10 units/ml, 100 units/ml
Disposable syringes: 10 units/ml, 25 units/2.5 ml, 2,500 units/2.5 ml

Indications and dosages

Deep vein thrombosis, pulmonary embolism
Adults: Initially, 5,000 to 10,000 units I.V. push, then adjust dose according to partial thromboplastin time (PTT) results and give dose I.V. q 4 hours (usually 4,000 to 5,000 units); or 5,000 units I.V. bolus, then 20,000 to 40,000 units in 24 hours by I.V. infusion pump. Wait 4 to 6 hours after bolus dose, and adjust hourly rate based on PTT.
Children: Initially, 50 units/kg I.V. bolus. Maintenance dosage is 50 to 100 units/kg I.V. drip q 4 hours. Constant infusion: 20,000 units/m^2 daily. Adjust dosage based on PTT.

Embolism prophylaxis, ◊post MI, ◊cerebral thrombosis in evolving stroke, ◊left ventricular thrombi
Adults: 5,000 units S.C. q 8 to 12 hours.

Open-heart surgery
Adults: (total body perfusion) 150 to 400 units/kg continuous I.V. infusion.

Disseminated intravascular coagulation
Adults: 50 to 100 units/kg I.V. q 4 hours as a single injection or constant infusion. Discontinue if no improvement in 4 to 8 hours.
Children: 25 to 50 units/kg I.V. q 4 hours, as a single injection or constant infusion. Discontinue if no improvement in 4 to 8 hours.

To maintain patency of I.V. indwelling catheters
Adults and children: 10 to 100 units as an I.V. flush (not intended for therapeutic use).

◊Unstable angina
Adults: Keep PTT 1.5 to 2 times control during first week of anginal pain.

◊Anticoagulation in blood transfusion and samples
Transfusions and samples: Mix 7,500 units and 100 ml of normal saline and add 6 to 8 ml of mixture to each 100 ml of whole blood or 70 to 150 units to each 10 to 20 ml of blood sample.

Note: Heparin dosing is highly individualized, depending on disease state, age, weight, and renal and hepatic status.

Pharmacodynamics

Anticoagulant action: Heparin accelerates formation of antithrombin III-thrombin complex; it inactivates thrombin and prevents conversion of fibrinogen to fibrin.

Pharmacokinetics

Absorption: Not absorbed from GI tract and must be given parenterally.
Distribution: Extensively bound to lipoprotein, globulins, and fibrinogen; it doesn't cross the placenta.
Metabolism: Although metabolism isn't completely described, drug is thought to be removed by the reticuloendothelial system, with some metabolism occurring in the liver.
Excretion: Little is known; a small fraction is excreted in urine as unchanged drug. Drug isn't excreted in breast milk. Plasma half-life is 1 to 2 hours.

Route	Onset	Peak	Duration
I.V.	Immediate	Unknown	Variable
S.C.	20-60 min	2-4 hr	Variable

Contraindications and precautions

Contraindicated in patients with hypersensitivity to drug. Conditionally contraindicated in patients with active bleeding; blood dyscrasia; or bleeding tendencies, such as hemophilia, thrombocytopenia, or hepatic disease with hypoprothrombinemia; suspected intracranial hemorrhage; suppurative thrombophlebitis; inaccessible ulcerative lesions (especially of GI tract) and open ulcerative wounds; extensive denudation of skin; ascorbic acid deficiency and other conditions that cause increased capillary permeability; during or after brain, eye, or spinal cord surgery; during spinal tap or spinal anesthesia; during continuous tube drainage of stomach or small intestine; in subacute bacterial endocarditis; shock; advanced renal disease; threatened abortion; or severe hypertension. Although heparin use is clearly hazardous in these conditions, its risks and its benefits must be evaluated.

Use cautiously in postpartum women or women during menses; in patients with mild hepatic or renal disease, alcoholism, or history of asthma, allergies, or GI ulcer; or in those with occupations that have a high incidence of accidents.

Interactions

Drug-drug. *Oral anticoagulants and platelet inhibitors:* Increases anticoagulant effect. Recommend monitoring INR, PT, and PTT.
Antihistamines, cardiac glycosides, nicotine, tetracyclines: May partially counteract the anticoagulant action of heparin. Dosage adjustment may be needed.
Drug-herb. *Motherwort or red clover:* May risk increased bleeding. Avoid use together.

Effects on diagnostic tests

Valid PT results in the presence of concurrent coumarin or indandione therapy can only be obtained when blood samples are drawn 4 to 6 hours after I.V. heparin dose or 12 to 24 hours after S.C. heparin dose. Continuous I.V. heparin dose doesn't affect reliability of PT result. Heparin interferes with sulfobromophthalein test, causing an upward shift in the absorption peak; heparin also causes falsely elevated thyroxine level results when competitive protein-binding methods of testing are used. Heparinized blood shouldn't be used for erythrocyte sedimentation rates, platelet counts, fragility tests, or tests involving complement or isoagglutinins.

Adverse reactions

Hematologic: ***hemorrhage*** (with excessive dosage), *overly prolonged clotting time,* ***thrombocytopenia.***
Other: irritation; mild pain; hematoma; ulceration; cutaneous or subcutaneous necrosis; ***"white clot" syndrome; hypersensitivity reactions*** (including chills, fever, pruritus, rhinitis, urticaria, ***anaphylactoid reactions***).

Overdose and treatment

The major sign of overdose is hemorrhage. Immediate withdrawal of drug usually allows the hemorrhage to resolve; however, severe hemorrhage may require treatment with protamine sulfate. Usually, 1 mg protamine sulfate neutralizes 90 units of bovine heparin or 115 units of porcine heparin.

Heparin administered by I.V. route disappears rapidly from the blood, so the protamine dose depends on when heparin was administered. Give protamine slowly by I.V. injection (over 3 minutes); no more than 50 mg should be given in any 10-minute period.

Heparin administered by S.C. route is slowly absorbed. Give protamine as a 25- to 50-mg loading dose, followed by constant infusion of the remainder of the calculated dose over 8 to 16 hours.

For severe bleeding, transfusions may be required.

Clinical considerations

- Many I.V. medications are incompatible with heparin, and may form precipitates if they come in contact with heparin.
- Avoid I.M. administration of other drugs, if possible, to prevent or minimize hematomas.
- Abrupt withdrawal may increase coagulability; heparin is usually followed by prophylactic oral anticoagulant therapy.

Therapeutic monitoring

- Obtain pretherapy baseline INR, PT, and PTT; measure PTT regularly. Anticoagulation is present when PTT values are 1½ to 2 times control values.
- Recommend monitoring platelet count and assessing patient regularly for signs and symptoms of abnormal bleeding.

Special populations

Pregnant patients. Heparin doesn't cross the placental barrier. Use heparin with caution during pregnancy, especially during the third trimester and postpartum period because of the increased risks of uteroplacental junction bleeding and maternal hemorrhage. Heparin therapy lasting longer than 1 month during pregnancy may result in maternal osteopenia and osteoporosis.
Breast-feeding patients. Heparin isn't excreted in breast milk.
Pediatric patients. Because of the risk of overdose, avoid heparin lock flush solutions containing heparin sodium 100 mg/ml for use in neonates, especially those with a low birthweight.
Geriatric patients. At least one manufacturer reports a greater risk of hemorrhage in women over age 60. May have increased heparin plasma levels and APTT may be prolonged.

Patient counseling

- Teach injection technique and methods of record-keeping if patient or family will be giving drug.
- Encourage compliance with medication schedule, follow-up appointments, and need for routine monitoring of blood studies; teach patient and family signs of bleeding, and stress importance of immediately reporting first sign of excess bleeding.
- Caution patient against trying to make up missed doses and against use of aspirin, moth-

erwort, red clover, and other OTC or herbal medications.

Instruct patient to inform dentist or other health care providers of his heparin therapy.

Advise consulting prescriber before taking any other drugs, including OTC products.

hepatitis A vaccine, inactivated

Havrix, Vaqta

Pharmacologic classification: vaccine
Therapeutic classification: viral vaccine
Pregnancy risk category C

How supplied

Available by prescription only
Injection: 720 ELISA units (EL.U.)/0.5 ml, 1,440 EL.U./1 ml (Havrix); 25 units/0.5 ml, 50 units/0.5 ml (Vaqta)

Indications and dosages

Immunization against disease caused by hepatitis A virus
Adults: 1,440 EL.U./1 ml (Havrix) I.M. as a single dose. Give booster dose of 1,440 EL.U./1 ml I.M. 6 to 12 months after initial dose. Or 50 units (Vaqta) I.M. and booster dose 6 months after initial dose.
Children age 2 to 18: 720 EL.U./1 ml (Havrix) I.M. as a single dose and booster dose 6 to 12 months after initial dose.
Children age 2 to 17: Single dose of 25 units (Vaqta) I.M. and booster dose 6 to 18 months after initial dose.

Pharmacodynamics

Immunostimulant action: Hepatitis A vaccine, inactivated, promotes active immunity to hepatitis A virus. Immunity isn't permanent or completely predictable.

Pharmacokinetics

No information available.

Route	Onset	Peak	Duration
I.M.	1-15 days	Unknown	6 mo

Contraindications and precautions

Contraindicated hypersensitivity to any component of vaccine. Use cautiously in patients with thrombocytopenia or bleeding disorders or in those taking anticoagulants; bleeding may occur after I.M. injection in these individuals.

Interactions

None significant.

Effects on diagnostic tests

A positive result in the absence of infection may occur in individuals who received hepatitis A vaccine and who are being evaluated by serology to detect IgM anti-HAV.

Adverse reactions

CNS: *malaise, fatigue,* headache, insomnia, photophobia, vertigo.
GI: *anorexia, nausea,* abdominal pain, diarrhea, dysgeusia, vomiting.
Hepatic: jaundice, hepatitis.
Musculoskeletal: arthralgia, myalgia.
Respiratory: pharyngitis, other upper respiratory tract infections.
Skin: pruritus, *rash*, urticaria, *induration, redness, swelling,* hematoma.
Other: *fever,* lymphadenopathy, hypertonic episode, elevation of CK.

Overdose and treatment

No information available.

Clinical considerations

As with any vaccine, administration of hepatitis A vaccine should be delayed, if possible, in patients with febrile illness.

Although anaphylaxis is rare, have epinephrine available to treat this reaction.

If vaccine is administered to immunosuppressed persons or those receiving immunosuppressive therapy, the expected immune response may not be obtained.

There is no data to support routine vaccination of individuals with chronic hepatitis B or C who lack evidence of chronic liver disease.

Persons who should receive the vaccine include people traveling to or living in areas of higher endemicity for hepatitis A (Africa, Asia [except Japan], the Mediterranean basin, Eastern Europe, the Middle East, Central and South America, Mexico, and parts of the Caribbean), military personnel, natives of Alaska and the Americas, persons engaging in high-risk sexual activity, and users of illicit injectable drugs. Also, certain institutional workers, child day-care workers, laboratory workers who handle live hepatitis A virus, and handlers of primate animals may benefit from immunization.

Therapeutic monitoring

Serologic confirmation of immunity isn't necessary.

Special populations

Breast-feeding patients. It's unknown if vaccine is excreted in breast milk. Administer cautiously in breast-feeding women.
Pediatric patients. Vaccine is well tolerated, highly immunogenic, and effective in children age 2 and older.

Patient counseling

Inform patient that vaccine won't prevent hepatitis caused by other agents such as hepatitis B virus, hepatitis C virus, hepatitis E virus, or other pathogens known to infect the liver.

hepatitis B immune globulin, human (HBIG)

H-BIG, Hep-B-Gammagee, HyperHep

Pharmacologic classification: immune serum
Therapeutic classification: hepatitis B prophylaxis
Pregnancy risk category C

How supplied

Available by prescription only
Injection: 1-ml, 4-ml, and 5-ml vials
Prefilled syringe: 0.5 ml

Indications and dosages

Hepatitis B exposure
Adults and children: 0.06 ml/kg I.M. within 7 days after exposure. Repeat 28 days after exposure.
Neonates born to HBsAg-positive women: 0.5 ml I.M. within 12 hours of birth. Initiation of HB vaccination is also indicated.

The American College of Obstetricians and Gynecologists recommends use of HBIG in pregnancy for postexposure prophylaxis. Hepatitis B immune globulin should only be given if clearly needed.

Pharmacodynamics

Prophylactic action: HBIG provides passive immunity to hepatitis B.

Pharmacokinetics

Absorption: Absorbed slowly after I.M. injection. Antibodies to hepatitis B surface antigen (HBsAg) appear in serum within 1 to 6 days, peak within 3 to 11 days, and persist for about 2 to 6 months.
Distribution: Although specific information isn't available, HBIG probably crosses the placenta, as do other immunoglobulins.
Metabolism: No information available.
Excretion: Serum half-life for antibodies to HBsAg is reportedly 21 days.

Route	Onset	Peak	Duration
I.M.	1-6 days	3-11 days	2 mo

Contraindications and precautions

Contraindicated in patients with history of anaphylactic reactions to immune serum or thimerosal allergy.

Interactions

Drug-drug. *Vaccination with live virus vaccines, such as measles, mumps, and rubella:* HBIG may interfere with immune response to vaccination. Administer live virus vaccines 2 weeks before or 3 months after HBIG whenever possible.

Effects on diagnostic tests

None reported.

Adverse reactions

Skin: urticaria, pain, tenderness (at injection site).
Other: ***anaphylaxis, angioedema.***

Overdose and treatment

Manufacturers report the only anticipated manifestation would be injection site pain and tenderness. No treatment has been identified.

Clinical considerations

- Epinephrine solution 1:1,000 should be available to treat allergic reactions.
- Administer drug I.M. only. Severe, even fatal, reactions may occur if administered I.V.
- HBIG may be given simultaneously, but at different sites, with hepatitis B vaccine.
- Store between 36° and 46° F (2° and 8° C). Don't freeze.
- HBIG hasn't been associated with a higher incidence of AIDS. The immune globulin is devoid of HIV. Immune globulin recipients don't develop antibodies to HIV.

Therapeutic monitoring

Monitor patient for adverse reactions.

Special populations

Pregnant patients. It's unknown if drug can cause harm to fetus; use only when potential risk from exposure to hepatitis B infection outweighs potential risk of adverse drug event.
Breast-feeding patients. It's unknown if HBIG is excreted in breast milk.

Patient counseling

- Explain that patient's chances of getting AIDS after receiving HBIG are very small.
- Inform patient that HBIG provides temporary protection against hepatitis B only.
- Tell patient what to expect after vaccination: local pain, swelling, and tenderness at the injection site. Recommend acetaminophen to relieve minor discomfort.
- Encourage patient to promptly report headache, skin changes, or difficulty breathing.

hepatitis B vaccine, recombinant

Engerix-B, Recombivax HB, Recombivax HB Dialysis Formulation

Pharmacologic classification: vaccine
Therapeutic classification: viral vaccine
Pregnancy risk category C

How supplied

Available by prescription only
Injection: 5 mcg HBsAg/0.5 ml (Recombivax

HB pediatric/adolescent formulation); 10 mcg HBsAg/0.5 ml (Engerix-B, pediatric/adolescent injection); 10 mcg HBsAg/ml (Recombivax HB); 20 mcg HBsAg/ml (Engerix-B); 40 mcg HBsAg/ml (Recombivax HB Dialysis Formulation)

Indications and dosages

Immunization against infection from all known subtypes of hepatitis B; primary preexposure prophylaxis against hepatitis B; postexposure prophylaxis (when given with hepatitis B immune globulin)

Engerix-B

Adults age 20 and older: Initially, give 20 mcg (1-ml adult formulation) I.M., followed by a second dose of 20 mcg I.M. 30 days later. Give a third dose of 20 mcg I.M. 6 months after the initial dose.

Neonates and children up to age 19: Initially, give 10 mcg (0.5-ml pediatric/adolescent formulation) I.M., followed by a second dose of 10 mcg I.M. 30 days later. Give a third dose of 10 mcg I.M. 6 months after the initial dose.

Adults undergoing dialysis or receiving immunosuppressant therapy: Initially, give 40 mcg I.M. (divided into two 20-mcg doses and administered at different sites). Follow with a second dose of 40 mcg I.M. in 30 days, a third dose after 2 months, and a final dose of 40 mcg I.M. 6 months after the initial dose.

Note: Alternative dosing schedule in certain populations (neonates born to infected mothers, persons recently exposed to the virus, and travelers to high-risk areas) who may receive the initial vaccine dose (20 mcg for adults and children over age 10, and 10 mcg for neonates and children up to age 10 for this dosing schedule) followed by a second dose in 1 month and the third dose after 2 months. For prolonged maintenance of protective antibody titers, a booster dose is recommended 12 months after the initial dose.

Recombivax HB

Adults age 20 and older: Initially, give 10 mcg (1-ml adult formulation) I.M., followed by a second dose of 10 mcg I.M. 30 days later. Give a third dose of 10 mcg I.M. 6 months after the initial dose.

Neonates and children up to age 19: Initially, give 5 mcg (0.5-ml pediatric/adolescent formulation) I.M., followed by a second dose of 5 mcg I.M. 30 days later. Give a third dose of 5 mcg I.M. 6 months after inital dose.

Neonates born to HBsAg-positive mothers: Initially, give 5 mcg (0.5-ml pediatric/adolescent formulation) I.M. with 0.5 ml hepatitis B immune globulin. Follow with a second dose of 5 mcg I.M. 30 days later. Give a third dose of 5 mcg I.M. 6 months after the initial dose.

Adults undergoing dialysis or receiving immunosuppressant therapy: Initially, give 40 mcg I.M. (1-ml dialysis formulation). Follow with a second dose of 40 mcg I.M. in 30 days, and give a final dose of 40 mcg I.M. 6 months after the initial dose.

Pharmacodynamics

Prophylactic action: Hepatitis B vaccine promotes active immunity to hepatitis B.

Pharmacokinetics

No information available.

Route	Onset	Peak	Duration
I.M.	2 weeks after last dose	> 6 mo	> 3 yr

Contraindications and precautions

Contraindicated in patients hypersensitive to yeast; recombinant vaccines are derived from yeast cultures.

Use cautiously in patients with active infections or compromised cardiac and pulmonary status or in those to whom a febrile or systemic reaction could pose a risk.

Interactions

Drug-drug. *Corticosteroids, immunosuppressants:* May impair the immune response to hepatitis B vaccine. Larger-than-usual doses of vaccine may be necessary to develop adequate circulating antibody levels.

Effects on diagnostic tests

None reported.

Adverse reactions

CNS: headache, dizziness, insomnia, paresthesia, neuropathy, transient malaise.
GI: nausea, pharyngitis, anorexia, diarrhea, vomiting.
Musculoskeletal: arthralgia, myalgia.
Skin: local inflammation, *soreness* (at injection site).
Other: slight fever, flulike symptoms.

Overdose and treatment

No information available.

Clinical considerations

- Have epinephrine solution 1:1,000 available.
- The Centers for Disease Control and Prevention reports that response to hepatitis B vaccine is significantly better after injection into the deltoid rather than the gluteal muscle.
- Hepatitis B vaccine may be administered S.C., but only to persons, such as hemophiliacs and patients with thrombocytopenia, who are at risk of hemorrhage from I.M. injection. Don't administer I.V.
- Hepatitis B vaccine may be given simultaneously, but at different sites, with hepatitis B immune globulin, influenza virus vaccine, *Haemophilus influenzae* type B conjugate vaccine, polyvalent pneumococcal vaccine, or DTP.

Therapeutic monitoring

- Although not necessary for most patients, serologic testing (to confirm immunity to hepatitis B after the three-dose regimen) is recommended for patients over age 50, those at high risk of needlestick injury (who might require postexposure prophylaxis), hemodialysis patients, immunocompromised patients, and those who inadvertently received one or more injections into the gluteal muscle.

Special populations

Pregnant patients. Use drug in pregnant women only when benefits outweigh risks.
Breast-feeding patients. Use drug with caution in breast-feeding women.
Pediatric patients. Routine immunization is recommended for all neonates, regardless of whether the mother tests positive or negative for HBsAg. It's usually well tolerated and highly immunogenic in children and infants of all ages. However, it's most effective in neonates weighing 4.4 lb (2 kg) or more. To minimize cumulative exposure to mercury in infants under age 6 months, especially neonates and those born prematurely, the use of thimerosal-free hepatitis B vaccine is recommended.

Patient counseling

- Tell patient that there's no risk of contracting HIV infection or AIDS from hepatitis B vaccine because it's synthetically derived.
- Explain that hepatitis B vaccine provides protection against hepatitis B only, not against hepatitis A or hepatitis C.
- Tell patient to expect some discomfort at injection site and possible fever, headache, or upset stomach. Recommend acetaminophen to relieve such effects. Encourage patient to report distressing adverse reactions.

hetastarch (HES, hydroxyethyl starch)

Hespan

Pharmacologic classification: amylopectin derivative
Therapeutic classification: plasma volume expander
Pregnancy risk category C

How supplied

Available by prescription only
Injection: 500 ml (6 g/100 ml in normal saline solution)

Indications and dosages

Plasma expander in shock and cardiopulmonary bypass surgery
Adults: 500 to 1,000 ml I.V. dependent on amount of blood lost and resultant hemoconcentration. Total dose usually shouldn't exceed 20 ml/kg, up to 1,500 ml/day. Up to 20 ml/kg (1.2 g/kg)/hour may be used in hemorrhagic shock; in burns or septic shock, rate should be reduced.
Leukapheresis adjunct
Hetastarch is an adjunct in leukapheresis to improve harvesting and increase the yield of granulocytes.
Adults: Hetastarch 250 to 700 ml is infused at a constant fixed ratio, usually 1:8 to venous whole blood during continuous flow centrifugation (CFC) procedures. Up to 2 CFC procedures weekly, with total number of 7 to 10 procedures using hetastarch, have been found safe and effective. Safety of larger numbers of procedures is unknown.

Note: Hetastarch can be used as a priming fluid in pump oxygenators for perfusion during extracorporeal circulation or as a cryoprotective agent for long-term storage of whole blood.

Pharmacodynamics

Plasma volume expanding action: Hetastarch has an average molecular weight of 450,000 and exhibits colloidal properties similar to human albumin. After an I.V. infusion of hetastarch 6%, the plasma volume expands slightly in excess of the volume infused because of the colloidal osmotic effect. Maximum plasma volume expansion occurs in a few minutes and decreases over 24 to 36 hours. Hemodynamic status may improve for 24 hours or longer.
Leukapheresis adjunctive action: Hetastarch enhances yield of granulocytes obtained by centrifugal means.

Pharmacokinetics

Absorption: No information available.
Distribution: Distributed in blood plasma.
Metabolism: Hetastarch molecules larger than 50,000 molecular weight are slowly enzymatically degraded to molecules that can be excreted.
Excretion: 40% of hetastarch molecules smaller than 50,000 molecular weight are excreted in urine within 24 hours. Hetastarch molecules that aren't hydroxyethylated are slowly degraded to glucose. About 90% of dose is eliminated from the body with an average half-life of 17 days; remainder has a half-life of 48 days.

Route	Onset	Peak	Duration
I.V.	Immediate	Immediate	Unknown

Contraindications and precautions

Contraindicated in patients with severe bleeding disorders, severe heart failure, or renal failure with oliguria and anuria.

Interactions

None reported.

Effects on diagnostic tests
None reported

Adverse reactions
CNS: headache.
CV: peripheral edema of lower extremities.
EENT: periorbital edema.
GI: nausea, vomiting.
Musculoskeletal: muscle pain.
Respiratory: wheezing.
Skin: urticaria.
Other: mild fever, chills.

Overdose and treatment
Signs and symptoms of overdose include the adverse reactions listed above. Stop infusion if an overdose occurs and treat supportively.

Clinical considerations
- When added to whole blood, hetastarch increases the erythrocyte sedimentation rate.
- Don't administer as a substitute for blood or plasma.
- Discard partially used bottle because it doesn't contain a preservative.
- Monitor I.V. site for signs of infiltration and phlebitis.

Therapeutic monitoring
- To avoid circulatory overload, carefully monitor patients with impaired renal function and those at high risk of pulmonary edema or heart failure. Hetastarch 6% in normal saline contains 77 mEq sodium and chloride per 500 ml.
- Recommend monitoring CBC, total leukocyte and platelet counts, leukocyte differential count, hemoglobin, hematocrit, PT, PTT, electrolyte, BUN, and creatinine levels.
- Assess vital signs and cardiopulmonary status to obtain baseline at start of infusion to prevent fluid overload.
- Observe patient for edema.

Special populations
Pregnant patients. Hetastarch shouldn't be used in pregnant women, especially during early pregnancy. Drug should be used only when benefit to mother outweighs risk to fetus.
Breast-feeding patients. Discontinue breast-feeding temporarily in women receiving hetastarch.
Pediatric patients. Safety and efficacy in children haven't been established.
Geriatric patients. Use hetastarch with caution in geriatric patients because of the potential for fluid overload; a lower dosage may be sufficient to produce desired plasma volume expansion.

Patient counseling
- Explain use and administration of drug to patient and family.
- Instruct patient to report adverse reactions promptly.

homatropine hydrobromide
AK-Homatropine, I-Homatrine, Isopto Homatropine, Minims Homatropine*

Pharmacologic classification: anticholinergic
Therapeutic classification: cycloplegic, mydriatic
Pregnancy risk category C

How supplied
Available by prescription only
Ophthalmic solution: 2%, 5%

Indications and dosages
Cycloplegic refraction
Adults: Instill 1 to 2 drops of 2% or 1 drop of 5% solution in eye; repeat in 5 to 10 minutes, p.r.n.
Children: Instill 1 drop of 2% solution in the eye; repeat at 10-minute intervals, p.r.n.
Uveitis
Adults: Instill 1 to 2 drops of 2% or 5% solution in eye up to q 3 or 4 hours.
Children: Instill 1 drop of 2% solution b.i.d. or t.i.d.

Pharmacodynamics
Cycloplegic and mydriatic actions: Anticholinergic action prevents the sphincter muscle of the iris and the muscle of the ciliary body from responding to cholinergic stimulation, resulting in unopposed adrenergic influence and producing pupillary dilation (mydriasis) and paralysis of accommodation (cycloplegia).

Pharmacokinetics
Absorption: Unknown.
Distribution: Unknown.
Metabolism: Unknown.
Excretion: Recovery from cycloplegic and mydriatic effects usually occurs within 1 to 3 days.

Route	Onset	Peak	Duration
Ophthalmic	Rapid	40-60 min	1-3 days

Contraindications and precautions
Contraindicated in patients with hypersensitivity to drug or other belladonna alkaloids such as atropine, and in those with glaucoma or those who have adhesions between the iris and lens.

Use cautiously in the elderly and in those with increased ocular pressure.

Interactions
Drug-drug. *Carbachol, cholinesterase inhibitors, pilocarpine:* Interference with the antiglaucoma effects of these drugs.

Effects on diagnostic tests
None reported.

Adverse reactions
CNS: confusion, somnolence, headache.
CV: tachycardia.
EENT: eye irritation, *blurred vision, photophobia,* increased intraocular pressure, transient stinging and burning, conjunctivitis, vascular congestion, edema.
GI: dry mouth.
Skin: dryness, rash.

Overdose and treatment
Signs and symptoms of overdose include flushed dry skin, dry mouth, blurred vision, ataxia, dysarthria, hallucinations, tachycardia, and decreased bowel sounds.

Treat accidental ingestion by emesis or activated charcoal. Use physostigmine to antagonize anticholinergic activity of homatropine in severe toxicity; propranolol may be used to treat symptomatic tachyarrhythmias unresponsive to physostigmine.

Clinical considerations
- Drug may produce symptoms of atropine sulfate poisoning, such as severe mouth dryness and tachycardia.
- Patient may be photophobic and may benefit from wearing dark glasses to minimize discomfort.

Therapeutic monitoring
Monitor patient for adverse reactions and to ascertain therapeutic result.

Special populations
Pediatric patients. Use drug cautiously in young children and infants. There's an increased chance of sensitivity in children with Down syndrome, spastic paralysis, or brain damage. Feeding intolerance may result.
Geriatric patients. Use drug cautiously in geriatric patients because of the potential risk of undiagnosed glaucoma and increased sensitivity to effects of drug.

Patient counseling
- Provide patient with information on correct method of administration.
- Inform patient that vision will be temporarily blurred after instillation, and advise caution when driving or operating machinery.
- Inform patient that drug may produce drowsiness.

hyaluronidase
Wydase

Pharmacologic classification: protein enzyme
Therapeutic classification: adjunctive agent
Pregnancy risk category C

How supplied
Available by prescription only
Injection (lyophilized powder): 150 USP units/vial, 1,500 USP units/vial
Injection (solution): 150 USP units/ml in 1-ml and 10-ml vials

Indications and dosages
Adjunct to increase absorption and dispersion of other injected drugs
Adults and children: Add 150 USP units to solution containing other medication.
Adjunct to increase absorption rate of fluids given by hypodermoclysis
Adults and children: Inject 150 USP units into the rubber tubing close to the needle of the running clysis solution. Generally, 150 USP units will facilitate absorption of 1 L or more of solution; individualize dosage administration and type of solution.
Adjunct in excretory urography
Adults and children: Administer 75 USP units S.C. over each scapula before administration of the contrast medium.

Pharmacodynamics
Diffusing action: Hyaluronidase is a spreading or diffusing substance that modifies the permeability of connective tissue through the hydrolysis of hyaluronic acid. Drug enhances the diffusion of substances injected S.C. as long as local interstitial pressure is adequate.

Pharmacokinetics
No information available.

Route	Onset	Peak	Duration
S.C.	Immediate	Unknown	1-2 days

Contraindications and precautions
Contraindicated in patients with hypersensitivity to drug.

Interactions
Drug-drug. *Local anesthetics:* May increase analgesia, hasten onset, and reduce local swelling, but may also increase systemic absorption, increase toxicity, and shorten duration of action.

Effects on diagnostic tests
None reported.

Adverse reactions
Skin: allergic reactions (rare).

Overdose and treatment
Up to 75,000 units have been administered without ill effect; local adverse effects would be anticipated. Treat symptomatically.

Clinical considerations
- Give skin test for sensitivity before use with an intradermal injection using about 0.02 ml of hyaluronidase solution; a wheal with pseudopods appearing within 5 minutes after injection and lasting for 20 to 30 minutes along with urticaria indicates a positive reaction.
- Because of the potential for allergic reactions, although rare, epinephrine, corticosteroids, and antihistamines should be available for emergency treatment.
- Avoid contact with eyes; if it occurs, flood with water immediately.
- Drug also may be used to diffuse local anesthetics at injection site, especially in nerve block anesthesia. It also has been used to enhance the diffusion of drugs in management of I.V. extravasation.

Therapeutic monitoring
Monitor patient for adverse drug events.

Special populations
Pregnant patients. Use drug during pregnancy only when clearly indicated.
Breast-feeding patients. It's unknown if drug is excreted in breast milk. Use drug with caution in breast-feeding women.
Pediatric patients. If administering drug for hypodermoclysis, take care to avoid overhydration. In children under age 3, clysis shouldn't exceed 200 ml; in premature neonates, clysis shouldn't exceed 25 ml/kg and the rate shouldn't exceed 2 ml/minute.

Patient counseling
Instruct patient to report unusual and significant adverse effects after injection.

hydralazine hydrochloride
Apresoline, Novo-Hylazin

Pharmacologic classification: peripheral vasodilator
Therapeutic classification: antihypertensive
Pregnancy risk category C

How supplied
Available by prescription only
Tablets: 10 mg, 25 mg, 50 mg, 100 mg
Injection: 20 mg/ml

Indications and dosages
Moderate to severe hypertension
Adults: Initially, 10 mg P.O. q.i.d. for 2 to 4 days, then increased to 25 mg q.i.d. for remainder of week. If necessary, increase dosage to 50 mg q.i.d. Maximum recommended dose is 200 mg daily, but some patients may require 300 to 400 mg daily.

For severe hypertension, 10 to 50 mg I.M. or 10 to 20 mg I.V. repeated, p.r.n. Switch to oral antihypertensives as soon as possible.

For hypertensive crisis associated with pregnancy, initially 5 mg I.V., followed by 5 to 10 mg I.V. q 20 to 30 minutes until adequate reduction in blood pressure is achieved (usual range, 5 to 20 mg).
Children: Initially, 0.75 mg/kg P.O. daily in four divided doses (25 mg/ m^2 daily); may increase gradually to 7.5 mg/kg daily.

I.M. or I.V. drug dosage is 0.4 to 1.2 mg/kg daily or 50 to 100 mg/ m^2 daily in four to six divided doses. Initial parenteral dose should not exceed 20 mg.

◇***Management of severe heart failure***
Adults: Initially, 50 to 75 mg P.O., then adjusted according to patient response. Most patients respond to 200 to 600 mg daily, divided q 6 to 12 hours, but doses as high as 3 g daily have been used.

Pharmacodynamics
Antihypertensive action: Hydralazine has a direct vasodilating effect on vascular smooth muscle, thus lowering blood pressure. The effect of hydralazine on resistance vessels (arterioles and arteries) is greater than that on capacitance vessels (venules and veins).

Pharmacokinetics
Absorption: Absorbed rapidly from GI tract after oral administration; peak plasma levels occur in 1 hour; bioavailability is 30% to 50%. Antihypertensive effect occurs 20 to 30 minutes after oral dose, 5 to 20 minutes after I.V. administration, and 10 to 30 minutes after I.M. administration. Food enhances absorption.
Distribution: Distributed widely throughout the body; drug is about 88% to 90% protein-bound.
Metabolism: Metabolized extensively in the GI mucosa and the liver. Hydralazine is subject to polymorphic acetylation. Slow acetylators have higher plasma levels, generally requiring lower doses.
Excretion: Mostly excreted in urine, primarily as metabolites; about 10% of an oral dose is excreted in feces. Antihypertensive effect persists 2 to 4 hours after an oral dose and 2 to 6 hours after I.V. or I.M. administration.

Route	Onset	Peak	Duration
P.O.	20-30 min	1-2 hr	2-4 hr
I.V.	5-20 min	10-80 min	2-6 hr
I.M.	10-30 min	1 hr	2-6 hr

Contraindications and precautions
Contraindicated in patients with hypersensitivity to drug, coronary artery disease, or mitral valvular rheumatic heart disease. Use cautiously in patients with suspected cardiac disease, CVA, or severe renal impairment, and in those receiving other antihypertensive drugs.

Interactions
Drug-drug. *Diuretics and other antihypertensives:* Increased effects of these drugs. Use with caution.
Diazoxide, MAO inhibitors: May cause severe hypotension. Use together cautiously.
Epinephrine: Decreased pressor response. Monitor patient closely.

Effects on diagnostic tests
None reported.

Adverse reactions
CNS: peripheral neuritis, *headache*, dizziness.
CV: orthostatic hypotension, *tachycardia*, edema, angina, *palpitations*.
GI: *nausea, vomiting, diarrhea, anorexia*, constipation.
Hematologic: ***neutropenia, leukopenia, agranulocytosis.***
Skin: rash.
Other: *lupus-like syndrome* (especially with high doses).

Overdose and treatment
Signs and symptoms of overdose include hypotension, tachycardia, headache, and skin flushing; arrhythmias and shock may occur.

After acute ingestion, empty stomach by emesis or gastric lavage and give activated charcoal to reduce absorption. Follow with symptomatic and supportive care.

Clinical considerations
- Incidence of drug-induced systemic lupus erythematosus (SLE) syndrome is greatest in patients receiving more than 200 mg/day for prolonged periods.
- Food enhances oral absorption and helps minimize gastric irritation.
- Some preparations contain tartrazine, which may precipitate allergic reactions, especially in aspirin-sensitive patients.
- Inject drug as soon as possible after draining through needle into syringe; drug changes color after contact with metal.
- Patients with renal impairment may respond to lower maintenance dosages of hydralazine.

Therapeutic monitoring
- Recommend performing CBC, lupus erythematosus (LE) cell preparation, and ANA titer determinations before therapy and at regular intervals during long-term therapy.
- With I.V. administration, recommend monitoring blood pressure every 5 minutes until stable, then every 15 minutes.
- Headache and palpitations may occur 2 to 4 hours after first oral dose but should subside spontaneously.
- Sodium retention can occur with long-term use.

Special populations
Breast-feeding patients. It's unknown if drug is excreted in breast milk. An alternative feeding method is recommended during therapy.
Pediatric patients. Drug has had limited use in children. Safety and efficacy in children haven't been established; use only if potential benefit outweighs risk.
Geriatric patients. Geriatric patients may be more sensitive to antihypertensive effects. Use with special caution in patients with history of stroke or impaired renal function; patients with renal impairment may respond to lower maintenance dosages.

Patient counseling
- Instruct patient that drug should be taken exactly as prescribed, even when feeling well; warn against discontinuing drug suddenly because severe rebound hypertension may occur.
- Explain adverse effects and advise patient to report unusual effects, especially symptoms of SLE (sore throat, fever, rash, and muscle and joint pain).
- Reassure patient that headaches and palpitations occurring 2 to 4 hours after initial dose usually subside spontaneously.
- Instruct patient to report weight gain that exceeds 5 lb (2.3 kg) weekly.
- Warn patient to seek medical approval before taking OTC cold preparations.

hydrochlorothiazide
Apo-Hydro*, Aquazide-H, Diuchlor H*, Esidrix, Hydro-chlor, Hydro-D, HydroDIURIL, Microzide, Mictrin, Neo-Codema*, Novo-Hydrazide*, Oretic, Urozide*

Pharmacologic classification: thiazide diuretic
Therapeutic classification: diuretic, antihypertensive
Pregnancy risk category B

How supplied
Available by prescription only
Capsules: 12.5 mg
Tablets: 25 mg, 50 mg, 100 mg
Solution: 50 mg/5 ml, 100 mg/ml

Indications and dosages

Edema

Adults: Initially, 25 to 200 mg P.O. daily for several days or until dry weight is attained. Maintenance dosage is 25 to 100 mg P.O. daily or intermittently. A few refractory cases may require up to 200 mg daily.

Children under age 6 months: 1 to 2 mg/kg P.O. daily divided b.i.d.

Children over age 6 months: Up to 3 mg/kg P.O. daily divided b.i.d.

Hypertension

Adults: 25 to 50 mg P.O. once daily or in divided doses. Daily dose increased or decreased based on blood pressure.

Pharmacodynamics

Diuretic action: Hydrochlorothiazide increases urinary excretion of sodium and water by inhibiting sodium reabsorption in the cortical diluting tubule of the nephron, thus relieving edema.

Antihypertensive action: Exact mechanism of antihypertensive effect of drug is unknown. It may result partially from direct arteriolar vasodilation and a decrease in total peripheral resistance.

Pharmacokinetics

Absorption: Absorbed from the GI tract; rate and extent of absorption vary with different formulations.

Distribution: Unknown.

Metabolism: None.

Excretion: Excreted unchanged in urine, usually within 24 hours; half-life is 5½ to 14¾ hours.

Route	Onset	Peak	Duration
P.O.	2 hr	4-5 hr	6-12 hr

Contraindications and precautions

Contraindicated in patients with anuria or hypersensitivity to other thiazides or other sulfonamide derivatives. Use cautiously in patients with severely impaired renal or hepatic function or progressive hepatic disease.

Interactions

Drug-drug. *Amphetamine, quinidine, methenamine compounds (such as methenamine mandelate):* Alkaline urine, decreased urinary excretion of some amines, decreased therapeutic efficacy. Monitor patient for drug effect.

Antihypertensive drugs: Increased hypotensive effect; this may be used to therapeutic advantage. Check blood pressure frequently.

Cholestyramine, colestipol: May bind hydrochlorothiazide, preventing its absorption. Give drugs 1 hour apart.

Diazoxide: Increased hyperglycemic, hypotensive, and hyperuricemic effects. Insulin dosage may require adjustment.

Lithium: Reduced renal clearance, elevating serum lithium levels. Reduction in lithium dosage by 50% may be necessary.

Effects on diagnostic tests

Hydrochlorothiazide may interfere with tests for parathyroid function and should be discontinued before such tests.

Adverse reactions

CNS: dizziness, vertigo, headache, paresthesia, weakness, restlessness.

CV: volume depletion and dehydration, orthostatic hypotension, allergic myocarditis, vasculitis.

GI: anorexia, nausea, ***pancreatitis,*** epigastric distress, vomiting, abdominal pain, diarrhea, constipation.

GU: polyuria, frequent urination, ***renal failure,*** interstitial nephritis.

Hematologic: ***aplastic anemia, agranulocytosis, leukopenia, thrombocytopenia,*** hemolytic anemia.

Hepatic: jaundice.

Metabolism: hypokalemia; asymptomatic hyperuricemia; hyperglycemia and impaired glucose tolerance; fluid and electrolyte imbalances, including dilutional hyponatremia, hypochloremia, metabolic alkalosis, hypercalcemia.

Musculoskeletal: muscle cramps.

Respiratory: respiratory distress, pneumonitis.

Skin: dermatitis, photosensitivity, rash, purpura, alopecia.

Other: hypersensitivity reactions; gout; ***anaphylactic reactions.***

Overdose and treatment

Clinical signs of overdose include GI irritation and hypermotility, diuresis, and lethargy, which may progress to coma.

Treatment is mainly supportive; monitor and assist respiratory, CV, and renal function as indicated. Monitor fluid and electrolyte balance. Induce vomiting with ipecac in conscious patient; otherwise, use gastric lavage to avoid aspiration. Don't give cathartics; these promote additional loss of fluids and electrolytes.

Clinical considerations

Recommendations for preparation and use of hydrochlorothiazide are the same as those for all thiazide diuretics.

Therapeutic monitoring

Drug may cause glucose intolerance in some people. Recommend monitoring blood glucose in diabetic patients. May require dose adjustment of insulin or oral antidiabetic medication.

Special populations

Breast-feeding patients. Drug is distributed in breast milk; safety and efficacy in breast-feeding women haven't been established.
Pediatric patients. Drug can be used in pediatric patients; single daily dose of 1mg/kg is recommended.
Geriatric patients. Geriatric and debilitated patients require close observation and may require reduced dosages. They're more sensitive to excess diuresis because of age-related changes in CV and renal function. Excess diuresis promotes orthostatic hypotension, dehydration, hypovolemia, hyponatremia, hypomagnesemia, and hypokalemia.

Patient counseling

- Instruct patient to take drug with food to avoid GI upset, to take drug in morning or early afternoon to avoid nocturia, and to avoid sudden postural changes.
- Encourage patient to use sun block to avoid photosensitivity reactions.
- Tell patient to consult doctor before taking OTC medications.

hydrocortisone (systemic)

Cortef, Cortenema, Hycort*, Hydrocortone

hydrocortisone acetate

Cortifoam

hydrocortisone cypionate

Cortef

hydrocortisone sodium phosphate

Hydrocortone Phosphate

hydrocortisone sodium succinate

A-hydroCort, Solu-Cortef

Pharmacologic classification: glucocorticoid, mineralocorticoid
Therapeutic classification: adrenocorticoid replacement
Pregnancy risk category C

How supplied

Available by prescription only
hydrocortisone
Tablets: 5 mg, 10 mg, 20 mg
Injection: 25 mg/ml, 50 mg/ml suspension
Enema: 100 mg/60 ml
hydrocortisone acetate
Injection: 25 mg/ml, 50 mg/ml suspension
Enema: 10% aerosol foam (provides 90 mg/application)
hydrocortisone cypionate
Oral suspension: 10 mg/5 ml
hydrocortisone sodium phosphate
Injection: 50 mg/ml solution
hydrocortisone sodium succinate
Injection: 100 mg/vial, 250 mg/vial, 500 mg/vial, 1,000 mg/vial

Indications and dosages

Severe inflammation, adrenal insufficiency
hydrocortisone
Adults: 5 to 30 mg P.O. b.i.d., t.i.d., or q.i.d. (as much as 80 mg P.O. q.i.d. may be given in acute situations).
Children: 2 to 8 mg/kg or 60 to 240 mg/ m^2 P.O. daily.
hydrocortisone acetate
Adults: 10 to 75 mg into joints or soft tissue at 2- or 3-week intervals. Dose varies with size of joint. In many cases, local anesthetics are injected with dose.
hydrocortisone sodium phosphate
Adults: 15 to 240 mg S.C., I.M., or I.V. daily in divided doses q 12 hours.
hydrocortisone sodium succinate
Adults: Initially, 100 to 500 mg I.M. or I.V., then 50 to 100 mg I.M. as indicated.
Shock (other than adrenal crisis)
hydrocortisone sodium phosphate
Children: 0.16 to 1 mg/kg I.M. daily or b.i.d.
hydrocortisone sodium succinate
Adults: 100 to 500 mg I.M. or I.V. q 2 to 6 hours.
Children: 0.16 to 1 mg/kg or 6 to 30 mg/ m^2 I.M. or I.V. daily to b.i.d.
Life-threatening shock
hydrocortisone sodium succinate
Adults: 0.5 to 2 g I.V. initially, repeated at 2- to 6-hour intervals, p.r.n. High-dose therapy should be continued only until patient's condition has stabilized. Therapy shouldn't be continued beyond 48 to 72 hours.
Adjunctive treatment of ulcerative colitis and proctitis
hydrocortisone
Adults: One enema (100 mg) nightly for 21 days.
hydrocortisone acetate (rectal foam)
Adults: 90 mg (1 applicatorful) once or twice daily for 2 or 3 weeks; decrease frequency to every other day thereafter.

Pharmacodynamics

Adrenocorticoid replacement action: Hydrocortisone is an adrenocorticoid with both glucocorticoid and mineralocorticoid properties. It's a weak anti-inflammatory agent but a potent mineralocorticoid, having potency similar to that of cortisone and twice that of prednisone. Hydrocortisone (or cortisone) is usually the drug of choice for replacement therapy in patients with adrenal insufficiency. It's usually not used for immunosuppressant activity because of the extremely large doses necessary and unwanted mineralocorticoid effects.

Hydrocortisone and hydrocortisone cypionate may be administered orally. Hydrocortisone sodium phosphate may be administered by I.M., S.C., or I.V. injection or by I.V. infusion, usually at 12-hour intervals. Hydrocortisone sodium succinate may be administered by I.M. or I.V. injection or I.V. infusion every 2 to 10 hours, depending on the clinical situation. Hydrocortisone acetate is a suspension that may be administered by intra-articular, intrasynovial, intrabursal, intralesional, or soft-tissue injection. It has a slow onset but a long duration of action. Injectable forms are usually used only when the oral dosage forms can't be used.

Pharmacokinetics

Absorption: Absorbed readily after oral administration. After oral and I.V. administration, peak effects occur in about 1 to 2 hours. The acetate suspension for injection has a variable absorption over 24 to 48 hours, depending on whether it's injected into an intra-articular space or a muscle, and the blood supply to that muscle.

Distribution: Removed rapidly from the blood and distributed to muscle, liver, skin, intestines, and kidneys. Hydrocortisone is bound extensively to plasma proteins (transcortin and albumin). Only the unbound portion is active. Adrenocorticoids are distributed into breast milk and through the placenta.

Metabolism: Metabolized in the liver to inactive glucuronide and sulfate metabolites.

Excretion: Inactive metabolites and small amounts of unmetabolized drug are excreted by the kidneys. Insignificant quantities of drug are excreted in feces. Biologic half-life of hydrocortisone is 8 to 12 hours.

Route	Onset	Peak	Duration
P.O., I.V., I.M., P.R.	Variable	Variable	Variable

Contraindications and precautions

Contraindicated in patients allergic to any component of the formulation, in those with systemic fungal infections, and in premature infants (with hydrocortisone sodium succinate).

Use hydrocortisone sodium phosphate or succinate cautiously in patients with a recent MI, GI ulcer, renal disease, hypertension, osteoporosis, diabetes mellitus, hypothyroidism, cirrhosis, diverticulitis, ulcerative colitis, recent intestinal anastomosis, thromboembolic disorders, seizures, myasthenia gravis, heart failure, tuberculosis, ocular herpes simplex, emotional instability, and psychotic tendencies.

Interactions

Drug-drug. *Antacids, cholestyramine, colestipol:* Decrease corticosteroid effect by adsorbing the corticosteroid, thereby decreasing the amount absorbed. May require dosage adjustment.

Oral anticoagulants: Decreased effects of oral anticoagulants by unknown mechanisms. Monitor PT and INR.

Barbiturates, phenytoin, rifampin: May decrease corticosteroid effects because of increased hepatic metabolism. May require increased corticosteroid dosage.

Cardiac glycosides: Increased risk of toxicity. Monitor patient closely.

Diuretic or amphotericin B: May result in hypokalemia. Recommend monitoring serum potassium levels.

Estrogens: Reduced metabolism of corticosteroids. Monitor patient for drug effect.

Isoniazid and salicylates: Increased metabolism of these drugs. Monitor patient carefully.

Ulcerogenic drugs (such as NSAIDs): Increased risk of GI ulceration. Avoid use together.

Effects on diagnostic tests

Hydrocortisone suppresses reactions to skin tests, causes false-negative results in nitroblue tetrazolium tests for systemic bacterial infections, and decreases ^{131}I uptake and protein-bound iodine levels in thyroid function tests.

Adverse reactions

Most adverse reactions to corticosteroids are dose- or duration-dependent.

CNS: *euphoria, insomnia,* psychotic behavior, pseudotumor cerebri, vertigo, headache, paresthesia, ***seizures.***

CV: ***heart failure,*** hypertension, edema, ***arrhythmias,*** thrombophlebitis, ***thromboembolism.***

EENT: cataracts, glaucoma.

GI: *peptic ulceration,* GI irritation, increased appetite, *pancreatitis,* nausea, vomiting.

GU: menstrual irregularities.

Metabolic: possible hypokalemia, hyperglycemia (requiring dosage adjustment in diabetics).

Musculoskeletal: muscle weakness, osteoporosis, growth suppression in children.

Skin: delayed wound healing, acne, various skin eruptions, easy bruising.

Other: hirsutism, susceptibility to infections; cushingoid state (moonface, buffalo hump, central obesity), carbohydrate intolerance, ***acute adrenal insufficiency with increased stress (infection, surgery, trauma) or abrupt withdrawal (after long-term therapy).***

After abrupt withdrawal: rebound inflammation, fatigue, weakness, arthralgia, fever, dizziness, lethargy, depression, fainting, orthostatic hypotension, dyspnea, anorexia, hypoglycemia. ***After prolonged use, sudden withdrawal may be fatal.***

Overdose and treatment

Acute ingestion, even in massive doses, is rarely a clinical problem. Toxic signs and symptoms rarely occur if drug is used for less than 3 weeks, even at large doses. However, chronic use causes adverse physiologic effects, including suppression of the hypothalamic-pituitary-adrenal axis, cushingoid appearance, muscle weakness, and osteoporosis.

Clinical considerations
Recommendations for use of hydrocortisone and for care and teaching of patients during therapy are the same as those for all systemic adrenocorticoids.

Therapeutic monitoring
Monitor patient for adverse reactions.

Special populations
Pediatric patients. Long-term use of hydrocortisone in children and adolescents may delay growth and maturation.

Patient counseling
- Caution patient to take medication as directed.
- Inform patient of potential adverse effects and instruct to contact prescriber immediately to report serious adverse events.

hydrocortisone (topical)
Acticort 100, Aeroseb-HC, Ala-Cort, Ala-Scalp, Anusol-HC, Bactine, Barriere-HC*, CaldeCORT, Cetacort, CortaGel, Cortaid, Cortate*, Cort-Dome, Cortizone, Dermacort, DermiCort, Dermolate, Dermtex HC, Emo-Cort*, Hi-Cor, Hydro-Tex, Hytone, LactiCare-HC, Nutracort, Penecort, Rectocort*, S-T Cort, Synacort, Texacort, Unicort*

hydrocortisone acetate
Anusol-HC, CaldeCORT, Cortaid, Cort-Dome, Cortef, Corticaine, Corticreme*, Cortoderm*, Gynecort, Hyderm*, Lanacort, Novohydrocort*, Orabase-HCA, Pharma-Cort, Rhulicort

hydrocortisone buteprate
Pandel

hydrocortisone butyrate
Locoid

hydrocortisone valerate
Westcort

Pharmacologic classification: glucocorticoid
Therapeutic classification: anti-inflammatory
Pregnancy risk category C

How supplied
Available by prescription only
hydrocortisone
Cream: 2.5%
Ointment: 0.5%, 1%, 2.5%
Lotion: 0.25%, 0.5%, 1%, 2%, 2.5%
Gel: 0.5%, 1%
Solution: 0.5%, 1%, 2.5%
Aerosol: 0.5%, 1%
Pledgets (saturated with solution): 0.5%, 1%
hydrocortisone acetate
Cream: 1%
Ointment: 0.5%, 1%
Lotion: 0.5%
Suppositories: 25 mg
Rectal foam: 10%
Paste: 0.5%
Solution: 1%
hydrocortisone buteprate
Cream: 0.1%
hydrocortisone butyrate
Cream, ointment, solution: 0.1%
hydrocortisone valerate
Cream, ointment: 0.2%
Available without a prescription
hydrocortisone
Cream: 0.5%, 1%
hydrocortisone acetate
Cream: 0.5%

Indications and dosages
Inflammation of corticosteroid-responsive dermatoses, including those on face, groin, armpits, and under breasts; seborrheic dermatitis of scalp
Adults and children: Apply cream, lotion, ointment, foam, or aerosol sparingly once daily to q.i.d.
Aerosol
Shake can well. Direct spray onto affected area from a distance of 15 cm (6 inches). Apply for only 3 seconds (to avoid freezing tissues). Apply to dry scalp after shampooing; no need to massage or rub medication into scalp after spraying. Apply daily until acute phase is controlled, then reduce dosage to once to three times weekly, p.r.n., to maintain control.
Rectal administration
Shake can well. Apply once daily or b.i.d. for 2 to 3 weeks, then every other day, p.r.n.
Dental lesions
Adults and children: Apply paste b.i.d. or t.i.d. and h.s.

Pharmacodynamics
Anti-inflammatory action: Hydrocortisone stimulates the synthesis of enzymes needed to decrease the inflammatory response. Hydrocortisone, a corticosteroid secreted by the adrenal cortex, is about 1.25 times more potent an anti-inflammatory agent than equivalent doses of cortisone, but both have twice the mineralocorticoid activity of the other glucocorticoids.

Hydrocortisone 0.5%, 1%, and hydrocortisone acetate 0.5% are available without a prescription for the temporary relief of minor skin irritation, itching, and rashes caused by eczema, insect bites, soaps, and detergents.

Hydrocortisone is also administered rectally as a retention enema for the temporary treatment of acute ulcerative colitis. Hydrocortisone acetate suspension is also available as a rectal suppository or aerosol foam suspension for the temporary treatment of inflammatory conditions of the rectum, such as hemorrhoids, cryptitis, proctitis, and pruritus ani.

Pharmacokinetics

Absorption: Absorption depends on potency of preparation, amount applied, and nature of skin at application site. It ranges from about 1% in areas with a thick stratum corneum (such as the palms, soles, elbows, and knees) to as high as 36% in areas where the stratum corneum is thinnest (face, eyelids, and genitals). Absorption increases in areas of skin damage, inflammation, or occlusion. Some systemic absorption occurs, especially through the oral mucosa.
Distribution: After topical application, drug is distributed throughout the local skin layers. Any drug absorbed into circulation is removed rapidly from the blood and distributed into muscle, liver, skin, intestines, and kidneys.
Metabolism: After topical administration, hydrocortisone is metabolized primarily in the skin. The small amount absorbed into systemic circulation is metabolized primarily in the liver to inactive compounds.
Excretion: Inactive metabolites are excreted by the kidneys, primarily as glucuronides and sulfates, but also as unconjugated products. Small amounts of metabolites are also excreted in feces.

Route	Onset	Peak	Duration
P.R., Topical	Unknown	Unknown	Unknown

Contraindications and precautions

Contraindicated in patients hypersensitive to drug.

Interactions

None significant.

Effects on diagnostic tests

None reported.

Adverse reactions

GU: glucosuria.
Metabolic: hyperglycemia.
Skin: burning, pruritus, irritation, dryness, erythema, folliculitis, hypertrichosis, hypopigmentation, acneiform eruptions, allergic contact dermatitis; *maceration, secondary infection, atrophy, striae, miliaria* (with occlusive dressings).
Other: ***hypothalamic-pituitary-adrenal axis suppression,*** Cushing's syndrome.

Overdose and treatment

No information available.

Clinical considerations

Recommendations for use of hydrocortisone are the same as those for all topical adrenocorticoids.

Therapeutic monitoring

Recommendations for therapeutic monitoring of hydrocortisone are the same as those for all topical adrenocorticoids.

Special populations

Recommendations are the same as those for all topical adrenocorticoids.

Patient counseling

Recommendations are the same as those for all topical adrenocorticoids.

hydromorphone hydrochloride

Dilaudid, Dilaudid-HP, Hydrostat IR

Pharmacologic classification: opioid
Therapeutic classification: analgesic, antitussive
Controlled substance schedule II
Pregnancy risk category C

How supplied

Available by prescription only
Tablets: 1 mg, 2 mg, 3 mg, 4 mg, 8 mg
Oral liquid: 5 mg/5 ml
Injection: 1 mg/ml, 2 mg/ml, 3 mg/ml, 4 mg/ml, 10 mg/ml
Suppository: 3 mg

Indications and dosages

Moderate to severe pain
Adults: 2 to 10 mg P.O. q 3 to 6 hours, p.r.n., or around the clock; or 2 to 4 mg I.M., S.C., or I.V. q 4 to 6 hours, p.r.n., or around the clock (give I.V. dose over 3 to 5 minutes); or 3 mg rectal suppository q 6 to 8 hours, p.r.n., or around the clock. (Give 1 to 14 mg Dilaudid-HP S.C. or I.M. q 4 to 6 hours.)

Note: Give hydromorphone hydrochloride in the smallest effective dose to minimize the development of tolerance and physical dependence. Dose must be individually adjusted based on patient's severity of pain, age, and size.

Cough
Adults: 1 mg P.O. q 3 to 4 hours, p.r.n.
Children age 6 to 12: 0.5 mg P.O. q 3 to 4 hours, p.r.n.

Pharmacodynamics

Antitussive action: Hydromorphone acts directly on the cough center in the medulla, producing an antitussive effect.
Analgesic action: Hydromorphone has analgesic properties related to opiate receptor affinity, and is recommended for moderate to severe pain. There's no intrinsic limit to the analgesic effect of hydromorphone, unlike other opioids.

Pharmacokinetics

Absorption: Well absorbed after oral, rectal, or parenteral administration.
Distribution: Unknown.
Metabolism: Metabolized primarily in the liver, where it undergoes conjugation with glucuronic acid.
Excretion: Excreted primarily in urine as the glucuronide conjugate. Duration of action is 4 to 5 hours.

Route	Onset	Peak	Duration
P.O.	30 min	1½-2 hr	4 hr
I.V.	10-15 min	15-30 min	2-3 hr
I.M.	15 min	½-1 hr	4-5 hr
S.C.	15 min	½-1½ hr	4 hr
P.R.	Unknown	Unknown	4 hr

Contraindications and precautions

Contraindicated in patients with hypersensitivity to drug, intracranial lesions associated with increased intracranial pressure, and whenever ventilator function is depressed, such as in status asthmaticus, COPD, cor pulmonale, emphysema, and kyphoscoliosis.

Use cautiously in geriatric or debilitated patients and in those with hepatic or renal disease, Addison's disease, hypothyroidism, prostatic hyperplasia, or urethral strictures.

Interactions

Drug-drug. *General anesthetics:* Severe CV depression may result. Avoid use together.
Anticholinergics: Use of drug with anticholinergics may cause paralytic ileus. Avoid use together.
Cimetidine: Increases respiratory and CNS depression, causing confusion, disorientation, apnea, or seizures; reduced dosage of hydromorphone is usually required.
Other CNS depressants (narcotic analgesics, general anesthetics, antihistamines, phenothiazines, barbiturates, benzodiazepines, sedative-hypnotics, tricyclic antidepressants, muscle relaxants): Increase respiratory and CNS depression, sedation, and hypotensive effects of drug. Use together with extreme caution.
Narcotic antagonist: Patients who become physically dependent on drug may experience acute withdrawal syndrome. Avoid use together.
Rifampin, phenytoin, digitoxin: Drug accumulation and enhanced effects may result. Monitor patient closely.
Drug-lifestyle. *Alcohol use:* Increases CNS effects of drug. Avoid use together.

Effects on diagnostic tests

Increased biliary tract pressure resulting from contraction of the sphincter of Oddi may interfere with hepatobiliary imaging studies.

Adverse reactions

CNS: *sedation, somnolence, clouded sensorium,* dizziness, *euphoria.*
CV: *hypotension,* bradycardia.
EENT: blurred vision, diplopia, nystagmus.
GI: *nausea, vomiting, constipation,* ileus.
GU: *urine retention.*
Respiratory: ***respiratory depression, bronchospasm.***
Other: induration (with repeated S.C. injections), physical dependence.

Overdose and treatment

The most common signs and symptoms of hydromorphone overdose are CNS depression, respiratory depression, and miosis (pinpoint pupils). Other acute toxic effects include hypotension, bradycardia, hypothermia, shock, apnea, cardiopulmonary arrest, circulatory collapse, pulmonary edema, and seizures.

To treat an acute overdose, first establish adequate respiratory exchange via a patent airway and ventilation as needed; administer a narcotic antagonist (naloxone) to reverse respiratory depression. (Because the duration of action of hydromorphone is longer than that of naloxone, repeated dosing is necessary.) Naloxone shouldn't be given unless patient has clinically significant respiratory or CV depression. Monitor vital signs closely.

If patient is seen within 2 hours of ingestion of an oral overdose, empty the stomach immediately by inducing emesis (ipecac syrup) or using gastric lavage. Use caution to avoid risk of aspiration. Administer activated charcoal via nasogastric tube for further removal of an oral overdose.

Provide symptomatic and supportive treatment (continued respiratory support, correction of fluid or electrolyte imbalance). Monitor laboratory values, vital signs, and neurologic status closely.

Contact the local or regional poison control center for further information.

Clinical considerations

Consider the recommendations relevant to all opioids as well as the following:

- Oral dosage form is particularly convenient for patients with chronic pain because tablets are available in several strengths, enabling patient to adjust his own dosage precisely.

■ Dilaudid-HP, a highly concentrated form (10 mg/ml), may be administered in smaller volumes, preventing discomfort associated with large-volume injections.

Therapeutic monitoring

Monitor patient for adverse reactions and response to dose adjustments.

Special populations

Breast-feeding patients. It's unknown if drug is excreted in breast milk; use with caution in breast-feeding women.
Geriatric patients. Lower doses are usually indicated for geriatric patients because they may be more sensitive to the therapeutic and adverse effects of drug.

Patient counseling

■ Instruct patient to take or ask for drug before pain becomes intense.
■ Warn patient to avoid hazardous activities that require mental alertness.
■ Advise patient to avoid alcohol.

hydroxychloroquine sulfate

Plaquenil Sulfate

Pharmacologic classification: 4-aminoquinoline
Therapeutic classification: antimalarial, anti-inflammatory
Pregnancy risk category C

How supplied

Available by prescription only
Tablets: 200 mg (155 mg base)

Indications and dosages

Suppressive prophylaxis of malarial attacks
Adults: 400 mg of sulfate (310 mg base) P.O. weekly on exactly the same day each week. (Begin 2 weeks before entering the endemic area and continue for 8 weeks after leaving.)
Infants and children: 5 mg, calculated as base per kilogram of body weight (shouldn't exceed the adult dose regardless of weight) on exactly the same day each week. Start 2 weeks before exposure. If unable to do so, give 10 mg base/kg in two divided doses 6 hours apart.
Treatment of acute attack of malaria
Adults: 800 mg (620 mg base) followed by 400 mg (310 mg base) in 6 to 8 hours and 400 mg (310 mg base) on each of 2 consecutive days.
Infants and children: Initial dose, 10 mg base/kg (but not exceeding a single dose of 620 mg base). Second dose, 5 mg base/kg (but not exceeding a single dose of 310 mg base), is given 6 hours after first dose. Third dose, 5 mg base/kg, is given 18 hours after second dose. Fourth dose, 5 mg base/kg, is given 24 hours after third dose.
Lupus erythematosus (chronic discoid and systemic)
Adults: 400 mg P.O. daily or b.i.d., continued for several weeks or months, based on response. Prolonged maintenance dosage is 200 to 400 mg P.O. daily.
◊***Rheumatoid arthritis***
Adults: Initially, 400 to 600 mg P.O. daily. When good response occurs (usually in 4 to 12 weeks), reduce dose by half.

Pharmacodynamics

Antimalarial action: Hydroxychloroquine binds to DNA, interfering with protein synthesis. It also inhibits DNA and RNA polymerases. It's active against asexual erythrocytic forms of *Plasmodium malariae, P. ovale, P. vivax,* and many strains of *P. falciparum.*
Amebicidal action: Mechanism of action is unknown.
Anti-inflammatory action: Mechanism of action is unknown. Drug may antagonize histamine and serotonin and inhibit prostaglandin effects by inhibiting conversion of arachidonic acid to prostaglandin F_2; it may also inhibit chemotaxis of polymorphonuclear leukocytes, macrophages, and eosinophils.

Pharmacokinetics

Absorption: Absorbed readily and almost completely.
Distribution: Bound to plasma proteins. It concentrates in the liver, spleen, kidneys, heart, and brain and is strongly bound in melanin-containing cells.
Metabolism: Metabolized by the liver to desethylchloroquine and desethyl hydroxychloroquine.
Excretion: Most of an administered dose is excreted unchanged in urine. Drug and its metabolites are excreted slowly in urine; unabsorbed drug is excreted in feces. Small amounts of drug may be present in urine for months after it's discontinued. Drug is excreted in breast milk.

Route	Onset	Peak	Duration
P.O.	Unknown	2-4½ hr	Unknown

Contraindications and precautions

Contraindicated in patients with hypersensitivity to drug, in long-term therapy for children, and in patients with retinal or visual field changes or porphyria. Use cautiously in patients with severe GI, neurologic, or blood disorders.

Interactions

Drug-drug. *Digoxin:* May increase serum digoxin levels. Monitor digoxin levels; patient requires close monitoring for signs of digitalis toxicity.

Kaolin or magnesium trisilicate: Decreased absorption of hydroxychloroquine. Give drugs at separate times.
Drug-lifestyle. *Prolonged, unprotected sun exposure:* May cause drug-induced dermatoses. Advise patient to take precautions.

Effects on diagnostic tests
Drug may cause inversion or depression of the T wave or widening of the QRS complex on ECG.

Adverse reactions
CNS: irritability, nightmares, ataxia, ***seizures***, psychosis, vertigo, nystagmus, dizziness, hypoactive deep tendon reflexes, ataxia, lassitude, headache.
EENT: visual disturbances (blurred vision; difficulty in focusing; reversible corneal changes; typically irreversible, sometimes progressive or delayed retinal changes, such as narrowing of arterioles; macular lesions; pallor of optic disk; optic atrophy; visual field defects; patchy retinal pigmentation, commonly leading to blindness), ototoxicity (irreversible nerve deafness, tinnitus, labyrinthitis).
GI: anorexia, abdominal cramps, diarrhea, nausea, vomiting.
Hematologic: ***agranulocytosis, leukopenia, thrombocytopenia, hemolysis (in patients with G6PD deficiency), aplastic anemia.***
Metabolic: weight loss.
Musculoskeletal: skeletal muscle weakness.
Skin: alopecia, bleaching of hair, pruritus, lichen planus eruptions, skin and mucosal pigmentary changes, pleomorphic skin eruptions.

Overdose and treatment
Symptoms of drug overdose may appear within 30 minutes after ingestion and may include headache, drowsiness, visual changes, CV collapse, and seizures followed by respiratory and cardiac arrest.

Treatment is symptomatic. Empty stomach by emesis or lavage. After lavage, activated charcoal in an amount at least five times the estimated amount of drug ingested may be helpful if given within 30 minutes of ingestion.

Ultra-short-acting barbiturates may help control seizures. Intubation may become necessary. Peritoneal dialysis and exchange transfusions may also be useful. Forced fluids and acidification of the urine are helpful after the acute phase.

Clinical considerations
☐ ***ALERT*** Dosage may be discussed in mg or mg-base; be aware of the difference.
- Administer drug immediately before or after meals on the same day each week to minimize gastric distress.
- Drug isn't effective for chloroquine-resistant strains of *P. falciparum*.

Therapeutic monitoring
- Monitor for blurred vision, increased sensitivity to light, hearing loss, pronounced GI disturbances, or muscle weakness.
- Baseline and periodic ophthalmologic examinations are necessary in prolonged or high-dosage therapy.

Special populations
Breast-feeding patients. Safety hasn't been established. Use with caution in breast-feeding women.
Pediatric patients. Children are extremely susceptible to toxicity; monitor closely for adverse effects. Don't use drug for long-term therapy in children and don't exceed recommended dose.

Patient counseling
To prevent drug-induced dermatoses, warn patient to avoid excessive sun exposure.

hydroxyprogesterone caproate
Hylutin, Prodrox

Pharmacologic classification: progestin
Therapeutic classification: progestin, antineoplastic
Pregnancy risk category X

How supplied
Available by prescription only
Injection: 250 mg/ml

Indications and dosages
Amenorrhea and uterine bleeding
Adults: 375 mg I.M. May be repeated at 4-week intervals, if needed. After 4 days of desquamation or if there's no bleeding within 21 days after administration, begin cyclic therapy with an estrogen.
Endometrial cancer
Adults: 1 g I.M. up to seven times weekly for 12 weeks or as indicated. Therapy is discontinued if relapse occurs or if no objective response is seen after 12 weeks of therapy.

Pharmacodynamics
Progestational action: Drug suppresses ovulation, causes thickening of cervical mucus, and induces sloughing of the endometrium. It inhibits growth progression of progestin-sensitive uterine cancer tissue by an unknown mechanism.

Pharmacokinetics
Absorption: Absorbed slowly after I.M. injection.
Distribution: Unknown.

Metabolism: Metabolism is primarily hepatic but is not well characterized.
Excretion: Excretion is primarily renal, but is not well characterized.

Route	Onset	Peak	Duration
I.M.	Unknown	Unknown	14 days

Contraindications and precautions
Contraindicated during pregnancy and in patients with hypersensitivity to drug, thromboembolic disorders, cerebral apoplexy, breast or genital organ cancer, undiagnosed abnormal vaginal bleeding, severe hepatic disease, or missed abortion.

Use cautiously in patients with diabetes mellitus, seizures, migraine, cardiac or renal disease, asthma, mental depression, or impaired liver function.

Interactions
Drug-drug. *Bromocriptine:* May cause amenorrhea or galactorrhea, thus interfering with the action of bromocriptine. Use of these drugs together isn't recommended.

Effects on diagnostic tests
Endocrine and liver function tests shouldn't be considered reliable until the drug has been discontinued for at least 60 days.

Adverse reactions
CNS: depression.
CV: thrombophlebitis, ***thromboembolism, CVA, pulmonary embolism,*** edema.
EENT: exophthalmos, diplopia.
GU: breakthrough bleeding, dysmenorrhea, amenorrhea, cervical erosion, abnormal secretions.
Hepatic: cholestatic jaundice.
Metabolic: changes in weight.
Skin: rash, acne, pruritus, melasma; irritation, pain (at injection site).
Other: breast tenderness, enlargement, or secretion.

Overdose and treatment
No information available.

Clinical considerations
Clinical considerations are the same as those relevant to all progestins.

Therapeutic monitoring
- Monitor diabetic patients during therapy for signs of decreased glucose tolerance.
- Patients receiving drug should have a full physical examination, including a gynecologic examination and a Papanicolaou test, every 6 to 12 months.

Special populations
Pregnant patients. Drug is contraindicated for use in pregnant women.

Breast-feeding patients. Drug is contraindicated for use in breast-feeding women.

Patient counseling
- Warn patient that edema and weight gain are likely.
- Remind patient that normal menstrual cycles may not resume for 2 to 3 months after discontinuing drug therapy.
- Advise patient of potential risks to the fetus if she becomes pregnant during therapy or is inadvertently exposed to drug during the first 4 months of pregnancy.

hydroxyurea
Droxia, Hydrea

Pharmacologic classification: antimetabolite (cell cycle-phase specific, S phase)
Therapeutic classification: antineoplastic
Pregnancy risk category NR

How supplied
Available by prescription only
Capsules: 200 mg, 300 mg, 400 mg, 500 mg

Indications and dosages
Dosage and indications for hydroxyurea may vary. Check current literature for recommended protocol.

Solid tumors
Adults: 80 mg/kg P.O. as a single dose q 3 days; or 20 to 30 mg/kg P.O. as a single daily dose.

Head and neck cancers, excluding the lip
Adults: 80 mg/kg P.O. as a single dose q 3 days.

Resistant chronic myelocytic leukemia
Adults: 20 to 30 mg/kg P.O. as a single daily dose.

Pharmacodynamics
Antineoplastic action: The exact mechanism of the cytotoxic action of hydroxyurea is unclear. Hydroxyurea inhibits DNA synthesis without, however, interfering with RNA or protein synthesis. Drug may act as an antimetabolite, inhibiting the incorporation of thymidine into DNA, and it may also damage DNA directly.

Pharmacokinetics
Absorption: Well absorbed after oral administration. Higher serum levels are achieved if drug is given as a large, single dose rather than in divided doses.
Distribution: Hydroxyurea crosses the blood-brain barrier.
Metabolism: About 50% of an oral dose is degraded in the liver.
Excretion: The remaining 50% is excreted in urine as unchanged drug. The metabolites are

excreted through the lungs as carbon dioxide and in urine as urea.

Route	Onset	Peak	Duration
P.O.	Unknown	2 hr	24 hr

Contraindications and precautions
Contraindicated in patients hypersensitive to drug and with marked bone marrow depression (leukopenia [less than 2,500 WBCs/mm^3], thrombocytopenia [less than 100,000 platelets/ mm^3], or severe anemia).

Use cautiously in patients with impaired renal function. Don't administer to pregnant women or women of childbearing age who may become pregnant unless potential benefit to patient outweighs possible risk to fetus.

Interactions
Drug-drug. *Didanosine, stavudine, indinavir:* Fatal pancreatitis has occurred with concomitant use of these drugs. Avoid use together.
Fluorouracil: Neurotoxicity may occur when these two agents are administered together. Avoid use together.

Effects on diagnostic tests
None reported.

Adverse reactions
CNS: hallucinations, headache, dizziness, disorientation, ***seizures***, malaise.
GI: *anorexia, nausea, vomiting, diarrhea,* stomatitis, constipation, ***fatal pancreatitis.***
GU: increased BUN and serum creatinine levels.
Hematologic: ***leukopenia, thrombocytopenia,*** anemia, *megaloblastosis,* ***bone marrow suppression,*** with rapid recovery (dose-limiting and dose-related).
Skin: rash, alopecia, erythema.
Other: fever, chills.

Overdose and treatment
Signs and symptoms of overdose include myelosuppression, ulceration of buccal and GI mucosa, facial erythema, maculopapular rash, disorientation, hallucinations, and impairment of renal tubular function.

Treatment is usually supportive and includes transfusion of blood components.

Clinical considerations
- Dose modification may be required following other chemotherapy or radiation therapy.
- Auditory and visual hallucinations and blood toxicity increase when decreased renal function exists.
- Avoid all I.M. injections when platelet counts are below 100,000/ mm^3.
- Store capsules in tight container at room temperature. Avoid exposure to excessive heat.
- Drug is currently under investigation for the treatment of sickle cell anemia. Widespread use of drug for this disease isn't recommended because of the potential for toxicity.

Therapeutic monitoring
- Recommend monitoring intake and output levels; patient must remain hydrated.
- Recommend obtaining BUN, uric acid, and serum creatinine levels routinely.
- Drug may exacerbate postirradiation erythema.

Special populations
Pregnant patients. Drug isn't to be administered to pregnant women or women of childbearing age who may become pregnant unless potential benefit to patient outweighs possible risk to fetus.
Breast-feeding patients. It's unknown if drug is excreted in breast milk. However, because of risk of serious adverse reactions, mutagenicity, and carcinogenicity in the infant, breast-feeding isn't recommended.
Pediatric patients. Children may require a lower dosage.
Geriatric patients. Geriatric patients may be more sensitive to effects of drug, requiring a lower dosage.

Patient counseling
- Emphasize importance of continuing drug therapy despite nausea and vomiting.
- Encourage daily fluid intake of 10 to 12 8-oz glasses to increase urine output and facilitate excretion of uric acid.
- Advise patient of potential for adverse reactions and instruct to report immediately postdose vomiting, and unusual bruising or bleeding.
- Advise patient to avoid exposure to people with infections and to report signs of infection immediately.

hydroxyzine hydrochloride
Anxanil, Apo-Hydroxyzine*, Atarax, Hydroxacen, Hyzine-50, Multipax*, Novo-Hydroxyzin*, Quiess, Vistacon, Vistazine-50

hydroxyzine pamoate
Vistaril

Pharmacologic classification: antihistamine (piperazine derivative)
Therapeutic classification: antianxiety, sedative, antipruritic, antiemetic, antispasmodic
Pregnancy risk category C

How supplied
Available by prescription only
hydroxyzine hydrochloride
Capsules: 10 mg, 25 mg, 50 mg

Tablets: 10 mg, 25 mg, 50 mg, 100 mg
Syrup: 10 mg/5 ml
Injection: 25 mg/ml, 50 mg/ml
hydroxyzine pamoate
Capsules: 25 mg, 50 mg, 100 mg
Oral suspension: 25 mg/5 ml

Indications and dosages

Anxiety, tension, hyperkinesia
Adults: 50 to 100 mg P.O. q.i.d.
Children over age 6: 50 to 100 mg P.O. daily in divided doses.
Children under age 6: 50 mg P.O. daily in divided doses.
Preoperative and postoperative adjunctive sedation, to control emesis, adjunct to asthma treatment
Adults: 25 to 100 mg I.M. q 4 to 6 hours.
Children: 1.1 mg/kg I.M. q 4 to 6 hours.

Pharmacodynamics

Anxiolytic and sedative actions: Hydroxyzine produces its sedative and antianxiety effects through suppression of activity at subcortical levels; analgesia occurs at high doses.
Antipruritic action: Drug is a direct competitor of histamine for binding at cellular receptor sites.
Other actions: Hydroxyzine is used as a preoperative and postoperative adjunct for its sedative, antihistaminic, and anticholinergic activity.

Pharmacokinetics

Absorption: Absorbed rapidly and completely after oral administration. Peak serum levels occur within 2 to 4 hours. Sedation and other clinical effects are usually noticed in 15 to 30 minutes.
Distribution: Not well understood.
Metabolism: Metabolized almost completely in the liver.
Excretion: Metabolites are excreted primarily in urine; small amounts of drug and metabolites are found in feces. Half-life of drug is 3 hours. Sedative effects can last for 4 to 6 hours, and antihistaminic effects can persist for up to 4 days.

Route	Onset	Peak	Duration
P.O.	15-30 min	2 hr	4-6 hr
I.M.	Unknown	Unknown	4-6 hr

Contraindications and precautions

Contraindicated in patients hypersensitive to drug and during early pregnancy.

Use cautiously with adjustments in dosage in geriatric or debilitated patients.

Interactions

Drug-drug. *Other anticholinergic drugs:* Cause additive anticholinergic effects. Monitor patient closely.
Barbiturates, opioids, tranquilizers, other CNS depressants: Increased CNS effects. Reduce dose of CNS depressants by 50%.
Epinephrine: Concurrent use blocks vasopressor action. If a vasoconstrictor is needed, use norepinephrine or phenylephrine.
Drug-lifestyle. *Alcohol use:* Additive effects. Advise patient to avoid alcohol use.

Effects on diagnostic tests

Drug therapy causes falsely elevated urinary 17-hydroxycorticosteroid levels. It also may cause false-negative skin allergen tests by attenuating or inhibiting the cutaneous response to histamine.

Adverse reactions

CNS: *drowsiness,* involuntary motor activity.
GI: *dry mouth.*
Other: marked discomfort at I.M. injection site, ***hypersensitivity reactions*** (wheezing, dyspnea, chest tightness).

Overdose and treatment

Signs and symptoms of overdose include excessive sedation and hypotension; seizures may occur.

Treatment is supportive only. For recent oral ingestion, empty gastric contents through emesis or lavage. Correct hypotension with fluids and vasopressors (phenylephrine or metaraminol). Don't give epinephrine because hydroxyzine may counteract its effect.

Clinical considerations

Carefully review patient's drug sensitivities and the use of CNS depressants for potential dose adjustments.

Therapeutic monitoring

Observe patient for excessive sedation, especially if he's receiving other CNS depressants.

Special populations

Pregnant patients. Drug isn't to be used during early pregnancy because of potential risk to the fetus. Safety and efficacy in pregnant women haven't been determined.
Breast-feeding patients. It's unknown if drug is excreted in breast milk. Safety hasn't been established in breast-feeding women.
Geriatric patients. Geriatric patients may experience greater CNS depression and anticholinergic effects. Lower doses are indicated.

Patient counseling

- Advise patient to avoid tasks that require mental alertness or physical coordination until CNS effects of drug are known.
- Advise patient against use of other CNS depressants with hydroxyzine unless prescribed. Advise him to avoid alcohol and alcohol-containing products.

■ Instruct patient to seek medical approval before taking OTC cold or allergy preparations that contain antihistamine, which may potentiate the effects of hydroxyzine.

hyoscyamine
Cystospaz

hyoscyamine sulfate
Anaspaz, Cystospaz-M, Levsin, Levsin Drops, Levsinex Timecaps, Neoquess

Pharmacologic classification: belladonna alkaloid
Therapeutic classification: anticholinergic
Pregnancy risk category C

How supplied
Available by prescription only
hyoscyamine
Tablets: 0.15 mg
hyoscyamine sulfate
Tablets: 0.125 mg
Capsules (extended-release): 0.375 mg
Tablets (extended-release): 0.375 mg
Oral solution: 0.125 mg/ml
Elixir: 0.125 mg/5 ml
Injection: 0.5 mg/ml

Indications and dosages
GI tract disorders caused by spasm; adjunctive therapy for peptic ulcers
Adults: 0.125 to 0.25 mg P.O. or S.L. q.i.d. before meals and h.s.; 0.375 to 0.75 mg P.O. (extended-release form) q 12 hours; or 0.25 to 0.5 mg I.M., I.V., or S.C. q 4 hours b.i.d. to q.i.d. (Substitute oral medication when symptoms are controlled.)
Children age 2 to 12: 0.033 mg at about 22 lb (10 kg); at about 44 lb (20 kg), 0.0625 mg; at about 88 lb (40 kg), 0.0938 mg; at about 110 lb (50 kg), 0.125 mg. May repeat q 4 hours, p.r.n. Maximum dose 0.75 mg/day.
Children under age 2: 0.0125 mg at about 5 lb (2.3 kg); at about 7.5 lb (3.4 kg), 0.0167 mg; at about 11 lb (5 kg), 0.02 mg; at about 15 lb (6.8 kg), 0.025 mg; at about 22 lb (10 kg), 0.033 mg; at about 33 lb (15 kg), 0.05 mg. May repeat q 4 hours, p.r.n. Maximum daily doses 0.075 mg, 0.1 mg, 0.125 mg, 0.15 mg, 0.2 mg, and 0.275 mg, respectively.
Endoscopy or hypotonic duodenography
Adults: 0.25 to 0.5 mg I.V., I.M., or S.C., 5 to 10 minutes before procedure.
Preoperative medication
Adults and children over age 2: 5 mcg/kg I.V., I.M., or S.C. 30-60 minutes prior to induction of anesthesia.

Pharmacodynamics
Antispasmodic and antiulcer action: Hyoscyamine competitively blocks acetylcholine at cholinergic neuroeffector sites, decreasing GI motility and inhibiting gastric acid secretion.

Pharmacokinetics
Absorption: Well absorbed when taken orally.
Distribution: Well distributed throughout the body and crosses the blood-brain barrier. About 50% of dose binds to plasma proteins.
Metabolism: Metabolized in the liver. Usual duration of effect is up to 4 hours with standard oral and parenteral administration and up to 12 hours for the extended-release preparation.
Excretion: Excreted in the urine.

Route	Onset	Peak	Duration
P.O.	20-30 min	½-1 hr	4-12 hr
P.O. (extended)	20-30 min	40-90 min	12 hr
I.V.	2 min	15-30 min	4 hr
I.M., S.C.	Unknown	15-30 min	4-12 hr
S.L.	5-20 min	½-1 hr	4 hr

Contraindications and precautions
Contraindicated in patients with glaucoma, obstructive uropathy, obstructive disease of the GI tract, severe ulcerative colitis, myasthenia gravis, hypersensitivity to anticholinergics, paralytic ileus, intestinal atony, unstable CV status in acute hemorrhage, or toxic megacolon.

Use cautiously in patients with autonomic neuropathy, hyperthyroidism, coronary artery disease, arrhythmias, heart failure, hypertension, hiatal hernia with reflux esophagitis, hepatic or renal disease, and ulcerative colitis. Also use cautiously in hot or humid environments where drug-induced heat stroke can occur.

Interactions
Drug-drug. *Amantadine:* Increased anticholinergic effects. Avoid use together.
Antacids, antidiarrheals: Decrease absorption of hyoscyamine. Hyoscyamine should be taken 1 hour before these agents.
Haloperidol or phenothiazines: Reduced antipsychotic effectiveness. Monitor patient carefully.
Phenothiazines: Increase adverse anticholinergic effects of hyoscyamine. Avoid use together.
Drug-herb. *Jimson weed:* May adversely effect CV function. Avoid use together.

Effects on diagnostic tests
None reported.

Adverse reactions

CNS: headache, insomnia, drowsiness, dizziness, nervousness, weakness; *confusion, excitement* (in geriatric patients).
CV: *palpitations,* tachycardia.
EENT: *blurred vision,* mydriasis, increased intraocular pressure, cycloplegia, photophobia.
GI: *dry mouth,* dysphagia, *constipation,* heartburn, loss of taste, nausea, vomiting, *paralytic ileus.*
GU: *urinary hesitancy, urine retention,* impotence.
Skin: urticaria, decreased sweating or possible anhidrosis, other dermal manifestations.
Other: fever, allergic reactions.

Overdose and treatment

Signs and symptoms of overdose include curare-like symptoms, such as respiratory paralysis; central stimulation followed by depression; and such psychotic symptoms as disorientation, confusion, hallucinations, delusions, anxiety, agitation, and restlessness. Peripheral effects may include dilated, nonreactive pupils; blurred vision; flushed, hot, dry skin; dryness of mucous membranes; dysphagia; decreased or absent bowel sounds; urine retention, hyperthermia; headache; tachycardia; hypertension; and increased respiration.

Treatment is primarily symptomatic and supportive, as needed. Maintain patent airway. If patient is alert, induce emesis (or use gastric lavage) and follow with a saline cathartic and activated charcoal to prevent further drug absorption. In severe cases, physostigmine may be administered to block antimuscarinic effects. Give fluids, as needed, to treat shock; diazepam to control psychotic symptoms; and pilocarpine (instilled into the eyes) to relieve mydriasis. If urine retention occurs, catheterization may be necessary.

Clinical considerations

- Consider the recommendations relevant to all anticholinergics.
- Hyoscyamine is administered P.O. Hyoscyamine sulfate usually is administered P.O. or S.L., but may be given I.V., I.M., or S.C. when therapeutic effect is needed or if oral administration isn't possible.

Therapeutic monitoring

Drug regimen is adjusted based on patient's response and tolerance.

Special populations

Breast-feeding patients. Drug may be excreted in breast milk, possibly resulting in infant toxicity. Avoid use in breast-feeding women. Drug may also decrease milk production.
Pediatric patients. Safety and efficacy for use in children haven't been reported.
Geriatric patients. Use drug cautiously in geriatric patients; lower doses are indicated.

Patient counseling

- Advise patient to avoid driving or performing other hazardous activities if drowsiness, dizziness, or blurred vision occurs.
- Advise patient to avoid using jimsonweed with hyoscyamine.
- Tell patient to drink fluids to avoid constipation.
- Instruct patient to report rash or other skin eruptions.
- Advise patient that extended-release tablets may not completely disintegrate and table fragments may be excreted in stools in some patients.
- Tell patient not to crush or chew extended-release tablets.

I

ibuprofen
Advil, Children's Advil, Medipren, Motrin, Motrin IB, Nuprin, PediaProfen, Rufen, Trendar

Pharmacologic classification: NSAID
Therapeutic classification: nonnarcotic analgesic, antipyretic, anti-inflammatory
Pregnancy risk category B (D, in third trimester)

How supplied
Available without a prescription
Tablets: 100 mg, 200 mg
Tablets (chewable): 50 mg, 100 mg
Oral suspension: 100 mg/5 ml
Available by prescription only
Tablets: 100 mg, 300 mg, 400 mg, 600 mg, 800 mg
Oral suspension: 100 mg/5 ml
Oral drops: 40 mg/ml

Indications and dosages
Arthritis, gout, and postextraction dental pain
Adults: 300 to 800 mg P.O. t.i.d. or q.i.d. Don't exceed 3,200 mg as total daily dose.
Primary dysmenorrhea
Adults: 400 mg P.O. q 4 to 6 hours.
Mild to moderate pain
Adults: 400 mg P.O. q 4 to 6 hours.
Children: 10 mg/kg P.O. q 6 to 8 hours; maximum dose, 40 mg/kg.
Juvenile arthritis
Children: 20 to 40 mg/kg/day P.O., divided into three or four doses. For mild disease, 20 mg/kg/day in divided doses.
Fever reduction
Adults: 200 to 400 mg P.O. q 4 to 6 hours, p.r.n. Don't exceed 1,200 mg/day or take more than 3 days.
Children age 6 months to 12 years: 5 mg/kg P.O. q 6 to 8 hours, p.r.n., if baseline temperature is 102.5° F (39.2° C) or below; 10 mg/kg P.O. q 6 to 8 hours, p.r.n., if baseline temperature is more than 102.5° F. Recommended daily maximum dose, 40 mg/kg.

Pharmacodynamics
Analgesic, antipyretic, and anti-inflammatory actions: Mechanisms of action are unknown; ibuprofen is thought to inhibit prostaglandin synthesis.

Pharmacokinetics
Absorption: Part of oral dose (80%) is absorbed from GI tract.
Distribution: Highly protein-bound.
Metabolism: Undergoes biotransformation in the liver.
Excretion: Excreted mainly in urine, with some biliary excretion. Plasma half-life ranges from 2 to 4 hours.

Route	Onset	Peak	Duration
P.O.	Variable	Variable	Variable

Contraindications and precautions
Contraindicated in patients with hypersensitivity to drug or in those who have the syndrome of nasal polyps, angioedema, and bronchospastic reaction to aspirin or other NSAIDs.

Use cautiously in patients with impaired renal or hepatic function, GI disorders, peptic ulcer disease, cardiac decompensation, hypertension, or known coagulation defects. Because chewable tablets contain aspartame, use cautiously in patients with phenylketonuria. Ibuprofen is contraindicated during the last trimester of pregnancy because it may cause problems with the fetus, or complications during delivery.

Interactions
Drug-drug. *ACE inhibitors:* Reduced response when used together; may result in acute reduction in renal function. Monitor patient closely.
Antacids: May decrease the absorption of ibuprofen. Patient should take drugs at separate times.
Anticoagulants, thrombolytic drugs (coumarin derivatives, heparin, streptokinase, urokinase): Increased anticoagulant effects. Dosage adjustment may be needed. Monitor coagulation studies.
Aspirin, carbenicillin, cefamandole, cefoperazone, dextran, dipyridamole, mezlocillin, piperacillin, plicamycin, salicylates, sulfinpyrazone, ticarcillin, valproic acid, corticosteroids, or other anti-inflammatory agents: Increased risk of bleeding or adverse GI reactions. Avoid use together.
Aspirin: May decrease the bioavailability of ibuprofen. Monitor patient for drug effect.
Coumarin derivatives, nifedipine, phenytoin, verapamil: Toxicity may occur with concurrent use; avoid use together.

Diuretics, antihypertensives: Concurrent use may decrease effectiveness of these drugs; diuretics may increase nephrotoxicity. Monitor patient closely.
Gold compounds, other anti-inflammatory agents, or acetaminophen: Increased nephrotoxicity may occur. Use with caution.
Insulin or oral antidiabetic agents: May potentiate hypoglycemic effects. Dosage adjustment may be needed.
Lithium, methotrexate: Decreased renal clearance of these drugs. Use together cautiously.

Effects on diagnostic tests
None reported.

Adverse reactions
CNS: *headache, dizziness,* nervousness, aseptic meningitis.
CV: *peripheral edema,* fluid retention, edema.
EENT: *tinnitus.*
GI: *epigastric distress, nausea, occult blood loss, peptic ulceration,* diarrhea, constipation, dyspepsia, flatulence, heartburn, decreased appetite.
GU: ***acute renal failure,*** azotemia, cystitis, hematuria.
Hematologic: prolonged bleeding time, anemia, ***neutropenia, pancytopenia, thrombocytopenia, aplastic anemia, leukopenia, agranulocytosis.***
Hepatic: elevated enzymes.
Respiratory: ***bronchospasm.***
Skin: pruritus, *rash,* urticaria, ***Stevens-Johnson syndrome.***

Overdose and treatment
Signs and symptoms of overdose include dizziness, drowsiness, paresthesia, vomiting, nausea, abdominal pain, headache, sweating, nystagmus, apnea, and cyanosis.

To treat drug overdose, empty stomach immediately by inducing emesis with ipecac syrup or by gastric lavage. Administer activated charcoal via nasogastric tube. Provide symptomatic and supportive measures (respiratory support and correction of fluid and electrolyte imbalances). Monitor laboratory parameters and vital signs closely. Alkaline diuresis may enhance renal excretion. Dialysis is of minimal value because ibuprofen is strongly protein-bound.

Clinical considerations
Consider the recommendations relevant to all NSAIDs as well as the following:
- Maximum results in arthritis may require 1 to 2 weeks of continuous therapy with ibuprofen. Improvement may be seen, however, within 7 days.
- Administer drug on an empty stomach, 1 hour before or 2 hours after meals for maximum absorption. However, it may be administered with meals to lessen GI upset.

Therapeutic monitoring
- Monitor auditory and ophthalmic functions periodically during ibuprofen therapy.
- Monitor cardiopulmonary status closely; monitor vital signs, especially heart rate and blood pressure.
- Observe for possible fluid retention.

Special populations
Pregnant patients. Drug shouldn't be used in third trimester unless specifically directed by a doctor.
Breast-feeding patients. Drug doesn't enter breast milk in significant quantities. However, manufacturer recommends alternative feeding methods during ibuprofen therapy.
Pediatric patients. Safety and efficacy in children under age 6 months haven't been established.
Geriatric patients. Patients over age 60 may be more susceptible to the toxic effects of ibuprofen, especially adverse GI reactions. Use lowest possible effective dose. The effect of drug on renal prostaglandins may cause fluid retention and edema, a significant drawback for geriatric patients, especially those with heart failure.

Patient counseling
- Instruct patient to seek medical approval before taking OTC medications.
- Advise patient not to self-medicate with ibuprofen for longer than 10 days for analgesic use and not to exceed maximum dose of six tablets (1.2 g) daily for self-medication. Caution patient not to take drug if fever lasts longer than 3 days, unless prescribed.
- Tell patient to report adverse reactions; they're usually dose-related.
- Instruct patient in safety measures to prevent injury. Caution him to avoid hazardous activities that require mental alertness until CNS effects of drug are known.
- Encourage patient to adhere to prescribed drug regimen and stress importance of medical follow-up.

ibutilide fumarate
Corvert

Pharmacologic classification: ibutilide derivative
Therapeutic classification: supraventricular antiarrhythmic
Pregnancy risk category C

How supplied
Available by prescription only
Injection: 0.1 mg/ml

Indications and dosages

Rapid conversion of atrial fibrillation or atrial flutter of recent onset to sinus rhythm

Adults weighing 132 lb (60 kg) or more: 1 mg I.V. over 10 minutes.

Adults weighing below 132 lb: 0.01 mg/kg I.V. over 10 minutes.

Note: Stop infusion if arrhythmia is terminated or if sustained or nonsustained ventricular tachycardia or marked prolongation of QT or QTc interval occurs. If arrhythmia doesn't terminate within 10 minutes after infusion ends, a second 10-minute infusion of equal strength may be administered.

Pharmacodynamics

Antiarrhythmic action: An antiarrhythmic drug with predominantly class III properties, ibutilide prolongs action potential duration in isolated cardiac myocytes and increases both atrial and ventricular refractoriness.

Pharmacokinetics

Absorption: Only given I.V.

Distribution: Highly distributed and about 40% protein-bound.

Metabolism: Not clearly defined.

Excretion: Excreted mainly in urine with the rest in feces; half-life of drug is about 6 hours.

Route	Onset	Peak	Duration
I.V.	Unknown	Unknown	Unknown

Contraindications and precautions

Contraindicated in patients with hypersensitivity to drug or its components and history of polymorphic ventricular tachycardia, such as torsades de pointes.

Use cautiously in patients with hepatic or renal dysfunction.

Interactions

Drug-drug. *Class Ia antiarrhythmic drugs (disopyramide, quinidine, procainamide) and other class III drugs (amiodarone, sotalol):* Increase the potential for prolonged refractoriness. Avoid concurrent administration and for at least five half-lives before administration of ibutilide and for 4 hours after ibutilide dosing. Supraventricular arrhythmias may mask the cardiotoxicity associated with excessive digoxin levels. Use cautiously.

Phenothiazines, tricyclic antidepressants, tetracyclic antidepressants, H_1-receptor antagonist antihistamines, and other drugs that prolong QT interval: Increase the risk for proarrhythmia. Patient requires ECG monitoring.

Effects on diagnostic tests

None reported.

Adverse reactions

CNS: headache.

CV: ventricular extrasystoles, nonsustained ventricular tachycardia, hypotension, bundle branch block, ***sustained ventricular tachycardia,*** AV block, hypertension, QT-segment prolongation, *bradycardia,* palpitation, tachycardia.

GI: nausea.

Overdose and treatment

Overdose could exaggerate the expected prolongation of repolarization seen at usual clinical doses. Treatment should be supportive and appropriate for the condition.

Clinical considerations

- Proper equipment and facilities, including cardiac monitoring, intracardiac pacing facilities, cardioverter-defibrillator, and medication for treatment of sustained ventricular tachycardia, should be available during and after drug administration.
- Hypokalemia and hypomagnesemia should be corrected before therapy begins to reduce the potential for proarrhythmia.
- Admixtures of the product, with approved diluents, are chemically and physically stable for 24 hours at room temperature and for 48 hours at refrigerated temperatures.

Therapeutic monitoring

- Patients with atrial fibrillation of more than 2 to 3 days' duration must be given adequate anticoagulants, generally for at least 2 weeks.
- Monitor patient's ECG continuously throughout drug administration and for at least 4 hours afterward or until QTc interval has returned to baseline because drug can induce or worsen ventricular arrhythmias in some patients. Longer monitoring is required if arrhythmic activity is noted.

Special populations

Breast-feeding patients. It's unknown if drug is excreted in breast milk; discourage breast-feeding during drug therapy.

Pediatric patients. Safety and efficacy in children under age 18 haven't been established.

Patient counseling

- Tell patient to report adverse reactions at once.
- Instruct patient to report discomfort at I.V. injection site.

idarubicin

Idamycin

Pharmacologic classification: antibiotic antineoplastic
Therapeutic classification: antineoplastic
Pregnancy risk category D

How supplied

Available by prescription only
Injection: 5 mg, 10 mg, 20 mg (lyophilized powder) in single-dose vials with 50-, 100-, or 200-mg lactose

Indications and dosages

Treatment of acute myelocytic leukemia in adults, including French-American-British classifications M1 through M7, in combination with other approved antileukemic agents

Adults: 12 mg/m^2 daily by slow I.V. injection (over 10 to 15 minutes) for 3 days. Administer in combination with cytarabine 100 mg/m^2 daily by continuous infusion for 7 days, or give cytarabine as a 25-mg/m^2 bolus followed by 200 mg/m^2 daily by continuous I.V. infusion for 5 days. A second course may be administered if needed.

≡ ***Dosage adjustment.*** If patient experiences severe mucositis, delay administration until recovery is complete and reduce dosage by 25%. Also, reduce dosage in patients with hepatic or renal impairment. Idarubicin shouldn't be given if bilirubin level is more than 5 mg/dl.

Dosage and indications may vary. Check current literature for recommended protocol.

Pharmacodynamics

Antineoplastic action: Idarubicin inhibits nucleic acid synthesis by intercalation and interacts with the enzyme topoisomerase II. It's highly lipophilic, which results in an increased rate of cellular uptake.

Pharmacokinetics

Absorption: Peak cellular levels are achieved within minutes of I.V. injection.
Distribution: Highly lipophilic and excessively tissue-bound (97%), with highest levels in nucleated blood and bone marrow cells. Its metabolite, idarubicinol, is detected in CSF; clinical significance of this is under evaluation.
Metabolism: Extensive extrahepatic metabolism is indicated. Metabolite has cytotoxic activity.
Excretion: Excreted predominantly by biliary excretion as its metabolite and, to a lesser extent, by renal elimination. Mean terminal half-life is 22 hours (range, 4 to 46 hours) when used as a single agent and 20 hours (range, 7 to 38 hours) when combined with cytarabine. Plasma levels of metabolite are sustained for longer than 8 days.

Route	Onset	Peak	Duration
I.V.	Unknown	Unknown	Unknown

Contraindications and precautions

No known contraindications. Use cautiously in patients with impaired renal or hepatic function and in those with bone marrow suppression induced by previous drug therapy or radiation therapy.

Interactions

None reported.

Effects on diagnostic tests

None reported.

Adverse reactions

CNS: *headache, changed mental status,* peripheral neuropathy, ***seizures.***
CV: ***heart failure,*** atrial fibrillation, chest pain, ***MI,*** asymptomatic decline in left ventricular ejection fraction, ***myocardial insufficiency, arrhythmias, hemorrhage, myocardial toxicity.***
GI: *nausea, vomiting, cramps, diarrhea, mucositis,* ***severe enterocolitis with perforation*** (rare).
GU: decreased renal function.
Hematologic: ***myelosuppression.***
Hepatic: changes in hepatic function.
Skin: *alopecia, rash, urticaria, bullous erythrodermatous rash on palms and soles,* hives (at injection site), erythema (at previously irradiated sites), tissue necrosis at injection site (if extravasation occurs).
Other: INFECTION, *fever,* hyperuricemia, hypersensitivity reactions.

Overdose and treatment

Severe and prolonged myelosuppression and possibly increased severity of GI toxicity are anticipated. Supportive treatment, including platelet transfusions, antibiotics, and treatment of mucositis, is required. Acute cardiac toxicity with severe arrhythmias and delayed cardiac failure may also occur. Peritoneal dialysis or hemodialysis isn't effective.

Clinical considerations

- Idarubicin shouldn't be mixed with other drugs unless specific compatibility data are available. Heparin causes precipitation. Degradation occurs with prolonged contact with alkaline solutions.
- Hyperuricemia may result from rapid lysis of leukemic cells; take appropriate preventive measures (including adequate hydration) before starting treatment.
- Systemic infections should be controlled before therapy begins.

▪ If extravasation or signs of extravasation occur, discontinue the infusion immediately and restart in another vein. Treat the site with intermittent ice packs for 30 minutes four times daily for 4 days.
▪ Follow usual chemotherapy mixing precautions. Vial is under negative pressure.
▪ Reconstituted solutions are stable for 3 days (72 hours) at room temperature (59° to 86° F [15° to 30° C]); 7 days, if refrigerated. Discard unused solutions appropriately.

Therapeutic monitoring
Frequently monitor CBC and hepatic and renal function.

Special populations
Breast-feeding patients. It's unknown if idarubicin is excreted in breast milk. To avoid risk of serious adverse reactions in the infant, discontinue breast-feeding before starting therapy with idarubicin.
Pediatric patients. Safety and efficacy in children haven't been established.

Patient counseling
▪ Instruct patient to recognize signs and symptoms of extravasation and to report them if they occur.
▪ Tell patient to report signs and symptoms of infection, including persistent fever or sore throat.
▪ Advise patient to minimize dangerous behavior that can cause bleeding and to report bleeding or abnormal bruising.

ifosfamide
Ifex

Pharmacologic classification: alkylating agent (cell cycle-phase nonspecific)
Therapeutic classification: antineoplastic
Pregnancy risk category D

How supplied
Available by prescription only
Injection: 1-g, 3-g vials

Indications and dosages
Germ cell testicular cancer, ◇lung cancer, ◇Hodgkin's and ◇malignant lymphoma, ◇breast cancer, ◇acute and ◇chronic lymphocytic leukemia, ◇ovarian cancer, ◇gastric cancer, ◇pancreatic cancer, ◇sarcomas
Adults: 1.2 g/m²/day I.V. for 5 days. Regimen is usually repeated q 3 weeks. Drug may be given by slow I.V. push, by intermittent infusion over at least 30 minutes, or by continuous infusion. Dosage and indications may vary. Check current literature for recommended protocol.

Pharmacodynamics
Antineoplastic action: Ifosfamide requires activation by hepatic microsomal enzymes to exert its cytotoxic activity. The active compound cross-links strands of DNA and also breaks the DNA chain.

Pharmacokinetics
Absorption: Not administered orally.
Distribution: Crosses the blood-brain barrier along with its metabolites.
Metabolism: About 50% of a dose is metabolized in the liver.
Excretion: Excreted primarily in the urine. The terminal half-life is reported to be about 7 hours at doses of 1.6 to 2.4 g/m²/day and about 15 hours at a single dose of 3.8 to 5 g/m².

Route	Onset	Peak	Duration
I.V.	Unknown	Unknown	Unknown

Contraindications and precautions
Contraindicated in patients with severe bone marrow suppression or hypersensitivity to drug. Use cautiously in patients with renal or hepatic impairment, compromised bone marrow reserve as indicated by granulocytopenia, bone marrow metastases, prior radiation therapy, or therapy with cytotoxic agents. Contraindicated in pregnancy due to possible embryotoxic and teratogenic effects on the fetus.

Interactions
Drug-drug. *Chloral hydrate, phenobarbital, phenytoin:* May increase the activity of ifosfamide by induction of hepatic microsomal enzymes, increasing the conversion of ifosfamide to its active form. Be alert for possible combined drug actions, desirable or undesirable, involving ifosfamide, even though it has been used successfully together with other drugs, including other cytotoxic drugs.

Effects on diagnostic tests
None reported.

Adverse reactions
CNS: *somnolence, confusion,* ***coma, seizures,*** ataxia, hallucinations, depressive psychosis, dizziness, disorientation, cranial nerve dysfunction.
GI: *nausea, vomiting.*
GU: *hemorrhagic cystitis, hematuria,* ***nephrotoxicity.***
Hematologic: ***leukopenia, thrombocytopenia, myelosuppression.***
Hepatic: elevated liver enzyme levels, liver dysfunction.
Other: *alopecia, metabolic acidosis,* infection, phlebitis.

Overdose and treatment
Signs and symptoms of overdose include myelosuppression, nausea, vomiting, alopecia, and hemorrhagic cystitis.

Treatment is usually supportive and includes transfusion of blood components, antiemetics, and bladder irrigation.

Clinical considerations
- Follow all established procedures for the safe handling, administration, and disposal of chemotherapeutic agents.
- Push fluids (3 L daily) and administer with mesna (Mesnex) to prevent hemorrhagic cystitis. Avoid giving drug at bedtime, because infrequent voiding during the night may increase the possibility of cystitis. Bladder irrigation with normal saline solution may decrease the possibility of cystitis.
- Drug can be further diluted with D_5W or normal saline solution for I.V. infusion. This solution is stable for 7 days at room temperature and 6 weeks at 41° F (5° C).
- Drug may be given by I.V. push injection in a minimum of 75 ml normal saline solution over 30 minutes.
- Infusing each dose over 2 hours or longer decreases the possibility of cystitis.

Therapeutic monitoring
- Assess patient for changes in mental status and cerebellar dysfunction. Dose may have to be decreased.
- Recommend monitoring CBC and renal and liver function tests.
- Sterile phlebitis may occur at the injection site; apply warm compresses.

Special populations
Pregnant patients. If the patient becomes pregnant while taking drug, she should be informed of the potential hazard to the fetus.
Breast-feeding patients. Drug is excreted in breast milk. Because of the potential for serious adverse reactions, mutagenicity, and carcinogenicity in the infant, breast-feeding isn't recommended.
Pediatric patients. Safety and efficacy in children haven't been established.

Patient counseling
- Tell patient to ensure adequate fluid intake to prevent bladder toxicity and to facilitate excretion of uric acid.
- Warn patient to avoid exposure to infections and to report signs of infection or unusual bleeding immediately.
- Reassure patient that hair should grow back after treatment has ended.
- Tell patient to contact prescriber immediately if blood appears in the urine.
- Advise both men and women to use contraceptive measures during therapy.

imipenem and cilastatin sodium
Primaxin I.M., Primaxin I.V.

Pharmacologic classification: carbapenem (thienamycin class), beta-lactam antibiotic
Therapeutic classification: antibiotic
Pregnancy risk category C

How supplied
Available by prescription only
Powder (for I.M. injection): 500-mg, 750-mg vial
Injection: 250-mg, 500-mg vials, ADD-Vantage, and infusion bottles

Indications and dosages
Mild to moderate lower respiratory tract, skin and skin-structure, or gynecologic infections
Adults weighing at least 154 lb (70 kg): 500 to 750 mg I.M. q 12 hours.
Mild to moderate intra-abdominal infections
Adults weighing at least 154 lb (70 kg): 750 mg I.M. q 12 hours.
Serious respiratory and urinary tract infections; intra-abdominal, gynecologic, bone, joint, or skin infections; bacterial septicemia; endocarditis
Adults weighing at least 154 lb (70 kg): 250 mg to 1 g by I.V. infusion q 6 to 8 hours. Maximum daily dose is 50 mg/kg/day or 4 g/day, whichever is less.
Children: 15 to 25 mg/kg q 6 hours.
≡ ***Dosage adjustment.*** In patients with renal failure and creatinine clearance of 6 to 20 ml/minute/1.73 m^2, 125 to 250 mg I.V. q 12 hours for most pathogens. There may be an increased risk of seizures when doses of 500 mg q 12 hours are administered to these patients. When creatinine clearance is 5 ml/minute/1.73 m^2 or less, imipenem shouldn't be given unless hemodialysis is instituted within 48 hours.

Note: In patients weighing less than 154 lb (70 kg) or those with impaired renal function, dosages vary. Check current literature for recommended protocol.

Pharmacodynamics
Antibacterial action: A bactericidal drug, imipenem inhibits bacterial cell wall synthesis. Its spectrum of antimicrobial activity includes many gram-positive, gram-negative, and anaerobic bacteria, including *Staphylococcus* and *Streptococcus* species, *Escherichia coli, Klebsiella, Proteus, Enterobacter* species, *Pseudomonas aeruginosa,* and *Bacteroides* species, including *B. fragilis.* Resistant bacteria include methicillin-resistant staphylococ-

ci, *Clostridium difficile,* and other *Pseudomonas* species.

Cilastatin inhibits the enzymatic breakdown of imipenem in the kidneys, making it effective in treating urinary tract infections.

Pharmacokinetics

Absorption: Following I.M. administration, imipenem blood levels peak within 2 hours; cilastatin levels reach their peak within 1 hour. After I.V. administration, peak levels of both agents appear in about 20 minutes. Imipenem is about 75% bioavailable and cilastatin is about 95% bioavailable after I.M. administration compared with I.V. administration.
Distribution: Distributed rapidly and widely. About 20% of imipenem is protein-bound; 40% of cilastatin is protein-bound.
Metabolism: Imipenem is metabolized by kidney dehydropeptidase I, resulting in low urine levels. Cilastatin inhibits this enzyme, thereby reducing metabolism of imipenem.
Excretion: About 70% of imipenem and cilastatin dose is excreted unchanged by the kidneys (when imipenem is combined with cilastatin) by tubular secretion and glomerular filtration. Imipenem is cleared by hemodialysis; therefore, a supplemental dose is required after this procedure. Half-life of drug is about 1 hour after I.V. administration. The prolonged absorption that occurs after I.M. administration results in a longer half-life (2 to 3 hours).

Route	Onset	Peak	Duration
I.M.	Unknown	1-2 hr	Unknown
I.V.	Unknown	Unknown	Unknown

Contraindications and precautions

Contraindicated in patients with hypersensitivity to drug. Imipenem and cilastatin sodium reconstituted with lidocaine hydrochloride for I.M. injection is contraindicated in patients with known hypersensitivity to local anesthetics of the amide type and in patients with severe shock or heart block.

Use cautiously in patients with impaired renal function, seizure disorders, or allergy to penicillins or cephalosporins.

Interactions

Drug-drug. *Chloramphenicol:* May impede the bactericidal effects of imipenem. Give chloramphenicol a few hours after imipenem and cilastatin.
Ganciclovir: Generalized seizures have occurred in several patients during combined imipenem and cilastatin and ganciclovir therapy. Monitor patient closely.
Probenecid: May prevent tubular secretion of cilastatin (but not imipenem) and prolong plasma cilastatin half-life.

Effects on diagnostic tests

None reported.

Adverse reactions

CNS: ***seizures***, dizziness, somnolence.
CV: hypotension.
GI: nausea, vomiting, diarrhea, *pseudomembranous colitis.*
Hematologic: ***agranulocytosis,*** thrombocytosis.
Hepatic: transient increases in liver enzymes.
Skin: rash, urticaria, pruritus, pain at injection site.
Other: ***hypersensitivity reactions (anaphylaxis),*** thrombophlebitis, fever.

Overdose and treatment

If overdose occurs, discontinue drug, treat symptomatically, and institute supportive measures as required. Although imipenem and cilastatin sodium are hemodialyzable, use of hemodialysis in treating drug overdose is questionable.

Clinical considerations

- Culture and sensitivity tests should be done before starting therapy.
- Drug may be physically incompatible with aminoglycosides; avoid mixing together.
- Drug isn't to be administered by direct I.V. bolus injection. Infuse 250- or 500-mg dose over 20 to 30 minutes; infuse 1-g dose over 40 to 60 minutes. If nausea occurs, slow infusion.
- Drug has broadest antibacterial spectrum of any available antibiotic. It's most valuable for empiric treatment of unidentified infections and for mixed infections that would otherwise require combination of antibiotics, possibly including an aminoglycoside.

Therapeutic monitoring

- Continue use of anticonvulsants in patients with known seizure disorders. Patients who exhibit CNS toxicity should receive phenytoin or benzodiazepines. Reduce dosage or discontinue drug if CNS toxicity continues.
- Prolonged use may result in overgrowth of nonsusceptible organisms. In addition, use of imipenem and cilastatin as a sole course of therapy has resulted in resistance during therapy.

Special populations

Breast-feeding patients. It's unknown if drug is distributed in breast milk. Administer cautiously to breast-feeding women.
Pediatric patients. Safety and efficacy in children under age 12 haven't been established; however, drug has been used in children age 3 months to 13 years. Dosage range is 15 to 25 mg/kg every 6 hours.
Geriatric patients. Administer cautiously to geriatric patients because they may also have renal dysfunction.

Patient counseling

- Advise patient of potential adverse reactions.

■ Instruct patient to report to prescriber immediately any serious adverse drug events.

imipramine hydrochloride

Apo-Imipramine*, Impril*, Novopramine*, Tofranil

imipramine pamoate

Tofranil-PM

Pharmacologic classification: dibenzazepine tricyclic antidepressant
Therapeutic classification: antidepressant
Pregnancy risk category B

How supplied

Available by prescription only
imipramine hydrochloride
Tablets: 10 mg, 25 mg, 50 mg
imipramine pamoate
Capsules: 75 mg, 100 mg, 125 mg, 150 mg

Indications and dosages

Depression
Adults: Initially, 75 to 100 mg P.O. daily in divided doses, with 25- to 50-mg increments, up to 200 mg. Alternatively, some patients can start with lower doses (25 mg P.O.) and dosage is adjusted slowly in 25-mg increments every other day. Maximum dose, 300 mg daily. Alternatively, entire dosage may be given h.s. Maximum dose is 200 mg/day for outpatients, 300 mg/day for inpatients, 100 mg/day for elderly patients.
◊ ***Childhood enuresis***
Children age 6 and older: 25 to 75 mg P.O. daily, 1 hour before bedtime. Usual dose 1.5 mg/kg/day in three divided doses. Maximum dose, 5 mg/kg/day.

Pharmacodynamics

Antidepressant action: Imipramine is thought to exert its antidepressant effects by inhibiting reuptake of norepinephrine and serotonin in CNS nerve terminals (presynaptic neurons), which results in increased levels and enhanced activity of these neurotransmitters in the synaptic cleft. Drug also has anticholinergic activity and is used to treat nocturnal enuresis in children over age 6.

Pharmacokinetics

Absorption: Absorbed rapidly from GI tract and muscle tissue after oral and I.M. administration.
Distribution: Distributed widely into the body, including the CNS and breast milk. Drug is 90% protein-bound. Steady state is achieved within 2 to 5 days. Therapeutic plasma levels (parent drug and metabolite) are thought to range from 150 to 300 ng/ml.
Metabolism: Metabolized by the liver to the active metabolite desipramine. A significant first-pass effect may explain variability of serum levels in different patients taking the same dosage.
Excretion: Mostly excreted in urine.

Route	Onset	Peak	Duration
P.O.	Unknown	½ to 2 hr	Unknown

Contraindications and precautions

Contraindicated during acute recovery phase of MI, in patients with hypersensitivity to drug, and in those receiving MAO inhibitors.

Use cautiously in patients at risk for suicide; in those with impaired renal or hepatic function, history of urine retention, angle-closure glaucoma, increased intraocular pressure, CV disease, hyperthyroidism, and in patients receiving thyroid medications.

Interactions

Drug-drug. *Barbiturates:* Induce imipramine metabolism and decrease therapeutic efficacy. Avoid use together.
Beta blockers, cimetidine, methylphenidate, oral contraceptives, propoxyphene: Inhibit imipramine metabolism, increasing plasma levels and toxicity. Use together cautiously.
Centrally acting antihypertensive drugs, such as clonidine, guanabenz, guanadrel, guanethidine, methyldopa, and reserpine: Decreased hypotensive effects of antihypertensives. Use cautiously.
CNS depressants, including analgesics, barbiturates, narcotics, tranquilizers, and anesthetics (oversedation); atropine or other anticholinergic drugs, including antihistamines, meperidine, phenothiazines, and antiparkinsonian agents: Oversedation, paralytic ileus, visual changes, and severe constipation. Avoid use together.
Disulfiram or ethchlorvynol: May cause delirium and tachycardia. Observe patient closely.
Haloperidol and phenothiazines: Decrease metabolism of imipramine, decreasing therapeutic efficacy. Monitor patient closely.
Metrizamide: Increased risk of seizures. Monitor patient closely.
Pimozide, thyroid medication, and antiarrhythmic agents (quinidine, disopyramide, procainamide: May increase incidence of arrhythmias and conduction defects. Avoid use together.
Sympathomimetics, including epinephrine, phenylephrine, phenylpropanolamine, and ephedrine (often found in nasal sprays): May increase blood pressure. Patient needs frequent blood pressure checks.
Warfarin: May prolong PT and cause bleeding. Monitor PT and INR.
Drug-lifestyle. *Alcohol use:* Additive CNS depressive effects. Advise patient to avoid alcohol use.

Heavy smoking: Induces imipramine metabolism and decreases therapeutic efficacy. Monitor patient for therapeutic effect.

Effects on diagnostic tests
None reported

Adverse reactions
CNS: *drowsiness, dizziness,* excitation, tremor, confusion, hallucinations, anxiety, ataxia, paresthesia, nervousness, EEG changes, ***seizures,*** extrapyramidal reactions.
CV: *orthostatic hypotension, tachycardia, ECG changes,* hypertension, ***MI, stroke, arrhythmias, heart block,*** *precipitation of heart failure.*
EENT: blurred vision, tinnitus, mydriasis.
GI: *dry mouth, constipation,* nausea, vomiting, anorexia, paralytic ileus, abdominal cramps.
GU: *urine retention,* gynecomastia (in males), testicular swelling, impotence.
Metabolic: increased or decreased serum glucose levels.
Skin: rash, urticaria, photosensitivity, pruritus.
Other: galactorrhea and breast enlargement (in females), altered libido, inappropriate antidiuretic hormone secretion syndrome, *diaphoresis,* ***hypersensitivity reaction.***
After abrupt withdrawal of long-term therapy: nausea, headache, malaise (does not indicate addiction).

Overdose and treatment
Drug overdose is frequently life-threatening, particularly when combined with alcohol. The first 12 hours after acute ingestion are a stimulatory phase characterized by excessive anticholinergic activity including agitation, irritation, confusion, hallucinations, hyperthermia, parkinsonian symptoms, seizure, urine retention, dry mucous membranes, pupillary dilatation, constipation, and ileus. This is followed by CNS depressant effects, including hypothermia, decreased or absent reflexes, sedation, hypotension, cyanosis, and cardiac irregularities, including tachycardia, conduction disturbances, and quinidine-like effects on the ECG.

Severity of overdose is best indicated by widening of the QRS complex, which usually represents a serum level in excess of 1,000 ng/ml; serum levels are usually not helpful. Metabolic acidosis may follow hypotension, hypoventilation, and seizures.

Treatment is symptomatic and supportive, including maintaining airway, stable body temperature, and fluid or electrolyte balance. Induce emesis if patient is conscious; follow with gastric lavage and activated charcoal to prevent further absorption. Dialysis is of little use.

Treat seizures with parenteral diazepam or phenytoin and arrhythmias with parenteral phenytoin or lidocaine. Quinidine, procainamide, and atropine aren't to be used during an overdose. Treat acidosis with sodium bicarbonate. Don't give barbiturates; these may enhance CNS and respiratory depressant effects.

Clinical considerations
Consider the recommendations relevant to all tricyclic antidepressants as well as the following:
- Drug may be used to treat nocturnal enuresis in children.
- Drug is associated with a high incidence of orthostatic hypotension.
- Discontinue drug at least 48 hours before surgical procedures.
- Drug shouldn't be withdrawn abruptly, but tapered gradually over time.

Therapeutic monitoring
- Monitor sitting and standing blood pressures after initial dose.
- Tolerance to sedative effects of drug usually develops over several weeks.

Special populations
Breast-feeding patients. Drug is excreted in breast milk in low levels. The potential benefit to the woman should outweigh possible risks to the infant.
Pediatric patients. Drug isn't recommended for treating depression in patients under age 12. Don't use pamoate salt for enuresis in children.
Geriatric patients. Recommended dose is 30 to 40 mg P.O. daily, not to exceed 100 mg daily. Initiate therapy at low doses (10 mg) and adjust slowly. Geriatric patients may be at greater risk for adverse cardiac reactions.

Patient counseling
- Tell patient to take drug exactly as prescribed.
- Explain that full effects of drug may not become apparent for up to 4 to 6 weeks after initiation of therapy.
- Warn patient not to discontinue drug abruptly, not to share drug with others, and not to drink alcoholic beverages while taking drug.
- Advise patient to take drug with food or milk if it causes stomach upset.
- Suggest relieving dry mouth with sugarless chewing gum or hard candy. Encourage good dental prophylaxis because persistent dry mouth may lead to increased incidence of dental caries.
- Encourage patient to report unusual or troublesome effects immediately, including confusion, movement disorders, rapid heartbeat, dizziness, fainting, or difficulty urinating.

immune globulin (gamma globulin, IG, immune serum globulin, ISG)

immune globulin for I.M. use (IGIM)

BayGam, Gammar

immune globulin for I.V. use (IGIV)

Gamimune N (5%, 10%), Gammagard S/D, Gammar-P IV, Iveegam, Panglobulin, Polygam S/D, Sandoglobulin, Venoglobulin-I, Venoglobulin-S

Pharmacologic classification: immune serum
Therapeutic classification: antibody production stimulator
Pregnancy risk category C

How supplied

Available by prescription only
IGIM
Injection: 2-ml, 10-ml vials
IGIV
I.V.: Gamimune N—5% and 10% solution in 10-ml, 50-ml, 100-ml, and 250-ml single-use vials; Gammagard S/D—2.5-g, 5-g, and 10-g single-use vials for reconstitution; Gammar-P IV—1-g, 2.5-g, and 5-g vials with diluent and 10-g vials with administration set and diluent; Iveegam—1-g, 2.5-g, and 5-g vials with diluent; Polygam S/D—2.5-g, 5-g, and 10-g single-use vials with diluent; Sandoglobulin—1-g, 3-g, 6-g, and 12-g vials or kits with diluent or bulk packs without diluent; Venoglobulin-I—2.5-g and 5-g vials with or without reconstitution kits with sterile water, 10-g vials with reconstitution kit and administration set, and 0.5-g vials with reconstitution kit; Venoglobulin-S—5% and 10% in 50-ml, 100-ml, and 200-ml vials.

Indications and dosages

Agammaglobulinemia, hypogammaglobulinemia, immune deficiency (IGIV)
Adults and children: For Gamimune N only, 100 to 200 mg/kg or 2 to 4 ml/kg I.V. infusion monthly. Infusion rate is 0.01 to 0.02 ml/kg/minute for 30 minutes. Rate can then be increased to maximum of 0.08 ml/kg/minute for remainder of infusion.

For Gammagard S/D only, initially 200 to 400 mg/kg I.V., followed by 100 mg/kg monthly. Initiate infusion at 0.5 ml/kg/hour, gradually increasing to maximum of 4 ml/kg/hour.

For Gammar-P IV only, 200 to 400 mg/kg q 3 to 4 weeks. Infusion rate is 0.01 ml/kg/minute, increasing to 0.02 ml/kg/minute after 15 to 30 minutes, with gradual increase to 0.06 ml/kg/minute.

For Iveegam only, 200 mg/kg I.V. monthly. If response is inadequate, doses may be increased up to 800 mg/kg or the drug may be administered more frequently. Infuse at 1 to 2 ml/minute.

For Polygam S/D only, 100 mg/kg I.V. monthly. An initial dose of 200 to 400 mg/kg may be administered. Initiate infusion at 0.5 ml/kg/hour, gradually increasing to maximum of 4 ml/kg/hour.

For Sandoglobulin and Panglobulin, 200 mg/kg I.V. monthly. Start with 0.5 to 1 ml/minute of a 3% solution; increase up to 2.5 ml/minute gradually after 15 to 30 minutes.

For Venoglobulin-I only, 200 mg/kg I.V. monthly; may be increased to 300 to 400 mg/kg and may be repeated more frequently than once monthly. Infuse at 0.01 to 0.02 ml/kg/minute for 30 minutes, then increase to 0.04 ml/kg/minute or higher, if tolerated.

For Venoglobulin-S only, 200 mg/kg I.V. monthly. Increase dose to 300 to 400 mg/kg monthly or administer more frequently if adequate IgI levels aren't achieved. Initiate infusion at 0.01 to 0.02 ml/kg/minute for 30 minutes, then increase 5% solutions to 0.04 ml/kg/minute and 10% solutions to 0.05 ml/kg/minute, if tolerated.

Hepatitis A exposure (IGIM)
Adults and children: 0.02 to 0.04 ml/kg I.M. as soon as possible after exposure. Up to 0.1 ml/kg may be given after prolonged or intense exposure.

Measles exposure (IGIM)
Adults and children: 0.2 to 0.25 ml/kg within 6 days after exposure.

Postexposure prophylaxis of measles (IGIM) for immunosuppressed patients
Adults and children: 0.5 ml/kg I.M. within 6 days after exposure.

Chickenpox exposure (IGIM)
Adults and children: 0.6 to 1.2 ml/kg I.M. as soon as exposed.

Rubella exposure in first trimester of pregnancy (IGIM)
Women: 0.55 ml/kg I.M. as soon as exposed.

Idiopathic thrombocytopenic purpura (IGIV)
Adults and children: Initially, 400 mg/kg daily of Sandoglobulin, Panglobulin, or Gamimune N (5% or 10%) I.V. for 2 to 5 consecutive days depending on platelet count and clinical response. Maintenance dosage is 400 to 1,000 mg/kg I.V. of Gamimune N 5%, 10%, or Sandoglobulin as a single infusion to maintain a platelet count greater than 30,000/mm^3.

Bone marrow transplantation (IGIV)
Adults over age 20: Gamimune N 10%, 500 mg/kg on day 7 and day 2 before transplantation; then weekly through 90 days after transplantation.

Pharmacodynamics
Immune action: Immune globulin provides passive immunity by increasing antibody titer. The mechanism by which IGIV increases platelet counts in idiopathic thrombocytopenic purpura isn't fully known.

Pharmacokinetics
Absorption: Slow I.M. absorption.
Distribution: Distributes evenly between intravascular and extravascular spaces.
Metabolism: Unknown.
Excretion: Serum half-life is reportedly 21 to 24 days in immunocompetent patients.

Route	Onset	Peak	Duration
I.V.	Unknown	2 days	Unknown

Contraindications and precautions
Contraindicated in patients hypersensitive to drug.

Interactions
Drug-drug. *Live virus vaccines:* Immune globulin may interfere with the immune response to live virus vaccines (such as measles, mumps, rubella). Live virus vaccines must not be given within 3 months after administration of immune globulin.

Effects on diagnostic tests
None reported.

Adverse reactions
CNS: faintness, headache, malaise.
CV: chest pain, chest tightness.
GI: nausea, vomiting.
GU: increased serum creatinine and BUN, oliguria, anuria, acute renal failure, acute tubular necrosis, proximal tubular nephropathy, osmotic nephrosis.
Musculoskeletal: hip pain, joint pain, muscle stiffness (at injection site).
Respiratory: dyspnea, shortness of breath.
Skin: erythema, urticaria.
Other: fever, ***anaphylaxis,*** chills, infusion reactions, aseptic meningitis syndrome, ***death.***

Overdose and treatment
Excessively rapid I.V. infusion rate can precipitate an anaphylactoid reaction.

Clinical considerations
- Obtain a thorough history of allergies and reactions to immunizations.
- Epinephrine solution 1:1,000 should be available to treat allergic reactions.
- Inject I.M. formulation into different sites, preferably into buttocks. Don't inject more than 3 ml per injection site.
- Don't give for hepatitis A exposure if 2 weeks or more have elapsed since exposure or after onset of clinical illness.
- Although pregnancy isn't a contraindication to use, it's unknown if immune globulin can cause fetal harm.
- Store Sandoglobulin and Gammagard S/D at room temperature not exceeding 77° F (25° C); Gamimune-N and Iveegam, at 36° to 46° F (2° to 8° C) but don't freeze; Gammar-P IV, at room temperature below 86° F (30° C) but don't freeze; Venoglobulin-I at room temperature below 86° F (30° C).
- Immune globulin has been studied in the treatment of various conditions, including Kawasaki disease, asthma, allergic disorders, autoimmune neutropenia, myasthenia gravis, and platelet transfusion rejection. It also has been used in the prophylaxis of infections in immunocompromised patients.
- Gamimune N can be diluted with D_5W.
- Reconstitute Gammagard S/D with diluent (sterile water for injection) and transfer device provided by manufacturer. Administration set (provided) contains a 15-micron in-line filter that must be used during administration.
- Reconstitute Sandoglobulin with diluent supplied (normal saline).

Therapeutic monitoring
Closely monitor blood pressure in patient receiving IGIV, especially if it's patient's first infusion of immune globulin.

Special populations
Breast-feeding patients. It's unknown if immune globulin is excreted in breast milk. Use with caution in breast-feeding women.

Patient counseling
- Explain that the patient's chances of getting AIDS or hepatitis after receiving immune globulin are minute because of stringent government standards that require testing for these viruses.
- Instruct patient to promptly report headache, skin changes, or difficulty breathing; decreased urine output; sudden weight gain; swelling; and shortness of breath.

indapamide
Lozol

Pharmacologic classification: thiazide-like diuretic
Therapeutic classification: diuretic, antihypertensive
Pregnancy risk category B

How supplied
Available by prescription only
Tablets: 1.25 mg, 2.5 mg

Indications and dosages

Edema of heart failure
Adults: 2.5 mg P.O. as a single daily dose taken in the morning; increase dose to 5 mg daily after 1 week if response is poor.
Hypertension
Adults: 1.25 mg P.O. as a single daily dose taken in the morning; increase dose to 2.5 mg daily after 4 weeks if response is poor. Maximum daily dose, 5 mg.

Pharmacodynamics

Diuretic action: Indapamide increases urinary excretion of sodium and water by inhibiting sodium reabsorption in the cortical diluting tubule of the nephron, thus relieving edema.
Antihypertensive action: Exact mechanism of antihypertensive effect of indapamide is unknown. This effect may result from direct arteriolar vasodilatation through calcium channel blockade. Drug also reduces total body sodium.

Pharmacokinetics

Absorption: Absorbed completely from the GI tract.
Distribution: Distributes widely into body tissues because of its lipophilicity; drug is 71% to 79% plasma protein-bound.
Metabolism: Indapamide undergoes significant hepatic metabolism.
Excretion: About 60% of drug dose is excreted in urine within 48 hours; about 16% to 23% is excreted in feces.

Route	Onset	Peak	Duration
P.O.	Unknown	2-5 hr	18 hr

Contraindications and precautions

Contraindicated in patients with anuria or hypersensitivity to other sulfonamide-derived drugs. Use cautiously in patients with severe impaired renal or hepatic function and progressive hepatic disease.

Interactions

Drug-drug. *Amphetamine, quinidine:* Indapamide turns urine slightly more alkaline and may decrease urinary excretion of some amines, such as alkaline urine. Monitor patient.
Other antihypertensive drugs: Indapamide potentiates hypotensive effects. This may be used to therapeutic advantage.
Cholestyramine and colestipol: May bind indapamide, preventing its absorption. Give drugs 1 hour apart.
Diazoxide: Increased hyperglycemic, hypotensive, and hyperuricemic effects of diazoxide. Monitor patient closely; insulin dose may need adjustment.
Lithium: Reduced renal clearance, elevating serum lithium levels. May necessitate reduction in lithium dosage by 50%.
Methenamine compounds (such as methenamine mandelate): Decreased therapeutic efficacy of these drugs. Monitor patient closely.

Effects on diagnostic tests

Indapamide therapy may interfere with tests for parathyroid function and should be discontinued before such tests are done.

Adverse reactions

CNS: headache, nervousness, dizziness, lightheadedness, weakness, vertigo, restlessness, drowsiness, fatigue, anxiety, depression, numbness of extremities, irritability, agitation.
CV: volume depletion and dehydration, orthostatic hypotension, palpitations, PVCs, irregular heartbeat, vasculitis.
EENT: rhinorrhea.
GI: anorexia, nausea, epigastric distress, vomiting, abdominal pain, diarrhea, constipation.
GU: nocturia, polyuria, frequent urination, impotence.
Metabolic: asymptomatic hyperuricemia; fluid and electrolyte imbalances, including dilutional hyponatremia and hypochloremia, metabolic alkalosis, hypokalemia; gout; weight loss.
Musculoskeletal: muscle cramps and spasms.
Skin: rash, pruritus, flushing.

Overdose and treatment

Clinical signs of overdose include GI irritation and hypermotility, diuresis, and lethargy, which may progress to coma.

Treatment is mainly supportive; monitor and assist respiratory, CV, and renal function as indicated. Monitor fluid and electrolyte balance. Induce vomiting with ipecac in conscious patient; otherwise, use gastric lavage to avoid aspiration. Don't give cathartics; these promote additional loss of fluids and electrolytes.

Clinical considerations

Clinical considerations for use of indapamide are the same as those for all thiazide and thiazide-like diuretics.

Therapeutic monitoring

Therapeutic monitoring considerations for use of indapamide are the same as those for all thiazide and thiazide-like diuretics.

Special populations

Breast-feeding patients. Drug is distributed into breast milk; its safety and effectiveness in breast-feeding women haven't been established.
Pediatric patients. Safety and efficacy in children haven't been established.
Geriatric patients. Geriatric and debilitated patients require close observation and may require reduced dosages. They're more sensitive to excess diuresis because of age-related changes in CV and renal function. Excess diuresis promotes orthostatic hypotension, de-

hydration, hypovolemia, hyponatremia, hypomagnesemia, and hypokalemia.

Patient counseling

Patient counseling considerations for use of indapamide are the same as those for all thiazide and thiazide-like diuretics.

indinavir sulfate

Crixivan

Pharmacologic classification: HIV protease inhibitor
Therapeutic classification: antiviral
Pregnancy risk category C

How supplied

Available by prescription only
Capsules: 200 mg, 333 mg, 400 mg

Indications and dosages

Treatment of patients with HIV infection when antiretroviral therapy is warranted
Adults: 800 mg P.O. q 8 hours with other antiretroviral agents. Indinavir shouldn't be used as monotherapy.
≡ ***Dosage adjustment.*** Reduce dosage to 600 mg P.O. q 8 hours in patients with mild to moderate hepatic insufficiency resulting from cirrhosis.

Pharmacodynamics

Antiviral action: Indinavir sulfate inhibits HIV protease, an enzyme required for the proteolytic cleavage of viral polyprotein precursors into individual functional proteins found in infectious HIV. By binding to the protease active site, indinavir prevents cleavage of the viral polyproteins, resulting in formation of immature noninfectious viral particles.

Pharmacokinetics

Absorption: Rapidly absorbed in GI tract when it is administered on an empty stomach. A meal high in calories, fat, and protein significantly interferes with drug absorption, whereas lighter meals don't.
Distribution: About 60% is plasma protein-bound.
Metabolism: Metabolized to at least seven metabolites. Cytochrome P-450 3A4 (CYP3A4) is the major enzyme responsible for formation of the oxidative metabolites.
Excretion: Less than 20% is excreted unchanged in urine.

Route	Onset	Peak	Duration
P.O.	Unknown	Unknown	Unknown

Contraindications and precautions

Contraindicated in patients with hypersensitivity to any component of drug. Use cautiously in patients with hepatic insufficiency resulting from cirrhosis.

Interactions

Drug-drug. *Cisapride, midazolam, triazolam:* Competition for CYP3A4 by indinavir could result in inhibition of the metabolism of these drugs and create the potential for serious or life-threatening events, such as arrhythmias or prolonged sedation. These drugs shouldn't be administered with indinavir.
HMG-CoA reductase inhibitors, such as atorvastatin, cerivastatin, lovastatin, and simvastatin: Increased risk of myopathy, including rhabdomyolysis. Use together cautiously.
Indinavir, didanosine: A normal gastric pH may be necessary for optimal absorption of indinavir. Administer these drugs and indinavir at least 1 hour apart on an empty stomach.
Ketoconazole, itraconazole: Causes an increase in the plasma levels of indinavir. Consider a dosage reduction of indinavir when administered together.
Rifabutin: Increased plasma levels. Reduced dosage of rifabutin is necessary.
Rifampin: Is a potent inducer of CYP3A4, which could markedly diminish plasma levels of indinavir; coadministration of indinavir and rifampin isn't recommended.

Effects on diagnostic tests

None reported.

Adverse reactions

CNS: malaise; headache, insomnia, dizziness, somnolence, asthenia, fatigue.
GI: abdominal pain, *nausea,* diarrhea, vomiting, acid regurgitation, anorexia, dry mouth, taste perversion.
GU: nephrolithiasis.
Hematologic: decreased hemoglobin, platelet count, or neutrophil count.
Hepatic: elevations in ALT, AST, and serum amylase; *hyperbilirubinemia,* jaundice.
Musculoskeletal: flank pain, back pain.

Overdose and treatment

Symptoms of acute or chronic overdose have been reported as renal and GI effects. Treatment is supportive, and the patient is observed closely. It's not known if indinavir is removed by hemodialysis or peritoneal dialysis.

Clinical considerations

- Dosage of indinavir is the same whether drug is used alone or in combination with other antiretroviral agents. However, antiretroviral activity of indinavir may be increased when used in combination with approved reverse transcriptase inhibitors.
- When administering with rifabutin, reduce the dose of rifabutin by half. However, when administering with ketoconazole, decrease dose of indinavir to 600 mg q 8 hours.

Therapeutic monitoring
- Recommend periodic measuring of HIV-RNA, CD4+.
- Drug may cause nephrolithiasis. If signs and symptoms of nephrolithiasis occur, consider stopping drug for 1 to 3 days during the acute phase. To prevent nephrolithiasis, patient should maintain adequate hydration.

Special populations
Breast-feeding patients. Drug may be excreted in breast milk. Because of the potential for indinavir to cause adverse effects in nursing infants and to prevent transmitting the infection to the infant, breast-feeding isn't recommended.
Pediatric patients. Safety and efficacy in children haven't been established.

Patient counseling
- Inform patient that indinavir isn't a cure for HIV infection. Opportunistic infections and other complications associated with HIV disease may continue to develop. Drug has also not been shown to reduce risk of transmitting HIV to others through sexual contact or blood contamination.
- Caution patient not to adjust dosage or discontinue indinavir therapy without medical approval.
- Advise patient that, if a dose of indinavir is missed, therapy should be resumed with the next dose and that a double dose shouldn't be taken.
- Instruct patient to take drug on an empty stomach with water 1 hour before or 2 hours after a meal. Alternatively, he may take it with other liquids (such as skim milk, juice, coffee, or tea) or with a light meal. Inform patient that a meal high in calories, fat, and protein reduces the absorption of indinavir.
- Tell patient to store capsules in the original container and to keep the desiccant in the bottle because the capsules are sensitive to moisture.
- Instruct patient to drink at least 1.5 L of fluid daily.

indomethacin, indomethacin sodium trihydrate
Apo-Indomethacin*, Indameth, Indochron E-R, Indocid*, Indocin, Indocin SR, Novomethacin*

Pharmacologic classification: NSAID
Therapeutic classification: nonnarcotic analgesic, antipyretic, anti-inflammatory
Pregnancy risk category NR

How supplied
Available by prescription only
Capsules: 25 mg, 50 mg
Capsules (sustained-release): 75 mg
Suspension: 25 mg/5 ml
Injection: 1-mg vials
Suppositories: 50 mg

Indications and dosages
Moderate to severe arthritis, ankylosing spondylitis
Adults: 25 mg P.O. b.i.d. or t.i.d. with food or antacids; dose may be increased by 25 to 50 mg daily q 7 days up to 200 mg daily; or 50 mg P.R. q.i.d. Alternatively, sustained-release capsules may be given: 75 mg to start, in the morning or h.s., followed, if necessary, by 75 mg b.i.d.
Acute gouty arthritis
Adults: 50 mg t.i.d. Reduce dose as soon as possible, then stop it. Don't use sustained-release capsules for this condition.
To close a hemodynamically significant patent ductus arteriosus in premature infants (I.V. form only)
Neonate age less than 48 hours: 0.2 mg/kg I.V. followed by 2 doses of 0.1 mg/kg at 12- to 24-hour intervals.
Neonate age 2 to 7 days: 0.2 mg/kg I.V. followed by 2 doses of 0.2 mg/kg at 12- to 24-hour intervals.
Neonate over age 7 days: 0.2 mg/kg I.V. followed by 2 doses of 0.25 mg/kg at 12- to 24-hour intervals.
Acute shoulder pain
Adults: 75 to 150 mg P.O. b.i.d. or t.i.d. with food or antacids; usual treatment is 7 to 14 days.
◊ ***Pericarditis***
Adults: 75 to 200 mg P.O. daily in three or four divided doses.
◊ ***Dysmenorrhea***
Adults: 25 mg P.O. t.i.d. with food or antacids.
◊ ***Bartter's syndrome***
Adults: 150 mg/day P.O. with food or antacids.
Children: 0.5 to 2 mg/kg in divided doses.

Pharmacodynamics
Analgesic, antipyretic, and anti-inflammatory actions: Exact mechanisms of action are unknown; indomethacin is thought to produce its analgesic, antipyretic, and anti-inflammatory effects by inhibiting prostaglandin synthesis and possibly by inhibiting phosphodiesterase.
Closure of patent ductus arteriosus: Mechanism of action is unknown, but is believed to be through inhibition of prostaglandin synthesis.

Pharmacokinetics
Absorption: Absorbed rapidly and completely from the GI tract.
Distribution: Highly protein-bound.
Metabolism: Metabolized in the liver.
Excretion: Excreted mainly in urine, with some biliary excretion.

Route	Onset	Peak	Duration
P.O., I.V., P.R.	Unknown	Unknown	Unknown

Contraindications and precautions

Contraindicated in patients with hypersensitivity to drug or history of aspirin- or NSAID-induced asthma, rhinitis, or urticaria; in pregnancy or in breast-feeding women. Also contraindicated in infants with untreated infection, active bleeding, coagulation defects or thrombocytopenia, congenital heart disease in those for whom patency of the ductus arteriosus is necessary for satisfactory pulmonary or systemic blood flow, necrotizing enterocolitis, or impaired renal function. Suppositories are contraindicated in patients with a history of proctitis or recent rectal bleeding.

Use cautiously in the elderly and in patients with history of GI disease, impaired renal or hepatic function, epilepsy, parkinsonism, CV disease, infection, mental illness, or depression.

Interactions

Drug-drug. *Anticoagulants and thrombolytic drugs (such as coumarin derivatives, heparin, streptokinase, urokinase):* May potentiate anticoagulant effects. Recommend monitoring PT, partial thromboplastin time (PTT), and INR.
Antihypertensives and diuretics: Concurrent use may decrease their effectiveness.
Aspirin, parenteral carbenicillin, cefamandole, cefoperazone, dextran, dipyridamole, mezlocillin, piperacillin, plicamycin, salicylates, sulfinpyrazone, ticarcillin, valproic acid, or other anti-inflammatory agents, corticotropin, or corticosteroids: Bleeding problems may occur. Monitor patient closely.
Aspirin: May decrease the bioavailability of indomethacin. Avoid use together.
Coumarin derivatives, nifedipine, phenytoin, verapamil: Toxicity may occur. Monitor patient carefully.
Gold compounds, other anti-inflammatory agents, acetaminophen: Increased nephrotoxicity may occur. Don't use together.
Insulin or oral antidiabetic agents: Concurrent use may potentiate hypoglycemic effects. Avoid use together.
Methotrexate, lithium: Indomethacin may decrease the renal clearance of these drugs. Monitor patient closely.
Triamterene and other diuretics: Potential nephrotoxicity. Avoid use together.
Drug-herb. *Senna:* May block diarrheal effects. Avoid use together.
Drug-lifestyle. *Alcohol use:* May increase GI adverse effects. Advise patient to avoid alcohol.

Effects on diagnostic tests

Drug therapy may interfere with dexamethasone suppression test results. It may also interfere with urinary 5-hydroxyindoleacetic acid determinations.

Adverse reactions

Oral and rectal forms
CNS: *headache, dizziness,* depression, drowsiness, confusion, somnolence, fatigue, peripheral neuropathy, ***seizures,*** psychic disturbances, syncope, *vertigo.*
CV: hypertension, *edema,* ***heart failure.***
EENT: blurred vision, corneal and retinal damage, hearing loss, tinnitus.
GI: *nausea,* anorexia, *diarrhea, peptic ulceration,* ***GI bleeding,*** constipation, dyspepsia, ***pancreatitis.***
GU: hematuria, ***acute renal failure,*** proteinuria, interstitial nephritis.
Hematologic: ***hemolytic anemia, aplastic anemia, agranulocytosis, leukopenia, thrombocytopenic purpura,*** iron-deficiency anemia.
Metabolic: hyperkalemia.
Skin: pruritus, urticaria, ***Stevens-Johnson syndrome.***
Other: hypersensitivity (rash, respiratory distress, ***anaphylaxis, angioedema***).
I.V. form
GU: proteinuria, interstitial nephritis.

Overdose and treatment

Signs and symptoms of overdose include dizziness, nausea, vomiting, intense headache, mental confusion, drowsiness, tinnitus, sweating, blurred vision, paresthesias, and seizures.

To treat overdose, empty stomach immediately by inducing emesis with ipecac syrup or by gastric lavage. Administer activated charcoal via nasogastric tube. Provide symptomatic and supportive measures (respiratory support and correction of fluid and electrolyte imbalances). Monitor laboratory parameters and vital signs closely. Dialysis may be of little value because indomethacin is strongly protein-bound.

Clinical considerations

Consider the recommendations relevant to all NSAIDs as well as the following:

- Don't mix oral suspension with liquids or antacids before administering.
- Patient should retain suppository in the rectum for at least 1 hour after insertion to ensure maximum absorption.
- Reconstitute 1 mg vial of I.V. dose with 1 to 2 ml of sterile water for injection or normal saline injection. Prepare solution immediately before use to prevent deterioration. Don't use solution if it's discolored or contains a precipitate.
- Use I.V. administration only for premature neonates with patent ductus arteriosus. Don't administer a second or third I.V. dose if anuria or marked oliguria exists.
- If ductus arteriosus reopens, a second course of one to three doses may be given. If ineffective, surgery may be necessary.

Therapeutic monitoring

- Monitor carefully for bleeding and for reduced urine output.
- Monitor cardiopulmonary status for significant changes. Watch for signs and symptoms of fluid overload. Check weight and intake and output daily.
- Monitor renal function studies before start of therapy and frequently during therapy to prevent adverse effects.
- Severe headache may occur. If headache persists, decrease dose.

Special populations

Breast-feeding patients. Drug is excreted in breast milk in levels similar to those in maternal plasma; avoid use in breast-feeding women.
Pediatric patients. Safety of long-term drug use in children under age 14 hasn't been established. Use of I.V. indomethacin in premature infants for patent ductus arteriosus is considered an alternative to surgery.
Geriatric patients. Patients over age 60 may be more susceptible to the toxic effects of indomethacin. The effect of drug on renal prostaglandins may cause fluid retention and edema, a significant drawback for geriatric patients and those with heart failure.

Patient counseling

- Instruct patient in proper administration of dosage form prescribed, such as suppository, sustained-release capsule, or suspension.
- Advise patient to seek medical approval before taking OTC medications.
- Caution patient to avoid hazardous activities that require alertness or concentration.
- Tell patient to report signs and symptoms of adverse reactions and to adhere to prescribed drug regimen.

infliximab

Remicade

Pharmacologic classification: monoclonal antibody IgG1k
Therapeutic classification: anti-inflammatory
Pregnancy risk category C

How supplied

Available by prescription only
Injection: 100 mg 20-ml vial

Indications and dosages

Reduction of signs and symptoms in patients with moderately to severely active Crohn's disease with inadequate response to conventional therapy
Adults: 5 mg/kg single I.V. infusion over a period of not less than 2 hours.

Reduction in the number of draining enterocutaneous fistulas in patients with fistulizing Crohn's disease
Adults: 5 mg/kg I.V. infused over a period of not less than 2 hours. Give additional doses of 5 mg/kg at 2 and 6 weeks after initial infusion.

Pharmacodynamics

Anti-inflammatory action: Drug is a monoclonal antibody that binds to human tumor necrosis factor (TNF)-alpha to neutralize its activity and inhibit its binding with receptors, reducing the infiltration of inflammatory cells and TNF-alpha production in inflamed areas of the intestine.

Pharmacokinetics

Absorption: Administered I.V.; absorption is incomplete.
Distribution: Not reported.
Metabolism: Not reported.
Excretion: Terminal half-life is 9½ days.

Route	Onset	Peak	Duration
I.V.	Unknown	Unknown	Unknown

Contraindications and precautions

Contraindicated in patients with hypersensitivity to murine proteins or other components of the drug. Use with caution in the elderly.

Interactions

None reported.

Effects on diagnostic tests

None reported.

Adverse reactions

CNS: *headache, fatigue,* dizziness, malaise, insomnia.
CV: hypertension, hypotension, flushing, tachycardia, chest pain.
EENT: pharyngitis, rhinitis, sinusitis, conjunctivitis, toothache.
GI: *nausea, abdominal pain,* vomiting, constipation, dyspepsia, flatulence, intestinal obstruction, oral pain, ulcerative stomatitis.
GU: dysuria, increased micturition frequency.
Hematologic: anemia, hematoma, ecchymosis.
Hepatic: elevated liver enzymes.
Musculoskeletal: myalgia, arthralgia, arthritis, back pain.
Respiratory: *upper respiratory tract infections,* bronchitis, coughing, dyspnea, flu syndrome, respiratory tract allergic reaction.
Skin: rash, pruritus, moniliasis, acne, alopecia, eczema, erythema, erythematous rash, maculopapular rash, papular rash, dry skin, increased sweating, urticaria.
Other: *fever,* chills, pain, peripheral edema, hot flashes, abscess.

Overdose and treatment
Single doses up to 20 mg/kg have been given without direct toxic effects. If overdose should occur, monitor patient for signs and symptoms of adverse events and give symptomatic treatment.

Clinical considerations
- Drug is incompatible with plasticized polyvinyl chloride equipment or devices; prepare only in glass infusion bottles or polypropylene or polyolefin infusion bags. Administer through polyethylene-lined administration sets with an in-line, sterile, nonpyrogenic, low-protein-binding filter (pore size of 1.2 mm or less).
- Vials don't contain antibacterial preservatives.
- Dilute total volume of reconstituted dose to 250 ml with normal saline injection. Infusion concentration range is 0.4 to 4 mg/ml. Infusion should begin within 3 hours of preparation and must be administered over a period of not less than 2 hours.
- Drug shouldn't be infused in the same I.V. line with other agents.

Therapeutic monitoring
- Infusion-related reactions such as fever, chills, pruritus, urticaria, dyspnea, hypotension, hypertension, and chest pain may occur. If an infusion reaction occurs, discontinue drug, notify doctor, and be prepared to give acetaminophen, antihistamines, corticosteroids, and epinephrine, as ordered.
- Monitor for development of lymphomas and infection. Patients with long duration of Crohn's disease and chronic exposure to immunosuppressant therapies are more susceptible to development of lymphomas and infections.
- Drug may affect normal immune responses. Autoimmune antibodies and lupus-like syndrome may develop; discontinue drug therapy. Symptoms can be expected to resolve.

Special populations
Breast-feeding patients. It's unknown if infliximab is excreted in breast milk. Discontinue either drug or breast-feeding.
Pediatric patients. Safety and efficacy of drug use in children haven't been established.
Geriatric patients. Use with caution in patients over age 65.

Patient counseling
- Tell patient about infusion-reaction symptoms and instruct to report adverse events.
- Inform patient of postinfusion side effects and instruct him to report them promptly.

influenza virus vaccine, 1999-2000 trivalent types A & B (purified surface antigen)
Fluvirin

influenza virus vaccine, 1999-2000 trivalent types A & B (subvirion or purified subvirion)
Fluogen, FluShield, Fluzone

influenza virus vaccine, 1999-2000 trivalent types A & B (whole virion)
Fluzone

Pharmacologic classification: vaccine
Therapeutic classification: viral vaccine
Pregnancy risk category C

How supplied
Available by prescription only
Injection: 0.5 ml prefilled syringe; 5-ml vials

Indications and dosages
Annual influenza prophylaxis in high-risk patients
Adults and children age 13 and older: 0.5 ml I.M. (whole virus or split virus).
Children age 9 to 12: 0.5 ml I.M. (split virus only).
Children age 3 to 8: 0.5 ml I.M. (split virus only).
Infants and children age 6 to 35 months: 0.25 ml I.M. (split virus only).

Note: Second dose may be given in previously unvaccinated children under age 9 at least 1 month after first dose.

Check package insert for annual changes and additional dosing recommendations.

Pharmacodynamics
Influenza prophylaxis: Vaccine promotes active immunity to influenza by inducing antibody production. Protection is provided only against those strains of virus from which the vaccine is prepared (or closely related strains).

Pharmacokinetics
Absorption: Duration of immunity varies widely.
Distribution: No information available.
Metabolism: No information available.
Excretion: No information available.

Route	Onset	Peak	Duration
I.M.	Unknown	Unknown	About 1 yr

Contraindications and precautions

Contraindicated in patients with hypersensitivity to chicken eggs or any component of the vaccine such as thimersol. Defer vaccination in patients with acute respiratory or other active infection and delay immunization in those with an active neurologic disorder.

Interactions

Drug-drug. *Corticosteroids or immunosuppressants:* Concurrent use may impair the immune response to the vaccine. Avoid use together.
Phenytoin and aminopyrine: Decreased serum phenytoin and aminopyrine levels. Monitor patient and drug levels.
Theophylline: Increased serum theophylline levels. Monitor theophylline levels.
Warfarin: Rare prolonged PT, GI bleeding, transient gross hematuria, and epistaxis. Monitor patient closely.

Effects on diagnostic tests

None reported.

Adverse reactions

CNS: malaise.
Musculoskeletal: myalgia.
Skin: erythema, induration, and *soreness at injection site.*
Other: ***anaphylaxis***, fever.

Note: Fever and malaise reactions occur most often in children and in others not exposed to influenza viruses. Severe reactions in adults are rare.

Overdose and treatment

No information available.

Clinical considerations

Patients with a known or suspected hypersensitivity to egg protein should have a skin test to assess sensitivity to vaccine. Administer a scratch test with 0.05 to 0.1 ml of a 1:100 dilution in normal saline solution for injection. Patients with positive skin test reactions shouldn't receive the influenza virus vaccine.

Epinephrine solution 1:1,000 should be available to treat allergic reactions.

Influenza vaccine shouldn't be administered to patients with active influenza infection. Such infection should be treated with amantadine.

To reduce the frequency of adverse reactions, use only the split-virus or purified surface antigen vaccine in children.

Pneumococcal vaccine, DTP, or live attenuated measles virus vaccine may be given simultaneously but at a different injection site.

Store vaccine between 36° and 46° F (2° and 8° C). Don't freeze.

Therapeutic monitoring

Monitor for adverse drug reactions.

Special populations

Pregnant patients. If given during pregnancy, the influenza vaccine should be given during the second trimester to avoid a coincidental association with spontaneous abortion, which is common in the first trimester.
Breast-feeding patients. Breast-feeding isn't a contraindication for receiving vaccine.
Pediatric patients. Influenza vaccine is contraindicated in children under age 6 months.
Geriatric patients. Annual vaccination is highly recommended for patients over age 65.

Patient counseling

Advise patient of potential injection site discomfort, fever, malaise, and muscle aches.

Encourage patient to report distressing adverse reactions promptly.

Warn patient that many cases of Guillain-Barré syndrome were reported after vaccination for the swine flu of 1976. This condition usually causes reversible paralysis and muscle weakness, but it can be fatal in some individuals. Influenza vaccines made after 1976 haven't been associated with as high an incidence of Guillain-Barré syndrome, but the condition still occurs, albeit rarely. Patients with history of Guillain-Barré syndrome have a greater risk for repeat episodes.

---

insulin (regular)

Humulin-R, Novolin R, Novolin R PenFill, Pork Regular Iletin II, Regular (Concentrated) Iletin II, Regular Insulin, Regular Purified Pork Insulin, Velosulin Human*, Velosulin BR

insulin (lispro)

Humalog

isophane insulin suspension (NPH)

Humulin N, NPH-N, Novolin N, Novolin N PenFill, Pork NPH Iletin II

insulin zinc suspension (lente)

Humulin L, Lente Iletin II, Lente L, Novolin L

extended zinc insulin suspension (ultralente)

Humulin U Ultralente, Ultralente*

isophane insulin suspension and insulin injection (70% isophane insulin and 30% insulin injection)

Humulin 70/30, Novolin 70/30, Novolin 70/30 PenFill

isophane insulin suspension and insulin injection (50% isophane insulin and 50% insulin injection)

Humulin 50/50

Pharmacologic classification: pancreatic hormone
Therapeutic classification: antidiabetic
Pregnancy risk category NR

How supplied

Available without a prescription
insulin (regular)
Injection (pork): 100 units/ml
Injection (human): 100 units/ml
isophane insulin suspension (NPH)
Injection (pork): 100 units/ml
Injection (human): 100 units/ml
insulin zinc suspension (lente)
Injection (pork): 100 units/ml
Injection (human): 100 units/ml
extended zinc insulin suspension (ultralente)
Injection (human): 100 units/ml

Available by prescription only
insulin (lispro)
Injection (human): 100 units/ml
Cartridge (human): 1.5 ml
regular (concentrated) Iletin II insulin
Injection (pork): 500 units/ml

Indications and dosages

Diabetic ketoacidosis (regular insulin)
Adults: Administer loading dose of 0.15 units/kg I.V. followed by 0.1 units/kg/hour as a continuous infusion. Decrease rate of insulin infusion when plasma glucose level reaches 300 mg/dl. Start infusion of D_5W separately from the insulin infusion when plasma glucose reaches 250 mg/dl. Thirty minutes before discontinuing insulin infusion, administer a dose of insulin S.C.; intermediate-acting insulin is recommended.

Alternative dosage schedule is 50 to 100 units I.V. and 50 to 100 units S.C. immediately; base subsequent doses on therapeutic response and glucose, acetone, or ketone levels monitored at 1- to 2-hour intervals, or 2.4 to 7.2 units I.V. loading dose followed by 2.4 to 7.2 units/hour.
Children: 0.5 to 1 unit/kg in two divided doses, one given I.V. and the other S.C., followed by 0.5 to 1 unit/kg I.V. q 1 to 2 hours; or 0.1 unit/kg I.V. bolus, then 0.1 unit/kg/hour continuous I.V. infusion until serum glucose decreases to 250 mg/dl; then start S.C. insulin.
Ketosis-prone and juvenile-onset diabetes mellitus, diabetes mellitus inadequately controlled by diet and oral antidiabetics
Adults and children: Individualized dosage adjusted based on patient's serum and urine glucose levels.
Hyperkalemia
Adults: 5 to 10 units of regular insulin with 50 ml of D_5W over 5 minutes. Alternatively, 25 units of regular insulin given S.C. and an infusion of 1,000 ml dextrose 10% in water with 90 mEq sodium bicarbonate; infuse 330 ml over 30 minutes and the balance over 3 hours.
Provocative test for growth hormone secretion
Adults: Rapid I.V. injection of regular insulin 0.05 to 0.15 units/kg.

Pharmacodynamics

Antidiabetic action: Insulin is used as a replacement for the physiologic production of endogenous insulin in patients with insulin-dependent diabetes mellitus (IDDM) and diabetes mellitus inadequately controlled by diet and oral hypoglycemic agents. Insulin increases glucose transport across muscle and fat-cell membranes to reduce blood glucose levels. It also promotes conversion of glucose to its storage form, glycogen; triggers amino acid uptake and conversion to protein in muscle cells and inhibits protein degradation; stimulates triglyceride formation and inhibits release of free fatty acids from adipose tissue; and stimulates lipoprotein lipase activity, which converts circulating lipoproteins to fatty acids. Insulin is available in various forms and these differ mainly in onset, peak, and duration of action. Characteristics of the various insulin preparations are compared in the following chart.

Pharmacokinetics

Absorption: Insulin must be given parenterally because it's destroyed in the GI tract. Commercially available preparations are formulated to differ in onset, peak, and duration after subcutaneous administration. They're classified as rapid-acting (½- to 1-hour onset), intermediate-acting (1- to 2-hour onset), and long-acting (4- to 8-hour onset). The accompanying chart summarizes major pharmacokinetic differences
Distribution: Distributed widely throughout the body.

COMPARING INSULIN PREPARATIONS

The table below lists the various forms of insulin and their times of onset, peak, and duration. Individual responses can vary.

Preparation	Purified†	Onset (hr)	Peak (hr)	Duration (hr)
Rapid-acting insulins				
insulin injection (regular, crystalline zinc)				
Regular Insulin	No	½	2½ to 5	8 hr
Pork Regular Iletin II	Yes	½	2 to 4	6 to 8
Velosulin BR Human	Yes	½	1 to 3	8
Regular Purified Pork Insulin	Yes	½	2½ to 5	8
Humulin R	N.A.	½	2 to 4	6 to 8
Novolin R/Novolin R PenFill	N.A.	½	2½ to 5	8
insulin injection (lispro)				
Humalog	Yes	< ½	½ to 1½	< 6
Intermediate-acting insulins				
isophane insulin suspension (NPH)				
NPH	No	1½	4 to 12	24
Pork NPH Iletin II	Yes	1 to 2	6 to 12	18 to 24
Humulin N	N.A.	1 to 2	6 to 12	18 to 24
Novolin N/Novolin N PenFill	N.A.	1½	4 to 12	24
insulin zinc suspension (lente)				
Lente Iletin II	Yes	1 to 3	6 to 12	18 to 24
Lente L	Yes	2½	7 to 15	22
Humulin L	N.A.	1 to 3	6 to 12	18 to 24
Novolin L	N.A.	2½	7 to 15	22
isophane (NPH) 70%, regular insulin 30%				
Humulin 70/30	N.A.	½	4 to 8	24
Novolin 70/30/Novolin 70/30 PenFill	N.A.	½	2 to 12	24
isophane (NPH) 50%, regular insulin 50%				
Humulin 50/50	N.A.	½	4 to 8	24
Long-acting insulins				
extended insulin zinc suspension (ultralente)				
Ultralente	No	4	10 to 30	36
Humulin U Ultralente	Yes	4 to 6	8 to 20	24 to 28

N.A. indicates not applicable.
† Purified insulins contain < 10 ppm proinsulin.

Metabolism: Some insulin is bound and inactivated by peripheral tissues, but the majority appears to be degraded in the liver and kidneys.
Excretion: Filtered by the renal glomeruli and undergoes some tubular reabsorption. Plasma half-life is about 9 minutes after I.V. administration.

Route	Onset	Peak	Duration
I.V.	Immediate	Unknown	Unknown
S.C. (rapid)	0.5-1.5 hr	2-3 hr	5-7 hr
(intermediate)	1-2.5 hr	4-15 hr	12-24 hr
(long-acting)	4-8 hr	10-30 hr	36 hr

Contraindications and precautions

No known contraindications.

Interactions

Drug-drug. *Anabolic steroids, beta blockers, clofibrate, fenfluramine, MAO inhibitors, salicylates, tetracycline:* Prolonged hypoglycemic effect. Monitor blood glucose carefully.
Corticosteroids, dextrothyroxine sodium, epinephrine, and thiazide diuretics: Diminish insulin response. Monitor for hyperglycemia.
Drug-herb. *Basil, bay, bee pollen, burdock, ginseng, glucomannian, horehound, marsh mallow, myrrh, sage:* May affect glycemic control. Monitor blood glucose carefully and avoid use together.
Drug-lifestyle. *Smoking:* Decreases absorption of insulin administered S.C. Advise patient to avoid smoking within 30 minutes of insulin injection.
Alcohol use: May cause a prolonged hypoglycemic effect. Advise patient to avoid alcohol.
Marijuana use: May increase insulin requirements. Advise patient to avoid marijuana use.

Effects on diagnostic tests

None reported.

Adverse reactions

Skin: urticaria, pruritus, swelling, redness, stinging, warmth at injection site.
Other: *lipoatrophy, lipohypertrophy,* hypersensitivity reactions ***(anaphylaxis,*** rash), ***hypoglycemia,*** hyperglycemia (rebound, or Somogyi, effect).

Overdose and treatment

Insulin overdose may produce signs and symptoms of hypoglycemia (tachycardia, palpitations, anxiety, hunger, nausea, diaphoresis, tremors, pallor, restlessness, headache, and speech and motor dysfunction).

Treatment is directed toward treating hypoglycemia and is based on patient's symptoms. If patient is responsive, give 10 to 15 g of a fast-acting oral carbohydrate. If patient's signs and symptoms persist after 15 minutes, give an additional 10 g carbohydrate. If patient is unresponsive, an I.V. bolus of dextrose 50% solution should immediately increase blood glucose. Some prefer to use dextrose 25% in water because it's less irritating should extravasation occur. A common infusion rate is based on glucose content: 10 to 20 mg/kg/minute. Parenteral glucagon or epinephrine S.C. may also be given; both drugs elevate blood glucose levels in a few minutes by stimulating glycogenolysis. Fluid and electrolyte imbalance may require I.V. fluids and electrolyte (such as potassium) replacement.

Clinical considerations

- Human insulin may be advantageous for non-insulin-dependent patients requiring intermittent or short-term therapy (such as pregnancy, surgery, infection, or total parenteral nutrition therapy), for patients with insulin resistance, or for those with lipoatrophy.
- Lente, semilente, and ultralente insulins may be mixed in any proportion.
- Regular insulin may be mixed with NPH or lente insulins in any proportion. However, in vitro binding occurs over time until an equilibrium is reached. Administer these mixtures either immediately after preparation or after stability occurs (15 minutes for NPH regular, 24 hours for lente regular) in order to minimize variability in patient response. Note that switching from separate injections to a prepared mixture also may alter the patient's response. When mixing two insulins, always draw regular insulin into the syringe first.
- Lispro insulin may be mixed with Humulin N or Humulin U and given within 15 minutes before a meal to prevent a hypoglycemic reaction. The effects of mixing lispro insulin with insulins of animal source or insulin preparations produced by other manufacturers haven't been studied and may require a change in dosage.
- Store insulin in cool area. Refrigeration is desirable but not essential, except with regular insulin concentrated.
- Administration route is S.C. because it allows slower absorption and causes less pain than I.M. injections. Ketosis-prone, juvenile-onset, severely ill, and newly diagnosed diabetics with very high blood glucose levels may require hospitalization and I.V. treatment with regular fast-acting insulin. Ketosis-resistant diabetics may be treated as outpatients with intermediate-acting insulin after they have received instructions on how to alter dosage according to self-performed urine or blood glucose determinations. Some patients, primarily pregnant or brittle diabetics, may use a dextrometer to perform fingerstick blood glucose tests at home.
- Injection sites should be rotated; however, unstable diabetics may achieve better control if injection site is rotated within same anatomic region.
- In pregnant diabetic women, insulin requirements increase, sometimes drastically, then decline immediately postpartum.
- Human insulin may be advantageous in patients allergic to pork forms. Humulin is synthesized by a genetically altered strain of *Escherichia coli*. Novolin brands are derived by enzymatic alteration of pork insulin.

Therapeutic monitoring

- With regular insulin concentrated, a secondary hypoglycemic reaction may occur 18 to 24 hours after injection. This may be caused by a repository effect of drug and the high concentration of insulin in the preparation (500 units/ml).
- Some patients may develop insulin resistance and require large insulin doses to control symp-

toms of diabetes. Iletin, II, Regular Purified Pork, 500 units/ml may be used for these patients.

- Patient should notify pharmacist several days before prescription refill is needed in case U-500 is not in stock. Give hospital pharmacy sufficient notice before refill of inhouse prescription.
- Never store U-500 insulin in same area with other insulin preparations because of danger of severe overdose if given accidentally to other patients. U-500 insulin must be administered with a U-100 syringe because no syringes are made for this drug.

Special populations

Pregnant patients. Monitor insulin use during pregnancy.
Breast-feeding patients. Monitor drug use closely in breast-feeding women.
Geriatric patients. There may be an increased incidence of hypoglycemia associated with insulin therapy and an increased potential for stroke and heart attack in older patients.

Patient counseling

- Instruct patient to strictly adhere to manufacturer's instructions regarding assembly, administration, and care of specialized delivery systems, such as insulin pumps.
- Emphasize importance of regular meal times and that meals must not be omitted.
- Teach patient that blood glucose monitoring is an essential guide to correct dosage and to therapeutic success.
- Emphasize importance of recognizing hypoglycemic symptoms because insulin-induced hypoglycemia is hazardous and may cause brain damage if prolonged.
- Advise patient to always wear a medical identification bracelet or pendant, to carry ample insulin supply and syringes on trips, to have carbohydrates (sugar or candy) on hand for emergency, and to note time-zone changes for dose schedule when traveling.
- Instruct patient not to change the order of mixing insulins or change the model or brand of syringe or needle. Be sure he knows when mixing two insulins, always to draw regular insulin into the syringe first.
- Inform patient that use of marijuana may increase insulin requirements.
- Inform patient that cigarette smoking decreases absorption of insulin administered S.C. Advise him not to smoke within 30 minutes after insulin injection.

interferon alfa-2a, recombinant

Roferon-A

interferon alfa-2b, recombinant

Intron A

Pharmacologic classification: biological response modifier
Therapeutic classification: antineoplastic
Pregnancy risk category C

How supplied

Available by prescription only
alfa-2a
Solution for injection: 3 million IU/vial, 9 million IU/vial, 9 million IU/multidose vial, 18 million IU/multidose vial, 36 million IU/multidose vial
Powder for injection with diluent: 18 million IU/multidose vial
alfa-2b
Powder for injection with diluent: 3 million IU/vial; 5 million IU/vial; 10 million IU/vial; 18 million IU/multidose vial; 25 million IU/vial; 50 million IU/vial
Solution for injection: 10 million IU/vial, 18 million IU/multidose vial, 25 million IU/vial

Indications and dosages

Hairy cell leukemia
alfa-2a
Adults: For induction, 3 million IU S.C. or I.M. daily for 16 to 24 weeks. For maintenance, 3 million IU S.C. or I.M. three times weekly.
alfa-2b
Adults: For induction and maintenance, 2 million IU/m^2 I.M. or S.C. three times weekly.
Condylomata acuminata
alfa-2b
Adults: 1 million IU per lesion, intralesionally, three times weekly for 3 weeks.
Kaposi's sarcoma
alfa-2a
Adults: For induction, 36 million IU S.C. or I.M. daily for 10 to 12 weeks; for maintenance, 36 million IU three times weekly.
alfa-2b
Adults: 30 million IU/m^2 S.C. or I.M. three times weekly. Maintain dose unless disease progresses rapidly or intolerance occurs.
Chronic hepatitis C
Adults: 3 million IU (alfa-2b) S.C. or I.M. three times weekly. If response occurs, continue therapy for 6 months. If no response by 16 weeks, discontinue therapy.
Chronic hepatitis B
Adults: 30 to 35 million IU (alfa-2b) S.C. or I.M. weekly either as 5 million IU daily or 10 million IU three times weekly for 16 weeks.

Pharmacodynamics

Antineoplastic action: Interferon alfa is a sterile protein product produced by recombinant DNA techniques applied to genetically engineered *Escherichia coli* bacteria. The interferons are naturally occurring small protein molecules produced and secreted by cells in response to viral infections or synthetic and biological inducers. Their exact mechanism of action is unknown but appears to involve direct antiproliferative action against tumor cells or viral cells to inhibit replication and modulation of host immune response by enhancing the phagocytic activity of macrophages and augmenting specific cytotoxicity of lymphocytes for target cells. To date, three major classes of interferons have been identified: alfa, beta, and gamma.

Pharmacokinetics

Absorption: More than 80% of dose is absorbed after I.M. or S.C. injection.
Distribution: Not applicable.
Metabolism: Appears to be metabolized in the liver and kidney.
Excretion: Reabsorbed from glomerular filtrate with minor biliary elimination.

Route	Onset	Peak	Duration
I.M., S.C.	Unknown	Unknown	Unknown

Contraindications and precautions

Contraindicated in patients hypersensitive to drug or to murine (mouse) immunoglobulin. Use cautiously in patients with CV or pulmonary disease, diabetes mellitus, coagulation disorders, or myelosuppression. Contraindicated in pregnant women and in male partners of pregnant women. Use cautiously in breast-feeding women; it isn't known if drug is excreted in breast milk.

Interactions

Drug-drug. *Blood dyscrasia-causing medications, bone marrow depressant therapy, radiation therapy:* Increased bone marrow depressant effects. Dosage reduction may be required.
CNS depressants: Enhanced CNS depression. Monitor patient closely.
Live virus vaccine: May potentiate replication of vaccine virus, increase adverse effects, and decrease patient's antibody response. Avoid use together.
Methylxanthines, such as aminophylline and theophylline: Increased half-life of these drugs, perhaps by interfering with cytochrome P-450 drug-metabolizing enzymes. Monitor patient closely.

Effects on diagnostic tests

None reported.

Adverse reactions

CNS: *dizziness, confusion,* paresthesia, numbness, lethargy, *depression, decreased mental status,* forgetfulness, ***coma,*** nervousness, insomnia, sedation, apathy, anxiety, irritability, fatigue, vertigo, gait disturbances, incoordination.
CV: hypotension, chest pain, ***arrhythmias,*** palpitations, syncope, ***heart failure,*** hypertension, edema, ***MI.***
EENT: *dryness or inflammation of the oropharynx,* rhinorrhea, sinusitis, conjunctivitis, earache, eye irritation.
GI: *anorexia, nausea, diarrhea, vomiting,* abdominal fullness, *abdominal pain,* flatulence, constipation, hypermotility, gastric distress, *weight loss, change in taste.*
GU: transient impotence.
Hematologic: ***leukopenia, mild thrombocytopenia.***
Hepatic: *hepatitis.*
Respiratory: *cough, dyspnea.*
Skin: diaphoresis, *rash, dryness, pruritus, partial alopecia,* urticaria, flushing.
Other: inflammation at injection site (rare), *flulike syndrome (fever, fatigue, myalgia, headache, chills, arthralgia),* excessive salivation, cyanosis, night sweats, hot flashes.

Overdose and treatment

No information available.

Clinical considerations

- When preparing antineoplastic agents for injection, take special precautions because of their potential for carcinogenicity and mutagenicity. Use of a biological containment cabinet is recommended. Don't shake vials.

□ ***ALERT*** Use S.C. administration route in patients whose platelet count is less than 50,000/mm³.

- Different brands of interferons may not be therapeutically interchangeable.
- Administration of drug at bedtime minimizes inconvenience of fatigue.
- When using interferon alfa-2b for condylomata acuminata by intralesional injection, use only the 10 million-IU vial reconstituted with 1 ml of diluent. Using other strengths or more diluent would produce a hypertonic solution. For administration, use a 25G to 30G needle and a tuberculin syringe. Up to five lesions may be treated simultaneously.
- The following indications aren't included in U.S. labeling, but drug may be used for these applications: chronic myelocytic leukemia; treatment of renal carcinoma or superficial bladder carcinoma; treatment of malignant lymphomas, especially nodular, poorly differentiated types; malignant melanoma; multiple myeloma; mycosis fungoides; papillomas; and laryngeal papillomatosis (interferon alfa-2b).

Therapeutic monitoring

- Almost all patients experience flulike symptoms at the beginning of therapy; these effects tend to diminish with continued therapy.
- Dosage reduction may be needed if headaches persist. Hypotension may result from fluid depletion; supportive treatment may be required.
- Recommend monitoring blood pressure, BUN, hematocrit, platelet count, ALT, AST, LD, alkaline phosphatase, serum bilirubin, creatinine, uric acid, total and differential leukocyte count, and ECG.
- Monitor for CNS adverse reactions, such as decreased mental status and dizziness. Periodic neuropsychiatric monitoring is recommended.

Special populations

Pregnant patients. Contraindicated in pregnancy. Women of childbearing age should use an effective method of contraception during therapy with interferon alpha preparations.
Breast-feeding patients. Drug has potential for serious adverse effects on breast-fed infants; a decision should be made whether to discontinue breast-feeding or discontinue drug.
Pediatric patients. Safety and efficacy in children under age 18 haven't been established.
Geriatric patients. Neurotoxicity and cardiotoxicity are more common in geriatric patients, especially those with underlying CNS or cardiac impairment.

Patient counseling

- Instruct patient the bone marrow depressant effects of interferon may result in increased incidence of microbial infection, delayed healing, and gingival bleeding. A decrease in salivary flow may also occur.
- Advise patient not to take a missed dose or to double the next dose, but to call for further instructions.
- Inform patient to store drug in refrigerator and to keep it from freezing.
- Caution patient against driving or performing tasks requiring alertness until response to medication is known.
- Advise patient to seek medical approval before taking OTC medications for colds, coughs, allergies, and similar disorders; explain that interferons commonly cause flulike symptoms and patient may need to take acetaminophen before each dose.
- Tell patient drug may cause temporary loss of some hair. Normal hair growth should return when drug is discontinued.
- Inform patient to avoid use of aspirin and chronic alcohol intake because these may increase risk of GI bleeding.

interferon beta-1a

Avonex

Pharmacologic classification: biological response modifier
Therapeutic classification: antiviral, immunoregulator
Pregnancy risk category C

How supplied

Available by prescription only
Lyophilized powder for injection: 33 mcg (6.6 million IU) of interferon beta-1a

Indications and dosages

To slow progression of physical disability and decrease the frequency of clinical exacerbations in relapsing multiple sclerosis
Adults: 30 mcg I.M. once weekly.

Pharmacodynamics

Antiviral and immunoregulator actions: The mechanisms by which interferon beta-1a exerts its actions in multiple sclerosis aren't clearly understood. However, it's known that the biological response-modifying properties of interferon beta-1a are mediated through its interactions with specific cell receptors found on the surface of human cells. The binding to these receptors induces the expression of a number of interferon-induced gene products that are believed to be the mediators of the biological actions of interferon beta-1a.

Pharmacokinetics

None known.

Route	Onset	Peak	Duration
I.M.	Unknown	Unknown	Unknown

Contraindications and precautions

Contraindicated in pregnancy and in patients with history of hypersensitivity to natural or recombinant interferon beta, human albumin, or any other component of the formulation. Use cautiously in patients with depression, seizure disorders, or severe cardiac conditions.

Interactions

None reported.

Effects on diagnostic tests

None reported.

Adverse reactions

CNS: malaise, *asthenia, headache, sleep difficulty, dizziness,* syncope, suicidal tendency, ***seizure,*** speech disorder, ataxia.
CV: chest pain, vasodilation.
EENT: otitis media, decreased hearing.
GI: *nausea, diarrhea, dyspepsia,* anorexia, abdominal pain.
GU: ovarian cyst, vaginitis.

Hematologic: anemia, elevated eosinophil levels, decreased hematocrit.
Hepatic: elevated AST levels.
Musculoskeletal: *muscle ache,* muscle spasm, arthralgia.
Respiratory: *upper respiratory tract infection,* sinusitis, dyspnea.
Skin: ecchymosis (at injection site), injection site reaction, urticaria, alopecia, nevus, herpes zoster, herpes simplex.
Other: *flulike symptoms, pain, fever, chills, infection,* hypersensitivity reaction.

Overdose and treatment
No information available.

Clinical considerations
- Exercise caution when administering drug to patients with preexisting seizure disorders.
- Store vials of drug in the refrigerator. If refrigeration is unavailable, drug can be stored at 77° F (25° C) for up to 30 days. Don't expose drug to high temperatures or freezing.

Therapeutic monitoring
- Recommend the following laboratory tests before initiating therapy and at periodic intervals thereafter: complete and differential WBC counts, platelet counts, and blood chemistries, including liver function tests.
- Use of interferon beta-1a may cause depression and suicidal ideation. It isn't known if these symptoms may be related to the underlying neurologic basis of multiple sclerosis, to interferon beta-1a treatment, or to a combination of both. Closely monitor patient for these symptoms and consider cessation of therapy if they occur.
- Monitor patient with cardiac disease, such as angina, heart failure, or arrhythmia, for worsening of clinical condition during initiation of therapy. Although drug doesn't have any known direct-acting cardiac toxicity, it does cause flulike symptoms, which may be stressful to patients with severe cardiac conditions.

Special populations
Pregnant patients. Discontinue therapy if pregnancy occurs.
Breast-feeding patients. It's unknown if drug is excreted in breast milk. Consider risks and benefits before continuing either breast-feeding or drug therapy.
Pediatric patients. Safety and effectiveness in children under age 18 haven't been established.

Patient counseling
- Caution patient not to change dosage or administration schedule. If a dose is missed, tell him to take it as soon as he remembers. The regular schedule may then be resumed, but two injections shouldn't be administered within 2 days of each other.
- Instruct patient how to store drug properly.
- Inform patient that flulike symptoms are common following initiation of therapy. Recommend use of acetaminophen to lessen the impact of these symptoms.
- Advise patient to report depression, suicidal ideation, or other adverse reactions.
- Advise women of childbearing age not to become pregnant while taking interferon beta-1a because of the abortifacient potential of drug. If pregnancy does occur, instruct patient to discontinue treatment and call immediately.

interferon beta-1b
Betaseron

Pharmacologic classification: biological response modifier
Therapeutic classification: antiviral, immunoregulator
Pregnancy risk category C

How supplied
Available by prescription only
Powder for injection, lyophilized: 9.6 million IU (0.3 mg)

Indications and dosages
Reduction of the frequency of exacerbations in relapsing-remitting multiple sclerosis
Adults: 8 million IU (0.25 mg) S.C. every other day.

Pharmacodynamics
Antiviral and immunoregulator actions: The mechanisms by which interferon beta-1b exerts its actions in multiple sclerosis aren't clearly understood. However, it's known that the biological response-modifying properties of interferon beta-1b are mediated through its interactions with specific cell receptors found on the surface of human cells. The binding to these receptors induces the expression of a number of interferon-induced gene products that are believed to be the mediators of the biological actions of interferon beta-1b.

Pharmacokinetics
Absorption: Serum levels are undetectable after the recommended dose.
Distribution: No information available.
Metabolism: No information available.
Excretion: No information available on patients with multiple sclerosis; however, in clinical studies involving healthy patients, elimination half-life ranged from 8 minutes to 4 hours.

Route	Onset	Peak	Duration
S.C.	Unknown	1-8 hr	Unknown

Contraindications and precautions
Contraindicated in patients hypersensitive to interferon beta or human albumin. Use cautiously in women of childbearing age; drug is contraindicated in pregnancy.

Interactions
None significant.

Effects on diagnostic tests
None reported.

Adverse reactions
CNS: *malaise,* depression, anxiety, emotional lability, depersonalization, ***suicidal tendencies,*** confusion, somnolence, *hypertonia, asthenia, migraine,* ***seizures,*** *headache, dizziness.*
CV: palpitations, hypertension, tachycardia, peripheral vascular disorder, hemorrhage.
EENT: laryngitis, *sinusitis, conjunctivitis,* abnormal vision.
GI: *diarrhea, constipation, abdominal pain, vomiting.*
GU: *menstrual disorders (bleeding or spotting, early or delayed menses, fewer days of menstrual flow, menorrhagia).*
Hematologic: *decreased WBC and absolute neutrophil counts.*
Hepatic: *elevated ALT levels; elevated bilirubin levels.*
Respiratory: dyspnea.
Skin: *inflammation, pain, and necrosis at injection site, alopecia.*
Other: *flulike symptoms (fever, chills, myalgia, diaphoresis);* breast pain, *pelvic pain; lymphadenopathy,* generalized edema, *myasthenia, diaphoresis,* Cushing's syndrome, diabetes insipidus, diabetes mellitus, hypothyroidism, SIADH secretion.

Overdose and treatment
No information available.

Clinical considerations
- Drug is being investigated in the treatment of AIDS, AIDS-related Kaposi's sarcoma, metastatic renal-cell carcinoma, malignant melanoma, cutaneous T-cell lymphoma, and acute hepatitis C as unlabeled uses.
- Inject drug immediately after preparation.
- Refrigerate drug or reconstituted product (up to 3 hours) at 36° to 46° F (2° to 8° C). Don't freeze.

Therapeutic monitoring
- Recommend performing the following laboratory tests before initiating therapy and at periodic intervals thereafter: hemoglobin, complete and differential WBC counts, platelet counts, and blood chemistries, including liver function tests.
- Drug use may cause depression and suicidal ideation. Other mental disorders have been observed and can include anxiety, emotional lability, depersonalization, and confusion. It's not known if these symptoms may be related to the underlying neurologic basis of multiple sclerosis, to interferon beta-1b treatment, or to a combination of both. Closely monitor patient with these symptoms and consider stopping therapy.

Special populations
Pregnant patients. Discontinue therapy if pregnancy occurs.
Breast-feeding patients. It's unknown if drug is excreted in breast milk. Consider risks and benefits before continuing either breast-feeding or drug therapy.
Pediatric patients. Safety and efficacy in children under age 18 haven't been established.

Patient counseling
- Caution patient to take protective measures (such as sunscreens, protective clothing) against exposure to ultraviolet light or sunlight until tolerance is determined.
- Teach patient how to self-administer S.C. injections, including solution preparation, use of aseptic technique, rotation of injection sites, and equipment disposal. Periodically reevaluate patient's technique.
- Instruct patient to rotate injection sites to minimize local reactions.
- Inform patient that flulike symptoms are common following initiation of therapy. Recommend taking drug at bedtime to help minimize the symptoms.
- Caution patient not to change dosage or schedule of administration without medical consultation.
- Advise patient to report depression or suicidal ideation.
- Inform women of childbearing age about abortifacient potential of drug.

interferon gamma-1b
Actimmune

Pharmacologic classification: biological response modifier
Therapeutic classification: antineoplastic
Pregnancy risk category C

How supplied
Available by prescription only
Injection: 100 mcg (3 million units)/0.5 ml in single-dose vials

Indications and dosages
To decrease the frequency and severity of serious infection of chronic granulomatous disease
Adults with body surface area over 0.5 m^2*:* 50 mcg/m^2 (1.5 million units/m^2) S.C. three times

weekly (such as Monday, Wednesday, and Friday).
Adults with body surface area of 0.5 m² *or less:* 1.5 mcg/kg S.C. three times weekly (such as Monday, Wednesday, and Friday).

Pharmacodynamics

Antineoplastic action: Interferon gamma-1b is a single-chain polypeptide containing 140 amino acids, produced by fermentation of genetically engineered *Escherichia coli.* It has potent phagocytic activity not seen with other interferons. Exact mechanism of action is unknown, but growing evidence suggests it interacts functionally with other interleukin molecules and all form part of a complex lymphokine network. A broad range of biological activities has been noted, including enhancement of oxidative metabolism of tissue macrophages, antibody-dependent cellular cytotoxicity, natural killer cell activity, and effects on Fc receptor expression on monocytes and major histocompatibility antigen expression. In chronic granulomatous disease, interferon gamma-1b provides enhancement of phagocyte function, including elevation of superoxide levels and improved killing of *Staphylococcus aureus.*

Pharmacokinetics

Absorption: About 90% is absorbed after S.C. injection.
Distribution: Unknown.
Metabolism: Unknown.
Excretion: Unknown. Mean elimination half-life after S.C. dosing is about 6 hours.

Route	Onset	Peak	Duration
P.O.	Unknown	7 hr	Unknown

Contraindications and precautions

Contraindicated in patients hypersensitive to drug or to genetically engineered products derived from *Escherichia coli.* Use cautiously in patients with CV disease (arrhythmias, heart failure, or ischemia), compromised CNS function, or seizure disorders and in those receiving myelosuppressive agents.

Interactions

Drug-drug. *Drugs that use this metabolic degradation pathway:* Interferon gamma-1b can decrease hepatic microsomal cytochrome P-450 levels, which could lead to decreased metabolism of drug. Use with caution.
Myelosuppressive agents: Additive effects. Use together cautiously.

Effects on diagnostic tests

None reported.

Adverse reactions

CNS: *fatigue,* decreased mental status, gait disturbance, dizziness.
GI: *nausea, vomiting, diarrhea,* abdominal pain.
GU: proteinuria.
Hematologic: ***neutropenia, thrombocytopenia.***
Hepatic: elevated liver enzyme levels (at high doses).
Metabolic: weight loss.
Musculoskeletal: back pain.
Skin: *rash; erythema, tenderness* (at injection site).
Other: flulike syndrome (headache, fever, chills, myalgia, arthralgia).

Overdose and treatment

No information available.

Clinical considerations

- Store drug in refrigerator immediately; don't freeze. Avoid excessive or vigorous agitation. Don't shake. Unopened or unentered vials shouldn't be left at room temperature longer than 12 hours before use. Don't return vials that exceed these limits to refrigerator; discard them.
- Each vial is designed for single use only.

Therapeutic monitoring

- If acute hypersensitivity reaction occurs, discontinue drug immediately and institute symptomatic and supportive treatment.
- Transient cutaneous rash hasn't required discontinuation of therapy.
- If severe adverse reactions occur, reduce dose by 50% or discontinue therapy until reaction subsides.

Special populations

Breast-feeding patients. It's unknown if drug is excreted in breast milk. Consider risks and benefits before continuing either breast-feeding or drug therapy.
Pediatric patients. Safety and efficacy haven't been established in children under age 1.

Patient counseling

Thoroughly review the patient information package insert with patient.

ipecac syrup

Pharmacologic classification: alkaloid emetic
Therapeutic classification: emetic
Pregnancy risk category C

How supplied

Available with and without a prescription
Syrup: 70 mg powdered ipecac/ml

Indications and dosages

To induce vomiting in poisoning
Adults: 15 to 30 ml P.O., followed by 200 to 300 ml of water.
Children age 1 or older: 15 ml P.O., followed by about 200 ml of water or milk.
Children under age 1: 5 to 10 ml P.O., followed by 100 to 200 ml of water or milk.
May repeat dose once after 20 minutes, if necessary.

Pharmacodynamics

Emetic action: Ipecac syrup directly irritates the GI mucosa and directly stimulates the chemoreceptor trigger zone through the effects of emetine and cephalin, its two alkaloids.

Pharmacokinetics

Absorption: Absorbed in significant amounts mainly when it doesn't produce emesis.
Distribution: Unknown.
Metabolism: Unknown.
Excretion: Emetine is excreted in urine slowly, over a period lasting up to 60 days.

Route	Onset	Peak	Duration
P.O.	20 min	Unknown	20-25 min

Contraindications and precautions

Contraindicated in semicomatose or unconscious patients or those with severe inebriation, seizures, shock, or loss of gag reflex. Don't give after ingestion of gasoline, kerosene, volatile oils, or caustic substances (lye).

Interactions

Drug-drug. *Activated charcoal:* May inactivate ipecac syrup and shouldn't be taken together. Activated charcoal may be given after patient vomits.
Antiemetics: Decreased effectiveness of ipecac. Avoid use together.
Drug-food. *Milk (or milk products):* May decrease therapeutic effectiveness of ipecac syrup. Avoid use together.
Carbonated beverages: May cause abdominal distention. Avoid use together.
Vegetable oil: Delays absorption. Don't take together.

Effects on diagnostic tests

None reported.

Adverse reactions

CNS: depression, *drowsiness.*
CV: ***arrhythmias,*** bradycardia, hypotension; atrial fibrillation, ***fatal myocarditis*** (with excessive doses).
GI: diarrhea.

Overdose and treatment

Clinical effects of overdose include diarrhea, persistent nausea or vomiting (longer than 30 minutes), stomach cramps or pain, arrhythmias, hypotension, myocarditis, difficulty breathing, and unusual fatigue or weakness.

Toxicity from chronic ipecac overdose usually involves use of the concentrated fluid extract in dosage appropriate for the syrup. Clinical effects of cardiotoxicity include tachycardia, T-wave depression, atrial fibrillation, depressed myocardial contractility, heart failure, and myocarditis. Other toxic effects include bloody stools and vomitus, hypotension, shock, seizures, and coma. Heart failure is the usual cause of death.

Treatment requires discontinuation of drug followed by symptomatic and supportive care, which may include digitalis and pacemaker therapy to treat cardiotoxic effects. However, no antidote exists for the cardiotoxic effects of ipecac, which may be fatal despite intensive treatment.

Clinical considerations

- Ipecac syrup usually empties the stomach completely within 30 minutes (in over 90% of patients); average emptying time is 20 minutes.

☐ ***ALERT*** Don't confuse ipecac syrup with ipecac fluidextract, which is rarely used but is 14 times more potent. Never store these two drugs together—the wrong drug could cause death.

- In antiemetic toxicity, ipecac syrup is usually effective if less than 1 hour has passed since ingestion of antiemetic.
- Ipecac syrup may be used in small amounts as an expectorant in cough preparations; however, this use has doubtful therapeutic benefit.

Therapeutic monitoring

- Little if any systemic toxicity occurs with doses of 30 ml or less.
- Drug may be abused by patients with eating disorders (such as bulimia or anorexia nervosa).

Special populations

Breast-feeding patients. Safety in breast-feeding women hasn't been established; possible risks must be weighed against benefits of drug.
Pediatric patients. Advise parents to keep ipecac syrup at home at all times but to keep it out of children's reach.

Patient counseling

- Instruct patient to take syrup with 1 or 2 glasses of water.
- Advise patient to take activated charcoal only after vomiting has stopped.

ipratropium bromide

Atrovent

Pharmacologic classification: anticholinergic
Therapeutic classification: bronchodilator
Pregnancy risk category B

How supplied

Available by prescription only
Inhaler: each metered dose supplies 18 mcg
Inhalation solution: 0.02%
Nasal spray: 0.03%, 0.06%

Indications and dosages

Bronchospasm in chronic bronchitis and emphysema
Adults: Usually, 2 inhalations (36 mcg) q.i.d.; patient may take additional inhalations, p.r.n., but shouldn't exceed 12 inhalations in 24 hours or 500 mcg q 6 to 8 hours via oral nebulizer.
Rhinorrhea associated with allergic and nonallergic perennial rhinitis
0.03% nasal spray
Adults and children age 12 and older: 2 sprays (42 mcg) per nostril b.i.d. or t.i.d.
Rhinorrhea associated with the common cold
0.06% nasal spray
Adults and children age 12 and older: 2 sprays (84 mcg) per nostril t.i.d. or q.i.d.
Children age 5 to 11: 2 sprays (84 mcg) per nostril three times daily.

Pharmacodynamics

Anticholinergic action: Ipratropium appears to inhibit vagally mediated reflexes by antagonizing the action of acetylcholine. Anticholinergics prevent the increases in intracellular concentration of cyclic guanosine monophosphate (cyclic GMP) that result from interaction of acetylcholine with the muscarinic receptor on bronchial smooth muscle.

The bronchodilation following inhalation is primarily a local, site-specific effect, not a systemic one.

Pharmacokinetics

Absorption: Not readily absorbed into the systemic circulation either from the surface of the lung or from the GI tract as confirmed by blood levels and renal excretion studies. Much of an inhaled dose is swallowed.
Distribution: Not applicable.
Metabolism: Metabolism is hepatic; elimination half-life is about 2 hours.
Excretion: Most of an administered dose is excreted unchanged in feces. Absorbed drug is excreted in urine and bile.

Route	Onset	Peak	Duration
Inhalation	Unknown	Unknown	Unknown
Intranasal	Unknown	Unknown	Unknown

Contraindications and precautions

Contraindicated in patients with hypersensitivity to drug or atropine or its derivatives and in those with a history of hypersensitivity to soya lecithin or related food products, such as soybeans and peanuts. Use cautiously in patients with angle-closure glaucoma, prostatic hyperplasia, and bladder-neck obstruction.

Interactions

Drug-drug. *Antimuscarinic agents, including ophthalmic preparations:* Concurrent use may produce additive effects. Avoid use together.
Fluorocarbon propellant-containing oral inhalants, such as adrenocorticoids, cromolyn, glucocorticoids, and sympathomimetics: Increased risk of fluorocarbon toxicity may result from too-closely timed administration of ipratropium and other fluorocarbon propellant–containing oral inhalants. A 5-minute interval between administration of such agents is recommended.
Drug-herb. *Jaborandi tree, pill-bearing spurge:* Products may decrease therapeutic effect of drug. Monitor patient closely.

Effects on diagnostic tests

None reported.

Adverse reactions

CNS: dizziness, headache, nervousness.
CV: palpitations, chest pain.
EENT: cough, blurred vision, rhinitis, sinusitis.
GI: nausea, GI distress, dry mouth.
Musculoskeletal: back pain.
Respiratory: *upper respiratory tract infection, bronchitis,* cough, dyspnea, pharyngitis, ***bronchospasm,*** increased sputum.
Skin: rash.
Other: pain, flulike symptoms.

Overdose and treatment

Acute overdose by inhalation is unlikely because ipratropium isn't well absorbed systemically after aerosol or oral administration.

Clinical considerations

- Because of delayed onset of bronchodilation, drug isn't recommended to treat acute respiratory distress.
- Initial nasal spray pump requires priming with seven actuations of the pump. If used regularly as recommended, no further priming is needed. If not used for more than 24 hours, the pump will require two actuations. If not used

for more than 7 days, the pump will require seven actuations to reprime.

Therapeutic monitoring

Monitor for adverse drug events and therapeutic effect.

Special populations

Breast-feeding patients. It's unknown if drug is excreted in breast milk. Although lipid-insoluble quaternary bases pass into breast milk, ipratropium is unlikely to reach the infant, especially when taken by aerosol. Use caution when administering to breast-feeding women.
Pediatric patients. Safety and efficacy in children under age 12 haven't been established.

Patient counseling

- Instruct patient on correct method of administration.
- Advise patient to allow 1 minute between inhalations.
- Instruct patient to take a missed dose as soon as possible, unless it is almost time for the next scheduled dose, in which case he should skip the missed dose. Warn him to never double the dose.
- Suggest sugarless hard candy, gum, ice, or saliva substitute to relieve dry mouth. Tell patient to report dry mouth to prescriber if it persists longer than 2 weeks.
- Instruct patient to call prescriber if he experiences no benefits within 30 minutes after administration, or if condition worsens.

irbesartan

Avapro

Pharmacologic classification: angiotensin II receptor antagonist
Therapeutic classification: antihypertensive
Pregnancy risk category C (D, in second and third trimesters)

How supplied

Available by prescription only
Tablets: 75 mg, 150 mg, 300 mg

Indications and dosages

Treatment of hypertension—alone, or in combination with other antihypertensives
Adults: Initially 150 mg P.O. once daily, increased to maximum of 300 mg once daily if necessary, without regard to food.
≡ ***Dosage adjustment.*** In volume- and salt-depleted patients, give 75 mg P.O. initially.

Pharmacodynamics

Antihypertensive action: Irbesartan blocks the vasoconstrictor and aldosterone-secreting effects of angiotensin II by selectively blocking the binding of angiotensin II to its receptor sites.

Pharmacokinetics

Absorption: Absorbed rapidly and completely. The average absolute bioavailability is 60% to 80% and is not affected by food.
Distribution: 90% bound to plasma proteins. It may cross the blood-brain barrier and placenta. Steady state is achieved within 3 days. Drug is widely distributed.
Metabolism: Metabolized by conjugation and oxidation. Cytochrome P-450 2C9 is the major enzyme responsible for formation of the oxidative metabolites. Metabolites don't appear to add appreciably to the pharmacologic activity.
Excretion: Excreted in the bile and urine. 20% is excreted in the urine and the rest in the feces. Drug may also be excreted in breast milk. Elimination half-life is 11 to 15 hours.

Route	Onset	Peak	Duration
P.O.	Unknown	1½-2 hr	24 hr

Contraindications and precautions

Contraindicated in patients who are hypersensitive to drug or its components and in pregnant or breast-feeding women.

Use cautiously in volume- or salt-depleted patients, in patients whose renal function may depend on the activity of the renin-angiotensin-aldosterone system (e.g., patients with severe heart failure), and in those with unilateral or bilateral renal artery stenosis.

Interactions

None reported.

Effects on diagnostic tests

None reported.

Adverse reactions

CNS: fatigue, anxiety, dizziness, headache.
CV: chest pain, edema, tachycardia.
EENT: pharyngitis, rhinitis, sinus abnormality.
GI: diarrhea, dyspepsia, abdominal pain, nausea, vomiting.
GU: urinary tract infection.
Musculoskeletal: musculoskeletal trauma or pain.
Respiratory: upper respiratory infection.
Skin: rash.

Overdose and treatment

No information available. The most likely signs and symptoms of an overdose are expected to be hypotension and tachycardia, and possibly bradycardia. Drug isn't removed by hemodialysis. If hypotension occurs, place patient in supine position and, if necessary, give an I.V. infusion of normal saline.

Clinical considerations

- Pharmacokinetics of drug aren't altered in patients with renal impairment or in patients on hemodialysis. Irbesartan isn't removed by hemodialysis. Dosage adjustment isn't necessary in patients with mild to severe renal impairment unless patient with renal impairment is also volume depleted.
- Dosage adjustment isn't necessary in patients with hepatic insufficiency.
- Patients not adequately treated by the maximum 300-mg once-daily dose are unlikely to derive additional benefit from a higher dose or twice-daily dosing.

Therapeutic monitoring

Monitor blood pressure regularly. A transient hypotensive response isn't a contraindication to further treatment. Therapy with irbesartan can usually be continued once blood pressure has stabilized.

Special populations

Pregnant patients. Contraindicated during pregnancy because of potential danger to the fetus. The patient should immediately call prescriber if pregnancy is suspected.
Breast-feeding patients. Because of the potential for serious adverse reactions in breast-fed infants, alternative feeding method should be used during drug therapy.
Pediatric patients. Safety and efficacy in children under age 18 haven't been established.

Patient counseling

- Instruct patient on the proper administration of the drug and the potential adverse reactions.
- Advise patient that if a dose is missed to take it as soon as possible, but not to double the dose.
- Warn patient about symptoms of hypotension and what to do.
- Caution patient not to discontinue drug without medical approval.

irinotecan hydrochloride

Camptosar

Pharmacologic classification: topoisomerase inhibitor
Therapeutic classification: antineoplastic
Pregnancy risk category D

How supplied

Available by prescription only
Injection: 20 mg/ml

Indications and dosages

Treatment of metastatic carcinoma of the colon or rectum in which the disease has recurred or progressed following fluorouracil (5-FU)-based therapy
Adults: Initially, 125 mg/m² I.V. infusion over 90 minutes. Recommended treatment regimen is 125 mg/m² I.V. administered once weekly for 4 weeks, followed by a 2-week rest period. Thereafter, additional courses of treatment may be repeated q 6 weeks (4 weeks on therapy, followed by 2 weeks off therapy). Subsequent doses may be adjusted to as high as 150 mg/m² or to as low as 50 mg/m² in 25- to 50-mg/m² increments depending on patient's tolerance. Treatment with additional courses may continue indefinitely in patients who attain a response or in those whose disease remains stable provided intolerable toxicity does not occur.

Pharmacodynamics

Antineoplastic action: Irinotecan is a derivative of camptothecin. Camptothecins interact specifically with the enzyme topoisomerase I, which relieves torsional strain in DNA by inducing reversible single-strand breaks. Irinotecan and its active metabolite bind to the topoisomerase I—DNA complex and prevent religation of these single-strand breaks.

Pharmacokinetics

Absorption: Only administered I.V.
Distribution: About 30% to 68% bound to plasma protein, whereas its active metabolite, SN-38, is about 95% bound.
Metabolism: Undergoes metabolic conversion in the liver to its active metabolite SN-38.
Excretion: A small amount of drug and SN-38 are excreted in urine. Terminal half-life of irinotecan is 6 hours in patients age 65 and older and 5½ hours in patients under age 65; mean terminal elimination half-life of SN-38 is about 10 hours.

Route	Onset	Peak	Duration
I.V.	Unknown	Unknown	Unknown

Contraindications and precautions

Contraindicated in patients with hypersensitivity to drug. Use cautiously in geriatric patients and in those who have previously received pelvic or abdominal irradiation because of increased risk of severe myelosuppression. Due to possible fetal risk, drug shouldn't be used during pregnancy.

Interactions

Drug-drug. *Other antineoplastic agents:* May cause additive adverse effects such as myelosuppression and diarrhea. Monitor patient closely.

Effects on diagnostic tests

None reported.

Adverse reactions

CNS: *insomnia, dizziness, asthenia, headache.*

CV: *vasodilation, edema.*
GI: DIARRHEA, *nausea, vomiting, anorexia, constipation, flatulence, stomatitis, dyspepsia, abdominal cramping and pain, abdominal enlargement.*
Hematologic: LEUKOPENIA, *anemia,* NEUTROPENIA.
Hepatic: *increased alkaline phosphatase, increased AST levels.*
Metabolic: *weight loss, dehydration.*
Musculoskeletal: *back pain.*
Respiratory: *dyspnea, increased coughing, rhinitis.*
Skin: *alopecia, sweating, rash.*
Other: *fever, pain, chills, minor infection.*

Overdose and treatment

The adverse effects of overdose are similar to those reported with the recommended dosage and regimen. There's no known antidote for drug overdose. Institute maximum supportive care to prevent dehydration because of diarrhea and to treat any infectious complications.

Clinical considerations

- Irinotecan must be diluted before infusion with D_5W injection (preferred) or normal saline injection to a final concentration range of 0.12 to 1.1 mg/ml.
- Drug solution is stable for up to 24 hours at room temperature of 77° F (25° C) and in ambient fluorescent lighting. Store solutions diluted in D_5W in refrigerator (35° to 46° F [2° to 8° C]) and protect from light; these are stable for 48 hours. However, because of possible microbial contamination during dilution, use admixture within 24 hours if refrigerated or within 6 hours if kept at room temperature. Refrigeration of admixtures using normal saline isn't recommended due to a low and sporadic incidence of visible particulates.
- Avoid freezing of drug and admixtures because drug may precipitate.
- Don't add other drugs to drug infusion.
- Irinotecan can induce severe forms of diarrhea.
- Routine administration of a colony-stimulating factor isn't necessary but may be helpful in patients experiencing significant neutropenia.

Therapeutic monitoring

- Careful monitoring of the WBC count with differential, hemoglobin, and platelet count is recommended before each dose of irinotecan.
- Temporarily discontinue therapy if neutropenic fever occurs or if the absolute neutrophil count drops below 500/mm^3. Reduce drug dose if there's a clinically significant decrease in the total WBC count (less than 2,000/mm^3), neutrophil count (less than 1,000/mm^3), hemoglobin (less than 8 g/dl), or platelet count (less than 100,000/mm^3). Consult manufacturer for dosage guidelines in these situations.

Special populations

Pregnant patients. Drug may be harmful to fetus.
Breast-feeding patients. It's unknown if drug is excreted in breast milk. Because of the potential for serious adverse reactions in breast-fed infants, discontinue breast-feeding during irinotecan therapy.
Pediatric patients. Safety and efficacy in children haven't been established.
Geriatric patients. Use caution when administering drug to geriatric patients, especially those with history of heart failure and hypotension.

Patient counseling

- Advise women of childbearing age to avoid pregnancy because drug may cause fetal harm.
- Inform patient about risk of diarrhea and when and how to treat it if it occurs.
- Tell patient to call prescriber if vomiting occurs, fever or evidence of infection develops, or symptoms of dehydration (fainting, lightheadedness, or dizziness) occur following drug administration.
- Warn patient that alopecia may occur.

iron dextran

DexFerrum, InFeD

Pharmacologic classification: parenteral iron supplement
Therapeutic classification: hematinic
Pregnancy risk category C

How supplied

Available by prescription only
Injection: 50 mg elemental iron/ml in 2-ml single dose vials

Indications and dosages

Iron-deficiency anemia
Adults and children: Dosage is highly individualized and is based on patient's weight and hemoglobin level. Drug is usually given I.M.; preservative-free solution can be given I.V. Check current literature for recommended protocol.

Pharmacodynamics

Hematinic action: Iron dextran is a complex of ferric hydroxide and dextran in a colloidal solution. After I.M. injection, 10% to 50% remains in the muscle for several months; remainder enters bloodstream, increasing plasma iron level for up to 2 weeks. Iron is an essential component of hemoglobin.

Pharmacokinetics

Absorption: I.M. doses are absorbed in two stages: 60% after 3 days, and up to 90% by 3 weeks. Remainder is absorbed over several months or longer.
Distribution: During first 3 days, local inflammation facilitates passage of drug into the lymphatic system; drug is then ingested by macrophages, which enter lymph and blood.
Metabolism: After I.M. or I.V. administration, iron dextran is cleared from plasma by reticuloendothelial cells of the liver, spleen, and bone marrow.
Excretion: In doses of 500 mg or less, half-life is 6 hours. Traces are excreted in breast milk, urine, bile, and feces. Drug can't be removed by hemodialysis.

Route	Onset	Peak	Duration
I.M., I.V.	Unknown	Unknown	Unknown

Contraindications and precautions

Contraindicated in patients with hypersensitivity to drug, in those with all types of anemia except iron-deficiency anemia, and in those with acute infectious renal disease. Use cautiously in patients with impaired hepatic function, rheumatoid arthritis, and other inflammatory diseases.

Interactions

Drug-herb. *Oregano:* Reduced iron absorption. Separate administration by at least 2 hours when given with iron supplements or iron-containing foods.

Effects on diagnostic tests

Large doses (more than 250 mg iron) may color the serum brown. Iron dextran may cause false elevations of serum bilirubin level and false reductions in serum calcium level. Iron dextran prevents meaningful measurement of serum iron level and total iron binding capacity for up to 3 weeks; I.M. injection may cause dense areas of activity on bone scans using technetium 99m diphosphonate, for 1 to 6 days.

Adverse reactions

CNS: headache, transitory paresthesia, dizziness, malaise.
CV: *hypotensive reaction, peripheral vascular flushing (with overly rapid I.V. administration),* bradycardia.
GI: nausea, anorexia.
Musculoskeletal: arthralgia, myalgia.
Respiratory: ***bronchospasm,*** dyspnea.
Skin: rash, urticaria, purpura. *brown skin discoloration (at I.M. injection site); local phlebitis (at I.V. injection site),* sterile abscess, necrosis, atrophy, fibrosis.
Other: *soreness, inflammation,* ***anaphylaxis,*** delayed sensitivity reactions, fever, chills.

Overdose and treatment

Injected iron has much greater bioavailability than oral iron, but data on acute overdose are limited.

Clinical considerations

- Discontinue oral iron before giving iron dextran.
- Administer a test dose of 0.5 ml iron dextrose I.M. or I.V. with monitoring for drug reactions including anaphylaxis. Keep epinephrine (0.5 ml of a 1:1,000 solution) readily available for such an emergency.
- I.V. use is controversial, and some health care facilities don't allow it. I.V. is route of choice if patient has insufficient muscle mass for deep injection, impaired absorption from muscle because of stasis or edema, a risk of uncontrolled I.M. bleeding from trauma (as in hemophilia), or need for massive and prolonged parenteral therapy (as in chronic substantial blood loss). Administer no more than 50 mg of iron/minute (1 ml/minute) if using drug undiluted. Vein must be flushed with 10 ml normal saline injection to minimize local irritation.

Therapeutic monitoring

- Monitor hemoglobin, hematocrit, and reticulocyte count during therapy. An increase of about 1 g/dl weekly in hemoglobin is usual.
- Monitor for tissue damage and adverse events.

Special populations

Breast-feeding patients. Traces of unmetabolized iron dextran are excreted in breast milk; impact on infant is unknown.
Pediatric patients. Drug isn't recommended for use in children under age 4 months.

Patient counseling

Warn patient of possibility of skin staining with I.M. injections.

isoniazid (INH)

Isotamine*, Laniazid, Laniazid C.T., Nydrazid, PMS Isoniazid*

Pharmacologic classification: isonicotinic acid hydrazine
Therapeutic classification: antitubercular
Pregnancy risk category C

How supplied

Available by prescription only
Tablets: 50 mg, 100 mg, 300 mg
Oral solution: 50 mg/5 ml
Injection: 100 mg/ml

Indications and dosages

Primary treatment against actively growing tubercle bacilli
Adults: 5 mg/kg P.O. or I.M. daily in a single dose, up to 300 mg/day, continued for 9 months to 2 years.
Infants and children: 10 mg/kg P.O. or I.M. daily in a single dose, up to 300 mg/day, continued for 18 months to 2 years. Concomitant administration of at least one other effective antitubercular drug is recommended.
Prophylaxis against tubercle bacilli of those closely exposed or with positive skin test
Adults: 300 mg P.O. daily single dose, continued for 6 months to 1 year.
Infants and children: 10 mg/kg P.O. daily single dose, up to 300 mg/day, continued for 6 months to 1 year.

Pharmacodynamics

Antitubercular action: INH interferes with lipid and DNA synthesis, thus inhibiting bacterial cell wall synthesis. Its action is bacteriostatic or bactericidal, depending on organism susceptibility and drug concentration at infection site. INH is active against *Mycobacterium tuberculosis, M. bovis,* and some strains of *M. kansasii.*

Resistance by *M. tuberculosis* develops rapidly when INH is used to treat tuberculosis, and it's usually combined with another antitubercular agent to prevent or delay resistance. During prophylaxis, however, resistance isn't a problem and isoniazid can be used alone.

Pharmacokinetics

Absorption: Rapidly and completely absorbed from the GI tract after oral administration. INH also is absorbed readily after I.M. injection.
Distribution: Distributed widely into body tissues and fluids, including ascitic, synovial, pleural, and cerebrospinal fluids; lungs and other organs; and sputum and saliva. Drug crosses the placenta and enters breast milk in levels similar to plasma.
Metabolism: Inactivated primarily in the liver by genetically controlled acetylation. Rate of metabolism varies individually; fast acetylators metabolize drug five times as rapidly as others. About 50% of blacks and whites are slow acetylators of INH, whereas more than 80% of Chinese, Japanese, and Eskimos are fast acetylators.
Excretion: About 75% of a dose is excreted in urine as unchanged drug and metabolites in 24 hours; some drug is excreted in saliva, sputum, feces, and breast milk. Plasma half-life in adults is 1 to 4 hours, depending on metabolic rate. Drug is removed by peritoneal dialysis or hemodialysis.

Route	Onset	Peak	Duration
P.O.	Unknown	1-2 hr	Unknown
I.M.	Unknown	Unknown	Unknown

Contraindications and precautions

Contraindicated in patients with acute hepatic disease or drug-associated hepatic damage. Use cautiously in the elderly and in patients with severe, non-INH-associated hepatic disease, seizure disorders (especially those taking phenytoin), severe renal impairment, or chronic alcoholism.

Interactions

Drug-drug. *Antacids:* Decreases oral absorption of INH. Give antacid at least one hour before INH.
Anticoagulants: May increase anticoagulant activity. Dosage adjustment may be needed.
Benzodiazepines (such as diazepam), carbamazepine, phenytoin: INH-induced inhibition of metabolism and elevation of serum levels, causing toxicity. Monitor patient closely.
Corticosteroids: May decrease INH efficacy. Monitor patient for drug effects.
Cycloserine: Increases hazard of CNS toxicity, drowsiness, and dizziness. Monitor patient for safety.
Disulfiram: May cause coordination difficulties and psychotic episodes. Patient requires close observation.
Rifampin: May accelerate INH metabolism to hepatotoxic metabolites. Use with caution.
Drug-lifestyle. *Alcohol use:* Increased incidence of INH-induced hepatitis and seizures. Advise patient to avoid alcohol.

Effects on diagnostic tests

INH alters results of urine glucose tests that use cupric sulfate method (Benedict's reagent, Diastix, or Chemstrip uG). Elevated liver function study results occur in about 15% of cases; most abnormalities are mild and transient, but some persist throughout treatment.

Adverse reactions

CNS: *peripheral neuropathy* (dose-related and especially in patients who are malnourished, alcoholic, diabetic, or slow acetylators), usually preceded by paresthesia of hands and feet, ***seizures,*** toxic encephalopathy, memory impairment, toxic psychosis.
EENT: optic neuritis, atrophy.
GI: nausea, vomiting, epigastric distress.
GU: gynecomastia.
Hematologic: ***agranulocytosis,*** hemolytic anemia, ***aplastic anemia,*** eosinophilia, ***thrombocytopenia,*** sideroblastic anemia.
Hepatic: ***hepatitis*** (occasionally severe and sometimes fatal, especially in elderly patients), jaundice, *elevated serum transaminase levels,* bilirubinemia.
Metabolic: hyperglycemia, metabolic acidosis, pyridoxine deficiency, hypocalcemia, hypophosphatemia.
Skin: irritation at I.M. injection site.
Other: rheumatic and lupuslike syndromes, ***hypersensitivity reactions*** (fever, rash, lymphadenopathy, vasculitis).

Overdose and treatment

Early signs of overdose include nausea, vomiting, slurred speech, dizziness, blurred vision, and visual hallucinations, occurring 30 minutes to 3 hours after ingestion; gross overdose causes CNS depression progressing from stupor to coma, with respiratory distress, intractable seizures, and death.

To treat, establish ventilation; control seizures with diazepam. Pyridoxine is administered to equal dose of INH. Initial dose is 1 to 4 g pyridoxine I.V., followed by 1 g every 30 minutes thereafter, until the entire dose is given. Clear drug with gastric lavage after seizure control and correct acidosis with parenteral sodium bicarbonate; force diuresis with I.V. fluids and osmotic diuretics, and, if necessary, enhance clearance of the drug with hemodialysis or peritoneal dialysis.

Clinical considerations

- At least 12 months of preventive therapy is recommended for patients with past tuberculosis and HIV-infected patients.
- If compliance is a problem, twice-weekly supervised drug administration may be effective. Recommended twice-weekly dose for adults is 15 mg/kg P.O., not to exceed 900 mg.
- Oral doses should be taken on empty stomach for maximum absorption, or with food if gastric irritation occurs.
- Aluminum-containing antacids or laxatives should be taken 1 hour after oral dose of INH.
- Drug may hinder stabilization of serum glucose level in patients with diabetes mellitus.
- Pyridoxine 50 mg P.O. daily is sometimes recommended to prevent peripheral neuropathy from large doses of INH. It may also be useful in patients at risk of developing peripheral neuropathy (malnourished patients, diabetics, and alcohol abusers). Pyridoxine (50 to 200 mg daily) has been used to treat drug-induced neuropathy.
- Because drug is dialyzable, patients undergoing hemodialysis or peritoneal dialysis may need dosage adjustments.

Therapeutic monitoring

- Monitor for adverse effects, especially hepatic dysfunction, CNS toxicity, and optic neuritis.
- Monitor blood, renal, and hepatic function studies before and periodically during therapy to minimize toxicity; assess visual function periodically.
- Hepatotoxicity appears to be age-related and may limit use for prophylaxis. Alcohol consumption and history of alcohol-related liver disease also increases risk of hepatotoxicity.
- Improvement is usually evident after 2 to 3 weeks of therapy.

Special populations

Pregnant patients. Safe use of drug during pregnancy hasn't been established. Potential benefits to the woman should be weighed against the risks to the fetus.

Breast-feeding patients. Drug is excreted in breast milk; use with caution in breast-feeding women and monitor infants for possible INH-induced toxicity.

Pediatric patients. Infants and children tolerate larger doses of drug.

Geriatric patients. Use with caution in geriatric patients; incidence of hepatic effects is increased after age 35. Drug prophylaxis in patients with a positive purified protein derivative (PPD) test may not be indicated in older patients because of risk of hepatotoxicity.

Patient counseling

- Instruct patient on the proper administration of drug and the potential for adverse reactions.
- Warn patient not to use alcohol.
- Urge patient to comply with and complete prescribed regimen.
- Advise patient not to discontinue drug without medical approval.
- Explain importance of follow-up appointments.

isoproterenol

Isuprel

isoproterenol hydrochloride

Isuprel, Isuprel Mistometer

isoproterenol sulfate

Medihaler-Iso

Pharmacologic classification: adrenergic
Therapeutic classification: bronchodilator, cardiac stimulant
Pregnancy risk category C

How supplied

Available by prescription only
isoproterenol
Nebulizer inhaler: 0.25%, 0.5%, 1%
isoproterenol hydrochloride
Aerosol inhaler: 120 mcg/metered spray, 131 mcg/metered spray
Injection: 20 mcg/ml, 200 mcg/ml
isoproterenol sulfate
Aerosol inhaler: 80 mcg/metered spray

Indications and dosages

Complete heart block after closure of ventricular septal defect
Adults: I.V. bolus, 0.02 to 0.06 mg (1 to 3 ml of a 1:50,000 dilution).
Children: I.V. bolus, 0.01 to 0.03 mg (0.5 to 1.5 ml of a 1:50,000 dilution).

Bronchospasm during mild acute asthma attacks
isoproterenol hydrochloride
Adults and children: Via aerosol inhalation, 1 inhalation initially, repeated, p.r.n. after 1 to 5 minutes, to maximum 6 inhalations daily. Maintenance dosage is 1 to 2 inhalations four to six times daily at 3- to 4-hour intervals. Via hand-bulb nebulizer, 5 to 15 deep inhalations of a 0.5% solution; if needed, may be repeated in 5 to 10 minutes. May be repeated up to five times daily.

Alternatively, 3 to 7 deep inhalations of a 1% solution, repeated once in 5 to 10 minutes if needed. May be repeated up to five times daily.

isoproterenol sulfate
Adults and children: For acute dyspneic episodes, 1 inhalation initially; repeated if needed after 2 to 5 minutes. Maximum 6 inhalations daily. Maintenance dosage is 1 to 2 inhalations up to six times daily.

Bronchospasm in COPD
isoproterenol hydrochloride
Adults and children: Via hand-bulb nebulizer: 5 to 15 deep inhalations of a 0.5% solution, or 3 to 7 deep inhalations of a 1% solution no more frequently than q 3 to 4 hours.

Bronchospasm during mild acute asthma attacks or in COPD
isoproterenol hydrochloride
Adults and children: Oral inhalation of 2 ml of 0.125% solution or 2.5 ml of 0.1% solution up to five times daily.

Acute asthma attacks unresponsive to inhalation therapy or control of bronchospasm during anesthesia
isoproterenol hydrochloride
Adults: 0.01 to 0.02 mg (0.5 to 1 ml of a 1:50,000 dilution) I.V. Repeat, if needed.

Emergency treatment of arrhythmias
isoproterenol hydrochloride
Adults: Initially, 0.02 to 0.06 mg I.V. bolus. Subsequent doses 0.01 to 0.2 mg I.V. Alternatively, 5 mcg/minute titrated to patient's response. Range, 2 to 20 mcg/minute. Alternatively, 0.2 mg I.M. or S.C.; subsequent doses 0.02 to 1 mg I.M. or 0.15 to 0.2 mg S.C. In extreme cases, 0.02 mg (0.1 of 1:5,000) intracardiac injection.
Children: May give half of initial adult dose.

Immediate temporary control of atropine-resistant hemodynamically significant bradycardia
isoproterenol hydrochloride
Adults: 2 to 10 mcg/minute I.V. infusion, titrated to patient's response.
Children: 0.1 mcg/kg/minute, titrated to patient's response. Maximum rate 1 mcg/kg/minute.

Heart block, Stokes-Adams attacks, and shock
isoproterenol hydrochloride
Adults and children: 0.5 to 5 mcg/minute by continuous I.V. infusion titrated to patient's response; or 0.02 to 0.06 mg I.V. boluses with 0.01 to 0.2 mg additional doses; or 0.2 mg I.M. or S.C. with 0.02 to 1 mg I.M. or 0.15 to 0.2 mg additional doses.

Pharmacodynamics

Bronchodilator action: Isoproterenol relaxes bronchial smooth muscle by direct action on $beta_2$-adrenergic receptors, relieving bronchospasm, increasing vital capacity, decreasing residual volume in lungs, and facilitating passage of pulmonary secretions. It also produces relaxation of GI and uterine smooth muscle via stimulation of $beta_2$ receptors. Peripheral vasodilation, cardiac stimulation, and relaxation of bronchial smooth muscle are the main therapeutic effects.
Cardiac stimulant action: Isoproterenol acts on $beta_1$-adrenergic receptors in the heart, producing a positive chronotropic and inotropic effect; it usually increases cardiac output. In patients with AV block, isoproterenol shortens conduction time and the refractory period of the AV node and increases the rate and strength of ventricular contraction.

Pharmacokinetics

Absorption: After injection or oral inhalation, absorption is rapid; after sublingual or rectal administration, absorption is variable and often unreliable.
Distribution: Distributed widely throughout the body.
Metabolism: Metabolized by conjugation in the GI tract and by enzymatic reduction in liver, lungs, and other tissues.
Excretion: Excreted primarily in urine as unchanged drug and its metabolites.

Route	Onset	Peak	Duration
I.V.	Immediate	Unknown	Few minutes
S.C.	Immediate	Unknown	2 hr
Oral inhaler	Immediate	Unknown	Unknown

Contraindications and precautions

Contraindicated in patients with tachycardia caused by digitalis intoxication, in patients with preexisting arrhythmias (other than those that may respond to treatment with isoproterenol), and in those with angina pectoris. Use cautiously in the elderly and in patients with impaired renal function, CV disease, coronary insufficiency, diabetes, hyperthyroidism, or a sensitivity to sympathomimetic amines.

Interactions

Drug-drug. *Beta blockers:* Antagonize cardiac-stimulating, bronchodilating, and vasodilating effects of isoproterenol. Monitor patient closely.

Cardiac glycoside, potassium-depleting drugs, or other drugs that affect cardiac rhythm: Arrhythmias may occur. Monitor patient's ECG.
Cyclopropane or halogenated hydrocarbon general anesthetics: Increased risk of arrhythmias. Avoid use together.
Epinephrine and other sympathomimetics: May cause additive CV reactions. Drugs may be used together if at least 4 hours elapse between administration of the two drugs. Use together cautiously.
Ergot alkaloids: May increase blood pressure. Use with caution.

Effects on diagnostic tests

Isoproterenol may reduce the sensitivity of spirometry in the diagnosis of asthma.

Adverse reactions

CNS: *headache, mild tremor,* weakness, dizziness, *nervousness,* insomnia, ***Stokes-Adams attacks.***
CV: palpitations, *tachycardia, anginal pain,* ***arrhythmias, cardiac arrest,*** *rapid increase and decrease in blood pressure.*
GI: *nausea, vomiting, heartburn.*
Metabolic: hyperglycemia.
Respiratory: ***bronchospasm,*** bronchitis, sputum increase, pulmonary edema.
Skin: diaphoresis.
Other: swelling of parotid glands (with prolonged use).

Overdose and treatment

Signs and symptoms of overdose include exaggeration of common adverse reactions, particularly arrhythmias, extreme tremors, nausea, vomiting, and profound hypotension.

Treatment includes symptomatic and supportive measures. Monitor vital signs closely. Sedatives (barbiturates) may be used to treat CNS stimulation. Use cardioselective beta blockers to treat tachycardia and arrhythmias. Use these agents with caution; they may induce asthmatic attack.

Clinical considerations

Consider the recommendations relevant to all adrenergics as well as the following:

- Drug doesn't replace administration of blood, plasma, fluids, or electrolytes in patients with blood volume depletion.
- Severe paradoxical airway resistance may follow oral inhalations.
- Hypotension must be corrected before isoproterenol is administered.
- Continuously monitor ECG during I.V. administration.
- Prescribed I.V. infusion rate should include specific guidelines for regulating flow or terminating infusion in relation to heart rate, premature beats, ECG changes, precordial distress, blood pressure, and urine flow. Because of danger of precipitating arrhythmias, rate of infusion is usually decreased or infusion may be temporarily discontinued if heart rate exceeds 110 beats/minute.
- Isoproterenol has also been used to aid diagnosis of coronary artery disease and of mitral regurgitation.

Therapeutic monitoring

- Carefully monitor response to therapy by frequent determinations of heart rate, ECG pattern, blood pressure, and central venous pressure, as well as (for patients in shock) urine volume, blood pH, and Pco_2 levels.
- Monitor patient for rebound bronchospasm when effects of drug end.
- If three to five treatments within 6 to 12 hours provide minimal or no relief, re-evaluate therapy.

Special populations

Pregnant patients. Administer drug during pregnancy only when clearly indicated.
Breast-feeding patients. It's unknown if drug is excreted in breast milk; therefore, use cautiously in breast-feeding women.
Pediatric patients. Use with caution in children.
Geriatric patients. Geriatric patients may be more sensitive to therapeutic and adverse effects of drug.

Patient counseling

- Urge patient to call prescriber if no relief is gained or condition worsens.
- Advise patient to store oral forms away from heat and light (not in bathroom medicine cabinet where heat and moisture will cause deterioration of the drug). Keep drug out of the reach of children.

Inhalation

- Give patient instructions on proper use of inhaler.
- Tell patient that saliva and sputum may appear red or pink after oral inhalation, because isoproterenol turns red on exposure to air.
- Advise patient to rinse mouth with water after drug is absorbed completely and between doses.

Sublingual

- Tell patient to allow sublingual tablet to dissolve under tongue, without sucking, and not to swallow saliva (may cause epigastric pain) until drug has been absorbed completely.
- Warn patient that frequent use of sublingual tablets may damage teeth due to acidity of drug.

isosorbide dinitrate

Apo-ISDN*, Coronex*, Dilatrate-SR, Iso-Bid, Isonate, Isordil, Isordil Titradose, Isotrate, Novosorbide*, Sorbitrate, Sorbitrate SA

Pharmacologic classification: nitrate
Therapeutic classification: antianginal, vasodilator
Pregnancy risk category C

How supplied

Available by prescription only
Tablets: 5 mg, 10 mg, 20 mg, 30 mg, 40 mg
Tablets (S.L.): 2.5 mg, 5 mg, 10 mg
Tablets (extended-release): 40 mg
Tablets (chewable): 5 mg, 10 mg
Capsules (extended-release): 40 mg

Indications and dosages

Treatment or prophylaxis of acute anginal attacks; treatment of chronic ischemic heart disease (by preload reduction)
Adults: S.L. form—2.5 to 10 mg under tongue for prompt relief of angina pain, repeated q 2 to 3 hours during acute phase, or q 4 to 6 hours for prophylaxis.

Chewable form—2.5 to 10 mg, p.r.n., for acute attack or q 2 to 3 hours for prophylaxis, but only after initial test dose of 5 mg to determine risk of severe hypotension.

Oral form—10 to 20 mg P.O. t.i.d. or q.i.d. for prophylaxis only (use smallest effective dose).

Extended-release forms—20 to 40 mg P.O. q 8 to 12 hours.

◇***Adjunctive treatment of heart failure***
Adults: 5 to 10 mg S.L. q 3 to 4 hours. Alternatively, give 20 to 40 mg P.O. (or chewable tablets) q 4 hours. Usually administered with vasodilators.

◇***Diffuse esophageal spasm without gastroesophageal reflux***
Adults: 10 to 30 mg P.O. q 4 hours.

Pharmacodynamics

Antianginal action: Drug reduces myocardial oxygen demand through peripheral vasodilation, resulting in decreased venous filling pressure (preload) and, to a lesser extent, decreased arterial impedance (afterload). These combined effects result in decreased cardiac work and, consequently, reduced myocardial oxygen demands. Drug also redistributes coronary blood flow from epicardial to subendocardial regions.
Vasodilating action: Drug dilates peripheral vessels (primarily venous), helping to manage pulmonary edema and heart failure caused by decreased venous return to the heart (preload). Arterial vasodilatory effects also decrease arterial impedance (afterload) and thus left ventricular work, benefiting the failing heart. These combined effects may help some patients with acute MI. (Use of isosorbide dinitrate in patients with heart failure and acute MI is currently unapproved.)

Pharmacokinetics

Absorption: Oral form is well absorbed from the GI tract but undergoes first-pass metabolism, resulting in bioavailability of about 50% (depending on dosage form used).
Distribution: Limited information is available on plasma protein binding and distribution of drug. Like nitroglycerin, it's distributed widely throughout the body.
Metabolism: Metabolized in the liver to active metabolites.
Excretion: Metabolites are excreted in the urine; elimination half-life is about 5 to 6 hours with oral administration; 2 hours with S.L. administration. About 80% to 100% of absorbed dose is excreted in urine within 24 hours. Duration of effect is longer than that of S.L. preparations.

Route	Onset	Peak	Duration
P.O.	30 min	Unknown	5-6 hr
S.L., P.O. (chewable)	3 min	Unknown	½-2 hr
P.O. (extended)	1 hr	Unknown	5-6 hr

Contraindications and precautions

Contraindicated in patients with hypersensitivity or idiosyncrasy to nitrates, severe hypotension, shock, or acute MI with low left ventricular filling pressure.

Use cautiously in patients with hypotension or blood volume depletion (such as from diuretic therapy).

Interactions

Drug-drug. *Antihypertensive drugs, calcium channel blockers, phenothiazines, vasodilators:* Additive hypotensive effects. Use with caution; check blood pressure frequently.
Drug-lifestyle. *Alcohol use:* Additive hypotensive effects. Advise patient to avoid alcohol.

Effects on diagnostic tests

Isosorbide dinitrate may interfere with serum cholesterol determination tests using the Zlatkis-Zak color reaction, causing a falsely decreased value.

Adverse reactions

CNS: *headache* (sometimes with throbbing), dizziness, weakness.
CV: *flushing, orthostatic hypotension, tachycardia, palpitations, ankle edema,* fainting.
GI: nausea, vomiting.
Skin: cutaneous vasodilation, rash.
Other: hypersensitivity reactions, sublingual burning.

Overdose and treatment

Clinical effects of overdose result primarily from vasodilation and methemoglobinemia and include hypotension, persistent throbbing headache, palpitations, visual disturbance, flushing of the skin and sweating (with skin later becoming cold and cyanotic), nausea and vomiting, colic and bloody diarrhea, orthostatism, initial hyperpnea, dyspnea, slow respiratory rate, bradycardia, heart block, increased intracranial pressure with confusion, fever, paralysis, and tissue hypoxia, which can lead to cyanosis, metabolic acidosis, coma, clonic seizures, and circulatory collapse. Death may result from circulatory collapse or asphyxia.

Treatment includes gastric lavage followed by administration of activated charcoal to remove remaining gastric contents. Monitor blood gas measurements and methemoglobin levels, as indicated. Supportive care includes respiratory support and oxygen administration, passive movement of extremities to aid venous return, recumbent positioning (Trendelenburg position, if necessary), maintenance of adequate body temperature, and administration of I.V. fluids.

An I.V. adrenergic agonist (such as phenylephrine) may be considered if further treatment is required. For methemoglobinemia, methylene blue (1 to 2 mg/kg I.V.) may be given. (Epinephrine and related compounds are contraindicated in isosorbide dinitrate overdose.)

Clinical considerations

- Store drug in a cool place, in a tightly closed container away from light.
- Maintenance of continuous 24-hour plasma levels may result in refractory tolerance. Dosing regimens should include dose-free intervals, which vary based on form of drug used.
- Drug may cause orthostatic hypotension. To minimize this, have patient change to upright position slowly, walk up and down stairs carefully, and lie down at first sign of dizziness.
- Don't discontinue drug abruptly because this may cause coronary vasospasm.
- Additional dose may be given before anticipated stress or at bedtime if angina is nocturnal.

Therapeutic monitoring

- Monitor blood pressure and intensity and duration of patient's response to drug.
- Drug may cause headache, especially at first. Dose may need to be reduced temporarily, but tolerance usually develops to this effect. In the interim, patient may relieve headache with aspirin or acetaminophen.

Special populations

Breast-feeding patients. It's unknown if drug is excreted in breast milk. Use cautiously in breast-feeding women.

Pediatric patients. Methemoglobinemia may occur in infants receiving large doses of isosorbide dinitrate.

Patient counseling

- Instruct patient to take medication regularly, as prescribed, and to keep it easily accessible at all times. Drug is physiologically necessary but not addictive.
- Warn patient that headache may occur initially, but may respond to usual headache remedies or dosage reduction. Assure patient that headache usually subsides gradually with continued treatment.
- Tell patient to take oral tablets on an empty stomach, either 30 minutes before or 1 to 2 hours after meals; to swallow oral tablets whole; and to chew chewable tablets thoroughly before swallowing.
- Advise patient to sit when self-administering S.L. tablets. He should lubricate tablet with saliva or place a few milliliters of fluid under tongue with tablet. If patient experiences tingling sensation with drug placed sublingually, he may try to hold tablet in buccal pouch. Dose may be repeated every 10 to 15 minutes for maximum of three doses. If no relief occurs, he should call or go to hospital emergency department.
- Warn patient to make positional changes gradually to avoid excessive dizziness.
- Instruct patient to avoid alcohol while taking drug because severe hypotension and CV collapse may occur.
- Advise patient to report blurred vision, dry mouth, or persistent headache.
- Caution patient not to stop long-term therapy abruptly.

isosorbide mononitrate

Imdur, ISMO, Monoket

Pharmacologic classification: nitrate
Therapeutic classification: antianginal
Pregnancy risk category C

How supplied

Available by prescription only
Tablets: 10 mg, 20 mg
Tablets (extended-release): 30 mg, 60 mg, 120 mg

Indications and dosages

Prevention of angina pectoris due to coronary artery disease (but not to abort acute anginal attacks)
Adults: 20 mg P.O. b.i.d., with doses 7 hours apart and first dose on awakening. For extended-release tablets, 30 to 60 mg P.O. once daily, on arising; after several days, dosage may be increased to 120 mg once daily; rarely, 240 mg may be required; extended-release tablets shouldn't be crushed or chewed.

Pharmacodynamics

Antianginal action: Drug is the major active metabolite of isosorbide dinitrate. It relaxes vascular smooth muscle and consequently dilates peripheral arteries and veins. Dilation of the veins promotes peripheral pooling of blood and decreases venous return to the heart, thereby reducing left ventricular end-diastolic pressure and pulmonary capillary wedge pressure (preload). Arteriolar relaxation reduces systemic vascular resistance, systolic arterial pressure, and mean arterial pressure (afterload). Dilation of the coronary arteries also occurs.

Pharmacokinetics

Absorption: Absolute bioavailability is almost 100%.
Distribution: Volume of distribution is about 0.6 L/kg. Less than 4% is bound to plasma proteins.
Metabolism: Drug isn't subject to first-pass metabolism in the liver.
Excretion: Less than 1% of isosorbide mononitrate is eliminated in urine. Overall elimination half-life of drug is about 5 hours.

Route	Onset	Peak	Duration
P.O.	Unknown	30-60 min	Unknown

Contraindications and precautions

Contraindicated in patients with hypersensitivity or idiosyncrasy to nitrates, severe hypotension, shock, or acute MI with low left ventricular filling pressure. Use cautiously in patients with hypotension or blood volume depletion (such as from diuretic therapy).

Interactions

Drug-drug. *Calcium channel blockers and organic nitrates:* Marked symptomatic orthostatic hypotension. Dose adjustments of either class of agents may be necessary.
Drug-lifestyle. *Alcohol use:* Increased vasodilation. Advise patient to avoid alcohol.

Effects on diagnostic tests

None reported.

Adverse reactions

CNS: *headache* (sometimes with throbbing), dizziness, weakness.
CV: *flushing, orthostatic hypotension, tachycardia, palpitations, ankle edema,* fainting.
GI: nausea, vomiting.
Musculoskeletal: arthralgia.
Respiratory: bronchitis, pneumonia, upper respiratory tract infection.
Skin: cutaneous vasodilation, rash.
Other: hypersensitivity reactions, sublingual burning.

Overdose and treatment

Symptoms of overdose may include increased intracranial pressure; persistent, throbbing headache; confusion; moderate fever; vertigo; palpitations; visual disturbances; nausea and vomiting (possibly with colic and even bloody diarrhea); syncope (especially with upright position); air hunger; dyspnea, later followed by reduced ventilatory effort; diaphoresis, with skin either flushed or cold and clammy; heart block and bradycardia; paralysis; coma; seizures; and death.

No specific antagonist to vasodilator effects of drug is known. However, drug is significantly removed from the blood during hemodialysis.

If drug is ingested, induce emesis or perform gastric lavage followed by activated charcoal administration. Because drug is rapidly and completely absorbed, however, gastric lavage may be effective only with recent ingestion. Treat severe hypotension and reflex tachycardia by elevating legs and administering I.V. fluids. Epinephrine is ineffective in reversing severe hypotension associated with overdose, and epinephrine and related compounds are contraindicated. Administer oxygen and artificial ventilation if necessary. Monitor methemoglobin levels as indicated.

Clinical considerations

- Drug-free interval sufficient to avoid tolerance to drug isn't completely defined. The recommended regimen involves two daily doses given 7 hours apart, with a gap of 17 hours between the second dose of 1 day and the first dose of the next day. Considering the relatively long half-life of drug, this result is consistent with those obtained for other organic nitrates.
- The asymmetric twice-daily regimen successfully avoids significant rebound or withdrawal effects. In studies of other nitrates, the incidence and magnitude of such phenomena appear to be highly dependent on the schedule of nitrate administration.
- Onset of action of oral drug isn't sufficiently rapid to be useful in aborting an acute anginal episode.

Therapeutic monitoring

- Benefits of drug in patients with acute MI or heart failure have not been established. Because effects of drug are difficult to terminate rapidly, its use isn't recommended in such patients. If it's used, however, careful clinical or hemodynamic monitoring must be performed to avoid the hazards of hypotension and tachycardia.
- Monitor blood pressure, especially in those susceptible to hypotension.
- Methemoglobinemia has occurred in patients receiving other organic nitrates and probably could occur as an adverse reaction. Significant methemoglobinemia has occurred in association with moderate overdoses of organic nitrates. Suspect methemoglobinemia in patients

who exhibit signs of impaired oxygen delivery despite adequate cardiac output and adequate Pao_2. Classically, methemoglobinemic blood is chocolate brown, without color change on exposure to air. Treatment of choice for methemoglobinemia is methylene blue, 1 to 2 mg/kg I.V.

Special populations

Breast-feeding patients. Excretion of drug in breast milk is unknown. Use caution when administering to breast-feeding women.
Pediatric patients. Safety and efficacy in children haven't been established.

Patient counseling

- Tell patient to follow prescribed dosing schedule carefully (two doses taken 7 hours apart) to maintain antianginal effect and to prevent tolerance.
- Warn patient that daily headaches sometimes accompany treatment with nitrates, including isosorbide mononitrate, and are a marker of drug activity. Patient shouldn't alter treatment schedule, because loss of headache may be associated with simultaneous loss of antianginal efficacy. Tell patient to treat headaches with aspirin or acetaminophen.
- Warn patient to avoid alcohol while taking drug because of increased risk of light-headedness.
- Tell patient to rise slowly from recumbent or seated position to avoid light-headedness caused by sudden decrease in blood pressure.

isotretinoin

Accutane

Pharmacologic classification: retinoic acid derivative
Therapeutic classification: antiacne, keratinization stabilizer
Pregnancy risk category X

How supplied

Available by prescription only
Capsules: 10 mg, 20 mg, 40 mg

Indications and dosages

Severe recalcitrant nodular acne
Adults and adolescents: 0.5 to 2 mg/kg P.O. daily given in two divided doses and continued for 15 to 20 weeks.
◇ ***Keratinization disorders resistant to conventional therapy,*** ◇ ***prevention of skin cancer***
Adults: Dosage varies with specific disease and severity of the disorder; dosages up to 2 to 4 mg/kg P.O. daily have been used. Consult current literature for specific recommendations.
◇ ***Squamous cell cancer of the head and neck***
Adults: 50 to 100 mg/m^2.

Pharmacodynamics

Antiacne action: Exact mechanism of action is unknown; isotretinoin decreases the size and activity of sebaceous glands, which decreases secretion and probably explains the rapid clinical improvement. A reduction in *Propionibacterium acnes* in the hair follicles occurs as a secondary result of decreased nutrients.
Keratinizing action: Isotretinoin has anti-inflammatory and keratinizing effects. The mechanism is unknown.

Pharmacokinetics

Absorption: When administered orally, drug is absorbed rapidly from the GI tract. Therapeutic range for isotretinoin hasn't been established.
Distribution: Distributed widely. In animals, it's found in most organs and is known to cross the placenta. In humans, degree of placental transfer and the degree of secretion in breast milk are unknown. Isotretinoin is 99.9% protein-bound, primarily to albumin.
Metabolism: Metabolized in the liver and possibly in the gut wall. The major metabolite is 4-oxo-isotretinoin, with tretinoin and 4-oxo-tretinoin also found in the blood and urine.
Excretion: Elimination process is not fully known, although renal and biliary pathways are known to be used.

Route	Onset	Peak	Duration
P.O.	Unknown	3 hr	Unknown

Contraindications and precautions

Contraindicated in women of childbearing age unless patient has had a negative serum pregnancy test within 2 weeks before beginning therapy, will begin drug therapy on day 2 or 3 of next menstrual period, and will comply with stringent contraceptive measures for 1 month before therapy, during therapy, and for at least 1 month after therapy. Severe fetal abnormalities may occur if used during pregnancy. Also contraindicated in patients hypersensitive to parabens, which are used as preservatives.

Interactions

Drug-drug. *Carbamazepine:* Decreased carbamazepine levels. Monitor patient carefully.
Medicated soaps and cleansers, medicated cover-ups, topical resorcinol peeling agents (benzoyl peroxide), and alcohol-containing preparations: Cumulative drying effect. Use cautiously.
Tetracyclines: May increase the potential for the development of pseudotumor cerebri. Avoid use together.
Vitamin A products: Additive toxic effect. Avoid use together.
Drug-lifestyle. *Alcohol use:* Increased plasma triglyceride levels.

Effects on diagnostic tests
None reported.

Adverse reactions
CNS: headache, fatigue, *pseudotumor cerebri* (benign intracranial hypertension).
EENT: *conjunctivitis, drying of mucous membranes,* corneal deposits, dry eyes, visual disturbances, *epistaxis, dry nose.*
GI: nonspecific GI symptoms, gum bleeding and inflammation, *nausea, vomiting,* anorexia, *dry mouth, abdominal pain.*
Hematologic: anemia, elevated platelet count.
Hepatic: elevated AST, ALT, and alkaline phosphatase levels.
Metabolic: hyperglycemia.
Musculoskeletal: *musculoskeletal pain (skeletal hyperostosis).*
Skin: *cheilosis, rash, dry skin, facial skin desquamation,* peeling of palms and toes, skin infection, photosensitivity, *cheilitis, pruritus, fragility, petechiae, nail brittleness,* thinning of hair.
Other: *hypertriglyceridemia.*

Overdose and treatment
Signs and symptoms of overdose are rare and would be extensions of adverse reactions.

Clinical considerations
- For women of childbearing age, a negative blood test for pregnancy must be obtained before therapy.
- Administer drug with or shortly after meals.
- Therapy usually lasts 15 to 20 weeks, followed by at least 8 weeks off drug before beginning a second course.
- Contact lenses may become uncomfortable during treatment; recommend use of artificial tears.
- Drug has been used in a limited number of patients to treat psoriasis (combined with psoralen and ultraviolet light); it has also been used to treat cutaneous neoplasms.

Therapeutic monitoring
- Monitor patient for visual problems.
- Pregnancy tests must be repeated monthly to avoid administration during pregnancy.

Special populations
Pregnant patients. Drug is a potent teratogen and shouldn't be taken during pregnancy.
Breast-feeding patients. It's unknown if drug is excreted in breast milk; breast-feeding isn't recommended during drug therapy.

Patient counseling
- Recommend taking drug with or shortly after meals to ease GI discomfort.
- Caution against alcohol ingestion, to reduce risk of hypertriglyceridemia.
- Warn patient to be cautious when driving, particularly at night because drug causes decreased night vision.
- Advise patient not to take vitamin supplements containing vitamin A while taking drug.
- Instruct patient to avoid prolonged exposure to sunlight or sun lamps to prevent photosensitivity.

isradipine
DynaCirc

Pharmacologic classification: calcium channel blocker
Therapeutic classification: antihypertensive
Pregnancy risk category C

How supplied
Available by prescription only
Capsules: 2.5 mg, 5 mg

Indications and dosages
Management of hypertension
Adults: Individualize dosage. Initially, 2.5 mg P.O. b.i.d. alone or with thiazide diuretic. Maximal response may require 2 to 4 weeks; therefore, dose adjustments of 5 mg daily should be made at 2- to 4-week intervals up to maximum of 20 mg daily. Doses of 10 mg or more per day haven't been shown to be more effective but rather to lead to increased incidence of adverse reactions. Same starting dose is used in geriatric, hepatic-impaired, and renal-impaired patients.

Pharmacodynamics
Antihypertensive action: A dihydropyridine calcium channel blocker, isradipine binds to calcium channels and inhibits calcium flux into cardiac and smooth muscle, which results in dilation of arterioles. This dilation reduces systemic resistance and lowers blood pressure while producing small increases in resting heart rate.

Pharmacokinetics
Absorption: About 90% to 95% is absorbed after oral administration.
Distribution: 95% bound to plasma protein.
Metabolism: Completely metabolized before elimination, with extensive first-pass metabolism.
Excretion: About 60% to 65% is excreted in urine; 25% to 30%, in feces.

Route	Onset	Peak	Duration
P.O.	Unknown	1½ hr	Unknown

Contraindications and precautions
Contraindicated in patients with hypersensitivity to drug. Use cautiously in patients with

heart failure, especially if combined with a beta blocker.

Interactions

Drug-drug. *Fentanyl anesthesia:* Severe hypotension has been reported with concomitant use of a beta blocker and a calcium channel blocker. Avoid use together.

Effects on diagnostic tests

None reported.

Adverse reactions

CNS: dizziness, *headache,* fatigue.
CV: edema, flushing, syncope, angina, tachycardia.
GI: nausea, diarrhea, abdominal discomfort, vomiting.
Respiratory: dyspnea.
Skin: rash.

Overdose and treatment

No well-documented cases of overdose have been reported; however, presumably excessive peripheral vasodilation with marked and prolonged systemic hypotension may occur. Provide symptomatic and supportive treatment, including active CV support, monitoring of input and output and cardiac and respiratory function, elevation of lower extremities, and fluid replacement, as needed. Use vasoconstrictors only when not specifically contraindicated.

Clinical considerations

- Drug has no significant effect on heart rate and no adverse effects on cardiac contractility, conduction or digitalis clearance, or lipid or renal function.
- Administration with food significantly increases the time to reach peak levels by about 1 hour. However, food has no effect on total bioavailability of drug.

Therapeutic monitoring

- Elevated liver function test results have been reported in some patients.
- Individualize dosage. Allow 2 to 4 weeks between dosage adjustments.

Special populations

Breast-feeding patients. It's unknown if isradipine is excreted in breast milk. Consider the potential risk of serious adverse reactions in the infant.
Pediatric patients. Safety and efficacy haven't been established in children under age 18.
Geriatric patients. No age-related problems have been reported.

Patient counseling

- Instruct patient to report irregular heartbeat, shortness of breath, swelling of hands or feet, pronounced dizziness, constipation, nausea, or hypotension.

itraconazole

Sporanox

Pharmacologic classification: synthetic triazole
Therapeutic classification: antifungal
Pregnancy risk category C

How supplied

Available by prescription only
Capsules: 100 mg
Injection: 10 mg/ml
Oral solution: 10 mg/ml

Indications and dosages

Treatment of blastomycosis (pulmonary and extrapulmonary), histoplasmosis (including chronic cavitary pulmonary disease and disseminated nonmeningeal histoplasmosis)
Adults: 200 mg P.O. once daily. If condition doesn't improve or shows evidence of progressive fungal disease, increase dose in 100-mg increments to maximum of 400 mg daily. Give doses of more than 200 mg/day in two divided doses. Alternatively, 200 mg I.V. b.i.d. for 4 doses, then decrease to 200 mg I.V. once daily for up to 14 days.
Aspergillosis (pulmonary and extrapulmonary) in patients who are intolerant of or refractory to amphotericin B therapy
Adults: 200 to 400 mg P.O. daily, or 200 mg I.V. b.i.d. for 4 doses, then decrease to 200 mg I.V. daily for up to 14 days.
Oropharyngeal candidiasis
Adults: 200 mg (20 ml) oral solution P.O. daily for 1 to 2 weeks.
Esophageal candidiasis
Adults: 100 mg (10 ml) oral solution P.O. daily for at least 3 weeks.
◇ ***Treatment of superficial mycoses (dermatophytoses, pityriasis versicolor, sebopsoriasis, candidiasis [vaginal, oral, or chronic mucocutaneous], onychomycosis), ◇systemic mycoses (candidiasis, cryptococcal infections [meningitis, disseminated], ◇dimorphic infections [paracoccidioidomycosis, coccidioidomycosis]), ◇subcutaneous mycoses (sporotrichosis, chromomycosis), ◇cutaneous leishmaniasis, ◇fungal keratitis, ◇alternariatoxicosis, and ◇zygomycosis***
Adults: 50 to 400 mg P.O. daily. Duration of therapy varies from 1 day to greater than 6 months, depending on the condition and mycologic response.

Note: Discontinue drug if clinical signs and symptoms develop that are consistent with liver disease and may be attributable to itraconazole.

Pharmacodynamics

Antifungal action: Itraconazole is a synthetic triazole antifungal agent. In vitro, itraconazole inhibits the cytochrome P-450 dependent synthesis of ergosterol, a vital component of fungal cell membranes.

Pharmacokinetics

Absorption: Oral bioavailability of drug is maximal when taken with food; absolute oral bioavailability is 55%.
Distribution: Plasma protein binding of drug is 99.8%; 99.5% for its metabolite, hydroxyitraconazole.
Metabolism: Extensively metabolized by the liver into a large number of metabolites, including hydroxyitraconazole, the major metabolite.
Excretion: Fecal excretion of parent drug varies between 3% and 18% of the dose. Renal excretion of parent drug is less than 0.03% of dose. About 40% of dose is excreted as inactive metabolites in the urine. Drug isn't removed by hemodialysis.

Route	Onset	Peak	Duration
P.O.	Unknown	Unknown	Unknown

Contraindications and precautions

Contraindicated in patients with hypersensitivity to drug, in patients receiving terfenadine and in breast-feeding women because drug is excreted in breast milk. Coadministration with cisapride is contraindicated because serious CV events (prolonged QT interval), including death, have occurred in patients taking itraconazole with cisapride.

Use cautiously in patients with hypochlorhydria or HIV infection and in those receiving medications that are highly protein-bound.

Interactions

Drug-drug. *Nonsedating antihistamines:* Rare instances of life-threatening arrhythmias and death. Don't use together.
Cisapride: Increased levels of cisapride, causing prolongation of the QT interval and, rarely, serious ventricular arrhythmias. Avoid use together.
Cyclosporine: Itraconazole may increase cyclosporine plasma levels. Reduce cyclosporine dosage by 50% when using itraconazole doses greater than 100 mg/day. Recommend monitoring cyclosporine levels.
Digoxin: Increased digoxin levels. Recommend monitoring digoxin levels.
H_2 antagonists, isoniazid, phenytoin, rifampin: May reduce plasma itraconazole levels. Monitor patient for drug effect.
HMG-CoA reductase inhibitors: Contraindicated during treatment with itraconazole. Don't use together.
Phenytoin: Altered phenytoin metabolism. Recommend monitoring phenytoin levels.
Sulfonylureas: Concurrent use may cause hypoglycemia. Recommend monitoring serum glucose.
Warfarin: Enhanced anticoagulant effect. Recommend monitoring PT.

Effects on diagnostic tests

None reported.

Adverse reactions

CNS: malaise, fatigue, headache, dizziness, somnolence.
CV: edema, hypertension.
GI: *nausea,* vomiting, diarrhea, abdominal pain, anorexia.
GU: albuminuria, impotence.
Hepatic: impaired hepatic function.
Metabolic: hypokalemia.
Skin: rash, pruritus.
Other: fever, decreased libido.

Overdose and treatment

In the event of accidental overdose, employ supportive measures, including gastric lavage with sodium bicarbonate. Itraconazole isn't removed by dialysis.

Clinical considerations

- In life-threatening situations, the recommended loading dose is 200 mg three times daily (600 mg/day) for first 3 days. Continue treatment for minimum of 3 months and until clinical parameters and laboratory tests indicate that the active fungal infection has subsided. An inadequate period of treatment may lead to recurrence of active infection.
- Instruct prescriber to obtain specimens for fungal cultures and other relevant laboratory studies (wet mount, histopathology, serology) before therapy to isolate and identify causative organisms. Therapy may be instituted before results of cultures and other laboratory studies are known; once results become available, adjust anti-infective therapy accordingly.
- The clinical course of histoplasmosis in HIV-infected patients is more severe and usually requires maintenance therapy to prevent relapse. Because hypochlorhydria has occurred in HIV-infected patients, absorption of itraconazole may be decreased.
- Itraconazole shouldn't be given to a patient with creatinine clearance under 30 ml per minute.

Therapeutic monitoring

Monitor hepatic enzyme test values in patients with preexisting hepatic function abnormalities.

Special populations

Pregnant patients. Drug shouldn't be administered during pregnancy due to potential risk to fetus.

Breast-feeding patients. Because drug is excreted in breast milk, its use is contraindicated in breast-feeding women.
Pediatric patients. Safety and efficacy in children haven't been established.

Patient counseling

- Instruct patient to take drug with food to enhance absorption.
- Tell patient to swish oral solution vigorously before swallowing.
- Tell patient to report signs and symptoms that may suggest liver dysfunction (jaundice, unusual fatigue, anorexia, nausea, vomiting, dark urine, pale stool) so appropriate laboratory testing can be performed.

ketamine hydrochloride

Ketalar

Pharmacologic classification: dissociative anesthetic
Therapeutic classification: I.V. anesthetic
Pregnancy risk category NR

How supplied

Available by prescription only
Injection: 10 mg/ml, 50 mg/ml, 100 mg/ml

Indications and dosages

Induction of general anesthesia, especially for short diagnostic or surgical procedures not requiring skeletal muscle relaxation; adjunct to other general anesthetics or low-potency agents, such as nitrous oxide
Adults and children: 1 to 4.5 mg/kg I.V. administered over 60 seconds; or 6.5 to 13 mg/kg I.M. To maintain anesthesia, repeat in increments of half to full initial dose.

Pharmacodynamics

Anesthetic action: Ketamine induces a profound sense of dissociation from the environment by direct action on the cortex and limbic system.

Pharmacokinetics

Absorption: Absorbed rapidly and well after I.M. injection.
Distribution: Rapidly enters the CNS.
Metabolism: Metabolized by the liver to an active metabolite with one-third the potency of parent drug.
Excretion: Excreted in urine.

Route	Onset	Peak	Duration
I.V.	30 sec	Unknown	5-10 min
I.M.	3-4 min	Unknown	12-25 min

Contraindications and precautions

Contraindicated in patients with schizophrenia or other acute psychosis because it may exacerbate the condition; in those with CV disease in whom a sudden increase in blood pressure would be harmful; and in patients allergic to drug.

Interactions

Drug-drug. *Halothane and enflurane:* Myocardial depression and hypotension. Avoid use together.
Barbiturates or narcotics: Concurrent use may cause prolonged recovery time. Monitor patient closely.
Tubocurarine and other nondepolarizing muscle relaxants: Increased neuromuscular effects; prolonged respiratory depression. Monitor patient closely.
Thyroid hormones: May cause hypertension and tachycardia. Monitor patient closely.

Effects on diagnostic tests

None reported.

Adverse reactions

CNS: tonic-clonic movements, hallucinations, confusion, excitement, dreamlike states, irrational behavior, psychic abnormalities.
CV: *hypertension; tachycardia;* hypotension, *bradycardia* (if used with halothane); ***arrhythmias.***
EENT: diplopia, nystagmus, laryngospasm.
GI: mild anorexia, nausea, vomiting, excessive salivation.
Respiratory: ***respiratory depression*** in high doses, *apnea* (if administered too rapidly).
Skin: transient erythema, measles-like rash.

Overdose and treatment

Clinical signs include respiratory depression. Support respiration, using mechanical ventilation if necessary.

Clinical considerations

- The effect of ketamine on blood pressure makes it particularly useful in hypovolemic patients as an induction agent that supports blood pressure.
- Barbiturates are incompatible in the same syringe.
- For direct injection, dilute 100 mg/ml concentration with an equal volume of sterile water for injection, normal saline, or D_5W. For continuous infusion, prepare a 1-mg/ml solution by adding 5 ml from the 100 mg/ml vial to 500 ml of D_5W or normal saline.
- Emergency reactions may be reduced by using lower dosage of ketamine with I.V. diazepam and can be treated with short- or ultrashort-acting barbiturates.

- Incidence of emergency reactions is lower in patients under age 15 or over age 65 and when drug is given I.M.
- Keep verbal, tactile, and visual stimulation to a minimum during induction and recovery.
- Dissociative and hallucinatory adverse effects have led to drug abuse.

Therapeutic monitoring

- Patients require physical support because of rapid induction; monitor vital signs perioperatively. Blood pressure begins to increase shortly after injection, peaks at 10% to 50% above preanesthetic levels, and returns to baseline within 15 minutes. Clinical signs of overdose include respiratory depression.
- Emergency reactions occur in 12% of patients, including dreams, visual imagery, hallucinations, and delirium and may occur for up to 24 hours postoperatively.

Special populations

Pediatric patients. Drug is safe and especially useful in managing minor surgical or diagnostic procedures or in repeated procedures that require large amounts of analgesia, such as the changing of burn dressings.
Geriatric patients. Use drug with caution, especially in patients with suspected stroke, hypertension, or cardiac disease.

Patient counseling

Warn patient to avoid tasks requiring motor coordination and mental alertness for 24 hours after anesthesia.

ketoconazole

Nizoral

Pharmacologic classification: imidazole derivative
Therapeutic classification: antifungal
Pregnancy risk category C

How supplied

Available by prescription only
Tablets: 200 mg
Cream: 2%
Shampoo: 2%

Indications and dosages

Severe fungal infections caused by susceptible organisms
Adults: Initially, 200 mg P.O. daily as a single dose. Dose may be increased to 400 mg once daily in patients who don't respond to lower dosage.
Children over age 2: 3.3 to 6.6 mg/kg P.O. daily as a single dose.
Topical treatment of tinea corporis, tinea cruris, tinea versicolor, and tinea pedis
Adults and children: Apply daily or b.i.d. for about 2 weeks; for tinea pedis, apply for 6 weeks.
Seborrheic dermatitis
Adults and children: Apply b.i.d. for about 4 weeks.
Dandruff
Adults: Apply for 1 minute, rinse, then reapply for 3 minutes. Shampoo twice weekly for 4 weeks with at least 3 days between shampoos.
Prostatic carcinoma; disseminated intravascular coagulation (DIC) associated with prostatic cancer
Adults: 400 mg P.O. q 8 hours.

Pharmacodynamics

Antifungal action: Drug is fungicidal and fungistatic, depending on concentrations. It inhibits demethylation of lanosterol, thereby altering membrane permeability and inhibiting purine transport. The in vitro spectrum of activity includes most pathogenic fungi. However, CSF concentrations following oral administration aren't predictable. It shouldn't be used to treat fungal meningitis, and specimens should be obtained for susceptibility testing before therapy. Currently available tests may not accurately reflect in vivo activity, so interpret results with caution.

Drug is used orally to treat disseminated or pulmonary coccidioidomycosis, paracoccidioidomycosis, or histoplasmosis; oral candidiasis; and candiduria (but low renal clearance may limit its usefulness).

It's also useful in some dermatophytoses, including tinea capitis, tinea cruris, tinea pedis, tinea manus, and tinea unguium (onychomycosis) caused by *Epidermophyton, Microsporum,* or *Trichophyton.*

Pharmacokinetics

Absorption: Converted to the hydrochloride salt before absorption. Absorption is erratic; it's decreased by raised gastric pH and may be increased in extent and consistency by food.
Distribution: Distributed into bile, saliva, cerumen, synovial fluid, and sebum; CSF penetration is erratic and considered minimal. It is 84% to 99% bound to plasma proteins.
Metabolism: Converted into several inactive metabolites in the liver.
Excretion: More than 50% of a dose is excreted in feces within 4 days; drug and metabolites are secreted in bile. About 13% is excreted unchanged in urine. It is probably excreted in breast milk. Half-life is biphasic, initially 2 hours, with a terminal half-life of 8 hours.

Route	Onset	Peak	Duration
P.O.	Unknown	1-4 hr	Unknown
Topical	Unknown	Unknown	Unknown

Contraindications and precautions

Contraindicated in patients with hypersensitivity to drug and in those taking astemizole, or cisapride due to potential for serious CV adverse events. Use oral form cautiously in patients with hepatic disease. Because CSF concentrations of ketoconazole are unpredictable following oral administration, don't use drug alone to treat fungal meningitis.

Interactions

Drug-drug. *Cyclosporine:* Drug may raise serum levels as a result of interference with metabolism. Monitor patient closely.
Drugs that raise gastric pH (antacids, antimuscarinic agents, cimetidine, famotidine, ranitidine): Decreased absorption of ketoconazole. Give 2 hours after ketoconazole.
Other hepatotoxic drugs: Drug may enhance toxicity. Monitor patient closely.
Oral sulfonylureas: Effects of sulfonylureas may be intensified. Monitor patient closely.
Phenytoin: Serum levels of both drugs may be altered. Monitor patient response to medication; monitor drug levels.
Rifampin: May decrease serum concentration of ketoconazole to ineffective levels. Monitor patient for drug effect.
*Tacrolimus:*Increased plasma levels of tacrolimus. Use with caution. Monitor renal function and tacrolimus level.
Warfarin: May enhance anticoagulant effect. Monitor PT and INR.
Drug-lifestyle. *Alcohol use:* May cause a disulfiram-like reaction. Advise patient to avoid alcohol.
Corticosteroids: May result in increased corticosteroid plasma levels. Monitor patient carefully.
Drug-herb. *Yew preparations:* Inhibit ketoconazole metabolism. Avoid use together.

Effects on diagnostic tests

None reported.

Adverse reactions

CNS: headache, nervousness, dizziness, somnolence, photophobia, ***suicidal tendencies,*** severe depression (with oral administration).
GI: *nausea, vomiting,* abdominal pain, diarrhea (with oral administration).
GU: gynecomastia with tenderness, impotence (with oral administration).
Hematologic: ***thrombocytopenia,*** hemolytic anemia, ***leukopenia*** (with oral administration).
Hepatic: elevated liver enzymes, ***fatal hepatotoxicity*** (with oral administration).
Skin: pruritus; severe irritation, stinging (with topical administration).
Other: fever, chills.

Overdose and treatment

Overdose may cause dizziness, tinnitus, headache, nausea, vomiting, or diarrhea; patients with adrenal hypofunction or patients on long-term corticosteroid therapy may show signs of adrenal crisis.

Treatment includes induced emesis and sodium bicarbonate lavage, followed by activated charcoal and a cathartic; supportive measures as needed.

Clinical considerations

- Identify organism, but don't delay therapy for laboratory test results.
- Give P.O. drug with citrus juice.
- P.O. drug requires acidity for absorption; administration adjustments needed for patients with achlorhydria.

Therapeutic monitoring

Advise prescriber to monitor for signs of hepatotoxicity: persistent nausea, unusual fatigue, jaundice, dark urine, and pale stools.

Special populations

Pregnant patients. Ketoconazole shouldn't be given to pregnant women.
Breast-feeding patients. Drug may be distributed in breast milk. Alternative feeding methods are recommended.
Pediatric patients. Safe use in children under age 2 hasn't been established. Consider use in pediatric patients only when the benefits outweigh the risks.

Patient counseling

- Instruct achlorhydric patients how to dissolve each tablet in 4 ml of 0.2N hydrochloric acid solution or take with 200 ml of 0.1N hydrochloric acid. Use a glass or plastic straw to avoid damaging tooth enamel. Follow each dose with glass of water.
- Tell patient to avoid driving or performing other hazardous activities if dizziness or drowsiness occur; these often occur early in treatment but abate as treatment continues.
- Caution patient not to alter dose or dosage interval or to discontinue drug without medical approval; therapy must continue until active fungal infection is completely eradicated, to prevent recurrence.
- Reassure patient that nausea will subside; to minimize reaction, patient may take drug with food or may divide dosage into two doses.
- Advise patient to avoid self-prescribed preparations for GI distress (such as antacids); some may alter gastric pH levels and interfere with drug action.
- Caution patient concerning drug-drug and drug-herb interactions.

ketoprofen

Actron, Orudis, Orudis KT, Oruvail

Pharmacologic classification: NSAID
Therapeutic classification: nonnarcotic analgesic, antipyretic, anti-inflammatory
Pregnancy risk category B

How supplied

Available by prescription only
Capsules: 25 mg, 50 mg, 75 mg
Capsules (extended-release): 100 mg, 150 mg, 200 mg
Available without a prescription
Tablets: 12.5 mg

Indications and dosages

Rheumatoid arthritis and osteoarthritis
Adults: Usual dose is 75 mg t.i.d. or 50 mg q.i.d. P.O. Maximum dose is 300 mg/day; or 200 mg (extended-release capsules) P.O. daily.
Mild to moderate pain; dysmenorrhea
Adults: 25 to 50 mg P.O. q 6 to 8 hours, p.r.n.
Temporary relief of mild aches and pain, fever (self-medication)
Adults: 12.5 mg q 4 to 6 hours. Don't exceed 75 mg in a 24-hour period.

Pharmacodynamics

Analgesic, antipyretic, and anti-inflammatory actions: Mechanisms of action are unknown; ketoprofen is thought to inhibit prostaglandin synthesis.

Pharmacokinetics

Absorption: Absorbed rapidly and completely from the GI tract.
Distribution: Highly protein-bound. Extent of body tissue fluid distribution isn't known, but therapeutic levels range from 0.4 to 6 mcg/ml.
Metabolism: Metabolized in the liver.
Excretion: Excreted in urine as parent drug and its metabolites.

Route	Onset	Peak	Duration
P.O., P.R.	1-2 hr	½-2 hr	3-4 hr

Contraindications and precautions

Contraindicated in patients with hypersensitivity to drug or history of aspirin-induced or NSAID-induced asthma, urticaria, or other allergic-type reactions. Use cautiously in patients with impaired renal or hepatic function, peptic ulcer disease, heart failure, hypertension, or fluid retention.

Interactions

Drug-drug. *Other drugs that inhibit platelet aggregation, such as aspirin, parenteral carbenicillin, cefamandole, cefoperazone, dextran, dipyridamole, mezlocillin, piperacillin, plicamycin, salicylates, sulfinpyrazone, ticarcillin, valproic acid, or other anti-inflammatory agents:* Bleeding problems may occur. Monitor patient for signs of bleeding.
Antihypertensive agents and diuretics: Decreased effectiveness of these drugs; increased nephrotoxic potential from diuretics. Don't use together.
Aspirin: Decreases the bioavailability of ketoprofen. Avoid use together.
Coumarin derivatives, heparin, streptokinase, urokinase, nifedipine, phenytoin, or verapamil: Toxicity may occur; increased risk of bleeding. Monitor patient, PT and INR closely.
Gold compounds, other anti-inflammatory agents, or acetaminophen: Increased nephrotoxicity. Avoid use together.
Insulin or oral antidiabetic agents: Because of the influence of prostaglandins on glucose metabolism, concurrent use may potentiate hypoglycemic effects. Monitor blood glucose levels.
Lithium and methotrexate: Decreased renal clearance of lithium and methotrexate. Monitor patient closely
Salicylates, anti-inflammatory agents, corticotropin, or corticosteroids: May cause GI ulceration and hemorrhage. Avoid use together.
Drug-lifestyle: *Alcohol use:* Increased GI adverse effects, including ulceration and hemorrhage. Advise patient to avoid alcohol.
Prolonged sun exposure: Increases the risk of photosensitive reaction. Advise patient to take precautions.

Effects on diagnostic tests

In vitro interactions with glucose determinations have been reported with glucose oxidase and peroxidase methods resulting in falsely elevated blood glucose concentrations.

Ketoprofen may interfere with serum iron determination (false increases or decreases depending on method used), and may cause falsely elevated serum bilirubin concentrations.

Adverse reactions

CNS: *headache, dizziness, CNS excitation* or depression.
EENT: tinnitus, visual disturbances.
GI: *nausea, abdominal pain, diarrhea, constipation, flatulence, peptic ulceration,* dyspepsia, anorexia, vomiting, stomatitis, ***peptic ulceration.***
GU: ***nephrotoxicity,*** elevated BUN.
Hematologic: prolonged bleeding time, ***thrombocytopenia, agranulocytosis.***
Hepatic: elevated liver enzymes.
Respiratory: dyspnea, ***bronchospasm, laryngeal edema.***
Skin: rash, photosensitivity, ***exfoliative dermatitis.***
Other: peripheral edema.

Overdose and treatment

Signs and symptoms of overdose include nausea and drowsiness. Induce emesis with ipecac syrup or empty stomach via gastric lavage; administer activated charcoal via nasogastric tube. Provide symptomatic and supportive measures (respiratory support and correction of fluid and electrolyte imbalances). Monitor laboratory parameters and vital signs closely. Hemodialysis may be useful in removing ketoprofen and assisting in care of renal failure.

Clinical considerations

- Consider the recommendations relevant to all NSAIDs.
- Administer tablets on an empty stomach either 30 minutes before or 2 hours after meals to ensure adequate absorption. However, capsules may be taken with foods or antacids to minimize GI distress.

Therapeutic monitoring

- Advise prescriber to monitor patient for CNS effects and possible photosensitivity reactions.
- Monitor laboratory test results for abnormalities.

Special populations

Breast-feeding patients. Most NSAIDs are distributed into breast milk; however, distribution of ketoprofen is unknown. Avoid use of ketoprofen in breast-feeding women.
Pediatric patients. Safe use in children under age 12 hasn't been established.
Geriatric patients. Patients over age 60 may be more susceptible to the toxic effects of ketoprofen. Use with caution. The effects of drug on renal prostaglandins may cause fluid retention and edema, a significant drawback for geriatric patients and those with heart failure. The manufacturer recommends that initial dose be reduced by 33% to 50% in geriatric patients.

Patient counseling

- Instruct patient in prescribed drug regimen and proper medication administration, to avoid alcoholic beverages during therapy, and to report adverse reactions.
- Tell patient to seek medical approval before taking OTC medications (especially aspirin and aspirin-containing products).
- Caution patient to avoid activities that require alertness or concentration; stress need for safety measures to prevent injury.
- Advise patient of potential photosensitivity reactions. Recommend use of sunscreen.

ketorolac tromethamine

Toradol

Pharmacologic classification: NSAID
Therapeutic classification: analgesic
Pregnancy risk category C

How supplied

Available by prescription only
Tablets: 10 mg
Injection: 15 mg/ml (1-ml cartridge), 30 mg/ml (1-ml and 2-ml cartridges)

Indications and dosages

Short-term management of pain
Adults under age 65: Dosage should be based on patient response; initially, 60 mg I.M. or 30 mg I.V. as a single dose, or multiple doses of 30 mg I.M. or I.V. q 6 hours. Maximum daily dose shouldn't exceed 120 mg.
≡***Dosage adjustment.*** In patients age 65 or older, renally impaired patients, and those weighing less than 110 lb (50 kg), 30 mg I.M. or 15 mg I.V. initially as a single dose, or multiple doses of 15 mg I.M. or I.V. q 6 hours. Maximum daily dose shouldn't exceed 60 mg.
Short-term management of moderately severe, acute pain when switching from parenteral to oral administration
Adults under age 65: 20 mg P.O. as a single dose followed by 10 mg P.O. q 4 to 6 hours, not to exceed 40 mg/day.
≡***Dosage adjustment.*** In patients age 65 or older, renally impaired patients, and those weighing less than 110 lb (50 kg) body weight, 10 mg P.O. as a single dose, followed by 10 mg P.O. q 4 to 6 hours, not to exceed 40 mg/day.

Pharmacodynamics

Analgesic action: Ketorolac is an NSAID that acts by inhibiting the synthesis of prostaglandins.

Pharmacokinetics

Absorption: Completely absorbed after I.M. administration. After oral administration, food delays absorption but doesn't decrease total amount of drug absorbed.
Distribution: Mean peak plasma levels occur about 30 minutes after a 50-mg dose and range from 2.2 to 3 mcg/ml. More than 99% of drug is protein-bound.
Metabolism: Metabolism is primarily hepatic; a para-hydroxy metabolite and conjugates have been identified; less than 50% of a dose is metabolized. Liver impairment doesn't substantially alter drug clearance.
Excretion: Primary excretion is in urine (more than 90%); the rest in feces. Terminal plasma half-life is 3¾ to 6⅓ hours (average 4½ hours) in young adults; it's substantially prolonged in patients with renal failure.

Route	Onset	Peak	Duration
P.O.	½-1 hr	½-1 hr	6-8 hr
I.V.	Immediate	Immediate	6-8 hr
I.M.	10 min	½-1 hr	6-8 hr

Contraindications and precautions

Contraindicated in patients with hypersensitivity to drug, active peptic ulcer disease, recent GI bleeding or perforation, advanced renal impairment, risk for renal impairment due to volume depletion, suspected or confirmed cerebrovascular bleeding, hemorrhagic diathesis, incomplete hemostasis, or high risk of bleeding.

Also contraindicated in patients with history of peptic ulcer disease or GI bleeding, past allergic manifestations to aspirin or other NSAIDs, and during labor and delivery or breast-feeding. In addition, drug is contraindicated as prophylactic analgesic before major surgery or intraoperatively when hemostasis is critical; in patients receiving aspirin, an NSAID, or probenecid; and in those requiring analgesics to be administered epidurally or intrathecally.

Use cautiously in patients with impaired renal or hepatic function.

Interactions

Drug-drug. *Diuretics:* Decreased efficacy of diuretic; increased risk of nephrotoxicity. Monitor patient closely.
Free (unbound) salicylates or warfarin: Increased blood levels of salicylates or warfarin. Use with extreme caution; monitor patient closely.
NSAIDs: Increased lithium levels and decreased methotrexate clearance, increasing its toxicity. Monitor patient closely.
Drug-lifestyle. *Alcohol use:* Increased GI effects, including ulceration and hemorrhage. Advise patient to avoid alcohol.

Effects on diagnostic tests

None reported.

Adverse reactions

CNS: *drowsiness, sedation,* dizziness, *headache.*
CV: edema, hypertension, palpitations, ***arrhythmias.***
GI: *nausea, dyspepsia, GI pain,* diarrhea, peptic ulceration, vomiting, constipation, flatulence, stomatitis.
GU: ***renal failure.***
Hematologic: decreased platelet adhesion, purpura, ***thrombocytopenia.***
Skin: pain (at injection site), pruritus, rash, diaphoresis.

Overdose and treatment

There is no experience with overdose in humans. Withhold drug and provide supportive treatment.

Clinical considerations

- Hypovolemia should be corrected before initiating therapy with ketorolac.
- The combined duration of ketorolac I.M., I.V., or P.O. shouldn't exceed 5 days. Oral use is only for continuation of I.V. or I.M. therapy.

Therapeutic monitoring

I.M. injections in patients with coagulopathies or those receiving anticoagulants may cause bleeding and hematoma at the site of injection.

Special populations

Breast-feeding patients. Because drug is distributed in breast milk, its use is contraindicated in breast-feeding women.
Pediatric patients. Drug isn't recommended for use in children because safety and efficacy haven't been established.
Geriatric patients. Use lower initial doses (30 mg I.M.) in patients over age 65 or weighing less than 110 lb. In clinical trials, elderly subjects have exhibited a longer terminal half-life of drug (average 7 hours in geriatric patients compared with 4½ hours in healthy young adults).

Patient counseling

- Instruct patient to avoid aspirin, aspirin-containing products, and alcoholic beverages during therapy.
- Warn patient that GI ulceration, bleeding, and perforation can occur at any time, with or without warning, in anyone taking NSAIDs on a long-term basis. Inform patient of signs and symptoms of GI bleeding.

ketorolac tromethamine (ophthalmic)

Acular

Pharmacologic classification: NSAID
Therapeutic classification: ophthalmic anti-inflammatory
Pregnancy risk category C

How supplied

Available by prescription only
Ophthalmic solution: 0.5%

Indications and dosages

Relief of ocular itching caused by seasonal allergic conjunctivitis
Adults: Instill 1 drop (0.25 mg) in conjunctival sac q.i.d. Efficacy hasn't been established beyond 1 week of continued use.

Pharmacodynamics

Anti-inflammatory action: Anti-inflammatory action of ketorolac tromethamine is thought to be a result, in part, of its ability to inhibit prostaglandin biosynthesis. Drug reduces prostaglandin E_2 levels in aqueous humor with ocular administration. It has also demonstrated analgesic and antipyretic activity because of the same mechanism of action.

Pharmacokinetics

No information available.

Route	Onset	Peak	Duration
Ophthalmic	Unknown	Unknown	Unknown

Contraindications and precautions
Contraindicated in patients hypersensitive to any component of the formulation and in those wearing soft contact lenses. Use cautiously in patients with hypersensitivity to other NSAIDs or aspirin and in those with bleeding disorders.

Interactions
None reported.

Effects on diagnostic tests
None reported.

Adverse reactions
EENT: *transient stinging and burning on instillation,* superficial keratitis, superficial ocular infections, ocular irritation.
Other: hypersensitivity reactions.

Overdose and treatment
Overdose will not ordinarily cause acute problems. If accidentally ingested, have the patient drink fluids to dilute.

Clinical considerations
- Ophthalmic solution has been safely administered in conjunction with other ophthalmic medications, such as antibiotics, beta blockers, carbonic anhydrase inhibitors, cycloplegics, and mydriatics.
- Store drug at controlled room temperature and protect from light.

Therapeutic monitoring
Monitor for adverse reactions, including superficial ocular infections and hypersensitivity reactions.

Special populations
Breast-feeding patients. Use cautiously in breast-feeding women.
Pediatric patients. Safety and efficacy in children haven't been established.

Patient counseling
- Teach patient how to administer eye drops and stress importance of not touching dropper to eye or surrounding area.
- Advise patient not to use more drops than prescribed and to use only as prescribed.

L

labetalol hydrochloride

Normodyne, Trandate

Pharmacologic classification: alpha and beta blocker
Therapeutic classification: antihypertensive
Pregnancy risk category C

How supplied

Available by prescription only
Tablets: 100 mg, 200 mg, 300 mg
Injection: 5 mg/ml in 20-, 40-, and 60-ml vials and 4- and 8-ml disposable syringes

Indications and dosages

Hypertension; ◇pheochromocytoma
Adults: 100 mg P.O. b.i.d. with or without a diuretic. Dosage may be increased by 100 mg b.i.d. q 2 or 3 days until optimum response is reached. Usual maintenance dosage is 200 to 600 mg b.i.d.; maximum daily dose is 2,400 mg.
Severe hypertension and hypertensive emergencies; ◇clonidine withdrawal hypertension
Adults: Initially, 20 to 80 mg I.V. bolus slowly over 2 minutes; may repeat injections of 40 to 80 mg q 10 minutes to maximum dose of 300 mg.

Alternatively, drug may be given as continuous I.V. infusion at an initial rate of 0.5 to 2 mg/minute until satisfactory response is obtained. Usual effective, cumulative dose is 50 to 200 mg although up to 300 mg may be required.

Oral dose following I.V. therapy: 200 mg P.O. followed by 200 to 400 mg in 6 to 12 hours (depending on blood pressure response); then increase in usual increments at 1-day intervals while patient is hospitalized to achieve desired effects.
◇Controlled hypotension during anesthesia
Adults: Initially, 10 to 30 mg I.V. bolus slowly; may repeat injections of 5 to 10 mg I.V., p.r.n.
≡*Dosage adjustment.* In geriatric patients, use a lower maintenance dosage of 100 to 200 mg P.O. b.i.d.

Pharmacodynamics

Antihypertensive action: Labetalol inhibits catecholamine access to both beta- and postsynaptic alpha-adrenergic receptor sites. Drug may also have a vasodilating effect.

Pharmacokinetics

Absorption: Oral absorption is high (90% to 100%); however, drug undergoes extensive first-pass metabolism in the liver and only about 25% of an oral dose reaches systemic circulation unchanged.
Distribution: Distributed widely throughout the body; about 50% protein-bound.
Metabolism: Orally administered drug is metabolized extensively in the liver and possibly in GI mucosa.
Excretion: About 5% of a dose is excreted unchanged in urine; remainder is excreted as metabolites in urine and feces (biliary elimination). Plasma half-life is about 5½ hours after I.V. administration or 6 to 8 hours after oral administration.

Route	Onset	Peak	Duration
P.O.	20 min	2-4 hr	8-12 hr
I.V.	2-5 min	5 min	2-4 hr

Contraindications and precautions

Contraindicated in patients with a history of obstructive airway disease such as bronchial asthma; overt cardiac failure; greater than first-degree heart block; cardiogenic shock; severe bradycardia; other conditions associated with severe and prolonged hypotension; and hypersensitivity to drug.

Use cautiously in patients with heart failure, hepatic failure, chronic bronchitis, emphysema, preexisting peripheral vascular disease, and pheochromocytoma.

Ejaculation failure and impotence in males and decreased libido have been reported.

Interactions

Drug-drug. *Beta-adrenergic agonists:* Labetalol may antagonize bronchodilation produced by these drugs. Avoid use together.
Cimetidine: May increase bioavailability of oral labetalol. If used together, labetalol dosage may require adjustment.
Diuretics and other antihypertensive agents: Labetalol may potentiate antihypertensive effects of these drugs. Patient requires close monitoring.
Glutethimide: May decrease bioavailability of oral labetalol, requiring adjustment in labetalol dosage.
Halothane: Synergistic antihypertensive effect and significant myocardial depression. Patient requires close monitoring.

Nitroglycerin: Labetalol blunts the reflex tachycardia produced by nitroglycerin without preventing its hypotensive effect. In patients with angina, additional antihypertensive effects may occur. Use with caution.
Tricyclic antidepressants: May increase incidence of labetalol-induced tremor. Avoid use together.

Effects on diagnostic tests

Drug may cause a false-positive increase of urine free and total catecholamine levels when measured by a nonspecific trihydroxindole fluorometric method.

Adverse reactions

CNS: vivid dreams, fatigue, headache, paresthesia, syncope, transient scalp tingling.
CV: *orthostatic hypotension, dizziness,* ***ventricular arrhythmias.***
EENT: nasal stuffiness.
GI: nausea, vomiting, diarrhea.
GU: sexual dysfunction, urine retention.
Musculoskeletal: muscle spasm, toxic myopathy.
Respiratory: dyspnea, ***bronchospasm.***
Skin: rash.

Overdose and treatment

Clinical signs of overdose include severe hypotension, bradycardia, heart failure, and bronchospasm.

After acute ingestion, empty stomach by induced emesis or gastric lavage, and give activated charcoal to reduce absorption. Subsequent treatment is usually symptomatic and supportive.

Clinical considerations

Consider the recommendations relevant to all beta blockers as well as the following:
- Unlike other beta blockers, labetalol doesn't decrease resting heart rate or cardiac output.
- Dosage may need to be reduced in patients with hepatic insufficiency and severe renal impairment.
- Dizziness, a troublesome adverse effect, tends to occur in early stages of treatment and in patients taking diuretics or receiving higher doses.
- Investigational uses include managing chronic stable angina pectoris, excessive sympathetic activity associated with tetanus, and uncontrolled hypertension before and during anesthesia.
- It may be more cost-effective for patient to take drug twice daily rather than once daily.
- For I.V. infusion, dilute labetalol injection to an appropriate concentration (such as 200 mg of drug added to 160 ml of solution to provide a concentration of 1 mg/ml). Administer using a controlled infusion device.
- Don't mix labetalol with 5% sodium bicarbonate injection because of incompatibility; avoid giving drug in same infusion line with other alkaline solutions (such as furosemide).
- Patients receiving I.V. labetalol infusion must be kept in the supine position during the infusion and for 3 hours after the infusion.
- Store tablets and injection at 36° to 86° F (2° to 30° C) and protect from light, moisture, and freezing.

Therapeutic monitoring

- Use specific radioenzyme or high-performance liquid chromatography assay techniques to reduce incidence of false-positive urine free and total catecholamine levels.
- Blood pressure must be closely monitored during and after I.V. infusion; after infusion, recommend monitoring blood pressure every 5 minutes for 30 minutes, then at 30-minute intervals for 2 hours, then hourly for 6 hours.
- During direct I.V. infusion, recommend monitoring blood pressure before and at 5-minute intervals after each injection; maximum hypotensive effect usually occurs in 5 to 15 minutes after each injection.

Special populations

Pregnant patients. Labetalol has been effective for management of hypertension associated with pregnancy and with reduced proteinuria and prevention of eclampsia. Rarely, transient hypotension, bradycardia, respiratory depression, and hypoglycemia have occurred in neonates.
Breast-feeding patients. Small amounts of drug are excreted in breast milk; use cautiously in breast-feeding women.
Pediatric patients. Safety and efficacy in children haven't been established; use drug only if potential benefit outweighs risk.
Geriatric patients. Geriatric patients may require lower maintenance dosages of labetalol because of increased bioavailability or delayed metabolism; they also may experience enhanced adverse effects. Use drug with caution in geriatric patients.

Patient counseling

- Advise patient that transient scalp tingling may occur during initiation of therapy but that it usually subsides quickly.
- Tell patient to take drug as prescribed to maintain adequate blood pressure control.

lactulose

Cephulac, Cholac, Chronulac, Constilac, Constulose, Duphalac, Enulose

Pharmacologic classification: disaccharide
Therapeutic classification: laxative
Pregnancy risk category B

How supplied

Available by prescription only

Pharmacist's Drug Handbook
Photoguide to tablets and capsules

This photoguide provides full-color photographs of some of the most commonly prescribed tablets and capsules in the United States. Shown in actual size, the drugs are organized alphabetically by trade or generic name for quick reference. Page numbers direct you to drug information.

Accupril
(page 972)

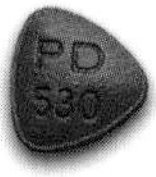

10 mg

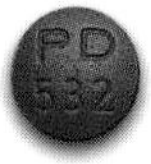

20 mg

Adalat CC
(extended-release)
(page 823)

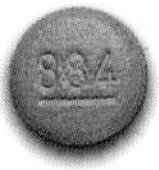

30 mg

Allegra
(page 499)

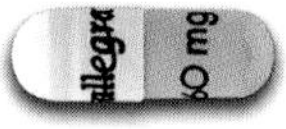

60 mg

Altace
(page 985)

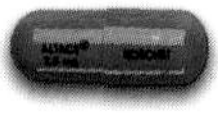

2.5 mg

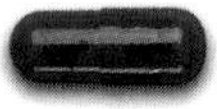

5 mg

Ambien
(page 1195)

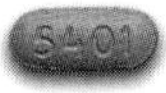

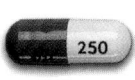

5 mg

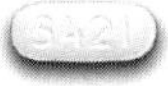

10 mg

amitriptyline hydrochloride
(page 123)

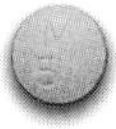

25 mg

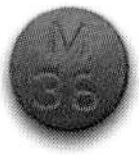

50 mg

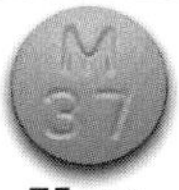

75 mg

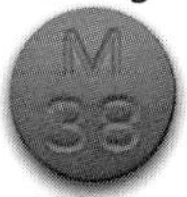

100 mg

amoxicillin trihydrate
(page 130)

250 mg

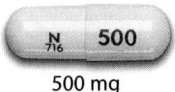

500 mg

Amoxil
(page 130)

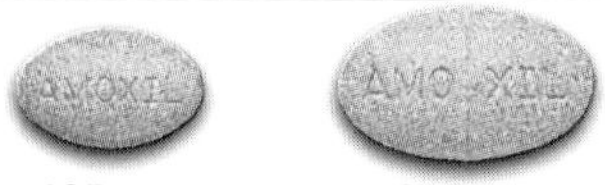

125 mg (chewable) | 250 mg (chewable)

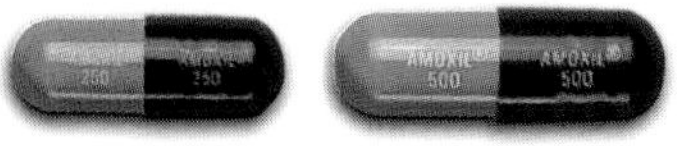

250 mg | 500 mg

atenolol
(page 157)

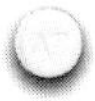

25 mg

Ativan
(page 687)

0.5 mg | 1 mg

Augmentin
(page 128)

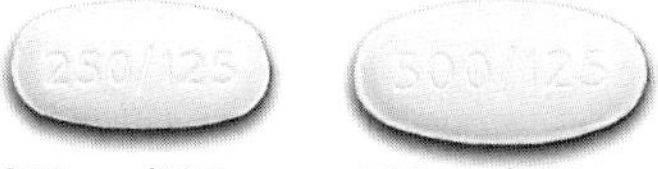

250 mg/125 mg | 500 mg/125 mg

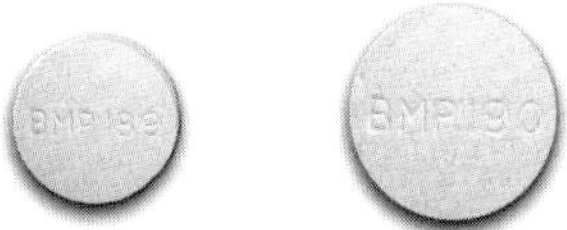

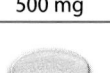

125 mg/31.25 mg (chewable) | 250 mg/62.5 mg (chewable)

Axid
(page 831)

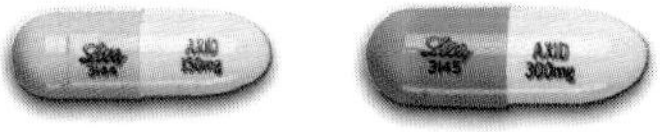

150 mg | 300 mg

Biaxin
(page 302)

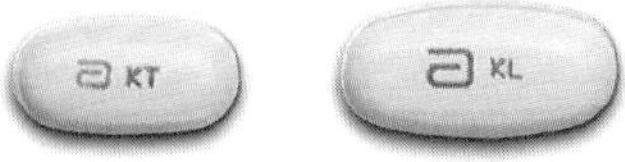

250 mg | 500 mg

Bumex
(page 205)

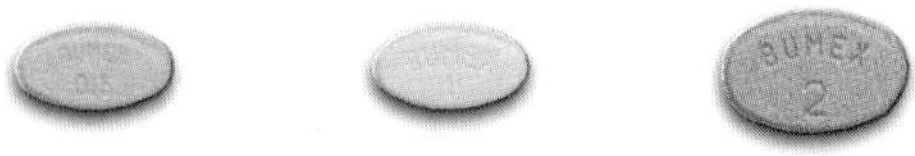

0.5 mg | 1 mg | 2 mg

BuSpar
(page 210)

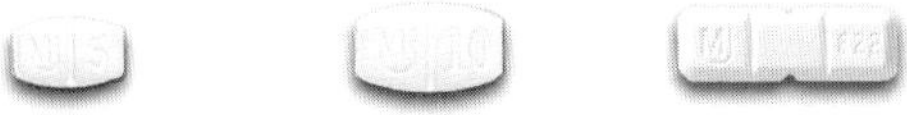

5 mg | 10 mg | 15 mg

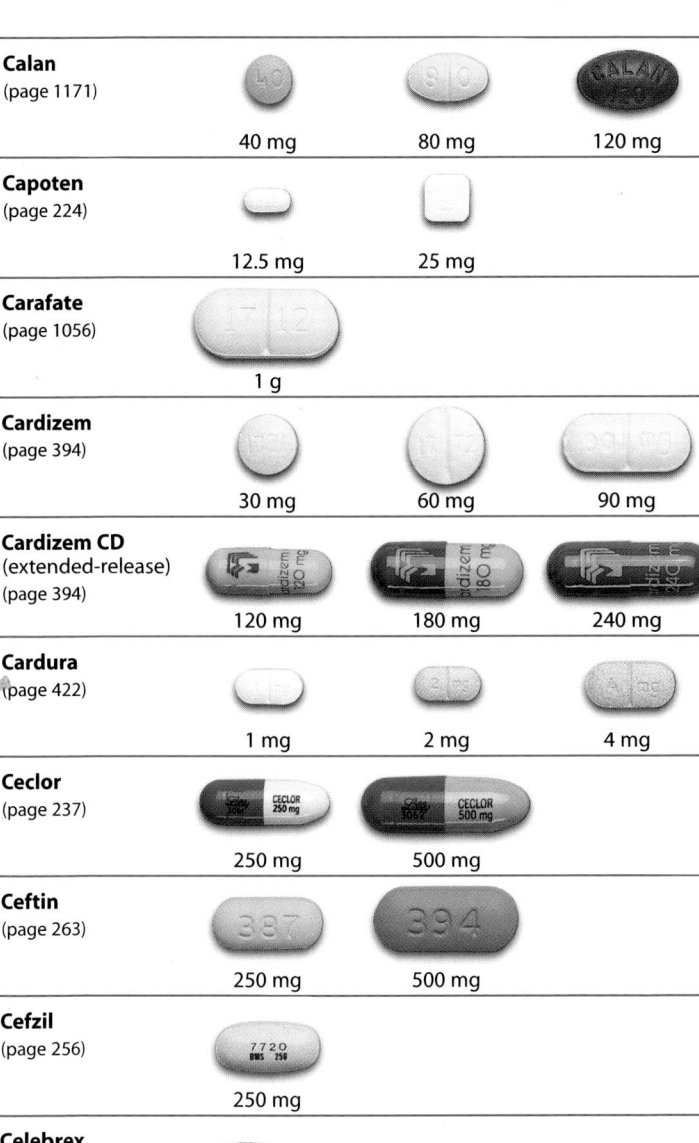

Calan
(page 1171)

40 mg | 80 mg | 120 mg

Capoten
(page 224)

12.5 mg | 25 mg

Carafate
(page 1056)

1 g

Cardizem
(page 394)

30 mg | 60 mg | 90 mg

Cardizem CD
(extended-release)
(page 394)

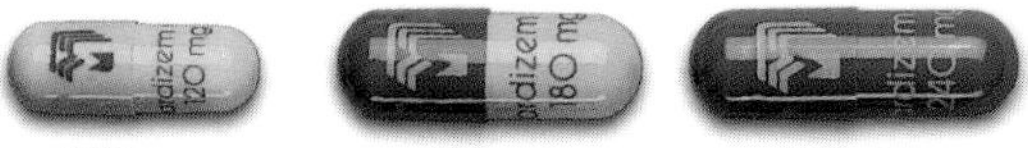

120 mg | 180 mg | 240 mg

Cardura
(page 422)

1 mg | 2 mg | 4 mg

Ceclor
(page 237)

250 mg | 500 mg

Ceftin
(page 263)

250 mg | 500 mg

Cefzil
(page 256)

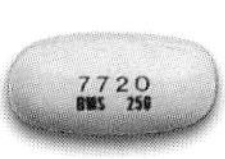

250 mg

Celebrex
(page 265)

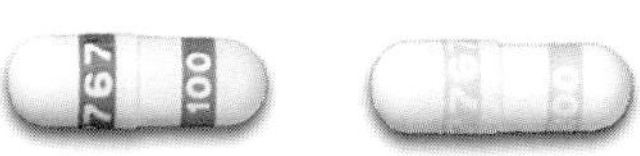

100 mg | 200 mg

cephalexin monohydrate
(page 267)

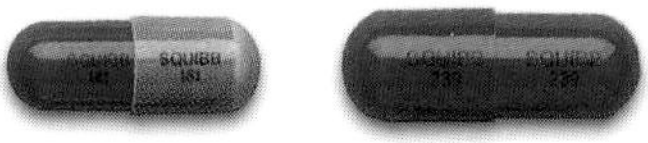

250 mg | 500 mg

cimetidine (page 290)	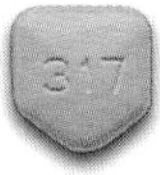 300 mg	 400 mg	
Cipro (page 292)	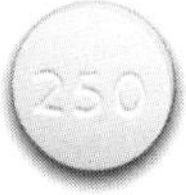 250 mg	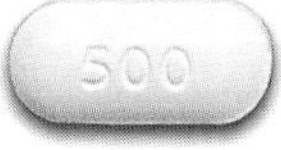 500 mg	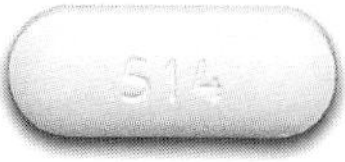 750 mg
Claritin (page 686)	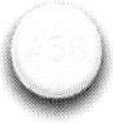 10 mg		
Compazine (page 946)	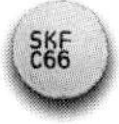 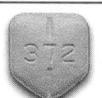 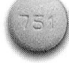 5 mg	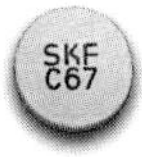 10 mg	
Cordarone (page 121)	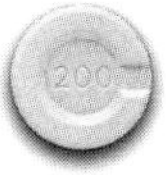 200 mg		
Coreg (page 233)	 3.125 mg	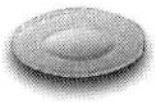 6.25 mg	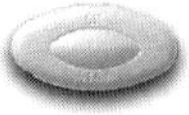 12.5 mg
	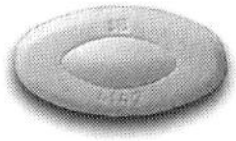 25 mg		
Coumadin (page 1183)	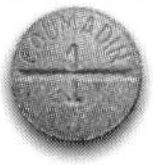 1 mg	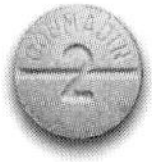 2 mg	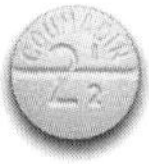 2.5 mg
	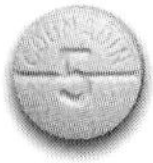 5 mg	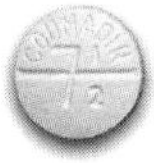 7.5 mg	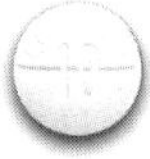 10 mg
Cozaar (page 689)	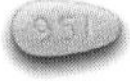 25 mg	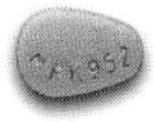 50 mg	
cyclobenzaprine hydrochloride (page 335)	 10 mg		

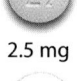

Darvocet-N 100
(page 1212)

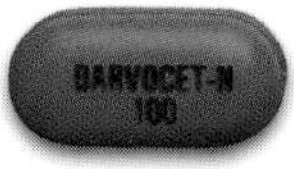

100 mg/650 mg

Daypro
(page 856)

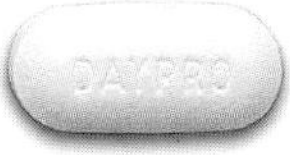

600 mg

Deltasone
(page 937)

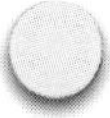

2.5 mg

5 mg

10 mg

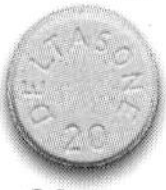

20 mg

Depakote
(page 1160)

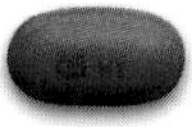

125 mg

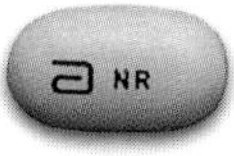

250 mg

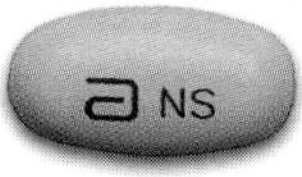

500 mg

Depakote Sprinkle
(delayed-release)
(page 1160)

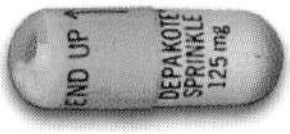

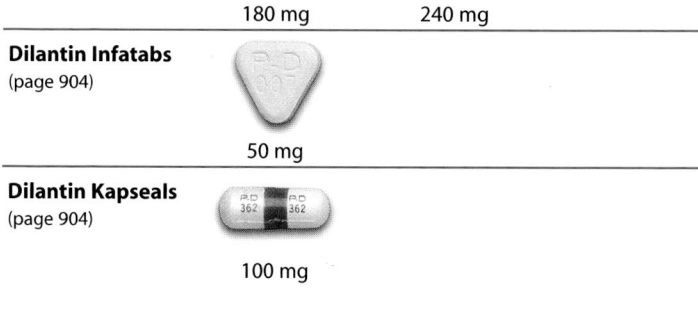

125 mg

DiaBeta
(page 548)

1.25 mg

2.5 mg

5 mg

Diflucan
(page 505)

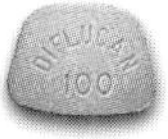

100 mg

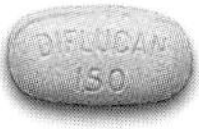

150 mg

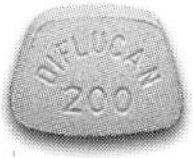

200 mg

Dilacor XR
(page 394)

180 mg

240 mg

Dilantin Infatabs
(page 904)

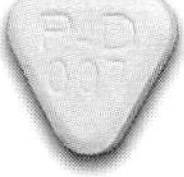

50 mg

Dilantin Kapseals
(page 904)

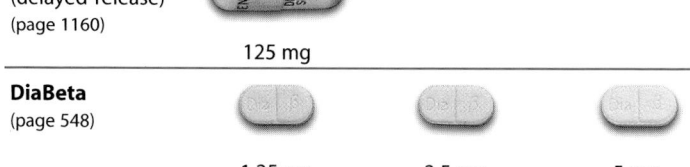

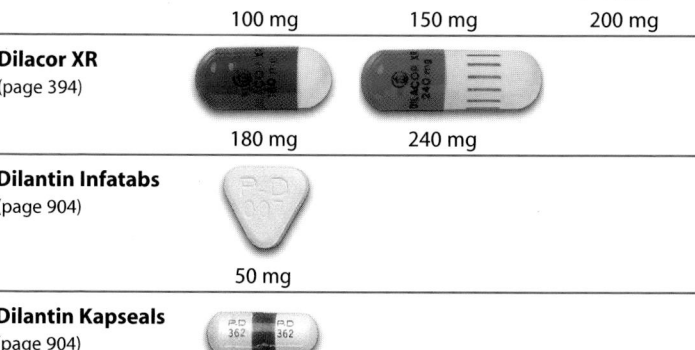

100 mg

doxepin hydrochloride
(page 423)

75 mg

Duricef
(page 238)

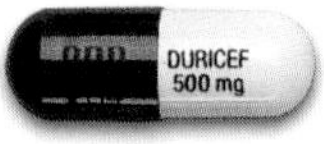

500 mg

E.E.S.
(page 457)

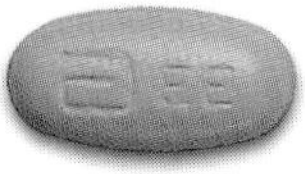

400 mg

Effexor
(page 1170)

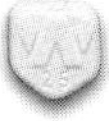

25 mg

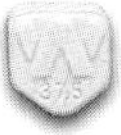

37.5 mg

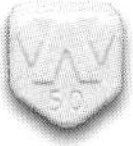

50 mg

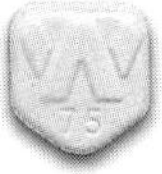

75 mg

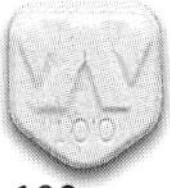

100 mg

Ery-Tab
(delayed-release)
(page 457)

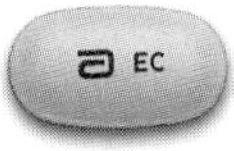

250 mg

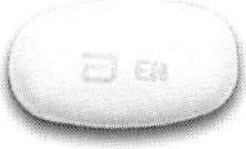

333 mg

Erythrocin Stearate Filmtab
(page 457)

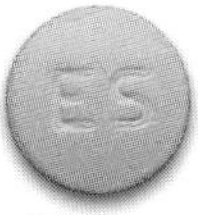

250 mg

Erythromycin Base Filmtab
(page 457)

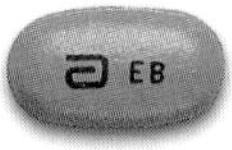

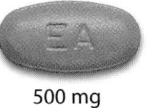

250 mg

500 mg

Estrace
(page 464)

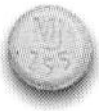

1 mg

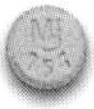

2 mg

Fiorinal with Codeine
(page 1212)

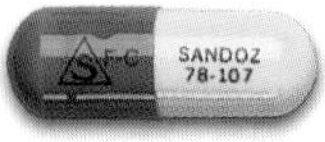

325 mg aspirin, 50 mg butalbital, 40 mg caffeine, 30 mg codeine phosphate

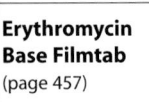

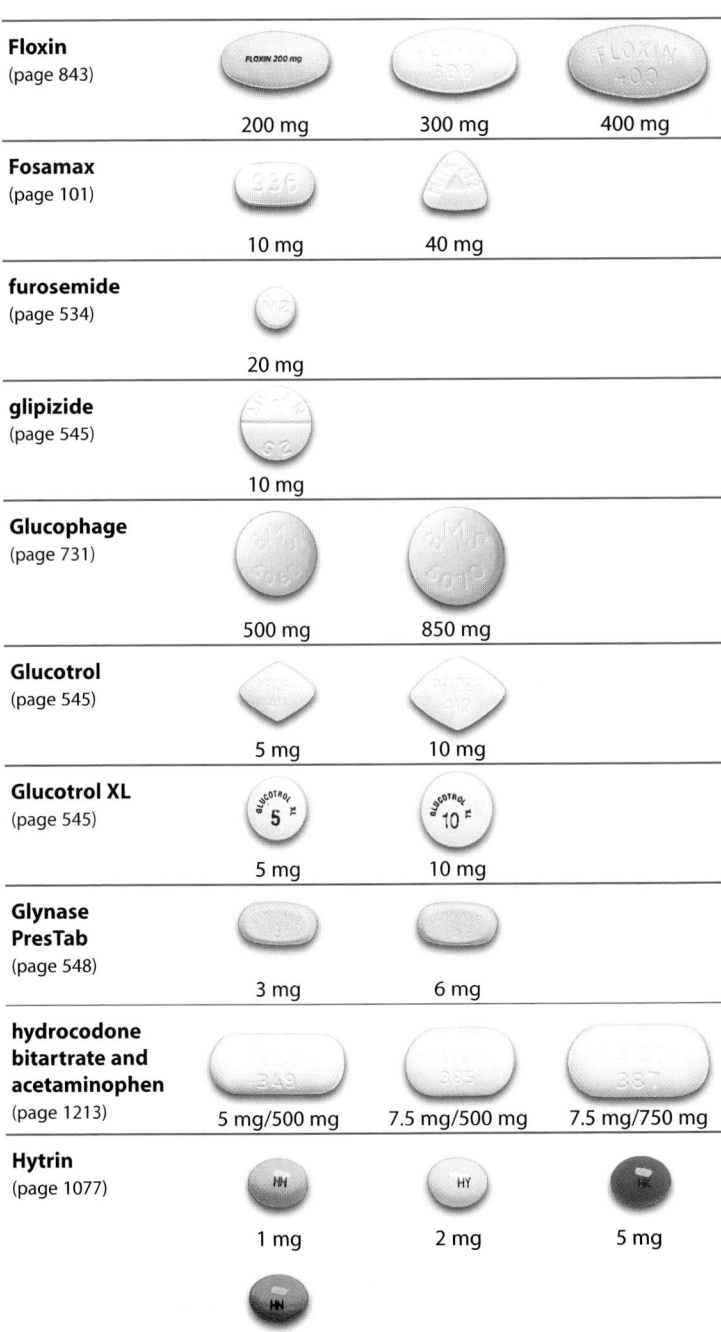

Floxin
(page 843)

200 mg | 300 mg | 400 mg

Fosamax
(page 101)

10 mg | 40 mg

furosemide
(page 534)

20 mg

glipizide
(page 545)

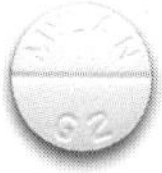

10 mg

Glucophage
(page 731)

500 mg | 850 mg

Glucotrol
(page 545)

5 mg | 10 mg

Glucotrol XL
(page 545)

5 mg | 10 mg

Glynase PresTab
(page 548)

3 mg | 6 mg

hydrocodone bitartrate and acetaminophen
(page 1213)

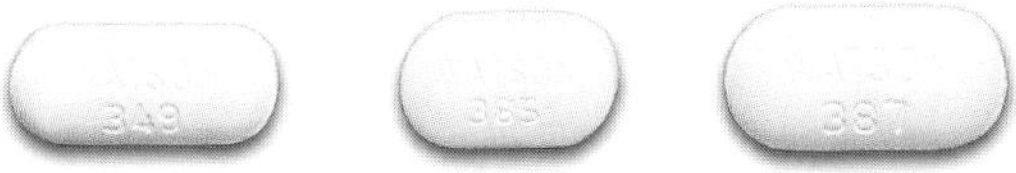

5 mg/500 mg | 7.5 mg/500 mg | 7.5 mg/750 mg

Hytrin
(page 1077)

1 mg | 2 mg | 5 mg

10 mg

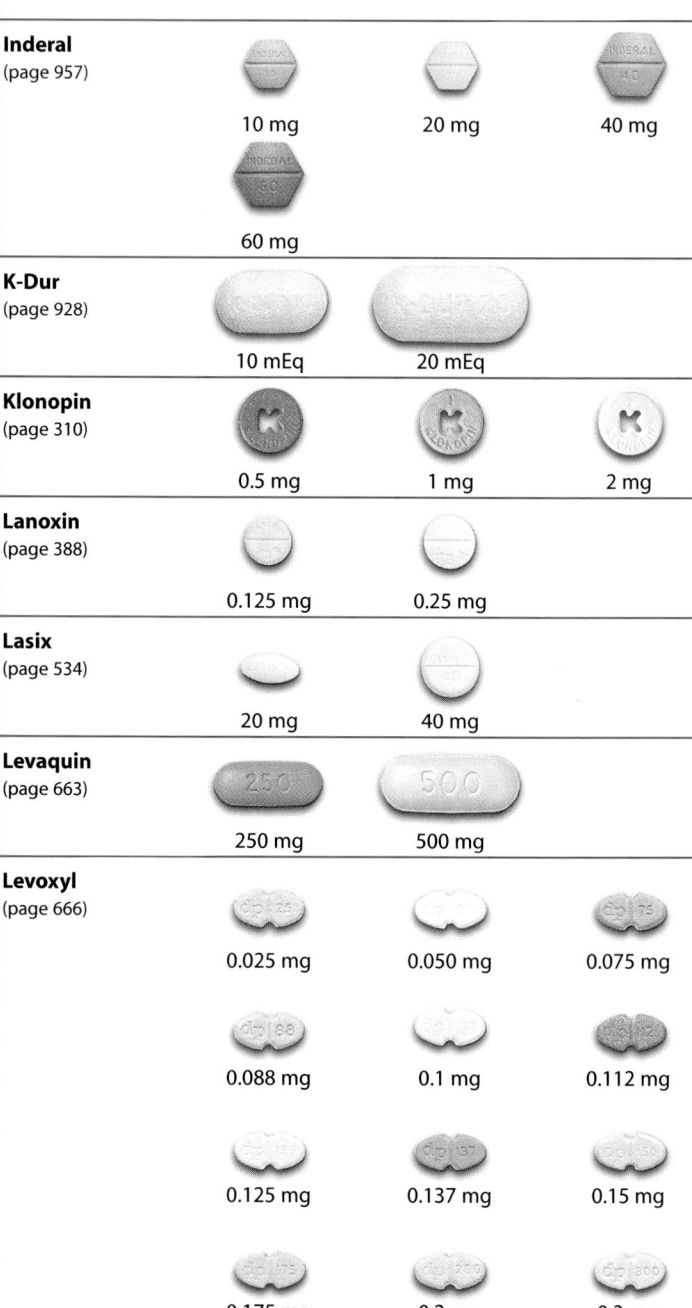

Inderal
(page 957)

10 mg | 20 mg | 40 mg

60 mg

K-Dur
(page 928)

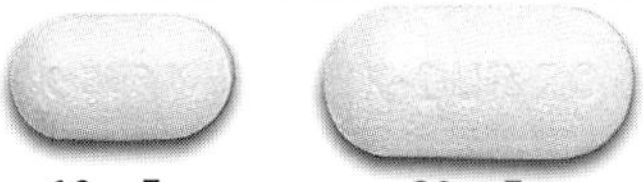

10 mEq | 20 mEq

Klonopin
(page 310)

0.5 mg | 1 mg | 2 mg

Lanoxin
(page 388)

0.125 mg | 0.25 mg

Lasix
(page 534)

20 mg | 40 mg

Levaquin
(page 663)

250 mg | 500 mg

Levoxyl
(page 666)

0.025 mg | 0.050 mg | 0.075 mg

0.088 mg | 0.1 mg | 0.112 mg

0.125 mg | 0.137 mg | 0.15 mg

0.175 mg | 0.2 mg | 0.3 mg

Lipitor
(page 158)

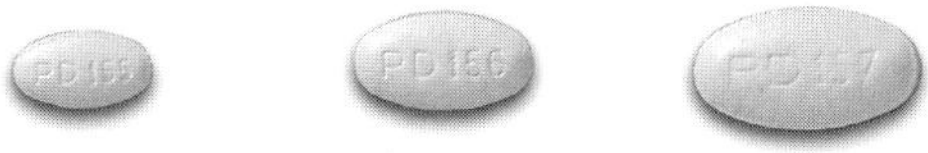

10 mg 20 mg 40 mg

Lodine
(page 481)

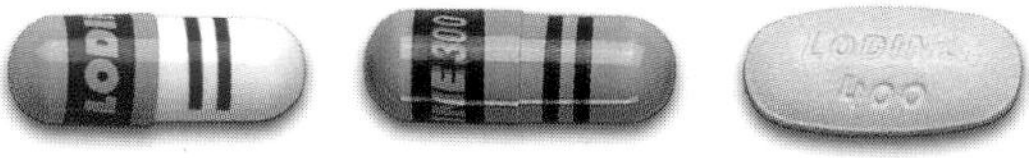

200 mg 300 mg 400 mg

Lopid
(page 541)

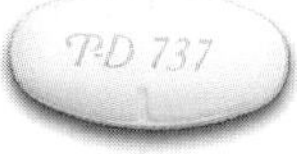

600 mg

Lorabid
(page 684)

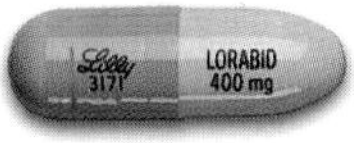

400 mg

Lorcet 10/650
(page 1212)

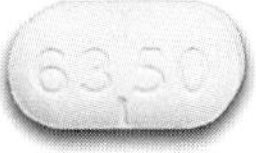

10 mg/650 mg

Lotensin
(page 178)

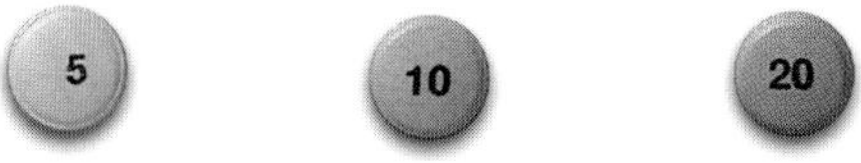

5 mg 10 mg 20 mg

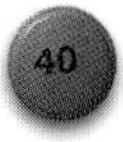

40 mg

Macrobid
(page 825)

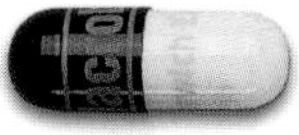

75/25 mg

methylphenidate hydrochloride
(page 747)

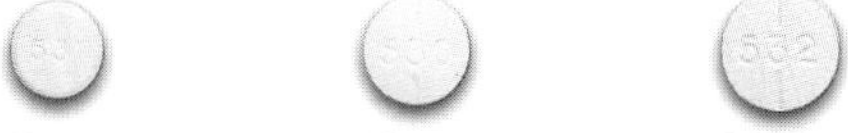

5 mg 10 mg 20 mg

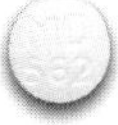

20 mg
(extended-release)

Mevacor
(page 690)

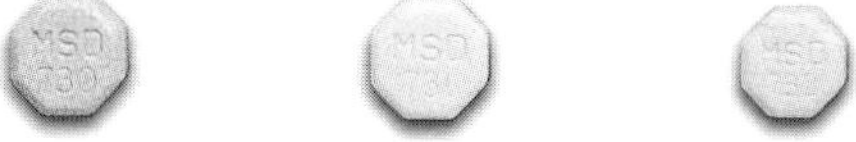

10 mg 20 mg 40 mg

Micro-K Extencaps
(controlled-release)
(page 928)

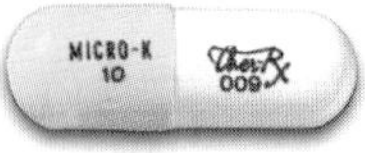

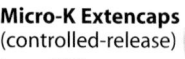

10 mEq (750 mg)

Micronase
(page 548)

2.5 mg | 5 mg

Monopril
(page 530)

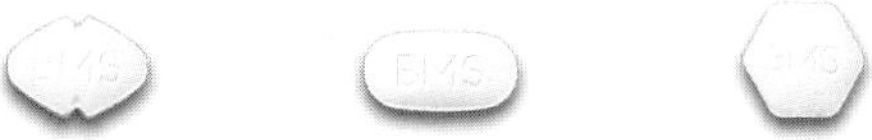

10 mg | 20 mg | 40 mg

Motrin
(page 589)

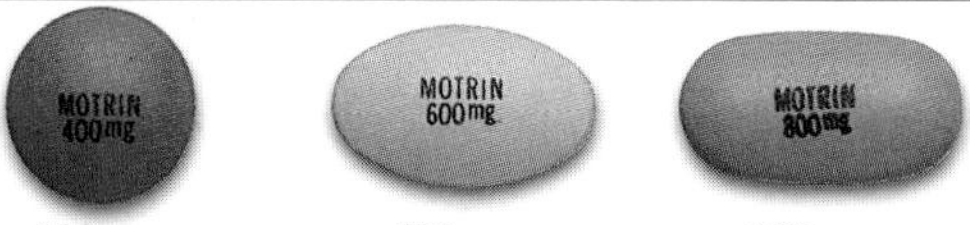

400 mg | 600 mg | 800 mg

Naprosyn
(page 805)

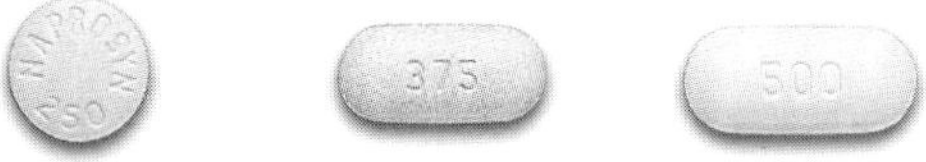

250 mg | 375 mg | 500 mg

naproxen
(page 805)

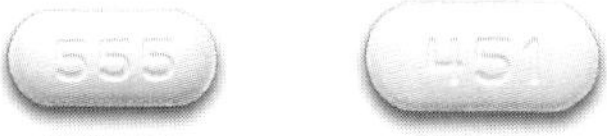

375 mg | 500 mg

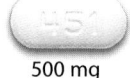

Nitrostat
(page 827)

0.3 mg | 0.4 mg | 0.6 mg

Nolvadex
(page 1070)

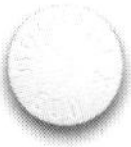

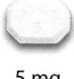

10 mg

nortriptyline hydrochloride
(page 838)

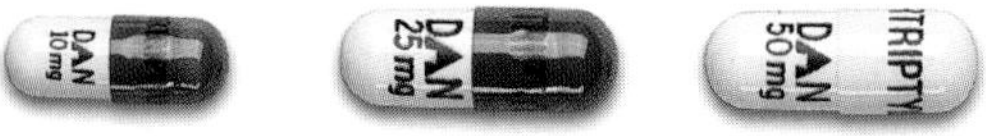

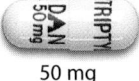

10 mg | 25 mg | 50 mg

Norvasc
(page 125)

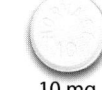

5 mg | 10 mg

Oruvail
(page 637)

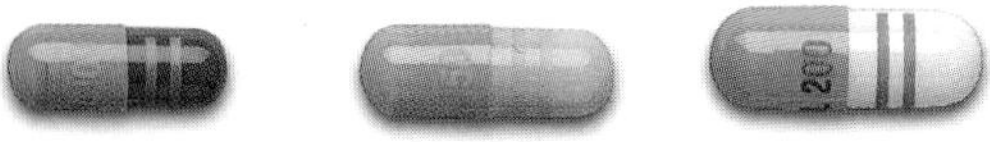

100 mg | 150 mg | 200 mg

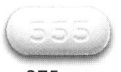

Pamelor
(page 838)

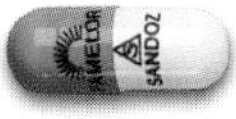

10 mg

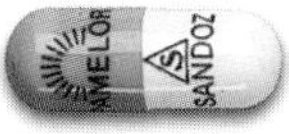

25 mg

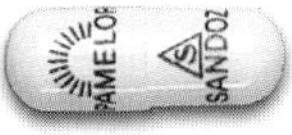

50 mg

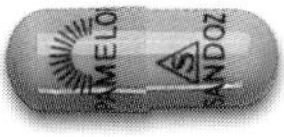

75 mg

Paxil
(page 873)

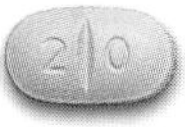

20 mg

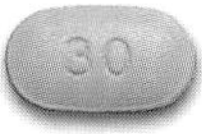

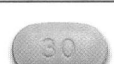

30 mg

PCE
(page 457)

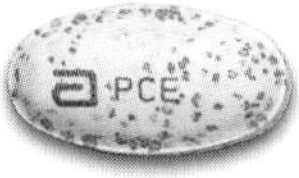

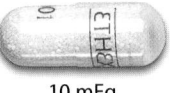

333 mg

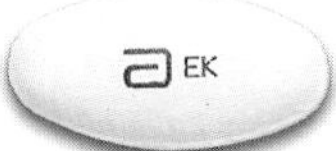

500 mg

Pepcid
(page 487)

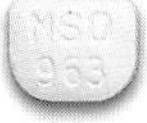

20 mg

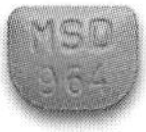

40 mg

Percocet 5/325
(page 1213)

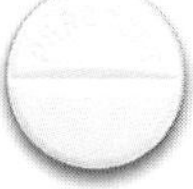
5 mg/325 mg

potassium chloride
(controlled-release)
(page 928)

10 mEq

Pravachol
(page 932)

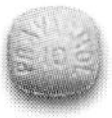
10 mg

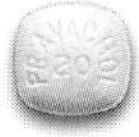
20 mg

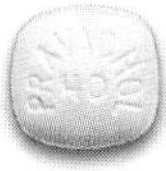
40 mg

Premarin
(page 471)

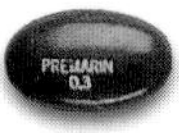

0.3 mg

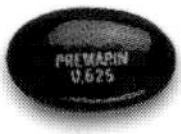

0.625 mg

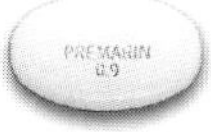

0.9 mg

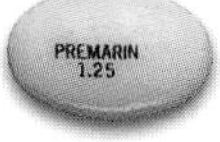

1.25 mg

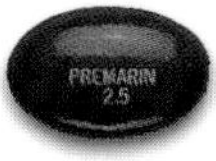

2.5 mg

Prevacid
(page 648)

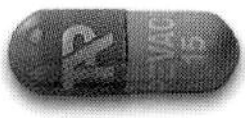
15 mg

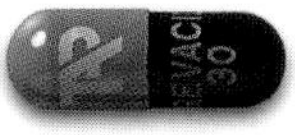
30 mg

Prilosec
(page 847)

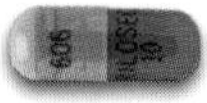
10 mg

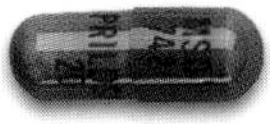

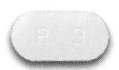
20 mg

Prinivil
(page 676)

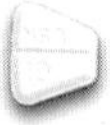
5 mg

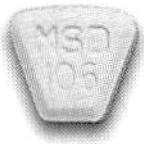

10 mg

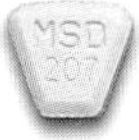

20 mg

Procardia XL
(extended-release)
(page 823)

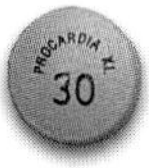

30 mg

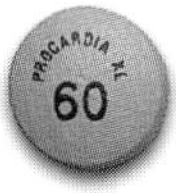

60 mg

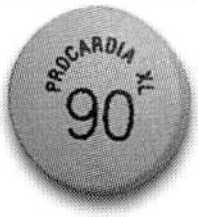

90 mg

propoxyphene napsylate with acetaminophen
(page 1213)

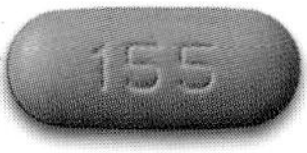

100 mg/650 mg

Provera
(page 710)

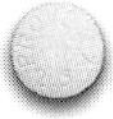
2.5 mg

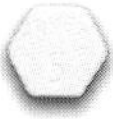
5 mg

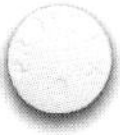
10 mg

Prozac
(page 515)

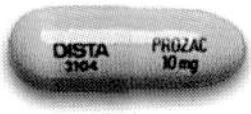

10 mg

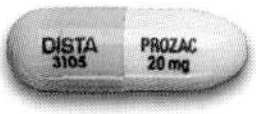

20 mg

Relafen
(page 794)

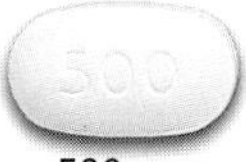

500 mg

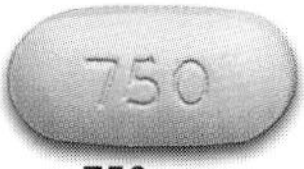

750 mg

Risperdal
(page 1003)

1 mg

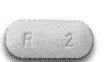

2 mg

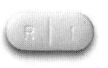

3 mg

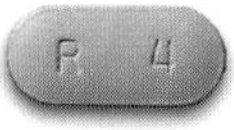

4 mg

Roxicet
(page 1213)

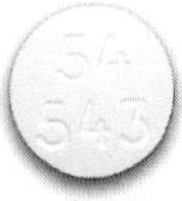
5 mg/325 mg

Serzone
(page 809)

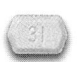

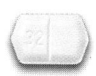

50 mg

100 mg

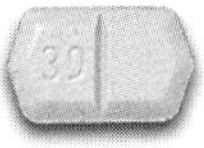

150 mg

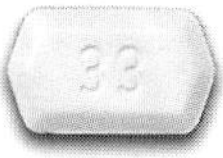

200 mg

Sinemet
(page 661)

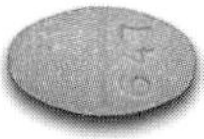
10 mg/100 mg

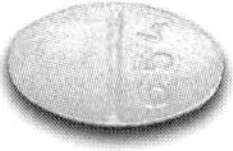
25 mg/250 mg

Sinemet CR
(extended-release)
(page 661)

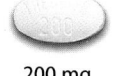

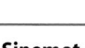

25 mg/100 mg

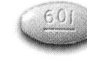

Slo-bid Gyrocaps
(extended-release)
(page 1092)

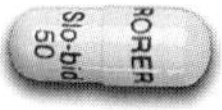

50 mg

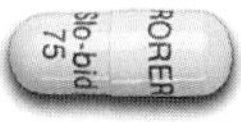

75 mg

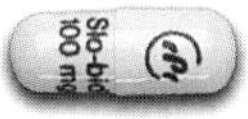

100 mg

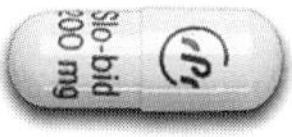

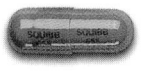

200 mg

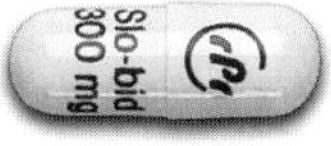

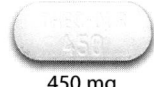

300 mg

Sumycin
(page 1087)

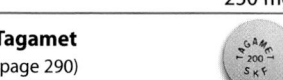

250 mg

Tagamet
(page 290)

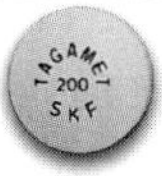

200 mg

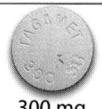

300 mg

Tenormin
(page 157)

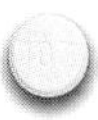
25 mg

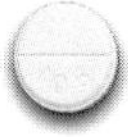

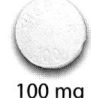
50 mg

100 mg

Theo-Dur
(extended-release)
(page 1092)

100 mg

200 mg

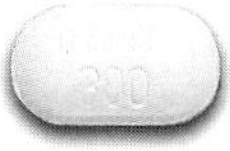

300 mg

450 mg

Ticlid
(page 1107)

250 mg

Toprol XL
(page 754)

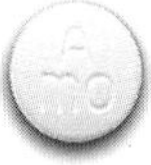

50 mg

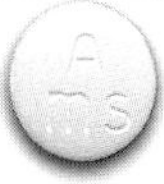

100 mg

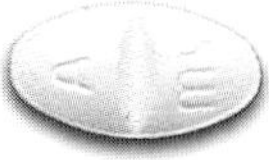

200 mg

Toradol
(page 638)

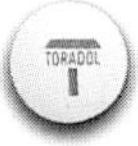

10 mg

Trental
(page 889)

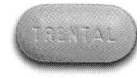

400 mg

Trimox
(page 130)

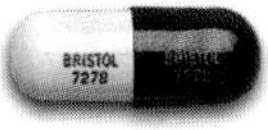

250 mg

500 mg

Tylenol with Codeine No. 3
(page 1213)

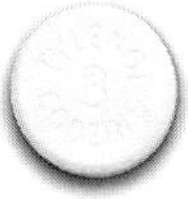

300 mg/30 mg

Ultram
(page 1129)

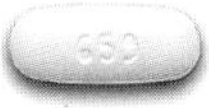

50 mg

Valium
(page 375)

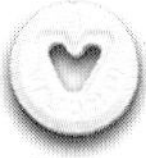

2 mg

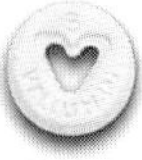

5 mg

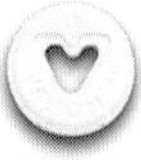

10 mg

Vasotec
(page 439)

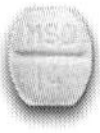

2.5 mg

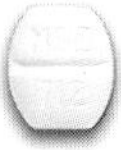

5 mg

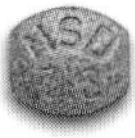

10 mg

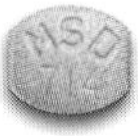

20 mg

Veetids
(page 881)

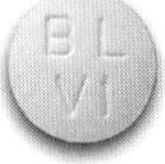

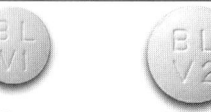

250 mg

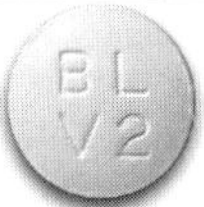

500 mg

verapamil hydrochloride
(sustained-release)
(page 1171)

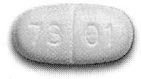

180 mg

Verelan
(extended-release)
(page 1171)

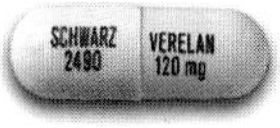

120 mg

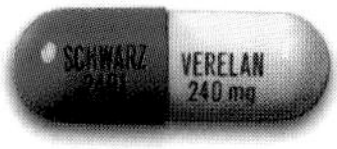

240 mg

Viagra
(page 1032)

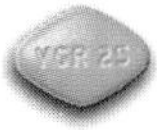

25 mg

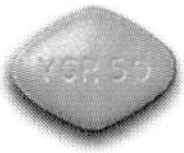

50 mg

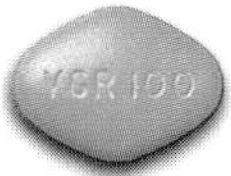

100 mg

Vioxx
(page 1010)

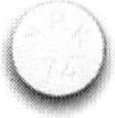
12.5 mg

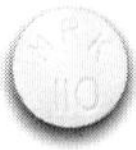

25 mg

Xanax
(page 105)

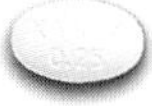
0.25 mg

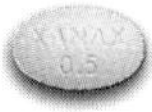
0.5 mg

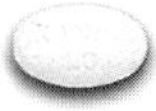
1 mg

Zantac
(page 986)

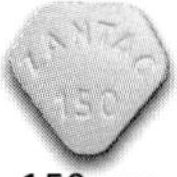

150 mg

300 mg

Zantac EFFERdose
(page 986)

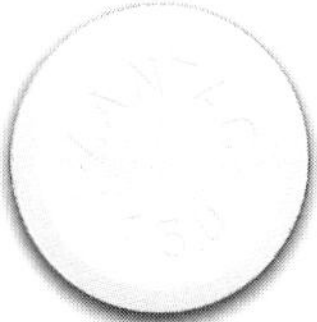
150 mg

Zestril
(page 676)

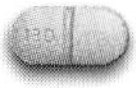

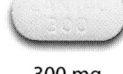
5 mg

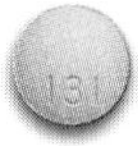

10 mg

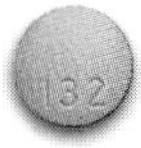

20 mg

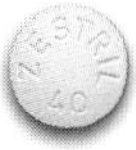

40 mg

Zithromax
(page 167)

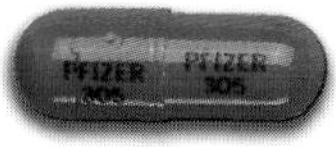

250 mg

Zocor
(page 1034)

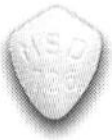

5 mg

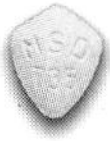

10 mg

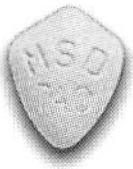

20 mg

Zoloft
(page 1029)

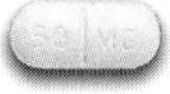

50 mg

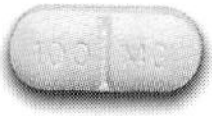

100 mg

Zovirax
(page 91)

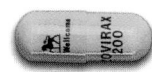

200 mg

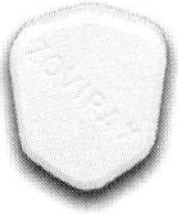

400 mg

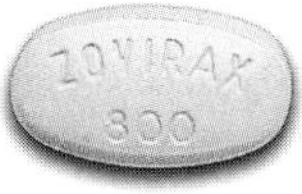

800 mg

Zyrtec
(page 271)

5 mg

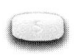

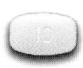

10 mg

Powder: 10 g/packet, 20 g/packet
Syrup: 10 g/15 ml
Rectal solution: 3.33 g/5 ml

Indications and dosages

Constipation
Adults: 10 to 20 g P.O. daily (may increase to 40 g if needed).
◊ *Children:* 5 g P.O. daily as single dose after breakfast.
To prevent and treat portal-systemic encephalopathy, including hepatic precoma and coma in patients with severe hepatic disease
Adults: Initially, 20 to 30 g (30 to 45 ml) P.O. t.i.d. or q.i.d., until two or three soft stools are produced daily. Usual dosage is 60 to 100 g daily in divided doses; can also be given by retention enema. Mix 200 g of lactulose with 700 ml of water or normal saline solution for retention for 60 minutes. May repeat q 4 to 6 hours. May repeat immediately if retention is less than 30 minutes.
Infants: Initially, 1.67 to 6.67 g P.O. daily in divided doses. Adjust doses q 1 to 2 days to produce two to three loose stools daily.
Older children and adolescents: Initially, 27 to 60 g P.O. daily in divided doses. Adjust doses q 1 to 2 days to produce two to three loose stools daily.
◊ ***After barium meal examination***
Adults: 3.3 to 6.7 g, P.O. b.i.d. for 1 to 4 weeks.
◊ ***To restore bowel movements after hemorrhoidectomy***
Adults: 10 g P.O. twice during day before surgery and for 5 days postoperatively.

Pharmacodynamics

Laxative action: Because lactulose is indigestible, it passes through the GI tract to the colon unchanged; there, it's digested by normally occurring bacteria. The weak acids produced in this manner increase the fluid content of the stool and cause distention, thus promoting peristalsis and bowel evacuation.

Lactulose also is used to reduce serum ammonia levels in patients with hepatic disease. Lactulose breakdown acidifies the colon, which, in turn, converts ammonia (NH_3) to ammonium ($NH4^+$), which isn't absorbed and is excreted in the stool. Furthermore, this "ion trapping" effect causes ammonia to diffuse from the blood into the colon, where it's excreted as well.

Pharmacokinetics

Absorption: Absorbed minimally.
Distribution: Distributed locally, primarily in the colon.
Metabolism: Metabolized by colonic bacteria (absorbed portion isn't metabolized).
Excretion: Mostly excreted in feces; absorbed portion is excreted in urine.

Route	Onset	Peak	Duration
P.O.	24-48 hr	Variable	Variable
P.R.	Unknown	Unknown	Unknown

Contraindications and precautions

Contraindicated in patients on a low-galactose diet. Use cautiously in patients with diabetes mellitus. Use cautiously in patients who may require electrocautery procedures during proctoscopy or colonoscopy.

Interactions

Drug-drug. *Neomycin and other antibiotics:* May theoretically decrease lactulose effectiveness by eliminating bacteria needed to digest it into the active form. Recommend monitoring for effect.
Nonabsorbable antacids: May decrease lactulose effectiveness by preventing a decrease in the pH of the colon. Avoid use together.

Effects on diagnostic tests

None reported.

Adverse reactions

GI: *abdominal cramps, belching, gaseous distention, flatulence,* nausea, vomiting, *diarrhea* (with excessive dosage).

Overdose and treatment

No cases of overdose have been reported. Clinical effects include diarrhea and abdominal cramps.

Clinical considerations

- After giving drug through nasogastric tube, flush tube with water to clear it and ensure passage of drug to stomach.
- Dilute drug with water or fruit juice to minimize its sweet taste.
- For oral administration, reconstitute powder by dissolving 10- to 20-g packet in 120 ml of water.
- For administration by retention enema, patient should retain drug for 30 to 60 minutes. If retained less than 30 minutes, repeat dose immediately. Begin oral therapy before discontinuing retention enemas.
- Don't administer drug with other laxatives because resulting loose stools may falsely indicate adequate dosage of lactulose.
- Store at 59° to 86° F (15° to 30° C); avoid freezing.

Therapeutic monitoring

- Monitor frequency and consistency of stools.
- Monitor serum potassium, chloride, and carbon dioxide in long-term treatment.

Special populations

Breast-feeding patients. It's unknown if drug is excreted in breast milk. Use with caution in breast-feeding women.
Geriatric patients. Monitor patient's serum electrolyte levels; geriatric patients are more sensitive to possible hypernatremia.

Patient counseling

- Advise patient to take drug with juice to improve taste.
- Instruct patient to contact doctor if unusual diarrhea condition occurs.

lamivudine (3TC)

Epivir, Epivir-HBV

Pharmacologic classification: synthetic nucleoside analogue
Therapeutic classification: antiviral
Pregnancy risk category C

How supplied

Available by prescription only
Epivir
Tablets: 150 mg
Oral solution: 10 mg/ml
Epivir-HBV
Tablets: 100 mg
Oral solution: 5 mg/ml

Indications and dosages

Treatment of patients with HIV infection (should be used in combination with other antiretroviral agents)
Adults weighing 110 lb (50 kg) or more and children age 16 and older: 150 mg P.O. b.i.d.
Adults weighing less than 110 lb (50 kg): 2 mg/kg P.O., b.i.d.
Children age 3 months to 16 years: 4 mg/kg P.O. b.i.d. Maximum dose is 150 mg b.i.d.
◊*Neonates 30 days and younger:* 2 mg/kg P.O. b.i.d
≡***Dosage adjustment.*** For adults and adolescents with renal failure, refer to the table below. In pediatric patients with renal failure, consider decreasing the dose or increasing the dosage interval.

Creatinine clearance (ml/min)	Recommended dosage
≥ 50	150 mg b.i.d.
30 to 49	150 mg once daily
15 to 29	150 mg first dose; then 100 mg once daily
5 to 14	150 mg first dose; then 50 mg once daily
< 5	50 mg first; then 25 mg once daily

Treatment of chronic hepatitis B associated with evidence of hepatitis B viral replication and active liver inflammation
Adults: 100 mg P.O. once daily. Safety and efficacy of treatment beyond 1 year haven't been established; optimum duration of treatment isn't known. Formulation and dosage of lamivudine in Epivir-HBV aren't appropriate for those dually infected with hepatitis B virus (HBV) and HIV; test patients for HIV before treatment is initiated. If lamivudine is administered to patients with HBV and HIV, use the higher dosage indicated for HIV therapy as part of an appropriate combination regimen.
≡***Dosage adjustment.*** In patients with renal impairment (age 16 and older), if creatinine clearance is 30 to 49 ml/minute, 100 mg P.O. on the first day, then 50 mg P.O. once daily thereafter. If clearance is 15 to 29 ml/minute, 100 mg on the first day, then 25 mg P.O. once daily thereafter. If clearance is 5 to 14 ml/minute, 35 mg on the first day, then 15 mg once daily thereafter. If creatinine clearance is less than 5 ml/minute, 35 mg on the first day, then 10 mg P.O. once daily thereafter.
◊***Post-exposure prophylaxis following occupational exposure to HIV***
Adults: 150 mg P.O. b.i.d. in combination with oral zidovudine (600 mg daily); oral indinavir (800 mg q 8 hours) or oral nelfinavir (750 mg P.O. t.i.d.) is added if risk of transmission is likely. Initiate within a few hours and continue for 28 days.

Pharmacodynamics

Antiviral action: Lamivudine inhibits HIV reverse transcription via viral DNA chain termination. RNA- and DNA-dependent DNA polymerase activities are also inhibited.

Pharmacokinetics

Absorption: Rapidly absorbed after oral administration in HIV-infected patients.
Distribution: Believed to be distributed into extravascular spaces. Volume of distribution is independent of dose and doesn't correlate with body weight. Less than 36% is bound to plasma proteins.
Metabolism: Metabolism is minor route of elimination. The only known metabolite is the trans-sulfoxide metabolite.
Excretion: Primarily eliminated unchanged in urine. Mean elimination half-life is 5 to 7 hours.

Route	Onset	Peak	Duration
P.O.	Unknown	1-3 hr	Unknown

Contraindications and precautions

Contraindicated in patients with hypersensitivity to drug. Use drug with extreme caution and only if there's no satisfactory alternative therapy in pediatric patients with history of pancreatitis or other significant risk factors for development of pancreatitis. Stop treatment with lamivudine immediately if clinical signs, symptoms, or laboratory abnormalities suggest pancreatitis.

Use cautiously in children with a history of prior therapy with nucleoside reverse transcriptase inhibitors, and in patients with impaired renal function; use dosage reduction.

Lactic acidosis and severe hepatomegaly with steatosis have been reported in patients receiving lamivudine. Stop treatment if signs of lactic acidosis or hepatotoxicity develop.

Interactions

Drug-drug. *Co-trimoxazole:* Decreased clearance of lamivudine may cause increased blood levels of lamivudine. Monitor patient closely.

Effects on diagnostic tests

None reported.

Adverse reactions

Adverse reactions are related to the combination therapy of lamivudine and zidovudine.
CNS: *malaise, headache, fatigue, neuropathy, dizziness, insomnia and other sleep disorders,* depressive disorders.
EENT: *nasal symptoms, sore throat.*
GI: *nausea, diarrhea, vomiting, anorexia,* abdominal pain, abdominal cramps, dyspepsia, ***pancreatitis*** (in children age 3 months to 12 years).
Hematologic: ***neutropenia,*** anemia, ***thrombocytopenia.***
Hepatic: elevated liver enzymes and bilirubin levels.
Musculoskeletal: *musculoskeletal pain,* myalgia, arthralgia.
Respiratory: *cough.*
Skin: rash.
Other: *fever, chills.*

Overdose and treatment

No information available.

Clinical considerations

- When used in treatment of HIV infection, drug must be administered with zidovudine. It isn't intended for use as monotherapy.
- Safety and efficacy of treatment of HBV for periods over 1 year or in patients with decompensated liver disease or organ transplant haven't been established.
- Monotherapy with lamivudine in patients with HIV-HBV co-infection in HBV dosage is inadequate and may lead to rapid emergence of HIV resistance. Counseling and testing for HIV infection before and periodically during treatment is recommended. Use higher dosage in combination with other appropriate antiretroviral agents.

Therapeutic monitoring

Monitor CBC, platelet count, and liver function studies throughout therapy.

Special populations

Pregnant patients. An Antiretroviral Pregnancy Registry has been established to monitor maternal-fetal outcomes of pregnant women exposed to lamivudine. Pregnant patients can be registered by calling 1-800-258-4263.
Breast-feeding patients. To avoid transmitting HIV to the infant, HIV-positive women shouldn't breast-feed.
Pediatric patients. Safety and efficacy in treatment of HIV infection haven't been established in children younger than 3 months.

Patient counseling

- Inform patient that long-term effects of drug are unknown.
- Stress importance of taking drug exactly as prescribed.
- Instruct parents of children receiving drug about signs and symptoms of pancreatitis and tell them to report these immediately.
- Inform patients receiving dosage of less than therapeutic levels for HIV treatment that HIV testing is recommended.

lamivudine/zidovudine

Combivir

Pharmacologic classification: reverse transcriptase inhibitor
Therapeutic classification: antiretroviral
Pregnancy risk category C

How supplied

Available by prescription only
Tablets: Each tablet contains 150 mg lamivudine and 300 mg zidovudine

Indications and dosages

Treatment of HIV infection
Adults and children over age 12 and weighing 110 lb (50 kg) or more: One tablet P.O. b.i.d.

Pharmacodynamics

Antiretroviral action: Lamivudine and zidovudine are phosphorylated intracellularly to active metabolites that inhibit reverse transcriptase by way of DNA chain termination. Both drugs are also weak inhibitors of mammalian DNA polymerase. Together, they have synergistic antiretroviral activity. Combination therapy with lamivudine and zidovudine aims to suppress or delay emergence of phenotypic and genotypic resistant strains that can occur with retroviral monotherapy, because more mutations are necessary to develop dual resistance.

Pharmacokinetics

Absorption: Both lamivudine and zidovudine are rapidly absorbed following oral administration with respective oral bioavailability of 86% and 64%.
Distribution: Both drugs are extensively distributed and exhibit low protein binding.
Metabolism: Only about 5% of lamivudine is metabolized whereas zidovudine is primarily (74%) metabolized in the liver.
Excretion: Lamivudine is primarily eliminated unchanged in the urine. Zidovudine and its major metabolite are primarily eliminated in the urine. Elimination half-lives of lamivudine and zidovudine are 5 to 7 hours and ½ to 3 hours, respectively. Because renal excretion is a principal route of elimination, dosage adjustments are necessary in patients with compromised renal function, making this fixed ratio combination unsuitable. Hemodialysis and peritoneal dialysis have negligible effect on the removal of zidovudine, but removal of its metabolite, GZDV, is enhanced. The effect of dialysis on lamivudine is unknown.

Route	Onset	Peak	Duration
P.O.	Unknown	Unknown	Unknown

Contraindications and precautions

Contraindicated in patients with known hypersensitivity to components of drug and in those with low body weight (less than 110 lb), those with creatinine clearance less than 50 ml/minute, or those experiencing dose-limiting adverse effects.

Use combination with caution in patients with bone marrow suppression or renal insufficiency. Lactic acidosis and severe hepatomegaly with steatosis have been reported in patients receiving lamivudine and zidovudine alone and in combination. Stop treatment if signs of lactic acidosis or hepatotoxicity develop. Hepatotoxic events may be more severe in patients with decompensated liver function due to hepatitis B. Myopathy and myositis associated with prolonged use of zidovudine may occur.

Interactions

Drug-drug. *Atovaquone, fluconazole, methadone, probenecid, and valproic acid coadministered with zidovudine:* Increased bioavailability of zidovudine. Dosage modification isn't needed.
Ganciclovir, interferon-alpha, and other bone marrow suppressive or cytotoxic agents: May increase hematologic toxicity of zidovudine. Most drug interaction studies haven't been completed. Use cautiously as with other reverse transcriptase inhibitors.
Nelfinavir, ritonavir: Decreased bioavailability of zidovudine may occur with concurrent administration. Dosage modification isn't needed.
Nelfinavir or co-trimoxazole coadministered with lamivudine: Increased bioavailability of lamivudine. Dosage modification isn't needed.

Effects on diagnostic tests

None reported.

Adverse reactions

CNS: *headache,* malaise, *fatigue, insomnia, dizziness, neuropathy,* depression.
GI: *nausea, diarrhea, vomiting, anorexia,* abdominal pain, abdominal cramps, dyspepsia, ***pancreatitis.***
EENT: *nasal signs and symptoms.*
Hematologic: ***neutropenia,*** anemia.
Musculoskeletal: *musculoskeletal pain,* myalgia, arthralgia, myopathy, myositis.
Respiratory: *cough.*
Skin: rash.
Other: *fever, chills.*

Overdose and treatment

Overdose (6 g) with lamivudine results in normal hematologic tests and no clinical signs or symptoms. Overdoses of zidovudine, with exposure up to 50 g, results in only nausea and vomiting. No antidote is known for lamivudine/zidovudine overdose.

Clinical considerations

- Don't use combination drug therapy in patients requiring dosage adjustments such as those with renal dysfunction or pediatric patients.
- Combination may be administered with or without food.

Therapeutic monitoring

- Monitor for bone marrow toxicity with frequent blood counts, particularly in patients with advanced HIV infection.
- Monitor for signs of lactic acidosis and hepatotoxicity.
- Monitor patient's fine motor skills and peripheral sensation for evidence of peripheral neuropathies.

Special populations

Pregnant patients. Contact 1-800-722-9292, extension 39437, for patients exposed to Combivir during pregnancy.
Breast-feeding patients. Although zidovudine is excreted in breast milk at levels similar to those in serum, it's unknown if lamivudine/zidovudine is excreted in breast milk.
Pediatric patients. Don't use in patients under age 12 because the fixed-dose combination treatment can't be adjusted for this patient group.
Geriatric patients. Safety and efficacy in patients over age 65 haven't been established.

Patient counseling

- Advise patient that combination drug therapy isn't a cure for HIV infection, and that he may continue to experience illness including opportunistic infections.
- Warn patient that transmission of HIV virus can still occur with drug therapy.
- Teach patient signs and symptoms of neutropenia and anemia, and instruct him to report such occurrences.
- Advise patient to consult his doctor before taking other medications.
- Warn patient to report abdominal pain immediately.
- Stress importance of taking combination drug therapy exactly as prescribed to reduce the development of resistance.

lamotrigine

Lamictal

Pharmacologic classification: phenyltriazine
Therapeutic classification: anticonvulsant
Pregnancy risk category C

How supplied

Available by prescription only
Tablets: 25 mg, 100 mg, 150 mg, 200 mg
Chewable tablets: 5 mg, 25 mg

Indications and dosages

Adjunct therapy in treatment of partial seizures caused by epilepsy and Lennox-Gastout syndrome
Adults and children age 16 and older (12 and older for Lennox-Gastaut syndrome): 50 mg P.O. daily for 2 weeks, followed by 100 mg daily in two divided doses for 2 weeks. Thereafter, usual maintenance dosage is 300 to 500 mg P.O. daily given in two divided doses. For patients also taking valproic acid, give 25 mg P.O. every other day for 2 weeks, followed by 25 mg P.O. daily for 2 weeks. Thereafter, increase 25 to 50 mg q 1 to 2 weeks. Effective maintenance dosage is 100 to 400 mg daily in 1 or 2 divided doses.
Adjunct treatment of Lennox-Gastaut syndrome in patients receiving hepatic-enzyme-inducing anticonvulsant drugs without concomitant valproic acid therapy
Children age 2 to 12 years: 0.6 mg/kg P.O. daily (rounded down to the nearest 5 mg) in two divided doses for 2 weeks. During subsequent 2 weeks, 1.2 mg/kg (rounded down to the nearest 5 mg) daily in two divided doses. Then, increase q 1 to 2 weeks by 1.2 mg/kg (rounded down to the nearest 5 mg) until effective daily dose of about 5 to 15 mg/kg (maximum of 400 mg/day in two divided doses) is reached.
Adjunct treatment of Lennox-Gastaut syndrome in patients receiving hepatic-enzyme-inducing anticonvulsant drugs with concomitant valproic acid therapy
Children age 2 to 12 years: 0.15 mg/kg P.O. daily (rounded down to the nearest 5 mg) in one or two divided doses for 2 weeks. If the initial calculated daily dose of lamotrigine is 2.5 to 5 mg, then a 5-mg dose should be administered on alternate days for the first 2 weeks. During subsequent 2 weeks, 0.3 mg/kg (rounded down to the nearest 5 mg) daily in one or two divided doses. Then, increase q 1 to 2 weeks by 0.3 mg/kg (rounded down to the nearest 5 mg) until effective daily dose of about 1 to 5 mg/kg (maximum of 200 mg/day in one or two divided doses) is reached.

Pharmacodynamics

Anticonvulsant action: Unknown. Possibly related to inhibition of release of glutamate and aspartate in the brain. This may occur by acting on voltage-sensitive sodium channels.

Pharmacokinetics

Absorption: Rapidly and completely absorbed from the GI tract with negligible first-pass metabolism. Absolute bioavailability is 98%.
Distribution: About 55% is bound to plasma proteins.
Metabolism: Metabolized predominantly by glucuronic acid conjugation; the major metabolite is an inactive 2-N-glucuronide conjugate.
Excretion: Excreted primarily in urine with only a small portion being excreted in feces.

Route	Onset	Peak	Duration
P.O.	Unknown	1½-4¾ hr	Unknown

Contraindications and precautions

Contraindicated in patients with hypersensitivity to drug. Use cautiously in patients with impaired renal, hepatic, or cardiac function.

Interactions

Drug-drug. *Carbamazepine, phenobarbital, phenytoin, primidone:* Decreased lamotrigine steady-state levels. Patient requires careful monitoring.
Folate inhibitors such as cotrimoxazole, methotrexate: May be affected by lamotrigine because it inhibits dihydrofolate reductase, an enzyme involved in the synthesis of folic acid. Patient requires close monitoring because drug may have an additive effect.
Valproic acid: Decreased lamotrigine clearance, which increases steady-state levels of drug. Monitor patient closely for toxicity.
Drug-lifestyle. *Sun exposure:* Possible photosensitivity reactions. Advise patient to take precautions.

Effects on diagnostic tests

None reported.

Adverse reactions

CNS: *dizziness, headache, ataxia, somnolence,* malaise, incoordination, insomnia, tremor, depression, anxiety, ***seizures,*** irritability, speech disorder, decreased memory, concentration disturbance, sleep disorder, emotional lability, vertigo, mind racing, ***suicide attempts.***
CV: palpitations.
EENT: *diplopia, blurred vision,* vision abnormality, nystagmus.
GI: *nausea, vomiting,* diarrhea, dyspepsia, abdominal pain, constipation, tooth disorder, anorexia, dry mouth, rectal hemorrhage, peptic ulcer.
GU: dysmenorrhea, vaginitis, amenorrhea, epistaxis, bronchitis.
Musculoskeletal: dysarthria, muscle spasm, neck pain.
Respiratory: rhinitis, pharyngitis, cough, dyspnea.
Skin: ***Stevens-Johnson syndrome,*** *rash,* pruritus, hot flashes, alopecia, acne, epidermal neurolyisis (rarely toxic), photosensitivity, contact dermatitis, dry skin, sweating.
Other: flulike syndrome, fever, infection, chills, peripheral edema, weight loss.

Overdose and treatment

Limited information available. Following a suspected overdose, treatment should be supportive. Induce emesis or perform gastric lavage, if necessary. It isn't known if hemodialysis is effective.

Clinical considerations

- Drug may be administered without regard to meals. Chewable tablets may be swallowed whole, chewed and swallowed with a small amount of water or diluted fruit juice or dispersed in about 5 ml of liquid for about 1 minute and consumed immediately.
- Don't discontinue drug abruptly because of risk of increasing seizure frequency. Instead, taper drug over at least 2 weeks.
- Stop drug immediately if drug-induced rash occurs.
- If lamotrigine is added to a multidrug regimen that includes valproate, reduce dose of lamotrigine and use a lower maintenance dosage in patients with severe renal impairment.

Therapeutic monitoring

- Evaluate patient for reduction in the frequency and duration of seizures.
- Check adjunct serum levels of anticonvulsant.

Special populations

Breast-feeding patients. Drug use in breast-feeding women isn't recommended.
Pediatric patients. Recommended use in children age 2 to 12 is very limited and must be carefully administered following the detailed guidelines provided with the medication. The incidence of severe, potentially life-threatening rash in pediatric patients is much higher than that reported in adults.
Geriatric patients. Safety and efficacy in patients over age 65 haven't been established.

Patient counseling

- Inform patient that rash may occur, especially during first 6 weeks of therapy and in pediatric patients. Combination therapy of valproic acid and lamotrigine is likely to precipitate a serious rash. Although it may resolve with continued therapy, tell patient to report rash immediately in case drug needs to be discontinued.
- Warn patient not to perform hazardous activities until CNS effects are known.
- Advise patient to take protective measures against photosensitivity reactions until tolerance is known.

lansoprazole

Prevacid

Pharmacologic classification: acid (proton) pump inhibitor
Therapeutic classification: antiulcer
Pregnancy risk category B

How supplied

Available by prescription only
Capsules (delayed-release): 15 mg, 30 mg

Indications and dosages

Short-term treatment of active duodenal ulcer
Adults: 15 mg P.O. daily before meals for 4 weeks.
Short-term treatment of erosive esophagitis
Adults: 30 mg P.O. daily before meals for up to 8 weeks. If healing doesn't occur, an additional 8 weeks of therapy may be needed.
Long-term treatment of pathologic hypersecretory conditions, including Zollinger-Ellison syndrome
Adults: Initially, 60 mg P.O. once daily. Increase dosage, p.r.n. Administer daily doses exceeding 120 mg in divided doses.
Maintenance of healed duodenal ulcer
Adults: 15 mg P.O. once daily.
Short-term treatment of gastric ulcer
Adults: 30 mg P.O. daily for up to 8 weeks.
Short-term treatment of symptomatic gastroesophageal reflux disease (GERD)
Adults: 15 mg P.O. daily for up to 8 weeks.
Helicobacter pylori ***eradication to reduce risk of duodenal ulcer recurrence***
Adults: In patients receiving dual therapy, 30 mg P.O. lansoprazole with 1 g P.O. amoxicillin, each given q 8 hours for 14 days. In patients receiving triple therapy, 30 mg P.O. lansopra-

zole with 1 g P.O. amoxicillin and 500 mg P.O. clarithromycin, all given q 12 hours for 10 to 14 days.

Pharmacodynamics

Antiulcer action: Lansoprazole inhibits activity of the acid (proton) pump and binds to hydrogen-potassium ATPase, located at the secretory surface of the gastric parietal cells, to block the formation of gastric acid.

Pharmacokinetics

Absorption: Rapidly absorbed with absolute bioavailability of more than 80%.
Distribution: 97% bound to plasma proteins.
Metabolism: Extensively metabolized in the liver.
Excretion: About two-thirds of dose is excreted in feces; one-third in urine.

Route	Onset	Peak	Duration
P.O.	Unknown	1¾ hr	Unknown

Contraindications and precautions

Contraindicated in patients with hypersensitivity to drug.

Interactions

Drug-drug. *Ampicillin esters, iron salts, ketoconazole:* Lansoprazole may interfere with the absorption of. these drugs. Monitor patient closely.
Sucralfate: Delays lansoprazole absorption. Give lansoprazole at least 30 minutes before sucralfate.
Theophylline: May cause mild increase in theophylline excretion. Use together cautiously. Dosage adjustment of theophylline may be necessary.
Drug-herb. *Male fern*: Inactivated in alkaline stomach environment. These shouldn't be given together.

Effects on diagnostic tests

None reported.

Adverse reactions

CNS: asthenia, headache, agitation, amnesia, anxiety, apathy, confusion, depression, dizziness or syncope, hallucinations, hemiplegia, aggravated hostility, malaise, nervousness, paresthesia, thinking abnormality.
CV: chest pain, edema, angina, *CVA,* hypertension or hypotension, *MI, shock,* palpitations, vasodilation, ***cardiospasm.***
EENT: amblyopia, deafness, eye pain, visual field deficits, otitis media, taste perversion, tinnitus.
GI: *diarrhea, nausea, abdominal pain,* halitosis, melena, anorexia, cholelithiasis, constipation, dry mouth, thirst, dyspepsia, dysphagia, eructation, esophageal stenosis, esophageal ulcer, esophagitis, fecal discoloration, flatulence, gastric nodules, fundic gland polyps, gastroenteritis, GI hemorrhage, hematemesis, increased appetite, increased salivation, rectal hemorrhage, stomatitis, tenesmus, ulcerative colitis.
GU: hematuria, impotence, kidney calculus, albuminuria, abnormal menses, gynecomastia, candidiasis, decreased libido, breast tenderness or breast enlargement.
Hematologic: anemia, hemolysis.
Hepatic: abnormal liver function tests.
Metabolic: diabetes mellitus, goiter, hyperglycemia, hypoglycemia, gout, weight gain or loss.
Musculoskeletal: arthritis, arthralgia, musculoskeletal pain, myalgia.
Respiratory: asthma, bronchitis, increased cough, dyspnea, epistaxis, hemoptysis, hiccups, pneumonia, upper respiratory tract inflammation.
Skin: acne, alopecia, pruritus, rash, urticaria.
Other: fever, flulike syndrome, infection.

Overdose and treatment

No adverse effects have been reported with drug overdose. Drug isn't removed from the circulation by hemodialysis. If required, treatment should be supportive.

Clinical considerations

- Dosage adjustment isn't necessary in the elderly or in patients with renal insufficiency; however, it may be required for patients with severe liver disease.
- Drug shouldn't be used as maintenance therapy for patients with duodenal ulcer disease or erosive esophagitis.
- Contents of capsule can be mixed with 40 ml of apple juice in a syringe and administered within 3 to 5 minutes via an nasogastric tube. Flush with additional apple juice to administer entire dose and maintain patency of the tube.

Therapeutic monitoring

Monitor liver function studies in long-term therapy.

Special populations

Breast-feeding patients. Because it isn't known if lansoprazole is excreted in breast milk, a decision to discontinue breast-feeding or using drug should be made.
Pediatric patients. Safety and efficacy in children haven't been established.
Geriatric patients. Although initial dosing regimen need not be altered for geriatric patients, subsequent doses over 30 mg/day shouldn't be administered unless additional gastric acid suppression is necessary.

Patient counseling

- Instruct patient to take drug before meals.
- Caution patient not to open, chew, or crush capsules; capsules should be swallowed whole.

latanoprost

Xalatan

Pharmacologic classification: prostaglandin analogue
Therapeutic classification: antiglaucoma; ocular antihypertensive
Pregnancy risk category C

How supplied

Available by prescription only
Ophthalmic solution: 0.005%

Indications and dosages

Increased intraocular pressure (IOP) in patients with ocular hypertension or open-angle glaucoma who are intolerant of other IOP-lowering medications or insufficiently responsive to another IOP-lowering medication
Adults: Instill 1 drop in the conjunctival sac of the affected eyes once daily in the evening.

Pharmacodynamics

Antiglaucoma and ocular antihypertensive actions: Exact mechanism of action unknown. Drug may lower IOP by increasing the outflow of aqueous humor.

Pharmacokinetics

Absorption: Absorbed through the cornea.
Distribution: Distribution volume is about 0.16 L/kg. The acid of latanoprost could be measured in aqueous humor during first 4 hours and in plasma only during first hour after local administration.
Metabolism: Hydrolyzed by esterases in the cornea to the biologically active acid. The active acid of drug reaching the systemic circulation is primarily metabolized by the liver.
Excretion: Metabolites are mainly eliminated in urine.

Route	Onset	Peak	Duration
Ophthalmic	2-4 hr	8-12 hr	Unknown

Contraindications and precautions

Contraindicated in patients with hypersensitivity to drug, benzalkonium chloride, or other ingredients in the product.

Use cautiously when administering to patients with impaired renal or hepatic function. Use with caution in patients with active ocular inflammation (iritis, uveitis), patients at risk for macular edema, aphakic patients, and pseudophakic patients.

Interactions

Drug-drug. *Thimerosal:* Precipitation occurs when eyedrops containing thimerosal are mixed with latanoprost. If such drugs are used together, administer them at least 5 minutes apart.
Topical beta-adrenergic blocking agents (betaxolol, carteolol, levobunolol, metipranolol, timolol), topical dipivefrin, topical epinephrine, an oral carbonic anhydrase inhibitor (acetazolamide), or a topical carbonic anhydrase inhibitor (dorzolamide): IOP-lowering effects of theses drugs may be additive. This may be a therapeutic advantage, but if using other topical drugs, separate administration times by 5 minutes.

Effects on diagnostic tests

None reported.

Adverse reactions

CV: chest pain; angina pectoris.
EENT: *blurred vision; burning; stinging;* itching; conjunctival hyperemia; foreign body sensation; increased pigmentation of iris; punctate epithelial keratopathy; dry eye; excessive tearing; photophobia; conjunctivitis; diplopia; eye pain or discharge; retinal artery embolus (rare); retinal detachment (rare); vitreous hemorrhage from diabetic retinopathy (rare); lid crusting, edema, erythema, discomfort, or pain; herpes simplex keratitis.
Musculoskeletal: muscle, joint, or back pain.
Respiratory: upper respiratory tract infection, asthma.
Skin: rash; allergic skin reaction.
Other: cold, flu.

Overdose and treatment

Apart from ocular irritation and conjunctival or episcleral hyperemia, ocular effects of latanoprost at high doses aren't known. Treatment should be symptomatic if overdose occurs.

Clinical considerations

- Latanoprost may gradually change eye color, increasing the amount of brown pigment in the iris. The change in iris color occurs slowly and may not be noticeable for several months to years. The increased pigmentation may be permanent.
- Protect drug from light; refrigerate unopened bottle.

Therapeutic monitoring

Monitor IOP-lowering effects of drug.

Special populations

Breast-feeding patients. It isn't known if drug is excreted in breast milk. Exercise caution when administering drug to breast-feeding women.
Pediatric patients. Safety and efficacy in children haven't been established.

Patient counseling

- Tell patient receiving treatment in only one eye about the potential for increased brown

pigmentation in the treated eye as well as heterochromia between the eyes.
- Teach patient to instill drops. Advise him to wash hands before and after instilling solution, and warn him not to touch dropper or tip to eye or surrounding tissue.
- Advise patient to apply light finger pressure on lacrimal sac for 1 minute after instillation to minimize systemic absorption of drug.
- Instruct patient to report ocular reactions, especially conjunctivitis and lid reactions.
- Tell patient using contact lenses to remove them before administration of the solution and not to reinsert the contact lenses for 15 minutes after administration.
- Advise patient that if more than one topical ophthalmic drug is being used, to administer the drugs at least 5 minutes apart.
- Stress importance of compliance with recommended therapy.

leflunomide

Arava

Pharmacologic classification: pyrimidine synthesis inhibitor
Therapeutic classification: antirheumatic agent
Pregnancy risk category X

How supplied

Available by prescription only
Tablets: 10 mg, 20 mg, 100 mg

Indications and dosages

To reduce signs and symptoms of active rheumatoid arthritis and to retard structural damage as evidenced by erosions and joint space narrowing seen on X-ray
Adults: 100 mg P.O. q 24 hours for 3 days, followed by 20 mg (maximum daily dose) P.O. q 24 hours. Dose may be decreased to 10 mg daily if higher dose isn't well tolerated.

Pharmacodynamics

Immunomodulatory action: Drug inhibits dihydroorotate dehydrogenase, an enzyme involved in de novo pyrimidine synthesis, and has antiproliferative activity and anti-inflammatory effects.

Pharmacokinetics

Absorption: Bioavailability is 80%. Without loading dose, peak plasma levels are reached in about 2 months.
Distribution: Extensively bound to plasma proteins (over 99%).
Metabolism: Metabolized to an active metabolite (M1), responsible for most of its activity.
Excretion: Leflunomide is eliminated by renal and direct biliary excretion. About 43% is excreted in the urine and 48% in the feces. Half-life of the active metabolite is about 2 weeks.

Route	Onset	Peak	Duration
P.O.	Unknown	6-12 hr	Unknown

Contraindications and precautions

Contraindicated in patients with known hypersensitivity to drug or its components and in women who are or may become pregnant or who are breast-feeding. Drug isn't recommended for patients with hepatic insufficiency, hepatitis B or C, severe immunodeficiency, bone marrow dysplasia, or severe uncontrolled infections. Drug isn't recommended for use by men attempting to father a child.

Vaccination with live vaccines isn't recommended. Consider the long half-life of drug when contemplating administration of a live vaccine after stopping drug treatment.

Be aware that the risk of malignancy, particularly lymphoproliferative disorders, increases with use of some immunosuppressants, including leflunomide. Use cautiously in patients with renal insufficiency.

Interactions

Drug-drug. *Activated charcoal and cholestyramine:* Decreased plasma levels of leflunomide. They are sometimes used for this effect in treating overdose.
Methotrexate and other hepatotoxic drugs: Increased risk of hepatotoxicity. Monitor liver enzymes as appropriate.
Rifampin: Increased level of active leflunomide metabolite. Use together cautiously.

Effects on diagnostic tests

None reported.

Adverse reactions

CNS: asthenia, dizziness, headache, paresthesia, malaise, migraine, sleep disorder, vertigo, neuritis, anxiety, depression, insomnia, neuralgia.
CV: angina pectoris, *hypertension*, chest pain, palpitation, tachycardia, vasculitis, vasodilation, varicose vein, peripheral edema.
EENT: pharyngitis, rhinitis, sinusitis, epistaxis, mouth ulcer, oral candidiasis, enlarged salivary glands, stomatitis, tooth disorder, dry mouth, blurred vision, cataract, conjunctivitis, eye disorder, gingivitis, taste perversion.
GI: anorexia, *diarrhea,* dyspepsia, gastroenteritis, nausea, abdominal pain, vomiting, cholelithiasis, colitis, constipation, esophagitis, flatulence, gastritis, melena.
GU: urinary tract infection, albuminuria, cystitis, dysuria, hematuria, menstrual disorder, pelvic pain, vaginal candidiasis, prostate disorder, urinary frequency.
Hematologic: anemia, ecchymosis, hyperlipidemia.
Hepatic: elevated liver enzymes.

Metabolic: increased CK, diabetes mellitus, hyperglycemia, hyperthyroidism, hypokalemia, weight loss.
Musculoskeletal: arthrosis, back pain, bursitis, muscle cramps, myalgia, bone necrosis, bone pain, arthralgia, leg cramps, joint disorder, neck pain, synovitis, tendon rupture, tenosynovitis.
Respiratory: bronchitis, increased cough, pneumonia, *respiratory infection*, asthma, dyspnea, lung disorder.
Skin: *alopecia*, eczema, pruritus, *rash*, dry skin, acne, contact dermatitis, fungal dermatitis, hair discoloration, hematoma, herpes simplex, herpes zoster, nail disorder, skin nodule, subcutaneous nodule, maculopapular rash, skin disorder, skin discoloration, skin ulcer, increased sweating.
Other: ***allergic reaction***, fever, flu syndrome, injury or accident, pain, abscess, cyst, hernia.

Overdose and treatment
No overdose has been reported in humans. If overdose occurs, activated charcoal (50 g every 6 hours for 24 hours) reduces plasma levels. Cholestyramine may also be administered as 8 g P.O. three times daily for 11 days.

Clinical considerations
- Leflunomide can cause fetal harm when administered to pregnant women; it's recommended that women planning to become pregnant discontinue leflunomide therapy and consult their doctor.
- Men planning to father a child should discontinue drug therapy and follow recommended leflunomide removal protocol (cholestyramine 8 g, P.O. t.i.d. for 11 days).
- Aspirin, other NSAIDs, and low-dose corticosteroids may be continued during treatment; however, combined use of drug with antimalarials, intramuscular or oral gold, penicillamine, azathioprine, or methotrexate hasn't been adequately studied.

Therapeutic monitoring
Monitor liver enzymes (ALT and AST) before starting therapy and monthly thereafter until stable. Frequency can then be decreased based on clinical situation.

Special populations
Breast-feeding patients. Drug shouldn't be used by breast-feeding women.
Pediatric patients. Safety in children and adolescents hasn't been established. Not recommended for children under age 18.
Geriatric patients. No significant differences noted compared with younger population.

Patient counseling
- Explain the need and frequency of required blood tests and monitoring.
- Instruct patient to use birth control during course of treatment and until it has been determined that drug is no longer active.
- Warn female patient to immediately notify doctor if signs or symptoms of pregnancy occur (such as late menses or breast tenderness).

letrozole
Femara

Pharmacologic classification: aromatase inhibitor
Therapeutic classification: hormone
Pregnancy risk category D

How supplied
Available by prescription only
Tablets: 2.5 mg

Indications and dosages
Metastatic breast cancer in postmenopausal women with disease progression following antiestrogen therapy
Adults and elderly: 2.5 mg P.O. as a single daily dose, without regard to meals.

Pharmacodynamics
Hormone action: Inhibits conversion of androgens to estrogens by competitive inhibition of the aromatase enzyme system. Decreased estrogens are likely to lead to decreased tumor mass or delayed progression of tumor growth in some women.

Pharmacokinetics
Absorption: Rapidly and completely absorbed. Food doesn't affect bioavailability. Steady-state plasma levels are reached in 2 to 6 weeks after daily dosing.
Distribution: Large volume of distribution (1.9 L/kg). It's weakly protein-bound.
Metabolism: Slowly metabolized to an inactive form. In human liver microsomes, letrozole strongly inhibits cytochrome P-450 isozyme 2A6 and moderately inhibits isozyme 2C19.
Excretion: The inactive glucuronide metabolite is eliminated in the urine.

Route	Onset	Peak	Duration
P.O.	Unknown	2 days	Unknown

Contraindications and precautions
Contraindicated in patients with known hypersensitivity to drug or its components. Avoid use in pregnant patients because drug may cause fetal harm.

Use cautiously in patients with severe liver impairment.

Interactions
None reported.

Effects on diagnostic tests
None reported.

Adverse reactions
CNS: headache, somnolence, dizziness, fatigue, asthenia.
CV: edema, hypertension, ***thromboembolism,*** chest pain.
GI: *nausea,* vomiting, constipation, diarrhea, abdominal pain, anorexia, dyspepsia.
Hematologic: hypercholesterolemia.
Metabolic: weight gain.
Musculoskeletal: *bone pain, extremities, and back pain,* arthralgias.
Respiratory: dyspnea, coughing.
Skin: hot flashes, rash, pruritus.
Other: viral infections.

Overdose and treatment
There have been no reports of overdose during clinical trials with letrozole. If overdose occurs, consider inducing emesis if patient is alert; provide supportive care and monitor vital signs frequently.

Clinical considerations
- No dosage adjustment is needed in patients with mild to moderate liver dysfunction or in renally impaired patients with creatinine clearance of 10 ml/minute or more.
- Patients treated with letrozole don't need glucocorticoid or mineralocorticoid replacement therapy. Letrozole significantly lowers serum estrone, estradiol, and estrone sulfate, but hasn't been shown to significantly affect adrenal corticosteroid synthesis, aldosterone synthesis, or synthesis of thyroid hormones.

Therapeutic monitoring
Monitor for decreased tumor progression.

Special populations
Breast-feeding patients. It's unknown if letrozole is excreted in breast milk. Use caution when administering letrozole to breast-feeding women.

Patient counseling
- Instruct patient to take drug exactly as prescribed.
- Tell patient that drug can be taken with or without food.
- Advise patient that drug treatment is chronic, and stress importance of follow-up appointments.
- Tell patient to inform doctor if pregnancy is suspected or is being planned.

leucovorin calcium (citrovorum factor or folinic acid)
Wellcovorin

Pharmacologic classification: formyl derivative (active reduced form of folic acid)
Therapeutic classification: vitamin, antidote
Pregnancy risk category C

How supplied
Available by prescription only
Tablets: 5 mg, 10 mg, 15 mg, 25 mg
Injection: 1-ml ampule (3 mg/ml with 0.9% benzyl alcohol, 5 mg/ml with methyl and propyl parabens); 50-mg, 100-mg, and 350-mg vials for reconstitution (contain no preservatives)

Indications and dosages
Overdose of folic acid antagonist
Adults and children: I.M., or I.V. dose equivalent to weight of antagonist given as soon as possible after the overdose.
Leucovorin rescue after large methotrexate dose in treatment of cancer
Adults and children: Administer 24 hours after last dose of methotrexate according to protocol. Initially, 10 mg/m² I.M. or I.V.; then give 10 mg/m² orally q 6 hours until serum methotrexate level is less than 5×10^{-8} M (0.05 micromolar). Adjust subsequent doses based upon serum creatinine and methotrexate levels.
Toxic effects of methotrexate used to treat severe psoriasis
Adults and children: 4 to 8 mg I.M. 2 hours after methotrexate dose.
Hematologic toxicity from pyrimethamine therapy
Adults and children: Dosage highly individualized depending on dosage of folic acid antagonist and patient's clinical status.
Prevention of toxicities in* Pneumocystis carinii *patients receiving trimetrexate glucuronate
Adults: 20 mg/m² P.O. or I.V. over 5 to 10 minutes q 6 hours (total daily dose of 80 mg/m²). If administered orally, round up to the next 25-mg dose. Leucovorin should be continued at least 72 hours after last trimetrexate dose. Adjust doses of both drugs based on hematologic response of the patient.
Advanced colorectal cancer
Adults: 200 mg /m² by slow I.V. injection over 3 minutes followed by 5-fluorouracil (5-FU) or 20 mg/m² by slow I.V. injection over 3 minutes followed by 5-FU. Repeat treatment for 5 days. May repeat course at 4-week intervals for two courses and then at 4- to 5-week intervals as long as the patient has recovered from

toxic effects of previous treatment. Dosage of 5-FU should be individualized.

Megaloblastic anemia from congenital enzyme deficiency

Adults and children: 3 to 6 mg I.M. daily.

Folate-deficient megaloblastic anemias

Adults and children: Up to 1 mg of leucovorin I.M. daily. Duration of treatment depends on hematologic response.

Pharmacodynamics

Reversal of folic acid antagonism: Leucovorin is a derivative of tetrahydrofolic acid, the reduced form of folic acid. Leucovorin performs as a cofactor in 1-carbon transfer reactions in the biosynthesis of purines and pyrimidines of nucleic acids. Impairment of thymidylate synthesis in patients with folic acid deficiency may account for defective DNA synthesis, megaloblast formation, and megaloblastic and macrocytic anemias. Leucovorin is a potent antidote for the hematopoietic and reticuloendothelial toxic effects of folic acid antagonists (trimethoprim, pyrimethamine, and methotrexate). "Leucovorin rescue" is used to prevent or decrease toxicity of massive methotrexate doses. Folinic acid rescues normal cells without reversing the oncolytic effect of methotrexate.

Pharmacokinetics

Absorption: After oral administration, leucovorin is absorbed rapidly. The increase in plasma and serum folate activity after oral administration is mainly from 5-methyltetrahydrofolate (the major transport and storage form of folate in the body).

Distribution: Tetrahydrofolic acid and its derivatives are distributed throughout the body; the liver contains about half of the total body folate stores.

Metabolism: Metabolized in the liver.

Excretion: Excreted by the kidneys as 10-formyl tetrahydrofolate and 5,10-methenyl tetrahydrofolate.

Route	Onset	Peak	Duration
P.O.	20-30 min	2-3 hr	3-6 hr
I.V.	5 min	10 min	3-6 hr
I.M.	10-20 min	< 1 hr	3-6 hr

Contraindications and precautions

Contraindicated in patients with pernicious anemia and other megaloblastic anemias that result from the lack of vitamin B_{12}.

Interactions

Drug-drug. *Fluorouracil:* When given together, leucovorin increases toxicity of fluorouracil. Use lower doses of fluorouracil.

Phenytoin: Decreased serum phenytoin levels and increased frequency of seizures. Although this interaction has occurred solely in patients receiving folic acid, it should be considered when leucovorin is administered. Adjust phenytoin dose.

Phenytoin, primidone: May decrease serum folate levels, producing symptoms of folate deficiency. Patient requires careful monitoring.

Effects on diagnostic tests

None reported.

Adverse reactions

Skin: hypersensitivity reactions (urticaria, ***anaphylactoid reactions***).

Overdose and treatment

Leucovorin is relatively nontoxic; no specific recommendations for overdose are reported. However, an excessive amount of leucovorin may nullify the chemotherapeutic effect of folic acid antagonists such as methotrexate.

Clinical considerations

- Drug administration continues until plasma methotrexate levels are less than 5×10^{-8} M.
- Don't use as sole treatment of pernicious anemia or vitamin B_{12} deficiency.
- To treat overdose of folic acid antagonists, use the drug within 1 hour; it isn't effective after a 4-hour delay.
- When giving more than 25 mg, administer drug parenterally.
- Reconstitute drug by adding 5 to 10 ml of sterile water for injection or bacteriostatic water for injection (which contains benzyl alcohol) to vial containing 50 or 100 mg of leucovorin, respectively. Solution will contain 10 mg/ml. Add 17 ml of sterile water for injection or bacteriostatic water for injection to vial containing 350 mg of leucovorin for a resulting concentration of 20 mg/ml. When parenteral doses greater than 10 mg/m^2 are necessary, only reconstitute with sterile water for injection. If reconstituted with sterile water for injection, use immediately. If reconstituted with bacteriostatic water for injection, use within 7 days.
- Leucovorin admixed with 10% dextrose injection, 0.9% sodium chloride injection, Ringer's or lactated Ringer's injection is stable for 24 hours when stored at room temperature and protected from light.
- Maximum rate of leucovorin infusion shouldn't exceed 160 mg/minute because of calcium concentration of solution.
- Store at room temperature in a light-resistant container, not in high-moisture areas.

Therapeutic monitoring

- Recommend monitoring patient for signs of drug allergy, such as rash, wheezing, pruritus, and urticaria.
- Monitor serum creatinine levels daily to detect possible renal function impairment.
- When used in combination with fluorouracil, monitor CBC and platelet count before each course of therapy and repeat weekly during

first two courses of therapy. Also, monitor serum electrolytes and liver function tests before each course of therapy for three courses and then before every other course.

Special populations
Breast-feeding patients. It's unknown if leucovorin is distributed into breast milk; use with caution in breast-feeding women.
Pediatric patients. Drug may increase frequency of seizures in susceptible children. Don't use diluents containing benzyl alcohol when reconstituting drug for neonates.

Patient counseling
Emphasize importance of taking leucovorin only under medical supervision.

leuprolide acetate
Lupron, Lupron Depot, Lupron Depot-Ped, Lupron Depot-3 Month, Lupron Depot-4 month

Pharmacologic classification: gonadotropin-releasing hormone
Therapeutic classification: antineoplastic; luteinizing hormone-releasing hormone (LHRH) analogue
Pregnancy risk category X

How supplied
Available by prescription only
Injection: 5 mg/ml in 2.8-ml multiple-dose vials
Suspension for depot injection: 3.75 mg, 7.5 mg, 11.25 mg, 15 mg, 22.5 mg, 30 mg

Indications and dosages
Dosage and indications may vary. Check current literature for recommended protocol. The four different depot preparations aren't interchangeable.
Management of advanced prostate cancer
Adults: 7.5 mg I.M. (depot injection) once monthly or 1 mg S.C. daily; or 22.5 mg I.M. (depot injection) q 3 months or 30 mg I.M. q 4 months (depot injection).
Treatment of endometriosis
Adults: 3.75 mg I.M. (depot injection) once monthly for a maximum of 6 months.
Correction of anemia associated with uterine fibroids before surgery
Adults: 3.75 mg I.M. q 1 month for up to 3 consecutive months in combination with iron therapy
◇ ***Central precocious puberty (CPP)***
Children (girls under age 8 and boys under age 9): Starting dose 0.3 mg/kg (minimum 7.5 mg), given as a single I.M. or S.C. dose (depot injection) q 4 weeks. An initial dose of 7.5 mg if weight is 55 lb (25 kg) or less; 11.25 mg if weight is 55 to 82½ lb (25 to 37.5 kg); and 15 mg if weight is more than 82½ lb (37.5 kg). Titrate upward in increments of 3.75 mg q 4 weeks until clinical or laboratory tests indicate no progression of the disease. If leuprolide acetate injection is used, initial dose is 50 mcg/kg S.C. daily. Titrate upward by 10 mcg/kg daily.

Pharmacodynamics
Antineoplastic action: Leuprolide is a synthetic analogue of LHRH. It inhibits gonadotropin secretion and androgen or estrogen synthesis. Because of this effect, leuprolide may inhibit the growth of hormone-dependent tumors.
Hormonal action: Because leuprolide lowers levels of sex hormones, it reduces the size of endometrial implants, resulting in decreased dysmenorrhea and pelvic pain in women with endometriosis.

Pharmacokinetics
Absorption: Leuprolide is a polypeptide molecule that's destroyed in the GI tract. After S.C. administration, drug is rapidly and essentially completely absorbed.
Distribution: Distribution in humans hasn't been determined, but high levels may distribute into kidney, liver, pineal, and pituitary tissue. About 7% to 15% of a dose is bound to plasma proteins.
Metabolism: Metabolism is unclear, but drug may be metabolized in the anterior pituitary and hypothalamus, similar to endogenous gonadotropin-releasing hormone.
Excretion: Plasma elimination half-life is 3 hours.

Route	Onset	Peak	Duration
I.M., S.C.	< 2-4 wk	1-2 mo	60-90 days

Contraindications and precautions
Contraindicated in patients hypersensitive to drug or other gonadotropin-releasing hormone analogues, during pregnancy or lactation, and in women with undiagnosed vaginal bleeding.

Use cautiously in patients with hypersensitivity to benzyl alcohol.

Interactions
None reported.

Effects on diagnostic tests
None reported.

Adverse reactions
CNS: *dizziness, depression, headache, pain,* insomnia, *asthenia..*
CV: ***arrhythmias,*** angina, ***MI,*** *peripheral edema, ECG changes,* hypertension, murmur.
GI: *nausea, vomiting,* anorexia, constipation.
GU: *impotence, vaginitis,* urinary frequency, hematuria, urinary tract infection, gynecomastia.
Hematologic: anemia.
Hepatic: elevated liver enzyme levels.

Metabolic: *weight gain or loss,* initially increased then decreased with continued therapy serum acid phosphatase and testosterone levels.
Musculoskeletal: transient bone pain during first week of treatment, joint disorder, myalgia, neuromuscular disorder.
Respiratory: dyspnea, sinus congestion, pulmonary fibrosis.
Skin: skin reactions at injection site, dermatitis.
Other: *hot flashes, androgen-like effects.*

Overdose and treatment
No information available.

Clinical considerations
- Experimental uses include male contraception, treatment of endocrine disorders, hypogonadism, delayed puberty, oligospermia, anovulation, and amenorrhea.
- When treating endometriosis, administer for a maximum of 6 months. Safety and efficacy of re-treatment are unknown.
- To reconstitute suspension containing 3.75, 7.5, 11.25, or 15 mg of drug/dose, add 1 ml of provided diluent to leuprolide acetate powder for injection using a 22G needle; 1.5 ml of provided diluent is added to the 22.5 or 30 mg drug/dose vial using a 23G needle. Shake well. Resulting suspension is milky. Use 22.5 and 30 mg concentration immediately.
- Use a 22G needle for monthly injection and a 23G needle for 3-month injection.
- A 0.5 ml low dose, U-100 insulin syringe may be used if necessary to replace manufacturer-provided syringes to inject leuprolide acetate injection; fill syringe to the 20-unit mark.
- Discard solution if particulate matter is visible or if the solution is discolored.
- Erythema or induration may develop at injection site.
- When treating prostate cancer, leuprolide may aggravate signs and symptoms of disease during first 1 to 2 weeks of therapy. Temporary paresthesia and weakness may occur during first week of therapy.
- No unusual adverse effects were observed in patients who had received 20 mg daily for 2 years.
- Refrigerate leuprolide vials for injection until used. Don't freeze. Vial in use may be stored at room temperature. Leuprolide powder for injection suspension may be stored at room temperature. Reconstituted suspension is stable for 24 hours.

Therapeutic monitoring
- Measure serum testosterone and acid phosphatase levels before and during therapy.
- Measure serum testosterone, prostate specific antigen, and prostatic acid phosphatase levels before and during therapy in patients with prostate cancer.
- Monitor liver function tests.

Special populations
Pregnant patients. Reversible suppression of fertility in males and females has occurred.

Patient counseling
- Reassure patient that bone pain is transient and will disappear after about 1 week.
- Inform patient that a temporary reaction of burning, itching, and swelling at injection site may occur. Tell him to report persistent reactions.
- Advise patient to continue taking drug even if he experiences a sense of well-being.
- Instruct women of childbearing age to use an effective nonhormonal method of contraception during therapy, and to discontinue drug and notify doctor if pregnancy occurs.

levalbuterol hydrochloride
Xopenex

Pharmacologic classification: beta$_2$ agonist
Therapeutic classification: bronchodilator
Pregnancy risk category C

How supplied
Available by prescription only
Solution for inhalation: 0.63 mg or 1.25 mg in 3-ml vials

Indications and dosages
To prevent or treat bronchospasm in patients with reversible obstructive airway disease
Adults and adolescents age 12 and older: 0.63 mg administered t.i.d. every 6 to 8 hours, by oral inhalation via a nebulizer. Patients with more severe asthma who don't respond adequately to a dose of 0.63 mg may benefit from a dosage of 1.25 mg t.i.d.

Pharmacodynamics
Bronchodilator action: Levalbuterol activates beta$_2$ receptors on airway smooth muscle, which leads the smooth muscle in all airways—from the trachea to the terminal bronchioles—to relax, thereby relieving bronchospasm and reducing airway resistance. Drug also inhibits the release of mediators from mast cells in the airway.

Pharmacokinetics
No information available.

Route	Onset	Peak	Duration
Inhalation	Unknown	Unknown	Unknown

Contraindications and precautions
Contraindicated in patients with a history of hypersensitivity to levalbuterol or racemic albuterol.

Use cautiously in patients with cardiovascular disorders, especially coronary insufficiency, hypertension, and arrhythmias. Also use cautiously in patients with seizure disorders, hyperthyroidism, or diabetes mellitus and in patients who are unusually responsive to sympathomimetic amines.

Interactions

Drug-drug. *Beta blockers:* May cause reduced pulmonary effect of the drug and, possibly, severe bronchospasm. Don't use together, if possible. If use together is necessary, consider a cardioselective beta blocker, but administer with caution.
Digoxin: Decreased digoxin levels (up to 22%). Monitor serum digoxin levels.
Loop or thiazide diuretics: May cause ECG changes and hypokalemia from concurrent administration of these non-potassium-sparing diuretics. Use together cautiously.
MAO inhibitors or tricyclic antidepressants: Potentiate the action of levalbuterol on the vascular system. Administer with extreme caution in patients being given MAO inhibitors or tricyclic antidepressants, or within 2 weeks of discontinuation of these drugs.
Other short-acting sympathomimetic aerosol bronchodilators or epinephrine: May cause increased adrenergic adverse effects. To avoid serious CV effects, use additional adrenergics with caution.

Effects on diagnostic tests

None reported.

Adverse reactions

CNS: dizziness, migraine, nervousness, tremor, anxiety, pain.
CV: tachycardia.
EENT: *rhinitis*, sinusitis, turbinate edema.
GI: dyspepsia.
Musculoskeletal: leg cramps.
Respiratory: increased cough, *viral infection.*
Other: flu syndrome, accidental injury.

Overdose and treatment

Signs and symptoms of overdose are those of excessive beta-receptor stimulation, including seizures, angina, hypertension or hypotension, tachycardia with rates up to 200 beats/minute, arrhythmias, nervousness, headache, tremor, dry mouth, palpitation, nausea, dizziness, fatigue, malaise, and sleeplessness. Hypokalemia may also occur. As with other sympathomimetics, abuse of levalbuterol may result in cardiac arrest and death.

Treatment consists of stopping the drug and giving symptomatic therapy. A cardioselective beta-receptor blocker may be used, but keep in mind that beta-receptor blockers can cause bronchospasm. It's unknown if dialysis is beneficial in managing levalbuterol overdose.

Clinical considerations

- Like other inhaled beta agonists, levalbuterol can produce paradoxical bronchospasm, which may be life-threatening. If this occurs, stop drug immediately and institute alternative therapy.
- Small, transient increases in blood glucose levels may occur after oral inhalation.
- Serum potassium levels may decrease slightly, but potassium supplementation is usually unnecessary.
- Keep unopened vials in foil pouch. Once the foil pouch is opened, use the vials within 2 weeks. If vials are removed from pouch but not used immediately, protect from light and excessive heat and use within 1 week.

Therapeutic monitoring

Recommend monitoring patient for clinical effect of drug and for worsening of symptoms.

Special populations

Pregnant patients. Use drug only if benefits outweigh risk to the fetus.
Breast-feeding patients. Plasma levels of levalbuterol are very low following inhalation of therapeutic dosages. It's unknown if drug is excreted in breast milk. Administer cautiously to breast-feeding women.
Pediatric patients. Safety and efficacy of levalbuterol in children under age 12 are unknown.
Geriatric patients. Safety and efficacy of levalbuterol are unknown in patients age 65 and older. In general, patients in this age group should be started at a dose of 0.63 mg.

Patient counseling

- Warn patient that he may experience paradoxical bronchospasm (difficulty breathing). Tell him to discontinue drug and contact his doctor immediately if this occurs.
- Inform patient that common adverse effects include palpitations, rapid heart rate, headache, dizziness, tremor, and nervousness.
- Inform patient that the effects of levalbuterol may last up to 8 hours.
- Warn patient not to increase dose or frequency without consulting his doctor.
- Advise patient to seek medical attention immediately if levalbuterol becomes less effective for treating signs and symptoms, signs and symptoms become worse, or he's using levalbuterol more frequently than usual.
- Caution patient to use other inhalants and antiasthma drugs only as directed while taking levalbuterol.
- Advise female patient to inform doctor about the use of levalbuterol if she becomes pregnant or is breast-feeding.
- Instruct patient not to use levalbuterol after the expiration date stamped on the container.
- Inform patient that once the foil pouch is opened, the vials should be used within 2 weeks. If opened pouch isn't used immediately, vials

should be protected from light and excessive heat, and used within 1 week.
- Tell patient to discard any vials containing discolored solution.

levobunolol hydrochloride

AKBeta, Betagan

Pharmacologic classification: beta blocker
Therapeutic classification: antiglaucoma
Pregnancy risk category C

How supplied

Available by prescription only
Ophthalmic solution: 0.25%, 0.5%

Indications and dosages

Chronic open-angle glaucoma and ocular hypertension
Adults: Instill 1 to 2 drops (0.5% solution) daily or 1 to 2 drops (0.25% solution) b.i.d. in eye.

Pharmacodynamics

Antiglaucoma action: Levobunolol is a nonselective beta-blocking agent that reduces intraocular pressure. Exact mechanisms are unknown, but the drug appears to reduce formation of aqueous humor.

Pharmacokinetics

Absorption: Systemic absorption is undetermined, but may occur.
Distribution: Unknown.
Metabolism: Unknown.
Excretion: Unknown.

Route	Onset	Peak	Duration
Ophthalmic	1 hr	2-6 hr	24 hr

Contraindications and precautions

Contraindicated in patients with hypersensitivity to drug, bronchial asthma, history of bronchial asthma or severe COPD, sinus bradycardia, second- or third-degree AV block, cardiac failure, and cardiogenic shock. Use cautiously in patients with chronic bronchitis, emphysema, diabetes mellitus, hyperthyroidism, and myasthenia gravis.

Interactions

Drug-drug. *Oral beta blockers:* Increased systemic effects. Monitor patient carefully.
Epinephrine, pilocarpine, or carbonic anhydrase inhibitors: Increased reductions in intraocular pressure. Use together cautiously.
Reserpine and catecholamine-depleting agents: Enhance the hypotensive and bradycardiac effects of these drugs. Monitor carefully.

Effects on diagnostic tests

None reported.

Adverse reactions

CNS: headache, depression, insomnia.
CV: slight reduction in resting heart rate.
EENT: *transient eye stinging and burning,* tearing, erythema, itching, keratitis, corneal punctate staining, photophobia; decreased corneal sensitivity (with long-term use).
GI: nausea.
Skin: urticaria.
Other: evidence of beta blockade and systemic absorption (*hypotension,* ***bradycardia,*** *syncope,* ***asthmatic attacks in patients with history of asthma, heart failure***).

Overdose and treatment

Overdose is extremely rare with ophthalmic use. However, usual symptoms include bradycardia, hypotension, bronchospasm, heart block, and cardiac failure.

After accidental ingestion, emesis is most effective if initiated within 30 minutes, providing patient isn't obtunded, comatose, or having seizures. Follow with activated charcoal. Treat bradycardia, conduction defects, and hypotension with I.V. fluids, glucagon, atropine, or isoproterenol. Treat bronchoconstriction with I.V. aminophylline, and seizures with I.V. diazepam.

Clinical considerations

□ ***ALERT*** Be aware that drug contains sodium metabisulfite which may precipitate an allergic reaction in susceptible individuals.
- Levobunolol is faster acting than timolol.
- Because levobunolol has little or no effect on pupil size, don't use drug alone in patients with angle-closure glaucoma; use in combination with a miotic.
- Store at 59° to 86° F (15° to 30° C) in light-resistant container.

Therapeutic monitoring

- Cardiac output is reduced in both healthy patients and those with heart disease. Drug may decrease heart rate and blood pressure and produces beta blockade in bronchi and bronchioles. No effect on pupil size or accommodation has been noted. Recommend monitoring for these effects.
- In some patients, a few weeks' treatment may be required to stabilize pressure-lowering response; determine intraocular pressure after 4 weeks of treatment.

Special populations

Geriatric patients. Use drug with caution in geriatric patients with cardiac or pulmonary disease who may experience exacerbation of symptoms, depending on extent of systemic absorption.

Patient counseling

- Warn patient not to touch dropper to eye or surrounding tissue.

- Show patient how to instill drug. Teach him to press lacrimal sac lightly for 1 minute after drug administration, to decrease chance of systemic absorption.
- Remind patient not to blink more than usual or to close eyes tightly during treatment.
- Tell patient to report severe reaction, although transient stinging and discomfort are common.

levodopa

Dopar, Larodopa

Pharmacologic classification: dopamine precursor
Therapeutic classification: antiparkinsonian
Pregnancy risk category C

How supplied

Available by prescription only
Tablets: 100 mg, 250 mg, 500 mg
Capsules: 100 mg, 250 mg, 500 mg

Indications and dosages

Parkinsonism
Levodopa is indicated in treating idiopathic, postencephalitic, arteriosclerotic parkinsonism, and symptomatic parkinsonism that may follow injury to the nervous system by carbon monoxide intoxication and manganese intoxication.
Adults: Initially, 0.5 to 1 g P.O. daily, given b.i.d., t.i.d., or q.i.d. with food; increase 100 to 750 mg daily q 3 to 7 days, as tolerated. The usual optimal dose is 3 to 6 g daily divided into three or more doses. Maximum recommended dose is 8 g daily; some patients may require more. A significant therapeutic response may not be obtained for 6 months. Larger dose requires close supervision.

Pharmacodynamics

Antiparkinsonian action: Precise mechanism hasn't been established. A small percentage of each dose crossing the blood-brain barrier is decarboxylated. The dopamine then stimulates dopaminergic receptors in the basal ganglia to enhance the balance between cholinergic and dopaminergic activity, resulting in improved modulation of voluntary nerve impulses transmitted to the motor cortex.

Pharmacokinetics

Absorption: Absorbed rapidly from the small intestine by an active amino acid transport system, with 30% to 50% reaching general circulation.
Distribution: Distributed widely to most body tissues, but not to the CNS, which receives less than 1% of dose because of extensive metabolism in the periphery.
Metabolism: Most (95%) is converted to dopamine by l-aromatic amino acid decarboxylase enzyme in the lumen of the stomach and intestines and on the first pass through the liver.
Excretion: Excreted primarily in urine; 80% of dose is excreted within 24 hours as dopamine metabolites. Half-life is 1 to 3 hours.

Route	Onset	Peak	Duration
P.O.	Unknown	1-3 hr	5 hr

Contraindications and precautions

Contraindicated in concurrent therapy with MAO inhibitors within 14 days, and in hypersensitivity to drug, acute angle-closure glaucoma, melanoma, or undiagnosed skin lesions.

Use cautiously in patients with severe renal, CV, hepatic, and pulmonary disorders; peptic ulcer; psychiatric illness; MI with residual arrhythmias; bronchial asthma; emphysema; and endocrine disorders.

Interactions

Drug-drug. *Amantadine, benztropine, procyclidine, trihexyphenidyl:* May increase the efficacy of levodopa.
Anesthetics or hydrocarbon inhalation: May cause arrhythmias because of increased endogenous dopamine concentration. Discontinue levodopa 6 to 8 hours before administration of anesthetics such as halothane.
Antacids containing calcium, magnesium, or sodium bicarbonate: May increase absorption of levodopa. Recommend administering antacids 1 hour after levodopa.
Anticholinergics: Used with levodopa may produce a mild synergy and increased efficacy. Gradual reduction in anticholinergic dosage is necessary.
Anticonvulsants (such as hydantoins, phenytoin), benzodiazepines, haloperidol, papaverine, phenothiazines, rauwolfia alkaloids, or thioxanthenes: May decrease therapeutic effects of levodopa. Patient requires monitoring for decreased effectiveness.
Antihypertensives: Increased hypotensive effect. Blood pressure must be monitored.
Bromocriptine: May produce additive effects. Reduced levodopa dosage may be necessary.
Methyldopa: May alter the antiparkinsonian effects of levodopa and may produce additive toxic CNS effects. Avoid use together.
MAO inhibitors: May cause a hypertensive crisis. Discontinue MAO inhibitors for 2 to 4 weeks before starting levodopa.
Pyridoxine: A small dose (10 mg) reverses the antiparkinsonian effects of levodopa. Don't give together.
Sympathomimetics: May increase the risk of arrhythmias. Dosage reduction of the sympathomimetic is recommended; the administration of carbidopa with levodopa reduces the tendency of sympathomimetics to cause dopamine-induced arrhythmias. Reduce levodopa dosage.

Tricyclic antidepressants: May increase sympathetic activity, with sinus tachycardia and hypertension. Avoid use together if possible.
Drug-herb. *Jimsonweed:* May adversely affect CV function. Avoid use together.
Kava: May increase parkinsonian symptoms. Avoid use together.
Rauwolfia: May decrease effectiveness of levodopa. Avoid use together.

Effects on diagnostic tests

Coombs' test occasionally becomes positive during extended therapy. Colorimetric test for uric acid has shown false elevations. False-positive results have been noted on tests for urine glucose using the copper-reduction method; false-negative results have occurred with the glucose oxidase method. Levodopa also may interfere with tests for urine ketones, urine norepinephrine and urine protein determinations.

Adverse reactions

CNS: *aggressive behavior; choreiform, dystonic, and dyskinetic movements; involuntary grimacing, head movements, myoclonic body jerks,* ***seizures,*** ataxia, tremor, muscle twitching; bradykinetic episodes; psychiatric disturbances; mood changes, nervousness, anxiety, disturbing dreams, euphoria, malaise, fatigue; severe depression, ***suicidal tendencies,*** dementia, delirium, hallucinations.
CV: *orthostatic hypotension,* cardiac irregularities, phlebitis.
EENT: blepharospasm, blurred vision, diplopia, mydriasis or miosis, activation of latent Horner's syndrome, oculogyric crises, excessive salivation.
GI: dry mouth, bitter taste, *nausea, vomiting, anorexia,* constipation, flatulence, diarrhea, abdominal pain.
GU: urinary frequency, urine retention, incontinence, darkened urine, priapism.
Hematologic: ***hemolytic anemia, leukopenia, agranulocytosis.***
Hepatic: elevated liver enzymes, ***hepatotoxicity.***
Metabolic: weight loss (at start of therapy).
Respiratory: hyperventilation, hiccups.
Other: dark perspiration.

Overdose and treatment

Signs and symptoms of overdose include spasm or closing of eyelids, irregular heartbeat, or palpitations. Treatment includes immediate gastric lavage, maintenance of an adequate airway, and judicious administration of I.V. fluids and may include antiarrhythmic drugs, if necessary. Pyridoxine 10 to 25 mg P.O. has been reported to reverse toxic and therapeutic effects of levodopa. (Its usefulness hasn't been established in acute overdose.)

Clinical considerations

- Give drug between meals and with low-protein snack to maximize drug absorption and minimize GI upset. Foods high in protein appear to interfere with transport of drug.
- Tablets and capsules may be crushed and mixed with applesauce or baby-food fruits for patients who have difficulty swallowing pills.
- Maximum effectiveness of drug may not occur for several weeks or months after therapy begins.
- Because of risk of precipitating a symptom complex resembling neuroleptic malignant syndrome, observe patient closely if levodopa dosage is reduced abruptly or discontinued.
- If restarting therapy after a long period of interruption, adjust drug dosage gradually to previous level.
- Patients undergoing surgery should continue levodopa as long as oral intake is permitted, usually 6 to 24 hours before surgery. Resume drug as soon as patient is able to take oral medication.
- Although controversial, a medically supervised period of drug discontinuance (drug holiday) may reestablish the effectiveness of a lower dose regimen.
- Combination of levodopa-carbidopa usually reduces amount of levodopa needed, thus reducing incidence of adverse reactions.
- Levodopa has also been used to relieve pain of herpes zoster, management of bone pain in metastatic disease, and management of hepatic coma.
- Protect drug from heat, light, and moisture. If preparation darkens, it has lost potency and should be discarded.

Therapeutic monitoring

- Recommend monitoring patient also receiving antihypertensive medication for possible drug interactions. Discontinue MAO inhibitors at least 2 weeks before levodopa therapy begins.
- Recommend monitoring vital signs, especially while adjusting dose.
- Recommend monitoring patient for muscle twitching and blepharospasm (twitching of eyelids), which may be an early sign of drug overdose.
- Patients on long-term therapy should be tested regularly for diabetes and acromegaly; check blood tests and liver and kidney function studies periodically for adverse effects. Leukopenia may require cessation of therapy.
- Monitor serum laboratory tests periodically. Coombs' test occasionally becomes positive during extended use. Expect uric acid elevation with colorimetric method but not with uricase method.
- Alkaline phosphatase, AST, ALT, LDH, bilirubin, BUN, and protein-bound iodine levels show transient elevations in patients receiving levodopa; WBC, hemoglobin level, and hematocrit show occasional reduction.

Special populations

Breast-feeding patients. Drug may inhibit lactation and shouldn't be used by breast-feeding women.

Pediatric patients. Safety of levodopa in children under age 12 hasn't been established.

Geriatric patients. Smaller doses may be required because of reduced tolerance to effects of drug. Geriatric patients, especially those with osteoporosis, should resume normal activity gradually, because increased mobility may increase risk of fractures. Geriatric patients are more likely to develop adverse effects, such as anxiety, confusion, or nervousness; those with preexisting heart disease are more susceptible to cardiac effects of levodopa.

Patient counseling

- Warn patient and family not to increase drug dose without specific instruction. (They may be tempted to do this as parkinsonian symptoms progress.)
- Explain that therapeutic response may not occur for up to 6 months.
- Advise patient and family that multivitamin preparations, fortified cereals, and certain OTC products may contain pyridoxine (vitamin B_6), which can reverse the effects of levodopa.
- Warn patient of possible dizziness and orthostatic hypotension, especially at start of therapy. Tell patient to change position slowly and dangle legs before getting out of bed. Instruct patient in use of elastic stockings to control this adverse reaction if appropriate.
- Inform patient of signs and symptoms of adverse reactions and therapeutic effects and need to report changes.
- Tell patient to take a missed dose as soon as possible; skip dose if next scheduled dose is within 2 hours, but not to double the dose.
- Advise patient not to take drug with food, and that eating something about 15 minutes after administration may help reduce GI upset.
- Warn patient of possible darkening of urine, sweat, and other body fluids.

levodopa-carbidopa

Sinemet 10-100, Sinemet 25-100, Sinemet 25-250, Sinemet CR 25-100, Sinemet CR 50-200

Pharmacologic classification: decarboxylase inhibitor/dopamine precursor combination
Therapeutic classification: antiparkinsonian
Pregnancy risk category C

How supplied

Available by prescription only
Tablets: 10 mg carbidopa with 100 mg levodopa (Sinemet 10-100), 25 mg carbidopa with 100 mg levodopa (Sinemet 25-100), 25 mg carbidopa with 250 mg levodopa (Sinemet 25-250)
Tablets (sustained-release): 50 mg carbidopa with 200 mg levodopa (Sinemet CR 50-200), 25 mg carbidopa with 100 mg levodopa (Sinemet CR 25-100)

Indications and dosages

Parkinsonism

Adults: Most patients respond to a 25 mg/100 mg combination (1 tablet P.O. t.i.d.). Dose may be increased q 1 or 2 days to maximum of 8 tablets or 1 tablet of 10 mg/100 mg t.i.d. or q.i.d. up to 2 tablets q.i.d.; or 1 sustained-release tablet b.i.d. at intervals at least 6 hours apart. Intervals may be adjusted based on patient response. Usual dose is 2 to 8 tablets daily in divided doses every 4 to 8 hours while awake.

Maintenance therapy must be carefully adjusted based on patient tolerance and desired therapeutic response.

Usual maintenance dosage is 3 to 6 tablets of 25 mg carbidopa/250 mg levodopa P.O. daily in divided doses. Don't exceed 8 tablets of 25 mg carbidopa/250 mg levodopa daily. Optimum daily dose must be determined by careful adjustment for each patient.

Daily dose of carbidopa should be 70 to 100 mg or more to suppress the peripheral metabolism of levodopa.

Pharmacodynamics

Decarboxylase-inhibiting action: Carbidopa inhibits the peripheral decarboxylation of levodopa, thus slowing its conversion to dopamine in extracerebral tissues. This results in an increased availability of levodopa for transport to the brain, where it undergoes decarboxylation to dopamine.

Pharmacokinetics

Absorption: A total of 40% to 70% of dose is absorbed after oral administration. Plasma levodopa levels are increased when carbidopa and levodopa are administered together because carbidopa inhibits the peripheral metabolism of levodopa.

Distribution: Carbidopa is distributed widely in body tissues except the CNS. Levodopa is also distributed into breast milk.

Metabolism: Carbidopa isn't metabolized extensively. It inhibits metabolism of levodopa in the GI tract, thus increasing its absorption from the GI tract and its level in plasma.

Excretion: Some (30%) of the dose is excreted unchanged in urine within 24 hours. When given with carbidopa, the amount of levodopa excreted unchanged in urine is increased by about 6%. Half-life is 1 to 2 hours.

Route	Onset	Peak	Duration
P.O.	Unknown	40-150 min	Unknown

Contraindications and precautions
Contraindicated in patients with hypersensitivity to drug, acute angle-closure glaucoma, melanoma, or undiagnosed skin lesions, and within 14 days of MAO inhibitor therapy.

Use cautiously in patients with severe CV, endocrine, pulmonary, renal, or hepatic disorders; peptic ulcer; psychiatric illness; MI with residual arrhythmias; bronchial asthma; emphysema; and well-controlled chronic open-angle glaucoma.

Interactions
Drug-drug. *Amantadine, benztropine, procyclidine, trihexyphenidyl:* May increase the efficacy of levodopa.
Anesthetics or hydrocarbon inhalation: May cause arrhythmias because of increased endogenous dopamine concentration. Discontinue levodopa 6 to 8 hours before administration of anesthetics such as halothane.
Antacids containing calcium, magnesium, or sodium bicarbonate: May increase absorption of levodopa. Give antacids 1 hour after levodopa.
Anticonvulsants (such as hydantoins, phenytoin), benzodiazepines, haloperidol, papaverine, phenothiazines, rauwolfia alkaloids, or thioxanthenes: May decrease therapeutic effects of levodopa. Recommend monitoring for decreased effectiveness.
Antihypertensives: Increased hypotensive effect. Blood pressure monitoring is necessary.
Bromocriptine: May produce additive effects. Reduced levodopa dosage may be necessary.
Methyldopa: May alter the antiparkinsonian effects of levodopa and may produce additive toxic CNS effects. Avoid use together.
MAO inhibitors: May cause a hypertensive crisis. Discontinue MAO inhibitors for 2 to 4 weeks before starting levodopa.
Molindone: May inhibit antiparkinsonian effects of levodopa by blocking dopamine receptors in the brain. Avoid use together.
Sympathomimetics: May increase the risk of arrhythmias. Dosage reduction of the sympathomimetic is recommended; the administration of carbidopa with levodopa reduces the tendency of sympathomimetics to cause dopamine-induced arrhythmias. Reduce levodopa dose.

Effects on diagnostic tests
Antiglobulin determinations (Coombs' test) are occasionally positive after long-term use. Thyroid function determinations may inhibit thyroid-stimulating hormone response to protirelin.

Serum and urine uric acid determinations may show false elevations. Urine glucose determinations using copper reduction method may show false-positive results; with the glucose oxidase method, false-negative results. Urine ketone determination using dip-stick method, urine norepinephrine determinations, and urine protein determinations using Lowery test may show false-positive results.

Adverse reactions
CNS: *choreiform, dystonic, dyskinetic movements; involuntary grimacing, head movements, myoclonic body jerks, ataxia,* tremor, muscle twitching; bradykinetic episodes; psychiatric disturbances, anxiety, disturbing dreams, euphoria, malaise, fatigue; severe depression, ***suicidal tendencies,*** dementia, delirium, hallucinations (may necessitate reduction or withdrawal of drug), confusion, insomnia, agitation.
CV: *orthostatic hypotension,* ***cardiac irregularities,*** phlebitis.
EENT: blepharospasm, blurred vision, diplopia, mydriasis or miosis, oculogyric crises, excessive salivation.
GI: *dry mouth,* bitter taste, *nausea, vomiting, anorexia,* constipation; flatulence; diarrhea; abdominal pain.
GU: urinary frequency, elevated BUN, urine retention, urinary incontinence, darkened urine, priapism.
Hematologic: ***hemolytic anemia, thrombocytopenia, leukopenia, agranulocytosis.***
Hepatic: elevated levels of ALT, AST, alkaline phosphatase, serum bilirubin, LD; ***hepatotoxicity.***
Metabolic: weight loss (at start of therapy); elevated levels of serum protein-bound iodine; elevated serum gonadotropin levels.
Respiratory: hyperventilation, hiccups.
Other: dark perspiration.

Overdose and treatment
There have been no reports of overdose with carbidopa. Signs and symptoms of levodopa overdose are irregular heartbeat and palpitations, severe continuous nausea and vomiting, spasm or closing of eyelids.

Treatment of overdose includes immediate gastric lavage and antiarrhythmic medication, if necessary. Pyridoxine isn't effective in reversing the actions of carbidopa and levodopa combinations.

Clinical considerations
- Muscle twitching and blepharospasm (twitching of eyelids) may be an early sign of overdose.
- If patient is being treated with levodopa, discontinue at least 8 hours before starting levodopa-carbidopa. Initial combination therapy should provide no more than 20% to 25% of previous levodopa dosage.
- The combination drug usually reduces the amount of levodopa needed by 75%, thereby reducing the incidence of adverse reactions.
- Sustained-release tablets may be split, but never crushed or chewed.
- For patients being transferred from conventional levodopa-carbidopa preparation to an

extended-release preparation, the extended-release tablet should provide 10% to 30% more levodopa daily.

- Pyridoxine (vitamin B_6) doesn't reverse beneficial effects of levodopa-carbidopa. Multivitamins can be taken without fear of losing control of symptoms.
- If therapy is interrupted temporarily, usual daily dosage may be given as soon as patient resumes oral medications.
- Maximum effectiveness of drug may not occur for several weeks or months after therapy begins.

Therapeutic monitoring

- Recommend carefully monitoring patients who also receive antihypertensive or hypoglycemic agents. Discontinue MAO inhibitors at least 2 weeks before therapy begins.
- Dosage adjustment is based on patient's response and tolerance to drug. Therapeutic and adverse reactions occur more rapidly with levodopa-carbidopa combination than with levodopa alone. Recommend observing and monitoring vital signs, especially while dosage is being adjusted.
- Test patients on long-term therapy regularly for diabetes and acromegaly; periodically repeat blood test and liver and kidney function studies.

Special populations

Breast-feeding patients. Because levodopa may inhibit lactation, don't use drug in breast-feeding women.
Pediatric patients. Safety of drug in children under age 18 hasn't been established.
Geriatric patients. Smaller doses may be required in geriatric patients because of their reduced tolerance to the effects of levodopa-carbidopa. Geriatric patients, especially those with osteoporosis, should resume normal activity gradually because increased mobility may increase the risk of fractures. Geriatric patients are especially vulnerable to CNS adverse effects, such as anxiety, confusion, or nervousness; those with preexisting heart disease are more susceptible to cardiac effects.

Patient counseling

- Instruct patient to report adverse reactions and therapeutic effects.
- Warn patient of possible dizziness or orthostatic hypotension, especially at start of therapy. Tell patient to change position slowly and dangle legs before getting out of bed. Elastic stockings may be helpful in some patients.
- Tell patient to take food shortly after taking drug to relieve gastric irritation.
- Inform patient that drug may cause urine or sweat to darken.
- Tell patient to take a missed dose as soon as possible, to skip a missed dose if next scheduled dose is within 2 hours, and never to double the dose.

levofloxacin

Levaquin

Pharmacologic classification: fluorinated carboxyquinolone
Therapeutic classification: broad-spectrum antibacterial
Pregnancy risk category C

How supplied

Available by prescription only
Tablets: 250 mg, 500 mg
Single-use vials: 500 mg
Infusion (premixed): 250 mg in 50 ml D_5W, 500 mg in 100 ml D_5W

Indications and dosages

***Acute maxillary sinusitis caused by susceptible strains of* Streptococcus pneumoniae, Moraxella catarrhalis, *or* Haemophilus influenzae**
Adults: 500 mg P.O. or I.V. daily for 10 to 14 days.
***Acute bacterial exacerbation of chronic bronchitis caused by* Staphylococcus aureus, S. pneumoniae, M. catarrhalis, H. influenzae, *or* H. parainfluenzae**
Adults: 500 mg P.O. or I.V. daily for 7 days.
***Community-acquired pneumonia caused by* S. aureus, S. pneumoniae, M. catarrhalis, H. influenzae, H. parainfluenzae, Klebsiella pneumoniae, Chlamydia pneumoniae, Legionella pneumoniae, *or* Mycoplasma pneumoniae**
Adults: 500 mg P.O. or I.V. daily for 7 to 14 days.
***Uncomplicated skin and skin structure infections (mild to moderate) caused by* S. aureus *or* Streptococcus pyogenes**
Adults: 500 mg P.O. or I.V. daily for 7 to 10 days.
≡ ***Dosage adjustment.*** If creatinine clearance is 20 to 49 ml/minute, initial dose is 500 mg and subsequent doses are half the initial dose. If creatinine clearance is 10 to 19 ml/minute, subsequent doses are half the initial dose and the interval is prolonged to q 48 hours.
***Complicated urinary tract infections (mild to moderate) caused by* Enterococcus faecalis, Enterobacter cloacae, Escherichia coli, K. pneumoniae, Proteus mirabilis, *or* Pseudomonas aeruginosa**
Adults: 250 mg P.O. or I.V. daily for 10 days.
***Acute pyelonephritis (mild to moderate) caused by* E. coli**
Adults: 250 mg P.O. or I.V. daily for 10 days.
≡ ***Dosage adjustment.*** If creatinine clearance is 10 to 19 ml/minute, dosage interval is increased to q 48 hours.

◇ ***Traveler's diarrhea***
Adults: 500 mg P.O. single dose in conjunction with loperamide hydrochloride.
◇ ***Prophylaxis of traveler's diarrhea***
Adults: 500 mg P.O. once daily during period of risk, for up to 3 weeks.

Pharmacodynamics

Antibacterial action: Drug inhibits bacterial DNA gyrase, an enzyme required for DNA replication, transcription, repair, and recombination in susceptible bacteria.

Pharmacokinetics

Absorption: The plasma level after I.V. administration is comparable to that observed for equivalent oral doses (on a mg/mg basis). Therefore, oral and I.V. routes can be considered interchangeable.
Distribution: Mean volume of distribution ranges from 89 to 112 L after single and multiple 500-mg doses, indicating widespread distribution into body tissues. Drug also penetrates well into lung tissues, generally twofold to fivefold higher than plasma levels.
Metabolism: Undergoes limited metabolism in humans. The only identified metabolites are the desmethyl and *N*-oxide metabolites, which have little relevant pharmacologic activity.
Excretion: Primarily excreted unchanged in the urine. Mean terminal half-life is about 6 to 8 hours.

Route	Onset	Peak	Duration
P.O., I.V.	Unknown	1-2 hr	Unknown

Contraindications and precautions

Contraindicated in patients with hypersensitivity to drug, its components, or quinolone antimicrobials. Safety and efficacy of levofloxacin in children, adolescents (under age 18), and pregnant and breast-feeding women haven't been established.

Use cautiously in patients with history of seizure disorders or other CNS diseases, such as cerebral arteriosclerosis, because quinolones can cause CNS stimulation and increased intracranial pressure. This may lead to seizures (lowered seizure threshold), toxic psychoses, tremors, restlessness, anxiety, light-headedness, confusion, hallucinations, paranoia, depression, nightmares, insomnia and, rarely, suicidal thoughts or acts. These can occur after the first dose.

Interactions

Drug-drug. *Antacids containing aluminum or magnesium, iron salts, products containing zinc, and sucralfate:* May interfere with GI absorption of levofloxacin. Administer these drugs at least 2 hours apart.
Antidiabetic agents: May alter blood glucose levels. Monitor glucose levels closely.
NSAIDs: May increase CNS stimulation. Patient requires monitoring for seizure activity.
Warfarin and derivatives: May cause increased effect of oral anticoagulant with some fluoroquinolones. Monitor PT and INR.
Theophylline: Coadministration may result in decreased clearance of theophylline. Monitor theophylline levels.
Drug-lifestyle. *Sun exposure:* Increased photosensitivity. Advise patient to take precautions.

Effects on diagnostic tests

None reported.

Adverse reactions

CNS: headache, insomnia, dizziness, encephalopathy, paresthesia, abnormal EEG, ***seizures.***
CV: chest pain, palpitations, vasodilation.
GI: nausea, diarrhea, constipation, vomiting, abdominal pain, dyspepsia, flatulence, ***pseudomembranous colitis.***
GU: vaginitis.
Hematologic: eosinophilia, hemolytic anemia, decreased lymphocyte count.
Metabolic: decreased glucose level.
Musculoskeletal: back pain, tendon rupture.
Respiratory: allergic pneumonitis.
Skin: rash, photosensitivity, pruritus, erythema multiforme, ***Stevens-Johnson syndrome.***
Other: pain, ***hypersensitivity reactions,*** injection site reaction, ***anaphylaxis, multisystem organ failure.***

Overdose and treatment

No information available. If acute overdose occurs, empty the stomach, maintain hydration, and observe. Drug isn't effectively removed by hemodialysis or peritoneal dialysis.

Clinical considerations

- If patient experiences symptoms of excessive CNS stimulation (restlessness, tremor, confusion, hallucinations), stop drug and institute seizure precautions.
- Ruptures of tendons and tendonitis have occurred with quinolone therapy. Discontinue drug if pain, inflammation, or rupture of a tendon occurs. These ruptures can occur after therapy has been stopped.
- For I.V. preparations, single-dose vial must be diluted to concentration of 5 mg/ml. Don't infuse other drugs through the same I.V. line.
- Because a rapid or bolus administration may result in hypotension, I.V. levofloxacin should only be administered by slow infusion over 60 minutes.

Therapeutic monitoring

Monitor blood glucose and renal, hepatic, and hematopoietic studies as indicated.

Special populations
Breast-feeding patients. Based on data from ofloxacin, it can be presumed that levofloxacin will be excreted in breast milk. Because of potential for serious adverse reactions in breast-fed infants, a decision should be made whether to discontinue breast-feeding or drug.
Pediatric patients. Safety and efficacy in children under age 18 haven't been established.
Geriatric patients. Dosage adjustment based on age alone isn't necessary.

Patient counseling
- Tell patient to take drug as prescribed, even if symptoms disappear.
- Advise patient to take drug with plenty of fluids and to avoid antacids, sucralfate, and products containing iron or zinc for at least 2 hours before and after each dose.
- Warn patient to avoid hazardous tasks until adverse CNS effects of drug are known.
- Advise patient to use sunblock and wear protective clothing when exposed to excessive sunlight.
- Tell patient to stop drug and report if rash or other signs of hypersensitivity develop.
- Tell patient to report pain or inflammation.
- Tell diabetic patient to monitor blood glucose levels and report if a hypoglycemic reaction occurs.

levonorgestrel implants
Norplant System

Pharmacologic classification:
progestin
Therapeutic classification:
contraceptive
Pregnancy risk category X

How supplied
Available by prescription only
Implants: 36 mg in each of six Silastic capsules; kits also include trocar, scalpel, forceps, syringe, two needles, package of skin closures, three packages of gauze sponges, stretch bandages, and surgical drape

Indications and dosages
Long-term (up to 5 years), reversible prevention of pregnancy
Adults: Six Silastic capsules containing 36 mg each for a total of 216 mg are surgically implanted in the superficial plane beneath the skin of a woman's upper arm during first 7 days of onset of menses.

Pharmacodynamics
Contraceptive action: Levonorgestrel is a synthetic, biologically active progestin, exhibiting no significant estrogenic activity. A continuous low dose of levonorgestrel is diffused through the wall of each capsule. Pregnancy is prevented by at least two mechanisms: inhibition of ovulation and thickening of the cervical mucus.

Pharmacokinetics
Absorption: 100% bioavailable. Plasma levels average 0.3 ng/ml over 5 years but are highly variable as a function of individual metabolism and body weight.
Distribution: Bound by the circulating protein sex hormone-binding globulin (SHBG).
Metabolism: Metabolized by the liver.
Excretion: Metabolites are excreted in the urine.

Route	Onset	Peak	Duration
Subdermal	24 hr	24 hr	Unknown

Contraindications and precautions
Contraindicated in patients with active thrombophlebitis or thromboembolic disorders, undiagnosed abnormal genital bleeding, acute liver disease, malignant or benign liver tumors, known or suspected breast cancer, known or suspected pregnancy, history of idiopathic intracranial hypertension, and hypersensitivity to levonorgestrel or components of the Norplant System.

Use cautiously in diabetic and prediabetic patients and in those with history of depression or hyperlipidemia.

Interactions
Drug-drug. *Carbamazepine, phenytoin:* Reduced efficacy of levonorgestrel. Patient should take additional precautions to avoid pregnancy.

Effects on diagnostic tests
None reported.

Adverse reactions
CNS: headache, nervousness, dizziness, depression, tingling, numbness.
GI: nausea, *abdominal discomfort,* appetite change.
GU: *amenorrhea, many days of bleeding or prolonged bleeding, spotting, irregular onset of bleeding, frequent onset of bleeding, scanty bleeding, cervicitis, vaginitis, leukorrhea, breast discharge.*
Metabolic: decreased thyroxine levels, increased T_3 uptake, weight gain.
Musculoskeletal: mastalgia, *musculoskeletal pain.*
Skin: dermatitis, acne, hirsutism, hypertrichosis, alopecia; infection, transient pain, itching (at implant site).
Other: adnexal enlargement, *removal difficulty.*

Overdose and treatment
Overdose can occur if more than six Silastic capsules are in situ, resulting in fluid retention with its associated effects and uterine bleed-

ing irregularities. All previously implanted capsules should be removed before insertion of a new set.

Clinical considerations

- The total implanted dose is 216 mg. Implantation of all six capsules should be performed during the first 7 days of menstrual cycle. Insertion is subdermal in the midportion of the inside of the upper arm, 8 to 10 cm above the elbow crease.
- Each capsule is 2.4 mm in diameter and 34 mm in length.
- Determine whether patient has allergies to the antiseptic or anesthetic to be used, or contraindications to progestin-only contraception.
- During insertion, special attention must be given to asepsis and correct placement of capsules; careful technique minimizes tissue trauma.
- Patients should receive a copy of patient information booklet and should be made aware of potential adverse reactions and of risks and benefits of the system and of other forms of contraception.
- Store at room temperature away from excess heat and moisture.

Therapeutic monitoring

- Patients should be reexamined at least yearly; examinations should focus on implant site, blood pressure, breasts, abdominal and pelvic organs, including cervical cytology, and related laboratory tests.
- Patient should be monitored for recurrent or abnormal vaginal bleeding.
- Patients with strong family history of breast cancer should be monitored for breast nodules.

Patient counseling

- Tell patient that altered bleeding patterns tend to become more regular after 9 to 12 months.
- Warn patient to report heavy bleeding.
- Advise patient to avoid bumping or wetting the insertion site for at least 3 days after insertion.
- Explain that some tenderness in the implant area may occur for 1 to 2 days.
- Tell patient that insertion usually takes 10 to 15 minutes and causes little or no discomfort because of the local anesthetic.
- Advise patient that, when laboratory studies are ordered, she should inform all health care providers that levonorgestrel implants are being used.
- Tell patient who takes phenytoin or carbamazepine that she may need to use additional contraceptive measures.
- Advise patient to thoroughly review patient information booklet.

levothyroxine sodium (T_4 or L-thyroxine sodium)

Eltroxin, Levo-T, Levothroid, Levoxine, Levoxyl, Synthroid

Pharmacologic classification: thyroid hormone
Therapeutic classification: thyroid hormone replacement
Pregnancy risk category A

How supplied

Available by prescription only
Tablets: 25 mcg, 50 mcg, 75 mcg, 88 mcg, 100 mcg, 112 mcg, 125 mcg, 137 mcg, 150 mcg, 175 mcg, 200 mcg, 300 mcg
Injection: 200 mcg/vial, 500 mcg/vial

Indications and dosages

Congenital hypothyroidism
Neonates: 37.5 mcg (25 to 50 mcg) P.O. daily.
Premature neonates under 4.4 lb (2 kg) and those at risk for cardiac failure: 25 mcg P.O. daily initially; dosage may be increased to 50 mcg daily in 4 to 6 weeks.
Children under age 1: Initially, 25 to 50 mcg P.O. daily.
Children age 1 and older: 3 to 5 mcg/kg P.O. daily until adult dose (150 mcg) is reached in early or mid-adolescence.
Myxedema coma
Adults: 300 to 500 mcg I.V. If no response occurs in 24 hours, give an additional 100 to 300 mcg I.V. in 48 hours. A maintenance dosage of 50 to 200 mcg may be given until condition stabilizes and drug can be given orally.
Thyroid hormone replacement for atrophy of gland, surgical removal, excessive radiation or antithyroid drugs, or congenital defect
Adults: For mild hypothyroidism—initially, 50 mcg P.O. daily, increased by 25 to 50 mcg P.O. daily q 2 to 4 weeks until desired response is achieved; may be administered I.V. or I.M. when P.O. ingestion is precluded for long periods. Usual dose is 100 to 200 mcg daily.

For severe hypothyroidism—12.5 to 25 mcg P.O. daily, increased by 25 to 50 mcg daily q 2 to 4 weeks until desired response is achieved.
Elderly: Start at 12.5 to 50 mcg P.O. daily and increase in 12.5- to 25-mcg increments q 3 to 8 weeks.
≡ ***Dosage adjustment.*** For patients with CV disease, start at 50 mcg daily and increase in 50-mcg increments at 2- to 4-week intervals.
Children: Therapy may be initiated at the full therapeutic dose. Incremental doses aren't usually needed.
Children over age 12: Over 150 mcg or 2 to 3 mcg/kg/day.

Children age 6 to 12: 100 to 150 mcg or 4 to 5 mcg/kg/day.
Children age 1 to 5: 75 to 100 mcg or 5 to 6 mcg/kg/day.
Children age 6 to 12 months: 50 to 75 mcg or 6 to 8 mcg/kg/day.
Children under age 6 months: 25 to 50 mcg or 8 to 10 mcg/kg/day.

Pharmacodynamics

Thyroid hormone replacement: Drug affects protein and carbohydrate metabolism, promotes gluconeogenesis, increases the use and mobilization of glycogen stores, stimulates protein synthesis, and regulates cell growth and differentiation.

Pharmacokinetics

Absorption: Between 50% and 80% is absorbed from the GI tract. Full effects don't occur for 1 to 3 weeks after oral therapy begins. After I.M. administration, absorption is variable and poor. After an I.V. dose in patients with myxedema coma, increased responsiveness may occur within 6 to 8 hours, but maximum therapeutic effect may not occur for up to 24 hours.
Distribution: Distribution isn't fully described; however, drug is distributed into most body tissues and fluids. The highest levels are found in the liver and kidneys; 99% is protein bound.
Metabolism: Metabolized in peripheral tissues, primarily in the liver, kidneys, and intestines. About 85% of metabolized levothyroxine is deiodinated.
Excretion: Fecal excretion eliminates 20% to 40% of levothyroxine. Half-life is 6 to 7 days.

Route	Onset	Peak	Duration
P.O.	24 hr	Unknown	Unknown
I.V.	Unknown	Unknown	Unknown
I.M.	Unknown	Unknown	Unknown

Contraindications and precautions

Contraindicated in patients with hypersensitivity to drug, acute MI and thyrotoxicosis uncomplicated by hypothyroidism, or uncorrected adrenal insufficiency.

Use cautiously in the elderly and in patients with renal impairment, angina pectoris, hypertension, ischemia, or other CV disorders.

Interactions

Drug-drug. *Anticoagulant:* May alter anticoagulant effect. An increase in levothyroxine dosage may necessitate a decrease in anticoagulant dosage.
Beta blockers: May decrease conversion of levothyroxine to liothyronine. Monitor patient.
Cholestyramine: May delay absorption of levothyroxine. Don't administer together.
Corticotropin: Concurrent use causes changes in thyroid status. Monitor patient; dose adjustment of both medications may be needed.
Estrogens: Increase levothyroxine requirements. Recommend monitoring for decreased levothyroxine effect.
Hepatic enzyme inducers such as phenytoin: May increase hepatic degradation of levothyroxine and increase dosage requirements of levothyroxine. Recommend adjusting dosages as needed.
Oral antidiabetic agents or insulin: Altered serum glucose levels. Recommend adjusting doses of these medications as needed.
Somatrem: May accelerate epiphyseal maturation. Avoid concurrent use in children if possible.
Theophylline: Decreased theophylline clearance can be expected in hypothyroid patients. Clearance returns to normal when euthyroid state is achieved.
Tricyclic antidepressants or sympathomimetics: May increase the effects of any or all of these drugs and may lead to coronary insufficiency or arrhythmias. Recommend monitoring closely if concurrent use is necessary.

Effects on diagnostic tests

Levothyroxine therapy alters radioactive iodine (^{131}I) thyroid uptake, protein-bound iodine levels, and liothyronine uptake.

Adverse reactions

CNS: *nervousness, insomnia, tremor,* headache.
CV: *tachycardia, palpitations,* ***arrhythmias,*** *angina pectoris,* ***cardiac arrest.***
GI: diarrhea, vomiting.
GU: menstrual irregularities.
Metabolic: weight loss.
Skin: diaphoresis, allergic skin reactions.
Other: heat intolerance, fever.

Overdose and treatment

Evidence of overdose includes signs and symptoms of hyperthyroidism, including weight loss, increased appetite, palpitations, nervousness, diarrhea, abdominal cramps, sweating, tachycardia, increased blood pressure, widened pulse pressure, angina, arrhythmias, tremor, headache, insomnia, heat intolerance, fever, and menstrual irregularities.

Treatment of overdose requires reduction of GI absorption and efforts to counteract central and peripheral effects, primarily sympathetic activity. Use gastric lavage or induce emesis (followed by activated charcoal up to 4 hours after ingestion). If the patient is comatose or is having seizures, inflate cuff on endotracheal tube to prevent aspiration. Treatment may include oxygen and artificial ventilation as needed to support respiration. It also should include appropriate measures to treat heart failure and to control fever, hypoglycemia, and fluid loss. Propranolol (or another beta blocker) may be used to combat many of the effects of increased sympathetic activity.

Levothyroxine should be gradually withdrawn over 2 to 6 days, then resumed at a lower dose.

Clinical considerations

- Levothyroxine has predictable effects because of standard hormonal content; therefore, it's the usual drug of choice for thyroid hormone replacement.
- Administer as a single dose before breakfast.
- Patient with history of lactose intolerance may be sensitive to Levothroid, which contains lactose.
- Synthroid 100- and 300-mcg tablets contain tartrazine, a dye that causes allergic reactions in susceptible individuals.
- When switching from levothyroxine to liothyronine, stop levothyroxine dosage when liothyronine treatment begins. After residual effects of levothyroxine have disappeared, liothyronine dosage can be increased in small increments. When switching from liothyronine to levothyroxine, begin levothyroxine therapy several days before withdrawing liothyronine to avoid relapse.
- Levothyroid powder for injection or levothyroxine sodium powder is reconstituted by adding 2 ml or 5 ml of 0.9% sodium chloride for injection to vial containing 200 or 500 mcg, respectively. Shake until a clear solution is obtained. Concentration is about 100 mcg/ml.
- Synthroid powder for injection is reconstituted by adding 5 ml of 0.9% sodium chloride for injection or bacteriostatic sodium chloride injection with benzyl alcohol to 200 or 500 mcg vial. Shake until a clear solution is obtained. Concentration is 40 or 100 mcg/ml, respectively. Use reconstituted solutions immediately and don't coadminister with other I.V. infusion solutions.
- Protect drug from moisture and light.

Therapeutic monitoring

- Recommend carefully observing patient for adverse effects during initial dose adjustment phase.
- Recommend monitoring patient for aggravation of concurrent diseases, such as Addison's disease or diabetes mellitus.
- Patient taking levothyroxine who requires ^{131}I uptake studies must discontinue drug 4 weeks before test.

Special populations

Breast-feeding patients. Minimal amounts of drug are excreted in breast milk. Use with caution in breast-feeding women.
Pediatric patients. Partial and temporary hair loss may occur during the first few months of therapy.
Geriatric patients. Geriatric patients are more sensitive to effects of drug. In patients over age 60, initial dosage should be 25% lower than usual recommended dosage.

Patient counseling

- Advise taking drug at same time each day; encourage morning dosing to avoid insomnia.
- Tell patient to report headache, diarrhea, nervousness, excessive sweating, heat intolerance, chest pain, increased pulse rate, or palpitations.
- Encourage patient to use the same product consistently because all brands don't have equal bioavailability.
- Advise patient to store drug in cool, dry place to prevent deterioration of product.
- Tell patient that replacement therapy is to be taken essentially for life, except in cases of transient hypothyroidism.

lidocaine (lignocaine)

Xylocaine

lidocaine hydrochloride

Anestacon, Dilocaine, L-Caine, Lidoderm Patch, Lidoject, LidoPen Auto-Injector, Nervocaine, Xylocaine, Xylocaine Viscous, Zilactin-L

Pharmacologic classification: amide derivative
Therapeutic classification: ventricular antiarrhythmic, local anesthetic
Pregnancy risk category B

How supplied

Available by prescription only
Injection: 5 mg/ml, 10 mg/ml, 15 mg/ml, 20 mg/ml, 40 mg/ml, 100 mg/ml, 200 mg/ml
Premixed solutions: 2 mg/ml, 4 mg/ml, 8 mg/ml in D_5W
Parenteral injection: 0.5%, 1 %, 1.5%, 2%, 4% (lidocaine with epinephrine combinations also available.)
Ointment: 5%
Topical solution: 2%, 4%
Jelly: 2%
Spray: 10%
Available without a prescription
Ointment: 2.5%
Liquid: 2.5%
Cream: 0.5%
Spray: 0.5%
Gel: 0.5%, 2.5%
Transdermal patch: 5%

Indications and dosages

Ventricular arrhythmias from MI, cardiac manipulation, or cardiac glycosides
Adults: 50 to 100 mg (1 to 1.5 mg/kg) I.V. bolus at 25 to 50 mg/minute. Repeat bolus (e.g., 25 to 50 mg or 0.5 to 0.75 mg/kg) q 5 to 10 minutes until arrhythmia subsides. Don't exceed 300-mg total bolus during a 1-hour period. Simultaneously, begin constant infusion of 1 to 4 mg/minute. If single bolus has been given, repeat smaller bolus (usually one-half ini-

tial bolus) 5 to 10 minutes after start of infusion to maintain therapeutic serum level. After 24 hours of continuous infusion, decrease rate by one half.
Elderly: Give half the bolus amount and use slower infusion rate.
≡ ***Dosage adjustment.*** Give half the bolus amount to lightweight patients and to those with heart failure or hepatic disease. Use slower infusion rate in those with heart failure or hepatic disease, or patients weighing less than 110 lb (50 kg).

For I.M. administration in all adults, 300 mg (4.3 mg/kg) in deltoid muscle has been used in early stages of acute MI. If necessary, may be repeated in 60 to 90 minutes.
Children: 0.5 to 1 mg/kg by I.V. bolus; may repeat bolus if needed not to exceed 3 to 5 mg/kg, followed by infusion of 10 to 50 mcg/kg/minute. In advanced cardiac life support, 1 mg/kg I.V. bolus, followed by an infusion of 20 to 50 mcg/kg/minute if needed after defibrillation or cardioversion.

◇ ***Status epilepticus***
Adults: 1 mg/kg I.V. bolus; then, if seizure continues, administer 0.5 mg/kg 2 minutes after first dose; infusion at 30 mcg/kg/minute may be used.

Local anesthesia of skin or mucous membranes, pain from dental extractions, stomatitis
Adults and children: Apply 2% to 5% solution or ointment or 15 ml of Xylocaine Viscous q 3 to 4 hours to oral or nasal mucosa.

Local anesthesia in procedures involving the male or female urethra
Adults: Instill about 15 ml (male) or 3 to 5 ml (female) into urethra.

Pain, burning, or itching caused by burns, sunburn, or skin irritation
Adults and children: Apply topical agent liberally.

Relief of pain associated with post-herpetic neuralgia
Adults: Apply 1 to 3 patches to intact skin, covering most painful area, once daily for up to 12 hours each day. Smaller areas of treatment are recommended in patients who are debilitated or have poor elimination. Excessive dosing by applying patch to larger areas or for longer than recommended wearing time could cause increased absorption of lidocaine and high lidocaine levels, leading to serious adverse effects.

Lidocaine hydrochloride injection used as procedural anesthetic
Adults: Lidocaine with epinephrine, 7 mg/kg (no more than 500 mg total); lidocaine without epinephrine, 4.4 mg/kg (no more than 300 mg total). For continuous epidural or caudal anesthesia, maximum doses shouldn't be administered at intervals less than 90 minutes. Maximum recommended dose in paracervical block is 200 mg total. For I.V. regional anesthesia, dose shouldn't exceed 4 mg/kg. See table below.
Children: Based on age and weight. For I.V. regional anesthesia, use dilute solutions (0.25% to 0.5%) not to exceed 3 mg/kg.

RECOMMENDED DOSAGES

	Injection (without epinephrine)		
Procedure	**Concentration (%)**	**Volume (ml)**	**Total dose (mg)**
Infiltration			
Percutaneous	0.5 or 1	1-60	5-300
I.V. regional	0.5	10-60	50-300
Peripheral nerve blocks			
Brachial	1.5	15-20	225-300
Dental	2	1-5	20-100
Intercostal	1	3	30
Paravertebral	1	3-5	30-50
Pudendal (each side)	1	10	100
Paracervical			
Obstetrical analgesia (each side)	1	10	100
Sympathetic nerve blocks			
Cervical (stellate ganglion)	1	5	50
Lumbar	1	5-10	50-100
Central neural blocks			
Epidural*			
Thoracic	1	20-30	200-300
Lumbar			
Analgesia	1	25-30	250-300
Anesthesia	1.5	15-20	225-300
	2	10-15	200-300
Caudal			
Obstetrical analgesia	1	20-30	200-300
Surgical anesthesia	1.5	15-20	225-300

*Dose determined by number of dermatomes to be anesthetized (2-3 ml/dermatome)

The suggested concentrations and volumes serve only as a guide. Other volumes and concentrations may be used as long as the total maximum recommended dose isn't exceeded.
≡ ***Dosage adjustment.*** Dosages are reduced for children, geriatric patients, debilitated pa-

tients, and patients with cardiac or liver disease.

Pharmacodynamics

Ventricular antiarrhythmic action: One of the oldest antiarrhythmics, lidocaine remains among the most widely used drugs for treating acute ventricular arrhythmias. Lidocaine is the drug of choice to treat ventricular tachycardia and fibrillation. As a class IB antiarrhythmic, it suppresses automaticity and shortens the effective refractory period and action potential duration of His-Purkinje fibers and suppresses spontaneous ventricular depolarization during diastole. Therapeutic levels don't significantly affect conductive atrial tissue and AV conduction.

Unlike quinidine and procainamide, lidocaine doesn't significantly alter hemodynamics when given in usual doses. Drug seems to act preferentially on diseased or ischemic myocardial tissue; exerting its effects on the conduction system, it inhibits reentry mechanisms and halts ventricular arrhythmias.

Local anesthetic action: As a local anesthetic, lidocaine acts to block initiation and conduction of nerve impulses by decreasing the permeability of the nerve cell membrane to sodium ions.

Pharmacokinetics

Absorption: Absorbed after oral administration; however, a significant first-pass effect occurs in the liver and only about 35% of drug reaches the systemic circulation. Oral doses high enough to achieve therapeutic blood levels result in an unacceptable toxicity, probably from high levels of lidocaine.

Distribution: Distributed widely throughout the body; it has a high affinity for adipose tissue. After I.V. bolus administration, an early, rapid decline in plasma levels occurs; this is associated mainly with distribution into highly perfused tissues, such as the kidneys, lungs, liver, and heart, followed by a slower elimination phase in which metabolism and redistribution into skeletal muscle and adipose tissue occur. The first (early) distribution phase occurs rapidly, calling for initiation of a constant infusion after an initial bolus dose. Distribution volume declines in patients with liver or hepatic disease, resulting in toxic levels with usual doses. About 60% to 80% of circulating drug is bound to plasma proteins. Usual therapeutic drug level is 1.5 to 5 mcg/ml. Although toxicity may occur within this range, levels greater than 5 mcg/ml are considered toxic and warrant dosage reduction.

Metabolism: Metabolized in the liver to two active metabolites. Less than 10% of a parenteral dose escapes metabolism and reaches the kidneys unchanged. Metabolism is affected by hepatic blood flow, which may decrease after MI and with heart failure. Liver disease also may limit metabolism.

Excretion: Half-life undergoes a biphasic process, with an initial phase of 7 to 30 minutes followed by a terminal half-life of 1½ to 2 hours. Elimination half-life may be prolonged in patients with heart failure or liver disease. Continuous infusions longer than 24 hours also may cause an apparent half-life increase.

Route	Onset	Peak	Duration
I.V.	Immediate	Immediate	10-20 min
I.M.	5-15 min	10 min	2 hr
Peripheral injection	Variable	Variable	Variable
Topical	30-60 sec	Unknown	Variable

Contraindications and precautions

Contraindicated in patients with hypersensitivity to amide-type local anesthetics, Stokes-Adams syndrome, Wolff-Parkinson-White syndrome, and severe degrees of SA, AV, or intraventricular block in absence of artificial pacemaker. Also contraindicated in patients with inflammation or infection in puncture region, septicemia, severe hypertension, spinal deformities, and neurologic disorders.

Use cautiously in geriatric patients; in patients with renal or hepatic disease, complete or second-degree heart block, sinus bradycardia, or heart failure; and in those weighing less than 110 lb.

Interactions

Drug-drug. *Beta blockers:* Enhanced sympathomimetic effects. Don't use with lidocaine and epinephrine.

Butyrophenones, phenothiazines: May reduce or reverse the pressor effects of epinephrine. Patient requires monitoring for drug effect.

Cimetidine or beta blockers: May cause lidocaine toxicity from reduced hepatic clearance. Avoid use together.

Cyclic antidepressants and MAO inhibitors: Prolonged and severe hypertension when lidocaine with epinephrine is used. Avoid use together.

Succinylcholine and high-dose lidocaine: May increase neuromuscular effects of succinylcholine. Use together cautiously.

Other antiarrhythmic agents, including phenytoin, procainamide, propranolol, and quinidine: May cause additive or antagonist effects as well as additive toxicity. Avoid use together.

Vasopressor drugs and ergot-type oxytoxic drugs: Severe, persistent hypertension or CVA. Avoid using lidocaine with epinephrine.

Drug-herb. *Pareira:* May add to or potentiate the effects of neuromuscular blockade. Avoid use together.

Effects on diagnostic tests

Because I.M. lidocaine therapy may increase CK levels, isoenzyme tests should be performed for differential diagnosis of acute MI.

Adverse reactions

CNS: anxiety, nervousness, lethargy, somnolence, paresthesia, muscle twitching; *confusion, tremor, stupor, restlessness, light-headedness,* hallucinations, *seizures* (with systemic form); apprehension, unconsciousness, confusion, tremors, stupor, restlessness, slurred speech, euphoria, depression, light-headedness, ***seizures*** (with topical use).
CV: bradycardia, CARDIAC ARREST; *hypotension, **new or worsened arrhythmias*** (with systemic form); hypotension, myocardial depression, ***arrhythmias*** (with topical use), edema, ***fatal episodes of bradycardia, asystole***.
EENT: *tinnitus, blurred or double vision* (with systemic form); tinnitus, blurred or double vision (with topical use).
GI: nausea, vomiting (with topical use).
Respiratory: ***respiratory arrest, status asthmaticus.***
Skin: dermatologic reactions, sensitization, diaphoresis (with topical use), rash (with topical use).
Other: ***anaphylaxis;*** soreness at injection site, sensation of cold (with systemic form).

Overdose and treatment

Clinical effects of overdose include signs and symptoms of CNS toxicity, such as seizures or respiratory depression, and CV toxicity (as indicated by hypotension).

Treatment includes general supportive measures and drug discontinuation. A patent airway should be maintained and other respiratory support measures carried out immediately. Diazepam or thiopental may be given to treat any seizures. To treat significant hypotension, vasopressors (including dopamine and norepinephrine) may be administered.

Clinical considerations

- Drug has been used investigationally to treat refractory status epilepticus.
- Don't administer lidocaine with epinephrine (for local anesthesia) to treat arrhythmias. Use solutions with epinephrine cautiously in CV disorders and in body areas with limited blood supply (ears, nose, fingers, toes).
- Patient receiving lidocaine I.M. will show a sevenfold increase in serum CK level. Such CK originates in skeletal muscle, not the heart. Test isoenzyme levels to confirm MI, if using I.M. route.
- When larger volumes are required for local anesthesia, use a solution containing epinephrine.
- For I.V. regional anesthesia, use 50 ml Xylocaine 0.5% injection.
- Preparations used for epidural, spinal, or caudal anesthesia should contain no bacteriostatic agents.
- I.V. infusions are prepared by adding 1 g of lidocaine (using 25 ml of a commercially available 4% or 5 ml of a 20% injection) to 1 L of 5% dextrose injection to provide a concentration of 1 mg/ml. Alternatively, 0.2% or 0.4% is available. In fluid-restricted patients, an 8 mg/ml concentration may be used. Don't add to blood transfusion assemblies.
- In many severely ill patients, seizures may be the first sign of toxicity. However, severe reactions are usually preceded by somnolence, confusion, and paresthesia. Regard all signs and symptoms of toxicity as serious, and promptly reduce dosage or discontinue therapy. Continued infusion could lead to seizures and coma. Give oxygen through nasal cannula, if not contraindicated. Keep oxygen and CPR equipment handy.
- Doses of up to 400 mg I.M. have been advocated in prehospital phase of acute MI.

□ ***ALERT*** Don't use solutions containing preservatives for spinal, epidural, or caudal block or I.V. injection.

□ ***ALERT*** Lidocaine injections additive syringes and single-use vials containing 40, 100, or 200 mg/ml are for I.V. infusion preparation and must be diluted before use.

- With epidural use, inject a 2- to 5-ml test dose at least 5 minutes before giving total dose to check for intravascular or subarachnoid injection. Motor paralysis and extensive sensory anesthesia indicate subarachnoid injection.
- Discard partially used vials containing no preservatives.

Therapeutic monitoring

- Patient requires constant cardiac monitoring when receiving I.V. lidocaine. Use infusion pump or microdrip system and timer to monitor infusion precisely. Never exceed infusion rate of 4 mg/minute, if possible. A faster rate greatly increases risk of toxicity.
- Recommend monitoring vital signs and serum electrolyte, BUN, and creatinine levels.
- Recommend monitoring ECG constantly if administering drug I.V., especially in patients with liver disease, heart failure, hypoxia, respiratory depression, hypovolemia, or shock, because these conditions may affect drug metabolism, excretion, or distribution volume, predisposing patient to drug toxicity.
- Recommend monitoring for signs of excessive depression of cardiac conductivity (such as sinus node dysfunction, PR interval prolongation, QRS complex widening, and appearance or exacerbation of arrhythmias). If they occur, reduce dosage or discontinue drug.
- Therapeutic serum levels range from 2 to 5 mcg/ml.

Special populations

Pediatric patients. Safety and efficacy in children haven't been established. Use of an I.M. autoinjector device isn't recommended.
Geriatric patients. Because of prevalence of concurrent disease states and declining organ system function in geriatric patients, use conservative lidocaine doses.

lindane (gamma benzene hexachloride)

G-well, Kwell, Scabene

Pharmacologic classification: chlorinated hydrocarbon insecticide
Therapeutic classification: scabicide, pediculicide
Pregnancy risk category B

How supplied

Available by prescription only
Lotion: 1%
Shampoo: 1%

Indications and dosages

Note: In no case should more than 2 oz be used by one person in one application.
Scabies
Adults and children: Apply a thin layer of cream or lotion and gently massage it on all skin surfaces, moving from the neck to the toes. For adults and children age 6 and older, 30 to 60 ml; for children under age 6, 30 ml. After 8 to 12 hours, remove drug by bathing and scrubbing well. Treatment may be repeated after 1 week if needed.
Pediculosis
Adults and children: Apply shampoo to clean, dry, affected area and wait 4 minutes. Then add a small amount of water and lather for 4 to 5 minutes; rinse thoroughly. Comb hair to remove nits. Treatment may be repeated after 1 week if needed.

Pharmacodynamics

Scabicide and pediculicide actions: Lindane is toxic to the parasitic mite *Sarcoptes scabiei* and its eggs, and to lice (*Pediculus capitis, Pediculus corporis*, and *Phthirus pubis*). Drug is absorbed through the organism's exoskeleton, causing death.

Pharmacokinetics

Absorption: About 10% of topical dose may be absorbed in 24 hours.
Distribution: Stored in body fat.
Metabolism: Metabolism occurs in the liver.
Excretion: Excreted in urine and feces.

Route	Onset	Peak	Duration
Topical	190 min	Unknown	Unknown

Contraindications and precautions

Contraindicated in patients hypersensitive to drug, with raw or inflamed skin, with seizure disorders, and in premature infants. Use cautiously in young patients (including infants).

Interactions

None reported. However, avoid using together with other oils or ointments.

Effects on diagnostic tests

None reported.

Adverse reactions

CNS: *dizziness, **seizures**.*
Skin: *irritation* (with repeated use).

Overdose and treatment

Accidental ingestion may cause extreme CNS toxicity; symptoms include CNS stimulation, dizziness, and seizures. To treat lindane ingestion, empty stomach by appropriate measures (emesis or lavage); follow with saline catharsis (do not use oil laxative). Treat seizures with pentobarbital, phenobarbital, or diazepam, as needed.

Clinical considerations

- Make sure patient's body is clean (scrubbed well) and dry before application.
- Avoid applying drug to acutely inflamed skin or raw, weeping surfaces.
- Avoid contact with face, eyes, mucous membranes, and urethral meatus.
- Place hospitalized patient in isolation with linen-handling precautions.

Therapeutic monitoring

- Recommend monitoring for need of retreatment.
- Recommend monitoring for signs of systemic toxicity.

Special populations

Pregnant patients. The Centers for Disease Control and Prevention (CDC) states that lindane isn't for use in pregnant women.
Breast-feeding patients. Because drug is secreted in breast milk in low levels, an alternative method of feeding may be used for 4 days if there's any concern.
Pediatric patients. Use cautiously, especially in infants and small children, who are much more susceptible to CNS toxicity. Discourage thumb-sucking in children using lindane, to prevent ingestion of drug. The CDC recommends other scabicide therapies for children under age 10.
Geriatric patients. Use reduced dose in geriatric patients because of their increased susceptibility to percutaneous absorption.

Patient counseling

- Explain correct use of drug.
- The CDC recommends that bathing before application be avoided because toxicity (such as seizures) has been associated with such application. If the patient does bathe, the skin should be allowed to dry and cool completely before application of lotion. Before application of shampoo, the hair should be washed with plain shampoo and dried.
- Warn patient that itching may continue for several weeks, even if treatment is effective, especially in scabies infestation.
- If drug contacts eyes, tell patient to flush with water and call for further instructions. He should avoid inhaling vapor.
- Explain that reapplication usually isn't necessary unless live mites are found; advise reapplication if drug is accidentally washed off, but caution against overuse.
- Tell patient he may use drug to clean combs and brushes, and to wash them thoroughly afterward; advise patient that all clothing and bed linen that may have been contaminated by him within the past 2 days should be machine-washed in hot water and dried in hot dryer or dry cleaned to avoid reinfestation or transmission of organism.
- Discourage repeated use of drug, which may irritate skin and cause systemic toxicity.
- Caution patient to avoid using with other oils or ointments.
- Advise patient that family and close contacts, including sexual contacts, should be treated at the same time.
- Warn patient not to use if open wounds, cuts, or sores are present on scalp or groin, unless directed by his doctor.

liothyronine sodium (T_3)

Cytomel, Triostat

Pharmacologic classification: thyroid hormone
Therapeutic classification: thyroid hormone replacement
Pregnancy risk category A

How supplied

Available by prescription only
Tablets: 5 mcg, 25 mcg, 50 mcg
Injection: 10 mcg/ml

Indications and dosages

Congenital hypothyroidism
Children: 5 mcg P.O. daily, increased by 5 mcg q 3 to 4 days until desired response occurs.
Myxedema
Adults: Initially, 5 mcg daily, increased by 5 to 10 mcg q 1 to 2 weeks. Maintenance dosage is 50 to 100 mcg daily.
Myxedema coma, precoma
Adults: Initially, 25 to 50 mcg I.V.; reassess after 4 to 12 hours, then switch to P.O. as soon as possible. Patients with known or suspected cardiac disease should receive 10 to 20 mcg I.V.
Nontoxic goiter
Adults: Initially, 5 mcg P.O. daily; may be increased by 5 to 10 mcg daily at intervals of 1 to 2 weeks until dosage of 25 mcg daily is reached. Thereafter, dosage may be increased by 12.5 to 25 mcg daily at intervals of 1 to 2 weeks until desired response is noted. Usual maintenance dosage is 75 mcg daily.
Adults older than 65: Initially, 5 mcg P.O. daily, increased by 5-mcg increments q 1 to 2 weeks until desired response is obtained
Children: Initially, 5 mcg P.O. daily, increased by 5-mcg increments at weekly intervals until desired response is achieved.
Thyroid hormone replacement
Adults: Initially, 25 mcg P.O. daily, increased by 12.5 to 25 mcg q 1 to 2 weeks until satisfactory response is achieved. Usual maintenance dosage is 25 to 75 mcg daily.
Liothyronine suppression test to differentiate hyperthyroidism from euthyroidism
Adults: 75 to 100 mcg daily for 7 days.

Pharmacodynamics

Thyroid hormone replacement: Liothyronine is usually a second-line drug in the treatment of hypothyroidism, myxedema, and cretinism. This component of thyroid hormone affects protein and carbohydrate metabolism, promotes gluconeogenesis, increases the utilization and mobilization of glycogen stores, stimulates protein synthesis, and regulates cell growth and differentiation. The major effect of liothyronine is to increase the metabolic rate of tissue. It may be most useful in syndromes of thyroid hormone resistance.

Pharmacokinetics

Absorption: 95% absorbed from the GI tract.
Distribution: Highly protein-bound. Its distribution hasn't been fully described.
Metabolism: Not fully understood.
Excretion: Half-life is 1 to 2 days.

Route	Onset	Peak	Duration
P.O.	Unknown	2-3 days	3 days
I.V.	Unknown	Unknown	Unknown

Contraindications and precautions

Contraindicated in patients with hypersensitivity to drug, acute MI uncomplicated by hypothyroidism, untreated thyrotoxicosis, or uncorrected adrenal insufficiency.

Use cautiously in the elderly and in patients with angina pectoris, hypertension, ischemia, other CV disorders, renal insufficiency, diabetes, or myxedema.

Interactions

Drug-drug. *Adrenocorticoids or corticotropin:* Altered thyroid status. Changes in liothyronine dosages may require dosage changes in the adrenocorticoid or corticotropin as well.
Anticoagulants: Altered PT and INR. Monitor for potential dosage adjustment.
Tricyclic antidepressants or sympathomimetics: May increase the effects of any or all of these medications, causing coronary insufficiency or arrhythmias. Use together cautiously.
Oral antidiabetic agents or insulin: May affect dosage requirements of these agents. Monitor for potential dosage adjustment.
Estrogens: Increased serum thyroxine-binding globulin levels. May increase liothyronine requirements.

Effects on diagnostic tests

Liothyronine therapy alters radioactive iodine (^{131}I) uptake, protein-bound iodine levels, and liothyronine uptake.

Adverse reactions

CNS: *nervousness, insomnia, tremor,* headache.
CV: *tachycardia,* ***arrhythmias,*** angina pectoris, ***cardiac decompensation and collapse.***
GI: diarrhea, vomiting.
GU: menstrual irregularities.
Metabolic: weight loss.
Musculoskeletal: accelerated bone maturation in infants and children.
Skin: diaphoresis, skin reactions.
Other: heat intolerance.

Overdose and treatment

Signs and symptoms of overdose include signs and symptoms of hyperthyroidism, including weight loss, increased appetite, palpitations, diarrhea, nervousness, abdominal cramps, sweating, headache, tachycardia, increased blood pressure, widened pulse pressure, angina, arrhythmias, tremor, insomnia, heat intolerance, fever, and menstrual irregularities.

Treatment of overdose reduces GI absorption and counteracts central and peripheral effects, primarily sympathetic activity. Use gastric lavage or induce emesis (followed by activated charcoal up to 4 hours after ingestion). If patient is comatose or having seizures, inflate the cuff on an endotracheal tube to prevent aspiration. Treatment may include oxygen and ventilation to maintain respiration. It also should include appropriate measures to treat heart failure and to control fever, hypoglycemia, and fluid loss. Propranolol (or another beta blocker) may be used to counteract many of the effects of increased sympathetic activity. Withdraw liothyronine gradually over 2 to 6 days, then resumed at a lower dose.

Clinical considerations

- Liothyronine may be preferred when rapid effect is desired or when GI absorption or peripheral conversion of levothyroxine to liothyronine is impaired.
- Oral absorption may be reduced in patients with heart failure.
- When switching from levothyroxine to liothyronine, discontinue levothyroxine and start liothyronine at low dosage, increasing in small increments after residual effects of levothyroxine have disappeared. When switching from liothyronine to levothyroxine, start levothyroxine several days before withdrawing liothyronine to avoid relapse.
- Discontinue drug 7 to 10 days before patient undergoes radioactive iodine uptake studies.

Therapeutic monitoring

Monitor thyroid studies to assess response to drug therapy.

Special populations

Breast-feeding patients. Minimal amounts of drug are excreted in breast milk. Use with caution in breast-feeding women.
Pediatric patients. Partial hair loss may occur during first few months of therapy. Reassure child and parents that this is temporary. Infants and children may experience an accelerated rate of bone maturation.
Geriatric patients. Geriatric patients are more sensitive to effects of the drug. In patients over age 60, initial dosage should be 25% lower than usual recommended dosage.

Patient counseling

- Tell patient to report headache, diarrhea, nervousness, excessive sweating, heat intolerance, chest pain, increased pulse rate, or palpitations.
- Advise patient not to store drug in warm, humid areas, such as the bathroom, to prevent deterioration of drug.
- Encourage patient to take drug at the same time each day, preferably in the morning, to avoid insomnia.

liotrix

Thyrolar

Pharmacologic classification: thyroid hormone
Therapeutic classification: thyroid hormone replacement
Pregnancy risk category A

How supplied

Available by prescription only
Tablets: Euthroid-1/2—levothyroxine sodium 30 mcg and liothyronine sodium 7.5 mcg
Euthroid-1—levothyroxine sodium 60 mcg and liothyronine sodium 15 mcg
Euthroid-2—levothyroxine sodium 120 mcg and liothyronine sodium 30 mcg
Euthroid-3—levothyroxine sodium 180 mcg and liothyronine sodium 45 mcg

Thyrolar-1/4—levothyroxine sodium 12.5 mcg and liothyronine sodium 3.1 mcg
Thyrolar-1/2—levothyroxine sodium 25 mcg and liothyronine sodium 6.25 mcg
Thyrolar-1—levothyroxine sodium 50 mcg and liothyronine sodium 12.5 mcg
Thyrolar-2—levothyroxine sodium 100 mcg and liothyronine sodium 25 mcg
Thyrolar-3—levothyroxine sodium 150 mcg and liothyronine sodium 37.5 mcg

Indications and dosages
Hypothyroidism
Dosages must be individualized to approximate deficit in patient's thyroid secretion.
Adults: Initially, 12.5 to 30 mg thyroid equivalent (usually, Thyrolar 1/4, Thyrolar 1/2, or Euthroid 1/2) P.O. daily; increased q 1 to 2 weeks until desired response is achieved.
Children over age 12: 2 to 3 mcg/kg/day.
Children age 6 to 12: 4 to 5 mcg/kg/day.
Children age 1 to 5: 5 to 6 mcg/kg/day.
Children age 6 to 12 months: 6 to 8 mcg/kg/day.
Children under age 6 months: 8 to 10 mcg/kg/day.

Pharmacodynamics
Thyroid stimulant and replacement: Liotrix affects protein and carbohydrate metabolism, promotes gluconeogenesis, increases the use and mobilization of glycogen stores, stimulates protein synthesis, and regulates cell growth and differentiation. The major effect of liotrix is to increase the metabolic rate of tissue. It's used to treat hypothyroidism (myxedema, cretinism, and thyroid hormone deficiency).

Liotrix is a synthetic preparation combining levothyroxine sodium and liothyronine sodium in a 4 to 1 ratio by weight. Such combination products were developed because circulating T_3 was assumed to result from direct release from the thyroid gland. About 80% of T_3 is known to be derived from deiodination of T_4 in peripheral tissues, and patients receiving only T_4 have normal serum T_3 and T_4 levels. Therefore, there's no clinical advantage to combining thyroid agents; such combination could result in excessive T_3 concentration.

Pharmacokinetics
Absorption: About 50% to 95% is absorbed from the GI tract.
Distribution: Distribution isn't fully understood.
Metabolism: Metabolized partially in peripheral tissues (liver, kidneys, and intestines).
Excretion: Excreted partially in feces.

Route	Onset	Peak	Duration
P.O.	Unknown	Unknown	Unknown

Contraindications and precautions
Contraindicated in patients with hypersensitivity to drug, acute MI uncomplicated by hypothyroidism, untreated thyrotoxicosis, or uncorrected adrenal insufficiency.

Use cautiously in the elderly and in patients with impaired renal function, ischemia, angina pectoris, hypertension, other CV disorders, myxedema, and diabetes mellitus or insipidus.

Interactions
Drug-drug. *Adrenocorticoids or corticotropin:* Altered thyroid status. Changes in liothyronine dosages may require dosage changes in the adrenocorticoid or corticotropin as well.
Anticoagulants: Altered PT and INR. Monitor for potential dosage adjustment.
Tricyclic antidepressants or sympathomimetics: Drug may increase the effects of any or all of these medications, causing coronary insufficiency or arrhythmias. Use together cautiously.
Oral antidiabetic agents or insulin: May affect dosage requirements of these agents. Monitor for potential dosage adjustment.
Beta blockers: May decrease the conversion of T_4 to T_3. Recommend monitoring for effect.
Cholestyramine: May delay absorption of T_4. Separate doses by 4 to 5 hours.
Estrogens: Increased serum thyroxine-binding globulin levels. May increase liothyronine requirements.
Hepatic enzyme inducers such as phenytoin: May increase hepatic degradation of T_4, resulting in increased requirements of T_4. Patient requires monitoring for drug effect.
Somatrem: May accelerate epiphyseal maturation. Recommend monitoring for effect.

Effects on diagnostic tests
Liotrix therapy alters radioactive iodine (^{131}I) thyroid uptake, protein-bound iodine levels, and T_3 uptake.

Adverse reactions
CNS: nervousness, insomnia, tremor, headache.
CV: *tachycardia,* ***arrhythmias,*** angina pectoris, ***cardiac decompensation and collapse.***
GI: diarrhea, vomiting.
GU: Menstrual irregularities.
Metabolic: weight loss.
Musculoskeletal: accelerated rate of bone maturation in infants and children.
Skin: diaphoresis, allergic skin reactions.
Other: heat intolerance.

Overdose and treatment
Evidence of overdose includes signs and symptoms of hyperthyroidism, including weight loss, increased appetite, palpitations, nervousness, diarrhea, abdominal cramps, sweating, tachycardia, increased pulse rate and blood pressure, angina, arrhythmias, tremor, headache, insomnia, heat intolerance, fever, and menstrual irregularities.

Treatment requires reduction of GI absorption and efforts to counteract central and peripheral effects, primarily sympathetic activity. Use gastric lavage or induce emesis, then follow with activated charcoal, if less than 4 hours since ingestion. If patient is comatose or having seizures, inflate the cuff on an endotracheal tube to prevent aspiration. Treatment may include oxygen and artificial ventilation as needed to maintain respiration. It should also include appropriate measures to treat heart failure and to control fever, hypoglycemia, and fluid loss. Propranolol (or atenolol, metoprolol, acebutolol, nadolol, or timolol) may be used to combat many of the effects of increased sympathetic activity. Withdraw thyroid therapy gradually over 2 to 6 days, then resume at a lower dosage.

Clinical considerations

- Note that T_4 is drug of choice for hypothyroidism. Hepatic conversion of T_4 to T_3 is usually adequate. Excessive exogenous supplementation of T_3 is usually associated with toxicity.
- The two commercially prepared liotrix brands contain different amounts of each ingredient; don't change from one brand to the other without considering the differences in potency.
- Initiate dosages at lower limits in geriatric patients, in patients with long-standing disease, other endocrinopathies, or CV disease, and in patients with severe hypothyroidism.
- Protect drug from heat and moisture.

Therapeutic monitoring

- Monitor patient's pulse rate and blood pressure.
- Monitor thyroid studies for clinical response to doses given and for dose adjustment.

Special populations

Breast-feeding patients. Minimal amounts of drug are excreted in breast milk. Use with caution in breast-feeding women.
Pediatric patients. Partial hair loss may occur during first few months of therapy. Reassure child and parents that this is temporary. Infants and children may experience accelerated rate of bone maturation.
Geriatric patients. Geriatric patients are more sensitive to effects of drug and may require a lower dosage.

Patient counseling

- Tell patient to report headache, diarrhea, nervousness, excessive sweating, heat intolerance, chest pain, increased pulse rate, or palpitations.
- Advise patient not to store liotrix in warm and humid areas, such as the bathroom.
- Encourage patient to take a single daily dose in the morning to avoid insomnia.

lisinopril

Prinivil, Zestril

Pharmacologic classification: ACE inhibitor
Therapeutic classification: antihypertensive
Pregnancy risk category C (D, second and third trimesters)

How supplied

Available by prescription only
Tablets: 5 mg, 10 mg, 20 mg, 40 mg

Indications and dosages

Mild to severe hypertension
Adults: Initially, 5 to 10 mg P.O. daily. Most patients are well controlled on 20 to 40 mg daily as a single dose. Doses up to 80 mg have been used.
Heart failure
Adults: Initially, 2.5 to 5 mg P.O. daily. Most patients are well controlled on 5 to 20 mg daily as a single dose.
Acute MI
Adults: Initially, 5 mg P.O.; then give 5 mg after 24 hours, 10 mg after 48 hours, and 10 mg daily for 6 weeks.

In patients with acute MI with low systolic blood pressure (less than 120 mm Hg), give 2.5 mg P.O. when treatment is started or during the first 3 days after an infarct. If hypotension occurs, a daily maintenance dosage of 5 mg may be given with temporary reductions to 2.5 mg, if needed.

≡ ***Dosage adjustment.*** In adults with renal failure, initially, 5 mg/day P.O. if creatinine clearance is between 10 and 30 ml/minute, and 2.5 mg/day P.O. if it's less than 10 ml/minute. Dosage may be adjusted upward until blood pressure is controlled or to maximum of 40 mg daily. Dosage for patients with heart failure who have a creatinine clearance of less than 30 ml/minute is 2.5 mg/day P.O. Adults with heart failure, hyponatremia (serum sodium less than 130 mEq/L), or moderate to severe renal impairment (creatinine clearance less than 30 ml/min) should receive an initial dose of 2.5 mg.

Pharmacodynamics

Antihypertensive action: Lisinopril inhibits angiotensin-converting enzyme (ACE), preventing the conversion of angiotensin I to angiotensin II, a potent vasoconstrictor. Reduced formation of angiotensin II decreases peripheral arterial resistance and aldosterone secretion, thereby reducing sodium and water retention and blood pressure.

Pharmacokinetics

Absorption: Variable absorption occurs after oral administration; an average of about 25%

of an oral dose has been absorbed by test subjects.
Distribution: Distributed widely in tissues. Plasma protein binding appears insignificant. Minimal amounts enter the brain. Preclinical studies indicate that it crosses the placenta.
Metabolism: Not metabolized.
Excretion: Excreted unchanged in the urine.

Route	Onset	Peak	Duration
P.O.	1 hr	7 hr	24 hr

Contraindications and precautions
ACE inhibitor therapy shouldn't be initiated in hypotensive patients who are at immediate risk of cardiogenic shock and require I.V. administration of a vasopressor agent.

Contraindicated in patients with hypersensitivity to ACE inhibitors or history of angioedema related to previous treatment with ACE inhibitor, and in patients during the second and third trimesters of pregnancy.

Use cautiously in patients at risk for hyperkalemia or in those with impaired renal function.

Interactions
Drug-drug. *Diuretics:* May cause excessive hypotension. Monitor blood pressure closely.
Indomethacin: May attenuate the hypotensive effect of lisinopril. Monitor patient closely.
Lithium: May increase plasma lithium levels. Monitor lithium levels.
Potassium-sparing diuretics, potassium supplements: May lead to hyperkalemia. Monitor serum potassium levels.
Drug-food. *Potassium-containing salt substitutes:* May lead to hyperkalemia. Monitor serum potassium levels.

Effects on diagnostic tests
None reported.

Adverse reactions
CNS: *dizziness, headache, fatigue, paresthesia.*
CV: hypotension, *orthostatic hypotension,* chest pain.
EENT: *nasal congestion.*
GI: *diarrhea,* nausea, dyspepsia.
GU: impotence.
Hematologic: ***neutropenia, agranulocytopenia.***
Metabolic: hyperkalemia.
Respiratory: *dry, persistent, tickling, nonproductive cough;* dyspnea.
Skin: rash.
Other: ***angioedema, anaphylaxis.***

Overdose and treatment
The most likely sign of overdose would be hypotension. Recommended treatment is I.V. infusion of normal saline solution.

Clinical considerations
Consider the recommendations relevant to all ACE inhibitors as well as the following:
- Drug absorption is unaffected by food.
- Discontinue diuretics 2 to 3 days before lisinopril therapy to reduce the risk of hypotension.
- If drug doesn't adequately control blood pressure, diuretics may be added.
- Lower dosage is necessary in patients with impaired renal function.
- Initiate drug therapy in the hospital for heart failure patients because of the risk of severe hypotension.
- Drug shouldn't be used after acute MI in patients at risk for severe hemodynamic deterioration or cardiogenic shock.
- Beneficial effects of lisinopril may require several weeks of therapy.

Therapeutic monitoring
- Review WBC and differential counts before treatment, every 2 weeks for 3 months, and periodically thereafter.
- Recommend monitoring patient's peak and trough blood pressures to assess clinical response.

Special populations
Breast-feeding patients. Drug may be distributed into breast milk, but effect on infant is unknown; use with caution in breast-feeding women.
Pediatric patients. Safety and efficacy in children haven't been established; use only if potential benefits outweigh risks.
Geriatric patients. Geriatric patients may require lower doses due to impaired drug clearance. They may also be more sensitive to hypotensive effects of drug.

Patient counseling
- Tell patient to report light-headedness, especially in first few days of treatment, so dose can be adjusted; signs of infection, such as sore throat or fever, because drug may decrease WBC count; facial swelling or difficulty breathing, because drug may cause angioedema; and loss of taste, which may necessitate discontinuation of drug.
- Advise patient to avoid sudden postural changes to minimize orthostatic hypotension.
- Warn patient to seek medical approval before taking OTC cold preparations.
- Instruct patient to avoid potassium-containing salt substitutes.
- Warn women of childbearing age of the need to avoid pregnancy during therapy.
- Instruct patient to report any adverse events including persistent dry cough.

lithium carbonate

Carbolith*, Duralith*, Eskalith, Eskalith CR, Lithane, Lithizine*, Lithobid, Lithonate, Lithotabs

lithium citrate

Cibalith-S

Pharmacologic classification: alkali metal
Therapeutic classification: antimanic, antipsychotic
Pregnancy risk category D

How supplied

Available by prescription only
lithium carbonate
Capsules: 150 mg, 300 mg, 600 mg
Tablets: 300 mg
Tablets (sustained-release): 300 mg, 450 mg
Tablets (film-coated): 300 mg
Tablets (extended-release, film-coated): 300 mg
lithium citrate
Syrup (sugarless): 300 mg/5 ml (with 0.3% alcohol)

Indications and dosages

Prevention or control of mania; prevention of depression in patients with bipolar illness
Adults: For acute episodes: 1.8 g or 30 ml of lithium citrate P.O. daily in two or three divided doses or 20 to 30 mg/kg/day in two or three divided doses to maintain lithium levels at 1 to 1.5 mEq/L.
≡ ***Dosage adjustment.*** In geriatric patients, 600 to 900 mg daily.
Adults: For maintenance dosage: 900 mg to 1.2 g or 15 to 20 ml of oral solution P.O. daily in two to four divided doses to maintain serum lithium concentration of 0.6 to 1.2 mEq/L. Usual maintenance dosage doesn't exceed 2.4 g daily.
◊ ***Major depression,*** ◊ ***schizoaffective disorder,*** ◊ ***schizophrenic disorder,*** ◊ ***alcohol dependence***
Adults: 300 mg lithium carbonate P.O. t.i.d. or q.i.d.
◊ ***Apparent mixed bipolar disorder in children***
Children: Initially, 15 to 60 mg/kg or 0.5 to 1.5 g/m^2 lithium carbonate P.O. daily in three divided doses. Don't exceed usual adult dosage. Adjust dosage based on patient response and serum lithium levels; usual dosage range is 150 to 300 mg daily in divided doses to maintain lithium levels of 0.5 to 1.2 mEq/L.
◊ ***Chemotherapy-induced neutropenia in children and patients with AIDS receiving zidovudine***
Adults and children: 300 to 1,000 mg P.O. daily.

Pharmacodynamics

Antimanic action: Lithium is thought to exert its antipsychotic and antimanic effects by competing with other cations for exchange at the sodium-potassium ion pump, thus altering cation exchange at the tissue level. It also inhibits adenyl cyclase, reducing intracellular levels of cAMP and, to a lesser extent, cyclic guanosine monophosphate (cGMP).

Pharmacokinetics

Absorption: Rate and extent of absorption vary with dosage form; absorption is complete within 6 hours of oral administration from conventional tablets and capsules.
Distribution: Distributed widely into the body, including breast milk; levels in thyroid gland, bone, and brain tissue exceed serum levels. Steady-state serum level achieved in 12 hours: therapeutic effect begins in 5 to 10 days and is maximal within 3 weeks. Therapeutic and toxic serum levels and therapeutic effects show good correlation. Therapeutic range is 0.6 to 1.2 mEq/L; adverse reactions increase as level reaches 1.5 to 2 mEq/L; such levels may be necessary in acute mania. Toxicity usually occurs at levels above 2 mEq/L.
Metabolism: Not metabolized.
Excretion: Excreted 95% unchanged in urine; about 50% to 80% of a given dose is excreted within 24 hours. Level of renal function determines elimination rate.

Route	Onset	Peak	Duration
P.O.	Unknown	½ to 3 hr	Unknown

Contraindications and precautions

Contraindicated if therapy can't be closely monitored and during pregnancy. Use cautiously in the elderly; in patients with thyroid disease, seizure disorders, renal or CV disease, severe dehydration or debilitation, or sodium depletion; and in those receiving neuroleptics, neuromuscular blockers, and diuretics.

Interactions

Drug-drug. *Antacids and other drugs containing aminophylline, caffeine, calcium, sodium, or theophylline:* May increase lithium excretion by renal competition for elimination, thus decreasing therapeutic effect of lithium. Monitor patient closely.
Carbamazepine, mazindol, methyldopa, phenytoin, tetracyclines: May increase lithium toxicity. Monitor patient closely.
Chlorpromazine: Decreased effects of chlorpromazine. Avoid administering together.
Electroconvulsive therapy (ECT): Acute neurotoxicity with delirium has occurred in patients receiving lithium and. ECT. Reduce lithium dosage or withdraw before ECT.
Fluoxetine: Increases lithium serum levels. Monitor patient closely.

Haloperidol: May result in severe encephalopathy characterized by confusion, tremors, extrapyramidal effects, and weakness. Use this combination with caution.
Indomethacin, phenylbutazone, piroxicam, other NSAIDs: Decreased renal excretion of lithium. May require a 30% reduction in lithium dosage.
Neuromuscular blocking agents, such as atracurium, pancuronium, and succinylcholine: May potentiate the effects of these drugs. Monitor patient closely.
Sympathomimetic agents, especially norepinephrine: Lithium may interfere with pressor effects of these drugs. Monitor patient closely.
Thiazide diuretics: May decrease renal excretion and enhance lithium toxicity. Diuretic dosage may need to be reduced by 30%.
Drug-food. *Dietary sodium:* May alter renal elimination of lithium. Increased sodium intake may increase elimination of drug; decreased intake may decrease elimination. Monitor serum lithium levels.
Drug-herb. *Parsley:* May promote or produce serotonin syndrome. Avoid use together.
Psyllium seed: Inhibited GI absorption. Avoid use together.
Drug-lifestyle. *Caffeine:* Interferes with effectiveness of drug. Advise patient to avoid caffeine use.

Effects on diagnostic tests
Drug causes false-positive test results on thyroid function tests.

Adverse reactions
CNS: tremors, drowsiness, headache, confusion, restlessness, dizziness, psychomotor retardation, lethargy, *coma,* blackouts, ***epileptiform seizures,*** EEG changes, worsened organic mental syndrome, impaired speech, ataxia, muscle weakness, incoordination.
CV: *reversible ECG changes,* ***arrhythmias,*** hypotension, ***bradycardia, peripheral vascular collapse (rare).***
EENT: tinnitus, blurred vision.
GI: dry mouth, metallic taste, nausea, vomiting, anorexia, diarrhea, *thirst,* abdominal pain, flatulence, indigestion.
GU: *polyuria,* glycosuria, renal toxicity with long-term use, decreased creatinine clearance, albuminuria.
Hematologic: *leukocytosis with WBC count of 14,000 to 18,000/mm^3* (reversible); elevated neutrophil count.
Metabolic: goiter, transient hyperglycemia, hypothyroidism (lowered T_3, T_4, and protein-bound iodine, but elevated ^{131}I uptake), hyponatremia.
Skin: pruritus, rash, diminished or absent sensation, drying and thinning of hair, psoriasis, acne, alopecia.
Other: ankle and wrist edema.

Overdose and treatment
Vomiting and diarrhea occur within 1 hour of acute ingestion (induce vomiting in noncomatose patients if it is not spontaneous). Death has occurred in patients ingesting 10 to 60 g of lithium; patients have ingested 6 g with minimal toxic effects. Serum lithium levels above 3.4 mEq/L are potentially fatal.

Overdose with chronic lithium ingestion may follow altered pharmacokinetics, drug interactions, or volume or sodium depletion; sedation, confusion, hand tremors, joint pain, ataxia, muscle stiffness, increased deep tendon reflexes, visual changes, and nystagmus may occur. Symptoms may progress to coma, movement abnormalities, tremors, seizures, and CV collapse.

Treatment is symptomatic and supportive; closely monitor vital signs. If emesis isn't feasible, treat with gastric lavage. Monitor fluid and electrolyte balance; correct sodium depletion with normal saline solution. Institute hemodialysis if serum level is above 3 mEq/L, and in severely symptomatic patients unresponsive to fluid and electrolyte correction, or if urine output decreases significantly. Serum rebound of tissue lithium stores (from high volume distribution) commonly occurs after dialysis and may necessitate prolonged or repeated hemodialysis. Peritoneal dialysis may help but is less effective.

Clinical considerations
- Lithium is used investigationally to increase WBC count in patients undergoing cancer chemotherapy. It has also been used investigationally to treat cluster headaches, aggression, organic brain syndrome, and tardive dyskinesia. Drug has been used to treat SIADH.
- EEG changes include diffuse slowing, widening of frequency spectrum, potentiation, and disorganization of background rhythm.
- Shake syrup formulation before administration.
- Discontinue drug before ECT therapy.
- Administer drug with food or milk to reduce GI upset.
- Expect lag of 1 to 3 weeks before beneficial effects of drug are noticed. Other psychotropic medications (such as chlorpromazine) may be necessary during interim period.
- Adjust fluid and salt ingestion to compensate if excessive loss occurs through protracted sweating or diarrhea. Patient should have fluid intake of 2,500 to 3,000 ml daily and a balanced diet with adequate salt intake.
- Lithane tablets contain tartrazine, a dye that may precipitate an allergic reaction in certain individuals, particularly asthmatics sensitive to aspirin.

Therapeutic monitoring
- Monitor baseline ECG, thyroid and renal studies, and electrolyte levels. Monitor lithi-

um blood levels 8 to 12 hours after first dose, usually before morning dose, two or three times weekly the first month, then weekly to monthly on maintenance therapy.

Determination of serum drug levels is crucial to safe use of drug. Don't use drug in patients who can't have regular serum drug level checks. Be sure patient or responsible family member can comply with instructions.

When lithium blood levels are below 1.5 mEq/L, adverse reactions usually remain mild.

Monitor fluid intake and output, especially when surgery is scheduled.

Observe patient for signs of edema or sudden weight gain.

Outpatient follow-up of thyroid and renal functions should occur every 6 to 12 months. Thyroid should be palpated to check for enlargement.

Check urine for specific gravity below 1.015, which may indicate diabetes insipidus.

Drug may alter glucose tolerance in diabetic patients. Monitor blood glucose levels closely.

Monitor serum levels and signs of impending toxicity.

Monitor drug dosing carefully when patient's initial manic symptoms begin to subside because the ability to tolerate high serum lithium levels decreases as symptoms resolve. Dose must be adjusted based upon lithium level, patient tolerance, and clinical response.

Special populations

Pregnant patients. Lithium has been used during pregnancy in life-threatening situations and severe disease when other therapies couldn't be used or were ineffective. Fetal toxicity includes increased risk of cardiovascular abnormalities, Down syndrome, clubfoot, meningomyelocele, transient hypothyroidism with goiter, transient nephrogenic diabetes insipidus, muscular hypotonia, and apnea.

Breast-feeding patients. Lithium level in breast milk is 33% to 50% that of maternal serum level. Women should avoid breast-feeding during treatment with lithium.

Pediatric patients. Drug isn't recommended for use in children under age 12.

Geriatric patients. Geriatric patients are more susceptible to chronic overdose and toxic effects, especially dyskinesias. These patients usually respond to a lower dosage.

Patient counseling

Explain that lithium has a narrow therapeutic margin of safety. A serum drug level that's even slightly high can be dangerous.

Warn patient and family to watch for signs of toxicity (diarrhea, vomiting, dehydration, drowsiness, muscle weakness, tremor, fever, and ataxia) and to expect transient nausea, polyuria, thirst, and discomfort during first few days. If toxic symptoms occur, tell patient to withhold one dose and report symptoms promptly.

Warn ambulatory patient to avoid activities that require alertness and good psychomotor coordination until CNS response to drug is determined.

Advise patient to maintain adequate water intake and adequate—but not excessive—salt in diet.

Explain importance of regular follow-up visits to measure lithium serum levels.

Tell patient to avoid large amounts of caffeine, which will interfere with effectiveness of drug.

Advise patient to seek medical approval before initiating weight-loss program.

Tell patient not to switch brands of lithium or take other prescription or OTC drugs without medical approval. Different brands may not provide equivalent effect.

Tell patient to take drug with food or milk.

Warn patient against stopping this drug abruptly.

Tell patient to explain to close friend or family members the signs of lithium overdose, in case emergency aid is needed.

Instruct patient to carry identification and instruction card with toxicity and emergency information.

lomefloxacin hydrochloride

Maxaquin

Pharmacologic classification: fluoroquinolone
Therapeutic classification: broad-spectrum antibiotic
Pregnancy risk category C

How supplied

Available by prescription only
Tablets: 400 mg

Indications and dosages

***Acute bacterial exacerbations of chronic bronchitis caused by* Haemophilus influenzae *or* Moraxella (Branhamella) catarrhalis**
Adults: 400 mg P.O. daily for 10 days.

***Uncomplicated urinary tract infections (cystitis) caused by* Escherichia coli, Klebsiella pneumoniae, Proteus mirabilis, *or* Staphylococcus saprophyticus**
Adults: 400 mg P.O. daily for 10 days.

***Complicated urinary tract infections caused by* E. coli, K. pneumoniae, P. mirabilis, *or* Pseudomonas aeruginosa*; possibly effective against infections caused by* Citrobacter diversus *or* Enterobacter cloacae**
Adults: 400 mg P.O. daily for 14 days.

Prophylaxis of infections after transurethral surgical procedures
Adults: 400 mg P.O. 2 to 6 hours before surgery as a single dose.
◇ ***Uncomplicated gonorrhea***
Adults: 400 mg P.O. as a single dose.
≡ ***Dosage adjustment.*** In adults with renal failure and creatinine clearance of 10 to 40 ml/minute/1.73 m^2, give loading dose of 400 mg P.O. on first day, followed by 200 mg P.O. daily for duration of therapy. Periodic determination of blood drug levels is recommended. Hemodialysis removes negligible amounts of drug.

Pharmacodynamics
Antibiotic action: Lomefloxacin inhibits bacterial DNA gyrase, an enzyme necessary for bacterial replication. Drug is bactericidal.

Pharmacokinetics
Absorption: Rapidly absorbed from the GI tract; absolute bioavailability is 95% to 98%. Food impairs absorption by reducing total amount absorbed and slowing absorption rate.
Distribution: Only 10% is bound to plasma proteins.
Metabolism: About 10% is metabolized in the liver.
Excretion: Mostly excreted unchanged in urine; about 10% is excreted as metabolites. Solubility in urine is pH dependent. About 10% of a dose appears unchanged in the feces. Half-life is 8 hours. Steady state is reached after 2 days of once-daily therapy.

Route	Onset	Peak	Duration
P.O.	Unknown	1½ hr	Unknown

Contraindications and precautions
Contraindicated in patients with hypersensitivity to drug or other fluoroquinolones. Use cautiously in patients with known or suspected CNS disorders, such as seizures or cerebral arteriosclerosis.

Interactions
Drug-drug. *Antacids, minerals, and sucralfate:* Bind with lomefloxacin in the GI tract and impair its absorption. Give antacids and sucralfate no less than 4 hours before or 2 hours after lomefloxacin.
Cimetidine: Other quinolones show substantially increased plasma half-lives. Monitor for toxicity.
Cyclosporine and warfarin: Other quinolones also increase the effects or serum levels of these drugs. Lomefloxacin hasn't been tested for these effects. Monitor for toxicity.
Probenecid: Decreases excretion of lomefloxacin. Don't administer together.
Drug-lifestyle. *Sun exposure:* Photosensitivity reactions may occur. Advise patient to take precautions.

Effects on diagnostic tests
None reported.

Adverse reactions
CNS: *dizziness, headache,* abnormal dreams, fatigue, malaise, asthenia, agitation, anorexia, anxiety, confusion, depersonalization, depression, increased appetite, insomnia, nervousness, somnolence, ***seizures, coma,*** hyperkinesia, tremor, vertigo, paresthesia.
CV: flushing, hypotension, hypertension, edema, syncope, ***arrhythmias,*** tachycardia, ***bradycardia,*** extrasystoles, cyanosis, angina pectoris, ***MI, cardiac failure, pulmonary embolism,*** cerebrovascular disorder, cardiomyopathy, phlebitis.
EENT: epistaxis, abnormal vision, conjunctivitis, eye pain, earache, tinnitus, tongue discoloration, taste perversion.
GI: *diarrhea, nausea,* thirst, dry mouth, pseudomembranous colitis, abdominal pain, dyspepsia, vomiting, flatulence, constipation, inflammation, dysphagia, bleeding.
GU: dysuria, hematuria, anuria, leukorrhea, epididymitis, orchitis, vaginitis, vaginal moniliasis, intermenstrual bleeding, perineal pain.
Hematologic: thrombocythemia, ***thrombocytopenia,*** lymphadenopathy, increased fibrinolysis.
Hepatic: elevated liver enzymes.
Metabolic: hypoglycemia.
Musculoskeletal: leg cramps, arthralgia, myalgia.
Respiratory: dyspnea, ***bronchospasm,*** respiratory disorder or infection, increased sputum, stridor.
Skin: pruritus, skin disorder, skin exfoliation, eczema, increased diaphoresis, rash, urticaria, *photosensitivity.*
Other: ***anaphylaxis,*** chest or back pain, chills, allergic reaction, facial edema, flulike symptoms, decreased heat tolerance, gout.

Overdose and treatment
Treatment of overdose includes emptying the stomach by induced vomiting or gastric lavage, observing patient closely, and providing supportive care. Drug isn't significantly removed by hemodialysis or peritoneal dialysis.

Clinical considerations
- Drug shouldn't be used for empiric treatment of acute exacerbations of chronic bronchitis when suspected pathogen is *Streptococcus pneumoniae* because this organism demonstrates resistance to drug. Because blood drug levels don't readily exceed the minimum inhibitory concentration against *Pseudomonas aeruginosa,* drug shouldn't be used to treat bacteremia caused by this organism, but it has been used successfully to treat complicated urinary tract *Pseudomonas* infections.
- Achilles and other tendon ruptures have been reported. Discontinue medication if pain, inflammation or tendon rupture occurs.

Therapeutic monitoring
Monitor renal and hepatic function tests and CBC in patients with impairments.

Special populations
Breast-feeding patients. It's unknown if drug is excreted in breast milk. Because of risk of serious adverse effects on the infant, a decision should be made whether to discontinue the drug or breast-feeding.
Pediatric patients. Because studies have shown that quinolones can cause arthropathy in immature animals, avoid using these drugs in children.

Patient counseling
- Remind patient to take all of drug prescribed, even after he feels better.
- Advise patient to take drug on an empty stomach.
- Tell patient to avoid hazardous tasks that require alertness, such as driving, until adverse CNS effects of drug are known.
- Instruct patient to avoid sunlight or artificial ultraviolet light, and to call immediately if signs of photosensitivity occur.
- Caution patient to avoid mineral supplements or vitamins with iron or minerals within the 2-hour period before or after taking drug.
- Tell patient that sucralfate or antacids containing magnesium or aluminum shouldn't be taken within 4 hours before or 2 hours after taking drug.
- Instruct patient to drink fluids liberally.

lomustine (CCNU)
CeeNU, CeeNU Dose Pack

Pharmacologic classification: alkylating agent, nitrosourea (cell cycle-phase nonspecific)
Therapeutic classification: antineoplastic
Pregnancy risk category D

How supplied
Available by prescription only
Capsules: 10 mg, 40 mg, 100 mg
Dose pack: 2 capsules lomustine 10 mg, 2 capsules lomustine 40 mg, 2 capsules lomustine 100 mg

Indications and dosages
Dosage and indications may vary. Check current literature for recommended protocol. Wait at least 6 weeks between repeat courses.
Brain tumors, Hodgkin's disease, lymphomas
Adults and children: 100 to 130 mg/m² P.O. as single dose q 6 weeks.
≡***Dosage adjustment.*** Reduce dose according to bone marrow depression using the following guidelines:

Repeat doses should not be given until WBC count is more than 4,000/mm³ and platelet count is more than 100,000/mm³. Hematologic toxicity is delayed and cumulative; do not give repeat courses before 6 weeks.

Nadir after prior dose		Percentage of prior dose to be given
WBCs/mm³	Platelets/mm³	
> 4,000	100,000	100%
3,000 to 3,999	75,000 to 99,999	100%
2,000 to 2,999	25,000 to 74,999	70%
< 2,000	< 25,000	50%

Pharmacodynamics
Antineoplastic action: Lomustine exerts its cytotoxic activity through alkylation, resulting in the inhibition of DNA and RNA synthesis. As with other nitrosourea compounds, lomustine is known to modify cellular proteins and alkylate proteins, resulting in an inhibition of protein synthesis. Cross-resistance exists between lomustine and carmustine.

Pharmacokinetics
Absorption: Rapidly and well absorbed across the GI tract after oral administration.
Distribution: Distributed widely into body tissues. Because of its high lipid solubility, drug and its metabolites cross the blood-brain barrier to a significant extent.
Metabolism: Metabolized rapidly and extensively in the liver. Some of the metabolites have cytotoxic activity.
Excretion: Metabolites are excreted primarily in urine, with smaller amounts excreted in feces and through the lungs. Plasma elimination of drug is biphasic, with an initial phase half-life of 6 hours and a terminal phase of 1 to 2 days. Extended half-life of the terminal phase is thought to be caused by enterohepatic circulation and protein-binding.

Route	Onset	Peak	Duration
P.O.	Unknown	Unknown	Unknown

Contraindications and precautions
Contraindicated in patients with hypersensitivity to drug. Use cautiously in patients with decreased platelet, WBC, or RBC counts and in those receiving other myelosuppressants.

Interactions
None reported.

Effects on diagnostic tests
None reported.

Adverse reactions
CNS: disorientation, lethargy, ataxia.
GI: *nausea, vomiting,* stomatitis.
GU: ***nephrotoxicity,*** progressive azotemia, ***renal failure.***
Hematologic: *anemia,* ***leukopenia,*** delayed up to 6 weeks, lasting 1 to 2 weeks; ***thrombocytopenia,*** delayed up to 4 weeks, lasting 1 to 2 weeks; ***bone marrow suppression,*** delayed up to 6 weeks.
Hepatic: ***hepatotoxicity.***
Respiratory: pulmonary fibrosis.
Skin: alopecia.
Other: ***secondary malignant disease.***

Overdose and treatment
Signs and symptoms of overdose include myelosuppression, nausea, and vomiting. Treatment is usually supportive, including antiemetics and transfusion of blood components.

Clinical considerations
- Drug has been used investigationally to treat bronchiogenic carcinoma, non-Hodgkin's lymphoma, malignant melanoma, breast cancer, renal cell carcinoma, and GI carcinoma.
- Give drug 2 to 4 hours after meals. Drug is more completely absorbed if taken when the stomach is empty. To avoid nausea, give antiemetic before administering.
- Anorexia may persist for 2 to 3 days after a given dose.
- Dosage adjustment may be required in event of decreased platelet, WBC, or RBC count.
- Avoid all I.M. injections when platelet count is below 100,000/mm^3.
- Use anticoagulants cautiously. Watch closely for signs of bleeding.
- Because drug crosses the blood-brain barrier, it may be used to treat primary brain tumors.

Therapeutic monitoring
- Monitor CBC weekly. Drug is usually not administered more than every 6 weeks; bone marrow toxicity is cumulative and delayed.
- Frequently assess renal and hepatic status.

Special populations
Breast-feeding patients. Metabolites of lomustine have been found in breast milk. Discontinue breast-feeding because of increased risk of serious adverse reactions, mutagenicity, and carcinogenicity in the infant.

Patient counseling
- Emphasize importance of continuing medication despite nausea and vomiting.
- Stress importance of taking the exact dose.
- Tell patient to immediately report if vomiting occurs shortly after a dose is taken.
- Advise patient to avoid exposure to people with infections.
- Caution patient to avoid alcoholic beverages for a short period after taking drug.
- Warn patient to avoid aspirin-containing products.
- Tell patient to promptly report a sore throat, fever, or unusual bruising or bleeding.
- Advise patient to use effective contraceptive measures during drug therapy.

loperamide hydrochloride
Imodium, Imodium A-D, Kaopectate II, Maalox Anti-Diarrheal, Pepto Diarrhea Control

Pharmacologic classification: piperidine derivative
Therapeutic classification: antidiarrheal
Pregnancy risk category B

How supplied
Available by prescription only
Capsules: 2 mg
Available without a prescription
Tablets: 2 mg
Solution: 1 mg/5 ml

Indications and dosages
Acute, nonspecific diarrhea
Adults and children over age 12: Initially, 4 mg P.O., then 2 mg after each unformed stool. Maximum dose, 16 mg daily.
Children age 9 to 11: 2 mg P.O. t.i.d. on first day.
Children age 6 to 8: 2 mg P.O. b.i.d. on first day.
Children age 2 to 5: 1 mg P.O. t.i.d. on first day.

Maintenance dosage is one-third to one-half the initial dose (0.1 mg/kg only after each unformed stool) not to exceed dose recommended on the first day. Discontinue if no improvement after 48 hours.

Chronic diarrhea
Adults: Initially, 4 mg P.O., then 2 mg after each unformed stool until diarrhea subsides. Adjust dose to individual response. Discontinue if 16 mg is used for at least 10 days.
◇ *Children:* 0.08 to 0.24 mg/kg daily in 2 to 3 divided doses.

Directions for patient self-medication
Adults: 4 teaspoons or 2 tablets P.O. after the first loose bowel movement, followed by 2 teaspoons or 1 tablet after each subsequent loose bowel movement. Don't exceed 8 mg daily.
Children age 9 to 11 (60 to 95 lb [27 to 43 kg]): 2 teaspoons or 1 tablet P.O after first loose bowel movement, followed by 1 teaspoon or ½ tablet after each subsequent loose bowel movement. Don't exceed 6 mg daily.
Children age 6 to 8 (48 to 59 lb [22 to 27 kg]): 2 teaspoons or 1 tablet P.O. after first loose bowel movement, followed by 1 teaspoon or ½ tablet after each subsequent loose bowel movement. Don't exceed 4 mg daily.

Pharmacodynamics
Antidiarrheal action: Loperamide reduces intestinal motility by acting directly on intestinal mucosal nerve endings; tolerance to antiperistaltic effect doesn't develop. Drug also may inhibit fluid and electrolyte secretion by an unknown mechanism. Although it's chemically related to opiates, it hasn't shown any physical dependence characteristics in humans, and it possesses no analgesic activity.

Pharmacokinetics
Absorption: Absorbed poorly from the GI tract.
Distribution: Distribution isn't well characterized.
Metabolism: Absorbed loperamide is metabolized in the liver.
Excretion: Excreted primarily in feces; less than 2% is excreted in urine.

Route	Onset	Peak	Duration
P.O.	Unknown	2½ to 5 hr	24 hr

Contraindications and precautions
Contraindicated in children under age 2 and in patients with hypersensitivity or when constipation must be avoided. Also, OTC use is contraindicated in patients with a fever exceeding 101° F (38.3° C) or if blood is present in the stool. Use cautiously in patients with hepatic impairment.

Interactions
Opioid analgesics: May cause severe constipation. Avoid use together.

Effects on diagnostic tests
None reported.

Adverse reactions
CNS: drowsiness, fatigue, dizziness.
GI: dry mouth; abdominal pain, distention, or discomfort; *constipation;* nausea; vomiting.
Skin: rash, ***hypersensitivity reactions.***

Overdose and treatment
Clinical effects of overdose include constipation, GI irritation, and CNS depression. Treatment is with activated charcoal if ingestion was recent. If patient is vomiting, activated charcoal may be given in a slurry when patient can retain fluids. Alternatively, gastric lavage may be performed, followed by administration of activated charcoal slurry. Monitor for CNS depression; treat respiratory depression with naloxone.

Clinical considerations
After administration via nasogastric tube, flush tube to clear it and ensure passage of drug to stomach.

Therapeutic monitoring
- Patient should be monitored for reduced stools or lack of improvement.
- Monitor fluid and electrolytes if severe diarrhea occurs.

Special populations
Breast-feeding patients. It's unknown if drug is excreted in breast milk. Use with caution.
Pediatric patients. Drug is approved for use in children age 2 and older; however, children may be more susceptible to untoward CNS effects.

Patient counseling
- Warn patient to take drug only as directed and not to exceed recommended dose.
- Caution patient to avoid driving and other tasks requiring alertness because drug may cause drowsiness and dizziness.
- Instruct patient to call if no improvement occurs in 48 hours or if fever develops.

loracarbef
Lorabid

Pharmacologic classification: synthetic beta-lactam antibiotic of carbacephem class
Therapeutic classification: antibiotic
Pregnancy risk category B

How supplied
Available by prescription only
Pulvules: 200 mg, 400 mg
Powder for oral suspension: 100 mg/5 ml, 200 mg/5 ml

Indications and dosages
Secondary bacterial infections of acute bronchitis
Adults and adolescents age 13 and older: 200 to 400 mg P.O. q 12 hours for 7 days.
Acute bacterial exacerbations of chronic bronchitis
Adults and adolescents 13 age and older: 400 mg P.O. q 12 hours for 7 days.
Pneumonia
Adults and adolescents age 13 and older: 400 mg P.O. q 12 hours for 14 days.
Pharyngitis or tonsillitis
Adults and adolescents age 13 and older: 200 mg P.O. q 12 hours for 10 days.
Children age 6 months to 12 years: 15 mg/kg P.O. daily in divided doses q 12 hours for 10 days.
Sinusitis
Adults and adolescents age 13 and older: 400 mg P.O. q 12 hours for 10 days.
Children age 6 months to 12 years: 15 mg/kg P.O. q 12 hours for 10 days.

Acute otitis media
Children age 6 months to 12 years: 30 mg/kg (oral suspension) P.O. daily in divided doses q 12 hours for 10 days.
Uncomplicated skin and skin-structure infections
Adults and adolescents age 13 and older: 200 mg P.O. q 12 hours for 7 days.
Impetigo
Children: 15 mg/kg P.O. daily in divided doses q 12 hours for 7 days.
Uncomplicated cystitis
Adults and adolescents age 13 and older: 200 mg P.O. daily for 7 days.
Uncomplicated pyelonephritis
Adults and adolescents age 13 and older: 400 mg P.O. q 12 hours for 14 days.
≡***Dosage adjustment.*** Adults and children with renal failure and creatinine clearance of 50 ml/minute or more don't require dose and interval changes. In patients with creatinine clearance of 10 to 49 ml/minute, half usual dose at same interval or normal recommended dose at twice the usual dosage interval; in those with creatinine clearance below 10 ml/minute, usual dose q 3 to 5 days. Hemodialysis patients should be given another dose after dialysis.

Pharmacodynamics
Antibiotic action: Loracarbef exerts its bactericidal action by binding to essential target proteins of the bacterial cell wall, leading to inhibition of cell-wall synthesis. Loracarbef is active against gram-positive aerobes, such as *Staphylococcus aureus, S. saprophyticus, Streptococcus pneumoniae,* and *S. pyogenes;* and gram-negative aerobes, such as *Escherichia coli, Haemophilus influenzae,* and *Moraxella (Branhamella) catarrhalis.*

Pharmacokinetics
Absorption: After oral administration, drug is about 90% absorbed from the GI tract. When pulvules are taken with food, peak plasma levels are 50% to 60% of those achieved on an empty stomach. (Effect of food on rate and extent of absorption of suspension form has not been studied to date.) Absorption of suspension form is greater than that of pulvule.
Distribution: About 25% of circulating drug is bound to plasma proteins.
Metabolism: Doesn't appear to be metabolized.
Excretion: Eliminated primarily in urine. Elimination half-life in patients with normal renal function averages 1 hour.

Route	Onset	Peak	Duration
P.O.	Unknown	½-1 hr	Unknown

Contraindications and precautions
Contraindicated in patients with hypersensitivity to drug or other cephalosporins and in patients with diarrhea caused by pseudomembranous colitis. Use cautiously in pregnant and breast-feeding women.

Interactions
Probenecid: Decreased excretion of loracarbef, causing increased plasma levels. Monitor for toxicity.

Effects on diagnostic tests
Drug can cause positive direct Coombs' test.

Adverse reactions
CNS: headache, somnolence, nervousness, insomnia, dizziness.
CV: vasodilation.
GI: diarrhea, nausea, vomiting, abdominal pain, anorexia, ***pseudomembranous colitis.***
GU: vaginal candidiasis, transient increases in BUN and creatinine levels.
Hematologic: ***transient thrombocytopenia, leukopenia,*** eosinophilia.
Hepatic: transient elevations in AST, ALT, and alkaline phosphatase levels.
Skin: rash, urticaria, pruritus, ***erythema multiforme.***
Other: hypersensitivity reactions, including ***anaphylaxis.***

Overdose and treatment
Toxic symptoms after overdose of beta-lactams, such as loracarbef, may include nausea, vomiting, epigastric distress, and diarrhea. Forced diuresis, peritoneal dialysis, hemodialysis, or hemoperfusion haven't been established as beneficial for an overdose of loracarbef. Hemodialysis is effective in hastening the elimination of loracarbef from plasma in patients with chronic renal failure.

Clinical considerations
- Consider the increased rate of absorption if oral suspension is to be substituted for pulvule. Pulvules shouldn't be substituted for oral suspension when treating otitis media.
- Pseudomembranous colitis has been reported with nearly all antibacterial agents and may range from mild to life-threatening. Therefore, diagnosis must be considered in patients with diarrhea subsequent to drug administration.
- To reconstitute powder for oral suspension, add 30 ml of water in two portions to the 50-ml bottle or 60 ml of water in two portions to the 100-ml bottle; shake after each addition.
- After reconstitution, oral suspension is stable for 14 days at room temperature (59° to 86° F [15° to 30° C]).

Therapeutic monitoring
- Culture and sensitivity tests should be done before giving first dose. Therapy may begin pending test results.
- Drug may cause overgrowth of nonsusceptible bacteria or fungi. Patient needs to be mon-

itored for signs and symptoms of superinfection.

Special populations

Breast-feeding patients. It isn't known if drug is excreted in breast milk. Use caution when administering drug to breast-feeding women.
Pediatric patients. Safety and efficacy in infants under age 6 months haven't been established.

Patient counseling

- Instruct patient to take drug at least 1 hour before or at least 2 hours after eating.
- Tell patient to take drug exactly as prescribed, even after he feels better.
- Inform patient that oral suspension can be stored at room temperature for 14 days. Instruct patient to discard unused portion after 14 days.

loratadine

Claritin

Pharmacologic classification: tricyclic antihistamine
Therapeutic classification: antihistaminic
Pregnancy risk category B

How supplied

Available by prescription only
Tablets: 10 mg
Tablets (rapidly distintegrating): 10 mg
Syrup: 1 mg/ml

Indications and dosages

Symptomatic treatment of seasonal allergic rhinitis and indicated for treatment of idiopathic chronic urticaria
Adults and children age 6 and older: 10 mg P.O. daily.
≡ ***Dosage adjustment.*** In patients with liver failure or glomerular filtration rate below 30 ml/ minute, adjust dose to 10 mg every other day.
◊ ***Perennial allergic rhinitis***
Adults: 10 mg P.O. daily.

Pharmacodynamics

Antihistaminic action: Loratadine is a long-acting tricyclic antihistamine with selective peripheral H_1-receptor antagonistic activity.

Pharmacokinetics

Absorption: Readily absorbed. Because loratadine's peak plasma level may be delayed by 1 hour with a meal, administer drug on an empty stomach.
Distribution: About 97% is bound to plasma protein. Drug doesn't readily cross the blood-brain barrier.
Metabolism: Extensively metabolized to an active metabolite (descarboethoxyloratadine). The specific enzyme systems responsible for metabolism haven't been identified.
Excretion: About 80% of total dose administered can be found equally distributed between urine and feces. Mean elimination half-life is 8½ hours for loratadine. Drug isn't eliminated by hemodialysis; it's unknown if drug is eliminated by peritoneal dialysis.

Route	Onset	Peak	Duration
P.O.	1-3 hr	8-10 hr	24 hr

Contraindications and precautions

Contraindicated in patients with hypersensitivity to drug. Use cautiously in patients with hepatic impairment and in breast-feeding women.

Interactions

Drug-drug. *Drugs known to inhibit hepatic metabolism:* Should be coadministered with caution until definitive interaction studies can be completed.
Drug-herb. *Licorice:* May prolong the QT interval and be potentially additive. Use together cautiously.

Effects on diagnostic tests

None reported.

Adverse reactions

CNS: headache, somnolence, fatigue.
GI: dry mouth.

Overdose and treatment

Somnolence, tachycardia, and headache have been reported with overdoses greater than 10 mg (40 to 180 mg). If overdose occurs, institute symptomatic and supportive measures promptly and maintain for as long as necessary.

Treatment consists of emesis (ipecac syrup), except in patients with impaired consciousness, followed by administration of activated charcoal to adsorb any remaining drug. If vomiting is unsuccessful or contraindicated, perform gastric lavage with normal saline. Saline cathartics also may be of value for rapid dilution of bowel contents.

Clinical considerations

- No information exists to indicate that drug abuse or dependency occurs.
- Store drug in a cool, dry place away from heat and direct sunlight.

Therapeutic monitoring

Monitor renal and hepatic function in patients with preexisting conditions.

Special populations
Breast-feeding patients. Loratadine passes easily into breast milk. Antihistamine therapy is contraindicated in breast-feeding women.
Pediatric patients. Safety and efficacy in children under age 6 haven't been established.

Patient counseling
- Instruct patient to take drug on an empty stomach at least 2 hours after a meal and to avoid eating for at least 1 hour after taking drug.
- Tell patient to take drug only once daily. Tell him to call if symptoms persist or worsen.
- Warn patient to stop taking drug 4 days before allergy skin tests to preserve accuracy of tests.

lorazepam
Apo-Lorazepam*, Ativan, Novo-Lorazem*

Pharmacologic classification: benzodiazepine
Therapeutic classification: antianxiety, sedative-hypnotic
Controlled substance schedule IV
Pregnancy risk category D

How supplied
Available by prescription only
Tablets: 0.5 mg, 1 mg, 2 mg
Tablets (S.L.):* 1 mg, 2 mg
Injection: 2 mg/ml, 4 mg/ml
Solution: 2 mg/ml

Indications and dosages
Anxiety, tension, agitation, irritability, especially in anxiety neuroses or organic (especially GI or CV) disorders
Adults: Initially, 2 to 3 mg P.O. daily in two to three divided doses. Usual range is 2 to 6 mg P.O. daily in divided doses; maximum dose, 10 mg/day.
Insomnia
Adults: 2 to 4 mg P.O. h.s.
Preoperatively
Adults: 0.05 mg/kg I.M. 2 hours before surgery (maximum, 4 mg). Alternatively, 0.044 mg/kg (maximum total dose, 2 mg) I.V. 15 to 20 minutes before surgery; in adults under age 50, dosage may be increased to 0.05 mg/kg (maximum, 4 mg) I.V. when increased lack of recall of preoperative events is desired.
◇***Management of nausea and vomiting associated with emetogenic cancer chemotherapy***
Adults: 2.5 mg P.O. the evening before chemotherapy and repeat just after the initiation of chemotherapy. Alternatively, 1.5 mg/m^2 (maximum 3 mg) I.V. over 5 minutes 45 minutes prior to chemotherapy.
≡***Dosage adjustment.*** Geriatric patients should initially receive 1 to 2 mg P.O. daily in divided doses. Then dosage is divided p.r.n.
◇***Status epilepticus***
Adults and children: 0.05 to 0.1 mg/kg I.V. Doses may be repeated at 10- to 15-minute intervals as necessary for seizure control. Alternatively, adults may be given 4 to 8 mg I.V.

Pharmacodynamics
Anxiolytic and sedative actions: Lorazepam depresses the CNS at the limbic and subcortical levels of the brain. It produces an antianxiety effect by influencing the effect of the neurotransmitter gamma-aminobutyric acid (GABA) on its receptor in the ascending reticular activating system, which increases inhibition and blocks both cortical and limbic arousal after stimulation of the reticular formation.

Pharmacokinetics
Absorption: When administered orally, is well absorbed through the GI tract.
Distribution: Distributed widely throughout the body. Drug is about 85% protein-bound.
Metabolism: Metabolized in the liver to inactive metabolites.
Excretion: Metabolites are excreted in urine as glucuronide conjugates.

Route	Onset	Peak	Duration
P.O.	1 hr	2 hr	12-24 hr
I.V.	5 min	1-1½ hr	6-8 hr
I.M.	15-30 min	1-1½ hr	6-8 hr

Contraindications and precautions
Contraindicated in patients with acute angle-closure glaucoma or hypersensitivity to drug, other benzodiazepines, or its vehicle (used in parenteral dosage form).

Use cautiously in patients with pulmonary, renal, or hepatic impairment and in elderly, acutely ill, or debilitated patients. Don't use in pregnant women, especially during the first trimester of pregnancy.

Interactions
Drug-drug. *Antidepressants, antihistamines, barbiturates, general anesthetics, MAO inhibitors, narcotics,* and *phenothiazines:* Lorazepam potentiates the CNS depressant effects of these drugs. Use together cautiously.
Cimetidine and possibly disulfiram: Diminished hepatic metabolism of lorazepam, which increases its plasma level. Avoid use together.
Scopolamine: Combined use of parenteral lorazepam and scopalamine may be associated with an increased incidence of hallucinations, irrational behavior, and increased sedation. Use together cautiously.

Drug-lifestyle. *Alcohol use*: Lorazepam potentiates the CNS depressant effects of alcohol. Avoid use together.
Heavy smoking: Accelerated lorazepam metabolism, thus lowering clinical effectiveness. Avoid use together.

Effects on diagnostic tests
None reported.

Adverse reactions
CNS: *drowsiness,* amnesia, insomnia, agitation, *sedation,* dizziness, weakness, unsteadiness, disorientation, depression, headache.
EENT: visual disturbances.
GI: abdominal discomfort, nausea, change in appetite.
Other: ***acute withdrawal syndrome*** (after sudden discontinuation in physically dependent persons).

Overdose and treatment
Signs and symptoms of overdose include somnolence, confusion, coma, hypoactive reflexes, dyspnea, labored breathing, hypotension, bradycardia, slurred speech, and unsteady gait or impaired coordination.

Treatment requires support of blood pressure and respiration until drug effects subside; monitor vital signs. Mechanical ventilatory assistance via endotracheal tube may be required to maintain a patent airway and support adequate oxygenation. Flumazenil, a specific benzodiazepine antagonist, may be useful. Use I.V. fluids and vasopressors such as dopamine and phenylephrine to treat hypotension, if necessary. If patient is conscious, induce emesis. Use gastric lavage if ingestion was recent, but only if an endotracheal tube is present to prevent aspiration. After emesis or lavage, administer activated charcoal with a cathartic as a single dose. Dialysis is of limited value.

Clinical considerations
Consider the following recommendations relevant to all benzodiazepines as well as the following:
- Lorazepam is one of the preferred benzodiazepines for patients with hepatic disease.
- Use lowest possible effective dose to avoid oversedation.
- Parenteral lorazepam appears to possess potent amnestic effects.
- For the oral concentrated solution, add dose to 30 ml or more of water, juice, or soda, or to semisolid foods.
- Oral drug is given in divided doses, with the largest dose given before bedtime.

□ ***ALERT*** Arteriospasm may result from intra-arterial injection of lorazepam. Don't administer by this route.
- For I.V. administration, dilute lorazepam with an equal volume of a compatible diluent, such as D_5W, sterile water for injection, or normal saline solution.
- Drug may be injected directly into a vein or into the tubing of a compatible I.V. infusion, such as normal saline solution or D_5W solution. The rate of lorazepam I.V. injection shouldn't exceed 2 mg/minute. Emergency resuscitative equipment should be available when administering I.V.
- Diluted lorazepam solutions must be given immediately.
- Don't use drug solutions if they're discolored or contain a precipitate.
- I.M. doses of lorazepam are given undiluted, deep into a large muscle mass.

Therapeutic monitoring
- Monitor hepatic function studies to prevent cumulative effects and to ensure adequate drug metabolism.
- Monitor renal function tests.

Special populations
Breast-feeding patients. Drug may be excreted in breast milk. Don't administer to breast-feeding women.
Pediatric patients. Safety of oral lorazepam in children under age 12 hasn't been established. Safety of sublingual or parenteral lorazepam in children under age 18 hasn't been established. Neonates haven't been closely observed for withdrawal symptoms when mother took lorazepam for a prolonged period during pregnancy.
Geriatric patients. Geriatric patients are more sensitive to CNS depressant effects of lorazepam. They may require supervision with ambulation and activities of daily living during initiation of therapy or after an increase in dose. Lower doses usually are effective in geriatric patients because of decreased elimination. Parenteral administration of drug is more likely to cause apnea, hypotension, bradycardia, and cardiac arrest in geriatric patients.

Patient counseling
- Caution patient not to make changes in drug regimen without specific instructions.
- Teach safety measures, as appropriate, to protect from injury, such as gradual position changes and supervised walking.
- Advise patient of possible retrograde amnesia after I.V. or I.M. use.
- Tell patient to avoid large amounts of caffeine-containing products, which may interfere with effectiveness of drug.
- Advise patient of potential for physical and psychological dependence with chronic use.
- Tell patient to discontinue drug slowly (over 8 to 12 weeks) after long-term therapy.

losartan potassium

Cozaar

Pharmacologic classification: angiotensin II receptor antagonist
Therapeutic classification: antihypertensive
Pregnancy risk category C (D second and third trimesters)

How supplied

Available by prescription only
Tablets: 25 mg, 50 mg

Indications and dosages

Hypertension
Adults: Initially, 25 to 50 mg P.O. daily. Maintenance dosage is 25 to 100 mg P.O. once daily or b.i.d.

Pharmacodynamics

Antihypertensive action: Losartan is an angiotensin II receptor antagonist; it blocks the vasoconstrictor and aldosterone-secreting effects of angiotensin II by selectively blocking the binding of angiotensin II to its receptor sites found in many tissues, including vascular smooth muscle.

Pharmacokinetics

Absorption: Well absorbed and undergoes substantial first-pass metabolism; systemic bioavailability is about 33%.
Distribution: Both losartan and its active metabolite are highly bound to plasma proteins, primarily albumin.
Metabolism: Cytochrome P-450 2C9 and 3A4 are involved in the biotransformation of drug to its metabolites.
Excretion: Drug and its metabolites are primarily excreted in feces with a small amount excreted in urine.

Route	Onset	Peak	Duration
P.O.	Unknown	1 hr	Unknown

Contraindications and precautions

Contraindicated in patients with hypersensitivity to drug. Use cautiously in patients with impaired renal or hepatic function.

Interactions

None significant.

Effects on diagnostic tests

None reported.

Adverse reactions

CNS: dizziness, insomnia.
EENT: nasal congestion, sinus disorder, sinusitis.
GI: diarrhea, dyspepsia.
Musculoskeletal: muscle cramps, myalgia, back or leg pain.
Respiratory: cough, upper respiratory infection.

Overdose and treatment

The most likely signs are hypotension and tachycardia; bradycardia could occur from parasympathetic stimulation. If symptomatic hypotension occurs, initiate supportive treatment. Neither losartan nor its active metabolite can be removed by hemodialysis.

Clinical considerations

- Use the lowest dose (25 mg) initially in patients with impaired hepatic function and in those who are intravascularly volume-depleted (receiving diuretic therapy).
- Drug can be used alone or in combination with other antihypertensive agents.
- If antihypertensive effect measured at trough (using once-daily dosing) is inadequate, a twice-daily regimen at the same total daily dose or an increased dose may give a more satisfactory response.
- Patients with severe heart failure whose renal function depends on the angiotensin-aldosterone system have experienced acute renal failure during therapy with ACE inhibitors. Manufacturer of losartan states that drug would be expected to do the same. Closely monitor patient, especially during first few weeks of therapy.

Therapeutic monitoring

- Monitor patient taking diuretics concurrently in treatment of hypertension for symptomatic hypotension.
- Monitor patient's renal function (serum creatinine and BUN levels).

Special populations

Pregnant patients. Drugs such as losartan that act directly on the renin-angiotensin system can cause fetal and neonatal morbidity and death when administered to pregnant women; these problems haven't been detected when exposure has been limited to the first trimester. If pregnancy is suspected, discontinue drug.
Breast-feeding patients. It isn't known if drug is excreted in breast milk. Because of the potential for adverse effects on the breast-fed infant, a decision should be made whether to discontinue the drug or breast-feeding, taking into account the importance of drug to the woman.
Pediatric patients. Safety and efficacy in children haven't been established.

Patient counseling

- Instruct patient not to discontinue drug abruptly.
- Tell patient to avoid sodium substitutes; these products may contain potassium, which can

cause hyperkalemia in patients taking losartan.

- Inform woman of childbearing age about the consequences of second- and third-trimester exposure to losartan; instruct her to call immediately if pregnancy is suspected.

lovastatin

Mevacor

Pharmacologic classification: lactone, HMG-CoA reductase inhibitor
Therapeutic classification: cholesterol-lowering agent
Pregnancy risk category X

How supplied

Available by prescription only
Tablets: 10 mg, 20 mg, 40 mg

Indications and dosages

Reduction of low-density lipoprotein and total cholesterol levels in patients with primary hypercholesterolemia (types IIa and IIb), atherosclerosis

Adults: Initially, 20 mg P.O. once daily with evening meal. For patients with severely elevated cholesterol levels (> 300 mg/dl), initial dose should be 40 mg. Recommended range is 20 to 80 mg in single or divided doses.

≡***Dosage adjustment.*** For patients also taking immunosuppressive drugs, 10 mg P.O. daily, not to exceed 20 mg daily.

Pharmacodynamics

Antilipemic action: Lovastatin, an inactive lactone, is hydrolyzed to the beta-hydroxy acid, which specifically inhibits 3-hydroxy-3-methylglutaryl-coenzyme A reductase (HMG-CoA reductase). This enzyme is an early (and rate-limiting) step in the synthetic pathway of cholesterol. At therapeutic doses, the enzyme isn't blocked, and biologically necessary amounts of cholesterol can still be synthesized.

Pharmacokinetics

Absorption: About 30% of an oral dose is absorbed in animals. Administration of drug with food improves plasma levels of total inhibitors by about 30%. Onset of action is about 3 days, with maximal therapeutic effects seen in 4 to 6 weeks.

Distribution: Less than 5% of an oral dose reaches the systemic circulation because of extensive first-pass hepatic extraction; the liver is the principal site of action for the drug. Both the parent compound and its principal metabolite are highly bound (more than 95%) to plasma proteins. Lovastatin can cross the placenta and the blood-brain barrier.

Metabolism: Converted to the active B hydroxy acid form in the liver. Other metabolites include the 6′ hydroxy derivative and two unidentified compounds.

Excretion: About 80% is excreted primarily in feces, about 10% in urine.

Route	Onset	Peak	Duration
P.O.	Unknown	2 hr	Unknown

Contraindications and precautions

Contraindicated in patients with hypersensitivity to drug, in those with active liver disease or conditions associated with unexplained persistent elevations of serum transaminase levels, in pregnant and breast-feeding women, and in women of childbearing age unless there's no risk of pregnancy.

Use cautiously in patients who consume excessive amounts of alcohol or have history of liver disease.

Interactions

Drug-drug. *Cholestyramine, colestipol:* May enhance lipid-reducing effects but may decrease bioavailability of lovastatin. Patient requires close monitoring.
Cyclosporine, erythromycin, gemfibrozil, niacin: May increase risk of severe myopathy or rhabdomyolysis. Use together cautiously.
Warfarin: Increased anticoagulant effect. Monitor PT and INR.
Isradipine: May increase clearance of lovastatin and its metabolites. Patient requires careful monitoring.
Itraconazole: Coadministration with lovastatin increases HMG-CoA reductase inhibitor levels. Therapy with lovastatin should be temporarily interrupted if systemic azole antifungal treatment is required.
Drug-lifestyle. *Sun exposure:* Photosensitivity reaction. Advise patient to take precautions.
Alcohol use: May increase hepatic effects. Advise patient to avoid alcohol use.

Effects on diagnostic tests

None reported.

Adverse reactions

CNS: headache, dizziness, peripheral neuropathy, insomnia.
CV: chest pain.
EENT: blurred vision.
GI: constipation, diarrhea, dyspepsia, flatulence, abdominal pain or cramps, heartburn, nausea, vomiting.
Hepatic: elevated serum transaminase levels, abnormal liver test results.
Musculoskeletal: muscle cramps, myalgia, myositis, ***rhabdomyolysis.***
Skin: rash, pruritus, alopecia.
Other: photosensitivity.

Overdose and treatment

No information available.

Clinical considerations

- Initiate drug therapy only after diet and other nonpharmacologic therapies have proved ineffective. Patient should be on a standard cholesterol-lowering diet and continue on this diet during therapy.
- Administer drug with evening meal; absorption is enhanced and cholesterol biosynthesis is greater in the evening.
- Therapeutic response occurs in about 2 weeks, with maximum effects in 4 to 6 weeks.
- Store tablets at room temperature in a light-resistant container.
- Don't exceed 20 mg/day if patient is receiving immunosuppressive drugs.

Therapeutic monitoring

- Patient must be monitored for signs of myositis; have patient report muscle aches and pains.
- Liver function tests are needed frequently during initiation of therapy and periodically thereafter.
- Monitor serum lipoprotein, triglycerides, and serum cholesterol periodically during therapy.

Special populations

Breast-feeding patients. An alternative feeding method is recommended during therapy with lovastatin.
Pediatric patients. Safety and efficacy in children haven't been established.

Patient counseling

- Stress importance of lowering cholesterol.
- Advise patient to restrict alcohol intake.
- Instruct patient to take drug with evening meal.
- Tell patient to report adverse reactions, particularly muscle aches and pains, and to take precautions with exposure to sun and other ultraviolet light until tolerance is determined.

loxapine hydrochloride

Loxitane C, Loxitane IM

loxapine succinate

Loxapac*, Loxitane

Pharmacologic classification: dibenzoxazepine
Therapeutic classification: antipsychotic
Pregnancy risk category NR

How supplied

Available by prescription only
Capsules: 5 mg, 10 mg, 25 mg, 50 mg
Oral concentrate: 25 mg/ml
Injection: 50 mg/ml

Indications and dosages

Psychotic disorders
Adults: Initially, 10 mg P.O. b.i.d. (in severe schizophrenia, 50 mg P.O. daily); usual therapeutic and maintenance dosage is 60 to 100 mg P.O. daily b.i.d. to q.i.d. or most patients (dose varies from patient to patient) or 12.5 to 50 mg I.M. q 4 to 6 hours or longer. Maximum daily dose, 250 mg. After desired symptom control, change to oral therapy. Don't administer drug I.V.

Pharmacodynamics

Antipsychotic action: Loxapine is the only tricyclic antipsychotic; it's structurally similar to amoxapine. Loxapine is thought to exert its antipsychotic effects by postsynaptic blockade of CNS dopamine receptors, thus inhibiting dopamine-mediated effects. Loxapine has many other central and peripheral effects; its most prominent adverse reactions are extrapyramidal.

Pharmacokinetics

Absorption: Absorbed rapidly and completely from the GI tract. First-pass metabolism results in lower systemic availability.
Distribution: Distributed widely into the body, including breast milk. Steady-state serum level is achieved within 3 to 4 days. Drug is 91% to 99% protein-bound.
Metabolism: Metabolized extensively by the liver, forming a few active metabolites; duration of action is 12 hours.
Excretion: Mostly excreted as metabolites in urine; some is excreted in feces by way of the biliary tract. About 50% is excreted in urine and feces within 24 hours.

Route	Onset	Peak	Duration
P.O., I.M.	½ hr	1½-3 hr	12 hr

Contraindications and precautions

Contraindicated in patients with hypersensitivity to dibenzoxazepines and in patients experiencing coma, severe CNS depression, or drug-induced depressed states. Use cautiously in patients with seizure or CV disorders, glaucoma, or history of urine retention.

Interactions

Drug-drug. *Aluminum- and magnesium-containing antacids and antidiarrheals:* Decrease loxapine absorption and its therapeutic effects. Separate administration times.
Antiarrhythmic agents, disopyramide, quinidine, and procainamide: Increased incidence of arrhythmias and conduction defects. Use together cautiously.
Atropine and other anticholinergic drugs, including antidepressants, antihistamines, MAO inhibitors, meperidine, phenothiazines, and antiparkinson agents: Oversedation, paralytic

ileus, visual changes, and severe constipation. Avoid use together.
Beta blockers: May inhibit loxapine metabolism, increasing plasma levels and toxicity. Use together cautiously.
Bromocriptine: Loxapine may antagonize therapeutic effect of bromocriptine on prolactin secretion. Monitor for effect.
CNS depressants, including analgesics, barbiturates, narcotics, tranquilizers, anesthetics (general, spinal, and epidural), and parenteral magnesium sulfate (oversedation, respiratory depression, and hypotension): Additive effects are likely after use of loxapine with these drugs. Use together cautiously.
Centrally acting antihypertensive drugs, such as clonidine, guanabenz, guanadrel, guanethidine, methyldopa, and reserpine: Loxapine may inhibit blood pressure response. Use together cautiously.
Dopamine: Decreased vasoconstricting effects of high-dose dopamine. Avoid use together.
Levodopa: Decreased effectiveness and increased toxicity of levodopa (by dopamine blockade). Avoid use together.
Lithium: May result in severe neurologic toxicity with an encephalitis-like syndrome and a decreased therapeutic response to loxapine. Avoid use together.
Nitrates: May cause hypotension. Use together cautiously.
Sympathomimetics, including epinephrine, phenylephrine, phenylpropanolamine, and ephedrine (often found in nasal sprays), and with appetite suppressants: Decreased stimulatory and pressor effects. Loxapine may cause epinephrine reversal, an inhibition of the vasopressor effect of epinephrine. Use together cautiously.
Drug-lifestyle. *Alcohol use*: Additive effects are likely. Avoid use together.

Effects on diagnostic tests
Drug causes false-positive test results for urinary porphyrins, urobilinogen, amylase, and 5-hydroxyindoleacetic acid (5-HIAA) because of darkening of urine by metabolites; it also causes false-positive urine pregnancy test results using human chorionic gonadotropin.

Adverse reactions
CNS: *extrapyramidal reactions, sedation, drowsiness,* ***seizures,*** numbness, confusion, syncope, *tardive dyskinesia,* pseudoparkinsonism, EEG changes, dizziness.
CV: *orthostatic hypotension, tachycardia,* ECG changes, hypertension.
EENT: *blurred vision,* nasal congestion.
GI: *dry mouth, constipation,* nausea, vomiting, paralytic ileus.
GU: *urine retention,* menstrual irregularities, gynecomastia.
Hematologic: ***leukopenia, agranulocytosis, thrombocytopenia.***
Hepatic: jaundice.
Metabolic: weight gain.
Skin: *mild photosensitivity,* allergic reactions, rash, pruritus.
Other: ***neuroleptic malignant syndrome.***

Overdose and treatment
CNS depression is characterized by deep, unarousable sleep and possible coma, hypotension or hypertension, extrapyramidal symptoms, abnormal involuntary muscle movements, agitation, seizures, arrhythmias, ECG changes, hypothermia or hyperthermia, and autonomic nervous system dysfunction. Treatment is symptomatic and supportive, including maintaining vital signs, airway, stable body temperature, and fluid and electrolyte balance.

Don't induce vomiting: drug inhibits cough reflex, and aspiration may occur. Use gastric lavage, then activated charcoal and saline cathartics; hemodialysis may be helpful. Regulate body temperature as needed. Treat hypotension with I.V. fluids; don't give epinephrine. Treat seizures with parenteral diazepam or barbiturates; arrhythmias with parenteral phenytoin (1 mg/kg with rate adjusted to blood pressure); and extrapyramidal reactions with benztropine at 1 to 2 mg or parenteral diphenhydramine at 10 to 50 mg.

Clinical considerations
- Tardive dyskinesia may occur, usually after prolonged use. It may not appear until months or years after treatment and may disappear spontaneously or persist for life.
- Avoid combining drug with alcohol or other depressants.
- Dilute liquid concentrate with orange or grapefruit juice just before giving.
- Dose of 10 mg is therapeutic equivalent of 100 mg chlorpromazine.
- Photosensitivity warnings may apply with loxapine.

Therapeutic monitoring
- Patient needs to be assessed periodically for abnormal body movement.
- Obtain baseline blood pressure measurements before starting therapy and monitor regularly.
- Periodic ophthalmic testing should be performed.

Special populations
Pediatric patients. Drug isn't recommended for children under age 16.
Geriatric patients. Geriatric patients are highly sensitive to antimuscarinic, hypotensive, and sedative effects of drug and have a higher risk of extrapyramidal adverse reactions, such as parkinsonism and tardive dyskinesia. Higher plasma levels develop in these patients and, therefore, they require lower initial dosage and more gradual dosage adjustment.

Patient counseling

- Warn patient against activities that require alertness and good psychomotor coordination until CNS response to drug is determined. Drowsiness and dizziness usually subside after first few weeks.
- Recommend sugarless gum or candy, mouthwash, ice chips, or artificial saliva to help alleviate dry mouth.
- Advise patient to get up slowly to avoid orthostatic hypotension.

Lyme disease vaccine (recombinant OspA)

LYMErix

Pharmacologic classification: vaccine, bacterial-recombinant
Therapeutic classification: biological
Pregnancy risk category C

How supplied

Avaialable by prescription only
Single-dose vials and prefilled syringes: 30 mcg/0.5 ml

Indications and dosages

Active immunization against Lyme disease
Children and adults age 15 to 70: 30 mcg I.M. in deltoid region; repeat dose at 1 and 12 months after first dose. Safety and efficacy of this vaccine are based on administration of second and third doses several weeks before the onset of the disease transmission season.

Pharmacodynamics

Lyme disease prophylaxis: The vaccine stimulates specific antibodies directed against *Borrelia burgdorferi* (a bacterial spirochete that causes Lyme disease). The vaccine contains lipoprotein OspA, an outer surface protein of *B. burgdorferi.*

Pharmacokinetics

No information available.

Route	Onset	Peak	Duration
I.M.	Unknown	Unknown	Unknown

Contraindications and precautions

Contraindicated in patients with known hypersensitivity to vaccine or its components. Don't administer vaccine to patients with treatment-resistant Lyme arthritis (antibiotic refractory) or moderate or severe febrile illness. Lyme disease vaccine shouldn't be given to patients receiving anticoagulants unless potential benefit outweighs risk of administration.

Use cautiously in immunosuppressed patients or in those receiving immunosuppressive therapy because the expected immune response may not occur. For patients receiving immunosuppressive therapy, consider deferring vaccination for 3 months after therapy.

Also use cautiously in persons who may have allergic reactions to packaging for the LYMErix syringe, which contains dry natural rubber. Note that the vial packaging doesn't contain rubber.

Interactions

None reported.

Effects on diagnostic tests

LYMErix vaccination may result in a positive IgG enzyme-linked immunosorbent assay in the absence of infection.

Adverse reactions

CNS: *headache, fatigue,* dizziness, depression, hypoesthesia, paresthesia.
GI: diarrhea, nausea.
Musculoskeletal: *arthralgia,* back pain, achiness, myalgia, arthritis, arthrosis, stiffness, tendinitis.
Respiratory: bronchitis, coughing, pharyngitis, rhinitis, sinusitis, upper respiratory tract infection.
Skin: *rash, injection site pain, redness, soreness, swelling,* injection site reaction, contact dermatitis.
Other: chills or rigors, fever, viral infection, flulike symptoms.

Overdose and treatment

No information available.

Clinical considerations

- Before immunization, review the patient's history for possible vaccine sensitivity, allergies, previous vaccination-related adverse reactions, and occurrence of any adverse-event related symptoms or signs. Epinephrine injection (1:1,000) and other appropriate agents used for control of immediate allergic reactions must be immediately available.
- Shake well before withdrawal and use. Inspect visually for particulate matter or discoloration before administration. With thorough agitation, LYMErix is a turbid white suspension. Discard if it appears otherwise. Use vaccine as supplied; no dilution or reconstitution is necessary. Discard any vaccine remaining in a single-dose vial.
- Packaging for vaccine prefilled syringe contains dry natural rubber, which may cause allergic reactions; packaging for the vial doesn't contain natural rubber.
- A separate sterile syringe and needle or a sterile disposable unit must be used for each patient to prevent transmission of infectious agents. Dispose of needles properly; don't recap.
- Administer vaccine by I.M. injection in the deltoid region. Don't inject I.V., intradermally, or subcutaneously.

■ No data are available on the immune response to vaccine when administered concurrently with other vaccines. When concomitant administration of other vaccines is required, they should be given with different syringes and at different injection sites.
■ It's recommended that vaccine not be administered to antibiotic-resistant Lyme arthritis patients.
■ As with other I.M. injections, vaccine shouldn't be given to individuals on anticoagulant therapy or with clotting disorders, unless the potential benefit clearly outweighs the risk of administration.
■ Store between 36° and 46° F (2° and 8° C). Don't freeze; discard if product has been frozen.

Therapeutic monitoring
Monitor for adverse reactions and report any such reactions to 1-800-822-7967.

Special populations
Pregnant patients. Health care providers are encouraged to register pregnant women who received the vaccine by calling 1-800-366-8900, ext. 5231.
Breast-feeding patients. It isn't known if vaccine is excreted in beast milk; use cautiously in breast-feeding women.
Pediatric patients. Safety and efficacy in children under age 15 haven't been evaluated. Avoid giving to this age group.
Geriatric patients. Vaccine isn't indicated for patients over age 70.

Patient counseling
■ Inform patient that this vaccine is specific for preventing, not treating, Lyme disease.
■ Inform patients, parents, or guardians of the benefits and risks of immunization with the vaccine, and of the importance of completing the immunization series.
■ Ask patient regarding the occurrence of any symptoms or signs after a previous dose of the same vaccine and advise him to report any adverse events.
■ Instruct patient to tell health care provider administering vaccine if he's taking anticoagulant drugs (warfarin, heparin) or other blood-thinning drugs such as aspirin.
■ Advise patient of ways to prevent other tick-borne diseases (wearing long-sleeved shirts, long pants, tucking pants into socks, and treating clothing with tick repellents). In addition, tell patient to carefully check himself when returning from endemic areas for the presence of ticks.
■ Instruct patient on the appropriate way to remove ticks (use fine-pointed tweezers to avoid squashing the tick during removal from skin).

lymphocyte immune globulin (antithymocyte globulin [equine], ATG)
Atgam

Pharmacologic classification: immunoglobulin
Therapeutic classification: immunosuppressive
Pregnancy risk category C

How supplied
Available by prescription only
Injection: 50 mg of equine IgG per ml, in 5-ml ampules

Indications and dosages
Prevention of acute renal allograft rejection
Adults and children: 15 mg/kg/day I.V. for 14 days, then same dosage every other day for next 14 days (to a total of 21 doses in 28 days). Administer the first dose of ATG within 24 hours before or after transplantation.
Treatment of acute renal allograft rejection
Adults and children: 10 to 15 mg/kg/day I.V. for 14 days; if necessary, same dosage may be given every other day for another 14 days (to a total of 21 doses in 28 days). Begin ATG therapy at the first sign of acute rejection.
Aplastic anemia
Adults and children: 10 to 20 mg/kg I.V. daily for 8 to 14 days, followed by alternate-day therapy for an additional 14 days (total of 21 doses in 28 days).
◇Skin allotransplantation
Adults: 10 mg/kg I.V. 24 hours before allograft; then 10 to 15 mg/kg every other day. Maintenance dosage is variable and can range from 5 to 40 mg/ kg/day, based on clinical response and clinical indicators of immunosuppressive activity. Therapy usually continues until allografts cover less than 20% of total body surface area; often, this requires 40 to 60 days of treatment.
Bone marrow allotransplantation; ◇graft-versus-host disease after bone marrow transplantation
Adults: 7 to 10 mg/kg I.V. every other day for six doses.

Pharmacodynamics
Immunosuppressive action: The exact mechanism hasn't been fully defined but may involve elimination of antigen-reactive T cells (T lymphocytes) in peripheral blood or alteration of T-cell function. The effects of antilymphocyte preparations, including ATG, on T cells are variable and complex. Whether the effects of ATG are mediated through a specific subset of T cells hasn't been determined.

Pharmacokinetics

Absorption: Peak plasma levels of equine IgG after I.V. administration of ATG vary, depending on patient's ability to catabolize foreign IgG.

Distribution: Distribution of ATG into body fluids and tissues hasn't been fully described. Because antilymphocyte serum reportedly is poorly distributed into lymphoid tissues (such as spleen, lymph nodes), it's likely that ATG is also poorly distributed into these tissues.

No information is available on transplacental distribution of ATG. However, such distribution is likely because other immunoglobulins cross the placenta. Virtually all transplacental passage of immunoglobulins occurs during the last 4 weeks of pregnancy.

Metabolism: Not known.

Excretion: Plasma half-life of equine IgG reportedly averages about 6 days (range 1.5 to 13 days). About 1% of a dose of ATG is excreted in urine, principally as unchanged equine IgG. In one report, mean urinary level of equine IgG was about 4 mcg/ml after about 21 doses of ATG over 28 days.

Contraindications and precautions

Contraindicated in patients hypersensitive to drug. An intradermal skin test is recommended at least 1 hour before first dose. Marked local swelling or erythema larger than 10 mm indicates an increased potential for severe systemic reaction, such as anaphylaxis. Severe reactions to skin test, such as hypotension, tachycardia, dyspnea, generalized rash, or anaphylaxis, usually preclude further administration of drug.

Use cautiously in patients receiving other immunosuppressive medications, such as corticosteroids or azathioprine.

Interactions

Drug-drug. *Other immunosuppressive therapy (azathioprine, corticosteroids, graft irradiation):* May intensify immunosuppression, an effect that can be used to therapeutic advantage; however, such therapy may increase vulnerability to infection and possibly the risk of lymphoma or lymphoproliferative disorders. Patient requires close monitoring.

Effects on diagnostic tests

None reported.

Adverse reactions

CNS: malaise, *seizures, headache.*
CV: ***hypotension,*** chest pain, thrombophlebitis, tachycardia, edema, iliac vein obstruction, renal artery stenosis.
EENT: ***laryngospasm.***
GI: *nausea, vomiting, diarrhea,* epigastric pain, abdominal distention, stomatitis.
Hematologic: **LEUKOPENIA, THROMBOCYTOPENIA,** ***hemolysis, aplastic anemia.***
Hepatic: elevated liver enzyme level.
Metabolic: hyperglycemia.
Musculoskeletal: *myalgia, arthralgia.*
Respiratory: hiccups, *dyspnea,* ***pulmonary edema.***
Skin: *rash, pruritus, urticaria.*
Other: *febrile reactions,* serum sickness, ***anaphylaxis,*** *infections,* night sweats, lymphadenopathy, *chills.*

Overdose and treatment

No information available.

Clinical considerations

- Drug has been used to treat aplastic anemia, lymphoma, agranulocytosis, and as an adjunct in bone marrow, cardiac allotransplantation, and skin allotransplantation.
- To minimize risks of leukopenia and infection, some clinicians recommend that azathioprine and corticosteroid dosages be reduced by 50% when ATG is used with these drugs for the prevention or treatment of renal allograft rejection.
- Some clinicians elect to administer prophylactic platelet transfusion in patients receiving drug for aplastic anemia because of high risk of thrombocytopenia.
- Dilute drug concentrate for injection before I.V. infusion. Dilute required dose of ATG in normal saline or 0.45% saline injection (usually 250 to 1,000 ml); final level preferably shouldn't exceed 1 mg of equine IgG per ml. Infuse over at least 4 hours.
- Infusion in dextrose or highly acidic solutions isn't recommended.
- Invert I.V. infusion solution container into which ATG concentrate is added to prevent contact of undiluted ATG with air inside the container. Refrigerate diluted solutions of ATG at 36° to 46° F (2° to 8° C) if administration is delayed. Reconstituted solutions shouldn't be used after 12 hours (including actual infusion time), even if stored at 36° to 46° F.
- Because of risk of severe systemic reaction (anaphylaxis), manufacturer recommends an intradermal skin test before administration of initial dose of ATG. The skin test procedure consists of intradermal injection of 0.1 ml of a 1:1,000 dilution of ATG concentrate for injection in normal saline injection (5 mcg of equine IgG). Administer a control test using normal saline injection in the other arm to facilitate interpretation of the results. If a wheal or area of erythema exceeding 10 mm in diameter (with or without pseudopod formation) and itching or marked local swelling develops, infusion of ATG requires extreme caution; severe and potentially fatal systemic reactions can occur in patients with a positive skin test. A systemic reaction to the skin test such as generalized rash, tachycardia, dyspnea, hypotension, or anaphylaxis rules out further administration of ATG. The predictive value of

the ATG skin test hasn't been clearly established, and an allergic reaction may occur despite a negative skin test.

- The manufacturer hasn't yet determined the total number of ATG doses (10 to 20 mg/kg per dose) that can be administered safely to a patient. Some renal allograft recipients have received up to 50 doses in 4 months; others, up to four 28-day courses of 21 doses each without an increased incidence of adverse effects.

Therapeutic monitoring

- Anaphylaxis may occur at any time during drug therapy and may be indicated by hypotension, respiratory distress, or pain in the chest, flank, or back. Recommend monitoring patient closely.
- Recommend observing patient receiving drug for signs of leukopenia, thrombocytopenia, and concurrent infection.
- Monitor peripheral blood levels of rosette-forming cells (RFCs) in order to guide therapy in allograft recipient (maintain RFCs at 10% of treatment level).
- Recommend monitoring patient for signs of infection during ATG therapy.

Special populations

Breast-feeding patients. Although it's unknown if drug is excreted in breast milk, other immunoglobulins are distributed into breast milk. Breast-feeding women should consider an alternative feeding method.
Pediatric patients. Safety and efficacy in children haven't been established. Drug has had limited use in children age 3 months to 19 years.

Patient counseling

Warn patient that a febrile reaction is likely.

M

magaldrate (aluminum magnesium hydroxide sulfate)

Iosopan, Lowsium, Magaldrate, Riopan

Pharmacologic classification: aluminum-magnesium salt
Therapeutic classification: antacid
Pregnancy risk category C

How supplied
Available without a prescription
Suspension: 540 mg/5 ml

Indications and dosages
Indigestion or hyperacidity associated with peptic ulcer, gastritis, peptic esophagitis, hiatal hernia
Adults: 5 to 10 ml (suspension) P.O. between meals and h.s. with water.

Pharmacodynamics
Antacid action: Magaldrate neutralizes gastric acid, reducing the direct acid irritant effect. This increases gastric pH, which inactivates pepsin. Magaldrate also enhances mucosal barrier integrity and improves gastroesophageal sphincter tone.

Pharmacokinetics
Absorption: Aluminum may be absorbed systemically. Magnesium also may be absorbed, posing a risk to patients with renal failure. Absorption is unrelated to mechanism of action.
Distribution: Distribution is primarily local.
Metabolism: None.
Excretion: Excreted in feces; some aluminum and magnesium may be excreted in breast milk. Duration of action is prolonged.

Route	Onset	Peak	Duration
P.O.	20 min	Unknown	20-180 min

Contraindications and precautions
Contraindicated in patients with severe renal disease. Use cautiously in patients with mild renal impairment.

Interactions
Drug-drug. *Enterically coated drugs:* Magaldrate may cause premature release of these drugs. Separate doses of magaldrate and all oral drugs by 1 to 2 hours.
Levodopa: Concurrent administration may increase levodopa absorption, increasing risk of toxicity. Separate administration times.
Phenothiazines (especially chlorpromazine), anticoagulants, antimuscarinics, coumadin, chenodiol, chlordiazepoxide, diazepam, digoxin, isoniazid, phosphates, quinolones, tetracycline, and vitamin A: Decreased absorption, thus lessening their effectiveness. Separate administration times.
Drug-herb. *Melatonin:* Additive inhibitory effects on the *N*-methyl-*D*-aspartate receptor. Avoid use together.

Effects on diagnostic tests
Magaldrate may antagonize effect of pentagastrin during gastric acid secretion tests.

Adverse reactions
GI: mild constipation, diarrhea.
GU: increased urine pH levels.
Metabolic: decreased serum potassium levels, increased serum gastrin levels.

Overdose and treatment
No information available.

Clinical considerations
- Shake suspension well; give with small amounts of water or fruit juice.
- After administration through nasogastric tube, flush tube with water to clear it and ensure passage of drug to stomach.
- Give drug at least 1 hour apart from enterically coated medications.
- Suspension contains saccharin and sorbitol.
- Most formulations contain less than 0.5 mg of sodium per tablet (or 5 ml of liquid).

Therapeutic monitoring
Monitor renal function and serum phosphate, potassium, and magnesium levels in patients with renal disease.

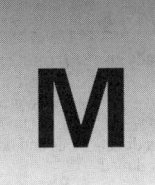

Special populations
Breast-feeding patients. Some aluminum and magnesium may be excreted in breast milk. However, no problems have been associated with use in breast-feeding women.
Pediatric patients. Use of drug as an antacid in children under age 6 requires a well-estab-

lished diagnosis because children typically give vague descriptions of symptoms.

Patient counseling

- Caution patient to take drug only as directed and 1 or 2 hours apart from other oral medications.
- Remind patient to shake suspension well or to chew tablets thoroughly.
- Warn patient not to take more than 18 teaspoonfuls in a 24-hour period.

magnesium hydroxide (milk of magnesia)

Milk of Magnesia, Phillips' Milk of Magnesia, Concentrated Phillips' Milk of Magnesia

Pharmacologic classification: magnesium salt
Therapeutic classification: antacid, antiulcer agent, laxative
Pregnancy risk category NR

How supplied

Available without a prescription
Tablets: 300 mg, 600 mg
Tablets (chewable): 311 mg
Liquid: 400 mg/5 ml, 800 mg/5 ml
Suspension (concentrated): 10 ml (equivalent to 30 ml of milk of magnesia)
Suspension: 77.5 mg/g

Indications and dosages

Constipation, bowel evacuation before surgery
Adults and children over age 6: 10 to 20 ml concentrated milk of magnesia P.O.; 15 to 60 ml milk of magnesia P.O.
Laxative
Adults: 30 to 60 ml P.O., usually h.s.
Children age 6 to 12: 15 to 30 ml P.O.
Children age 2 to 6: 5 to 15 ml P.O.
Antacid
Adults: 5 to 15 ml (liquid) P.O., p.r.n., up to q.i.d.; 2.5 to 7.5 ml (liquid concentrate) P.O., p.r.n., up to q.i.d.; 2 to 4 tablets P.O., p.r.n., up to q.i.d.
Children: 2.5 to 5 ml P.O., p.r.n.

Pharmacodynamics

Antiulcer action: Magnesium hydroxide neutralizes gastric acid, decreasing the direct acid irritant effect. This increases pH, which, in turn, leads to pepsin inactivation. Magnesium hydroxide also enhances mucosal barrier integrity and improves gastric and esophageal sphincter tone.
Antacid action: Drug reacts rapidly with hydrochloric acid in the stomach to form magnesium chloride and water.
Laxative action: Magnesium hydroxide produces its laxative effect by increasing the osmotic gradient in the gut and drawing in water, causing distention that stimulates peristalsis and bowel evacuation.

Pharmacokinetics

Absorption: About 15% to 30% may be absorbed systemically (posing a potential risk to patients with renal failure).
Distribution: None.
Metabolism: None.
Excretion: Unabsorbed drug is excreted in feces; absorbed drug is excreted rapidly in urine.

Route	Onset	Peak	Duration
P.O.	½-3 hr	Variable	Variable

Contraindications and precautions

Contraindicated in patients with abdominal pain, nausea, vomiting, or other symptoms of appendicitis or acute surgical abdomen and in those with myocardial damage, heart block, fecal impaction, rectal fissures, intestinal obstruction or perforation, renal disease, and patients about to deliver.

Use cautiously in patients with rectal bleeding.

Interactions

Drug-drug. *Chlordiazepoxide, chlorpromazine, dicumarol, digoxin, iron salts, isoniazid:* Use of magnesium hydroxide with aluminum hydroxide may decrease the absorption rate of these drugs. Separate administration times.
Enteric-coated tablets: Premature release of enterically coated drugs. Separate administration times.
Quinolones and tetracyclines: Decreased absorption. Separate administration times.

Effects on diagnostic tests

None reported.

Adverse reactions

GI: *abdominal cramping, nausea, diarrhea,* laxative dependence (with long-term or excessive use).
Metabolic: fluid and electrolyte disturbances (with daily use).

Overdose and treatment

No information available.

Clinical considerations

- Give drug at least 1 hour apart from enterically coated medications; shake suspension well.
- After administration of the drug through nasogastric tube, flush tube with water to clear it.

Therapeutic monitoring
Recommend monitoring for signs and symptoms of hypermagnesemia, especially if patient has impaired renal function.

Special populations
Breast-feeding patients. Some magnesium may be excreted in breast milk, but no problems have been reported with use by breast-feeding women.
Pediatric patients. Use as an antacid in children under age 6 requires a well-established diagnosis because children tend to give vague descriptions of symptoms.

Patient counseling
- Caution patient to avoid overuse to prevent laxative dependence.
- Instruct patient to shake suspension well or to chew tablets well.
- Encourage patient using drug as a laxative to maintain adequate fluid intake, diet, and exercise.

magnesium sulfate

Pharmacologic classification: mineral/electrolyte
Therapeutic classification: anticonvulsant
Pregnancy risk category A

How supplied
Available by prescription only
Parenteral injection: 10%, 12.5%, 50%
Injection for I.V. use: 4% (4, 20, and 40 g); 8% (4g)
Parenteral injection for I.V. use: 1% (1 and 10 g) in 5% dextrose; 2% (10 and 20 g) in 5% dextrose

Indications and dosages
Hypomagnesemic seizures
Adults: 1 g I.V. or I.M. Alternatively, 1 to 2 g (as 10% solution) I.V. over 15 minutes, then 1 g I.M. q 4 to 6 hours, based on patient's response and magnesium blood levels.
Seizures secondary to hypomagnesemia in acute nephritis
Children: 0.2 ml/kg of 50% solution I.M. q 4 to 6 hours, p.r.n., or 100 to 200 mg/kg as a 1% to 3% solution I.V. given slowly over 1 hour with the first half of dose in the first 15 to 20 minutes. Also, 0.1 to 0.2 ml/kg of 20% solution (20 to 40 mg/kg) I.M. Titrate dosage according to magnesium blood levels and seizure response.
Life-threatening arrhythmias
Adults: For patient with sustained ventricular tachycardia or torsades de pointes, give 1 to 6 g I.V. over several minutes followed by 3 to 20 mg/minute I.V. infusion for 5 to 48 hours depending on patient response and serum magnesium levels. For patients with paroxysmal atrial tachycardia, give 3 to 4 g I.V. over 30 seconds.
Prevention or control of seizures in preeclampsia or eclampsia
Adults: Initially, 4 g I.V. in 250 ml D_5W and 4 to 5 g deep I.M. into each buttock (using undiluted 50% magnesium sulfate injection); then 4 to 5 g deep I.M. into alternate buttock q 4 hours, p.r.n. Alternatively, 4 g I.V. as a loading dose followed by 1 to 3 g hourly as an I.V. infusion. Maximum daily dose, 30 to 40 g. Alternatively, 8 to 15 g (depending on weight of patient—8 g for 100-lb [45-kg] patient and 15 g for 198-lb [90-kg] patient); 4 g of magnesium sulfate (as magnesium sulfate injection or magnesium sulfate in 5% dextrose) is given I.V. and the remaining dose is given I.M. using undiluted 50% magnesium sulfate injection. Dosage over next 24 hours based on serum concentration and urinary excretion of magnesium following the initial dose. Subsequent doses should be sufficient to replace magnesium excreted in urine, about 65% of the initial dose administered I.M. q 6 hours.
≡ ***Dosage adjustment.*** In severe renal insufficiency, maximum dose is 20 g in 48 hours.
Barium poisoning, ◇asthma
Adults: 1 to 2 g I.V.
◇Management of preterm labor
Adults: 4 to 6 g I.V. over 20 minutes as a loading dose, followed by maintenance infusions of 2 to 4 g/hour for 12 to 24 hours as tolerated after contractions subside.
Mild hypomagnesemia
Adults: 1 to 3 g I.M. q 6 hours for 4 doses; or 5 g in 1 L of D_5W or dextrose 5% in normal saline solution I.V. over 3 hours.
Reduction of CV morbidity and mortality associated with acute myocardial infarction
Adults: 2 g I.V. over 5 to 15 minutes, followed by infusion of 18 g over 24 hours (12.5 mg/min). Initiate therapy as soon as possible, but no longer than 6 hours after MI.

Pharmacodynamics
Anticonvulsant action: Magnesium sulfate has CNS and respiratory depressant effects. It acts peripherally, causing vasodilation; moderate doses cause flushing and sweating, whereas high doses cause hypotension. It prevents or controls seizures by blocking neuromuscular transmission.

Drug is sometimes used in pregnant women to prevent or control preeclamptic or eclamptic seizures; it also is used to treat hypomagnesemic seizures in adults, and in children with acute nephritis.

Pharmacokinetics
Absorption: Effective anticonvulsant serum levels are 2.5 to 7.5 mEq/L.
Distribution: Magnesium sulfate is distributed widely throughout the body.
Metabolism: None.

Excretion: Excreted unchanged in urine; some is excreted in breast milk.

Route	Onset	Peak	Duration
I.V.	1-2 min	Rapid	½ hr
I.M.	1 hr	Unknown	3-4 hr

Contraindications and precautions
Parenteral administration of drug contraindicated in patients with heart block or myocardial damage. Use cautiously in patients with impaired renal function and in women in labor. Don't give in toxemia of pregnancy during the 2 hours preceding delivery.

Interactions
Drug-drug. *Antidepressants, antipsychotics, anxiolytics, barbiturates, general anesthetics, hypnotics, or narcotics:* May increase CNS depressant effects. Reduced dosages may be required.
Cardiac glycosides: Changes in cardiac conduction in digitalized patients may lead to heart block if I.V. calcium is administered. Avoid use together, if possible.
Succinylcholine or tubocurarine: Potentiated and prolonged neuromuscular blocking action of these drugs. Use with caution.
Drug-lifestyle. *Alcohol use:* Increased CNS depressant effects. Avoid use together.

Effects on diagnostic tests
None reported.

Adverse reactions
CNS: drowsiness, *depressed reflexes,* flaccid paralysis.
CV: *hypotension, flushing,* ***circulatory collapse,*** depressed cardiac function.
Metabolic: hypocalcemia.
Respiratory: ***respiratory paralysis.***
Skin: diaphoresis.
Other: hypothermia.

Overdose and treatment
Signs and symptoms of overdose with magnesium sulfate include a sharp decrease in blood pressure and respiratory paralysis, ECG changes (increased PR, QRS, and QT intervals), heart block, and asystole.

Treatment requires artificial ventilation and I.V. calcium salt to reverse respiratory depression and heart block. Usual dose is 5 to 10 mEq of calcium (10 to 20 ml of a 10% calcium gluconate solution).

Clinical considerations
☐ ***ALERT*** Read label closely to ensure proper dosage and concentration is given.
- I.V. bolus must be injected slowly to avoid respiratory or cardiac arrest.
- If available, administer by constant infusion pump; maximum infusion rate is 150 mg/minute. Rapid drip causes feeling of heat.
- Discontinue drug as soon as needed effect is achieved.
- Level of magnesium sulfate for I.V. administration shouldn't exceed 20% at a rate no greater than 150 mg/minute (1.5 ml of a 10% concentration or equivalent). For I.M. administration in adults, levels of 25% or 50% are generally used; in infants and children, levels shouldn't exceed 20% (200 mg/ml).
- Respiratory rate must be 16 breaths per minute or more before each dose. Keep I.V. calcium gluconate 20% on hand.
- To calculate grams of magnesium in a percentage of solution: X% = X g/100 ml (for example, 25% = 25 g/100 ml = 250 mg/ml).

Therapeutic monitoring
- Monitor serum magnesium level and clinical status to avoid overdose.
- When giving repeated doses, test knee jerk reflex before each dose; if absent, discontinue magnesium. Use of drug beyond this point risks respiratory center failure.
- When used as a tocolytic agent, patient requires monitoring for magnesium toxicity and of I.V. fluids infused to avoid circulatory overload.
- After use in toxemic women within 24 hours before delivery, newborn requires observation for signs of magnesium toxicity, including neuromuscular and respiratory depression.

Special populations
Breast-feeding patients. Drug is excreted in breast milk; in patients with normal renal function, all magnesium sulfate is excreted within 24 hours of discontinuing drug. Alternative feeding method is recommended during therapy.
Pediatric patients. Drug isn't indicated for pediatric use.

mannitol
Osmitrol, Resectisol

Pharmacologic classification: osmotic diuretic
Therapeutic classification: diuretic
Pregnancy risk category C

How supplied
Available by prescription only
Injection: 5%, 10%, 15%, 20%, 25%
Urogenital solution: 5 g/100 ml distilled water

Indications and dosages
Test dose for marked oliguria or suspected inadequate renal function
Adults and children over age 12: 200 mg/kg or 12.5 g as a 15% or 20% solution I.V. over 3 to 5 minutes. Response is adequate if 30 to 50 ml urine/hour is excreted over 2 to 3 hours. May repeat test dose one time if response is inadequate the first time.

◊ *Children under age 12:* 0.2 g/kg or 6 g/m² I.V. over 3 to 5 minutes.
Treatment of oliguria
Adults and children over age 12: 50 to 100 g as a 15% to 20% solution I.V. over 90 minutes to several hours.
Children under age 12: 2 g/kg or 60 g/ m² I.V.
Prevention of oliguria or acute renal failure
Adults and children over age 12: 50 to 100 g followed by a 5% to 10% solution I.V. Exact level is determined by fluid requirements.
Treatment of edema and ascites
Adults and children over age 12: 100 g as a 10% to 20% solution I.V. over 2 to 6 hours.
◊ *Children under age 12:* 2 g/kg or 60 g/m² I.V. as a 15% to 20% solution over 2 to 6 hours.
To reduce intraocular pressure or intracranial pressure
Adults and children over age 12: 1.5 to 2 g/kg as a 15% to 25% solution I.V. over 30 to 60 minutes (administer 60 to 90 minutes before surgery if used preoperatively).
◊ *Children under age 12:* 2 g/kg or 60 g/m² I.V. as a 15% to 20% solution over 30 to 60 minutes.
To promote diuresis in drug intoxication
Adults and children over age 12: 25 g loading dose followed by an infusion maintaining 100 to 500 ml urine output/hour and positive fluid balance (of 1 to 2 L). For patients with barbiturate poisoning, give 0.5 g/kg followed by a 5% to 10% solution. Alternatively, 1 L of 10% solution during first hour. Subsequent dosing based on urine output, urine pH, and fluid balance.
◊ *Children under age 12:* 2 g/kg or 60 g/m² of 5% to 10% solution as needed.
Urologic irrigation
Adults: 2.5% to 5 % irrigating solution via indwelling urethral catheter.

Pharmacodynamics
Diuretic action: Mannitol increases the osmotic pressure of glomerular filtrate, inhibiting tubular reabsorption of water and electrolytes, thus promoting diuresis. This action also promotes urinary elimination of certain drugs. This effect is useful for prevention and management of acute renal failure or oliguria. This action is also useful for reduction of intracranial or intraocular pressure because mannitol elevates plasma osmolality, enhancing flow of water into extracellular fluid.

Pharmacokinetics
Absorption: Not absorbed from the GI tract. I.V. mannitol lowers intracranial pressure in 15 minutes and intraocular pressure in 30 to 60 minutes; it produces diuresis in 1 to 3 hours.
Distribution: Remains in the extracellular compartment. It doesn't cross the blood-brain barrier.
Metabolism: Metabolized minimally to glycogen in the liver.
Excretion: Filtered by the glomeruli; half-life in adults with normal renal function is about 100 minutes.

Route	Onset	Peak	Duration
I.V.	¼-1 hr	1-3 hr	3-8 hr

Contraindications and precautions
Contraindicated in patients with hypersensitivity to drug and in those with anuria, severe pulmonary congestion, frank pulmonary edema, severe heart failure, severe dehydration, metabolic edema, progressive renal disease or dysfunction, or active intracranial bleeding except during craniotomy. Use cautiously in pregnant patients.

Interactions
Drug-drug. *Cardiac glycosides:* May enhance the possibility of digitalis toxicity. Monitor serum digoxin levels.
Diuretics, including carbonic anhydrase inhibitors: Increased effects of these drugs. Patient requires close monitoring.
Lithium: Enhanced renal excretion of lithium and lower serum lithium levels. Monitor lithium levels.

Effects on diagnostic tests
Drug therapy may interfere with tests for inorganic phosphorus level or blood ethylene glycol.

Adverse reactions
CNS: ***seizures,*** dizziness, headache.
CV: edema, thrombophlebitis, hypotension, hypertension, ***heart failure,*** tachycardia, angina-like chest pain.
EENT: blurred vision, rhinitis, dry mouth.
GI: thirst, nausea, vomiting, *diarrhea.*
GU: urine retention.
Metabolic: fluid and electrolyte imbalance, dehydration.
Skin: urticaria.
Other: local pain, fever, chills.

Overdose and treatment
Signs and symptoms of overdose include polyuria, cellular dehydration, hypotension, and CV collapse.

Discontinue infusion and institute supportive measures. Hemodialysis removes mannitol and decreases serum osmolality.

Clinical considerations
- For maximum pressure reduction during surgery, give drug 1 to 1½ hours preoperatively.
- Administer drug I.V. via an in-line filter with great care to avoid extravasation.
- Don't administer with whole blood; agglutination will occur.

- Mannitol solutions commonly crystallize at low temperatures; place crystallized solutions in a hot water bath, shake vigorously to dissolve crystals, and cool to body temperature before use. Don't use solutions with undissolved crystals.
- Fluid administration shouldn't exceed 1 L per day in excess of urine output.
- Store drug at 59° to 86° F (15° to 30° C) and protect from freezing.

Therapeutic monitoring
Use with extreme caution in patients with compromised renal function; monitoring should include: vital signs (including CVP) hourly and input and output, weight, renal function, fluid balance, and serum and urinary sodium and potassium levels daily.

Special populations
Breast-feeding patients. Safety of drug in breast-feeding women hasn't been established.
Pediatric patients. Dosage for children under age 12 hasn't been established.
Geriatric patients. Geriatric or debilitated patients require close observation and may require lower dosages. Excessive diuresis promotes rapid dehydration, leading to hypovolemia, hypokalemia, and hyponatremia.

Patient counseling
- Tell patient he may feel thirsty or experience mouth dryness, and emphasize importance of drinking only the amount of fluids provided.
- With initial doses, warn patient to change position slowly, especially when rising from lying or sitting position, to prevent dizziness from orthostatic hypotension.
- Instruct patient to immediately report pain in the chest, back, or legs; shortness of breath; or apnea.

measles, mumps, and rubella virus vaccine, live
M-M-R II

Pharmacologic classification: vaccine
Therapeutic classification: viral vaccine
Pregnancy risk category C

How supplied
Available by prescription only
Injection: Single-dose vial containing not less than 1,000 $TCID_{50}$ (tissue culture infective doses) of attenuated measles virus derived from Enders' attenuated Edmonston strain (grown in chick embryo culture); 20,000 $TCID_{50}$ of the Jeryl Lynn (B level) mumps strain (grown in chick embryo culture); and 1,000 $TCID_{50}$ of the Wistar RA 27/3 strain of rubella virus (propagated in human diploid cell culture)

Indications and dosages
Measles, mumps, and rubella immunization
Adults (born after 1957): Two doses of 0.5 ml S.C. in outer aspect of upper arm, given at least 1 month apart.
Children: Initially, 0.5 ml S.C. in outer aspect of upper arm at age 12 to 15 months; second dose at age 4 to 6 years. Second dose may be given earlier if at least 4 weeks have elapsed since first dose and both doses are given beginning at or after age 12 months.

Pharmacodynamics
Measles, mumps, and rubella prophylaxis: This vaccine promotes active immunity to measles (rubeola), mumps, and German measles (rubella) by inducing production of antibodies.

Pharmacokinetics
Absorption: Antibodies are usually evident 2 to 3 weeks after injection. Duration of vaccine-induced immunity is expected to be lifelong.
Distribution: No information available.
Metabolism: No information available.
Excretion: No information available.

Route	Onset	Peak	Duration
S.C.	Unknown	Unknown	< 11 yr

Contraindications and precautions
Contraindicated in immunosuppressed patients; in those with cancer, blood dyscrasias, gamma globulin disorders, fever, active untreated tuberculosis, or anaphylactic or anaphylactoid reactions to neomycin or eggs; in those receiving corticosteroid or radiation therapy; and in pregnant women. Use cautiously in patients with history of cerebral injury, individual or family history of seizures, or any other condition in which stress resulting from fever should be avoided.

Interactions
Drug-drug. *Immune serum globulin or transfusions of blood or blood products:* May interfere with the immune response to the vaccine. Whenever possible, defer vaccination for 3 months in these situations.
Immunosuppressive agents: May interfere with the response to vaccine. Avoid use together if possible.

Effects on diagnostic tests
Measles, mumps, and rubella vaccine may temporarily decrease the response to tuberculin skin testing. If a tuberculin skin test is necessary, administer it either before or simultaneously with this vaccine.

Adverse reactions
CNS: syncope, malaise, headache.

EENT: otitis media, conjunctivitis, sore throat.
GI: diarrhea, vomiting.
Respiratory: cough.
Skin: urticaria, rash.
Other: fever, regional lymphadenopathy, ***anaphylaxis,*** vasculitis, erythema at injection site.

Overdose and treatment

No information available.

Clinical considerations

- Drug can be given to patient with HIV infection who doesn't have severe immunosuppression.
- Obtain a thorough history of allergies, especially to antibiotics, eggs, chicken, or chicken feathers, and of reactions to immunizations.
- Perform a skin test to assess vaccine sensitivity (against a control of normal saline solution in the opposing extremity) in patients with history of anaphylactoid reactions to egg ingestion. Administer a prick (intracutaneous) or scratch test with a 1:10 dilution. Read results after 5 to 30 minutes. A positive reaction is a wheal with or without pseudopodia and surrounding erythema.
- Epinephrine solution 1:1,000 should be available to treat allergic reactions.
- Most adults born before 1957 are believed to have been infected with naturally occurring disease, and vaccination isn't necessary; however, vaccination should be offered if they are considered susceptible.
- Use only the diluent supplied. Discard reconstituted solution after 8 hours.
- Drug shouldn't be administered I.V. Use a 25G, ⅝-inch needle and inject S.C., preferably into the outer aspect of the upper arm. Use a sterile syringe free of preservatives, antiseptics, and detergents for each injection, because these substances may inactivate the live virus vaccine.
- Solution may be used if red, pink, or yellow, but it must be clear.
- Vaccine shouldn't be given less than 1 month before or after immunization with other live virus vaccines—except for monovalent or trivalent live oral poliovirus vaccine or poliovirus vaccine, inactivated, which may be administered simultaneously at separate sites using separate syringes.
- Vaccine may not offer any protection when given within a few days after exposure to natural measles, mumps, or rubella.
- Give passive immunization with immune serum globulin, if necessary, when immediate protection against measles is required in patients who cannot receive the measles vaccine component. Don't administer any live virus vaccine component simultaneously with immune serum globulin.
- Revaccination is unnecessary if the child received two doses of vaccine at least 1 month apart, beginning after the first birthday.
- Store vaccine at 36° to 46° F (2° to 8° C) and protect from light.

Therapeutic monitoring

Patient should be observed for allergic reactions.

Special populations

Breast-feeding patients. No data are available regarding distribution of measles or mumps virus components in breast milk. Some reports have demonstrated transfer of rubella virus or virus antigen into breast milk in about 68% of women. Few adverse effects have been associated with breast-feeding after immunization with rubella-containing vaccines. The risk-benefit ratio suggests that breast-feeding women may be immunized with the rubella component, if necessary.
Pediatric patients. Children under age 15 months may not respond to one, two, or all three of vaccine components, because retained maternal antibodies may interfere with immune response. However, vaccination at age 12 months is recommended if child lives in a high-risk area, because the benefits outweigh the risk of a slightly lower efficacy of vaccine.

Patient counseling

- Tell patient what to expect after vaccination: tingling sensations in the extremities or joint aches and pains that may resemble arthritis, beginning several days to several weeks after vaccination. These symptoms usually resolve within 1 week. Other effects include pain and inflammation at the injection site and a low-grade fever, a rash, or difficulty breathing. Recommend acetaminophen to alleviate adverse reactions, such as fever.
- Tell patient to report distressing adverse reactions.
- Advise women of childbearing age not to become pregnant for 3 months after receiving vaccine.

measles and rubella virus vaccine, live, attenuated

M-R-Vax II

Pharmacologic classification: vaccine
Therapeutic classification: viral vaccine
Pregnancy risk category C

How supplied

Available by prescription only
Injection: Single-dose vial containing not less than 1,000 $TCID_{50}$ (tissue culture infective doses) each of attenuated measles virus derived from Enders' attenuated Edmonston strain (grown in chick embryo culture) and the Wistar RA 27/3 strain of rubella virus (propagated in human diploid cell culture)

Note: 10-dose and 50-dose vials are available to government agencies and institutions only.

Indications and dosages

Measles and rubella immunization

Adults and children age 15 months and older: 0.5 ml in outer aspect of the upper arm. For adequate protection against measles, a two-dose schedule is recommended (at least 1 month between doses).

Pharmacodynamics

Measles and rubella prophylaxis: Vaccine promotes active immunity to measles (rubeola) and German measles (rubella) virus by inducing production of antibodies.

Pharmacokinetics

Absorption: Antibodies are usually detectable 2 to 3 weeks after injection. Duration of vaccine-induced immunity is expected to be lifelong.
Distribution: No information available.
Metabolism: No information available.
Excretion: No information available.

Route	Onset	Peak	Duration
S.C.	Unknown	Unknown	< 11 yr

Contraindications and precautions

Contraindicated in immunosuppressed patients; in those with cancer, blood dyscrasias, gamma globulin disorders, fever, active untreated tuberculosis, or anaphylactic or anaphylactoid reactions to eggs or neomycin; in those receiving corticosteroid or radiation therapy; and in pregnant women. Use cautiously in patients with history of cerebral injury, individual or family history of seizures, or any other condition in which stress resulting from fever should be avoided.

Interactions

Drug-drug. *Immune serum globulin or transfusions of blood or blood products:* May interfere with the immune response to the vaccine. Whenever possible, defer vaccination for 3 months in these situations.
Immunosuppressants: May interfere with response to vaccine. Avoid use together if possible.

Effects on diagnostic tests

Measles and rubella vaccine may temporarily decrease response to tuberculin skin testing. If a tuberculin skin test is necessary, administer it either before or simultaneously with measles and rubella vaccine.

Adverse reactions

CNS: syncope, malaise, headache.
EENT: sore throat.
GI: vomiting, diarrhea.
Respiratory: cough.
Skin: rash.
Other: fever, lymphadenopathy, erythema, burning, or stinging (at injection site); vasculitis, ***anaphylaxis.***

Overdose and treatment

No information available.

Clinical considerations

- Drug can be given to patient with HIV infection who doesn't have severe immunosuppression.
- Obtain a thorough history of allergies, especially to antibiotics, eggs, chicken, or chicken feathers, and of reactions to immunizations.
- Skin testing is necessary to assess vaccine sensitivity (against a control of normal saline solution in the opposing extremity) in patients with history of anaphylactoid reactions to eggs. Administer a prick (intracutaneous) or scratch test with a 1:10 dilution. Read results after 5 to 30 minutes. A positive reaction is a wheal with or without pseudopodia and surrounding erythema.
- Epinephrine solution 1:1,000 should be available to treat allergic reactions.
- Drug shouldn't be administered I.V. Use a 25G, ⅝-inch needle and inject S.C., preferably into the outer aspect of the upper arm.
- Use a sterile syringe free of preservatives, antiseptics, and detergents for each injection because these substances may inactivate the live virus vaccine.
- Use only diluent supplied. Discard reconstituted solution after 8 hours.
- Solution may be used if red, pink, or yellow, but it must be clear.
- Vaccine shouldn't be given less than 1 month before or after immunization with other live virus vaccines, except for mumps virus vaccine and monovalent or trivalent live oral poliovirus vaccine, and poliovirus vaccine, inactivated, which may be administered simultaneously.
- Vaccine may not offer protection when given within a few days' exposure to natural measles or rubella.
- According to Centers for Disease Control and Prevention recommendations, measles, mumps and rubella (MMR) is the preferred vaccine.
- Passive immunization is given with immune serum globulin when immediate protection against measles is required in patients who can't receive the measles vaccine component. Don't administer either vaccine component simultaneously with immune serum globulin.
- Store vaccine at 36° to 46° F (2° to 8° C) and protect from light.
- Revaccination is usually given between 4 to 6 years of age. Measles virus vaccine, live, MMR II, or MR-VAX II may be used.

Therapeutic monitoring
Patient should be monitored for adverse allergic reaction.

Special populations
Breast-feeding patients. No data are available regarding distribution of measles and rubella virus components in breast milk. Some reports have demonstrated transfer of rubella virus or virus antigen into breast milk in about 68% of patients. Few adverse effects have been associated with breast-feeding after immunization with rubella-containing vaccines. The risk-benefit ratio suggests that breast-feeding women may be immunized with the rubella component, if necessary.
Pediatric patients. Children under age 15 months may not respond to one or both of the vaccine components because retained maternal antibodies may interfere with the immune response; revaccination is recommended after age 15 months.

Patient counseling
- Tell patient to expect tingling sensations in the extremities or joint aches and pains that may resemble arthritis, beginning several days to several weeks after vaccination. These symptoms usually resolve within 1 week. Other effects include pain and inflammation at the injection site and a low-grade fever, rash, or difficulty breathing. Recommend acetaminophen for relief of fever.
- Encourage patient to report distressing adverse reactions.
- Advise women of childbearing age not to become pregnant for 3 months after receiving the vaccine.

measles virus vaccine, live, attenuated
Attenuvax

Pharmacologic classification: vaccine
Therapeutic classification: viral vaccine
Pregnancy risk category C

How supplied
Available by prescription only
Injection: Single-dose vial containing not less than 1,000 $TCID_{50}$ (tissue culture infective doses) per 0.5 ml of attenuated measles virus derived from Enders' attenuated Edmonston strain grown in chick embryo culture.
Note: 10-dose and 50-dose vials are available to government agencies and institutions only.

Indications and dosages
Immunization
Adults and children age 15 months and older: 0.5 ml (1,000 units) S.C. in outer aspect of the upper arm. Administer two doses at least 1 month apart. For children, usual schedule is the first dose at age 15 months and a second dose at the entry of school (age 4 to 6 years).

Pharmacodynamics
Measles prophylaxis: Measles virus vaccine promotes active immunity to measles virus by inducing production of antibodies.

Pharmacokinetics
Absorption: Antibodies are usually evident 2 to 3 weeks after injection. Duration of vaccine-induced immunity is at least 13 to 16 years and probably lifelong in most immunized persons.
Distribution: No information available.
Metabolism: No information available.
Excretion: No information available.

Route	Onset	Peak	Duration
S.C.	Few days	Unknown	≥ 13 yr

Contraindications and precautions
Contraindicated in immunosuppressed patients; in those with cancer, blood dyscrasias, gamma globulin disorders, fever, active untreated tuberculosis, or anaphylactic or anaphylactoid reactions to neomycin or eggs; in those receiving corticosteroid or radiation therapy; and in pregnant patients. Use cautiously in patients with history of cerebral injury, individual or family history of seizures, or any other condition where stress resulting from fever should be avoided.

Interactions
Drug-drug. *Immune serum globulin or transfusions of blood or blood products:* May interfere with the immune response to the vaccine. Whenever possible, defer vaccination for 3 months in these situations.
Immunosuppressants: May interfere with the response to vaccine. Avoid use together if possible.
Meningococcal vaccine: Administration of meningococcal vaccine with measles virus vaccine can result in a reduced seroconversion rate to meningococci. Avoid administration together.

Effects on diagnostic tests
Measles vaccine temporarily may decrease the response to tuberculin skin testing. If a tuberculin skin test is necessary, administer it either before or simultaneously with the measles vaccine.

Adverse reactions
CNS: ***febrile seizures*** (in susceptible children).
GI: anorexia.
Hematologic: ***leukopenia.***
Skin: rash, erythema, swelling, tenderness (at injection site).
Other: fever, lymphadenopathy, ***anaphylaxis.***

Overdose and treatment
No information available.

Clinical considerations
■ Obtain a thorough history of allergies, especially to antibiotics, eggs, chicken, or chicken feathers, and of reactions to immunizations.
■ Measles vaccine shouldn't be given less than 1 month before or after immunization with other live virus vaccines, except for mumps virus vaccine, rubella virus vaccine, or monovalent or trivalent live oral poliovirus vaccine or poliovirus vaccine, inactivated, which may be administered simultaneously.
■ Vaccine may offer some protection when given within a few days after exposure to natural measles and substantial protection when given a few days before exposure.
■ According to Centers for Disease Control and Prevention recommendations, measles, mumps, and rubella (MMR) is the preferred vaccine.
■ Passive immunization is given with immune serum globulin if immediate protection against measles is required in patients who can't receive the measles vaccine.
■ Patients with a history of anaphylactoid reactions to eggs should first have a skin test to assess vaccine sensitivity (against a control of normal saline solution in the other arm). Administer a prick (intracutaneous) or scratch test with a 1:10 dilution. Read results after 5 to 30 minutes. A positive reaction is a wheal with or without pseudopodia and surrounding erythema.
■ Patients who received measles vaccine live when under age 1 year should be considered susceptible to measles, and therefore should be revaccinated.
■ Epinephrine solution 1:1,000 should be available to treat allergic reactions.
■ Drug shouldn't be administered I.V. Use a 25G, ⅝-inch needle and inject S.C., preferably into the outer aspect of the upper arm. Use a sterile syringe free of preservatives, antiseptics, and detergents for each injection, because these substances may inactivate the live virus vaccine.
■ Use diluent supplied. Discard reconstituted solution after 8 hours.
■ Store vaccine at 35° to 46° F (2° to 8° C), and protect from light. Solution may be used if red, pink, or yellow, but it must be clear.

Special populations
Breast-feeding patients. It's unknown if vaccine is excreted in breast milk. Use with caution in breast-feeding women.
Pediatric patients. Children under age 15 months may not respond to the vaccine, because retained maternal antibodies may interfere with the immune response, revaccination is recommended after age 15 months.

Patient counseling
■ Tell patient to expect pain and inflammation at the injection site, fever, rash, general malaise, or difficulty breathing. Recommend acetaminophen for relief of fever.
■ Encourage patient to report distressing adverse reactions.
■ Advise women of childbearing age not to become pregnant for 3 months after receiving the vaccine.

mebendazole
Vermox

Pharmacologic classification: benzimidazole
Therapeutic classification: anthelmintic
Pregnancy risk category C

How supplied
Available by prescription only
Tablets (chewable): 100 mg

Indications and dosages
Pinworm infestations
Adults and children over age 2: 100 mg P.O. as a single dose. If infection persists 2 weeks later, repeat treatment.
◊***Other roundworm, whipworm, and hookworm infestations, off label trichostrongylosis***
Adults and children over age 2: 100 mg P.O. b.i.d. for 3 days. If infection persists 3 weeks later, repeat treatment. Alternatively, for treatment of hookworm, whipworm, or roundworm, 500 mg P.O. as a single dose.
◊***Trichinosis***
Adults: 200 to 400 mg P.O. t.i.d. for 3 days, then 400 to 500 mg t.i.d. for 10 days.
◊***Capillariasis***
Adults: 200 mg P.O. b.i.d. for 20 days.
◊***Toxocariasis***
Adults and children: 200 to 400 mg P.O. daily divided into 2 doses for 5 days.
◊***Dracunculiasis***
Adults: 400 to 800 mg P.O. daily for 6 days.
◊***Mansonella perstans infestations***
Adults: 100 mg P.O. b.i.d. for 30 days.
◊***Angiostrongylus cantonensis infestations***
Adults and children: 100 mg P.O. b.i.d. for 5 days.
◊***Onchocerciasis***
Adults: 1 g P.O. b.i.d. for 28 days.
◊***Treatment of hydatid disease (echinococcosis)***
Adults: 40 mg/kg P.O. for 1 to 6 months. Alternatively, sequential 2-week courses of 50 mg/kg daily; 200 mg/kg daily; and 50 mg/kg daily for 21 to 30 days.
◊***Angiostrongylus costaricensis***
Adults and children: 600 to 1,200 mg P.O. daily divided t.i.d. for 10 days.

Pharmacodynamics

Anthelmintic action: Mebendazole inhibits uptake of glucose and other low-molecular-weight nutrients in susceptible helminths, depleting the glycogen stores they need for survival and reproduction. It has a broad spectrum and may be useful in mixed infections. It's considered a drug of choice in the treatment of ascariasis, capillariasis, enterobiasis, trichuriasis, and uncinariasis; it has been used investigationally to treat echinococciasis, onchocerciasis, and trichinosis.

Pharmacokinetics

Absorption: About 5% to 10% of an administered dose is absorbed. Absorption varies widely among patients.
Distribution: Highly bound to plasma proteins; it crosses the placenta.
Metabolism: Metabolized to inactive 2-amino-5(6)-benzimidazolyl phenylketone.
Excretion: Most of a dose is excreted in feces; 2% to 10% is excreted in urine in 48 hours as either unchanged drug or the 2-amine metabolite. Half-life is 3 to 9 hours. It's unknown if drug is excreted in breast milk.

Route	Onset	Peak	Duration
P.O.	Unknown	2-4 hr	Variable

Contraindications and precautions

Contraindicated in patients with hypersensitivity to drug.

Interactions

Drug-drug. *Anticonvulsants, including carbamazepine and phenytoin:* May enhance the metabolism of mebendazole and decrease its efficacy. Patient requires monitoring for clinical effect.
Cimetidine: Inhibits mebendazole metabolism and may result in increased plasma levels of drug. Use together cautiously.

Effects on diagnostic tests

None reported.

Adverse reactions

GI: occasional, transient abdominal pain and diarrhea in massive infection and expulsion of worms.
Other: fever.

Overdose and treatment

Signs and symptoms of overdose may include GI disturbances and altered mental status. No specific recommendations exist; treatment is supportive. After recent ingestion (within 4 hours), empty stomach by induced emesis or gastric lavage. Follow with activated charcoal to decrease absorption.

Clinical considerations

- Tablets may be chewed, swallowed whole, or crushed and mixed with food.
- Laxatives, enemas, or dietary restrictions are unnecessary.
- Collect stool specimens in a clean, dry container and transfer to a properly labeled container to send to laboratory; ova may be destroyed by toilet bowl water, urine, and some drugs.
- Store drug at 59° to 77° F (15° to 25° C) in well-closed container; product expires 3 years from date of manufacture.

Therapeutic monitoring

High-dose treatment of hydatid disease and trichinosis is investigational. Frequently monitor WBC counts to detect drug toxicity, especially during initial therapy.

Special populations

Breast-feeding patients. Safety in breast-feeding women hasn't been established.
Pediatric patients. Give drug to children under age 2 only when potential benefits justify risks.

Patient counseling

- Teach patient and family members personal hygiene measures to prevent reinfection: washing perianal area and changing undergarments and bedclothes daily; washing hands and cleaning fingernails before meals and after defecation; and sanitary disposal of feces.
- Advise patient to bathe often, by showering, if possible.
- Advise patient to keep hands away from mouth, to keep fingernails short, and to wear shoes to avoid hookworm; explain that ova are easily transmitted directly and indirectly by hands, food, or contaminated articles. Washing clothes in household washing machine will destroy ova.
- Instruct patient to handle bedding carefully because shaking will send ova into the air, and to disinfect toilet facilities and vacuum or damp-mop floors daily to reduce number of ova.
- Encourage patient's family and contacts to be checked for infestation and treated, if necessary

mechlorethamine hydrochloride (nitrogen mustard)

Mustargen

Pharmacologic classification: alkylating agent (cell cycle-phase nonspecific)
Therapeutic classification: antineoplastic
Pregnancy risk category D

How supplied

Available by prescription only
Injection: 10-mg vials

Indications and dosages

Dosage and indications may vary. Check current literature for recommended protocols.

Hodgkin's disease, bronchogenic carcinoma, chronic lymphocytic leukemia, chronic myelocytic leukemia, lymphosarcoma, polycythemia vera

Adults: 0.4 mg/kg I.V. per course of therapy as a single dose or 0.1 to 0.2 mg/kg on 2 to 4 successive days q 3 to 6 weeks. Give through running I.V. infusion. Dose reduced in prior radiation therapy or chemotherapy to 0.2 to 0.4 mg/kg. Dose based on ideal or actual body weight, whichever is less.

Intracavitary doses for neoplastic effusions

Adults: 0.2 to 0.4 mg/kg.

Treatment of advanced Hodgkin's disease (MOPP regimen)

Adults: 6 mg/ m^2 given I.V. on days 1 and 8 of 28-day cycle. In subsequent cycles, dose is based on leukocyte count.

Pharmacodynamics

Antineoplastic action: Mechlorethamine exerts its cytotoxic activity through the basic processes of alkylation. Drug causes cross-linking of DNA strands, single-strand breakage of DNA, abnormal base pairing, and interruption of other intracellular processes, resulting in cell death.

Pharmacokinetics

Absorption: Well absorbed after oral administration; however, because drug is very irritating to tissue, it must be administered I.V. After intracavitary administration, mechlorethamine is absorbed incompletely, probably from deactivation by body fluids in the cavity.

Distribution: Doesn't cross the blood-brain barrier.

Metabolism: Undergoes rapid chemical transformation and reacts quickly with various cellular components before being deactivated.

Excretion: Metabolites are excreted in urine. Less than 0.01% of an I.V. dose is excreted unchanged in urine.

Route	Onset	Peak	Duration
I.V., Intracavitary	Few seconds, few minutes	Unknown	Unknown

Contraindications and precautions

Contraindicated in patients with hypersensitivity to drug and with known infectious diseases. Use cautiously in patients with severe anemia or depressed neutrophil or platelet count and in those who have recently undergone chemotherapy or radiation therapy.

Interactions

None reported.

Effects on diagnostic tests

None reported.

Adverse reactions

CNS: weakness, vertigo.

EENT: tinnitus; deafness (with high doses).

GI: *nausea, vomiting, anorexia* (beginning within minutes, lasting 8 to 24 hours).

GU: menstrual irregularities, impaired spermatogenesis.

Hematologic: ***thrombocytopenia, lymphocytopenia, agranulocytosis,*** nadir of myelosuppression occurring by days 4 to 10 and lasting 10 to 21 days; mild anemia begins in 2 to 3 weeks.

Hepatic: jaundice.

Metabolic: hyperuricemia.

Skin: *alopecia,* rash, sloughing, severe irritation (if drug extravasates or touches skin).

Other: precipitation of herpes zoster, ***anaphylaxis,*** *thrombophlebitis,* amyloidosis.

Overdose and treatment

Signs and symptoms of overdose include severe leukopenia, anemia, thrombocytopenia, and a hemorrhagic diathesis with subsequent delayed bleeding. Death may follow.

Treatment is usually supportive and includes transfusion of blood components and antibiotic treatment of complicating infections.

Clinical considerations

- Avoid contact with skin or mucous membranes. Wear gloves when preparing solution and during administration to prevent accidental skin contact. If contact occurs, wash with copious amounts of water.
- To prevent hyperuricemia with resulting uric acid nephropathy, allopurinol may be given; keep patient well hydrated.
- Drug has been used topically to treat mycosis fungoides.
- To reconstitute powder, use 10 ml of sterile water for injection or normal saline solution to give a concentration of 1 mg/ml.
- When reconstituted, drug is a clear colorless solution. Don't use if solution is discolored or if droplets of water are visible within vial before reconstitution.
- Solution is very unstable. Prepare immediately before infusion and use within 15 minutes. Discard unused solution.
- Dilution of drug into a large volume of I.V. solution isn't recommended, because it may react with the diluent and isn't stable for a prolonged period.
- Drug may be administered I.V. push over a few minutes into the tubing of a freely flowing I.V. infusion. Following administration, flush vein for 2.5 minutes with running I.V. solution or inject 5 to 10 ml of solution into sidearm.
- Treatment of extravasation includes local injections of a 1/6 M sodium thiosulfate solu-

tion. Prepare solution by mixing 4 ml of sodium thiosulfate 10% with 6 ml of sterile water for injection. Also, apply ice packs for 6 to 12 hours to minimize local reactions.

- During intracavitary administration, patient should be turned from side to side every 15 minutes for 1 hour to distribute drug.
- Avoid all I.M. injections when platelet count is low.

Therapeutic monitoring

- Monitor uric acid levels, CBC, and liver function tests.
- Use anticoagulants cautiously. Watch closely for signs of bleeding.

Special populations

Breast-feeding patients. It isn't known if drug is excreted in breast milk. However, because of the potential for serious adverse reactions, mutagenicity, and carcinogenicity in the infant, breast-feeding isn't recommended.

Patient counseling

- Tell patient to avoid exposure to people with infections.
- Advise patient that adequate fluid intake is very important to facilitate excretion of uric acid.
- Reassure patient that hair should grow back after treatment has ended.
- Tell patient to promptly report signs or symptoms of bleeding or infection.
- Advise patient to use contraception while using drug.

meclizine hydrochloride

Antivert, Antivert/25, Antrizine, Bonine, Dizmiss, Meclizine, Meni-D, Ru-Vert-M

Pharmacologic classification: piperazine-derivative antihistamine
Therapeutic classification: antiemetic, antivertigo
Pregnancy risk category B

How supplied

Available with or without a prescription
Tablets: 12.5 mg, 25 mg, 50 mg
Tablets (chewable): 25 mg
Capsules: 25 mg

Indications and dosages

Dizziness
Adults and children age 12 or older: 25 to 100 mg P.O. daily in divided doses. Dosage varies with patient response.
Motion sickness
Adults and children age 12 or older: 25 to 50 mg P.O. 1 hour before travel; may repeat dose daily for duration of journey.

Pharmacodynamics

Antiemetic action: Meclizine probably inhibits nausea and vomiting by centrally decreasing sensitivity of labyrinth apparatus that relays stimuli to the chemoreceptor trigger zone and stimulates the vomiting center in the brain.
Antivertigo action: Drug decreases labyrinth excitability and conduction in vestibular-cerebellar pathways.

Pharmacokinetics

Absorption: Well absorbed.
Distribution: Well distributed throughout the body and crosses the placenta.
Metabolism: Probably metabolized in the liver.
Excretion: Half-life is about 6 hours. Drug is excreted unchanged in feces; metabolites are found in urine.

Route	Onset	Peak	Duration
P.O.	1 hr	Unknown	8-24 hr

Contraindications and precautions

Contraindicated in patients hypersensitive to drug. Use cautiously in patients with asthma, glaucoma, or prostatic hyperplasia.

Interactions

Drug-drug. *CNS depressants, such as barbiturates, sleeping agents, tranquilizers, and antianxiety agents:* Additive sedative. Use together cautiously.
Other ototoxic medications, such as aminoglycosides, cisplatin, loop diuretics, salicylates, and vancomycin: Meclizine may mask signs of ototoxicity. Avoid use together.
Drug-lifestyle. *Alcohol use*: Additive sedative and CNS depressant effects. Advise patient to avoid alcohol use.

Effects on diagnostic tests

Discontinue meclizine 4 days before diagnostic skin tests to avoid preventing, reducing, or masking test response.

Adverse reactions

CNS: *drowsiness,* restlessness, excitation, nervousness, auditory and visual hallucinations.
CV: hypotension, palpitations, tachycardia.
EENT: blurred vision, diplopia, tinnitus, dry nose and throat.
GI: dry mouth, constipation, anorexia, nausea, vomiting, diarrhea.
GU: urine retention, urinary frequency.
Skin: urticaria, rash.

Overdose and treatment

Signs and symptoms of moderate overdose may include hyperexcitability alternating with drowsiness. Seizures, hallucinations, and respiratory paralysis may occur in profound overdose. Anticholinergic symptoms, such as dry mouth, flushed skin, fixed and dilated pupils, and GI symptoms, are common, especially in children.

Treat overdose by administering gastric lavage to empty stomach contents; emesis with ipecac syrup may be ineffective. Treat hypotension with vasopressors, and control seizures with diazepam or phenytoin. Don't give stimulants.

Clinical considerations

Consider the recommendations relevant to all antihistamines as well as the following:

- Tablets may be placed in mouth and allowed to dissolve without water, or they may be chewed or swallowed whole.
- Abrupt withdrawal of drug after long-term use may cause paradoxical reactions or sudden reversal of improved state.

Therapeutic monitoring

Recommend monitoring patient for excessive CNS effects.

Special populations

Breast-feeding patients. Safety in breast-feeding women hasn't been established.
Pediatric patients. Safety and efficacy for use in children haven't been established. Don't use in children under age 12; infants and children under age 6 may experience paradoxical hyperexcitability.
Geriatric patients. Geriatric patients are usually more sensitive to adverse effects of antihistamines and are especially likely to experience a greater degree of dizziness, sedation, hyperexcitability, dry mouth, and urine retention than younger patients.

Patient counseling

Instruct patient to avoid activities that require mental alertness and physical coordination, such as driving and operating dangerous machinery.

medroxyprogesterone acetate

Amen, Curretab, Cycrin, Depo-Provera, Provera

Pharmacologic classification: progestin
Therapeutic classification: progestin, antineoplastic
Pregnancy risk category X

How supplied

Available by prescription only
Tablets: 2.5 mg, 5 mg, 10 mg
Injection: 150 mg/ml, 400 mg/ml

Indications and dosages

Abnormal uterine bleeding from hormonal imbalance
Adults: 5 to 10 mg P.O. daily for 5 to 10 days beginning on day 16 to 21 of menstrual cycle. If patient has received estrogen, then 10 mg P.O. daily for 10 days beginning on day 16 of cycle. If bleeding is controlled satisfactorily, give 2 subsequent cycles of combination therapy.
Secondary amenorrhea
Adults: 5 to 10 mg P.O. daily for 5 to 10 days, preferably beginning on day 16 to 21 of menstrual cycle. If patient has received estrogen, then 10 mg P.O. daily for 10 days.
Endometrial or renal carcinoma (adjunct)
Adults: 400 to 1,000 mg I.M. weekly. If disease improves or stabilizes in a few weeks or months, 400 mg/month.
◊ ***Paraphilia in males***
Adults: Initially, 200 mg I.M. b.i.d. or t.i.d. or 500 mg I.M. weekly. Adjust dosage based on response.
Contraception in females
Adults: 150 mg I.M. q 3 months; give first injection on first 5 days of menstrual cycle.

Pharmacodynamics

Progestational action: Parenteral medroxyprogesterone suppresses ovulation, causes thickening of cervical mucus, and induces sloughing of the endometrium.
Antineoplastic action: Drug may inhibit growth progression of progestin-sensitive endometrial or renal cancer tissue by an unknown mechanism.

Pharmacokinetics

Absorption: Absorption is slow after I.M. administration.
Distribution: Not well characterized.
Metabolism: Primarily hepatic; not well characterized.
Excretion: Primarily renal; not well characterized.

Route	Onset	Peak	Duration
P.O., I.M.	Unknown	Unknown	Unknown

Contraindications and precautions

Contraindicated in patients with hypersensitivity to drug, active thromboembolic disorders, or past history of thromboembolic disorders or of cerebral vascular disease or apoplexy, breast cancer, undiagnosed abnormal vaginal bleeding, missed abortion, or hepatic dysfunction, and during pregnancy. Tablets are also contraindicated in patients with liver dysfunction or known or suspected malignant disease of the genital organs.

Use cautiously in patients with diabetes mellitus, seizures, migraines, cardiac or renal disease, asthma, or mental depression.

Interactions

Drug-drug. *Aminoglutethimide:* May increase the hepatic metabolism of medroxyprogesterone, possibly decreasing its therapeutic effect. Avoid use together.
Bromocriptine: Progestins may cause amenorrhea or galactorrhea, thus interfering with the action of bromocriptine. Avoid use together.

Effects on diagnostic tests

None reported.

Adverse reactions

CNS: depression.
CV: thrombophlebitis, ***pulmonary embolism,*** edema, ***thromboembolism, CVA.***
EENT: exophthalmos, diplopia.
GU: breakthrough bleeding, dysmenorrhea, amenorrhea, cervical erosion, abnormal secretions, breast tenderness, enlargement, or secretion.
Hepatic: cholestatic jaundice.
Metabolic: changes in weight.
Skin: rash, pain, induration, sterile abscesses, acne, pruritus, melasma, alopecia, hirsutism.

Overdose and treatment

No information available.

Clinical considerations

Consider the recommendations relevant to all progestins as well as the following:

- Parenteral form is for I.M. administration only. Inject deep into large muscle mass, preferably the gluteal muscle. Monitor for development of sterile abscesses. Suspension must be shaken vigorously immediately before each use to ensure complete suspension of drug.
- Drug has been used to treat obstructive sleep apnea and to manage paraphilia.
- When used as a long-acting contraceptive in females, rule out pregnancy before initiating therapy.
- Store drug between 59° to 86° F (15° and 30° C); avoid freezing.

Therapeutic monitoring

Monitor serum glucose in diabetic patient.

Special populations

Breast-feeding patients. Detectable amounts of drug have been identified in breast milk. Infants exposed to drug via breast milk have been studied for developmental and behavioral effects through puberty; no adverse effects have been noted.

Patient counseling

- Tell patient not to take drug if she becomes pregnant.
- Advise patient to report chest pain, difficulty breathing, or leg pain.
- Warn patient about signs of CVA.

megestrol acetate

Megace

Pharmacologic classification: progestin
Therapeutic classification: antineoplastic
Pregnancy risk category X

How supplied

Available by prescription only
Tablets: 20 mg, 40 mg
Suspension: 200 mg/5 ml

Indications and dosages

Dosage and indications may vary. Check current literature for recommended protocol.
Palliative treatment of breast carcinoma
Adults: 40 mg (tablets) P.O. q.i.d.
Palliative treatment of endometrial carcinoma
Adults: 10 to 80 mg (tablets) P.O. q.i.d.
Anorexia, cachexia, or weight loss in patients with AIDS
Adults: 800 mg (suspension) P.O. daily; 100 to 400 mg for AIDS-related cachexia.
◊***Anorexia or cachexia in patients with neoplastic disease***
Adults: 480 to 600 mg P.O. daily.

Pharmacodynamics

Antineoplastic action: Megestrol inhibits growth and causes regression of progestin-sensitive breast and endometrial cancer tissue by an unknown mechanism.
Treatment of anorexia, cachexia, or weight loss: Mechanism for weight gain is unknown. Megestrol may stimulate appetite by interfering with the production of mediators such as cachectin.

Pharmacokinetics

Absorption: Well absorbed across the GI tract after oral administration.
Distribution: Appears to be stored in fatty tissue and is highly bound to plasma proteins.
Metabolism: Completely metabolized in the liver.
Excretion: Metabolites are eliminated primarily through the kidneys.

Route	Onset	Peak	Duration
P.O.	Unknown	Unknown	Unknown

Contraindications and precautions

Contraindicated in patients hypersensitive to drug and during pregnancy (especially first 4 months). Use cautiously in patients with history of thrombophlebitis.

Interactions

Drug-drug. *Bromocriptine:* May cause amenorrhea or galactorrhea, interfering with the action of bromocriptine. Use of these drugs together isn't recommended.

Effects on diagnostic tests
None reported.

Adverse reactions
CV: thrombophlebitis, hypertension, edema, chest pain.
GI: increased appetite, nausea, vomiting, diarrhea, flatulence.
GU: breakthrough menstrual bleeding, impotence, decreased libido.
Hepatic: hepatomegaly.
Metabolic: weight gain, hyperglycemia.
Musculoskeletal: carpal tunnel syndrome.
Respiratory: ***pulmonary embolism,*** dyspnea, pneumonia, cough, pharyngitis.
Skin: alopecia, rash, pruritus, candidiasis.

Overdose and treatment
No information available.

Clinical considerations
- Recommendations for administration of megestrol and for care and teaching of the patient during therapy are the same as those for all progestins.
- Investigational uses include prevention of contraception, treatment of prostatic hypertrophy, endometriosis, and endometrial hyperplasias.
- Store tablets between 59° and 86° F (15° and 30° C) and oral suspension at 77° F (25° C) or less.

Therapeutic monitoring
Monitor hemapoietic function and liver function.

Patient counseling
Recommendations for care and teaching of the patient during therapy are the same as those for all progestins.

melphalan (phenylalanine mustard)
Alkeran

Pharmacologic classification: alkylating agent (cell cycle-phase nonspecific)
Therapeutic classification: antineoplastic
Pregnancy risk category D

How supplied
Available by prescription only
Tablets (scored): 2 mg
Powder for injection: 50 mg

Indications and dosages
Dosage and indications may vary. Check current literature for recommended protocol.

Multiple myeloma
Adults: 6 mg P.O. daily for 2 to 3 weeks; then stop therapy for 4 weeks. When WBC and platelet count begin to increase, start maintenance dosage of 2 mg P.O. daily. Alternatively, give 0.15 mg/kg/day P.O. for 7 days or 0.25 mg/kg/day P.O. for 4 days at 4- to 6-week intervals, usually with prednisone; monitor patient's blood counts. Other dosing methods: 10 mg P.O. for 7 to 10 days. When platelet and leukocyte counts exceed 100,000/µL and 4000/µL, respectively, initiate maintenance therapy at 2 mg P.O. daily. Dose adjusted by 1 to 3 mg based on hematologic response.

For I.V. administration, give 16 mg/m^2 over 15 to 20 minutes once at 2-week intervals for four doses. Monitor patient's blood counts and reduce dose as necessary. After satisfactory recovery, repeat dose at 4-week intervals.

Epithelial ovarian cancer
Adults: 200 mcg/kg/day P.O. for 5 days, repeated q 4 to 5 weeks if blood counts return to normal.

≡ ***Dosage adjustment.*** I.V. melphalan dose is reduced by 50% in patients with renal impairment to reduce severe leukopenia and drug-related death.

Pharmacodynamics
Antineoplastic action: Melphalan exerts its cytotoxic activity by forming cross-links of strands of DNA and RNA and inhibiting protein synthesis.

Pharmacokinetics
Absorption: Absorption from GI tract is incomplete and variable. One study found that absorption ranged from 25% to 89% after an oral dose of 0.6 mg/kg.
Distribution: Distributes rapidly and widely into total body water. Drug is initially 50% to 60% bound to plasma proteins and eventually increases to 80% to 90% over time.
Metabolism: Extensively deactivated by the process of hydrolysis.
Excretion: Elimination has been described as biphasic, with an initial half-life of 8 minutes and a terminal half-life of 2 hours. Melphalan and its metabolites are excreted primarily in urine, with 10% of an oral dose excreted as unchanged drug.

Route	Onset	Peak	Duration
P.O., I.V.	Unknown	Unknown	Unknown

Contraindications and precautions
Contraindicated in patients with hypersensitivity to drug and in those whose disease is known to be resistant to drug. Patients hypersensitive to chlorambucil may have cross-sensitivity to melphalan.

Use cautiously in patients with impaired renal function, severe leukopenia, thrombocytopenia, anemia, or chronic lymphocytic leukemia.

Interactions

Drug-drug. *Cimetidine:* Inhibits GI absorption. Avoid administration together.
Cyclosporine, cisplatin: May increase nephrotoxicity. Monitor renal function closely in patients receiving melphalan and cyclosporine together or melphalan and cisplatin together.
Interferon alpha: May cause a decrease in melphalan serum levels. Patient requires careful monitoring.
Drug-food. *Food:* Reduces bioavailability of melphalan. Advise patient to take drug on an empty stomach.

Effects on diagnostic tests

None reported.

Adverse reactions

CNS: transient paralysis, peripheral neuritis.
CV: hypotension, tachycardia, edema, thrombosis, phlebitis, ***pulmonary embolism.***
GI: nausea, vomiting, diarrhea, oral ulceration.
Hematologic: ***thrombocytopenia, leukopenia, bone marrow suppression, hemolytic anemia.***
Hepatic: ***hepatotoxicity.***
Respiratory: ***pneumonitis, pulmonary fibrosis,*** dyspnea, ***bronchospasm.***
Skin: pruritus, alopecia, urticaria.
Other: ***anaphylaxis,*** hypersensitivity, ***secondary malignancy,*** vesiculation and tissue necrosis.

Overdose and treatment

Signs and symptoms of overdose include myelosuppression, hypocalcemia, severe nausea, vomiting, ulceration of the mouth, decreased consciousness, seizures, muscular paralysis, and cholinomimetic effects.

Treatment is usually supportive and includes transfusion of blood components.

Clinical considerations

- Be aware that fever may enhance elimination of the drug.
- Use anticoagulants, aspirin, and aspirin-containing products cautiously.
- Oral dose may be taken all at one time.
- Administer drug on an empty stomach because absorption is decreased by food.
- Discontinue therapy temporarily or reduce dosage if WBC count goes below 3,000/mm^3 or platelet count goes below 100,000/mm^3.
- Avoid I.M. injections when platelet count is less than 100,000/mm^3.
- Consider dosage reduction in patients with renal failure receiving I.V. melphalan.
- Increased bone marrow suppression was observed in patients with BUN levels of 30 mg/dl or more.
- Follow procedure for proper handling and disposal of antineoplastic drugs.
- Reconstitute powder for injection by adding 10 ml of provided diluent to 50-mg vial using a 20G or larger needle; produces a concentration of 5 mg/ml. Add diluent rapidly and shake vial until solution is clear. Don't refrigerate because a precipitate may form. Immediately, dilute further in 0.9% sodium chloride for injection to provide a solution concentration not exceeding 0.45 mg/ml. Administer over 15 to 20 minutes; infuse solution within 60 minutes from time of reconstitution.

Therapeutic monitoring

- Frequent hematologic monitoring, including CBC, is necessary for accurate dosage adjustments and prevention of toxicity.
- Monitor renal function, especially if BUN is greater than 30 mg/dL.

Special populations

Breast-feeding patients. It isn't known if melphalan is excreted in breast milk. However, because of risk of serious adverse reactions, mutagenicity, and carcinogenicity in the infant, breast-feeding isn't recommended.

Patient counseling

- Instruct patient to continue taking drug despite nausea and vomiting.
- Tell patient to call immediately if vomiting occurs shortly after taking a dose.
- Explain that adequate fluid intake is important to facilitate excretion of uric acid.
- Instruct patient to avoid exposure to people with infections.
- Reassure patient that hair should grow back after treatment has ended.
- Tell patient to promptly report signs and symptoms of infection or bleeding.
- Advise women of childbearing age to avoid becoming pregnant while receiving drug therapy.

meningococcal polysaccharide vaccine

Menomune-A/C/Y/W-135

Pharmacologic classification: vaccine
Therapeutic classification: bacterial vaccine
Pregnancy risk category C

How supplied

Available by prescription only
Injection: A killed bacterial vaccine in single-dose, 10-dose, and 50-dose vials with vial of diluent

Indications and dosages

Meningococcal meningitis prophylaxis
Adults and children over age 2: 0.5 ml S.C.
◇ *Children age 3 to 18 months:* 0.5 ml S.C. for 2 doses 3 months apart.

Pharmacodynamics
Meningitis prophylaxis: Vaccine promotes active immunity to meningitis caused by *Neisseria meningitidis.*

Pharmacokinetics
No information available.

Route	Onset	Peak	Duration
S.C.	Unknown	Unknown	3 yr

Contraindications and precautions
Contraindicated in immunosuppressed patients with hypersensitivity to thimerosal. Defer vaccination in patients with acute illness. Avoid use during pregnancy unless clearly needed.

Interactions
Drug-drug. *Vaccines containing whole-cell pertussis or whole-cell typhoid antigens:* Combined endotoxin effect. Don't use together.

Effects on diagnostic tests
None reported.

Adverse reactions
CNS: headache, malaise.
GU: nephropathy.
Musculoskeletal: muscle cramps.
Other: *pain, tenderness, erythema, induration* (at injection site); ***anaphylaxis,*** chills, fever.

Overdose and treatment
No information available.

Clinical considerations
- Obtain a thorough history of patient's allergies and reactions to immunizations.
- Don't give meningitis vaccine intradermally, I.M., or I.V.; safety and efficacy haven't been established.
- Epinephrine solution 1:1,000 should be available to treat allergic reactions.
- Booster responses to second doses of vaccine are poor and unpredictable.
- In a child age 3 to 6 months, vaccine may provide short-term protection against serotype A meningococcal disease.
- In a child as young as 6 months, vaccine may provide short-term protection against serotype C meningococcal disease.
- Older children and adults in high-risk exposure areas should consider revaccination every 3 to 5 years.
- Children under age 4 vaccinated in high-risk exposure areas should be revaccinated 2 to 3 years after primary immunization.
- The 50-dose vial of vaccine is intended for jet injector administration only and generally shouldn't be administered using syringes and needles. Discard any unused vaccine.
- Reconstitute vaccine with diluent provided. Shake until dissolved. Discard reconstituted solution after 5 days.
- Store vaccine between 36° and 46° F (2° and 8° C).
- Protective antibody levels may be achieved within 10 to 14 days after vaccination.

Therapeutic monitoring
Recommend monitoring patient for adverse allergic reactions.

Special populations
Breast-feeding patients. It isn't known if vaccine is excreted in breast milk. Use with caution in breast-feeding women.
Pediatric patients. Vaccine isn't recommended for children under age 2, but has been used investigationally in children age 3 to 24 months.

Patient counseling
- Tell patient that pain and inflammation may occur at injection site. Recommend acetaminophen to alleviate adverse reactions, such as fever.
- Encourage patient to report distressing adverse reactions.
- Advise patient on use of contraceptives, if necessary.
- Explain that vaccine will provide immunity only to meningitis caused by one type of bacteria.

menotropins
Humegon, Pergonal

Pharmacologic classification: gonadotropin
Therapeutic classification: ovulation stimulant, spermatogenesis stimulant
Pregnancy risk category X

How supplied
Available by prescription only
Injection: 75 IU of luteinizing hormone (LH) and 75 IU of follicle-stimulating hormone (FSH) activity per ampule; 150 IU of LH and 150 IU of FSH activity per ampule

Indications and dosages
Production of follicular maturation
Adults: 75 IU each of FSH and LH I.M. daily for 9 to 12 days, followed by 10,000 USP units chorionic gonadotropin (CG) I.M. 1 day after last dose of menotropins; may repeat for two more menstrual cycles if evidence of ovulation, but pregnancy doesn't occur. Then, if ovulation or follicular development doesn't occur, increase to 150 IU each of FSH and LH I.M. daily for 9 to 12 days, followed by 10,000 USP units CG I.M. 1 day after last dose of menotropins; may repeat for two menstrual cycles if evidence of ovulation, but pregnancy doesn't occur.

Note: If the ovaries are abnormally enlarged or if total urinary estrogen excretion is > 100

mcg daily, or if urinary estriol excretion is >50 mcg daily, hold CG dose because hyperstimulation syndrome is more likely to occur.
Stimulation of spermatogenesis
Adults: After 5,000 USP units of CG I.M. 3 times weekly for 4 to 6 months of treatment; 1 ampule (75 IU FSH/LH) I.M. three times weekly (given with 2,000 USP units CG twice weekly) for at least 4 months. If no improvement occurs after 4 months, treatment may continue with 75 IU FSH/LH three times weekly or 150 IU FSH/LH three times weekly. Dosage of CG doesn't change.

Pharmacodynamics
Ovulation stimulant action: Menotropins causes growth and maturation of the ovarian follicle in women who don't have primary ovarian failure by mimicking the action of endogenous LH and FSH. Additional treatment with CG is usually required to achieve ovulation.
Spermatogenesis stimulant action: Menotropins causes spermatogenesis when coadministered with CG in men with primary or secondary pituitary hypofunction.

Pharmacokinetics
Absorption: Must be administered parenterally for effectiveness.
Distribution: Unknown.
Metabolism: Not fully known.
Excretion: Excreted in urine.

Route	Onset	Peak	Duration
I.M.	9-12 days	Unknown	Unknown

Contraindications and precautions
Contraindicated in patients hypersensitive to drug; in women with primary ovarian failure, uncontrolled thyroid or adrenal dysfunction, pituitary tumor, abnormal uterine bleeding, uterine fibromas, or ovarian cysts or enlargement; in pregnant women; and in men with normal pituitary function, primary testicular failure, or infertility disorders other than hypogonadotropic hypogonadism.

Interactions
None reported.

Effects on diagnostic tests
None reported.

Adverse reactions
CNS: headache, malaise, dizziness.
CV: ***stroke,*** tachycardia.
GI: nausea, vomiting, diarrhea, abdominal cramps, bloating.
GU: *ovarian enlargement with pain and abdominal distention, ovarian hyperstimulation syndrome* (sudden severe abdominal pain, distention, nausea, vomiting, weight gain, and dyspnea followed by hypovolemia, hemoconcentration, electrolyte imbalance, pleural effusion, ascites, and hemoperitoneum), gynecomastia, ovarian cysts, ectopic pregnancy.
Musculoskeletal: musculoskeletal aches, joint pains.
Respiratory: ***atelectasis, acute respiratory distress syndrome, pulmonary embolism, pulmonary infarction, arterial occlusion,*** dyspnea, tachypnea.
Skin: rash.
Other: fever, multiple births, ***hypersensitivity and anaphylactic reactions,*** chills.

Overdose and treatment
The most common dose-related adverse effect appears to be ovarian hyperstimulation syndrome. Drug should be discontinued. Symptomatic and supportive care include bed rest, fluid and electrolyte replacement, and analgesics.

Clinical considerations
- Drug is administered by I.M. route only.
- Reconstitute drug with 1 to 2 ml of sterile saline injection. Use immediately and discard any unused portion.
- Pregnancies that follow ovulation induced with menotropins show a relatively high frequency of multiple births.
- Store drug at 37° to 86° F (3° to 30° C).

Therapeutic monitoring
Recommend monitoring patient at least every other day for enlarged ovaries or hyperstimulation syndrome during and for 2 weeks after therapy.

Special populations
Breast-feeding patients. Drug isn't indicated for use in breast-feeding women.

Patient counseling
- Teach patient signs and tests that indicate time of ovulation, such as increase in basal body temperature and increase in the appearance and volume of cervical mucus.
- Warn patient to immediately report symptoms of ovarian hyperstimulation syndrome, such as abdominal distention and pain, dyspnea, and vaginal bleeding.
- Warn patient multiple births are possible. Ectopic pregnancy and congenital malformations have been reported in pregnancies following treatment.
- Encourage daily intercourse from day before CG is given until ovulation occurs.
- Advise patient that she should be examined at least every other day for signs of excessive ovarian stimulation during therapy and for 2 weeks after treatment is discontinued.

meperidine hydrochloride (pethidine hydrochloride)

Demerol

Pharmacologic classification: opioid
Therapeutic classification: analgesic, adjunct to anesthesia
Controlled substance schedule II
Pregnancy risk category C

How supplied

Available by prescription only
Tablets: 50 mg, 100 mg
Liquid: 50 mg/5 ml
Injection: 10 mg/ml, 25 mg/ml, 50 mg/ml, 75 mg/ml, 100 mg/ml

Indications and dosages

Moderate to severe pain
Adults: 50 to 150 mg P.O., I.M., or S.C. q 3 to 4 hours; or continuous infusion of 15 to 35 mg/hour.
Children: 1.1 to 1.8 mg/kg P.O., I.M., or S.C. q 3 to 4 hours or 175 mg/ m^2 daily in six divided doses. Maximum single dose for children shouldn't exceed 100 mg.
Preoperatively
Adults: 50 to 100 mg I.M. or S.C. 30 to 90 minutes before surgery.
Children: 1 to 2 mg/kg I.M. or S.C. 30 to 90 minutes before surgery. Don't exceed adult dose.
Support of anesthesia
Adults: Repeated slow I.V. injections of fractional doses (10 mg/ml) or continuous I.V. infusion of 1 mg/ml. Titrate dose to meet patient's needs.
Obstetric analgesia
Adults: 50 to 100 mg I.M. or S.C. when pain becomes regular; may repeat at 1- to 3-hour intervals.

Pharmacodynamics

Analgesic action: Meperidine is a narcotic agonist with actions and potency similar to those of morphine, with principal actions at the opiate receptors. It's recommended for the relief of moderate to severe pain.

Pharmacokinetics

Absorption: Given orally, drug is only half as effective as it is parenterally.
Distribution: Distributed widely throughout the body and is 60% to 80% bound to plasma proteins.
Metabolism: Metabolized primarily by hydrolysis in the liver to an active metabolite, normeperidine.
Excretion: About 30% is excreted in urine as the *N*-demethylated derivative; about 5% is excreted unchanged. Excretion is enhanced by acidifying the urine. Half-life of parent compound is 3 to 5 hours and the half-life of metabolite is 8 to 21 hours.

Route	Onset	Peak	Duration
P.O.	15 min	1-1½ hr	2-4 hr
I.V.	1 min	5-7 min	2-4 hr
I.M.	10-15 min	30-50 min	2-4 hr
S.C.	10-15 min	40-60 min	2-4 hr

Contraindications and precautions

Contraindicated in patients with hypersensitivity to drug and in those who have received MAO inhibitors within the past 14 days.

Use cautiously in geriatric or debilitated patients and in those with increased intracranial pressure, head injury, asthma, other respiratory conditions, supraventricular tachycardia, seizures, acute abdominal conditions, renal or hepatic disease, hypothyroidism, Addison's disease, urethral stricture, and prostatic hyperplasia.

Interactions

Drug-drug. *Anticholinergics:* May cause paralytic ileus. Patient requires close monitoring.
Cimetidine: May increase respiratory and CNS depression, causing confusion, disorientation, apnea, or seizures. Reduce dosage of meperidine.
Other CNS depressants, such as narcotic analgesics, general anesthetics, antihistamines, barbiturates, benzodiazepines, muscle relaxants, phenothiazines, sedative-hypnotics, and tricyclic antidepressants: Potentiate respiratory and CNS depression, sedation, and hypotensive effects of drugs. Use together cautiously.
General anesthetics: Severe CV depression may result from use together. Use together cautiously.
Isoniazid: Meperidine can potentiate adverse effects of isoniazid. Avoid use together.
MAO inhibitors: May precipitate unpredictable and occasionally fatal reactions, even in patients who may receive MAO inhibitors within 14 days of receiving meperidine. Avoid use together.
Narcotic antagonist: Patients who become physically dependent on drug may experience acute withdrawal syndrome if given a narcotic antagonist. Avoid use together.
Drug-herb. *Parsley:* May promote or produce serotonin syndrome. Avoid use together.
Drug-lifestyle. *Alcohol use:* Potentiates respiratory and CNS depression, sedation, and hypotensive effects of drug. Avoid use together.

Effects on diagnostic tests

Drug increases plasma amylase or lipase levels through increased biliary tract pressure; levels may be unreliable for 24 hours after meperidine administration.

Adverse reactions

CNS: *sedation, somnolence, clouded sensorium, euphoria, dizziness,* paradoxical excitement, tremor, ***seizures*** (with large doses), headache, hallucinations, syncope, *light-headedness.*
CV: *hypotension,* bradycardia, tachycardia, ***cardiac arrest, shock.***
GI: *constipation,* ileus, dry mouth, *nausea, vomiting,* biliary tract spasms.
GU: *urine retention.*
Respiratory: ***respiratory depression, respiratory arrest.***
Skin: pruritus, urticaria, *diaphoresis.*
Other: physical dependence, muscle twitching; phlebitis (after I.V. delivery); pain (at injection site); local tissue irritation, induration (after S.C. injection).

Overdose and treatment

The most common signs and symptoms of meperidine overdose are CNS depression, respiratory depression, skeletal muscle flaccidity, cold and clammy skin, mydriasis, bradycardia, and hypotension. Other acute toxic effects include hypothermia, shock, apnea, cardiopulmonary arrest, circulatory collapse, pulmonary edema, and seizures.

To treat acute overdose, first establish adequate respiratory exchange via a patent airway and ventilation as needed; administer a narcotic antagonist (naloxone) to reverse respiratory depression. (Because the duration of action of meperidine is longer than that of naloxone, repeated dosing is necessary.) Naloxone shouldn't be given unless the patient has clinically significant respiratory or CV depression. Monitor vital signs.

If patient presents within 2 hours of ingestion of an oral overdose, empty the stomach immediately by inducing emesis (ipecac syrup) or using gastric lavage. Use caution to avoid risk of aspiration. Administer activated charcoal via nasogastric tube for further removal of meperidine, and acidify urine to help remove drug.

Provide symptomatic and supportive treatment (continued respiratory support, correction of fluid or electrolyte imbalance). Monitor laboratory values, vital signs, and neurologic status closely.

Clinical considerations

Consider the recommendations relevant to all opioids as well as the following:

- Drug may be administered to patients allergic to morphine.
- Commercial preparations contain sodium metabisulfite, which may cause allergic reactions in susceptible individuals.
- Question patient carefully regarding possible use of MAO inhibitors within the past 14 days.
- Concentration of 10 mg/ml should only be used with compatible infusion device and doesn't require further dilution.
- Because drug toxicity commonly appears after several days of treatment, this drug isn't recommended for treatment of chronic pain.
- Meperidine may be given slowly through an I.V., preferably as a diluted solution. S.C. injection is very painful. During I.V. administration, tachycardia may occur, possibly as a result of atropine-like effects of the drug.
- Oral dose is less than half as effective as parenteral dose. Give I.M. if possible. When changing from parenteral to oral route, increase dosage.
- Syrup has local anesthetic effect. Give with water.
- Alternating meperidine with a peripherally active non-opioid analgesic, such as aspirin, acetaminophen or NSAIDs, may improve pain control while allowing lower opioid dosages.
- Injectable meperidine is compatible with sodium chloride and D_5W solutions and their combinations, and with lactated Ringer's and sodium lactate solution.

Therapeutic monitoring

Meperidine and its active metabolite normeperidine accumulate. Monitor patient for neurotoxic effects, especially in burn patients and those with poor renal function, sickle cell anemia, or cancer.

Special populations

Breast-feeding patients. Drug is excreted in breast milk; use with caution in breast-feeding women.
Pediatric patients. Drug shouldn't be administered to infants under age 6 months.
Geriatric patients. Lower doses are usually indicated for geriatric patients, because they may be more sensitive to the therapeutic and adverse effects of drug.

Patient counseling

- Caution patient about CNS drug effects. Warn patient to avoid driving and other potentially hazardous activities that require mental alertness until CNS effects of drug are known.
- Advise patient to avoid alcohol.
- Tell patient to take drug before pain becomes intense.

mephenytoin

Mesantoin

Pharmacologic classification: hydantoin derivative
Therapeutic classification: anticonvulsant
Pregnancy risk category NR

How supplied

Available by prescription only
Tablets: 100 mg

Indications and dosages

Generalized tonic-clonic or complex-partial seizures

Adults: 50 to 100 mg P.O. daily; may increase by 50 to 100 mg at weekly intervals; usual maintenance dosage is 200 to 600 mg daily administered in three equally divided doses. Doses up to 800 mg/day may be required.

Children: Initial dose is 50 to 100 mg P.O. daily. May increase slowly by 50 to 100 mg at weekly intervals. Dosage must be adjusted individually. Usual maintenance dosage is 100 to 400 mg/day (or 3 to 15 mg/kg/day or 100 to 450 mg/m^2/day) administered in three equally divided doses.

Pharmacodynamics

Anticonvulsant action: Like other hydantoin derivatives, mephenytoin stabilizes the neuronal membranes and limits seizure activity either by increasing efflux or by decreasing influx of sodium ions across cell membranes in the motor cortex during generation of nerve impulses. Like phenytoin, mephenytoin appears to have antiarrhythmic effects.

Mephenytoin is used for prophylaxis of tonic-clonic (grand mal), psychomotor, focal, and jacksonian-type partial seizures in patients refractory to less toxic agents. It's usually combined with phenytoin, phenobarbital, or primidone; phenytoin is preferred because it causes less sedation than barbiturates. Mephenytoin also is used with succinimides to control combined absence and tonic-clonic disorders; combined use with oxazolidinediones, paramethadione or trimethadione isn't recommended because of the increased hazard of blood dyscrasias.

Pharmacokinetics

Absorption: Absorbed from the GI tract.

Distribution: Distributed widely throughout the body; good seizure control without toxicity occurs when serum levels of drug and major metabolite reach 25 to 40 mcg/ml.

Metabolism: Metabolized by the liver.

Excretion: Excreted in urine.

Route	Onset	Peak	Duration
P.O.	30 min	Unknown	24-48 hr

Contraindications and precautions

Contraindicated in patients with hydantoin hypersensitivity.

Interactions

Drug-drug. *Oral anticoagulants, antihistamines, chloramphenicol, cimetidine, diazepam, diazoxide, disulfiram, isoniazid, phenylbutazone, salicylates, sulfamethizole, or valproate:* Therapeutic effects and toxicity of mephenytoin may be increased by use with these medications. Patient requires close monitoring.

Oral contraceptives: Decreased effects of oral contraceptives. Recommend alternative means of contraception.

Folic acid: Therapeutic effects of mephenytoin may be decreased. Use together cautiously.

Drug-lifestyle. *Alcohol use:* May reduce therapeutic effects of drug. Avoid use together.

Effects on diagnostic tests

None reported.

Adverse reactions

CNS: ataxia, *drowsiness,* fatigue, irritability, choreiform movements, depression, tremor, insomnia, dizziness (usually transient).

EENT: conjunctivitis, diplopia, nystagmus, gingival hyperplasia (with prolonged use).

GI: nausea and vomiting (with prolonged use).

Hematologic: ***leukopenia, neutropenia, agranulocytosis, thrombocytopenia,*** eosinophilia, leukocytosis.

Hepatic: elevated liver function tests.

Musculoskeletal: polyarthropathy.

Respiratory: ***pulmonary fibrosis.***

Skin: rash, ***exfoliative dermatitis, Stevens-Johnson syndrome, fatal dermatitides.***

Other: edema, lymphadenopathy.

Overdose and treatment

Signs of acute mephenytoin toxicity may include restlessness, dizziness, drowsiness, nausea, vomiting, nystagmus, ataxia, dysarthria, tremor, and slurred speech; hypotension, respiratory depression, and coma may follow. Death may result from respiratory and circulatory depression.

Treat overdose with gastric lavage or emesis and follow up with supportive treatment. Carefully monitor vital signs and fluid and electrolyte balance. Forced diuresis is of little or no value. Hemodialysis or peritoneal dialysis may be helpful.

Clinical considerations

- Decreased alertness and coordination are most pronounced at start of treatment. Patient may need help with walking and other activities for first few days.
- Drug shouldn't be discontinued abruptly. Transition from mephenytoin to other anticonvulsant drug should progress over 6 weeks.
- When patient is receiving phenobarbital, continue phenobarbital until the transition to the other anticonvulsant is completed. Then attempt a gradual withdrawal of phenobarbital.
- Safe use of mephenytoin during pregnancy hasn't been established. Use drug during pregnancy only when clearly needed.

Therapeutic monitoring

- CBC and platelet counts should be performed before therapy, after 2 weeks of initial therapy, and after 2 weeks on maintenance dosage; they should be repeated every month for 1 year

and, subsequently, at 3-month intervals. If neutrophil count declines to 1,600 to 2,500/mm^3, obtain CBC every 2 weeks.
- Discontinue drug if neutrophil count is less than 1,600/mm^3.

Special populations
Breast-feeding patients. Safe use during breast-feeding hasn't been established. Alternative feeding method is recommended.
Pediatric patients. Children usually require from 100 to 400 mg/day.

Patient counseling
- Tell patient never to discontinue drug or change dosage except as prescribed and to avoid alcohol, which decreases effectiveness of drug and increases sedative effects.
- Explain that follow-up laboratory tests are essential for safe use.
- Instruct patient to report unusual changes immediately (cutaneous reaction, sore throat, glandular swelling, fever, mucous membrane swelling).

meprobamate
Apo-Meprobamate*, Equanil, MB-Tab, Meprospan, Miltown, Neuramate

Pharmacologic classification: carbamate
Therapeutic classification: antianxiety
Controlled substance schedule IV
Pregnancy risk category D

How supplied
Available by prescription only
Tablets: 200 mg, 400 mg, 600 mg
Capsules (sustained-release): 200 mg, 400 mg

Indications and dosages
Anxiety and tension
Adults: 1.2 to 1.6 g P.O. daily in three or four equally divided doses. Maximum dose, 2.4 g daily (sustained-release capsules, 400 to 800 mg b.i.d.).
Children age 6 to 12: 100 to 200 mg P.O. b.i.d. or t.i.d. Alternatively, 25 mg/kg/day or 700 mg/m^2/day in two or three divided doses. Sustained-release capsules, 200 mg b.i.d. Not recommended for children under age 6.
Preoperative sedation and relief of anxiety
Adults: 400 mg P.O.
Children: 200 mg P.O.

Pharmacodynamics
Anxiolytic action: While the cellular mechanism is unknown, drug causes nonselective CNS depression similar to that seen with use of barbiturates. Meprobamate acts at multiple sites in the CNS, including the thalamus, hypothalamus, limbic system, and spinal cord, but not the medulla or reticular activating system.

Pharmacokinetics
Absorption: Well absorbed after oral administration. Sedation usually occurs within 1 hour.
Distribution: Distributed throughout the body; 20% is protein-bound. Drug is excreted in breast milk at two to four times the serum level; meprobamate crosses the placenta.
Metabolism: Metabolized rapidly in the liver to inactive glucuronide conjugates. Half-life of drug is 6 to 17 hours.
Excretion: Metabolites of drug and 10% to 20% of a single dose as unchanged drug are excreted in urine.

Route	Onset	Peak	Duration
P.O.	Unknown	Unknown	Unknown

Contraindications and precautions
Contraindicated in patients hypersensitive to meprobamate or related compounds, such as carisoprodol, mebutamate, tybamate, and carbromal, and in those with porphyria. Avoid use of drug during first trimester of pregnancy and in breast-feeding women.

Use cautiously in geriatric or debilitated patients and in those with impaired renal or hepatic function, seizure disorders, or suicidal tendencies.

Interactions
Drug-drug. *Antihistamines, barbiturates, narcotics, tranquilizers, or other CNS depressants:* Potentiated effects. Use together cautiously.
Drug-lifestyle. *Alcohol use:* Potentiated effects. Use together cautiously.

Effects on diagnostic tests
Drug therapy may falsely elevate urinary 17-ketosteroids, 17-ketogenic steroids (as determined by the Zimmerman reaction), and 17-hydroxycorticosteroid levels (as determined by the Glenn-Nelson technique).

Adverse reactions
CNS: *drowsiness,* ataxia, dizziness, slurred speech, headache, syncope, vertigo, ***seizures.***
CV: palpitations, tachycardia, hypotension, ***arrhythmias.***
GI: nausea, vomiting, diarrhea.
Hematologic: *aplastic anemia, thrombocytopenia, agranulocytosis.*
Skin: pruritus, urticaria, erythematous maculopapular rash, *hypersensitivity reactions.*
After abrupt withdrawal of long-term therapy: severe generalized tonic-clonic seizures may occur.

Overdose and treatment
Signs and symptoms of overdose include drowsiness, lethargy, ataxia, coma, hypotension, shock, and respiratory depression.

Treatment of overdose is supportive and symptomatic, including maintaining adequate ventilation and a patent airway, with mechanical ventilation, if needed.

Treat hypotension with fluids and vasopressors as needed. Empty gastric contents by emesis or lavage if ingestion was recent, followed by activated charcoal and a cathartic. Treat seizures with parenteral diazepam. Peritoneal dialysis and hemodialysis may effectively remove drug. Serum levels of more than 100 mcg/ml may be fatal.

Clinical considerations

- Safety precautions are needed; such as raised bed rails, especially for geriatric patients, when initiating treatment or increasing the dose. Patient may need assistance when walking.
- Drug abuse and addiction may occur.
- Withdraw drug gradually; otherwise, withdrawal symptoms may occur if patient has been taking drug for a long time.
- Store drug at 59° to 86° F (15° to 30° C); expires 2 to 5 years from date of manufacture.

Therapeutic monitoring

- Frequent assessment of level of consciousness and vital signs is needed.
- Periodic evaluation of CBC is recommended during long-term therapy.
- Monitor hepatic and renal function.

Special populations

Breast-feeding patients. Drug is found in breast milk at two to four times the serum level. Don't use in breast- feeding women.
Pediatric patients. Safety hasn't been established in children under age 6.
Geriatric patients. Geriatric patients may have more pronounced CNS effects. Use lowest dose possible.

Patient counseling

- Tell patient to avoid alcohol and other CNS depressants, such as antihistamines, narcotics, and tranquilizers, while taking drug, unless prescribed.
- Advise patient not to increase dose or frequency and not to abruptly discontinue or decrease dose unless prescribed.
- Tell patient to avoid tasks that require mental alertness or physical coordination until CNS effects of drug are known.
- Recommend sugarless candy or gum or ice chips to relieve dry mouth.
- Advise patient to report sore throat, fever, or unusual bleeding or bruising.
- Inform patient of potential for physical or psychological dependence with chronic use.

mercaptopurine (6-MP)

Purinethol

Pharmacologic classification: antimetabolite (cell cycle-phase specific, S phase)
Therapeutic classification: antineoplastic
Pregnancy risk category D

How supplied

Available by prescription only
Tablets (scored): 50 mg

Indications and dosages

Dosage and indications may vary. Check current literature for recommended protocols.

Acute lymphoblastic leukemia (in children), chronic myelocytic leukemia
Adults: 2.5 mg/kg P.O. daily as a single dose, increase to 5 mg/kg daily (only if, after 4 weeks, there's no clinical improvement or signs of toxicity). Alternatively, 80 to 100 mg/m^2/day. Maintenance dosage is 1.5 to 2.5 mg/kg daily.
Children: 2.5 mg/kg P.O. daily. Alternatively, 70 mg/m^2 per day. Maintenance dosage is 1.5 to 2.5 mg/kg daily.

◇***Acute myeloblastic leukemia***
Adults: 500 mg/m^2/day P.O. in combination with other therapies.

Pharmacodynamics

Antineoplastic action: Mercaptopurine is converted intracellularly to its active form, which exerts its cytotoxic antimetabolic effects by competing for an enzyme required for purine synthesis. This results in inhibition of DNA and RNA synthesis. Cross-resistance exists between mercaptopurine and thioguanine.

Pharmacokinetics

Absorption: Absorption after an oral dose is incomplete and variable; about 50% of a dose is absorbed. Peak serum levels occur in 2 hours.
Distribution: Distributes widely into total body water. Drug crosses the blood-brain barrier, but the CSF level is too low for treatment of meningeal leukemias.
Metabolism: Extensively metabolized in the liver. It appears to undergo extensive first-pass metabolism, contributing to its low bioavailability.
Excretion: Excreted in urine.

Route	Onset	Peak	Duration
P.O.	Unknown	Unknown	Unknown

Contraindications and precautions

Contraindicated in patients whose disease has shown resistance to drug. Use cautiously in pregnancy or after chemotherapy or radiation therapy in patients with depressed neutrophil or platelet counts and in those with impaired renal or hepatic function.

Interactions

Drug-drug. *Allopurinol at doses of 300 to 600 mg/day:* Increased toxic effects of mercaptopurine, especially myelosuppression. Reduce dosage by 25% to 30% when administering with allopurinol.
Other hepatotoxic drugs: Increased potential for hepatotoxicity. Use together cautiously.
Co-trimoxazole: Enhanced marrow suppression. Use together cautiously.
Warfarin: Decreased anticoagulant activity of warfarin with use together. Monitor PT and INR.

Effects on diagnostic tests

Drug may also cause falsely elevated serum glucose and uric acid values when sequential multiple analyzer is used.

Adverse reactions

GI: *nausea, vomiting, anorexia, painful oral ulcers, diarrhea,* ***pancreatitis,*** *GI ulceration.*
Hematologic: ***leukopenia, thrombocytopenia,*** anemia (all may persist several days after drug is stopped).
Hepatic: *jaundice,* ***hepatotoxicity.***
Metabolic: hyperuricemia.
Skin: rash, hyperpigmentation.

Overdose and treatment

Signs and symptoms of overdose include myelosuppression, nausea, vomiting, and hepatic necrosis.

Treatment is usually supportive and includes transfusion of blood components and antiemetics. Hemodialysis is thought to be of marginal use because of the rapid intracellular incorporation of mercaptopurine into active metabolites with long persistence.

Clinical considerations

- Investigational uses include prevention of rejection of homografts, treatment of various autoimmune diseases, treatment of Crohn's disease, and treatment of chronic active hepatitis.
- Drug is sometimes called 6-mercaptopurine or 6-MP.
- Dose modifications may be required following chemotherapy or radiation therapy, in depressed neutrophil or platelet count, and in impaired hepatic or renal function.
- Hepatic dysfunction is reversible when drug is stopped. Recommend watching for jaundice, clay-colored stools, and frothy dark urine. Stop drug if hepatic tenderness occurs. Monitor hepatic function during initiation of therapy.
- Avoid all I.M. injections when platelet count is less than 100,000/mm^3.
- Store tablets at room temperature and protect from light.

Therapeutic monitoring

- Monitor weekly blood counts; watch for precipitous decline.
- Monitor intake and output. Push fluids (3 L/day).
- Monitor hepatic function and hematologic values weekly during therapy.
- Monitor serum uric acid levels. If allopurinol is necessary, use very cautiously.
- Observe patient for signs of bleeding and infection.

Special populations

Breast-feeding patients. It isn't known if drug is excreted in breast milk. However, because of the potential for serious adverse reactions, mutagenicity, and carcinogenicity in the infant, breast-feeding isn't recommended.
Pediatric patients. Adverse GI reactions are less common in children than in adults.

Patient counseling

- Warn patient that improvement may take 2 to 4 weeks or longer.
- Tell patient to continue medication despite nausea and vomiting.
- Instruct patient to immediately report vomiting that occurs shortly after taking a dose.
- Warn patient to avoid alcoholic beverages while taking drug.
- Urge patient to ensure adequate fluid intake to increase urine output and facilitate the excretion of uric acid.
- Advise patient to avoid exposure to people with infections. Tell patient to immediately report signs of unusual bleeding or infection.
- Advise women of childbearing age not to become pregnant while taking drug.

meropenem

Merrem I.V.

Pharmacologic classification: carbapenem derivative
Therapeutic classification: antibiotic
Pregnancy risk category B

How supplied

Available by prescription only
Powder for injection: 500 mg/15 ml, 500 mg/20 ml, 500 mg/100 ml, 1 g/15 ml, 1 g/30 ml, 1 g/100 ml

Indications and dosages

Complicated appendicitis and peritonitis caused by viridans group streptococci, **Escherichia coli, Klebsiella pneumoniae, Pseudomonas aeruginosa, Bacteroides fragilis, B. thetaiotaomicron,** ***and*** **Peptostreptococcus** ***species; bacterial meningitis caused by*** **Streptococcus pneumoni-**

ae, Haemophilus influenzae, *and* Neisseria meningitidis
Recommended concentration not to exceed 50 mg/ml
Adults: Administer 1 g I.V. q 8 hours over 15 to 30 minutes as I.V. infusion or over about 3 to 5 minutes as I.V. bolus injection (5 to 20 ml).
Children age 3 months and older weighing 110 lb (50 kg) or less: Give 20 mg/kg (intra-abdominal infection) or 40 mg/kg (bacterial meningitis) q 8 hours over 15 to 30 minutes as I.V. infusion or over about 3 to 5 minutes as I.V. bolus injection (5 to 20 ml).

Note: For children weighing more than 110 lb, give 1 g q 8 hours for treating intra-abdominal infections and 2 g q 8 hours for treating meningitis.

≡***Dosage adjustment.*** In adults with renal failure, give 1 g q 12 hours if creatinine clearance is 26 to 50 ml/minute, 500 mg q 12 hours if it's 10 to 25 ml/minute, and 500 mg q 24 hours if it's less than 10 ml/minute. There's no clinical experience in children with renal impairment.

Pharmacodynamics
Antibiotic action: Meropenem inhibits cell wall synthesis in bacteria. It readily penetrates the cell wall of most gram-positive and gram-negative bacteria to reach penicillin-binding protein targets.

Pharmacokinetics
Absorption: Only given I.V.
Distribution: Distributed into most body fluids and tissues, including CSF. It's only about 2% bound to plasma protein.
Metabolism: Thought to undergo minimal metabolism. One inactive metabolite has been identified.
Excretion: Excreted unchanged primarily in urine. Elimination half-life of drug in adults with normal renal function and children age 2 and older is about 1 hour and 1½ hours in children age 3 months to 2 years.

Route	Onset	Peak	Duration
I.V.	Unknown	1 hr	Unknown

Contraindications and precautions
Contraindicated in patients with hypersensitivity to any component of drug or other drugs in the same class and in those who have demonstrated anaphylactic reactions to beta-lactams. Use cautiously in patients with history of seizure disorders or impaired renal function.

Interactions
Drug-drug. *Probenecid:* Competes with meropenem for active tubular secretion and thus inhibits the renal excretion of meropenem. Avoid use together.

Effects on diagnostic tests
None reported.

Adverse reactions
CNS: headache, syncope, insomnia, agitation, delirium, confusion, dizziness, ***seizure,*** nervousness, paresthesia, hallucinations, somnolence, anxiety, depression.
CV: ***heart failure, cardiac arrest, MI, pulmonary embolism,*** tachycardia, chest pain, hypertension, ***bradycardia,*** hypotension.
GI: diarrhea, nausea, vomiting, constipation, abdominal pain or enlargement, oral moniliasis, anorexia.
GU: dysuria, ***kidney failure,*** increased creatinine clearance or BUN levels, presence of RBCs in urine.
Hematologic: anemia, increased or decreased platelet count, increased eosinophil count, prolonged or shortened PT and INR or partial thromboplastin time, positive direct or indirect Coombs' test, decreased hemoglobin or hematocrit, decreased WBC count.
Hepatic: ***hepatic failure,*** cholestatic jaundice, jaundice, flatulence, ileus; increased levels of ALT, AST, alkaline phosphatase, LD, and bilirubin.
Musculoskeletal: back pain.
Respiratory: ***apnea, hypoxia,*** respiratory disorder, dyspnea.
Skin: rash, pruritus, urticaria, sweating.
Other: ***hypersensitivity and anaphylactic reactions;*** inflammation, pain, edema, phlebitis, or thrombophlebitis at injection site; bleeding events, pain, ***sepsis, shock,*** fever, peripheral edema.

Overdose and treatment
Signs and symptoms and treatment of overdose are unknown. If overdose occurs, discontinue drug and give general supportive treatment until renal elimination occurs. Meropenem and its metabolite are readily dialyzable and effectively removed by hemodialysis.

Clinical considerations
- Don't use to treat methicillin-resistant staphylococci.
- Obtain specimen for culture and sensitivity tests before giving first dose. Therapy may begin pending test results.
- Serious and occasionally fatal hypersensitivity (anaphylactic) reactions have been reported in patients receiving therapy with beta-lactams. Before therapy is initiated, ascertain whether previous hypersensitivity reactions to penicillins, cephalosporins, other beta-lactams, and other allergens have occurred.
- Discontinue drug immediately if an allergic reaction occurs. Serious anaphylactic reactions require immediate emergency treatment with epinephrine, oxygen, I.V. steroids, and airway management. Other therapy may also be required as indicated by the patient's condition.

■ Seizures and other CNS adverse reactions associated with meropenem therapy commonly occur in patients with CNS disorders, bacterial meningitis, and compromised renal function.
■ If seizures occur during meropenem therapy, decrease dosage or discontinue meropenem.
■ For I.V. bolus administration, add 10 ml of sterile water for injection to 500 mg/20 ml vial size or 20 ml to 1 g/30 ml vial size to provide concentration of 50 mg/ml. Shake to dissolve and let stand until clear.
■ For I.V. infusion, infusion vials (500 mg/100 ml and 1 g/100 ml) may be directly reconstituted with a compatible infusion fluid to provide a concentration of 2.5 to 50 mg/ml. Alternatively, an injection vial may be reconstituted, then the resulting solution added to an I.V. container and further diluted with an appropriate infusion fluid. ADD-Vantage vials shouldn't be used.
■ For ADD-Vantage vials, reconstitute only with half 0.45% saline injection, normal saline injection, or 5% dextrose injection in 50-, 100-, or 250-ml Abbott ADD-Vantage flexible diluent containers. Follow manufacturer guidelines closely when using ADD-Vantage vials.
■ Don't mix with or physically add meropenem to solutions containing other drugs. Infuse drug over 15 to 30 minutes.
■ Use freshly prepared solutions of meropenem immediately whenever possible. Stability of drug varies with type of drug used (injection vial, infusion vial, or ADD-Vantage container). Consult manufacturer's literature for details.

Therapeutic monitoring
■ Drug may cause overgrowth of nonsusceptible bacteria or fungi. Recommend monitoring patient for signs and symptoms of superinfection.
■ Periodic assessment of organ system functions, including renal, hepatic, and hematopoietic, is recommended during prolonged therapy.

Special populations
Breast-feeding patients. It isn't known if drug is excreted in breast milk; use cautiously in breast-feeding women.
Pediatric patients. Safety and efficacy haven't been established in children under age 3 months.
Geriatric patients. Use cautiously in geriatric patients because of decreased renal function. Dosage adjustment is recommended in patients with advanced age whose creatinine clearance levels are less than 50 ml/minute.

Patient counseling
■ Tell patient to report pain, inflammation or swelling at I.V. site to health care provider.
■ Advise breast-feeding patient of risk of transmitting drug to infant through breast milk.
■ Instruct patient to report adverse reactions or symptoms of superinfection to doctor.

mesalamine (5-aminosalicylic acid)
Asacol, Pentasa, Rowasa

Pharmacologic classification: salicylate
Therapeutic classification: anti-inflammatory
Pregnancy risk category B

How supplied
Available by prescription only
Capsules (controlled-release): 250 mg
Tablets (delayed-release): 400 mg
Suppositories: 500 mg
Rectal suspension: 4 g/60 ml, in units of 7 disposable bottles

Indications and dosages
Active mild to moderate distal ulcerative colitis, proctosigmoiditis, proctitis
Adults: 800 mg (delayed-release tablets) P.O. t.i.d. for 6 weeks or 1 g (controlled-release capsules) q.i.d. for up to 8 weeks.

Alternatively, use 1 rectal suppository b.i.d. for 3 to 6 weeks. For maximum benefit, the suppository should be retained for 1 to 3 hours or longer. Usual dosage of mesalamine suspension enema in 60-ml units is one rectal instillation (4 g) once daily, preferably h.s., retained for about 8 hours.

◇Lower doses of suspension enemas of 4 g q 2 to 3 nights or 1 g daily have been effective.
◇***Maintenance of remission of ulcerative colitis***
Adults: 1.6 g P.O. daily in divided doses for 6 months. Alternatively, 60 ml (4 g) rectal suspension q 2 to 3 nights or 1 to 3 g rectal suspension daily.

Pharmacodynamics
Anti-inflammatory action: Mechanism of action of mesalamine (and sulfasalazine) is unknown, but appears to be topical rather than systemic. Mucosal production of arachidonic acid (AA) metabolites, both through cyclooxygenase pathways (such as prostaglandins [PGs]) and lipoxygenase pathways (such as leukotrienes [LTs] and hydroxyeicosatetraenoic acids [HETEs]) is increased in patients with chronic inflammatory bowel disease; possibly, mesalamine may diminish inflammation by blocking cyclooxygenase and inhibiting PG production in the colon.

Sulfasalazine is split by bacterial action in the colon into sulfapyridine (SP) and mesalamine (5-ASA). The mesalamine component is considered therapeutically active in ulcerative colitis.

Pharmacokinetics

Absorption: Drug administered rectally as a suppository or suspension enema is poorly absorbed from the colon. Extent of absorption depends on retention time, with considerable individual variation. Oral tablets are coated with an acrylic resin that delays the release of drug until tablet is beyond the terminal ileum. About 72% of a dose reaches the colon; 28% of a dose is absorbed. Absorption isn't affected by food. Capsules are formulated to release therapeutic levels throughout the GI tract. About 20% to 30% is absorbed.
Distribution: Maximum plasma levels of oral mesalamine and *N*-acetyl 5-aminosalicylic acid are about twice as high as those seen with sulfasalazine therapy. At steady state, about 10% to 30% of daily 4-g rectal dose can be recovered in cumulative 24-hour urine collections.
Metabolism: Undergoes acetylation, but site is unknown. Most absorbed drug is excreted in urine as the *N*-acetyl-5-ASA metabolite. Elimination half-life of drug is ½ to 1½ hours; half-life of acetylated metabolite is 5 to 10 hours. Steady-state plasma levels show no accumulation of either free or metabolized drug during repeated daily administrations.
Excretion: After rectal administration, drug is mostly excreted in the feces as parent drug and metabolite. After oral administration, drug is mostly excreted in the urine as metabolite.

Route	Onset	Peak	Duration
P.O., P.R.	Unknown	3-12 hr	Unknown

Contraindications and precautions

Contraindicated in patients hypersensitive to drug, its components (sulfite in rectal preparation), or salicylates. Use cautiously in patients with impaired renal function.

Interactions

None reported.

Effects on diagnostic tests

None reported.

Adverse reactions

CNS: headache, dizziness, fatigue, malaise, asthenia, chills, anxiety, depression, hyperesthesia, paresthesia, tremor.
CV: chest pain.
GI: abdominal pain, cramps, discomfort, flatulence, diarrhea, rectal pain, bloating, nausea, *pancolitis, **pancreatitis,*** vomiting, constipation, eructation.
GU: dysuria, hematuria, urinary urgency.
Musculoskeletal: arthralgia, myalgia, back pain.
Respiratory: wheezing.
Skin: itching, rash, urticaria, hair loss.
Other: ***anaphylaxis*** (rare), fever, hypertonia.

Overdose and treatment

No information available.

Clinical considerations

- Drug has been used to treat Crohn's disease.
- Rectal suspension contains potassium metabisulfite, which may produce an allergic reaction in susceptible individuals.
- While effects of drug may be evident in 3 to 21 days, usual course of therapy is 3 to 6 weeks depending on symptoms and sigmoidoscopic findings. Clinical studies haven't determined whether suspension enema will modify relapse rates after the 6-week, short-term treatment.

Therapeutic monitoring

Monitor renal function studies during therapy.

Special populations

Breast-feeding patients. It isn't known if drug or its metabolites are excreted in breast milk. Avoid breast-feeding during therapy.
Pediatric patients. Safety and efficacy for use in children haven't been established.

Patient counseling

- Tell patient to swallow tablets whole and not to crush or chew them.
- Tell patient to retain suppository as long as possible (at least 1 to 3 hours) for maximum effectiveness.
- Instruct patient in correct use of rectal suspension:
  - — Shake bottle well to make sure the suspension is homogeneous.
  - —Remove the protective sheath from the applicator tip. Holding the bottle at the neck will not cause medication to be discharged.
  - —To administer, lie on the left side (to facilitate migration into the sigmoid colon) with the lower leg extended and the upper right leg flexed forward for balance; or may use the knee-chest position.
  - —Gently insert the applicator tip in the rectum, pointing toward the umbilicus.
  - —Steadily squeeze the bottle to discharge the preparation into the colon.
- Patient instructions are included with every 7 units.

mesna

Mesnex

Pharmacologic classification: thiol derivative
Therapeutic classification: uroprotectant
Pregnancy risk category B

How supplied

Available by prescription only
Injection: 100 mg/ml in 2- and 10-ml ampules

Indications and dosages

Prevention of ifosfamide-induced hemorrhagic cystitis

Adults: Calculate daily dose as 60% of the ifosfamide dose. Administer in three equally divided bolus doses: Give first dose at time of ifosfamide injection. Subsequent doses are given at 4 and 8 hours following ifosfamide. Alternatively, administer dose in four divided doses just before ifosfamide dose, then at 4, 8, and 12 hours after ifosfamide; or, at time of ifosfamide dose and then at 3, 6, and 9 hours after ifosfamide dose

Protocols that use 1.2 g/m^2 ifosfamide would employ 240 mg/m^2 mesna at 0, 4, and 8 hours after ifosfamide.

◊ Continuous mesna I.V. infusion is given at 100% ifosfamide dosage and may be mixed in the same I.V. solution. Continue regimen as long as ifosfamide is given; it may have to continue for additional 8 to 24 hours as a result of shorter mesna half-life.

◊ ***Prophylaxis in bone marrow recipients receiving cyclophosphamides***

Adults: 60% to 160% of the cyclophosphamide daily dose given in three to five divided doses or by continuous infusion. Alternatively, in patients receiving cyclophosphamide, 50 to 60 mg/kg I.V. daily for 2 to 4 days; give 10 mg/kg I.V. loading dose of mesna followed by 60 mg/kg by way of continuous I.V. infusion over 24 hours. Give mesna regimen with each cyclophosphamide dose and continue for an additional 24 hours.

Pharmacodynamics

Uroprotectant action: Mesna disulfide is reduced to mesna in the kidney and reacts with the urotoxic metabolites of ifosfamide to detoxify the drug and protect the urinary system.

Pharmacokinetics

Absorption: Administered I.V.
Distribution: Remains in the vascular compartment; doesn't distribute through tissues.
Metabolism: Rapidly metabolized to mesna disulfide, its only metabolite.
Excretion: In the kidneys, 33% of the dose is eliminated in the urine in 24 hours; half-life of mesna and mesna disulfide are ½ and 1¼ hours, respectively.

Route	Onset	Peak	Duration
I.V.	Unknown	Unknown	Unknown

Contraindications and precautions

Contraindicated in patients hypersensitive to mesna or thiol-containing compounds.

Interactions

None reported.

Effects on diagnostic tests

Mesna may produce a false-positive test for urinary ketones. A red-violet color will return to violet with the addition of glacial acetic acid.

Adverse reactions

CNS: headache, fatigue.
CV: hypotension.
GI: soft stools, nausea, vomiting, diarrhea, dysgeusia.
Musculoskeletal: limb pain.
Other: *allergy.*

Note: Because mesna is used with ifosfamide and other chemotherapeutic agents, it's difficult to determine adverse reactions attributable solely to mesna.

Overdose and treatment

No information available. There's no known antidote.

Clinical considerations

- The parent form of the drug has been administered orally by preparing extemporaneous oral solutions by mixing injection with flavored syrup to produce a concentration of 20 to 50 mg/ml. Solutions are stable for 7 days at 75° F (24° C). If carbonated beverages, apple juice, or orange juice is used, solution is stable for at least 24 hours at 41° F (5° C).
- Patients receiving mesna for ifosfamide-induced hemorrhagic cystitis should be adequately hydrated (2 L of oral or I.V. fluid before and during ifosfamide therapy).
- Mesnex multidose vials may be stored and used for up to 8 days.
- Discard unused mesna from open ampules. It will form an inactive oxidation product (dimesna) upon exposure to oxygen.
- Dilute appropriate dose in 5% dextrose injection, normal saline solution injection, or lactated Ringer's injection to a level of 20 mg/ml. Once diluted, solution is stable for 24 hours at room temperature. However, the manufacturer recommends refrigerating the solution and using within 6 hours (contains no preservatives).
- Infuse I.V. solution over 15 to 30 minutes.
- Mesna is physically incompatible with cisplatin or carboplatin. Don't add mesna to cisplatin infusions.
- Store drug at 59° to 86° F (15° to 30° C); expires 5 years from date of manufacture.

Therapeutic monitoring

Recommend monitoring morning urine specimen for erythrocytes, which may precede hemorrhagic cystitis.

Special populations

Breast-feeding patients. It isn't known if mesna is excreted in breast milk.
Pediatric patients. Safety in children hasn't been established. However, drug has been used

for prophylaxis of ifosfamide-induced hemorrhagic cystitis in infants and children age 4 to 16 and for prophylaxis of cyclophosphamide-induced hemorrhagic cystitis in children age 5 months and older. Note: Multidose vials contain benzyl alcohol.

Patient counseling
Instruct patient to report hematuria or allergy immediately.

mesoridazine besylate
Serentil

Pharmacologic classification: phenothiazine (piperidine derivative)
Therapeutic classification: antipsychotic
Pregnancy risk category NR

How supplied
Available by prescription only
Tablets: 10 mg, 25 mg, 50 mg, 100 mg
Oral concentrate: 25 mg/ml (0.6% alcohol)
Injection: 25 mg/ml

Indications and dosages
Psychoneurotic manifestations (anxiety)
Adults and children over age 12: 10 mg P.O. t.i.d. up to maximum of 150 mg/day.
Psychotic disorders
Adults and children over age 12: Initially, 50 mg P.O. t.i.d. to maximum of 400 mg/day; or 25 mg I.M. repeated in 30 to 60 minutes, p.r.n., not to exceed 200 mg I.M. daily.
Alcoholism
Adults and children over age 12: 25 mg P.O. b.i.d., up to maximum of 200 mg/day.
Behavioral problems associated with chronic brain syndrome
Adults and children over age 12: 25 mg P.O. t.i.d., up to maximum of 300 mg/day.

Pharmacodynamics
Antipsychotic action: Mesoridazine, a metabolite of thioridazine, is thought to exert its antipsychotic effects by postsynaptic blockade of CNS dopamine receptors, thereby inhibiting dopamine-mediated effects.

Drug has many other central and peripheral effects; it produces both alpha and ganglionic blockade and counteracts histamine- and serotonin-mediated activity. Its most prominent adverse reactions are antimuscarinic and sedative; it causes fewer extrapyramidal effects than other antipsychotics.

Pharmacokinetics
Absorption: Appears to be well absorbed from the GI tract following oral administration. I.M. dosage form is absorbed rapidly.
Distribution: Distributed widely into the body, including breast milk. Steady-state serum level is achieved within 4 to 7 days. Drug is 91% to 99% protein-bound.
Metabolism: Metabolized extensively by the liver; no active metabolites are formed.
Excretion: Mostly excreted as metabolites in urine; some excreted in feces via biliary tract.

Route	Onset	Peak	Duration
P.O., I.M.	Unknown	2-4 hr	4-6 hr

Contraindications and precautions
Contraindicated in patients with hypersensitivity to drug or in those experiencing severe CNS depression or comatose states.

Interactions
Drug-drug. *Aluminum- and magnesium-containing antacids and antidiarrheals:* Decreased absorption. Separate administration times.
Antiarrhythmic agents, disopyramide, procainamide, quinidine: Increased incidence of arrhythmias and conduction defects. Avoid use together.
Atropine and other anticholinergic drugs, including antidepressants, antihistamines, MAO inhibitors, meperidine, phenothiazines, and antiparkinson agents: Oversedation, paralytic ileus, visual changes, and severe constipation. Use together cautiously.
Beta blockers: May inhibit mesoridazine metabolism, increasing plasma levels and toxicity. Monitor patient for signs of toxicity.
Bromocriptine: Mesoridazine may antagonize therapeutic effect of bromocriptine on prolactin secretion. Use together cautiously.
CNS depressants, including analgesics, barbiturates, opioids, tranquilizers, and general, spinal, or epidural anesthetics, or parenteral magnesium sulfate: Oversedation, respiratory depression, and hypotension. Avoid use together.
Centrally acting antihypertensive drugs, such as clonidine, guanabenz, guanadrel, guanethidine, methyldopa, and reserpine: Mesoridazine may inhibit blood pressure response to these drugs. Recommend monitoring blood pressure frequently.
High-dose dopamine: Decreased vasoconstricting effects. Recommend monitoring for clinical effects.
Levodopa: Decreased effectiveness and increased toxicity of levodopa. Use together cautiously.
Lithium: May result in severe neurologic toxicity with an encephalitis-like syndrome and a decreased therapeutic response to mesoridazine. Avoid use together.
Metrizamide: Increased risk of seizures. Use together cautiously.
Nitrates: Hypotension. Recommend monitoring blood pressure.

Phenobarbital: Enhanced renal excretion of mesoridazine. Patient requires monitoring for clinical effects.
Phenytoin: Mesoridazine may inhibit metabolism and increase toxicity of phenytoin. Decreased phenytoin dosage may be necessary.
Propylthiouracil: Increased risk of agranulocytosis. Monitor hemapoeitic studies.
Sympathomimetics, including epinephrine, phenylephrine, phenylpropanolamine, and ephedrine (often found in nasal sprays), or appetite suppressants: May decrease their stimulatory and pressor effects. Use together cautiously.
Drug-food. *Caffeine:* Increased metabolism of drug. Use together cautiously.
Drug-lifestyle. *Alcohol use:* Additive effects. Advise patient to avoid alcohol.
Sun exposure: Increased risk of photosensitivity reactions. Recommend patient use sun screen or limit exposure.
Heavy smoking: Increased metabolism. Advise patient to avoid smoking.

Effects on diagnostic tests

Mesoridazine causes false-positive test results for urinary porphyrins, urobilinogen, amylase, and 5-hydroxyindoleacetic acid, because of darkening of urine by metabolites; it also causes false-positive urine pregnancy test results using human chorionic gonadotropin.

Adverse reactions

CNS: extrapyramidal reactions, *tardive dyskinesia, sedation, drowsiness, tremor, rigidity, weakness, EEG changes, dizziness.*
CV: *hypotension, tachycardia, ECG changes.*
EENT: *ocular changes, blurred vision, retinitis pigmentosa, nasal congestion.*
GI: *dry mouth, constipation, nausea, vomiting.*
GU: *urine retention, menstrual irregularities, gynecomastia, inhibited ejaculation.*
Hematologic: ***leukopenia, agranulocytosis, aplastic anemia,*** eosinophilia, ***thrombocytopenia.***
Hepatic: jaundice, abnormal liver function test results.
Metabolic: weight gain, elevated tests for protein-bound iodine.
Skin: *mild photosensitivity, allergic reactions, pain at I.M. injection site, sterile abscess, rash.*
Other: ***neuroleptic malignant syndrome.***
After abrupt withdrawal of long-term therapy: gastritis, nausea, vomiting, dizziness, tremor, feeling of warmth or cold, diaphoresis, tachycardia, headache, insomnia.

Overdose and treatment

CNS depression is characterized by deep, unarousable sleep and possible coma, hypotension or hypertension, extrapyramidal symptoms, abnormal involuntary muscle movements, agitation, seizures, arrhythmias, ECG changes, hypothermia or hyperthermia, and autonomic nervous system dysfunction.

Treatment is symptomatic and supportive, including maintaining vital signs, airway, stable body temperature, and fluid and electrolyte balance.

Don't induce vomiting; drug inhibits cough reflex, and aspiration may occur. Use gastric lavage, then activated charcoal and saline cathartics; dialysis doesn't help. Regulate body temperature as needed. Treat hypotension with I.V. fluids; don't give epinephrine. Treat seizures with parenteral diazepam or barbiturates; arrhythmias, with parenteral phenytoin (15 mg to 18 mg/kg not exceeding 50 mg/min, with rate titrated to blood pressure); treat extrapyramidal reactions with benztropine at 1 to 2 mg or parenteral diphenhydramine at 10 to 50 mg.

Clinical considerations

- Recommendations for administration of mesoridazine, for care and teaching of the patient during therapy, and for use in geriatric patients and breast-feeding women are the same as those for all phenothiazines.
- I.M. form is irritating.

Therapeutic monitoring

- Recommend monitoring vital signs, especially during parenteral therapy.
- Monitor hematopoietic and liver function studies.

Special populations

Pediatric patients. Drug isn't recommended for children under age 12.

Patient counseling

- Warn patient to avoid activities that require alertness and good psychomotor coordination until CNS effects of drug are known. Tell patient that drowsiness and dizziness usually subside after a few weeks.
- Advise patient to change position slowly.
- Warn patient to avoid alcohol while taking this drug.
- Instruct patient to relieve dry mouth with sugarless gum or hard candy.
- Advise patient to use sunblock and to wear protective clothing to avoid photosensitivity reactions.

metaproterenol sulfate

Alupent, Metaprel

Pharmacologic classification: adrenergic
Therapeutic classification: bronchodilator
Pregnancy risk category C

How supplied

Available by prescription only

Tablets: 10 mg, 20 mg
Syrup: 10 mg/5 ml
Aerosol inhaler: 0.65 mg/metered spray
Nebulizer inhaler: 0.4%, 0.6%, 5% solution

Indications and dosages

Bronchial asthma and reversible bronchospasm

Oral

Adults and children over age 9 or weighing more than 60 lb (27 kg): 20 mg P.O. t.i.d. or q.i.d.
Children age 6 to 9 or weighing less than 60 lb: 10 mg P.O. t.i.d. or q.i.d.

Children under age 6: 1.3 to 2.6 mg/kg P.O. daily in divided doses.

Inhalation

Adults and children age 12 and older: Administered by metered aerosol, 2 or 3 inhalations q 3 to 4 hours with at least 2 minutes between inhalations; no more than 12 inhalations in 24 hours. Administered by hand-bulb nebulizer, 10 inhalations of an undiluted 5% solution or, alternatively, administered by intermittent positive pressure breathing, 0.3 ml (range, 0.2 to 0.3 ml of a 5% solution diluted in about 2.5 ml of a normal saline solution or 2.5 ml of a commercially available 0.4% or 0.6% solution for nebulization).
Children age 6 to 11: 0.1 ml (range 0.1 to 0.2 ml) of 5% solution diluted with normal saline solution to final volume of 3 ml. Administer by nebulizer.

Note: To relieve acute bronchospasm, usually don't need to repeat more than q 4 hours. If part of bronchospastic pulmonary disease treatment regimen, administer 3 to 4 times daily.

Pharmacodynamics

Bronchodilator action: Metaproterenol relaxes bronchial smooth muscle and peripheral vasculature by stimulating $beta_2$-adrenergic receptors, thus decreasing airway resistance by way of bronchodilation. It has lesser effect on $beta_1$ receptors and has little or no effect on alpha-adrenergic receptors. In high doses, it may cause CNS and cardiac stimulation, resulting in tachycardia, hypertension, or tremors.

Pharmacokinetics

Absorption: Well-absorbed from the GI tract.
Distribution: Widely distributed throughout the body.
Metabolism: Extensively metabolized on first pass through the liver.
Excretion: Excreted in urine, mainly as glucuronic acid conjugates.

Route	Onset	Peak	Duration
P.O.	15 min	1 hr	1-4 hr
Inhalation	1 min	1 hr	1-2½ hr
Nebulizer	5-30 min	1 hr	1-2½ hr

Contraindications and precautions

Contraindicated in patients with hypersensitivity to drug or its ingredients, in use during anesthesia with cyclopropane or halogenated hydrocarbon general anesthetics, and in those with tachycardia and arrhythmias associated with tachycardia, peripheral or mesenteric vascular thrombosis, profound hypoxia, or hypercapnia.

Use cautiously in patients with hypertension, hyperthyroidism, heart disease, diabetes, or cirrhosis and in those receiving cardiac glycosides.

Interactions

Drug-drug. *Beta blockers, especially propranolol:* Antagonize bronchodilating effects of metaproterenol. Avoid use together.
General anesthetics (especially chloroform, cyclopropane, halothane, and trichloroethylene), cardiac glycosides, levodopa, theophylline derivatives, or thyroid hormones: May increase the potential for cardiac effects, including severe ventricular tachycardia, arrhythmias, and coronary insufficiency. Use together cautiously.
MAO inhibitors or tricyclic antidepressants: May potentiate their CV actions. Use together cautiously.
Other sympathomimetics: May produce additive effects and toxicity. Use together cautiously.
Xanthines, other sympathomimetics, other CNS-stimulating drugs: Increased CNS stimulation. Monitor patient closely.

Effects on diagnostic tests

Drug may reduce sensitivity of spirometry in diagnosis of asthma.

Adverse reactions

CNS: *nervousness, weakness, drowsiness, tremor, vertigo, headache.*
CV: *tachycardia, hypertension, palpitations,* ***cardiac arrest (with excessive use).***
GI: *vomiting, nausea, heartburn, dry mouth.*
Respiratory: ***paradoxical bronchiolar constriction with excessive use,*** cough, dry and irritated throat.
Skin: rash, ***hypersensitivity reactions.***

Overdose and treatment

Signs and symptoms of overdose include exaggeration of common adverse reactions, particularly nausea and vomiting, arrhythmias, angina, hypertension, and seizures.

Treatment includes supportive and symptomatic measures. Monitor vital signs closely. Support CV status. Use cardioselective $beta_1$-adrenergic blockers (acebutolol, atenolol, metoprolol) to treat symptoms with extreme caution; they may induce severe bronchospasm or asthmatic attack.

Clinical considerations

Consider the recommendations relevant to all adrenergics as well as the following:

- Adverse reactions are dose-related and characteristic of sympathomimetics, and may persist a long time because of the long duration of action of metaproterenol.
- Excessive or prolonged use may lead to decreased effectiveness.
- Avoid simultaneous administration of adrenocorticoid inhalation aerosol. Allow at least 5 minutes to lapse between using the two aerosols.
- Aerosol treatments may be used with oral tablet dosing.
- Store tablets and oral solution at 59° to 86° F (15° to 30° C) in tight, light-resistant containers. Store oral inhalation and nebulizer solution at 50° to 86° F (15° to 30° C).

Therapeutic monitoring

Monitor patient for signs and symptoms of toxic effects, such as nausea and vomiting, tremors, and arrhythmias.

Special populations

Pediatric patients. Oral inhalation in children under age 12 isn't recommended because safety and efficacy haven't been established. Safety and efficacy of oral preparations in children under age 6 haven't been established.
Geriatric patients. Geriatric patients may be more sensitive to the therapeutic and adverse effects of drug.

Patient counseling

- Instruct patient to use only as directed and to take no more than two inhalations at one time with 1- to 2-minute intervals between. Remind patient to save applicator; refills may be available.
- Tell patient to take missed dose if remembered within 1 hour. If beyond 1 hour, patient should skip dose and resume regular schedule. The patient shouldn't double the dose.
- Tell patient to store drug away from heat and light, and safely out of reach of children.
- Inform patient to immediately report if no relief occurs or condition worsens.
- Warn patient to avoid simultaneous use of adrenocorticoid aerosol and to allow at least 5 minutes to lapse between using the two aerosols.
- Tell patient that he may experience bad taste in mouth after using oral inhaler.
- Instruct patient to shake container, exhale through nose as completely as possible, then administer aerosol while inhaling deeply through mouth, and hold breath for 10 seconds before exhaling slowly. Patient should wait 1 to 2 minutes before repeating inhalations.
- Tell patient that drug may have shorter duration of action after prolonged use. Advise patient to report failure to respond to usual dose.
- Warn patient not to increase dose or frequency unless prescribed; serious adverse reactions are possible.

metaraminol bitartrate

Aramine

Pharmacologic classification: adrenergic
Therapeutic classification: vasopressor
Pregnancy risk category C

How supplied

Available by prescription only
Injection: 10 mg/ml parenteral

Indications and dosages

Prevention of hypotension
Adults: 2 to 10 mg I.M. or S.C. At least 10 minutes should elapse prior to repeat dosing.
Children: 0.1 mg/kg or 3 mg/m^2 S.C. or I.M.
Hypotension in severe shock
Adults: 0.5 to 5 mg direct I.V. followed by I.V. infusion. If necessary, mix 15 to 100 mg (up to 500 mg has been used) in 500 ml normal saline solution or D_5W; titrate infusion based on blood pressure response.
Children: 0.01 mg/kg or 0.3 mg/m^2 direct I.V. followed by I.V. infusion (dilution of 1 mg in 25 ml of diluent) if necessary, of 0.4 mg/kg or 12 mg/m^2 diluted and titrated to maintain desired blood pressure.
◇ ***Priapism***
Adults: 1 to 2 mg injected into corpus cavernosum of the penis.

Pharmacodynamics

Vasopressor action: Drug acts predominantly by direct stimulation of alpha-adrenergic receptors, which constrict both capacitance and resistance blood vessels, resulting in increased total peripheral resistance; increased systolic and diastolic blood pressure; decreased blood flow to vital organs, skin, and skeletal muscle; and constriction of renal blood vessels, which reduces renal blood flow. It also has a direct stimulating effect on $beta_1$ receptors of the heart, producing a positive inotropic response, and an indirect effect, releasing norepinephrine from its storage sites, which, with repeated use, may result in tachyphylaxis. Metaraminol also acts as a weak or false neurotransmitter by replacing norepinephrine in sympathetic nerve endings. Its main effects are vasoconstriction and cardiac stimulation. It doesn't usually cause CNS stimulation but may cause contraction of pregnant uterus and uterine blood vessels because of its alpha-adrenergic effects.

Pharmacokinetics

Absorption: Pressor effects may persist 20 to 90 minutes, depending on route of administration and patient variability.

Distribution: Not completely known.
Metabolism: In vitro tests suggest that metaraminol is not metabolized. Effects appear to be terminated by uptake of drug into tissues and by urinary excretion.
Excretion: Excreted in urine; may be accelerated by acidifying urine.

Route	Onset	Peak	Duration
I.V.	1-2 min	Unknown	20 min
I.M.	10 min	Unknown	< 90 min
S.C.	5-20 min	Unknown	< 90 min

Contraindications and precautions
Contraindicated in patients with hypersensitivity to drug and in those receiving anesthesia with cyclopropane and halogenated hydrocarbon anesthetics.

Use cautiously in patients with cardiac or thyroid disease, hypertension, peripheral vascular disease, cirrhosis, history of malaria, or sulfite sensitivity; in those receiving cardiac glycosides; and during pregnancy.

Interactions
Drug-drug. *Alpha blockers:* Pressor effects may be decreased, but not completely blocked. Use together cautiously.
General anesthetics, cardiac glycosides, levodopa, maprotiline, other sympathomimetics, or thyroid hormones: Increased cardiac effects may result. Use together cautiously.
Atropine: Blocks the reflex bradycardia caused by metaraminol and enhances its pressor response. Use together cautiously.
Beta blockers: Mutual inhibition of therapeutic effects with increased potential for hypertension, and excessive bradycardia with possible heart block. Avoid use together.
Doxapram, ergot alkaloids, mazindol, methylphenidate, or trimethaphan: Pressor effects may be increased. Use together cautiously.
Guanadrel, guanethidine, rauwolfia alkaloids, and diuretics used as antihypertensives: Decreased hypotensive effects. Monitor blood pressure frequently.
MAO inhibitors: May prolong and intensify cardiac stimulant and vasopressor effects. Don't administer metaraminol until 14 days after MAO inhibitors have been discontinued.

Effects on diagnostic tests
None reported.

Adverse reactions
CNS: apprehension, dizziness, headache, tremor.
CV: hypertension; hypotension; palpitations; ***arrhythmias,*** including sinus or ***ventricular tachycardia; cardiac arrest.***
GI: nausea.
Skin: flushing, diaphoresis.
Other: abscess, necrosis, sloughing upon extravasation.

Overdose and treatment
Signs and symptoms of overdose include severe hypertension, arrhythmias, seizures, cerebral hemorrhage, acute pulmonary edema, and cardiac arrest.

Treatment requires discontinuation of drug followed by supportive and symptomatic measures. Monitor vital signs closely. Use atropine for reflex bradycardia and propranolol for tachyarrhythmias. Use a sympatholytic agent to relieve hypertension.

Clinical considerations
Consider the recommendations relevant to all adrenergics as well as the following:
- Commercial preparations contain sodium bisulfite, which may cause allergic reactions in susceptible individuals.
- Correct blood volume depletion before administration. Metaraminol isn't a substitute for blood, plasma, fluids, or electrolyte replacement.
- Drug must be diluted before I.V. use. Preferred solutions for dilution are normal saline solution or dextrose 5% injection. Select injection site carefully. I.V. route is preferred, using large veins. Avoid extravasation. Monitor infusion rate; use of infusion-controlling device preferred. Withdraw drug gradually; recurrent hypotension may follow abrupt withdrawal.
- When administering I.M. or S.C., allow at least 10 minutes to elapse before administering additional doses because maximum effect isn't immediately apparent.
- To treat extravasation, infiltrate site promptly with 10 to 15 ml normal saline solution containing 5 to 10 mg phentolamine, using fine needle.
- Cumulative effect possible after prolonged use. Excessive vasopressor response may persist after drug is withdrawn.
- Keep emergency drugs on hand to reverse effect of metaraminol: atropine for reflex bradycardia, phentolamine for extravasation, and propranolol for tachyarrhythmias.
- Don't mix in bag or syringe with other medications.

Therapeutic monitoring
- Blood pressure, heart rate and rhythm should be checked during and after metaraminol administration until patient is stable.
- Monitor diabetic patients closely. Insulin adjustments may be needed.
- Fluid and electrolyte status must be monitored carefully.

Special populations
Breast-feeding patients. It isn't known if drug is excreted in breast milk. Use cautiously in breast-feeding women.

Pediatric patients. Because safety hasn't been fully established, use cautiously.
Geriatric patients. Geriatric patients may be more sensitive to effects of drug.

Patient counseling

- Ask patient about sulfite allergy before giving drug; vials contain sodium bisulfite.
- Inform patient that he'll need frequent assessment of vital signs.
- Advise patient to report adverse reactions.

metformin hydrochloride

Glucophage

Pharmacologic classification: biguanide
Therapeutic classification: antidiabetic
Pregnancy risk category B

How supplied

Available by prescription only
Tablets: 500 mg, 850 mg, 1,000 mg

Indications and dosages

Adjunct to diet and exercise to lower blood glucose in patients with non-insulin-dependent diabetes mellitus
Adults: Initially, give 500 mg P.O. b.i.d. with morning and evening meals or 850 mg P.O. once daily with morning meal. When 500-mg dose is used, increase dose by 500 mg weekly to maximum dose of 2,500 mg daily, p.r.n. Alternatively, 500 mg P.O. b.i.d. May be increased to 850 mg P.O. b.i.d. after 2 weeks. When 850-mg dose is used, increase dose 850 mg every other week to maximum daily dose of 2,550 mg, p.r.n.

Note: If patient requires more than 2 g daily, administer in three divided doses.

Pharmacodynamics

Antidiabetic action: Drug decreases hepatic glucose production and intestinal absorption of glucose and improves insulin sensitivity (increases peripheral glucose uptake and utilization).

Pharmacokinetics

Absorption: Absorbed from GI tract with absolute bioavailability being about 50% to 60%. Food decreases the extent and slightly delays absorption.
Distribution: Negligibly bound to plasma proteins. It partitions into erythrocytes, most likely as a function of time.
Metabolism: Not metabolized.
Excretion: 90% is excreted in urine. Elimination half-life in plasma is about 6¼ hours and 17½ hours in blood.

Route	Onset	Peak	Duration
P.O.	Unknown	Unknown	Unknown

Contraindications and precautions

Contraindicated in patients with heart failure, hypersensitivity to drug, renal disease, or metabolic acidosis. Drug should be temporarily withheld in patients undergoing radiologic studies involving parenteral administration of iodinated contrast materials because use of such products may result in acute renal dysfunction. Discontinue drug if a hypoxic state develops. Avoid use in patients with hepatic disease.

Use cautiously in geriatric, debilitated, or malnourished patients and in those with adrenal or pituitary insufficiency because of increased susceptibility to developing hypoglycemia.

Interactions

Drug-drug. *Calcium channel blockers, corticosteroids, estrogens, isoniazid, nicotinic acid, oral contraceptives, phenothiazines, phenytoin, sympathomimetics, thiazides or other diuretics, and thyroid agents:* May produce hyperglycemia. Monitor patient's glycemic control. Metformin dosage may need to be increased.
Cationic drugs such as amiloride, cimetidine, digoxin, morphine, procainamide, quinidine, quinine, ranitidine, triamterene, trimethoprim, and vancomycin: Potential to compete for common renal tubular transport systems, which may increase metformin plasma levels. Monitor patient's blood glucose level.
Nifedipine: Increased metformin plasma levels. Monitor patient closely. Metformin dosage may need to be decreased.

Effects on diagnostic tests

None reported.

Adverse reactions

GI: unpleasant or metallic taste, diarrhea, nausea, vomiting, abdominal bloating, flatulence, anorexia.
Hematologic: ***megaloblastic anemia.***
Metabolic: ***lactic acidosis.***
Skin: rash, dermatitis.

Overdose and treatment

Hypoglycemia hasn't been observed with ingestion of up to 85 g of metformin, although lactic acidosis has occurred. Hemodialysis may be useful for removing accumulated drug from patients in whom metformin overdose is suspected.

Clinical considerations

- Give drug with meals; give once-daily dose with breakfast, twice-daily dose with breakfast and dinner.
- When transferring patients from standard oral hypoglycemic agents other than chlorpropamide to metformin, no transition period is necessary. When transferring patients from chlorpropamide, exercise care during the first

2 weeks because of prolonged retention of chlorpropamide in the body, increasing risk of hypoglycemia during this time.

- If patient doesn't respond to 4 weeks of maximum dose of metformin, add an oral sulfonylurea while continuing metformin at the maximum dose. If patient still doesn't respond after several months of concomitant therapy at maximum doses, discontinue both agents and initiate insulin therapy.
- Incidence of drug-induced lactic acidosis is very low. Reported cases have occurred primarily in diabetic patients with significant renal insufficiency, multiple concomitant medical or surgical problems, and multiple concomitant medications. Risk of lactic acidosis increases with advanced age and degree of renal impairment.
- Discontinue drug immediately if patient develops conditions associated with hypoxemia or dehydration because of risk of lactic acidosis associated with these conditions.
- Suspend therapy temporarily for surgical procedures (except minor procedures not associated with restricted intake of food and fluids) or radiologic procedures involving parenteral administration of iodinated contrast, and don't restart until patient's oral intake has resumed and renal function is normal.

Therapeutic monitoring

- Patient's renal function is assessed before beginning therapy and then annually thereafter. If renal impairment is detected, another antidiabetic agent should be prescribed.
- Monitor patient's blood glucose level regularly to evaluate effectiveness.
- Patient requires close monitoring during times of increased stress, such as infection, fever, surgery, or trauma. Insulin therapy may be required in these situations.
- Monitor patient's hematologic status for megaloblastic anemia. Patients with inadequate vitamin B_{12} or calcium intake or absorption appear to be predisposed to developing subnormal vitamin B_{12} levels. These patients should have serum vitamin B_{12} levels checked routinely at 2- to 3-year intervals.
- Monitor glycosylated hemoglobin q 3 months to monitor continued response.

Special populations

Breast-feeding patients. It isn't known if metformin is excreted in breast milk. Because of the potential for serious adverse effects in nursing infants, drug shouldn't be administered to breast-feeding women.

Pediatric patients. Safety and efficacy in pediatric patients haven't been established. Studies in maturity-onset diabetes of the young haven't been conducted.

Geriatric patients. Because aging is associated with decreased renal function, administer cautiously to geriatric patients.

Patient counseling

- Instruct patient to discontinue drug immediately and report unexplained hyperventilation, myalgia, malaise, unusual somnolence, or other nonspecific symptoms of early lactic acidosis.
- Warn patient not to consume excessive amounts of alcohol while taking metformin.
- Instruct patient about nature of diabetes, importance of following therapeutic regimen, adhering to specific diet, weight reduction, exercise and personal hygiene programs; and avoiding infection. Explain how and when to perform self-monitoring of blood glucose level, and teach recognition of hypoglycemia and hyperglycemia.
- Tell patient not to change drug dosage without medical approval. Encourage him to report abnormal blood glucose levels.
- Advise patient not to take other medications, including OTC drugs, without medical approval.
- Instruct patient to carry medical identification regarding diabetic status.

methadone hydrochloride

Dolophine, Methadose, Physeptone*

Pharmacologic classification: opioid
Therapeutic classification: analgesic, narcotic detoxification adjunct
Controlled substance schedule II
Pregnancy risk category C

How supplied

Available by prescription only
Tablets: 5 mg, 10 mg, 40 mg for oral solution (for narcotic abstinence syndrome)
Oral solution: 5 mg/5 ml, 10 mg/5 ml, 10 mg/ml (concentrate)
Injection: 10 mg/ml

Indications and dosages

Severe pain
Adults: 2.5 to 10 mg P.O., I.M., or S.C. q 3 to 4 hours, p.r.n., or around-the-clock.
◇ *Children:* 0.7 mg/kg P.O. q 4 to 6 hours
Relief of severe, chronic pain
Adults: 5 to 20 mg P.O. q 6 to 8 hours.
Narcotic abstinence syndrome
Adults: 15 to 20 mg P.O. daily (highly individualized).

Maintenance dosage is 20 to 120 mg P.O. daily. Adjust dose, p.r.n. Daily doses above 120 mg require special state and federal approval. If patient feels nauseated, give one-fourth of total P.O. dose in two injections, S.C. or I.M. Treatment is 30 (short-term) to 180 (long-term) days.

Pharmacodynamics

Analgesic action: Methadone is an opiate agonist that has analgesic activity via an affinity for the opiate receptors similar to that of morphine. It's recommended for severe, chronic pain and is also used in detoxification and maintenance of patients with opiate abstinence syndrome.

Pharmacokinetics

Absorption: Well absorbed from the GI tract. Oral administration delays onset and prolongs duration of action as compared to parenteral administration.
Distribution: Highly bound to tissue protein, which may explain its cumulative effects and slow elimination.
Metabolism: Metabolized primarily in the liver by N-demethylation.
Excretion: Half-life is prolonged (7 to 11 hours) in patients with hepatic dysfunction. Urinary excretion, the major route, is dose-dependent. Methadone metabolites are also excreted in the feces via the bile.

Route	Onset	Peak	Duration
P.O.	½-1 hr	½-2 hr	4-6 hr
I.M.	10-20 min	1-2 hr	4-5 hr

Contraindications and precautions

Contraindicated in patients with hypersensitivity to drug. Use cautiously in geriatric or debilitated patients and in those with severe renal or hepatic impairment, acute abdominal conditions, hypothyroidism, Addison's disease, prostatic hyperplasia, urethral stricture, head injury, increased intracranial pressure, asthma, or other respiratory disorders.

Interactions

Drug-drug. *Other CNS depressants, such as narcotic analgesics, general anesthetics, antidepressants, antihistamines, barbiturates, benzodiazepines, muscle relaxants, phenothiazines, and sedative-hypnotics:* Potentiated respiratory and CNS depression, sedation, and hypotensive effects. Use together cautiously.
Cimetidine: Increased respiratory and CNS depression, causing confusion, disorientation, apnea, or seizures. Such use usually requires reduced dosage of methadone.
Opioid antagonist: Patients who become physically dependent on drug may experience acute withdrawal syndrome if given with methadone. Use with caution, and monitor closely.
Rifampin: May reduce blood level of methadone. Monitor patient.
Drug-lifestyle. *Alcohol use:* Potentiated respiratory and CNS depression, sedation, and hypotensive effects. Avoid use together.

Effects on diagnostic tests

None reported.

Adverse reactions

CNS: *sedation, somnolence, clouded sensorium, euphoria, dizziness, choreic movements,* ***seizures*** (with large doses), headache, insomnia, agitation, *light-headedness,* syncope.
CV: *hypotension,* ***bradycardia, shock, cardiac arrest,*** palpitations, edema.
EENT: visual disturbances.
GI: *nausea, vomiting, constipation, ileus, dry mouth, anorexia, biliary tract spasm,* increased plasma amylase levels.
GU: *urine retention, decreased libido.*
Respiratory: ***respiratory depression, respiratory arrest.***
Skin: *diaphoresis,* pruritus, urticaria.
Other: physical dependence; pain at injection site; tissue irritation, induration (after S.C. injection).

Overdose and treatment

The most common signs and symptoms of drug overdose are CNS depression, respiratory depression, and miosis (pinpoint pupils). Others include hypotension, bradycardia, hypothermia, shock, apnea, cardiopulmonary arrest, circulatory collapse, pulmonary edema, and seizures. Toxicity may result from accumulation of drug over several weeks.

To treat acute overdose, first establish adequate respiratory exchange by way of a patent airway and ventilation as needed; administer an opioid antagonist (naloxone) to reverse respiratory depression. Because the duration of action of methadone is longer than that of naloxone, repeated naloxone dosing is necessary. The antagonist naloxone shouldn't be given unless the patient has clinically significant respiratory or CV depression. Monitor vital signs closely.

If patient is seen within 2 hours of ingestion of an oral overdose, empty the stomach immediately by inducing emesis (ipecac syrup) or using gastric lavage. Use caution to avoid risk of aspiration. Administer activated charcoal through nasogastric tube for further removal of drug in an oral overdose.

Provide symptomatic and supportive treatment (continued respiratory support, correction of fluid or electrolyte imbalance). Monitor laboratory values, vital signs, and neurologic status closely.

Clinical considerations

Consider the recommendations relevant to all opioids as well as the following:

- Verify that patient is in a methadone maintenance program for management of narcotic addiction and, if so, at what dosage, and continue that program appropriately.
- Dispersible tablets may be dissolved in 4 oz (120 ml) of water or fruit juice; oral concentrate must be diluted to at least 30 ml, but when used for detoxification, must be diluted with at least 3 oz (90 ml) of water before administration.

☐ ***ALERT*** Diluents used for diluting methadone and levomethadyl acetate should differ in col-

or and taste in any specific clinic setting to avoid confusion.
- Oral liquid form (not tablets) is legally required and is the only form available in drug maintenance programs.
- Regimented scheduling (around-the-clock) is beneficial in severe, chronic pain. When used for severe, chronic pain, tolerance may develop with long-term use, requiring a higher dose to achieve the same degree of analgesia.
- Patient treated for narcotic abstinence syndrome usually requires an additional analgesic if pain control is necessary.
- Physical and psychological tolerance or dependence may occur. Be aware of potential for abuse.

Therapeutic monitoring
Patient requires observation for increased sedation, respiratory depression, stabilization of symptoms of withdrawal, or for pain relief.

Special populations
Breast-feeding patients. Methadone is excreted in breast milk; it may cause physical dependence in breast-feeding infants of women on methadone maintenance therapy.
Pediatric patients. Drug isn't recommended for use in children. Safe use as maintenance drug in adolescent addicts hasn't been established.
Geriatric patients. Lower doses are usually indicated for geriatric patients because they may be more sensitive to the therapeutic and adverse effects of drug.

Patient counseling
- If appropriate, tell patient that constipation is often severe during maintenance with methadone. Instruct him to take a stool softener or other laxative.
- Caution patient to avoid activities that require full alertness, such as driving and operating machinery, because of potential for drowsiness.

methamphetamine hydrochloride
Desoxyn, Desoxyn Gradumets

Pharmacologic classification: amphetamine
Therapeutic classification: CNS stimulant, short-term adjunctive anorexigenic agent, sympathomimetic amine
Controlled substance schedule II
Pregnancy risk category C

How supplied
Available by prescription only
Tablets: 5 mg
Tablets (extended-release): 5 mg, 10 mg, 15 mg

Indications and dosages
Attention deficit hyperactivity disorder
Children age 6 and older: Initially, 5 mg P.O. once daily or b.i.d., with 5-mg increments weekly, p.r.n. Usual effective dose is 20 to 25 mg daily.
Short-term adjunct in exogenous obesity
Adults: 2.5 to 5 mg P.O. b.i.d. to t.i.d. 30 minutes before meals or 10 to 15 mg/day (extended-release) P.O. in morning. Don't use for more than a few weeks.

Pharmacodynamics
CNS stimulant action: Amphetamines are sympathomimetic amines with CNS stimulant activity; in hyperactive children, they have a paradoxical calming effect.
Anorexigenic action: Anorexigenic effects are thought to occur in the hypothalamus, where decreased smell and taste acuity decreases appetite; they may involve other systemic and metabolic effects. They may be tried for short-term control of refractory obesity, with caloric restriction and behavior modification.

The cerebral cortex and reticular activating system appear to be the primary sites of activity; amphetamines release nerve terminal stores of norepinephrine, promoting nerve impulse transmission. At high dosages, effects are mediated by dopamine.

Amphetamines are used to treat narcolepsy and as adjuncts to psychosocial measures in attention deficit disorder in children. The precise mechanisms of action in these conditions are unknown.

Pharmacokinetics
Absorption: Rapidly absorbed from the GI tract after oral administration.
Distribution: Widely distributed throughout the body. Drug crosses the placenta and enters breast milk.
Metabolism: Metabolized in the liver to at least seven metabolites.
Excretion: Excreted in urine.

Route	Onset	Peak	Duration
P.O.	Unknown	Unknown	24 hr

Contraindications and precautions
Contraindicated in patients with moderate to severe hypertension, hyperthyroidism, symptomatic CV disease, advanced arteriosclerosis, glaucoma, hypersensitivity or idiosyncrasy to sympathomimetic amines, or history of drug abuse; within 14 days of MAO inhibitor therapy; and in agitated patients.

Use cautiously in geriatric, debilitated, asthenic, or psychopathic patients and in those with history of suicidal or homicidal tendencies.

Interactions

Drug-drug. *Acetazolamide, antacids, or sodium bicarbonate:* Enhances reabsorption of methamphetamine and prolongs duration of action. Patient requires close monitoring.
General anesthesia: Increased risk of arrhythmias. Patient requires close monitoring.
Antihypertensives: May antagonize their effects. Patient requires close monitoring.
Ascorbic acid: Enhances methamphetamine excretion and shortens duration of action. May need to increase methamphetamine dose.
Barbiturates: Antagonize methamphetamine by CNS depression: Avoid use together.
Other CNS stimulants: Additive effects. Avoid use together.
Insulin: Drug may alter insulin requirements. Monitor serum glucose.
MAO inhibitors (or drugs with MAO-inhibiting activity, such as furazolidone) or within 14 days of such therapy: May cause hypertensive crisis. Avoid use together.
Phenothiazines or haloperidol: Decreased methamphetamine effects. Patient requires close monitoring.
Drug-food. *Caffeine:* Additive effects. Avoid use together.
Drug-herb. *Melatonin:* Enhances monoaminergic effects of methamphetamine and may exacerbate insomnia. Avoid use together.

Effects on diagnostic tests

Drug may interfere with urinary steroid determinations.

Adverse reactions

CNS: *nervousness, insomnia, irritability,* talkativeness, dizziness, headache, hyperexcitability, tremor, euphoria.
CV: hypertension, *tachycardia, palpitations,* ***arrhythmias.***
EENT: blurred vision, mydriasis.
GI: dry mouth, metallic taste, diarrhea, constipation, anorexia.
GU: impotence, altered libido.
Metabolic: elevated plasma corticosteroid levels.
Skin: urticaria.

Overdose and treatment

Symptoms of overdose include increasing restlessness, tremor, hyperreflexia, tachypnea, confusion, aggressiveness, hallucinations, and panic; fatigue and depression usually follow the excitement stage. Other symptoms may include arrhythmias, shock, alterations in blood pressure, nausea, vomiting, diarrhea, and abdominal cramps; death is usually preceded by seizures and coma.

Treat overdose symptomatically and supportively: if ingestion is recent (within 4 hours), use gastric lavage or emesis and sedate with barbiturate; monitor vital signs and fluid and electrolyte balance. I.V. phentolamine is suggested for treatment of severe acute hypertension. Chlorpromazine is useful in decreasing CNS stimulation and sympathomimetic effects. Urinary acidification may enhance excretion. Saline catharsis (magnesium citrate) may hasten GI evacuation of unabsorbed long-acting forms. Hemodialysis or peritoneal dialysis may be effective in severe cases.

Clinical considerations

Consider the recommendations relevant to all amphetamines as well as the following:
- Drug isn't recommended for first-line treatment of obesity.
- Don't crush long-acting dosage forms.
- Rapid withdrawal after prolonged use may lead to depression, somnolence, and increased appetite.

Therapeutic monitoring

When treating behavioral disorders in children, consider a periodic discontinuation of the drug to evaluate effectiveness and the need for continued therapy.

Special populations

Breast-feeding patients. Amphetamines are excreted in breast milk. An alternative method of feeding should be used.
Pediatric patients. Drug isn't recommended for weight reduction in children under age 12.
Geriatric patients. Geriatric or debilitated patients may be especially sensitive to effects of methamphetamine. Use drug with caution.

Patient counseling

- Warn patient that potential for abuse is high. Discourage use to combat fatigue.
- Advise patient to avoid caffeine-containing drinks and alcohol, to take drug 1 hour before next meal, and to take last daily dose at least 6 hours before bedtime to prevent insomnia. Sustained-release (long-acting) forms should be taken at the start of the day.
- Warn patient not to increase dosage unless prescribed.
- Inform patient that methamphetamine may impair ability to engage in potentially hazardous activities, such as operating machinery or driving a motor vehicle.

methimazole

Tapazole

Pharmacologic classification: thyroid hormone antagonist
Therapeutic classification: antihyperthyroid
Pregnancy risk category D

How supplied

Available by prescription only
Tablets: 5 mg, 10 mg

Indications and dosages

Hyperthyroidism, preparation for thyroidectomy, thyrotoxic crisis

Adults: 15 mg P.O. daily if mild; 30 to 40 mg P.O. daily if moderately severe; 60 mg P.O. daily if severe; all are given in three equally divided doses q 8 hours. Continue until patient is euthyroid, then start maintenance dosage of 5 to 15 mg daily. Continue initial dosage for 2 months.

Children: 0.4 mg/kg/day P.O. divided q 8 hours. Continue until patient is euthyroid, then start maintenance dosage of 0.2 mg/kg/day divided q 8 hours.

Pharmacodynamics

Antithyroid action: In treating hyperthyroidism, methimazole inhibits synthesis of thyroid hormone by interfering with the incorporation of iodide into tyrosyl. Methimazole also inhibits the formation of iodothyronine. As preparation for thyroidectomy, methimazole inhibits synthesis of the thyroid hormone and causes a euthyroid state, reducing surgical problems during thyroidectomy; as a result, the mortality for a single-stage thyroidectomy is low. Iodide reduces the vascularity of the gland, making it less friable. For treating thyrotoxic crisis (thyrotoxicosis), propylthiouracil (PTU) theoretically is preferred over methimazole because it inhibits peripheral deiodination of thyroxine to triiodothyronine.

Pharmacokinetics

Absorption: Absorbed rapidly from the GI tract (80% to 95% bioavailable).

Distribution: Readily crosses the placenta and is distributed into breast milk. Drug is concentrated in the thyroid, and isn't protein-bound.

Metabolism: Undergoes hepatic metabolism.

Excretion: About 80% of drug and its metabolites are excreted renally; 7% is excreted unchanged. Half-life is between 5 and 13 hours.

Route	Onset	Peak	Duration
P.O.	< 5 days	½-1 hr	Unknown

Contraindications and precautions

Contraindicated in patients with hypersensitivity to drug and in breast-feeding women. Use cautiously in pregnant women.

Interactions

Drug-drug. *Anticoagulants:* Antivitamin K action of methimazole potentiates the action of anticoagulants. Monitor PT and INR.

Other bone marrow depressant agents: Increased risk of agranulocytosis. Monitor CBC.

Other hepatotoxic agents: Increases the risk of hepatotoxicity. Monitor liver function tests and use together cautiously.

Iodinated glycerol, lithium, potassium iodide: May potentiate hypothyroid and goitrogenic effects. Use together cautiously.

PTU and adrenocorticoids or corticotropin: May require a dosage adjustment of the steroid when thyroid status changes. Patient requires careful monitoring.

Effects on diagnostic tests

None reported.

Adverse reactions

CNS: headache, drowsiness, vertigo, paresthesia, neuritis, neuropathies, CNS stimulation, depression.

GI: diarrhea, nausea, vomiting (may be dose-related), salivary gland enlargement, loss of taste, epigastric distress.

GU: nephritis.

Hematologic: ***agranulocytosis, leukopenia, thrombocytopenia, aplastic anemia.***

Hepatic: jaundice, hepatic dysfunction, ***hepatitis.***

Metabolic: hypothyroidism (mental depression; cold intolerance; hard, nonpitting edema; hypoprothrombinemia and bleeding).

Musculoskeletal: arthralgia, myalgia.

Skin: rash, urticaria, discoloration, pruritus, erythema nodosum, exfoliative dermatitis, lupus-like syndrome.

Other: fever, lymphadenopathy.

Overdose and treatment

Signs and symptoms of overdose include nausea, vomiting, epigastric distress, fever, headache, arthralgia, pruritus, edema, and pancytopenia. Treatment is supportive; perform gastric lavage or induce emesis, if possible. If bone marrow depression develops, fresh whole blood, corticosteroids, and anti-infectives may be required.

Clinical considerations

- Best response occurs if dosage is administered around-the-clock and given at the same time each day with respect to meals.
- Doses of more than 40 mg/day increase the risk of agranulocytosis.
- A beta blocker, most often propranolol, is given to manage the peripheral signs of hyperthyroidism, primarily tachycardia.
- Euthyroid state may take several months to develop.
- Sulfonamide-type adverse reactions can occur.

Therapeutic monitoring

- Monitor CBC in patients with signs and symptoms of illness.
- Monitor LFTs, especially if hepatic dysfunction is suspected.

Special populations

Pregnant patients. Drug can induce goiter and hypothyroidism in developing fetus. The manufacturer states that the drug may be used ju-

diciously to treat hyperthyroidism complicated by pregnancy.
Breast-feeding patients. Patient should discontinue breast-feeding before beginning therapy because drug is excreted in breast milk. However, if breast-feeding is necessary, PTU is the preferred antithyroid agent.

Patient counseling
- Tell patient to take drug at regular intervals around-the-clock and to take it at the same time each day in relation to meals.
- If GI upset occurs, advise patient to take drug with meals.
- Tell patient to promptly report fever, sore throat, malaise, unusual bleeding, yellowing of eyes, nausea, or vomiting.
- Advise patient not to store drug in bathroom; heat and humidity cause it to deteriorate.
- Tell patient to inform other doctors and dentists of drug use.
- Teach patient how to recognize the signs of hyperthyroidism and hypothyroidism and what to do if they occur.

methocarbamol
Robaxin

Pharmacologic classification: carbamate derivative of guaifenesin
Therapeutic classification: skeletal muscle relaxant
Pregnancy risk category C

How supplied
Available by prescription only
Tablets: 500 mg, 750 mg
Tablets (film-coated): 500 mg, 750 mg
Injection: 100 mg/ml parenteral in 10 ml vial

Indications and dosages
Adjunct in acute, painful musculoskeletal conditions
Adults: 1.5 g P.O. q.i.d. for 2 to 3 days. Maintenance dosage, 4 to 4.5 g P.O. daily in three to six divided doses. Alternatively, 1 g I.M. or I.V. For severe conditions, I.M. or I.V. doses may be administered at 8-hour intervals. Maximum dosage, 3 g daily I.M. or I.V. for 3 consecutive days. Patient may resume I.M. or I.V. use after drug-free interval of 2 days.
Supportive therapy in tetanus management
Adults: 1 to 2 g I.V. push (300 mg/minute) and an additional 1 to 2 g may be added to I.V. solution. Total initial I.V. dosage, 3 g. Repeat I.V. infusion of 1 to 2 g q 6 hours until nasogastric tube can be inserted. Total adult P.O. dose may be up to 24 g daily to manage tetanus.
Children: 15 mg/kg or 500 mg/m^2 I.V. Don't inject faster than 180 mg/m^2 /minute. May be repeated q 6 hours, if necessary, to total dosage of 1.8 g/m^2 daily for 3 consecutive days.

Pharmacodynamics
Skeletal muscle relaxant action: Drug doesn't relax skeletal muscle directly. Its effects appear to be related to its sedative action; however, the exact mechanism of action is unknown.

Pharmacokinetics
Absorption: Rapidly and completely absorbed from the GI tract.
Distribution: Widely distributed throughout the body.
Metabolism: Extensively metabolized in liver by way of dealkylation and hydroxylation. Half-life of drug is between 1 and 2 hours.
Excretion: Rapidly and almost completely excreted in urine, mainly as its glucuronide and sulfate metabolites (40% to 50%), as unchanged drug (10% to 15%), and the rest as unidentified metabolites.

Route	Onset	Peak	Duration
P.O.	30 min	2 hr	Unknown
I.V.	Immediate	Immediate	Unknown
I.M.	Unknown	Unknown	Unknown

Contraindications and precautions
Contraindicated in patients with hypersensitivity to drug, impaired renal function (injectable form), or seizure disorder (injectable form). Safe use of methocarbamol in regard to fetal development hasn't been established. Therefore, drug shouldn't be used in women who are or may become pregnant, especially during early pregnancy, unless the benefits outweigh the possible hazards.

Interactions
Drug-drug. *Anticholinesterase agents:* In patients with myasthenia gravis, severe weakness may result if given methocarbamol. Avoid use together.
Other CNS depressant drugs, including anxiolytics, narcotics, psychotics, and tricyclic antidepressants: May cause additive CNS depression. Use together cautiously.
Drug-lifestyle. *Alcohol use:* May cause additive CNS depression. Avoid use together.

Effects on diagnostic tests
Methocarbamol therapy alters results of laboratory tests for urine 5-hydroxyindoleacetic acid (5-HIAA) using quantitative method of Udenfriend (false-positive) and for urine vanillylmandelic acid (false-positive when Gitlow screening test used; no problem when quantitative method of Sunderman used).

Adverse reactions
CNS: drowsiness, dizziness, light-headedness, headache, syncope, mild muscular incoordination (with I.M. or I.V. use), ***seizures*** (with I.V. use only), vertigo.

CV: flushing, hypotension, ***bradycardia*** (with I.M. or I.V. use).
EENT: blurred vision, conjunctivitis, nystagmus, diplopia.
GI: nausea, GI upset, metallic taste.
GU: hematuria (with I.V. use only), discoloration of urine.
Skin: urticaria, pruritus, rash.
Other: thrombophlebitis, extravasation (with I.V. use only), fever, ***anaphylactic reactions*** (with I.M. or I.V. use).

Overdose and treatment
Signs and symptoms of overdose include extreme drowsiness, nausea and vomiting, and arrhythmias.

Treatment includes symptomatic and supportive measures. If ingestion is recent, empty stomach by emesis or gastric lavage (may reduce absorption). Maintain adequate airway; monitor urine output and vital signs; and administer I.V. fluids, if needed.

Clinical considerations
- Don't administer S.C. Give I.V. undiluted at a rate not exceeding 300 mg per minute. May also be given by I.V. infusion after diluting in D_5W or normal saline solution.
- For I.V. administration, dilute 1 g of drug with up to 250 ml of 5% dextrose or normal saline injection. Don't refrigerate I.V. solution because precipitate and haze may occur.
- Methocarbamol solutions containing 4 mg/ml in sterile water for injection, 5% dextrose, or normal saline injection are stable for 6 days at room temperature.
- Inspect all solutions before administration for particles and haze.
- Patient should be supine during and for at least 10 to 15 minutes after I.V. injection.
- To give via nasogastric tube, crush tablets and suspend in water or normal saline solution.
- When used in tetanus, follow manufacturer's instructions.
- Patient's urine may turn black, blue, brown, or green if left standing.
- Patient needs assistance in walking after parenteral administration.
- Extravasation of I.V. solution may cause thrombophlebitis and sloughing from hypertonic solution.
- Oral administration should replace parenteral use as soon as feasible.
- Adverse reactions after oral administration are usually mild and transient and subside with dosage reduction.
- For I.M. administration, don't give more than 500 mg in each gluteal region.
- Store at 59° to 86° F (15° to 30° C). Avoid freezing injection.

Therapeutic monitoring
Recommend monitoring vital signs during I.V. or I.M. administration.

Special populations
Breast-feeding patients. Drug is excreted in breast milk in small amounts. Patient shouldn't breast-feed during treatment with methocarbamol.
Pediatric patients. For children under age 12, use only as recommended for tetanus.
Geriatric patients. Lower doses are indicated, because geriatric patients are more sensitive to effects of drug.

Patient counseling
- Tell patient urine may turn black, blue, green, or brown.
- Warn patient drug may cause drowsiness. Patient should avoid hazardous activities that require alertness until degree of CNS depression can be determined.
- Advise patient to make position changes slowly, particularly from recumbent to upright position, and to dangle legs before standing.
- Advise patient to avoid alcoholic beverages and use OTC cold or cough preparations carefully because some contain alcohol.
- Tell patient to store drug away from heat and light (not in bathroom medicine cabinet) and safely out of reach of children.
- Tell patient to take missed dose if remembered within 1 hour. Beyond 1 hour, patient should skip that dose and resume regular schedule. He shouldn't double the dose.
- Inform athletes that skeletal muscle relaxants are banned in competition and tested for by the U.S. Olympic Committee and the National Collegiate Athletic Association.

methohexital sodium
Brevital Sodium, Brietal Sodium*

Pharmacologic classification: barbiturate
Therapeutic classification: I.V. anesthetic
Controlled substance schedule IV
Pregnancy risk category B

How supplied
Available by prescription only
Injection: 500 mg, 2.5 g, 5 g powder for injection

Indications and dosages
Induction of anesthesia; anesthesia for short procedures (such as electroconvulsive therapy [ECT])
Dosage is highly individualized.
Adults and children: For induction of anesthesia, a 1% solution is administered at a rate of about 1 ml/5 seconds, possibly with inhalant anesthetics or skeletal muscle relaxants, or both. Induction dose may vary from 50 to 120 mg or more but averages about 70 mg; it usually provides anesthesia for 5 to 7 minutes. Main-

tenance of anesthesia may be achieved via intermittent injections of about 20 to 40 mg (2 to 4 ml of 1% solution), as needed, usually q 4 to 7 minutes; or by continuous I.V. infusion of a 0.2% solution (average rate of about 3 ml of a 0.2% solution per minute [1 drop/second]).

Pharmacodynamics

Anesthetic action: Methohexital produces anesthesia by direct depression of the polysynaptic midbrain reticular activating system; drug decreases presynaptic (via decreased neurotransmitter release) and postsynaptic excitation. These effects may be subsequent to increased gamma-aminobutyric acid (GABA), enhancement of effects of GABA, or a direct effect on GABA receptor sites.

Pharmacokinetics

Absorption: Only given I.V.; an ultrashort-acting barbiturate.
Distribution: Distributes throughout the body; highest initial levels occur in vascular areas of the brain, primarily gray matter.
Metabolism: Metabolized extensively in the liver.
Excretion: Excretion of metabolites occurs via the kidneys through glomerular filtration. Duration of action depends on tissue redistribution.

Route	Onset	Peak	Duration
I.V.	Immediate	30 sec-2 min	Unknown

Contraindications and precautions

Contraindicated in patients with acute intermittent or variegate porphyria or known hypersensitivity to drug and whenever general anesthesia is contraindicated.

Use cautiously in patients with circulatory, cardiac, renal, hepatic, endocrine, or pulmonary dysfunction; severe anemia; marked obesity or status asthmaticus (use extremely cautiously) because drug worsens these conditions. Also, use cautiously in patients with a full stomach because it blocks airway reflexes and may predispose the patient to aspiration.

Interactions

Drug-drug. *Antihistamines, benzodiazepines, hypnotics, narcotics, phenothiazines, and sedatives:* Potentiated effects. Use together cautiously.
Ketamine: Profound respiratory depression. Use together cautiously.
Drug-lifestyle. *Alcohol use*: Potentiated CNS depressant effects. Avoid use together.

Effects on diagnostic tests

None reported.

Adverse reactions

CNS: skeletal muscle hyperactivity, anxiety, restlessness, headache, emergence delirium, alteration of EEG patterns.
CV: transient hypotension, tachycardia, ***circulatory depression, peripheral vascular collapse.***
GI: abdominal pain, nausea, vomiting, excessive salivation.
Respiratory: ***respiratory arrest, respiratory depression, apnea, laryngospasm, bronchospasm,*** hiccups.
Skin: pain, swelling; ulceration, necrosis (on extravasation).
Other: thrombophlebitis, pain (at injection site); injury to adjacent nerves; ***hypersensitivity reaction.***

Note: Drug must be discontinued if peripheral vascular collapse, respiratory arrest, or hypersensitivity reaction occurs.

Overdose and treatment

Clinical signs include respiratory depression, respiratory arrest, hypotension, and shock. Treat supportively, using, as needed, mechanical ventilation and I.V. fluids or vasopressors (dopamine, phenylephrine) for hypotension. Monitor vital signs closely.

Clinical considerations

- Maintenance of patent airway and adequate ventilation must be ensured during induction and maintenance of anesthesia.
- Solutions used should be clear and colorless. Prepare according to manufacturer directions.
- Solutions prepared with sterile water for injection are stable for at least 6 weeks at room temperature.
- Solutions in 5% dextrose injection or in normal saline injection aren't stable beyond 24 hours.
- Avoid extravasation or intra-arterial injection because of possible tissue necrosis and gangrene.
- Drug is physically incompatible with lactated Ringer's solution; with acidic solutions, such as atropine, metocurine, and succinylcholine; and with silicone. Avoid contact with rubber stoppers or parts of syringes that have been treated with silicone. The preferred diluent is sterile water, but D_5W or normal saline may be used. Don't use bacteriostatic diluents.
- Store powder for injection at room temperature less than 77° F (25° C).

Therapeutic monitoring

Recommend close monitoring of patient's vital signs, respiratory status, and cardiac monitor during drug administration.

Special populations

Breast-feeding patients. Use cautiously in breast-feeding women.
Pediatric patients. Safety and efficacy in children haven't been established.
Geriatric patients. Lower doses may be indicated.

methotrexate, methotrexate sodium

Folex, Mexate, Mexate-AQ, Rheumatrex Dose Pack

Pharmacologic classification: antimetabolite (cell cycle-phase specific, S phase)
Therapeutic classification: antineoplastic
Pregnancy risk category X

How supplied

Available by prescription only
Tablets (scored): 2.5 mg
Injection: 20-mg, 25-mg, 50-mg, 100-mg, 250-mg, 1-g vials, lyophilized powder, preservative-free; 25-mg/ml vials, preservative-free solution; 2.5-mg/ml, 25-mg/ml vials, lyophilized powder, preserved

Indications and dosages

Dosage and indications may vary. Check current literature for recommended protocols.
Trophoblastic tumors (choriocarcinoma, hydatidiform mole)
Adults: 15 to 30 mg P.O. or I.M. daily for 5 days. Repeat after 1 or more weeks, according to response or toxicity.
◊*Adults:* 10 to 15 mg via the hypogastric artery until toxicity or therapeutic response occurs; 3 to 5 courses are usually needed.
Acute lymphoblastic leukemia
Adults and children: 3.3 mg/ m² P.O. daily for 4 to 6 weeks or until remission occurs; then 20 to 30 mg/m² P.O. or I.M. twice weekly or 2.5 mg/kg I.V. q 14 days. (Used in combination with prednisone.)
Prophylaxis against meningeal leukemia
12 mg/m² or 15 mg intrathecally—consult specific references for intervals and dosing.
Meningeal leukemia
Adults and children: 12 mg/ m² intrathecally to a maximum dose of 15 mg q 2 to 5 days until CSF is normal. Alternatively, 12 mg/m² once weekly for 2 weeks, then once monthly. Use only vials of powder with no preservatives; dilute using normal saline solution injection without preservatives. Use only new vials of drug and diluent. Use immediately after reconstitution.
Burkitt's lymphoma (stage I or II)
Adults: 10 to 25 mg P.O. daily for 4 to 8 days with 7- to 10-day rest intervals.
Lymphosarcoma (stage III; malignant lymphoma)
Adults: 0.625 to 2.5 mg/kg daily P.O., I.M., or I.V.
Mycosis fungoides (advanced)
Adults: 2.5 to 10 mg P.O. daily or 50 mg I.M. weekly; or 25 mg I.M. twice weekly for several weeks to months.
Psoriasis (severe)
Adults: Initially, a 5- to 10-mg test dose should be given 1 week before therapy. Then, 2.5 to 5 mg P.O. at 12-hour intervals for three doses each week or at 8-hour intervals for four doses each week. May increase by 2.5 mg/week, not to exceed 25 to 30 mg/week. Alternatively, 10 to 25 mg P.O., I.M., or I.V. as single weekly dose. May increase by 2.5 to 5 mg/week, not to exceed 50 mg/week. Alternatively, 2.5 mg P.O. daily for 5 days followed by a 2-day rest period. Dosage shouldn't exceed 6.25 mg/day. Improvement within 4 weeks should be noted with optimum results in 2 to 3 months.
Rheumatoid arthritis (severe, refractory)
Adults: 7.5 to 20 mg weekly P.O. in single or divided doses.
◊*Adults:* 7.5 to 15 mg I.M. once weekly.
Adjunct treatment in osteosarcoma
Adults: Give 12 g/m² as a 4-hour I.V. infusion.
◊***Head and neck carcinoma***
Adults: 40 to 60 mg/m² I.V. once weekly. Response limited to 4 months.

Pharmacodynamics

Antineoplastic action: Methotrexate exerts its cytotoxic activity by tightly binding with dihydrofolic acid reductase, an enzyme crucial to purine metabolism, resulting in an inhibition of DNA, RNA, and protein synthesis.

Pharmacokinetics

Absorption: Absorption across the GI tract appears to be dose related. Lower doses are essentially completely absorbed, while absorption of larger doses is incomplete and variable. I.M. doses are absorbed completely.
Distribution: Distributed widely throughout the body, with the highest levels found in the kidneys, gallbladder, spleen, liver, and skin. Drug crosses the blood-brain barrier but doesn't achieve therapeutic levels in the CSF. About 50% of the drug is bound to plasma protein.
Metabolism: Metabolized only slightly in the liver.
Excretion: Excreted primarily into urine as unchanged drug. Elimination has been described as biphasic, with a first phase half-life averaging 1.5 to 3.5 hours and a terminal phase half-life of 8 to 15 hours.

Route	Onset	Peak	Duration
P.O.	Unknown	1-2 hr	Unknown
I.V.	Unknown	Immediate	Unknown
I.M.	Unknown	½-1 hr	Unknown
Intrathecal	Unknown	Unknown	Unknown

Contraindications and precautions

Contraindicated in patients hypersensitive to drug and during pregnancy or breast-feeding. Also contraindicated in patients with psoriasis or rheumatoid arthritis who also have alcoholism, alcoholic liver, chronic liver disease, immunodeficiency syndromes, or preexisting blood dyscrasias.

Use cautiously in very young or geriatric or debilitated patients and in those with impaired renal or hepatic function, bone marrow suppression, aplasia, leukopenia, thrombocytopenia, anemia, folate deficiency, infection, peptic ulcer, or ulcerative colitis. Drug exits slowly from third space compartments resulting in a prolonged terminal plasma half-life and risk of toxicity.

Interactions

Drug-drug. *Probenecid:* Increases the therapeutic and toxic effects of methotrexate. Combined use of these agents requires a lower dosage of methotrexate.

NSAIDs, salicylates, sulfonamides, and sulfonylureas: May increase the therapeutic and toxic effects of methotrexate by displacing methotrexate from plasma proteins, increasing the levels of free methotrexate. Avoid use together if possible.

Immunizations: May not be effective when given during methotrexate therapy. Vaccines shouldn't be given during methotrexate therapy.

Phenytoin: Increased risk of seizures. Patient requires careful monitoring.

Folic acid: May decrease the effectiveness of methotrexate. Use together cautiously

Pyrimethamine: Similar pharmacologic action. Avoid use together.

Oral antibiotics, such as chloramphenicol, tetracycline, and nonabsorbable broad-spectrum antibiotics: May decrease absorption of the drug. Use together cautiously.

Other potentially hepatotoxic drugs, such as retinoids, azathiopine, and sulfasalazine; MTX: Increased risk of hepatoxicity. Monitor patient closely.

Drug-lifestyle. *Sun exposure:* Increased risk of photosensitivity reactions. Advise patient to take precautions.

Effects on diagnostic tests

Methotrexate may alter results of the laboratory assay for folate by inhibiting the organism used in the assay, thus interfering with the detection of folic acid deficiency.

Adverse reactions

CNS: *arachnoiditis* (within hours of intrathecal use), subacute ***neurotoxicity*** (may begin a few weeks later), ***necrotizing demyelinating leukoencephalopathy*** (may occur a few years later), malaise, fatigue, dizziness, headache, drowsiness, ***seizures.***

EENT: pharyngitis, gingivitis, blurred vision.

GI: stomatitis, diarrhea, abdominal distress, anorexia, GI ulceration and bleeding, enteritis, *nausea, vomiting.*

GU: nephropathy, *tubular necrosis,* ***renal failure,*** hyperuricemia, hematuria, menstrual dysfunction, defective spermatogenesis, cystitis.

Hematologic: WBC and platelet count nadirs occurring on day 7; anemia, ***leukopenia, thrombocytopenia*** (all dose-related).

Hepatic: acute toxicity (elevated transaminase level), ***chronic toxicity*** *(cirrhosis, hepatic fibrosis).*

Metabolic: diabetes.

Musculoskeletal: arthralgia, myalgia, osteoporosis (in children, with long-term use).

Respiratory: ***pulmonary fibrosis, pulmonary interstitial infiltrates, pneumonitis;*** dry, nonproductive cough.

Skin: alopecia, *urticaria, pruritus, hyperpigmentation, erythematous rash, ecchymoses, psoriatic lesions (aggravated by exposure to sun), rash, photosensitivity.*

Other: fever, chills, reduced resistance to infection, soft tissue necrosis, osteonecrosis, ***septicemia, sudden death.***

Overdose and treatment

Signs and symptoms of overdose include myelosuppression, anemia, nausea, vomiting, dermatitis, alopecia, and melena.

The antidote for hematopoietic toxicity of methotrexate (diagnosed or anticipated) is calcium leucovorin, started as soon as possible and within 1 hour after the administration of methotrexate. The dosage of leucovorin should produce plasma levels higher than those of methotrexate. Since leucovorin blunts therapeutic response of methotrexate, consult specific disease protocol for details.

Clinical considerations

- Methotrexate has been used to treat breast cancer, bladder carcinoma, and various solid tumors. In addition, it has been used investigationally for its immunosuppressive and anti-inflammatory effects in various conditions.
- Methotrexate may be given undiluted by I.V. push injection.
- Drug can be diluted to a higher volume with normal saline solution for I.V. infusion.
- Use reconstituted solutions of preservative-free drug within 24 hours after mixing.
- For intrathecal administration, use preservative-free formulations only. Dilute with unpreserved normal saline.
- Dose modification may be required in impaired hepatic or renal function, bone marrow depression, aplasia, leukopenia, thrombocytopenia, or anemia. Use cautiously in infection, peptic ulcer, ulcerative colitis, and in very young, old, or debilitated patients.
- GI adverse reactions may require drug discontinuation.
- Rash, redness, or ulcerations in mouth or pulmonary adverse reactions may signal serious complications.

■ Alkalinize urine by giving sodium bicarbonate tablets to prevent precipitation of drug, especially with high doses. Maintain urine pH at more than 6.5. Reduce dose if BUN level is 20 to 30 mg/dl or serum creatinine level is 1.2 to 2 mg/dl. Stop drug if BUN level is more than 30 mg/dl or serum creatinine level is more than 2 mg/dl.
■ Avoid all I.M. injections in patients with thrombocytopenia.
■ Leucovorin rescue is necessary with high-dose protocols (doses greater than 100 mg).

Therapeutic monitoring

■ Monitor uric acid levels.
■ Recommend monitoring intake and output daily. Force fluids (2 to 3 L daily).
■ Watch for increases in AST, ALT, and alkaline phosphatase levels, which may signal hepatic dysfunction. Methotrexate shouldn't be used when the potential for "third spacing" exists.
■ Recommend monitoring for bleeding (especially GI) and infection.
■ Recommend monitoring temperature daily, and watch for cough, dyspnea, and cyanosis.

Special populations

Breast-feeding patients. Drug is excreted in breast milk. To avoid risk of serious adverse reactions, mutagenicity, and carcinogenicity in the infant, discontinue breast-feeding during therapy.

Patient counseling

■ Emphasize importance of continuing drug despite nausea and vomiting. Advise patient to call immediately if vomiting occurs shortly after taking a dose.
■ Encourage patient to maintain adequate fluid intake to increase urine output, to prevent nephrotoxicity, and to facilitate excretion of uric acid.
■ Instruct patients also taking leucovorin to take exactly as prescribed to avoid potentially serious adverse effects.
■ Warn patient to avoid alcoholic beverages during therapy.
■ Caution patient to avoid conception during and immediately after therapy because of possible abortion or congenital anomalies.
■ Tell patient to avoid prolonged exposure to sunlight and to use a highly protective sunscreen when exposed to sunlight.
■ Teach patient good mouth care to prevent superinfection of oral cavity.
■ Advise patient that hair should grow back after treatment has ended.
■ Recommend salicylate-free analgesics for pain relief or fever reduction.
■ Tell patient to avoid exposure to people with infections and to report signs of infection immediately.
■ Advise patient to report unusual bruising or bleeding promptly.

methoxsalen

8-MOP, Oxsoralen, Oxsoralen-Ultra

Pharmacologic classification: psoralen derivative
Therapeutic classification: pigmenting, antipsoriatic
Pregnancy risk category C

How supplied

Available by prescription only
Capsules: 10 mg
Lotion: 1%

Indications and dosages

Induction of repigmentation in vitiligo
Adults and children over age 12: 20 mg P.O. (maximum 0.6 mg/kg) 2 to 4 hours before measured periods of exposure to sunlight or ultraviolet (UV) light on alternate days. Alternatively, for small, well-defined lesions, apply lotion 1 to 2 hours before exposure to UV light, no more than once weekly. Wear gloves while applying lotion.
Psoriasis
Adults: Give dose P.O. 1.5 to 2 hours before exposure to high-intensity ultraviolet A light, two or three times weekly, at least 48 hours apart. Dosage is based on patient's weight.
◊ ***Cutaneous T-cell lymphoma***
Adults: 0.6 mg/kg P.O. If serum methoxsalen level is less than 50 ng/ml, give initial dose and an additional 10 mg after 24 hours.

Pharmacodynamics

Pigmenting action: Exact mechanism of action of methoxsalen isn't known; it's dependent on the presence of functioning melanocytes and UV light. Methoxsalen may stimulate the enzymes that catalyze melanin precursors. Also, the inflammatory response generated may stimulate melanin production.
Antipsoriatic action: Methoxsalen probably exerts its antipsoriatic effects by inhibiting DNA synthesis and decreasing cell proliferation. Cell-regulating, leukocyte, and vascular effects may also be involved in this action.

Oral dosage form produces greater erythemic and melanogenic effects, whereas the topical preparation causes a more intense photosensitizing response.

Pharmacokinetics

Absorption: Following oral administration, drug is absorbed well but variably. Food increases both absorption and peak concentration. Extent of topical absorption hasn't been determined. Skin sensitivity to UV light occurs in about 1 to 2 hours, reaches a maximum effect in 1 to 4 hours, and persists for 3 to 8

hours. Topical administration yields a UV sensitivity in 1 to 2 hours, which may persist for several days. Oxsoralen-Ultra dose form is absorbed more completely and at a faster rate than other dose forms.
Distribution: Distributed throughout the body, with epidermal cells preferentially taking up drug; 75% to 91% is bound to serum proteins, most commonly albumin. Distribution across the placenta or in breast milk is unknown.
Metabolism: Activated by long-wavelength UV light and is metabolized in the liver.
Excretion: Excreted almost entirely as metabolites in the urine, with 80% to 90% eliminated within the first 8 hours.

Route	Onset	Peak	Duration
P.O.	Unknown	1½-3 hr	Unknown
Topical	Unknown	Unknown	Unknown

Contraindications and precautions
Contraindicated in patients sensitive to psoralen compounds and in patients with diseases associated with photosensitivity (such as porphyria, acute lupus erythematosus, xeroderma, or hydromorphic and polymorphic light eruptions). Also contraindicated in patients with melanoma, invasive squamous cell carcinoma, and aphakia.

Oxsoralen capsules contain tartrazine; use cautiously in patients with tartrazine or aspirin sensitivity. Also use cautiously in patients with familial history of sunlight allergy, GI diseases, or chronic infection.

Interactions
Drug-drug. *Other photosensitizing drugs, including coal tar products, griseofulvin, nalidixic acid, phenothiazines, sulfonamides, tetracyclines, thiazides, and trioxsalen:* Additive photosensitizing effect. Advise patient to take skin precautions.
Drug-food. *Foods containing furocoumarin, such as carrots, celery, figs, limes, mustard, parsley, and parsnips:* May cause an additive effect. Use together cautiously.
Drug-lifestyle. *Sun exposure:* Increased risk of photosensitivity reactions. Advise patient to take precautions.

Effects on diagnostic tests
None reported.

Adverse reactions
CNS: dizziness, headache, depression, nervousness, trouble sleeping.
EENT: cataracts.
GI: *nausea,* abdominal discomfort, diarrhea.
Hepatic: abnormal liver function tests.
Musculoskeletal: leg cramps.
Skin: burns, blistering, peeling, swelling of extremities, itching, erythema, photosensitivity.
Other: ***toxic hepatitis.***

Note: Discontinue drug if signs of overexposure to sunlight occur.

Overdose and treatment
Signs and symptoms of overdose include serious burning and blistering of skin, which may occur from overdose of drug or overexposure to UV light. Treat acute oral overdose with gastric lavage, which, however, is effective only in the first 2 to 3 hours. Place patient in a darkened room for 8 to 24 hours or until cutaneous reactions subside. Treat burns as necessary.

Clinical considerations
- Refer to UVAR photopheresis procedure guide or other published protocols and references.
- Never dispense lotion to patient. It should be applied only by medically trained staff under controlled conditions.
- Wear gloves when applying lotion to patient.
- Temporary withdrawal of therapy is the recommended procedure in case of burning or blistering of the skin.
- Oxsoralen-Ultra shouldn't be used interchangeably with regular Oxsoralen because it exhibits significantly greater bioavailability.
- Treatment regimen of psoralens and ultraviolet radiation in the range of 320 to 400 nm wavelength (UVA) is known as PUVA. Preleukemia and acute myeloid leukemia have been associated with PUVA therapy.
- Initial UV light exposure times should be based on minimum phototoxic dose (MPD) for the specific light source being used.
- When sunlight is the UV source, initial sunlight exposures after methoxsalen administration shouldn't exceed 15, 20, or 25 minutes for patients with light, medium, or dark skin colors, respectively.
- Patient should wear UVA protective glasses for several hours after treatment.
- Store drug at 59° to 86° F (15° to 30° C) in well-closed, light-resistant container.

Therapeutic monitoring
- CBC with differential, antinuclear antibody, liver function, BUN, and creatinine tests should be performed at baseline and repeated every 6 months.
- Periodic ophthalmologic examinations are recommended during therapy.

Special populations
Breast-feeding patients. It isn't known if drug is excreted in breast milk; use cautiously in breast-feeding women.
Pediatric patients. Avoid use in children under age 12.

Patient counseling
- Teach patient how and when to use product; tell patient to wear gloves to avoid photosensitization and possible burns. Stress adherence

to correct dosage schedule. If a dose is missed, patient shouldn't increase the next dose. If more than one dose is missed, a proportionately lower dose should be given when therapy is resumed.
- Advise patient to take drug with food and milk to reduce GI irritation and, possibly, increase absorption; and to avoid foods containing furocoumarin, such as carrots, celery, figs, and mustard.
- Tell patient to use proper protective precautions, including sunglasses and sunscreens. However, sunscreens may be only partially effective. Tell patient to protect skin for 8 hours after oral administration.
- Explain that drug may take several months to work. Tell patient not to increase the dose or UV light exposure during this time.

methylcellulose

Citrucel, Methylcellulose Tablets

Pharmacologic classification: adsorbent
Therapeutic classification: bulk-forming laxative
Pregnancy risk category C

How supplied

Available without a prescription
Powder: 105 mg/g, 364 mg/g
Tablets: 500 mg

Indications and dosages

Chronic constipation
Adults: Maximum dose is 6 g P.O. daily, divided into 0.45 to 3 g/dose.
Children age 6 to 12: Maximum dose is 3 g P.O. daily, divided into 0.45 to 1.5 g/dose.

Pharmacodynamics

Laxative action: Methylcellulose adsorbs intestinal fluid and serves as a source of indigestible fiber, stimulating peristaltic activity.

Pharmacokinetics

Absorption: Not absorbed.
Distribution: Distributed locally, in the intestine.
Metabolism: None.
Excretion: Excreted in feces.

Route	Onset	Peak	Duration
P.O.	12-24 hr	< 3 days	Variable

Contraindications and precautions

Contraindicated in patients with abdominal pain, nausea, vomiting, or other symptoms of appendicitis or acute surgical abdomen and in those with intestinal obstruction or ulceration, disabling adhesions, or difficulty swallowing.

Interactions

Drug-drug. *Oral medications:* When used together, methylcellulose may absorb other medications. Separate administration times by at least 1 hour.

Effects on diagnostic tests

None reported.

Adverse reactions

GI: *nausea, vomiting, diarrhea* (with excessive use)*; esophageal, gastric, small intestinal, or colonic strictures* (when drug is chewed or taken in dry form); abdominal cramps, especially in severe constipation; laxative dependence (with long-term or excessive use).

Overdose and treatment

No information available.

Clinical considerations

- Administer drug with water or juice (at least 8 oz).
- Drug may absorb oral medications; schedule at least 1 hour apart from all other drugs.
- Bulk laxatives most closely mimic natural bowel function and don't promote laxative dependence.
- Drug is especially useful in patients with postpartum constipation, chronic laxative abuse, irritable bowel syndrome, diverticular disease, or colostomies; in debilitated patients; and to empty colon before barium enema examinations.

Therapeutic monitoring

Patient should be monitored for clinical response.

Special populations

Breast-feeding patients. Because drug isn't absorbed, use probably poses no risk to breast-feeding infants.

Patient counseling

- Instruct patient to take other oral medications 1 hour before or after methylcellulose.
- Explain that full effect of drug may not occur for 2 to 3 days.

methyldopa

Aldomet, Apo-Methyldopa*, Dopamet*, Novomedopa*

Pharmacologic classification: centrally acting antiadrenergic
Therapeutic classification: antihypertensive
Pregnancy risk category B (oral); C (I.V.)

How supplied

Available by prescription only
Tablets: 125 mg, 250 mg, 500 mg

Injection (as methyldopate hydrochloride): 250 mg/5 ml in 5-ml vials

Indications and dosages

Moderate to severe hypertension

Adults: Initially, 250 mg P.O. b.i.d. or t.i.d. in first 48 hours, then increased or decreased, p.r.n., q 2 days. Alternatively, 250 to 500 mg I.V. q 6 hours (maximum dose, 1 g q 6 hours). Adjust dosage if other antihypertensive drugs are added to or deleted from therapy.

Maintenance dosage is 500 mg to 2 g P.O. daily in two to four divided doses. Maximum recommended daily dose is 3 g. I.V. infusion dose is 250 to 500 mg given over 30 to 60 minutes q 6 hours. Maximum I.V. dose, 1 g q 6 hours.

Children: Initially, 10 mg/kg P.O. daily or 300 mg/m^2 P.O. daily in two to four divided doses; or 20 to 40 mg/kg I.V. daily or 0.6 to 1.2 g/m^2 I.V. daily in four divided doses. Increase dosage at least q 2 days until desired response occurs. Maximum daily dose is 65 mg/kg, 2 g/m^2, or 3 g, whichever is least.

Pharmacodynamics

Antihypertensive action: Exact mechanism of antihypertensive effect is unknown; it's thought to be caused by a metabolite of methyldopa, alpha-methylnorepinephrine, which stimulates central inhibitory alpha-adrenergic receptors, decreasing total peripheral resistance; drug may act as a false neurotransmitter. Drug may also reduce plasma renin activity.

Pharmacokinetics

Absorption: Absorbed partially from the GI tract. Absorption varies, but usually about 50% of an oral dose is absorbed. No correlation exists between plasma level and antihypertensive effect. After I.V. administration, blood pressure usually begins to decrease in 4 to 6 hours.
Distribution: Distributed throughout the body and is bound weakly to plasma proteins.
Metabolism: Metabolized extensively in the liver and intestinal cells.
Excretion: Drug and its metabolites are excreted in urine; unabsorbed drug is excreted unchanged in feces. Elimination half-life is about 2 hours.

Route	Onset	Peak	Duration
P.O.	Unknown	4-6 hr	12-48 hr
I.V.	Unknown	4-6 hr	10-16 hr

Contraindications and precautions

Contraindicated in patients with hypersensitivity to drug or active hepatic disease (such as acute hepatitis) and active cirrhosis. Also contraindicated if previous methyldopa therapy has been associated with liver disorders. Use cautiously in patients with impaired hepatic function, in those receiving MAO inhibitors, and in breast-feeding women.

Interactions

Drug-drug. *Anesthetics*: Increased effects. Patients undergoing surgery may require reduced dosages of anesthetics.
Other antihypertensive agents: Potentiated antihypertensive effects. Use together cautiously.
Diuretics: May increase hypotensive effect of methyldopa. Use together cautiously.
Haloperidol: May produce dementia and sedation. Use together cautiously.
Oral iron therapy: May decrease hypotensive effects and increase serum levels of levodopa. Use together cautiously.
Lithium: May increase risk of lithium toxicity. Monitor lithium levels.
Phenothiazines or tricyclic antidepressants: May cause a reduction in antihypertensive effects. Patient's blood pressure should be monitored.
Phenoxybenzamine: May cause reversible urinary incontinence. Avoid use together.
Sympathomimetic amines such as phenylpropanolamine: Potentiated pressor effects. Use together cautiously.
Tolbutamide: Methyldopa may impair tolbutamide metabolism. Monitor serum glucose levels.
Drug-herb. *Capsicum:* May reduce antihypertensive effectiveness of drug. Avoid use together.

Effects on diagnostic tests

Methyldopa may cause falsely high levels of urine catecholamines, interfering with the diagnosis of pheochromocytoma. A positive direct antiglobulin (Coombs') test may also occur.

Adverse reactions

CNS: *sedation, headache, weakness, dizziness,* decreased mental acuity, paresthesia, parkinsonism, involuntary choreoathetoid movements, psychic disturbances, depression, nightmares.
CV: ***bradycardia,*** *orthostatic hypotension, aggravated angina,* ***myocarditis,*** edema.
EENT: *nasal congestion.*
GI: nausea, vomiting, diarrhea, *pancreatitis, dry mouth,* constipation.
GU: gynecomastia, amenorrhea, decreased libido, impotence, altered serum creatinine, altered urine uric acid.
Hematologic: ***hemolytic anemia, thrombocytopenia, leukopenia, bone marrow depression.***
Hepatic: ***hepatic necrosis,*** abnormal liver function tests, *hepatitis.*
Skin: rash.
Other: galactorrhea, drug-induced fever.

Overdose and treatment

Clinical signs of overdose include sedation, hypotension, impaired atrioventricular conduction, and coma.

After recent (within 4 hours) ingestion, empty stomach by induced emesis or gastric lavage. Give activated charcoal to reduce absorption; then treat symptomatically and supportively. In severe cases, hemodialysis may be considered.

Clinical considerations

- Patients with impaired renal function may require smaller maintenance dosages of drug.
- Multiple dosing may decrease patient compliance, but b.i.d. dosing may provide adequate control with decreased cost.
- Methyldopate hydrochloride is administered I.V.; I.M. or S.C. administration isn't recommended because of unpredictable absorption.
- Patients receiving methyldopa may become hypertensive after dialysis because drug is dialyzable.
- Sedation and drowsiness usually disappear with continued therapy; bedtime dosage will minimize this effect. Orthostatic hypotension may indicate a need for dosage reduction. Some patients tolerate receiving the entire daily dose in the evening or h.s.
- Tolerance may develop after 2 to 3 weeks.
- Signs of hepatotoxicity may occur 2 to 4 weeks after therapy begins.
- For I.V. use, add required dose of drug to 100 ml of 5% dextrose injection. Alternatively, a concentration of 100 mg/ml may be used. ADD-Vantage vials contain 50 mg/ml and should be reconstituted per manufacturer direction. Administer I.V. infusion over 30 to 60 minutes.

Therapeutic monitoring

- At the initiation of, and periodically throughout therapy, monitor hemoglobin, hematocrit, and RBC count for hemolytic anemia; also monitor liver function tests.
- Take blood pressure in supine, sitting, and standing positions during dosage adjustment; take blood pressure at least every 30 minutes during I.V. infusion until patient is stable.
- Monitor intake and output and daily weights to detect sodium and water retention; voided urine exposed to air may darken because of the breakdown of methyldopa or its metabolites.
- Monitor for signs and symptoms of drug-induced depression.

Special populations

Pregnant patients. Methyldopa is the most extensively used hypotensive agent in pregnant women.
Breast-feeding patients. Drug is distributed into breast milk; the American Academy of Pediatrics considers methyldopa to be compatible with breast-feeding.
Pediatric patients. Safety and efficacy in children haven't been established; use only if potential benefits outweigh risks.
Geriatric patients. Dosage reductions may be necessary in geriatric patients because they're more sensitive to sedation and hypotension.

Patient counseling

- Teach patient signs and symptoms of adverse effects, such as "jerky" movements, and about the need to report them; he should also report excessive weight gain (5 lb [2.25 kg] weekly), signs of infection, or fever.
- Teach patient to minimize adverse effects by taking drug at bedtime until tolerance develops to sedation, drowsiness, and other CNS effects; by avoiding sudden position changes to minimize orthostatic hypotension; and by using ice chips, hard candy, or gum to relieve dry mouth.
- Warn patient to avoid hazardous activities that require mental alertness until sedative effects subside.
- Instruct patient to call for instructions before taking OTC cold preparations.

methylergonovine maleate

Methergine

Pharmacologic classification: ergot alkaloid
Therapeutic classification: oxytocic
Pregnancy risk category C

How supplied

Available by prescription only
Tablets: 0.2 mg
Injection: 0.2 mg/ml ampule

Indications and dosages

Prevention and treatment of postpartum hemorrhage due to uterine atony or subinvolution
Adults: 0.2 mg I.M. or I.V. q 2 to 4 hours for maximum five doses. Following initial I.M. or I.V. dose, may give 0.2 to 0.4 mg P.O. q 6 to 12 hours for maximum 7 days. Decrease dose if severe cramping occurs.
◊***Diagnosis of coronary artery spasm***
Adults: 0.1 to 0.4 mg I.V.

Pharmacodynamics

Oxytocic action: Drug stimulates contractions of uterine and vascular smooth muscle. The intense uterine contractions are followed by periods of relaxation. Drug produces vasoconstriction primarily of capacitance blood vessels, causing increased central venous pressure and elevated blood pressure. Drug increases the amplitude and frequency of uterine contractions and tone, which therefore impedes uterine blood flow.

Pharmacokinetics

Absorption: Absorption is rapid, with 60% of an oral dose appearing in the bloodstream.
Distribution: Distribution appears to be rapidly distributed into tissues.
Metabolism: Extensive first-pass metabolism precedes hepatic metabolism.

Excretion: Excreted primarily in the feces, with a small amount in urine.

Route	Onset	Peak	Duration
P.O.	5-10 min	30 min	3 hr
I.V.	Immediate	Unknown	45 min
I.M.	2-5 min	Unknown	3 hr

Contraindications and precautions
Contraindicated in patients with hypertension, toxemia, or sensitivity to ergot preparations and in pregnant women. Use cautiously in patients with renal or hepatic disease, sepsis, or obliterative vascular disease and during the first stage of labor.

Interactions
Drug-drug. *Other ergot alkaloids and sympathomimetic amines:* Enhanced vasoconstrictor potential. Use together cautiously.
Local anesthetics with vasoconstrictors (lidocaine with epinephrine): Enhanced vasoconstriction. Use together cautiously.
Drug-lifestyle. *Smoking (nicotine):* Enhanced vasoconstriction caused by drug. Avoid use together.

Effects on diagnostic tests
None reported.

Adverse reactions
CNS: dizziness, headache, ***seizures, CVA*** (with I.V. use), hallucinations.
CV: hypertension, transient chest pain, palpitations, hypotension.
EENT: tinnitus, nasal congestion, foul taste.
GI: *nausea, vomiting, diarrhea.*
GU: hematuria.
Musculoskeletal: leg cramps.
Respiratory: dyspnea.
Skin: diaphoresis.
Other: thrombophlebitis.

Overdose and treatment
Signs and symptoms of overdose include seizures and gangrene with nausea, vomiting, diarrhea, dizziness, fluctuations in blood pressure, weak pulse, chest pain, tingling, and numbness and coldness in extremities.

Treatment of oral overdose requires that the patient drink tap water, milk, or vegetable oil to delay absorption, then follow with gastric lavage or emesis, then activated charcoal and cathartics. Treat seizures with anticonvulsants and hypercoagulability with heparin; use vasodilators to improve blood flow as required. Gangrene may require surgical amputation.

Clinical considerations
- Contractions begin 5 to 15 minutes after P.O. administration, 2 to 5 minutes after I.M. injection, and immediately following I.V. injection; continue 3 hours or more after P.O. or I.M. administration, 45 minutes after I.V.
- Don't administer I.V. routinely because of the possibility of inducing sudden hypertensive and CV accidents.
- If I.V. administration is considered essential as a life-saving measure, dilute the desired dose with normal saline injection to a volume of 5 ml and give slowly over no less than 60 seconds.
- Store tablets in tightly closed, light-resistant containers. Discard if discolored.
- Store I.V. solutions below 77° F (25° C). Administer only if solution is clear and colorless.

Therapeutic monitoring
Patient requires monitoring of blood pressure, pulse rate, uterine response, and observation for sudden change in vital signs or frequent periods of uterine relaxation, character and amount of vaginal bleeding.

Special populations
Breast-feeding patients. Ergot alkaloids inhibit lactation. Drug is excreted in breast milk, and ergotism has been reported in breast-fed infants.

Patient counseling
- Advise smoking cessation during therapy.
- Warn patient of adverse reactions.

methylphenidate hydrochloride
Ritalin, Ritalin-SR

Pharmacologic classification: piperidine CNS stimulant
Therapeutic classification: CNS stimulant (analeptic)
Controlled substance schedule II
Pregnancy risk category NR

How supplied
Available by prescription only
Tablets: 5 mg, 10 mg, 20 mg
Tablets (sustained-release): 20 mg

Indications and dosages
Attention deficit hyperactivity disorder (ADHD)
Children age 6 and older: Initially 5 mg P.O. daily before breakfast and lunch, increased in 5- to 10-mg increments weekly, p.r.n., until an optimum daily dose of 2 mg/kg is reached, not to exceed 60 mg/day. Alternatively, initial dose of 0.25 mg/kg P.O. daily. Usual effective daily dose, 20 to 30 mg. Discontinue if there's no response in 1 month.
Narcolepsy
Adults: 10 mg P.O. b.i.d. or t.i.d. 30 to 45 minutes before meals. Dosage varies with patient needs; average dose is 40 to 60 mg/day.

When using sustained-release tablets, calculate regular dose in q 8-hour intervals and administer as such.

Pharmacodynamics

Analeptic action: The cerebral cortex and reticular activating system appear to be the primary sites of activity; methylphenidate releases nerve terminal stores of norepinephrine, promoting nerve impulse transmission. At high doses, effects are mediated by dopamine.

Drug is used to treat narcolepsy and as an adjunctive to psychosocial measures in ADHD. Like amphetamines, it has a paradoxical calming effect in hyperactive children.

Pharmacokinetics

Absorption: Absorbed rapidly and completely after oral administration.
Distribution: Unknown.
Metabolism: Metabolized by the liver.
Excretion: Excreted in urine.

Route	Onset	Peak	Duration
P.O.	Unknown	2-5 hr	Unknown

Contraindications and precautions

Contraindicated in patients with hypersensitivity to drug, glaucoma, motor tics, family history of or diagnosis of Tourette syndrome, or history of marked anxiety, tension, or agitation.

Use cautiously in patients with history of seizures, drug abuse, hypertension, or EEG abnormalities.

Interactions

Drug-drug. *Anticonvulsants (phenobarbital, phenytoin, primidone), coumarin anticoagulants, phenylbutazone, and tricyclic antidepressants:* Methylphenidate may inhibit metabolism and increase the serum levels of these drugs. Patient may need dosage adjustment if concomitant therapy is necessary.
Bretylium and guanethidine: Decreased hypotensive effects. Patient requires monitoring for clinical effect.
MAO inhibitors (or drugs with MAO-inhibiting activity) or within 14 days of such therapy: May cause severe hypertension. Avoid use together.
Drug-lifestyle. *Caffeine:* May enhance CNS stimulant effects of methylphenidate and decrease effectiveness of drug in ADHD. Avoid use together.

Effects on diagnostic tests

None reported.

Adverse reactions

CNS: *nervousness, insomnia, Tourette syndrome, dizziness, headache, akathisia, dyskinesia,* ***seizures,*** drowsiness.
CV: *palpitations, angina, tachycardia, changes in blood pressure and pulse rate,* ***arrhythmias.***
GI: nausea, abdominal pain, anorexia.
Hematologic: ***thrombocytopenia, thrombocytopenic purpura, leukopenia,*** anemia.
Metabolic: weight loss.
Skin: rash, urticaria, ***exfoliative dermatitis, erythema multiforme.***

Overdose and treatment

Symptoms of overdose may include euphoria, confusion, delirium, coma, toxic psychosis, agitation, headache, vomiting, dry mouth, mydriasis, self-injury, fever, diaphoresis, tremors, hyperreflexia, hyperpyrexia, muscle twitching, seizures, flushing, hypertension, tachycardia, palpitations, and arrhythmias.

Treat overdose symptomatically and supportively: use gastric lavage or emesis in patients with intact gag reflex. Maintain airway and circulation. Closely monitor vital signs and fluid and electrolyte balance. Maintain patient in cool room, monitor temperature, minimize external stimulation, and protect him against self-injury. External cooling blankets may be needed.

Clinical considerations

- Methylphenidate is the drug of choice for ADHD. Therapy is usually discontinued after puberty.
- If paradoxical aggravation of symptoms occurs during therapy, reduce dosage or discontinue drug.
- Drug may decrease seizure threshold in seizure disorders.
- Intermittent drug-free periods when stress is least evident (weekends, school holidays) may help prevent development of tolerance and permit decreased dosage when drug is resumed. Sustained-release form allows convenience of single, at-home dosing for school children.
- Drug has abuse potential; discourage use to combat fatigue. Some abusers dissolve tablets and inject drug.
- After high-dose and long-term use, abrupt withdrawal may unmask severe depression. Lower dosage gradually to prevent acute rebound depression.
- Drug impairs ability to perform tasks requiring mental alertness.
- Be sure patient obtains adequate rest; fatigue may result as drug wears off.
- Discourage methylphenidate use for analeptic effect; CNS stimulation superimposed on CNS depression may cause neuronal instability and seizures.
- Don't administer drug to women of childbearing age unless potential benefits outweigh the possible risks.
- Store drug in tight, light-resistant containers.

Therapeutic monitoring

- Recommend monitoring initiation of therapy closely; drug may precipitate Tourette syndrome.

■ Recommend checking vital signs regularly for increased blood pressure or other signs of excessive stimulation; avoid late-day or evening dosing, especially of long-acting dosage forms, to minimize insomnia.
■ Monitor CBC, differential, and platelet counts when patient is taking drug long-term.
■ Recommend monitoring height and weight; drug has been associated with growth suppression.

Special populations

Pediatric patients. Drug isn't recommended for ADHD in children under age 6. It has been associated with growth suppression; all patients should be monitored.

Patient counseling

■ Explain rationale for therapy and the risks and benefits that may be anticipated.
■ Tell patient to avoid drinks containing caffeine to prevent added CNS stimulation and not to alter dosage unless prescribed.
■ Advise narcoleptic patient to take first dose on awakening; advise ADHD patient to take last dose several hours before bedtime to avoid insomnia.
■ Tell patient not to chew or crush sustained-release dosage forms.
■ Warn patient not to use drug to mask fatigue, to be sure to obtain adequate rest, and to call if excessive CNS stimulation occurs.
■ Advise patient to avoid hazardous activities that require mental alertness until degree of sedative effect is determined.

methylprednisolone (systemic)

Medrol

methylprednisolone acetate

depMedalone-40, depMedalone-80, Depoject-40, Depoject-80, Depo-Medrol, Depo-Pred-40, Depo-Pred-80, Duralone-40, Duralone-80, Medralone, Rep-Pred-40, Rep-Pred-80

methylprednisolone sodium succinate

A-methaPred, Solu-Medrol

Pharmacologic classification: glucocorticoid
Therapeutic classification: anti-inflammatory, immunosuppressant
Pregnancy risk category C

How supplied

Available by prescription only
methylprednisolone
Tablets: 2 mg, 4 mg, 8 mg, 16 mg, 24 mg, 32 mg
methylprednisolone acetate
Injection: 20 mg/ml, 40 mg/ml, 80 mg/ml suspension
methylprednisolone sodium succinate
Injection: 40 mg, 125 mg, 500 mg, 1,000 mg, 2,000 mg/vial

Indications and dosages

Multiple sclerosis
Methylprednisolone (systemic)
Adults: 200 mg P.O. daily for 1 week, followed by 80 mg every other day for 1 month.
Inflammation
methylprednisolone
Adults: 2 to 60 mg P.O. daily in four divided doses, depending on disease being treated.
Children: 0.117 to 1.66 mg/kg daily or 3.3 to 50 mg/m^2 P.O. daily in three to four divided doses.
methylprednisolone acetate
Adults: 10 to 80 mg I.M. daily; or 4 to 80 mg into joints and soft tissue, p.r.n., q 1 to 5 weeks; or 20 to 60 mg intralesionally.
methylprednisolone sodium succinate
Adults: 10 to 250 mg I.M. or I.V. q 4 hours.
Children: 0.03 to 0.2 mg/kg or 1 to 6.25 mg m^2 I.M. or I.V. daily in 1 or 2 divided doses.
Shock
methylprednisolone sodium succinate
Adults: 100 to 250 mg I.V. at 2- to 6-hour intervals or 30 mg/kg I.V. initially and repeat q 4 to 6 hours, p.r.n. Alternatively, after original I.V. push dose, 30 mg/kg I.V. infusion q 12 hours for 24 to 48 hours.
◊ ***Severe lupus nephritis***
Adults: 1 g I.V. over 1 hour for 3 days. Therapy is then continued orally at 0.5 mg/kg/day
Children: 30 mg/kg I.V. every other day for 6 doses.
◊ ***Treatment or minimization of motor and sensory defects caused by acute spinal cord injury***
Adults: Initially, 30 mg/kg I.V. over 15 minutes followed in 45 minutes by I.V. infusion of 5.4 mg/kg/hour for 23 hours.
◊ ***Adjunct to moderate-severe* Pneumocystis carinii *pneumonia***
Adults and children over age 13: 30 mg I.V. b.i.d. for 5 days; 30 mg I.V. daily for 5 days; 15 mg I.V. daily for 11 days (or until completion of anti-infective regimen).

Pharmacodynamics

Anti-inflammatory action: Methylprednisolone stimulates the synthesis of enzymes needed to decrease the inflammatory response. It suppresses the immune system by reducing activity and volume of the lymphatic system, thus producing lymphocytopenia (primarily of T lymphocytes), decreasing immunoglobulin and complement levels, decreasing passage of immune complexes through basement membranes, and possibly by depressing reactivity of tissue to antigen-antibody interactions.

Drug is an intermediate-acting glucocorticoid. It has essentially no mineralocorticoid activity but is a potent glucocorticoid, with five times the potency of an equal weight of hydrocortisone. It's used primarily as an anti-inflammatory agent and immunosuppressant.

Methylprednisolone may be administered orally. Methylprednisolone sodium succinate may be administered by I.M. or I.V. injection or by I.V. infusion, usually at 4- to 6-hour intervals.

Methylprednisolone acetate suspension may be administered by intra-articular, intrasynovial, intrabursal, intralesional, or soft tissue injection. It has a slow onset but a long duration of action. Injectable forms are usually used only when the oral dosage forms can't be used.

Pharmacokinetics

Absorption: Absorbed readily after oral administration.
Distribution: Distributed rapidly to muscle, liver, skin, intestines, and kidneys. Adrenocorticoids are distributed into breast milk and through the placenta.
Metabolism: Metabolized in the liver to inactive glucuronide and sulfate metabolites.
Excretion: Inactive metabolites and small amounts of unmetabolized drug are excreted by the kidneys. Insignificant quantities of drug are excreted in feces. Biological half-life of methylprednisolone is 18 to 36 hours.

Route	Onset	Peak	Duration
P.O.	Rapid	2-3 hr	30-36 hr
I.V.	Rapid	Immediate	7 days
I.M.	6-48 hr	4-8 days	1-4 wk
Intra-articular	Rapid	7 days	1-5 wk

Contraindications and precautions

Contraindicated in patients allergic to any component of the formulation, in those with systemic fungal infections, and in premature infants (acetate and succinate).

Use cautiously in patients with renal disease, GI ulceration, hypertension, osteoporosis, diabetes mellitus, hypothyroidism, cirrhosis, diverticulitis, nonspecific ulcerative colitis, recent intestinal anastomoses, thromboembolic disorders, seizures, myasthenia gravis, heart failure, tuberculosis, emotional instability, ocular herpes simplex, and psychotic tendencies.

Interactions

Drug-drug. *Amphotericin B or diuretic therapy:* May enhance hypokalemia. Monitor serum potassium.
Antacids, cholestyramine, colestipol: Decreased corticosteroid effect. Separate administration times.
Anticholinesterase: Profound weakness. Use together cautiously.
Oral anticoagulants: Decreased effectiveness. Monitor PT and INR.
Barbiturates, phenytoin, rifampin: May cause decreased corticosteroid effects because of increased hepatic metabolism. Recommend monitoring patient for potential dosage adjustment.
Cyclosporine: Levels of cyclosporine may increase. Use together cautiously.
Estrogens: Reduced metabolism of corticosteroids. Patient may require dosage adjustment.
Insulin or oral antidiabetic agent: Hyperglycemia. Dosage adjustment may be needed.
Isoniazid and salicylates: Increased metabolism. May require dosage adjustment of isoniazid or salicylates.
Ulcerogenic drugs such as NSAIDs: Increased risk of GI ulceration. Use together cautiously.
Vaccines: Decreased effectiveness of vaccines. Vaccine shouldn't be administered during steroid therapy.

Effects on diagnostic tests

Drug suppresses reactions to skin tests; causes false-negative results in the nitroblue tetrazolium test for systemic bacterial infections, and decreases ^{131}I uptake and protein-bound iodine levels in thyroid function tests.

Adverse reactions

Most adverse reactions to corticosteroids are dose-dependent or duration-dependent.
CNS: *euphoria, insomnia,* psychotic behavior, pseudotumor cerebri, vertigo, headache, paresthesia, ***seizures.***
CV: ***heart failure,*** hypertension, edema, ***arrhythmias,*** thrombophlebitis, ***thromboembolism, fatal arrest or circulatory collapse*** (following rapid administration of large I.V. doses).
EENT: cataracts, glaucoma.
GI: *peptic ulceration,* GI irritation, increased appetite, ***pancreatitis,*** nausea, vomiting.
GU: menstrual irregularities, increased urine glucose and calcium levels.
Metabolic: hypokalemia, hyperglycemia, hypocalcemia, decreased serum thyroxine and triiodothyronine levels, carbohydrate intolerance, growth suppression in children, cushingoid state (moonface, buffalo hump, central obesity).
Musculoskeletal: muscle weakness, osteoporosis.
Skin: delayed wound healing, acne, various skin eruptions.
Other: hirsutism, susceptibility to infections, *acute adrenal insufficiency that may occur with increased stress (infection, surgery, or trauma) or abrupt withdrawal after long-term therapy.*
After abrupt withdrawal: rebound inflammation, fatigue, weakness, arthralgia, fever, dizziness, lethargy, depression, fainting, orthostatic hypotension, dyspnea, anorexia, hypoglycemia. ***After prolonged use, sudden withdrawal may be fatal.***

Overdose and treatment
Acute ingestion, even in massive doses, is rarely a clinical problem. Toxic signs and symptoms rarely occur if drug is used for less than 3 weeks, even at large doses. However, chronic use causes adverse physiologic effects, including suppression of the hypothalamus-pituitary-adrenal axis, cushingoid appearance, muscle weakness, and osteoporosis.

Clinical considerations
- Recommendations for use of methylprednisolone and for care and teaching of patients during therapy are the same as those for all systemic adrenocorticoids.
- Methylprednisolone sodium succinate is reconstituted for I.V. or I.M. use with bacteriostatic water for injection containing 0.9% benzyl alcohol. Reconstitute per manufacturer instruction. I.V. bolus administration is over at least 1 minute. For I.V. infusion, further dilute with compatible I.V. solution (such as normal saline solution, 5% dextrose). Reconstituted should be clear. Discard after 48 hours.
- Store drug at 68° to 77° F (20° to 25° C); avoid freezing methylprednisolone acetate.

Therapeutic monitoring
Monitor patient for adverse effects.

Special populations
Pediatric patients. Chronic use of adrenocorticoids in children and adolescents may delay growth and maturation.
Geriatric patients. In geriatric patients, compare the risks and benefits of steroid use; lower doses are recommended. Monitor blood pressure, blood glucose, and electrolyte levels at least every 6 months.

Patient counseling
- Tell patient not to stop drug abruptly or without doctor's consent.
- Instruct patient to take oral form of drug with food.
- Teach patient early signs of adrenal insufficiency: fatigue, muscular weakness, joint pain, fever, anorexia, nausea, dyspnea, dizziness and fainting.
- Tell patient to carry a card identifying need for supplemental systemic steroids during stress. Medication, dose, and name of doctor should be on card.
- Teach patient on long-term therapy to notify doctor of sudden weight gain or swelling.
- Tell patient on long-term therapy to consult with doctor about the need for vitamin D or calcium supplement, or a physical exercise program.
- Warn patient to avoid exposure to infections (such as chicken pox or measles) and to contact doctor if such exposure occurs.

metoclopramide hydrochloride
Apo-Metoclop*, Clopra, Maxeran*, Maxolon, Octamide PFS, Reclomide, Reglan

Pharmacologic classification: para-aminobenzoic acid (PABA) derivative
Therapeutic classification: antiemetic, GI stimulant
Pregnancy risk category B

How supplied
Available by prescription only
Tablets: 5 mg, 10 mg
Syrup: 5 mg/5 ml
Injection: 5 mg/ml
Solution: 10 mg/ml

Indications and dosages
Prevention or reduction of nausea and vomiting induced by highly emetogenic chemotherapy
Adults: 1 to 2 mg/kg I.V. q 2 hours for two doses, beginning 30 minutes before emetogenic chemotherapy drug administration, then q 3 hours for three doses. ◇ Some clinicians have used up to 2.75 mg/kg I.V. infusion to control nausea/vomiting. Diphenhydramine 50 mg I.M. may be necessary to control extrapyramidal symptoms at this dose.
Facilitation of small-bowel intubation and to aid in radiologic examinations
Adults: 10 mg I.V. as a single dose over 1 to 2 minutes.
Children age 6 to 14: 2.5 to 5 mg I.V.
Children under age 6: 0.1 mg/kg I.V.
Delayed gastric emptying secondary to diabetic gastroparesis
Adults: 10 mg P.O. 30 minutes before meals and h.s. for 2 to 8 weeks, depending on response; or 10 mg I.M. or I.V. over 2 minutes.
Gastroesophageal reflux
Adults: 10 to 15 mg P.O. q.i.d., p.r.n., taken 30 minutes before meals and h.s. for up to 12 weeks.
Geriatric patients may only require 5 mg per dose.
Postoperative nausea and vomiting
Adults: 10 to 20 mg I.M. near end of surgical procedure, repeated q 4 to 6 hours, p.r.n.
≡ ***Dosage adjustment.*** If creatinine clearance is less than 40 ml/minute, initial doses should be 50% of usual recommended doses and adjusted as tolerated.

Pharmacodynamics
Antiemetic action: Metoclopramide inhibits dopamine receptors in the chemoreceptor trigger zone of the brain to inhibit or reduce nausea and vomiting.

GI stimulant action: Drug relieves esophageal reflux by increasing lower esophageal sphincter tone and reduces gastric stasis by stimulating motility of the upper GI tract, thus reducing gastric emptying time.

Pharmacokinetics

Absorption: After oral administration, drug is absorbed rapidly and thoroughly from the GI tract. After I.M. administration, about 74% to 96% of drug is bioavailable.
Distribution: Distributed to most body tissues and fluids, including the brain. Drug crosses the placenta and is distributed in breast milk.
Metabolism: Not metabolized extensively; a small amount is metabolized in the liver.
Excretion: Mostly excreted in urine and feces. Hemodialysis and renal dialysis remove minimal amounts.

Route	Onset	Peak	Duration
P.O.	½-1 hr	1-2 hr	1-2 hr
I.V.	1-3 min	Unknown	1-2 hr
I.M.	10-15 min	Unknown	1-2 hr

Contraindications and precautions

Contraindicated in patients in whom stimulation of GI motility might be dangerous (such as those with hemorrhage, obstruction, or perforation) and in those with hypersensitivity to drug, pheochromocytoma, or seizure disorders. Use cautiously in patients with history of depression, Parkinson's disease, and hypertension.

Interactions

Drug-drug. *Acetaminophen, aspirin, diazepam, levodopa, lithium, tetracycline:* Increased absorption of these drugs. Patient requires careful monitoring.
Anticholinergics and opiates: May antagonize effect of metoclopramide on GI motility. Avoid use together if possible.
Antihypertensives and CNS depressants (such as sedatives and tricyclic antidepressants): May lead to increased CNS depression. Patient requires careful monitoring.
Butyrophenone antipsychotics and phenothiazine: May potentiate extrapyramidal reactions. Avoid use together if possible.
Cyclosporine: Increased absorption, possibly increasing its immunosuppressive and toxic effects. Patient requires careful monitoring.
Digoxin: Decreased absorption. Monitor serum digoxin levels.
MAO inhibitors: Increased blood pressure. Use together cautiously.
Drug-lifestyle. *Alcohol use:* May lead to increased CNS depression. Avoid use together.

Effects on diagnostic tests

None reported.

Adverse reactions

CNS: *restlessness, anxiety, drowsiness, fatigue, lassitude, depression, akathisia, insomnia, confusion,* ***suicidal ideation, seizures,*** hallucinations, headache, dizziness, extrapyramidal symptoms, tardive dyskinesia, dystonic reactions.
CV: transient hypertension, hypotension, supraventricular tachycardia, ***bradycardia.***
GI: nausea, bowel disturbances, diarrhea.
GU: urinary frequency, incontinence, prolactin secretion, loss of libido.
Hematologic: ***neutropenia, agranulocytosis.***
Respiratory: ***bronchospasm.***
Skin: rash, urticaria.
Other: fever, porphyria.

Overdose and treatment

Clinical effects of overdose (which is rare) include drowsiness, dystonia, seizures, and extrapyramidal effects.

Treatment includes administration of antimuscarinics, antiparkinsonian agents, or antihistamines with antimuscarinic activity (such as 50 mg diphenhydramine, given I.M.).

Clinical considerations

- Drug has been used investigationally to treat anorexia nervosa, dizziness, migraine, intractable hiccups, and to promote postpartum lactation; oral dose form is being used investigationally to treat nausea and vomiting.
- Don't use drug for more than 12 weeks.
- Metoclopramide is photosensitive and will degrade when exposed to light. Protect all forms from light. Store at 59° to 86° F (15° to 30° C).
- Drug may be used to facilitate nasoduodenal tube placement.
- When oral concentrate is used, dilute with water, juice, carbonated beverages, or mix with semisolid food.
- Diphenhydramine may be used to counteract extrapyramidal effects of high-dose metoclopramide.
- For I.V. push administration, use undiluted and inject over a 1- to 2-minute period. For I.V. infusion, dilute with 50 ml of D_5W, dextrose 5% in 0.45% saline injection, Ringer's injection, or lactated Ringer's injection, and infuse over at least 15 minutes. Solution is stable for 48 hours when stored at 39° to 86° F (4° to 30° C) and protected from light or for 24 hours when exposed to normal light.
- Drug is incompatible with cisplatin, methotrexate, cephalosporins, chloramphenicol, and sodium bicarbonate. Consult specific references for compatibility information.
- Administer by I.V. infusion 30 minutes before chemotherapy.

Therapeutic monitoring

Monitor renal and hepatic studies.

Special populations

Breast-feeding patients. Because drug is distributed in breast milk, use caution when administering to breast-feeding women.
Pediatric patients. Children have an increased incidence of adverse CNS effects.
Geriatric patients. Use drug with caution, especially if patient has impaired renal function; dosage may need to be decreased. Geriatric patients are more likely to experience extrapyramidal symptoms and tardive dyskinesia.

Patient counseling

- Warn patient to avoid driving for 2 hours after each dose because drug may cause drowsiness. Until extent of CNS effect is known, advise patient not to consume alcohol.
- Tell patient to report twitching or involuntary movement.
- Instruct patient to take medication 30 minutes before each meal.

metolazone

Mykrox, Zaroxolyn

Pharmacologic classification: quinazoline derivative (thiazide-like) diuretic
Therapeutic classification: diuretic, antihypertensive
Pregnancy risk category B

How supplied

Available by prescription only
Tablets: 2.5 mg, 5 mg, 10 mg
Tablets (rapid-acting): 0.5 mg (Mykrox)

Indications and dosages

Tablets
Edema (heart failure)
Adults: 5 to 10 mg P.O. daily.
Edema (renal disease)
Adults: 5 to 20 mg P.O. daily.
Hypertension
Adults: 2.5 to 10 mg P.O. daily; maintenance dosage based on patient's blood pressure. If using stepped-care approach, initial dose is 1.25 to 2.5 mg.
Rapid-acting tablets
Hypertension
Adults: 0.5 mg P.O. once daily; may be increased to maximum of 1 mg daily.

Pharmacodynamics

Diuretic action: Metolazone increases urinary excretion of sodium and water by inhibiting sodium reabsorption in the cortical diluting tubule of the nephron, thus relieving edema. Metolazone may be more effective in edema associated with impaired renal function than thiazide or thiazide-like diuretics.
Antihypertensive action: Exact mechanism of antihypertensive effect of metolazone is unknown; it may result from direct arteriolar vasodilatation. Metolazone also reduces total body sodium levels and total peripheral resistance.

Pharmacokinetics

Absorption: About 65% of a given dose of metolazone is absorbed after oral administration to healthy subjects; in cardiac patients, absorption falls to 40%. However, rate and extent of absorption vary among preparations.
Distribution: Metolazone is 50% to 70% erythrocyte-bound and about 33% protein-bound.
Metabolism: Insignificant.
Excretion: About 70% to 95% of metolazone is excreted unchanged in urine. Half-life is about 14 hours in healthy subjects; it may be prolonged in patients with decreased creatinine clearance.

Route	Onset	Peak	Duration
P.O.	1 hr	2-8 hr	12-24 hr

Contraindications and precautions

Contraindicated in patients with anuria, hepatic coma or precoma, or hypersensitivity to thiazides or other sulfonamide-derived drugs. Use cautiously in patients with impaired renal or hepatic function.

Interactions

Drug-drug. *Amphetamine and quinidine:* Decreased urinary excretion. Monitor patient closely.
Other antihypertensive drugs: Potentiated effects. This may be used to therapeutic advantage.
Cholestyramine and colestipol: May bind metolazone, preventing its absorption. Give drugs 1 hour apart.
Diazoxide: Metolazone may potentiate hyperglycemic, hypotensive, and hyperuricemic effects of diazoxide. Use together cautiously.
Digoxin: Increased risk of digoxin toxicity. Monitor electrolytes.
Furosemide: Excessive volume and electrolyte depletion. Monitor fluid and electrolytes.
Insulin or sulfonylurea: Increased requirements in diabetic patients. Monitor patient closely.
Lithium: Elevated serum lithium levels. May necessitate a 50% reduction in lithium dosage.
Methenamine mandelate: Decreased therapeutic effect. Monitor patient closely.
Drug-lifestyle. *Sun exposure:* Increased risk of photosensitivity reactions. Recommend patient use adequate protection or avoid excessive sun exposure.

Effects on diagnostic tests

Drug therapy may interfere with tests for parathyroid function and should be discontinued before such tests.

Adverse reactions

CNS: *dizziness, headache, fatigue, vertigo, paresthesia, weakness, restlessness, drowsiness, anxiety, depression, nervousness, blurred vision.*
CV: volume depletion and dehydration, orthostatic hypotension, palpitations, vasculitis.
GI: anorexia, nausea, ***pancreatitis,*** epigastric distress, vomiting, abdominal pain, diarrhea, constipation, dry mouth.
GU: nocturia, polyuria, frequent urination, impotence.
Hematologic: ***aplastic anemia, agranulocytosis, leukopenia.***
Hepatic: jaundice, ***hepatitis.***
Metabolic: hyperglycemia and glucose tolerance impairment; fluid and electrolyte imbalances, including hypokalemia, dilutional hyponatremia and hypochloremia, metabolic alkalosis, hypercalcemia.
Musculoskeletal: muscle cramps.
Skin: dermatitis, photosensitivity, rash, purpura, pruritus, urticaria.

Overdose and treatment

Clinical signs of overdose include orthostatic hypotension, dizziness, electrolyte abnormalities, GI irritation and hypermotility, diuresis, and lethargy, which may progress to coma.

Treatment is mainly supportive; monitor and assist respiratory, CV, and renal function as indicated. Monitor fluid and electrolyte balance. Induce vomiting with ipecac in conscious patient; otherwise, use gastric lavage to avoid aspiration. Don't give cathartics; these promote additional loss of fluids and electrolytes.

Clinical considerations

Consider the recommendations relevant to all thiazide and thiazide-like diuretics as well as the following:

- Drug is effective in patients with decreased renal function.
- Metolazone is used as an adjunct in furosemide-resistant edema.
- Drug has been used with furosemide to induce diuresis in patients who didn't respond to either diuretic alone.
- Rapid-acting form (Mykrox) isn't interchangeable with other forms of metolazone. Dosage and uses vary.
- Store at room temperature in tight, light-resistant containers.

Therapeutic monitoring

Monitor renal and hepatic function, electrolytes (potassium, sodium, chloride, calcium), and serum glucose.

Special populations

Breast-feeding patients. Drug may be distributed in breast milk. Safety and efficacy in breast-feeding women haven't been established.
Pediatric patients. Safety and efficacy in children haven't been established.
Geriatric patients. Geriatric and debilitated patients require close observation and may require reduced dosages. They are more sensitive to excess diuresis because of age-related changes in CV and renal function. Excess diuresis promotes orthostatic hypotension, dehydration, hypovolemia, hyponatremia, hypomagnesemia, and hypokalemia.

Patient counseling

- Tell patient to take drug in the morning to prevent nocturia.
- Advise patient to avoid sudden posture changes and to rise slowly to avoid orthostatic hypotension.
- Instruct patient to use a sunblock to prevent photosensitivity reactions.

metoprolol succinate

Toprol XL

metoprolol tartrate

Lopressor

Pharmacologic classification: beta blocker
Therapeutic classification: antihypertensive, adjunctive treatment of acute MI
Pregnancy risk category C

How supplied

Available by prescription only
Tablets: 50 mg, 100 mg
Tablets (extended-release): 50 mg, 100 mg, 200 mg
Injection: 1 mg/ml in 5-ml ampules or prefilled syringes

Indications and dosages

Mild to severe hypertension
Adults: Initially, 50 to 100 mg P.O. daily in single or divided doses; usual maintenance dosage is 100 to 450 mg daily. Alternatively, 50 to 100 mg P.O. extended-release tablets daily (maximum dose, 400 mg daily). Dosages may be increased weekly or as needed to desired effect.
Early intervention in acute MI
Adults: 2.5 to 5 mg rapid I.V. injections at 2 to 5 minute intervals up to a total of 15 mg over 10 to 15 minutes. Then give 50 mg P.O. 15 minutes after the last I.V. dose, and continue 50 mg P.O. every 6 hours for 48 hours. Maintenance dosage, 100 mg, b.i.d., P.O.
◇***Atrial tachyarrythmias following AMI***
Adults: 2.5 to 5 mg I.V. q 2 to 5 minutes to control rate up to 15 mg over a 10- to 15-minute period. Discontinue when therapeutic efficacy is achieved or if systolic blood pressure is

less than 100 mm Hg or heart rate is less than 50 bpm.

Angina

Adults: 100 mg P.O. per day in two divided doses. Maintenance dosage, 100 to 400 mg daily. Alternatively, 100 mg P.O. extended-release tablets daily (maximum dose, 400 mg daily). Dosages may be increased weekly or p.r.n.

Pharmacodynamics

Antihypertensive action: Metoprolol is classified as a cardioselective $beta_1$ antagonist; exact mechanism of antihypertensive effect of metoprolol is unknown. Drug may reduce blood pressure by blocking adrenergic receptors, thus decreasing cardiac output; by decreasing sympathetic outflow from the CNS; or by suppressing renin release.

Action after acute MI: The exact mechanism by which metoprolol decreases mortality after MI is unknown. In patients with MI, metoprolol reduces heart rate, systolic blood pressure, and cardiac output. Drug also appears to decrease the occurrence of ventricular fibrillation in these patients.

Pharmacokinetics

Absorption: Orally administered metoprolol is absorbed rapidly and almost completely from GI tract; food enhances absorption.

Distribution: Distributed widely throughout the body; about 12% is protein-bound.

Metabolism: Metabolized in the liver.

Excretion: About 95% of a given dose of metoprolol is excreted in urine within 72 hours, largely as metabolites.

Route	Onset	Peak	Duration
P.O.	15 min	1 hr	6-12 hr
P.O. (extended)	15 min	6-12 hr	24 hr
I.V.	5 min	20 min	5-8 hr

Contraindications and precautions

Contraindicated in patients with hypersensitivity to drug or other beta blockers. Also contraindicated in patients with sinus bradycardia, heart block greater than first-degree, cardiogenic shock, or overt cardiac failure when used to treat hypertension or angina. When used to treat MI, drug also is contraindicated in patients with heart rate less than 45 beats/minute, second- or third-degree heart block, PR interval of 0.24 second or longer with first-degree heart block, systolic blood pressure less than 100 mm Hg, or moderate to severe cardiac failure.

Use cautiously in patients with diabetes mellitus, impaired hepatic or respiratory function, diabetes, or heart failure.

Interactions

Drug-drug. *Cardiac glycosides:* Enhanced bradycardia. Monitor patient closely.

Diuretics or other antihypertensive agents: Potentiated antihypertensive effects. Monitor patient carefully.

Sympathomimetic agents: Antagonized beta-adrenergic effects of sympathomimetic agents. Monitor for drug effect.

Verapamil: May decrease bioavailability of metoprolol when given with antiarrhythmic agents. Monitor patient for drug effect.

Effects on diagnostic tests

None reported.

Adverse reactions

CNS: *fatigue, dizziness,* depression.

CV: ***bradycardia,*** *hypotension,* ***heart failure.***

GI: nausea, diarrhea.

Respiratory: dyspnea, ***bronchospasm.***

Skin: rash.

Overdose and treatment

Clinical signs of overdose include severe hypotension, bradycardia, heart failure, and bronchospasm.

After acute ingestion, empty stomach by induced emesis or gastric lavage, and give activated charcoal to reduce absorption. Subsequent treatment is usually symptomatic and supportive.

Clinical considerations

Consider the recommendations relevant to all beta blockers as well as the following:

- Metoprolol may be administered daily as a single dose or in divided doses. If a dose is missed, patient should take only the next scheduled dose.
- Administer drug with meals to enhance absorption.
- Reduce dosage in patients with impaired hepatic function.
- Avoid late-evening doses to minimize insomnia.
- Store drug at 59° to 86° F (15° to 30° C).

Therapeutic monitoring

- Patient requires monitoring of heart rate, blood pressure, and ECG during I.V. administration.
- Blood pressure should be checked during dosage adjustment and every 3 to 6 months when on maintenance therapy.
- Recommend observing patient for signs of mental depression.

Special populations

Breast-feeding patients. Metoprolol is distributed into breast milk. An alternative feeding method is recommended during therapy.

Pediatric patients. Safety and efficacy in children haven't been established. No dosage recommendation exists for children.

Geriatric patients. Geriatric patients may require lower maintenance dosages of metoprolol because of delayed metabolism; they may also experience enhanced adverse effects. Use with caution.

Patient counseling

- Instruct patient to take drug exactly as prescribed and to take it with meals.
- Inform patient not to stop drug abruptly and to notify the doctor for adverse reactions. Inform him that drug must be withdrawn gradually over 1 to 2 weeks.

metronidazole

Apo-Metronidazole*, Flagyl, Flagyl ER, Metric-21, Novonidazol*, Protostat

metronidazole hydrochloride

Flagyl I.V., Flagyl I.V. RTU, Metro I.V.

Pharmacologic classification: nitroimidazole
Therapeutic classification: antibacterial, antiprotozoal, amebicide
Pregnancy risk category B

How supplied

Available by prescription only
Tablets: 250 mg, 500 mg
Tablets (film-coated): 250 mg, 500 mg
Tablet (extended-release, film-coated): 750 mg
Capsules: 375 mg
Powder for injection: 500-mg single-dose vials
Injection: 500 mg/dl ready to use

Indications and dosages

Amebic hepatic abscess
Adults: 500 to 750 mg P.O. t.i.d. for 5 to 10 days. Alternatively, 2.4 g P.O. daily for 1 to 2 days or 500 mg I.V. q 6 hours for 10 days.
Children: 30 to 50 mg/kg P.O. daily (in three doses) for 5 to 10 days. Alternatively, 1.3 g/m^2 P.O. daily in three divided doses for 5 to 10 days.
Intestinal amebiasis
Adults: 750 mg P.O. t.i.d. for 5 to 10 days. Centers for Disease Control and Prevention recommends addition of iodoquinol 650 mg P.O. t.i.d. for 20 days. Alternatively, 2.4 g P.O. daily for 1 to 2 days or 500 mg I.V. q 6 hours for 10 days.
◊ *Children:* 30 to 50 mg/kg P.O. daily (in three divided doses) for 5 to 10 days. Follow this therapy with oral iodoquinol. Alternatively, 1.3 g/m^2 P.O. daily in three divided doses for 5 to 10 days.
Trichomoniasis
Adults (both men and women concurrently): 375-mg capsule P.O. b.i.d. for 7 days, or 500-mg tablet P.O. b.i.d. for 7 days or a single dose of 2 g P.O. or divided into two doses given on same day.
◊ *Children:* 15 mg/kg P.O. daily (in three doses) for 7 to 10 days. Alternatively, 40 mg/kg P.O. as a single dose. Dose shouldn't exceed 2 g.
◊ *Infants over age 4 weeks:* 10 to 30 mg/kg P.O. daily for 5 to 8 days.
Refractory trichomoniasis
Adults (women): 500 mg P.O. b.i.d. for 7 days. If repeated failure, 2 g P.O. daily for 3 to 5 days. Alternatively (for repeated failure), 2 to 3.5 g P.O. daily for 3 to 21 days depending on in vitro susceptibility testing.
Bacterial infections caused by anaerobic microorganisms
Adults: Loading dose is 15 mg/kg I.V. infused over 1 hour (about 1 g for a 154-lb [70-kg] adult). Maintenance dosage is 7.5 mg/kg I.V. or P.O. q 6 hours (about 500 mg for a 154-lb adult). Administer first maintenance dose 6 hours after the loading dose. Maximum dose shouldn't exceed 4 g daily. Continue therapy for 7 days to 3 weeks.
◊ ***Giardiasis***
Adults: 250 mg P.O. t.i.d. for 5 days, or 2 g once daily for 3 days. If coexistent amebiasis, 750 mg P.O. t.i.d. for 5 to 10 days.
Children: 5 mg/kg P.O. t.i.d. for 5 to 7 days.
Prevention of postoperative infection in contaminated or potentially contaminated colorectal surgery
Adults: 15 mg/kg infused over 30 to 60 minutes and completed about 1 hour before surgery. Then 7.5 mg/kg infused over 30 to 60 minutes at 6 and 12 hours after initial dose. If used with oral neomycin or oral kanamycin, 750 mg P.O. b.i.d. to t.i.d. beginning 2 days before surgery. Alternatively, 500 mg to 1 g I.V. 1 hour before surgery followed by 500 mg I.V. at 8 and 16 hours postoperatively.
◊ ***Bacterial vaginosis***
Adults: 500 mg P.O. b.i.d. for 7 days; or 2 g P.O. as a single dose. Alternatively, 750 mg (extended-release) P.O. daily for 7 days. If during pregnancy, 250 mg P.O. t.i.d. for 7 days or 2 g P.O. as a single dose.
Pelvic inflammatory disease
Adults: 500 mg I.V. q 12 hours in conjunction with I.V. ofloxacin or I.V. ciprofloxacin and I.V. or oral doxycycline.
◊ ***Pelvic inflammatory disease (ambulatory patients)***
Adults: 500 mg P.O. b.i.d. for 14 days (given with 400 mg b.i.d. of ofloxacin).
◊ ***Infection with* Clostridium difficile**
Adults: 750 mg to 2 g P.O. daily, in three to four divided doses for 7 to 14 days. Alternatively, 500 to 750 mg I.V. q 6 to 8 hours when oral dosing isn't feasible.
◊ **Helicobacter pylori *associated with peptic ulcer disease***
Adults: 250 to 500 mg P.O. t.i.d. to q.i.d. (in combination with other medications). Continue for 7 to 14 days depending on regimen used.

Children: 15 to 20 mg/kg P.O. daily, divided in two doses for 4 weeks (in combination with other medications).
◇ ***Amebiasis caused by* Dientamoeba fragilis**
Children: 250 mg P.O. t.i.d. for 7 days.
◇ **Entamoeba polecki *infection***
Adults: 750 mg P.O. t.i.d. for 10 days.
Children: 35 to 50 mg/kg P.O. daily in three divided doses for 10 days.
◇ ***Dracunculiasis caused by* Dracunculus medinensis *(guinea worm infection)***
Adults: 250 mg P.O. t.i.d. for 10 days
Children: 25 mg/kg daily P.O. in three divided doses (up to 750 mg daily) for 10 days.
◇ ***Balantidiasis caused by* Balantidium coli**
Adults: 750 mg P.O. t.i.d. for 5 days
Children: 35 to 50 mg/kg P.O. daily in three divided doses for 5 days.
◇ ***Symptomatic* Blastocystis hominis *infection***
Adults: 750 mg P.O. t.i.d. for 10 days.
◇ ***Active Crohn's disease***
Adults: 400 mg P.O. b.i.d. For refractory perineal disease, 20 mg/kg (1 to 1.5 g) in three to five divided doses daily.
◇ ***Prophylaxis in sexual assault victims***
Adults: 2 g P.O. in combination with other medications.

Pharmacodynamics

Bactericidal, amebicidal, and trichomonacidal actions: The nitro group of metronidazole is reduced inside the infecting organism; this reduction product disrupts DNA and inhibits nucleic acid synthesis. Drug is active in intestinal and extraintestinal sites. It's active against most anaerobic bacteria and protozoa, including *Bacteroides fragilis, B. melaninogenicus, Fusobacterium, Veillonella, Clostridium, Peptococcus, Peptostreptococcus, Entamoeba histolytica, Trichomonas vaginalis, Giardia lamblia*, and *Balantidium coli.*

Pharmacokinetics

Absorption: About 80% of an oral dose is absorbed; food delays the rate but not the extent of absorption.
Distribution: Distributed into most body tissues and fluids, including CSF, bone, bile, saliva, pleural and peritoneal fluids, vaginal secretions, seminal fluids, middle ear fluid, and hepatic and cerebral abscesses. CSF levels approach serum levels in patients with inflamed meninges; they reach about 50% of serum levels in patients with uninflamed meninges. Less than 20% of metronidazole is bound to plasma proteins. It readily crosses the placenta.
Metabolism: Metabolized to an active 2-hydroxymethyl metabolite and also to other metabolites.
Excretion: About 60% to 80% of dose is excreted as parent compound or its metabolites. About 20% of a metronidazole dose is excreted unchanged in urine; about 6% to 15% is excreted in feces. Half-life of drug is 6 to 8 hours in adults with normal renal function; its half-life may be prolonged in patients with impaired hepatic function.

Route	Onset	Peak	Duration
P.O.	Unknown	2 hr	Unknown
I.V.	Immediate	1 hr	Unknown

Contraindications and precautions

Contraindicated in patients with hypersensitivity to drug or other nitroimidazole derivatives. Use cautiously in patients with history of blood dyscrasia or alcoholism, hepatic disease, retinal or visual field changes, or CNS disorders and in those receiving hepatotoxic drugs.

Interactions

Drug-drug. *Oral anticoagulants:* Prolonged PT and INR. Monitor for this effect.
Barbiturates and phenytoin: Reduced antimicrobial effectiveness of metronidazole. May require higher doses of metronidazole.
Cimetidine: Decreased clearance of metronidazole. Patient requires monitoring for adverse effects.
Disulfiram: May precipitate psychosis and confusion. Avoid use together.
Lithium: May increase lithium levels. Monitor serum lithium levels.
Drug-lifestyle. *Alcohol use:* May cause disulfiram-like reaction (nausea, vomiting, headache, abdominal cramps, and flushing) with drug. Avoid use together.

Effects on diagnostic tests

Drug may interfere with the chemical analyses of aminotransferases and triglyceride, leading to falsely decreased values.

Adverse reactions

CNS: vertigo, headache, ataxia, dizziness, syncope, incoordination, confusion, irritability, depression, weakness, insomnia, ***seizures,*** peripheral neuropathy.
CV: ECG change (flattened T wave), edema (with I.V. RTU preparation).
GI: abdominal cramping, stomatitis, metallic taste, epigastric distress, nausea, vomiting, anorexia, diarrhea, constipation, proctitis, dry mouth.
GU: darkened urine, polyuria, dysuria, cystitis, dyspareunia, dryness of vagina and vulva, vaginal candidiasis, decreased libido.
Hematologic: ***transient leukopenia, neutropenia.***
Musculoskeletal: fleeting joint pain.
Skin: flushing, rash.
Other: overgrowth of nonsusceptible organisms, especially *Candida* (glossitis, furry

tongue); fever; thrombophlebitis (after I.V. infusion); sometimes resembling serum sickness.

Overdose and treatment

Clinical signs of overdose include nausea, vomiting, ataxia, seizures, and peripheral neuropathy.

There's no known antidote for metronidazole; treatment is supportive. If patient doesn't vomit spontaneously, induced emesis or gastric lavage is indicated for an oral overdose; activated charcoal and a cathartic may be used. Diazepam or phenytoin may be used to control seizures.

Clinical considerations

- Injection contains 28 mEq of sodium per gram of metronidazole.
- Trichomoniasis should be confirmed by wet smear and amebiasis by culture before giving metronidazole.
- When preparing powder for injection, follow manufacturer's instructions carefully; use solution prepared from powder within 24 hours. I.V. solutions must be prepared in three steps: reconstitution with 4.4 ml of normal saline solution injection (with or without bacteriostatic water); dilution with lactated Ringer's injection, D_5W, or normal saline solution; and neutralization with sodium bicarbonate, 5 mEq per 500 mg metronidazole. Final concentration should be 8 mg/ml or less.
- Administer I.V. form by slow infusion only; if used with a primary I.V. fluid system, discontinue the primary fluid during the infusion; don't give by I.V. push.

□ ***ALERT*** Infuse drug over at least 1 hour. Don't give I.V. push.

Therapeutic monitoring

- Monitor patient on I.V. drug for candidiasis.
- When treating amebiasis, recommend monitoring number and character of stools. Send fecal specimens to the laboratory promptly; infestation is detectable only in warm specimens. Repeat fecal studies at 3-month intervals to ensure elimination of organisms.

Special populations

Pregnant patients. If indicated during pregnancy for trichomoniasis, the 7-day regimen is preferred over the single-dose regimen. Avoid treatment with metronidazole during the first trimester.

Breast-feeding patients. Patient should discontinue breast-feeding while taking drug.

Pediatric patients. Neonates may eliminate drug more slowly than older infants and children.

Patient counseling

- Inform patient that drug may cause metallic taste and discolored (red-brown) urine.
- Tell patient to take tablets with meals to minimize GI distress and that tablets may be crushed to facilitate swallowing.
- Counsel patient on need for medical follow-up after discharge.
- Advise patient to report adverse effects.
- Tell patient to avoid alcohol and alcohol-containing medications during therapy and for at least 48 hours after the last dose to prevent disulfiram-like reaction.

Amebiasis patients

- Explain that follow-up examinations of stool specimens are necessary for 3 months after treatment is discontinued, to ensure elimination of amebae.
- To help prevent reinfection, instruct patient and family members in proper hygiene, including disposal of feces and hand washing after defecation and before handling, preparing, or eating food, and about the risks of eating raw food and the control of contamination by flies.
- Encourage other household members and suspected contacts to be tested and, if necessary, treated.

Trichomoniasis patients

- Teach correct personal hygiene, including perineal care.
- Explain that asymptomatic sexual partners of patients being treated for trichomoniasis should be treated simultaneously to prevent reinfection; patient should refrain from intercourse during therapy or have partner use condom.

metronidazole (topical)

MetroCream, MetroGel, MetroGel-Vaginal, Noritate

Pharmacologic classification: nitroimidazole
Therapeutic classification: antiprotozoal, antibacterial
Pregnancy risk category B

How supplied

Available by prescription only
Topical gel: 0.75%, 1%
Topical cream: 0.75%
Vaginal gel: 0.75%

Indications and dosages

Topical treatment of acne rosacea, ◇pressure ulcer, inflammatory papules or pustules

Adults: Apply a thin film b.i.d. to affected area during the morning and evening (once daily for Noritate 1% topical gel). Significant results should be seen within 3 weeks and continue for first 9 weeks of therapy.

Topical treatment of bacterial vaginosis

Adults: One applicator b.i.d., vaginally, for 5 days or once at bedtime (nonpregnant women).

◊ ***Treatment of decubitus pressure ulcer***
Adults: Prepare a 1% aqueous solution or suspension from crushed metronidazole tablets (sterilized); apply t.i.d.

Pharmacodynamics
Anti-inflammatory action: Although its exact mechanism of action is unknown, topical metronidazole probably exerts an anti-inflammatory effect through its antibacterial and antiprotozoal actions.

Pharmacokinetics
Absorption: Under normal conditions, serum levels of metronidazole after topical administration are negligible.
Distribution: Less than 20% bound to plasma proteins.
Metabolism: Unknown.
Excretion: Unknown after topical or intravaginal application.

Route	Onset	Peak	Duration
Topical	Unknown	Unknown	Unknown
Intravaginal	Unknown	6-12 hr	Unknown

Contraindications and precautions
Contraindicated in patients hypersensitive to drug or its ingredients (such as parabens) and other nitroimidazole derivatives. Use cautiously in patients with history of blood dyscrasia. Use vaginal form cautiously in patients with history of CNS disease because risk of seizures or peripheral neuropathy exists.

Interactions
Drug-drug. *Oral anticoagulants:* May potentiate anticoagulant effect. Patient requires close monitoring for adverse effects.
Drug-lifestyle. *Alcohol use:* May cause disulfiram-like reaction. Avoid use together.

Effects on diagnostic tests
None reported.

Adverse reactions
CNS: dizziness, light-headedness, headache (with vaginal form).
EENT: lacrimation (if topical gel is applied around the eyes).
GI: decreased appetite, cramps, pain, nausea, diarrhea, constipation, metallic or bad taste in mouth (with vaginal form).
GU: *cervicitis, vaginitis,* urinary frequency (with vaginal form).
Skin: rash, *transient redness, dryness, mild burning, stinging* (with vaginal form).
Other: overgrowth of nonsusceptible organisms (with vaginal form).

Overdose and treatment
No information available. Overdose after topical application is unlikely.

Clinical considerations
Topical metronidazole therapy hasn't been associated with the adverse reactions observed with parenteral or oral metronidazole therapy (including disulfiram-like reaction following alcohol ingestion). However, some of the drug can be absorbed following topical use. Limited clinical experience hasn't shown any of these adverse effects.

Therapeutic monitoring
Recommend monitoring for clinical effect.

Special populations
Breast-feeding patients. Drug is excreted in breast milk. A decision should be made whether to discontinue drug or breast-feeding, after assessing the importance of drug to the woman.
Pediatric patients. Safety hasn't been established in children.

Patient counseling
- Advise patient to cleanse area thoroughly before applying the drug. Patient may use cosmetics after applying the drug.
- Instruct patient to avoid use of drug on eyelids and to apply it cautiously if drug must be used around the eyes.
- If local reactions occur, advise patient to apply drug less frequently or to discontinue use and call for specific instructions.

mexiletine hydrochloride
Mexitil

Pharmacologic classification: lidocaine analogue, sodium channel antagonist
Therapeutic classification: ventricular antiarrhythmic
Pregnancy risk category C

How supplied
Available by prescription only
Capsules: 150 mg, 200 mg, 250 mg

Indications and dosages
Life-threatening documented ventricular arrhythmias, including ventricular tachycardia
Adults: 200 mg P.O. q 8 hours. May increase or decrease dose in increments of 50 to 100 mg q 8 hours every 2 to 3 days if satisfactory control isn't obtained. Alternatively, give a loading dose of 400 mg with maintenance dosage of 200 mg P.O. q 8 hours. Some patients may respond well to 450 mg q 12 hours. Maximum daily dose shouldn't exceed 1,200 mg.
◊ ***Diabetic neuropathy***
Adults: 150 mg P.O. daily for 3 days; then, 300 mg P.O. daily for 3 days followed by 10 mg/kg daily.

Pharmacodynamics

Antiarrhythmic action: Mexiletine is structurally similar to lidocaine and exerts similar electrophysiologic and hemodynamic effects. A class IB antiarrhythmic, it suppresses automaticity and shortens the effective refractory period and action potential duration of His-Purkinje fibers and suppresses spontaneous ventricular depolarization during diastole. At therapeutic serum levels, the drug doesn't affect conductive atrial tissue or AV conduction.

Unlike quinidine and procainamide, mexiletine doesn't significantly alter hemodynamics when given in usual doses. Its effects on the conduction system inhibit reentry mechanisms and halt ventricular arrhythmias. Drug doesn't have a significant negative inotropic effect.

Pharmacokinetics

Absorption: About 90% is absorbed from the GI tract. Absorption rate decreases with conditions that speed gastric emptying.
Distribution: Widely distributed throughout the body. About 50% to 60% of circulating drug is bound to plasma proteins. Usual therapeutic drug level is 0.5 to 2 mcg/ml. Although toxicity may occur within this range, levels above 2 mcg/ml are considered toxic and are associated with an increased frequency of adverse CNS effects, warranting dosage reduction.
Metabolism: Metabolized in the liver to relatively inactive metabolites. Less than 10% of a parenteral dose escapes metabolism and reaches the kidneys unchanged. Metabolism is affected by hepatic blood flow, which may be reduced in patients who are recovering from MI and in those with heart failure. Liver disease also limits metabolism.
Excretion: In healthy patients, half-life of drug is 10 to 12 hours. Elimination half-life may be prolonged in patients with heart failure or liver disease. Urinary excretion increases with urine acidification and slows with urine alkalinization.

Route	Onset	Peak	Duration
P.O.	½-2 hr	2-3 hr	Unknown

Contraindications and precautions

Contraindicated in patients with cardiogenic shock or preexisting second- or third-degree AV block in the absence of an artificial pacemaker. Use cautiously in patients with hypotension, heart failure, first-degree heart block, ventricular pacemaker, preexisting sinus node dysfunction, or seizure disorders.

Interactions

Drug-drug. *Ammonium chloride:* Enhances mexiletine excretion. Patient requires careful monitoring.
Antacids containing aluminum-magnesium hydroxide, atropine, and narcotics: May delay mexiletine absorption. Separate administration times.
High-dose antacids, carbonic anhydrase inhibitors, sodium bicarbonate: Decreases mexiletine excretion. Patient requires careful monitoring.
Cimetidine: May decrease mexiletine metabolism, resulting in increased serum levels. Patient requires careful monitoring.
Metoclopramide: May increase absorption. Patient requires careful monitoring.
Phenobarbital, phenytoin, rifampin: May induce hepatic metabolism of mexiletine and thus reduce serum drug levels. Patient requires careful monitoring.
Theophylline: Increased serum theophylline levels. Monitor serum theophylline levels.

Effects on diagnostic tests

None reported.

Adverse reactions

CNS: *tremor, dizziness, blurred vision, diplopia, confusion,* light-headedness, incoordination, changes in sleep habits, paresthesia, weakness, fatigue, speech difficulties, tinnitus, depression, *nervousness, headache.*
CV: ***new or worsened arrhythmias,*** palpitations, chest pain, nonspecific edema, angina.
GI: *nausea, vomiting, upper GI distress, heartburn, diarrhea, constipation, dry mouth, changes in appetite, abdominal pain.*
Hepatic: *altered liver function tests.*
Skin: rash.

Overdose and treatment

Clinical effects of overdose are primarily extensions of adverse CNS effects. Seizures are the most serious effect.

Treatment usually involves symptomatic and supportive measures. In acute overdose, emesis induction or gastric lavage should be performed. Urine acidification may accelerate drug elimination. If patient has bradycardia and hypotension, atropine may be given.

Clinical considerations

- Administer dosage with meals, if possible.
- Because of proarrhythmic effects, drug is generally not recommended for non-life-threatening arrhythmias.
- Avoid administering drug within 1 hour of antacids containing aluminum-magnesium hydroxide.
- When changing from lidocaine to mexiletine, stop infusion when first mexiletine dose is given. Keep infusion line open, however, until arrhythmia appears to be satisfactorily controlled.
- When transferring patient from another Class I oral antiarrhythmic, initial dose of 200 mg should be initiated 6 to 12 hours after last dose of quinidine; 3 to 6 hours after last dose of procainamide; 6 to 12 hours after last dose of

disopyramide; and 8 to 12 hours after last dose of tocainide.

- Patient whose condition isn't controlled by dosing every 8 hours may respond to dosing every 6 hours.
- Many patients who respond well to mexiletine (300 mg or less every 8 hours) can be maintained on an every 12-hour schedule. The same total daily dose is divided into twice-daily doses, which improves patient compliance.
- Tremor (usually a fine hand tremor) is commonly evident in patients taking higher doses of mexiletine.

Therapeutic monitoring

- Recommend monitoring blood pressure and heart rate and rhythm for significant change.
- Monitor hepatic function tests.

Special populations

Breast-feeding patients. Drug is excreted in breast milk. Alternative feeding method should be used during therapy.
Geriatric patients. Most geriatric patients require reduced dosages because of reduced hepatic blood flow and consequent decreased metabolism. Geriatric patients also may be more susceptible to CNS adverse effects.

Patient counseling

- Tell patient to take drug with food to reduce risk of nausea.
- Instruct patient to report if the following occur: unusual bleeding or bruising; signs of infection, such as fever, sore throat, stomatitis, or chills; or fatigue.

mezlocillin sodium

Mezlin

Pharmacologic classification: extended-spectrum penicillin, acyclaminopenicillin
Therapeutic classification: antibiotic
Pregnancy risk category B

How supplied

Available by prescription only
Injection: 1 g, 2 g, 3 g, 4 g
Infusion: 2 g, 3 g, 4 g
Pharmacy bulk package: 20 g

Indications and dosages

Infections caused by susceptible organisms
Adults: 200 to 300 mg/kg I.V. or I.M. daily given in four to six divided doses. Usual dosage is 3 g q 4 hours or 4 g q 6 hours. For serious infections, up to 24 g daily may be administered. Therapy is usually 10 to 14 days.
Children under age 12: For mild to moderate infection, 50 to 100 mg/kg daily in four divided doses. For more severe infections, 200 to 300 mg/kg per day I.M. or I.V. in divided doses q 4 to 6 hours.
◇*Neonates age 7 days and under:* 75 mg/kg q 12 hours I.V. or I.M.
Neonates age 8 days and older: 75 mg/kg q 8 hours (if weight less than 4.4 lb [2 kg]) or q 6 hours (if weight over 4.4 lb [2 kg]) I.V. or I.M.
Uncomplicated urinary tract infections
Adults: 100 to 125 mg/kg daily I.M. or I.V. in divided doses q 6 hours or 1.5 to 2 g q 6 hours.
Complicated urinary tract infections
Adults: 150 to 200 mg/kg I.V. daily divided into q 6 hour doses or 3 g q 6 hours.
***Uncomplicated gonococcal urethritis caused by* Neisseria gonorrhoeae**
Adults: 1 to 2 g I.M. or I.V. with 1 g of oral probenecid.
Surgical prophylaxis
Adults: 4 g I.V. 30 minutes to 1.5 hours before surgery and repeat I.V. 6 and 12 hours later.
≡***Dosage adjustment.*** In adult patients with renal failure with creatinine clearance of 10 to 30 ml/minute, give 3 g q 6 to 8 hours for life-threatening or serious infection. For urinary tract infection (UTI), give 1.5 g q 6 to 8 hours. If creatinine clearance is less than 10 ml/minute, give 2 g q 6 to 8 hours for life-threatening or serious infection. For UTI, give 1.5 g q 8 hours.

Patients on hemodialysis should be given 3 to 4 g after each dialysis session, then q 12 hours. Patients on peritoneal dialysis may receive 3 g q 12 hours.

Pharmacodynamics

Antibiotic action: Mezlocillin is bactericidal; it adheres to bacterial penicillin-binding proteins, thereby inhibiting bacterial cell wall synthesis.

Extended-spectrum penicillins are more resistant to inactivation by certain beta-lactamases, especially those produced by gram-negative organisms, but are still liable to inactivation by certain others.

Spectrum of activity of drug includes many gram-negative aerobic and anaerobic bacilli, many gram-positive and gram-negative aerobic cocci, and some gram-positive aerobic and anaerobic bacilli, but a large number of these organisms are resistant to mezlocillin. Mezlocillin may be effective against some strains of carbenicillin-resistant and ticarcillin-resistant gram-negative bacilli. Mezlocillin shouldn't be used as sole therapy because of the rapid development of resistance. Some clinicians believe that there's no evidence that it has any advantages over ticarcillin or carbenicillin, at least with respect to cure rates. Drug is less active against *Pseudomonas aeruginosa* than other members of this class, such as piperacillin.

Pharmacokinetics

Absorption: Well absorbed.
Distribution: Distributed widely. It penetrates minimally into CSF with uninflamed menin-

ges, crosses the placenta, and is 16% to 42% protein-bound.
Metabolism: Partially metabolized; about 15% of a dose is metabolized to inactive metabolites.
Excretion: Excreted primarily (39% to 72%) in urine by glomerular filtration and renal tubular secretion; up to 30% of a dose is excreted in bile, and some is excreted in breast milk. Elimination half-life in adults is ¾ to 1½ hours; in extensive renal impairment, half-life is extended to 2 to 14 hours. Mezlocillin is removed by hemodialysis but not by peritoneal dialysis.

Route	Onset	Peak	Duration
I.V.	Immediate	Immediate	Unknown
I.M.	Unknown	45-90 min	Unknown

Contraindications and precautions

Contraindicated in patients with hypersensitivity to drug or other penicillins. Use cautiously in patients with bleeding tendencies, uremia, hypokalemia, or allergy to cephalosporins.

Interactions

Drug-drug. *Aminoglycoside antibiotics:* Synergistic bactericidal effect against *Pseudomonas aeruginosa, Escherichia coli, Klebsiella, Citrobacter, Enterobacter, Serratia*, and *Proteus mirabilis*. This is a therapeutic advantage.
Clavulanic acid: Synergistic bactericidal effect against certain beta-lactamase-producing bacteria. This is a therapeutic advantage.
Methotrexate: Delayed elimination and elevated serum levels of methotrexate. Monitor patient closely.
Probenecid: Blocks tubular secretion of penicillins, raising their serum levels. Monitor patient carefully.
Vecuronium bromide: Prolonged neuromuscular blockade. Monitor patient closely.

Effects on diagnostic tests

Drug alters tests for urinary or serum proteins; it interferes with turbidimetric methods that use sulfosalicylic acid, trichloroacetic acid, acetic acid, or nitric acid. Positive Coombs' tests have been reported in patients taking carbenicillin disodium.

Adverse reactions

CNS: neuromuscular irritability, ***seizures.***
GI: nausea, diarrhea, vomiting, abnormal taste sensation, pseudomembranous colitis.
GU: interstitial nephritis.
Hematologic: *bleeding* (with high doses), ***neutropenia, thrombocytopenia,*** eosinophilia, ***leukopenia, hemolytic anemia.***
Metabolic: *hypokalemia.*
Other: *hypersensitivity reactions* (***anaphylaxis,*** edema, fever, chills, rash, pruritus, urticaria), overgrowth of nonsusceptible organisms, *pain at injection site, vein irritation, phlebitis.*

Overdose and treatment

Signs of overdose include neuromuscular sensitivity or seizures; a 4- to 6-hour hemodialysis will remove 20% to 30% of mezlocillin.

Clinical considerations

Consider the recommendations relevant to all penicillins as well as the following:
☐ ***ALERT*** Beware of sound-alikes: methicillin and mezlocillin.
- Mezlocillin may be more suitable than carbenicillin or ticarcillin for patients on salt-free diets; mezlocillin contains only 1.85 mEq of sodium per gram.
- Drug is almost always used with another antibiotic, such as an aminoglycoside, in life-threatening infections.
- For I.M. reconstitution, for each gram, add 3 to 4 ml of sterile water for injection or 1% lidocaine without epinephrine and dissolve.
- Inject I.M. dose slowly over 12 to 15 seconds to minimize pain. Don't exceed 2 g per site.
- For direct I.V. injection, add 9 to 10 ml of sterile water for injection, 5% dextrose injection, normal saline injection to each gram of mezlocillin. Shake vigorously and inject desired dose over 3 to 5 minutes. Don't exceed 100 mg/ml concentration. For I.V. infusion, further dilute in 50 to 100 ml of a compatible I.V. solution (such as normal saline or 5% dextrose) and infuse over 30 minutes. Reconstitute ADD-Vantage vial according to manufacturer instructions.
- Mezlocillin is incompatible with aminoglycosides and shouldn't be infused in the same I.V. line or solution.
- Solutions are stable for 24 hours to 7 days depending on solution used and storage temperature.
- If precipitate forms during refrigerated storage, warm to 98.6° F (37° C) in warm water bath and shake well. Solution should be clear.
- Because drug is partially dialyzable, dosage may need adjustment in patients undergoing hemodialysis.

Therapeutic monitoring

- Monitor serum potassium level and liver function studies.
- Recommend monitoring patient with high serum levels for seizures.

Special populations

Breast-feeding patients. Drug is excreted in breast milk; safe use in breast-feeding women hasn't been established. Alternative feeding method is recommended during therapy.
Geriatric patients. Half-life may be prolonged in geriatric patients because of impaired renal function.

Patient counseling
- Instruct patient to report adverse reactions promptly.
- Tell patient to alert health care provider if discomfort occurs.
- Caution patient to limit salt intake during mezlocillin therapy because of high sodium content of drug.

miconazole nitrate
Femizol-M, Micatin, Monistat 3, Monistat 7, Monistat-Derm

Pharmacologic classification: imidazole derivative
Therapeutic classification: antifungal
Pregnancy risk category B

How supplied
Available by prescription only
Vaginal suppositories: 200 mg
Vaginal cream: 2%
Cream: 2%
Available without a prescription
Cream: 2%
Powder: 2%
Spray: 2%
Vaginal cream: 2%
Vaginal suppositories: 100 mg, 200 mg

Indications and dosages
Cutaneous or mucocutaneous fungal infections caused by susceptible organisms
Topical use
Adults and children: Apply to affected areas b.i.d. for 2 to 4 weeks.
Treatment of pityriasis (tinea vericolor)
Adults and children over age 2: Apply cream to affected area once daily.
Vaginal use
Adults: Insert 200-mg suppository h.s. for 3 days, or 100-mg suppository or 1 applicatorful of vaginal cream h.s. for 7 days.

Pharmacodynamics
Antifungal action: Miconazole is both fungistatic and fungicidal, depending on drug concentration, in *Coccidioides immitis, Candida albicans, Cryptococcus neoformans, Histoplasma capsulatum, Candida tropicalis, C. parapsilosis, Paracoccidioides brasiliensis, Sporothrix schenckii, Aspergillus flavus, Microsporum canis, Curvularia, Pseudallescheria boydii,* dermatophytes, and some gram-positive bacteria. Miconazole causes thickening of the fungal cell wall, altering membrane permeability; it also may kill the cell by interference with peroxisomal enzymes, causing accumulation of peroxide within the cell wall. It attacks virtually all pathogenic fungi.

Pharmacokinetics
Absorption: About 50% of an oral dose is absorbed; however, no oral dosage form is currently available. A small amount of drug is systemically absorbed after vaginal administration.
Distribution: Penetrates well into inflamed joints, vitreous humor, and the peritoneal cavity. Distribution into sputum and saliva is poor, and CSF penetration is unpredictable. Over 90% is bound to plasma proteins.
Metabolism: Metabolized in the liver, predominantly to inactive metabolites.
Excretion: Elimination is triphasic; terminal half-life is about 24 hours. Between 10% and 14% of an oral dose is excreted in urine; 50%, in feces. Up to 1% of a vaginal dose is excreted in urine; 14% to 22% of an I.V. dose is excreted in urine. It's unknown if it's excreted in breast milk.

Route	Onset	Peak	Duration
Topical, Intravaginal	Unknown	Unknown	Unknown

Contraindications and precautions
Topical form contraindicated in patients with hypersensitivity to drug. Use cautiously in patients with hepatic insufficiency.

Interactions
Drug-drug. *Amphotericin B:* May antagonize the effects of amphotericin B. Monitor patient carefully.
Phenytoin: Increased phenytoin levels. Monitor phenytoin levels.
Warfarin: Increased anticoagulant effect. Monitor PT and INR.

Effects on diagnostic tests
None reported.

Adverse reactions
CNS: headache.
GU: vulvovaginal burning, pruritus, or irritation with vaginal cream; pelvic cramps.
Skin: irritation, burning, maceration, allergic contact dermatitis.

Overdose and treatment
No information available.

Clinical considerations
- Clean affected area before applying cream. After application, massage area gently until cream disappears.
- Continue topical therapy for at least 1 month; improvement should begin in 1 to 2 weeks. If no improvement occurs by 4 weeks, reevaluate diagnosis.
- Insert vaginal applicator high into vagina, except in pregnancy.

Therapeutic monitoring
Recommend monitoring patient for clinical effects.

Special populations
Pregnant patients. The 7-day vaginal treatment is preferred in pregnant women.
Breast-feeding patients. Safety hasn't been established in breast-feeding women.
Pediatric patients. Safety in children under age 1 hasn't been established.

Patient counseling
- Teach patient the symptoms of fungal infection, and explain treatment rationale.
- Encourage patient to adhere to prescribed regimen and follow-up visits and to report adverse effects.
- Teach patient correct procedure for intravaginal or topical applications.
- To prevent vaginal reinfection, teach correct perineal hygiene and recommend that patient abstain from sexual intercourse during therapy.

midazolam hydrochloride
Versed

Pharmacologic classification: benzodiazepine
Therapeutic classification: preoperative sedative, agent for conscious sedation, adjunct for induction of general anesthesia, amnesic agent
Controlled substance schedule IV
Pregnancy risk category D

How supplied
Available by prescription only
Injection: 1 mg/ml in 2-ml, 5-ml, and 10-ml vials; 5 mg/ml in 1-ml, 2-ml, 5-ml, and 10-ml vials; 5 mg/ml in 2-ml disposable syringe
Syrup: 2 mg/ml in 118 ml bottle

Indications and dosages
Preoperative sedation (to induce sleepiness or drowsiness and relieve apprehension)
Adults under age 60: 0.07 to 0.08 mg/kg I.M. about ½ to 1 hour before surgery. May be administered with atropine or scopolamine and reduced doses of narcotics.
≡ ***Dosage adjustment.*** Reduce dosage in patients over age 60, those with COPD, those considered to be high-risk surgical patients, and those who have received concomitant narcotics or other depressants.
Conscious sedation
Adults under age 60: Initially, 1 to 2.5 mg I.V. administered over at least 2 minutes; repeat in 2 minutes, if needed, in small increments of initial dose over at least 2 minutes to achieve desired effect. Total dose up to 5 mg may be used. Additional doses to maintain desired level of sedation may be given by slow titration in increments of 25% of dose used to reach the sedation endpoint.
Adults age 60 and older: 1.5 mg or less over at least 2 minutes. If additional titration is needed, give at a rate not exceeding 1 mg over 2 minutes. Total doses exceeding 3.5 mg aren't usually necessary.
Induction of general anesthesia
Unpremedicated adults under age 55: 0.3 to 0.35 mg/kg I.V. over 20 to 30 seconds if patient hasn't received preanesthesia medication, or 0.15 to 0.35 mg/kg (usually 0.25 mg/kg) I.V. over 20 to 30 seconds if patient has received preanesthesia medication. Additional increments of 25% of the initial dose may be needed to complete induction.
Unpremedicated adults age 55 and older: Initially, 0.3 mg/kg. For debilitated patients, initial dose is 0.2 to 0.25 mg/kg. For premedicated patients, 0.15 mg/kg may be sufficient.
Continuous infusion for sedation of intubated and mechanically ventilated patients as a component of anesthesia or during treatment in a critical-care setting
Adults: If a loading dose is necessary to rapidly initiate sedation, give 0.01 to 0.05 mg/kg slowly or infused over several minutes, with dose repeated at 10- to 15-minute intervals until adequate sedation is achieved. For maintenance of sedation, usual infusion rate is 0.02 to 0.10 mg/kg/hour (1 to 7 mg/hour). Titrate infusion rate to the desired amount of sedation. Drug can be titrated up or down by 25% to 50% of the initial infusion rate to achieve optimal sedation without oversedation.
Children: After a loading dose of 0.05 to 0.2 mg/kg over 2 to 3 minutes in intubated patients only, an infusion may be initiated at 0.06 to 0.12 mg/kg/ hour (1 to 2 mcg/kg/minute). Dose may be titrated up or down by 25% of the initial or subsequent infusion rate to obtain optimal sedation.
Neonates: Use only on intubated neonates. No loading dose is used in neonates. Neonates under age 32 weeks' gestation receive infusion rates of 0.03 mg/kg/hour (0.5 mcg/kg/minute). In neonates over age 32 weeks' gestation, infusion rates are 0.06 mg/kg/hour (1 mcg/kg/ minute). Infusion may be run more rapidly in the first few hours to obtain a therapeutic blood level. Rate of infusion should be frequently and carefully reassessed to administer the lowest possible amount of drug.
Sedation, anxiolysis and amnesia before diagnostic, therapeutic or endoscopic procedures or before induction of anesthesia in pediatric patients
Children age 6 months to 16 years: 250 to 500 mcg/kg P.O. up to 20 mg or up to 1 mg/kg. Lower doses may provide adequate therapeutic effect for children age 6 months to 16 years or cooperative patients. Alternatively, 100 to

150 mcg/kg I.M. (up to 500 mcg/kg may be necessary) not to exceed 10 mg.
Children age 6 months to 5 years: Initially 50 to 100 mcg/kg I.V. up to 600 mcg/kg (usual dose doesn't exceed 6 mg).
Children age 6 to 12: 25 to 50 mcg/kg I.V. up to 400 mcg/kg (usual dose doesn't exceed 10 mg).
Children age 13 to 16: 0.07 to 0.08 mg/kg I.M. ½ to 1 hour before surgery; for conscious sedation, 1 to 2.5 mg I.V. over at least 2 minutes.

Pharmacodynamics

Sedative and anesthetic actions: Although exact mechanism is unknown, midazolam, like other benzodiazepines, is thought to facilitate the action of gamma-aminobutyric acid (GABA) to provide a short-acting CNS depressant action.
Amnesic action: Mechanism of action by which midazolam causes amnesia isn't known.

Pharmacokinetics

Absorption: Absorption after I.M. administration appears to be 80% to 100%.
Distribution: Drug has a large volume of distribution and is about 97% protein-bound. Drug crosses the placenta and enters fetal circulation.
Metabolism: Metabolized in the liver.
Excretion: Metabolites are excreted in urine. Half-life of drug is 1¼ to 12⅓ hours.

Route	Onset	Peak	Duration
P.O.	10-20 min	1-2 hr	2-6 hr
I.V.	1½-5 min	Rapid	2-6 hr
I.M.	15 min	15-60 min	2-6 hr

Contraindications and precautions

Contraindicated in patients with hypersensitivity to drug or acute angle-closure glaucoma and in those experiencing shock, coma, or acute alcohol intoxication. Use cautiously in patients with uncompensated acute illnesses and in geriatric or debilitated patients.

Interactions

Drug-drug. *Antidepressants, antihistamines, barbiturates, narcotics, tranquilizers, and other CNS and respiratory depressants:* Potentiated effects. Use together cautiously.
Erythromycin: May decrease plasma clearance of midazolam. Close monitoring of patient is needed.
Droperidol, fentanyl, and narcotics: Potentiate the hypnotic effect of midazolam. Patient requires careful monitoring.
Inhaled anesthetics: Midazolam may decrease the needed dose of inhaled anesthetics by depressing respiratory drive. Anesthesia dosage may require adjustment.
Isoniazid: May decrease the metabolism of midazolam. Close monitoring of patient is needed.
Drug-food. *Grapefruit juice:* Increased bioavailability of oral syrup form of drug. Avoid use together.
Drug-lifestyle. *Alcohol use:* Potentiated effects of alcohol. Advise patient to avoid alcohol.

Effects on diagnostic tests

None reported.

Adverse reactions

CNS: headache, oversedation, drowsiness, amnesia.
CV: variations in blood pressure (hypotension) and pulse rate, ***cardiac arrest.***
GI: *nausea,* vomiting.
Respiratory: *hiccups, **decreased respiratory rate, apnea, respiratory arrest.***
Other: *pain, tenderness (at injection site).*

Overdose and treatment

Signs and symptoms of overdose include confusion, stupor, coma, respiratory depression, and hypotension.

Treatment is supportive. Maintain patent airway, and ensure adequate ventilation with mechanical support, if necessary. Monitor vital signs. Use I.V. fluids or ephedrine to treat hypotension. Flumazenil, a specific benzodiazepine-receptor antagonist, is indicated for complete or partial reversal of the sedative effects.

Clinical considerations

Consider the recommendations relevant to all benzodiazepines as well as the following:

- Individualized dosages are advised, using the smallest effective dose possible. Use with extreme caution and reduced dosage in geriatric and debilitated patients.
- Medical personnel who administer midazolam should be familiar with airway management. Close monitoring of cardiopulmonary function is required. Continuously monitor patients who have received midazolam to detect potentially life-threatening respiratory depression.
- Laryngospasm and bronchospasm may occur rarely; countermeasures should be available.
- Midazolam can be mixed in the same syringe with morphine, meperidine, atropine, and scopolamine.
- Syrup form must be given only to patients visually monitored by health care professionals.
- Solutions of D_5W, normal saline solution, and lactated Ringer's solution are compatible with midazolam.
- Before I.V. administration, ensure the immediate availability of oxygen and resuscitative equipment. Apnea and death have been reported with rapid I.V. administration. Avoid intra-arterial injection because the hazards of

this route are unknown. Avoid extravasation. Administer I.V. dose slowly to prevent respiratory depression.

- Know that there is a potential for adverse effects, such as hypotension, metabolic acidosis, and kernicterus, related to neonate metabolism of benzyl alcohol. Take into account the amount of benzyl alcohol when giving high doses of drugs, including midazolam, containing the preservative.
- Administer I.M. dose deep into a large muscle mass to prevent tissue injury.
- Don't use solution that's discolored or contains a precipitate.

Therapeutic monitoring

Hypotension occurs more frequently in patients premedicated with narcotics. Monitor vital signs closely.

Special populations

Breast-feeding patients. It isn't known if drug is excreted in breast milk; use with caution in breast-feeding women.
Pediatric patients. The safety and efficacy of oral solution in children under age 6 months haven't been established. Monitor the amount of benzyl alcohol when used in neonates.
Geriatric patients. Geriatric or debilitated patients, especially those with COPD, are at significantly increased risk for respiratory depression and hypotension. Lower doses are indicated. Use with caution. Oral dose forms aren't recommended for geriatric use.

Patient counseling

- Advise patient to postpone tasks that require mental alertness or physical coordination until the effects of the drug have worn off.
- Instruct patient as necessary in safety measures, such as supervised walking and gradual position changes, to prevent injury.
- Advise patient to contact health care provider before taking OTC drugs.

miglitol

Glyset

Pharmacologic classification: alpha-glucosidase inhibitor
Therapeutic classification: antidiabetic
Pregnancy risk category B

How supplied

Avaialable by prescription only
Tablets: 25 mg, 50 mg, 100 mg

Indications and dosages

Monotherapy adjunct to diet to improve glycemic control in patients with type 2 diabetes (non-insulin dependent diabetes mellitus—NIDDM) mellitus whose hyperglycemia can't be managed with diet alone, or in combination with a sulfonylurea when diet plus either miglitol or sulfonylurea alone don't result in adequate glycemic control
Adults: 25 mg P.O. t.i.d. at the start (with the first bite) of each main meal; dose may be increased after 4 to 8 weeks to 50 mg P.O. t.i.d. The dose may then be further increased after 3 months, based on the glycosylated hemoglobin level, to a maximum of 100 mg P.O. t.i.d.

Pharmacodynamics

Antidiabetic action: Miglitol lowers blood glucose through reversible inhibition of the enzymes alpha-glucosidases in the brush border of the small intestine. Alpha-glucosidases are responsible for the conversion of oligosaccharides and disaccharides to glucose. Inhibition of these enzymes results in delayed glucose absorption and a lowering of postprandial blood glucose. In contrast to sulfonylureas, miglitol has no effect on insulin secretion.

Pharmacokinetics

Absorption: Demonstrates saturable absorption at high doses. A 25-mg dose is completely absorbed, whereas a dose of 100 mg is only 50% to 70% absorbed.
Distribution: Distributes primarily into the extracellular fluid. Protein binding is negligible (less than 4%).
Metabolism: Not metabolized.
Excretion: Eliminated primarily by renal excretion. More than 95% of a given dose is recovered in the urine as unchanged drug. The elimination half-life is about 2 hours.

Route	Onset	Peak	Duration
P.O.	Unknown	2 - 3 hr	Unknown

Contraindications and precautions

Miglitol is contraindicated in patients with hypersensitivity to the drug or any of its components. Also contraindicated in patients with diabetic ketoacidosis, inflammatory bowel disease, colonic ulceration, or partial intestinal obstruction, and in patients predisposed to intestinal obstruction or those with chronic intestinal diseases associated with marked disorders of digestion or absorption, or with conditions that may deteriorate as a result of increased gas formation in the intestine.

Drug isn't recommended in patients with significant renal dysfunction (serum creatinine more than 2.0 mg/dl). Use cautiously in patients also receiving insulin or oral sulfonylureas.

Interactions

Drug-drug. *Digoxin, propranolol, ranitidine:* May decrease the bioavailability of these drugs. Monitor patient for loss of drug efficacy; dose adjustment may be needed.

Intestinal absorbents, such as charcoal, and digestive enzyme preparations, such as amylase and pancreatin: May reduce the effectiveness of miglitol. Avoid use together.

Effects on diagnostic tests
None reported.

Adverse reactions
GI: *Abdominal pain, diarrhea, flatulence.*
Metabolic: decreased serum iron.
Skin: rash.

Overdose and treatment
Overdose may result in transient increases in gastrointestinal adverse reactions. No serious systemic reactions are expected in the event of an overdose.

Clinical considerations
- An increased risk of hypoglycemia can occur when used in combination with insulin or sulfonylureas; dosage adjustments of these drugs may be needed.
- The management of type 2 diabetes should also include diet control, exercise program, and regular testing of urine and blood glucose.
- Give miglitol with the first bite of each main meal.
- Mild to moderate hypoglycemia may be treated with a form of dextrose such as glucose tablets or gel. Severe hypoglycemia may require I.V. glucose or glucagon administration.

Therapeutic monitoring
- During treatment initiation and dosage titration, one-hour postprandial plasma glucose may be used to determine therapeutic response.
- Monitor patients for an increased frequency of hypoglycemia.
- Monitor blood glucose regularly, especially during situations of increased stress, such as infection, fever, surgery, and trauma.
- Besides having glucose levels checked regularly, monitor glycosylated hemoglobin every 3 months for evaluating long-term glycemic control.

Special populations
Breast-feeding patients. Although the amount of miglitol excreted in breast milk is low, it's recommended that miglitol not be administered to breast-feeding women.
Pediatric patients. Safety and efficacy of miglitol in children haven't been established.
Geriatric patients. No significant differences in the safety and effectiveness of miglitol have been observed in placebo-controlled clinical trials between older and younger patients.

Patient counseling
- Instruct patient about the importance of adhering to dietary, weight reduction and exercise instructions and to have blood glucose and glycosylated hemoglobin tested regularly.
- Inform patient that treatment with miglitol relieves symptoms but doesn't cure diabetes.
- Teach patient to recognize signs and symptoms of hyperglycemia and hypoglycemia.
- Instruct patient to treat hypoglycemia with glucose tablets and to have a source of glucose readily available to treat symptoms of hypoglycemia when miglitol is taken with a sulfonylurea or insulin.
- Advise patient to seek medical advice promptly during periods of stress such as fever, trauma, infection, or surgery because medication requirements may change.
- Instruct patient to take miglitol three times a day with the first bite of each main meal.
- Show patient how and when to perform self-monitoring of glucose levels.
- Advise patient that adverse GI effects are most common during the first few weeks of therapy and should improve over time.
- Urge patient to carry medical identification at all times.

milrinone lactate
Primacor

Pharmacologic classification: bipyridine phosphodiesterase inhibitor
Therapeutic classification: inotropic vasodilator
Pregnancy risk category C

How supplied
Available by prescription only
Solution: 1 mg/ml in 10-ml and 20-ml vials
Cartridge: 5 ml
Injection, premixed: 200 mEq/ml in 5% dextrose

Indications and dosages
Short-term I.V. therapy for heart failure
Adults: Initial loading dose of 50 mcg/kg I.V. over 10 minutes, followed by continuous infusion/maintenance dosage of 0.375 to 0.75 mcg/kg/minute. Adjust infusion dose based on hemodynamic and clinical response.
≡ ***Dosage adjustment.*** For patients with renal impairment, refer to the following table.

Creatinine clearance (ml/min/1.73 m^2)	Infusion rate (mcg/kg/min)
5	0.20
10	0.23
20	0.28
30	0.33
40	0.38
50	0.43

Note: If hypotension occurs, administration of milrinone should be reduced or temporarily discontinued until patient's condition stabilizes.

Pharmacodynamics

Inotropic and vasodilator actions: Milrinone is a selective inhibitor of peak III cAMP phosphodiesterase isozyme in cardiac and vascular muscle. This inhibitory action is consistent with cAMP-mediated increases in intracellular ionized calcium and contractile force in cardiac muscle, as well as with cAMP-dependent contractile protein phosphorylation and relaxation in vascular muscle. In addition to increasing myocardial contractility, milrinone improves diastolic function, shown by improvements in left ventricular diastolic relaxation.

Pharmacokinetics

Absorption: Not applicable.
Distribution: About 70% is bound to human plasma protein.
Metabolism: About 12% is metabolized to a glucuronide metabolite.
Excretion: After I.V. administration, about 90% is excreted unchanged in urine within 8 hours.

Route	Onset	Peak	Duration
I.V.	5-15 min	1-2 hr	3-6 hr

Contraindications and precautions

Contraindicated in patients with hypersensitivity to drug, severe aortic or pulmonic valvular disease in place of surgical correction, or during the acute phase of an MI.

Use cautiously in patients with atrial fibrillation or flutter.

Interactions

None reported.

Effects on diagnostic tests

None reported.

Adverse reactions

CNS: headache.
CV: ***ventricular arrhythmias, ventricular ectopic activity, nonsustained ventricular tachycardia,*** **SUSTAINED VENTRICULAR TACHYCARDIA, VENTRICULAR FIBRILLATION,** hypotension, angina.

Overdose and treatment

Hypotension may occur with milrinone overdose because of its vasodilator effect. No specific antidote is known, but general measures for circulatory support should be taken.

Clinical considerations

- Drug therapy isn't recommended for patients in acute phase of post-MI; clinical studies in this population are lacking.
- Duration of therapy depends on patient responsiveness. Patients have been maintained on infusions of milrinone for up to 5 days.
- Milrinone must be further diluted before I.V. administration. Acceptable diluents include 0.45% sodium chloride or normal saline solution or D_5W. Prepare the 100 mcg/ml, 150 mcg/ml, or 200 mcg/ml solutions by adding 180 ml, 113 ml, or 80 ml to the 20-mg (20-ml) vial. Add one-half of the diluent amounts to the 10-ml vial to achieve same concentration.
- When furosemide is injected into an I.V. line containing milrinone, an immediate chemical interaction occurs, as evidenced by the formation of a precipitate. Therefore, furosemide shouldn't be administered in an I.V. line that contains milrinone.

Therapeutic monitoring

Monitor renal function and fluid and electrolyte changes during milrinone therapy. Correct hypokalemia with potassium supplements before or during use of milrinone.

Special populations

Breast-feeding patients. Excretion of drug into breast milk isn't known. Use caution when administering drug to breast-feeding women.
Pediatric patients. Safety and efficacy in children haven't been established.

mineral oil

Fleet Enema Mineral Oil, Kondremul*, Kondremul Plain, Lansoÿl*, Milkinol, Neo-Cultol, Nujol*, Petrogalar Plain

Pharmacologic classification: lubricant oil
Therapeutic classification: laxative
Pregnancy risk category C

How supplied

Available without a prescription
Jelly: 180 ml
Emulsion: 2.5 ml/5 ml, 1.4 g/5 ml
Suspension: 2.75 ml/5 ml, 4.75 ml/5 ml
Rectal oil enema: 120 ml

Indications and dosages

Constipation, preparation for bowel studies or surgery
Adults and children age 12 and older: 15 to 45 ml P.O. as a single dose or in divided doses, or 120-ml enema.
Children age 6 to 11: 5 to 15 ml P.O. daily as a single dose or in divided doses, or 30- to 60-ml enema.
Children age 2 to 6: 30- to 60-ml enema.

Pharmacodynamics
Laxative action: Mineral oil acts mainly in the colon, lubricating the intestine and retarding colonic fluid absorption.

Pharmacokinetics
Absorption: Absorbed minimally; with emulsified drug form, significant absorption occurs.
Distribution: Distributed locally, primarily in the colon.
Metabolism: None.
Excretion: Excreted in feces.

Route	Onset	Peak	Duration
P.O.	6-8 hr	Variable	Variable
P.R.	2-15 min	Unknown	Unknown

Contraindications and precautions
Contraindicated in patients with abdominal pain, nausea, vomiting, or other symptoms of appendicitis or acute surgical abdomen and in those with fecal impaction or intestinal obstruction or perforation. Contraindicated in patients with colostomy, ileostomy, ulcerative colitis, and diverticulitis. Use cautiously in geriatric, debilitated, and young patients.

Interactions
Drug-drug. *Stool softeners such as docusate:* Increase mineral oil absorption to potentially toxic levels. Avoid use together.
Fat-soluble vitamins (A, D, E, and K), anticoagulants, oral contraceptives, cardiac glycosides, and sulfonamides: Impaired absorption of these medications and vitamins, thus lessening their therapeutic effects. Avoid administration together and monitor patient for vitamin deficiency.

Effects on diagnostic tests
None reported.

Adverse reactions
GI: *nausea; vomiting; diarrhea* (with excessive use); abdominal cramps, especially in severe constipation; decreased absorption of nutrients and fat-soluble vitamins, resulting in deficiency; slowed healing after hemorrhoidectomy.
Respiratory: ***lipid pneumonia.***
Skin: anal pruritus, anal irritation, hemorrhoids, perianal discomfort.
Other: laxative dependence (with long-term or excessive use).

Overdose and treatment
No information available.

Clinical considerations
- Avoid administering drug to patients lying flat because if drug is aspirated into the lungs, pneumonitis may result.
- Drug shouldn't be given with food because this may delay gastric emptying, resulting in delayed drug action and increased aspiration risk. Separate administration by at least 2 hours.
- To improve taste, give emulsion and suspension with fruit juice or carbonated beverages.
- Prescribe cleansing enema 30 minutes to 1 hour after retention enema.
- Reduce or divide dose or use emulsified drug form to avoid leakage through anal sphincter.
- Mineral oil may impair absorption of fat-soluble vitamins (A, D, E, and K).

Therapeutic monitoring
Recommend monitoring patient for clinical effect.

Special populations
Pediatric patients. Mineral oil isn't recommended for children under age 6 because of risk of aspiration. Enema form is contraindicated in under age 2.
Geriatric patients. Because of increased aspiration risk, use caution when administering drug to geriatric patients.

Patient counseling
- Instruct patient not to take mineral oil with stool softeners.
- Warn patient that mineral oil may leak through anal sphincter, especially with repeated use or with enema form. Undergarment protection may be desired.

minocycline hydrochloride
Dynacin, Minocin

Pharmacologic classification: tetracycline
Therapeutic classification: antibiotic
Pregnancy risk category NR

How supplied
Available by prescription only
Capsules: 50 mg, 100 mg
Tablets: 50 mg, 100 mg
Suspension: 50 mg/5 ml
Injection: 100 mg/vial

Indications and dosages
Infections caused by sensitive organisms
Adults: Initially, 200 mg P.O., I.V.; then 100 mg q 12 hours or 50 mg P.O. q 6 hours.
Children over age 8: Initially, 4 mg/kg P.O., I.V.; then 4 mg/kg P.O. daily, divided q 12 hours. Give I.V. in 500 to 1,000 ml solution without calcium, over 6 hours.
Gonorrhea in patients sensitive to penicillin
Adults: Initially, 200 mg P.O., then 100 mg q 12 hours for 4 days.

Syphilis in patients sensitive to penicillin
Adults: Initially, 200 mg P.O.; then 100 mg q 12 hours for 10 to 15 days.
Meningococcal carrier state
Adults: Initially, 200 mg P.O., then 100 mg P.O. q 12 hours for 5 days.
***Uncomplicated urethral, endocervical, or rectal infection caused by* Chlamydia trachomatis *or* Ureaplasma urealyticum**
Adults: 100 mg P.O. q 12 hours for at least 7 days.
Uncomplicated gonococcal urethritis in men
Adults: 100 mg P.O. q 12 hours for 5 days.
Mycobacterium marinum
Adults: 100 mg P.O. q 12 hours for 6 to 8 weeks.
Cholera
Adults: Initially, 200 mg P.O.; then 100 mg P.O. q 12 hours for 72 hours.
Acne
Adults: 50 mg P.O. daily to t.i.d.
◊ ***Treatment of multibacillary leprosy***
Adults: 100 mg P.O. daily with clofazimine and ofloxacin for 6 months, followed by 100 mg P.O. daily for an additional 18 months in conjunction with clofazimine.
◊ ***Nocardiosis***
Adults: Usual dose for 12 to 18 months.
◊ ***Sclerosis agent for pleural effusions***
Adults: 300 mg mixed in 40 to 50 ml sodium chloride injection, instilled through a thoracostomy tube.
◊ ***Nongonococcal urethritis caused by* C. trachomatis *or mycoplasma***
Adults: 100 mg P.O. daily in one or two divided doses for 1 to 3 weeks.

Pharmacodynamics

Antibacterial action: Minocycline is bacteriostatic; it binds reversibly to ribosomal units, thus inhibiting bacterial protein synthesis.

Minocycline is active against many gram-negative and gram-positive organisms, *Mycoplasma, Rickettsia, Chlamydia,* and spirochetes; it may be more active against staphylococci than other tetracyclines.

The potential vestibular toxicity and cost of minocycline limit its usefulness. It may be more active than other tetracyclines against *Nocardia asteroides;* it's also effective against *Mycobacterium marinum* infections. It has been used for meningococcal meningitis prophylaxis because of its activity against *Neisseria meningitidis.*

Pharmacokinetics

Absorption: About 90% to 100% is absorbed after oral administration.
Distribution: Widely distributed into body tissues and fluids, including synovial, pleural, prostatic, and seminal fluids, bronchial secretions, saliva, and aqueous humor; CSF penetration is poor. Drug crosses the placenta, and is 55% to 88% protein-bound.
Metabolism: Metabolized partially.
Excretion: Excreted primarily unchanged in urine by glomerular filtration. Plasma half-life is 11 to 22 hours in adults with normal renal function. Some drug is excreted in breast milk.

Route	Onset	Peak	Duration
P.O.	Unknown	1-4 hr	Unknown
I.V.	Immediate	Immediate	Unknown

Contraindications and precautions

Contraindicated in patients with hypersensitivity to drug or other tetracyclines. Use cautiously in patients with impaired renal or hepatic function, in children under age 8, and during the last half of pregnancy.

Interactions

Drug-drug. *Antacids containing aluminum, calcium, or magnesium or with laxatives containing magnesium, oral iron products, or sodium bicarbonate:* Decreases oral absorption of minocycline because of chelation. Administer drugs at separate times.
Oral anticoagulants: Increased effects. Decreased anticoagulant dose may be necessary.
Oral contraceptives: May be less effective when administered with minocycline. Advise patient to use alternative method of birth control.
Digoxin: Increased bioavailability. Decreased digoxin dose may be necessary.
Penicillins: Tetracyclines may antagonize bactericidal effects of penicillin. Give penicillin 2 to 3 hours before minocycline.
Drug-food. *Foods, milk, and other dairy products:* May decrease absorption of minocycline. Avoid use together.
Drug-lifestyle. *Sun exposure:* Increased risk of photosensitivity reactions. Advise patient to use sunscreen and limit sun exposure.

Effects on diagnostic tests

Drug causes false-negative results in urine glucose tests using glucose oxidase reagent (Clinistix or glucose enzymatic test strip). Minocycline causes false elevations in fluorometric test results for urinary catecholamines.

Adverse reactions

CNS: headache, ***intracranial hypertension (pseudotumor cerebri),*** light-headedness, dizziness, vertigo.
CV: pericarditis.
EENT: dysphagia, glossitis.
GI: *anorexia, epigastric distress, oral candidiasis, nausea, vomiting, diarrhea,* enterocolitis, inflammatory lesions in anogenital region.
GU: increased BUN level.
Hematologic: ***neutropenia,*** eosinophilia, ***thrombocytopenia,*** hemolytic anemia.
Hepatic: elevated liver enzymes.

Skin: *maculopapular and erythematous rashes, photosensitivity, increased pigmentation, urticaria.*
Other: hypersensitivity reactions ***(anaphylaxis);*** permanent discoloration of teeth, enamel defects, and bone growth retardation if used in children under age 8; superinfection; *thrombophlebitis.*

Overdose and treatment
Signs of overdose are usually limited to GI tract; give antacids or empty stomach by gastric lavage if ingestion occurred within the preceding 4 hours.

Clinical considerations
Consider the recommendations relevant to all tetracyclines as well as the following:
□ ***ALERT*** Beware of sound-alikes: minocin, niacin, and mithracin.
□ ***ALERT*** Check expiration date. Outdated or deteriorated tetracyclines have been associated with reversible nephrotoxicity (Fanconi's syndrome).
- Reconstitute 100 mg powder with 5 ml sterile water for injection, with further dilution of 500 to 1,000 ml for I.V. infusion to a concentration of 100 to 200 mcg/ml. Infuse over 6 hours.
- Reconstituted solution is stable for 24 hours at room temperature. Use final diluted solution immediately.
- Avoid mixing with solutions containing calcium because a precipitate may form (Ringer's injection and lactated Ringer's injection are compatible).

Therapeutic monitoring
Monitor renal and hepatic function in prolonged therapy.

Special populations
Breast-feeding patients. Avoid use in breast-feeding women.
Pediatric patients. Drug isn't recommended for use in children under age 9.

Patient counseling
- Tell patient to take entire amount of medication prescribed, even after he feels better.
- Instruct patient to take oral form of drug with a full glass of water. Drug may be taken with food. Tell patient not to take within 1 hour of bedtime to avoid esophageal irritation or ulceration.
- Warn patient to avoid driving or other hazardous tasks due to possible adverse CNS effects.
- Caution patient to avoid direct sunlight and ultraviolet light, wear protective clothing, and use sunscreen. Photosensitivity reactions may occur within a few minutes to several hours after exposure. Photosensitivity persists for some time after discontinuation of therapy.

minoxidil (systemic)
Loniten

Pharmacologic classification: peripheral vasodilator
Therapeutic classification: antihypertensive
Pregnancy risk category C

How supplied
Available by prescription only
Tablets: 2.5 mg, 10 mg

Indications and dosages
Severe hypertension
Adults and children over age 12: Initially, 2.5 to 5 mg P.O. as a single daily dose. Dose may be increased at 3-day intervals (minimum) to 10 mg, 20 mg, and then 40 mg. If rapid control is necessary, dose may be adjusted q 6 hours. Effective dosage range is usually 10 to 40 mg daily in one to two divided doses. Maximum dose is 100 mg/day.
Children under age 12: 0.2 mg/kg (maximum 5 mg) as an initial single daily dose. Effective dosage range is usually 0.25 to 1 mg/kg daily in one or two doses. If necessary, dose is increased after at least 3-day intervals in increments of 50% to 100% until optimal response is attained. If rapid control is necessary, dose may be adjusted q 6 hours. Maximum dose is 50 mg/day.

Pharmacodynamics
Antihypertensive action: Drug produces its antihypertensive effect by a direct vasodilating effect on vascular smooth muscle; the effect on resistance vessels (arterioles and arteries) is greater than that on capacitance vessels (venules and veins).

Pharmacokinetics
Absorption: Absorbed rapidly and almost completely from the GI tract.
Distribution: Distributed widely into body tissues; it isn't bound to plasma proteins.
Metabolism: About 90% of a given dose is metabolized.
Excretion: Excreted primarily in urine. Average plasma half-life is 4¼ hours.

Route	Onset	Peak	Duration
P.O.	½ hr	2-3 hr	2-5 days

Contraindications and precautions
Contraindicated in patients with pheochromocytoma or hypersensitivity to drug. Use cautiously in patients with impaired renal function or after acute MI.

Interactions

Drug-drug. *Diuretics or guanethidine:* May cause profound orthostatic hypotension. Avoid use together.

Effects on diagnostic tests

None reported.

Adverse reactions

CV: *edema, tachycardia, pericardial effusion and tamponade,* ***heart failure,*** ECG changes, rebound hypertension.
GI: nausea, vomiting.
GU: *breast tenderness.*
Metabolic: *weight gain.*
Skin: rash, ***Stevens-Johnson syndrome.***
Other: *hypertrichosis (elongation, thickening, and enhanced pigmentation of fine body hair).*

Overdose and treatment

Signs of overdose include hypotension, tachycardia, headache, and skin flushing.

After acute ingestion, empty stomach by induced emesis or gastric lavage, and give activated charcoal to reduce absorption. Further treatment is usually symptomatic and supportive. Administer normal saline solution I.V. to maintain blood pressure. Avoid sympathomimetic drugs, such as epinephrine and norepinephrine, because of their excessive cardiac stimulating action.

Clinical considerations

- Drug therapy is usually given with other antihypertensive drugs, such as diuretics, beta blockers, or sympathetic nervous system suppressants.
- Patients with renal failure or on dialysis may require smaller maintenance dosages of minoxidil. Because minoxidil is removed by dialysis, it's recommended that, on the day of dialysis, the drug be administered immediately after dialysis if dialysis is at 9 a.m.; if dialysis is after 3 p.m., the daily dose is given at 7 a.m. (8 hours before dialysis).
- After blood pressure is stabilized, patient should be reevaluated every 3 to 6 months.

Therapeutic monitoring

- Recommend monitoring blood pressure and pulse after administration; assessing intake, output, and body weight for sodium and water retention.
- Recommend monitoring of patient for heart failure, pericardial effusion, and cardiac tamponade; have phenylephrine, dopamine, and vasopressin on hand to treat hypotension.

Special populations

Breast-feeding patients. Drug is excreted in breast milk. An alternative feeding method is recommended during therapy.
Pediatric patients. Because of limited experience in children, use with caution. Cautious drug adjustment is necessary.
Geriatric patients. Geriatric patients may be sensitive to antihypertensive effects of drug. Dosage adjustment may be necessary because of altered drug clearance. Monitor orthostatic blood pressure in geriatric patients.

Patient counseling

- Explain that drug is usually taken with other antihypertensive medications; emphasize importance of taking drug as prescribed.
- Caution patient to report the following cardiac symptoms promptly: increased heart rate (over 20 beats/minute over normal), rapid weight gain, shortness of breath, chest pain, severe indigestion, dizziness, light-headedness, or fainting.
- Tell patient to call prescriber for instructions before taking OTC cold preparations.
- Advise patient that hypertrichosis will disappear 1 to 6 months after stopping drug.

minoxidil (topical)

Rogaine

Pharmacologic classification: direct-acting vasodilator
Therapeutic classification: hair-growth stimulant
Pregnancy risk category C

How supplied

Available without a prescription
Topical solution: 2%, 5% in 60-ml bottle

Indications and dosages

Male-pattern baldness (alopecia androgenetica), diffuse hair loss or thinning in women, ◇adjunct to hair transplantation
Adults: Apply 1 ml to affected area b.i.d. for 4 months or longer.
◇Alopecia areata
Adults: 1 ml of 1%, 3%, or 5% solution applied to scalp b.i.d.

Pharmacodynamics

Hair-growth stimulation: Exact mechanism by which drug promotes hair growth is unknown. It may alter androgen metabolism in the scalp, or it may exert a local vasodilatation and enhance the microcirculation around the hair follicle. It may also directly stimulate the hair follicle.

Pharmacokinetics

Absorption: Poorly absorbed through intact skin. About 0.3% to 4.5% of a topically applied dose reaches the systemic circulation.
Distribution: Serum levels are generally negligible.
Metabolism: Metabolism is not fully described.

Excretion: Eliminated primarily by the kidneys. About 95% of a topically applied dose is eliminated after 4 days.

Route	Onset	Peak	Duration
Topical	Unknown	Unknown	Unknown

Contraindications and precautions
Contraindicated in patients hypersensitive to drug or any component of the solution or during pregnancy. Use cautiously in patients with renal, cardiac, or hepatic disease and in those over age 50 and in breast-feeding women.

Interactions
None reported.

Effects on diagnostic tests
None reported.

Adverse reactions
CNS: headache, dizziness, faintness, lightheadedness.
CV: edema, chest pain, hypertension, hypotension, palpitations, increased or decreased pulse rate, ***heart failure.***
EENT: sinusitis.
GI: diarrhea, nausea, vomiting.
GU: urinary tract infection, renal calculi, urethritis.
Metabolic: weight gain.
Musculoskeletal: back pain, tendinitis.
Respiratory: bronchitis, upper respiratory infection.
Skin: irritant dermatitis, allergic contact dermatitis, eczema, hypertrichosis, local erythema, pruritus, dry skin or scalp, flaking, alopecia, exacerbation of hair loss.

Overdose and treatment
None reported. However, if topical use produces systemic adverse effects, wash application site thoroughly with soap and water and treat symptoms, as appropriate. Treatment is symptomatic. Clinical signs of oral overdose include hypotension, tachycardia, headache, and skin flushing.

After acute ingestion, empty stomach by induced emesis or gastric lavage, and give activated charcoal to reduce absorption. Further treatment is usually symptomatic and supportive.

Clinical considerations
- Before treatment with topical minoxidil, patient should have a history and physical examination and should be advised of potential risks; a risk-benefit decision should be made. Patients with cardiac disease should realize that adverse effects may be especially serious. Alert patient to possibility of tachycardia and fluid retention, and monitor for increased heart rate, weight gain, or other systemic effects.
- Don't use with other topical agents such as corticosteroids, retinoids, and petrolatum or agents that enhance percutaneous absorption. Rogaine is for topical use only; each milliliter contains 20 or 50 mg minoxidil and accidental ingestion could cause adverse systemic effects.
- The alcohol base will burn and irritate the eye and other sensitive surfaces (eye, abraded skin, and mucous membranes). If topical minoxidil contacts sensitive areas, flush copiously with cool water.
- The 5% topical solution shouldn't be used in women.
- Self-medication should cease and a clinician consulted if there is no hair growth in 8 months for women and 12 months for men using the 2% solution and in 4 months in men using the 5% solution.

Therapeutic monitoring
- Before starting treatment, recommend checking that patient has a normal, healthy scalp. Local abrasion or dermatitis may increase absorption and the risk of adverse effects.
- Recommend monitoring patient 1 month after starting topical drug therapy and at least every 6 months afterward. Discontinue topical minoxidil if systemic effects occur.

Special populations
Breast-feeding patients. Topical minoxidil shouldn't be administered to breast-feeding women.
Pediatric patients. Safety and efficacy haven't been established for patients under age 18.

Patient counseling
- Tell patient to avoid inhaling the spray.
- Teach patient to apply topical minoxidil as follows: Dry hair and scalp before application. Apply dose of 1 ml to the total affected areas twice daily. Total daily dose shouldn't exceed 2 ml. If the fingertips are used to apply the drug, wash the hands afterward.
- Encourage patient to carefully review patient information leaflet, which is included with each package and in the full product information.
- Inform patient that 4 months of use may be required before results become apparent.

mirtazapine
Remeron

Pharmacologic classification: piperazinoazepine
Therapeutic classification: tetracyclic antidepressant
Pregnancy risk category C

How supplied
Available by prescription only
Tablets: 15 mg, 30 mg, 45 mg

Indications and dosages

Depression

Adults: initially, 15 mg P.O. h.s. Maintenance dosage ranges from 15 mg to 45 mg daily. Dosage adjustments should be made at intervals no less than 1 to 2 weeks apart.

Pharmacodynamics

Antidepressant action: Unknown.

Pharmacokinetics

Absorption: Rapidly and completely absorbed from the GI tract. Absolute bioavailability of drug is about 50%.
Distribution: About 85% is bound to plasma protein.
Metabolism: Extensively metabolized in the liver.
Excretion: Predominantly eliminated in urine (75%) with 15% being excreted in feces. Half-life is between 20 and 40 hours.

Route	Onset	Peak	Duration
P.O.	Unknown	2 hr	Unknown

Contraindications and precautions

Contraindicated in patients with hypersensitivity to drug. Coadministration with MAO inhibitors is contraindicated.

Use cautiously in patients with CV or cerebrovascular disease, seizure disorders, suicidal ideation, impaired hepatic and renal function, or history of mania or hypomania. Also, use cautiously in patients with conditions that predispose them to hypotension, such as dehydration, hypovolemia, or treatment with antihypertensive medication, and in pregnancy.

Interactions

Drug-drug. *Diazepam and other CNS depressants:* May cause additive CNS effects. Avoid use together.
MAO inhibitors or within 14 days of initiating or discontinuing therapy with MAO inhibitors: Potential for serious, and sometimes fatal, reactions. Avoid use together.
Drug-lifestyle. *Alcohol use:* Additive CNS effects. Avoid use together.

Effects on diagnostic tests

None reported.

Adverse reactions

CNS: *somnolence,* dizziness, asthenia, abnormal dreams, abnormal thinking, tremor, confusion.
CV: edema.
GI: nausea, *increased appetite, dry mouth, constipation.*
GU: urinary frequency.
Hematologic: ***agranulocytosis*** (rare).
Metabolic: *weight gain.*
Musculoskeletal: back pain, myalgia.
Respiratory: dyspnea.
Other: flu syndrome, peripheral edema.

Overdose and treatment

Overdose may result in disorientation, drowsiness, impaired memory, and tachycardia. If overdose occurs, treat as for any antidepressant overdose. If patient is unconscious, establish an airway and provide adequate oxygenation. Consider gastric lavage, induced emesis, or both; also consider activated charcoal. Monitor cardiac and vital signs and provide general symptomatic and supportive measures.

Clinical considerations

- Use with caution in patients with increased intraocular pressure, history of urinary retention, or history of narrow-angle glaucoma because of anticholinergic properties.
- There should be a drug-free interval of at least 2 weeks when switching from MAO-inhibitor therapy to mirtazapine or from mirtazapine to an MAO inhibitor.

Therapeutic monitoring

- Although incidence of agranulocytosis is rare, discontinue drug and recommend monitoring patient closely if he develops a sore throat, fever, stomatitis, or other signs of infection together with a low WBC count.
- Patient requires close observation because it isn't known if mirtazapine causes physical or psychological dependence.

Special populations

Breast-feeding patients. It isn't known if drug is excreted in breast milk; use cautiously in breast-feeding women.
Pediatric patients. Safety and efficacy in children haven't been established.
Geriatric patients. Administer mirtazapine cautiously to geriatric patients because pharmacokinetic studies reveal a decreased clearance in the elderly.

Patient counseling

- Caution patient not to perform hazardous activities if somnolence occurs with drug use.
- Instruct patient not to use alcohol or other CNS depressants while taking drug because of additive effect.
- Tell patient to report signs and symptoms of infection such as fever, chills, sore throat, mucous membrane ulceration, or other possible signs of infection including any flulike complaints.
- Stress importance of compliance with mirtazapine therapy.
- Instruct patient not to take any other medication without medical approval.
- Tell women of childbearing age to report suspected pregnancy immediately.

misoprostol

Cytotec

Pharmacologic classification: prostaglandin E_1 analogue
Therapeutic classification: antiulcer, gastric mucosal protectant
Pregnancy risk category X

How supplied

Available by prescription only
Tablets: 100 mcg, 200 mcg

Indications and dosages

Prevention of gastric ulcer induced by NSAIDs

Adults: 200 mcg P.O. q.i.d with meals and h.s. Reduce dosage to 100 mcg P.O. q.i.d. in patients who cannot tolerate this dosage.

◇***Duodenal or gastric ulcer***

Adults: 100 to 200 mcg P.O. q.i.d. with meals and h.s. for 4 to 8 weeks.

Pharmacodynamics

Antiulcer action: Misoprostol enhances the production of gastric mucous and bicarbonate, and decreases basal, nocturnal, and stimulated gastric acid secretion.

Pharmacokinetics

Absorption: Rapidly absorbed after oral administration.
Distribution: Less than 90% bound to plasma proteins.
Metabolism: Rapidly de-esterified to misoprostol acid, the biologically active metabolite. The de-esterified metabolite undergoes further oxidation in several body tissues.
Excretion: About 15% of an oral dose appears in the feces; the balance is excreted in urine. Terminal half-life is 20 to 40 minutes.

Route	Onset	Peak	Duration
P.O.	30 min	10-15 min	3 hr

Contraindications and precautions

Contraindicated in pregnant and breast-feeding women and in those with a known allergy to prostaglandins.

Interactions

None significant.

Effects on diagnostic tests

Misoprostol produces a modest decrease in basal pepsin secretion.

Adverse reactions

CNS: headache.
GI: *diarrhea, abdominal pain, nausea, flatulence, dyspepsia, vomiting, constipation.*
GU: hypermenorrhea, dysmenorrhea, spotting, cramps, menstrual disorders.

Overdose and treatment

There has been little clinical experience with overdose. Cumulative daily doses of 1,600 mcg have been administered, with only minor GI discomfort noted. Treatment should be supportive.

Clinical considerations

- Drug has been used for treatment and prophylaxis of reflux esophagitis, alcohol-induced gastritis, hemorrhagic gastritis, fat malabsorption in cystic fibrosis, and NSAID-induced nephropathy.
- Misoprostol shouldn't be prescribed for a woman of childbearing age unless she:
  – needs NSAID therapy and is at high risk for development of gastric ulcers.
  – is capable of complying with effective contraception practices.
  – has received both oral and written warnings regarding the hazards of misoprostol therapy, the risk of possible contraception failure, and the hazards this drug would pose to other women of childbearing age who might take this drug by mistake.
  – has had a negative serum pregnancy test within 2 weeks before beginning therapy and she'll begin therapy on the second or third day of her next normal menstrual period.
- Diarrhea is usually dose-related and develops within the first 2 weeks of therapy. It can be minimized by administering the drug after meals and at bedtime, and by avoiding magnesium-containing antacids.

Therapeutic monitoring

Recommend monitoring patient for GI distress, especially diarrhea.

Special populations

Pregnant patients. Drug shouldn't be routinely used in women of child-bearing age unless they're at high risk for development of ulcers or complications from NSAID-induced ulcers.
Breast-feeding patients. Breast-feeding isn't recommended because of potential for drug-induced diarrhea in infant.
Pediatric patients. Safety hasn't been established in children under age 18.

Patient counseling

- Explain importance of not giving drug to anyone else.
- Make sure patient understands that a miscarriage could result if drug is taken by a pregnant woman.
- Advise patient to take drug as prescribed for duration of therapy.

mitomycin (mitomycin-C; MTC)
Mutamycin

Pharmacologic classification: antineoplastic antibiotic (cell cycle-phase nonspecific)
Therapeutic classification: antineoplastic
Pregnancy risk category NR

How supplied
Available by prescription only
Injection: 5-mg, 20-mg, 40-mg vials

Indications and dosages
Dosage and indications may vary. Check current literature for recommended protocol. Not indicated as a single-agent primary therapy.
Stomach and pancreatic adenocarcinoma (in conjunction with other chemotherapeutic agents); cancer of ◇breast, ◇colon, ◇rectum, ◇head, ◇neck, ◇lung, ◇cervix
Adults: 20 mg/m² as a single dose. Repeat cycle q 6 to 8 weeks, adjusting dose, if needed, according to the following table:

Nadir after prior dose: WBCs/mm³	Nadir after prior dose: Platelets/mm³	Percentage of prior dose to be given
> 4,000	> 100,000	100%
3,000 to 3,999	75,000 to 99,999	100%
2,000 to 2,999	25,000 to 74,999	70%
< 2,000	< 25,000	50%

◻ ALERT Stop drug if WBC count is less than 4,000/mm³ or platelet count is less than 150,000/mm³. No repeat dose should be given until blood counts go above these levels. If disease progresses after two courses of therapy, discontinue use.
◇Bladder cancer
Adults: 20 to 60 mg intravesically once per week for 8 weeks.

Pharmacodynamics
Antineoplastic action: Mitomycin exerts its cytotoxic activity by a mechanism similar to that of the alkylating agents. The drug is converted to an active compound which forms cross-links between strands of DNA, inhibiting DNA synthesis. Mitomycin also inhibits RNA and protein synthesis to a lesser extent.

Pharmacokinetics
Absorption: Because of its vesicant nature, drug must be administered I.V.
Distribution: Distributes widely into body tissues; animal studies show that the highest levels are found in the kidneys followed by the muscle, eyes, lungs, intestines, and stomach. It doesn't cross the blood-brain barrier.
Metabolism: Metabolized by hepatic microsomal enzymes; deactivated in the kidneys, spleen, brain, and heart.
Excretion: Excreted in urine. A small portion is eliminated in bile and feces.

Route	Onset	Peak	Duration
I.V.	Unknown	Unknown	Unknown

Contraindications and precautions
Contraindicated in patients with hypersensitivity to drug, thrombocytopenia, coagulation disorders, or an increase in bleeding tendency due to other causes. Contraindicated as primary therapy as a single agent to replace surgery or radiotherapy.

Interactions
Drug-drug. *Vinca alkaloids:* Acute shortness of breath and severe bronchospasm have occurred following use of vinca alkaloids in patients who had previously or simultaneously received mitomycin. Patient requires careful monitoring.

Effects on diagnostic tests
None reported.

Adverse reactions
CNS: headache, neurologic abnormalities, confusion, drowsiness, fatigue.
EENT: blurred vision.
GI: *nausea, vomiting, anorexia, diarrhea.*
Hematologic: ***thrombocytopenia, leukopenia*** (may be delayed up to 8 weeks and may be cumulative with successive doses), ***microangiopathic hemolytic anemia, characterized by thrombocytopenia, renal failure,*** and hypertension.
Respiratory: ***interstitial pneumonitis,*** pulmonary edema, dyspnea, nonproductive cough, adult respiratory distress syndrome.
Skin: *reversible alopecia.*
Other: desquamation, induration, pruritus, pain at injection site; ***septicemia;*** cellulitis, ulceration, sloughing with extravasation; fever; pain.

Overdose and treatment
Signs and symptoms of overdose include myelosuppression, nausea, vomiting, and alopecia.

Treatment is usually supportive and includes transfusion of blood components, antiemetics, and antibiotics for infections that may develop.

Clinical considerations

□ ***ALERT*** Don't confuse this drug with mitoxantrone. Question any unfamiliar color of the drug.

- To reconstitute 5-mg vial, use 10 ml of sterile water for injection; to reconstitute 20-mg vial, use 40 ml of sterile water for injection; to reconstitute a 40-mg vial, use 80 ml sterile water for injection, to give a concentration of 0.5 mg/ml. Allow to stand at room temperature until complete dissolution occurs.
- Drug may be administered by I.V. push injection slowly over 5 to 10 minutes into the tubing of a freely flowing I.V. infusion.
- Drug can be further diluted to 100 to 150 ml with normal saline solution or D_5W for I.V. infusion (over 30 to 60 minutes or longer).
- Reconstituted solution remains stable for 1 week at room temperature and for 2 weeks if refrigerated.
- Mitomycin has been used intra-arterially to treat certain tumors, for example, into hepatic artery for colon cancer. It has also been given as a continuous daily infusion.
- Ulcers caused by extravasation develop late and dorsal to the extravasation site. Apply cold compresses for at least 12 hours.

Therapeutic monitoring

- Observe patient for evidence of renal toxicity. Don't give to patient with a serum creatinine over 1.7 mg/dl.
- Continue CBC and blood studies at least 7 weeks after therapy is stopped. Monitor for signs of bleeding.

Special populations

Breast-feeding patients. It isn't known if drug is excreted in breast milk. To avoid risk of serious adverse reactions, mutagenicity, and carcinogenicity in the infant, breast-feeding isn't recommended.

Patient counseling

- Tell patient to avoid exposure to people with infections.
- Warn patient not to receive immunizations during therapy and for several weeks afterward. Members of the same household shouldn't receive immunizations during the same period.
- Reassure patient that hair should grow back after treatment has been discontinued.
- Tell patient to call promptly if he develops a sore throat or fever or notices unusual bruising or bleeding.

mitoxantrone hydrochloride

Novantrone

Pharmacologic classification: antibiotic antineoplastic
Therapeutic classification: antineoplastic
Pregnancy risk category D

How supplied

Available by prescription only
Injection: 2 mg mitoxantrone base/ml in 10-ml, 12.5-ml, 15-ml vials

Indications and dosages

Initial treatment in combination with other approved drugs for acute nonlymphocytic leukemia

Adults: For induction (in combination chemotherapy), 12 mg/m^2 daily by I.V. infusion on days 1 to 3, and 100 mg/m^2 of cytosine arabinoside by continuous I.V. infusion (over 24 hours) on days 1 to 7 for 7 days.

Most complete remissions follow initial course of induction therapy. A second course may be given if antileukemic response is incomplete: give mitoxantrone for 2 days and cytosine for 5 days using the same daily dosage levels. Withhold second course of therapy until toxicity clears if severe or life-threatening nonhematologic toxicity occurs.

Combined initial therapy for pain related to advanced hormone-refractory prostate cancer

Adults: 12 to 14 mg/m^2 I.V. infusion over 15 to 30 minutes q 21 days.

Pharmacodynamics

Antineoplastic action: Mechanism of action isn't completely established. It's a DNA-reactive agent that has cytocidal effects on proliferating and nonproliferating cells, suggestive of lack of cell-phase specificity.

Pharmacokinetics

Absorption: Only administered by I.V. infusion.
Distribution: 78% plasma protein-bound.
Metabolism: Metabolized by the liver.
Excretion: Excretion is via renal and hepatobiliary systems; 6% to 11% of dose is excreted in urine within 5 days: 65% is unchanged drug; 35% is two inactive metabolites. Within 5 days, 25% of dose is excreted in feces.

Route	Onset	Peak	Duration
I.V.	Unknown	Unknown	Unknown

Contraindications and precautions

Contraindicated in patients hypersensitive to mitoxantrone. Use cautiously in patients with prior exposure to anthracyclines or other cardiotoxic drugs. Contraindicated in pregnancy unless potential benefits outweigh potential hazards to fetus.

Interactions
None reported.

Effects on diagnostic tests
None reported.

Adverse reactions
CNS: ***seizures,*** headache.
EENT: conjunctivitis, temporary blue color to sclera.
CV: ***heart failure, arrhythmias,*** tachycardia.
GI: *bleeding, abdominal pain, diarrhea, nausea, mucositis, vomiting,* stomatitis.
GU: ***renal failure.***
Hematologic: ***myelosuppression.***
Hepatic: jaundice.
Metabolic: hyperuricemia.
Respiratory: *dyspnea, cough.*
Skin: *alopecia, petechiae, ecchymoses.*
Other: ***sepsis,*** *fungal infections, fever.*

Overdose and treatment
Accidental overdoses have occurred and have caused severe leukopenia with infection. Monitor hematologic parameters and treat symptomatically. Antimicrobial therapy may be necessary.

Clinical considerations
◻ ***ALERT*** Don't confuse this drug with mitomycin. Question any unfamiliar color of the drug.
- Safety of administration by routes other than I.V. hasn't been established. Don't use intrathecally.
- To prepare, dilute solutions to at least 50 ml with either normal saline solution or D_5W. Inject slowly into tubing of a freely running I.V. solution of normal saline solution or D_5W over not less than 3 minutes. Discard unused infusion solutions appropriately. Don't mix for infusion with heparin; a precipitate may form. Specific compatibility data aren't available.
- For I.V. infusion over 15 to 30 minutes, further dilute solution.
- After penetration of container, undiluted mitoxantrone concentration may be stored no longer than 7 days at room temperature or 14 days if refrigerated.
- If extravasation occurs, discontinue I.V. and restart in another vein. Mitoxantrone is a nonvesicant and the possibility of severe local reactions is minimal.
- Urine may appear blue-green for 24 hours after administration.
- Bluish discoloration of sclera may occur; this may be a sign of myelosuppression.

Therapeutic monitoring
- Close and frequent monitoring of hematologic and chemical laboratory parameters, including serial CBC and liver function tests, with frequent patient observation is recommended.
- Hyperuricemia may result from rapid lysis of tumor cells. Monitor serum uric acid levels. Institute hypouricemic therapy before antileukemic therapy.
- Transient elevations of AST and ALT have occurred 4 to 24 days after mitoxantrone therapy.

Special populations
Breast-feeding patients. It isn't known if drug is excreted in breast milk. Because of potential for serious adverse reactions in infants, discontinue breast-feeding before therapy.
Pediatric patients. Safety and efficacy in children haven't been established.

Patient counseling
- Tell patient urine may appear blue-green for 24 hours after administration and sclera may appear bluish.
- Advise patient to call promptly if signs and symptoms of myelosuppression develop, such as fever, sore throat, easy bruising, or excessive bleeding.
- Advise patient to use contraception; tell patient to report if pregnancy is suspected.
- Tell patient to drink fluids to minimize uric acid nephropathy.

mivacurium chloride
Mivacron

Pharmacologic classification: nondepolarizing neuromuscular blocker
Therapeutic classification: skeletal muscle relaxant
Pregnancy risk category C

How supplied
Available by prescription only
Injection: 2 mg/ml in 5-ml and 10-ml vials
Infusion: 0.5 mg/ml, in 50 ml D_5W

Indications and dosages
Adjunct to general anesthesia, to facilitate endotracheal intubation, and to provide skeletal muscle relaxation during surgery or mechanical ventilation
Dosage is highly individualized. All times of onset and duration of neuromuscular blockade are averages and considerable individual variation is normal.
Adults: Usually, 0.15 mg/kg I.V. push over 5 to 15 seconds provides adequate muscle relaxation within 2 to 3 minutes for endotracheal intubation. Clinically sufficient neuromuscular blockade usually lasts about 15 to 20 minutes. Alternatively, 0.2 mg/kg over 30 seconds or 0.25 mg/kg in doses of 0.15 mg/kg and 0.1 mg/kg 30 seconds later. Spontaneous recovery

usually occurs in 25 to 35 minutes. Supplemental doses of 0.1 mg/kg I.V. q 15 to 25 minutes usually maintain muscle relaxation. Alternatively, maintain neuromuscular blockade with a continuous infusion of 4 mcg/kg/minute started simultaneously with initial dose, or 9 to 10 mcg/kg/minute started after evidence of spontaneous recovery of initial dose. When used with isoflurane or enflurane anesthesia, dosage is usually reduced about 35% to 40%.
≡ ***Dosage adjustment.*** Infusion rate needs to be reduced by 50% in end-stage renal and liver patients.
Children age 2 to 12: 0.20 mg/kg I.V. push administered over 5 to 15 seconds.

Neuromuscular blockade is usually evident in less than 2 minutes. Although supplemental doses of 0.1 mg/kg I.V. q 15 minutes usually maintain muscle relaxation in adults, maintenance dosages are usually required more frequently in children. Alternatively, maintain neuromuscular blockade with a continuous infusion titrated to effect. Most children respond to 5 to 31 mcg/kg/minute (average, 14 mcg/kg/minute).

Pharmacodynamics

Neuromuscular blocking action: Mivacurium competes with acetylcholine for receptor sites at the motor end-plate. Because this action may be antagonized by cholinesterase inhibitors, mivacurium is considered a competitive antagonist. Drug is a mixture of three stereoisomers, each possessing neuromuscular blocking activity: the cis-trans isomer (36% of the total) and the trans-trans isomer (57% of the total) are about 10 times as potent as the cis-cis isomer (only 6% of the total). The isomers don't interconvert in vivo.

Pharmacokinetics

Absorption: Absorption is rapid.
Distribution: Volume of distribution is small, indicating that drug isn't extensively distributed to tissues.
Metabolism: Rapidly hydrolyzed by plasma pseudocholinesterase to inactive components.
Excretion: Metabolites are excreted in bile and urine. Of the highly active isomers, the cis-trans and trans-trans isomers each have an elimination half-life of less than 2.3 minutes. The less active cis-cis isomer, which is only a small portion of the total drug, has an elimination half-life of 55 minutes.

Route	Onset	Peak	Duration
I.V.	1-2 min	2-5 min	20-35 min

Contraindications and precautions

Contraindicated in patients with hypersensitivity to drug. Use cautiously in patients with significant CV disease, metastatic cancer, severe electrolyte disturbances, or neuromuscular disease; in those who may be adversely affected by the release of histamine; and in those in whom neuromuscular blockade reversibility is difficult, such as patients with myasthenia gravis or myasthenic syndrome. Use with extreme caution in patients with reduced plasma cholinesterase activity; may cause prolonged neuromuscular blockade.

Interactions

Drug-drug. *Alkaline solutions such as barbiturate solutions:* May form a precipitate. Drug shouldn't be administered through the same I.V. line with any of these drugs.
Aminoglycosides (gentamicin, kanamycin, neomycin, streptomycin), bacitracin, colistimethate, colistin, magnesium salts, polymyxin B, or tetracyclines: May result in increased muscle weakness. Patient requires close monitoring.
Carbamazepine and phenytoin: May prolong the time to maximal block or shorten the duration of blockade with neuromuscular blockers. Patient requires close monitoring.
Oral contraceptives, glucocorticosteroids, or MAO inhibitors: Plasma cholinesterase activity may be diminished by chronic use. Patient requires close monitoring.
Quinidine or inhalational anesthetics (especially enflurane, isoflurane): May enhance the activity or prolong action. Patient requires close monitoring.

Effects on diagnostic tests

None reported.

Adverse reactions

CNS: dizziness.
CV: *flushing, tachycardia,* ***bradycardia, arrhythmias,*** *hypotension.*
Musculoskeletal: prolonged muscle weakness, muscle spasms.
Respiratory: ***bronchospasm,*** wheezing, ***respiratory insufficiency or apnea.***
Skin: rash, urticaria, erythema.
Other: phlebitis.

Overdose and treatment

Overdose may result in prolonged neuromuscular blockade. Maintain a patent airway and control respirations until patient recovers neuromuscular function. Antagonists shouldn't be administered until there's some evidence of spontaneous recovery. In clinical trials, administration of 0.03 to 0.064 mg/kg neostigmine methylsulfate or 0.5 mg/kg edrophonium chloride to patients with spontaneous recovery of muscle function resulted in increased muscle strength of about 10% recovery to about 95% recovery within 10 minutes.

Clinical considerations

- When mivacurium is administered I.V. push to adults receiving anesthetic combinations of nitrous oxide and opiates, neuromuscular blockade usually lasts 15 to 20 minutes; most patients recover 95% of muscle strength in 25 to 30 minutes.

- Duration of drug effect is increased about 150% in patients with end-stage renal disease and 300% in patients with hepatic dysfunction.
- Adjust dosage to ideal body weight in obese patients (patients 30% or more above their ideal weight) because of reported prolonged neuromuscular blockade.
- A nerve stimulator and train-of-four monitoring are recommended to document antagonism of neuromuscular blockade and recovery of muscle strength. Before attempting pharmacologic reversal with neostigmine methylsulfate or edrophonium chloride, some evidence of spontaneous recovery should be evident.
- Experimental evidence suggests that acid-base and electrolyte balance may influence actions of and response to nondepolarizing neuromuscular blockers. Alkalosis may counteract paralysis; acidosis may enhance it.
- Mivacurium, like other neuromuscular blockers, doesn't have an effect on consciousness or pain threshold. To avoid patient distress, this drug shouldn't be administered until the patient's consciousness is obtunded by the general anesthetic.
- Drug is compatible with D_5W, normal saline solution injection, dextrose 5% in normal saline solution injection, lactated Ringer's injection, and dextrose 5% in lactated Ringer's injection. Diluted solutions are stable for 24 hours at room temperature.
- When diluted as directed, mivacurium is compatible with alfentanil, fentanyl, sufentanil, droperidol, and midazolam.
- Drug is available as premixed infusion in D_5W. After removing the protective outer wrap, check container for minor leaks by squeezing the bag before administering. Don't add other drugs to the container, and don't use the container in series connections.

Therapeutic monitoring

Recommend monitoring vital signs and respirations until patient is fully recovered from neuromuscular blockade (as evidenced by hand grip, head lift, and ability to cough).

Special populations

Breast-feeding patients. It isn't known if drug is excreted in breast milk. Use with caution in breast-feeding women.

Pediatric patients. As with other neuromuscular blockers, dosage requirements for children are higher on a mg/kg basis as compared with adults. Onset and recovery of neuromuscular blockade occur more rapidly in children.

modafinil

Provigil

Pharmacologic classification: nonamphetamine CNS stimulant
Therapeutic classification: analeptic
Controlled substance schedule IV
Pregnancy risk category C

How supplied

Available by prescription only
Tablets: 100 mg, 200 mg

Indications and dosages

Improvement of wakefulness in patients with excessive daytime sleepiness associated with narcolepsy

Adults: 200 mg P.O. daily, given as a single dose in the morning.

≡ ***Dosage adjustment.*** In patients with severe hepatic impairment, 100 mg P.O. daily, given as a single dose in the morning.

Pharmacodynamics

CNS stimulant action: The exact mechanism of action in which modafinil promotes wakefulness is unknown. Modafinil has wake-promoting actions like sympathomimetic agents including amphetamines, but modafinil is structurally distinct from amphetamines and doesn't appear to alter the release of either dopamine or norepinephrine to produce CNS stimulation.

Pharmacokinetics

Absorption: Absorption is rapid.
Distribution: Well distributed in body tissue and is moderately bound to plasma protein (about 60%), primarily albumin.
Metabolism: Primarily metabolized (about 90%) in the liver, with subsequent renal elimination of the metabolites.
Excretion: Less than 10% is renally excreted as unchanged drug.

Route	Onset	Peak	Duration
P.O.	Unknown	2-4 hr	Unknown

Contraindications and precautions

Contraindicated in patients with known hypersensitivity to drug. Don't use in patients with history of left ventricular hypertrophy or ischemic ECG changes, chest pain, arrhythmias, or other clinically significant manifestations of mitral valve prolapse in association with CNS stimulant use.

Use with caution in patients with recent history of MI or unstable angina and in those with history of psychosis. Use cautiously, and in reduced dosages, in patients with severe hepatic impairment, with or without cirrhosis. Also use cautiously in patients concurrently treated with monoamine oxidase inhibitors and those with a history of psychosis.

Interactions

Drug-drug. *Itraconazole, ketoconazole, or other inhibitors of CYP3A4; carbamazepine, phenobarbital, rifampin, or other inducers of CYP3A4:* Alter levels of modafinil. Patient requires close monitoring.
Cyclosporine, theophylline: Reduced serum levels. Use together cautiously.
Diazepam, phenytoin, propranolol, or other agents metabolized by CYP2C19: Increased serum levels of drugs metabolized by this enzyme. Use together cautiously. Dosage adjustment may be necessary.
Methylphenidate: May delay absorption of modafinil by about 1 hour when administered together. Separate dosage administration times are recommended.
Phenytoin and warfarin: Increased serum levels of these drugs. Monitor patient closely for signs of toxicity.
Steroidal contraceptives: Reduced contraceptive effectiveness. Recommend alternative or concomitant method of contraception during modafinil therapy and for 1 month after drug is discontinued.
Tricyclic antidepressants, such as clomipramine and desipramine: Levels are increased by modafinil. Dosage reduction of these agents may be necessary.

Effects on diagnostic tests

None reported.

Adverse reactions

CNS: *headache,* nervousness, dizziness, syncope, depression, anxiety, cataplexy, insomnia, paresthesia, dyskinesia, hypertonia, confusion, amnesia, emotional lability, ataxia, tremor.
CV: hypotension, hypertension, vasodilation, ***arrhythmias,*** chest pain.
EENT: *rhinitis,* pharyngitis, epistaxis, amblyopia, abnormal vision, mouth ulcer, gingivitis, thirst.
GI: *nausea,* diarrhea, dry mouth, anorexia, vomiting.
GU: abnormal urine, urine retention, abnormal ejaculation, albuminuria.
Hematologic: eosinophilia.
Hepatic: abnormal liver function.
Metabolic: hyperglycemia.
Musculoskeletal: joint disorder, neck pain, rigid neck.
Respiratory: lung disorder, dyspnea, asthma.
Skin: herpes simplex, dry skin.
Other: chills, fever.

Overdose and treatment

No specific antidote to a modafinil overdose exists. In an overdose, initiate supportive care as appropriate, including cardiovascular monitoring. If there are no contraindications, consider induced emesis or gastric lavage. There are no data to suggest the utility of dialysis or urinary acidification or alkalinization in enhancing drug elimination.

Clinical considerations

- Safety and efficacy of dosage in patients with severe renal impairment haven't been determined.
- Although dosages of 400 mg daily as a single dose have been well tolerated, there's no consistent evidence that this dosage confers additional benefit beyond the 200-mg dose.
- Even though food has no effect on overall bioavailability, the absorption of modafinil may be delayed by about 1 hour if given with food.

Therapeutic monitoring

- Monitor patient for misuse or abuse.
- Monitor LFTs before and during drug therapy.

Special populations

Breast-feeding patients. It isn't known if modafinil is excreted in breast milk. Because many drugs are excreted in breast milk, administer modafinil cautiously to a breast-feeding woman.
Pediatric patients. Safety and efficacy in patients under age 16 haven't been established.
Geriatric patients. Safety and efficacy in patients over age 65 haven't been established. In geriatric patients, a lower dosage may be considered because elimination of drug and its metabolites may be reduced.

Patient counseling

- Advise female patient to notify physician if she becomes pregnant or intends to become pregnant during therapy.
- Caution patient regarding the potential increased risk of pregnancy when using steroidal contraceptives (including depot or implantable contraceptives) with modafinil tablets. Recommend alternative or concomitant method of contraception during modafinil therapy and for 1 month after drug is discontinued.
- Advise female patient to notify doctor if breast-feeding an infant.
- Instruct patient to avoid taking any prescription or OTC drugs before consulting with her health care provider because of the potential for interactions between modafinil and other drugs.
- Advise patient to avoid alcohol while taking modafinil.
- Tell patient to notify doctor if he develops a rash, hives, or a related allergic reaction.
- Modafinil may impair judgment. Advise patient to use caution while driving or during other activities requiring alertness until effects are known.

moexipril hydrochloride

Univasc

Pharmacologic classification: ACE inhibitor
Therapeutic classification: antihypertensive
Pregnancy risk category C (D second and third trimesters)

How supplied

Available by prescription only
Tablets: 7.5 mg, 15 mg

Indications and dosages

Hypertension

Adults: Initially, 7.5 mg P.O. once daily before meals for patients not receiving diuretics. If control isn't adequate, dose can be increased or divided dosing may be attempted. Recommended dosage range is 7.5 to 30 mg daily, administered in one or two divided doses 1 hour before meals. For patients receiving diuretics, give 3.75 mg P.O. once daily before meals. Make subsequent dosage adjustments according to blood pressure response.

≡ ***Dosage adjustment.*** If creatinine clearance is 40 ml/min per 1.73 m^2 or less, start dose at 3.75 mg P.O. daily, and adjust dose to a maximum of 15 mg daily. If concomitant diuretic therapy is needed, a loop diuretic is preferred.

Pharmacodynamics

Antihypertensive action: Exact mechanism is unknown. The action of moexipril is thought to result primarily from suppression of the renin-angiotensin-aldosterone system. A metabolite of moexipril, moexiprilat, inhibits angiotensin-converting enzymes (ACE) and thereby inhibits the production of angiotensin II (a potent vasoconstrictor and stimulator of aldosterone secretion). Other mechanisms may also be involved.

Pharmacokinetics

Absorption: Incompletely absorbed from the GI tract with a bioavailability of about 13%. Food significantly decreases bioavailability of drug.
Distribution: Metabolite is about 50% protein-bound.
Metabolism: Metabolized extensively to the active metabolite, moexiprilat.
Excretion: Excreted primarily in feces with a small amount being excreted in urine. Half-life of drug is over 2 to 9 hours.

Route	Onset	Peak	Duration
P.O.	½ hr	2-3 hr	2-5 days

Contraindications and precautions

Contraindicated in patients with hypersensitivity to drug, history of angioedema related to previous treatment with an ACE inhibitor, and during pregnancy. Use cautiously in patients with impaired renal function, heart failure, or renal artery stenosis and in breast-feeding women.

Interactions

Drug-drug. *Diuretics:* Increased risk of excessive hypotension.. Diuretic or lower dose of moexipril may be necessary.
Lithium: Lithium toxicity. Avoid use together.
Potassium-sparing diuretics, potassium supplements: Increased risk of hyperkalemia. Monitor serum potassium closely.
Drug-food. *Sodium substitutes containing potassium:* Increased risk of hyperkalemia. Monitor serum potassium closely.

Effects on diagnostic tests

None reported.

Adverse reactions

CNS: *dizziness,* headache, fatigue.
CV: peripheral edema, hypotension, orthostatic hypotension, chest pain, flushing.
EENT: pharyngitis, rhinitis, sinusitis.
GI: diarrhea, dyspepsia, nausea.
GU: urinary frequency.
Hematologic: ***neutropenia.***
Metabolic: hyperkalemia.
Musculoskeletal: myalgia.
Respiratory: *dry, persistent, tickling, nonproductive cough;* upper respiratory tract infection.
Skin: rash.
Other: ***anaphylactoid reactions, angioedema,*** flu syndrome, pain.

Overdose and treatment

Although no information is available on overdose of moexipril, it's believed that signs and symptoms would be similar to those of other ACE inhibitors with hypotension being the principal adverse reaction. Because the hypotensive effect of moexipril is achieved through vasodilation and effective hypovolemia, it's reasonable to treat moexipril overdose by infusion of normal saline solution. In addition, renal function and serum potassium should be monitored.

Clinical considerations

- Because angioedema associated with involvement of the tongue, glottis, or larynx may cause a fatal airway obstruction, have appropriate therapy, such as S.C. epinephrine 1:1,000 (0.3 to 0.5 ml) available as well as equipment to ensure a patent airway.
- In patients undergoing major surgery or anesthesia with agents that produce hypotension, moexipril may block the compensatory renin release. Hypotension can be treated with volume expansion.

Therapeutic monitoring

- Patient requires monitoring for hypotension. Excessive hypotension can occur when drug is given with diuretics. Diuretic therapy may be discontinued 2 to 3 days before starting moexipril to decrease potential for excessive hypotensive response. If drug doesn't adequately control blood pressure, diuretic therapy may be restarted with caution.
- Recommend measuring blood pressure at trough (just before a dose) to verify adequate blood pressure control. Be aware that drug is less effective in reducing trough blood pressures in blacks than in nonblacks.
- Renal function must be assessed before treatment and periodically throughout therapy. Monitor serum potassium levels.
- Other ACE inhibitors have been associated with agranulocytosis and neutropenia. Monitor CBC with differential counts before therapy, especially in patients who have collagen vascular disease with impaired renal function.

Special populations

Breast-feeding patients. It isn't known if drug is excreted in breast milk; use with caution in breast-feeding women.
Pediatric patients. Safety and efficacy in children haven't been established.

Patient counseling

- Instruct patient to take drug on an empty stomach; meals, particularly those high in fat, can impair absorption.
- Tell patient to avoid sodium substitutes; these products may contain potassium, which can cause hyperkalemia in patients taking this drug.
- Inform patient that light-headedness can occur, especially during the first few days of therapy. Tell him to rise slowly to minimize this effect and to report symptoms. If fainting occurs, tell patient to stop drug and call immediately.
- Instruct patient to use caution in hot weather and during exercise. Inadequate fluid intake, vomiting, diarrhea, and excessive perspiration can lead to light-headedness and syncope.
- Advise patient to report signs of infection, such as fever and sore throat. Also tell patient to report the following signs or symptoms: easy bruising or bleeding; swelling of tongue, lips, face, eyes, mucous membranes, or extremities; difficulty swallowing or breathing; and hoarseness.
- Tell female patient to report suspected pregnancy immediately. Drug will need to be discontinued.

molindone hydrochloride

Moban

Pharmacologic classification: dihydroindolone
Therapeutic classification: antipsychotic
Pregnancy risk category NR

How supplied

Available by prescription only
Tablets: 5 mg, 10 mg, 25 mg, 50 mg, 100 mg
Oral concentrate: 20 mg/ml

Indications and dosages

Psychotic disorders
Adults: 50 to 75 mg P.O. daily in 3 to 4 divided doses, increased 100 mg daily in 3 to 4 days to a maximum of 225 mg daily. Maintenance dosage for mild disease is 5 to 15 mg t.i.d. or q.i.d., moderate disease is 10 to 25 mg t.i.d. or q.i.d., and severe disease is up to 225 mg daily.
◇ ***Behavioral complications associated with mental retardation, mentally retarded schizophrenic child***
Children age 3 to 5: 1 to 2.5 mg P.O. daily as a single dose.

Pharmacodynamics

Antipsychotic action: Molindone is unrelated to all other antipsychotic drugs; it's thought to exert its antipsychotic effects by postsynaptic blockade of CNS dopamine receptors, thereby inhibiting dopamine-mediated effects.

Molindone has many other central and peripheral effects; it also produces alpha and ganglionic blockade. Its most prominent adverse reactions are extrapyramidal.

Pharmacokinetics

Absorption: Data are limited, but absorption appears rapid.
Distribution: Distributed widely into the body.
Metabolism: Metabolized extensively.
Excretion: Most of drug is excreted as metabolites in urine; some is excreted in feces by way of the biliary tract. Overall, 90% of a given dose is excreted within 24 hours.

Route	Onset	Peak	Duration
P.O.	Unknown	1½ hr	24-36 hr

Contraindications and precautions

Contraindicated in patients with hypersensitivity to drug and in those experiencing coma or severe CNS depression. Use cautiously in patients at risk for seizures or when high physical activity is harmful to patient.

Interactions

Drug-drug. *Antiarrhythmic agents, disopyramide, procainamide, or quinidine:* Increased

incidence of arrhythmias and conduction defects. Avoid use together.
Centrally acting antihypertensive drugs, such as clonidine, guanabenz, guanadrel, guanethidine, methyldopa, and reserpine: Mesoridazine may inhibit blood pressure response to these drugs. Blood pressure should be monitored carefully.
Atropine and other anticholinergic drugs, including antidepressants, antihistamines, MAO inhibitors, meperidine, phenothiazines, and antiparkinson agents: Oversedation, paralytic ileus, visual changes, and severe constipation. Use together cautiously.
Beta blockers: May inhibit molindone metabolism, increasing plasma levels and toxicity. Monitor patient for toxicity.
Bromocriptine: Molindone may antagonize therapeutic effect of bromocriptine on prolactin secretion. Use together cautiously.
CNS depressants, including analgesics, barbiturates, opioids, tranquilizers, and general, spinal, or epidural anesthetics, or parenteral magnesium sulfate: Oversedation, respiratory depression, and hypotension. Avoid use together.
High-dose dopamine: Decreased vasoconstricting effects. Monitor patient for clinical effects.
Levodopa: Decreased effectiveness and increased toxicity of levodopa. Use together cautiously.
Metrizamide: Increased risk of seizures. Use together cautiously.
Nitrates: Hypotension. Recommend monitoring blood pressure.
Phenytoin and tetracycline: Molindone may inhibit absorption. Patient requires careful monitoring.
Propylthiouracil: Increased risk of agranulocytosis. Monitor hematopoietic studies.
Sympathomimetics, including epinephrine, ephedrine (often found in nasal sprays), phenylephrine, phenylpropanolamine, or appetite suppressants: May decrease their stimulatory and pressor effects. Use together cautiously.
Drug-lifestyle. *Alcohol use:* Additive effects. Avoid use together.
Sun exposure: Increased risk of photosensitivity reactions. Recommend patient use sunscreen and avoid excessive exposure to the sun.

Effects on diagnostic tests
Drug causes false-positive results in urine pregnancy tests using human chorionic gonadotropin and has additive potential for causing seizures with metrizamide myelography.

Adverse reactions
CNS: *extrapyramidal reactions, tardive dyskinesia, sedation, drowsiness, depression, euphoria, pseudoparkinsonism, EEG changes, dizziness.*
CV: *orthostatic hypotension, tachycardia, ECG changes.*
EENT: *blurred vision.*
GI: *dry mouth, constipation, nausea.*
GU: *urine retention, menstrual irregularities, gynecomastia, inhibited ejaculation.*
Hematologic: ***leukopenia,*** leukocytosis.
Hepatic: jaundice, abnormal liver function test results.
Skin: *mild photosensitivity,* ***allergic reactions.***
Other: ***neuroleptic malignant syndrome*** (rare).

Overdose and treatment
CNS depression is characterized by deep, unarousable sleep and possible coma, hypotension or hypertension, extrapyramidal symptoms, abnormal involuntary muscle movements, agitation, seizures, arrhythmias, ECG changes, hypothermia or hyperthermia, and autonomic nervous system dysfunction.

Treatment is symptomatic and supportive, including maintaining vital signs, airway, stable body temperature, and fluid-electrolyte balance.

Don't induce vomiting; drug inhibits cough reflex, and aspiration may occur. Use gastric lavage, then activated charcoal and saline cathartics; dialysis doesn't help. Regulate body temperature as needed. Treat hypotension with I.V. fluids; don't give epinephrine. Treat seizures with parenteral diazepam or barbiturates; arrhythmias, with parenteral phenytoin; extrapyramidal reactions, with benztropine at 1 to 2 mg or parenteral diphenhydramine at 10 to 50 mg.

Clinical considerations
- Some commercial preparations contain sodium metabisulfite, which may cause severe allergic reaction in susceptible individuals.
- Drug may cause GI distress and should be administered with food or fluids.
- Dilute concentrate in 2 to 4 oz of liquid, preferably soup, water, juice, carbonated drinks, milk, or puddings.
- Drug may cause pink to brown discoloration of urine.
- Protect liquid form from light and store at 59° to 86° F (15° to 30° C).

Therapeutic monitoring
- Monitor for CNS adverse effects, especially drowsiness and extrapyramidal symptoms.
- Monitor CBC and LFTs in long-term therapy.

Special populations
Pediatric patients. Drug isn't recommended for children under age 12.
Geriatric patients. Lower doses are recommended; 30% to 50% of usual dose may be effective. Geriatric patients are at greater risk for tardive dyskinesia and other extrapyramidal effects.

Patient counseling

- Explain risks of dystonic reaction and tardive dyskinesia to patient and advise him to report abnormal body movements.
- Warn patient to avoid spilling liquid preparation on the skin; rash and irritation may result.
- Advise patient to avoid temperature extremes (hot or cold baths, sunlamps, or tanning beds) because drug may cause thermoregulatory changes.
- Suggest sugarless gum or candy, ice chips, or artificial saliva to relieve dry mouth.
- Warn patient not to take drug with antacids or antidiarrheals; not to drink alcoholic beverages or take other drugs that cause sedation; not to stop taking drug or take any other drug except as instructed; and to take drug exactly as prescribed, without doubling after missing a dose.
- Warn patient about sedative effect. Tell him to report difficult urination, sore throat, dizziness, or fainting.
- Advise patient to get up slowly from a recumbent or seated position to minimize effects of light-headedness.
- Tell patient that drug may contain sodium metabisulfite, which can cause an allergic reaction to those with a sulfite allergy.

montelukast sodium

Singulair

Pharmacologic classification: leukotriene receptor antagonist
Therapeutic classification: antiasthmatic
Pregnancy risk category B

How supplied

Available by prescription only
Tablets: 10 mg
Tablets (chewable): 5 mg

Indications and dosages

For prophylaxis and chronic treatment of asthma

Adults and adolescents: 10 mg P.O. once daily in evening.
Children age 6 to 14: 5 mg (chewable tablet) P.O. once daily in the evening.

Pharmacodynamics

Antiasthmatic action: Montelukast causes inhibition of airway cysteinyl leukotriene receptors. Drug binds with high affinity and selectivity to the $cysLT_1$ receptor, and inhibits the physiologic action of the cysteinyl leukotriene LTD_4. This receptor inhibition reduces early- and late-phase bronchoconstriction resulting from antigen challenge.

Pharmacokinetics

Absorption: Rapidly absorbed after oral administration with mean oral bioavailability of 64%. Food doesn't affect absorption of drug. For chewable tablet, mean oral bioavailability is 73%.
Distribution: Minimally distributed to the tissues with a steady-state volume of distribution of 8 to 11 L. Over 99% is bound to plasma proteins.
Metabolism: Extensively metabolized, but plasma levels of metabolites at therapeutic doses are undetectable. In vitro studies with human liver microsomes demonstrate metabolism involvement by cytochromes P-450 3A4 and 2C9.
Excretion: About 86% of an oral dose is metabolized and excreted in the feces, indicating drug and its metabolites are excreted almost exclusively in the bile. Half-life is 2¾ to 5½ hours.

Route	Onset	Peak	Duration
P.O. (film-coated)	Unknown	3-4 hr	Unknown
P.O. (chewable)	Unknown	2-2½ hr	Unknown

Contraindications and precautions

Contraindicated in patients with hypersensitivity to drug or its components. Also contraindicated in patients with acute asthmatic attacks or status asthmaticus. Although airway function is improved in patients with known aspirin hypersensitivity, these patients should avoid aspirin and NSAIDs.

Interactions

Drug-drug. *Phenobarbital, rifampin:* Increased metabolism of drug. Patient requires close monitoring.

Effects on diagnostic tests

None reported.

Adverse reactions

CNS: *headache,* dizziness, fatigue, asthenia.
EENT: nasal congestion, dental pain.
GI: dyspepsia, infectious gastroenteritis, abdominal pain.
Respiratory: cough, influenza.
Skin: rash.
Other: fever, trauma.

Overdose and treatment

No information is available on treatment of drug overdose. Provide supportive measures for overdose such as removal of unabsorbed material from the GI tract and clinical monitoring.

Clinical considerations

- Although dose of inhaled corticosteroids may be reduced gradually, montelukast shouldn't be abruptly substituted for inhaled or oral corticosteroids.

- Drug shouldn't be used as monotherapy for management of exercise-induced bronchospasm.
- No added benefit is achieved with doses above 10 mg daily.

Therapeutic monitoring

Monitor patient for worsening asthmatic symptoms.

Special populations

Breast-feeding patients. It isn't known if drug is excreted in breast milk. Use cautiously in breast-feeding women.
Pediatric patients. Safety and efficacy in children under age 6 haven't been established.
Geriatric patients. No difference in safety and effectiveness of drug has been reported between geriatric and younger patient populations.

Patient counseling

- Advise patient to take drug daily, even if asymptomatic, and to contact doctor if asthma isn't well controlled.
- Warn patient that drug isn't beneficial in acute asthma attacks, or in exercise-induced bronchospasm, and advise him to keep appropriate rescue medications available.
- Advise patient with known aspirin sensitivity not to take aspirin and NSAIDs.
- Warn patient with phenylketonuria that chewable tablet contains phenylalanine, a component of aspartame.
- Advise patients to seek medical attention if short-acting bronchodilators are needed more often than usual or prescribed.

moricizine hydrochloride

Ethmozine

Pharmacologic classification: sodium channel blocker
Therapeutic classification: antiarrhythmic
Pregnancy risk category B

How supplied

Available by prescription only
Tablets: 200 mg, 250 mg, 300 mg

Indications and dosages

Treatment of documented, life-threatening ventricular arrhythmias when benefit of treatment outweighs risks
Adults: Dosage must be individualized. Usual range is 600 to 900 mg P.O. daily, given q 8 hours in equally divided doses. Dosage may be adjusted within this range in increments of 150 mg daily at 3-day intervals until desired effect is obtained. Hospitalization is recommended for initiation of therapy because patient will be at high risk. Patients whose arrhythmias are well controlled during q 8-hour dosing may receive the same dose daily, divided q 12 hours to increase compliance.
≡ ***Dosage adjustment.*** For patients with hepatic impairment and significant renal dysfunction, give 600 mg or less daily. Monitor ECG before increasing dose.

Pharmacodynamics

Antiarrhythmic action: Although moricizine is chemically related to the neuroleptic phenothiazines, it has no demonstrated dopaminergic activities. It does have potent local anesthetic activity and myocardial membrane-stabilizing effects. A Class I antiarrhythmic agent, it reduces the fast inward current carried by sodium ions. In patients with ventricular tachycardia, moricizine prolongs AV conduction but has no significant effect on ventricular repolarization. Intra-atrial conduction or atrial effective refractory periods aren't consistently affected and moricizine has minimal effect on sinus cycle length and sinus node recovery time. This may be significant in patients with sinus node dysfunction.

In patients with impaired left ventricular function, moricizine has minimal effects on measurements of cardiac performance: cardiac index, stroke volume, pulmonary artery wedge pressure, systemic or pulmonary vascular resistance, and ejection fraction either at rest or during exercise. A small but consistent increase in resting blood pressure and heart rate are seen. Moricizine has no effect on exercise tolerance in patients with ventricular arrhythmias, heart failure, or angina pectoris.

Moricizine has antiarrhythmic activity similar to that of disopyramide, propranolol, and quinidine. Arrhythmia "rebound" isn't noted after discontinuation of therapy.

Pharmacokinetics

Absorption: Administration within 30 minutes of mealtime delays absorption and lowers peak plasma levels but has no effect on extent of absorption.
Distribution: 95% plasma protein-bound.
Metabolism: Undergoes significant first-pass metabolism resulting in an absolute bioavailability of about 38%. At least 26 metabolites have been identified with no single one representing at least 1% of the administered dose. It has been shown to induce its own metabolism.
Excretion: About 56% is excreted in feces, 39% in urine; some is also recycled through enterohepatic circulation.

Route	Onset	Peak	Duration
P.O.	2 hr	½-2 hr	10-24 hr

Contraindications and precautions

Contraindicated in patients with cardiogenic shock and in those with hypersensitivity to drug, preexisting second- or third-degree AV block or right bundle branch block when associated with left hemiblock (bifascicular block), unless an artificial pacemaker is present. Discontinue breast-feeding or drug because drug is excreted in breast milk.

Use cautiously in patients with impaired renal or hepatic function, sick sinus syndrome, coronary artery disease, or left ventricular function.

Interactions

Drug-drug. *Cimetidine:* Decreased moricizine clearance by 49% when used together; no significant changes in efficacy or tolerance have been observed. Patients should receive decreased doses of cimetidine (not more than 600 mg/day).
Digoxin: Prolongs the PR interval. Patient requires careful monitoring.
Propranolol: May produce a small additive increase in the PR interval. Monitor patient carefully.
Theophylline: Theophylline clearance increases and plasma half-life decreases. Monitor theophylline levels.

Effects on diagnostic tests

None reported.

Adverse reactions

CNS: *dizziness, headache, fatigue,* hyperesthesia, anxiety, asthenia, nervousness, paresthesia, sleep disorders.
CV: ***proarrhythmic events (ventricular tachycardia, premature ventricular contractions, supraventricular arrhythmias),*** ECG abnormalities (including *conduction defects, sinus pause, junctional rhythm,* or ***AV block***), ***heart failure,*** palpitations, chest pain, ***cardiac death,*** hypotension, hypertension, vasodilation, cerebrovascular events.
EENT: blurred vision.
GI: *nausea, vomiting, abdominal pain, dyspepsia, diarrhea, dry mouth.*
GU: urine retention, urinary frequency, dysuria.
Musculoskeletal: musculoskeletal pain.
Respiratory: dyspnea.
Skin: diaphoresis, rash.
Other: drug-induced fever, thrombophlebitis.

Overdose and treatment

Symptoms of overdose include emesis, lethargy, coma, syncope, hypotension, conduction disturbances, exacerbation of heart failure, MI, sinus arrest, arrhythmias, and respiratory failure. No specific antidote has been identified.

Treatment should be supportive and include careful monitoring of cardiac, respiratory, and CNS changes. Gastric evacuation with care to avoid aspiration may be used as well.

Clinical considerations

- When switching from another antiarrhythmic to moricizine, withdraw previous therapy one to two half-lives before starting moricizine. Initiate moricizine 6 to 12 hours after last dose of quinidine and disopyramide; 3 to 6 hours after last dose of procainamide; 8 to 12 after encainide, propaferone, tocainide, or mexiletine; and 12 to 24 hours after flecainide.
- Initial dose for patients with renal or hepatic impairment is 600 mg daily or lower. Monitor patient (with ECG) before making dosage adjustments.

Therapeutic monitoring

- Electrolyte imbalances should be corrected before starting therapy; hypokalemia, hyperkalemia, or hypomagnesemia may alter effects of drug.
- Monitor patient for increased dizziness and nausea with 12-hour dosing.

Special populations

Breast-feeding patients. Excreted in breast milk. Because of the potential for adverse reactions in the breast-fed infant, a decision whether to continue therapy must be made.
Pediatric patients. Safety and efficacy in children haven't been established.

Patient teaching

Instruct patient to take drug as prescribed to maintain adequate arrhythmia control.

morphine hydrochloride*

Morphitec*, M.O.S.*

morphine sulfate

Astramorph PF, Duramorph, Epimorph*, Infumorph, MS Contin, MSIR, MS/L, MS/S, OMS Concentrate, Oramorph SR, RMS Uniserts, Roxanol, Statex*

Pharmacologic classification: opioid
Therapeutic classification: narcotic analgesic
Controlled substance schedule II
Pregnancy risk category C

How supplied

Available by prescription only
morphine hydrochloride*
Tablets: 10 mg, 20 mg, 40 mg, 60 mg
Syrup: 1 mg/ml, 5 mg/ml, 10 mg/ml, 20 mg/ml, 50 mg/ml
Suppositories: 20 mg, 30 mg
morphine sulfate
Tablets: 15 mg, 30 mg
Tablets (extended-release): 15 mg, 30 mg, 60 mg, 100 mg
Tablets (soluble): 10 mg, 15 mg, 30 mg

Capsules: 15 mg, 30 mg
Oral solution: 10 mg/5 ml, 20 mg/5 ml, 20 mg/ml, 100 mg/5 ml
Injection (with preservative): 1 mg/ml, 2 mg/ml, 3 mg/ml, 4 mg/ml, 5 mg/ml, 8 mg/ml, 10 mg/ml, 15 mg/ml, 25 mg/ml, 50 mg/ml
Injection (without preservative): 500 mcg/ml, 1 mg/ml, 10 mg/ml, 15 mg/ml, 25 mg/ml
Suppositories: 5 mg, 10 mg, 20 mg, 30 mg

Indications and dosages

Severe pain
Adults: 10 mg q 4 hours S.C. or I.M., or 10 to 30 mg P.O., or 10 to 20 mg P.R. q 4 hours, p.r.n., or around the clock. May be injected slow I.V. (over 4 to 5 minutes) 2.5 to 15 mg diluted in 4 to 5 ml water for injection. May also administer controlled-release tablets 15 to 30 mg q 12 hours. As an intermittent epidural injection, 5 mg via an epidural catheter q 24 hours. For continuous epidural infusion (device not implanted surgically), initial dose is 2.4 mg per 24 hours. May increase 1 to 2 mg daily, as needed. For a surgically implanted device, 3.5 to 7.5 mg daily or 4.5 to 10 mg daily if opiate tolerant. Intrathecal dose is one-tenth epidural dose, 0.2 to 1 mg may provide adequate relief in patients not tolerant to opiates.
Children: 0.1 to 0.2 mg/kg S.C. or I.M. q 4 hours. Maximum dose is 15 mg. May also give 0.05 to 0.1 mg/kg I.V. very slowly. In some situations, morphine may be administered by continuous I.V. infusion or by intraspinal and intrathecal injection.
Severe chronic pain associated with cancer
Adults: Initial loading dose of 15 mg followed by 0.8 to 10 mg /hour continuous I.V. or ◇S.C. infusion. Titrate to effect.
Children: 0.025 to 2.6 mg/kg/hour by I.V. infusion or 0.025 to 1.79 mg/kg/hour by ◇S.C. infusion.
Preoperative sedation and adjunct to anesthesia
Adults: 8 to 10 mg I.M., S.C., or I.V.
Postoperative analgesia
Children: 0.01 to 0.04 mg/kg/hour by continuous I.V. infusion.
◇0.015 to 0.02 mg/kg/hour by continuous IV infusion.
Control of pain associated with acute MI
Adults: Initially, 2 to 15 mg I.M., S.C., or I.V. Additional doses of 1 to 4 mg I.V. may be given q 5 minutes, p.r.n.
Control of angina pain
Adults: 2 to 5 mg I.V. q 5 to 30 minutes, p.r.n., in pain unrelieved by three doses of sublingual nitroglycerin.
Adjunctive treatment of acute pulmonary edema
Adults: 10 to 15 mg I.V. at a rate not exceeding 2 mg/minute.
Analgesia during labor
Adults: 10 mg I.M. or S.C.

Pharmacodynamics

Analgesic action: Morphine is the principal opium alkaloid, the standard for opiate agonist analgesic activity. Mechanism of action is thought to be via the opiate receptors, altering patient's perception of pain. Morphine is particularly useful in severe, acute pain or severe, chronic pain. Morphine also has a central depressant effect on respiration and on the cough reflex center.

Pharmacokinetics

Absorption: Variable absorption is from the GI tract.
Distribution: Distributed widely through the body.
Metabolism: Metabolized primarily in the liver. One metabolite, morphine 6-glucuromide, is active.
Excretion: Excreted in the urine and bile. Morphine 6-glucuromide may accumulate after continuous dosing in patients with renal failure, leading to enhanced and prolonged opiate activity.

Route	Onset	Peak	Duration
P.O.	1 hr	1-2 hr	4-12 hr
I.V.	5 min	20 min	4-5 hr
I.M.	10-30 min	30-60 min	4-5 hr
S.C.	10-30 min	50-90 min	4-5 hr
P.R.	20-30 min	20-60 min	4-5 hr
Epidural	15-60 min	15-60 min	24 hr
Intrathecal	15-60 min	30-60 min	24 hr

Contraindications and precautions

Contraindicated in patients with hypersensitivity to drug or conditions that would preclude administration of opioids by I.V. route (acute bronchial asthma or upper airway obstruction).

Use cautiously in geriatric or debilitated patients and in those with head injury, increased intracranial pressure, seizures, pulmonary disease, prostatic hyperplasia, hepatic or renal disease, acute abdominal conditions, hypothyroidism, Addison's disease, or urethral strictures.

Interactions

Drug-drug. *General anesthetics:* Severe CV depression may result. Use together cautiously.
Anticholinergics: May cause paralytic ileus. Monitor patient carefully.
Cimetidine: Increased respiratory and CNS depression. Reduced dosage of morphine is usually necessary.
Other CNS depressants, such as narcotic analgesics, general anesthetics, antihistamines, barbiturates, benzodiazepines, MAO inhibitors, muscle relaxants, phenothiazines, sedative-hypnotics, and tricyclic antidepressants: Potentiate respiratory and CNS depression, sedation, and hypotensive effects of drug. Use together cautiously.

Narcotic antagonist: Patients who become physically dependent on this drug may experience acute withdrawal syndrome if given a narcotic antagonist. Avoid use together.
Drug-lifestyle. *Alcohol use:* Potentiates effects of drug. Avoid use together.

Effects on diagnostic tests
None reported.

Adverse reactions
CNS: *sedation, somnolence, clouded sensorium, euphoria,* ***seizures*** (with large doses), *dizziness, nightmares (with long-acting oral forms),* light-headedness, hallucinations, nervousness, depression, syncope.
CV: *hypotension,* ***bradycardia, shock, cardiac arrest,*** tachycardia, hypertension.
GI: *nausea, vomiting, constipation, ileus, dry mouth, biliary tract spasms, anorexia,* increases plasma amylase levels.
GU: *urine retention, decreased libido.*
Hematologic: ***thrombocytopenia.***
Respiratory: ***respiratory depression, apnea, respiratory arrest.***
Skin: pruritus, skin flushing (with epidural administration); *diaphoresis; edema.*
Other: *physical dependence.*

Overdose and treatment
Rapid I.V. administration may result in overdose because of the delay in maximum CNS effect (30 minutes). The most common signs and symptoms of morphine overdose is respiratory depression with or without CNS depression, and miosis (pinpoint pupils). Other acute toxic effects include hypotension, bradycardia, hypothermia, shock, apnea, cardiopulmonary arrest, circulatory collapse, pulmonary edema, and seizures.

To treat acute overdose, first establish adequate respiratory exchange by way of a patent airway and ventilation, as needed; administer a narcotic antagonist (naloxone) to reverse respiratory depression. (Because duration of action of morphine is longer than that of naloxone, repeated naloxone dosing is necessary.) Naloxone shouldn't be given in the absence of clinically significant respiratory or CV depression. Monitor vital signs closely.

If patient is seen within 2 hours of ingestion of an oral overdose, empty the stomach immediately by inducing emesis (ipecac syrup) or using gastric lavage. Use caution to avoid risk of aspiration. Administer activated charcoal via nasogastric tube for further removal of drug in an oral overdose.

Provide symptomatic and supportive treatment (continued respiratory support, correction of fluid or electrolyte imbalance). Monitor laboratory parameters, vital signs, and neurologic status closely.

Clinical considerations
Consider the recommendations relevant to all opioids as well as the following:

□ ***ALERT*** Don't confuse morphine with hydromorphone. Teach patient not to crush extended-release tablets.

- Morphine is the drug of choice in relieving pain of MI; it may cause transient decrease in blood pressure.
- Regimented scheduling (around-the-clock) is beneficial in severe, chronic pain.
- Oral solutions of various levels are available, as well as a new intensified oral solution.
- There's a greater fluctuation in pain control with extended-release preparations.
- Note the disparity between oral and parenteral doses.

□ ***ALERT*** For continuous epidural or intrathecal infusion, morphine is administered via a controlled-infusion device. Take care when refilling the reservoir of such devices to ensure that medication is instilled into the proper port. A technical error could result in life-threatening respiratory depression.

- Morphine sulfate 10 or 25 mg/ml injections are intended for use with continuous, controlled microinfusion devices.
- For I.V. administration, morphine 25 mg/ml is diluted to a concentration of 0.1 to 1 mg/ml in 5% dextrose. A higher concentration may be used for patients with a fluid restriction.
- Long-term therapy in patients with advanced renal disease may lead to toxicity as a result of accumulation of the active metabolite.
- Some morphine injections contain sulfites which may cause allergic-type reactions.
- For S.L. administration, measure oral solution with tuberculin syringe, and administer dose a few drops at a time to allow maximal sublingual absorption and to minimize swallowing.
- Refrigeration of rectal suppositories isn't necessary. In some patients, rectal and oral absorption may not be equivalent.
- Preservative-free preparations are available for epidural and intrathecal administration. The use of the epidural route is increasing.
- Morphine may worsen or mask gallbladder pain.

Therapeutic monitoring
- Epidural morphine has proven to be an excellent analgesic for patients with postoperative pain. After epidural administration, monitor closely for respiratory depression up to 24 hours after the injection. Check respiratory rate and depth according to protocol (such as every 15 minutes for 2 hours, then hourly for 18 hours). Some clinicians advocate a dilute naloxone infusion of 5 to 10 mcg/kg/hour during the first 12 hours to minimize respiratory depression without altering pain relief.
- Careful monitoring of patient's vital signs during morphine administration is needed.

Special populations
Breast-feeding patients. Morphine is excreted in breast milk. A woman should wait 2 to 3 hours after last dose before breast-feeding to avoid sedating the infant.
Pediatric patients. Safety and efficacy of epidural and intrathecal dosing in children haven't been established. Safety and efficacy of morphine use in neonates haven't been established. Children may be more sensitive to opiates on a body-weight basis.
Geriatric patients. Lower doses are usually indicated for geriatric patients, who may be more sensitive to the therapeutic and adverse effects of drug.

Patient counseling
- Tell patient that oral liquid form of morphine may be mixed with a glass of fruit juice immediately before it's taken, if desired, to improve the taste.
- Tell patient taking long-acting morphine tablets to swallow them whole. Tablets shouldn't be broken, crushed, or chewed before swallowing.

mumps virus vaccine, live
Mumpsvax

Pharmacologic classification: vaccine
Therapeutic classification: viral vaccine
Pregnancy risk category C

How supplied
Available by prescription only
Injection: single-dose vial containing not less than 20,000 $TCID_{50}$ (tissue culture infective doses) of attenuated mumps virus derived from Jeryl Lynn mumps strain (grown in chick embryo culture) and vial of diluent

Indications and dosages
Immunization
Adults and children over age 1: 1 vial (0.5 ml) S.C. in outer aspect of the upper arm.

Pharmacodynamics
Mumps prophylactic action: Vaccine promotes active immunity to mumps.

Pharmacokinetics
Absorption: Antibodies usually are evident 2 to 3 weeks after injection. Duration of vaccine-induced immunity is at least 20 years and probably lifelong.
Distribution: No information available.
Metabolism: No information available.
Excretion: No information available.

Route	Onset	Peak	Duration
S.C.	Unknown	Unknown	> 15 yr

Contraindications and precautions
Contraindicated in immunosuppressed patients; in those with cancer, blood dyscrasias, gamma globulin disorders, fever, untreated active tuberculosis, or anaphylactic or anaphylactoid reactions to neomycin or eggs; in those receiving corticosteroid or radiation therapy; and in pregnant women.

Interactions
Drug-drug. *Immune serum globulin or transfusions of blood or blood products:* May interfere with immune response to vaccine. If possible, defer vaccination for 3 months in these situations.
Immunosuppressive agents: May interfere with response to vaccine. Avoid use together.

Effects on diagnostic tests
Vaccine temporarily may decrease the response to tuberculin skin testing. If a tuberculin skin test is necessary, administer it either before or simultaneously with mumps vaccine.

Adverse reactions
CNS: *malaise, **febrile seizures*** (rare).
GI: *diarrhea.*
Skin: *rash.*
Other: *slight fever, mild allergic reactions, mild lymphadenopathy, injection-site reaction.*

Overdose and treatment
No information available.

Clinical considerations
- Mumps vaccine shouldn't be used in delayed hypersensitivity (anergy) skin testing.
- Obtain a thorough history of patient's allergies, especially to antibiotics, eggs, chicken, or chicken feathers, and of reactions to immunizations.
- Skin testing is done to assess vaccine sensitivity (against a control of normal saline solution in the opposite arm) in patients with history of anaphylactoid reactions to egg ingestion. Administer an intradermal or scratch test with a 1:10 dilution. Read results after 5 to 30 minutes. A positive reaction is a wheal with or without pseudopodia and surrounding erythema. If sensitivity test is positive, consider desensitization.
- The FDA requires the manufacturer, lot number, date of administration, and name, address, and title of person administering the vaccine be documented.
- Vaccine can be used in HIV-infected patiets who don't have severe immunosuppression.
- Have epinephrine solution 1:1,000 available to treat allergic reactions.
- Don't administer vaccine I.V. Use a 25G, ⅝-inch needle and inject S.C., preferably into the outer aspect of the upper arm.
- Use only diluent supplied. Discard reconstituted solution after 8 hours.

- Store in refrigerator and protect from light. Solution may be used if red, pink, or yellow, but it must be clear.
- Don't give vaccine less than 1 month before or after immunization with other live virus vaccines—except for live, attenuated measles virus vaccine, live rubella virus vaccine, or monovalent or trivalent live oral poliovirus vaccine or poliovirus vaccine, inactivated, which may be administered simultaneously.
- Vaccine doesn't offer protection when given after exposure to natural mumps.
- Revaccination is recommended at 4 to 6 years of age.

Therapeutic monitoring
Recommend monitoring patient for allergic response.

Special populations
Breast-feeding patients. It isn't known if vaccine is excreted in breast milk. No problems have been reported. Use vaccine cautiously in breast-feeding women.
Pediatric patients. Vaccine isn't recommended for children under age 1 because retained maternal mumps antibodies may interfere with immune response.

Patient counseling
- Tell patient that he may experience pain and inflammation at the injection site and a low-grade fever, rash, or general malaise.
- Encourage patient to report distressing adverse reactions.
- Recommend acetaminophen to alleviate adverse reactions, such as fever.
- Tell women of childbearing age to avoid pregnancy for 3 months after vaccination. Provide contraceptive information, if necessary.

mupirocin (pseudomonic acid A)
Bactroban

mupirocin calcium
Bactroban Nasal

Pharmacologic classification: antibiotic
Therapeutic classification: topical antibacterial
Pregnancy risk category B

How supplied
Available by prescription only
Ointment: 2% (1-g single-use tubes, 15 g, 30 g)
Cream: 2%
Ointment for intranasal use: 2%

Indications and dosages
***Topical treatment of impetigo due to* Staphylococcus aureus, *beta-hemolytic* Streptococcus, *and* Streptococcus pyogenes**
Adults and children: Apply a small amount to affected area t.i.d. for 1 to 2 weeks. The area treated may be covered with a gauze dressing, if desired.
***Eradication of nasal colonization of methicillin-resistant* S. aureus**
Adults: Apply one-half of a single-use tube to each nostril b.i.d. for 5 days. Press and release the sides of the nose repeatedly for 1 minute to disperse the medication through the nares.

Pharmacodynamics
Antibacterial action: Mupirocin is structurally unrelated to other agents and is produced by fermentation of the organism *Pseudomonas fluorescens.* Mupirocin inhibits bacterial protein synthesis by reversibly and specifically binding to bacterial isoleucyl transfer-RNA synthetase. Mupirocin shows no cross-resistance with chloramphenical. erythromycin, gentamicin, lincomycin, methicillin, neomycin, novobiocin, penicillin, streptomycin, or tetracycline.

Pharmacokinetics
Absorption: Normal subjects showed no absorption after 24-hour application under occlusive dressings.
Distribution: Highly protein-bound (about 95%). A substantial decrease in activity can be expected in the presence of serum (as in exudative wounds).
Metabolism: Slightly metabolized locally in the skin to monic acid.
Excretion: Eliminated locally by desquamation of the skin.

Route	Onset	Peak	Duration
Topical	Unknown	Unknown	Unknown

Contraindications and precautions
Contraindicated in patients hypersensitive to drug. Use cautiously in patients with burns or impaired renal function.

Interactions
None reported.

Adverse reactions
CNS: headache (with nasal use).
EENT: rhinitis, pharyngitis, taste perversion, burning (with nasal use).
Respiratory: upper respiratory congestions, cough (with nasal use).
Skin: burning, pruritus, stinging, rash, pain, erythema (with topical administration).

Overdose and treatment
No information available.

Clinical considerations
- If sensitivity or chemical irritation occurs, discontinue treatment and institute appropriate alternative therapy.
- When used on burns or to treat extensive open wounds, absorption of polyethylene glycol vehicle is possible and may result in serious renal toxicity.

Therapeutic monitoring
- Patients not showing a clinical response within 3 to 5 days should be re-evaluated.
- Monitor for superinfection. Use of antibiotics (prolonged or repeated) may result in bacterial or fungal overgrowth of nonsusceptible organisms.

Special populations
Breast-feeding patients. It isn't known if drug is excreted in breast milk. Use with caution.

Patient counseling
- Advise patient to wash and dry affected areas thoroughly. Then apply thin film rubbing in gently.
- Tell patient to use single-use tube for nasal application for one application only, then discard tube. Apply one-half of the ointment from the tube into one nostril and the remaining into the other nostril, in the morning and evening.
- Warn patient to avoid contact around eyes and mucous membranes.

mycophenolate mofetil
CellCept Intravenous

Pharmacologic classification: mycophenolic acid derivative
Therapeutic classification: immunosuppressive
Pregnancy risk category C

How supplied
Available by prescription only
Capsules: 250 mg
Tablets: 500 mg
Powder for injection: 500 mg

Indications and dosages
Prophylaxis of organ rejection in patients receiving allogeneic renal transplants
Adults: 1 g P.O. or I.V. b.i.d. Use in combination with corticosteroids and cyclosporine.
Prophylaxis of organ rejection in patients receiving cardiac transplants
Adults: 1.5 g P.O. or I.V. b.i.d. Use in combination with corticosteroids and cyclosporine.

Pharmacodynamics
Immunosuppressive action: Mycophenolate inhibits proliferative responses of T- and B-lymphocytes, suppresses antibody formation by B-lymphocytes, and may inhibit recruitment of leukocytes into sites of inflammation and graft rejection.

Pharmacokinetics
Absorption: Absorbed from the GI tract. Absolute bioavailability of drug and active metabolite is 94%.
Distribution: About 97% is bound to plasma protein.
Metabolism: Undergoes complete presystemic metabolism to mycophenolic acid.
Excretion: Primarily excreted in urine with a small amount excreted in feces. Half-life is about 18 hours.

Route	Onset	Peak	Duration
P.O.	Unknown	½-1¼ hr	7½-18 hr
I.V.	Unknown	Unknown	10-17 hr

Contraindication and precautions
Contraindicated in patients with hypersensitivity to drug, mycophenolic acid, or any component of drug product. Drug shouldn't be used during pregnancy unless the benefits outweigh the risks. Use cautiously in patients with GI disorders.

Interactions
Drug-drug. *Acyclovir and ganciclovir:* Increase risk of toxicity for both drugs. Monitor patient closely.
Antacids with magnesium and aluminum hydroxides: Decreased absorption of mycophenolate mofetil. Administer drugs separately.
Cholestyramine: May interfere with enterohepatic recirculation, causing a decrease in mycophenolate bioavailability. Don't administer together.
Oral contraceptives: Mycophenolate may affect efficacy of oral contraceptives. Advise patient to use alternative contraceptives measures.

Effects on diagnostic tests
None reported.

Adverse reactions
CNS: *astenia, tremor,* insomnia, dizziness, *headache.*
CV: *chest pain, hypertension, edema.*
GI: *diarrhea, constipation, nausea, dyspepsia, vomiting, oral moniliasis, abdominal pain.*
GU: *urinary tract infection, hematuria,* kidney tubular necrosis.
Hematologic: *anemia,* ***leukopenia,*** **THROMBOCYTOPENIA,** hypochromic anemia, leukocytosis.
Metabolic: *hypercholesterolemia, hypophosphatemia, hypokalemia,* hyperkalemia, hyperglycemia.
Musculoskeletal: *back pain.*
Respiratory: *dyspnea, cough,* pharyngitis, bronchitis, pneumonia.
Skin: *acne,* rash.

Other: *pain, fever, sepsis, possible immunosuppression-induced infection or lymphoma.*

Overdose and treatment

Although there's no reported experience of overdose in humans, does of 4 to 5 g/day compared with 3 g/day caused an increase in nausea, vomiting, or diarrhea and occasional hematologic abnormalities in some patients. Treatments includes use of bile acid sequestrants to increase the excretion of drug.

Clinical considerations

- Avoid doses exceeding 1 g b.i.d. in patients with severe chronic renal impairment (glomerular filtration rate below 25 ml/minute) outside the immediate post-transplant period.
- Because of potential teratogenic effects, don't open capsules and don't crush tablets. Also avoid inhalation of direct contact with skin or mucous membranes of the powder contained in the capsules. If such contact occurs, wash thoroughly with soap and water, rinse eyes with plain water.
- Immunosuppression-induced infection or lymphoma may occur.
- Don't administer I.V. solution by rapid or bolus method; it must be given over 2 hours or more.
- Reconstitute by injecting 14 ml 5% dextrose injection into a 500 mg vial; shake and inspect for particles or discoloration (solution is slightly yellow). Discard if particles or discoloration is present. To prepare a 1-g dose, further dilute two reconstituted vials in 140 ml of 5% dextrose injection. To prepare a 1.5-g dose, further dilute three reconstituted vials in 210 ml of 5% dextrose injection. The final concentration of both preparations is 6 mg/ml. Drug is incompatible with other I.V. infusion solutions and must be administered through an exclusive site.
- Use solution within 4 hours of reconstitution and dilution. Store at 77° F (25° C).

Therapeutic monitoring

- Monitor patient's CBC regularly. If neutropenia develops, interrupt therapy, reduce dose, perform appropriate diagnostic tests, or give additional treatment.

Special populations

Breast-feeding patients. It isn't known if drug is excreted in breast milk. Use in breast-feeding women isn't recommended.
Pediatric patients. Safety and efficacy in children haven't been established.

Patient counseling

- Warn patient not to open capsules or crush tablets; instruct him to swallow them whole on an empty stomach.
- Instruct patient of need for repeated appropriate laboratory tests during drug therapy.
- Give patient complete dosage instructions and inform him of increased risk of lymphoproliferative diseases and other malignancies.
- Explain that drug is used with other drug therapies. Stress importance of not interrupting or stopping these drugs without medical approval.
- Inform women that a pregnancy test should be done within 1 week before beginning therapy and that effective contraception must be used before, during, and for 6 weeks after therapy is completed, even when there's history of infertility (unless due to hysterectomy). Also, two forms of contraception must be used simultaneously unless abstinence is chosen. If pregnancy occurs despite these measures, she must contact her doctor immediately.

N

nabumetone

Relafen

Pharmacologic classification: NSAID
Therapeutic classification: antiarthritic
Pregnancy risk category C

How supplied

Available by prescription only
Tablets: 500 mg, 750 mg

Indications and dosages

Acute and chronic treatment of rheumatoid arthritis or osteoarthritis
Adults: Initially, 1,000 mg P.O. daily as a single dose or in divided doses b.i.d. Adjust dosage based on patient response. Maximum recommended daily dose, 2,000 mg.

Pharmacodynamics

Anti-inflammatory action: Nabumetone probably acts by inhibiting the synthesis of prostaglandins. Drug also has analgesic and antipyretic action.

Pharmacokinetics

Absorption: Well absorbed from the GI tract. After absorption, about 35% is rapidly transformed to 6-methoxy-2-naphthylacetic acid (6MNA), the principal active metabolite; the balance is transformed to unidentified metabolites. Administration with food increases the absorption rate and peak levels of 6MNA but doesn't change total drug absorbed.
Distribution: 6MNA is more than 99% bound to plasma proteins.
Metabolism: 6MNA is metabolized to inactive metabolites in the liver.
Excretion: Metabolites are excreted primarily in urine. About 9% appears in the feces. Elimination half-life is about 24 hours. Half-life is increased in patients with renal failure.

Route	Onset	Peak	Duration
P.O.	Unknown	2-4 hr	Unknown

Contraindications and precautions

Contraindicated in patients with hypersensitivity reactions, history of aspirin- or NSAID-induced asthma, urticaria, or other allergic-type reactions and during third trimester of pregnancy.

Use cautiously in patients with impaired renal or hepatic function, heart failure, hypertension, conditions that predispose to fluid retention, and history of peptic ulcer disease.

Interactions

Drug-drug. *Drugs that are highly bound to plasma proteins, such as warfarin:* Nabumetone may displace drug. Use together with caution.

Effects on diagnostic tests

None reported.

Adverse reactions

CNS: *dizziness, headache,* fatigue, insomnia, nervousness, somnolence.
CV: vasculitis, edema.
EENT: *tinnitus.*
GI: *diarrhea, dyspepsia, abdominal pain, constipation, flatulence, nausea,* dry mouth, gastritis, stomatitis, anorexia, vomiting, ***bleeding,*** ulceration.
Respiratory: dyspnea, pneumonitis.
Skin: *pruritus, rash,* increased diaphoresis.

Overdose and treatment

After an accidental overdose, empty the stomach by induced emesis or lavage. Activated charcoal may limit the amount of drug absorbed.

Clinical considerations

- Consider the recommendations relevant to all NSAIDs.
- Because NSAIDs impair the synthesis of renal prostaglandins, they can decrease renal blood flow and lead to reversible renal function impairment, especially in patients with preexisting renal failure, liver dysfunction, and heart failure; in geriatric patients; and in those taking diuretics. Monitor these patients closely during therapy.

Therapeutic monitoring

During long-term therapy, periodically monitor renal and liver function, CBC, and hematocrit. Monitor carefully for signs and symptoms of GI bleeding.

Special populations

Breast-feeding patients. The active metabolite of nabumetone, 6MNA, has been found in the milk of laboratory rats. Because of risk of serious toxicity to the infant, use in breast-feeding women isn't recommended.

Pediatric patients. Safety and efficacy in children haven't been established.
Geriatric patients. No differences in safety or efficacy have been noted in geriatric patients.

Patient counseling

- Tell patient to take drug with food, milk, or antacids to enhance drug absorption.
- Stress importance of follow-up examinations to detect adverse GI effects.
- Teach patient signs and symptoms of GI bleeding, and tell him to report them immediately.
- Advise patient to limit alcohol intake because of risk of additive GI toxicity.

nadolol

Corgard

Pharmacologic classification: beta blocker
Therapeutic classification: antihypertensive, antianginal
Pregnancy risk category C

How supplied

Available by prescription only
Tablets: 20 mg, 40 mg, 80 mg, 120 mg, 160 mg

Indications and dosages

Hypertension
Adults: Initially, 20 to 40 mg P.O. once daily. Dosage may be increased in 40- to 80-mg increments daily at 2- to 14-day intervals until optimum response occurs. Usual maintenance dosage is 40 or 80 mg once daily. Doses of up to 240 or 320 mg daily may be necessary. Rarely, up to 640 mg daily.
Long-term prophylactic management of chronic stable angina pectoris
Adults: Initially, 40 mg P.O. once daily. Dosage may be increased in 40- to 80-mg increments daily at 3- to 7-day intervals until optimum response occurs. Usual maintenance dosage is 40 or 80 mg once daily. Doses of up to 160 or 240 mg daily may be needed.
◇***Arrhythmias***
Adults: 60 to 160 mg P.O. daily.
◇***Prophylaxis of vascular headache***
Adults: 20 to 40 mg P.O. once daily; may gradually increase to 120 mg daily, if necessary.
≡***Dosage adjustment.*** For renally impaired patients, refer to the following table.

Creatinine clearance (ml/min/1.73 m²)	Dosing interval
> 50	q 24 hr
31 to 50	q 24 to 36 hr
10 to 30	q 24 to 48 hr
< 10	q 40 to 60 hr

Pharmacodynamics

Antihypertensive action: Mechanism of antihypertensive effect is unknown. Drug may reduce blood pressure by blocking adrenergic receptors, thus decreasing cardiac output; by decreasing sympathetic outflow from the CNS; or by suppressing renin release.
Antianginal action: Nadolol decreases myocardial oxygen consumption, thus relieving angina, by blocking catecholamine-induced increases in heart rate, myocardial contraction, and blood pressure.

Pharmacokinetics

Absorption: 30% to 40% of a dose of nadolol is absorbed from the GI tract. Absorption isn't affected by food.
Distribution: Distributed throughout the body; drug is about 30% protein-bound.
Metabolism: Not metabolized.
Excretion: Most of a given dose is excreted unchanged in urine; the remainder is excreted in feces. Plasma half-life is about 20 hours. Antihypertensive and antianginal effects persist for about 24 hours.

Route	Onset	Peak	Duration
P.O.	Unknown	2-4 hr	Unknown

Contraindications and precautions

Contraindicated in patients with bronchial asthma, sinus bradycardia and greater than first-degree heart block, and cardiogenic shock. Use cautiously in patients with hyperthyroidism, heart failure, diabetes, chronic bronchitis, emphysema, and impaired renal or hepatic function and in those receiving general anesthesia before undergoing surgery.

Interactions

Drug-drug. *Other antiarrhythmic agents:* May have additive or antagonistic cardiac effects and additive toxic effects. Use together cautiously.
Antimuscarinic agents, such as atropine: May antagonize nadolol-induced bradycardia. Use together cautiously.
Diuretics, other antihypertensive agents and, at high doses, the neuromuscular blocking effect of tubocurarine and related agents: Potentiated antihypertensive effects. Use together cautiously
Sympathomimetic agents, such as isoproterenol and epinephrine: Antagonized effects of these agents. Use together cautiously.
Drug-lifestyle. *Cocaine use:* Inhibited therapeutic effects of nadolol. Discourage use together.

Effects on diagnostic tests

None reported.

Adverse reactions

CNS: fatigue, dizziness.

CV: ***bradycardia,*** *hypotension,* ***heart failure,*** peripheral vascular disease, rhythm and conduction disturbances.
GI: nausea, vomiting, diarrhea, abdominal pain, constipation, anorexia.
Respiratory: *increased airway resistance.*
Skin: rash.
Other: fever.

Overdose and treatment
Signs of overdose include severe hypotension, bradycardia, heart failure, and bronchospasm.

After acute ingestion, empty patient's stomach by induced emesis or gastric lavage, and give activated charcoal to reduce absorption. Magnesium sulfate may be given orally as a cathartic. Subsequent treatment is usually symptomatic and supportive.

Clinical considerations
Consider the recommendations relevant to all beta blockers as well as the following:
- Dosage adjustments may be necessary in patients with renal impairment.
- Nadolol has been used as an antiarrhythmic agent and as a prophylactic agent for migraine headaches.
- If long-term therapy is used, gradually decrease dose over 1 to 2 weeks before discontinuing drug. Abrupt withdrawal can exacerbate angina and cause an MI.

Therapeutic monitoring
- Careful monitoring of blood pressure during initial dosing and adjustment is needed; once condition is stabilized, monitoring is done at 3- to 6-month intervals.
- Monitor patient for reflex bradycardia, which may be treated with atropine.
- Monitor patients with hyperthyroidism and diabetes carefully; symptoms may be masked by drug therapy.

Special populations
Breast-feeding patients. Drug is excreted in breast milk; an alternative feeding method is recommended during therapy.
Pediatric patients. Safety and efficacy in children haven't been established; use only if potential benefit outweighs risk.
Geriatric patients. Geriatric patients may require lower maintenance dosages of nadolol because of increased bioavailability or delayed metabolism; they also may experience enhanced adverse effects.

Patient counseling
Tell patient not to discontinue nadolol abruptly. Drug should be tapered.

nafcillin sodium
Nafcil, Nallpen, Unipen

Pharmacologic classification: penicillinase-resistant penicillin
Therapeutic classification: antibiotic
Pregnancy risk category B

How supplied
Available by prescription only
Capsules: 250 mg
Tablets: 500 mg
Injection: 500 mg, 1 g, 2 g
Pharmacy bulk package: 10 g
I.V. infusion piggyback: 1 g, 2 g

Indications and dosages
Systemic infections caused by susceptible organisms (methicillin-sensitive* Staphylococcus aureus*)
Adults: 250 to 500 mg P.O. q 4 to 6 hours for mild to moderate infections and 1 g q 4 to 6 hours for more severe infections. Alternatively, 500 mg I.M. q 4 hours or 500 to 1,000 mg I.V. q 4 hours depending on severity of the infection.
Children over age 1 month: 50 to 100 mg/kg P.O. daily, divided into doses given q 6 hours. Alternatively, 50 to 200 mg/kg/day I.M. or I.V. in divided doses q 4 to 6 hours depending on the severity of the infection.
Neonates: 30 to 40 mg/kg/day P.O. divided equally into three to four doses; or 20 mg/kg daily I.M. in two equally divided doses. Alternatively, 40 mg/kg/day I.M. in two equally divided doses q 12 hours if neonate is less than 7 days old and 60 to 200 mg/kg/day in equally divided doses q 8 hours if neonate is 7 to 28 days old. For mild to moderate infection, may give 50 to 100 mg/kg/day I.V. in divided doses q 6 hours. For more severe infections, 100 to 200 mg/kg/day I.V. divided q 4 to 6 hours. Alternatively, 25 mg/kg I.V. q 12 hours (if less than 7 days old and under 4.4 lb [2 kg]) or q 8 hours (if less than 7 days old and over 4.4 lb or over 7 days old and less than 4.4 lb) or q 6 hours (if over 7 days old and over 4.4 lb).
Meningitis
Neonates under age 7 days and under 4.4 lb: 50 mg/kg I.V. q 12 hours.
Neonates under age 7 days and over 4.4 lb: 50 mg/kg I.V. q 8 hours.
Neonates over age 7 days and under 4.4 lb: 50 mg/kg I.V. q 8 hours.
Neonates over age 7 days and over 4.4 lb: 50 mg/kg I.V. q 6 hours.
Acute or chronic osteomyelitis caused by susceptible organism
Adults: 1 to 2 g I.V. q 4 hours for 4 to 8 weeks.
Meningitis caused by susceptible organisms
Adults: 100 to 200 mg/kg/day I.V. in divided doses q 4 to 6 hours.

Native valve endocarditis caused by susceptible organisms
Adults: 2 g I.V. q 4 hours for 4 to 6 weeks in combination with gentamicin.

Pharmacodynamics
Antibiotic action: Nafcillin is bactericidal; it adheres to bacterial penicillin-binding proteins, thus inhibiting bacterial cell wall synthesis.

Nafcillin resists the effects of penicillinases—enzymes that inactivate penicillin—and is active against many strains of penicillinase-producing bacteria; this activity is most important against penicillinase-producing staphylococci; some strains may remain resistant. Nafcillin is also active against a few gram-positive aerobic and anaerobic bacilli but has no significant effect on gram-negative bacilli.

Pharmacokinetics
Absorption: Absorbed erratically and poorly from the GI tract; Food decreases absorption.
Distribution: Distributed widely; CSF penetration is poor but enhanced by meningeal inflammation. Drug crosses the placenta and is 70% to 90% protein-bound.
Metabolism: Metabolized primarily in the liver; it undergoes enterohepatic circulation. Dosage adjustment isn't necessary for patients in renal failure.
Excretion: Excreted primarily in bile; about 25% to 30% is excreted in urine unchanged. It may also be excreted in breast milk. Elimination half-life in adults is ½ to 1½ hours.

Route	Onset	Peak	Duration
P.O.	Unknown	½-2 hr	Unknown
I.V.	Immediate	Immediate	Unknown
I.M.	Unknown	½-1 hr	Unknown

Contraindications and precautions
Contraindicated in patients with hypersensitivity to drug or other penicillins. Use cautiously in patients with GI distress or sensitivity to cephalosporins.

Interactions
Drug-drug. *Aminoglycosides:* Produce synergistic bactericidal effects against *S. aureus.* However, the drugs are physically and chemically incompatible and are inactivated when mixed or given together. Don't mix in same solution.
Cyclosporines: Subtherapeutic cyclosporine levels. Cyclosporine levels should be monitored.
Hepatotoxic medications: May increase the risk of hepatotoxicity. Patient requires careful monitoring.
Drug-food. *Fruit juice or carbonated beverages:* Acidity may inactivate drug. Don't give together.

Effects on diagnostic tests
Nafcillin alters tests for urinary and serum proteins; turbidimetric urine and serum proteins are often falsely positive or elevated in tests using sulfosalicylic acid or trichloroacetic acid.

Adverse reactions
GI: *nausea,* vomiting, diarrhea, **Pseudomonas** ***colitis.***
Hematologic: ***transient leukopenia, neutropenia, granulocytopenia, thrombocytopenia*** with high doses.
Other: hypersensitivity reactions (chills, fever, rash, pruritus, urticaria, ***anaphylaxis***), vein irritation, thrombophlebitis.

Overdose and treatment
Signs and symptoms of overdose include neuromuscular irritability or seizures. There are no specific recommendations. Treatment is supportive. After recent ingestion (4 hours or less), empty stomach by induced emesis or gastric lavage; follow with activated charcoal to reduce absorption. Nafcillin isn't appreciably removed by hemodialysis.

Clinical considerations
Consider the recommendations relevant to all penicillins as well as the following:
- Give drug with water only; acid in fruit juice or carbonated beverage may inactivate drug.
- Give dose on empty stomach; food decreases absorption.
- Drug is incompatible with aminoglycosides.
- Infuse I.V. nafcillin for short time periods (24 to 48 hours) if possible to avoid risk of thrombophlebitis.
- If used to treat infections caused by group A beta-hemolytic streptococci, continue therapy for at least 10 days to decrease risk of rheumatic fever or glomerulonephritis.

Therapeutic monitoring
Renal, hepatic, and hematologic systems should be evaluated periodically during prolonged nafcillin therapy.

Special populations
Breast-feeding patients. Nafcillin is excreted into breast milk; use drug with caution in breast-feeding women.
Pediatric patients. Nafcillin that's been reconstituted with bacteriostatic water for injection with benzyl alcohol shouldn't be used in neonates because of toxicity.
Geriatric patients. Half-life may be prolonged in geriatric patients because of impaired hepatic and renal function.

Patient counseling
Tell patient to report severe diarrhea or allergic reactions promptly.

nalbuphine hydrochloride

Nubain

Pharmacologic classification: narcotic agonist-antagonist, opioid partial agonist
Therapeutic classification: analgesic, adjunct to anesthesia
Pregnancy risk category NR

How supplied

Available by prescription only
Injection: 1.5 mg/ml, 10 mg/ml, 20 mg/ml

Indications and dosages

Moderate to severe pain
Adults: 10 to 20 mg S.C., I.M., or I.V. q 3 to 6 hours, p.r.n., or around the clock. Maximum dose, 160 mg/day.
Supplement to anesthesia
Adults: 0.3 mg/kg to 3 mg/kg I.V. over 10 to 15 minutes; maintenance dosage, 0.25 to 0.5 mg/kg I.V.

Pharmacodynamics

Analgesic action: Analgesia is believed to result from action of drug at opiate receptor sites in the CNS, relieving moderate to severe pain. The narcotic antagonist effect may result from competitive inhibition at opiate receptors. Like other opioids, nalbuphine causes respiratory depression, sedation, and miosis. In patients with coronary artery disease or MI, it appears to produce no substantial changes in heart rate, pulmonary artery or wedge pressure, left ventricular end-diastolic pressure, pulmonary vascular resistance, or cardiac index.

Pharmacokinetics

Absorption: When administered orally, drug is about one-fifth as effective as an analgesic as it is when given I.M., apparently because of first-pass metabolism in the GI tract and liver.
Distribution: Not appreciably bound to plasma proteins.
Metabolism: Metabolized in the liver.
Excretion: Excreted in urine and to some degree in bile.

Route	Onset	Peak	Duration
I.V.	2-3 min	30 min	3-6 hr
I.M.	15 min	1 hr	3-6 hr
S.C.	15 min	Unknown	3-6 hr

Contraindications and precautions

Contraindicated in patients with hypersensitivity to drug. Use cautiously in patients with history of drug abuse, emotional instability, head injury, increased intracranial pressure, impaired ventilation, MI accompanied by nausea and vomiting, upcoming biliary surgery, and hepatic or renal disease.

Interactions

Drug-drug. *General anesthetics:* May cause severe CV depression. Avoid use together.
Barbiturate anesthetics, such as thiopental: Additive CNS and respiratory depressant effects and, possibly, apnea. Use together very cautiously.
Cimetidine: May increase narcotic nalbuphine toxicity. A narcotic antagonist may be needed if toxicity occurs.
Other CNS depressants (antihistamines, barbiturates, benzodiazepines, muscle relaxants, narcotic analgesics, phenothiazines, sedative-hypnotics, tricyclic antidepressants): Potentiated respiratory and CNS depression, sedation, and hypotensive effects. Reduced doses of nalbuphine are usually necessary.
Digitoxin, phenytoin, rifampin: Drug accumulation and enhanced effects may result. Patient requires careful monitoring for toxicity.
Narcotic antagonist: Patients who become physically dependent on drug may experience acute withdrawal syndrome if given high doses of a narcotic antagonist. Use with caution, and monitor closely.

Effects on diagnostic tests

Drug may interfere with enzymatic tests for detection of opioids.

Adverse reactions

CNS: *headache, sedation, dizziness, vertigo,* nervousness, depression, restlessness, crying, euphoria, hostility, unusual dreams, confusion, hallucinations, speech difficulty, delusions.
CV: hypertension, hypotension, tachycardia, ***bradycardia.***
EENT: blurred vision, *dry mouth.*
GI: cramps, dyspepsia, bitter taste, *nausea, vomiting,* constipation, biliary tract spasms.
GU: urinary urgency.
Respiratory: ***respiratory depression,*** dyspnea, asthma, ***pulmonary edema.***
Skin: pruritus, burning, urticaria, *clamminess.*

Overdose and treatment

The most common signs and symptoms of nalbuphine overdose are CNS depression, respiratory depression, and miosis (pinpoint pupils). Other acute toxic effects include hypotension, bradycardia, hypothermia, shock, apnea, cardiopulmonary arrest, circulatory collapse, pulmonary edema, and seizures.

To treat acute overdose, first establish adequate respiratory exchange via a patent airway and ventilation as needed; administer a narcotic antagonist (naloxone) to reverse respiratory depression. Because the duration of action of nalbuphine is longer than that of naloxone, repeated naloxone dosing is necessary. Naloxone shouldn't be given in the absence of clinically significant respiratory or CV depression. Monitor vital signs closely.

Provide symptomatic and supportive treatment, such as continued respiratory support and correction of fluid or electrolyte imbalance. Monitor laboratory values, vital signs, and neurologic status closely.

Clinical considerations

Consider the recommendations relevant to all opioid (narcotic) agonist-antagonists as well as the following:

- Some commercial preparations contain sodium metabisulfite which may cause allergic reactions in susceptible individuals.
- Drug is incompatible with diazepam and pentobarbital.
- Nalbuphine may obscure the signs and symptoms of an acute abdominal condition or worsen gallbladder pain.
- Drug may cause orthostatic hypotension in ambulatory patients.
- Before administration, visually inspect all parenteral products for particulate matter and discoloration.
- Parenteral administration of drug provides better analgesia than oral administration. Give I.V. doses by slow I.V. injection, preferably in diluted solution. Rapid I.V. injection increases the incidence of adverse effects.
- Drug causes respiratory depression, which at 10 mg is equal to the respiratory depression produced by 10 mg of morphine.
- Store at 59° to 86° F (15° to 30° C) and protect from light.

Therapeutic monitoring

- When drug is used during labor and delivery, neonate must be observed for signs of respiratory depression.
- Drug also acts as a narcotic antagonist; it may precipitate abstinence syndrome in narcotic-dependent patients. Give 25% of usual dose in these patients and monitor for signs and symptoms of withdrawal.

Special populations

Breast-feeding patients. It isn't known if drug is excreted in breast milk. Use with caution in breast-feeding women.
Pediatric patients. Safety in children under age 18 hasn't been established.
Geriatric patients. Lower doses are usually indicated for geriatric patients, who may be more sensitive to therapeutic and adverse effects of drug.

Patient counseling

Instruct patient to avoid driving or operating machinery because drug may cause dizziness and fatigue.

naloxone hydrochloride

Narcan

Pharmacologic classification: narcotic (opioid) antagonist
Therapeutic classification: narcotic antagonist
Pregnancy risk category B

How supplied

Available by prescription only
Injection: 0.4 mg/ml, 1 mg/ml with preservatives, and 0.02 mg/ml, 0.4 mg/ml paraben-free

Indications and dosages

Known or suspected narcotic-induced respiratory depression, including that caused by natural and synthetic narcotics, methadone, nalbuphine, pentazocine, and propoxyphene
Adults: 0.4 to 2 mg I.V., S.C., or I.M., repeated q 2 to 3 minutes, p.r.n. If no response is observed after 10 mg have been administered, question diagnosis of narcotic-induced toxicity. Also, 0.4 mg I.V. loading dose followed by 0.4 mg/hour infusion.
Children: 0.01 mg/kg I.V.; give a subsequent dose of 0.1 mg/kg if needed. Dosage for continuous infusion is 0.024 to 0.16 mg/kg/hour. If I.V. route not available, dose may be given I.M. or S.C. in divided doses. Alternatively, 0.1 mg/kg I.V. q. 2 to 3 minutes, p.r.n., in neonates and children up to age 5 and 2 mg I.V. q 2 to 3 minutes, p.r.n., in children age 6 and older.
Postoperative narcotic depression
Adults: 0.1 to 0.2 mg I.V. q 2 to 3 minutes, p.r.n., until desired response is obtained. Alternatively, 0.005 mg/kg I.V. and repeat in 15 minutes, p.r.n., or administer 0.01 mg/kg I.M. for the second dose. May give continuous infusion at 0.0037 mg/kg/hour.
Children: 0.005 to 0.01 mg/kg dose I.M., I.V., or S.C., repeated q 2 to 3 minutes, p.r.n., until desired degree of reversal is obtained.
Neonates (asphyxia neonatorum): 0.01 mg/kg I.V. into umbilical vein repeated q 2 to 3 minutes, p.r.n.
Drug level for use in neonates and children is 0.02 mg/ml.
◇***Naloxone challenge for diagnosing opiate dependence***
Adults: 0.16 mg I.M. naloxone; if no signs of withdrawal after 20 to 30 minutes, give second dose of 0.24 mg I.V.
◇***Opiate addiction***
Adults: 200 mg to 3 g P.O. daily.

Pharmacodynamics

Narcotic (opioid) antagonism: Naloxone is essentially a pure antagonist. In patients who have received an opioid agonist or other analgesic with narcotic-like effects, naloxone antagonizes most of the opioid effects, especially respiratory depression, sedation, and hypotension. Because the duration of action of naloxone in most cases is shorter than that of the opioid, opiate effects may return as those of naloxone dissipate. Naloxone doesn't produce tolerance or physical or psychological dependence. The precise mechanism of action is unknown, but is thought to involve competitive antagonism of more than one opiate receptor in the CNS.

Pharmacokinetics

Absorption: Rapidly inactivated after oral administration; therefore, it's given parenterally. The duration of action is longer after I.M. use and higher doses, when compared with I.V. use and lower doses.
Distribution: Rapidly distributed into body tissues and fluids.
Metabolism: Rapidly metabolized in the liver, primarily by conjugation.
Excretion: Excreted in urine. Plasma half-life has been reported to be from 60 to 90 minutes in adults and 3 hours in neonates.

Route	Onset	Peak	Duration
I.V.	1-2 min	5-15 min	Variable
I.M., S.C.	2-5 min	5-15 min	Variable

Contraindications and precautions

Contraindicated in patients with hypersensitivity to drug. Use cautiously in patients with cardiac irritability and opiate addiction. When given to a narcotic addict, naloxone may produce an acute abstinence syndrome. Use with caution, and monitor closely.

Interactions

Drug-drug. *Cardiotoxic drugs:* May have serious CV effects if also given naloxone. Use together cautiously.

Effects on diagnostic tests

None reported.

Adverse reactions

CNS: ***tremors, seizures.***
CV: tachycardia, hypertension (with higher-than-recommended doses); hypotension; ***ventricular fibrillation; cardiac arrest.***
GI: nausea, vomiting (with higher-than-recommended doses).
Respiratory: ***pulmonary edema.***
Skin: diaphoresis.
Other: withdrawal symptoms (in narcotic-dependent patients with higher-than-recommended doses).

Overdose and treatment

No serious adverse reactions to naloxone overdose are known except those of acute abstinence syndrome in narcotic-dependent persons.

Clinical considerations

Consider the recommendations relevant to all narcotic antagonists as well as the following:

- Before administration, visually inspect all parenteral products for particulate matter and discoloration.
- Take a careful drug history to rule out possible narcotic addiction, to avoid inducing withdrawal symptoms (apply cautions also to the baby of an addicted mother).
- Because duration of activity of naloxone is shorter than that of most narcotics, vigilance and repeated doses are usually necessary in the management of an acute narcotic overdose in a nonaddicted patient.
- Naloxone isn't effective in treating respiratory depression caused by nonopioid drugs.
- Naloxone can be diluted in dextrose 5% or normal saline solution. Use within 24 hours after mixing.
- Naloxone is the safest drug to use when cause of respiratory depression is uncertain.
- Naloxone may be administered by continuous I.V. infusion, which is necessary in many cases to control the adverse effects of epidurally administered morphine. Usual dose is 2 mg in 500 ml of D_5W or normal saline solution.
- Don't mix drug with preparations containing bisulfite, metabisulfite, long-chain, or high molecular weight anions, or any solution having an alkaline pH.
- Injections are stable at pH of 2.5 to 5.

Therapeutic monitoring

Avoid depending on drug too much; don't neglect attention to the airway, breathing, and circulation. Maintain adequate respiratory and CV status at all times. Respiratory "overshoot" may occur; monitor for respiratory rate higher than before respiratory depression. Respiratory rate increases in 1 to 2 minutes, and effect lasts 1 to 4 hours.

Special populations

Breast-feeding patients. It isn't known if drug is excreted in breast milk.
Geriatric patients. Lower doses are usually indicated for geriatric patients, because they may be more sensitive to therapeutic and adverse effects of drug.

naltrexone hydrochloride

ReVia

Pharmacologic classification: narcotic (opioid) antagonist
Therapeutic classification: narcotic detoxification adjunct
Pregnancy risk category C

How supplied

Available by prescription only
Tablets: 50 mg

Indications and dosages

Adjunct for maintenance of opioid-free state in detoxified individuals

Adults: Don't attempt treatment until naloxone challenge is negative (0.2 mg I.V., if no signs of withdrawal after 30 seconds, give additional 0.6 mg I.V.; alternatively, administer 0.8 mg S.C. and observe for 20 minutes for signs of withdrawal). Don't attempt treatment until patient has remained opioid-free for 7 to 10 days, verified by analyzing urine for opioids. Initially, 25 mg P.O. If no withdrawal signs occur within 1 hour, administer an additional 25 mg. Alternatively, 10- to 12.5-mg initial dose followed by 10- to 12.5-mg incremental increases daily to 50 mg, or 5 mg initially with incremental 10-mg increases hourly to 50 mg. Once patient has been started on 50 mg q 24 hours, flexible maintenance schedule may be used. From 50 to 150 mg may be given daily, depending on the schedule prescribed, but the average daily dose is 50 mg.

Alcoholism (short-term therapy)

Adults: 50 mg P.O. daily.

Pharmacodynamics

Opioid antagonism: Naltrexone is essentially a pure opiate (narcotic) antagonist. Like naloxone, it has little or no agonist activity. Its precise mechanism of action is unknown, but it's thought to involve competitive antagonism of more than one opiate receptor in the CNS. When administered to patients who haven't recently received opiates, it exhibits little or no pharmacologic effect. At oral doses of 30 to 50 mg daily, it produces minimal analgesia, only slight drowsiness, and no respiratory depression. However, pharmacologic effects, including psychotomimetic effects, increased systolic or diastolic blood pressure, respiratory depression, and decreased oral temperature, which are suggestive of opiate agonist activity, have reportedly occurred in a few patients. In patients who have received single or repeated large doses of opiates, naltrexone attenuates or produces a complete but reversible block of the pharmacologic effects of the narcotic. Naltrexone doesn't produce physical or psychological dependence, and tolerance to its antagonist activity reportedly doesn't develop.

Pharmacokinetics

Absorption: Well absorbed after oral administration. It undergoes extensive first-pass hepatic metabolism (only 5% to 20% of an oral dose reaches the systemic circulation unchanged).

Distribution: About 21% to 28% protein-bound. Extent and duration of antagonist activity of drug appear directly related to plasma and tissue levels of drug. It's widely distributed throughout the body, but considerable interindividual variation exists.

Metabolism: Oral naltrexone undergoes extensive first-pass hepatic metabolism. Its major metabolite is believed to be a pure antagonist also, and may contribute to its efficacy. Drug and hepatic metabolites may undergo enterohepatic recirculation.

Excretion: Excreted primarily by the kidneys. Elimination half-life is about 4 hours; that of its major active metabolite is about 13 hours.

Route	Onset	Peak	Duration
P.O.	15-30 min	12 hr	24 hr

Contraindications and precautions

Contraindicated in patients receiving opioid analgesics, in opioid-dependent patients, in patients in acute opioid withdrawal, in those with positive urine screen for opioids, or in those with acute hepatitis or liver failure. Also contraindicated in patients with hypersensitivity to drug.

Use cautiously in patients with mild hepatic disease or history of hepatic impairment.

Interactions

Drug-drug. *Drugs that alter hepatic metabolism:* May increase or decrease serum naltrexone levels. Monitor patient for this effect.

Opioid-containing medications, such as cough and cold preparations, antidiarrheals, and opioid analgesics: Attenuated opioid activity. Avoid use together.

Effects on diagnostic tests

None known.

Adverse reactions

CNS: *insomnia, anxiety, nervousness, headache,* depression, dizziness, fatigue, somnolence, ***suicidal ideation.***

GI: *nausea, vomiting,* anorexia, *abdominal pain,* constipation, increased thirst.

GU: delayed ejaculation, decreased potency.

Hematologic: lymphocytosis.

Hepatic: ***hepatotoxicity.***

Musculoskeletal: *muscle and joint pain.*

Skin: rash.

Other: chills.

Overdose and treatment

Overdose hasn't been documented. Test subjects have received 800 mg/day (16 tablets) for up to 1 week and shown no evidence of toxicity. In case of overdose, provide symptomatic and supportive treatment in a closely supervised environment. Contact your local or regional poison control center for further information.

Clinical considerations

Consider the recommendations relevant to all narcotic (opioid) antagonists as well as the following:

- Naltrexone has been used investigationally for the treatment of methadone dependence.
- A naloxone (Narcan) challenge test may be given to the patient before naltrexone use.

Naloxone (0.8 mg S.C. or I.V., incremental doses) is administered and the patient closely monitored for signs and symptoms of opiate withdrawal. If acute abstinence signs and symptoms are present, don't administer naltrexone. If inconclusive results, may repeat challenge with 1.6 mg IV.

- Before administration, a careful drug history should be taken to rule out possible narcotic use. Don't attempt treatment until the patient has been opiate-free for 7 to 10 days. Verify self-reporting of abstinence from narcotics by urinalysis. No withdrawal signs or symptoms should be reported by patient or be evident.
- Because naltrexone can precipitate potentially severe opiate withdrawal, it shouldn't be used in patients receiving opiates or in nondetoxified patients physically dependent on opiates.
- Drug can cause hepatocellular injury if given at higher-than-recommended doses. Naltrexone can cause or exacerbate signs and symptoms of abstinence in anyone not completely opioid-free.

Therapeutic monitoring

Perform liver function tests before naltrexone use to establish a baseline and to evaluate possible drug-induced hepatotoxicity every 1 month for 6 months. In an emergency requiring analgesia that can only be achieved by administering opiates, a patient who has been receiving naltrexone may need a higher dose than usual of narcotic, and the resulting respiratory depression may be deeper and more prolonged.

Special populations

Breast-feeding patients. It isn't known if drug is excreted in breast milk. Use drug with caution in breast-feeding women, especially because of its known hepatotoxicity.
Pediatric patients. Safety of naltrexone in pediatric patients under age 18 hasn't been established.
Geriatric patients. Use in geriatric patients isn't documented, but reduced dosage would probably be needed.

Patient counseling

- Inform patient that opioid medications, such as cough and cold preparations, antidiarrheal products, and narcotic analgesics may not be effective; recommend nonnarcotic alternative if available.
- Warn patient not to self-administer narcotics while taking naltrexone because serious injury, coma, or death may result.
- Explain that drug has no tolerance or dependence liability.
- Tell patient to report withdrawal signs and symptoms (tremors, vomiting, bone or muscle pains, sweating, abdominal cramps).
- Tell patient to carry an identification card that alerts medical personnel that naltrexone is taken, and to inform new doctor that he's receiving drug.

nandrolone decanoate

Androlone-D 200, Deca-Durabolin, Hybolin Decanoate-50, Hybolin Decanoate-100, Neo-Durabolic

Pharmacologic classification: anabolic steroid
Therapeutic classification: erythropoietic (nandrolone decanoate), anabolic (nandrolone decanoate)
Controlled substance schedule III
Pregnancy risk category X

How supplied

Available by prescription only
nandrolone decanoate
Injection: 50 mg/ml, 100 mg/ml, 200 mg/ml (in oil)

Indications and dosages

Anemia associated with renal insufficiency
nandrolone decanoate
Adults: 100 to 200 mg I.M. weekly in males; 50 to 100 mg/week in females.
Children age 2 to 13: 25 to 50 mg I.M. q 3 to 4 weeks.

Pharmacodynamics

Androgenic action: Nandrolone exerts inhibitory effects on hormone-responsive breast tumors and metastases.
Erythropoietic action: Nandrolone stimulates kidney production of erythropoietin, leading to increases in red blood cell mass and volume.
Anabolic action: Nandrolone may reverse corticosteroid-induced catabolism and promote tissue development in severely debilitated patients.

Pharmacokinetics

***Absorption*:** Well absorbed.
Distribution: Slowly released from I.M. depot following injection and is hydrolyzed to free nandrolone by plasma esterase.
Metabolism: Metabolized in the liver.
Excretion: Both the unchanged drug and its metabolites are excreted in the urine. The elimination half-life of nandrolone is 6 to 8 days.

Route	Onset	Peak	Duration
I.M. (decanoate)	Unknown	3-6 days	Unknown

Contraindications and precautions

Contraindicated in patients with hypersensitivity to anabolic steroids, in men with breast cancer or prostate cancer, in patients with nephrosis, in those experiencing the nephrotic phase of nephritis, in women with breast cancer and hypercalcemia, during pregnancy, or in breast-feeding women.

Use cautiously in patients with renal, cardiac, or hepatic disease; diabetes; epilepsy; migraine; or other conditions that may be aggravated by fluid retention.

Interactions

Drug-drug. *Adrenocorticosteroids or adrenocorticotropic hormone:* Increased potential for fluid and electrolyte retention. Patient requires monitoring for this effect.
Insulin or oral antidiabetic drugs: Decreased blood glucose levels; may require adjustment of antidiabetic agents or insulin.
Warfarin-type anticoagulants: Increases in PT and INR. Monitor PT and INR.

Effects on diagnostic tests

None reported.

Adverse reactions

CNS: excitation, insomnia, habituation, depression.
CV: edema.
GI: nausea, vomiting, diarrhea.
GU: bladder irritability, *hypoestrogenic effects in women (flushing; diaphoresis; vaginitis, including itching, dryness, and burning; vaginal bleeding; nervousness; emotional lability; menstrual irregularities), excessive hormonal effects in men (prepubertal-premature epiphyseal closure,* acne, priapism, *growth of body and facial hair,* phallic enlargement; postpubertal-testicular atrophy, oligospermia, decreased ejaculatory volume, impotence, gynecomastia, epididymitis), androgenic effects in women (acne, edema, *weight gain, hirsutism,* hoarseness, clitoral enlargement, *decreased breast size,* changes in libido, male-pattern baldness, *oily skin or hair*).
Hematologic: elevated serum lipid levels, suppression of clotting factors.
Hepatic: reversible jaundice, ***peliosis hepatitis,*** elevated liver enzyme levels, ***liver cell tumors.***
Metabolic: increased serum sodium, potassium, calcium and phosphate; abnormal results of fasting plasma glucose, glucose tolerance, and metyrapone tests; decreased thyroid function test results and 17-ketosteroid levels.
Skin: pain and induration at injection site.

Overdose and treatment

No information available.

Clinical considerations

- Administer nandrolone injections I.M. deeply into the gluteal muscle.
- An adequate iron intake is necessary for maximum response when patient is receiving nandrolone decanoate injections.
- Therapy should be intermittent, if possible.
- Duration is dependent on patient response and occurrence of adverse reactions.
- Surgically induced anephric patients may be less responsive to effect on anemia.

Therapeutic monitoring

- Monitor liver function tests, urine and serum calcium (in women with breast cancer), serum lipids and cholesterol, and CBC periodically.
- Prepubertal males and females should have X-ray studies every 6 months to evaluate bone age.

Special populations

Breast-feeding patients. It isn't known if anabolic steroids are excreted in breast milk. Because of the potential for serious adverse reactions in breast-fed infants, a decision to discontinue breast-feeding or drug should be made.
Pediatric patients. The adverse effects of giving androgens to young children aren't fully understood, but the risk of serious disturbances (premature epiphyseal closure, masculinization of females, or precocious development in males) exists; weigh the possible benefits before instituting therapy in young children.
Geriatric patients. Observe elderly men for the development of prostatic hypertrophy and prostatic carcinoma.

Patient counseling

- Instruct diabetic patient to monitor glucose closely because glucose tolerance may be altered.
- Tell women to report menstrual irregularities, acne, deepening of voice, male-pattern baldness, or hirsutism.
- Tell patient to notify doctor if persistent GI upset, nausea, vomiting, changes in skin color, or ankle swelling occur.

naphazoline hydrochloride

AK-Con, Albalon Liquifilm, Allerest, Clear Eyes, Comfort Eye Drops, Degest 2, Nafazair, Naphcon, Naphcon Forte, VasoClear, Vasocon

Pharmacologic classification: sympathomimetic
Therapeutic classification: decongestant, vasoconstrictor
Pregnancy risk category C

How supplied

Available by prescription only
Ophthalmic solution: 0.1%

Available without a prescription
Ophthalmic solution: 0.012%, 0.02%, 0.025% (generic), 0.03%
Nasal drops or sprays: 0.05% (solution)

Indications and dosages
Ocular congestion, irritation, itching
Adults: Instill 1 to 3 drops (0.1% solution) q 3 to 4 hours or 1 to 2 drops (0.012% to 0.03% solution) in eye daily to q.i.d for 3 to 4 days.
Nasal congestion
Adults and children over age 12: 1 or 2 drops or sprays (0.05% solution), p.r.n. May repeat doses q 3 to 6 hours. Treatment not to exceed 3 to 5 days.
Children age 6 to 12: 1 to 2 drops or sprays (0.025% solution), p.r.n.

Pharmacodynamics
Decongestant action: Naphazoline produces vasoconstriction by local and alpha-adrenergic action on blood vessels of the conjunctiva or nasal mucosa; therefore, it reduces blood flow and nasal congestion.

Pharmacokinetics
Absorption: Well absorbed intranasally.
Distribution: Unknown.
Metabolism: Unknown.
Excretion: Unknown.

Route	Onset	Peak	Duration
Ophthalmic	10 min	Unknown	2-6 hr
Nasal	10 min	Unknown	2-6 hr

Contraindications and precautions
Contraindicated in patients with hypersensitivity to ingredients of drug and in those with acute angle-closure glaucoma. Use of 0.1% solution is contraindicated in children. Use cautiously in patients with hyperthyroidism, cardiac disease, hypertension, or diabetes mellitus.

Interactions
Drug-drug. *MAO inhibitors:* May result in an increased adrenergic response and hypertensive crisis. Avoid use together.

Effects on diagnostic tests
None reported.

Adverse reactions
CNS: headache, dizziness, nervousness, weakness (with ophthalmic form).
CV: hypertension, ***cardiac irregularities.***
EENT: transient eye stinging, pupillary dilation, eye irritation, photophobia, blurred vision, increased intraocular pressure, keratitis, lacrimation (with ophthalmic form); rebound nasal congestion (with excessive or long-term use), sneezing, stinging, dryness of mucosa (with nasal administration).
GI: nausea (with ophthalmic form).
Other: diaphoresis (with ophthalmic form); systemic effects in children after excessive or long-term use, marked sedation (with nasal administration).

Overdose and treatment
Signs and symptoms of overdose include CNS depression, sweating, decreased body temperature, bradycardia, shocklike hypotension, decreased respiration, CV collapse, and coma.

Activated charcoal or gastric lavage may be used initially to treat accidental ingestion; administer early before sedation occurs. Monitor vital signs and ECG, as ordered. Treat seizures with I.V. diazepam.

Clinical considerations
- Naphazoline is the most widely used ocular decongestant.
- Don't shake container.

Therapeutic monitoring
Monitor patient for blurred vision, pain, or lid edema.

Special populations
Pediatric patients. Use in infants and children may result in CNS depression, leading to coma and marked reduction in body temperature. Although drug is available without a prescription, parents shouldn't use nasal solution containing 0.025% naphazoline hydrochloride in children under age 6, and 0.05% naphazoline hydrochloride in children under age 12.
Geriatric patients. Use drug with caution in geriatric patients with severe cardiac disease or poorly controlled hypertension and in diabetics prone to diabetic ketoacidosis.

Patient counseling
- Teach patient how to instill ophthalmic or nasal medication; tell him not to share drug with others.
- Advise patient to report blurred vision, eye pain, or lid swelling that occurs when using ophthalmic product.
- Inform patient using ophthalmic solution that photophobia may follow pupil dilation; tell patient to report this effect promptly.
- Warn patient not to exceed recommended dosage; rebound nasal congestion and conjunctivitis also may occur with frequent or prolonged use.
- Tell patient to call if nasal congestion persists after 5 days of using nasal solution.

naproxen

Naprosyn, EC-Naprosyn

naproxen sodium

Aleve, Anaprox, Naprelan

Pharmacologic classification: NSAID
Therapeutic classification: nonnarcotic analgesic, antipyretic, anti-inflammatory
Pregnancy risk category B

How supplied

Available by prescription only
naproxen
Tablets: 250 mg, 375 mg, 500 mg
Tablets (delayed-release): 375 mg, 500 mg
Oral suspension: 125 mg/5 ml
naproxen sodium
Tablets (film-coated): 275 mg, 550 mg
Tablets (extended-release): 375 mg, 500 mg

Note: 220 mg, 275 mg, 550 mg of naproxen sodium = 200 mg, 250 mg, or 500 mg of naproxen, respectively.

Available without a prescription
naproxen sodium
Tablets or capsules: 220 mg

Indications and dosages

Mild to moderately severe musculoskeletal or soft tissue irritation
naproxen
Adults: 250 to 500 mg P.O. b.i.d. Alternatively, 250 mg in the morning and 500 mg in the evening; 375 to 500 mg P.O. b.i.d. (delayed release), or 750 to 1,000 mg P.O. daily (controlled release).
naproxen sodium
Adults: 275 to 550 mg P.O. b.i.d. Alternatively, 275 mg in the morning and 550 mg in the evening; 825 to 1,100 mg (extended-release) P.O. once daily.
Mild to moderate pain; primary dysmenorrhea
naproxen
Adults: 500 mg P.O. to start, followed by 250 mg P.O. q 6 to 8 hours, p.r.n. Maximum daily dose shouldn't exceed 1.25 g naproxen. Or, 1,000 mg P.O. daily (controlled release); patients requiring greater analgesia, a 1,500 mg dose may be used for a limited period.
naproxen sodium
Adults: 550 mg P.O. to start, followed by 275 mg P.O. q 6 to 8 hours, p.r.n. Maximum daily dose is 1.375 g naproxen sodium.
Self-medication: 220 mg q 8 to 12 hours. Maximum daily dose is 440 mg for adults age 65 and older, or three tablets for adults under age 65. Don't self-medicate for more than 10 days.
Acute gout
naproxen
Adults: 750 mg P.O. initially, then 250 mg q 8 hours until episode subsides. Or, 1,000 mg to 1,500 mg (using naproxen sodium controlled-release tablets) P.O. daily on the first day, then 1,000 mg P.O. daily until attack subsides.
naproxen sodium
Adults: 825 mg P.O. initially, then 275 mg q 8 hours until attack has subsided.
Juvenile rheumatoid arthritis
naproxen
Children: 10 mg/kg/day P.O. in two divided doses.

Pharmacodynamics

Analgesic, antipyretic, and anti-inflammatory actions: Mechanisms of action are unknown; naproxen is thought to inhibit prostaglandin synthesis.

Pharmacokinetics

Absorption: Absorbed rapidly and completely from the GI tract.
Distribution: Highly protein-bound. It crosses the placenta and is distributed into the milk.
Metabolism: Metabolized in the liver.
Excretion: Excreted in urine. Half-life is 10 to 20 hours.

Route	Onset	Peak	Duration
P.O.	1 hr	2-4 hr	7 hr

Contraindications and precautions

Contraindicated in patients with hypersensitivity to drug or asthma, rhinitis, or nasal polyps. Use cautiously in the elderly and in patients with history of peptic ulcer disease or renal, CV, GI, or hepatic disease.

Interactions

Drug-drug. *Acetaminophen, gold compounds, or other anti-inflammatory agents:* Increased nephrotoxicity. Monitor renal function tests.
Anticoagulants and thrombolytic drugs, such as coumadin derivatives, heparin, streptokinase, and urokinase: May potentiate anticoagulant effects. Monitor PT and INR.
Antihypertensive agents and diuretics: Decreased effects of these drugs. Using together may increase risk of nephrotoxicity. Avoid use together.
Anti-inflammatory agents, corticotropin, salicylates, or corticosteroids: May cause increased GI adverse reactions, including ulceration and hemorrhage. Use together very cautiously.
Aspirin, parenteral carbenicillin, cefamandole, cefoperazone, dextran, dipyridamole, mezlocillin, piperacillin, plicamycin, sulfinpyrazone, ticarcillin, valproic acid, salicylates, or other anti-inflammatory agents: Bleeding problems. Use together very cautiously.
Aspirin: May decrease the bioavailability of naproxen. Patient requires monitoring for effect.
Coumadin derivatives, nifedipine, phenytoin, or verapamil: Increased risk of toxicity. Patient requires close monitoring.

Insulin or oral antidiabetic agents: May potentiate hypoglycemic effects. Monitor serum glucose.
Lithium and methotrexate: Increased nephrotoxicity may occur. Monitor renal function tests.

Effects on diagnostic tests
Naproxen and its metabolites may interfere with urinary 5-hydroxyindoleacetic acid and 17-hydroxy-corticosteroid determinations.

Adverse reactions
CNS: *headache, drowsiness, dizziness,* vertigo.
CV: *edema,* palpitations.
EENT: visual disturbances, *tinnitus,* auditory disturbances.
GI: *epigastric distress, occult blood loss, nausea,* ***peptic ulceration,*** constipation, dyspepsia, heartburn, diarrhea, stomatitis, thirst.
GU: nephrotoxicity.
Hematologic: ***thrombocytopenia,*** eosinophilia, ***agranulocytosis, neutropenia.***
Hepatic: elevated liver enzyme levels.
Respiratory: dyspnea.
Skin: *pruritus, rash,* urticaria, ecchymosis, diaphoresis, purpura.

Overdose and treatment
Signs and symptoms of overdose include drowsiness, heartburn, indigestion, nausea, and vomiting.

To treat overdose of naproxen, empty stomach immediately by inducing emesis with ipecac syrup or by gastric lavage. Administer activated charcoal via nasogastric tube. Provide symptomatic and supportive measures (respiratory support and correction of fluid and electrolyte imbalances). Monitor laboratory parameters and vital signs closely. Hemodialysis is ineffective in naproxen removal.

Clinical considerations
Consider the recommendations relevant to all NSAIDs as well as the following:
- Use lowest possible effective dose; 250 mg of naproxen is equivalent to 275 mg of naproxen sodium.
- Relief usually begins within 2 weeks after beginning therapy with naproxen.
- Institute safety measures to prevent injury resulting from possible CNS effects.

Therapeutic monitoring
- Recommend monitoring fluid balance. Monitor for signs and symptoms of fluid retention, especially significant weight gain.
- Monitor LFTs, renal function tests, CBC, bleeding times in long-term therapy.

Special populations
Breast-feeding patients. Because they're excreted in breast milk, avoid using naproxen and naproxen sodium during breast-feeding.
Pediatric patients. Safety of naproxen in children under age 2 hasn't been established. Safety of naproxen sodium in children hasn't been established. No age-related problems have been reported.
Geriatric patients. Patients over age 60 are more sensitive to the adverse effects (especially GI toxicity) of drug. The effect of naproxen on renal prostaglandins may cause fluid retention and edema. This may be significant in geriatric patients, especially those with heart failure.

Patient counseling
- Caution patient to avoid taking naproxen with OTC drugs.
- Teach patient signs and symptoms of possible adverse reactions and tell him to report them promptly.
- Instruct patient to check his weight every 2 to 3 days and to report any gain of 3 lb (1.4 kg) or more within 1 week.
- Instruct patient in safety measures; advise him to avoid activities that require alertness until CNS effects are known.
- Warn patient against combining naproxen (Naprosyn) with naproxen sodium (Anaprox) because both agents circulate in the blood as naproxen anion.
- Teach patient not to break or crush controlled or delayed-release tablets.

naratriptan hydrochloride
Amerge

Pharmacologic classification: selective 5-hydroxytryptamine$_1$ (5-HT$_1$) receptor subtype agonist
Therapeutic classification: antimigraine
Pregnancy risk category C

How supplied
Available by prescription only
Tablets: 1 mg, 2.5 mg

Indications and dosages
Treatment of acute migraine headache attacks with or without aura
Adults: 1 or 2.5 mg P.O. as a single dose. Dose should be individualized, depending on the possible benefit of the 2.5-mg dose and the greater risk of adverse events. If headache returns or if only partial response occurs, may repeat dose after 4 hours, for maximum dose of 5 mg within 24 hours.
≡ ***Dosage adjustment.*** In patients with mild to moderate renal or hepatic impairment, consider a lower initial dose; don't exceed maximum dose of 2.5 mg over a 24-hour period. Don't use in patients with severe renal or hepatic impairment.

Pharmacodynamics

Antimigraine action: Naratriptan binds with high affinity to 5-HT_{1D} and 5-HT_{1B} receptors. One theory suggests that activation of 5-$HT_{1D/1B}$ receptors located on intracranial blood vessels leads to vasoconstriction, which is associated with the migraine relief. Another hypothesis suggests that activation of 5-$HT_{1D/1B}$ receptors on sensory nerve endings in the trigeminal system results in the inhibition of proinflammatory neuropeptide release.

Pharmacokinetics

Absorption: Well absorbed with about 70% oral bioavailability.
Distribution: Steady-state volume of distribution is 170 L. Plasma protein binding is 28% to 31%.
Metabolism: In vitro, naratriptan is metabolized by many P-450 cytochrome isoenzymes to inactive metabolites.
Excretion: Predominantly eliminated in urine, with 50% of dose recovered unchanged and 30% as metabolites. Mean elimination half-life is 6 hours.

Route	Onset	Peak	Duration
P.O.	Unknown	2-3 hr	Unknown

Contraindications and precautions

Contraindicated in patients with hypersensitivity to drug or its components and in those with history, symptoms, or signs of ischemic cardiac, cerebrovascular (such as stroke or transient ischemic attack), or peripheral vascular syndromes (such as ischemic bowel disease). Also contraindicated in patients with significant underlying CV diseases, including angina pectoris, MI, and silent myocardial ischemia. Drug shouldn't be given to patients with uncontrolled hypertension because of potential increase in blood pressure.

Contraindicated in patients with severe renal (creatinine clearance less than 15 ml/minute) or hepatic (Child-Pugh grade C) impairment and in those with hemiplegic or basilar migraine.

Drug or other 5-HT_1 agonists are also contraindicated in patients with potential risk factors for coronary artery disease, such as hypertension, hypercholesterolemia, obesity, diabetes, strong family history of coronary artery disease, women with surgical or physiologic menopause, men over age 40, or smokers.

Interactions

Drug-drug. *Ergot-containing or ergot-type drugs or other 5-HT_1 agonists:* Prolonged vasospastic reactions. Use of these drugs within 24 hours of naratriptan is contraindicated.
Oral contraceptives: Increased naratriptan levels. Patient requires close monitoring.
Selective serotonin reuptake inhibitors (SSRIs), such as fluoxetine, fluvoxamine, paroxetine, and sertraline: Weakness, hyperreflexia, and incoordination when coadministered with 5-HT_1 agonists. Use together cautiously.
Drug-lifestyle. *Smoking:* Increased clearance of naratriptan by 30%. Advise patient to avoid smoking.

Effects on diagnostic tests

None reported.

Adverse reactions

CNS: paresthesia, dizziness, drowsiness, malaise, fatigue, vertigo.
CV: palpitations, increased blood pressure, tachyarrhythmias, ***abnormal ECG changes (PR, QT prolongation, ST/T wave abnormalities, premature ventricular contractions, atrial flutter and/or fibrillation),*** syncope.
EENT: ear, nose and throat infections, photophobia.
GI: nausea, hyposalivation, vomiting.
Other: warm or cold temperature sensations; pressure, tightness, heaviness sensations.

Overdose and treatment

A significant increase in blood pressure has been observed with an overdose, occurring between 30 minutes and 6 hours after ingestion of drug. Blood pressure returned to normal within 8 hours without pharmacologic intervention in some patients, whereas in others antihypertensive patients, drug treatment was necessary.

No specific antidote exists. Perform ECG monitoring for evidence of ischemia. Monitor patient for at least 24 hours after an overdose or while symptoms persist. The effect of hemodialysis or peritoneal dialysis on drug is unknown.

Clinical considerations

- Use drug only when a clear diagnosis of migraine has been established. It's not intended for prophylactic therapy of migraines or for use in the management of hemiplegic or basilar migraine.
- Safety and effectiveness haven't been established for cluster headaches.

Therapeutic monitoring

- First dose should be given in a medically equipped facility for patients at risk for coronary artery disease but determined to have a satisfactory CV evaluation. Consider ECG monitoring.
- Periodic cardiac reevaluation in patients who have or develop risk factors for coronary artery disease is necessary.

Special populations

Pregnant patients. To monitor fetal outcomes of patients exposed to naratriptan during pregnancy, call 1-800-722-9292, ext. 39441.

Breast-feeding patients. Use with caution in breast-feeding women.
Pediatric patients. Safety and efficacy in children under age 18 haven't been established.
Geriatric patients. Don't use drug in geriatric patients.

Patient counseling
- Tell patient that drug is intended to relieve, and not prevent, migraine headaches.
- Instruct patient not to use drug if pregnancy is suspected or during pregnancy itself.
- Teach patient to alert doctor of risk factors for coronary artery disease.
- Instruct patient to take dose soon after headache starts. If there's no response to the first tablet, tell patient to seek medical approval before taking second tablet.
- Tell patient that if more relief is needed after the first tablet, such as when a partial response occurs or if the headache returns, he may take a second tablet but not sooner than 4 hours after the first tablet. Inform him not to exceed two tablets within 24 hours.

nedocromil sodium
Tilade

Pharmacologic classification: pyranoquinoline
Therapeutic classification: anti-inflammatory respiratory inhalant
Pregnancy risk category B

How supplied
Available by prescription only
Inhalation aerosol: 1.75 mg per actuation in 16.2-g canister (U.S.); 2 mg per actuation in 16.2-g canister (Canada)

Indications and dosages
Maintenance therapy in mild to moderate bronchial asthma
Adults and children age 6 and older: 2 inhalations q.i.d., preferably at regular intervals; may gradually decrease dosing interval to b.i.d.

Pharmacodynamics
Anti-inflammatory and antiallergic action: Drug inhibits activation and release of inflammatory mediators from various cell types in the lumen and mucosa of the bronchial tree. These mediators, which include the leukotrienes, histamine, and prostaglandins, are preformed or derived from arachidonic acid metabolism. A range of human cells associated with asthma may be involved. As a result, nedocromil exhibits specific anti-inflammatory properties when administered topically to the bronchial mucosa. It has demonstrated a significant inhibitory effect on allergen-induced early and late asthmatic reactions and on bronchial hyperresponsiveness. Nedocromil also may affect sensory nerves in the lung. The result is inhibition of bradykinin-induced bronchoconstriction.

Pharmacokinetics
Absorption: 2% to 3% of amount swallowed after nedocromil inhalation is absorbed. From 6% to 9% of nedocromil deposited in the lungs is completely absorbed.
Distribution: Distributed to plasma only. About 89% is reversibly bound to plasma proteins when plasma levels range between 0.5 and 50 mcg/ml.
Metabolism: Not metabolized.
Excretion: Rapidly excreted unchanged in the bile and urine. Half-life is about 1½ to 3⅓ hours.

Route	Onset	Peak	Duration
Inhalation	Unknown	30 min	3½ hr

Contraindications and precautions
Contraindicated in patients hypersensitive to the formulation or in patients experiencing an acute asthmatic attack or acute bronchospasm.

Interactions
None reported.

Effects on diagnostic tests
None reported.

Adverse reactions
CV: chest pain.
CNS: headache, dysphagia, fatigue.
GI: nausea, vomiting, dyspepsia, abdominal pain, dry mouth, *unpleasant taste.*
Respiratory: upper respiratory tract infection, rhinitis, cough, pharyngitis, increased sputum, bronchitis, dyspnea, ***bronchospasm.***

Overdose and treatment
Because nedocromil doesn't pass the blood-brain barrier, symptoms of overdose probably require nothing more than observing patient and stopping drug when appropriate.

Clinical considerations
- Dosage may be reduced to two inhalations three times daily and then twice daily after several weeks, when patient's asthma is under control.
- In maintenance therapy, drug must be used regularly, even during symptom-free periods, to achieve benefit.
- Reduced severity of clinical symptoms or need for accessory therapy is a sign of improvement that usually occurs in the first 2 weeks of therapy if patient responds to therapy.
- When nedocromil is added to an existing regimen of bronchodilators, or given with inhaled or oral corticosteroids, a reduction in dosage of the steroid or bronchodilator may be achieved

in some patients. However, reduction should be gradual and under close medical supervision to avoid exacerbating asthma.

- Don't exceed 14 mg within 24 hours.
- In some patients, bronchospasm may be prevented by a single dose of nedocromil before activities that precipitate asthma, such as exercise or exposure to cold air, pollutants, or allergens.

Therapeutic monitoring
Monitor patient for response to therapy.

Special populations
Breast-feeding patients. It isn't known if drug is excreted in breast milk. Use cautiously when administering drug to breast-feeding women.
Pediatric patients. Safety and efficacy haven't been established for children under age 6.

Patient counseling
- Warn patient that drug has no direct bronchodilating action and can't replace bronchodilators during an acute asthmatic attack.
- Tell patient that drug is an adjunct to the regular bronchodilator regimen and may reduce the need for corticosteroids or bronchodilators.
- Emphasize that drug should be taken regularly for best results. Most patients report benefits after 1 week of use; some require longer treatment before improvement occurs.
- Teach patient how to use the inhaler. Instruct him to shake canister immediately before use and to invert it just before actuation. Prime inhaler with 3 actuations before first use or if unused for more than 7 days.
- Advise patient to clean inhaler at least twice weekly and to remove canister before rinsing inhaler in hot running water. Allow inhaler to air dry overnight.

nefazodone hydrochloride
Serzone

Pharmacologic classification: phenylpiperazine
Therapeutic classification: antidepressant
Pregnancy risk category C

How supplied
Available by prescription only
Tablets: 50 mg, 100 mg, 150 mg, 200 mg, 250 mg

Indications and dosages
Depression
Adults: Initially, 200 mg/day P.O. divided into two doses. Dosage increased in 100- to 200-mg/day increments at intervals of no less than 1 week, p.r.n. Usual dosage range, 300 to 600 mg/day.

≡ ***Dosage adjustment.*** In adults age 65 and older, dosage is 50 mg P.O. b.i.d. initially. Increase slowly as needed. Usual dose is 200 to 400 mg per day.

Pharmacodynamics
Antidepressive action: Action of drug isn't precisely defined. It inhibits neuronal uptake of serotonin and norepinephrine. It also occupies central 5-HT_1 (serotonin) and $alpha_1$-adrenergic receptors.

Pharmacokinetics
Absorption: Rapidly and completely absorbed but, because of extensive metabolism, its absolute bioavailability is only about 20%.
Distribution: More than 99% is bound to plasma proteins.
Metabolism: Extensively metabolized by n-dealkylation and aliphatic and aromatic hydroxylation.
Excretion: Excreted in urine. Half-life of drug is 2 to 4 hours.

Route	Onset	Peak	Duration
P.O.	Unknown	1 hr	Unknown

Contraindications and precautions
Contraindicated in patients with hypersensitivity to drug or other phenylpiperazine antidepressants. Don't use within 14 days of MAO inhibitor therapy or in coadministration with astemizole or cisapride.

Use cautiously in patients with CV or cerebrovascular disease that could be exacerbated by hypotension (such as history of MI, angina, or CVA) and conditions that would predispose patients to hypotension (such as, dehydration, hypovolemia, and antihypertensive drug treatment). Use cautiously in patients with history of mania.

Interactions
Drug-drug. *Alprazolam and triazolam:* Potentiated effects of these drugs. Don't administer together. However, if necessary, dosages of alprazolam and triazolam may need to be reduced greatly.
Astemizole or cisapride: May cause decreased metabolism of these drugs, leading to increased levels and cardiotoxicity. Avoid use together.
CNS active drugs: May alter CNS activity. Use together cautiously.
Digoxin: Increased serum digoxin levels. Use together cautiously and monitor digoxin levels.
MAO inhibitors: May cause severe excitation, hyperpyrexia, seizures, delirium, or coma. Avoid use together.
Other highly plasma protein-bound drugs: May increase incidence and severity of adverse reactions. Monitor patient closely.

Effects on diagnostic tests
None reported.

Adverse reactions
CNS: *headache, somnolence, dizziness, asthenia,* insomnia, *light-headedness, confusion,* memory impairment, paresthesia, abnormal dreams, decreased concentration, ataxia, incoordination, taste perversion, psychomotor retardation, tremor, hypertonia.
CV: orthostatic hypotension, vasodilation, hypotension, peripheral edema.
EENT: *blurred vision, abnormal vision,* pharyngitis, tinnitus, visual field defect.
GI: *dry mouth, nausea, constipation,* dyspepsia, diarrhea, increased appetite, vomiting, thirst.
GU: urinary frequency, urinary tract infection, urine retention, vaginitis, breast pain.
Musculoskeletal: neck rigidity, arthralgia.
Respiratory: cough.
Skin: pruritus, rash.
Other: infection, flu syndrome, chills, fever.

Overdose and treatment
Common symptoms associated with overdose of nefazodone include nausea, vomiting, and somnolence. Other drug-associated adverse reactions may occur. Provide symptomatic and supportive treatment in the case of hypotension or excessive sedation. Use gastric lavage if needed.

Clinical considerations
- Allow at least 1 week after stopping drug before giving patient an MAO inhibitor. Also, allow at least 14 days before patient is started on nefazodone after MAO inhibitor therapy has been stopped.
- Drug therapy may precipitate mania or hypomania in patients with bipolar or other affective disorders.

Therapeutic monitoring
- Patient needs to be monitored for suicidal tendencies. Only a minimum supply of drug should be allowed.
- Monitor LFTs in patients with hepatic dysfunction.

Special populations
Breast-feeding patients. It isn't known if nefazodone is excreted in breast milk; use caution when administering drug to breast-feeding women.
Pediatric patients. Safety and efficacy in children under age 18 haven't been established.
Geriatric patients. Because of increased systemic exposure to nefazodone, begin treatment at half the usual dose, but increase dose over the same dosage range as in younger patients. Observe usual precautions in geriatric patients who have ongoing medical illnesses or are receiving other drugs.

Patient counseling
- Warn patient not to engage in hazardous activities until CNS effects are known.
- Instruct men that if prolonged or inappropriate erections occur, to should stop drug immediately and seek medical attention.
- Instruct women to report suspected pregnancy or if planning to become pregnant during therapy.
- Instruct patient not to drink alcoholic beverages during therapy.
- Tell patient to report rash, hives, or a related allergic reaction.
- Inform patient that several weeks of therapy may be required to obtain the full antidepressant effect. Once improvement is seen, advise patient not to discontinue drug until directed.

nelfinavir mesylate
Viracept

Pharmacologic classification: HIV protease inhibitor
Therapeutic classification: antiviral
Pregnancy risk category B

How supplied
Available by prescription only
Tablets: 250 mg
Powder: 50 mg/g of powder

Indications and dosages
Treatment of HIV infection when antiretroviral therapy is warranted
Adults: 750 mg P.O. t.i.d with meal or light snack.
Children age 2 to 13: 20 to 30 mg/kg/dose P.O. t.i.d. with meal or light snack; don't exceed 750 mg t.i.d. Recommended pediatric dose given t.i.d. is shown in the following table.

Body weight (kg)	No. of level 1-g scoops	No. of level teaspoons	No. of tablets
7 to < 8.5	4	1	-
8.5 to < 10.5	5	1.25	-
10.5 to < 12	6	1.5	-
12 to < 14	7	1.75	-
14 to < 16	8	2	-
16 to < 18	9	2.25	-
18 to < 23	10	2.5	2
≥ 23	15	3.75	3

◊ *Children age 2 to 13 years weighing 50 to 116 lb (23 to 53 kg):* 25 to 30 mg/kg P.O. t.i.d. up to 1,250 or 1,500 mg per dose.
◊ ***Post-exposure prophylaxis following occupational exposure to HIV***
Adults: 750 mg P.O. t.i.d. in combination with oral zidovudine and lamivudine for 4 weeks.

Pharmacodynamics
Antiviral action: Inhibition of the protease enzyme prevents cleavage of the viral polyprotein, resulting in the production of an immature, noninfectious virus.

Pharmacokinetics
Absorption: Absolute bioavailability isn't determined. Food increases absorption of drug.
Distribution: Apparent volume of drug distribution is 2 to 7 L/kg. More than 98% of drug is bound to plasma protein.
Metabolism: Metabolized in the liver by multiple cytochrome P-450 isoforms, including CYP3A.
Excretion: Terminal half-life is 3½ to 5 hours. Drug is primarily excreted in the feces.

Route	Onset	Peak	Duration
P.O.	Unknown	2-4 hr	Unknown

Contraindications and precautions
Contraindicated in patients with hypersensitivity to any component of drug. Use cautiously in patients with hepatic dysfunction or hemophilia types A and B.

Interactions
Drug-drug. *Amiodarone, cisapride, ergot derivatives, midazolam, quinidine, or triazolam:* Increased plasma levels of these drugs, which may increase risk for serious or life-threatening adverse events. Avoid use together.
Anti-HIV protease inhibitors, such as indinavir or saquinavir: May increase plasma levels of both drugs. Use together cautiously.
Carbamazepine, phenobarbital, and phenytoin: May reduce the effectiveness of nelfinavir by decreasing nelfinavir plasma levels. Use together cautiously.
HMG-CoA inhibitors such as lovastatin, simvastatin: May increase plasma levels of antilipemic agents. Avoid using together.
Oral contraceptives: Nelfinavir may decrease plasma levels of oral contraceptives. Advise patient to use appropriate contraceptive measures during therapy.
Drugs primarily metabolized by CYP3A, such as dihydropyridine or calcium channel blockers: May result in increased levels of these drugs and decreased plasma level of nelfinavir. Use together cautiously.
Rifabutin: Increased rifabutin plasma levels. Reduce dose of rifabutin to one-half the usual dose.
Rifampin: Decreased nelfinavir plasma levels. Don't use together.
Ritonavir: May increase concentration of nelfinavir. Use together cautiously.
Sildenafil: May increase adverse effects of sildenafil. Use together cautiously.

Effects on diagnostic tests
None reported.

Adverse reactions
CNS: anxiety, depression, dizziness, emotional lability, hyperkinesia, insomnia, malaise, migraine headache, paresthesia, ***seizures,*** sleep disorders, somnolence, ***suicidal ideation.***
EENT: iritis, eye disorders, pharyngitis, rhinitis, sinusitis.
GI: abdominal pain, nausea, *diarrhea,* flatulence, anorexia, dyspepsia, epigastric pain, GI bleeding, ***pancreatitis,*** mouth ulceration, vomiting.
GU: sexual dysfunction, kidney calculus, urine abnormality.
Hematologic: anemia, ***leukopenia, thrombocytopenia.***
Hepatic: ***hepatitis.***
Metabolic: dehydration, diabetes mellitus, hyperlipidemia, hyperuricemia, hypoglycemia.
Musculoskeletal: back pain, arthralgia, arthritis, cramps, myalgia, myasthenia, myopathy.
Respiratory: dyspnea.
Skin: rash, dermatitis, folliculitis, fungal dermatitis, pruritus, sweating, urticaria.
Other: fever, redistribution or accumulation of body fat.

Overdose and treatment
Information is limited. Unabsorbed drug may be removed by emesis or gastric lavage; activated charcoal may also be used. Dialysis isn't beneficial.

Clinical considerations
- Decision to use drug is based on surrogate marker changes in patients who received drug in combination with nucleoside analogues or alone for up to 24 weeks. There are no results from controlled trials evaluating the effect on survival or incidence of opportunistic fungal infections.
- Drug dosage is same whether used alone or in combination with other antiretroviral agents.
- Antiretroviral activity may be increased when used in combination with approved reverse transcriptase inhibitors.
- Administer oral powder in children unable to take tablets; may mix oral powder with water, milk, formula, soy formula, soy milk, or dietary supplements.
- Don't reconstitute with water in its original container.
- Use reconstituted powder within 6 hours.
- Acidic foods or juice aren't recommended due to bitter taste.

Therapeutic monitoring

- Recommend monitoring CBC with differential (especially neutrophils) and chemistries; low incidences of laboratory abnormalities were reported in clinical studies. Increases in alkaline phosphatase, amylase, CK, LD, AST, ALT, and GGT may occur; monitor closely.
- Recommend monitoring patient for toxicity and disease progression.

Special populations

Pregnant patients. Use only when clearly needed. To monitor maternal-fetal outcomes, register patient by calling 1-800-258-4263.
Breast-feeding patients. It isn't known if drug is excreted in breast milk. Although safety hasn't been established, advise HIV-infected women not to breast-feed in order to avoid HIV transmission to the infant.
Pediatric patients. Safety and efficacy haven't been established in children under age 2.

Patient counseling

- Advise patient to take drug with food.
- Inform patient that drug isn't a cure for HIV infection.
- Tell patient that long-term effects of drug are currently unknown and that there's evidence that drug reduces risk of HIV transmission to others.
- Advise patient to take drug daily as prescribed and not to alter dose or discontinue drug without medical approval.
- If patient misses a dose, tell him to take the dose as soon as possible and return to his normal schedule. If a dose is skipped, advise patient not to double the dose.
- Tell patient that diarrhea is the most common adverse effect and that it can be controlled with loperamide, if necessary.
- Explain to patient that body fat may accumulate or redistribute during therapy.
- Instruct patient taking oral contraceptives to use alternate or additional contraceptive measures.
- Advise patient to report use of other prescribed or OTC drugs.

neomycin sulfate

Mycifradin, Myciguent, Neo-Tabs

Pharmacologic classification: aminoglycoside
Therapeutic classification: antibiotic
Pregnancy risk category D

How supplied

Available by prescription only
Tablets: 500 mg
Oral solution: 125 mg/5 ml
Otic suspension: 5 mg/ml (with polymyxin B sulfate 10,000 units/ml and hydrocortisone 1%)
Available without a prescription
Cream: 0.5%
Ointment: 0.5%

Indications and dosages

***Infectious diarrhea caused by enteropathogenic* Escherichia coli**
Adults: 50 mg/kg P.O. daily in four divided doses for 2 to 3 days.
Children: 50 to 100 mg/kg P.O. daily divided q 4 to 6 hours for 2 to 3 days.
Suppression of intestinal bacteria preoperatively
Adults: 1 g P.O. q 1 hour for four doses, then 1 g q 4 hours for rest of 24 hours. A saline cathartic should precede therapy.
Children: 40 to 100 mg/kg P.O. daily divided q 4 to 6 hours. First dose should be preceded by saline cathartic.
For 2- to 3-day regimen
Adults and children: 88 mg/kg P.O. in six equally divided doses at 4-hour intervals. Alternatively, for 8 a.m. surgery, 1 g of neomycin and 1 g of erythromycin base P.O. at 1 p.m., 2 p.m., and 11 p.m. on the day preceding surgery.
Adjunctive treatment in hepatic coma
Adults: 1 to 3 g P.O. q.i.d. for 5 to 6 days; 200 ml of 1% or 100 ml of 2% solution as enema retained for 20 to 60 minutes q 6 hours.
Children: 50 to 100 mg/kg P.O. daily in divided doses for 5 to 6 days.
◊ ***Treatment of hypercholesterolemia***
Adults: 500 mg to 2 g P.O. daily in two or three divided doses.
External ear canal infection
Adults and children: 2 to 5 drops into ear canal t.i.d. or q.i.d. for 7 to 10 days.
Topical bacterial infections, burns, wounds, skin grafts, following surgical procedure, lesions, pruritus, trophic ulcerations, and edema
Adults and children: Rub in small amount gently b.i.d., t.i.d., or as directed.
≡ ***Dosage adjustment.*** Use reduced dosage in adults and children with renal failure. Specific recommendations aren't available.

Pharmacodynamics

Antibiotic action: Neomycin is bactericidal; it binds directly to the 30S ribosomal subunit, thus inhibiting bacterial protein synthesis. Its spectrum of action includes many aerobic gram-negative organisms and some aerobic gram-positive organisms. Drug is far less active against many gram-negative organisms than are amikacin, gentamicin, netilmicin, and tobramycin. Given orally or as retention enema, neomycin inhibits ammonia-forming bacteria in the GI tract, reducing ammonia and improving neurologic status of patients with hepatic encephalopathy. It's rarely given systemically because of its high potential for ototoxicity and nephrotoxicity. The FDA recently revoked licensing of the parenteral preparation for this reason.

Pharmacokinetics

Absorption: Absorbed poorly (about 3%) after oral administration, although oral administration is enhanced in patients with impaired GI motility or mucosal intestinal ulcerations. Neomycin isn't absorbed through intact skin; it may be absorbed from wounds, burns, or skin ulcers.
Distribution: Crosses the placenta. Oral administration restricts distribution to the GI tract.
Metabolism: Not metabolized.
Excretion: Excreted primarily in urine by glomerular filtration. Elimination half-life in adults is 2 to 3 hours; in severe renal damage, half-life may extend to 24 hours. After oral administration, neomycin is excreted primarily unchanged in feces.

Route	Onset	Peak	Duration
P.O.	Unknown	1-4 hr	8 hr
Topical	Unknown	Unknown	Unknown

Contraindications and precautions

Contraindicated in patients hypersensitive to drug. Oral form contraindicated in patients sensitive to other aminoglycosides and in those with intestinal obstruction.

Use oral form cautiously in the elderly and in patients with impaired renal function, neuromuscular disorders, or ulcerative bowel lesions. Don't administer drug parenterally. Use topical form cautiously in patients with extensive dermatologic conditions.

Interactions

Drug-drug. *Oral anticoagulants*: Potentiated effects of anticoagulant. Dosage adjustment of anticoagulants may be necessary.

Effects on diagnostic tests

None reported.

Adverse reactions

EENT: *ototoxicity* (with oral administration).
GI: nausea, vomiting, diarrhea, malabsorption syndrome, *Clostridium difficile*-associated colitis (with oral administration).
GU: ***nephrotoxicity*** (with oral administration).
Skin: *rash, contact dermatitis,* urticaria (with topical administration).
Other: ***neuromuscular blockade*** (with topical administration).

Overdose and treatment

Signs of overdose include ototoxicity, nephrotoxicity, and neuromuscular toxicity. Remove drug by hemodialysis or peritoneal dialysis; treatment with calcium salts or anticholinesterases reverses neuromuscular blockade. After recent ingestion (4 hours or less), empty the stomach by induced emesis or gastric lavage; follow with activated charcoal to reduce absorption.

Clinical considerations

Consider the recommendations relevant to all aminoglycosides, as well as the following:
- In hepatic coma, decrease dietary protein and reassess neurologic status frequently.

Preoperative bowel contamination
- Provide low-residue diet and cathartic immediately before administration of oral neomycin; follow-up enemas may be necessary to completely empty bowel.

Topical therapy
- Don't apply to more than 20% of body surface.
- Don't apply to any body surface of patient with decreased renal function without considering risk/benefit ratio.

Otic therapy
- Reculture persistent drainage.
- Drug is best used in combination with other antibiotics.
- Avoid touching ear with dropper.

Therapeutic monitoring

- Recommend monitoring patient for hypersensitivity or contact dermatitis.
- Monitor renal function during drug therapy.
- Patient's hearing should be evaluated before and during prolonged drug therapy.
- Recommend monitoring for superinfection.

Patient counseling

- Instruct patient to report adverse reactions promptly.
- Encourage adequate fluid intake.

neostigmine bromide

neostigmine methylsulfate

Prostigmin

Pharmacologic classification: cholinesterase inhibitor
Therapeutic classification: muscle stimulant
Pregnancy risk category C

How supplied

Available by prescription only
Tablets: 15 mg
Injection: 0.5 mg/ml, 1 mg/ml

Indications and dosages

Antidote for nondepolarizing neuromuscular blocking agents
Adults: 0.5 to 2 mg slow I.V. Repeat, p.r.n.; maximum total dose, 5 mg. Give 0.6 to 1.2 mg atropine sulfate I.V. before antidote dose if patient is bradycardic.

Neonates, infants, and children: 0.04 mg/kg/dose I.V. with atropine sulfate (0.02 mg/kg atropine) with each dose of neostigmine.
Prevention of postoperative abdominal distention and bladder atony
Adults: 0.25 mg I.M. or S.C. q 4 to 6 hours for 2 to 3 days.
Treatment of postoperative abdominal distention and bladder atony
Adults: 0.5 to 1 mg S.C. or I.M.; if for urinary retention and there's no response in 1 hour, catheterize patient and repeat dose q 3 hours for five doses after bladder is emptied.
◇***Diagnosis of myasthenia gravis***
Adults: 0.022 mg/kg I.M. Give atropine 0.011 mg/kg I.V. with dose or I.M. 30 minutes before dose. If cholinergic reaction occurs, discontinue test and give atropine sulfate 0.4 to 0.6 mg I.V. If the results are inconclusive, retest on another day using 0.031 mg/kg I.M. of neostigmine preceded by atropine 0.01 mg/kg.
Children: 0.025 to 0.04 mg/kg I.M. preceded by 0.011 mg/kg S.C. of atropine sulfate.
Symptomatic control of myasthenia gravis
Adults: 0.5 to 2.5 mg S.C., I.V., or I.M. Oral dose can range from 15 to 375 mg/day (average 150 mg in 24 hours). Subsequent dosages must be individualized, based on response and tolerance of adverse effects. Therapy may be required day and night.
Children: 7.5 to 15 mg P.O. t.i.d. or q.i.d. Alternatively, 0.333 mg/kg or 10 mg/m^2 P.O. 6 times daily.
Neonates: 0.1 to 0.2 S.C. or 0.03 mg/kg I.M. q 2 to 4 hours or 1 to 4 mg P.O. q 2 to 3 hours. Gradual dose reduction as symptoms improve.
◇***Supraventricular tachycardia from tricyclic antidepressant overdose***
Children: 0.5 to 1 mg I.V. followed by 0.25 to 0.5 mg q 1 to 3 hours, p.r.n.
◇***Decrease small bowel transit time during radiography***
Adults: 0.5 to 0.75 mg S.C.

Pharmacodynamics
Muscle stimulant action: Neostigmine blocks hydrolysis of acetylcholine by cholinesterase, resulting in acetylcholine accumulation at cholinergic synapses, which leads to increased cholinergic receptor stimulation at the myoneural junction.

Pharmacokinetics
Absorption: Poorly absorbed (1% to 2%) from GI tract after oral administration.
Distribution: About 15% to 25% of dose binds to plasma proteins.
Metabolism: Hydrolyzed by cholinesterases and metabolized by microsomal liver enzymes. Duration of effect varies considerably, depending on patient's physical and emotional status and on disease severity.
Excretion: About 80% of dose is excreted in urine as unchanged drug and metabolites in the first 24 hours after administration.

Route	Onset	Peak	Duration
P.O.	45-75 min	1-2 hr	2-4 hr
I.V.	4-8 min	1-2 hr	2-4 hr
I.M., S.C.	20-30 min	1-2 hr	2-4 hr

Contraindications and precautions
Contraindicated in patients with hypersensitivity to cholinergics or to bromide and in those with peritonitis or mechanical obstruction of the intestine or urinary tract. Use cautiously in patients with bronchial asthma, bradycardia, seizure disorders, recent coronary occlusion, vagotonia, hyperthyroidism, arrhythmias, and peptic ulcer.

Interactions
Drug-drug. *Atropine, corticosteroids, magnesium, procainamide, quinidine:* May reverse cholinergic effect of neostigmine on muscle. Patient requires observation for drug effect.
Other cholinergic drugs: May cause additive toxicity. Avoid use together.
Succinylcholine: May result in prolonged respiratory depression. Patient requires careful monitoring.

Effects on diagnostic tests
None reported.

Adverse reactions
CNS: dizziness, convulsions, headache, muscle weakness, loss of consciousness, drowsiness.
CV: ***bradycardia,*** hypotension, tachycardia, AV block, syncope, ***cardiac arrest.***
EENT: blurred vision, lacrimation, miosis.
GI: *nausea, vomiting, diarrhea, abdominal cramps,* excessive salivation, flatulence, increased peristalsis.
GU: urinary frequency.
Musculoskeletal: *muscle cramps,* muscle fasciculations, arthralgia.
Respiratory: ***bronchospasm,*** dyspnea, ***respiratory depression, respiratory arrest,*** increased secretions.
Skin: rash, urticaria, diaphoresis, flushing.
Other: hypersensitivity reactions ***(anaphylaxis).***

Overdose and treatment
Signs and symptoms of overdose include headache, nausea, vomiting, diarrhea, blurred vision, miosis, excessive tearing, bronchospasm, increased bronchial secretions, hypotension, incoordination, excessive sweating, muscle weakness, cramps, fasciculations, paralysis, bradycardia or tachycardia, excessive salivation, and restlessness or agitation.

Support respiration; bronchial suctioning may be performed. Discontinue drug immediately. Atropine may be given to block muscarinic effects of neostigmine but won't counter paralytic effects of drug on skeletal muscle. Avoid atropine overdose, because it may lead to bronchial plug formation.

Clinical considerations

- If muscle weakness is severe, determine if this stems from drug toxicity or from exacerbation of myasthenia gravis. A test dose of edrophonium I.V. will aggravate drug-induced weakness but will temporarily relieve weakness resulting from the disease.
- Hospitalized patients may be able to manage a bedside supply of tablets to take themselves.
- Give drug with food or milk to reduce the chance for GI adverse effects.
- In diagnosis of myasthenia gravis, discontinue all anticholinergics for at least 8 hours before neostigmine administration.
- When administering drug to patient with myasthenia gravis, schedule largest dose before anticipated periods of fatigue. If patient has dysphagia, schedule this dose 30 minutes before each meal.
- Stop all other cholinergic drugs during neostigmine therapy because of risk of additive toxicity.
- When administering neostigmine to prevent abdominal distention and GI distress, insertion of a rectal tube may be indicated to help passage of gas.
- Administering atropine together with neostigmine can relieve or eliminate adverse reactions; these symptoms may indicate neostigmine overdose and will be masked by atropine.
- Patients may develop resistance to drug.

Therapeutic monitoring

Recommend monitoring patient's vital signs, particularly the pulse.

Special populations

Breast-feeding patients. Neostigmine may be excreted in breast milk, possibly resulting in infant toxicity. Evaluate patient's clinical status to see if breast-feeding or drug should be discontinued.
Pediatric patients. Safety and efficacy in children haven't been fully established.
Geriatric patients. Geriatric patients may be more sensitive to effects of neostigmine. Use with caution.

Patient counseling

Instruct patient to observe and record changes in muscle strength.

nevirapine

Viramune

Pharmacologic classification: nonnucleoside reverse transcriptase inhibitor
Therapeutic classification: antiviral
Pregnancy risk category C

How supplied

Available by prescription only
Tablets: 200 mg
Oral suspension: 50 mg/5 ml

Indications and dosages

Treatment of patients with HIV-1 infection
Adults and adolescents: 200 mg P.O. daily for first 14 days, followed by 200 mg P.O. q. 12 hours in combination with other antiretroviral agents.
Treatment in children infected with HIV-1 (in combination with other antiretroviral agents)
Children age 2 months to 8 years: 4 mg/kg P.O. once daily for first 14 days, followed by 7 mg/kg P.O. q 12 hours thereafter. Maximum daily dose shouldn't exceed 400 mg.
Children age 8 and older: 4 mg/kg P.O. once daily for first 14 days, followed by 4 mg/kg P.O. q 12 hours thereafter. Maximum daily dose shouldn't exceed 400 mg. Alternatively, children may receive 120 mg/m^2 P.O. daily for first 14 days, followed by 120 to 200 mg/m^2 q 12 hours.
◇*Neonates:* 5 mg/kg P.O. daily for first 14 days followed by 120 mg/m^2 q 12 hours for next 14 days, then 200 mg/m^2 q 12 hours.

Pharmacodynamics

Antiviral action: Nevirapine binds directly to reverse transcriptase and blocks the RNA-dependent and DNA-dependent DNA polymerase activities by causing a disruption of the catalytic site of the enzyme.

Pharmacokinetics

Absorption: Readily absorbed.
Distribution: Widely distributed, crosses the placenta, and excreted in breast milk. It's about 60% bound to plasma proteins.
Metabolism: Extensively metabolized in the liver.
Excretion: Metabolites are primarily excreted in urine; a small amount of drug is excreted in feces.

Route	Onset	Peak	Duration
P.O.	Unknown	4 hr	Unknown

Contraindications and precautions

Contraindicated in patients with hypersensitivity to drug. Use cautiously in patients with impaired renal or hepatic function because the pharmacokinetics of nevirapine haven't been evaluated in these patient groups.

Interactions
Drug-drug. *Drugs extensively metabolized by P-450 CYP3A:* Nevirapine may lower the plasma levels of these drugs. Dosage adjustment of these drugs may be required.
Ketoconazole: Decreased ketoconazole levels. Avoid using together.
Protease inhibitors or oral contraceptives: Decreased plasma levels of these drugs. Don't administer together.

Effects on diagnostic tests
None reported.

Adverse reactions
CNS: headache, peripheral neuropathy, paresthesia.
GI: nausea, diarrhea, abdominal pain, ulcerative stomatitis.
Hematologic: *decreased neutrophil count,* eosinophilia.
Hepatic: ***hepatitis,*** abnormal liver function test results, ***hepatotoxicity.***
Metabolic: myalgia.
Skin: *rash,* ***Stevens-Johnson syndrome,*** facial edema, epidermic necrolysis.
Other: fever.

Overdose and treatment
No information available.

Clinical considerations
- Nevirapine is generally used in three-drug combination regimens.
- Use of a 200-mg dose as a lead-in period has been shown to decrease the evidence of a rash.
- Resistant virus emerges rapidly when drug is administered as monotherapy. Therefore, always administer in combination with at least one other antiretroviral agent.
- Discontinue drug if patient develops a severe rash or a rash accompanied by fever, blistering, oral lesions, conjunctivitis, swelling, muscle or joint aches, or general malaise. If rash occurs during the initial 14 days, don't increase dosage until it has resolved. Most rashes occur within the first 6 weeks of therapy.
- Drug must be stopped temporarily in patients experiencing moderate or severe liver function test abnormalities (excluding GGT) until they've returned to baseline. May restart drug at half the previous dose level. If moderate or severe liver function test abnormalities recur, discontinue drug therapy. Monitor LFTs closely.
- If therapy is interrupted for more than 7 days, restart therapy as if being given for the first time.
- If disease progresses during therapy, alternative antiretroviral therapy must be considered.

Therapeutic monitoring
- Monitor clinical chemistry tests, including liver function tests, before initiating therapy and regularly throughout therapy.
- Patient should be monitored for development of rash.

Special populations
Breast-feeding patients. Drug is excreted in breast milk. HIV-infected women shouldn't breast-feed.
Pediatric patients. Safety and efficacy in children haven't been established.

Patient counseling
- Inform patient that drug isn't a cure for HIV infection, and the illnesses associated with advanced HIV-1 infection may still occur. Also tell patient that drug doesn't reduce risk of transmission of HIV-1 to others through sexual contact or blood contamination.
- Instruct patient to report rash immediately. Therapy may need to be stopped temporarily.
- Stress importance of taking drug exactly as prescribed. If a dose is missed, tell patient to take the next dose as soon as possible. However, if a dose is skipped, he shouldn't double the next dose.
- Tell patient not to use other medications without medical approval.
- Advise women of childbearing age to avoid oral contraceptives and other hormonal methods of birth control as a method of contraception during therapy.

niacin (vitamin B_3, nicotinic acid)
Niaspan, Nico-400, Nicobid, Nicotinex, Slo-Niacin

Pharmacologic classification: B-complex vitamin
Therapeutic classification: vitamin B_3, antilipemic, peripheral vasodilator
Pregnancy risk category A (C if greater than RDA)

How supplied
Available by prescription only
Capsules: 500 mg
Extended-release tablets: 500 mg, 750 mg and 1,000 mg; and 21-day starter pack (7 each) 375 mg, 500 mg, and 750 mg.
Available without a prescription
Tablets: 25 mg, 50 mg, 100 mg, 125 mg, 250 mg, 400 mg, 500 mg
Tablets (timed-release): 250 mg, 500 mg, 750 mg
Capsules (timed-release): 125 mg, 250 mg, 300 mg, 400 mg, 500 mg, 750 mg
Elixir: 50 mg/5 ml

Indications and dosages

Pellagra

Adults: 300 to 500 mg in divided doses P.O., depending on severity of niacin deficiency. Maximum recommended daily dose is 500 mg; should be divided into 10 doses, 50 mg each.
Children: Up to 300 mg P.O. daily, depending on severity of niacin deficiency.

To prevent recurrence after symptoms subside, advise adequate nutrition and adequate supplements to meet RDA.

Peripheral vascular disease and circulatory disorders

Adults: 100 to 150 mg P.O. three to five times daily. Alternatively, 1,000 to 2,000 g once daily at bedtime.

Adjunctive treatment of hyperlipidemias, especially those associated with hypercholesterolemia

Adults: 1.5 to 6 g P.O. daily in two to four divided doses with or after meals; maximum dose is 9 g daily. Alternatively, initial dose is 100 mg P.O. t.i.d., increasing by 300 mg/day at 4- to 7-day intervals or 500 mg P.O. t.i.d. with gradual increase to desired effect.

Hartnup disease

Adults: 50 to 200 mg P.O. daily in divided doses.

Dietary supplement

Adults: 10 to 20 mg P.O. daily.

Pharmacodynamics

Vitamin replacement action: As a vitamin, niacin functions as a coenzyme essential to tissue respiration, lipid metabolism, and glycogenolysis. Niacin deficiency causes pellagra, which manifests as dermatitis, diarrhea, and dementia; administration of niacin cures pellagra. Niacin lowers cholesterol and triglyceride levels by an unknown mechanism.
Vasodilating action: Niacin acts directly on peripheral vessels, dilating cutaneous vessels and increasing blood flow, predominantly in the face, neck, and chest.
Antilipemic action: Mechanism of action is unknown. Nicotinic acid inhibits lipolysis in adipose tissues, decreases hepatic esterification of triglyceride, and increases lipoprotein lipase activity. It reduces serum cholesterol and triglyceride levels.

Pharmacokinetics

Absorption: Absorbed rapidly from the GI tract. Cholesterol and triglyceride levels decrease after several days.
Distribution: Coenzymes are distributed widely in body tissues; niacin is distributed in breast milk.
Metabolism: Metabolized by the liver to active metabolites.
Excretion: Excreted in urine.

Route	Onset	Peak	Duration
P.O.	Unknown	45 min	Unknown

Contraindications and precautions

Contraindicated in patients with hepatic dysfunction, active peptic ulcer, severe hypotension, arterial hemorrhage, or hypersensitivity to drug. Use cautiously in patients with history of liver disease, peptic ulcer, allergy, gout, gallbladder disease, diabetes mellitus, or coronary artery disease.

Interactions

Drug-drug. *Aspirin:* May decrease the metabolic clearance of nicotinic acid. Use together cautiously.
Sympathetic blocking agents: May cause added vasodilation and hypotension. Use together cautiously.

Effects on diagnostic tests

Niacin therapy alters fluorometric test results for urine catecholamines and results for urine glucose tests using cupric sulfate (Benedict's reagent).

Adverse reactions

Most reactions are dose-dependent.
CV: *excessive peripheral vasodilation,* hypotension, atrial fibrillation, ***arrhythmias.***
EENT: toxic amblyopia.
GI: *nausea, vomiting, diarrhea,* possible activation of peptic ulceration, epigastric or substernal pain.
Hepatic: ***hepatic dysfunction.***
Metabolic: hyperglycemia, hyperuricemia.
Skin: *flushing,* pruritus, dryness, tingling.

Overdose and treatment

Niacin is a water-soluble vitamin; these seldom cause toxicity in patients with normal renal function.

Clinical considerations

- RDA of niacin in men is 19 mg; in women, 15 mg; and in children, 5 to 20 mg.
- Megadoses of niacin aren't usually recommended.
- Monitor hepatic function and blood glucose levels during initial therapy.
- Aspirin may reduce flushing response.

Therapeutic monitoring

Monitor hepatic function and blood glucose levels during initial therapy.

Special populations

Breast-feeding patients. There have been no reports of problems in breast-feeding women taking normal daily doses as dietary requirement.

Patient counseling

- Explain disease process and rationale for therapy; stress that use of niacin to treat hyperlipidemia or to dilate peripheral vessels is not simply "taking a vitamin," but serious medicine. Emphasize importance of complying with therapy.
- Instruct patient not to substitute sustained-release (timed) tablets for intermediate-release tablets in equivalent doses. Severe hepatic toxicity, including necrosis, has occurred.
- Explain that cutaneous flushing and warmth commonly occur in the first 2 hours; this will cease on continued therapy.
- Advise patient not to make sudden postural changes to minimize effects of orthostatic hypotension.
- Instruct patient to avoid hot liquids when initially taking drug to reduce flushing response.
- Advise patient to take drug with meals to minimize GI irritation.

nicardipine hydrochloride

Cardene, Cardene SR

Pharmacologic classification: calcium channel blocker
Therapeutic classification: antianginal, antihypertensive
Pregnancy risk category C

How supplied

Available by prescription only
Capsules: 20 mg, 30 mg
Capsules (extended-release): 30 mg, 45 mg, 60 mg
Injection: 2.5 mg/ml in 10-ml ampules

Indications and dosages

Hypertension; management of chronic stable angina
Adults: Initially, 20 mg P.O. t.i.d. Adjust dosage based on patient response. Usual dosage range, 20 to 40 mg t.i.d. Extended-release capsules (for hypertension only) can be initiated at 30 mg b.i.d. Usual dose, 30 to 60 mg b.i.d.
Short-term management of hypertension when oral therapy isn't feasible or possible
Adults: Initially, 5 mg/hour I.V. infusion; titrate infusion upward by 2.5 mg/hour q 5 to 15 minutes up to a maximum of 15 mg/hour, p.r.n. Maintenance infusion is 3 mg/ hour. When transferring to oral therapy, give P.O. of conventional capsule 1 hour before discontinuing infusion.

Note: If patient is already taking nicardipine and requires short-term I.V. management of hypertension, give 0.5 mg/hour if dose is 20 mg q 8 hours; 1.2 mg/hour if dose is 30 mg q 8 hours; and 2.2 mg/hour if dose is 40 mg q 8 hours.

Pharmacodynamics

Antihypertensive and antianginal action: Nicardipine inhibits the transmembrane flux of calcium ions into cardiac and smooth muscle cells. Drug appears to act specifically on vascular muscle, and may cause a smaller decrease in cardiac output than other calcium channel blockers because of its vasodilatory effect.

Pharmacokinetics

Absorption: Completely absorbed after oral administration. Absorption may be decreased if drug is taken with food. Therapeutic serum levels are 28 to 50 ng/ml.
Distribution: Extensively (more than 95%) bound to plasma proteins.
Metabolism: A substantial first-pass effect reduces absolute bioavailability to about 35%. Drug is extensively metabolized in the liver, and the process is saturable. Increasing dosage yields nonlinear increases in plasma levels.
Excretion: Elimination half-life of drug is about 8½ hours after steady-state levels are reached.

Route	Onset	Peak	Duration
P.O. (immediate)	½-11½ min	Unknown	Unknown
P.O. (sustained)	20 min	1-4 hr	12 hr
I.V.	Immediate	Immediate	Unknown

Contraindications and precautions

Contraindicated in patients with hypersensitivity to drug and in those with advanced aortic stenosis. Use cautiously in patients with impaired renal or hepatic function, cardiac conduction disturbances, hypotension, or heart failure.

Interactions

Drug-drug. *Cimetidine:* Higher plasma levels of nicardipine. Patient requires monitoring for increased effects.
Cyclosporine: Increased plasma levels of cyclosporine. Careful monitoring is recommended.
Digoxin: Increased plasma levels of cardiac glycosides. Monitor serum digoxin level.
Fentanyl anesthesia: Severe hypotension. Frequent monitoring of blood pressure is necessary.
Drug-food. *Grapefruit juice:* Increased bioavailability of drug. Advise patient to avoid taking drug with grapefruit juice.

Effects on diagnostic tests

None reported.

Adverse reactions

CNS: dizziness, light-headedness, headache, paresthesia, asthenia.
CV: *peripheral edema, palpitations,* angina, tachycardia.

GI: nausea, abdominal discomfort, dry mouth.
Skin: rash, *flushing.*

Overdose and treatment
Overdose may produce hypotension, bradycardia, drowsiness, confusion, and slurred speech. Treatment is supportive, with vasopressors administered as needed. I.V. calcium gluconate may be useful to counteract the effects of drug.

Clinical considerations
Consider the recommendations relevant to all calcium channel blockers as well as the following:
- Allow at least 3 days between oral dosage changes to ensure achievement of steady-state plasma levels.
- When treating patients with chronic stable angina, S.L. nitroglycerin, prophylactic nitrate therapy, and beta blockers may be continued.
- In patients with hepatic dysfunction, therapy should begin at 20 mg P.O. twice daily; carefully adjust subsequent dosage based on patient response.
- Dilute solution in ampule before I.V. infusion. Recommended dilution is 0.1 mg/ml in dextrose or saline solution.
- When used I.V., change I.V. site every 12 hours to minimize venous irritation.

Therapeutic monitoring
- When treating hypertension, recommend measuring blood pressure during times of plasma level trough (about 8 hours after dose, or immediately before subsequent doses). Because of prominent effects that may occur during plasma level peaks, measure blood pressure 1 to 2 hours after conventional dose and 2 to 4 hours after extended-release dose. Base dosage adjustment on blood pressure 2 to 4 hours after oral dose.
- Recommend monitoring blood pressure during I.V. administration because nicardipine I.V. decreases peripheral resistance.

Special populations
Breast-feeding patients. Substantial levels of drug have been found in the milk of animals given nicardipine. Breast-feeding isn't recommended.
Pediatric patients. Safety in children under age 18 hasn't been established.

Patient counseling
- Tell patient to take oral form of drug exactly as prescribed.
- Advise patient to report chest pain to physician immediately. Some patients may experience increased frequency, severity, or duration of chest pain at the beginning of therapy or during dosage adjustments.

nicotine
Habitrol, Nicoderm, Nicotrol, Nicotrol NS, ProStep

Pharmacologic classification: nicotinic cholinergic agonist
Therapeutic classification: smoking cessation aid
Pregnancy risk category D

How supplied
Available with and without a prescription
Transdermal system: Designed to release nicotine at a fixed rate
Habitrol: 21 mg/day, 14 mg/day, 7 mg/day
Nicoderm: 21 mg/day, 14 mg/day, 7 mg/day
Nicotrol: 15 mg/day
ProStep: 22 mg/day, 11 mg/day
Nasal spray: metered spray pump
Nicotrol NS: 10 mg/ml
Available by prescription only
Nicotrol inhaler: 10 mg cartridge, supplying 4 mg of nicotine

Indications and dosages
Relief of nicotine withdrawal symptoms in patients attempting smoking cessation
Adults: One transdermal system applied to a nonhairy part of the upper trunk or upper outer arm. Dosage varies slightly with product selected.
Habitrol, Nicoderm
Initially, apply one 21-mg/day system daily for 6 weeks. After 24 hours, remove system and apply a new system to a different site. Then, taper dosage to 14 mg/day for 2 to 4 weeks. Finally, taper dosage to 7 mg/day if necessary. Nicotine substitution and gradual withdrawal should take 8 to 12 weeks.
≡***Dosage adjustment.*** Patients who weigh less than 100 lb (45 kg), have CV disease, or who smoke less than half a pack of cigarettes daily should start therapy with the 14-mg/day system.
Nicotrol
Adults: Apply one 15-mg/day system daily for 6 weeks. Apply system upon waking and remove h.s. because patch provides systemic delivery over 16 hours.
Nicotrol NS
Adults: Initially, 1 or 2 doses/hour (1 dose = 2 sprays—one in each nostril). Encourage patient to use at least the recommended minimum of 8 doses/day. Maximum recommended dose is 40 mg or 80 sprays/day. Duration of treatment shouldn't exceed 3 months with gradual dose reduction during those 3 months.
ProStep
Adults: Initially, apply one 22-mg/day system daily for 4 to 8 weeks. After 24 hours, remove system and apply a new system to a different site. In patients weighing less than 100 lb (45 kg), start therapy with the 11-mg/day system;

those who have successfully stopped smoking during this period may discontinue drug. If therapy was initiated with the 22-mg/day system, treatment may continue for an additional 2 to 4 weeks at lower dosage (11 mg/day). Nicotine substitution and gradual withdrawal should take 6 to 12 weeks.

Nicotrol inhaler

Adults: Initial dose is 6 to 16 cartridges daily. Best effect is achieved with continuous puffing. Recommended treatment is up to 3 months and, if needed, gradual reduction over the next 6 to 12 weeks.

Pharmacodynamics

Nicotinic cholinergic action: Nicotine transdermal system and nasal spray provide nicotine, the chief stimulant alkaloid found in tobacco products, which stimulates nicotinic acetylcholine receptors in the CNS, neuromuscular junction, autonomic ganglia, and adrenal medulla.

Pharmacokinetics

Absorption: Rapidly absorbed.
Distribution: Plasma protein-binding of drug is below 5%.
Metabolism: Metabolized by the liver, kidney, and lungs. Over 20 metabolites have been identified. Primary metabolites are cotinine (15%) and trans-3-hydroxycotinine (45%).
Excretion: Excreted primarily in urine as metabolites; about 10% is excreted unchanged. With high urine flow rates or acidified urine, up to 30% can be excreted unchanged.

Route	Onset	Peak	Duration
Transdermal	Unknown	3-9 hr	Unknown
Intranasal	Unknown	4 to 15 min	Unknown
Inhalation	Unknown	15 min	Unknown

Contraindications and precautions

Contraindicated in patients with hypersensitivity to nicotine or any components. Also contraindicated in nonsmokers and in patients with recent MI, life-threatening arrhythmias, and severe or worsening angina pectoris.

Use cautiously in patients with hyperthyroidism, pheochromocytoma, insulin-dependent diabetes, or peptic ulcer disease.

Interactions

Drug-drug. *Acetaminophen, caffeine, imipramine, oxazepam, pentazocine, propranolol, theophylline:* Cessation of smoking may decrease induction of hepatic enzymes responsible for metabolizing certain drugs. Dosage reduction of such drugs may be necessary.
Adrenergic antagonists, such as labetalol and prazosin, or adrenergic agonists, such as isoproterenol and phenylephrine: Cessation of smoking may decrease levels of circulating catecholamines. Dosage adjustment of such drugs may be necessary.
Insulin: Cessation of smoking may increase the amount of subcutaneous insulin absorbed. Adjust insulin dosage.
Drug-herb. *Blue cohosh:* Increases effects of nicotine. Don't use together.

Effects on diagnostic tests

None reported.

Adverse reactions

CNS: somnolence, dizziness, *headache, insomnia,* paresthesia, abnormal dreams, nervousness.
CV: hypertension.
EENT: pharyngitis, sinusitis.
GI: abdominal pain, constipation, dyspepsia, nausea, diarrhea, vomiting, dry mouth.
GU: dysmenorrhea.
Musculoskeletal: back pain, myalgia.
Respiratory: increased cough.
Skin: *local or systemic erythema, pruritus, burning at application site,* cutaneous hypersensitivity, rash, diaphoresis.

Overdose and treatment

Overdose could produce symptoms associated with acute nicotine poisoning, including nausea, vomiting, diarrhea, weakness, respiratory failure, hypotension, and seizures. Treat symptomatically. Barbiturates or benzodiazepines may be used to treat seizures, and atropine may attenuate excessive salivation or diarrhea. Administer fluids to treat hypotension; increase urine flow to enhance elimination of drug.

Clinical considerations

- Transdermal nicotine has been used investigationally to manage ulcerative colitis.
- Discourage use of transdermal system for more than 3 months. Chronic nicotine consumption by any route can be dangerous and habit-forming.
- Patients who can't stop cigarette smoking during the initial 4 weeks of therapy will probably not benefit from continued use of drug. Patients who were unsuccessful may benefit from counseling to identify factors that led to the unsuccessful attempt. Encourage patient to minimize or eliminate the factors that contributed to treatment failure and to try again, possibly after some interval, before the next attempt.
- Health care workers' exposure to the nicotine within the transdermal systems should be minimal; however, avoid unnecessary contact with the system. After contact, wash hands with water alone because soap can enhance absorption.
- Nicotrol NS isn't recommended in patients with chronic nasal disorders or severe reactive airway disease.

■ Increased cough is a common occurrence in patients using the inhaler.
■ Although use of nicotine replacement therapy isn't recommended in recent MI patients, it may be considered preferable to cigarette smoking in patients experiencing withdrawal.

Therapeutic monitoring
Monitor patient for correct use of system to prevent overdose or failure of program.

Special populations
Breast-feeding patients. Nicotine passes freely into breast milk and is readily absorbed after oral administration. Weigh the infant's risk of exposure to nicotine against his risk of exposure from continued smoking by the woman.
Pediatric patients. Safety and efficacy in children haven't been established. Note that the amount of nicotine contained in a patch could prove fatal to a child if ingested; even used patches contain a substantial amount of residual nicotine. Patients should take care to ensure that both used and unused transdermal systems and metered spray bottles are kept out of the reach of children.

Patient counseling
■ Tell patient to discontinue use of patch and to immediately report a generalized rash or persistent or severe local skin reactions, such as pruritus, edema, or erythema.
■ Make sure patient understands that nicotine can evaporate from the transdermal system once it's removed from its protective packaging. The patch shouldn't be altered in any way (folded or cut) before it's applied. It should be applied promptly after removal of the system's protective packaging. Tell patient not to store patch at temperatures above 86° F (30° C).
■ Teach patient how to dispose of transdermal system. After removal, fold the patch in half, bringing the adhesive sides together. If the system comes in a protective pouch, dispose of the used patch in the pouch that contained the new system. Careful disposal is necessary to prevent accidental poisoning of children or pets.
■ Be sure that patient reads and understands the patient information that's dispensed with drug when the prescription is filled.
■ Inform patient to refrain from smoking while using the system; he may experience adverse effects from the increased nicotine levels.
■ Explain that patient is likely to experience nasal irritation, which may become less bothersome with continued use of Nicotrol NS.

nicotine polacrilex (nicotine resin complex)
Nicorette

Pharmacologic classification: nicotinic agonist
Therapeutic classification: smoking cessation aid
Pregnancy risk category X

How supplied
Available with and without a prescription
Chewing gum: 2 mg, 4 mg nicotine resin complex per square

Indications and dosages
Aid in managing nicotine dependence
Serves as a temporary aid to smokers seeking to give up smoking while participating in a behavior modification program under medical supervision. Generally, a smoker with the "physical" type of nicotine dependence is most likely to benefit from use of nicotine chewing gum.
Adults: Chew one piece of gum slowly and intermittently for 30 minutes whenever the urge to smoke occurs. Most patients require about 9 to 12 pieces of gum daily during first month. Patients using the 2-mg strength shouldn't exceed 24 pieces of gum daily if unsupervised or 30 pieces if supervised; those using the 4-mg strength shouldn't exceed 24 pieces of gum daily.

Pharmacodynamics
Nicotine replacement action: Nicotine is an agonist at the nicotinic receptors in the peripheral nervous system and CNS and produces both behavioral stimulation and depression. It acts on the adrenal medulla to aid in overcoming physical dependence on nicotine during withdrawal from habitual smoking.

CV effects of nicotine are usually dose-dependent. Nonsmokers have experienced CNS-mediated symptoms of hiccuping, nausea, and vomiting, even with a small dose. A smoker chewing a 2-mg piece of gum every hour usually doesn't experience CV adverse effects.

Pharmacokinetics
Absorption: Bound to ion-exchange resin and is released only during chewing. The blood level depends upon the vigor with which the gum is chewed.
Distribution: Distribution into tissues hasn't been fully characterized. It crosses the placenta and is excreted in breast milk.
Metabolism: Metabolized mainly by the liver and less so by the kidneys and lungs. Main metabolites are cotinine and nicotine-1'-*N*-oxide.

Excretion: Both nicotine and its metabolites are excreted in urine, with about 10% to 20% excreted unchanged. Excretion of nicotine is increased in acid urine and by high urine output.

Route	Onset	Peak	Duration
P.O.	Unknown	15-30 min	Unknown

Contraindications and precautions

Contraindicated in nonsmokers; in patients with recent MI, life-threatening arrhythmias, severe or worsening angina pectoris, or active temporomandibular joint disease; and during pregnancy.

Use cautiously in patients with hyperthyroidism, pheochromocytoma, insulin-dependent diabetes, peptic ulcer disease, history of esophagitis, oral or pharyngeal inflammation, or dental conditions that might be exacerbated by chewing gum.

Interactions

Drug-drug. *Adrenergic agonists or adrenergic blockers:* Nicorette gum and smoking can increase the circulating levels of cortisol and catecholamines. Dose adjustments may be necessary.
Imipramine, pentazocine, and theophylline: Smoking cessation either with or without nicotine substitutes may reverse increased metabolism of smoking. Dose adjustments may be necessary.
Propoxyphene: Smoking cessation may reduce the first-pass metabolism of propoxyphene. Dose adjustments may be necessary.
Drug-herb. *Blue cohosh:* May increase effects of nicotine. Don't use together.
Drug-food. *Caffeine:* Smoking may increase the metabolism of caffeine. Monitor for effect.
Food and beverages: Inhibited absorption. Advise patient to avoid eating and drinking 15 minutes before and during chewing of gum.

Effects on diagnostic tests

None reported.

Adverse reactions

CNS: dizziness, light-headedness, irritability, insomnia, headache, paresthesia.
CV: atrial fibrillation.
EENT: throat soreness, jaw muscle ache (from chewing).
GI: nausea, vomiting, indigestion, eructation, anorexia, excessive salivation.
Other: hiccups, sweating.

Overdose and treatment

The risk of overdose is minimized by early nausea and vomiting that result from excessive nicotine intake. Poisoning manifests as nausea, vomiting, salivation, abdominal pain, diarrhea, cold sweats, headache, dizziness, disturbed hearing and vision, mental confusion, and weakness.

Treatment includes emesis—give ipecac syrup if it hasn't occurred. A saline cathartic will speed the passage of the gum through the GI tract. Give gastric lavage followed by activated charcoal in unconscious patients. Provide supportive treatment of respiratory paralysis and CV collapse as needed.

Clinical considerations

- Patients most likely to benefit from Nicorette gum are smokers with a high physical dependence. Typically, they smoke over 15 cigarettes daily; prefer brands of cigarettes with high nicotine levels; usually inhale the smoke; smoke the first cigarette within 30 minutes of arising; and find the first morning cigarette the hardest to give up.
- Patient may initiate reduction by reducing actual pieces of gum chewed or length of time gum is chewed.
- Smoking cessation generally takes 2 to 3 months with gradual dose reduction.
- Although nicotine replacement therapy isn't recommended in patients with recent MI, it may be considered preferable to cigarette smoking in patients experiencing nicotine withdrawal.

Therapeutic monitoring

Recommend patient be reevaluated at least monthly to determine therapy response.

Special populations

Breast-feeding patients. Nicotine passes freely into breast milk and is readily absorbed after oral administration. Weigh the infant's risk of exposure to nicotine from a transdermal patch against his risk of exposure from continued smoking by the mother.

Patient counseling

- Instruct patient to chew gum slowly and intermittently for about 30 minutes to promote slow and even buccal absorption of nicotine. Fast chewing allows faster absorption and produces more adverse reactions. After about 15 chews, advise the patient to "park" the gum between the cheek and gum for a few minutes.
- At the initial visit, instruct patient to chew one piece of gum whenever the urge to smoke occurs instead of having a cigarette. Most patients will require about 10 pieces of gum daily during first month of treatment.
- Tell patient who has successfully abstained to gradually withdraw gum use after 3 months; he shouldn't use gum for longer than 6 months.
- Inform patient that gum is sugar-free and usually doesn't stick to dentures.

nifedipine

Adalat, Adalat CC, Procardia, Procardia XL

Pharmacologic classification: calcium channel blocker
Therapeutic classification: antianginal
Pregnancy risk category C

How supplied

Available by prescription only
Capsules: 10 mg, 20 mg
Tablets (extended-release): 30 mg, 60 mg, 90 mg

Indications and dosages

Management of Prinzmetal's or variant angina or chronic stable angina pectoris
Adults: Starting dose is 10 mg P.O. t.i.d. Usual effective dosage range is 10 to 20 mg t.i.d. Some patients may require up to 30 mg q.i.d. Alternatively, 30 to 60 mg (extended-release preparation) P.O. daily. Doses are gradually increased at 7 to 14 day intervals or more frequently, if necessary. Maximum daily dose for capsules is 180 mg; for extended-release tablets, 120 mg.
Hypertension
Adults: Initially, 30 to 60 mg P.O. once daily (extended-release tablets). Adjust dosage at 7- to 14-day intervals based on patient tolerance and response. Maximum daily dose is 120 mg.
◇***Quick reduction of blood pressure***
Adults: 10 to 20 mg q 20 to 30 minutes; capsule should be bitten and then swallowed.

Pharmacodynamics

Antianginal action: Nifedipine dilates systemic arteries, resulting in decreased total peripheral resistance and modestly decreased systemic blood pressure with a slightly increased heart rate, decreased afterload, and increased cardiac index. Reduced afterload and the subsequent decrease in myocardial oxygen consumption probably account for the value of nifedipine in treating chronic stable angina. In Prinzmetal's angina, nifedipine inhibits coronary artery spasm, increasing myocardial oxygen delivery.

Pharmacokinetics

Absorption: About 90% of a dose is absorbed rapidly from the GI tract after oral administration; however, only about 65% to 70% of drug reaches the systemic circulation because of a significant first-pass effect in the liver. Therapeutic serum levels are 25 to 100 ng/ml.
Distribution: About 92% to 98% of circulating nifedipine is bound to plasma proteins.
Metabolism: Metabolized in the liver.
Excretion: Excreted in urine and feces as inactive metabolites. Elimination half-life is 2 to 5 hours.

Route	Onset	Peak	Duration
P.O.	20 min	½-1 hr	4-8 hr
P.O. (extended)	20 min	6 hr	24 hr

Contraindications and precautions

Contraindicated in patients with hypersensitivity to drug. Use cautiously in the elderly and in patients with heart failure or hypotension. Use extended-release form cautiously in patients with GI narrowing.

Use with caution in patients with unstable angina who aren't currently taking a beta blocker because a higher incidence of MI has been reported.

Interactions

Drug-drug. *Beta blockers:* May exacerbate angina, heart failure, and hypotension. Use together cautiously.
Cimetidine: May decrease metabolism of nifedipine. Use together cautiously.
Digoxin: May cause increased serum digoxin levels. Monitor serum digoxin level.
Fentanyl: May cause excessive hypotension. Use together cautiously.
Hypotensive agents: May precipitate excessive hypotension. Use together cautiously.
Phenytoin: Drug may increase phenytoin levels. Monitor phenytoin levels.
Drug-food. *Grapefruit juice:* Increased bioavailability of drug. Advise patient to avoid taking drug with grapefruit juice.

Effects on diagnostic tests

None reported.

Adverse reactions

CNS: *dizziness, light-headedness, flushing, headache, weakness,* syncope, nervousness.
CV: *peripheral edema,* hypotension, palpitations, ***heart failure, MI, pulmonary edema.***
EENT: nasal congestion.
GI: *nausea,* diarrhea, constipation, abdominal discomfort; increase in serum levels of alkaline phosphate, LD, AST, and ALT.
Metabolic: hypokalemia.
Musculoskeletal: muscle cramps.
Respiratory: dyspnea, cough.
Skin: rash, pruritus.
Other: fever.

Overdose and treatment

Clinical effects of overdose are extensions of pharmacologic effects of the drug, primarily peripheral vasodilation and hypotension.

Treatment includes such basic support measures as hemodynamic and respiratory monitoring. If patient requires blood pressure support by a vasoconstrictor, norepinephrine may be administered. Elevate extremities and correct any fluid deficit.

Clinical considerations

- Nifedipine has been used investigationally to treat Raynaud's phenomenon and preterm labor.

□ ALERT Warn patient not to switch brands. Procardia XL and Adalat CC aren't therapeutically equivalent because of major differences in their pharmacokinetics.

- Initial doses or dosage increase may exacerbate angina briefly. Reassure patient that this symptom is temporary.
- Nifedipine isn't available in S.L. form. No advantage has been found in S.L. or intrabuccal use.
- Although rebound effect hasn't been observed when drug is stopped, reduce dosage slowly.

Therapeutic monitoring

Recommend monitoring blood pressure regularly, especially if patient is also taking beta blockers or antihypertensives.

Special populations

Geriatric patients. Use drug with caution in geriatric patients because they may be more sensitive to effects of drug and duration of effect may be prolonged. Orthostatic blood pressures should be monitored.

Patient counseling

- Instruct patient to swallow capsules whole without breaking, crushing, or chewing them unless instructed otherwise.
- Tell patient that he may experience annoying hypotensive effects during adjustment of dose and urge compliance with therapy.

nisoldipine

Sular

Pharmacologic classification: calcium channel blocker
Therapeutic classification: antihypertensive
Pregnancy risk category C

How supplied

Available by prescription only
Tablets (extended-release): 10 mg, 20 mg, 30 mg, 40 mg

Indications and dosages

Hypertension
Adults: Initially, 20 mg P.O. once daily, then increased by 10 mg/week or at longer intervals, p.r.n. Usual maintenance dosage, 20 to 40 mg once daily. Don't exceed 60 mg daily.

≡ ***Dosage adjustment.*** In patients over age 65 or those with hepatic dysfunction, give starting dose of 10 mg P.O. once daily. Monitor blood pressure closely during any dosage adjustment.

Pharmacodynamics

Antihypertensive action: Nisoldipine prevents the entry of calcium ions into vascular smooth muscle cells, causing dilation of the arterioles, which in turn decreases peripheral vascular resistance.

Pharmacokinetics

Absorption: Relatively well absorbed from GI tract. High-fat foods significantly affect release of drug from the coat-core formulation.
Distribution: About 99% is bound to plasma protein.
Metabolism: Extensively metabolized with five major metabolites identified.
Excretion: Excreted in urine; half-life ranges from 7 to 12 hours.

Route	Onset	Peak	Duration
P.O.	Unknown	6-12 hr	24 hr

Contraindications and precautions

Contraindicated in patients with hypersensitivity to dihydropyridine calcium channel blockers. Use cautiously in patients receiving beta blockers or in those who have compromised ventricular or hepatic function and heart failure.

Interactions

Drug-drug. *Cimetidine:* Increased bioavailability of nisoldipine as well as increasing peak level. Use together cautiously.
Quinidine: Decreased bioavailability, but not peak level of nisoldipine. Recommend monitoring blood pressure.
Drug-food. *High-fat meals or grapefruit juice:* May decrease absorption. Advise patient not to take drug with these foods.

Effects on diagnostic tests

None reported.

Adverse reactions

CNS: *headache,* dizziness.
CV: vasodilation, palpitations, chest pain, *peripheral edema.*
EENT: pharyngitis, sinusitis.
GI: nausea.
Skin: rash.

Overdose and treatment

Overdose with similar drugs leads to pronounced hypotension. Treatment should focus on CV support, including monitoring of CV and respiratory function, elevation of extremities, and judicious use of calcium infusion, pressor agents, and fluids.

Clinical considerations
Extended-release form of drug makes it unsuitable for use in hypertensive emergency.

Therapeutic monitoring
■ Patient requires careful monitoring. Some patients, especially those with severe obstructive coronary artery disease, have increased frequency, duration, or severity of angina or even acute MI after initiation of calcium channel blocker therapy or at time of dosage increase.
■ Blood pressure must be monitored regularly, especially during initial administration and adjustment of drug.

Special populations
Breast-feeding patients. It isn't known if drug is excreted in breast milk. Use of drug in breast-feeding women isn't recommended.
Pediatric patients. Safety and efficacy in children haven't been established.
Geriatric patients. Geriatric patients may have two- to three-fold higher plasma levels than younger patients, requiring cautious dosing.

Patient counseling
■ Tell patient to take drug exactly as prescribed, even if he feels better.
■ Advise patient to swallow tablet whole and not to chew, divide, or crush tablets, unless instructed otherwise.
■ Tell patient not to take drug with a high-fat meal or with grapefruit products.
■ Advise patient to rise slowly from supine position to avoid dizziness and hypotension, especially at beginning of therapy.

nitrofurantoin macrocrystals
Macrobid, Macrodantin

nitrofurantoin microcrystals
Furadantin

Pharmacologic classification: nitrofuran
Therapeutic classification: urinary tract anti-infective
Pregnancy risk category B

How supplied
Available by prescription only
macrocrystals
Capsules: 25 mg, 50 mg, 100 mg
Capsules (dual-release): 100 mg
microcrystals
Suspension: 25 mg/5 ml

Indications and dosages
Initial or recurrent urinary tract infections caused by susceptible organisms
Adults and children over age 12: 50 to 100 mg P.O. q.i.d. or 100 mg dual-release capsules q 12 hours for 7 days.
Children age 1 month to 12 years: 5 to 7 mg/kg/24 hours P.O. daily, divided q.i.d.
Long-term suppression therapy
Adults: 50 to 100 mg P.O. daily h.s. as a single dose.
Children: As low as 1 mg/kg/day P.O. in a single dose or two divided doses.

Pharmacodynamics
Antibacterial action: Nitrofurantoin has bacteriostatic action in low levels and possible bactericidal action in high levels. Although its exact mechanism of action is unknown, it may inhibit bacterial enzyme systems interfering with bacterial carbohydrate metabolism. Drug is most active at an acidic pH.

Spectrum of activity includes many common gram-positive and gram-negative urinary pathogens, including *Escherichia coli, Staphylococcus aureus,* enterococci, and certain strains of *Klebsiella,* and *Enterobacter.* Organisms that usually resist nitrofurantoin include *Acinetobacter, Proteus, Providencia, Pseudomonas,* and *Serratia.*

Pharmacokinetics
Absorption: When administered orally, drug is well absorbed (mainly by the small intestine) from GI tract. Presence of food aids dissolution of drug and speeds absorption. The macrocrystal form exhibits slower dissolution and absorption; it causes less GI distress.
Distribution: Crosses into bile and placenta. 60% binds to plasma proteins. Plasma half-life is about 20 minutes. Peak urine levels occur in about 30 minutes when drug is given as microcrystals, somewhat later when given as macrocrystals.
Metabolism: Metabolized partially in the liver.
Excretion: About 30% to 50% of dose is eliminated by glomerular filtration and tubular secretion into urine as unchanged drug within 24 hours. Some drug may be excreted in breast milk.

Route	Onset	Peak	Duration
P.O.	Unknown	Unknown	Unknown

Contraindications and precautions
Contraindicated in pregnant women at term (38 to 42 weeks' gestation), during labor and delivery, or when the onset of labor is imminent. Contraindicated in children age 1 month and under and in patients with moderate to severe renal impairment, anuria, oliguria, or creatinine clearance under 60 ml/minute.

Use cautiously in patients with impaired renal function, anemia, diabetes mellitus, electrolyte abnormalities, vitamin B deficiency, debilitating disease, or G6PD deficiency.

Interactions

Drug-drug. *Anticholinergic drugs:* Enhance bioavailability. Monitor patient carefully.
Magnesium trisilicate antacids: May decrease nitrofurantoin absorption. Separate administration times.
Probenecid and sulfinpyrazone: Reduced renal excretion of nitrofurantoin. Monitor for increased toxicity and decreased clinical effect.
Quinolone derivatives, such as cinoxacin, ciprofloxacin, nalidixic acid and norfloxacin: May antagonize anti-infective effects. Monitor patient for decreased clinical effect
Drug-food. *Food*: Enhances bioavailability of nitrofurantoin. Give drug with food.

Effects on diagnostic tests

Nitrofurantoin may cause false-positive results in urine glucose tests using cupric sulfate reagents (such as Benedict's test, Fehling's solution, or Clinitest) because it reacts with these reagents.

Adverse reactions

CNS: ***peripheral neuropathy,*** headache, dizziness, drowsiness, *ascending polyneuropathy* (with high doses or renal impairment).
GI: *anorexia, nausea, vomiting,* abdominal pain, *diarrhea.*
GU: overgrowth of nonsusceptible organisms in the urinary tract.
Hematologic: ***hemolysis in patients with G6PD deficiency*** (reversed after stopping drug), ***agranulocytosis, thrombocytopenia.***
Hepatic: ***hepatitis, hepatic necrosis,*** elevated bilirubin and alkaline phosphatase.
Respiratory: ***pulmonary sensitivity reactions*** (cough, chest pain, fever, chills, dyspnea, pulmonary infiltration with consolidation or pleural effusion), ***asthmatic attacks in patients with history of asthma.***
Skin: maculopapular, erythematous, or eczematous eruption; pruritus; urticaria; *exfoliative dermatitis;* **Stevens-Johnson syndrome.**
Other: hypersensitivity reactions ***(anaphylaxis),*** transient alopecia, drug fever, decreased serum glucose.

Overdose and treatment

Acute overdose may result in nausea and vomiting. Treat symptomatically. No specific antidote is known. Increase fluid intake to promote urinary excretion of drug. Nitrofurantoin is dialyzable.

Clinical considerations

- Obtain culture and sensitivity tests before starting therapy, and repeat as needed.
- Oral suspension may be mixed with water, milk, fruit juice, and formulas.
- Drug may turn urine brown or rust-yellow.
- Continue treatment for at least 3 days after sterile urine specimens have been obtained.
- Long-term therapy may cause overgrowth of nonsusceptible organisms, especially *Pseudomonas.*

Therapeutic monitoring

- Monitor CBC regularly.
- Monitor fluid intake and output and pulmonary status.

Special populations

Breast-feeding patients. Safety hasn't been established. Although drug is excreted in low levels in breast milk, no adverse reactions have been reported, except in infants with G6PD deficiency, in whom hemolytic anemia may develop.
Pediatric patients. Contraindicated in infants under age 1 month because their immature enzyme systems increase risk of hemolytic anemia.

Patient counseling

- Instruct patient to take drug with food or milk to minimize GI distress. Have patient report any unpleasant side effects.
- Caution patient that drug may cause false-positive results in urine glucose tests using cupric sulfate reduction method (Clinitest) but not in glucose oxidase test (glucose enzymatic test strip, Diastix, or Chemstrip uG).
- Emphasize that bedtime dose is important because drug will remain in bladder longer.
- Warn patient that drug may turn urine brown or rust-yellow.

nitrofurazone

Furacin

Pharmacologic classification: synthetic antibacterial nitrofuran derivative
Therapeutic classification: topical antibacterial
Pregnancy risk category C

How supplied

Available by prescription only
Topical solution: 0.2%
Ointment: 0.2% soluble dressing
Cream: 0.2%

Indications and dosages

Adjunct for major burns (especially when resistance to other anti-infectives occurs); prevention of skin graft infection before or after surgery
Adults and children: Apply directly to lesion or to dressings used to cover affected area daily or as indicated, depending on severity of burn. Apply once daily or q few days, depending on dressing technique.

Pharmacodynamics

Antibacterial action: Exact mechanism of action is unknown. However, it appears that drug inhibits bacterial enzymes involved in carbohydrate metabolism. Nitrofurazone has a broad spectrum of activity against gram-positive and gram-negative organisms.

Pharmacokinetics

Absorption: Limited drug absorption with topical use.
Distribution: None.
Metabolism: None.
Excretion: None.

Route	Onset	Peak	Duration
Topical	Unknown	Unknown	Unknown

Contraindications and precautions

Contraindicated in patients hypersensitive to drug. Use cautiously in patients with known or suspected renal impairment.

Interactions

None reported.

Effects on diagnostic tests

None reported.

Adverse reactions

Skin: *erythema, pruritus,* burning, edema, severe reactions (vesiculation, denudation, ulceration), *allergic contact dermatitis.*

Overdose and treatment

Discontinue use and cleanse area with mild soap and water.

Clinical considerations

- Investigationally, drug has been administered orally for the treatment of refractory African trypanosomiasis, acute bacillary dysentry, and testicular tumors. Diluted nitrofurazone solution with 6 to 10 parts of sterile water has been used for bladder irrigation.
- Avoid contact with eyes and mucous membranes.
- If undiluted solution is cloudy, warm to 122° to 140° F (50° to 60° C).
- Solutions for wet dressings are prepared by diluting nitrofurazone solution with distilled water (equal parts of each).
- Use diluted solutions within 24 hours after preparation; discard diluted solution that becomes cloudy.

Therapeutic monitoring

Monitor patient for overgrowth of nonsusceptible organisms, including fungi and *Pseudomonas.*

Special populations

Breast-feeding patients. Safety in breast-feeding women hasn't been established. Potential benefits to woman must be weighed against risks to infant.

Patient counseling

- Teach patient proper application of drug and to apply directly on lesion or place on gauze.
- Tell patient to avoid exposure of drug to direct sunlight, excessive heat, strong fluorescent lighting, and alkaline materials.

nitroglycerin (glyceryl trinitrate)

Oral, extended-release
Niong, Nitro-Bid, Nitrocine, Nitroglyn

Sublingual
Nitroquick, Nitrostat

Translingual
Nitrolingual

I.V.
Nitro-Bid IV, Tridil

Topical
Nitro-Bid, Nitrol

Transdermal
Deponit, Minitran, Nitro-Derm, Nitrodisc, Nitro-Dur, Transderm-Nitro

Transmucosal
Nitrogard

Pharmacologic classification: nitrate
Therapeutic classification: antianginal, vasodilator
Pregnancy risk category C

How supplied

Available by prescription only
Tablets (S.L.): 0.15 mg, 0.3 mg, 0.4 mg, 0.6 mg
Tablets (buccal, controlled-release): 1 mg, 2 mg, 3 mg
Capsules (sustained-release): 2.5 mg, 6.5 mg, 9 mg, 13 mg
Aerosol (lingual): 0.4 mg/metered spray
I.V.: 0.5 mg/ml, 0.8 mg/ml, 5 mg/ml
I.V. premixed solutions in dextrose: 100 mcg/ml, 200 mcg/ml, 400 mcg/ml
Topical: 2% ointment
Transdermal: 0.1-mg, 0.2-mg, 0.3-mg, 0.4-mg, 0.6-mg/hour systems, 0.8-mg/hour systems

Indications and dosages

Prophylaxis against chronic anginal attacks
Adults: 2.5 to 9 mg P.O. q 8 to 12 hours; or 2% ointment. Start with ½-inch ointment, in-

creasing with ½-inch increments until headache occurs, then decreasing to previous dose. Range of dosage with ointment is 0.5 to 4 inches q 4 to 6 hours. Usual dose is 1 to 2 inches. Alternatively, transdermal disc or pad may be applied to hairless site once daily. However, to prevent tolerance, topical forms shouldn't be worn overnight.

Relief of acute angina pectoris, prophylaxis to prevent or minimize anginal attacks when taken immediately before stressful events
Adults: One S.L. tablet dissolved under the tongue or in the buccal pouch immediately on indication of anginal attack. May repeat q 5 minutes for 15 to 30 minutes for a maximum of three doses. Or, using Nitrolingual spray, spray one or two doses into mouth, preferably onto or under the tongue. May repeat q 3 to 5 minutes to a maximum of three doses within a 15-minute period. Or, transmucosally, 1 to 3 mg q 3 to 5 hours during waking hours.

Hypertension, heart failure, angina
Nitroglycerin is indicated to control hypertension associated with surgery, to treat heart failure associated with MI, to relieve angina pectoris in acute situations, and to produce controlled hypotension during surgery (by I.V. infusion).
Adults: Initial infusion rate is 5 mcg/minute. May be increased by 5 mcg/minute q 3 to 5 minutes until a response is noted. If a 20-mcg/minute rate does not produce desired response, dosage may be increased by as much as 10 to 20 mcg/minute q 3 to 5 minutes.

Acute MI
Adults: Initially, 12.5 to 25 mcg I.V. followed by an infusion at 10 to 20 mcg/minute; increase 5 to 10 mcg/minute q 5 to 10 minutes as needed. Maximum dose is 200 mcg/minute. Decrease or discontinue if mean arterial pressure is under 80 mm Hg or systolic blood pressure under 90 mm Hg.

◇ ***Hypertensive crisis***
Adults: Infuse at 5 to 100 mcg/minute I.V.

Pharmacodynamics
Antianginal action: Nitroglycerin relaxes vascular smooth muscle of both the venous and arterial beds, resulting in a net decrease in myocardial oxygen consumption. It also dilates coronary vessels, leading to redistribution of blood flow to ischemic tissue. Systemic and coronary vascular effects of drug, which may vary slightly with the various nitroglycerin forms, probably account for its value in treating angina.
Vasodilating action: Nitroglycerin dilates peripheral vessels, making it useful (in I.V. form) in producing controlled hypotension during surgical procedures and in controlling blood pressure in perioperative hypertension. Because peripheral vasodilation decreases venous return to the heart (preload), nitroglycerin also helps to treat pulmonary edema and heart failure. Arterial vasodilation decreases arterial impedance (afterload), thereby decreasing left ventricular work and aiding the failing heart. These combined effects may prove valuable in treating some patients with acute MI.

Pharmacokinetics
Absorption: Well-absorbed from the GI tract. However, because it undergoes first-pass metabolism in the liver, it's incompletely absorbed into the systemic circulation. Onset of action for oral preparations is slow (except for sublingual tablets). After sublingual administration, absorption from the oral mucosa is relatively complete. Nitroglycerin also is well absorbed after topical administration as an ointment or transdermal system.
Distribution: Distributed widely throughout the body. About 60% of circulating drug is bound to plasma proteins.
Metabolism: Metabolized in the liver and serum to 1,3 glyceryl dinitrate; 1,2 glyceryl dinitrate; and glyceryl mononitrate. Dinitrate metabolites have a slight vasodilatory effect.
Excretion: Metabolites are excreted in urine; elimination half-life is about 1 to 4 minutes.

Route	Onset	Peak	Duration
P.O.	20-45 min	Unknown	3-8 hr
Buccal	3 min	Unknown	3-5 hr
S.L.	1-3 min	Unknown	½-1 hr
I.V.	Immediate	Immediate	3-5 min
Translingual	2-4 min	Unknown	½-1 hr
Topical	30 min	Unknown	2-12 hr
Transdermal	30 min	Unknown	24 hr

Contraindications and precautions
Contraindicated in patients with hypersensitivity to nitrates and in those with early MI (S.L. form), severe anemia, increased intracranial pressure, angle-closure glaucoma, orthostatic hypotension, and allergy to adhesives (transdermal form). I.V. form is contraindicated in patients with hypersensitivity to I.V. form, cardiac tamponade, restrictive cardiomyopathy, or constrictive pericarditis. Extended-release preparations shouldn't be used in patients with organic or functional GI hypermotility or malabsorption syndrome.

Use cautiously in patients with hypotension or volume depletion.

Interactions
Drug-drug. *Antihypertensive drugs or phenothiazines:* May cause additive hypotensive effects. Use together cautiously.
Ergot alkaloids: May precipitate angina. Avoid use together.
Sildenafil: Potentiates hypotensive effects of nitrates. Don't use together.
Drug-lifestyle. *Alcohol use:* May cause additive hypotensive effects. Don't use together.

Effects on diagnostic tests
Nitroglycerin may interfere with serum cholesterol determination tests using the Zlatkis-Zak color reaction, resulting in falsely decreased values.

Adverse reactions
CNS: *headache, sometimes with throbbing; dizziness;* weakness.
CV: *orthostatic hypotension, tachycardia, flushing, palpitations,* fainting.
GI: nausea, vomiting, sublingual burning.
Skin: cutaneous vasodilation, contact dermatitis (patch), rash.
Other: ***hypersensitivity reactions.***

Overdose and treatment
Clinical effects of overdose result primarily from vasodilation and methemoglobinemia and include hypotension, persistent throbbing headache, palpitations, visual disturbances, flushing of the skin, sweating (with skin later becoming cold and cyanotic), nausea and vomiting, colic, bloody diarrhea, orthostasis, initial hyperpnea, dyspnea, slow respiratory rate, bradycardia, heart block, increased intracranial pressure with confusion, fever, paralysis, tissue hypoxia (from methemoglobinemia) leading to cyanosis, and metabolic acidosis, coma, clonic seizures, and circulatory collapse. Death may result from circulatory collapse or asphyxia.

Treatment includes gastric lavage followed by administration of activated charcoal to remove remaining gastric contents. Monitor blood gas measurements and methemoglobin levels, as indicated. Supportive care includes respiratory support and oxygen administration, passive movement of the extremities to aid venous return, and recumbent positioning.

Clinical considerations
□ ***ALERT*** Don't confuse Nitro-Bid with Nicobid or nitroglycerin with nitroprusside.
- Ask all patients about the use of sildenafil (Viagra) before using nitrates.
- Use only S.L. and translingual forms to relieve acute angina attack.
- S.L. dose may be administered before anticipated stress or at bedtime if angina is nocturnal.
- To apply ointment, spread in uniform thin layer to hairless part of skin except distal parts of arms or legs, because absorption won't be maximal at these sites. Don't rub in. Cover with plastic film to aid absorption and to protect clothing. If using Tape-Surrounded Appli-Ruler (TSAR) system, keep TSAR on skin to protect patient's clothing and ensure that ointment remains in place. If serious adverse effects develop in patients using ointment or transdermal system, remove product at once or wipe ointment from skin. Be sure to avoid contact with ointment.
- Be sure to remove transdermal patch before defibrillation. Because of patch's aluminum backing, electric current may cause patch to explode.
- When terminating transdermal nitroglycerin treatment for angina, gradually reduce dosage and frequency of application over 4 to 6 weeks.
- Administration as I.V. infusion requires special nonabsorbent tubing supplied by manufacturer, because regular plastic tubing may absorb up to 80% of drug. Prepare infusion in a glass bottle or container.
- If drug causes headache, which is especially likely with initial doses, aspirin or acetaminophen may be indicated. Dosage may need to be reduced temporarily.
- Drug may cause orthostatic hypotension. To minimize this, patient should change to upright position slowly, go up and down stairs carefully, and lie down at the first sign of dizziness.
- To prevent withdrawal symptoms, reduce dosage gradually after long-term use of oral or topical preparations.
- Nitrate tolerance may develop.

Therapeutic monitoring
- When administering drug to patients during initial days after acute MI, recommend monitoring hemodynamic and clinical status carefully.
- Recommend monitoring blood pressure and intensity and duration of patient's response to drug.

Special populations
Pediatric patients. Methemoglobinemia may occur in infants receiving large doses of nitroglycerin.

Patient counseling
- Instruct patient to take medication regularly, as prescribed, and to keep S.L. form accessible at all times. Drug is physiologically necessary but not addictive.
- Teach patient to take oral tablet on empty stomach, either 30 minutes before or 1 to 2 hours after meals, to swallow oral tablets whole, and to chew chewable tablets thoroughly before swallowing.
- Instruct patient to take S.L. tablet at first sign of angina attack. Tell him to wet tablet with saliva, place it under the tongue until completely absorbed, and sit down and rest. If no relief occurs after three tablets, he should call or go to hospital emergency room. If he complains of tingling sensation with drug placed sublingually, he may try holding tablet in buccal pouch.
- Advise patient to store S.L. tablets in original container or other container specifically approved for this use away from heat and light. Keep cap to bottle tightly closed.
- Instruct patient to place transmucosal tablet under upper lip or in buccal pouch, to let it dis-

solve slowly over a 3- to 5-hour period, and not to chew or swallow tablet. Advise him that dissolution rate may increase if he touches tablet with tongue or drinks hot liquids.
- If patient is receiving nitroglycerin lingual aerosol (Nitrolingual), instruct him how to use this device correctly. Remind him not to inhale spray but to release it onto or under the tongue. Also tell him not to swallow immediately after administering the spray but to wait about 10 seconds before swallowing.
- Caution patient to use care when wearing transdermal patch near a microwave oven because leaking radiation may heat metallic backing of patch and cause burns.
- Warn patient that headache may follow initial doses but that this symptom may respond to usual headache remedies or dosage reduction (dose should be reduced only with medical approval). Assure patient that headache usually subsides gradually with continued treatment.
- Instruct patient to avoid alcohol while taking drug because severe hypotension and CV collapse may occur.
- Warn patient that drug may cause dizziness or flushing and to move to an upright position slowly.
- Tell patient to report blurred vision, dry mouth, or persistent headache.

nitroprusside sodium

Nipride*, Nitropress

Pharmacologic classification: vasodilator
Therapeutic classification: antihypertensive
Pregnancy risk category C

How supplied

Available by prescription only
Injection: 50 mg/2-ml, 50 mg/5-ml vials

Indications and dosages

Hypertensive emergencies
Adults and children: Initial dose is 0.25 to 3 mcg/kg/minute. I.V. infusion titrated to blood pressure, with a range of 0.3 to 10 mcg/kg/minute. Maximum infusion rate is 10 mcg/kg/minute for 10 minutes. If an adequate blood pressure response isn't achieved at this rate, discontinue infusion.
Acute heart failure
Adults and children: I.V. infusion titrated to cardiac output and systemic blood pressure. Same dosage range as for hypertensive emergencies.

Pharmacodynamics

Antihypertensive action: Nitroprusside acts directly on vascular smooth muscle, causing peripheral vasodilation.

Pharmacokinetics

Absorption: Administered by I.V. route. I.V. infusion of nitroprusside reduces blood pressure almost immediately.
Distribution: Unknown.
Metabolism: Metabolized rapidly in erythrocytes and tissues to a cyanide radical and then converted to thiocyanate in the liver.
Excretion: Excreted primarily as metabolites in urine. Blood pressure returns to pretreatment level 1 to 10 minutes after completion of infusion.

Route	Onset	Peak	Duration
I.V.	1-2 min	Immediate	10 min

Contraindications and precautions

Contraindicated in patients with hypersensitivity to drug, compensatory hypertension (such as in arteriovenous shunt or coarctation of the aorta), inadequate cerebral circulation, congenital optic atrophy, or tobacco-induced amblyopia.

Use cautiously in patients with renal or hepatic disease, increased intracranial pressure, hypothyroidism, hyponatremia, or low vitamin B_{12} levels.

Interactions

Drug-drug. *General anesthetics, particularly enflurane and halothane:* Potentiated hypotensive effects. Patient requires careful blood pressure monitoring.
Nitroprusside: May potentiate antihypertensive effects of other antihypertensive medications. Use together cautiously.
Pressor agents such as epinephrine: May cause an increase in blood pressure during nitroprusside therapy. Patient requires careful blood pressure monitoring.
Sildenafil: Potentiates hypotensive effects of nitrates. Don't use together.

Effects on diagnostic tests

None reported.

Adverse reactions

CNS: *headache, dizziness, loss of consciousness, apprehension,* ***increased intracranial pressure,*** *restlessness.*
CV: ***bradycardia,*** *hypotension, tachycardia, palpitations, ECG changes.*
GI: *nausea, abdominal pain, ileus.*
GU: *increased serum creatinine.*
Metabolic: ***acidosis, methemoglobinemia,*** *hypothyroidism.*
Musculoskeletal: *muscle twitching,*
Skin: pink color, flushing, rash, diaphoresis.
Other: ***thiocyanate toxicity, cyanide toxicity,*** *venous streaking, irritation at infusion site.*

Overdose and treatment

Signs and symptoms of overdose include the adverse reactions listed above and increased tolerance to the antihypertensive effects of drug.

Treat overdose by giving nitrites to induce methemoglobin formation. Discontinue drug and administer amyl nitrite inhalations for 15 to 30 seconds each minute until a 3% sodium nitrite solution can be prepared. Administer amyl nitrite cautiously to minimize risk of additional hypotension secondary to vasodilation. Then administer the sodium nitrite solution by I.V. infusion at a rate not exceeding 2.5 to 5 ml/minute up to a total dose of 10 to 15 ml. Follow with I.V. sodium thiosulfate infusion (12.5 g in 50 ml of D_5W solution) over 10 minutes. If necessary, repeat infusions of sodium nitrite and sodium thiosulfate at half the initial doses. Further treatment involves symptomatic and supportive care.

Clinical considerations

- Ask all patients about the use of sildenafil (Viagra) before using nitrates.
- Drug also may be used to produce controlled hypotension during anesthesia, to reduce bleeding from surgical procedure.
- Hypertensive patients are more sensitive to nitroprusside than normotensive patients. Also, patients taking other antihypertensive drugs are extremely sensitive to nitroprusside. Nitroprusside has been used in patients with acute MI, refractory heart failure, and severe mitral regurgitation.
- The goal of therapy is to reduce the mean arterial pressure by 25% within minutes to 2 hours.
- Prepare solution using D_5W solution; don't use bacteriostatic water for injection or sterile saline solution for reconstitution; because of light sensitivity, foil-wrap I.V. solution (but not tubing). Fresh solutions have faint brownish tint; discard after 24 hours.
- The concentrated solution is further diluted in 250, 500, or 1,000 ml 5% dextrose injection to produce a concentration of 200, 100, or 50 mcg/ml, respectively.
- Infuse drug with infusion pump.
- Drug is best run piggyback through a peripheral line with no other medications; don't adjust rate of main I.V. line while drug is running because even small boluses can cause severe hypotension.

Therapeutic monitoring

- Recommend monitoring blood pressure at least every 5 minutes at start of infusion and every 15 minutes thereafter during infusion.
- Nitroprusside can cause cyanide toxicity; therefore, check serum thiocyanate levels every 72 hours; levels above 100 mcg/ml are associated with cyanide toxicity, which can produce profound hypotension, metabolic acidosis, dyspnea, ataxia, and vomiting. If such symptoms occur, discontinue infusion and reevaluate therapy.

Special populations

Breast-feeding patients. It isn't known if drug is distributed into breast milk; administer with caution to breast-feeding women.
Geriatric patients. Geriatric patients may be more sensitive to antihypertensive effects of drug.

Patient counseling

Advise patient to report CNS symptoms, such as headache or dizziness, promptly.

nizatidine

Axid, Axid AR

Pharmacologic classification: H_2-receptor antagonist
Therapeutic classification: antiulcer
Pregnancy risk category B

How supplied

Available by prescription only
Capsules: 150 mg, 300 mg
Available without a prescription
Capsules: 75 mg

Indications and dosages

Treatment of active duodenal ulcer, gastric ulcer
Adults: 300 mg P.O. once daily h.s. Alternatively, may give 150 mg P.O. b.i.d. for up to 8 weeks.
Maintenance therapy for duodenal ulcer patients
Adults: 150 mg P.O. once daily h.s. for up to 1 year.
Gastroesophageal reflux disease
Adults: 150 mg P.O. b.i.d. up to 12 weeks.
Heartburn (self-medication)
Adults and children age 12 and older: One 75-mg capsule P.O. 30 to 60 minutes before meals; use up to b.i.d. not to exceed continuous therapy for 2 weeks.
≡ ***Dosage adjustment.*** In adults with renal impairment, refer to this table.

Creatinine clearance (ml/min)	Active duodenal ulcer	Maintenance
20 to 50	150 mg/day	150 mg q other day
< 20	150 mg q other day	150 mg q 3 days

Pharmacodynamics

Antiulcer action: Nizatidine is a competitive, reversible inhibitor of H_2 receptors, particularly those in the gastric parietal cells.

Pharmacokinetics

Absorption: Well absorbed (more than 90%) after oral administration. Absorption may be slightly enhanced by food, and slightly impaired by antacids.
Distribution: About 35% is bound to plasma protein.
Metabolism: Probably undergoes hepatic metabolism. About 40% of excreted drug is metabolized; the remainder is excreted unchanged.
Excretion: More than 90% of an oral dose is excreted in urine within 12 hours. Renal clearance is about 500 ml/minute, which indicates excretion by active tubular secretion. Less than 6% of an administered dose is eliminated in the feces. Elimination half-life is 1 to 2 hours. Moderate to severe renal impairment significantly prolongs half-life and decreases clearance of nizatidine. In anephric persons, half-life is 3½ to 11 hours; plasma clearance is 7 to 14 L/hour.

Route	Onset	Peak	Duration
P.O.	½ hr	½-3 hr	12 hr

Contraindications and precautions

Contraindicated in patients hypersensitive to H_2-receptor antagonists. Use cautiously in patients with impaired renal function.

Interactions

Drug-drug. *High doses of aspirin (3,900 mg/day) with nizatidine (150 mg twice-daily):* Increases serum salicylate levels. Monitor salicylate levels.
Drug-food. *Tomato-based mixed-vegetable juices:* May decrease potency of drug when used together. Advise patient not to use together.

Effects on diagnostic tests

False-positive tests for urobilinogen may occur during nizatidine therapy.

Adverse reactions

CNS: somnolence.
CV: *arrhythmias.*
Hematologic: eosinophilia.
Hepatic: hepatocellular injury, elevated liver function tests.
Metabolic: hyperuricemia.
Skin: *diaphoresis,* rash, urticaria.
Other: fever.

Overdose and treatment

Expected clinical effects of overdose are cholinergic, including lacrimation, salivation, emesis, miosis, and diarrhea. Treatment may include use of activated charcoal, emesis, or lavage, with clinical monitoring and supportive therapy.

Clinical considerations

- Because drug is excreted primarily by the kidneys, reduce dosage in patients with moderate to severe renal insufficiency.
- Nizatidine is partially metabolized in the liver. In patients with normal renal function and uncomplicated hepatic dysfunction, the disposition of nizatidine is similar to that in patients with normal hepatic function.
- For patients on maintenance therapy, consider that effects of continuous drug therapy for over 1 year aren't known.

Therapeutic monitoring

Monitor LFTs in prolonged therapy and BUN and creatinine in patients with renal impairment.

Special populations

Breast-feeding patients. Use with caution in breast-feeding women. Consider that nizatidine is secreted and concentrated in the milk of lactating rats.
Pediatric patients. Safety and efficacy in children haven't been established.
Geriatric patients. Safety and efficacy appear similar to those in younger patients. However, consider that geriatric patients have reduced renal function.

Patient counseling

- Advise patient not to smoke, as this may increase gastric acid secretion and worsen the disease.
- Tell patient not to mix drug with tomato-based mixed-vegetable juices.
- Urge patient to avoid cigarette smoking which can increase gastric acid secretion and worsen disease.
- Advise patient to report abdominal pain and blood in stools or emesis to doctor immediately.

norepinephrine bitartrate (formerly levarterenol bitartrate)

Levophed

Pharmacologic classification: adrenergic (direct-acting)
Therapeutic classification: vasopressor
Pregnancy risk category C

How supplied

Available by prescription only
Injection: 1 mg/ml parenteral

Indications and dosages

To maintain blood pressure in acute hypotensive states
Adults: Initially, 8 to 12 mcg/minute I.V. infusion, then titrated to maintain desired blood pressure; maintenance dosage, 2 to 4 mcg/minute.

Children: Initially, 2 mcg/minute or 2 mcg/m²/minute I.V. infusion, then titrated to maintain desired blood pressure. For advanced cardiac life support, initial infusion rate is 0.1 mcg/kg/minute.

◊ ***GI bleeding***

Adults: 8 mg in 250 ml normal saline solution given intraperitoneally, or 8 mg in 100 ml normal saline solution given via a nasogastric tube q hour for 6 to 8 hours then q 2 hours for 4 to 6 hours.

Pharmacodynamics

Vasopressor action: Norepinephrine acts predominantly by direct stimulation of alpha-adrenergic receptors, constricting both capacitance and resistance blood vessels. This results in increased total peripheral resistance; increased systolic and diastolic blood pressure; decreased blood flow to vital organs, skin, and skeletal muscle; and constriction of renal blood vessels, which reduces renal blood flow. It also has a direct stimulating effect on $beta_1$ receptors of the heart, producing a positive inotropic response. Its main therapeutic effects are vasoconstriction and cardiac stimulation.

Pharmacokinetics

Absorption: Pressor effect occurs rapidly after infusion, is of short duration, and stops within 1 to 2 minutes after infusion is stopped.

Distribution: Localizes in sympathetic nerve tissues. It crosses the placenta but not the blood-brain barrier.

Metabolism: Metabolized in the liver and other tissues to inactive compounds.

Excretion: Excreted in urine primarily as sulfate and glucuronide conjugates. Small amounts are excreted unchanged in urine.

Route	Onset	Peak	Duration
I.V.	Immediate	Immediate	1-2 min after infusion ends

Contraindications and precautions

Contraindicated in patients with mesenteric or peripheral vascular thrombosis, profound hypoxia, hypercapnia, or hypotension resulting from blood volume deficit and during cyclopropane and halothane anesthesia.

Use cautiously in patients with sulfite allergies or in those receiving MAO inhibitors or triptyline- or imipramine-type antidepressants.

Interactions

Drug-drug. *General anesthetics:* Norepinephrine may cause increased arrhythmias. Use together cautiously.

Atropine: Blocks the reflex bradycardia caused by norepinephrine and enhances its pressor effects. Use together cautiously.

Tricyclic antidepressants, some antihistamines, parenteral ergot alkaloids, guanethidine, MAO inhibitors, and methyldopa: Severe, prolonged hypertension. Avoid use together.

Beta blockers: May result in an increased potential for hypertension; propranolol may be used to treat arrhythmias occurring during norepinephrine administration. Use together cautiously.

Furosemide or other diuretics: May decrease arterial responsiveness. Monitor blood pressure for effect.

Effects on diagnostic tests

None reported.

Adverse reactions

CNS: anxiety, weakness, dizziness, tremor, restlessness, insomnia.

CV: ***bradycardia, severe hypertension, arrhythmias.***

Respiratory: respiratory difficulties, ***asthmatic episodes.***

Other: ***anaphylaxis,*** irritation or necrosis with extravasation.

Overdose and treatment

Signs and symptoms of overdose include severe hypertension, photophobia, retrosternal or pharyngeal pain, intense sweating, vomiting, cerebral hemorrhage, seizures, and arrhythmias. Monitor vital signs closely.

Treatment includes supportive and symptomatic measures. Use atropine for reflex bradycardia, phentolamine for extravasation, and propranolol for tachyarrhythmias.

Clinical considerations

Besides those relevant to all adrenergics as well as the following:

- Correct blood volume depletion before administration. Norepinephrine isn't a substitute for blood, plasma, fluid, or electrolyte replacement.
- Select injection site carefully. Administration by I.V. infusion requires an infusion pump or other device to control flow rate. If possible, infuse into antecubital vein of the arm or the femoral vein. Change injection sites for prolonged therapy. Must be diluted before use with 5% dextrose or with saline (dilution with saline alone isn't recommended). Monitor infusion rate. Withdraw drug gradually; recurrent hypotension may follow abrupt withdrawal.
- Prepare infusion solution by adding 4 mg norepinephrine to 1 L of 5% dextrose. The resultant solution contains 4 mcg/ml.
- To treat extravasation, infiltrate site promptly with 10 to 15 ml saline solution containing 5 to 10 mg phentolamine, using a fine needle.
- Some clinicians add phentolamine (5 to 10 mg) to each liter of infusion solution as a preventive against sloughing, should extravasation occur.
- In patients with previously normal blood pressure, adjust flow rate to maintain blood

pressure at low normal (usually 80 to 100 mm Hg systolic); in hypertensive patients, maintain systolic no more than 40 mm Hg below preexisting pressure level.
- Avoid contact of drug with iron salts, alkalies, or oxidizing agents.
- Protect solution from light. Discard solution that's discolored or contains a precipitate.

Therapeutic monitoring
- Recommend monitoring intake and output. Norepinephrine reduces renal blood flow, which may cause decreased urine output initially.
- Patient should be observed constantly during administration of norepinephrine. Obtain baseline blood pressure and pulse before therapy, and repeat every 2 minutes until stabilization; repeat every 5 minutes during drug administration.
- In addition to vital signs, recommend monitoring patient's mental state, skin temperature of extremities, and skin color (especially earlobes, lips, and nail beds).

Special populations
Pediatric patients. Use with caution in children.
Geriatric patients. Drug hasn't been evaluated systematically in patients age 65 or older. No specific dosage recommendations.

Patient counseling
- Inform patient of need for frequent monitoring of vital signs.
- Advise patient to report adverse reactions.

norethindrone
Micronor, Nor-Q.D.

norethindrone acetate
Aygestin, Norlutate*

Pharmacologic classification: progestin
Therapeutic classification: contraceptive
Pregnancy risk category X

How supplied
Available by prescription only
norethindrone
Tablets: 0.35 mg
norethindrone acetate
Tablets: 5 mg

Indications and dosages
Amenorrhea, abnormal uterine bleeding, endometriosis
norethindrone acetate
Adults: 2.5 to 10 mg P.O. daily on days 5 to 10 of second half of menstrual cycle.
Endometriosis
norethindrone acetate
Adults: 5 mg P.O. daily for 14 days, then increase by 2.5 mg/day q 2 weeks up to 15 mg/day. Daily therapy may be continued consecutively for 6 to 9 months; if breakthrough bleeding occurs, temporarily discontinue therapy.
Contraception
Adults: 0.35 mg norethindrone P.O. daily, beginning day 1 of menstrual cycle and continuing uninterrupted thereafter.

Pharmacodynamics
Contraceptive action: Norethindrone suppresses ovulation, causes thickening of cervical mucus, and induces sloughing of the endometrium.

Pharmacokinetics
Absorption: Well absorbed after oral administration.
Distribution: Distributed into bile and breast milk and is about 80% protein-bound.
Metabolism: Primarily metabolized in the liver, where it undergoes extensive first-pass metabolism.
Excretion: Excreted primarily in feces. Elimination half-life is 5 to 14 hours.

Route	Onset	Peak	Duration
P.O.	Unknown	Unknown	Unknown

Contraindications and precautions
Contraindicated in patients with thromboembolic disorders, cerebral apoplexy, or history of these conditions; hypersensitivity to drug; breast cancer, undiagnosed abnormal vaginal bleeding; severe hepatic disease; missed abortion; and during pregnancy.

Use cautiously in patients with diabetes mellitus, seizures, migraine, cardiac or renal disease, asthma, or mental depression.

Interactions
Drug-drug. *Bromocriptine:* Amenorrhea or galactorrhea, thus interfering with the action of bromocriptine. Don't use together.

Effects on diagnostic tests
None reported.

Adverse reactions
CNS: depression.
CV: thrombophlebitis, ***pulmonary embolism,*** edema, ***thromboembolism, CVA.***
EENT: exophthalmos, diplopia, retinal thrombosis.
GU: breakthrough bleeding, dysmenorrhea, amenorrhea, cervical erosion, abnormal secretions, breast tenderness, enlargement, or secretion.
Hepatic: cholestatic jaundice.

Metabolic: changes in weight, decreased pregnanediol excretion, increased serum alkaline phosphatase and amino acid levels, glucose tolerance.
Skin: melasma, rash, acne, pruritus.

Overdose and treatment
No information available.

Clinical considerations
Recommendations for administration of norethindrone, and for care and teaching of the patient during therapy, are the same as those for all progestins.
☐ ***ALERT*** Norethindrone acetate is twice as potent as norethindrone. Norethindrone acetate shouldn't be used for contraception.
- Use as a test for pregnancy isn't appropriate; drug may cause birth defects and masculinization of female fetus.
- Preliminary estrogen treatment is usually needed in menstrual disorders.

Therapeutic monitoring
- Monitor LFTs in patients with hepatic impairment.
- Observe patient for signs of edema. Blood pressure must be monitored.

Patient counseling
- Recommendations for care and teaching of the patient during therapy are the same as those for all progestins.
- FDA regulations require that patient reads package insert explaining possible adverse reactions, before receiving first dose.
- Tell patient to use drug at same time of day every day of the year when used as a contraceptive.
- Tell patient with visual disturbances or migraine to stop drug and notify doctor immediately.
- Inform patient of procedure if drug dose is missed.

norfloxacin (ophthalmic)
Chibroxin

Pharmacologic classification: fluoroquinolone
Therapeutic classification: broad-spectrum antibiotic
Pregnancy risk category C

How supplied
Available by prescription only
Ophthalmic solution: 0.3% in 5-ml containers

Indications and dosages
Conjunctivitis caused by susceptible strains of bacteria
Adults and children age 1 and older: 1 or 2 drops in the affected eye q.i.d. for up to 7 days. If condition warrants, 2 drops may be applied q 2 hours during the waking hours of first day of treatment.

Pharmacodynamics
Antibiotic action: Ophthalmic norfloxacin inhibits bacterial DNA gyrase, an enzyme necessary for bacterial replication. Drug is bacteriostatic or bactericidal, depending on level.

Pharmacokinetics
Absorption: Systemic absorption of ophthalmic norfloxacin is limited.
Distribution: No information available.
Metabolism: No information available.
Excretion: No information available.

Route	Onset	Peak	Duration
Ophthalmic	Unknown	Unknown	Unknown

Contraindications and precautions
Contraindicated in patients with a history of hypersensitivity to norfloxacin or other fluoroquinolone antibiotics. Don't inject drug into eye.

Interactions
Drug-food. *Caffeine*. Systemically administered drug interferes with metabolism of caffeine. Use cautiously in patients receiving these drugs.

Effects on diagnostic tests
None reported.

Adverse reactions
EENT: local burning or discomfort, itching, chemosis, photophobia, conjunctival hyperemia, white crystalline precipitates, lid margin crusting, bad or bitter taste in mouth, ***hypersensitivity reactions.***
GI: nausea.

Overdose and treatment
A topical overdose of the drug may be flushed from the eye with warm tap water.

Clinical considerations
Drug is indicated for treatment of conjunctivitis when caused by susceptible bacteria. Known susceptible strains include *Acinetobacter calcoaceticus, Aeromonas hydrophila, Haemophilus influenzae, Proteus mirabilis, Serratia marcescens, Staphylococcus aureus, S. epidermidis, S. warnerii, Streptococcus pneumoniae,* and *Pseudomonas aeruginosa.*

Therapeutic monitoring
Monitor for overgrowth of nonsusceptible organisms including fungi.

Special populations
Breast-feeding patients. It's unknown if drug is excreted in breast milk. Use with caution in breast-feeding women.

Patient counseling
- Teach patient how to instill drug correctly. Remind him not to touch the tip of the bottle with his hands and to avoid contact of the tip with the eye or surrounding tissue.
- Instruct patient not to share washcloths or towels with other family members to avoid spreading infection. Tell him not to share drug with others.
- Advise patient to wash hands before and after instilling solution.
- Tell patient to store drug at room temperature and to protect it from light.
- Advise patient not to wear contact lenses during therapy.

norfloxacin (systemic)
Noroxin

Pharmacologic classification: fluoroquinolone
Therapeutic classification: broad-spectrum antibiotic
Pregnancy risk category C

How supplied
Available by prescription only
Tablets: 400 mg

Indications and dosages
Complicated and uncomplicated urinary tract infections caused by various gram-negative and gram-positive bacteria
Adults: For complicated infection, 400 mg P.O. b.i.d. for 10 to 21 days; for uncomplicated infection, 400 mg P.O. b.i.d. for 3 to 10 days. Don't exceed 800 mg/day. Patients with creatinine clearance less than 30 ml/minute should receive 400 mg/day for appropriate duration of therapy.
Uncomplicated gonorrhea
Adults: 800 mg P.O. as a single dose.
Prostatitis
Adults: 400 mg P.O. q 12 hours for 28 days.
◊ ***Gastroenteritis***
Adults: 400 mg P.O. b.i.d. for 5 days.
◊ ***Treatment of traveler's diarrhea***
Adults: 400 mg P.O. b.i.d. for up to 3 days.

Pharmacodynamics
Antibacterial action: Norfloxacin is generally bactericidal. It inhibits DNA gyrase, blocking DNA synthesis. Spectrum of activity includes most aerobic gram-positive and gram-negative urinary pathogens, including *Pseudomonas aeruginosa.*

Pharmacokinetics
Absorption: About 30% to 40% of dose is absorbed from the GI tract; as dose increases, percentage of absorbed drug decreases. Food may reduce absorption.
Distribution: Distributed into renal tissue, liver, gallbladder, prostatic fluid, testicles, seminal fluid, bile, and sputum. From 10% to 15% binds to plasma proteins.
Metabolism: Unknown.
Excretion: Most of systemically absorbed drug is excreted by the kidneys, with about 30% appearing in feces. In patients with normal renal function, plasma half-life is 3 to 4 hours; up to 8 hours in severe renal impairment.

Route	Onset	Peak	Duration
P.O.	Unknown	½-2 hr	Unknown

Contraindications and precautions
Contraindicated in patients with hypersensitivity to fluoroquinolones. Use cautiously in patients with renal impairment or conditions predisposing them to seizure disorders, such as cerebral arteriosclerosis.

Interactions
Drug-drug. *Antacids:* Decreased absorption. Administer drugs at separate times.
Multivitamins containing divalent or trivalent cations: May interfere with absorption of norfloxacin. Administer drugs at separate times.
Nitrofurantoin: Antagonizes antibacterial activity of norfloxacin. Monitor patient for clinical effect.
Probenecid: May increase serum norfloxacin levels. Monitor patient for toxicity.
Warfarin: Prolonged PT. Monitor PT and INR.
Xanthine derivatives, such as aminophylline and theophylline: May increase theophylline level. Monitor for xanthine-related toxicities.
Drug-food. *Food:* Interferes with absorption of norfloxacin. Give drug 1 hour before meals or 2 hours after meals.
Drug-lifestyle. *Sun exposure:* May cause photosensitivity reaction. Advise patient to take precautions.

Effects on diagnostic tests
None reported.

Adverse reactions
CNS: fatigue, somnolence, headache, dizziness, ***seizures,*** depression, insomnia.
GI: nausea, constipation, flatulence, heartburn, dry mouth, abdominal pain, diarrhea, vomiting, anorexia.
GU: increased serum creatinine and BUN levels, crystalluria.
Hematologic: eosinophilia, neutropenia, decreased hematocrit.
Hepatic: transient elevations of AST, ALT, and alkaline phosphatase.
Musculoskeletal: back pain, tendinitis.

Skin: photosensitivity.
Other: hypersensitivity reactions (rash, ***anaphylactoid reaction***), fever; hyperhidrosis.

Overdose and treatment
No information available.

Clinical considerations
- Culture and sensitivity tests should be obtained before starting therapy, and repeated as needed throughout therapy.
- Patient should be well hydrated before and during therapy to avoid crystalluria.

Therapeutic monitoring
- Monitor baseline and follow-up BUN, creatinine clearance, CBC, and liver function tests.
- Recommend observing patient for signs and symptoms of resistant infection or reinfection.

Special populations
Breast-feeding patients. Safety in breast-feeding women hasn't been established; alternative feeding method is recommended during treatment with norfloxacin.
Pediatric patients. Contraindicated in children because animal studies suggest a potential risk of arthropathy.

Patient counseling
- Instruct patient to continue taking drug as directed, even if he feels better.
- Advise patient to take drug 1 hour before or 2 hours after meals and antacids.
- Warn patient that drug may cause dizziness that impairs his ability to perform tasks that require alertness and coordination.
- Instruct patient to avoid excessive exposure to sunlight.

norgestrel
Ovrette

Pharmacologic classification: progestin
Therapeutic classification: contraceptive
Pregnancy risk category X

How supplied
Available by prescription only
Tablets: 0.075 mg

Indications and dosages
Contraception
Adults: 1 tablet P.O. daily, beginning on first day of menstruation.

Pharmacodynamics
Contraceptive action: Norgestrel suppresses ovulation and causes thickening of cervical mucus.

Pharmacokinetics
Absorption: Well absorbed after oral administration.
Distribution: No information available.
Metabolism: No information available.
Excretion: No information available.

Route	Onset	Peak	Duration
P.O.	Unknown	Unknown	Unknown

Contraindications and precautions
Contraindicated in patients with thromboembolic disorders, cerebral apoplexy, or history of these conditions; hypersensitivity to drug; breast cancer; undiagnosed abnormal vaginal bleeding; severe hepatic disease; missed abortion; and during pregnancy.

Use cautiously in patients with renal or cardiac disease, diabetes mellitus, migraine, seizures, asthma, or mental depression.

Interactions
Drug-drug. *Bromocriptine:* May cause amenorrhea or galactorrhea, interfering with the action of bromocriptine. Don't administer together.

Effects on diagnostic tests
None reported.

Adverse reactions
CNS: ***cerebral thrombosis or hemorrhage,*** migraine, depression.
CV: thrombophlebitis, ***pulmonary embolism,*** edema, ***thromboembolism, CVA.***
EENT: exophthalmos, diplopia.
GU: *breakthrough bleeding, change in menstrual flow,* dysmenorrhea, spotting, amenorrhea, cervical erosion, breast tenderness, enlargement, or secretion.
Hepatic: cholestatic jaundice, increased serum alkaline phosphatase.
Metabolic: increased amino acid levels, changes in weight, decreased pregnanediol excretion, glucose tolerance.
Skin: melasma, rash, acne, pruritus.

Overdose and treatment
No information available.

Clinical considerations
Besides those relevant to all progestins as well as the following:
- Failure rate of the progestin-only contraceptive is about three times higher than that of the combination contraceptives.
- Ovrette tablets contain tartrazine. Use cautiously in patients with tartrazine or aspirin sensitivity.

Therapeutic monitoring
Monitor LFTs in patients with hepatic impairment or during prolonged therapy.

Special populations

Breast-feeding patients. If possible, advise breast-feeding women not to use oral contraceptives until infant is completely weaned because drug may interfere with lactation by decreasing the quantity and quality of breast milk. Recommend other means of contraception.

Patient counseling

- Tell patient to take drug at the same time every day, even during menstruation. Norgestrel is also known as the "minipill."
- Advise patient of increased risk of serious CV adverse reactions associated with heavy smoking, especially while taking oral contraceptives.
- Tell patient that risk of pregnancy increases with each tablet missed. If one tablet is missed, she should take it as soon as she remembers and then take the next tablet at the regular time. If two tablets are missed, she should take one as soon as she remembers and then take the next regular dose at the usual time; she should use a nonhormonal method of contraception in addition to norgestrel until 14 tablets have been taken. If three or more tablets are missed, she should discontinue drug and use a nonhormonal method of contraception until after her period. Instruct patient to do a pregnancy test if her menstrual period doesn't occur within 45 days.
- Advise patient to report excessive bleeding or bleeding between menstrual cycles immediately.
- Instruct patient to use a second method of birth control for the first cycle on norgestrel, or for 3 weeks after starting the hormonal contraceptive, to ensure full protection.
- Advise patient who wishes to become pregnant to wait at least 3 months after discontinuing norgestrel, to prevent birth defects.

nortriptyline hydrochloride

Aventyl, Pamelor

Pharmacologic classification: tricyclic antidepressant
Therapeutic classification: antidepressant
Pregnancy risk category NR

How supplied

Available by prescription only
Capsules: 10 mg, 25 mg, 50 mg, 75 mg
Solution: 10 mg/5 ml (4% alcohol)

Indications and dosages

Depression, ◇***panic disorder***
Adults: 25 mg P.O. t.i.d. or q.i.d., gradually increasing to a maximum of 150 mg/day. Alternatively, entire dosage may be given h.s.
Elderly or adolescents: 30 to 50 mg P.O. daily or in divided doses.

Pharmacodynamics

Antidepressant action: Drug is thought to exert its antidepressant effects by inhibiting reuptake of norepinephrine and serotonin in CNS nerve terminals (presynaptic neurons), which results in increased levels and enhanced activity of these neurotransmitters in the synaptic cleft. Nortriptyline inhibits reuptake of serotonin more actively than norepinephrine; it's less likely than other tricyclic antidepressants to cause orthostatic hypotension.

Pharmacokinetics

Absorption: Absorbed rapidly from the GI tract after oral administration.
Distribution: Distributed widely into the body, including the CNS and breast milk, and is 95% protein-bound. Steady-state serum levels are achieved within 2 to 4 weeks. Therapeutic serum level ranges from 50 to 150 ng/ml.
Metabolism: Metabolized by the liver; a significant first-pass effect may account for variability of serum levels in different patients taking the same dosage.
Excretion: Mostly excreted in urine; some in feces, via the biliary tract.

Route	Onset	Peak	Duration
P.O.	Unknown	7-8½ hr	Unknown

Contraindications and precautions

Contraindicated during acute recovery phase of MI and in patients with hypersensitivity to drug or MAO therapy within past 14 days. Use cautiously in patients with history of urine retention or seizures, glaucoma, suicidal tendencies, CV disease, or hyperthyroidism and in those receiving thyroid medication.

Interactions

Drug-drug. *Centrally acting antihypertensive drugs, such as clonidine, guanabenz, guanadrel, guanethidine, methyldopa, and reserpine:* Decreased hypotensive effects. Monitor blood pressure.
Atropine and other anticholinergic drugs, including antihistamines, meperidine, phenothiazines, and antiparkinson agents: Oversedation, paralytic ileus, visual changes, and severe constipation. Use together cautiously.
Barbiturates: Induce nortriptyline metabolism and decrease therapeutic efficacy. Patient requires close monitoring.
Beta blockers, cimetidine, methylphenidate, oral contraceptives, and propoxyphene: May inhibit nortriptyline metabolism, increasing plasma levels. Monitor patient for toxicity.
CNS depressants, including analgesics, barbiturates, narcotics, tranquilizers, and anesthetics (oversedation): Additive effects. Use together cautiously.
Disulfiram or ethchlorvynol: May cause delirium and tachycardia. Avoid use together.

Metrizamide: Increased risk of seizures. Avoid use together, if possible.
Phenothiazines and haloperidol: Decreased nortryptyline metabolism. Patient requires close monitoring.
Pimozide, thyroid medications, or antiarrhythmic agents, such as disopyramide, procainamide and quinidine: May increase incidence of arrhythmias and conduction defects. Use together cautiously.
Sympathomimetics, including epinephrine, phenylephrine, phenylpropanolamine, and ephedrine (often found in nasal sprays): May increase blood pressure. Use together cautiously.
Warfarin: May increase PT and cause bleeding. Monitor PT and INR.
Drug-lifestyle. *Heavy smoking:* Induces nortriptyline metabolism and decreases therapeutic efficacy. Advise patient to avoid smoking.
Alcohol use: Additive effects. Advise patient to avoid alcohol use.

Effects on diagnostic tests
None reported.

Adverse reactions
CNS: *drowsiness, dizziness, **seizures,*** tremor, weakness, confusion, headache, nervousness, EEG changes, extrapyramidal reactions, insomnia, nightmares, hallucinations, paresthesia, ataxia, agitation.
CV: *tachycardia,* hypertension, hypotension, ***MI,*** heart block, ***stroke,*** prolonged conduction time (elongation of QT and PR intervals, flattened T waves on ECG).
EENT: *blurred vision,* tinnitus, mydriasis.
GI: dry mouth, *constipation,* nausea, vomiting, anorexia, paralytic ileus.
GU: *urine retention*, elevated liver function test.
Hematologic: ***bone marrow depression, agranulocytosis,*** eosinophilia, ***thrombocytopenia.***
Metabolic: increased serum glucose levels.
Skin: rash, urticaria, photosensitivity.
Other: *diaphoresis, **hypersensitivity reaction.***
After abrupt withdrawal of long-term therapy: nausea, headache, malaise (doesn't indicate addiction).

Overdose and treatment
The first 12 hours after acute ingestion are a stimulatory phase characterized by excessive anticholinergic activity, including agitation, irritation, confusion, hallucinations, hyperthermia, parkinsonian symptoms, seizures, urine retention, dry mucous membranes, pupillary dilation, constipation, and ileus. This is followed by CNS depressant effects, including hypothermia; decreased or absent reflexes; sedation; hypotension; cyanosis; and cardiac irregularities, including tachycardia, conduction disturbances, and quinidine-like effects on the ECG.

Severity of overdose is best indicated by prolonging QRS complex beyond 100 ms, which usually indicates a serum level above 1,000 ng/ml. Metabolic acidosis may follow hypotension, hypoventilation, and seizures.

Treatment is symptomatic and supportive, including maintaining a patent airway, stable body temperature, and fluid and electrolyte balance. Induce emesis with ipecac syrup if patient is conscious; follow with gastric lavage and activated charcoal to prevent further absorption. Dialysis is usually ineffective. Consider use of cardiac glycosides or physostigmine if serious CV abnormalities or cardiac failure occurs. Treat seizures with parenteral diazepam or phenytoin; arrhythmias with parenteral phenytoin or lidocaine; and acidosis with sodium bicarbonate. Don't use quinidine, procainamide or disopyramide to treat arrhythmias, since these agents can further depress myocardial conduction and contractility. Don't give barbiturates; these may enhance CNS and respiratory depressant effects.

Clinical considerations
Consider the recommendations relevant to all tricyclic antidepressants as well as the following:
- Drug may be administered at bedtime to reduce daytime sedation. Tolerance to sedative effects usually develops over the initial weeks of therapy.
- Withdraw drug gradually over a few weeks; however, it should be discontinued at least 48 hours before surgical procedures.
- Drug is available in liquid form.
- In patients with bipolar disorders, drug may cause symptoms of the manic phase to emerge.

Therapeutic monitoring
Monitor plasma notriptyline concentration if dose is over 100 mg/day.

Special populations
Breast-feeding patients. Nortriptyline is excreted in breast milk in low levels; potential benefit to woman should outweigh potential harm to infant.
Pediatric patients. Drug isn't recommended for children. Lower dosages may be indicated for adolescents.
Geriatric patients. Lower dosages may be indicated. Geriatric patients are at greater risk for adverse cardiac effects. Nortriptyline is less likely to cause hypotension than other TCAs.

Patient counseling
- Explain that patient may not see full effects of drug therapy for up to 4 weeks after start of therapy.
- Warn patient about sedative effects.

- Recommend taking full daily dose at bedtime to prevent daytime sedation.
- Instruct patient to avoid drinking alcoholic beverages, doubling doses after missing one, and discontinuing drug abruptly, unless instructed.
- Warn patient about possible dizziness. Tell patient to lie down for about 30 minutes after each dose at start of therapy and to avoid sudden orthostatic changes, to prevent dizziness. Orthostatic hypotension is usually less severe than with amitriptyline.
- Urge patient to report unusual reactions promptly: confusion, movement disorders, fainting, rapid heartbeat, or difficulty urinating.
- Tell patient to store drug away from children.
- Suggest relieving dry mouth with sugarless chewing gum or candy.
- Advise patient to avoid activities that require physical and mental alertness, such as driving a car or operating machinery.

nystatin

Mycostatin, Nilstat

Pharmacologic classification: polyene macrolide
Therapeutic classification: antifungal
Pregnancy risk category B

How supplied

Available by prescription only
Tablets: 500,000 units
Suspension: 100,000 units/ml
Powder for suspension: 50-, 150-, 500-million units; 1-, 2-, 5-billion units
Vaginal suppositories: 100,000 units
Cream: 100,000 units/g
Ointment: 100,000 units/g
Powder: 100,000 units/g
Lozenges: 200,000 units

Indications and dosages

GI infections
Adults: 500,000 to 1 million units as oral tablets, t.i.d.
Oropharyngeal candidiasis
Adults and children: 400,000 to 600,000 units of oral suspension q.i.d. Alternatively, give 200,000 to 400,000 units (lozenges) four to five times daily for up to 14 days; allow to dissolve in mouth.
Infants: 200,000 units of oral suspension q.i.d.
Neonates and premature infants: 100,000 units of oral suspension q.i.d.
Oropharyngeal candidiasis in HIV-infected patients
Adults: 500,000 to 1,000,000 units 3 to 5 times daily as oral suspension or tablets (dissolved in mouth). Alternatively, oral lozenges may be used.
Cutaneous or mucocutaneous candidal infections
Topical use: Apply to affected areas b.i.d. or t.i.d. until healing is complete (about 2 weeks).
Vaginal use: 100,000 units, as vaginal tablets, inserted high into vagina daily or b.i.d. for 14 days.
For prevention of thrush in the neonate, 100,000 - to 200,000-unit vaginal tablets daily for 3 to 6 weeks before delivery.
Candidal diaper dermatitis
Infants: 100,000 units of oral suspension P.O. q.i.d. as an adjunct to topical nystatin therapy.

Pharmacodynamics

Antifungal action: Nystatin is both fungistatic and fungicidal. It binds to sterols in the fungal cell membrane, altering its permeability and allowing leakage of intracellular components. It acts against various yeasts and fungi, including *Candida albicans.*

Pharmacokinetics

Absorption: Not absorbed from GI tract, nor through intact skin or mucous membranes.
Distribution: No detectable amount is available for tissue distribution.
Metabolism: No detectable amount is systemically available for metabolism.
Excretion: Oral nystatin is excreted almost entirely unchanged in feces.

Route	Onset	Peak	Duration
P.O., Topical, Intravaginal	Unknown	Unknown	Unknown

Contraindications and precautions

Contraindicated in patients with hypersensitivity to drug.

Interactions

None reported.

Effects on diagnostic tests

None reported.

Adverse reactions

GI: transient nausea, diarrhea (usually with large oral dosage), vomiting (with oral administration or vaginal tablets).
Skin: occasional contact dermatitis from preservatives in some forms (with topical administration or vaginal tablets).

Overdose and treatment

Overdose may result in nausea, vomiting, and diarrhea. Treatment is unnecessary because toxicity is negligible.

Clinical considerations

- Avoid hand contact with drug; hypersensitivity is rare but can occur.

■ For treatment of oral candidiasis, patient should have a clean mouth, and should hold suspension in mouth for several minutes before swallowing; for infant thrush, medication should be swabbed on oral mucosa.
■ May give immunosuppressed patient vaginal tablets (100,000 units) orally to provide prolonged drug contact with oral mucosa; alternatively, use clotrimazole troche.
■ For candidiasis of the feet, patient should dust powder on shoes and stockings as well as feet for maximal contact and effectiveness.
■ Avoid occlusive dressings or ointment on moist covered body areas that favor yeast growth.
■ To prevent maceration, use cream on intertriginous areas, and powder on moist lesions.
■ Clean affected skin gently before topical application; cool, moist compresses applied for 15 minutes between applications help soothe dry skin.
■ Cleansing douches may be used by nonpregnant women for esthetic reasons; they should use preparations that don't contain antibacterials, which may alter flora and promote reinfection.
■ Protect drug from light, air, and heat.
■ Drug is ineffective in systemic fungal infection.

Therapeutic monitoring

Recommend monitoring patient for proper use of medication and for clinical effect.

Special populations

Breast-feeding patients. Safety in breast-feeding women hasn't been established.

Patient counseling

■ Teach patient signs and symptoms of candidal infection. Inform patient about predisposing factors: use of antibiotics, oral contraceptives, and corticosteroids; diabetes; infected sexual partners; and tight-fitting pantyhose and undergarments.
■ Teach good oral hygiene. Explain that overuse of mouthwash and poorly fitting dentures, especially in geriatric patients, may alter flora and promote infection.
■ Tell patient to continue using vaginal cream through menstruation; emphasize importance of washing applicator thoroughly after each use.
■ Advise patient to change stockings and undergarments daily; teach good skin care.
■ Teach patient how to administer each dosage form prescribed.
■ Tell patient to continue drug for at least 48 hours after symptoms clear, to prevent reinfection.

O

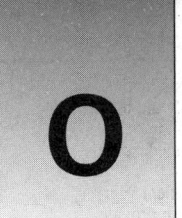

octreotide acetate

Sandostatin, Sandostatin LAR

Pharmacologic classification: synthetic octapeptide
Therapeutic classification: somatotropic hormone
Pregnancy risk category B

How supplied

Available by prescription only
Injection: 0.05 mg/ml, 0.1 mg/ml, and 0.5mg/ml in 1-ml ampules; 0.2 mg/ml and 1 mg/ml in 5-ml multidose vials
Injection suspension, extended-release: 10 mg/2 ml, 20 mg/2 ml, 30 mg/2 ml

Indications and dosages

Symptomatic treatment of flushing and diarrhea associated with carcinoid tumors
Adults: Initially, 100 to 600 mcg daily S.C. in two to four divided doses for first 2 weeks of therapy (usual daily dose, 300 mcg). Subsequent dosage based on individual response. 50 to 500 mcg I.V. and repeat, p.r.n.; prolonged I.V. infusion (e.g. 50 mcg/hour) infused over 8 to 24 hours also may be used. Also, 20 mg I.M. of suspension q 4 weeks for 2 months (after using injection for at least 2 weeks). Continue S.C. injection of immediate release for at least first 2 weeks of therapy with long-acting formulation. After 2 months, increase dose to 30 mg or decrease to 10 mg I.M. q 4 weeks as needed.
Prevention of carcinoid crisis associated with surgery
Adults: 250 to 500 mcg S.C. 1 to 2 hours before induction of anesthesia.
Symptomatic treatment of watery diarrhea associated with vasoactive intestinal peptide-secreting tumors (VIPomas)
Adults: Initially, 200 to 300 mcg daily S.C. in two to four divided doses for first 2 weeks of therapy. Subsequent dosage based on individual response, but usually won't exceed 450 mcg daily. Also, 10 to 30 mg I.M. of suspension based on growth hormone concentration, insulin-like growth factor 1 (IGF-1), and symptom control q 4 weeks for 2 months (after using injection for at least 2 weeks). Continue S.C. injection of immediate release for at least first 2 weeks of therapy with long-acting formulation. After 2 months, increase dose to 30 mg or decrease to 10 mg I.M. q 4 weeks as needed.
Acromegaly
Adults: Initially, 50 mcg t.i.d. S.C. Subsequent dosage based on individual response. Usual dosage is 100 to 200 mcg S.C. t.i.d. but some patients may require up to 500 mcg t.i.d. for maximum effectiveness. Patients currently receiving S.C. Sandostatin may be switched directly to Sandostatin LAR in a dose of 20 mg I.M. of suspension q 4 weeks for 3 months (after using S.C. injection for at least 2 weeks). After 3 months of receiving Sandostatin LAR, dosage adjustment is based on growth hormone concentration, IGF-1, and symptom control. Dose ranges from 10 to 40 mg I.M. q 4 weeks.

Pharmacodynamics

Antidiarrheal action: Octreotide mimics the action of naturally occurring somatostatin and decreases the secretion of gastroenterohepatic peptides that may contribute to the adverse signs and symptoms seen in patients with metastatic carcinoid tumors and VIPomas. It isn't known if drug affects the tumor directly.

Pharmacokinetics

Absorption: Absorbed rapidly and completely after injection.
Distribution: Distributed to the plasma, where it binds to serum lipoprotein and albumin.
Metabolism: Eliminated from the plasma at a slower rate than the naturally occurring hormone. Apparent half-life is about 1½ hours, with a duration of effect of up to 12 hours.
Excretion: About 35% appears unchanged in urine.

Route	Onset	Peak	Duration
S.C.	½ hr	½ hr	< 12 hr

Contraindications and precautions

Contraindicated in patients hypersensitive to drug or its components.

Interactions

Drug-drug. *Cyclosporine*: Decreased plasma levels of cyclosporine. Monitor patient closely.
Insulin, oral antidiabetic agents (sulfonylureas), oral diazoxide: Medication interactions. Dosage adjustments may be required.
Other drugs used to control symptoms of the disease, such as beta blockers, calcium channel blockers, and electrolyte-controlling agents:

Medication interactions. Use with octreotide may require dosage adjustment of these medications.

Effects on diagnostic tests
None reported.

Adverse reactions
CNS: dizziness, light-headedness, fatigue, headache.
CV: ***sinus bradycardia,*** conduction abnormalities, ***arrhythmias.***
EENT: blurred vision.
GI: *nausea, diarrhea, abdominal pain or discomfort, loose stools,* vomiting, fat malabsorption, gallstones or biliary sludge, flatulence, constipation.
GU: pollakiuria, urinary tract infection.
Metabolic: hyperglycemia, hypoglycemia, hypothyroidism, suppressed secretion of growth hormone and of gastroenterohepatic peptides gastrin, glucagon, insulin, motilin, pancreatic polypeptide, secretin, and VIP.
Musculoskeletal: backache, joint pain.
Skin: flushing, edema, wheals, erythema or pain at injection site, alopecia, pain or burning at S.C. injection site.
Other: flulike symptoms.

Overdose and treatment
Doses of 1,000 mcg have been administered as an I.V. bolus in volunteers without adverse effects. Drug may produce metabolic changes in certain patients.

Clinical considerations
- Fluid and electrolyte balance may be altered after initiation of octreotide therapy.
- Half-life may be altered in patients with end-stage renal failure who are undergoing dialysis. Dosage adjustment may be necessary.
- Octreotide suspension must be given under clinical supervision. Suspension is for I.M. use only into the gluteal muscle and should be stored refrigerated at 36° to 46° F (2° to 8° C) and protected from light. Warm to room temperature for 30 to 60 minutes before mixing.
- I.V. injection may be given undiluted for carcinoid crisis. For I.V. infusion, dilute drug in 50 to 200 ml of normal saline or 5% dextrose injection. Infuse over 15 to 30 minutes. Drug remains stable for 24 hours. Store ampules in the refrigerator. Drug may be stored at room temperature for 14 days. Injection is incompatible with total parenteral nutrition solution.

Therapeutic monitoring
- Monitor baseline and periodic tests of thyroid function because long-term effects of drug on hypothalamic-pituitary function aren't known.
- Monitor laboratory values during therapy, such as urinary 5-hydroxyindoleacetic acid, plasma serotonin, plasma substance P for carcinoid tumors, and plasma VIP for VIPomas.
- Mild, transient hypoglycemia or hyperglycemia may occur during therapy. Recommend observing patient for signs of glucose imbalance and monitoring closely.
- Drug may alter fat absorption and aggravate fat malabsorption. Monitor periodic assessment of 72-hour fecal fat and serum carotene.
- Drug may decrease vitamin B_{12} levels during chronic treatment. Monitor patient's vitamin B_{12} levels.
- Patients with acromegaly are more likely to experience GI side effects and bradycardia. Recommend monitoring closely.

Special populations
Breast-feeding patients. It isn't known if drug is excreted in breast milk.
Pediatric patients. Doses of 1 to 10 mcg/kg appear to be well tolerated in children.

Patient counseling
Because drug may cause gallstones, tell patient to report abdominal discomfort promptly.

ofloxacin
Floxin, Ocuflox

Pharmacologic classification: fluoroquinolone
Therapeutic classification: antibiotic
Pregnancy risk category C

How supplied
Available by prescription only
Tablets: 200 mg, 300 mg, 400 mg
Injection: 200 mg in 50 ml D_5W; 400 mg in water for injection in 10-ml single-use vials; 400 mg in 100 ml D_5W.
Ophthalmic solution: 0.3%
Otic solution: 0.3%

Indications and dosages
Conjunctivitis caused by known organism
Adults and children over age 1: Instill 1 to 2 drops in conjunctival sac q 2 to 4 hours, while awake, for first 2 days and then q.i.d. for up to 5 additional days.
Bacterial keratitis
Adults and children over age 1: 1 to 2 drops in affected eye q 30 minutes while awake and q 4 to 6 hours after retiring for 2 days. On day 3, apply 1 to 2 drops to the affected eye q 1 hour while awake for an additional 4 to 6 days. Then, 1 to 2 drops q.i.d. until clinical cure is achieved.
Acute bacterial exacerbations of chronic bronchitis and pneumonia caused by susceptible organisms, mild to moderate skin and skin-structure infections, and community-acquired pneumonia
Adults: 400 mg P.O. or I.V. q 12 hours for 10 days.

Sexually transmitted diseases, such as acute uncomplicated urethral and cervical gonorrhea, nongonococcal urethritis and cervicitis, and mixed infections of urethra and cervix
Adults: For acute uncomplicated gonorrhea, 400 mg P.O. or I.V. once as a single dose; for cervicitis and urethritis, 300 mg P.O. or I.V. q 12 hours for 7 days.
Urinary tract infections
Adults: For cystitis caused by *Escherichia coli* or *Klebsiella pneumoniae,* 200 mg P.O. or I.V. q 12 hours for 3 days; for cystitis caused by other organisms, 200 mg P.O. or I.V. q 12 hours for 7 days.
Complicated urinary tract infections
Adults: 200 mg P.O. or I.V. q 12 hours for 10 days.
Prostatitis
Adults: 300 mg P.O. or I.V. q 12 hours for 6 weeks or longer. Change I.V. administration to P.O. after 10 days.
Pelvic inflammatory disease
Adults: 400 mg P.O. q. 12 hours in combination with metronidazole for 14 days. Alternatively, 400 mg I.V. q 12 hours in combination with metronidazole.
Otitis externa
Adults and children over age 12: 10 drops into affected ear b.i.d. for 10 days.
Children age 1 to 12: 5 drops instilled into affected ear b.i.d. for 10 days.
Acute otitis media in pediatric patients with tympanostomy tubes
Children age 1 to 12: Instill 5 drops into affected ear b.i.d. for 10 days.
Chronic supportive otitis media with perforated tympanic membrane
Adults and children age 12 and older: Instill 10 drops into affected ear b.i.d. for 14 days.
◊***Adjunct in* Brucella *infections***
Adults: 400 mg P.O. daily for 6 weeks.
◊***Peritonitis in patients receiving continuous ambulatory peritoneal dialysis***
Adults: 400 mg P.O. loading dose, then 300 mg P.O. daily for 7 to 10 days.
◊***Typhoid fever***
Adults: 200 to 400 mg P.O. q 12 hours for 7 to 14 days.
◊***Antituberculosis agent (adjunct)***
Adults: 300 mg P.O. daily.
◊***Treatment of postoperative sternotomy or soft-tissue wounds caused by* Mycobacterium fortuitum**
Adults: 300 to 600 mg P.O. daily for 3 to 6 months.
◊***Acute Q fever pneumonia***
Adults: 600 mg P.O. daily for up to 16 days.
◊***Mediterranean spotted fever***
Adults: 200 mg P.O. q 12 hours for 7 days.
◊***Traveler's diarrhea***
Adults: 300 mg P.O. b.i.d. for 3 days.
≡***Dosage adjustment.*** In patients with renal failure and creatinine clearance of 50 ml/minute or less, adjust dosage. Give initial dose as recommended; additional doses as follows: If creatinine clearance is 10 to 50 ml/minute, no dosage adjustment at 24-hour intervals; if less than 10 ml/ minute, 50% of recommended dose q 24 hours.

Maximum daily dose in patients with hepatic function disorders is 400 mg.

Pharmacodynamics

Antibacterial action: Ofloxacin interferes with DNA gyrase, which is needed for synthesis of bacterial DNA. Spectrum of action includes many gram-positive and gram-negative aerobic bacteria including Enterobacteriaceae and *Pseudomonas aeruginosa.* Also, drug has some in vitro activity against chlamydia, mycoplasma, mycobacterium, plasmodium, and rickettsia.

Pharmacokinetics

Absorption: Well absorbed after oral administration. Because oral bioavailability of ofloxacin is about 98%, oral and I.V. dosages are the same.
Distribution: Widely distributed to body tissues and fluids.
Metabolism: Less than 10% of a single dose is metabolized.
Excretion: 70% to 80% excreted unchanged in urine; less than 5% in feces.

Route	Onset	Peak	Duration
P.O.	Unknown	½-2 hr	Unknown
I.V.	Unknown	Immediate	Unknown
Ophthalmic	Unknown	Unknown	Unknown

Contraindications and precautions

Contraindicated in patients with hypersensitivity to drug or other fluoroquinolones. Use oral and I.V. forms cautiously in patients with seizure disorders, CNS diseases such as cerebral arteriosclerosis, hepatic disorders, or renal failure and during pregnancy.

Interactions

Drug-drug. *Antacids:* Interferes with GI absorption of ofloxacin, resulting in decreased serum levels. Separate administration by 2 to 4 hours.
Antidiabetic agents: May affect blood glucose levels, causing hypoglycemia or hyperglycemia. Monitor patient closely.
Theophylline: May increase serum theophylline levels. Monitor patient closely and adjust theophylline dosage as needed.
Warfarin: May have prolonged PT and INR. Monitor PT and INR.
Drug-lifestyle. *Sun exposure:* May cause photosensitivity reactions. Advise patient to take precautions.

Effects on diagnostic tests
None reported.

Adverse reactions
CNS: dizziness; headache, fatigue, lethargy, malaise, drowsiness, sleep disorders, nervousness, insomnia, visual disturbances, ***seizures*** (with oral or I.V. form).
CV: chest pain (with oral or I.V. form).
EENT: *transient ocular burning or discomfort,* stinging, redness, itching, photophobia, lacrimation, eye dryness (with ophthalmic form).
GI: *nausea,* ***pseudomembranous colitis,*** anorexia, abdominal pain or discomfort, diarrhea, vomiting, constipation, dry mouth, flatulence, dysgeusia (with oral or I.V. form).
GU: vaginitis, vaginal discharge, genital pruritus (with oral or I.V. form).
Hepatic: elevated liver enzymes.
Metabolic: increased blood glucose levels.
Musculoskeletal: trunk pain (with oral or I.V. form).
Skin: rash, pruritus, photosensitivity (with oral or I.V. form).
Other: hypersensitivity reactions ***(anaphylactoid reaction),*** fever, phlebitis (with oral or I.V. form).

Overdose and treatment
In case of overdose, empty the stomach and maintain hydration. Observe patient and treat symptomatically.

Clinical considerations
- Give I.V. ofloxacin by slow infusion only; don't give I.M., S.C., intrathecally, or by intraperitoneal injection. Administer over at least 60 minutes and avoid rapid or bolus injection. Compatible with most common I.V. solutions, including D_5W injection, normal saline injection, dextrose 5% in normal saline injection, dextrose 5% in 0.45% saline injection, 5% dextrose in lactated Ringer's solution, and 5% sodium bicarbonate injection. Dilute 20 to 40 mg/ml vials to solution containing 4 mg/ml.
- Administer drug I.V. for no longer than 10 days; after 10 days, change I.V. to P.O.
- Drug isn't recommended for syphilis.

Therapeutic monitoring
- Periodic assessment of organ system functions during prolonged therapy is necessary.
- Monitor for overgrowth of nonsusceptible organisms.
- Monitor renal and hepatic studies and CBC in prolonged therapy.

Special populations
Breast-feeding patients. Safety hasn't been established in breast-feeding women. Ofloxacin is excreted in breast milk in levels similar to those found in plasma.
Pediatric patients. Safety and efficacy in children under age 18 haven't been established. Similar drugs have caused arthropathy in juvenile animals.

Patient counseling
- Tell patient to drink fluids liberally.
- Advise patient to separate doses of antacids, vitamins, and ofloxacin by 2 hours.
- Tell patient drug may be taken without regard to meals.
- Warn patient that dizziness and lightheadedness may occur. Advise caution when driving or operating hazardous machinery until effects of drug are known.
- Warn patient that hypersensitivity reactions may follow first dose; he should discontinue drug at first sign of rash or other allergic reaction and notify doctor immediately.
- Advise patient to avoid prolonged exposure to direct sunlight and to use a sunscreen when outdoors.

olanzapine
Zyprexa

Pharmacologic classification: thienobenzodiazepine derivative
Therapeutic classification: antipsychotic
Pregnancy risk category C

How supplied
Available by prescription only
Tablets: 2.5 mg, 5 mg, 7.5 mg, 10 mg

Indications and dosages
Management of signs and symptoms of psychotic disorders
Adults: Initially, 5 to 10 mg P.O. once daily. Adjust dosage in 5-mg daily increments at intervals of not less than 1 week. Most patients respond to 10 mg/day; do not exceed 20 mg/day.

Pharmacodynamics
Unknown. Drug acts as an antagonist at dopamine (D_{1-4}) and serotonin ($5\text{-}HT_{2A/2C}$) receptors; it may also exhibit antagonist-binding at adrenergic, cholinergic, and histaminergic receptors.

Pharmacokinetics
Absorption: Food doesn't affect rate or extent of absorption. About 40% of dose is eliminated by first pass metabolism.
Distribution: Distributes extensively throughout the body, with a volume of distribution of about 1,000 L. Drug is 93% protein-bound, primarily to albumin and $alpha_1$-acid glycoprotein.
Metabolism: Metabolized by direct glucuronidation and cytochrome P-450-mediated oxidation.
Excretion: About 57% appears in urine and 30% in feces as metabolites. Only 7% of dose

is recovered in urine unchanged. Elimination half-life ranges from 21 to 54 hours.

Route	Onset	Peak	Duration
P.O.	Unknown	6 hr	Unknown

Contraindications and precautions

Contraindicated in patients with known hypersensitivity to drug. Use cautiously in patients with heart disease, cerebrovascular disease, conditions that predispose to hypotension (gradual titration of therapy minimizes the risk), history of seizures or conditions that might lower the seizure threshold, and hepatic impairment. Also, use cautiously in geriatric patients, in those with history of paralytic ileus, significant prostatic hypertrophy, or narrow-angle glaucoma, or those at risk for aspiration pneumonia.

Interactions

Drug-drug. *Antihypertensives and diazepam:* May potentiate hypotensive effects. Monitor blood pressure closely.
Carbamazepine, omeprazole, rifampin: May cause increased clearance of olanzapine. Recommend monitoring patient for clinical effect.
Fluvoxamine: May inhibit olanzapine elimination. Monitor for toxicity.
Levodopa and dopamine agonists: May cause antagonized effects of these agents. Use together cautiously.
Drug-lifestyle. *Alcohol use:* May potentiate hypotensive effects. Advise patient to avoid alcohol use.
Drug-herb. *Nutmeg:* May cause a loss of symptom control in patients taking these drugs or interfere with existing therapy for psychiatric illnesses. Avoid use together.

Effects on diagnostic tests

None reported.

Adverse reactions

CNS: *somnolence, agitation, insomnia, headache, nervousness, hostility, parkinsonism, dizziness,* anxiety, personality disorder, *akathisia,* hypertonia, tremor, amnesia, articulation impairment, euphoria, stuttering, dystonic/dyskinetic events, tardive dyskinesia, ***suicide attempt.***
CV: orthostatic hypotension, tachycardia, chest pain, hypotension, edema.
EENT: amblyopia, blepharitis, corneal lesion.
GI: constipation, dry mouth, abdominal pain, increased appetite, increased salivation, nausea, vomiting, thirst.
GU: premenstrual syndrome, hematuria, metrorrhagia, urinary incontinence, urinary tract infection.
Hematologic: increased eosinophil count.
Hepatic: increased ALT, AST, gamma glutamyltransferase.
Metabolic: weight gain or loss, increased CK, serum prolactin.
Musculoskeletal: joint pain, extremity pain, back pain, neck rigidity, twitching.
Respiratory: *rhinitis,* increased cough, pharyngitis, dyspnea.
Skin: vesiculobullous rash.
Other: fever, intentional injury, flu syndrome.

Overdose and treatment

Symptoms of overdose may include drowsiness and slurred speech. There's no specific antidote to olanzapine; treatment should be symptomatic. Monitor patient for hypotension, circulatory collapse, obtundation, seizures, or dystonic reactions. Gastric lavage with activated charcoal and sorbitol may be effective. Drug isn't removed by dialysis. Avoid epinephrine, dopamine, or other sympathomimetics with beta-agonist activity.

Clinical considerations

□ ***ALERT*** Zyrtec is an antihistamine; Zyprexa is an antipsychotic. But they look alike, sound alike, and have similar dosing. Store separately.

- Initial therapy of 5 mg may be used in patients who are debilitated, predisposed to hypotension, or have an alteration in metabolism because of their smoking status, gender, or age or who are pharmacologically sensitive to drug.
- Efficacy for long-term use (more than 6 weeks) hasn't been established.

Therapeutic monitoring

- Monitor patient for signs of neuroleptic malignant syndrome (hyperpyrexia, muscle rigidity, altered mental status, autonomic instability), a rare but frequently fatal adverse reaction that can occur with the administration of antipsychotic drugs. Drug should be stopped immediately and patient monitored and treated.
- Monitor baseline and periodic liver function tests.

Special populations

Breast-feeding patients. Drug is excreted in breast milk. Advise breast-feeding women to seek alternative feeding methods during therapy.
Pediatric patients. Safety and efficacy in children under age 18 haven't been established.
Geriatric patients. Drug may be initiated at lower dose because clearance may be decreased in geriatric patients. Half-life is 1½ times greater in this population.

Patient counseling

- Warn patient to avoid hazardous tasks until adverse CNS effects of drug are known.
- Caution patient against exposure to extreme heat; drug may impair ability of the body to reduce core temperature.
- Advise patient to avoid alcohol.

- Tell patient to rise slowly to avoid orthostatic hypotension.
- Advise patient to use ice chips or sugarless candy or gum to relieve dry mouth.
- Inform patient not to take prescription or OTC drugs without medical approval because of potential drug interactions.

olsalazine sodium

Dipentum

Pharmacologic classification: salicylate
Therapeutic classification: anti-inflammatory
Pregnancy risk category C

How supplied

Available by prescription only
Capsules: 250 mg

Indications and dosages

Maintenance of remission of ulcerative colitis in patients intolerant of sulfasalazine
Adults: 1 g P.O. daily in two divided doses.

Pharmacodynamics

Anti-inflammatory action: Mechanism of action is unknown but appears to be topical rather than systemic. Drug is converted to mesalamine (5-aminosalicylic acid; 5-ASA) in the colon. Presumably, mesalamine diminishes inflammation by blocking cyclooxygenase and inhibiting prostaglandin production in the colon.

Pharmacokinetics

Absorption: After oral administration, about 2.4% of a single dose is absorbed.
Distribution: Once metabolized to 5-ASA, drug is absorbed slowly from the colon, resulting in very high local levels.
Metabolism: 0.1% is metabolized in the liver; remainder will reach the colon, where it's rapidly converted to 5-ASA by colonic bacteria.
Excretion: Less than 1% is recovered in urine.

Route	Onset	Peak	Duration
P.O.	Unknown	1 hr	Unknown

Contraindications and precautions

Contraindicated in patients hypersensitive to salicylates. Use cautiously in patients with existing renal disease.

Interactions

Drug-drug. *Warfarin:* Increased PT. Monitor PT and INR.

Effects on diagnostic tests

None reported.

Adverse reactions

CNS: headache, depression, vertigo, dizziness, fatigue.
GI: *diarrhea,* nausea, *abdominal pain,* dyspepsia, bloating, anorexia, stomatitis.
Musculoskeletal: arthralgia.
Skin: rash, itching.

Overdose and treatment

Decreased motor activity and diarrhea can occur. Treat overdose symptomatically and supportively.

Clinical considerations

Diarrhea from drug therapy is difficult to distinguish from underlying condition.

Therapeutic monitoring

Monitor CBC with differential and liver function tests periodically.

Special populations

Breast-feeding patients. It's unknown if drug is excreted in breast milk. Use with caution in breast-feeding women.
Pediatric patients. Safety and efficacy in children haven't been established.

Patient counseling

- Advise patient to take drug with food and in evenly divided doses.
- Inform patient to call doctor if diarrhea develops.

omeprazole

Prilosec

Pharmacologic classification: substituted benzimidazole
Therapeutic classification: gastric acid suppressant
Pregnancy risk category C

How supplied

Available by prescription only
Capsules (delayed-release): 10 mg, 20 mg, 40 mg

Indications and dosages

Active duodenal ulcer
Adults: 20 mg P.O. daily for 4 to 8 weeks.
Helicobacter pylori ***eradication to reduce risk of duodenal ulcer recurrence***
Triple therapy (omeprazole/clarithromycin/amoxicillin)
Adults: 20 mg P.O. b.i.d. plus 500 mg clarithromycin P.O. b.i.d. plus 1,000 mg amoxicillin P.O. b.i.d. for 10 days. In patients with an ulcer present at the time of initiation of therapy, an additional 18 days of omeprazole 20 mg once daily is recommended alone for ulcer healing and symptom relief.

Note: Refer to entries on clarithromycin and amoxicillin.
Dual therapy (omeprazole/clarithromycin)
Adults: 40 mg q morning plus 500 mg clarithromycin t.i.d. for 14 days followed by 14 days of omeprazole 20 mg daily.
Note: Refer to entry on clarithromycin.
Severe erosive esophagitis; symptomatic, poorly responsive gastroesophageal reflux disease (GERD)
Adults: 20 mg P.O. daily for 4 to 12 weeks. Patients with GERD should have failed initial therapy with an H_2 antagonist. May continue with maintenance dosage of 20 mg daily for up to 1 year.
Pathological hypersecretory conditions (such as Zollinger-Ellison syndrome)
Adults: Initial dosage is 60 mg P.O. daily; adjust dosage based on patient response. Administer daily doses exceeding 80 mg in divided doses. Doses up to 120 mg t.i.d. have been administered. Continue therapy as long as clinically indicated.
Gastric ulcer
Adults: 40 mg P.O. daily for 4 to 8 weeks.
≡ ***Dosage adjustment.*** Dosage adjustments aren't required for patients with impaired renal function; however, they may be needed in those with hepatic impairment. Dosage adjustments may be necessary in Asian patients because of increased bioavailability of drug in this population.

Pharmacodynamics
Antisecretory action: Omeprazole inhibits the activity of the acid (proton) pump, H^+/K^+ adenosine triphosphatase (ATPase), located at the secretory surface of the gastric parietal cell. This blocks the formation of gastric acid.

Pharmacokinetics
Absorption: Omeprazole is acid-labile, and the formulation contains enteric-coated granules that permit absorption after drug leaves the stomach. Absorption is rapid. Bioavailability is about 40% because of instability in gastric acid as well as a substantial first-pass effect. Bioavailability increases slightly with repeated dosing, possibly because of drug's effect on gastric acidity.
Distribution: About 95% protein-bound.
Metabolism: Primarily metabolized in the liver.
Excretion: Primarily excreted by the kidneys. Plasma half-life is ½ to 1 hour, but drug effects may persist for days.

Route	Onset	Peak	Duration
P.O.	1 hr	2 hr	< 3 days

Contraindications and precautions
Contraindicated in patients hypersensitive to drug or its components.

Interactions
Drug-drug. *Ampicillin esters, iron derivatives, itraconazole, ketoconazole:* Poor bioavailability because optimal absorption of these drugs requires a low gastric pH. Avoid use together.
Diazepam, phenytoin, propranolol, theophylline, warfarin: Effects may be impaired by omeprazole. Patient requires monitoring closely for decreased effect or toxicity.
Drug-herb. *Male fern:* Inactivated in alkaline environments. Advise patient concerning this effect.
Pennyroyal: May change the rate of formation of toxic metabolites of pennyroyal. Don't use together.

Effects on diagnostic tests
Serum gastrin levels rise in most patients during first 2 weeks of therapy.

Adverse reactions
CNS: headache, dizziness, asthenia.
GI: diarrhea, abdominal pain, nausea, vomiting, constipation, flatulence.
Musculoskeletal: back pain.
Respiratory: cough, upper respiratory infection.
Skin: rash.

Overdose and treatment
Reports of overdose are rare. Symptoms include confusion, drowsiness, blurred vision, tachycardia, nausea, vomiting, diaphoresis, dry mouth, and headache. Doses up to 360 mg daily have been well tolerated. Dialysis is of little value because of the extent of binding to plasma proteins. Treatment should be symptomatic and supportive.

Clinical considerations
- Drug increases its own bioavailability with repeated administration. It is labile in gastric acid; less of it is lost to hydrolysis because drug elevates gastric pH.
- Capsules shouldn't be crushed.

Therapeutic monitoring
- Recommend monitoring patient for clinical effects of therapy.
- Monitor LFTs in patients with hepatic impairment.

Special populations
Breast-feeding patients. It isn't known if drug is excreted in breast milk. Avoid breast-feeding during therapy.
Pediatric patients. Safety in children hasn't been established.

Patient counseling
- Explain importance of taking drug exactly as prescribed.
- Tell patient to take 30 minutes before meals and not to crush capsules.

ondansetron hydrochloride

Zofran

Pharmacologic classification: serotonin (5-HT_3) receptor antagonist
Therapeutic classification: antiemetic
Pregnancy risk category B

How supplied

Available by prescription only
Tablets: 4 mg, 8 mg
Injection: 2 mg/ml in 20-ml multidose vials, 2-ml single-dose vials
Injection, premixed: 32 mg/50 ml in 5% dextrose single-dose vial
Oral solution: 4 mg/5 ml
Orally disintegrating tablets: 4 mg, 8 mg

Indications and dosages

Prevention of nausea and vomiting associated with initial and repeat courses of emetogenic cancer chemotherapy, including high-dose cisplatin
Adults and children age 4 and older: Three I.V. doses of 0.15 mg/kg with first dose infused over 15 minutes beginning 30 minutes before start of chemotherapy, with subsequent doses of 0.15 mg/kg administered 4 and 8 hours after first dose. In adults, may also administer as a single dose of 32 mg, infused over 15 minutes, 30 minutes before start of chemotherapy.
Adults and children over age 12: Initially, 8 mg P.O. starting 30 minutes before start of chemotherapy, with a repeat dose after the first dose, then q 12 hours for 1 to 2 days after completion of chemotherapy.
Children age 4 to 11: Initially, 4 mg given P.O. 30 minutes before start of chemotherapy with subsequent doses 4 and 8 hours after initial dose. Then 4 mg given P.O. q 8 hours for 1 to 2 days after completion of chemotherapy.
Prevention of radiation-induced nausea and vomiting
Adults: 8 mg P.O. t.i.d. First dose should be 1 to 2 hours before radiation treatment. Patients receiving single, high-dose radiation to abdomen should continue q 8-hour dosing for 1 to 2 days.
Prevention of postoperative nausea and vomiting
Adults: 16 mg P.O. 1 hour before anesthesia or 4 mg I.V. immediately before anesthesia or soon after operation. Alternatively, 4 mg I.M. undiluted as a single injection.
Children age 2 to 12 weighing more than 88 lb (40 kg): 4 mg I.V. as a single dose.
Children age 2 to 12 weighing 40 kg or less: 0.1 mg/kg I.V. as a single dose.
≡ ***Dosage adjustment.*** In patients with severe hepatic impairment, total daily dose shouldn't exceed 8 mg.

Pharmacodynamics

Antiemetic action: Not well known. Ondansetron isn't a dopamine-receptor antagonist. Because serotonin receptors of the 5-HT_3 type occur peripherally on vagal nerve terminals and centrally in the chemoreceptor trigger zone, it's uncertain if antiemetic action is mediated centrally, peripherally, or both.

Pharmacokinetics

Absorption: Absorption is variable with oral administration; bioavailability is 50% to 60%.
Distribution: 70% to 76% protein-bound.
Metabolism: Extensively metabolized by hydroxylation on the indole ring, followed by glucuronide or sulfate conjugation.
Excretion: 5% recovered in urine as parent compound. Half-life in adults is 3½ to 6 hours.

Route	Onset	Peak	Duration
P.O.	Unknown	2 hr	Unknown
I.V.	Unknown	Unknown	Unknown

Contraindications and precautions

Contraindicated in patients hypersensitive to drug. Use cautiously in patients with hepatic failure. Orally disintegrating tablet contains aspartame; use cautiously in patients with phenylketonuria.

Interactions

Drug-herb. *Horehound:* May enhance serotonergic effects. Don't use together.

Effects on diagnostic tests

None reported.

Adverse reactions

CNS: *headache, malaise, fatigue, dizziness, sedation,* anxiety/agitation, oculogyric crisis.
CV: chest pain, hypotension.
GI: *diarrhea, constipation,* abdominal pain, xerostomia.
GU: urine retention, gynecologic disorders.
Hepatic: transient elevation of AST and ALT.
Musculoskeletal: *musculoskeletal pain.*
Respiratory: ***hypoxia.***
Skin: rash, injection-site reaction.
Other: chills, fever, ***anaphylaxis***.

Overdose and treatment

Doses more than 10 times recommended dose have been given without incident. If overdose is suspected, manage with supportive therapy.

Clinical considerations

- Drug may be administered I.V. undiluted over 2 to 5 minutes.
- For infusion, dilute drug of 50 ml in compatible solution and infuse over 15 minutes.
- Ondansetron is stable at room temperature for 48 hours after dilution with normal saline, D_5W, 5% dextrose and normal saline, 5% dextrose and 0.45% saline, or 3% saline.

Therapeutic monitoring
- Monitor liver function if repeated doses.
- For patients undergoing abdominal surgery, monitor for ileus and/or gastric distension.

Special populations
Breast-feeding patients. It's unknown if drug is excreted in breast milk. Use with caution in breast-feeding women.
Pediatric patients. Little information available for use in children age 3 and under for preventing chemotherapy-induced nausea and vomiting, and in children under age 2 for preventing postoperative nausea and vomiting.
Geriatric patients. No age-related problems have been reported.

Patient counseling
Advise patient to alert doctor if adverse effects occur.

opium tincture, deodorized (laudanum)

opium tincture, camphorated (paregoric)

Pharmacologic classification: opiate
Therapeutic classification: antidiarrheal
Controlled substance schedule II or III (depending on amount of opium contained in product)
Pregnancy risk category B (D for high doses or long term)

How supplied
Available by prescription only
opium tincture
Alcoholic solution: Equivalent to morphine 10 mg/ml
opium tincture, camphorated
Alcoholic solution: Each 5 ml contains morphine, 2 mg; anise oil, 0.2 ml; benzoic acid, 20 mg; camphor, 20 mg; glycerin, 0.2 ml; and ethanol to make 5 ml

Indications and dosages
Acute, nonspecific diarrhea
Don't confuse doses of opium tincture and camphorated opium tincture.
Adults: 0.6 ml opium tincture (range, 0.3 to 1 ml) P.O. q.i.d. (maximum dose, 6 ml daily); or 5 to 10 ml camphorated opium tincture daily, b.i.d., t.i.d., or q.i.d. until diarrhea subsides.
Children: 0.25 to 0.5 ml/kg camphorated opium tincture daily, b.i.d., t.i.d., or q.i.d. until diarrhea subsides.
Severe opiate withdrawal symptoms in neonates
Neonates: Camphorated opium tincture or a 1:25 dilution of opium tincture in water, administered as 0.2 ml P.O. q 3 hours. Adjust dosage to control withdrawal symptoms. Increase dosage by 0.05 ml q 3 hours until symptoms are controlled. Once symptoms are stabilized for 3 to 5 days, gradually decrease dosage over a 2-to 4-week period.

Pharmacodynamics
Antidiarrheal action: Opium contains several ingredients. The most active, morphine, increases GI smooth-muscle tone, inhibits motility and propulsion, and diminishes secretions. By inhibiting peristalsis, the drug delays passage of intestinal contents, increasing water resorption and relieving diarrhea.

Pharmacokinetics
Absorption: Absorbed variably from the gut.
Distribution: Although opium alkaloids are distributed widely in the body, the low doses used to treat diarrhea act primarily in the GI tract. Camphor crosses the placenta.
Metabolism: Metabolized rapidly in the liver.
Excretion: Opium is excreted in urine; opium alkaloids (especially morphine) enter breast milk.

Route	Onset	Peak	Duration
P.O.	Unknown	Unknown	4-5 hr

Contraindications and precautions
Contraindicated in patients with acute diarrhea caused by poisoning until toxic material is removed from GI tract or in those with diarrhea caused by organisms that penetrate intestinal mucosa. Use cautiously in patients with asthma, prostatic hyperplasia, hepatic disease, and history of opium dependence.

Interactions
Drug-drug. *Other CNS depressants:* Additive effect. Use together cautiously.
Metoclopramide: May antagonize the effects of metoclopramide. Avoid use together.

Effects on diagnostic tests
Opium tincture and camphorated opium tincture may prevent delivery of technetium-99m disofenin to the small intestine during hepatobiliary imaging tests; delay test until 24 hours after last dose.

Adverse reactions
CNS: dizziness, light-headedness.
GI: nausea, vomiting, increased serum amylase and lipase levels.
Other: physical dependence (after long-term use).

Overdose and treatment
Signs and symptoms of overdose include drowsiness, hypotension, seizures, and apnea. Empty stomach by induced emesis or gastric lavage; maintain patent airway. Use naloxone to treat respiratory depression. Monitor patient

for signs and symptoms of CNS or respiratory depression.

Clinical considerations

- Mix drug with sufficient water to ensure passage to stomach.

□ ***ALERT*** Opium tincture, deodorized (laudanum) is 25 times more potent than camphorated opium tincture (paregoric); take care not to confuse these drugs. Camphorated opium tincture is more dilute, and teaspoon doses are easier to measure than dropper quantities of opium tincture.

- When camphorated opium tincture is added to water, a milky fluid forms.
- Risk of physical dependence on drug increases with long-term use.
- Don't refrigerate drug.

Therapeutic monitoring

Recommend monitoring vital signs and bowel function.

Special populations

Breast-feeding patients. Because opium alkaloids, especially morphine, are excreted in breast milk, possible risks must be weighed against benefits.
Pediatric patients. Opium tincture has been used to treat withdrawal symptoms in infants whose mothers are narcotic addicts.

Patient counseling

- Warn patient that physical dependence may result from long-term use.
- Advise patient to use caution when driving a car or performing other tasks requiring alertness because drug may cause drowsiness, dizziness, and blurred vision.
- Instruct patient to report diarrhea that persists longer than 48 hours because drug is indicated only for short-term use.
- Advise patient to take drug with food if it causes nausea, vomiting, or constipation.
- Instruct patient to call prescriber immediately if he has difficulty breathing or shortness of breath.
- Instruct patient to drink adequate fluids while diarrhea persists.

orlistat

Xenical

Pharmacologic classification: lipase inhibitor
Therapeutic classification: antiobesity drug
Pregnancy risk category B

How supplied

Available by prescription only
Capsules: 120 mg

Indications and dosages

Management of obesity, including weight loss and weight maintenance in conjunction with a reduced-calorie diet; reduction of risk of weight regain after prior weight loss
Adults: 120 mg P.O. t.i.d. with each main meal containing fat (during or up to 1 hour after the meal).

Pharmacodynamics

Antiobesity action: As a reversible inhibitor of lipases, orlistat forms a bond with the active site of gastric and pancreatic lipases. These inactivated enzymes are unavailable to hydrolyze dietary fat, in the form of triglycerides, into absorbable free fatty acids and monoglycerides. Because the undigested triglycerides aren't absorbed, the resulting caloric deficit may have a positive effect on weight control. The recommended dose of 120 mg t.i.d. inhibits dietary fat absorption by about 30%.

Pharmacokinetics

Absorption: Systemic exposure to orlistat is minimal because only a small amount of the drug is absorbed.
Distribution: More than 99% binds to plasma proteins; lipoproteins and albumin are major binding proteins.
Metabolism: Primarily metabolized within the GI wall.
Excretion: Most of unabsorbed drug is excreted in feces.

Route	Onset	Peak	Duration
P.O.	Unknown	8 hr	Unknown

Contraindications and precautions

Contraindicated in patients with chronic malabsorption syndrome, cholestasis, or known hypersensitivity to orlistat or to any component of this drug. Also, exclude organic causes of obesity such as hypothyroidism before starting patient on orlistat therapy.

Use cautiously in patients with a history of hyperoxaluria or calcium oxalate nephrolithiasis or a risk of anorexia nervosa or bulimia.

Use cautiously in patients receiving cyclosporine therapy because of the potential changes in cyclosporine absorption related to the variations in dietary intake.

Interactions

Drug-drug. *Fat-soluble vitamins such as vitamin E and beta-carotene:* Absorption may be decreased by drug. Separate administration times by 2 hours.
Pravastatin: May cause slightly increased pravastatin levels and additive lipid-lowering effects of drug. Monitor patient carefully.
Warfarin: May cause possible change in coagulation parameters. Monitor PT and INR.

Effects on diagnostic tests
None reported.

Adverse reactions
CNS: *headache,* dizziness, fatigue, sleep disorder, anxiety, depression.
CV: pedal edema.
EENT: otitis, tooth and gingival disorders.
GI: *oily spotting, flatus with discharge, fecal urgency, fatty or oily stool, oily evacuation, increased defecation, abdominal pain,* fecal incontinence, nausea, infectious diarrhea, rectal pain, vomiting.
GU: menstrual irregularity, vaginitis, urinary tract infection.
Musculoskeletal: *back pain,* pain in lower extremities, arthritis, myalgia, joint disorder, tendonitis.
Respiratory: *influenza, upper respiratory tract infection,* lower respiratory tract infection.
Skin: rash, dry skin.

Overdose and treatment
If an overdose occurs, discontinue drug and observe patient for 24 hours. Systemic effects attributable to the lipase-inhibiting properties of orlistat should be rapidly reversible.

Clinical considerations
- Drug is recommended for use in patients with an initial body mass index (BMI) of 30 kg/m^2 or more, or 27 kg/m^2 or more and other risk factors, such as hypertension, diabetes, or dyslipidemia.
- Advise patients to adhere to dietary guidelines. GI effects may increase when patient takes orlistat with foods that are high in fat—specifically, when more than 30% of their total daily calories come from fat.
- Orlistat has been shown to reduce absorption of some fat-soluble vitamins and beta-carotene. To ensure adequate nutrition, encourage patient to take a multivitamin supplement that contains fat-soluble vitamins during orlistat therapy.
- It's unknown if orlistat is safe and effective to use in patients for more than 2 years.
- As with any weight loss agent, the potential for misuse in certain patient populations, such as patients with anorexia nervosa or bulimia, exists.

Therapeutic monitoring
In diabetic patients, improved metabolic control may accompany weight loss, so the dosage of their oral antidiabetic (such as, sulfonylureas and metformin) or insulin may need to be reduced. Monitor serum glucose.

Special populations
Pregnant patients. Not recommended for use in pregnant women; effects on fetus aren't known.
Breast-feeding patients. It's unknown if orlistat is secreted in breast milk; therefore, breast-feeding women shouldn't take the drug.
Pediatric patients. Safety and efficacy in pediatric patients haven't been established.
Geriatric patients. It isn't known if patients age 65 and older respond differently to the drug than younger patients.

Patient counseling
- Advise patient to follow a nutritionally balanced, reduced-calorie diet that derives only 30% of its calories from fat. The daily intake of fat, carbohydrate, and protein should be distributed over three main meals. If a meal is occasionally missed or contains no fat, tell the patient the dose of orlistat can be omitted.
- To ensure adequate nutrition, advise patient to take a daily multivitamin supplement that contains fat-soluble vitamins at least 2 hours before or after the administration of orlistat, such as at bedtime.
- Tell patient with diabetes that weight loss may improve his glycemic control, so the dosage of his oral antidiabetic (such as sulfonylureas and metformin) or insulin may need to be reduced while he's taking the drug.
- Tell women to inform their doctor if pregnancy or breast-feeding is planned.

orphenadrine citrate
Banflex, Flexoject, Flexon, Myolin, Myotrol, Norflex

orphenadrine hydrochloride
Disipal*

Pharmacologic classification: diphenhydramine analogue
Therapeutic classification: skeletal muscle relaxant
Pregnancy risk category C

How supplied
Available by prescription only
Tablets: 50 mg, 100 mg
Tablets (extended-release): 100 mg
Injection: 30 mg/ml parenteral

Indications and dosages
Adjunct in painful, acute musculoskeletal conditions
Adults: 100 mg P.O. b.i.d., or 60 mg I.V. or I.M. q 12 hours. If used in combination with acetylsalicylic acid and caffeine, 25 to 50 mg P.O. t.i.d. to q.i.d.
◊ ***Leg cramps***
Adults: 100 mg P.O. h.s.

Pharmacodynamics
Skeletal muscle relaxant action: Orphenadrine doesn't relax skeletal muscle directly. Atropine-

like central action on cerebral motor centers or on the medulla may be the mechanism by which it reduces skeletal muscle spasm. Its reported analgesic effect may add to its skeletal muscle relaxant properties.

Pharmacokinetics

Absorption: Rapidly absorbed from the GI tract.
Distribution: Widely distributed throughout the body.
Metabolism: Pathway unknown, but drug is almost completely metabolized to at least eight metabolites.
Excretion: Excreted in urine, mainly as its metabolites. Small amounts are excreted unchanged. Half-life is about 14 hours.

Route	Onset	Peak	Duration
P.O.	1 hr	2 hr	4-6 hr
I.V., I.M.	Unknown	Unknown	Unknown

Contraindications and precautions

Contraindicated in patients with hypersensitivity to drug; glaucoma; prostatic hyperplasia; pyloric, duodenal, or bladder neck obstruction; myasthenia gravis; and peptic ulceration.

Use cautiously in geriatric or debilitated patients or in those with tachycardia, cardiac disease, arrhythmias, or sulfite allergy.

Interactions

Drug-drug. *Other anticholinergic agents:* May increase anticholinergic effects. Use together cautiously.
MAO inhibitors: May increase CNS adverse effects. Use together cautiously.
Propoxyphene or CNS depressants, such as antipsychotics, anxiolytics, and tricyclic antidepressants: May produce additive CNS effects. Concurrent use requires reduction of both agents.
Drug-lifestyle. *Alcohol use:* Additive CNS effects. Advise patient to avoid combined use.

Effects on diagnostic tests

None reported.

Adverse reactions

CNS: weakness, *drowsiness,* light-headedness, confusion, agitation, tremor, headache, dizziness, hallucinations.
CV: palpitations, tachycardia, syncope.
EENT: dilated pupils, blurred vision, difficulty swallowing, increased intraocular pressure.
GI: constipation, *dry mouth,* nausea, vomiting, epigastric distress.
GU: urinary hesitancy, urine retention.
Hematologic: ***aplastic anemia.***
Skin: urticaria, pruritus.
Other: ***anaphylaxis.***

Overdose and treatment

Signs and symptoms of overdose include dry mouth, blurred vision, urine retention, tachycardia, confusion, paralytic ileus, deep coma, seizures, shock, respiratory arrest, arrhythmias, and death.

Treatment includes symptomatic and supportive measures. If ingestion is recent, induce emesis or gastric lavage followed by activated charcoal. Monitor vital signs and fluid and electrolyte balance.

Clinical considerations

- When giving drug I.V., inject slowly over 5 minutes. Keep patient supine during and 5 to 10 minutes after injection. Paradoxical initial bradycardia may occur when giving I.V.; usually disappears in 2 minutes.
- Some commercially available orphenadrine citrate injection formulations may contain sodium bisulfite, a sulfite that can cause allergic-type reactions, including anaphylaxis.

Therapeutic monitoring

- Monitor periodic blood, urine, and liver function tests during prolonged therapy.
- Recommend monitoring vital signs, especially intake and output, noting urine retention

Special populations

Pediatric patients. Safety and efficacy in children under age 12 haven't been established.
Geriatric patients. Geriatric patients may be more sensitive to effects of drug.

Patient counseling

- Suggest ice chips, sugarless gum, hard candy, or saliva substitutes to relieve dry mouth.
- Tell patient to avoid hazardous activities that require alertness or physical coordination until CNS depressant effects can be determined.
- Warn patient to avoid alcoholic beverages and to use cough and cold preparations cautiously, because some contain alcohol.
- Tell patient to store drug away from heat and light (not in bathroom medicine cabinet) and safely out of reach of children.
- Instruct patient to take missed dose if remembered within 1 hour. If beyond 1 hour, patient should skip that dose and return to regular schedule. He shouldn't double the dose.

oseltamivir phosphate

Tamiflu

Pharmacologic classification: influenza virus neuraminidase inhibitor
Therapeutic classification: antiviral
Pregnancy risk category: C

How supplied

Available by prescription only.
Capsules: 75 mg

Indications and dosages

Treatment of uncomplicated, acute influenza A and B infection in adults symptomatic for 2 days or less.

Adults: 75 mg P.O. twice daily for 5 days, beginning within 2 days of symptom onset.

≡ ***Dosage adjustment.*** For patients with renal impairment (creatinine clearance less than 30 ml/min), 75 mg P.O. once daily for 5 days, beginning within 2 days of symptom onset.

Pharmacodynamics

Antiviral action: Oseltamivir is hydrolyzed in the liver to its active form, oseltamivir carboxylase. Oseltamivir carboxylase inhibits the enzyme neuraminidase within the influenza virus particles. This action is thought to inhibit viral replication, possibly by interfering with viral particle aggregation and release from the host cell.

Pharmacokinetics

Absorption: Well absorbed after oral administration. More than 75% of the administered dose reaches the systemic circulation as oseltamivir carboxylase. Peak level of oseltamivir is 65.2 ng/ml whereas that of oseltamivir carboxylase is 348 ng/ml.

Distribution: Serum protein binding is low for both oseltamivir (42%) and oseltamivir carboxylase (3%). Volume of distribution of oseltamivir carboxylase is 23 to 26 L.

Metabolism: Oseltamivir is extensively metabolized by hepatic esterases to its active component, oseltamivir carboxylase. Oseltamivir is neither a substrate nor an inhibitor of cytochrome P-450 oxidases.

Excretion: Oseltamivir carboxylase is almost entirely eliminated in the urine by way of glomerular filtration and tubular secretion. Less than 20% of the orally administered dose is eliminated in feces.

Route	Onset	Peak	Duration
P.O.	Unknown	Unknown	Unknown

Contraindications and precautions

Contraindicated in patients with hypersensitivity to any of the components of the formulation. Use cautiously in patients with chronic cardiac disease, chronic respiratory disease, or any acute medical illness requiring hospitalization. The efficacy of oseltamivir hasn't been established in these settings.

Interactions

None reported.

Effects on diagnostic tests

None reported.

Adverse reactions

CNS: dizziness, insomnia, headache, vertigo.

GI: abdominal pain, diarrhea, nausea, vomiting.

Respiratory: bronchitis, cough.

Other: fatigue.

Overdose and treatment

Single doses as high as 1,000 mg have been associated with only nausea and vomiting. The entire 5-day course of therapy provides a total dose of 750 mg.

Clinical considerations

- Oseltamivir doesn't appear to interfere with normal humoral antibody response to influenza infection.
- There's no evidence supporting prophylactic use of oseltamivir.
- Efficacy of oseltamivir against influenza virus type A and B has been demonstrated in clinical trials. There's no evidence supporting the use of oseltamivir in the treatment of other viral infections.
- Administration of oseltamivir with meals may alleviate gastrointestinal side effects.
- Nausea and vomiting are the most frequently occurring side effects.
- Store oseltamivir at controlled room temperature (59° to 86° F [15° to 30° C]).

Therapeutic monitoring

Recommend monitoring patient for adverse GI effects and clinical response of medication.

Special populations

Breast-feeding patients. It's unknown if drug is excreted in breast milk. The potential benefits and potential risks of oseltamivir therapy on the breast-fed infant must be considered.

Pediatric patients. Safety and efficacy in children haven't been established.

Geriatric patients: Dosage reduction isn't required for geriatric patients, unless creatinine clearance is less than 30 ml/min.

Patient counseling

- Advise patient to contact his health care professional as soon as possible to begin treatment within 2 days of onset of flu symptoms.
- Tell patient to complete the full 5 days of treatment, even if he feels better.
- Inform patient that oseltamivir may be taken with or without meals. Side effects of nausea or vomiting may be relieved by taking oseltamivir with food or milk.
- Advise patient that if a dose is missed, it should be taken as soon as possible. The patient should skip the dose, however, if the next dose is due within 2 hours.
- Tell patient that drug isn't a replacement for the influenza virus vaccine. If patient is at risk for influenza, he should continue to receive the vaccine each fall.

oxacillin sodium

Bactocill

Pharmacologic classification: penicillinase-resistant penicillin
Therapeutic classification: antibiotic
Pregnancy risk category B

How supplied

Available by prescription only
Capsules: 250 mg, 500 mg
Oral solution: 250 mg/5 ml (after reconstitution)
Injection: 250 mg, 500 mg, 1 g, 2 g, 4 g
Pharmacy bulk package: 10 g
I.V. infusion: 1 g, 2 g, 4 g

Indications and dosages

***Systemic infections caused by* Staphylococcus aureus**
Adults and children weighing over 88 lb (40 kg): 500 mg P.O. q. 4 to 6 hours for mild to moderate infections. Dose is 1 g P.O. q. 4 to 6 hours when changing from IV to P.O. therapy. Alternatively, 250 to 500 mg I.M. or I.V. q 4 to 6 hours. For more severe infections, 1 g or more I.V. or I.M. q 4 to 6 hours. Serious infections are treated for 1 to 2 weeks.
Children over age 1 month weighing less than 88 lb: 50 to 100 mg/kg P.O. daily, divided into doses given q 4 to 6 hours; 50 to 200 mg/kg I.M. or I.V. daily, divided into doses given q 4 to 6 hours. Doses vary based on severity of infection.
Acute or chronic osteomyelitis caused by susceptible organisms
Adults: 1.5 to 2 g I.V. q 4 hours for 4 to 8 weeks or I.V. dose for 5 to 28 days followed by P.O. dose for 3 to 6 weeks for a total of 6 weeks of therapy.
Treatment of native valve endocarditis caused by methicillin-susceptible staphylococci
Adults: 2 g I.V. q 4 hours for 4 to 6 weeks in combination with gentamicin for the first 3 to 5 days.
Treatment of prosthetic valve endocarditis caused by methicillin-susceptible staphylococci
Adults: 2 g I.V. q 4 hours for 6 weeks or longer in combination with gentamicin and rifampin.
≡***Dosage adjustment.*** In adults with creatinine clearance below 10 ml/minute, 1 g I.M. or I.V. q 4 to 6 hours.

Pharmacodynamics

Antibiotic action: Oxacillin is bactericidal; it adheres to bacterial penicillin-binding proteins, thus inhibiting bacterial cell wall synthesis. Oxacillin resists the effects of penicillinases—enzymes that inactivate penicillin—and is thus active against many strains of penicillinase-producing bacteria; this activity is most important against penicillinase-producing staphylococci; some strains may remain resistant. Oxacillin is also active against a few gram-positive aerobic and anaerobic bacilli but has no significant effect on gram-negative bacilli.

Pharmacokinetics

Absorption: Absorbed rapidly but incompletely from the GI tract; it's stable in an acid environment. Food decreases absorption.
Distribution: Distributed widely. CSF penetration is poor but enhanced by meningeal inflammation. Oxacillin crosses the placenta, and is 89% to 94% protein-bound.
Metabolism: Metabolized partially.
Excretion: Excreted primarily in urine by renal tubular secretion and glomerular filtration; it's also excreted in breast milk and in small amounts in bile. Elimination half-life in adults is ½ to 1 hour, extended to 2 hours in severe renal impairment. Dosage adjustments aren't required in patients with creatinine clearance less than 10 ml/minute.

Route	Onset	Peak	Duration
P.O.	Unknown	½-2 hr	Unknown
I.V.	Immediate	Immediate	Unknown
I.M.	Unknown	½ hr	Unknown

Contraindications and precautions

Contraindicated in patients with hypersensitivity to drug or other penicillins. Use cautiously in patients with other drug allergies (especially to cephalosporins), in neonates, and in infants.

Interactions

Drug-drug. *Aminoglycosides:* Produces synergistic bactericidal effects against *S. aureus.* This is a therapeutic effect.
Probenecid: Blocks renal tubular secretion of penicillins, increasing their serum levels. Use together cautiously.
Drug-food. *Food:* Decreases absorption. Drug should be taken on an empty stomach.
Fruit juice and carbonated beverages: Interfere with absorption. Drug should be taken with water.

Effects on diagnostic tests

Oxacillin alters tests for urinary and serum proteins; turbidimetric urine and serum proteins are often falsely positive or elevated in tests using sulfosalicylic acid or trichloroacetic acid.

Oxacillin may falsely decrease serum aminoglycoside levels.

Adverse reactions

CNS: neuropathy, neuromuscular irritability, ***seizures,*** lethargy, hallucinations, anxiety, confusion, agitation, depression, dizziness, fatigue.
GI: oral lesions, nausea, vomiting, diarrhea, enterocolitis, ***pseudomembranous colitis.***

GU: interstitial nephritis, nephropathy.
Hematologic: ***thrombocytopenia,*** eosinophilia, ***hemolytic anemia, neutropenia,*** anemia, ***agranulocytosis.***
Hepatic: elevated liver enzymes.
Other: hypersensitivity reactions (fever, chills, rash, urticaria, ***anaphylaxis,*** overgrowth of nonsusceptible organisms, *thrombophlebitis*).

Overdose and treatment

Signs of overdose include neuromuscular sensitivity or seizures. There are no specific recommendations. Treatment is supportive. After recent ingestion (within 4 hours), empty the stomach by induced emesis or gastric lavage; follow with activated charcoal to reduce absorption. Oxacillin isn't appreciably removed by peritoneal dialysis or hemodialysis.

Clinical considerations

Consider the recommendations relevant to all penicillins as well as the following:

- Coagulase-negative staphylococci causing prosthetic valve endocarditis is methicillin-resistant.
- When given for group A beta-hemolytic streptococci, continue therapy for at least 10 days to decrease risk of glomerulonephritis and rheumatic fever.
- Give oral drug with water only; acid in fruit juice or carbonated beverage may inactivate drug.
- Give oral dose on empty stomach; food decreases absorption.
- Except in osteomyelitis, don't give I.M. or I.V. unless patient can't take oral dose.
- For oral preparation, add amount of water specified on bottle to provide a solution of 250 mg/5 ml. Add water in 2 parts and shake vigorously.
- For I.M. preparation, add 1.4, 2.8, 5.7, 11.4, or 21.8 ml of sterile water for injection or 0.45% sodium chloride or normal saline injection to vial containing 250 mg, 500 mg, 1 g, 2 g, or 4 g, respectively. Final solution concentration is 250 mg/1.5 ml.
- For intermittent I.V. injection, use sterile water for injection or normal saline injection; add 5 ml to 250-mg vial to equal 50 mg/ml. Add 5 ml, 10 ml, 20 ml, or 40 ml to vials containing 500 mg, 1 g, 2 g, or 4 g, respectively, and 93 ml to 10-g pharmacy bulk package to produce a concentration of 100 mg/ml. Inject slowly over 10 minutes. For continuous I.V. infusion, further dilute with compatible solution to 0.5 to 40 mg/ml concentration. Infuse over 30 to 60 minutes. Drug loses 10% of potency within 6 hours of dilution.
- Thaw commercial solutions of drug at room temperature or in refrigerator.
- Oxacillin is incompatible with aminoglycosides in the same I.V. infusion.

Therapeutic monitoring

Monitor renal and hepatic function and hematologic function; watch for elevated AST and ALT and report significant changes.

Special populations

Breast-feeding patients. Oxacillin is excreted into breast milk. Use drug with caution in breast-feeding women.
Pediatric patients. Elimination of oxacillin is reduced in neonates. Transient hematuria, azotemia, and albuminuria have occurred in some neonates receiving oxacillin. Monitor renal function closely.
Geriatric patients. Half-life of drug may be prolonged in geriatric patients because of impaired renal function. Geriatric patients are at increased risk for thrombophlebitis during I.V. infusion.

Patient counseling

- Explain need to take oral preparations without food and to follow with water only, not fruit juice or carbonated beverages.
- Tell patient to report allergic reactions or severe diarrhea promptly.
- Emphasize importance of completing the full course of therapy.

oxaprozin

Daypro

Pharmacologic classification: NSAID
Therapeutic classification: nonnarcotic analgesic, antipyretic, anti-inflammatory
Pregnancy risk category C

How supplied

Available by prescription only
Caplets: 600 mg

Indications and dosages

Management of acute or chronic osteoarthritis or rheumatoid arthritis
Adults: Initially, 1,200 mg P.O. daily. Individualize to smallest effective dosage to minimize adverse reactions. Smaller patients or those with mild symptoms may require only 600 mg daily. Maximum daily dose is 1,800 mg or 26 mg/kg, whichever is lower, in divided doses.
≡ ***Dosage adjustment.*** For patients with renal impairment or on hemodialysis, initial dose is 600 mg P.O. daily.

Pharmacodynamics

Analgesic, antipyretic, and anti-inflammatory actions: Exact mechanism of action isn't clearly defined. It inhibits several steps along the arachidonic acid pathway of prostaglandin synthesis. One of the modes of action is presumed to be a result of the inhibition of cyclooxygenase activity and prostaglandin synthesis at the site of inflammation.

Pharmacokinetics

Absorption: Demonstrates high oral bioavailability (95%). Food may reduce the rate of absorption, but extent of absorption is unchanged.
Distribution: About 99.9% bound to albumin in plasma.
Metabolism: Primarily metabolized in the liver by microsomal oxidation (65%) and glucuronic acid conjugation (35%).
Excretion: Glucuronide metabolites are excreted in urine (65%) and feces (35%). Elimination half-life in adults is 42 to 50 hours.

Route	Onset	Peak	Duration
P.O.	Unknown	3-5 hr	Unknown

Contraindications and precautions

Contraindicated in patients with hypersensitivity to drug or with the syndrome of nasal polyps, angioedema, and bronchospastic reaction to aspirin or other NSAIDs.

Use cautiously in patients with renal or hepatic dysfunction, history of peptic ulcer, hypertension, CV disease, or conditions predisposing to fluid retention.

Interactions

Drug-drug. *Oral anticoagulants:* May increase the risk of bleeding. Monitor PT and INR.
Aspirin: Oxaprozin displaces salicylates from plasma protein binding, increasing the risk of salicylate toxicity. Avoid use together.
Beta blockers such as metoprolol: May cause a transient increase in blood pressure after 14 days of therapy. Recommend monitoring blood pressure.
Drug-lifestyle. *Sun exposure:* May cause photosensitivity reactions. Advise patient to take precautions.

Effects on diagnostic tests

None reported.

Adverse reactions

CNS: depression, sedation, somnolence, confusion, sleep disturbances.
EENT: tinnitus, blurred vision.
GI: *nausea, dyspepsia, diarrhea, constipation,* abdominal pain or distress, anorexia, flatulence, vomiting, ***hemorrhage,*** stomatitis, ulcer.
GU: dysuria, urinary frequency.
Hematologic: prolonged bleeding time.
Hepatic: elevated liver function test results (with chronic use), ***severe hepatic dysfunction*** (rare).
Skin: *rash,* photosensitivity.

Overdose and treatment

No information specific to oxaprozin overdose is available. Common symptoms of acute overdose with other NSAIDs, including lethargy, drowsiness, nausea, vomiting, and epigastric pain, are generally reversible with supportive care. GI bleeding and coma have occurred after NSAID overdose. Hypertension, acute renal failure, and respiratory depression are rare. Gut decontamination may be indicated in symptomatic patients seen within 4 hours of ingestion or after a large overdose (5 to 10 times the usual dose). This is accomplished by emesis or activated charcoal with an osmotic cathartic.

Clinical considerations

- Serious GI toxicity, including peptic ulceration and bleeding, can occur in patients taking NSAIDs despite the absence of GI symptoms. Patients at risk for development of peptic ulceration and bleeding are those with history of serious GI events, alcoholism, smoking, or other factors associated with peptic ulcer disease.
- Dosages exceeding 1,200 mg/day should be used for patients who weigh more than 110 lb (50 kg), who have normal renal and hepatic function, who are at low risk of peptic ulceration, and whose severity of disease justifies maximal therapy.
- Most patients tolerate once-daily dosing. Divided doses may be tried in patients unable to tolerate single doses.

Therapeutic monitoring

- Elevations of liver function tests can occur after chronic use. These abnormal findings may persist, worsen, or resolve with continued therapy. Rarely, patients may progress to severe hepatic dysfunction. Periodically monitor liver function tests in patients receiving long-term therapy, and closely monitor patients with abnormal test results.
- Anemia may occur in patients receiving oxaprozin. Monitor hemoglobin level or hematocrit in patients with prolonged therapy at intervals appropriate for their clinical situation.

Special populations

Breast-feeding patients. Studies of oxaprozin excretion in breast milk haven't been conducted. Use cautiously in breast-feeding women.
Pediatric patients. Safety and efficacy in children haven't been established.
Geriatric patients. Geriatric patients may need a reduced dose because of low body weight or disorders associated with aging. Geriatric patients are less likely than younger patients to tolerate adverse reactions associated with oxaprozin.

Patient counseling

- Warn patient to immediately report signs and symptoms of GI bleeding or visual or auditory adverse reactions.
- Tell patient to take drug with milk or meals if adverse GI reactions occur.

■ Because photosensitivity reactions may occur, advise patient to use a sunblock, wear protective clothing, and avoid prolonged exposure to sunlight.

oxazepam

Apo-Oxazepam*, Novoxapam*, Ox-pam*, Serax

Pharmacologic classification: benzodiazepine
Therapeutic classification: antianxiety agent, sedative-hypnotic
Controlled substance schedule IV
Pregnancy risk category D

How supplied

Available by prescription only
Tablets: 15 mg
Capsules: 10 mg, 15 mg, 30 mg

Indications and dosages

Alcohol withdrawal, severe anxiety
Adults: 15 to 30 mg P.O. t.i.d. or q.i.d.
Tension, mild to moderate anxiety
Adults: 10 to 15 mg P.O. t.i.d. or q.i.d.
≡ ***Dosage adjustment.*** In older adults, give 10 mg P.O. t.i.d.; then increase to 15 mg t.i.d. or q.i.d., p.r.n.

Pharmacodynamics

Anxiolytic and sedative-hypnotic actions: Oxazepam depresses the CNS at the limbic and subcortical levels of the brain. It produces an antianxiety effect by enhancing the effect of the neurotransmitter gamma-aminobutyric acid on its receptor in the ascending reticular activating system, which increases inhibition and blocks both cortical and limbic arousal.

Pharmacokinetics

Absorption: When administered orally, oxazepam is well absorbed through the GI tract.
Distribution: Distributed widely throughout the body, and is 85% to 95% protein-bound.
Metabolism: Metabolized in the liver to inactive metabolites.
Excretion: Metabolites are excreted in urine as glucuronide conjugates. Half-life of drug is 5¾ to 11 hours.

Route	Onset	Peak	Duration
P.O.	Unknown	3 hr	Unknown

Contraindications and precautions

Contraindicated in patients with psychosis or hypersensitivity to drug. Use cautiously in geriatric or debilitated patients; in those with history of drug abuse; and in those in whom a decrease in blood pressure is associated with cardiac problems.

Interactions

Drug-drug. *General anesthetics, antidepressants, antihistamines, barbiturates, MAO inhibitors, narcotics, and phenothiazines:* Potentiate the CNS depressant effects of these drugs. Avoid use together, if possible.
Antacids: May decrease rate of oxazepam absorption. Separate administration times of these drugs.
Cimetidine and possibly disulfiram: Diminished hepatic metabolism of oxazepam, which increases its plasma level. Monitor patient carefully.
Levodopa: Inhibited therapeutic effects of levodopa. Monitor patient closely.
Drug-lifestyle. *Heavy smoking:* Accelerates oxazepam metabolism, lowering clinical effectiveness. Avoid use together.
Alcohol use: Potentiated CNS depressant effects. Avoid use together.

Effects on diagnostic tests

None reported.

Adverse reactions

CNS: *drowsiness, lethargy,* dizziness, vertigo, headache, syncope, tremor, slurred speech, changes in EEG patterns.
CV: edema.
GI: nausea.
GU: altered libido.
Hematologic: ***leukopenia*** (rare).
Hepatic: ***hepatic dysfunction.***
Skin: rash.

Overdose and treatment

Signs and symptoms of overdose include somnolence, confusion, coma, hypoactive reflexes, dyspnea, labored breathing, hypotension, bradycardia, slurred speech, and unsteady gait or impaired coordination.

Support blood pressure and respiration until the effects of the drug have subsided; monitor vital signs. Mechanical ventilatory assistance via endotracheal tube may be required to maintain a patent airway and support adequate oxygenation. Flumazenil, a specific benzodiazepine antagonist, may be useful. As needed, use I.V. fluids and vasopressors, such as dopamine and phenylephrine, to treat hypotension. If the patient is conscious, induce emesis. Use gastric lavage if ingestion was recent, but only if an endotracheal tube is present to prevent aspiration. After emesis or lavage, administer activated charcoal with a cathartic as a single dose. Dialysis is of limited value.

Clinical considerations

Consider the recommendations relevant to all benzodiazepines as well as the following:
■ Oxazepam tablets contain tartrazine dye; check patient's history for allergy to this substance.

■ Store drug in a cool, dry place away from light.
■ Use of drug for greater than 4 months hasn't been established.
■ Gradually reduce dosage (over 8 to 12 weeks) after long-term use.

Therapeutic monitoring
Monitor hepatic and renal function studies to ensure normal function.

Special populations
Breast-feeding patients. The breast-fed infant of a woman who uses oxazepam may become sedated, have feeding difficulties, or lose weight. Avoid use in breast-feeding women.
Pediatric patients. Safety in children under age 6 hasn't been established. Closely observe neonate for withdrawal symptoms if mother took oxazepam for a prolonged period during pregnancy.
Geriatric patients. Geriatric patients are more susceptible to the CNS depressant effects of oxazepam. Some may require supervision with ambulation and activities of daily living during initiation of therapy or after an increase in dose. Lower doses are usually effective in geriatric patients because of decreased elimination.

Patient counseling
■ Advise patient not to change part of drug regimen without medical approval.
■ Instruct patient in safety measures, such as gradual position changes and supervised ambulation, to prevent injury.
■ Because sleepiness may not occur for up to 2 hours after taking oxazepam, tell patient to wait before taking an additional dose.
■ Advise patient of potential for physical and psychological dependence with chronic use of oxazepam.
■ Tell patient not to discontinue drug suddenly if he's been taking it for prolonged periods.

oxybutynin chloride
Ditropan, Ditropan XL

Pharmacologic classification: synthetic tertiary amine
Therapeutic classification: antispasmodic
Pregnancy risk category B

How supplied
Available by prescription only
Tablets: 5 mg
Tablets (extended release): 5 mg, 10 mg, 15 mg
Syrup: 5 mg/5 ml

Indications and dosages
For relief of symptoms of bladder instability associated with voiding in patients with uninhibited and reflex neurogenic bladder
Adults: 5 mg P.O. b.i.d. to t.i.d. to maximum of 5 mg q.i.d.
Children over age 5: 5 mg P.O. b.i.d. to maximum of 5 mg t.i.d.

Pharmacodynamics
Antispasmodic action: Oxybutynin reduces the urge to void, increases bladder capacity, and reduces the frequency of contractions to the detrusor muscle. Drug exerts a direct spasmolytic action and an antimuscarinic action on smooth muscle.

Pharmacokinetics
Absorption: Absorbed rapidly
Distribution: No data available.
Metabolism: Metabolized by the liver.
Excretion: Excreted principally in urine.

Route	Onset	Peak	Duration
P.O.	½-1 hr	3-4 hr	6-10 hr

Contraindications and precautions
Contraindicated in patients with hypersensitivity to drug, myasthenia gravis, GI obstruction, glaucoma, adynamic ileus, megacolon, severe colitis, ulcerative colitis when megacolon is present, or obstructive uropathy; in geriatric or debilitated patients with intestinal atony; and in hemorrhaging patients with unstable CV status.

Use cautiously in the elderly and in patients with impaired renal or hepatic function, autonomic neuropathy, or reflux esophagitis.

Interactions
Drug-drug. *CNS depressants:* Additive sedative effects. Use together cautiously.
Digoxin: May increase digoxin levels. Monitor serum digoxin levels.
Haloperidol: Worsening of schizophrenia, decreased serum levels of haloperidol, and development of tardive dyskinesia may occur with coadministration. Use together cautiously, if at all.
Phenothiazine: Increased incidence of anticholinergic adverse effects. Monitor patient closely.

Effects on diagnostic tests
None reported.

Adverse reactions
CNS: dizziness, insomnia, restlessness, hallucinations, asthenia.
CV: *palpitations, tachycardia,* vasodilation.
EENT: mydriasis, cycloplegia, decreased lacrimation, amblyopia.
GI: nausea, vomiting, *constipation, dry mouth,* decreased GI motility.

GU: *urinary hesitancy, urine retention,* suppressed lactation.
Skin: rash.
Other: decreased diaphoresis, fever.

Overdose and treatment

Signs and symptoms of overdose include restlessness, excitement, psychotic behavior, flushing, hypotension, circulatory failure, and fever. In severe cases, paralysis, respiratory failure, and coma may occur. Treatment requires gastric lavage. Activated charcoal may be administered as well as a cathartic. Physostigmine may be considered to reverse symptoms of anticholinergic intoxication. Treat hyperpyrexia symptomatically with ice bags or other cold applications and alcohol sponges. Maintain artificial respiration if paralysis of respiratory muscles occurs.

Clinical considerations

- Discontinue drug periodically to determine whether patient still requires medication.
- Store drug in tight, light-resistant container at 59° to 86° F (15° to 30° C); drug expires 4 years from date of manufacture.

Therapeutic monitoring

Recommend monitoring patient with hepatic and renal disease carefully.

Special populations

Breast-feeding patients. It isn't known if drug is excreted in breast milk. Use caution when administering to breast-feeding women.
Pediatric patients. Dosage guidelines haven't been established for children under age 5.
Geriatric patients. Geriatric patients may be more sensitive to the antimuscarinic effects. Drug is contraindicated in geriatric and debilitated patients with intestinal atony.

Patient counseling

- Instruct patient regarding medication and dosage schedule; tell him to take a missed dose as soon as possible and not to double the doses.
- Tell patient not to crush or chew extended-release tablets. They may be administered without regard to food. Extended-release tablets don't disintegrate and are eliminated in feces.
- Warn patient about possibility of decreased mental alertness or visual changes.
- Remind patient to use drug cautiously when in warm climates to minimize risk of heatstroke that may occur because of decreased sweating.

oxycodone hydrochloride

OxyContin, OxyFAST, Oxy IR, Roxicodone, Supeudol*

Pharmacologic classification: opioid
Therapeutic classification: analgesic
Controlled substance schedule II
Pregnancy risk category C

How supplied

Available by prescription only
Tablets: 5 mg
Tablets (sustained-release): 10 mg, 20 mg, 40 mg, 80 mg
Capsules: 5 mg
Oral solution: 5 mg/ml, 20 mg/ml

Indications and dosages

Moderate to severe pain
Adults: 5 mg P.O. q 6 hours
Chronic pain
Adults: Initially, 10-mg sustained-release tablet P.O. q 12 hours; may increase dose q 1 to 2 days. Dosing frequency shouldn't be increased.

Pharmacodynamics

Analgesic action: Oxycodone acts on opiate receptors, providing analgesia for moderate to moderately severe pain. Episodes of acute pain, rather than chronic pain, appear to be more responsive to treatment with oxycodone.

Pharmacokinetics

Absorption: After oral administration.
Distribution: Rapidly distributed.
Metabolism: Metabolized in the liver.
Excretion: Excreted principally by the kidneys.

Route	Onset	Peak	Duration
P.O.	10-15 min	1 hr	3-12 hr

Contraindications and precautions

Contraindicated in patients with hypersensitivity to drug. Use cautiously in geriatric or debilitated patients and in those with head injury, increased intracranial pressure, seizures, asthma, COPD, prostatic hyperplasia, severe hepatic or renal disease, acute abdominal conditions, urethral stricture, hypothyroidism, Addison's disease, or arrhythmias.

Interactions

Drug-drug. *General anesthetics:* Severe CV depression. Use together with extreme caution.
Anticholinergics: May cause paralytic ileus. Use together cautiously.
Anticoagulants: Oxycodone products containing aspirin may increase effects of anticoagulant. Monitor clotting times, and use together cautiously.
Other CNS depressants, such as general anesthetics, antihistamines, barbiturates, benzodiazepines, muscle relaxants, narcotic analgesics,

phenothiazines, sedative-hypnotics, and tricyclic antidepressants: Potentiate respiratory and CNS depression, sedation, and hypotensive effects of drug. Use together with extreme caution.
Cimetidine: May increase respiratory and CNS depression, causing confusion, disorientation, apnea, or seizures. Avoid use together.
Digitoxin, phenytoin, rifampin: Drug accumulation and enhanced effects may result from use with other drugs that are extensively metabolized in the liver. Monitor patient closely.
Opioid agonist-antagonist or a single dose of an antagonist: Patients who become physically dependent on oxycodone may experience acute withdrawal syndrome. Avoid use together in this situation.
Drug-lifestyle. *Alcohol use:* Potentiates respiratory and CNS depression, sedation, and hypotensive effects of drug. Advise patient to avoid combined use.

Effects on diagnostic tests
None reported.

Adverse reactions
CNS: *sedation, somnolence, clouded sensorium, euphoria, dizziness, light-headedness,* ***seizures.***
CV: *hypotension,* ***bradycardia.***
GI: *nausea, vomiting, constipation,* ileus, increased plasma amylase and lipase and liver enzyme levels.
GU: *urine retention.*
Hepatic: increased liver enzyme levels.
Respiratory: ***respiratory depression.***
Skin: *diaphoresis,* pruritus, rash.
Other: physical dependence.

Overdose and treatment
The most common signs and symptoms of a severe overdose are CNS depression, respiratory depression, and miosis, or pinpoint pupils. Other acute toxic effects include hypotension, bradycardia, hypothermia, shock, apnea, cardiopulmonary arrest, circulatory collapse, pulmonary edema, and convulsions.

To treat acute overdose, first establish adequate respiratory exchange via a patent airway and ventilation as needed; administer a narcotic antagonist (naloxone) to reverse respiratory depression. Because the duration of action of oxycodone is longer than that of naloxone, repeated naloxone dosing is necessary. Naloxone shouldn't be given unless patient has clinically significant respiratory or CV depression. Monitor vital signs closely.

If patient presents within 2 hours of ingestion of an oral overdose, empty the stomach immediately by inducing emesis (ipecac syrup) or using gastric lavage. Use caution to avoid any risk of aspiration. Administer activated charcoal via nasogastric tube for further removal of the drug in an oral overdose.

Provide symptomatic and supportive treatment, including continued respiratory support and correction of fluid or electrolyte imbalance. Monitor laboratory values, vital signs, and neurologic status closely.

Dialysis may be helpful if combination products with aspirin or acetaminophen are involved.

Clinical considerations
Consider the recommendations relevant to all opioids as well as the following:
- Some commercial preparations contain sodium metabisulfite, which may cause an allergic reaction in susceptible individuals.
- Single-agent oxycodone solution or tablets are ideal for patients who can't take aspirin or acetaminophen.
- The extended-release preparation isn't intended for preoperative or immediate postoperative pain in patients not already taking the drug.
- Oxycodone has high abuse potential.
- Drug may obscure signs and symptoms of an acute abdominal condition or worsen gallbladder pain.
- Consider prescribing a stool softener for patients on long-term therapy.
- The 80 mg sustained-release tablets are for opioid-tolerant patients only.
- Patients being transferred from 5 to 25 mg daily conventional dose should receive 10 to 20 mg q 12 hours of the extended-release preparation. If conventional dose is 30 to 45 mg or 50 to 60 mg daily, the extended-release dose is 20 to 30 mg q 12 hours or 30 to 40 mg q 12 hours, respectively.
- The extended-release preparation isn't intended for preoperative or immediate postoperative pain in patients not already taking the drug.

Therapeutic monitoring
Recommend monitoring patient for relief of pain and development of tolerance to drug's effects.

Special populations
Breast-feeding patients. It's unknown if drug is excreted in breast milk. Use with caution in breast-feeding women.
Pediatric patients. Dosage may be individualized for children; however, safety and effectiveness in children haven't been established.
Geriatric patients. Lower doses are usually indicated for geriatric patients, who may be more sensitive to the therapeutic and adverse effects of drug.

Patient counseling
- For full analgesic effect, teach patient to take drug before onset of intense pain.
- Warn patient about possibility of decreased alertness or visual changes.

oxymetazoline hydrochloride

Afrin, Allerest 12 Hour Nasal Spray, Chlorphed-LA, Dristan Long Lasting, Duramist Plus, Duration, 4-Way Long Lasting Spray, Neo-Synephrine 12 Hour Nasal Spray, Nostrilla Long Acting Nasal Decongestant, NTZ Long Acting Decongestant Nasal Spray, OcuClear, Sinarest 12 Hour Nasal Spray, Sinex Long-Acting, Visine L.R.

Pharmacologic classification: sympathomimetic
Therapeutic classification: decongestant, vasoconstrictor
Pregnancy risk category C

How supplied

Available without a prescription
Nasal solution: 0.025% (drops) for children
Nasal drops or spray: 0.05%
Ophthalmic solution: 0.025%

Indications and dosages

Nasal congestion
Adults and children over age 6: Apply 2 to 3 drops or sprays of 0.05% solution in each nostril q 10 to 12 hours. Use no more than 3 to 5 days. Dosage for younger children hasn't been established.
Relief of minor eye redness
Adults and children over age 6: Apply 1 to 2 drops in the conjunctival sac up to q.i.d. (space at least 6 hours apart).

Pharmacodynamics

Decongestant action: Oxymetazoline produces local vasoconstriction of arterioles through alpha receptors to reduce blood flow and nasal congestion.

Pharmacokinetics

Absorption: Occasional systemic absorption may occur.
Distribution: Unknown.
Metabolism: Unknown.
Excretion: Unknown.

Route	Onset	Peak	Duration
Ophthalmic	5 min	Unknown	6 hr
Nasal	5-10 min	6 hr	< 12 hr

Contraindications and precautions

Contraindicated in patients with hypersensitivity to drug. Ophthalmic form contraindicated in patients with angle-closure glaucoma.

Use cautiously in patients with hyperthyroidism, cardiac disease, or hypertension and in those receiving MAO inhibitors. Use nasal solution cautiously in patients with diabetes mellitus. Use ophthalmic form cautiously in those with eye disease, infection, or injury.

Interactions

Drug-drug. *Local anesthetics:* Can increase absorption of ophthalmic form. Monitor patient closely.
Beta blockers: Can increase systemic adverse effects. Monitor patient carefully.
Tricyclic antidepressants: May potentiate the pressor effects from significant systemic absorption of the decongestant. Monitor patient carefully.

Effects on diagnostic tests

None reported.

Adverse reactions

CNS: headache, insomnia; drowsiness, dizziness, possible sedation (with nasal form); lightheadedness, nervousness (with ophthalmic form).
CV: palpitations; ***CV collapse,*** hypertension (with nasal form); tachycardia, ***bradycardia,*** irregular heartbeat (with ophthalmic form).
EENT: rebound nasal congestion or irritation with excessive or long-term use, dryness of nose and throat, increased nasal discharge, stinging, sneezing (with nasal form); *transient stinging upon instillation,* blurred vision, reactive hyperemia, keratitis, lacrimation, increased intraocular pressure (with ophthalmic form).
Other: systemic effects in children (with excessive or long-term use, with nasal form); trembling (with ophthalmic form).

Overdose and treatment

Signs and symptoms of overdose include somnolence, sedation, sweating, CNS depression with hypertension, bradycardia, decreased cardiac output, rebound hypertension, CV collapse, depressed respirations, and coma.

If ingested, emesis isn't recommended, unless given early, because of rapid onset of sedation. Activated charcoal or gastric lavage may be used initially. Monitor vital signs and ECG. Treat seizures with I.V. diazepam.

Clinical considerations

Excessive dosing may irritate nasal mucosa and cause rebound congestion (nasal) or rebound hyperemia (ophthalmic).

Therapeutic monitoring

Monitor for adverse reactions in patients with CV disease, diabetes mellitus, or prostatic hypertrophy because systemic absorption can occur.

Special populations

Pediatric patients. Children may exhibit increased adverse effects from systemic absorption; 0.05% nasal solution is contraindicated in children under age 6; 0.025% nasal solution

should be used in children under age 2 only under medical direction and supervision.
Geriatric patients. Use drug with caution in geriatric patients with cardiac disease, poorly controlled hypertension, or diabetes mellitus.

Patient counseling

- Emphasize that only one person should use dropper bottle or nasal spray.
- Advise patient not to exceed recommended dosage and to use drug only when needed.
- Tell patient to discontinue drug and report symptoms that persist after 3 days of self-medication.
- Tell patient that nasal mucosa may sting, burn, or become dry.
- Warn patient that excessive use may cause bradycardia, hypotension, dizziness, and weakness.
- Show patient how to apply drug. Have him bend head forward and sniff spray briskly or apply light pressure on lacrimal sac after instillation of eyedrop.

oxymorphone hydrochloride

Numorphan

Pharmacologic classification: opioid
Therapeutic classification: analgesic
Controlled substance schedule II
Pregnancy risk category C

How supplied

Available by prescription only
Injection: 1 mg/ml, 1.5 mg/ml
Suppository: 5 mg

Indications and dosages

Moderate to severe pain
Adults: 1 to 1.5 mg I.M. or S.C. q 4 to 6 hours, p.r.n., or around the clock; 0.5 mg I.V. q 4 to 6 hours, p.r.n., or around the clock; or 1 suppository administered P.R. q 4 to 6 hours, p.r.n., or around the clock.

Note: Parenteral administration of drug is also indicated for preoperative medication, for support of anesthesia, for obstetric analgesia, and for relief of anxiety in dyspnea associated with acute left-sided heart failure and pulmonary edema.

Pharmacodynamics

Analgesic action: Oxymorphone effectively relieves moderate to severe pain by way of agonist activity at the opiate receptors. It has little or no antitussive effect.

Pharmacokinetics

Absorption: Well absorbed after P.R., S.C., I.M., or I.V. administration.
Distribution: Widely distributed.
Metabolism: Primarily metabolized in the liver.
Excretion: Excreted primarily in the urine as oxymorphone conjugates.

Route	Onset	Peak	Duration
I.V.	5-10 min	15-30 min	3-4 hr
I.M.	10-15 min	½-1½ hr	3-6 hr
S.C.	10-20 min	1-1½ hr	3-6 hr
P.R.	15-30 min	2 hr	3-6 hr

Contraindications and precautions

Contraindicated in patients with hypersensitivity to drug. Use cautiously in geriatric or debilitated patients and in those with head injury, increased intracranial pressure, seizures, asthma, COPD, acute abdomen conditions, prostatic hyperplasia, severe renal or kidney disease, urethral stricture, respiratory depression, Addison's disease, arrhythmias, or hypothyroidism.

Interactions

Drug-drug. *General anesthetics:* Severe CV depression. Use together with extreme caution.
Anticholinergics: May cause paralytic ileus. Use together cautiously.
Cimetidine: May increase respiratory and CNS depression, causing confusion, disorientation, apnea, or seizures. Avoid use together.
CNS depressants, such as general anesthetics, antihistamines, barbiturates, benzodiazepines, muscle relaxants, opiates, phenothiazines, sedative-hypnotics, and tricyclic antidepressants: Potentiate respiratory and CNS depression, sedation, and hypotensive effects of drug. Use together with extreme caution.
Digitoxin, phenytoin, rifampin: Drug accumulation and enhanced effects may result from use with other drugs that are extensively metabolized in the liver. Monitor patient closely.
Opioid agonist-antagonist or a single dose of an antagonist: Patients who become physically dependent on oxycodone may experience acute withdrawal syndrome. Avoid use together in this situation.
Drug-lifestyle. *Alcohol use:* Potentiates respiratory and CNS depression, sedation, and hypotensive effects of drug. Advise patient to avoid combined use.

Effects on diagnostic tests

None reported.

Adverse reactions

CNS: *sedation, somnolence, clouded sensorium, euphoria,* dizziness, ***seizures*** (with large doses), light-headedness, headache.
CV: *hypotension,* ***bradycardia.***
GI: *nausea, vomiting, constipation,* ileus, increased plasma amylase levels.
GU: *urine retention.*
Respiratory: ***respiratory depression.***
Skin: pruritus.
Other: physical dependence.

Overdose and treatment

The most common signs and symptoms of oxymorphone overdose are CNS depression, including extreme somnolence progressing to stupor and coma; respiratory depression; and miosis, or pinpoint pupils. Other acute toxic effects include hypotension, bradycardia, hypothermia, shock, apnea, cardiopulmonary arrest, circulatory collapse, pulmonary edema, and seizures.

To treat acute overdose, first establish adequate respiratory exchange via a patent airway and ventilation, as needed; administer a narcotic antagonist (naloxone) to reverse respiratory depression. Because duration of action of drug is longer than that of naloxone, repeated naloxone dosing is necessary. Naloxone shouldn't be given unless patient has clinically significant respiratory or CV depression. Monitor vital signs closely.

Provide symptomatic and supportive treatment, including continued respiratory support and correction of fluid or electrolyte imbalance. Monitor laboratory values vital signs, and neurologic status closely.

Clinical considerations

Consider the recommendations relevant to all opioids as well as the following:

- An opiate antagonist and oxygen should be available after I.V. administration.
- Refrigerate oxymorphone suppositories.
- Drug is well absorbed P.R. and is an alternative to opioids with more limited dosage forms.
- Drug may worsen gallbladder pain.

Therapeutic monitoring

Recommend monitoring vital signs and respiratory status.

Special populations

Breast-feeding patients. It isn't known if drug is excreted in breast milk. Use with caution in breast-feeding women.
Pediatric patients. Don't use in children under age 12.
Geriatric patients. Lower doses are usually indicated for geriatric patients, who may be more sensitive to the therapeutic and adverse effects of drug.

Patient counseling

- Tell patient to ask for drug before pain is intense.
- Caution ambulatory patient about getting out of bed and walking. Patient should avoid driving or other potentially hazardous activities until CNS effects are known.
- Instruct patient to store suppositiories in the refrigerator.
- Advise patient to avoid alcohol.

oxytocin

Pitocin

Pharmacologic classification: exogenous hormone
Therapeutic classification: oxytocic, lactation stimulant
Pregnancy risk category C

How supplied

Available by prescription only
Injection: 10-units/ml ampules, vials, and closed injection system

Indications and dosages

Induction of labor
Adults: Initially, no more than 0.5 to 1 milliunits/minute I.V. infusion. Rate of infusion may be increased slowly (1 to 2 milliunits/minute at 30 to 60 minute intervals until a response is observed). Decrease rate when labor is firmly established.
Augmentation of labor
Adults: Initially, 2 milliunits/minute I.V. infusion. Rate of infusion may be increased slowly to maximum of 20 milliunits/minute.
Reduction of postpartum bleeding after expulsion of placenta
Adults: 20 to 40 milliunits/minute I.V. infusion to total of 10 units (or 10 units I.M.) after delivery of the placenta.
To induce abortion
Adults: 10 units mixed in 500 ml D_5W or normal saline solution I.V. at 10 to 100 milliunits/minute (not to exceed 30 units in 12 hours)
◇ ***Oxytocin challenge test to assess fetal distress in high-risk pregnancies greater than 31 weeks' gestation***
Adults: Prepare solution by adding 5 to 10 units oxytocin to 1 L of 5% dextrose injection, yielding a solution of 5 to 10 milliunits per ml. Infuse 0.5 milliunits/minute, gradually increasing at 15-minute intervals to maximum infusion of 20 milliunits/minute. Discontinue infusion when three moderate uterine contractions occur in a 10-minute interval. Response of fetal heart rate to test may be used to evaluate prognosis.

Pharmacodynamics

Oxytocic action: Oxytocin increases the sodium permeability of uterine myofibrils, indirectly stimulating the contraction of uterine smooth muscle. The threshold for response is lowered in the presence of high estrogen levels. Uterine response increases with the length of the pregnancy and increases further during active labor. Response mimics labor contractions.

Pharmacokinetics

Absorption: Destroyed in the GI tract.

Distribution: Distributed throughout the extracellular fluid; small amounts may enter the fetal circulation.
Metabolism: Metabolized rapidly in the kidneys and liver. In early pregnancy, a circulating enzyme, oxytocinase, can inactivate the drug.
Excretion: Only small amounts are excreted in the urine as oxytocin. Half-life is 3 to 5 minutes.

Route	Onset	Peak	Duration
I.V.	Immediate	Unknown	1 hr
I.M.	3-5 min	Unknown	2-3 hr

Contraindications and precautions
Contraindicated when cephalopelvic disproportion is present or when delivery requires conversion, as in transverse lie; in fetal distress when delivery isn't imminent; prematurity and other obstetric emergencies; and in patients with severe toxemia, hypertonic uterine patterns, hypersensitivity to drug, total placenta previa, and vasoprevia.

Use cautiously during first and second stages of labor and in patients with history of cervical or uterine surgery (including cesarean section), grand multiparity, uterine sepsis, traumatic delivery, overdistended uterus, and invasive cervical cancer.

Interactions
Drug-drug. *Cyclopropane anesthesia:* May modify CV effects of oxytocin. Use together cautiously.
Thiopental anesthesia: Delays the induction of anesthesia. Use together cautiously.
Sympathomimetics: May increase pressor effects, possibly resulting in postpartum hypertension. Avoid use together.

Effects on diagnostic tests
None reported.

Adverse reactions
Maternal
CNS: ***subarachnoid hemorrhage*** (from hypertension), ***seizures or coma*** (from water intoxication).
CV: *hypertension,* increased heart rate, systemic venous return, and cardiac output, ***arrhythmias.***
GI: nausea, vomiting.
GU: tetanic uterine contractions, ***abruptio placentae, impaired uterine blood flow,*** pelvic hematoma, ***increased uterine motility, uterine rupture, postpartum hemorrhage.***
Hematologic: ***afibrinogenemia*** (may be related to postpartum bleeding).
Other: hypersensitivity reactions ***(anaphylaxis), water retention.***
Fetal
CNS: ***infant brain damage.***
EENT: retinal hemorrhage.
CV: ***bradycardia, premature ventricular contractions, arrhythmias.***
Hepatic: ***jaundice.***
Respiratory: ***anoxia, asphyxia.***
Other: ***death, low Apgar scores.***

Overdose and treatment
Signs and symptoms of overdose include hyperstimulation of the uterus, causing tetanic contractions and possible uterine rupture, cervical laceration, abruptio placentae, impaired uterine blood flow, amniotic fluid embolism, and fetal trauma. Drug has a very short half-life; halt therapy and initiate supportive care.

Clinical considerations
- Drug must be administered by I.V. infusion, not I.V. bolus injection. Use an infusion device.
- When administering oxytocin challenge test, monitor fetal heart rate and uterine contractions immediately before and during infusion. If fetal heart rate doesn't change during test, repeat in 1 week. If late deceleration in fetal heart rate is noted, consider terminating pregnancy.
- During long infusions, recommend watching for signs of water intoxication.
- Have magnesium sulfate (20% solution) available for relaxation of the myometrium.
- Drug isn't recommended for routine I.M. use. However, 10 units may be administered I.M. after delivery of the placenta to control postpartum uterine bleeding.
- I.V. infusion rates up to 6 milliunits/minute produce maternal plasma concentration similar to spontaneous labor. Rates exceeding 9 to 10 milliunits/minute are rarely needed.
- Solution containing 10 milliunits/ml may be prepared by adding 10 units of oxytocin to 1 L of normal saline solution or D_5W. Solution containing 20 milliunits/ml may be prepared by adding 10 units of oxytocin to 500 ml of normal saline solution or D_5W.
- Oxytocin injection is incompatible with fibrinolysin, norepinephrine bitartrate, prochlorperazine edisylate, and warfarin sodium.
- Discontinue drug if prolonged uterine contractions are prolonged (more than 90 seconds), if intrauterine pressure rises, or if uterine motility interferes with fetal heart rate.

Therapeutic monitoring
- Uterine contractions, heart rate, blood pressure, intrauterine pressure, fetal heart rate, and character of blood loss should be recorded every 15 minutes.
- Drug may produce an antidiuretic effect; fluid intake and output should be monitored.

Special populations
Breast-feeding patients. Minimal amounts of drug enter breast milk. Risks must be evaluated.

Patient counseling
- Explain possible adverse effects of drug.

paclitaxel

Taxol

Pharmacologic classification: novel antimicrotubule
Therapeutic classification: antineoplastic
Pregnancy risk category D

How supplied

Available by prescription only
Injection: 30 mg/5 ml, 100 mg/16.7 ml, 300 mg/50 ml

Indications and dosages

Metastatic ovarian cancer after failure of first-line or subsequent chemotherapy
Adults: 135 or 175 mg/m² I.V. over 3 hours q 3 weeks. Subsequent courses shouldn't be repeated until neutrophil count is at least 1,500 cells/mm³ and platelet count is at least 100,000 cells/mm³.
Breast carcinoma after failure of combination chemotherapy for metastatic disease or relapse within 6 months of adjuvant chemotherapy (prior therapy should have included an anthracycline unless clinically contraindicated)
Adults: 175 mg/m² I.V. over 3 hours q 3 weeks.
AIDS-related Kaposi's sarcoma
Adults: 135 mg/m² I.V. over 3 hours; repeat every 3 weeks as tolerated. Or, 100 mg/m² I.V. over 3 hours; repeat every 2 weeks as tolerated.

Pharmacodynamics

Antineoplastic action: Paclitaxel prevents depolymerization of cellular microtubules, inhibiting the normal reorganization of the microtubule network necessary for mitosis and other vital cellular functions.

Pharmacokinetics

Absorption: Unknown.
Distribution: About 89% to 98% of paclitaxel is bound to serum proteins.
Metabolism: May be metabolized in the liver.
Excretion: Excretion isn't fully understood.

Route	Onset	Peak	Duration
I.V.	Unknown	Unknown	Unknown

Contraindications and precautions

Contraindicated in patients with hypersensitivity to drug or polyoxyethylated castor oil, a vehicle used in drug solution, and in those with baseline neutrophil counts less than 1,500/mm³. Use cautiously in patients who have received radiation therapy.

Interactions

Drug-drug. *Cisplatin:* Possible additive myelosuppression. When given together, administer paclitaxel before cisplatin.
Cyclosporine, dexamethasone, diazepam, etoposide, ketoconazole, quinidine, teniposide, verapamil, vincristine: May inhibit paclitaxel metabolism. Use together cautiously.

Effects on diagnostic tests

None reported.

Adverse reactions

CNS: *peripheral neuropathy.*
CV: *bradycardia, hypotension, abnormal ECG.*
GI: *nausea, vomiting, diarrhea, mucositis.*
Hematologic: NEUTROPENIA, LEUKOPENIA, THROMBOCYTOPENIA, anemia, *bleeding.*
Hepatic: *elevated liver enzyme levels.*
Musculoskeletal: *myalgia, arthralgia.*
Other: *hypersensitivity reactions* ***(anaphylaxis),*** *alopecia, phlebitis, cellulitis at injection site, infections.*

Overdose and treatment

Primary complications of overdose include bone marrow suppression, peripheral neurotoxicity, and mucositis and acute ethanol toxicity in pediatric patients. No specific antidote for paclitaxel overdose is known.

Clinical considerations

- Severe hypersensitivity reactions characterized by dyspnea, hypotension, angioedema, and generalized urticaria have occurred in 2% of patients receiving paclitaxel. To reduce the incidence or severity of these reactions, pretreat patient with corticosteroids such as dexamethasone; antihistamines such as diphenhydramine; and H_2-receptor antagonists, such as cimetidine or ranitidine.
- Don't rechallenge patients who experience severe hypersensitivity reactions to paclitaxel.
- In patients who experience severe neutropenia (neutrophil count less than 500 cells/mm³ for 1 week or longer) or severe peripheral neu-

ropathy during drug therapy, reduce dosage by 20% for subsequent courses. Incidence and severity of neurotoxicity and hematologic toxicity increase with dose, especially more than 190 mg/m^2.

- If significant conduction abnormalities develop during drug administration, administer appropriate therapy and monitor cardiac function continuously during subsequent drug therapy.
- Use caution during preparation and administration of paclitaxel. Use of gloves is recommended. If solution contacts skin, wash skin immediately and thoroughly with soap and water. If drug contacts mucous membranes, flush membranes thoroughly with water. Mark all waste materials with CHEMOTHERAPY HAZARD labels.
- Concentrate must be diluted before infusion. Compatible solutions include normal saline injection, D_5W, dextrose 5% in normal saline injection, and 5% dextrose in lactated Ringer's injection. Dilute to a final concentration of 0.3 to 1.2 mg/ml. Diluted solutions are stable for 27 hours at room temperature.
- Prepare and store infusion solutions in glass containers. Undiluted concentrate shouldn't contact polyvinyl chloride I.V. bags or tubing. Store diluted solution in glass or polypropylene bottles, or use polypropylene or polyolefin bags. Administer through polyethylene-lined administration sets, and use an in-line filter with a microporous membrane not exceeding 0.22 microns.

Therapeutic monitoring

- Bone marrow toxicity is the most frequent and dose-limiting toxicity. Frequent blood count monitoring is necessary during therapy. Packed RBC or platelet transfusions may be necessary in severe cases. Institute bleeding precautions as appropriate.
- Continuously monitor patient for 30 minutes after initiating the infusion. Continue close monitoring throughout infusion.

Special populations

Pregnant patients. Advise women of childbearing age to avoid becoming pregnant during therapy with paclitaxel because of potential harm to the fetus.
Breast-feeding patients. Because of potential for serious adverse reactions in breast-fed infants, breast-feeding should be discontinued during paclitaxel therapy.
Pediatric patients. Safety and efficacy in children haven't been established.

Patient counseling

- Tell patient to watch for signs and symptoms of infection, and bleeding, and to take temperature daily.
- Teach patient to recognize and immediately report signs and symptoms of peripheral neuropathy, such as tingling, burning, or numbness in the extremities. Although mild symptoms are common, severe symptoms occur infrequently. Dosage reduction may be necessary.
- Warn patient that alopecia occurs in almost all patients.

palivizumab

Synagis

Pharmacologic classification: recombinant monoclonal antibody $IgG1_K$
Therapeutic classification: RSV prophylaxis agent
Pregnancy risk category C

How supplied

Available by prescription only
Injection: 100-mg single use vial

Indications and dosages

Prevention of serious lower respiratory tract disease caused by respiratory syncytial virus (RSV) in children at high risk
Children: 15 mg/kg I.M. monthly throughout RSV season. Administer first dose before beginning of RSV season.

Pharmacodynamics

RSV prophylaxis agent action: Drug exhibits neutralizing and fusion-inhibitory activity against RSV, which inhibits RSV replication.

Pharmacokinetics

Absorption: Not reported.
Distribution: Not reported.
Metabolism: Not reported.
Excretion: Half-life of drug is about 18 days.

Route	Onset	Peak	Duration
I.M.	Unknown	Unknown	Unknown

Contraindications and precautions

Contraindicated in children with a history of severe prior reaction to the drug or its components. Administer with caution in patients with thrombocytopenia or any coagulation disorder.

Interactions

None reported.

Effects on diagnostic tests

None reported.

Adverse reactions

CNS: nervousness.
EENT: *otitis media, rhinitis,* pharyngitis, sinusitis, conjunctivitis, oral candidiasis.
GI: diarrhea, vomiting, gastroenteritis.
Hematologic: anemia.

Hepatic: liver function abnormality (increased ALT, AST).
Respiratory: *upper respiratory infection,* cough, wheeze, bronchiolitis, *apnea,* pneumonia, bronchitis, asthma, croup, dyspnea.
Skin: *rash,* fungal dermatitis, eczema, seborrhea.
Other: pain, hernia, failure to thrive, injection site reaction, viral infection, flu syndrome.

Overdose and treatment
No information available.

Clinical considerations
- Patients should receive monthly doses throughout RSV season, even if RSV infection develops. In the northern hemisphere, RSV season typically lasts from November to April.
- To reconstitute, slowly add 1 ml of sterile water for injection into a 100-mg vial. Gently swirl the vial for 30 seconds to avoid foaming. Don't shake vial. Let reconstituted solution stand at room temperature for 20 minutes.
- Vial doesn't contain preservative and should be administered within 6 hours of reconstitution.
- Administer drug in anterolateral aspect of thigh. Don't use gluteal muscle routinely as an injection site because of risk of damage to sciatic nerve. Injection volumes over 1 ml should be given as a divided dose. Don't administer I.V.
- Drug is intended for prophylaxis only. Not used for treatment of present RSV infection.

Therapeutic monitoring
Anaphylactoid reactions following administration of drug have not been observed, but can occur following the administration of proteins. If anaphylaxis or severe allergic reaction occurs, administer epinephrine (1:1,000) and provide supportive care as required.

Special populations
Pregnant patients. It isn't known if drug causes fetal harm. Not recommended for use in pregnant women.

Patient counseling
- Explain to parent or caregiver that drug is used to prevent RSV, not to treat it.
- Advise parent or caregiver that monthly injections are recommended throughout RSV season (November to April in the northern hemisphere).
- Advise parent or caregiver to report adverse reactions immediately.

pamidronate disodium
Aredia

Pharmacologic classification: bisphosphonate, pyrophosphate analogue
Therapeutic classification: antihypercalcemic
Pregnancy risk category C

How supplied
Available by prescription only
Injection: 30 mg/vial, 60 mg/vial, 90 mg/vial

Indications and dosages
Moderate to severe hypercalcemia associated with malignancy (with or without metastases)
Adults: Dosage depends on severity of hypercalcemia. Serum calcium levels should be corrected for serum albumin. Corrected serum calcium (CCa) is calculated using the following formula:

$$\underset{(\text{mg/dl})}{\text{CCa}} = \underset{(\text{mg/dl})}{\text{serum Ca}} + \underset{(\text{g/dl})}{0.8\,(4 - \text{serum albumin})}$$

Repeat doses shouldn't be given sooner than 7 days to allow for full response of initial dose.
≡ ***Dosage adjustment.*** Patients with moderate hypercalcemia (CCa levels of 12 to 13.5 mg/dl) may receive 60 to 90 mg by I.V. infusion over 24 hours. Patients with severe hypercalcemia (CCa levels of more than 13.5 mg/dl) may receive 90 mg as the initial dose.
Paget's disease
Adults: 30 mg I.V. daily over 4 hours for 3 consecutive days for total dose of 90 mg.
Osteolytic bone lesions of multiple myeloma
Adults: 90 mg I.V. daily over 4 hours once monthly.

Pharmacodynamics
Antihypercalcemic action: Pamidronate inhibits the resorption of bone. Drug adsorbs to hydroxyapatite crystals in bone and may directly block the dissolution of calcium phosphate. Drug apparently doesn't inhibit bone formation or mineralization.

Pharmacokinetics
Absorption: Onset is rapid; duration of action up to 6 months in bone.
Distribution: After I.V. administration in animals, about 50% to 60% of a dose is rapidly absorbed by bone; drug is also taken up by the kidneys, liver, spleen, teeth, and tracheal cartilage.
Metabolism: None.

Excretion: Excreted by the kidneys; an average of 51% of a dose is excreted in urine within 72 hours of administration.

Route	Onset	Peak	Duration
I.V.	Unknown	Unknown	Unknown

Contraindications and precautions

Contraindicated in patients hypersensitive to drug or other bisphosphonates, such as etidronate. Use with extreme caution in patients with impaired renal function.

Interactions

Drug-drug. *Solutions that contain calcium:* Pamidronate may form a precipitate when mixed together. Don't mix together.

Effects on diagnostic tests

None reported.

Adverse reactions

CNS: ***seizures,*** fatigue, headache, somnolence.
CV: atrial fibrillation, syncope, tachycardia, *hypertension.*
GI: *abdominal pain, anorexia, constipation, nausea, vomiting,* GI hemorrhage.
Hematologic: ***leukopenia, thrombocytopenia,*** *anemia.*
Metabolic: *hypophosphatemia, hypokalemia, hypomagnesemia, hypocalcemia.*
Musculoskeletal: *bone pain.*
Other: *fever, infusion-site reaction, generalized pain.*

Overdose and treatment

Symptomatic hypocalcemia could result from overdose; treat with I.V. calcium. In one reported case, a 209-lb (95-kg) woman who received 285 mg daily for 3 days experienced hyperpyrexia (103° F [39.4° C]), hypotension, and transient taste perversion. Fever and hypotension were rapidly corrected with corticosteroids.

Clinical considerations

- Reconstitute vial with 10 ml sterile water for injection. Once drug is completely dissolved, add to 1,000 ml 0.45% or normal saline solution injection or D_5W. Don't mix with infusion solutions that contain calcium, such as Ringer's injection or lactated Ringer's injection. Administer in a single I.V. solution, in a separate line from all other drugs. Visually inspect for precipitate before administering.
- Injection solution is stable for 24 hours when refrigerated. Give only by I.V. infusion. Animal studies have shown evidence of nephropathy when drug is given as a bolus.
- Consider retreatment if hypercalcemia recurs; allow a minimum of 7 days to elapse before retreatment to allow for full response to the initial dose.

Therapeutic monitoring

- Because drug can cause electrolyte disturbances, careful monitoring of serum electrolytes (especially calcium, phosphate, and magnesium) is essential. Short-term administration of calcium may be necessary in patients with severe hypocalcemia. Also monitor creatinine, CBC, differential, hematocrit, and hemoglobin levels.
- Carefully monitor patients with preexisting anemia, leukopenia, or thrombocytopenia during first 2 weeks after therapy.
- Monitor patient's temperature. In trials, 27% of patients experienced a slightly elevated temperature for 24 to 48 hours after therapy.

Special populations

Breast-feeding patients. It's unknown if drug is excreted in breast milk. Use with caution in breast-feeding women.
Pediatric patients. Safety and efficacy in children haven't been established.

Patient counseling

Instruct patient to report adverse reactions immediately.

pancuronium bromide

Pavulon

Pharmacologic classification: nondepolarizing neuromuscular blocker
Therapeutic classification: skeletal muscle relaxant
Pregnancy risk category C

How supplied

Available by prescription only
Injection: 1 mg/ml, 2 mg/ml parenteral

Indications and dosages

Adjunct to anesthesia to induce skeletal muscle relaxation, facilitate intubation and ventilation, and weaken muscle contractions in induced seizures
Dose depends on anesthetic used, individual needs, and response. Doses are representative and must be adjusted.
Adults and children over age 1 month: Initially, 0.04 to 0.1 mg/kg I.V.; then 0.01 mg/kg q 25 to 60 minutes if needed.

Pharmacodynamics

Skeletal muscle relaxant action: Pancuronium prevents acetylcholine (ACh) from binding to the receptors on the motor end-plate, blocking depolarization. It may increase heart rate through direct blocking effect on the ACh receptors of the heart; increase is dose-related. Pancuronium causes little or no histamine release and no ganglionic blockade.

Pharmacokinetics

Absorption: Onset and duration are dose-related. After 0.06 mg/kg dose, effects begin to subside in 35 to 45 minutes. Repeated doses may increase the magnitude and duration of action.
Distribution: 87% bound to plasma proteins.
Metabolism: Metabolism is unknown; small amounts may be metabolized by the liver.
Excretion: Mainly excreted unchanged in urine; some through biliary excretion.

Route	Onset	Peak	Duration
I.V.	30-45 sec	3-4½ min	35-65 min

Contraindications and precautions

Contraindicated in patients with hypersensitivity to bromides or preexisting tachycardia and in those for whom even a minor increase in heart rate is undesirable.

Use cautiously in geriatric or debilitated patients and in those with impaired renal, pulmonary, or hepatic function; respiratory depression; myasthenia gravis; myasthenic syndrome of lung or bronchogenic cancer; dehydration; thyroid disorders; collagen diseases; porphyria; electrolyte disturbances; hyperthermia; or toxemic states. Also use large doses cautiously in patients undergoing cesarean section.

Interactions

Drug-drug. *Aminoglycoside antibiotics, beta blockers, clindamycin, depolarizing neuromuscular blocking agents, furosemide, general anesthetics, lincomycin, lithium, other nondepolarizing neuromuscular blocking agents, parenteral magnesium salts, polymyxin antibiotics, potassium-depleting agents, quinidine or quinine, thiazide diuretics:* The effects of pancuronium may be potentiated. Use cautiously during surgical and postoperative periods.
Opioid analgesics: May increase respiratory depression. Use with extreme caution and reduce dose of pancuronium.
Succinylcholine: May enhance and prolong neuromuscular blocking effects of pancuronium. Allow effects of succinylcholine to subside before administering pancuronium.

Effects on diagnostic tests

None reported.

Adverse reactions

CV: tachycardia, increased blood pressure.
Respiratory: *prolonged, dose-related respiratory insufficiency or apnea.*
Skin: transient rashes.
Musculoskeletal: residual muscle weakness.
Other: excessive salivation, allergic or idiosyncratic hypersensitivity reactions.

Overdose and treatment

Signs and symptoms of overdose include prolonged respiratory depression, apnea, and CV collapse.

Use a peripheral nerve stimulator to monitor response and to evaluate neuromuscular blockade. Maintain an adequate airway and manual or mechanical ventilation until patient can maintain adequate ventilation unassisted. Neostigmine, edrophonium, or pyridostigmine may be used to reverse effects.

Clinical considerations

- Administration requires direct medical supervision, with emergency respiratory support available.
- Store drug in refrigerator and not in plastic container or syringes. Plastic syringes may be used to administer dose.
- Don't mix in same syringe or give through same needle with barbiturates or other alkaline solutions.
- Reduce dosage when ether or other inhalation anesthetics that enhance neuromuscular blockade are used.
- Large doses may increase frequency and severity of tachycardia.
- Drug doesn't relieve pain or affect consciousness; be sure to assess need for analgesic or sedative.

Therapeutic monitoring

Monitor baseline electrolyte levels, intake and output, and vital signs, especially heart rate and respiration.

Special populations

Breast-feeding patients. It's unknown if drug is excreted in breast milk. Use with caution in breast-feeding women.
Pediatric patients. Dosage for neonates under age 1 month must be carefully individualized. For infants over age 1 month and children, see adult dosage.
Geriatric patients. The usual adult dose must be individualized depending on response.

Patient counseling

Explain all events and procedures to patient because he can still hear.

papaverine hydrochloride

Cerespan, Genabid, Pavabid, Pavacels, Pavacot, Pavagen, Pavarine, Pavased, Pavatine, Pavatym, Paverolan

Pharmacologic classification: benzylisoquinoline derivative, opiate alkaloid
Therapeutic classification: peripheral vasodilator
Pregnancy risk category C

How supplied

Available by prescription only
Capsules (sustained-release): 150 mg
Injection: 30 mg/ml

Indications and dosages

Relief of cerebral and peripheral ischemia associated with arterial spasm and myocardial ischemia; treatment of coronary occlusion and certain cerebral angiospastic states

Adults: 75 to 300 mg P.O. three to five times daily or 150 to 300 mg sustained-release preparations q 8 to 12 hours; 30 to 120 mg I.M. or I.V. q 3 hours, as indicated. In treatment of extrasystoles, give two doses 10 minutes apart.
Children: 6 mg/kg I.M. or I.V. q.i.d.

◇***Impotence***

Adults: 2.5 to 60 mg injected intracavernously.

Pharmacodynamics

Vasodilating action: Papaverine relaxes smooth muscle directly by inhibiting phosphodiesterase, increasing the level of cyclic adenosine monophosphate. There's considerable controversy regarding the clinical effectiveness of papaverine. Some clinicians find little objective evidence of any clinical value.

Pharmacokinetics

Absorption: About 54% of orally administered papaverine is bioavailable. Half-life varies from ½ hour to 24 hours, but levels can be maintained by giving drug at 6-hour intervals. Sustained-release forms are sometimes absorbed poorly and erratically.
Distribution: Tends to localize in adipose tissue and in the liver; the remainder is distributed throughout the body. About 90% of drug is protein-bound.
Metabolism: Metabolized by the liver.
Excretion: Excreted in urine as metabolites.

Route	Onset	Peak	Duration
P.O.	Unknown	1-2 hr	Unknown
I.V., I.M.	Unknown	Unknown	Unknown

Contraindications and precautions

I.V. use is contraindicated in patients with Parkinson's disease or complete AV block. Use cautiously in patients with glaucoma or hepatic dysfunction.

Interactions

Drug-drug. *CNS depressants:* The effects of papaverine may be potentiated. Avoid use together.
Levodopa: Papaverine may decrease the antiparkinsonian effects and exacerbate such symptoms as rigidity and tremors. Don't use together.
Morphine: May have a synergic response. Monitor patient closely.
Drug-lifestyle. *Heavy smoking:* Interferes with the therapeutic effect of papaverine. Advise patient to avoid smoking.

Effects on diagnostic tests

None reported.

Adverse reactions

CNS: *headache,* vertigo, drowsiness, sedation, malaise.
CV: *increased heart rate, increased blood pressure* (with parenteral use), depressed AV and intraventricular conduction, *arrhythmias.*
GI: constipation, *nausea,* anorexia, abdominal pain, diarrhea.
Hepatic: *hepatitis* (jaundice, eosinophilia, abnormal liver function tests), *cirrhosis.*
Respiratory: increased depth and rate of respiration.
Skin: *diaphoresis, flushing,* rash.

Overdose and treatment

Signs and symptoms of overdose include drowsiness, weakness, nystagmus, diplopia, incoordination, and lassitude, progressing to coma with cyanosis and respiratory depression.

To slow drug absorption, give activated charcoal, tap water, or milk; then evacuate stomach contents by gastric lavage or emesis, and follow with catharsis. If coma and respiratory depression occur, take appropriate measures; maintain blood pressure. Hemodialysis may be helpful.

Clinical considerations

- Papaverine is an opiate; however, it has strikingly different pharmacologic properties than other drugs in this group.
- Drug may be given orally, I.M. or, when immediate effect is needed, by slow I.V. injection. Inject I.V. slowly over 1 to 2 minutes; arrhythmias and fatal apnea may follow rapid injection.
- Papaverine injection is incompatible with lactated Ringer's injection; a precipitate will form.

Therapeutic monitoring

Monitor for fibrotic changes, such as indurations and lumpy areas in the penis.

Special populations

Breast-feeding patients. Safety in breast-feeding women hasn't been established.
Pediatric patients. Children's doses are administered parenterally.
Geriatric patients. Geriatric patients are at greater risk of papaverine-induced hypothermia.

Patient counseling

- Advise patient to avoid sudden postural changes to minimize possible orthostatic hypotension.
- Instruct patient to report nausea, abdominal distress, anorexia, constipation, diarrhea, jaundice, rash, sweating, tiredness, or headache.

paricalcitol

Zemplar

Pharmacologic classification: Vitamin D analogue
Therapeutic classification: hyperparathyroidism agent
Pregnancy risk category C

How supplied

Available by prescription only
Injection: 5 mcg/ml, 1-ml and 2-ml vials

Indications and dosages

Prevention and treatment of secondary hyperparathyroidism associated with chronic renal failure
Adults: 0.04 to 0.1 mcg/kg (2.8 to 7 mcg) I.V. bolus no more frequently than every other day during dialysis. Doses as high as 0.24 mcg/kg (16.8 mcg) have been safely administered. If satisfactory response isn't observed, dosage may be increased by 2 to 4 mcg at 2- to 4-week intervals.

Pharmacodynamics

Parathyroid action: A synthetic vitamin D analogue shown to reduce parathyroid hormone (PTH) levels.

Pharmacokinetics

Absorption: Administered I.V.
Distribution: Not reported.
Metabolism: Not reported.
Excretion: Eliminated primarily by heptobiliary excretion, 74% in the feces and 16% in the urine. Half-life is about 15 hours.

Route	Onset	Peak	Duration
I.V.	Immediate	Unknown	15 hr

Contraindications and precautions

Contraindicated in patients with evidence of vitamin D toxicity, hypercalcemia, or hypersensitivity to drug or its ingredients. Use cautiously in patients taking digitalis compounds. Patients taking digoxin are at greater risk for digitalis toxicity during drug therapy secondary to potential for hypercalcemia.

Interactions

None reported.

Effects on diagnostic tests

None reported.

Adverse reactions

CNS: light-headedness, malaise.
CV: palpitation.
GI: dry mouth, GI bleeding, *nausea,* vomiting.
Hepatic: reduced serum total alkaline phosphatase level.
Respiratory: pneumonia.
Other: chills, edema, fever, flu syndrome, sepsis.

Overdose and treatment

Overdose may cause hypercalcemia. Symptoms include weakness, headache, nausea, vomiting, constipation, anorexia, pancreatitis, ectopic calcification, cardiac arrhythmias, and death. Treatment should include correcting electrolyte abnormalities, assessing cardiac abnormalities, and hemodialysis or peritoneal dialysis against a calcium-free dialysate.

Clinical considerations

- As the PTH level is decreased, paricalcitol dose may need to be decreased. Acute overdose of paricalcitol may cause hypercalcemia, which may require emergency attention.
- Appropriate types of phosphate-binding compounds may be needed to control serum phosphorus levels in patients with chronic renal failure; avoid excessive use of aluminum-containing compounds.
- Store drug at room temperature (59° to 86°F [15° to 30° C]).
- Drug is only administered as an I.V. bolus. Discard unused portion.
- Inspect drug for particulate matter and discoloration before use.

Therapeutic monitoring

- Monitor for ECG abnormalities.
- Monitor patient for symptoms of hypercalcemia. Immediately notify doctor if hypercalcemia is suspected.
- Monitor serum calcium and phosphorus levels twice weekly when dose is being adjusted, and then monitor monthly. PTH level should be measured every 3 months during therapy.

Special populations

Breast-feeding patients. It isn't known if drug is excreted in breast milk. Exercise caution when administering to breast-feeding women.
Pediatric patients. Safety and efficacy in children haven't been established.
Geriatric patients. No significant difference in safety and efficacy has been reported in patients over age 65.

Patient counseling

- Stress importance of adhering to a dietary regimen of calcium supplementation and phosphorus restriction during drug therapy.
- Caution against use of phosphate or vitamin D-related compounds during drug therapy.
- Instruct patient with chronic renal failure to take phosphate-binding compounds as prescribed but to avoid excessive use of aluminum-containing compounds.
- Alert patient to early symptoms of hypercalcemia and vitamin D intoxication, such as weakness, headache, somnolence, nausea, vom-

iting, dry mouth, constipation, muscle pain, bone pain, and metallic taste.
- Instruct patient to promptly report adverse reactions.
- Remind patient taking digoxin to watch for signs of digitalis toxicity.

paroxetine hydrochloride
Paxil

Pharmacologic classification: selective serotonin reuptake inhibitor
Therapeutic classification: antidepressant
Pregnancy risk category C

How supplied
Available by prescription only
Tablets: 10 mg, 20 mg, 30 mg, 40 mg
Suspension: 10 mg/5 ml

Indications and dosages
Depression
Adults: Initially, 20 mg P.O. daily, preferably in the morning. Increase dosage by 10 mg/day at 1-week intervals, to maximum of 50 mg daily, if necessary.
Obsessive-compulsive disorder (OCD)
Adults: Initially, 20 mg P.O. daily, preferably in the morning. Increase dosage by 10 mg/day at 1-week intervals to target dose of 40 mg/day. Maximum dose, 60 mg/day.
Generalized social phobia (social anxiety disorder)
Adults: 20 mg P.O. daily.
Panic disorder
Adults: Initially, 10 mg P.O. daily, preferably in the morning. Increase dosage by 10 mg/day at 1-week intervals, to target dose of 40 mg/day. Maximum dose, 60 mg/day.
≡ ***Dosage adjustment.*** For geriatric or debilitated patients or patients with severe hepatic or renal disease, 10 mg P.O. daily, preferably in the morning. Increase dosage by 10 mg/day at 1-week intervals, p.r.n., to maximum of 40 mg daily.
◇ ***Diabetic neuropathy***
Adults: 10 to 60 mg P.O. daily.
◇ ***Headaches***
Adults: 10 to 50 mg P.O. daily.
◇ ***Premature ejaculation***
Adults: 20 mg P.O. daily.

Pharmacodynamics
Antidepressant action: Action is presumed to be linked to potentiation of serotonergic activity in the CNS, resulting from inhibition of neuronal reuptake of serotonin.

Pharmacokinetics
Absorption: Completely absorbed after oral dosing.
Distribution: Distributed throughout the body, including the CNS, with only 1% remaining in the plasma. About 93% to 95% of paroxetine is bound to plasma protein.
Metabolism: About 36% is metabolized in the liver. The principal metabolites are polar and conjugated products of oxidation and methylation, which are readily cleared.
Excretion: About 64% is excreted in urine (2% as parent compound and 62% as metabolite).

Route	Onset	Peak	Duration
P.O.	Unknown	2-8 hr	Unknown

Contraindications and precautions
Contraindicated in patients taking MAO inhibitors or within 14 days of discontinuing MAO inhibitors. Use cautiously in patients with history of seizures or mania; in those with severe, concurrent systemic illness; or in those at risk for volume depletion and those with hypersensitivity to SSRIs.

Interactions
Drug-drug. *Cimetidine:* Decreases hepatic metabolism of paroxetine, leading to risk of toxicity. Dosage adjustments may be necessary.
Digoxin: Paroxetine may decrease levels. Monitor patient closely.
MAO inhibitors: May increase risk of serious, sometimes fatal, adverse reactions. Avoid use together.
Phenobarbital, phenytoin: Reduces plasma levels of drug. Dosage adjustment may be necessary.
Procyclidine: Increases procyclidine levels. Monitor patient for excessive anticholinergic effects.
Theophylline: Paroxetine may increase levels. Monitor patient closely.
Tryptophan: May increase the incidence of adverse reactions. Avoid use together.
Warfarin: Increased risk of bleeding. Monitor INR.
Drug-lifestyle. *Alcohol use:* May increase risk of CNS adverse effects. Advise patient to avoid alcohol during treatment.
Drug-herb. *St. John's wort:* May result in sedative-hypnotic intoxication. Don't use together.

Effects on diagnostic tests
None reported.

Adverse reactions
CNS: *somnolence, dizziness, insomnia, tremor, nervousness,* anxiety, paresthesia, confusion, *headache,* agitation, decreased levels, abnormal dreams.
CV: palpitations, vasodilation, orthostatic hypotension, chest pain.
EENT: lump or tightness in throat, dysgeusia, visual disturbances, double vision.

GI: *dry mouth, nausea, constipation, diarrhea,* flatulence, vomiting, dyspepsia, increased or decreased appetite, abdominal pain.
GU: ejaculatory disturbances, male genital disorders (including anorgasmia, erectile difficulties, delayed ejaculation or orgasm, impotence, and sexual dysfunction), urinary frequency, other urinary disorders, female genital disorders (including anorgasmia, difficulty with orgasm).
Musculoskeletal: myopathy, myalgia, myasthenia, *asthenia.*
Skin: *diaphoresis,* rash, pruritus.
Other: decreased libido, yawning.

Overdose and treatment

Signs and symptoms of overdose may include nausea, vomiting, dizziness, sweating, facial flushing, drowsiness, sinus tachycardia, and dilated pupil. Treatment should consist of general measures used in management of overdose with any antidepressant. Perform gastric evacuation by emesis, lavage, or both. In most cases, 20 to 30 g of activated charcoal may then be administered every 4 to 6 hours during the first 24 to 48 hours after ingestion. Supportive care, frequent monitoring of vital signs, and careful observation are indicated. ECG and cardiac function monitoring are warranted with evidence of any abnormality.

Take special caution with a patient who currently receives or recently received paroxetine if the patient ingests an excessive quantity of a tricyclic antidepressant. In such cases, accumulation of the parent tricyclic and its active metabolite may increase the possibility of clinically significant sequelae and extend the time needed for close medical observation.

Clinical considerations

- At least 14 days should elapse between discontinuation of an MAO inhibitor and initiation of drug therapy. Similarly, at least 14 days should elapse between discontinuation of paroxetine and initiation of an MAO inhibitor.
- If signs of psychosis occur or increase, reduce dosage. Monitor patients for suicidal tendencies and allow them only a minimum supply of drug.

Therapeutic monitoring

Hyponatremia may occur with paroxetine use, especially in geriatric patients, those taking diuretics, and those who are otherwise volume depleted. Monitor serum sodium levels.

Special populations

Breast-feeding patients. Drug is excreted in breast milk. Use with caution in breast-feeding women.
Pediatric patients. Safety and efficacy in children haven't been established.
Geriatric patients. Use cautiously and in lower dosages in geriatric patients.

Patient counseling

- Caution patient not to operate hazardous machinery, including automobiles, until reasonably certain that paroxetine therapy doesn't affect ability to engage in such activity.
- Tell patient that he may notice improvement in 1 to 4 weeks but that he must continue with the prescribed regimen to obtain continued benefits.
- Instruct patient to contact health care provider before taking other medications, including OTC preparations, while receiving paroxetine therapy.
- Tell patient to abstain from alcohol while taking paroxetine.

pegaspargase (PEG-L-asparaginase)

Oncaspar

Pharmacologic classification: modified version of the enzyme l-asparaginase
Therapeutic classification: antineoplastic
Pregnancy risk category C

How supplied

Available by prescription only
Injection: 750 IU/ml in single-use vial

Indications and dosages

Acute lymphoblastic leukemia (ALL) in patients who require L-asparaginase but have developed hypersensitivity to the native forms of L-asparaginase
Adults and children with body surface area of at least 0.6 m²: 2,500 IU/m² I.M. or I.V. q 14 days.
Children with body surface area less than 0.6 m²: 82.5 IU/kg I.M. or I.V. q 14 days.

Note: Moderate to life-threatening hypersensitivity reactions necessitate discontinuation of L-asparaginase treatment.

Pharmacodynamics

Antineoplastic action: Pegaspargase is a modified version of the enzyme L-asparaginase, which exerts its cytotoxic activity by inactivating the amino acid asparagine. Because leukemic cells can't synthesize their own asparagine, protein synthesis and eventually synthesis of DNA and RNA are inhibited.

Pharmacokinetics

No information available.

Route	Onset	Peak	Duration
I.M., I.V.	Unknown	Unknown	Unknown

Contraindications and precautions

Contraindicated in patients with pancreatitis or a history of pancreatitis; in those who have had significant hemorrhagic events associated with prior L-asparaginase therapy; and in those with previous serious allergic reactions, such as generalized urticaria, bronchospasm, laryngeal edema, hypotension, or other unacceptable adverse reactions to pegaspargase.

Use cautiously in patients with hepatic dysfunction and during pregnancy.

Interactions

Drug-drug. *Aspirin, dipyridamole, heparin, NSAIDs, warfarin:* May cause imbalances in coagulation factors, predisposing the patient to bleeding or thrombosis. Use together cautiously.
Methotrexate: During its inhibition of protein synthesis and cell replication, pegaspargase may interfere with the action of such drugs that require cell replication for their lethal effects. Monitor for decreased effectiveness.
Protein-bound drugs: Depletion of serum protein by pegaspargase may increase the toxicity of these drugs. Monitor for toxicity. Pegaspargase may interfere with the enzymatic detoxification of other drugs, particularly in the liver. Use caution when administering together.

Effects on diagnostic tests

None reported.

Adverse reactions

CNS: seizures, headache, paresthesia, ***status epilepticus,*** somnolence, coma, mental status changes, dizziness, emotional lability, mood changes, parkinsonism, confusion, disorientation, fatigue.
CV: hypotension, tachycardia, chest pain, subacute bacterial endocarditis, hypertension.
EENT: epistaxis.
GI: nausea, vomiting, abdominal pain, anorexia, diarrhea, constipation, indigestion, flatulence, GI pain, mucositis, ***pancreatitis (sometimes fulminant and fatal),*** increased serum amylase and lipase levels, severe colitis.
GU: increased BUN level, increased creatinine level, increased urinary frequency, hematuria, severe hemorrhagic cystitis, renal dysfunction, renal failure.
Hematologic: ***thrombosis;*** prolonged PT, prolonged partial thromboplastin time, decreased antithrombin III; ***DIC;*** decreased fibrinogen; hemolytic anemia; ***leukopenia; pancytopenia; agranulocytosis; thrombocytopenia;*** increased thromboplastin; easy bruising; ecchymoses; ***hemorrhage*** (may be fatal).
Hepatic: jaundice, abnormal liver function test results, bilirubinemia, increased ALT and AST, ascites, hypoalbuminemia, fatty changes in liver, ***liver failure.***
Metabolic: hyperuricemia, hyperglycemia, hypoglycemia, hyponatremia, uric acid nephropathy, hypoproteinemia, proteinuria, weight loss, metabolic acidosis, increased blood ammonia level.
Musculoskeletal: arthralgia, myalgia, musculoskeletal pain, joint stiffness, cramps.
Respiratory: cough, ***severe bronchospasm,*** upper respiratory tract infection.
Skin: itching, alopecia, fever blister, purpura, hand whiteness, fungal changes, nail whiteness and ridging, erythema simplex, petechial rash, injection pain or reaction, localized edema.
Other: hypersensitivity reactions, including ***anaphylaxis,*** rash, erythema, edema, pain, fever, chills, urticaria, dyspnea, or bronchospasm; pain in extremities; peripheral edema; malaise; night sweats; mouth tenderness; infection; ***sepsis, septic shock.***

Overdose and treatment

Only three cases of overdose (10,000 IU/m^2 as an I.V. infusion) have been reported. One patient experienced a slight increase in liver enzymes, a rash developed in another, and the third experienced no adverse effects. No other information is available.

Clinical considerations

□ ***ALERT*** Hypersensitivity reactions to pegaspargase, including life-threatening anaphylaxis, may occur during therapy, especially in patients with known hypersensitivity to other forms of L-asparaginase. As a precaution, observe patient for 1 hour and have resuscitation equipment and other agents necessary to treat anaphylaxis available.

- I.M. is the preferred administration route because it has a lower incidence of hepatotoxicity, coagulopathy, and GI and renal disorders than the I.V. route.
- Drug shouldn't be administered if it has ever been frozen. Although there may not be an apparent change in appearance of drug, its activity is destroyed after freezing.
- Avoid excessive agitation; don't shake. Keep refrigerated at 36° to 46° F (2° to 8° C). Don't use if cloudy, if precipitate is present, or if stored at room temperature for more than 48 hours. Don't freeze. Discard unused portions. Use only one dose per vial; don't reenter the vial. Don't save unused drug for later administration.
- When administering I.M., limit volume at a single injection site to 2 ml. If the volume to be administered is greater than 2 ml, use multiple injection sites.
- When administered I.V., give over 1 to 2 hours in 100 ml of normal saline solution or 5% dextrose injection through an infusion that is already running.
- Pegaspargase should be the sole induction agent only when a combined regimen using other chemotherapeutic agents is inappropriate because of toxicity or other specific patient-related factors or in patients refractory to other therapy.

▪ Pegaspargase may be a contact irritant, and the solution must be handled and administered with care. Gloves are recommended. Avoid inhalation of vapors and contact with skin or mucous membranes, especially those of the eyes. In case of contact, wash with copious amounts of water for at least 15 minutes.

Therapeutic monitoring

▪ A decrease in circulating lymphoblasts is common after initiating therapy. This may be accompanied by a marked increase in serum uric acid. As a guide to the effects of therapy, monitor patient's peripheral blood count and bone marrow.
▪ Obtain frequent serum amylase determinations to detect early evidence of pancreatitis. Monitor blood glucose during therapy because hyperglycemia may occur.
▪ When using pegaspargase with hepatotoxic chemotherapy, monitor patient for liver dysfunction.
▪ Pegaspargase may affect some plasma proteins; therefore, monitoring of fibrinogen, PT, and partial thromboplastin time may be indicated.

Special populations

Breast-feeding patients. Because of potential for serious adverse reactions in breast-fed infants, a decision must be made whether to discontinue breast-feeding or drug, taking into account the importance of drug to the woman.
Pediatric patients. Safety and efficacy in infants under age 1 haven't been established.

Patient counseling

▪ Tell patient to report hypersensitivity reactions immediately.
▪ Instruct patient not to take other drugs, including OTC preparations, without obtaining medical approval; pegaspargase increases the risk of bleeding when given with certain drugs, such as aspirin, and may increase the toxicity of other medications.
▪ Instruct patient to report signs and symptoms of infection (fever, chills, malaise); drug may have immunosuppressive activity.

penbutolol sulfate

Levatol

Pharmacologic classification: beta blocker
Therapeutic classification: antihypertensive
Pregnancy risk category C

How supplied

Available by prescription only
Tablets: 20 mg

Indications and dosages

Treatment of mild to moderate hypertension
Adults: 20 mg P.O. once daily. Usually given with other antihypertensive agents, such as thiazide diuretics. Dosages as high as 40 to 80 mg daily and as low as 10 mg daily have been effective.

Pharmacodynamics

Antihypertensive action: Penbutolol blocks both $beta_1$- and $beta_2$-adrenergic receptors. Its antihypertensive effects may be related to its peripheral antiadrenergic effects that lead to decreased cardiac output, a central effect that leads to decreased sympathetic tone, or decreased renin secretion by the kidneys.

Pharmacokinetics

Absorption: Almost completely absorbed after oral administration.
Distribution: 80% to 98% is bound to plasma proteins.
Metabolism: Metabolized by the liver. Several metabolites have been identified; some retain partial pharmacologic activity.
Excretion: Average elimination half-life of the parent drug is 5 hours; some metabolites persist for 20 hours or more. Most metabolites are excreted in urine.

Route	Onset	Peak	Duration
P.O.	1 hr	1½-3 hr	24 hr

Contraindications and precautions

Contraindicated in patients with hypersensitivity to drug or other beta blockers and in those with sinus bradycardia, cardiogenic shock, overt cardiac failure, greater than first-degree heart block, bronchial asthma, bronchospastic disease, or chronic bronchitis.

Use cautiously in patients with heart failure controlled by drug therapy, diabetes, or history of bronchospastic disease.

Interactions

Drug-drug. *Clonidine:* May cause paradoxical hypertension when combined with beta blockers. Also, beta blockers may enhance rebound hypertension when clonidine is withdrawn. Monitor patient closely.
Doxazosin, prazocin, terazocin: Beta blockers may enhance the "first dose" orthostatic hypotension seen with these drugs. Use together cautiously.
Insulin or oral antidiabetic agents: Beta blockers may alter hypoglycemic response. Monitor patient closely.
Lidocaine: Penbutolol may increase the volume of distribution of lidocaine in normal patients, increasing the loading dose requirements in some patients.
Oral calcium antagonists: May enhance the hypotensive effects of beta blockers as well as

predispose the patient to bradycardia and arrhythmias. Monitor patient closely.
Reserpine or other catecholamine-depleting drugs: Decreased hypotensive response. Monitor patient closely.

Effects on diagnostic tests
Drug may interfere with glucose or insulin tolerance tests.

Adverse reactions
CNS: *dizziness,* headache, fatigue, insomnia, asthenia.
CV: chest pain, ***bradycardia, heart failure.***
GI: nausea, diarrhea, dyspepsia.
GU: impotence.
Respiratory: cough, dyspnea.
Skin: excessive diaphoresis.

Note: Consider the potential for adverse effects associated with other beta blockers.

Overdose and treatment
Signs of overdose may include bradycardia, bronchospasm, heart failure, and severe hypotension.

After emptying the stomach by lavage (for acute oral ingestion), administer symptomatic and supportive care. Bradycardia may be treated with atropine or cautious use of isoproterenol. Cardiac glycosides, glucagon hydrochloride, dobutamine, and diuretics may be useful in treating heart failure, and vasopressors, such as epinephrine or alpha-adrenergic agonists, may be used to counter severe hypotension. In refractory cases of hypotension, administration of glucagon hydrochloride may be useful. Treat bronchospasm with aminophylline or isoproterenol.

Clinical considerations
Consider the recommendations relevant to all beta blockers as well as the following:

- Like other beta blockers, penbutolol may cause patients to exhibit hypersensitivity to catecholamines upon withdrawal.
- To discontinue drug, slowly taper dosage over a period of 1 to 2 weeks, especially in patients with ischemic heart disease. If symptoms of angina develop, immediately reinstitute therapy, at least temporarily, and take steps to control the patient's unstable angina.

Therapeutic monitoring
Advise checking patient's apical pulse before giving drug. If extremes in pulse rate are detected, drug should be withheld and doctor notified immediately.

Special populations
Breast-feeding patients. It isn't known if penbutolol is excreted in breast milk. Use with caution in breast-feeding women.
Pediatric patients. Safety and efficacy in children haven't been established.
Geriatric patients. No difference has been found in plasma half-life in healthy geriatric patients compared with patients on renal dialysis.

Patient counseling
- Advise patient not to discontinue drug abruptly because sudden withdrawal of other beta blockers has precipitated angina and MI.
- Tell patient to report adverse effects immediately, particularly slow heart rate, chest congestion, cough, wheezing, or shortness of breath from mild exertion.
- Teach patient about disease and therapy. Explain why it's important to continue taking drug, even when feeling well.
- Inform patient to contact health care provider before taking OTC medications.

penicillamine
Cuprimine, Depen

Pharmacologic classification: chelating agent
Therapeutic classification: heavy metal antagonist, antirheumatic
Pregnancy risk category NR

How supplied
Available by prescription only
Capsules: 125 mg, 250 mg
Tablets: 250 mg

Indications and dosages
Wilson's disease
Adults: 250 mg P.O. q.i.d. 0.5 to 1 hour before meals and at least 2 hours after evening meal. Adjust dosage to achieve urinary copper excretion of 0.5 to 1 mg daily. Dose over 2 g is seldom necessary.
Cystinuria
Adults: 250 mg P.O. daily in four divided doses, then gradually increasing dosage. Usual dose, 2 g daily (range, 1 to 4 g daily). Adjust dosage to achieve urinary cystine excretion of less than 100 mg daily when renal calculi are present, or 100 to 200 mg daily when no calculi are present.
Rheumatoid arthritis,* ◊*Felty's syndrome
Adults: Initially, 125 to 250 mg P.O. daily, with increases of 125 to 250 mg daily at 1- to 3-month intervals if necessary. Maximum dose is 1.5 g daily.
◊***Adjunctive treatment of heavy metal poisoning***
Adults: 500 to 1,500 mg P.O. daily for 1 to 2 months.
◊***Primary biliary cirrhosis***
Adults: Initially, 250 mg P.O. daily, with increases of 250 mg q 2 weeks. Maximum dose, 1 g daily in divided doses.

Pharmacodynamics

Antirheumatic action: Mechanism of action in rheumatoid arthritis is unknown; penicillamine depresses circulating IgM rheumatoid factor (but not total circulating immunoglobulin levels) and depresses T-cell but not B-cell activity. It also depolymerizes some macroglobulins (such as rheumatoid factor).

Chelating agent action: Penicillamine forms stable, soluble complexes with copper, iron, mercury, lead, and other heavy metals that are excreted in urine; it's particularly useful in chelating copper in patients with Wilson's disease. Penicillamine also combines with cystine to form a complex more soluble than cystine alone, thereby reducing free cystine below the level of urinary stone formation.

Pharmacokinetics

Absorption: Well absorbed after oral administration.

Distribution: Limited data available.

Metabolism: Metabolized by liver to inactive compounds.

Excretion: Only small amounts of penicillamine are excreted unchanged; after 24 hours, about 50% of drug is excreted in urine and about 50% in feces.

Route	Onset	Peak	Duration
P.O.	Unknown	3 hr	Unknown

Contraindications and precautions

Contraindicated in patients with known hypersensitivity to drug, history of penicillamine-related aplastic anemia or agranulocytosis, or significant renal or hepatic insufficiency; in pregnant women; and in patients receiving gold salts, immunosuppressants, antimalarials, or phenylbutazone because of the increased risk of serious hematologic effects.

Use cautiously in patients allergic to penicillin (cross reaction is rare); in those who receive a second course of therapy and who may have become sensitized and are more likely to have allergic reactions; and in patients in whom proteinuria associated with Goodpasture's syndrome develops.

Interactions

Drug-drug. *Antacids, iron salts:* Decrease absorption of penicillamine. Separate administration times.

Antimalarial or cytotoxic agents, gold therapy, oxyphenbutazone, phenylbutazone: Both are associated with serious hematologic and renal effects. Don't use together.

Digoxin: Levels may be decreased when given together. Monitor serum digoxin levels closely.

Effects on diagnostic tests

Drug therapy may cause positive test results for antinuclear antibody with or without clinical systemic lupus erythematosus-like syndrome.

Adverse reactions

EENT: oral ulcerations, glossitis, cheilosis, tinnitus, optic neuritis.

GI: anorexia, nausea, vomiting, dyspepsia, alteration in sense of taste (salty and sweet), metallic taste, diarrhea, dysgeusia, *hypogeusia.*

Hematologic: eosinophilia, leukopenia, ***thrombocytopenia, aplastic anemia, agranulocytosis,*** thrombotic thrombocytopenic purpura, hemolytic anemia or iron deficiency anemia, lupus-like syndrome, bone marrow suppression.

Hepatic: cholestatic jaundice, ***pancreatitis,*** hepatic dysfunction.

Respiratory: pneumonitis, Goodpasture's syndrome.

Musculoskeletal: arthralgia, myasthenia gravis (with prolonged use).

Skin: *pruritus; erythematous rash;* intensely pruritic rash with scaly, macular lesions on trunk; pemphigoid reactions; urticaria; ***exfoliative dermatitis;*** increased skin friability; purpuric or vesicular ecchymoses; wrinkling.

Other: *proteinuria,* lymphadenopathy, alopecia, drug fever, thyroiditis.

Note: Discontinue drug if patient has signs of hypersensitivity or drug fever, usually in conjunction with other allergic signs and symptoms (if Wilson's disease, may rechallenge); or if the following occur: rash developing 6 months or more after start of therapy; pemphigoid reaction; hematuria or proteinuria with hemoptysis or pulmonary infiltrates; gross or persistent microscopic hematuria or proteinuria greater than 2 g/day in patients with rheumatoid arthritis; platelet count less than 100,000/mm^3 or leukocyte count less than 3,500/mm^3, or if either shows three consecutive decreases, even within normal range.

Overdose and treatment

There are no reports of significant drug overdose. Induce emesis unless unconscious or gag reflex is absent; otherwise empty stomach by gastric lavage and then administer activated charcoal and sorbitol. Thereafter, treat supportively. Treat seizures with diazepam (or pyridoxine if previously successful). Hemodialysis will remove penicillamine.

Clinical considerations

□ ***ALERT*** Beware of sound-alikes: There are various types of penicillin, plus polycillin and penicillamine. Don't confuse these various drugs.

- About one-third of patients receiving drug experience an allergic reaction. Monitor patient for signs and symptoms of allergic reaction.

■ Patients with Wilson's disease or cystinuria may require daily pyridoxine (vitamin B_6) supplementation.
■ Prescribe drug to be taken 1 hour before or 2 hours after meals or other medications to facilitate absorption.
■ For initial treatment of Wilson's disease, administer 10 to 40 mg of sulfurated potash with each meal during penicillamine therapy for 6 months to 1 year; then it should be discontinued.

Therapeutic monitoring
■ Recommend performing urinalyses and CBC including differential blood count every 2 weeks for 6 months, then monthly.
■ Recommend performing kidney and liver functions studies, usually every 6 months.
■ Report fever or allergic reactions, such as rash, joint pain, and easy bruising, immediately. Check routinely for proteinuria, and handle patient carefully to avoid skin damage.

Special populations
Breast-feeding patients. Safety hasn't been established in breast-feeding patients; alternative feeding method is recommended during therapy.
Pediatric patients. Check for possible iron deficiency resulting from chronic use. Safety and efficacy of penicillamine in juvenile rheumatoid arthritis haven't yet been established.
Geriatric patients. Lower doses may be indicated. Monitor renal and hepatic function closely. Toxicity may be more common in the elderly.

Patient counseling
■ Provide health education for patients with Wilson's disease, rheumatoid arthritis, or cystinuria. Explain disease process and rationale for therapy and explain that clinical results may not be evident for 3 months.
■ Stress importance of immediate reporting of fever, chills, sore throat, bruising, bleeding, or allergic reaction.
■ Tell patient to take drug on an empty stomach 30 minutes to 1 hour before meals or 2 hours after ingesting food, antacids, mineral supplements, vitamins, or other medications. Tell patient to drink large amounts of water, especially at night.
■ Advise patient taking penicillamine for Wilson's disease to maintain a low-copper (less than 2 mg daily) diet by excluding foods with high copper content, such as chocolate, nuts, liver, and broccoli. Also, sulfurated potash may be administered with meals to minimize copper absorption.
■ Advise patient receiving drug for rheumatoid arthritis that an exacerbation of disease may occur during therapy. This usually can be controlled by concurrent use of NSAIDs.

penicillin G benzathine
Bicillin L-A, Megacillin, Permapen

penicillin G benzathine and procaine
Bicillin C-R

penicillin G potassium
Pfizerpen

penicillin G procaine
Ayercillin*, Bicillin C-R, Crysticillin A.S., Pfizerpen-AS, Wycillin

penicillin G sodium

Pharmacologic classification: natural penicillin
Therapeutic classification: antibiotic
Pregnancy risk category B

How supplied
Available by prescription only
penicillin G benzathine
Suspension: 250,000 units/5 ml*; 500,000 units/ml*
Injection: 300,000 units/ml; 600,000 units/ml; 1.2 million units/2 ml; 2.4 million units/4 ml
penicillin G benzathine and procaine
Injection: 300,000 units/ml; 600,000 units/ml; 1.2 million units/2 ml; 2.4 million units/4 ml
penicillin G potassium
Powder for injection: 1 million units, 5 million units, 10 million units, 20 million units
Injection (premixed, frozen): 1 million units/50 ml, 2 million units/50 ml, 3 million units/50 ml
penicillin G procaine
Injection: 600,000 units/ml, 1.2 million units/2 ml, 2.4 million units/2 ml
penicillin G sodium
Powder for injection: 1 million units*, 5 million units, 10 million units*

Indications and dosages
Congenital syphilis
penicillin G benzathine
Children under age 2: 50,000 units/kg I.M. as a single injection.
Group A streptococcal upper respiratory infections, ◇diphtheria, ◇yaws, pinta, and bejel
penicillin G benzathine
Adults: 1.2 million units I.M. as a single injection.
Children weighing 60 lb (27 kg) or more: 900,000 units I.M. in a single injection.
Children weighing less than 60 lb: 300,000 to 600,000 units I.M. in a single injection.

Prophylaxis of poststreptococcal rheumatic fever
penicillin G benzathine
Adults and children: 1.2 million units I.M. once monthly.
Syphilis of less than 1 year's duration
penicillin G benzathine
Adults: 2.4 million units I.M. in a single dose.
Syphilis of more than 1 year's duration
penicillin G benzathine
Adults: 2.4 million units I.M. weekly for 3 successive weeks.
Moderate to severe systemic infections
penicillin G potassium, sodium
Adults: 12 to 24 million units I.M. or I.V. daily, given in divided doses q 4 hours.
Children: 25,000 to 300,000 units/kg I.M. or I.V. daily, given in divided doses q 4 hours.
Moderate to severe systemic infections, pneumococcal pneumonia
penicillin G procaine
Adults: 600,000 to 1.2 million units I.M. daily as a single dose or q 6 to 12 hours.
Children: 300,000 units I.M. daily as a single dose.
Uncomplicated gonorrhea
penicillin G procaine
Adults and children over age 12: 1 g probenecid, P.O. then 30 minutes later, 4.8 million units of penicillin G procaine I.M., divided into two injection sites.
≡ ***Dosage adjustment.*** For patients with renal failure, refer to following dosing chart.

Creatinine clearance (ml/min)	Dosage (after full loading dose)
10 to 50	50% of usual dose q 4 to 5 hr; or, give usual dose q 8 to 12 hr
< 10	50% of usual dose q 8 to 12 hr; or, give usual dose q 12 to 18 hr

Pharmacodynamics

Antibiotic action: Penicillin G is bactericidal; it adheres to penicillin-binding proteins, inhibiting bacterial cell wall synthesis. Penicillin G's spectrum of activity includes most nonpenicillinase-producing strains of gram-positive and gram-negative aerobic cocci; spirochetes, and some gram-positive aerobic and anaerobic bacilli.

Pharmacokinetics

Penicillin G is available as four salts, each having the same bactericidal action, but designed to offer greater oral stability (potassium salt) or to prolong duration of action by slowing absorption after I.M. injection (benzathine and procaine salts).
Absorption: Sodium and potassium salts of penicillin G are absorbed rapidly after I.M. injection; peak serum levels occur within 15 to 30 minutes. Absorption of other salts is slower. Peak serum levels of penicillin G procaine occur at 1 to 4 hours, with drug detectable in serum for 1 to 2 days; peak serum levels of penicillin G benzathine occur at 13 to 24 hours, with serum levels detectable for 1 to 4 weeks.
Distribution: Distributed widely into synovial, pleural, pericardial, and ascitic fluids and bile, and into liver, skin, lungs, kidneys, muscle, intestines, tonsils, maxillary sinuses, saliva, and erythrocytes. CSF penetration is poor but is enhanced in patients with inflamed meninges. Penicillin G crosses the placenta; it is 45% to 68% protein-bound.
Metabolism: Between 16% and 30% of an I.M. dose of penicillin G is metabolized to inactive compounds.
Excretion: Excreted primarily in urine by tubular secretion; 20% to 60% of dose is recovered in 6 hours. Some drug is excreted in breast milk. Elimination half-life in adults is about ½ to 1 hour. Severe renal impairment prolongs half-life; penicillin G is removed by hemodialysis and is only minimally removed by peritoneal dialysis.

Route	Onset	Peak	Duration
I.V, I.M.	Varies	Varies	Varies

Contraindications and precautions

Contraindicated in patients with hypersensitivity to drug or other penicillins. Use cautiously in patients with drug allergies (especially to cephalosporins or imipenem). Penicillin G potassium is contraindicated in patients with renal failure.

Interactions

Drug-drug. *Aminoglycosides:* Produce synergistic therapeutic effects; however, drugs are physically and chemically incompatible and are inactivated when mixed or given together. Don't use together.
Clavulanate: Appears to enhance effect of penicillin G against certain beta-lactamase-producing bacteria. Monitor patient.
Heparin or oral anticoagulants: May increase the risk of bleeding. Monitor patient and PT/INR closely.
Methotrexate: Delayed elimination and elevating serum levels of methotrexate. Don't use together.
NSAIDs: Prolong penicillin half-life. Monitor patient closely.
Oral contraceptives: Penicillins may decrease effectiveness. Advise patient to use alternative method of birth control.
Potassium-sparing diuretics: Use with penicillin may cause hyperkalemia. Monitor patient.
Probenecid: Blocks tubular secretion of penicillin, increasing its serum levels. Monitor patient closely.

Sulfinpyrazone: Prolongs penicillin half-life. Monitor patient closely.

Effects on diagnostic tests

Penicillin G alters test results for urine and serum protein levels; it interferes with turbidimetric methods using sulfosalicylic acid, trichloracetic acid, acetic acid, and nitric acid. Penicillin G doesn't interfere with tests using bromophenol blue (Albustix, Albutest, Multistix).

Penicillin G alters urine glucose testing using cupric sulfate (Benedict's reagent); use Diastix, Chemstrip uG, or glucose enzymatic test strip instead. Penicillin G may cause falsely elevated results of urine specific gravity tests in patients with low urine output and dehydration, and falsely elevated Norymberski and Zimmermann test results for 17-ketogenic steroids; it causes false-positive CSF protein test results (Folin-Ciocalteau method) and may cause positive Coombs' test results.

Penicillin G may falsely decrease serum aminoglycoside levels. Adding beta-lactamase to the sample inactivates the penicillin, rendering the assay more accurate. Alternatively, the sample can be spun down and frozen immediately after collection.

Adverse reactions

CNS: neuropathy, ***seizures*** (with high doses), lethargy, hallucinations, anxiety, confusion, agitation, depression, dizziness, fatigue.
GI: nausea, vomiting, enterocolitis, pseudomembranous colitis.
GU: interstitial nephritis, nephropathy.
Hematologic: eosinophilia, hemolytic anemia, ***thrombocytopenia,*** leukopenia, anemia, ***agranulocytosis.***
Other: hypersensitivity reactions (maculopapular and ***exfoliative dermatitis,*** chills, fever, edema, ***anaphylaxis),*** pain and sterile abscess at injection site; overgrowth of nonsusceptible organisms (with penicillin G potassium and procaine); possible severe potassium poisoning with high doses (hyperreflexia, ***seizures, coma),*** thrombophlebitis (with penicillin G potassium only).

Overdose and treatment

Signs of overdose include neuromuscular irritability or seizures. No specific recommendations are available. Penicillin G can be removed by hemodialysis.

Clinical considerations

□ ***ALERT*** Beware of sound-alikes: There are various types of penicillin, plus polycillin and penicillamine. Don't confuse these various drugs.
□ ***ALERT*** Penicillin G benzathine, penicillin G procaine: Never give I.V. Inadvertent I.V. administration has caused cardiac arrest and death.
Consider the recommendations relevant to all penicillins as well as the following:

- Have emergency equipment on hand to manage possible anaphylaxis.
- Because penicillins are dialyzable, patients undergoing hemodialysis may need dosage adjustments.
- Administer by deep I.M. injection in upper outer quadrant of buttock. In infants and small children, use the midlateral aspect of thigh.
- Drug can be administered as a continuous infusion for meningitis.

Therapeutic monitoring

- Monitor patient closely for possible hypernatremia with sodium salt or hyperkalemia with potassium salt.
- Patients with poor renal function are predisposed to high blood levels, which may cause seizures. Monitor renal function.

Special populations

Breast-feeding patients. Drug is excreted in breast milk; use in breast-feeding women may sensitize infant to penicillin.
Geriatric patients. Half-life is prolonged in geriatric patients because of impaired renal function.

Patient counseling

- Tell patient to report adverse reactions promptly.
- Warn patient that I.M. injection may be painful, but that ice may be applied to the site to ease discomfort.

penicillin V

penicillin V potassium

Betapen-VK, Ledercillin VK, Nadopen-V*, Pen Vee K, PVF K*, V-Cillin K, Veetids

Pharmacologic classification: natural penicillin
Therapeutic classification: antibiotic
Pregnancy risk category B

How supplied

Available by prescription only
penicillin V
Tablets: 250 mg, 500 mg
Solution: 125 mg/5 ml, 250 mg/5 ml (after reconstitution)
penicillin V potassium
Tablets: 125 mg, 250 mg, 500 mg
Tablets (film-coated): 250 mg, 500 mg
Solution: 125 mg/5 ml, 250 mg/5 ml (after reconstitution)

Indications and dosages

Mild to moderate susceptible infections
Adults and children age 12 and older: 125 to 500 mg (200,000 to 800,000 units) P.O. q 6 hours.

Children age 1 month to 12 years: 15 to 56 mg/kg P.O. daily, divided into doses given q 6 to 8 hours.

Endocarditis prophylaxis for dental surgery

Adults: 2 g P.O. 30 to 60 minutes before procedure, then 1 g 6 hours later.

Children weighing less than 66 lb (30 kg): Half the adult dose.

Necrotizing ulcerative gingivitis

Adults: 250 to 500 mg P.O. q 6 to 8 hours.

◊***Lyme disease***

Adults: 250 to 500 mg P.O. q.i.d. for 10 to 20 days.

◊***Prophylaxis for pneumococcal infection***

Adults: 250 mg P.O. b.i.d.

Children over age 5: 125 mg P.O. b.i.d.

Pharmacodynamics

Antibiotic action: Penicillin V is bactericidal; it adheres to penicillin-binding proteins, inhibiting bacterial cell wall synthesis. Penicillin V's spectrum of activity includes most non-penicillinase-producing strains of gram-positive and gram-negative aerobic cocci; spirochetes; and some gram-positive aerobic and anaerobic bacilli.

Pharmacokinetics

Absorption: Has greater acid stability and is absorbed more completely than penicillin G after oral administration. About 60% to 75% of an oral dose of penicillin V is absorbed.

Distribution: Distributed widely into synovial, pleural, pericardial, and ascitic fluids and bile, and into liver, skin, lungs, kidneys, muscle, intestines, tonsils, maxillary sinuses, saliva, and erythrocytes. CSF penetration is poor but is enhanced in patients with inflamed meninges. Penicillin V crosses the placenta, and is 75% to 89% protein-bound.

Metabolism: Between 35% and 70% of a dose is metabolized to inactive compounds.

Excretion: Excreted primarily in urine by tubular secretion; 26% to 65% of dose is recovered in 6 hours. Some drug is excreted in breast milk. Elimination half-life in adults is ½ hour. Severe renal impairment prolongs half-life.

Route	Onset	Peak	Duration
P.O.	Unknown	½-1 hr	Unknown

Contraindications and precautions

Contraindicated in patients with hypersensitivity to drug or other penicillins. Use cautiously in patients with drug allergies (especially to cephalosporins or imipenem).

Interactions

Drug-drug. *Aminoglycosides:* Drugs are physically and chemically incompatible and are inactivated when given together. Avoid use together.

Anticoagulants and heparin: Can increase risk of bleeding. Monitor patient and PT and INR closely.

Estrogen-containing oral contraceptives: Efficacy may be decreased. Recommend additional form of contraceptive during penicillin therapy.

Probenecid: Higher serum levels of penicillin. Probenecid may be used for this purpose.

Sulfinpyrazone: Prolongs penicillin half-life. Monitor patient closely.

Effects on diagnostic tests

Penicillin V alters test results for urine and serum protein levels; it interferes with turbidimetric methods using sulfosalicylic acid, trichloracetic acid, acetic acid, and nitric acid. Penicillin V doesn't interfere with tests using bromophenol blue (Albustix, Albutest, Multistix). Penicillin V may falsely decrease serum aminoglycoside levels.

Adverse reactions

CNS: neuropathy.

GI: *epigastric distress,* vomiting, diarrhea, *nausea,* black "hairy" tongue.

GU: nephropathy.

Hematologic: eosinophilia, hemolytic anemia, leukopenia, ***thrombocytopenia.***

Other: hypersensitivity reactions (rash, urticaria, fever, laryngeal edema, ***anaphylaxis),*** overgrowth of nonsusceptible organisms.

Overdose and treatment

Signs of overdose include neuromuscular sensitivity or seizures. No specific recommendations are available. Treatment is supportive. After recent ingestion (within 4 hours), empty stomach by induced emesis or gastric lavage; follow with activated charcoal to reduce absorption.

Clinical considerations

□ ***ALERT*** Beware of sound-alikes; there are various types of penicillin, plus polycillin and penicillamine. Don't confuse these various drugs.

Consider the recommendations relevant to all penicillins as well as the following:

- Give oral dose 1 hour before or 2 hours after meals for maximum absorption.
- After reconstitution, oral solution is stable for 14 days if refrigerated.

Therapeutic monitoring

With large doses or prolonged therapy, bacterial or fungal superinfection may occur.

Special populations

Breast-feeding patients. Penicillin V is excreted in breast milk; use in breast-feeding women may sensitize the infant to penicillins.

Geriatric patients. Half-life may be prolonged in geriatric patients because of impaired renal function.

Patient counseling

- Instruct patient to take entire amount of medication exactly as prescribed, even if he feels better.
- Advise patient to report rash, fever, or chills.

pentamidine isethionate

NebuPent, Pentacarinat, Pentam 300

Pharmacologic classification: diamidine derivative
Therapeutic classification: antiprotozoal
Pregnancy risk category C

How supplied

Available by prescription only
Injection: 300-mg vials
Solution for inhalation: 300 mg

Indications and dosages

***Pneumonia caused by* Pneumocystis carinii**
Adults and children over age 4 months: 3 to 4 mg/kg I.V. once a day for 14 to 21 days.
◇ ***Primary or secondary prevention of* P. carinii *pneumonia***
Adults and children: 300 mg by inhalation once q 4 weeks. Aerosol form of drug should be administered by the Respirgard II jet nebulizer.
◇ ***Trypanosomiasis***
Adults: 4 mg/kg I.M. once daily for 10 days. Alternatively, 3 to 4 mg/kg I.V. once daily or every other day, to a total of 7 to 10 doses.
◇ ***Leishmaniasis***
Adults: 2 to 4 mg/kg I.M. daily or every other day up to 15 doses. Alternatively, 4 mg/kg I.V. 3 times weekly for 5 to 25 weeks or longer, depending on response.

Pharmacodynamics

Antiprotozoal action: Mechanism is unknown. However, pentamidine may work by inhibiting synthesis of RNA, DNA, proteins, or phospholipids. It may also interfere with several metabolic processes, particularly certain energy-yielding reactions and reactions involving folic acid. Spectrum of activity includes *P. carinii* and *Trypanosoma* organisms.

Pharmacokinetics

Absorption: Daily I.M. doses (4 mg/kg) produce surprisingly few plasma level fluctuations. Little information exists regarding pharmacokinetics with I.V. administration. Absorption is limited after aerosol administration.
Distribution: Appears to be extensively tissue-bound. CNS penetration is poor. Extent of plasma protein-binding is unknown.
Metabolism: Unknown.
Excretion: Mostly unchanged in urine. Tissue-binding may explain drug's appearance in urine 6 to 8 weeks after therapy ends.

Route	Onset	Peak	Duration
I.V.	Unknown	1 hr	Unknown
I.M., Inhalation	Unknown	½ hr	Unknown

Contraindications and precautions

Contraindicated in patients with a history of hypersensitivity to drug. Use cautiously in patients with hepatic or renal dysfunction, hypertension, hypotension, hyperglycemia, hypoglycemia, hypocalcemia, leukopenia, thrombocytopenia, or anemia. Use with caution in patients with ventricular tachycardia, pancreatitis, or Stevens-Johnson syndrome.

Interactions

Drug-drug. *Aminoglycosides, amphotericin B, capreomycin, cisplatin, colistin, foscarnet, methoxyflurane, polymyxin B, vancomycin:* Pentamidine may have additive nephrotoxic effects. Closely monitor patient; avoid use together if possible.

Effects on diagnostic tests

None reported.

Adverse reactions

CNS: confusion, hallucinations, *fatigue, dizziness,* headache.
CV: *hypotension,* ***ventricular tachycardia,*** chest pain.
GI: nausea, metallic taste, decreased appetite, pharyngitis, vomiting, diarrhea, abdominal pain, anorexia, bad taste in mouth.
GU: *elevated serum creatinine, acute renal failure.*
Hematologic: ***leukopenia, thrombocytopenia,*** anemia.
Hepatic: elevated liver function tests.
Metabolic: ketoacidosis, *hypoglycemia,* hyperglycemia, hyperkalemia, hypocalcemia, hypomagnesemia.
Musculoskeletal: myalgia.
Respiratory: *cough,* ***bronchospasm,*** *shortness of breath, congestion,* pneumothorax.
Skin: *rash, sterile abscess,* ***Stevens-Johnson syndrome.***
Other: anaphylactoid reaction, *pain or induration at injection site, night sweats, chills,* edema.

Overdose and treatment

No information available.

Clinical considerations

□ ***ALERT*** To minimize risk of hypotension, patient should be supine during I.V. administration. Because sudden, severe hypotension may develop after I.M. injection or during I.V.

infusion, closely monitor blood pressure during infusion and several times thereafter until patient is stable.
- Keep emergency drugs and equipment, including emergency airway, vasopressors, and I.V. fluids, on hand.
- Make sure patient is adequately hydrated before administering drug; dehydration may lead to hypotension and renal toxicity.
- To minimize risk of hypotensive reactions during I.V. administration, give infusions over 1 to 2 hours. To prepare drug for I.V. infusion, add 3 to 5 ml of sterile water for injection or D_5W at 72° to 86° F (22° to 30° C) to 300-mg vial to yield 100 mg/ml or 60 mg/ml, respectively. Withdraw desired dose and dilute further into 50 to 250 ml of D_5W; infuse over at least 60 minutes. Diluted solution remains stable for 48 hours.
- To prepare drug for I.M. injection, add 3 ml of sterile water for injection at at 72° to 86° F (22° to 30° C) to 300-mg vial to yield 100 mg/ml. Withdraw desired dose and inject deep I.M.
- When inhalation solution is used for prophylaxis against PCP, high-risk individuals include patients infected with HIV with a history of PCP; patients who have never had an episode of PCP but whose $CD4^+$ T cells are less than 20% of total lymphocytes; or whose $CD4^+$ T-cell count is less than $200/mm^3$.
- To administer by inhalation, dilute dose in 6 ml of sterile water and deliver at 6 L/minute from a 50-p.s.i. compressed air source until reservoir is dry. Alternate delivery systems (other than the Respirgard II) are under investigation but are currently not recommended.
- If wheezing or cough develops during pentamidine aerosol therapy, patient may benefit by pretreatment with a bronchodilator at least 5 minutes before pentamidine administration.

Therapeutic monitoring
- Monitor daily blood glucose, BUN, and serum creatinine levels.
- Monitor periodic electrolyte levels, CBC, platelet count, and liver function tests.
- Observe patient for signs and symptoms of hypoglycemia.

Special populations
Pregnant patients. Avoid using aerosol form in pregnant women.
Breast-feeding patients. It isn't known if drug is distributed in breast milk.
Pediatric patients. Safety and efficacy of inhalation therapy haven't been clearly established in children age 16 or under.

Patient counseling
- Instruct patient to use aerosol device until the chamber is empty; this may take up to 45 minutes.
- Instruct patient to complete the full course of therapy, even if he feels better.

pentazocine hydrochloride
Talwin*, Talwin-Nx (with naloxone hydrochloride)

pentazocine lactate
Talwin

Pharmacologic classification: narcotic agonist-antagonist, opioid partial agonist
Therapeutic classification: analgesic, adjunct to anesthesia
Controlled substance schedule IV
Pregnancy risk category NR (C for Talwin-Nx)

How supplied
Available by prescription only
Tablets: 50 mg
Injection: 30 mg/ml

Indications and dosages
Moderate to severe pain
Adults: 50 to 100 mg P.O. q 3 to 4 hours, p.r.n., or around the clock. Maximum oral dose, 600 mg daily. Or, 30 mg I.M., I.V., or S.C. q 3 to 4 hours, p.r.n., or around the clock. Maximum parenteral dose, 360 mg daily. Doses above 30 mg I.V. or 60 mg I.M. or S.C. not recommended.

For patients in labor, give 30 mg I.M. or 20 mg I.V. in 2- to 3-hour intervals.

Pharmacodynamics
Analgesic action: Exact mechanism of action is unknown. It's believed to be a competitive antagonist at some receptors, and an agonist at others, resulting in relief of moderate pain.

Pentazocine can produce respiratory depression, sedation, miosis, and antitussive effects. It also may cause psychotomimetic and dysphoric effects. In patients with coronary artery disease, it elevates mean aortic pressure, left ventricular end-diastolic pressure, and mean pulmonary artery pressure. In patients with acute MI, I.V. pentazocine increases systemic and pulmonary arterial pressures and systemic vascular resistance.

Pharmacokinetics
Absorption: Well absorbed after oral or parenteral administration. However, orally administered drug undergoes first-pass metabolism in the liver and less than 20% of a dose reaches the systemic circulation unchanged. Bioavailability is increased in patients with hepatic dysfunction; patients with cirrhosis absorb 60% to 70% of drug.
Distribution: Appears to be widely distributed in the body.
Metabolism: Metabolized in the liver, mainly by oxidation and secondarily by glucuronida-

tion. Metabolism may be prolonged in patients with impaired hepatic function.
Excretion: Duration of effect is 3 hours. There's considerable interpatient variability in its urinary excretion. Small amounts of drug are excreted in feces after oral or parenteral administration.

Route	Onset	Peak	Duration
P.O.	15-30 min	1-3 hr	2-3 hr
I.V.	2-3 min	15-30 min	2-3 hr
I.M., S.C.	10-20 min	30-60 min	2-3 hr

Contraindications and precautions

Contraindicated in patients with hypersensitivity to drug or its components and in children under age 12. Use cautiously in patients with impaired renal or hepatic function, acute MI, head injury, increased intracranial pressure, or respiratory depression.

Interactions

Drug-drug. *Barbiturates such as thiopental:* Pentazocine may produce additive CNS and respiratory depressant effects and, possibly, apnea. Use together cautiously.
Cimetidine: May increase pentazocine toxicity. Monitor patient closely.
General anesthetics: May cause severe CV depression. Use together cautiously.
Narcotic agonist-antagonists: Patient may become physically dependent on pentazocine. Use with caution; monitor closely.
Other CNS depressants, such as antihistamines, barbiturates, benzodiazepines, muscle relaxants, narcotic analgesics, phenothiazines, sedative-hypnotics, and tricyclic antidepressants: Potentiates respiratory and CNS depression of drug; reduced doses of pentazocine usually are necessary.
Drug-lifestyle. *Alcohol use:* Potentiates respiratory and CNS depression of drug. Discourage patient from alcohol use during therapy.

Effects on diagnostic tests

None reported.

Adverse reactions

CNS: *sedation,* visual disturbances, hallucinations, drowsiness, *dizziness, light-headedness,* confusion, *euphoria,* headache, syncope, psychotomimetic effects.
CV: circulatory depression, ***shock,*** hypertension, hypotension.
EENT: dry mouth, blurred vision, nystagmus.
GI: *nausea, vomiting,* constipation, taste alteration.
GU: urine retention.
Hematologic: WBC depression.
Respiratory: ***respiratory depression,*** dyspnea, apnea.
Skin: induration, nodules, sloughing, and sclerosis of injection site; diaphoresis; pruritus.
Other: hypersensitivity reactions ***(anaphylaxis),*** physical and psychological dependence.

Overdose and treatment

The signs of pentazocine hydrochloride overdose haven't been defined because of a lack of clinical experience with overdose. If overdose should occur, use all supportive measures (oxygen, I.V. fluids, vasopressors) as necessary. Consider mechanical ventilation. Parenteral naloxone is an effective antagonist for respiratory depression because of pentazocine.

Clinical considerations

Consider the recommendations relevant to all opioid (narcotic) agonist-antagonists as well as the following:

- Tablets aren't well absorbed.
- Don't mix in same syringe with soluble barbiturates.
- Drug possesses narcotic antagonist properties. May precipitate abstinence syndrome in narcotic-dependent patients.
- Talwin-Nx, the available oral pentazocine, contains the narcotic antagonist naloxone, which prevents illicit I.V. use.
- Use S.C. route only when necessary. Severe tissue damage is possible at injection site.

Therapeutic monitoring

- Pentazocine may obscure the signs and symptoms of an acute abdominal condition or worsen gallbladder pain.
- Drug may cause orthostatic hypotension in ambulatory patients. Have patient sit down to relieve symptoms.

Special populations

Breast-feeding patients. It's unknown if drug is excreted in breast milk; use with caution in breast-feeding women.
Pediatric patients. Use of drug isn't recommended in children under age 12.
Geriatric patients. Lower doses are usually indicated for geriatric patients, who may be more sensitive to the therapeutic and adverse effects of drug.

Patient counseling

- Tell patient to report rash, confusion, disorientation, or other serious adverse effects.
- Warn patient that Talwin-Nx is for oral use only. Severe reactions may result if tablets are crushed, dissolved, and injected.

pentobarbital sodium

Nembutal

Pharmacologic classification: barbiturate
Therapeutic classification: anticonvulsant, sedative-hypnotic
Controlled substance schedule II (suppositories schedule III)
Pregnancy risk category D

How supplied

Available by prescription only
Elixir: 18.2 mg/5 ml
Capsules: 50 mg, 100 mg
Injection: 50 mg/ml, 1-ml and 2-ml disposable syringes; 2-ml, 20-ml, and 50-ml vials
Suppositories: 30 mg, 60 mg, 120 mg, 200 mg

Indications and dosages

Sedation
Adults: 20 to 40 mg P.O. b.i.d., t.i.d., or q.i.d.
Children: 2 to 6 mg/kg P.O. daily in divided doses, to maximum of 100 mg/dose.
Insomnia
Adults: 100 mg P.O. h.s. or 150 to 200 mg deep I.M.; 120 to 200 mg P.R.
Children: 2 to 6 mg/kg I.M., up to maximum of 100 mg/dose. Or 30 mg P.R. (age 2 months to 1 year), 30 to 60 mg P.R. (age 1 to 4), 60 mg P.R. (age 5 to 12), 60 to 120 mg P.R. (age 12 to 14).
Preanesthetic medication
Adults: 150 to 200 mg I.M. or P.O. in two divided doses.
Seizures
Adults: Initially, 100 mg I.V.; after 1 minute, additional doses may be given, up to a total of from 200 to 500 mg I.V. Maximum dose, 500 mg.
Children: 50 mg initially; after 1 minute additional small doses may be given until desired effect is obtained.

Pharmacodynamics

Sedative-hypnotic action: Exact cellular site and mechanisms of action are unknown. Pentobarbital acts throughout the CNS as a nonselective depressant with a fast onset of action and short duration of action. Particularly sensitive to this drug is the reticular activating system, which controls CNS arousal. Pentobarbital decreases both presynaptic and postsynaptic membrane excitability by facilitating the action of gamma-aminobutyric acid (GABA).
Anticonvulsant action: Pentobarbital suppresses the spread of seizure activity produced by epileptogenic foci in the cortex, thalamus, and limbic systems by enhancing the effect of GABA. Both presynaptic and postsynaptic excitability are decreased, and the seizure threshold is raised.

Pharmacokinetics

Absorption: Absorbed rapidly after oral or rectal administration. Serum levels needed for sedation and hypnosis are 1 to 5 mcg/ml and 5 to 15 mcg/ml, respectively.
Distribution: Distributed widely throughout the body. About 35% to 45% is protein-bound. Drug accumulates in fat with long-term use.
Metabolism: Metabolized in the liver by penultimate oxidation.
Excretion: About 99% of pentobarbital is eliminated as glucuronide conjugates and other metabolites in the urine. Terminal half-life ranges from 35 to 50 hours. Duration of action is 3 to 4 hours.

Route	Onset	Peak	Duration
P.O.	20 min	½-1 hr	1-4 hr
I.V.	Immediate	Immediate	15 min
I.M.	10-25 min	Unknown	Unknown
P.R.	20 min	Unknown	1-4 hr

Contraindications and precautions

Contraindicated in patients with hypersensitivity to barbiturates or porphyria or with severe respiratory disease when dyspnea or obstruction is evident. Use cautiously in geriatric or debilitated patients and in those with acute or chronic pain, mental depression, suicidal tendencies, history of drug abuse, or impaired hepatic function.

Interactions

Drug-drug. *Antidepressants, antihistamines, narcotics, sedative-hypnotics, tranquilizers:* Pentobarbital may potentiate or add to CNS and respiratory depressant effects. Use together cautiously.
Corticosteroids, digitoxin (not digoxin), doxycycline, oral contraceptives and other estrogens, theophylline and other xanthines: Enhanced hepatic metabolism of these drugs. Monitor patient closely.
Disulfiram, MAO inhibitors, valproic acid: Decrease metabolism of pentobarbital and increase its toxicity. Barbiturate dose may need adjustment.
Griseofulvin: Decreased absorption of griseofulvin. Monitor effectiveness of griseofulvin.
Rifampin: May decrease pentobarbital levels by increasing hepatic metabolism. Avoid use together.
Warfarin and other oral anticoagulants: Pentobarbital enhances the enzymatic degradation. Patients may require increased doses of the anticoagulants.
Drug-herb: *Kava:* May cause additive effects. Avoid use together.
Drug-lifestyle. *Alcohol use:* Pentobarbital may potentiate or add to CNS and respiratory depressant effects. Advise patient to avoid alcohol use.

Effects on diagnostic tests

Pentobarbital may cause a false-positive phentolamine test. Physiologic effects of drug may impair the absorption of cyanocobalamin ^{57}Co; it may decrease serum bilirubin levels in neonates, epileptic patients, and patients with congenital nonhemolytic unconjugated hyperbilirubinemia. EEG patterns show a change in low-voltage, fast activity; changes persist for a time after discontinuation of therapy.

Adverse reactions

CNS: *drowsiness, lethargy, hangover,* paradoxical excitement in elderly patients, somnolence, syncope, hallucinations.
CV: bradycardia, hypotension.
GI: nausea, vomiting.
Hematologic: exacerbation of porphyria.
Respiratory: ***respiratory depression.***
Skin: rash, urticaria, **STEVENS-JOHNSON SYNDROME.**
Other: ***angioedema,*** physical and psychological dependence.

Overdose and treatment

Signs and symptoms of overdose include unsteady gait, slurred speech, sustained nystagmus, somnolence, confusion, respiratory depression, pulmonary edema, areflexia, and coma. Typical shock syndrome with tachycardia and hypotension may occur. Jaundice, hypothermia followed by fever, and oliguria also may occur. Serum levels greater than 10 mcg/ml may produce profound coma; levels greater than 30 mcg/ml may be fatal.

To treat, maintain and support ventilation and pulmonary function as necessary; support cardiac function and circulation with vasopressors and I.V. fluids, as needed. If patient is conscious and gag reflex is intact, induce emesis (if ingestion was recent) by administering ipecac syrup. If emesis is contraindicated, perform gastric lavage while a cuffed endotracheal tube is in place to prevent aspiration. Follow with administration of activated charcoal or sodium chloride cathartic. Measure intake and output, vital signs, and laboratory parameters. Maintain body temperature.

Alkalinization of urine may be helpful in removing drug from the body. Hemodialysis may be useful in severe overdose.

Clinical considerations

Consider the recommendations relevant to all barbiturates as well as the following:

- Reserve I.V. injection for emergency treatment. Be prepared for emergency resuscitative measures.
- Avoid I.V. administration at a rate exceeding 50 mg/minute to prevent hypotension and respiratory depression.
- High-dose therapy for elevated intracranial pressure may require mechanically assisted ventilation.
- Administer I.M. dose deep into large muscle mass. Don't administer more than 5 ml into any one site.
- Discard solution that's discolored or contains precipitate.
- Administration of full loading doses over short periods of time to treat status epilepticus will require ventilatory support in adults.
- To ensure accuracy of dosage, don't divide suppositories.
- Nembutal tablets contain tartrazine dye, which may cause allergic reactions in susceptible persons.
- To prevent rebound of rapid-eye-movement sleep after prolonged therapy, discontinue gradually over 5 to 6 days.

Therapeutic monitoring

- Inspect patient's skin. Skin eruptions may precede potentially fatal reactions to barbiturate therapy.
- In some patients, high fever, stomatitis, headache or rhinitis may precede skin eruptions.

Special populations

Pregnant patients. Advise pregnant women of potential hazard to fetus or neonate when taking pentobarbital late in pregnancy. Withdrawal symptoms can occur.
Breast-feeding patients. Pentobarbital is excreted in breast milk. Don't administer to breast-feeding women.
Pediatric patients. Barbiturates may cause paradoxical excitement in children. Use with caution.
Geriatric patients. Usually require lower doses because of increased susceptibility to CNS depressant effects of pentobarbital. Confusion, disorientation, and excitability may occur in geriatric patients. Use with caution.

Patient counseling

- Tell patient not to take drug continuously for longer than 2 weeks.
- Drug has no analgesic effect and may cause restlessness or delirium in patients with pain.
- Caution patient about performing activities that require mental alertness or physical coordination.

pentostatin (2′-deoxycoformycin; DCF)

Nipent

Pharmacologic classification: antimetabolite (adenosine deaminase inhibitor)
Therapeutic classification: antineoplastic
Pregnancy risk category D

How supplied

Available by prescription only
Powder for injection: 10 mg/vial

Indications and dosages

Alpha-interferon-refractory hairy cell leukemia
Adults: 4 mg/m^2 I.V. every other week.

Pharmacodynamics

Antileukemic action: Pentostatin inhibits the enzyme adenosine deaminase (ADA), causing an increase in intracellular levels of deoxyadenosine triphosphate. This increase leads to cell damage and death. Because ADA is most active in cells of the lymphoid system (especially malignant T cells), drug is useful in treating leukemias.

Pharmacokinetics

Absorption: Achieves response in 3 to 24 months; duration of pharmacologic action is more than 1 week after a single dose.
Distribution: Plasma protein-binding is low (about 4%); distribution half-life is about 11 minutes.
Metabolism: Unknown.
Excretion: More than 90% is excreted in urine. Clearance depends on renal function; mean terminal half-life is about 6 hours in patients with normal renal function; increases to 18 hours or more in patients with renal impairment (creatinine clearance less than 50 ml/minute).

Route	Onset	Peak	Duration
I.V.	Unknown	Unknown	Unknown

Contraindications and precautions

Contraindicated in patients hypersensitive to drug.

Interactions

Drug-drug. *Fludarabine:* Increases the risk of severe or fatal pulmonary toxicity. Don't use together.
Vidarabine: Increases the incidence or severity of adverse effects associated with either drug. Don't use together.

Effects on diagnostic tests

None reported.

Adverse reactions

CNS: *headache, neurologic symptoms,* anxiety, confusion, depression, dizziness, insomnia, nervousness, paresthesia, somnolence, abnormal thinking, *fatigue.*
CV: ARRHYTHMIAS, abnormal ECG, thrombophlebitis, peripheral edema, HEMORRHAGE.
EENT: abnormal vision, conjunctivitis, ear pain, eye pain, epistaxis, pharyngitis, rhinitis, sinusitis.
GI: *nausea, vomiting, anorexia, diarrhea,* weight loss, constipation, flatulence, stomatitis, abdominal pain.
GU: hematuria, dysuria, increased BUN and creatinine levels.
Hematologic: ***myelosuppression,*** **LEUKOPENIA,** *anemia,* **THROMBOCYTOPENIA,** lymphadenopathy.
Hepatic: *elevated liver enzyme levels.*
Musculoskeletal: myalgia, arthralgia, asthenia.
Respiratory: *cough, bronchitis,* dyspnea, lung edema, pneumonia.
Skin: ecchymosis, petechiae, *rash,* eczema, dry skin, herpes simplex or zoster, maculopapular rash, vesiculobullous rash, pruritus, seborrhea, discoloration, diaphoresis.
Other: *fever,* **INFECTION,** *pain, hypersensitivity reactions, chills,* sepsis, ***death, neoplasm,*** chest pain, back pain, flulike syndrome, malaise.

Overdose and treatment

High dosage of pentostatin (20 to 50 mg/m^2 in divided doses over 5 days) has been associated with deaths from severe CNS, hepatic, pulmonary, and renal toxicity. No specific antidote is known. If overdose occurs, treat symptoms and provide supportive care.

Clinical considerations

- Use drug only in patients who have hairy cell leukemia refractory to alpha interferon, when disease progresses after a minimum of 3 months of treatment with alpha interferon or doesn't respond after 6 months of therapy.
- Optimal duration of therapy is unknown. Current recommendations call for two additional courses of therapy after a complete response. If patient hasn't had a partial response after 6 months of therapy, discontinue drug. If patient has had only a partial response, continue drug for another 6 months; if patient has had a complete response, continue for two courses of therapy.
- Store powder for injection in the refrigerator (36° to 46° F [2° to 8° C]). Use reconstituted and diluted solutions within 8 hours because drug contains no preservative.
- Follow appropriate guidelines for proper handling, administration, and disposal of chemotherapeutic agents. Treat all spills and waste products with 5% sodium hypochlorite solution. Wear protective clothing and polyethylene gloves. To prepare and administer: Add 5 ml sterile water for injection to the vial containing pentostatin powder for injection. Mix thoroughly to make a solution of 5 mg/ml. Administer drug by I.V. bolus injection, or dilute further in 25 or 50 ml of D_5W or normal saline injection and infuse over 20 to 30 minutes.
- Be sure patient is adequately hydrated before therapy. Administer 500 to 1,000 ml of D_5W in 0.45% saline injection. Give 500 ml of D_5W after drug is given.

Therapeutic monitoring

- Before therapy, assess renal function with a serum creatinine or creatinine clearance assay; repeat determinations periodically.

- Perform baseline and periodic determinations of CBC.
- Bone marrow aspirates and biopsies may be required at 2- to 3-month intervals to assess response to treatment.

Special populations

Breast-feeding patients. It isn't known if drug is excreted in breast milk. Because of the risk of serious toxicity to the breast-feeding infant, either the drug or breast-feeding should be discontinued.
Pediatric patients. Safety in children and adolescents hasn't been established.

Patient counseling

- Warn patient to avoid contact with infected persons.
- Tell patient to immediately report signs of infection or unusual bleeding.

pentoxifylline

Trental

Pharmacologic classification: xanthine derivative
Therapeutic classification: hemorrheologic
Pregnancy risk category C

How supplied

Available by prescription only
Tablets (extended-release): 400 mg

Indications and dosages

Intermittent claudication from chronic occlusive vascular disease
Adults: 400 mg P.O. t.i.d. with meals.

Pharmacodynamics

Hemorrheologic action: Pentoxifylline improves capillary blood flow by increasing erythrocyte flexibility and reducing blood viscosity.

Pharmacokinetics

Absorption: Absorbed almost completely from the GI tract but undergoes first-pass hepatic metabolism. Absorption is slowed by food.
Distribution: Unknown; drug is bound to erythrocyte membrane.
Metabolism: Metabolized extensively by erythrocytes and the liver.
Excretion: Metabolites are excreted principally in urine; less than 4% of drug is excreted in feces. Half-life of unchanged drug is about ½ to ¾ hour; half-life of metabolites is about 1 to 1½ hours.

Route	Onset	Peak	Duration
P.O.	Unknown	1 hr	Unknown

Contraindications and precautions

Contraindicated in patients who are intolerant to pentoxifylline or methylxanthines, such as caffeine, theophylline, and theobromine, and in patients with recent cerebral or retinal hemorrhage.

Use cautiously in geriatric patients.

Interactions

Drug-drug. *Antihypertensives:* May increase hypotensive response; blood pressure must be monitored closely.
Oral anticoagulants such as warfarin or drugs that inhibit platelet aggregation: When used with pentoxifylline, may have bleeding abnormalities. Monitor PT and INR.
Theophylline: Levels may increase when given with pentoxifylline. Monitor patient closely.
Drug-lifestyle. *Smoking:* Vasoconstriction may result. Advise patient to avoid smoking, as it may worsen his condition.

Effects on diagnostic tests

None reported.

Adverse reactions

CNS: headache, dizziness.
CV: angina, chest pain.
GI: dyspepsia, nausea, vomiting, flatus, bloating.

Overdose and treatment

Signs of overdose include flushing, hypotension, seizures, somnolence, loss of consciousness, fever, and agitation. There's no known antidote. Empty stomach by gastric lavage and use activated charcoal; treat symptoms and support respiration and blood pressure.

Clinical considerations

- If GI and CNS adverse effects occur, decrease dosage to twice daily. If adverse effects persist, discontinue drug.
- Drug is useful in patients who aren't good candidates for surgery.
- Don't crush or break extended-release tablets; make sure patient swallows them whole.

Therapeutic monitoring

Monitor blood pressure regularly, especially in patients taking antihypertensive agents; also monitor INR, especially in patients taking anticoagulants such as warfarin.

Special populations

Breast-feeding patients. Pentoxifylline enters breast milk. Alternative feeding method is recommended during therapy.
Pediatric patients. Safety and efficacy haven't been established for children under age 18.
Geriatric patients. Geriatric patients may have increased bioavailability and decreased excretion of drug and are at higher risk for toxicity;

adverse reactions may be more common in the elderly.

Patient counseling

- Explain need for continuing therapy for at least 8 weeks; warn patient not to discontinue drug during this period without medical approval.
- Advise patient to take drug with meals to minimize GI distress.
- Tell patient to report GI or CNS adverse reactions; they may require dosage reduction.

pergolide mesylate

Permax

Pharmacologic classification: dopaminergic agonist
Therapeutic classification: antiparkinsonian
Pregnancy risk category B

How supplied

Available by prescription only
Tablets: 0.05 mg, 0.25 mg, 1 mg

Indications and dosages

Adjunct to levodopa-carbidopa in the management of Parkinson's disease
Adults: Initially, 0.05 mg P.O. daily for first 2 days. Gradually increase dosage by 0.1 to 0.15 mg every third day over next 12 days of therapy. Subsequent dosage can be increased by 0.25 mg every third day until optimum response occurs. Mean therapeutic daily dose is 3 mg.

Drug is usually administered in divided doses t.i.d. Gradual reductions in levodopa-carbidopa dosage may be made during dosage adjustment.

Pharmacodynamics

Antiparkinsonian action: Pergolide stimulates dopamine receptors at both D_1 and D_2 sites. It acts by directly stimulating postsynaptic receptors in the nigrostriatal system.

Pharmacokinetics

Absorption: Well absorbed after oral administration. Half-life is about 24 hours.
Distribution: About 90% bound to plasma proteins.
Metabolism: Metabolized to at least 10 different compounds, some of which retain some pharmacologic activity.
Excretion: Excreted primarily by the kidneys.

Route	Onset	Peak	Duration
P.O.	Unknown	Unknown	Unknown

Contraindications and precautions

Contraindicated in patients hypersensitive to drug or to ergot alkaloids. Use cautiously in patients susceptible to arrhythmias and underlying psychiatric disorders.

Interactions

Drug-drug. *Dopamine antagonists, including butyrophenones, metoclopramide, phenothiazines, and thioxanthines:* May antagonize the effects of pergolide. Monitor patient closely.
Drugs known to affect protein binding: Pergolide is extensively protein-bound; exercise caution if pergolide is coadministered.

Effects on diagnostic tests

None reported.

Adverse reactions

CNS: headache, asthenia, *dyskinesia, dizziness, hallucinations, dystonia, confusion, somnolence,* insomnia, anxiety, depression, tremor, abnormal dreams, personality disorder, psychosis, abnormal gait, akathisia, extrapyramidal syndrome, incoordination, akinesia, hypertonia, neuralgia, speech disorder, twitching, paresthesia.
CV: *orthostatic hypotension,* vasodilation, palpitations, hypotension, syncope, hypertension, ***arrhythmias, MI.***
EENT: *rhinitis,* epistaxis, abnormal vision, diplopia, eye disorder.
GI: dry mouth, taste perversion, abdominal pain, *nausea, constipation,* diarrhea, dyspepsia, anorexia, vomiting.
GU: urinary frequency, urinary tract infection, hematuria.
Musculoskeletal: chest, neck, and back pain, arthralgia; bursitis; myalgia.
Skin: rash, diaphoresis.
Other: flulike syndrome; chills; infection; facial, peripheral, or generalized edema; weight gain; dyspnea; anemia.

Overdose and treatment

Some cases of overdose revealed symptoms of hallucinations, involuntary movements, palpitations, and arrhythmias.

Provide supportive treatment. Monitor cardiac function and protect the patient's airway. Antiarrhythmics and sympathomimetics may be necessary to support CV function. Adverse CNS effects may be treated with dopaminergic antagonists such as phenothiazines. If indicated, gastric lavage or induced emesis may be used to empty the stomach of its contents. Orally administered activated charcoal may be useful in attenuating absorption.

Clinical considerations

In early clinical trials, 27% of patients who attempted pergolide therapy didn't finish the trial because of adverse effects (primarily hallucinations and confusion).

Therapeutic monitoring
Monitor blood pressure. Symptomatic orthostatic or sustained hypotension may occur especially at the start of therapy.

Special populations
Breast-feeding patients. Safety in breast-feeding women hasn't been established.
Pediatric patients. Safety in children hasn't been established.

Patient counseling
- Inform patient of potential for adverse effects. Warn patient to avoid activities that could expose him to injury secondary to orthostatic hypotension and syncope.
- Caution patient to rise slowly to avoid orthostatic hypotension, particularly at the beginning of therapy.

perindopril erbumine
Aceon

Pharmacologic classification: angiotensin converting enzyme (ACE) inhibitor
Therapeutic classification: antihypertensive
Pregnancy risk category C (first trimester) and D (second and third trimesters)

How supplied
Available by prescription only
Tablets: 2 mg, 4 mg, 8 mg

Indications and dosages
Treatment of essential hypertension
Adults: Initially, 4 mg P.O. once daily. Increase dosage until blood pressure is controlled or to a maximum of 16 mg per day; usual maintenance dosage, 4 to 8 mg once daily; may be given in two divided doses.
Elderly: Initially, 4 mg P.O. daily as one dose or in two divided doses. Dosage increases exceeding 8 mg per day should only be made under close medical supervision.
≡ ***Dosage adjustment.*** For renally impaired patients, initially, 2 mg P.O. daily with a maximum maintenance dosage of 8 mg/day.
≡ ***Dosage adjustment.*** For patients taking diuretics, initially, 2 to 4 mg P.O. daily as one dose or in two divided doses with close medical supervision for several hours and until blood pressure has stabilized. Adjust dosage based on patient's blood pressure response.

Pharmacodynamics
Antihypertensive action: Perindopril erbumine is a prodrug that's converted by the liver to the active metabolite perindoprilat. Perindoprilat is thought to lower blood pressure through inhibition of angiotensin-converting enzyme (ACE) activity, thereby preventing the conversion of angiotensin I to angiotensin II, a potent vasoconstrictor. Inhibition of ACE results in decreased vasoconstriction, and decreased aldosterone, reducing sodium and water retention and lowering blood pressure.

Pharmacokinetics
Absorption: Rapidly absorbed following oral administration. The absolute oral bioavailability of perindopril is around 75%. Plasma concentration of perindopril and perindoprilat are increased about twofold in the elderly.
Distribution: Perindopril and perindoprilat are about 60% and 10% to 20% bound to plasma proteins, respectively. Therefore, drug interactions resulting from effects on protein binding aren't anticipated.
Metabolism: Extensively metabolized by the liver to the active ACE inhibitor perindoprilat.
Excretion: About 4% to 12% of a given dose of perindopril is excreted in the urine as unchanged drug. Clearance of the drug is reduced in the elderly, and patients with heart failure or renal insufficiency.

Route	Onset	Peak	Duration
P.O.	Unknown	1 hr	Unknown

Contraindications and precautions:
Contraindicated in patients with known hypersensitivity to perindopril or to any other ACE inhibitor. Also contraindicated in patients with a history of angioedema secondary to ACE inhibitors. Don't use drug in pregnant women.

Use cautiously in patients with a history of angioedema unrelated to ACE inhibitor therapy. Also use cautiously in patients with impaired renal function, heart failure, ischemic heart disease, cerebrovascular disease or renal artery stenosis, and in patients with collagen vascular disease, such as systemic lupus erythematosus or scleroderma.

Interactions
Drug-drug. *Diuretics:* Additive hypotensive effect. Monitor patient closely.
Potassium-sparing diuretics, such as amiloride, spironolactone, and triamterene; potassium supplements; other drugs capable of increasing serum potassium, such as cyclosporine, heparin, and indomethacin: Additive hyperkalemic effect. Use together cautiously and monitor serum potassium frequently.
Lithium: Increased serum lithium and symptoms of lithium toxicity can occur. Use together cautiously and monitor serum lithium concentration. Use of a diuretic may further increase the risk of lithium toxicity.
Drug-food. *Salt substitutes containing potassium:* May increase risk of hyperkalemia. Use together cautiously.

Effects on diagnostic tests
None reported.

Adverse reactions
CNS: dizziness, asthenia, sleep disorder, paresthesia, depression, somnolence, nervousness, *headache.*
CV: palpitation, edema, chest pain, abnormal ECG.
EENT: rhinitis, sinusitis, ear infection, pharyngitis, tinnitus.
GI: dyspepsia, diarrhea, abdominal pain, nausea, vomiting, flatulence.
GU: proteinuria, urinary tract infection, male sexual dysfunction, menstrual disorder.
Hepatic: increased ALT.
Metabolic: triglyceride increase.
Musculoskeletal: back pain, hypertonia, neck pain, joint pain, myalgia, arthritis, low or upper extremity pain.
Respiratory: cough, upper respiratory infection.
Skin: rash.
Other: viral infection, fever, injury, seasonal allergy, angioedema.

Overdose and treatment
Hypotension would be the most likely manifestation of perindopril overdose. Treatment should be symptomatic and supportive. Discontinue perindopril and observe patient closely. Treat dehydration, electrolyte imbalances, and hypotension using established protocols.

Clinical considerations
- Angioedema involving the face, extremities, lips, tongue, glottis and larynx has been reported in patients treated with perindopril. Discontinue drug and observe patient until the swelling disappears. If swelling is confined to the face and lips, it will probably resolve without treatment, but antihistamines may be useful in relieving symptoms. Angioedema associated with involvement of the tongue, glottis or larynx may cause fatal airway obstruction. Appropriate therapy, such as subcutaneous epinephrine solution should be promptly administered.
- Patients with a history of angioedema unrelated to ACE inhibitor therapy may be at increased risk of angioedema while receiving an ACE inhibitor.
- Excessive hypotension can occur when drug is given with diuretics. If possible, discontinue diuretic therapy 2 to 3 days before starting perindopril to decrease potential for excessive hypotensive response. If it isn't possible to discontinue the diuretic, consider starting with a lower dose of perindopril and/or decreasing the dose of diuretic.
- Monitor patients at risk for hypotension closely during initiation of therapy and for the first 2 weeks of treatment, and whenever the dose of perindopril or concomitant diuretic is increased.
- If severe hypotension occurs, place patient in supine position and treat symptomatically.
- Hypotension can also occur when initiating therapy or adjusting doses in patients who have been volume- or salt-depleted as a result of prolonged diuretic therapy, dietary salt restriction, dialysis, diarrhea, or vomiting. Volume and salt depletion should be corrected before starting drug.
- ACE inhibitors have rarely been associated with a syndrome of cholestatic jaundice, fulminant hepatic necrosis, and death. Discontinue drug in patients in whom jaundice or marked elevations of hepatic enzymes develop during therapy.

Therapeutic monitoring
- Monitor CBC with differential before therapy, especially in renally impaired patients with systemic lupus erythematosus or scleroderma.
- Monitor renal function before and periodically throughout therapy. Drug shouldn't be used in patients with a creatinine clearance less than 30 ml/minute.
- Monitor serum potassium levels closely.

Special populations
Pregnant patients. Advise women of childbearing age of the consequences of second- and third-trimester exposure to drug. Advise them to notify health care provider immediately if pregnancy is suspected.
Breast-feeding patients. It isn't known if drug is excreted in breast milk. Use with caution in breast-feeding women.
Pediatric patients. Safety and efficacy in children haven't been established.
Geriatric patients. Plasma concentrations of both perindopril and perindoprilat in patients over age 70 are about twice those observed in younger patients. With the exception of dizziness and possibly rash, adverse effects don't appear to be increased in the elderly. Administer doses above 8 mg/day with caution and under close medical supervision.

Patient counseling
- Inform patient that angioedema, including laryngeal edema, can occur during therapy, especially with the first dose. Advise patient to stop taking the drug and immediately report any signs or symptoms suggestive of angioedema, such as swelling of face, extremities, eyes, lips, tongue, hoarseness, or difficulty in swallowing or breathing.
- Advise patient to promptly report to doctor any sign of infection, such as sore throat or fever, or jaundice (yellowing of eyes or skin).
- Caution patient that light-headedness may occur, especially during the first few days of therapy. Advise patient to report light-headedness and, if fainting occurs, to discontinue the

drug and consult a health care provider promptly.

■ Caution patient that inadequate fluid intake or excessive perspiration, diarrhea, or vomiting can lead to an excessive decrease in blood pressure.

permethrin

Elimite, Nix

Pharmacologic classification: synthetic pyrethroid
Therapeutic classification: scabicide, pediculocide
Pregnancy risk category B

How supplied

Available by prescription only
Elimite
Cream: 5%
Available without a prescription
Nix
Lotion: 1%

Indications and dosages

Pediculosis
Adults and children: Apply sufficient volume to saturate the hair and scalp. Allow drug to remain on the hair for 10 minutes before rinsing.
Scabies
Adults and children: Thoroughly massage into skin from head to soles. Treat infants on the hairline, neck, scalp, temple, and forehead. Remove cream by washing after 8 to 14 hours. One application usually is curative.

Pharmacodynamics

Scabicidal action: Permethrin acts on the parasites' nerve cell membranes to disrupt the sodium channel current and thereby paralyze them.

Pharmacokinetics

Absorption: Not entirely investigated but probably less than 2% of the amount applied.
Distribution: Systemic distribution is unknown.
Metabolism: Rapidly metabolized by ester hydrolysis to inactive metabolites.
Excretion: Metabolites are excreted in urine. Residue on hair is detectable for up to 10 days.

Route	Onset	Peak	Duration
Topical	10-15 min	Unknown	10 days

Contraindications and precautions

Contraindicated in patients hypersensitive to pyrethrins or chrysanthemums.

Interactions

None reported.

Effects on diagnostic tests

None reported.

Adverse reactions

Skin: pruritus, *burning, stinging,* edema, tingling, numbness or scalp discomfort, mild erythema, scalp rash.

Overdose and treatment

For accidental ingestion, perform gastric lavage and use general supportive measures.

Clinical considerations

■ A single treatment is usually effective. Although combing of nits isn't required for effectiveness, drug package supplies a fine-toothed comb.

■ Permethrin is at least as effective as lindane (Kwell) in treating head lice.

Therapeutic monitoring

A second application may be necessary if lice are observed 7 days after the initial application.

Special populations

Breast-feeding patients. It isn't known if permethrin is excreted in breast milk. Consider discontinuing breast-feeding temporarily or not using the medication.
Pediatric patients. Safety and efficacy for use in children under age 2 haven't been established.

Patient counseling

■ Tell patient or caregiver to wash hair with shampoo, rinse it thoroughly, and then towel dry.

■ Tell patient or caregiver to apply sufficient volume to saturate the hair and scalp.

■ Instruct patient to report itching, redness, or swelling of the scalp.

■ Advise patient that drug is for external use only and to avoid contact with mucous membranes.

perphenazine

Apo-Perphenazine*, Trilafon

Pharmacologic classification: phenothiazine (piperazine derivative)
Therapeutic classification: antipsychotic; antiemetic
Pregnancy risk category NR

How supplied

Available by prescription only
Tablets: 2 mg, 4 mg, 8 mg, 16 mg
Oral concentrate: 16 mg/5 ml
Injection: 5 mg/ml

Indications and dosages

Psychosis
Adults: Initially, 8 to 16 mg P.O. b.i.d., t.i.d., or q.i.d., increasing to 64 mg daily. Alterna-

tively, administer 5 to 10 mg I.M.; change to P.O. as soon as possible.

Mental disturbances, acute alcoholism, nausea, vomiting, hiccups

Adults: 5 to 10 mg I.M., p.r.n. Maximum dose is 15 mg daily in ambulatory patients; 30 mg daily in hospitalized patients; or 8 to 16 mg P.O. daily in divided doses.

Perphenazine may be given slowly by I.V. drip at a rate of 1 mg/2 minutes with continuous blood pressure monitoring (rarely used). A maximum of 5 mg I.V. diluted to 0.5 mg/ml with normal saline solution may be given for severe hiccups or vomiting. Oral preparation may be given 8 to 16 mg P.O. b.i.d. for outpatients; 8 to 32 mg P.O. b.i.d. for inpatients.

Pharmacodynamics

Antipsychotic action: Perphenazine is thought to exert its antipsychotic effects by postsynaptic blockade of CNS dopamine receptors, thus inhibiting dopamine-mediated effects; antiemetic effects are attributed to dopamine receptor blockade in the medullary chemoreceptor trigger zone. Perphenazine has many other central and peripheral effects: it produces both alpha and ganglionic blockade and counteracts histamine- and serotonin-mediated activity. Its most serious adverse reactions are extrapyramidal.

Pharmacokinetics

Absorption: Rate and extent of absorption vary with administration route: oral tablet absorption is erratic and variable; oral concentrate absorption is much more predictable. I.M. drug is absorbed rapidly.

Distribution: Distributed widely into the body, including breast milk. Drug is 91% to 99% protein-bound.

Metabolism: Metabolized extensively by the liver, but no active metabolites are formed.

Excretion: Mostly excreted in urine via the kidneys; some in feces via the biliary tract.

Route	Onset	Peak	Duration
P.O., I.V., I.M.	½-1 hr	2-4 hr	Unknown

Contraindications and precautions

Contraindicated in patients with hypersensitivity to drug; in patients experiencing coma; in those with CNS depression, blood dyscrasia, bone marrow depression, liver damage, or subcortical damage; and in those receiving large doses of CNS depressants.

Use cautiously in geriatric or debilitated patients; in those with alcohol withdrawal, psychic depression, suicidal tendencies, adverse reaction to other phenothiazines, impaired renal function, respiratory disorders; and in patients receiving other CNS depressants or anticholinergics.

Interactions

Drug-drug. *Aluminum- and magnesium-containing antacids and antidiarrheals, phenobarbital:* Pharmacokinetic alterations and subsequent decreased therapeutic response to perphenazine. Don't use together.

Antiarrhythmic agents, disopyramide, procainamide, quinidine: Increased incidence of arrhythmias and conduction defects. Don't use together.

Appetite suppressants; sympathomimetics, such as ephedrine, epinephrine, phenylephrine, and phenylpropanolamine: May decrease their stimulatory and pressor effects. Monitor patient closely.

Atropine or other anticholinergic drugs: Oversedation, paralytic ileus, visual changes, and severe constipation. Avoid use together.

Beta blockers: May inhibit perphenazine metabolism, increasing plasma levels and toxicity. Don't use together.

Bromocriptine: Perphenazine may antagonize therapeutic effect. Avoid use together.

Centrally acting antihypertensive drugs, such as clonidine, guanabenz, guanadrel, guanethidine, methyldopa, and reserpine: Perphenazine may inhibit blood pressure response. Avoid use together.

CNS depressants, general, spinal, or epidural anesthetics, or parenteral magnesium sulfate: Additive effects are likely if perphenazine is used. Avoid use together.

High-dose dopamine: Decreased vasoconstricting effects. Don't use together.

Levodopa: Decreased effectiveness and increased toxicity . Don't use together.

Lithium: May result in severe neurologic toxicity with an encephalitis-like syndrome, and a decreased therapeutic response to perphenazine. Don't use together.

Metrizamide: Increased risk of seizures. Don't use together.

Nitrates: Hypotension. Monitor blood pressure.

Phenytoin: Perphenazine may inhibit metabolism and increase toxicity. Don't use together.

Propylthiouracil: Increases risk of agranulocytosis. Monitor CBC results.

Drug-lifestyle. *Alcohol use:* Additive effects are likely. Advise patient to avoid alcohol.

Heavy smoking: Decreased therapeutic response to perphenazine. Advise patient to avoid smoking.

Sun exposure: Photosensitivity reactions may occur. Advise patient to take precautions.

Drug-food. *Caffeine:* Decreases therapeutic response to perphenazine. Instruct patient to avoid foods and beverages that contain caffeine.

Effects on diagnostic tests

Perphenazine causes false-positive test results for urinary porphyrins, urobilinogen, amylase, and 5-hydroxyindoleacetic acid because of darkening of urine by metabolites; it also causes false-positive urine pregnancy test results using human chorionic gonadotropin.

Adverse reactions

CNS: *extrapyramidal reactions, tardive dyskinesia,* sedation, pseudoparkinsonism, EEG changes, dizziness, adverse behavioral effects, ***seizures,*** drowsiness.
CV: *orthostatic hypotension,* tachycardia, ECG changes, ***cardiac arrest.***
EENT: ocular changes, *blurred vision,* nasal congestion.
GI: *dry mouth, constipation,* nausea, vomiting, diarrhea, ileus.
GU: *urine retention,* dark urine, menstrual irregularities, gynecomastia, inhibited ejaculation.
Hematologic: leukopenia, galactorrhea, hyperglycemia, hypoglycemia, ***agranulocytosis,*** eosinophilia, ***hemolytic anemia, thrombocytopenia.***
Hepatic: jaundice, abnormal liver function test results.
Skin: *mild photosensitivity,* allergic reactions, pain at I.M. injection site, sterile abscess.
Other: weight gain, SIADH, ***neuroleptic malignant syndrome.***
After abrupt withdrawal of long-term therapy: gastritis, nausea, vomiting, dizziness, tremor, feeling of warmth or cold, diaphoresis, tachycardia, headache, insomnia.

Overdose and treatment

CNS depression is characterized by deep, unarousable sleep and possible coma, hypotension, or hypertension, extrapyramidal symptoms, dystonia, abnormal involuntary muscle movements, agitation, seizures, arrhythmias, ECG changes, hypothermia or hyperthermia, and autonomic nervous system dysfunction.

Treatment is symptomatic and supportive, including maintaining vital signs, airway, stable body temperature, and fluid and electrolyte balance.

Induce vomiting in a conscious patient with ipecac syrup even if spontaneous vomiting has occurred. Don't induce vomiting in patients with impaired consciousness. Use gastric lavage, then activated charcoal and sodium chloride cathartics; dialysis is usually ineffective. Regulate body temperature as needed. Treat hypotension with I.V. fluids: Don't give epinephrine. Treat seizures with parenteral diazepam or barbiturates; arrhythmias with parenteral phenytoin (1 mg/kg with rate titrated to blood pressure); and extrapyramidal reactions with benztropine at 1 to 2 mg or parenteral diphenhydramine at 10 to 50 mg.

Clinical considerations

Consider the recommendations relevant to all phenothiazines as well as the following:

- Oral formulations may cause stomach upset; administer with food or fluid.
- Dilute the concentrate in 2 to 4 oz (60 to 120 ml) of liquid (water, caffeine-free carbonated drinks, fruit juice (not apple), tomato juice, milk, or puddings). Dilute every 5 ml of concentrate with 60 ml of suitable fluid. Shake oral concentrate before administration.
- Liquid formulation may cause rash upon contact with skin.
- I.M. injection may cause skin necrosis; avoid extravasation.
- Administer I.M. injection deep into upper outer quadrant of buttocks. Massaging the injection site may prevent formation of abscesses.
- Don't administer drug for injection if it's excessively discolored or contains precipitate.

Therapeutic monitoring

Monitor blood pressure before and after parenteral administration.

Special populations

Breast-feeding patients. Drug is widely distributed, including in breast milk; use with caution. Potential benefits to the woman should outweigh the potential harm to the infant.
Pediatric patients. Drug isn't recommended for children under age 12.
Geriatric patients. Use lower doses in geriatric patients. Dose must be titrated to effects; 30% to 50% of the usual dose may be effective. Geriatric patients are at greater risk for adverse effects, especially tardive dyskinesia and other extrapyramidal effects.

Patient counseling

- Explain the risks of dystonic reactions and tardive dyskinesia, and tell patient to report abnormal body movements.
- Tell patient to avoid spilling the liquid; contact with skin may cause rash and irritation.
- Warn patient not to take extremely hot or cold baths and to avoid exposure to temperature extremes, sun lamps, or tanning beds; drug may cause thermoregulatory changes.
- Advise patient to take drug exactly as prescribed and not to double the dose for missed doses.
- Instruct patient not to stop taking drug suddenly; any adverse reactions may be alleviated by a dosage reduction. Patient should promptly report difficulty urinating, sore throat, dizziness, or fainting.
- Tell patient to avoid hazardous activities that require alertness until effect of drug is established. Reassure patient that sedative effects of drug should become tolerable in several weeks.
- Explain which fluids are appropriate for diluting the concentrate (not apple juice or caffeine-containing drinks); explain dropper technique of measuring dose.

■ Recommend sugarless hard candy or chewing gum, ice chips, or artificial saliva to relieve dry mouth.

phenazopyridine hydrochloride

Azo-Standard, Baridium, Phenazo*, Prodium, Pyridiate, Pyridium, Urogesic

Pharmacologic classification: azo dye
Therapeutic classification: urinary analgesic
Pregnancy risk category B

How supplied

Available by prescription only
Tablets: 100 mg, 200 mg
Available without prescription
Tablets: 95 mg

Indications and dosages

Pain with urinary tract irritation or infection
Adults: 200 mg P.O. t.i.d. Give drug after meals.

Pharmacodynamics

Analgesic action: Phenazopyridine has a local anesthetic effect on urinary tract mucosa via an unknown mechanism.

Pharmacokinetics

Absorption: Not described.
Distribution: Traces of drug are thought to enter CSF and cross the placenta.
Metabolism: Metabolized in the liver.
Excretion: Excreted by the kidneys; 65% is excreted unchanged in urine. Average time of total excretion of drug is 20½ hours.

Route	Onset	Peak	Duration
P.O.	Unknown	Unknown	Unknown

Contraindications and precautions

Contraindicated in patients with hypersensitivity to drug, glomerulonephritis, severe hepatitis, uremia, pyelonephritis during pregnancy, or renal insufficiency.

Interactions

None significant.

Effects on diagnostic tests

Drug may alter results of Diastix, Chemstrip uG, glucose enzymatic test strip, Acetest, and Ketostix. Clinitest should be used to obtain accurate urine glucose test results.

Drug may also interfere with Ehrlich's test for urine urobilinogen; phenolsulfonphthalein excretion tests of kidney function; sulfobromophthalein excretion tests of liver function; and urine tests for protein, steroids, or bilirubin.

Adverse reactions

CNS: headache.
GI: nausea, GI disturbances.
Hematologic: hemolytic anemia, methemoglobinemia.
Skin: rash, pruritus.
Other: ***anaphylactoid reactions.***

Overdose and treatment

Signs and symptoms of overdose include methemoglobinemia (most obvious as cyanosis), along with renal and hepatic impairment and failure.

To treat overdose of phenazopyridine, empty stomach immediately by inducing emesis with ipecac syrup or by gastric lavage. Administer methylene blue, 1 to 2 mg/kg I.V., or 100 to 200 mg ascorbic acid P.O. to reverse methemoglobinemia. Provide symptomatic and supportive measures (respiratory support and correction of fluid and electrolyte imbalances). Monitor laboratory parameters and vital signs closely. Contact local or regional poison information center for specific instructions.

Clinical considerations

■ Drug colors urine red or orange; it may stain fabrics.
■ Use only as an analgesic.
■ May be used with an antibiotic to treat urinary tract infections.
■ Discontinue drug in 2 days with concurrent antibiotic use.

Therapeutic monitoring

■ Monitor patient for anaphlyactoid reactions.
■ Evaluate response to medication therapy; assess urinary function, such as output, complaints of burning, pain, and frequency.
■ Monitor vital signs, especially temperature.

Special populations

Breast-feeding patients. Safety in breast-feeding women hasn't been established.
Geriatric patients. Use with caution in geriatric patients because of possible decreased renal function.

Patient counseling

■ Instruct patient in measures to prevent urinary tract infection.
■ Tell patient that stains on clothing may be removed with a 0.25% solution of sodium dithionate or hydrosulfite.
■ Advise patient to take a missed dose as soon as possible and not to double the doses.
■ Instruct patient to report symptoms that worsen or don't resolve.
■ Encourage patient to force fluids (if not contraindicated). Monitor intake and output.

phenobarbital

Barbita

phenobarbital sodium

Luminal

Pharmacologic classification: barbiturate
Therapeutic classification: anticonvulsant, sedative-hypnotic
Controlled substance schedule IV
Pregnancy risk category D

How supplied

Available by prescription only
Tablets: 15 mg, 16 mg, 30 mg, 32 mg, 60 mg, 65 mg, 100 mg
Capsules: 16 mg
Elixir: 15 mg/5 ml; 20 mg/5 ml
Injection: 30 mg/ml, 60 mg/ml, 65 mg/ml, 130 mg/ml

Indications and dosages

All forms of epilepsy except absence seizures, febrile seizures in children
Adults: 60 to 100 mg P.O. daily, divided t.i.d. or given as single dose h.s. Alternatively, give 200 to 300 mg I.M. or I.V. and repeat q 6 hours, p.r.n.
Children: 1 to 6 mg/kg P.O. daily, usually divided q 12 hours. It can, however, be administered once daily. Alternatively, give 4 to 6 mg/kg I.V. or I.M. daily and monitor patient's blood levels.
Status epilepticus
Adults and children: 10 to 20 mg/kg I.V. over 10 to 15 minutes; don't exceed 60 mg/min. Repeat if necessary.
Sedation
Adults: 30 to 120 mg P.O., I.M., or I.V. daily in two or three divided doses. Maximum dose, 400 mg/24 hours.
Children: 8 to 32 mg P.O. daily.
Insomnia
Adults: 100 to 200 mg P.O. or 100 to 320 mg I.M.
Preoperative sedation
Adults: 100 to 200 mg I.M. 60 to 90 minutes before surgery.
Children: 1 to 3 mg/kg I.V. or I.M. 60 to 90 minutes before surgery.

Pharmacodynamics

Anticonvulsant action: Phenobarbital suppresses the spread of seizure activity produced by epileptogenic foci in the cortex, thalamus, and limbic systems by enhancing the effect of gamma-aminobutyric acid (GABA). Both presynaptic and postsynaptic excitability are decreased; also, phenobarbital raises the seizure threshold.

Sedative-hypnotic action: Phenobarbital acts throughout the CNS as a nonselective depressant with a slow onset of action and a long duration of action. Particularly sensitive to this drug is the reticular-activating system, which controls CNS arousal. Phenobarbital decreases both presynaptic and postsynaptic membrane excitability by facilitating the action of GABA. The exact cellular site and mechanisms of action are unknown.

Pharmacokinetics

Absorption: Well absorbed after oral and rectal administration, with 70% to 90% reaching the bloodstream. Absorption after I.M. administration is 100%. After oral administration peak levels in the CNS are achieved at 1 to 3 hours. A serum level of 10 mcg/ml is needed to produce sedation; 40 mcg/ml usually produces sleep. Levels of 20 to 40 mcg/ml are considered therapeutic for anticonvulsant therapy.
Distribution: Distributed widely throughout the body. Phenobarbital is about 25% to 30% protein-bound.
Metabolism: Metabolized by the hepatic microsomal enzyme system.
Excretion: About 25% to 50% of a phenobarbital dose is eliminated unchanged in urine; remainder is excreted as metabolites of glucuronic acid. Half-life of drug is 5 to 7 days.

Route	Onset	Peak	Duration
P.O.	1 hr	8-12 hr	10-12 hr
I.V.	5 min	½ hr	4-10 hr
I.M.	> 5 min	> ½ hr	4-10 hr

Contraindications and precautions

Contraindicated in patients with barbiturate hypersensitivity, history of manifest or latent porphyria, hepatic dysfunction, respiratory disease with dyspnea or obstruction, and nephritis.

Use cautiously in geriatric or debilitated patients and in those with acute or chronic pain, depression, suicidal tendencies, history of drug abuse, blood pressure alterations, CV disease, shock, or uremia.

Interactions

Drug-drug. *Antidepressants, antihistamines, narcotics, phenothiazines, sedative-hypnotics, tranquilizers:* Phenobarbital may add to or potentiate CNS and respiratory depressant effects. Don't use together.
Corticosteroids, digitoxin (not digoxin), doxycycline, oral contraceptives and other estrogens, theophylline and other xanthines: Drug enhances hepatic metabolism. Avoid use together; monitor patient closely.
Disulfiram, MAO inhibitors, valproic acid: Decrease the metabolism of phenobarbital and can increase its toxicity. Monitor patient for toxicity.

Griseofulvin: Phenobarbital impairs the effectiveness of griseofulvin by decreasing absorption from the GI tract. Administer drugs at separate times.
Rifampin: May decrease phenobarbital levels by increasing hepatic metabolism. Monitor levels closely.
Warfarin and other oral anticoagulants: Phenobarbital enhances the enzymatic degradation. May require increased doses of the anticoagulant.
Drug-lifestyle. *Alcohol use:* Phenobarbital may add to or potentiate CNS and respiratory depressant effects. Avoid use together.

Effects on diagnostic tests

Phenobarbital may cause a false-positive phentolamine test. The physiologic effects of drug may impair the absorption of cyanocobalamin ^{57}Co; it may decrease serum bilirubin levels in neonates and epileptics, and in patients with congenital nonhemolytic unconjugated hyperbilirubinemia. Barbiturates may increase sulfobromophthalein retention. EEG patterns show a change in low-voltage, fast activity; changes persist for a time after discontinuation of therapy.

Adverse reactions

CNS: *drowsiness, lethargy, hangover,* paradoxical excitement in elderly patients, somnolence.
CV: bradycardia, hypotension.
GI: nausea, vomiting.
Hematologic: exacerbation of porphyria.
Respiratory: ***respiratory depression, apnea.***
Skin: rash, ***erythema multiforme, Stevens-Johnson syndrome,*** urticaria; pain, swelling, thrombophlebitis, necrosis, nerve injury at injection site.
Other: ***angioedema,*** physical and psychological dependence.

Overdose and treatment

Signs and symptoms of phenobarbital overdose include unsteady gait, slurred speech, sustained nystagmus, somnolence, confusion, respiratory depression, pulmonary edema, areflexia, and coma. Typical shock syndrome with tachycardia and hypotension along with jaundice, oliguria, and chills followed by fever may occur.

Treatment aims to maintain and support ventilation and pulmonary function as necessary; and to support cardiac function and circulation with vasopressors and I.V. fluids as needed. If patient is conscious and gag reflex is intact, induce emesis (if ingestion was recent) by administering ipecac syrup. If emesis is contraindicated, perform gastric lavage while a cuffed endotracheal tube is in place to prevent aspiration. Follow with administration of activated charcoal or sodium chloride cathartic. Measure intake and output, vital signs, and laboratory parameters. Maintain body temperature.

Alkalinization of urine may be helpful in removing drug from the body; hemodialysis may be useful in severe overdose. Oral activated charcoal may enhance phenobarbital elimination regardless of its route of administration.

Clinical considerations

Consider the recommendations relevant to all barbiturates as well as the following:
- Oral solution may be mixed with water or juice to improve taste.
- Reconstitute powder for injection with 2.5 to 5 ml sterile water for injection. Roll vial in hands; don't shake.
- Use a larger vein for I.V. administration to prevent extravasation.
- Avoid I.V. administration at a rate exceeding 60 mg/minute to prevent hypotension and respiratory depression. It may take up to 30 minutes after I.V. administration to achieve maximum effect.
- Administer a parenteral dose within 30 minutes of reconstitution because phenobarbital hydrolyzes both in solution and on exposure to air.
- Administer I.M. dose deep into a large muscle mass to prevent tissue injury.
- Don't use injectable solution if it contains a precipitate.
- Administration of full loading doses over short periods of time to treat status epilepticus will require ventilatory support in adults.

Therapeutic monitoring

- Keep emergency resuscitation equipment on hand when administering phenobarbital intravenously.
- Full therapeutic effects aren't seen for 2 to 3 weeks, except when loading dose is used.

Special populations

Breast-feeding patients. Phenobarbital passes into breast milk; avoid administering to breast-feeding women.
Pediatric patients. Paradoxical hyperexcitability may occur in children. Use with caution.
Geriatric patients. Geriatric patients are more sensitive to effects of drug and usually require lower doses. Confusion, disorientation, and excitability may occur in geriatric patients.

Patient counseling

- Advise patient of the potential for physical and psychological dependence with prolonged use.
- Caution patient not to stop taking drug suddenly because this could cause a withdrawal reaction.

■ Advise patient to avoid driving and other hazardous activities that require alertness until the adverse CNS effects of drug are known.

phentermine hydrochloride

Adipex-P, Anoxine-AM, Dapex, Ionamin, Obe-Nix, Obephen, Obermine, Obestin-30, Parmine, Phentrol

Pharmacologic classification: amphetamine congener
Therapeutic classification: short-term adjunctive anorexigenic, indirect-acting sympathomimetic amine
Controlled substance schedule IV
Pregnancy risk category X

How supplied

Available by prescription only
Capsules: 8 mg, 18.75 mg, 30 mg, 37.5 mg
Tablets: 8 mg, 37.5 mg
Capsules (resin complex): 15 mg, 30 mg, 37.5 mg

Indications and dosages

Short-term adjunct in exogenous obesity
Adults: 8 mg P.O. t.i.d. ½ hour before meals; or 15 to 37.5 mg P.O. daily before breakfast; or 15 to 30 mg P.O. daily before breakfast (resin complex).

Pharmacodynamics

Anorexigenic action: Phentermine is an indirect-acting sympathomimetic amine; it causes fewer and less severe adverse reactions from CNS stimulation than do amphetamines, and its potential for addiction is lower. Anorexigenic effects are thought to follow direct stimulation of the hypothalamus; they may involve other CNS and metabolic effects.

Pharmacokinetics

Absorption: Absorbed readily after oral administration.
Distribution: Distributed widely throughout the body.
Metabolism: Unknown.
Excretion: Excreted in urine.

Route	Onset	Peak	Duration
P.O.	Unknown	Unknown	12-14 hr

Contraindications and precautions

Contraindicated in patients with hyperthyroidism, moderate to severe hypertension, advanced arteriosclerosis, symptomatic CV disease, glaucoma, or hypersensitivity or idiosyncrasy to sympathomimetic amines; within 14 days of MAO inhibitor therapy; and in agitated patients.

Use cautiously in patients with mild hypertension.

Interactions

Drug-drug. *Acetazolamide, antacids, sodium bicarbonate:* Increase renal reabsorption of phentermine and prolong its duration of action. Monitor patient closely.
General anesthetics: May result in arrhythmias. Monitor patient closely.
Guanethidine and other antihypertensive agents: Phentermine may decrease hypotensive effect. Don't use together.
Haloperidol and phenothiazines: Decrease phentermine effects. Avoid use together.
Insulin: Phentermine may alter requirements in diabetic patients. Monitor serum glucose levels and patient closely.
MAO inhibitors: May cause hypertensive crisis. Don't use together or within 14 days after MAO inhibitor has been discontinued.
Drug-food. *Caffeine:* May cause additive CNS stimulation. Avoid use together.

Effects on diagnostic tests

None reported.

Adverse reactions

CNS: overstimulation, headache, euphoria, dysphoria, dizziness, *insomnia.*
CV: *palpitations, tachycardia,* increased blood pressure.
GI: dry mouth, dysgeusia, constipation, diarrhea, other GI disturbances.
GU: impotence, dysuria, polyuria, urinary frequency.
Skin: urticaria.
Other: altered libido.

Overdose and treatment

Signs and symptoms of acute overdose include restlessness, tremor, hyperreflexia, fever, tachypnea, dizziness, confusion, aggressive behavior, hallucinations, blood pressure changes, arrhythmias, nausea, vomiting, diarrhea, and cramps. Fatigue and depression usually follow CNS stimulation; seizures, coma, and death may follow.

Treat overdose symptomatically and supportively; sedation may be necessary. Chlorpromazine may antagonize CNS stimulation. Acidification of urine may hasten excretion. Monitor vital signs and fluid and electrolyte balance.

Clinical considerations

Besides those relevant to all amphetamines, consider the following recommendations:

■ Intermittent courses of treatment (6 weeks on, followed by 4 weeks off) are as effective as continuous use.

■ Greatest weight loss occurs in the first weeks of therapy and diminishes in succeeding weeks. When such tolerance to drug effect develops, discontinue drug instead of increasing the dosage.

Therapeutic monitoring
Monitor patient for tolerance and dependence.

Special populations
Pregnant patients. Safety hasn't been established for use in pregnant women; give to pregnant women only if clearly needed.
Pediatric patients. Phentermine isn't recommended for children under age 12.

Patient counseling
- Advise patient to take morning dose 2 hours after breakfast, and to avoid caffeine-containing drinks.
- Tell patient to take last daily dose at least 6 hours before bedtime to prevent insomnia.
- Warn patient not to take drug more frequently than prescribed.
- Advise patient that drug may produce dizziness, fatigue, or drowsiness.
- Tell patient to contact health care provider if palpitations occur.

phentolamine mesylate
Regitine

Pharmacologic classification: alpha blocker
Therapeutic classification: antihypertensive for pheochromocytoma, cutaneous vasodilator
Pregnancy risk category C

How supplied
Available by prescription only
Injection: 5 mg/ml in 1-ml vials

Indications and dosages
Aid for diagnosis of pheochromocytoma
Adults: 5 mg I.V. or I.M.
Children: 1 mg I.V., or 3 mg I.M.
Control or prevention of paroxysmal hypertension immediately before or during pheochromocytomectomy
Adults: 5 mg I.M. or I.V. 1 to 2 hours preoperatively, repeated as necessary; 5 mg I.V. during surgery if indicated.
Children: 1 mg I.M. or I.V. 1 to 2 hours preoperatively, repeated as necessary; 1 mg I.V. during surgery if indicated.
Prevention or treatment of dermal necrosis and sloughing of extravasation after I.V. administration of norepinephrine or ◇dopamine
Adults: Inject 5 to 10 mg in 10 ml of normal saline solution into the affected area, or add 10 mg to each liter of I.V. fluids containing norepinephrine.
Children: 0.1 to 0.2 mg/kg injected into affected area, up to a maximum of 10 mg per dose, following extravasation of dopamine.
◇Adjunctive treatment of left-sided heart failure secondary to acute MI
Adults: 170 to 400 mcg/minute by I.V. infusion.
◇Treatment adjunct for males with impotence (neurogenic or vascular)
Adults: 0.5 to 1 mg by intracavernosal injection. Usually administered with 30 mg papaverine injection.
◇Hypertensive crisis from sympathomimetic amines
Adults: 5 to 15 mg I.V.

Pharmacodynamics
Antihypertensive action: Phentolamine competitively antagonizes endogenous and exogenous amines at presynaptic and postsynaptic alpha-adrenergic receptors, decreasing both preload and afterload.
Cutaneous vasodilation action: Phentolamine blocks epinephrine- and norepinephrine-induced vasoconstriction.

Pharmacokinetics
Absorption: Antihypertensive effect is immediate after I.V. administration.
Distribution: Unknown.
Metabolism: Unknown.
Excretion: About 10% of a given dose is excreted unchanged in urine; excretion of remainder is unknown. Drug has a short duration of action; plasma half-life is 19 minutes after I.V. administration.

Route	Onset	Peak	Duration
I.V.	Immediate	Unknown	Unknown
I.M.	Unknown	Unknown	Unknown

Contraindications and precautions
Contraindicated in patients with angina, coronary artery disease, MI or history of MI, or hypersensitivity to drug. Use cautiously in patients with peptic ulcer or gastritis.

Interactions
Drug-drug. *Ephedrine and epinephrine*: Phentolamine antagonizes vasoconstrictor and hypertensive effects. Don't use together.

Effects on diagnostic tests
None reported.

Adverse reactions
CNS: *dizziness, weakness, flushing,* ***cerebrovascular occlusion,*** cerebrovascular spasm.
CV: *hypotension,* ***shock, arrhythmias,*** tachycardia, ***MI.***
EENT: *nasal congestion.*
GI: *diarrhea, nausea, vomiting.*

Overdose and treatment
Signs and symptoms of overdose include hypotension, dizziness, fainting, tachycardia, vomiting, lethargy, and shock.

Treat supportively and symptomatically. Use norepinephrine if necessary to increase the blood pressure. Don't use epinephrine; it stimulates both alpha and beta receptors and causes vasodilation and a further decrease in blood pressure.

Clinical considerations
Consider the recommendations relevant to all alpha blockers as well as the following:
- Usual doses of phentolamine have little effect on the blood pressure of normal individuals or patients with essential hypertension.
- Before test for pheochromocytoma, have patient rest in supine position until blood pressure is stabilized. When phentolamine is administered I.V., inject dose rapidly after effects of the venipuncture on the blood pressure have passed. A marked decrease in blood pressure is seen immediately, with the maximum effect seen within 2 minutes. Record blood pressure immediately after the injection, at 30-second intervals for the first 3 minutes, and at 1-minute intervals for the next 7 minutes. When drug is administered I.M., maximum effect occurs within 20 minutes. Record blood pressure every 5 minutes for 30 to 45 minutes after injection.
- A positive test response occurs when patient's blood pressure decreases at least 35 mm Hg systolic and 25 mm Hg diastolic; a negative test response occurs when the patient's blood pressure remains unchanged, is elevated, or decreases less than 35 mm Hg systolic and 25 mm Hg diastolic.
- When possible, withdraw sedatives, analgesics, and all other medication at least 24 hours (preferably 48 to 72 hours) before the phentolamine test. Withdraw antihypertensive drugs and don't perform test until blood pressure returns to pretreatment levels; withdraw rauwolfia drugs at least 4 weeks before test.
- Drug has been used to treat hypertension resulting from clonidine withdrawal and to treat the reaction to sympathetic amines or other drugs or foods in patients taking MAO inhibitors.
- Drug has also been used in patients with MI associated with left-sided heart failure in an attempt to reduce infarct size and decrease left ventricular ejection impedance. It also has been used to treat supraventricular premature contractions.

Therapeutic monitoring
Monitor vital signs closely.

Special populations
Breast-feeding patients. It isn't known if drug is excreted in breast milk. Because of possible adverse reactions in the infant, discontinue either breast-feeding or drug based on the importance of drug to the woman.
Pediatric patients. Administer cautiously.
Geriatric patients. Administer cautiously.

Patient counseling
- Teach patient about phentolamine test, if indicated.
- Tell patient to report adverse effects at once.
- Tell patient not to take sedatives or narcotics for at least 24 hours before phentolamine test.

phenylephrine hydrochloride
Nasal products
Alconefrin 12, Alconefrin 25, Neo-Synephrine, Nostril, Rhinall, Sinex

Parenteral
Neo-Synephrine

Ophthalmic
AK-Dilate, AK-Nefrin, Isopto Frin, Mydfrin, Neo-Synephrine, Prefrin Liquifilm, Relief Phenoptic

Pharmacologic classification: adrenergic
Therapeutic classification: vasoconstrictor
Pregnancy risk category C

How supplied
Available by prescription only
Injection: 10 mg/ml parenteral
Ophthalmic solution: 0.12%, 2.5%, 10%
Available without a prescription
Nasal solution: 0.125%, 0.16%, 0.25%, 0.5%, 1%
Nasal spray: 0.25%, 0.5%, 1%

Indications and dosages
Hypotensive emergencies during spinal anesthesia
Adults: Initially, 0.1 to 0.2 mg I.V.; subsequent doses should also be low (0.1 mg).
Prevention of hypotension during spinal or inhalation anesthesia
Adults: 2 to 3 mg S.C. or I.M. 3 to 4 minutes before anesthesia.
Mild to moderate hypotension
Adults: 1 to 10 mg S.C. or I.M.; initial dose shouldn't exceed 5 mg. Additional doses may be given in 1 to 2 hours if needed. Or, 0.1 to 0.5 mg slow I.V. injection; initial dose shouldn't exceed 0.5 mg. Additional doses may be given q 10 to 15 minutes.
Children: 0.1 mg/kg or 3 mg/m^2 I.M. or S.C.
Paroxysmal supraventricular tachycardia
Adults: Initially, 0.5 mg rapid I.V.; subsequent doses may be increased in increments of 0.1 to 0.2 mg. Maximum dose shouldn't exceed 1 mg.
Prolongation of spinal anesthesia
Adults: 2 to 5 mg added to anesthetic solution.

Adjunct in the treatment of severe hypotension or shock
Adults: 0.1 to 0.18 mcg/minute I.V. infusion. After blood pressure stabilizes, maintain at 0.04 to 0.06 mcg/minute, adjusted to patient response.
Vasoconstrictor for regional anesthesia
Adults: 1 mg phenylephrine added to 20 ml local anesthetic.
Mydriasis (without cycloplegia)
Adults: Instill 1 or 2 drops 2.5% or 10% solution in eye before procedure. May be repeated in 10 to 60 minutes if needed.
Posterior synechia (adhesion of iris)
Adults: Instill 1 drop of 10% solution in eye 3 or more times daily with atropine sulfate.
Diagnosis of Horner's or Raeder's syndrome
Adults: Instill a 1% or 10% solution in both eyes.
Initial treatment of postoperative malignant glaucoma
Adults: Instill 1 drop of a 10% solution with 1 drop of a 1% to 4% atropine sulfate solution 3 or more times daily.
Nasal, ◊sinus, or eustachian tube congestion
Adults and children over age 12: Apply 2 to 3 drops or 1 to 2 sprays of 0.25% to 1% solution instilled in each nostril; or a small quantity of 0.5% nasal jelly applied into each nostril. Apply jelly or spray to nasal mucosa.
Children age 6 to 12: Apply 2 to 3 drops or 1 to 2 sprays in each nostril.
Children under age 6: Apply 2 to 3 drops or sprays of 0.125% or 0.16% solution in each nostril.

Note: Drops, spray, or jelly can be given q 4 hours, p.r.n.
Conjunctival congestion
Adults: 1 to 2 drops of 0.08% to 0.25% solution applied to conjunctiva q 3 to 4 hours, p.r.n.

Pharmacodynamics

Vasopressor action: Phenylephrine acts predominantly by direct stimulation of alpha-adrenergic receptors, which constrict resistance and capacitance blood vessels, resulting in increased total peripheral resistance; increased systolic and diastolic blood pressure; decreased blood flow to vital organs, skin, and skeletal muscle; and constriction of renal blood vessels, reducing renal blood flow. Its main therapeutic effect is vasoconstriction.

It may also act indirectly by releasing norepinephrine from its storage sites. Phenylephrine doesn't stimulate beta receptors except in large doses, when it activates $beta_1$ receptors. Tachyphylaxis (tolerance) may follow repeated injections.

Other alpha-adrenergic effects include action on the dilator muscle of the pupil (producing contraction) and local decongestant action in the arterioles of the conjunctiva (producing constriction).

Phenylephrine acts directly on alpha-adrenergic receptors in the arterioles of conjunctiva nasal mucosa, producing constriction. Its vasoconstricting action on skin, mucous membranes, and viscera slows the vascular absorption rate of local anesthetics, which prolongs their action, localizes anesthesia, and decreases the risk of toxicity.

Phenylephrine may cause contraction of pregnant uterus and constriction of uterine blood vessels.

Pharmacokinetics

Absorption: Variable depending on route of administration.
Distribution: Unknown.
Metabolism: Metabolized in the liver and intestine by MAO.
Excretion: Unknown.

Route	Onset	Peak	Duration
I.V.	Immediate	Unknown	15-20 min
I.M.	10-15 min	Unknown	½-2 hr
S.C.	10-15 min	Unknown	50-60 min
Ophthalmic	Rapid	10-90 min	3-7 hr
Nasal	Rapid	Unknown	½-4 hr

Contraindications and precautions

All forms are contraindicated in patients with hypersensitivity to drug. Injected form is also contraindicated in those with severe hypertension or ventricular tachycardia. Ophthalmic form is also contraindicated in patients with angle-closure glaucoma and in those who wear soft contact lenses.

Use all forms cautiously in the elderly and in patients with hyperthyroidism or cardiac disease. Use nasal and ophthalmic forms cautiously in patients with type I diabetes mellitus, hypertension, or advanced arteriosclerotic changes and in children who have low body weight. Use injectable form cautiously in patients with severe atherosclerosis, bradycardia, partial heart block, myocardial disease, or allergy to sulfites.

Interactions

Drug-drug. *Alpha blockers, antihypertensives, diuretics used as antihypertensives, guanadrel or guanethidine, nitrates, rauwolfia alkaloids:* Decreased pressor response (hypotension). Recommend monitoring blood pressure closely.
Cardiac glycosides; epinephrine or other sympathomimetics; general anesthetics, such as cycloproprane and halothane, guanadrel or guanethidine, levodopa, MAO inhibitors, tricyclic antidepressants: Phenylephrine may increase risk of arrhythmias, including tachycardia. Monitor patient closely.

Cycloplegic antimuscarinic drugs: Mydriatic response to phenylephrine is increased. Avoid use together.
Doxapram, ergot alkaloids, MAO inhibitors, mazindol, methyldopa, oxytocics: Pressor effects are potentiated when phenylephrine is used concomitantly. Monitor patient closely.
Levodopa: The mydriatic response to phenylephrine is decreased. Avoid use together.
Nitrates: May reduce antianginal effects. Avoid use together.
Thyroid hormones: May increase effects of either drug. Avoid use together.

Effects on diagnostic tests
Drug may cause false-normal tonometry readings.

Adverse reactions
CNS: *headache;* excitability (with injected form); brow ache (with ophthalmic form); tremor, dizziness, nervousness (with nasal form).
CV: bradycardia, ***arrhythmias,*** hypertension (with injected form); *hypertension* (with 10% solution), tachycardia, palpitations, ***PVCs, MI*** (with ophthalmic form); *palpitations, tachycardia,* ***PVCs,*** hypertension, pallor (with nasal form).
EENT: transient eye burning or stinging on instillation, blurred vision, increased intraocular pressure, keratitis, lacrimation, reactive hyperemia of eye, allergic conjunctivitis, rebound miosis (with ophthalmic form); transient burning or stinging, dryness of nasal mucosa, rebound nasal congestion with continued use (with nasal form).
GI: nausea (with nasal form).
Skin: pallor, dermatitis (with ophthalmic form).
Other: tachyphylaxis (may occur with continued use), ***anaphylaxis, asthmatic episodes,*** decreased organ perfusion (with prolonged use), tissue sloughing with extravasation (with injected form); trembling, diaphoresis (with ophthalmic form).

Overdose and treatment
Signs and symptoms of overdose include exaggeration of common adverse reactions, palpitations, paresthesia, vomiting, arrhythmias, and hypertension.

To treat, discontinue drug and provide symptomatic and supportive measures. Monitor vital signs closely. Use atropine sulfate to block reflex bradycardia; phentolamine to treat excessive hypertension; and propranolol to treat cardiac arrhythmias, or levodopa to reduce an excessive mydriatic effect of an ophthalmic preparation as necessary.

Clinical considerations
Consider the recommendations relevant to all adrenergics as well as the following:

- Give I.V. through large veins, and monitor flow rate. To treat extravasation ischemia, infiltrate site promptly and liberally with 10 to 15 ml of NaCl solution containing 5 to 10 mg of phentolamine through fine needle. Topical nitroglycerin has also been used.
- During I.V. administration, pulse, blood pressure, and central venous pressure should be monitored every 2 to 5 minutes. Control flow rate and dosage to prevent excessive increases. I.V. overdoses can induce ventricular arrhythmias.
- Hypovolemic states should be corrected before administration of drug; phenylephrine shouldn't be used in place of fluid, blood, plasma, and electrolyte replacement.
- Phenylephrine is chemically incompatible with butacaine, sulfate, alkalies, ferric salts, and oxidizing agents and metals.

Ophthalmic
- Apply digital pressure to lacrimal sac during and for 1 to 2 minutes after instillation to prevent systemic absorption.
- Prolonged exposure to air or strong light may cause oxidation and discoloration. Don't use if solution is brown or contains precipitate.
- To prevent contamination, don't touch applicator tip to any surface. Instruct patient in proper technique.

Nasal
- After use, rinse tip of spray bottle or dropper with hot water and dry with clean tissue. Wipe tip of nasal jelly container with clean, damp tissues.

Therapeutic monitoring
- Prolonged or chronic use may result in rebound congestion and chronic swelling of nasal mucosa.
- To reduce risk of rebound congestion, use weakest effective dose.

Special populations
Breast-feeding patients. It isn't known if drug is excreted in breast milk; use with caution in breast-feeding women.
Pediatric patients. Infants and children may be more susceptible than adults to effects of drug. Because of the risk of precipitating severe hypertension, only ophthalmic solutions containing 0.5% or less should be used in infants under age 1. The 10% ophthalmic solution is contraindicated in infants. Most manufacturers recommend that the 0.5% nasal solution not be used in children under age 12 except under medical supervision, and the 0.25% nasal solution shouldn't be used in children under age 6 except under medical supervision.
Geriatric patients. Effects may be exaggerated in geriatric patients. In patients over age 50, phenylephrine (ophthalmic solution) appears to alter the response of the dilator mus-

cle of the pupil; rebound miosis may occur the day after drug is administered

Patient counseling

- Tell patient to store away from heat, light, and humidity (not in bathroom medicine cabinet) and out of children's reach.
- Warn patient to use only as directed. If using OTC product, patient should follow directions on label and not use more often or in larger doses than prescribed or recommended.
- Caution patient not to exceed recommended dosage regardless of formulation; patient shouldn't double, decrease, or omit doses, or change dosage intervals, unless so instructed.
- Tell patient to contact health care provider if drug provides no relief in 2 days after using phenylephrine ophthalmic solution or 3 days after using the nasal solution.
- Explain that systemic absorption from nasal and conjunctival membranes can occur. Patient should report systemic reactions, such as dizziness and chest pain, and discontinue drug.

Ophthalmic

- Instruct patient not to use if solution is brown or contains a precipitate.
- Tell patient to wash hands before applying and to use finger to apply pressure to lacrimal sac during and for 1 to 2 minutes after instillation to decrease systemic absorption.
- Inform patient that after applying drops, pupils will become unusually large. Advise patient to use sunglasses to protect eyes from sunlight and other bright lights, and to report if effects persist 12 hours or more.

Nasal

- After use, tell patient to rinse tip of spray bottle or dropper with hot water and dry with clean tissue or wipe tip of nasal jelly container with clean, damp tissues.
- Instruct patient to blow nose gently (with both nostrils open) to clear nasal passages well, before using medication.
- Teach patient correct method of instillation:

—Drops: Tilt head back while sitting or standing up, or lie on bed and hang head over side. Stay in position a few minutes to permit medication to spread through nose.

—Spray: With head upright, squeeze bottle quickly and firmly to produce 1 or 2 sprays into each nostril; wait 3 to 5 minutes, blow nose and repeat dose.

—Jelly: Place in each nostril and sniff it well back into nose.

- Tell patient that increased fluid intake helps keep secretions liquid.
- Warn patient to avoid using nonprescription medications with phenylephrine to prevent possible hazardous interactions.

phenytoin, phenytoin sodium, phenytoin sodium (extended)

Dilantin, Dilantin Kapseals, Dilantin Infatab, Dilantin-125

phenytoin sodium (prompt)

Pharmacologic classification: hydantoin derivative
Therapeutic classification: anticonvulsant
Pregnancy risk category D

How supplied

Available by prescription only
phenytoin
Tablets (chewable): 50 mg
Oral suspension: 30 mg/5 ml,* 125 mg/5 ml
phenytoin sodium
Injection: 50 mg/ml
phenytoin sodium (extended)
Capsules: 30 mg, 100 mg
phenytoin sodium (prompt)
Capsules: 100 mg

Indications and dosages

Generalized tonic-clonic seizures, status epilepticus, nonepileptic seizures (post-head trauma, Reye's syndrome)
Adults: Loading dose is 10 to 15 mg/kg I.V. slowly, not to exceed 50 mg/minute; oral loading dose consists of 1 g divided into three doses (400 mg, 300 mg, 300 mg) given at 2-hour intervals. Maintenance dosage once controlled is 300 mg P.O. daily (extended only); initially use a dose divided t.i.d. (extended or prompt).
Children: Loading dose is 15 to 20 mg/kg I.V. at 50 mg/minute, or P.O. divided q 8 to 12 hours; then start maintenance dosage of 4 to 8 mg/kg P.O. or I.V. daily, divided q 12 hours.
Neuritic pain (migraine, trigeminal neuralgia, and Bell's palsy)
Adults: 200 to 600 mg P.O. daily in divided doses.
Skeletal muscle relaxant
Adults: 200 to 600 mg P.O. daily, p.r.n.
◊ ***Ventricular arrhythmias unresponsive to lidocaine or procainamide, and arrhythmias induced by cardiac glycosides***
Adults: 50 to 100 mg I.V. q 10 to 15 minutes, p.r.n., not to exceed 15 mg/kg. Infusion rate should never exceed 50 mg/minute (slow I.V. push).
Alternate method: 100 mg I.V. q 15 minutes until adverse effects develop, arrhythmias are controlled, or 1 g has been given. Also may administer entire loading dose of 1 g I.V. slowly at 25 mg/minute. Can be diluted in normal saline solution. I.M. dosage isn't recommended because of pain and erratic absorption.

Prophylactic control of seizures during neurosurgery
Adults: 100 to 200 mg I.V. at intervals of about 4 hours during perioperative and postoperative periods.

Pharmacodynamics
Anticonvulsant action: Like other hydantoin derivatives, phenytoin stabilizes neuronal membranes and limits seizure activity by either increasing efflux or decreasing influx of sodium ions across cell membranes in the motor cortex during generation of nerve impulses. Phenytoin exerts its antiarrhythmic effects by normalizing sodium influx to Purkinje's fibers in patients with cardiac glycoside-induced arrhythmias. It's indicated for generalized tonic-clonic (grand mal) and partial seizures.
Other actions: Phenytoin inhibits excessive collagenase activity in patients with epidermolysis bullosa.

Pharmacokinetics
Absorption: Absorbed slowly from the small intestine; absorption is formulation-dependent and bioavailability may differ among products. Extended-release capsules give peak serum levels at 4 to 12 hours; prompt-release products peak at 1½ to 3 hours. I.M. doses are absorbed erratically; about 50% to 75% of I.M. dose is absorbed in 24 hours.
Distribution: Distributed widely throughout the body; therapeutic plasma levels are 10 to 20 mcg/ml, although in some patients, they occur at 5 to 10 mcg/ml. Lateral nystagmus may occur at levels above 20 mcg/ml; ataxia usually occurs at levels above 30 mcg/ml; significantly decreased mental capacity occurs at 40 mcg/ml. Phenytoin is about 90% protein-bound, less so in uremic patients.
Metabolism: Metabolized by the liver to inactive metabolites.
Excretion: Excreted in urine and exhibits dose-dependent (zero-order) elimination kinetics; above a certain dosage level, small increases in dosage disproportionately increase serum levels.

Route	Onset	Peak	Duration
P.O.	Unknown	1½-12 hr	Unknown
I.V.	Immediate	1-2 hr	Unknown
I.M.	Unknown	Unknown	Unknown

Contraindications and precautions
Contraindicated in patients with hydantoin hypersensitivity, sinus bradycardia, SA block, second- or third-degree AV block, or Adams-Stokes syndrome.

Use cautiously in geriatric or debilitated patients; in those with hepatic dysfunction, hypotension, myocardial insufficiency, diabetes, or respiratory depression; and in those receiving hydantoin derivatives.

Interactions
Drug-drug. *Allopurinol, amiodarone, benzodiazepines, chloramphenicol, chlorpheniramine, cimetidine, diazepam, disulfiram, fluconazole, ibuprofen, imipramine, isoniazid, metronidazole, miconazole, omeprazole, phenacemide, phenylbutazone, salicylates, succinimides, trimethoprim, or valproic acid:* Therapeutic effects of phenytoin may be increased. Monitor patient carefully.
Antacids, antineoplastics, barbiturates, calcium, calcium gluconate, carbamazepine, charcoal, diazoxide, folic acid, loxapine, nitrofurantoin, pyridoxine, rifampin, sucralfate, or theophylline: Therapeutic effects of phenytoin may be decreased. Monitor levels.
Antipsychotic agents: May attenuate therapeutic effects of phenytoin. Monitor patient closely.
APAP, amiodarone, carbamazepine, corticosteroids, cyclosporine, dicumarol, digitoxin, disopyramide, dopamine, doxycycline, estrogens, furosemide, haloperidol, levodopa, mebendazole, meperidine, methadone, metyrapone, oral contraceptives, phenothiazines, quinidine, or sulfonylureas: Phenytoin may decrease the effects of these drugs by stimulating hepatic metabolism. Monitor patient.
Drug-lifestyle. *Alcohol use:* Therapeutic effects of phenytoin may be decreased. Don't use together.
Drug-food. *Oral tube feedings with Osmolite or Isocal:* May interfere with absorption of oral phenytoin. Enteral feedings should be stopped for 2 hours before and 2 hours after phenytoin administration.

Effects on diagnostic tests
Phenytoin may raise blood glucose levels by inhibiting pancreatic insulin release; it may decrease serum levels of protein-bound iodine and may interfere with the 1-mg dexamethasone suppression test.

Adverse reactions
CNS: *ataxia, slurred speech,* dizziness, insomnia, nervousness, twitching, headache, *mental confusion, decreased coordination.*
CV: periarteritis nodosa, hypotension.
EENT: *nystagmus, diplopia,* blurred vision, *gingival hyperplasia* (especially in children).
GI: *nausea, vomiting,* constipation.
Hematologic: ***thrombocytopenia, leukopenia, agranulocytosis, pancytopenia,*** macrocythemia, megaloblastic anemia.
Hepatic: *toxic hepatitis.*
Skin: scarlatiniform or morbilliform rash; bullous, *exfoliative,* or purpuric dermatitis; ***Stevens-Johnson syndrome;*** lupus erythematosus; *hirsutism;* ***toxic epidermal necrolysis;*** photosensitivity; pain, necrosis, and inflammation at injection site; discoloration of skin ("purple glove syndrome") if given by I.V. push in back of hand.

Other: lymphadenopathy, hyperglycemia, osteomalacia, hypertrichosis.

Overdose and treatment

Early signs and symptoms of overdose may include drowsiness, nausea, vomiting, nystagmus, ataxia, dysarthria, tremor, and slurred speech; hypotension, arrhythmias, respiratory depression, and coma may follow. Death is caused by respiratory and circulatory depression. Estimated lethal dose in adults is 2 to 5 g.

Treat overdose with gastric lavage or emesis and follow with supportive treatment. Carefully monitor vital signs and fluid and electrolyte balance. Forced diuresis is of little or no value. Hemodialysis or peritoneal dialysis may be helpful.

Clinical considerations

Consider the recommendations relevant to all hydantoin derivatives as well as the following:

- Only extended-release capsules are approved for once-daily dosing; all other forms are given in divided doses every 8 to 12 hours.
- If suspension is used, shake well.
- Avoid I.M. administration; it's painful and drug absorption is erratic.
- Mix I.V. doses in normal saline solution and use within 30 minutes; mixtures with D_5W will precipitate. Don't refrigerate solution; don't mix with other drugs. In-line filter is recommended.
- Abrupt withdrawal may precipitate status epilepticus.
- If using I.V. bolus, use slow (50 mg/minute) I.V. push or constant infusion; too-rapid I.V. injection may cause hypotension and circulatory collapse. Don't use I.V. push in veins on back of hand; larger veins are needed to prevent discoloration associated with purple glove syndrome.
- Phenytoin commonly is abbreviated as DPH (diphenylhydantoin), an older drug name.

Therapeutic monitoring

- Monitoring of serum levels is essential because of dose-dependent excretion.
- When giving I.V., continuous monitoring of ECG, blood pressure, and respiratory status is essential.

Special populations

Breast-feeding patients. Drug is excreted in breast milk; an alternative feeding method is recommended during therapy.

Pediatric patients. Special pediatric-strength suspension (30 mg/5 ml) is available in Canada only. Take extreme care to use correct strength. Don't confuse with adult strength (125 mg/5 ml).

Geriatric patients. Geriatric patients metabolize and excrete phenytoin slowly; therefore, they may require lower doses.

Patient counseling

- Tell patient to use same brand of phenytoin consistently. Changing brands may change therapeutic effect.
- Instruct patient to take drug with food or milk to minimize GI distress.
- Warn patient not to discontinue drug, except with medical supervision; to avoid hazardous activities that require alertness until CNS effect is determined; and to avoid alcoholic beverages.
- Encourage patient to wear a medical identification bracelet or necklace.
- Stress good oral hygiene to minimize overgrowth and sensitivity of gums.

physostigmine salicylate

Antilirium

physostigmine sulfate

Eserine, Isopto Eserine

Pharmacologic classification: cholinesterase inhibitor
Therapeutic classification: antimuscarinic antidote, antiglaucoma
Pregnancy risk category C

How supplied

Available by prescription only
Injection: 1 mg/ml
Ophthalmic ointment: 0.25%

Indications and dosages

Anticholinergic toxicity from drugs and plants

Adults: 0.5 to 2 mg I.M. or I.V. given slowly (not to exceed 1 mg/minute I.V.). Dosage individualized and repeated, p.r.n., q 20 minutes until response or adverse effects occur.

Children: Reserve for life-threatening situations only. Initial pediatric I.V. or I.M. dose of physostigmine salicylate is 0.02 mg/kg. Dosage may be repeated at 5- to 10-minute intervals to maximum of 2 mg if no adverse cholinergic signs are present.

Postanesthesia care

Adults: 0.5 to 1 mg I.M. or I.V. given slowly (not to exceed 1 mg/minute I.V.). Dosage individualized and repeated, p.r.n., q 10 to 30 minutes.

Open-angle glaucoma

Adults: Instill 2 drops into eye up to q.i.d., or apply ointment to lower fornix up to t.i.d.

Pharmacodynamics

Antimuscarinic action: Physostigmine competitively blocks acetylcholine hydrolysis by cholinesterase, resulting in acetylcholine accumulation at cholinergic synapses; that antagonizes the muscarinic effects of overdose with antidepressants and anticholinergics. With ophthalmic use, miosis and ciliary muscle contraction increase aqueous humor outflow and decrease intraocular pressure.

Pharmacokinetics

Absorption: Well absorbed from the GI tract, mucous membranes, and subcutaneous tissues when given I.M. or I.V., with effects peaking within 5 minutes. After ophthalmic use, drug may be absorbed orally after passage through the nasolacrimal duct.
Distribution: Distributed widely and crosses the blood-brain barrier.
Metabolism: Cholinesterase hydrolyzes physostigmine relatively quickly. Duration of effect is 1 to 2 hours after I.V. administration, 12 to 48 hours after ophthalmic use.
Excretion: Only a small amount of drug is excreted in urine. Exact mode of excretion is unknown.

Route	Onset	Peak	Duration
Ophthalmic	10-30 min	Unknown	12-48 hr

Contraindications and precautions

Injected form contraindicated in patients with mechanical obstruction of the intestine or urogenital tract, asthma, gangrene, diabetes, CV disease, or vagotonia and in those receiving choline esters or depolarizing neuromuscular blockers.

Ophthalmic form is contraindicated in patients with intolerance to physostigmine, active uveitis, or corneal injury. Use injectable form cautiously during pregnancy.

Interactions

Drug-drug. *Succinylcholine:* May prolong respiratory depression. Monitor patient closely.
Systemic cholinergic agents: May cause additive toxicity. Monitor patient closely.
Drug-herb. *Jaborandi tree and pill-bearing spurge:* May have additive effect when used together. Use with caution to avoid risk of toxicity.

Effects on diagnostic tests

None reported.

Adverse reactions

CNS: weakness; headache (with ophthalmic form); ***seizures,*** *restlessness, excitability* (with injected form).
CV: slow or irregular heartbeat (with ophthalmic form); bradycardia, hypotension (with injected form).
EENT: blurred vision, eye pain, burning, redness, stinging, eye irritation, twitching of eyelids, watering of eyes (with ophthalmic form); miosis (with injected form).
GI: nausea, vomiting, diarrhea; epigastric pain, *excessive salivation* (with injected form).
GU: loss of bladder control (with ophthalmic form); urinary urgency (with injected form).
Respiratory: ***bronchospasm,*** bronchial constriction, shortness of breath, dyspnea (with injected form).
Other: diaphoresis.

Overdose and treatment

Signs and symptoms of overdose include headache, nausea, vomiting, diarrhea, blurred vision, miosis, myopia, excessive tearing, bronchospasm, increased bronchial secretions, hypotension, incoordination, excessive sweating, muscle weakness, bradycardia, excessive salivation, restlessness or agitation, and confusion.

Support respiration; bronchial suctioning may be performed. Discontinue drug immediately. Atropine may be given to block muscarinic effects of physostigmine. Avoid atropine overdose because it may cause bronchial plug formation.

Clinical considerations

Consider the recommendations relevant to all cholinesterase inhibitors as well as the following:

- Observe solution for discoloration. Don't use if darkened.
- Atropine sulfate injection should always be available as an antagonist and antidote for most of the effects of physostigmine. Monitor vital signs.
- The commercially available formulation of physostigmine salicylate injection contains sodium bisulfite, a sulfite that can cause allergic-type reactions including anaphylaxis and life-threatening or less severe asthmatic episodes in certain susceptible individuals.

Ophthalmic

- Have patient lie down or tilt his head back to facilitate administration of eyedrops.
- Wait at least 5 minutes before administering any other eyedrops.
- Gently pinch patient's nasal bridge for 1 to 2 minutes after administering each dose of eyedrops to minimize systemic absorption.
- After applying ointment, have patient close eyelids and roll eyes.

Therapeutic monitoring

- Monitor vital signs; patient should be observed for evidence of bronchoconstriction.
- Monitor patient for tolerance to drug.
- Cardiac monitoring is recommended.

Special populations

Breast-feeding patients. Safety and efficacy in breast-feeding women haven't been established.
Geriatric patients. Use caution when administering to geriatric patients because they may be more sensitive to effects of drug.

Patient counseling

Ophthalmic

- Teach patient how to administer ophthalmic ointment or solution.

- Instruct patient not to close his eyes tightly or blink unnecessarily after instilling the ophthalmic solution.
- Warn patient that he may experience blurred vision and difficulty seeing after initial doses.
- Instruct patient to report abdominal cramps, diarrhea, or excessive salivation.

pilocarpine hydrochloride

Adsorbocarpine, Akarpine, Isopto Carpine, Minims Pilocarpine*, Miocarpine*, Ocusert Pilo, Pilocar, Pilopine HS

pilocarpine nitrate

P.V. Carpine Liquifilm

Pharmacologic classification: cholinergic agonist
Therapeutic classification: miotic
Pregnancy risk category C

How supplied

Available by prescription only
pilocarpine hydrochloride
Ophthalmic solution: 0.25%, 0.5%, 1%, 2%, 3%, 4%, 5%, 6%, 8%, 10%
Gel: 4%
Releasing-system insert: 20 mcg/hour, 40 mcg/hour
pilocarpine nitrate
Solution: 1%, 2%, 4%

Indications and dosages

Chronic open-angle glaucoma; before, or instead of, emergency surgery in acute narrow-angle glaucoma
Adults and children: Instill 1 or 2 drops of a 1% to 4% solution in the lower conjunctival sac q 4 to 12 hours (dosage should be based on periodic tonometric readings) or apply ½-inch ribbon of 4% gel (Pilopine HS) h.s.

Alternatively, apply one Ocusert Pilo System (20 or 40 mcg/hour) q 7 days.

Emergency treatment of acute narrow-angle glaucoma
Adults and children: 1 drop of 2% solution q 5 minutes for three to six doses, followed by 1 drop q 1 to 3 hours until pressure is controlled.

To counteract mydriatic effects of sympathomimetic agents
Adults: 1 drop of 1% solution in affected eye.

Pharmacodynamics

Miotic action: Pilocarpine stimulates cholinergic receptors of the sphincter muscles of the iris, resulting in miosis. It also produces ciliary muscle contraction, resulting in accommodation with deepening of the anterior chamber, and vasodilation of conjunctival vessels of the outflow tract.

Pharmacokinetics

Absorption: With the Ocusert Pilo System, 0.3 to 7 mg of pilocarpine are released during the initial 6-hour period; during the remainder of the 1-week insertion period, the release rate is within ± 20% of the rated value.
Distribution: Unknown.
Metabolism: Unknown.
Excretion: Duration of effect of pilocarpine drops is 4 to 6 hours.

Route	Onset	Peak	Duration
Ophthalmic	10-30 min	30-85 min	4-8 hr

Contraindications and precautions

Contraindicated in patients with hypersensitivity to drug or when cholinergic effects such as constriction are undesirable (such as acute iritis, some forms of secondary glaucoma, pupillary block glaucoma, acute inflammatory disease of the anterior chamber).

Use cautiously in patients with acute cardiac failure, bronchial asthma, peptic ulcer, hyperthyroidism, GI spasm, urinary obstruction, and Parkinson's disease.

Interactions

Drug-drug. *Demecarium, echothiophate, isoflurophate:* Decrease the pharmacologic effects of pilocarpine. Avoid use together.
Epinephrine derivatives and timolol: Pilocarpine can enhance reductions in intraocular pressure. Monitor patient closely.

Effects on diagnostic tests

None reported.

Adverse reactions

CV: hypertension, tachycardia.
EENT: periorbital or supraorbital headache, *myopia,* ciliary spasm, *blurred vision,* conjunctival irritation, transient stinging and burning, keratitis, lens opacity, retinal detachment, lacrimation, changes in visual field, *brow pain.*
GI: nausea, vomiting, diarrhea, salivation.
Respiratory: ***bronchoconstriction, pulmonary edema.***
Other: hypersensitivity reactions, diaphoresis.

Overdose and treatment

Signs and symptoms of overdose include flushing, vomiting, bradycardia, bronchospasm, increased bronchial secretion, sweating, tearing, involuntary urination, hypotension, and tremors. Vomiting is usually spontaneous with accidental ingestion; if not, induce emesis and follow with activated charcoal or a cathartic. Treat dermal exposure by washing the areas twice with water. Use epinephrine to treat the CV responses. Atropine sulfate is the antidote of choice. Flush the eye with water or sodium chloride to treat a local overdose. Doses up to 20 mg are generally considered nontoxic.

Clinical considerations
Drug may be used alone or with mannitol, urea, glycerol, or acetazolamide. It also may be used to counteract effects of mydriatic and cycloplegic agents after surgery or ophthalmoscopic examination and may be used alternately with atropine to break adhesions.

Therapeutic monitoring
Patients with dark eyes may require stronger solutions or more frequent installation because eye pigment may absorb drug.

Patient counseling
- Warn patient that vision will be temporarily blurred, that miotic pupil may make surroundings appear dim and reduce peripheral field of vision, and that transient brow ache and myopia are common at first; assure patient that adverse effects subside 10 to 14 days after therapy begins.
- Instruct patient to check for the presence of the pilocarpine ocular system at bedtime and upon rising.
- Tell patient that if systems in both eyes are lost, they should be replaced as soon as possible. If one system is lost, it may either be replaced with a fresh system or the system remaining in the other eye may be removed and both replaced with fresh systems so that both systems will subsequently be replaced on the same schedule.
- Instruct patient that if the Ocusert System falls out of the eye during sleep, he should wash hands, then rinse Ocusert in cool tap water and reposition it in the eye. Don't use the insert if it's deformed.
- Inform patient that systems should be replaced every 7 days.
- Tell patient to use caution in night driving and other activities in poor illumination because miotic pupil diminishes side vision and illumination.
- Teach patient the correct way to instill drops and to apply light finger pressure on lacrimal sac for 1 minute after administration to minimize systemic absorption.
- Instruct patient to apply gel at bedtime because it will cause blurred vision.

pilocarpine hydrochloride
Salagen

Pharmacologic classification: cholinergic agonist
Therapeutic classification: antixerostomia
Pregnancy risk category C

How supplied
Available by prescription only
Tablets: 5 mg

Indications and dosages
Treatment of symptoms of xerostomia from salivary gland hypofunction caused by radiotherapy for cancer of the head and neck
Adults: 5 mg P.O. t.i.d. Dosage may be increased to 10 mg P.O. t.i.d., p.r.n.

Pharmacodynamics
Antixerostomia action: Oral pilocarpine increases secretion of the salivary glands, which eliminates dryness.

Pharmacokinetics
Absorption: Pilocarpine is absorbed in the GI tract. A high-fat meal may decrease rate of absorption.
Distribution: Unknown.
Metabolism: Inactivation of pilocarpine is believed to occur at neuronal synapses and probably in plasma.
Excretion: Drug and its minimally active or inactive degradation products are excreted in urine.

Route	Onset	Peak	Duration
P.O.	20 min	1 hr	3-5 hr

Contraindications and precautions
Contraindicated in patients with uncontrolled asthma or known hypersensitivity to pilocarpine and when miosis is undesirable, such as in acute iritis and narrow-angle glaucoma.

Use cautiously in patients with CV disease, controlled asthma, chronic bronchitis, COPD, cholelithiasis, biliary tract disease, nephrolithiasis, and cognitive or psychiatric disturbances.

Interactions
Drug-drug. *Beta-adrenergic antagonists:* May increase risk of conduction disturbances. Use together cautiously.
Drugs with anticholinergic effects: May antagonize anticholinergic effects of oral pilocarpine. Use together cautiously.
Drugs with parasympathomimetic effects: May result in additive pharmacologic effects. Monitor patient closely.

Effects on diagnostic tests
None reported.

Adverse reactions
CNS: *dizziness, headache,* tremor.
CV: hypertension, tachycardia.
EENT: *rhinitis,* lacrimation, amblyopia, pharyngitis, voice alteration, conjunctivitis, epistaxis, sinusitis, abnormal vision.
GI: *nausea,* dyspepsia, diarrhea, abdominal pain, vomiting, dysphagia, taste perversion.
GU: *urinary frequency.*
Musculoskeletal: *asthenia,* myalgia.
Skin: *flushing,* rash, pruritis.
Other: *sweating, chills,* edema.

Overdose and treatment
Taking 100 mg of oral pilocarpine is considered potentially fatal. Treatment is with atropine titration (0.5 mg to 1 mg S.C. or I.V.) and supportive measures to maintain respiration and circulation. Epinephrine (0.3 mg to 1 mg S.C. or I.M.) may also be useful during severe CV depression or bronchoconstriction. It isn't known if pilocarpine is dialyzable.

Clinical considerations
Patient should undergo careful examination of the fundus before therapy is initiated because retinal detachment has been reported with pilocarpine use in patients with preexisting retinal disease.

Therapeutic monitoring
Monitor patient for signs and symptoms of pilocarpine toxicity characterized by an exaggeration of its parasympathomimetic effects; these include headache, visual disturbance, lacrimation, sweating, respiratory distress, GI spasm, nausea, vomiting, diarrhea, AV block, tachycardia, bradycardia, hypotension, hypertension, shock, mental confusion, cardiac arrhythmia, and tremors.

Special populations
Breast-feeding patients. It's unknown if drug is excreted in breast milk. Because of the potential for serious adverse reactions in nursing infants, a decision should be made whether to discontinue breast-feeding or drug, taking into account the importance of drug to the woman.
Pediatric patients. Safety and efficacy in children haven't been established.

Patient counseling
- Warn patient that drug may cause visual disturbances, especially at night, that could impair his ability to drive safely.
- Tell patient to drink plenty of fluids to prevent dehydration if drug causes excessive sweating. If adequate fluid intake can't be maintained, tell patient to notify doctor.

pimozide
Orap

Pharmacologic classification:
diphenylbutylpiperidine
Therapeutic classification:
antipsychotic
Pregnancy risk category C

How supplied
Available by prescription only
Tablets: 1 mg, 2 mg

Indications and dosages
Suppression of severe motor and phonic tics in patients with Tourette syndrome
Adults: Initially, 1 to 2 mg/day P.O. in divided doses. Then, increase dosage, p.r.n., every other day. Maximum dose 0.2 mg/kg/day or 10 mg/day.
Children over age 12: 0.05 mg/kg P.O. h.s.; increase at 3-day intervals to maximum of 0.2 mg/kg. Maximum dose, 10 mg/day.

Pharmacodynamics
Antipsychotic action: Mechanism of action in Tourette syndrome is unknown; it's thought to exert its effects by postsynaptic or presynaptic blockade, or both, of CNS dopamine receptors, inhibiting dopamine-mediated effects. Pimozide also has anticholinergic, antiemetic, and anxiolytic effects and produces mild alpha blockade.

Pharmacokinetics
Absorption: Absorbed slowly and incompletely from the GI tract; bioavailability is about 50%.
Distribution: Distributed widely into the body.
Metabolism: Metabolized by the liver, mainly by cytochrome P-450 3A and to a lesser extent 1A2; a significant first-pass effect exists.
Excretion: About 40% of a given dose is excreted in urine as parent drug and metabolites in 3 to 4 days; about 15% is excreted in feces via the biliary tract within 3 to 6 days.

Route	Onset	Peak	Duration
P.O.	Unknown	4-12 hr	Unknown

Contraindications and precautions
Contraindicated in patients with hypersensitivity to drug, in treating simple tics or tics other than those associated with Tourette syndrome, concurrent drug therapy known to cause motor and phonic tics, congenital long QT syndrome or history of arrhythmias, patients with severe toxic CNS depression or experiencing coma.

Use cautiously in patients with impaired renal or hepatic function, glaucoma, prostatic hyperplasia, seizure disorders, or EEG abnormalities.

Interactions
Drug-drug. *Amphetamines, methylphenidate, pemoline:* May induce Tourette-like tic and may exacerbate existing tics. Avoid use together.
Anticonvulsants, such as carbamazepine, phenobarbital, and phenytoin: May induce seizures; an anticonvulsant dosage increase may be required.
Antidepressants, disopyramide, other antiarrhythmics, other antipsychotics, phenothiazines, procainamide, quinidine,: May further depress cardiac conduction and prolong QT interval,

resulting in serious arrhythmias. Use with caution and monitor patient closely.
CNS depressants: May cause additive CNS depressant effects. Avoid use together.
Drugs that inhibit CYP-450 isoenzyme 3A (azole fungal agents, macrolide antibiotics, protease inhibitors): Inhibit metabolism of pimozide. Don't use together.
Drug-food. *Grapefruit juice:* May inhibit metabolism of pimozide. Don't use together.
Drug-lifestyle. *Alcohol use:* Additive CNS depressant effects. Discourage alcohol use.

Effects on diagnostic tests
Pimozide causes quinidine-like ECG effects, including prolongation of QT interval and flattened T waves.

Adverse reactions
CNS: *parkinsonian-like symptoms,* drowsiness, headache, insomnia, ***neuroleptic malignant syndrome,*** extrapyramidal reactions, *tardive dyskinesia, sedation, adverse behavioral effects.*
CV: *ECG changes (prolonged QT interval),* hypotension, hypertension, tachycardia.
EENT: visual disturbances.
GI: *dry mouth, constipation.*
GU: impotence, urinary frequency.
Musculoskeletal: muscle rigidity.
Skin: rash, diaphoresis.

Overdose and treatment
Signs of overdose include severe extrapyramidal reactions, hypotension, respiratory depression, coma, and ECG abnormalities, including prolongation of QT interval, inversion or flattening of T waves, and new appearance of U waves.

Treat with gastric lavage. Maintain blood pressure with I.V. fluids, plasma expanders, or norepinephrine. Don't use epinephrine. Don't induce vomiting because of the potential for aspiration. Treat extrapyramidal symptoms with parenteral diphenhydramine. Monitor for adverse effects for at least 4 days because of prolonged half-life (55 hours) of drug.

Clinical considerations
- Obtain baseline ECG before therapy begins and then periodically to monitor CV effects.
- Assess patient periodically for abnormal body movement.
- Extrapyramidal reactions develop in about 10% to 15% of patients at normal doses. They're especially likely to occur during early days of therapy.
- If excessive restlessness and agitation occur, therapy with a beta blocker, such as propranolol or metoprolol, may be helpful.

Therapeutic monitoring
Maintain patient's serum potassium level within normal range; decreased potassium levels increase risk of arrhythmias. Monitor potassium level in patients with diarrhea and those taking diuretics.

Special populations
Pediatric patients. Use and efficacy in children under age 12 are limited. Dosage should be kept at the lowest possible level. Use of drug in children for any disorder other than Tourette syndrome isn't recommended.
Geriatric patients. Cardiac toxicity and tardive dyskinesia are more likely to develop in geriatric patients, even at normal doses.

Patient counseling
- Inform patient of risks, signs, and symptoms of dystonic reactions and tardive dyskinesia.
- Advise patient to take pimozide exactly as prescribed, not to double dose for missed doses, not to share drug with others, and not to stop taking it suddenly.
- Explain that therapeutic effect of drug may not be apparent for several weeks.
- Urge patient to report unusual effects promptly.
- Recommend use of sugarless hard candy or chewing gum, ice chips, or artificial saliva to relieve dry mouth.
- To prevent dizziness at start of therapy, tell patient to lie down for 30 minutes after taking each dose and to avoid sudden changes in posture, especially when rising to upright position.
- To minimize daytime sedation, suggest taking entire daily dose at bedtime.
- Warn patient to avoid hazardous activities that require alertness until effects of drug are known.

pindolol
Visken

Pharmacologic classification: beta blocker
Therapeutic classification: antihypertensive
Pregnancy risk category B

How supplied
Available by prescription only
Tablets: 5 mg, 10 mg

Indications and dosages
Hypertension
Adults: Initially, 5 mg P.O. b.i.d. increased by 10 mg/day q 3 to 4 weeks up to maximum of 60 mg/day. Usual dosage is 10 to 30 mg daily, given in two or three divided doses. In some patients, once-daily dosing may be possible.
◊***Angina***
Adults: 15 to 40 mg daily P.O. in three or four divided doses.

Pharmacodynamics

Antihypertensive action: Exact mechanism of antihypertensive action is unknown. Pindolol doesn't consistently affect cardiac output or renin release, and its other mechanisms such as decreased peripheral resistance probably contribute to its hypotensive effect. Because pindolol has some intrinsic sympathomimetic activity (beta-agonist sympathomimetic activity), it may be useful in patients in whom bradycardia develops with other beta blockers. It's a nonselective beta blocker, inhibiting both $beta_1$ and $beta_2$ receptors.

Pharmacokinetics

Absorption: After oral administration, pindolol is absorbed rapidly from the GI tract. Food doesn't reduce bioavailability but may increase the rate of GI absorption.
Distribution: Distributed widely throughout the body and is 40% to 60% protein-bound.
Metabolism: About 60% to 65% of a given dose of pindolol is metabolized by the liver.
Excretion: In adults with normal renal function, 35% to 50% of a given dose is excreted unchanged in urine; half-life is about 3 to 4 hours.

Route	Onset	Peak	Duration
P.O.	Unknown	1-2 hr	24 hr

Contraindications and precautions

Contraindicated in patients with hypersensitivity to drug, bronchial asthma, severe bradycardia, heart block greater than first degree, cardiogenic shock, or overt cardiac failure.

Use cautiously in patients with heart failure, nonallergic bronchospastic disease, diabetes, hyperthyroidism, and impaired renal or hepatic function.

Interactions

Drug-drug. *Antihypertensive agents:* Pindolol may potentiate the antihypertensive effects. Monitor patient closely.

Effects on diagnostic tests

None reported.

Adverse reactions

CNS: *insomnia, fatigue, dizziness, nervousness,* vivid dreams, weakness, paresthesia.
CV: *edema,* bradycardia, ***heart failure,*** chest pain.
GI: *nausea,* abdominal discomfort.
Musculoskeletal: *muscle pain, joint pain.*
Respiratory: *increased airway resistance,* dyspnea.
Skin: rash, pruritus.
Other: elevated serum transaminase, alkaline phosphatase, lactic dehydrogenase, and uric acid levels.

Overdose and treatment

Signs of overdose include severe hypotension, bradycardia, heart failure, and bronchospasm.

After acute ingestion, empty stomach by induced emesis or gastric lavage; give activated charcoal to reduce absorption. Subsequent treatment is usually symptomatic and supportive.

Clinical considerations

- Consider the recommendations relevant to all beta blockers.
- Maximum therapeutic response may not be seen for 2 weeks or more.

Therapeutic monitoring

- Always check patient's apical pulse rate before giving drug. Notify doctor and withhold medication if pulse rate extremes are found.
- Monitor blood pressure frequently.

Special populations

Breast-feeding patients. Pindolol is excreted in breast milk; an alternative feeding method is recommended during therapy.
Pediatric patients. Safety and efficacy of pindolol in children haven't been established; use only if potential benefit outweighs risk.
Geriatric patients. Geriatric patients may require lower maintenance dosages of pindolol because of increased bioavailability or delayed metabolism; they also may experience enhanced adverse effects. Half-life of drug may be increased in geriatric patients.

Patient counseling

- Instruct patient to take drug exactly as prescribed.
- Advise patient not to stop drug abruptly and to report adverse effects.

pioglitazone hydrochloride

Actos

Pharmacologic classification: thiazolidinedione
Therapeutic classification: antidiabetic
Pregnancy risk category C

How supplied

Available by prescription only
Tablets: 15 mg, 30 mg, 45 mg

Indications and dosages

Monotherapy adjunct to diet and exercise to improve glycemic control in patients with type 2 diabetes mellitus, or combination therapy with a sulfonylurea, metformin, or insulin when diet and exercise plus the single agent doesn't result in adequate glycemic control
Adults: Initially, 15 or 30 mg P.O. once daily. For patients who respond inadequately to the

initial dose, dose may be increased in increments; maximum dose is 45 mg/day. If used in combination therapy, maximum dose shouldn't exceed 30 mg/day.

Pharmacodynamics

Antidiabetic action: Pioglitazone lowers blood glucose levels by decreasing insulin resistance in the periphery and in the liver, resulting in increased insulin-dependent glucose disposal and decreased glucose output by the liver. Pioglitazone is a potent and highly selective agonist for receptors found in insulin-sensitive tissues, such as adipose tissue, skeletal muscle, and liver. Activation of these receptors modulates the transcription of a number of insulin-responsive genes involved in the control of glucose and lipid metabolism.

Pharmacokinetics

Absorption: When taken on an empty stomach, pioglitazone is rapidly absorbed and is measurable in the serum within 30 minutes. Food delays the time to peak serum levels slightly (to 3 to 4 hours), but doesn't affect the overall extent of absorption.
Distribution: Pioglitazone and its metabolites are extensively protein-bound (more than 98%), primarily to serum albumin.
Metabolism: Extensively metabolized by the liver. Three metabolites, M-II, M-III and M-IV, are pharmacologically active.
Excretion: About 15% to 30% of the dose is recovered in the urine, primarily as metabolites and their conjugates. The majority of an oral dose is excreted into the bile and eliminated in the feces. The half-life of pioglitazone ranges from 3 to 7 hours.

Route	Onset	Peak	Duration
P.O.	Unknown	2 hr	Unknown

Adverse reactions

CNS: headache.
CV: *edema* (in combination with insulin).
EENT: sinusitis, pharyngitis.
Hematologic: anemia.
Metabolic: hypoglycemia (with combination therapy), aggravated diabetes mellitus, weight gain.
Musculoskeletal: myalgia.
Respiratory: upper respiratory infection.
Other: tooth disorder, decreased triglycerides, increased high-density lipoprotein cholesterol.

Interactions

Drug-drug. *Ketoconazole:* May inhibit the metabolism of pioglitazone. Monitor patient's blood glucose levels more frequently.
Oral contraceptives: May reduce plasma levels of oral contraceptives, resulting in less effective contraception. Advise patients taking pioglitazone and oral contraceptives to consider additional birth control measures.

Effects on diagnostic tests

None reported.

Overdose and treatment

In the event of overdose, initiate supportive treatment appropriate to patient's clinical signs and symptoms to reverse hypoglycemia.

Contraindications and precautions

Contraindicated in patients with known hypersensitivity to pioglitazone or its components. Drug shouldn't be used in patients with type 1 diabetes mellitus or for the treatment of diabetic ketoacidosis, in patients with clinical evidence of active liver disease or serum ALT levels greater than 2½ times the upper limit of normal, or in those who experienced jaundice while taking troglitazone. Don't use in patients with New York Heart Association Class III or IV heart failure.

Use cautiously in patients with edema or heart failure.

Clinical considerations

- Because ovulation may resume in premenopausal, anovulatory women with insulin resistance, contraceptive measures may need to be considered.
- Patients with normal liver enzyme levels who are switched from troglitazone to pioglitazone should undergo a 1-week washout period before starting pioglitazone.
- Management of type 2 diabetes should include diet control. Because caloric restrictions, weight loss, and exercise help improve insulin sensitivity and help make drug therapy effective, these measures are essential for proper diabetes management.

Therapeutic monitoring

- Monitor for hypoglycemia in patients receiving pioglitazone with insulin or a sulfonylurea and adjust dosage of these agents as needed.
- Besides having blood glucose levels checked regularly, patients should also have glycosylated hemoglobin checked periodically to evaluate therapeutic response to drug.
- Liver enzyme levels should be measured at the start of therapy, every 2 months for the first year of therapy, and periodically thereafter. Liver function tests also should be performed in patients in whom signs and symptoms of liver dysfunction, such as nausea, vomiting, abdominal pain, fatigue, anorexia, or dark urine develop. Drug should be discontinued if jaundice develops or if results of liver functions tests show ALT elevations greater than three times the upper limit of normal.
- Patients with heart failure should be monitored for increased edema during pioglitazone therapy.
- While patient is receiving this drug, hemoglobin levels and hematocrit may decrease,

usually during the first 4 to 12 weeks of therapy.

Special populations

Pregnant patients. Use drug in pregnancy only if the benefit justifies the risk to the fetus. Insulin is the preferred antidiabetic for use during pregnancy.
Breast-feeding patients. It isn't known if drug is excreted in breast milk. Pioglitazone shouldn't be administered to breast-feeding women.
Pediatric patients. Safety and efficacy of pioglitazone in children haven't been evaluated.
Geriatric patients. No significant differences in safety and efficacy of pioglitazone have been seen between patients age 65 and older and younger patients.

Patient counseling

- Instruct patient to adhere to dietary instructions and to have blood glucose levels and glycosylated hemoglobin tested regularly.
- Inform patient taking pioglitazone with insulin or oral antidiabetics of the signs and symptoms of hypoglycemia.
- Advise patient to notify health care provider during periods of stress, such as during fever, trauma, infection, or surgery, because medication requirements may change.
- Tell patient to report unexplained nausea, vomiting, abdominal pain, fatigue, anorexia, or dark urine immediately because these may indicate potential liver problems.
- Inform patient that pioglitazone can be taken with or without meals. If a dose is missed, the dose shouldn't be doubled the following day.
- Advise anovulatory, premenopausal women with insulin resistance that therapy with pioglitazone may cause resumption of ovulation and contraceptive measures may need to be considered.

pipecuronium bromide

Arduan

Pharmacologic classification: nondepolarizing neuromuscular blocker
Therapeutic classification: skeletal muscle relaxant
Pregnancy risk category C

How supplied

Available by prescription only
Injection: 10 mg/vial

Indications and dosages

To provide skeletal muscle relaxation during surgery as an adjunct to general anesthesia

Adults and children: Dosage is highly individualized. The following doses may serve as a guide, assuming that patient isn't obese and has normal renal function. Initially, doses of 70 to 85 mcg/kg I.V. are used to provide conditions considered ideal for endotracheal intubation and will maintain paralysis for 1 to 2 hours. If succinylcholine is used for endotracheal intubation, initial doses of pipecuronium 50 mcg/kg will provide good relaxation for 45 minutes or more. Maintenance dosages of 10 to 15 mcg/kg provide relaxation for about 50 minutes.

≡ ***Dosage adjustment.*** For patients with renal failure, refer to this table.

Creatinine clearance (ml/min)	Dose (mcg/kg)
100	85
80	70
60	55
40	50

Pharmacodynamics

Muscle relaxant action: Like other nondepolarizing muscle relaxants, pipecuronium competes with acetylcholine for receptor sites at the motor end plate. Because this action may be antagonized by cholinesterase inhibitors, it's considered a competitive antagonist.

Pharmacokinetics

Absorption: No information available regarding use of drug by any route other than I.V.
Distribution: Volume of distribution (V_d) is about 0.25 L/kg and increases in patients with renal failure. Other conditions associated with increased V_d, including edema, old age, and CV disease, may delay onset.
Metabolism: Only about 20% to 40% of an administered dose is metabolized, probably in the liver. One metabolite (3-desacetyl pipecuronium) has about 50% of the neuromuscular blocking activity of the parent drug.
Excretion: Primarily excreted by the kidneys. In preliminary studies, the half-life of drug has been estimated at 1¾ hours; it may increase to 4 hours or more in patients with severe renal disease.

Route	Onset	Peak	Duration
I.V.	1-2 min	5 min	24 min

Contraindications and precautions

Contraindicated in patients with hypersensitivity to drug. Use cautiously in patients with renal failure.

Interactions

Drug-drug. *Aminoglycosides, such as gentamicin, kanamycin, neomycin and streptomycin; bacitracin; colistimethate sodium; colistin; polymyxin B; tetracyclines:* Use of pipecuronium in high doses has been associ-

ated with muscle weakness; this weakness may worsen in the presence of a nondepolarizing neuromuscular blocking agent. Use together cautiously.
Magnesium salts: May enhance and prolong neuromuscular blockade. Monitor patient closely.
Quinidine, volatile inhalational anesthetics: May intensify or prolong the action of nondepolarizing neuromuscular blocking agents. Monitor patient closely.

Effects on diagnostic tests
None reported.

Adverse reactions
CV: hypotension, bradycardia, hypertension, myocardial ischemia, *CVA,* thrombosis, atrial fibrillation, ***ventricular extrasystole.***
GU: anuria.
Musculoskeletal: prolonged muscle weakness.
Respiratory: dyspnea, respiratory depression, ***respiratory insufficiency or apnea.***
Skin: rash, urticaria.
Other: increased creatinine levels.

Overdose and treatment
No cases of overdose have been reported. Provide supportive treatment, and ventilate patient as necessary. Closely monitor vital signs.

Antagonists such as neostigmine shouldn't be used until there's some evidence of spontaneous recovery of neuromuscular function. A nerve stimulator is recommended to document antagonism of neuromuscular blockade.

Edrophonium 0.5 mg/kg isn't as effective as neostigmine 0.04 mg/kg in reversing the effects of pipecuronium. Higher doses of edrophonium and pyridostigmine haven't been studied.

Clinical considerations
- Experimental evidence suggests that acid-base balance may influence the actions of pipecuronium. Alkalosis may counteract the paralysis and acidosis may enhance it. Electrolyte disturbances may also influence response.
- Because of its prolonged duration of action, drug is recommended only for procedures that take 90 minutes or longer.
- Adjust dosage to ideal body weight in obese patients.
- Store powder at room temperature or in the refrigerator (36° to 86° F [2° to 30° C]).
- Reconstitute with 10 ml solution before use to yield a solution of 1 mg/ml. Large volumes of diluent or addition of drug to a hanging I.V. solution isn't recommended.
- When reconstituted with sterile water for injection or other compatible I.V. solutions, such as normal saline injection, D_5W, lactated Ringer's injection, and dextrose 5% in saline, drug is stable for 24 hours if refrigerated.
- If reconstituted with solution other than bacteriostatic water for injection, discard unused portions of drug.
- When reconstituted with bacteriostatic water for injection, drug is stable for 5 days at room temperature or in the refrigerator. Note that bacteriostatic water contains benzyl alcohol and isn't intended for use in neonates.

Therapeutic monitoring
- Monitor respirations closely until patient is fully recovered from neuromuscular blockade, as evidenced by tests of muscle strength (such as hand grip, head lift, and ability to cough).
- Monitor patient for bradycardia during anesthesia.

Special populations
Breast-feeding patients. There's no information regarding the distribution of drug in breast milk. Use with caution in breast-feeding women.
Pediatric patients. Drug isn't recommended for use in patients under age 3 months. Limited evidence suggests that children age 1 to 14 under balanced anesthesia or halothane anesthesia may be less sensitive than adults.

Patient counseling
Reassure patient and family that patient will be monitored at all times.

piperacillin sodium
Pipracil

Pharmacologic classification: extended-spectrum penicillin, acylaminopenicillin
Therapeutic classification: antibiotic
Pregnancy risk category B

How supplied
Available by prescription only
Injection: 2 g, 3 g, 4 g
Infusion: 2 g, 3 g, 4 g
Pharmacy bulk package: 40 g

Indications and dosages
Infections caused by susceptible organisms
Adults and children over age 12: Serious infection: 12 to 18 g/day I.V. in divided doses q 4 to 6 hours; uncomplicated urinary tract infection (UTI) and community-acquired pneumonia: 6 to 8 g/day I.V. in divided doses q 6 to 12 hours; complicated UTI: 8 to 16 g/day I.V. in divided doses q 6 to 8 hours; uncomplicated gonorrhea: 2 g I.M. as a single dose. Maximum daily dose, 24 g.
Prophylaxis of surgical infections
Adults: Intra-abdominal surgery: 2 g I.V. before surgery, 2 g during surgery, and 2 g q 6

hours after surgery for no more than 24 hours; vaginal hysterectomy: 2 g I.V. before surgery, 2 g 6 hours after first dose then 2 g 12 hours after second dose; cesarean section: 2 g I.V. after cord is clamped, then 2 g q 4 hours for two doses; abdominal hysterectomy: 2 g I.V. before surgery, 2 g in postanesthesia care unit, and 2 g after 6 hours.

≡ ***Dosage adjustment.*** For adult patients with renal failure, refer to the following table.

Creatinine clearance (ml/min)	Urinary tract infection Uncomplicated	Complicated	Serious systemic infection
20 to 40	*	3 g q 8 hr	4 g q 8 hr
< 20	3 g q 12 hr	3 g q 12 hr	4 g q 12 hr

*No dosage adjustment necessary.

Pharmacodynamics

Antibiotic action: Piperacillin is bactericidal; it adheres to bacterial penicillin-binding proteins, inhibiting bacterial cell wall synthesis.

Extended-spectrum penicillins are more resistant to inactivation by certain beta-lactamases, especially those produced by gram-negative organisms, but are still liable to inactivation by certain others. Because of the potential for rapid development of bacterial resistance, it shouldn't be used as a sole agent in the treatment of an infection.

The spectrum of activity of piperacillin includes many gram-negative aerobic and anaerobic bacilli, many gram-positive and gram-negative aerobic cocci, and some gram-positive aerobic and anaerobic bacilli. Piperacillin may be effective against some strains of carbenicillin-resistant and ticarcillin-resistant gram-negative bacilli. Piperacillin is more active against *Pseudomonas aeruginosa* than are other extended-spectrum penicillins.

Pharmacokinetics

Absorption: Peak plasma levels occur 30 to 50 minutes after an I.M. dose.

Distribution: Distributed widely after parenteral administration. It penetrates minimally into uninflamed meninges and slightly into bone and sputum. Piperacillin is 16% to 22% protein-bound; it crosses the placenta.

Metabolism: None significant.

Excretion: Excreted primarily (42% to 90%) in urine by renal tubular secretion and glomerular filtration; it's also excreted in bile and in breast milk. Elimination half-life in adults is about ½ to 1½ hours; in extensive renal impairment, half-life is extended to about 2 to 6 hours; in combined hepatorenal dysfunction, half-life may extend from 11 to 32 hours. Drug is removed by hemodialysis but not by peritoneal dialysis.

Route	Onset	Peak	Duration
I.V.	Immediate	Immediate	Unknown
I.M.	Unknown	30-50 min	Unknown

Contraindications and precautions

Contraindicated in patients with hypersensitivity to drug or other penicillins. Use cautiously in patients with other drug allergies (especially to cephalosporins), bleeding tendencies, uremia, or hypokalemia.

Interactions

Drug-drug. *Aminoglycoside antibiotics:* Synergistic bactericidal effects against *Pseudomonas aeruginosa, Escherichia coli, Citrobacter, Enterobacter, Klebsiella, Serratia,* and *Proteus mirabilis.* The drugs are physically and chemically incompatible and are inactivated when mixed or given together. Don't administer together.

Clavulanic acid, sulbactam, tazobactam: Synergistic bactericidal effect against certain beta-lactamase-producing bacteria. May be used for this advantage.

Methotrexate: Large doses of penicillins may interfere with renal tubular secretion, delaying elimination and elevating serum levels of methotrexate. Monitor patient closely.

Oral contraceptives: Penicillins may decrease efficacy. Recommend additional form of contraceptive while on penicillin therapy.

Probenecid: Blocks tubular secretion of piperacillin, raising serum levels of drug. Probenecid may be used for this purpose.

Effects on diagnostic tests

Piperacillin may falsely decrease serum aminoglycoside levels. Piperacillin may cause positive Coombs' tests.

Adverse reactions

CNS: ***seizures,*** headache, dizziness, fatigue.

GI: nausea, diarrhea, vomiting, pseudomembranous colitis, elevations in liver function studies.

GU: interstitial nephritis.

Hematologic: *bleeding* (with high doses), neutropenia, eosinophilia, leukopenia, ***thrombocytopenia.***

Other: *hypokalemia,* hypernatremia, hypersensitivity reactions (edema, fever, chills, rash, pruritus, urticaria, ***anaphylaxis***), overgrowth of nonsusceptible organisms, pain at injection site, vein irritation, phlebitis, prolonged muscle relaxation.

Overdose and treatment

Signs of overdose include neuromuscular hypersensitivity or seizures resulting from CNS irritation by high drug levels. A 4- to 6-hour session of hemodialysis removes 10% to 50% of piperacillin.

Clinical considerations

Consider the recommendations relevant to all penicillins as well as the following:

- Piperacillin is almost always used with another antibiotic such as an aminoglycoside in life-threatening situations.
- Drug may be administered by direct I.V. injection, given slowly over at least 5 minutes; chest discomfort occurs if injection is given too rapidly.
- Patients with cystic fibrosis are most susceptible to fever or rash from piperacillin.
- Because drug is dialyzable, patients undergoing hemodialysis may need dosage adjustments.
- Use reduced dosage in patients with creatinine clearance less than 40 ml/minute.

Therapeutic monitoring

- Monitor serum electrolytes, especially potassium.
- Monitor neurologic status. High serum levels of this drug may cause seizures.
- Monitor CBC, differential, and platelets. Drug may cause thrombocytopenia. Observe patient carefully for signs of occult bleeding.

Special populations

Breast-feeding patients. Drug is excreted in breast milk; use with caution in breast-feeding women.
Pediatric patients. Safety of piperacillin in children under age 12 hasn't been established.
Geriatric patients. Half-life may be prolonged in geriatric patients because of impaired renal function.

Patient counseling

- Tell patient to report adverse effects or discomfort at I.V. site.
- Instruct patient to limit salt intake while on therapy.
- Drug may be more suitable than carbenicillin or ticarcillin for patients on salt-free diets; piperacillin contains only 1.85 mEq of sodium per gram.

piperacillin sodium and tazobactam sodium

Zosyn

Pharmacologic classification: extended-spectrum penicillin/beta-lactamase inhibitor
Therapeutic classification: antibiotic
Pregnancy risk category B

How supplied

Available by prescription only
Powder for injection (equivalent to piperacillin/tazobactam in a ratio of 8 to 1): 2.25 g, 3.375 g, 4.5 g

Indications and dosages

***Treatment of moderate to severe infections caused by piperacillin-resistant, piperacillin/tazobactam-susceptible, beta-lactamase-producing strains of microorganisms in the following conditions: appendicitis (complicated by rupture or abscess) and peritonitis caused by* Escherichia coli, Bacteroides fragilis, B. ovatus, B. thetaiotaomicron, B. vulgatus; *skin and skin structure infections caused by* Staphylococcus aureus; *postpartum endometritis or pelvic inflammatory disease caused by* E. coli; *moderately severe community-acquired pneumonia caused by* Haemophilus influenzae**

Adults: 3.375 g (3.0 g piperacillin/0.375 g tazobactam) q 6 hours as a 30-minute I.V. infusion.

≡ ***Dosage adjustment.*** For patients with renal dysfunction, refer to the following table.

Creatinine clearance (ml/min)	Recommended dosage
> 40	12 g/1.5 g/day in divided doses of 3.375 g q 6 hr
20 to 40	8 g/1 g/day in divided doses of 2.25 g q 6 hr
< 20	6 g/0.75 g/day in divided doses of 2.25 g q 8 hr

Note: Discontinue therapy if hypersensitivity reactions or bleeding signs and symptoms occur.

Pharmacodynamics

Antibiotic action: Piperacillin is an extended-spectrum penicillin that inhibits cell wall synthesis during microorganism multiplication; tazobactam increases piperacillin effectiveness by inactivating beta-lactamases, which destroy penicillins.

Pharmacokinetics

Absorption: Unknown.
Distribution: Both piperacillin and tazobactam are about 30% bound to plasma proteins.
Metabolism: Piperacillin is metabolized to a minor microbiologically active desethyl metabolite. Tazobactam is metabolized to a single metabolite that lacks pharmacologic and antibacterial activities.
Excretion: Both piperacillin and tazobactam are eliminated via the kidneys by glomerular filtration and tubular secretion. Piperacillin is excreted rapidly as unchanged drug (68% of dose) and tazobactam is excreted as unchanged drug (80%) in the urine. Piperacillin, tazobac-

tam, and desethyl piperacillin also are secreted into the bile.

Route	Onset	Peak	Duration
I.V.	Immediate	Immediate	Unknown

Contraindications and precautions

Contraindicated in patients with hypersensitivity to drug or other penicillins. Use cautiously in patients with drug allergies (especially to cephalosporins), bleeding tendencies, uremia, or hypokalemia.

Interactions

Drug-drug. *Aminoglycosides:* Can result in substantial inactivation of the aminoglycoside. Don't mix in the same I.V. container.
Heparin, oral anticoagulants, and other drugs that may affect the blood coagulation system or the thrombocyte function: Prolonged effectiveness. Monitor PT and INR closely.
Probenecid: Increases blood levels of piperacillin/tazobactam. Probenecid may be used for this reason.
Vecuronium: Prolonged neuromuscular blockade of vecuronium. Monitor patient closely.

Effects on diagnostic tests

As with other penicillins, piperacillin/tazobactam may result in a false-positive reaction for urine glucose using a copper-reduction method such as Clinitest. Glucose tests based on enzymatic glucose oxidase reactions (such as Diastix or glucose enzymatic test strip) are recommended.

Adverse reactions

CNS: *headache, insomnia,* agitation, dizziness, anxiety.
CV: hypertension, tachycardia, chest pain, edema.
EENT: rhinitis.
GI: *diarrhea, nausea, constipation,* vomiting, dyspepsia, stool changes, abdominal pain.
GU: interstitial nephritis.
Hematologic: leukopenia, anemia, eosinophilia, ***thrombocytopenia.***
Respiratory: dyspnea.
Skin: rash (including maculopapular, bullous, urticarial, and eczematoid), pruritus.
Other: fever; pain; moniliasis; inflammation, phlebitis at I.V. site; ***anaphylaxis.***

Overdose and treatment

No information available.

Clinical considerations

- Obtain specimen for culture and sensitivity tests before giving first dose. Therapy may begin pending results.
- Pseudomembranous colitis has been reported with nearly all antibacterial agents, including piperacillin/tazobactam, and may range in severity from mild to life-threatening. Therefore, consider this diagnosis in patients presenting with diarrhea after piperacillin/tazobactam administration.
- Bacterial and fungal superinfection may occur and warrants appropriate measures.
- Use piperacillin/tazobactam in combination with an aminoglycoside to treat infections caused by *Pseudomonas aeruginosa.*
- Piperacillin/tazobactam contains 2.35 mEq (54 mg) of sodium per gram of piperacillin in the combination product. This should be considered in patients who require restricted sodium intake.
- Reconstitute piperacillin/tazobactam with 5 ml of diluent per 1 g of piperacillin. Appropriate diluents include sterile or bacteriostatic water for injection, normal saline injection, bacteriostatic normal saline injection, D_5W, dextrose 5% in normal saline solution injection, or dextran 6% in normal saline injection. Don't use lactated Ringer's injection. Shake until dissolved. Further dilution can be made to a final desired volume.
- Infuse over at least 30 minutes. Discontinue primary infusion during administration if possible. Don't mix with other drugs.
- Use single-dose vials immediately after reconstitution. Discard unused drug after 24 hours if held at room temperature; 48 hours if refrigerated. Once diluted, drug is stable in I.V. bags for 24 hours at room temperature or 1 week if refrigerated.

Therapeutic monitoring

- Perform periodic electrolyte determinations in patients with low potassium reserves; hypokalemia can occur when patient with potentially low potassium reserves receives cytotoxic therapy or diuretics.
- As with other semisynthetic penicillins, piperacillin has been associated with increased incidence of fever and rash in patients with cystic fibrosis.

Special populations

Pregnant patients: Safety for use during pregnancy hasn't been established.
Breast-feeding patients. Piperacillin is excreted in low levels in breast milk; tazobactam levels haven't been studied. Use with caution when administering piperacillin/tazobactam to breast-feeding women.
Pediatric patients. Safety and efficacy in children under age 12 haven't been established.

Patient counseling

- Instruct patient to report adverse effects.
- Advise patient to report discomfort at I.V. site. Inform patient that I.V. site will need to be changed every 48 hours.

pirbuterol acetate

Maxair

Pharmacologic classification: beta-adrenergic agonist
Therapeutic classification: bronchodilator
Pregnancy risk category C

How supplied

Available by prescription only
Inhaler: 0.2 mg per inhalation

Indications and dosages

Prevention and reversal of bronchospasm; asthma
Adults and children age 12 and over: 1 or 2 inhalations (0.2 to 0.4 mg) repeated q 4 to 6 hours. Not to exceed 12 inhalations daily.

Pharmacodynamics

Bronchodilating action: Pirbuterol stimulates $beta_2$-adrenergic receptors and increases the activity of intracellular adenylate cyclase, an enzyme that catalyzes the conversion of adenosine triphosphate to cyclic adenosine monophosphate (cAMP). Elevated cellular cAMP is associated with bronchodilation and inhibition of the cellular release of mediators of immediate hypersensitivity.

Pharmacokinetics

Absorption: Negligible serum levels are achieved after inhalation of the usual dose.
Distribution: Pirbuterol acts locally.
Metabolism: Metabolized in the liver.
Excretion: About 50% of an inhaled dose is recovered in urine as the parent drug and metabolites.

Route	Onset	Peak	Duration
Inhalation	5 min	½-1 hr	5 hr

Contraindications and precautions

Contraindicated in patients with hypersensitivity to pirbuterol. Use cautiously in patients with CV disorders, hyperthyroidism, diabetes, or seizure disorders and in those sensitive to sympathomimetic amines.

Interactions

Drug-drug. *MAO inhibitors or tricyclic antidepressants:* May enhance the vascular effects of beta-adrenergic agonists. Administer cautiously.
Propranolol and other beta blockers: May decrease the bronchodilating effects of beta agonists. Avoid use together.

Effects on diagnostic tests

None reported.

Adverse reactions

CNS: tremor, nervousness, dizziness, insomnia, headache, vertigo.
CV: tachycardia, palpitations, chest tightness.
EENT: dry or irritated throat, dry mouth, cough.
GI: nausea, vomiting, diarrhea.

Overdose and treatment

Anginal pain, hypertension, and tachycardia may result from overdose. Treatment is generally supportive. Sedatives or barbiturates may be necessary to counter any adverse CNS effects; cautious use of beta blockers may be useful to counter cardiac effects.

Clinical considerations

- Consider the recommendations relevant to all adrenergics.
- Don't administer to patients who are receiving other beta-adrenergic bronchodilators.

Therapeutic monitoring

Monitor for adverse effects, and lack of effectiveness of medication.

Special populations

Breast-feeding patients. It isn't known if pirbuterol is excreted in breast milk. Use with caution in breast-feeding women.
Pediatric patients. Use in children under age 12 isn't recommended.

Patient counseling

- Warn patient not to exceed recommended maximum dose of 12 inhalations daily. He should seek medical attention if a previously effective dosage doesn't control symptoms because this may signify a worsening of disease.
- Tell patient to promptly report increased bronchospasm after using drug.
- Teach patient how to use metered dose inhaler correctly. Have him shake container, exhale through the nose; administer aerosol while inhaling deeply on mouthpiece of inhaler; hold breath for a few seconds, then exhale slowly. Tell him to allow at least 2 minutes between inhalations and to wait at least 5 minutes before using his steroid inhalant, if he's also taking inhalational corticosteroids.

piroxicam

Apo-Piroxicam*, Feldene, Novo-Pirocam*

Pharmacologic classification: NSAID
Therapeutic classification: nonnarcotic analgesic, antipyretic, anti-inflammatory
Pregnancy risk category B (D in third trimester or near delivery)

How supplied

Available by prescription only
Capsules: 10 mg, 20 mg

Indications and dosages

Osteoarthritis and rheumatoid arthritis

Adults: 20 mg P.O. once daily. If desired, the dose may be divided.

◊ ***Juvenile rheumatoid arthritis***

Children weighing 33 to 67 lb (15 to 30 kg): 5 mg P.O.

Children weighing 68 to 100 lb (31 to 45 kg): 10 mg P.O.

Children weighing 101 to 121 lb (46 to 55 kg): 15 mg P.O.

Pharmacodynamics

Analgesic, antipyretic, and anti-inflammatory actions: Exact mechanisms of action are unknown, but piroxicam is thought to inhibit prostaglandin synthesis.

Pharmacokinetics

Absorption: Absorbed rapidly from the GI tract. Food delays absorption.

Distribution: Highly protein-bound.

Metabolism: Metabolized in the liver.

Excretion: Excreted in urine. Its long half-life (about 50 hours) allows for once-daily dosing.

Route	Onset	Peak	Duration
P.O.	1 hr	3-5 hr	48-72 hr

Contraindications and precautions

Contraindicated in patients with hypersensitivity to drug or with bronchospasm or angioedema precipitated by aspirin or NSAIDs, and in pregnant or breast-feeding women.

Use cautiously in the elderly and in patients with GI disorders, history of renal, peptic ulcer, or cardiac disease, hypertension, or conditions predisposing to fluid retention.

Interactions

Drug-drug. *Acetaminophen, diuretics, gold compounds, or other anti-inflammatory agents:* Increased nephrotoxicity may occur. Avoid use together.

Anticoagulants and thrombolytic drugs, such as coumarin derivatives, heparin, and other highly protein-bound drugs: May potentiate anticoagulant effects. Monitor PT, INR, and patient closely.

Antihypertensive agents and diuretics: Piroxicam may decrease effectiveness. Monitor patient closely.

Anti-inflammatory agents, corticosteroids, corticotropin, salicylates: May cause increased GI adverse effects. Avoid use together.

Aspirin, cefamandole, cefoperazone, dextran, dipyridamole, mezlocillin, piperacillin, plicamycin, salicylates, sulfinpyrazone, ticarcillin, valproic acid, and other anti-inflammatory agents: Increased risk of bleeding. Monitor PT, INR, and patient closely.

Coumarin derivatives, nifedipine, phenytoin, verapamil: Toxicity may occur. Avoid use together.

Insulin or oral antidiabetic agents: May potentiate hypoglycemic effects. Monitor serum glucose levels closely.

Lithium, methotrexate: Increased plasma lithium and methotrexate levels. Monitor patient for toxicity.

Drug-lifestyle. *Sun exposure:* May cause photosensitivity reaction. Advise patient to take precautions.

Alcohol use: Increased GI toxicity. Decreased plasma levels of piroxicam. Advise patient to avoid alcohol use.

Effects on diagnostic tests

None reported.

Adverse reactions

CNS: headache, drowsiness, dizziness, somnolence, vertigo.

CV: peripheral edema.

EENT: auditory disturbances.

GI: *epigastric distress, nausea, occult blood loss,* ***peptic ulceration, severe GI bleeding,*** diarrhea, constipation, abdominal pain, dyspepsia, flatulence, anorexia, stomatitis.

GU: *nephrotoxicity,* elevated BUN level.

Hematologic: prolonged bleeding time, anemia, leukopenia, ***aplastic anemia, agranulocytosis,*** eosinophilia, ***thrombocytopenia.***

Hepatic: elevated liver enzymes.

Skin: pruritus, rash, urticaria, *photosensitivity.*

Overdose and treatment

To treat piroxicam overdose, empty stomach immediately by inducing emesis with ipecac syrup or by gastric lavage. Administer activated charcoal via nasogastric tube. Provide symptomatic and supportive measures, such as respiratory support and correction of fluid and electrolyte imbalances. Monitor laboratory parameters and vital signs closely.

Clinical considerations

Consider the recommendations relevant to all NSAIDs as well as the following:

- Drug is usually administered as a single dose.
- Adverse skin reactions are more common with piroxicam than with other NSAIDs; photosensitivity reactions are the most common.

Therapeutic monitoring

- Effectiveness of piroxicam usually isn't seen for at least 2 weeks after therapy begins. Evaluate response to drug as evidenced by reduced symptoms.
- Check renal, hepatic, and auditory functions and CBC periodically during prolonged therapy. Discontinue drug if abnormalities are found.

Special populations

Pregnant patients. Drug hasn't been proven safe to the fetus.

Breast-feeding patients. Piroxicam may inhibit lactation. Because piroxicam is distrib-

uted into breast milk at 1% of maternal serum levels, use an alternative feeding method during drug therapy. Avoid use in breast-feeding women.
Pediatric patients. Safety of long-term piroxicam in children hasn't been established.
Geriatric patients. Patients over age 60 are more sensitive to the adverse effects of piroxicam. Use with caution. Through its effect on renal prostaglandins, piroxicam may cause fluid retention and edema. This may be significant in geriatric patients and those with heart failure.

Patient counseling
- Advise patient to seek medical approval before taking OTC medications.
- Caution patient to avoid hazardous activities requiring alertness until CNS effects are known. Instruct patient in safety measures to prevent injury.
- Instruct patient in signs and symptoms of adverse effects. Tell patient to report them immediately.
- Encourage patient to comply with recommended medical follow-up.

plasma protein fraction
Plasmanate, Plasma-Plex, Plasmatein, Protenate

Pharmacologic classification: blood derivative
Therapeutic classification: plasma volume expander
Pregnancy risk category C

How supplied
Available by prescription only
Injection: 50 mg/ml (5% solution in 50-ml, 250-ml, 500-ml vials)

Indications and dosages
Shock
Adults: Varies with patient's condition and response, but usually 250 to 500 ml (12.5 to 25 g protein) I.V., not to exceed 10 ml/minute.
Infants and young children: Initially, 6.6 to 33 ml/kg (0.33 to 1.65 g/kg of protein) infused at a rate of up to 5 to 10 ml/minute. Subsequent dosage is based on patient's condition.
Hypoproteinemia
Adults: 1,000 to 1,500 ml I.V. daily. Maximum infusion rate, 8 ml/minute (500 ml infused in 30 to 45 minutes).

Pharmacodynamics
Plasma-expanding action: Plasma protein fraction (PPF) supplies colloid to the blood and expands plasma volume. It causes fluid to shift from interstitial spaces into the circulation and slightly increases the plasma protein level. It's comprised mostly of albumin, but may contain up to 17% alpha and beta globulins and not more than 1% gamma globulin.

Pharmacokinetics
The pharmacokinetics of PPF are similar to its chief constituent, albumin (about 83% to 90%).
Absorption: Not adequately absorbed from the GI tract.
Distribution: Albumin accounts for about 50% of plasma proteins. It's distributed into the intravascular space and extravascular sites, including skin, muscle, and lungs. In patients with reduced circulating blood volumes, hemodilution secondary to albumin administration persists for many hours; in patients with normal blood volume, excess fluid and protein are lost from the intravascular space within a few hours.
Metabolism: Although albumin is synthesized in the liver, the liver isn't involved in clearance of albumin from the plasma in healthy individuals.
Excretion: Little is known about albumin excretion in healthy individuals. Administration of albumin decreases hepatic albumin synthesis and increases albumin clearance if plasma oncotic pressure is high. In certain pathologic states, the liver, kidneys, or intestines may provide elimination mechanisms.

Route	Onset	Peak	Duration
I.V.	Immediate	Immediate	Unknown

Contraindications and precautions
Contraindicated in patients with severe anemia or heart failure and in those undergoing cardiac bypass. Use cautiously in patients with impaired renal or hepatic function, low cardiac reserve, or restricted salt intake.

Interactions
None significant.

Effects on diagnostic tests
None reported.

Adverse reactions
CNS: headache.
CV: hypotension (after rapid infusion or intra-arterial administration), ***vascular overload*** (after rapid infusion), tachycardia.
GI: nausea, vomiting, hypersalivation.
Respiratory: dyspnea, ***pulmonary edema.***
Skin: rash.
Other: flushing, chills, fever, back pain, increased plasma protein levels.

Overdose and treatment
Rapid infusion can cause circulatory overload and pulmonary edema. Watch patient for signs of hypervolemia; monitor blood pressure and central venous pressure. Treatment is symptomatic.

Clinical considerations

- Don't use solution that's cloudy, contains sediment, or has been frozen. Store at room temperature; freezing may break bottle and allow bacterial contamination.
- Use opened solution promptly, discarding unused portion after 4 hours; solution contains no preservatives and becomes unstable.
- One unit is usually considered to be 250 ml of the 5% concentration.
- Avoid rapid I.V. infusion. Rate is individualized according to patient's age, condition, and diagnosis. Maximum dose is 250 g/48 hours; don't give faster than 10 ml/minute. Decrease infusion rate to 5 to 8 ml/minute as plasma volume approaches normal.
- PPF is also used in treatment of shock resulting from burns; dosage depends on the extent and severity of burn.
- No cross-matching is required. PPF shouldn't be administered with the same administration set of solutions containing protein hydrosylates, amino acid solutions, or alcohol.
- If patient is dehydrated, give additional fluids either P.O. or I.V.
- Each liter contains 130 to 160 mEq of sodium before dilution with any additional I.V. fluids; a 250-ml container of the 5% concentration contains about 33 to 40 mEq sodium.

Therapeutic monitoring

- Monitor blood pressure frequently; slow or stop infusion if hypotension suddenly occurs. Vital signs should return to normal gradually.
- Observe patient for signs of vascular overload, such as heart failure, pulmonary edema, and widening pulse pressure indicating increased cardiac output, and signs of hemorrhage or shock after surgery or trauma; be alert for bleeding sites not evident at lower blood pressure.
- Monitor intake and output (watch especially for decreased output), hemoglobin, hematocrit, and serum protein and electrolyte levels to help determine ongoing dosage.

Patient counseling

- Explain use and administration to patient and family.
- Instruct patient to report adverse effects.

plicamycin

Mithracin

Pharmacologic classification: antibiotic antineoplastic (cell cycle-phase nonspecific)
Therapeutic classification: antineoplastic, hypocalcemic
Pregnancy risk category X

How supplied

Available by prescription only
Injection: 2,500-mcg vials

Indications and dosages

Dosage and indications may vary. Check current literature for recommended protocol.

Hypercalcemia
Adults: 25 mcg/kg I.V. daily over 4 to 6 hours for 3 to 4 days. Repeat at intervals of 1 week, p.r.n.

Testicular cancer
Adults: 25 to 30 mcg/kg I.V. daily over 4 to 6 hours for up to 10 days (based on ideal body weight or actual weight, whichever is less).

◇***Paget's disease***
Adults: 15 mcg/kg I.V. daily over 4 to 6 hours for up to 10 days.

Pharmacodynamics

Antineoplastic action: Plicamycin exerts its cytotoxic activity by intercalating between DNA base pairs and also binding to the outside of the DNA molecule. The result is inhibition of DNA-dependent RNA synthesis.
Hypocalcemic action: The exact mechanism by which plicamycin lowers serum calcium levels is unknown. Plicamycin may block the hypercalcemic effect of vitamin D or may inhibit the effect of parathyroid hormone upon osteoclasts, preventing osteolysis. Both mechanisms reduce serum calcium levels.

Pharmacokinetics

Absorption: Not administered orally.
Distribution: Distributed mainly into the Kupffer's cells of the liver, into renal tubular cells, and along formed bone surfaces. Drug also crosses the blood-brain barrier and achieves appreciable levels in the CSF.
Metabolism: Poorly understood.
Excretion: Eliminated primarily through the kidneys.

Route	Onset	Peak	Duration
I.V.	1-2 days	3 days	7-10 days

Contraindications and precautions

Contraindicated in patients with thrombocytopenia, bone marrow suppression, or coagulation and bleeding disorders and in women who are or who may become pregnant.

Use cautiously in patients with impaired renal or hepatic function.

Interactions

None reported.

Effects on diagnostic tests

None reported.

Adverse reactions

CNS: drowsiness, weakness, lethargy, headache, malaise.
GI: *nausea, vomiting,* anorexia, diarrhea, stomatitis.
GU: increased BUN and serum creatinine levels.

Hematologic: ***leukopenia, thrombocytopenia; bleeding syndrome*** (from epistaxis to generalized hemorrhage).
Hepatic: ***elevated liver enzymes levels,*** hepatotoxicity.
Skin: facial flushing, rash.
Other: *decreased serum calcium,* potassium, and phosphorus levels; ***death;*** fever; cellulitis with extravasation; phlebitis.

Overdose and treatment
Signs of overdose include myelosuppression, electrolyte imbalance, and coagulation disorders. Treatment is usually supportive and includes transfusion of blood components and appropriate symptomatic therapy. Monitor patient's renal and hepatic status closely.

Clinical considerations
- Facial flushing is an early indication of bleeding. The first evidence of bleeding may manifest in epistaxis.
- To reconstitute drug, use 4.9 ml of sterile water to give a concentration of 500 mcg/ml. Reconstitute drug immediately before administration, and discard unused solution.
- Drug may be further diluted with normal saline solution or D_5W to a volume of 1,000 ml and administered as an I.V. infusion over 4 to 6 hours.
- Although drug may be administered by I.V. push injection, it's discouraged because of the higher incidence and greater severity of GI toxicity. Nausea and vomiting are greatly diminished as infusion rate is decreased.
- Infusions of plicamycin in 1,000 ml D_5W are stable for up to 24 hours.
- If I.V. infiltrates, stop infusion immediately and apply ice packs before restarting an I.V. in other arm.
- Give antiemetics before administering drug, to reduce nausea.
- Therapeutic effect in hypercalcemia may not be seen for 24 to 48 hours, and may last 3 to 15 days.
- Avoid drug contact with skin or mucous membranes.
- Store lyophilized powder in refrigerator.

Therapeutic monitoring
- Monitor LD, AST, ALT, alkaline phosphatase, BUN, creatinine, potassium, calcium, and phosphorus levels.
- Monitor platelet count and PT before and during therapy.
- Check serum calcium levels. Monitor patient for tetany, carpopedal spasm, Chvostek's sign, and muscle cramps because a sharp drop in calcium levels is possible.
- Observe for signs of bleeding.

Special populations
Pregnant patients. Drug may cause fetal toxicity. Drug is contraindicated for use during pregnancy. Advise patient to use contraceptive measures during therapy and to notify doctor immediately if she becomes pregnant or suspects she is pregnant.
Breast-feeding patients. It isn't known if drug is excreted in breast milk. However, because of potential for serious adverse reactions, mutagenicity, and carcinogenicity in the infant, breast-feeding isn't recommended.

Patient counseling
- Tell patient to use salicylate-free medication for pain relief or fever reduction.
- Instruct patient to avoid exposure to people with infections and to immediately report signs of infection or unusual bleeding.
- Inform patient that he and household members shouldn't receive immunizations during therapy and for several weeks after therapy.

pneumococcal vaccine, polyvalent
Pneumovax 23, Pnu-Imune 23

Pharmacologic classification: vaccine
Therapeutic classification: bacterial vaccine
Pregnancy risk category C

How supplied
Available by prescription only
Injection: 25 mcg each of 23 polysaccharide isolates of *Streptococcus pneumoniae* per 0.5-ml dose, in 1-ml and 5-ml vials and disposable syringes.

Indications and dosages
Pneumococcal immunization
Adults and children over age 2: 0.5 ml I.M. or S.C. as a one-time dose.

Pharmacodynamics
Pneumonia prophylaxis: Pneumococcal vaccine promotes active immunity against the 23 most prevalent pneumococcal types.

Pharmacokinetics
Absorption: Protective antibodies are produced within 3 weeks after injection.
Distribution: No information available.
Metabolism: No information available.
Excretion: No information available.

Route	Onset	Peak	Duration
I.M., S.C.	2-3 wk	Unknown	5 yr

Contraindications and precautions
Contraindicated in patients hypersensitive to drug or its components (phenol). Also contraindicated in patients with Hodgkin's disease who have received extensive chemotherapy or nodal irradiation.

Interactions
Drug-drug. *Corticosteroids, other immunosuppressants:* May impair the immune response to vaccine; therefore, vaccination should be avoided.

Effects on diagnostic tests
None reported.

Adverse reactions
GI: nausea, vomiting.
Musculoskeletal: myalgia.
Respiratory: difficulty breathing.
Other: adenitis, ***anaphylaxis,*** arthralgia, headache, rash, itching, serum sickness, *slight fever, soreness at injection site,* severe local reaction associated with revaccination within 3 years, general weakness.

Overdose and treatment
No information available.

Clinical considerations
- Obtain a thorough history of patient's allergies and reactions to immunizations.
- Persons with asplenia who received the 14-valent vaccine should be revaccinated with the 23-valent vaccine.
- Epinephrine solution 1:1,000 should be available to treat allergic reactions.
- Use the deltoid or midlateral thigh. Don't inject I.V. Avoid intradermal administration because this may cause severe local reactions.
- Polyvalent pneumococcal vaccine also may be administered to children to prevent pneumococcal otitis media.
- Candidates for pneumococcal vaccine include adults and children age 2 or older with chronic illness, asplenia, or splenic dysfunction; and those with sickle-cell anemia and HIV infection.
- Vaccine also is recommended for patients awaiting organ transplants, those receiving radiation therapy or cancer chemotherapy, persons in nursing homes and orphanages, and bedridden individuals.
- If different sites and separate syringes are used, pneumococcal vaccine may be administered simultaneously with influenza, DTP, poliovirus, or *Haemophilus* b polysaccharide vaccines.
- Store vaccine at 36° to 46° F (2° to 8° C). Reconstitution or dilution is unnecessary.

Therapeutic monitoring
- Check immunization history to avoid revaccination within 3 years.
- Severe local reaction has been associated with revaccination done within a 3-year period.

Special populations
Breast-feeding patients. It's unknown if vaccine is excreted in breast in milk. Use with caution in breast-feeding women.
Pediatric patients. Children under age 2 don't respond satisfactorily to pneumococcal vaccine. Safety and efficacy of vaccine haven't been established.
Geriatric patients. Vaccine is recommended for all adults over age 65.

Patient counseling
- Tell patient to expect redness, soreness, swelling, and pain at the injection site after vaccination. Fever, joint or muscle aches and pains, rash, itching, general weakness, or difficulty breathing may also develop.
- Encourage patient to report distressing adverse reactions promptly.
- Advise patient to use acetaminophen to relieve adverse reactions.

poliovirus vaccine, live, oral, trivalent (Sabin vaccine, TOPV)
Orimune

poliovirus vaccine, inactivated (IPV)
IPOL

Pharmacologic classification: vaccine
Therapeutic classification: viral vaccine
Pregnancy risk category C

How supplied
Available by prescription only
Orimune
Oral vaccine: Mixture of three viruses (types 1, 2, and 3), grown in monkey kidney tissue culture, in 0.5-ml single-dose Dispettes
IPOL
Injectable suspension: 40 D antigen units of type 1 (Mahoney), 8D antigen units of type 2 (MEF-1), and 32 D antigen units of type 3 (Saukett) per 0.5 ml

Indications and dosages
Poliovirus immunization (primary series)
IPOL
Adults (at increased risk of exposure to poliovirus): 0.5 ml I.M or S.C. at 4- to 8-week intervals for two doses; third dose is administered 6 to 12 months after second dose; total of three 0.5-ml doses are given. Booster vaccination of one additional dose may be administered to adults who have completed the three-dose primary series of IPV or OPV or combination of IPV and OPV, and who are at a high risk for exposure to poliovirus.
Infants and children: 0.5 ml I.M. or S.C. at age 2 months and 4 months; third dose is administered at age 6 to 18 months; and fourth dose at age 4 to 6 years.

Poliovirus immunization (primary series)
Orimune
Infants and children age 6 weeks and older: 0.5-ml doses P.O. at age 2, 4, and 6 to 18 months. A fourth dose at age 4 to 6 years or before entering school may be given unless third primary dose was administered on or after fourth birthday.
Adults age 18 and older: Use IPV whenever possible. If fewer than 4 weeks are available before prevention is needed, a single dose of OPV or IPV may be given.
IPV/OPV regimen for primary immunization when IPV cannot be given
Infants and children: 2 doses of IPV given I.M. or S.C. at age 2 and 4 months, and OPV given P.O. at ages 12 to 18 months and 4 to 6 years.

Pharmacodynamics
Polio prophylaxis: TOPV promotes immunity to poliomyelitis by inducing humoral and secretory antibodies and antibodies in the lymphatic tissue of the GI tract.

Pharmacokinetics
Absorption: Immunity is thought to be lifelong.
Distribution: No information available.
Metabolism: No information available.
Excretion: No information available.

Route	Onset	Peak	Duration
P.O.	7-10 days	21 days	Years
S.C., I.M.	Unknown	Unknown	Years

Contraindications and precautions
Oral vaccine is contraindicated in immunosuppressed patients, in those with cancer or immunoglobulin abnormalities, and in those receiving radiation, antimetabolite, alkylating agent, or corticosteroid therapy. These patients should receive IPV. Injectable vaccine is contraindicated in patients hypersensitive to neomycin, streptomycin, or polymyxin B.

Use cautiously in siblings of children with known immunodeficiency syndrome.

Interactions
Drug-drug. *Corticosteroids or other immunosuppressants:* Use of OPV with these drugs may impair the immune response to the vaccine. Defer vaccination with OPV until the immunosuppressant is stopped or, alternatively, inactivated poliovirus vaccine may be used.
Immune serum globulin and transfusions of blood or blood products: May also interfere with the immune response to poliovirus vaccine. Defer vaccination for 3 months in these situations.

Effects on diagnostic tests
OPV may temporarily decrease the response to tuberculin skin testing. If a tuberculin test is necessary, administer either before, simultaneously with, or at least 8 weeks after OPV.

Adverse reactions
Other: crying, decreased appetite, *fever,* hypersensitivity reactions, ***poliomyelitis,*** sleepiness, erythema, induration, *pain* (at injection site).

Overdose and treatment
No information available.

Clinical considerations
□ ***ALERT*** Parenteral form should be administered to immunodeficient patients or those with altered immune status because they may be at risk for development of the disease if live virus vaccine is administered.
- Obtain a thorough history of patient's allergies, especially to antibiotics, and of reactions to immunizations.
- IPV regimen is currently recommended for routine primary immunization in healthy infants.
- OPV is no longer recommended for routine immunizations but is recommended for outbreak control.
- Vaccine isn't effective in modifying or preventing existing or incubating poliomyelitis.
- OPV isn't for parenteral use. Dose may be administered directly or mixed with distilled water, chlorine-free tap water, simple syrup USP, or milk. It also may be placed on bread, cake, or a sugar cube.
- Keep vaccine frozen until used. It may be refrigerated up to 30 days once thawed, if unopened. Opened vials may be refrigerated up to 7 days.
- Color change from pink to yellow has no effect on the efficacy of the vaccine as long as the vaccine remains clear. Yellow color results from storage at low temperatures.

Therapeutic monitoring
- Have epinephrine 1:1,000 nearby in case of a rapid allergic reaction.
- Advise checking parents' immunization history when they bring in a child for the vaccine; this is an excellent time for parents to receive booster immunizations.

Special populations
Breast-feeding patients. Breast-feeding doesn't interfere with successful immunization; hence, no interruption in the feeding schedule is necessary.

Pediatric patients. Poliovirus vaccine shouldn't be administered to neonates under age 6 weeks.

Patient counseling

- Inform patient that risk of vaccine-associated paralysis is extremely small for vaccines, susceptible family members, and other close contacts (about 1 case per 2.6 million patients receiving the vaccines).
- Encourage patient to report distressing adverse reactions promptly.

polyethylene glycol-electrolyte solution (PEG-ES)

Colovage, CoLyte, GoLYTELY, NuLytely, OCL

Pharmacologic classification: polyethylene glycol 3350 nonabsorbable solution
Therapeutic classification: laxative and bowel evacuant
Pregnancy risk category C

How supplied

Available by prescription only
Powder for oral solution: Polyethylene glycol (PEG) 3350 (6 g), anhydrous sodium sulfate (568 mg), sodium chloride (146 mg), potassium chloride (74.5 mg/100 ml) (Colovage); PEG 3350 (120 g), sodium sulfate (3.36 g), sodium chloride (2.92 g), potassium chloride (1.49 g/2 L) (CoLyte); PEG 3350 (236 g), sodium sulfate (22.74 g), sodium bicarbonate (6.74 g), sodium chloride (5.86 g), potassium chloride (2.97 g/4.8 L) (GoLYTELY); PEG 3350 (420 g), sodium bicarbonate (5.72 g), sodium chloride (11.2 g), potassium chloride (1.48 g/4 L) (NuLytely); PEG 3350 (6 g), sodium sulfate decahydrate (1.29 g), sodium chloride (146 mg), potassium chloride (75 mg), polysorbate-80 (30 mg/100 ml) (OCL)

Indications and dosages

Bowel preparation before GI examination
Adults: 240 ml P.O. q 10 minutes until 4 L are consumed or the rectal effluent is clear. Typically, administer 4 hours before examination, allowing 3 hours for drinking and 1 hour for bowel evacuation.
Children age 3 weeks to 18 years: 25 to 40 ml/kg for 4 to 10 hours.
◊***Management of acute iron overdose***
Children under age 3: 0.5 L/hour.

Note: If a patient experiences severe bloating, distention, or abdominal pain, slow or temporarily discontinue administration until symptoms abate.

Pharmacodynamics

Laxative and bowel evacuant actions: PEG-ES acts as an osmotic agent. With sodium sulfate as the major sodium source, active sodium absorption is markedly reduced. Diarrhea results, which rapidly cleans the bowel, usually within 4 hours.

Pharmacokinetics

Absorption: PEG-ES is a nonabsorbable solution.
Distribution: Not applicable because drug isn't absorbed.
Metabolism: Not applicable because drug isn't absorbed.
Excretion: Excreted via the GI tract.

Route	Onset	Peak	Duration
P.O.	1 hr	Variable	Variable

Contraindications and precautions

Contraindicated in patients with GI obstruction or perforation, gastric retention, toxic colitis, ileus, or megacolon.

Interactions

Drug-drug. *Oral medication given within 1 hour before start of therapy:* May be flushed from the GI tract and not absorbed. Medications shouldn't be given during this time period.

Effects on diagnostic tests

Patient preparation for barium enema may be less satisfactory with this solution because it may interfere with the barium coating of the colonic mucosa using the double-contrast technique.

Adverse reactions

GI: ***nausea, bloating, cramps, vomiting, abdominal fullness,*** anal irritation.
Skin: urticaria, dermatitis.
Other: rhinorrhea, ***anaphylaxis.***

Overdose and treatment

No information available.

Clinical considerations

- Drug may be given via a nasogastric tube (at 20 to 30 ml/minute, or 1.2 to 1.8 L/hour) to patients unwilling or unable to drink the preparation. The first bowel movement should occur within 1 hour.
- Tap water may be used to reconstitute the solution. Shake container vigorously several times to ensure powder is completely dissolved. After reconstitution to 4 L with water, the solution contains PEG 3350 17.6 mmol/L, sodium 125 mmol/L, sulfate 40 mmol/L (Colyte 80 mmol/L), chloride 35 mmol/L, bicarbonate 20 mmol/L, and potassium 10 mmol/L (1 mmol/L = 1 mEq/L).
- Store reconstituted solution in refrigerator (chilling before administration improves palatability); use within 48 hours.

■ Don't add flavorings or additional ingredients to solution before use.

Therapeutic monitoring
■ If administered to semiconscious patient or to patients with impaired gag reflex, take care to prevent aspiration.
■ Monitor intake and output. No major shifts in fluid or electrolyte balance have been reported.

Special populations
Pediatric patients: Consult doctor; no dosing information is available for pediatric patients.

Patient counseling
■ Instruct patient to fast about 3 to 4 hours before ingesting the solution.
■ Tell patient never to take solid foods less than 2 hours before solution is administered. Also inform him that no foods except clear liquids are permitted after administration of solution until the examination is completed.

polysaccharide-iron complex
Ferrex-150, Fe-Tinic 150, Hytinic, Niferex, Niferex-150, Nu-Iron, Nu-Iron 150

Pharmacologic classification: oral iron supplement
Therapeutic classification: hematinic
Pregnancy risk category NR

How supplied
Available without a prescription
Tablets (film-coated): 50 mg
Capsules: 150 mg
Solution: 100 mg/5 ml

Indications and dosages
Treatment of uncomplicated iron-deficiency anemia
Adults and children age 12 and older: 150 to 300 mg P.O. daily as capsules or tablets or 1 to 2 teaspoonfuls of elixir P.O. daily.
Children age 6 to 12: 150 mg to 300 mg P.O. daily as tablets or 1 teaspoonful of elixir P.O. daily.
Children age 2 to 6: ½ teaspoonful of elixir P.O. daily.

Pharmacodynamics
Hematinic action: Polysaccharide-iron complex provides elemental iron, an essential component in the formation of hemoglobin.

Pharmacokinetics
Absorption: Although iron is absorbed from entire length of GI tract, the duodenum and proximal jejunum are the primary absorption sites. Up to 10% of iron is absorbed by healthy individuals; patients with iron-deficiency anemia may absorb up to 60%. Enteric coating has decreased absorption because they're designed to release iron past points in GI tract of highest absorption. Food may decrease absorption by 33% to 50%.
Distribution: Iron is transported through GI mucosal cells directly into the blood where it's immediately bound to a carrier protein, transferrin, and transported to the bone marrow for incorporation into hemoglobin. Iron is highly protein-bound.
Metabolism: Iron is liberated by the destruction of hemoglobin, but is conserved and reused by the body.
Excretion: Healthy individuals lose only small amounts of iron each day. Men and postmenopausal women lose about 1 mg/day and premenopausal women about 1.5 mg/day. Loss usually occurs in nails, hair, feces, and urine; trace amounts are lost in bile and sweat.

Route	Onset	Peak	Duration
P.O.	Few days	2-10 days	2 mo

Contraindications and precautions
Contraindicated in patients with hypersensitivity to any component of drug and in those with hemochromatosis and hemosiderosis.

Interactions
Drug-drug. *Antacids, cholestyramine resin, cimetidine, tetracycline, vitamin E:* Decrease iron absorption. Separate doses by 2 to 4 hours.
Chloramphenicol: Causes a delayed response to iron therapy. Monitor patient carefully.
Fluoroquinolones, levodopa, methyldopa, penicillamine: Iron decreases absorption of these drugs, possibly resulting in decreased serum levels or efficacy. Monitor patient.
Vitamin C: May increase iron absorption. Drugs may be given together.
Drug-food. *Dairy products, eggs, whole-grain breads and cereals, tea, and coffee:* Decrease iron absorption. Separate doses by 2 to 4 hours.
Foods high in vitamin C: May increase iron absorption. May be taken with these foods.
Drug-herb. *Oregano:* May reduce iron absorption. Oregano and iron supplements or iron-containing foods should be taken at least 2 hours apart.

Effects on diagnostic tests
Iron overload may decrease uptake of technetium-99m and, thus, interfere with skeletal imaging. Polysaccaride iron complex may interfere with test for occult blood in stool; guaiac and orthotoluidine tests may yield false-positive results.

Adverse reactions
Although nausea, constipation, black stools, and epigastric pain are common adverse reac-

tions associated with iron therapy, few, if any, occur with polysaccharide-iron complex. Iron-containing liquids may cause temporary staining of teeth.

Overdose and treatment

The lethal dose of iron is between 200 and 250 mg/kg; fatalities have occurred with lower doses. Symptoms may follow ingestion of 20 to 60 mg/kg. Clinical signs of acute overdose may occur as follows:

Between ½ and 8 hours after ingestion, patient may experience lethargy, nausea and vomiting, green then tarry stools, weak and rapid pulse, hypotension, dehydration, acidosis, and coma. If death doesn't immediately ensue, symptoms may clear for about 24 hours.

At 12 to 48 hours, symptoms may return, accompanied by diffuse vascular congestion, pulmonary edema, shock, seizures, anuria, and hyperthermia. Death may follow.

Treatment requires immediate support of airway, respiration, and circulation. Induce emesis with ipecac in conscious patients with intact gag reflex; for unconscious patients, empty stomach by gastric lavage. Follow emesis with lavage, using 1% sodium bicarbonate solution, to convert iron to less irritating, poorly absorbed form. (Phosphate solutions have been used, but carry risk of other adverse effects.) Perform radiographic evaluation of abdomen to determine continued presence of excess iron; if serum iron levels exceed 350 mg/dl, deferoxamine may be used for systemic chelation.

Survivors are likely to sustain organ damage, including pyloric or antral stenosis, hepatic cirrhosis, CNS damage, and intestinal obstruction.

Clinical considerations

- Administer iron with juice (preferably orange juice) or water, but not with milk or antacids.
- Polysaccharide-iron complex is nontoxic and there are relatively few, if any, of the GI adverse effects associated with other iron preparations.
- Oral iron may turn stools black. This unabsorbed iron is harmless; however, it could mask melena.

Therapeutic monitoring

Monitor hemoglobin level, hematocrit, and reticulocyte counts during therapy.

Special populations

Breast-feeding patients. Iron supplements are often recommended for breast-feeding women; no adverse effects have been documented.

Pediatric patients. Overdose of iron may be fatal in children; treat patient immediately.

Geriatric patients. Because iron-induced constipation is common in geriatric patients, stress proper diet to minimize this adverse effect. Geriatric patients may need higher doses of iron because reduced gastric secretions and achlorhydria may lower capacity for iron absorption.

Patient counseling

- Inform parents that as few as three or four tablets can cause serious iron poisoning in children.
- If patient misses a dose, tell him to take it as soon as he remembers but not to double the dose.
- Advise patient to avoid certain foods that may impair oral iron absorption, including yogurt, cheese, eggs, milk, whole-grain breads and cereals, tea, and coffee.
- Teach patient dietary measures to follow for preventing constipation.

potassium salts, oral

potassium acetate

potassium bicarbonate

K+ Care ET, K-Electrolyte, K-Ide, Klor-Con/EF, K-Lyte, K-Vescent

potassium chloride

Apo-K*, Cena-K, Gen-K, K-8, K-10*, Kalium Durules*, Kaochlor S-F, Kaon-Cl, Kaon-Cl-10, Kato, Kay Ciel, K+ Care, KCL*, K-Dur, K-Ide, K-Lease, K-Long*, K-Lor, Klor-Con, Klorvess, Klotrix, K-Lyte/Cl Powder, K-Med 900*, K-Norm, K-Sol, K-Tab, Micro-K Extencaps, Micro-K 10 Extencaps, Potasalan, Rum-K, Slow-K, Ten-K

potassium gluconate

Pharmacologic classification: potassium supplement
Therapeutic classification: therapeutic agent for electrolyte balance
Pregnancy risk category C

How supplied

Available by prescription only

potassium acetate
Vials: 2 mEq/ml in 20-, 50-, and 100-ml vials, 4 mEq/ml in 50-ml vials

potassium bicarbonate
Tablets (effervescent): 20 mEq, 25 mEq, 50 mEq
Liquid: 15 mEq/15 ml, 20 mEq/15 ml, 30 mEq/15 ml, 40 mEq/15 ml

potassium chloride
Tablets (sustained-release): 6.7 mEq, 8 mEq, 10 mEq, 20 mEq
Powder: 15 mEq/package, 20 mEq/package, and 25 mEq/package
Injection: 1.5 mEq/ml; 2 mEq/ml

potassium gluconate
Liquid: 15 mEq/15 ml, 20 mEq/15 ml

Indications and dosages

Hypokalemia

Adults and children: 40- to 100-mEq tablets divided into 2 to 4 doses daily. Use I.V. potassium chloride when oral replacement isn't feasible or when hypokalemia is life-threatening. Dosage up to 20 mEq/hour in concentration of 60 mEq/L or less. Further dose based on serum potassium determinations. Don't exceed total daily dose of 150 mEq (3 mEq/kg in children).

Further doses are based on serum potassium levels and blood pH. I.V. potassium replacement should be carried out only with ECG monitoring and frequent serum potassium determinations.

Prevention of hypokalemia

Adults and children: Initially, 20 mEq of potassium supplement P.O. daily, in divided doses. Adjust dosage, p.r.n., based on serum potassium levels.

Potassium replacement

Adults and children: Potassium chloride should be diluted in a suitable I.V. solution (not more than 40 mEq/L) and administered at rate not exceeding 20 mEq/hour. Don't exceed total dose of 400 mEq/day (3 mEq/kg/day or 40 mEq/m^2/day for children). I.V. potassium replacement should be carried out only with ECG monitoring and frequent serum potassium determinations.

◇Acute MI

Adults: High dose—80 mEq/L at a rate of 1.5 mL/kg/hour for 24 hours in combination with an I.V. infusion of 25% dextrose and 50 units/L regular insulin. Low dose—40 mEq/L at a rate of 1 mL/kg/hour for 24 hours, in combination with an I.V. infusion of 10% dextrose and 20 units/L regular insulin.

Pharmacodynamics

Potassium replacement action: Potassium is necessary for maintaining intracellular tonicity, maintaining a balance with sodium across cell membranes, transmitting nerve impulses, maintaining cellular metabolism, contracting cardiac and skeletal muscle, and maintaining acid-base balance and normal renal function.

Pharmacokinetics

Absorption: Potassium is well absorbed from the GI tract. It should be taken with meals and sipped slowly over a 5- to 10-minute period to decrease irritation. Potassium bicarbonate doesn't correct hypochloremic alkalosis.

Distribution: The normal serum levels of potassium range from 3.8 to 5 mEq/L. Plasma potassium levels up to 7.7 mEq/L may be normal in neonates. Up to 60 mEq/L of potassium may be found in gastric secretions and diarrhea fluid.

Metabolism: None significant.

Excretion: Potassium is excreted largely by the kidneys. Small amounts of potassium may be excreted via the skin and intestinal tract, but intestinal potassium usually is reabsorbed. A healthy patient on a potassium-free diet will excrete 40 to 50 mEq of potassium daily.

Route	Onset	Peak	Duration
P.O., I.V.	Varies	Varies	Varies

Contraindications and precautions

Contraindicated in patients with severe renal impairment with oliguria, anuria, or azotemia; in those with untreated Addison's disease; and in those with acute dehydration, heat cramps, hyperkalemia, hyperkalemic form of familial periodic paralysis, and conditions associated with extensive tissue breakdown.

Use cautiously in patients with cardiac or renal disease.

Interactions

Drug-drug. *Anticholinergics:* May increase the chance of GI irritation and ulceration when used with potassium. Monitor patient carefully.

Digitalized patients with severe or complete heart block: Potential for arrhythmias. Potassium shouldn't be given to these patients.

Potassium-containing products: May cause hyperkalemia within 1 to 2 days. Monitor serum potassium levels closely.

Potassium-sparing diuretics, ACE inhibitors such as captopril: Can cause severe hyperkalemia. Use with extreme caution. Monitor serum potassium levels closely.

Drug-food. *Salt substitutes containing potassium salts:* Can cause severe hyperkalemia. Avoid use together.

Effects on diagnostic tests

None reported.

Adverse reactions

CNS: paresthesia of the extremities, listlessness, mental confusion, weakness or heaviness of legs, flaccid paralysis.

CV: hypotension, ***arrhythmias, cardiac arrest,*** heart block, ECG changes.

GI: nausea, vomiting, abdominal pain, diarrhea.

Respiratory: ***respiratory paralysis.***

Other: pain and redness at infusion site, fever, hyperkalemia.

Overdose and treatment

Signs and symptoms of overdose include an increased serum potassium level and characteristic ECG changes, including tall peaked T waves, depression of ST segment, disappearance of P wave, prolonged QT interval, and widening and slurring of the QRS complex. Late clinical signs include weakness, paralysis of voluntary muscles, respiratory distress, and dysphagia. These may precede severe or fatal cardiac toxicity. Hyperkalemia produces symptoms paradoxically similar to those of hypokalemia.

Treatment of potassium overdose includes discontinuation of the potassium supplement and, if necessary, lavage of the GI tract. In patients with a potassium level greater then 6.5 mEq/L, supportive therapy may include the following interventions (with continuous ECG monitoring):

Infuse 40 to 160 mEq sodium bicarbonate I.V. over a 5-minute interval; repeat in 10 to 15 minutes if ECG abnormalities persist.

Infuse 300 to 500 ml of dextrose 10% to 25% over 1 hour. Insulin (5 to 10 units per 20 g of dextrose) should be added to the infusion or, ideally, administered as a separate injection.

Patients with absent P waves or broad QRS complex who aren't receiving cardiotonic glycosides should immediately be given 0.5 g to 1 g of calcium gluconate or another calcium salt I.V. over a 2-minute period (with continuous ECG monitoring) to antagonize the cardiotoxic effect of the potassium. May be repeated in 1 to 2 minutes if ECG abnormalities persist.

To remove potassium from the body, use sodium polystyrene sulfonate resin, hemodialysis, or peritoneal dialysis. Administer potassium-free I.V. fluids when hyperkalemia is associated with water loss.

Clinical considerations

☐ ***ALERT*** Give parenteral potassium by slow infusion only, never by I.V. push or I.M. Dilute I.V. potassium preparations with large volume of parenteral solutions.
- In patients receiving cardiac glycosides, removing potassium too rapidly may result in digitalis toxicity.
- Don't crush sustained-released potassium products.
- Don't give potassium during immediate postoperative period until urine flow is established.
- Give oral potassium supplements with extreme caution because its many forms deliver varying amounts of potassium. Patient may tolerate one product better than another.
- Potassium gluconate doesn't correct hypokalemic hypochloremic alkalosis.
- Enteric-coated tablets aren't recommended because of the potential for GI bleeding and small-bowel ulcerations.
- Tablets in wax matrix sometimes lodge in esophagus and cause ulceration in cardiac patients who have esophageal compression resulting from enlarged left atrium. In such patients and in those with esophageal or GI stasis or obstruction, use liquid form.
- Drug is often used orally with diuretics that cause potassium excretion. Potassium chloride is most useful because diuretics waste chloride ions. Hypokalemic alkalosis is treated best with potassium chloride.

Therapeutic monitoring

- Monitor ECG, pH, serum potassium levels, and other electrolytes during therapy.
- Monitor serum potassium, BUN, and serum creatinine levels; pH; and intake and output.

Special populations

Breast-feeding patients. Potassium supplements pass into the breast milk. Safety in breast-feeding hasn't been established; therefore, use potassium only when the benefits to the breast-feeding woman outweigh the risk to the infant.
Pediatric patients. Use cautiously in pediatric patients.

Patient counseling

- Tell patient potassium is available only with a prescription because the wrong amount may cause severe reactions.
- Suggest diluting liquid potassium product in at least 4 to 8 oz (120 to 240 ml) of water; to take it after meals; and to sip liquid potassium slowly to minimize GI irritation.
- Tell patient to dissolve powder, soluble tablets, or granules completely in at least 4 oz (120 ml) of water or juice, and to allow fizzing to finish before drinking.
- Instruct patient not to crush or chew sustained-release capsules; contents of capsule can be opened and sprinkled onto applesauce or other soft food.
- Tell patient to stop taking drug immediately and report the following reactions: confusion; irregular heartbeat; numbness of feet, fingers or lips; shortness of breath; anxiety, excessive tiredness or weakness of legs; unexplained diarrhea; nausea and vomiting; stomach pain; or bloody or black stools. Such reactions are rare.
- Tell patient that expelling a whole tablet in the stool (sustained-release tablet) is normal. The body eliminates the shell after absorbing the potassium.
- Warn patient to avoid salt substitutes except when prescribed.

pramipexole dihydrochloride

Mirapex

Pharmacologic classification: nonergot dopamine agonist
Therapeutic classification: antiparkinsonian
Pregnancy risk category C

How supplied

Available by prescription only
Tablets: 0.125 mg, 0.25 mg, 0.5 mg, 1 mg, 1.5 mg

Indications and dosages

Treatment of idiopathic Parkinson's disease
Adults: Initially, 0.375 mg P.O. daily given in three divided doses; don't increase more than q 5 to 7 days. Increase dose by 0.75 mg in divided doses weekly until maximum dose of 1.5 mg t.i.d. is reached after 7 weeks of therapy.

Maintenance dosing ranges from 1.5 to 4.5 mg daily administered in three divided doses.
≡ ***Dosage adjustment.*** In patients with impaired renal function and creatinine clearance of 35 to 59 ml/minute, initial dose is 0.125 mg P.O. b.i.d. and maintenance maximum dose is 1.5 mg b.i.d. For patients with creatinine clearance of 15 to 34 ml/minute, initial dose is 0.125 mg P.O. daily and maintenance maximum dose is 1.5 mg daily.

Pharmacodynamics
Antiparkinsonian action: Drug is thought to stimulate dopamine (D_2 and D_3) receptors in striatum; in animal studies, pramipexole influences striatal neuronal firing rates via activation of dopamine receptors in the striatum and the substantia nigra, the site of neurons that send projections to the striatum.

Pharmacokinetics
Absorption: Absolute bioavailability of drug is more than 90%, suggesting that it's well absorbed and undergoes little presystemic metabolism. Food doesn't affect extent of absorption but time of maximum plasma level is increased by about 1 hour when drug is taken with meals.
Distribution: Extensively distributed, with a volume of distribution of about 500 L. About 15% is bound to plasma proteins. Drug also is distributed into RBCs. Terminal half-life is 8 to 12 hours; steady state is reached within 2 days of dosing.
Metabolism: About 90% of dose is excreted unchanged in urine.
Excretion: Excreted mainly in urine. Nonrenal routes may contribute to a small extent to elimination, although no metabolites have been identified in plasma or urine. Drug is secreted by the renal tubules, probably by the organic transport system.

Route	Onset	Peak	Duration
P.O.	Rapid	2 hr	8-12 hr

Contraindications and precautions
Contraindicated in patients with hypersensitivity to drug or its components. Use with caution in patients who have renal impairment, such as the elderly, because dosing may need to be adjusted.

Interactions
Drug-drug. *Butyrophenones, metoclopramide, phenothiazines, thiothixenes:* May diminish the effectiveness of pramipexole. Monitor patient closely.
Cimetidine, diltiazem, quinidine, quinine, ranitidine, triamterene, verapamil: Decrease oral clearance of pramipexole. Adjust dose as needed.
Levodopa: Increased maximum plasma levels of levodopa. Adjust levodopa dose as needed.

Effects on diagnostic tests
None reported.

Adverse reactions
CNS: *dizziness,* somnolence, *insomnia*, hallucinations, *confusion*, amnesia, hypesthesia, dystonia, akathisia, thought abnormalities, myoclonus, *asthenia, dyskinesia, extrapyramidal syndrome, dream abnormalities*, gait abnormalities, hypertonia, paranoid reaction, delusions, sleep disorders, including sudden sleep onset resembling narcolepsy.
CV: chest pain, peripheral edema, *orthostatic hypotension.*
EENT: accommodation abnormalities, diplopia, dry mouth, rhinitis, vision abnormalities.
GI: anorexia, *constipation*, dysphagia, nausea.
GU: impotence, urinary frequency, urinary tract infection, urinary incontinence.
Musculoskeletal: arthritis, twitching, bursitis, myasthenia.
Respiratory: dyspnea, pneumonia.
Skin: skin disorders.
Other: general edema, malaise, fever, unevaluable reaction, decreased libido, *accidental injury.*

Overdose and treatment
No known antidote; if signs of CNS stimulation occur, a phenothiazine or other butyrophenone neuroleptic agent may be given. Management of overdose may require general supportive measures with gastric lavage, I.V. fluids, and ECG monitoring.

Clinical considerations
- If drug needs to be discontinued, it should be tapered over a 1-week period.
- Drug may cause orthostatic hypotension, especially during dose escalation; monitor patient carefully.
- Adjust dosage gradually. Increase dosage to achieve maximum therapeutic effect, balanced against the main adverse effects of dyskinesia, hallucinations, somnolence, and dry mouth.

Therapeutic monitoring
Neuroleptic malignant syndrome (elevated temperature, muscular rigidity, altered consciousness, and autonomic instability) without obvious cause has occurred in association with rapid dose reduction or withdrawal of or changes in antiparkinsonian therapy.

Special populations
Pediatric patients. Safety and efficacy in children haven't been established.
Breast-feeding patients. It isn't known if drug is excreted in breast milk. Use with caution.
Geriatric patients. Drug clearance decreases with age because half-life and clearance are about 40% longer and 30% lower, respectively, in patients age 65 or older.

Patient counseling

- Tell patient to take drug only as prescribed.
- Instruct patient not to rise rapidly after sitting or lying down because of risk of orthostatic hypotension.
- Caution patient not to drive a car or operate complex machinery until response to drug is known.
- Tell patient to use caution before taking drug with other CNS depressants.
- Advise patient to take drug with food if nausea develops.
- Tell patient not to stop taking drug abruptly.

pravastatin sodium

Pravachol

Pharmacologic classification: HMG-CoA reductase inhibitor
Therapeutic classification: antilipemic
Pregnancy risk category X

How supplied

Available by prescription only
Tablets: 10 mg, 20 mg, 40 mg

Indications and dosages

Reduction of low-density lipoprotein and total cholesterol levels in patients with primary hypercholesterolemia (types IIa and IIb), primary prevention of coronary events
Adults: Initially, 10 to 20 mg P.O. daily h.s. Adjust dosage q 4 weeks based on patient tolerance and response; maximum daily dose is 40 mg. Most elderly patients respond to a daily dose of 20 mg or less.

Pharmacodynamics

Antilipemic action: Pravastatin inhibits the enzyme 3-hydroxy-3-methylglutaryl-coenzyme A (HMG-CoA) reductase. This hepatic enzyme is an early (and rate-limiting) step in the synthetic pathway of cholesterol.

Pharmacokinetics

Absorption: Rapidly absorbed. Average oral absorption is 34%, with absolute bioavailability of 17%. Although food reduces bioavailability, drug effects are the same if drug is taken with meals or 1 hour before meals.
Distribution: Plasma levels of drug are proportional to dose, but don't necessarily correlate perfectly with lipid-lowering effects. About 50% is bound to plasma proteins. Drug undergoes extensive first-pass extraction, possibly because of an active transport system into hepatocytes.
Metabolism: Metabolized by the liver; at least six metabolites have been identified. Some are active.
Excretion: Excreted by the liver and kidneys.

Route	Onset	Peak	Duration
P.O.	Unknown	1-1½ hr	Unknown

Contraindications and precautions

Contraindicated in patients with hypersensitivity to drug; in those with active liver disease or conditions that cause unexplained, persistent elevations of serum transaminase levels; in pregnant and breast-feeding women; and in women of childbearing age unless there's no risk of pregnancy.

Use cautiously in patients who consume large quantities of alcohol or have history of liver disease.

Interactions

Drug-drug. *Cholestyramine, colestipol:* May decrease plasma levels of pravastatin. Administer pravastatin 1 hour before or 4 hours after these drugs.
Drugs that decrease levels or activity of endogenous steroids, such as cimetidine, ketoconazole, and spironolactone: May increase risk of endocrine dysfunction. No intervention appears necessary; take complete drug history in patients who develop endocrine dysfunction.
Erythromycin; fibric acid derivatives, such as clofibrate and gemfibrozil; high doses of niacin (1 g or more nicotinic acid daily); immunosuppressive agents such as cyclosporine: May increase risk of rhabdomyolysis. Monitor patient closely if drugs must be given together.
Gemfibrozil: Decreases protein-binding and urinary clearance of pravastatin. Avoid use together.
Hepatotoxic drugs: May increase risk of hepatotoxicity. Avoid use together.
Drug-lifestyle. *Chronic alcohol abuse:* May increase risk of hepatotoxicity. Monitor patient closely.
Sun exposure: Photosensitivity reaction may occur. Advise patient to take precautions.

Effects on diagnostic tests

None reported.

Adverse reactions

CNS: headache, dizziness, fatigue.
CV: chest pain.
EENT: rhinitis.
GI: vomiting, diarrhea, heartburn, abdominal pain, constipation, flatulence, nausea.
GU: renal failure secondary to myoglobinuria, urinary abnormality.
Hepatic: AST, ALT levels are increased
Musculoskeletal: myositis, myopathy, *localized muscle pain,* myalgia, ***rhabdomyolysis.***
Respiratory: cough, influenza, common cold.
Skin: rash.
Other: flulike symptoms, photosensitivity; thyroid function test is abnormal; CK, alkaline phosphatase, and bilirubin levels are increased.

Overdose and treatment
No information available. Treat symptomatically.

Clinical considerations
- Discontinue drug temporarily in patient with an acute condition that suggests a developing myopathy or in patient with risk factors that may predispose him to development of renal failure secondary to rhabdomyolysis, including severe acute infection; severe endocrine, metabolic, or electrolyte disorders; hypotension; major surgery; or uncontrolled seizures.
- Initiate drug therapy only after diet and other nonpharmacologic therapies have proved ineffective. Patients should continue a cholesterol-lowering diet during therapy.
- Give drug in the evening, preferably at bedtime. Drug may be given without regard to meals.
- Dosage adjustments should be made about every 4 weeks. May reduce dosage if cholesterol levels fall below target range.

Therapeutic monitoring
Watch for signs of myositis. Rarely, myopathy and marked elevations of CK, possibly leading to rhabdomyolysis and renal failure secondary to myoglobinuria, have been reported.

Special populations
Breast-feeding patients. Drug is excreted in breast milk. Women shouldn't breast-feed while taking pravastatin.
Pediatric patients. Safety and efficacy in children under age 18 haven't been established.
Geriatric patients. Maximum effectiveness is usually evident with daily doses of 20 mg or less.

Patient counseling
- Teach patient appropriate dietary management (restricting total fat and cholesterol intake), weight control, and exercise. Explain importance of these interventions in controlling serum lipids.
- Tell patient to report adverse reactions, particularly muscle aches and pains.

prazosin hydrochloride
Minipress

Pharmacologic classification: alpha blocker
Therapeutic classification: antihypertensive
Pregnancy risk category C

How supplied
Available by prescription only
Capsules: 1 mg, 2 mg, 5 mg

Indications and dosages
Hypertension
Adults: Initially, 1 mg P.O. b.i.d. or t.i.d.; gradually increased to maximum of 20 mg daily. Usual maintenance dosage is 6 to 15 mg daily in divided doses. If other antihypertensive agents or diuretics are added to prazosin therapy, reduce dose of prazosin to 1 or 2 mg t.i.d. and then gradually increase as necessary.
◇***Benign prostatic hyperplasia (BPH)***
Adults: Initially, 2 mg P.O. b.i.d. Dosage may range from 1 to 9 mg/day.

Pharmacodynamics
Antihypertensive action: Prazosin selectively and competitively inhibits alpha-adrenergic receptors, causing arterial and venous dilation, reducing peripheral vascular resistance and blood pressure.
Hypertrophic action: Alpha blockade of prazosin in nonvascular smooth muscle causes relaxation, notably in prostatic tissue, reducing urinary symptoms in men with BPH.

Pharmacokinetics
Absorption: Absorption from the GI tract is variable. Full antihypertensive effect may not occur for 4 to 6 weeks.
Distribution: Distributed throughout the body and is highly protein-bound (about 97%).
Metabolism: Metabolized extensively in the liver.
Excretion: Over 90% of a given dose is excreted in feces via bile; remainder is excreted in urine. Plasma half-life is 2 to 4 hours. Antihypertensive effect lasts less than 24 hours.

Route	Onset	Peak	Duration
P.O.	½-1½ hr	2-4 hr	7-10 hr

Contraindications and precautions
No known contraindications. Use cautiously in patients receiving antihypertensive medications and in those with chronic renal failure.

Interactions
Drug-drug. *Diuretics or other antihypertensive agents:* Hypotensive effects of prazosin may be increased when administered concurrently. Avoid use together.
Highly protein-bound drugs: Because prazosin is highly bound to plasma proteins, it may interact with other highly protein-bound drugs. Monitor patient.
Drug-herb. *Butcher's broom:* May cause reduction of drug effects. Don't use together.

Effects on diagnostic tests
Prazosin alters results of screening tests for pheochromocytoma and causes increases in levels of the urinary metabolite of norepinephrine and vanillylmandelic acid.

Adverse reactions

CNS: *dizziness,* headache, drowsiness, nervousness, paresthesia, weakness, *"first-dose syncope,"* depression.
CV: orthostatic hypotension, *palpitations.*
EENT: blurred vision, tinnitus, conjunctivitis, nasal congestion, epistaxis.
GI: vomiting, diarrhea, abdominal cramps, liver function test abnormalities, constipation, *nausea.*
GU: priapism, impotence, urinary frequency, incontinence.
Musculoskeletal: arthralgia, myalgia.
Respiratory: dyspnea.
Other: pruritus, edema, fever, transient decrease in leukocyte count and increased serum uric acid and BUN levels.

Overdose and treatment

Overdose is manifested by hypotension and drowsiness. After acute ingestion, empty stomach by induced emesis or gastric lavage, and give activated charcoal to reduce absorption. Further treatment is usually symptomatic and supportive. Prazosin isn't dialyzable.

Clinical considerations

Consider the recommendations relevant to all alpha blockers as well as the following:

- First-dose syncope (dizziness, light-headedness, and syncope) may occur within ½ to 1 hour after initial dose; it may be severe, with loss of consciousness, if initial dose exceeds 2 mg. Effect is transient and may be diminished by giving drug at bedtime, by limiting the initial dose of prazosin to 1 mg, by subsequently increasing the dosage gradually, and by introducing other antihypertensive agents into the patient's regimen cautiously; it's more common during febrile illness and more severe if patient has hyponatremia. Always increase dosage gradually and have patient sit or lie down if he experiences dizziness.
- Drug has been used to treat vasospasm associated with Raynaud's syndrome. It also has been used with diuretics and cardiac glycosides to treat severe heart failure, to manage the signs and symptoms of pheochromocytoma preoperatively, and to treat ergotamine-induced peripheral ischemia.

Therapeutic monitoring

Monitor patient's blood pressure and heart rate frequently; the effect of prazosin is most pronounced on diastolic blood pressure.

Special populations

Pregnant patients: Use only when potential benefits outweigh risks to fetus. Safety hasn't been established for use during pregnancy.
Breast-feeding patients. Small amounts of prazosin are excreted in breast milk; an alternative feeding method is recommended during therapy.
Pediatric patients. Safety and efficacy in children haven't been established; use only when potential benefit outweighs risk.
Geriatric patients. Geriatric patients may be more sensitive to hypotensive effects and may require lower doses because of altered drug metabolism.

Patient counseling

- Teach patient about his disease and therapy, and explain that he must take drug exactly as prescribed, even when feeling well; advise him never to discontinue drug suddenly because severe rebound hypertension may occur.
- Advise patient to promptly report malaise or unusual adverse effects.
- Tell patient to avoid hazardous activities that require mental alertness until tolerance develops to sedation, drowsiness, and other CNS effects; to avoid sudden position changes to minimize orthostatic hypotension; and to use ice chips, candy, or gum to relieve dry mouth.
- Warn patient to seek medical approval before taking OTC cold preparations.

prednisolone (systemic)

Delta-Cortef, Prelone

prednisolone acetate

Key-Pred-25, Predalone-50, Predate, Predcor-50

prednisolone sodium phosphate

Pediapred

prednisolone tebutate

Hydeltra-T.B.A., Nor-Pred T.B.A., Predate TBA, Predcor-TBA

Pharmacologic classification: glucocorticoid, mineralocorticoid
Therapeutic classification: anti-inflammatory, immunosuppressant
Pregnancy risk category C

How supplied

Available by prescription only
prednisolone
Tablets: 5 mg
Syrup: 15 mg/5 ml
prednisolone acetate
Injection: 25 mg/ml, 50 mg/ml suspension
prednisolone sodium phosphate
Oral liquid: 6.7 mg (5 mg base)/5 ml
prednisolone tebutate
Injection: 20 mg/ml suspension

Indications and dosages

Severe inflammation, modification of body's immune response to disease
Adults: 2.5 to 15 mg P.O. b.i.d., t.i.d., or q.i.d.
Children: 0.14 to 2 mg/kg or 4 to 6 mg/m^2 daily in divided doses.
prednisolone acetate
Adults: 2 to 30 mg I.M. q 12 hours.
Children: 0.04 to 0.25 mg/kg or 1.5 to 7.5 mg/m^2 I.M. 1 or 2 times daily.
prednisolone sodium phosphate
Adults: Initially, 5 to 60 mg P.O. daily.
Children: 0.14 to 2 mg/kg P.O. daily in 3 to 4 divided doses or 40 to 60 mg/m^2 daily.
prednisolone tebutate
Adults: 4 to 40 mg into joints and lesions, p.r.n.

Pharmacodynamics

Anti-inflammatory action: Prednisolone stimulates the synthesis of enzymes needed to decrease the inflammatory response. It suppresses the immune system by reducing activity and volume of the lymphatic system, thus producing lymphocytopenia (primarily of T-lymphocytes), decreasing immunoglobulin and complement levels, decreasing passage of immune complexes through basement membranes, and possibly by depressing reactivity of tissue to antigen-antibody interactions.

The mineralocorticoids regulate electrolyte homeostasis by acting renally at the distal tubules to enhance the reabsorption of sodium ions (and thus water) from the tubular fluid into the plasma and enhance the excretion of both potassium and hydrogen ions.

Prednisolone is an adrenocorticoid with both glucocorticoid and mineralocorticoid properties. It's a weak mineralocorticoid with only half the potency of hydrocortisone but is a more potent glucocorticoid, having four times the potency of equal weight of hydrocortisone. It's used primarily as an anti-inflammatory agent and an immunosuppressant. It isn't used for mineralocorticoid replacement therapy because of the availability of more specific and potent agents.

Prednisolone and prednisolone sodium phosphate may be administered orally. Prednisolone acetate and tebutate are suspensions that may be administered by intra-articular, intrasynovial, intrabursal, intralesional, or soft-tissue injection. They have a slow onset but a long duration of action.

Pharmacokinetics

Absorption: Absorbed readily after oral administration. Acetate and tebutate suspensions for injection have a variable absorption, depending on whether they're injected into an intra-articular space or a muscle. Systemic absorption occurs slowly after intra-articular injection.
Distribution: Removed rapidly from the blood and distributed to muscle, liver, skin, intestines, and kidneys. Drug is extensively bound to plasma proteins (transcortin and albumin). Only the unbound portion is active. Adrenocorticoids are distributed into breast milk and through the placenta.
Metabolism: Metabolized in the liver to inactive glucuronide and sulfate metabolites.
Excretion: The inactive metabolites, and small amounts of unmetabolized drug, are excreted in urine. Insignificant quantities of drug are excreted in feces. Biologic half-life of prednisolone is 18 to 36 hours.

Route	Onset	Peak	Duration
P.O.	Rapid	1-2 hr	3-36 hr
I.V.	Rapid	1 hr	Unknown
I.M.	Rapid	1 hr	4 wk

Contraindications and precautions

Contraindicated in patients with hypersensitivity to drug or its ingredients and systemic fungal infections.

Use cautiously in patients with a recent MI, GI ulcer, renal disease, hypertension, osteoporosis, diabetes mellitus, hypothyroidism, cirrhosis, diverticulitis, nonspecific ulcerative colitis, recent intestinal anastamoses, thromboembolic disorders, seizures, myasthenia gravis, heart failure, tuberculosis, ocular herpes simplex, emotional instability, or psychotic tendencies.

Interactions

Drug-drug. *Amphotericin B or diuretics:* May enhance hypokalemia, which may increase the risk of toxicity in patients also receiving cardiac glycosides. Monitor patient closely.
Antacids, cholestyramine, colestipol: Decrease effect of prednisolone. Avoid use together.
Barbiturates, phenytoin, and rifampin: May cause decreased corticosteroid effects. Increase corticosteroid dose as ordered.
Estrogens: May reduce the metabolism of prednisolone. Monitor patient closely.
Insulin or oral antidiabetic agents: Hyperglycemia may occur. May require dosage adjustment in diabetic patients.
Isoniazid and salicylates: Increased metabolism of these drugs. Monitor patient closely.
NSAIDs: May increase risk of GI ulceration. Give together cautiously.
Oral anticoagulants: Prednisolone rarely may decrease the effects of oral anticoagulants. Monitor PT and INR closely.

Effects on diagnostic tests

Prednisolone suppresses reactions to skin tests and causes false-negative results in the nitroblue tetrazolium test for systemic bacterial infections.

Adverse reactions

Most adverse reactions to corticosteroids are dose- or duration-dependent.

CNS: *euphoria, insomnia,* psychotic behavior, pseudotumor cerebri, vertigo, headache, paresthesia, ***seizures.***

CV: ***heart failure, thromboembolism,*** hypertension, edema, ***arrhythmias,*** thrombophlebitis.

EENT: cataracts, glaucoma.

Endocrine: menstrual irregularities, cushingoid state (moonface, buffalo hump, central obesity).

GI: *peptic ulceration,* GI irritation, increased appetite, pancreatitis, nausea, vomiting.

Musculoskeletal: muscle weakness, osteoporosis.

Skin: delayed wound healing, acne, various skin eruptions.

Other: altered thyroid studies, decreased calcium levels, increased urine glucose and calcium levels and serum cholesterol levels; hirsutism, susceptibility to infections; hypokalemia, hyperglycemia, and carbohydrate intolerance; growth suppression in children; ***acute adrenal insufficiency may occur with increased stress (infection, surgery, or trauma) or abrupt withdrawal after long-term therapy.***

After abrupt withdrawal: rebound inflammation, fatigue, weakness, arthralgia, fever, dizziness, lethargy, depression, fainting, orthostatic hypotension, dyspnea, anorexia, hypoglycemia. ***After prolonged use, sudden withdrawal may be fatal.***

Overdose and treatment

Acute ingestion, even in massive doses, is rarely a clinical problem. Toxic signs and symptoms rarely occur if drug is used for less than 3 weeks, even at large dosage ranges. However, chronic use causes adverse physiologic effects, including suppression of the hypothalamic-pituitary-adrenal axis, cushingoid appearance, muscle weakness, and osteoporosis.

Clinical considerations

□ ***ALERT*** Don't confuse prednisolone with prednisone.

- Recommendations for use of prednisolone and for care and teaching of patients are the same as those for all systemic adrenocorticoids.
- Determine if patient is sensitive to other corticosteroid medications.
- Always adjust to lowest effective dose.

Therapeutic monitoring

- Monitor patient's weight, blood pressure, and serum electrolytes.
- Watch for signs of depression or psychotic episodes, especially in high-dose therapy.

Special populations

Pediatric patients. Chronic use of adrenocorticoids or corticotropin may suppress growth and maturation in children and adolescents.

Geriatric patients: Geriatric patients may be more susceptible to osteoporosis with long-term use.

Patient counseling

- Instruct patient not to abruptly discontinue drug.
- Teach patient the signs of early adrenal insufficiency: fatigue, muscular weakness, joint pain, fever, anorexia, nausea, dyspnea, dizziness, and fainting.
- Patient should carry a medical identification card.
- Unless contraindicated, patient should follow low-sodium diet that's high in potassium and protein.

prednisolone acetate (ophthalmic)

AK-Tate, Econopred Ophthalmic, Ocu-Pred-A, Predair A, Pred Forte, Pred Mild Ophthalmic

prednisolone sodium phosphate

AK-Pred, Inflamase Forte, Inflamase Mild Ophthalmic, I-Pred, Ocu-Pred, Predair

Pharmacologic classification: corticosteroid
Therapeutic classification: ophthalmic anti-inflammatory
Pregnancy risk category C

How supplied

Available by prescription only
prednisolone acetate
Suspension: 0.12%, 0.125%, 1%
prednisolone sodium phosphate
Solution: 0.125%, 0.5%, 1%

Indications and dosages

Inflammation of palpebral and bulbar conjunctiva, cornea, and anterior segment of globe; corneal injury; graft rejection

Adults and children: Instill 1 or 2 drops in eye. In severe conditions, may be used hourly, tapering to discontinuation as inflammation subsides. In mild conditions, may be used four to six times daily.

Pharmacodynamics

Anti-inflammatory action: Corticosteroids stimulate the synthesis of enzymes needed to decrease the inflammatory response. Prednisolone, a synthetic corticosteroid, has about four times the anti-inflammatory potency of an equal weight of hydrocortisone. Prednisolone acetate is poorly soluble and therefore has a slower onset of action, but a longer duration of action, when applied in a liquid suspension. The sodium phosphate salt is highly soluble and has a rapid onset but short duration of action.

Pharmacokinetics

Absorption: After ophthalmic administration, is absorbed through the aqueous humor. Systemic absorption rarely occurs.
Distribution: After ophthalmic application, is distributed throughout local tissue layers. Any drug that's absorbed into circulation is rapidly removed from the blood and distributed into muscle, liver, skin, intestines, and kidneys.
Metabolism: After ophthalmic administration, corticosteroids are primarily metabolized locally. The small amount that's absorbed into systemic circulation is metabolized primarily in the liver to inactive compounds.
Excretion: Inactive metabolites are excreted by the kidneys, primarily as glucuronides and sulfates, but also as unconjugated products. Small amounts of metabolites are excreted in feces.

Route	Onset	Peak	Duration
Ophthalmic	Unknown	Unknown	Unknown

Contraindications and precautions

Contraindicated in patients with acute, untreated, purulent ocular infections; acute superficial herpes simplex (dendritic keratitis); vaccinia, varicella, or other viral or fungal eye diseases; or ocular tuberculosis.

Use cautiously in patients with corneal abrasions that may be contaminated (especially with herpes).

Interactions

None reported.

Effects on diagnostic tests

None reported.

Adverse reactions

EENT: increased intraocular pressure; thinning of cornea, interference with corneal wound healing, increased susceptibility to viral or fungal corneal infection, corneal ulceration; with excessive or long-term use: discharge, discomfort, foreign body sensation, glaucoma exacerbation, cataracts, visual acuity and visual field defects, optic nerve damage.
Other: systemic effects and adrenal suppression with excessive or long-term use.

Overdose and treatment

No information available.

Clinical considerations

Shake suspension and check dosage before administering. Store in tightly covered container.

Therapeutic monitoring

Patients on long-term therapy should have frequent tonometric examinations.

Patient counseling

- Teach patient correct way to instill medication.
- Advise patient to wash hands before and after applying, and warn him not to touch tip of dropper to eye or surrounding area.
- Advise patient to apply light pressure on lacrimal sac for 1 minute after instillation.
- Warn patient not to share medication or towels with family members.
- Tell patient to report if no improvement occurs within several days or if he experiences pain, itching or swelling of the eye.

prednisone

Apo-Prednisone*, Deltasone, Meticorten, Sterapred, Winpred*

Pharmacologic classification: adrenocorticoid
Therapeutic classification: anti-inflammatory, immunosuppressant
Pregnancy risk category C

How supplied

Available by prescription only
Tablets: 1 mg, 2.5 mg, 5 mg, 10 mg, 20 mg, 25 mg, 50 mg
Tablets (film-coated): 5 mg
Oral solution: 5 mg/5 ml
Oral solution (concentrate): 5 mg/ml

Indications and dosages

Severe inflammation, modification of body's immune response to disease
Adults: 5 to 60 mg P.O. daily in single dose or divided doses. Maximum daily dose, 250 mg. Maintenance dosage given once daily or every other day. Dosage must be individualized.
Children: 0.14 mg/kg or 4 to 6 mg/m^2 P.O. daily in divided doses; alternatively, may use the following dosage schedule:
Children age 11 to 18: 20 mg P.O. q.i.d.
Children age 5 to 10: 15 mg P.O. q.i.d.
Children age 18 months to 4 years: 7.5 to 10 mg P.O. q.i.d.
Acute exacerbations of multiple sclerosis
Adults: 200 mg P.O. daily for 1 week, then 80 mg every other day for 1 month.
Advanced pulmonary or extrapulmonary tuberculosis
Adults: 40 to 60 mg P.O. daily, tapered over 4 to 8 weeks.

◊***Adjunct to anti-infective therapy in the treatment of moderate to severe* Pneumocystis carinii *pneumonia***
Adults or children over age 13 with AIDS: 40 mg P.O. b.i.d. for 5 days; then 40 mg. P.O. once daily for 5 days; then 20 mg P.O. once daily for 11 days (or until completion of the concurrent anti-infective regimen).

Pharmacodynamics

Immunosuppressant action: Prednisone stimulates the synthesis of enzymes needed to decrease the inflammatory response. It suppresses the immune system by reducing activity and volume of the lymphatic system, producing lymphocytopenia (primarily of T-lymphocytes), decreasing immunoglobulin and complement levels, decreasing passage of immune complexes through basement membranes, and possibly by depressing reactivity of tissue to antigen-antibody interactions.
Anti-inflammatory action: Prednisone is one of the intermediate-acting glucocorticoids, with greater glucocorticoid activity than cortisone and hydrocortisone, but less anti-inflammatory activity than betamethasone, dexamethasone, and paramethasone. Prednisone is about four to five times more potent as an anti-inflammatory agent than hydrocortisone, but it has only half the mineralocorticoid activity of an equal weight of hydrocortisone. Prednisone is the oral glucocorticoid of choice for anti-inflammatory or immunosuppressant effects.

For patients who can't swallow tablets, liquid forms are available. The oral concentrate (5 mg/ml) may be diluted in juice or another flavored diluent or mixed in semisolid food such as applesauce before administration.

Pharmacokinetics

Absorption: Absorbed readily after oral administration.
Distribution: Distributed rapidly to muscle, liver, skin, intestines, and kidneys. Prednisone is extensively bound to plasma proteins (transcortin and albumin). Only the unbound portion is active. Adrenocorticoids are distributed into breast milk and through the placenta.
Metabolism: Metabolized in the liver to the active metabolite prednisolone, which, in turn, is then metabolized to inactive glucuronide and sulfate metabolites.
Excretion: The inactive metabolites and small amounts of unmetabolized drug are excreted by the kidneys. Insignificant quantities of drug are also excreted in feces. Biologic half-life of prednisone is 18 to 36 hours.

Route	Onset	Peak	Duration
P.O.	Variable	1-2 hr	Variable

Contraindications and precautions

Contraindicated in patients with hypersensitivity to drug or systemic fungal infections.

Use cautiously in patients with GI ulcer, renal disease, hypertension, osteoporosis, diabetes mellitus, hypothyroidism, cirrhosis, diverticulitis, nonspecific ulcerative colitis, recent intestinal anastamoses, thromboembolic disorders, seizures, myasthenia gravis, heart failure, tuberculosis, ocular herpes simplex, emotional instability, and psychotic tendencies.

Interactions

Drug-drug. *Amphotericin B or diuretic therapy:* Prednisone may enhance hypokalemia. Monitor serum potassium levels.
Antacids, cholestyramine, colestipol: Decrease the amount of prednisone absorbed. Monitor patient closely.
Barbiturates, phenytoin, rifampin: May cause decreased effects because of increased hepatic metabolism. Monitor patient closely.
Cardiac glycosides: Increase the risk of toxicity in patients concurrently receiving cardiac glycosides. Monitor patient closely.
Estrogens: May reduce the metabolism of prednisone by increasing the level of transcortin. Monitor patient closely.
Insulin or oral antidiabetic agents: Hyperglycemia; requiring dosage adjustment.
Isoniazid and salicylates: Prednisone increases the metabolism of isoniazid and salicylates. Monitor patient for lack of effect.
NSAIDs: May increase the risk of GI ulceration. Give together cautiously.
Oral anticoagulants: Use of prednisone may decrease effects. Monitor PT and INR closely.

Effects on diagnostic tests

Prednisone suppresses reactions to skin tests and causes false-negative results in the nitroblue tetrazolium test for systemic bacterial infections.

Adverse reactions

Most adverse reactions to corticosteroids are dose- or duration-dependent.
CNS: *euphoria, insomnia,* psychotic behavior, pseudotumor cerebri, vertigo, headache, paresthesia, ***seizures.***
CV: hypertension, edema, ***arrhythmias,*** thrombophlebitis, ***thromboembolism, heart failure.***
EENT: cataracts, glaucoma.
Endocrine: menstrual irregularities, cushingoid state (moonface, buffalo hump, central obesity).
GI: *peptic ulceration,* GI irritation, increased appetite, pancreatitis, nausea, vomiting.
Musculoskeletal: muscle weakness, osteoporosis.
Skin: delayed wound healing, acne, various skin eruptions.

Other: altered thyroid tests, increased urine glucose and calcium levels and serum cholesterol; decreased serum calcium levels; hirsutism, susceptibility to infections; hypokalemia, hyperglycemia, and carbohydrate intolerance; growth suppression in children; ***acute adrenal insufficiency may occur with increased stress (infection, surgery, or trauma) or abrupt withdrawal after long-term therapy.***
After abrupt withdrawal: rebound inflammation, fatigue, weakness, arthralgia, fever, dizziness, lethargy, depression, fainting, orthostatic hypotension, dyspnea, anorexia, hypoglycemia. ***After prolonged use, sudden withdrawal may be fatal.***

Overdose and treatment
Acute ingestion, even in massive doses, is rarely a clinical problem. Toxic signs and symptoms rarely occur if drug is used for less than 3 weeks, even at large dosage ranges. However, chronic use causes adverse physiologic effects, including suppression of the hypothalamic-pituitary-adrenal axis, cushingoid appearance, muscle weakness, and osteoporosis.

Clinical considerations
- Recommendations for use of prednisone and for care and teaching of patients are the same as those for all systemic adrenocorticoids.
- Determine whether patient is sensitive to other corticosteroid medication.
- For better results and less toxicity, give a once-daily dose in the morning.

Therapeutic monitoring
- Advise monitoring patient's blood pressure, sleep patterns, and serum potassium levels.
- Advise weighing patient daily.
- Watch for depression or psychotic episodes, especially in high-dose therapy.

Special populations
Pediatric patients. Chronic use of prednisone in drug or adolescents may delay growth and maturation.
Geriatric patients: Geriatric patients may be more susceptible to osteoporosis with long-term therapy.

Patient counseling
- Tell patient not to discontinue drug abruptly or without doctor's consent.
- Instruct patient to take drug with food or milk.
- Instruct patient to carry a card identifying his need for supplemental systemic glucocorticosteroids during stress.

primaquine phosphate

Pharmacologic classification: 8-aminoquinoline
Therapeutic classification: antimalarial
Pregnancy risk category C

How supplied
Available by prescription only
Tablets: 26.3 mg (15-mg base)

Indications and dosages
Radical cure of relapsing vivax malaria, eliminating symptoms and infection completely, and prevention of relapse
Adults: 15 mg (base) P.O. daily for 14 days (26.3-mg tablet equals 15 mg of base), or 79 mg (45-mg base) once weekly for 8 weeks.
Children: 0.3 mg (base)/kg/day for 14 days, or 0.9 mg (base)/kg/day once weekly for 8 weeks.
◇ **Pneumocystis carinii** ***pneumonia***
Adults: 15 to 30 mg (base) P.O. daily.

Pharmacodynamics
Antimalarial action: Primaquine disrupts the parasitic mitochondria, thereby interrupting metabolic processes requiring energy.

Spectrum of activity includes preerythrocytic and exoerythrocytic forms of *Plasmodium falciparum, P. malariae, P. ovale,* and *P. vivax.* Nifurtimox (Lampit), an investigational agent available from the Centers for Disease Control and Prevention, is preferred for intracellular parasites.

Pharmacokinetics
Absorption: Well absorbed from the GI tract.
Distribution: Distributed widely into the liver, lungs, heart, brain, skeletal muscle, and other tissues.
Metabolism: Carboxylated rapidly in the liver.
Excretion: Only a small amount is excreted unchanged in urine. Plasma half-life is 4 to 10 hours.

Route	Onset	Peak	Duration
P.O.	Unknown	1-3 hr	Unknown

Contraindications and precautions
Contraindicated in patients with systemic diseases in which granulocytopenia may develop (such as lupus erythematosus or rheumatoid arthritis) and in those taking bone marrow suppressants and potentially hemolytic drugs.

Use cautiously in patients with previous idiosyncratic reaction (manifested by hemolytic anemia, methemoglobinemia, or leukopenia) and in those with family or personal history of favism, erythrocytic G6PD deficiency, or nicotinamide adenine dinucleotide (NADH) methemoglobin reductase deficiency.

Interactions

Drug-drug. *Magnesium and aluminum salts:* May decrease GI absorption. Administer drugs at separate times.
Quinacrine: May potentiate the toxic effects of primaquine. Don't use together.

Effects on diagnostic tests

None reported.

Adverse reactions

GI: nausea, vomiting, epigastric distress, abdominal cramps.
Hematologic: leukopenia, ***hemolytic anemia in G6PD deficiency,*** methemoglobinemia in NADH methemoglobin reductase deficiency.

Overdose and treatment

Signs and symptoms of overdose include abdominal distress, vomiting, CNS and CV disturbances, cyanosis, methemoglobinemia, leukocytosis, leukopenia, and anemia. Treatment is symptomatic.

Clinical considerations

□ ***ALERT*** Drug dosage may be discussed in mg or mg-base. Be aware of the difference.
- Primaquine is often used with a fast-acting antimalarial, such as chloroquine.
- Before starting therapy, screen patients for possible G6PD deficiency.
- Light-skinned patients taking more than 30 mg daily, dark-skinned patients taking more than 15 mg daily, and patients with severe anemia or suspected sensitivity should have frequent blood studies and urine examinations. A sudden decrease in hemoglobin levels or erythrocyte or leukocyte counts, or a marked darkening of the urine suggests impending hemolytic reaction.

Therapeutic monitoring

Perform periodic blood studies and urinalyses to monitor for impending hemolytic reactions.

Special populations

Pregnant patients. Safety for use during pregnancy hasn't been established.
Breast-feeding patients. Safety in breast-feeding women hasn't been established.

Patient counseling

- Teach patient signs and symptoms of adverse reactions and to report them if they occur.
- Advise patient to check urine color at each voiding and to report if urine darkens, becomes tinged with red, or decreases in volume.
- Tell patient to take drug with meals to minimize gastric irritation and not to take with antacids, which may decrease absorption.
- Advise patient to complete entire course of therapy.

primidone

Myidone, Mysoline, Sertan

Pharmacologic classification: barbiturate analogue
Therapeutic classification: anticonvulsant
Pregnancy risk category NR

How supplied

Available by prescription only
Tablets: 50 mg, 250 mg
Suspension: 250 mg/5 ml

Indications and dosages

Generalized tonic-clonic seizures, focal seizures, complex-partial (psychomotor) seizures
Adults and children age 8 and older: 100 to 125 mg P.O. h.s. on days 1 to 3; 100 to 125 mg P.O. b.i.d. on days 4 to 6; 100 to 125 mg P.O. t.i.d. on days 7 to 9; and maintenance dosage of 250 mg P.O. t.i.d. on day 10. May require up to 2 g/day.
Children under age 8: 50 mg P.O. h.s. on days 1 to 3; 50 mg P.O. b.i.d. on days 4 to 6; 100 mg P.O. t.i.d. on days 7 to 9; and maintenance dosage of 125 to 250 mg P.O. t.i.d. on day 10.
Benign familial tremor (essential tremor)
Adults: 750 mg P.O. daily.

Pharmacodynamics

Anticonvulsant action: Primidone acts as a nonspecific CNS depressant used alone or with other anticonvulsants to control refractory tonic-clonic seizures and to treat psychomotor or focal seizures. Mechanism of action is unknown; some activity may be from phenobarbital, an active metabolite.

Pharmacokinetics

Absorption: Absorbed readily from the GI tract. Phenobarbital appears in plasma after several days of continuous therapy; most laboratory assays detect both phenobarbital and primidone. Therapeutic levels are 5 to 12 mcg/ml for primidone and 10 to 30 mcg/ml for phenobarbital.
Distribution: Distributed widely throughout the body.
Metabolism: Metabolized slowly by the liver to phenylethylmalonamide (PEMA) and phenobarbital; PEMA is the major metabolite.
Excretion: Excreted in urine; substantial amounts are excreted in breast milk.

Route	Onset	Peak	Duration
P.O.	Unknown	3-4 hr	Unknown

Contraindications and precautions

Contraindicated in patients with phenobarbital hypersensitivity or porphyria.

Interactions

Drug-drug. *Acetazolamide and succinimides:* Coadministration may decrease levels of primidone. Monitor levels.
Carbamazepine, phenytoin: May decrease effects of primidone and increase its conversion to phenobarbital. Monitor serum levels to prevent toxicity.
CNS depressants: Cause excessive depression in patients taking primidone. Don't use together.
Drug-lifestyle. *Alcohol use:* Causes excessive depression in patients taking primidone. Advise patient to avoid alcohol use.

Effects on diagnostic tests

None reported.

Adverse reactions

CNS: *drowsiness, ataxia,* emotional disturbances, vertigo, hyperirritability, fatigue, paranoia.
EENT: *diplopia,* nystagmus.
GI: anorexia, nausea, vomiting, abnormalities in liver function test results.
GU: impotence, polyuria.
Hematologic: megaloblastic anemia, ***thrombocytopenia.***
Skin: morbilliform rash.

Overdose and treatment

Signs and symptoms of overdose resemble those of barbiturate intoxication; they include CNS and respiratory depression, areflexia, oliguria, tachycardia, hypotension, hypothermia, and coma. Shock may occur.

Treat overdose supportively: In conscious patient with intact gag reflex, induce emesis with ipecac; follow in 30 minutes with repeated doses of activated charcoal. Use lavage if emesis isn't feasible. Alkalinization of urine and forced diuresis may hasten excretion. Hemodialysis may be necessary. Monitor vital signs and fluid and electrolyte balance.

Clinical considerations

Consider the recommendations relevant to all barbiturates as well as the following:

- Abrupt withdrawal of drug may cause status epilepticus; reduce dosage gradually.
- Barbiturates impair ability to perform tasks requiring mental alertness such as driving a car.

Therapeutic monitoring

Recommend performing a CBC and liver function tests every 6 months.

Special populations

Breast-feeding patients. Considerable amounts of drug are excreted in breast milk; use an alternative feeding method during therapy.
Pediatric patients. Primidone may cause hyperexcitability in children under age 6.
Geriatric patients. Reduce dose in geriatric patients; many have decreased renal function.

Patient counseling

- Explain rationale for therapy and the potential risks and benefits.
- Teach patient signs and symptoms of adverse reactions.
- Instruct patient not to discontinue drug or to alter dosage without medical approval.
- Explain that barbiturates may render oral contraceptives ineffective; advise patient to consider a different birth control method.
- Advise patient to avoid hazardous tasks that require mental alertness until degree of sedative effect is determined. Tell the patient that dizziness and incoordination are common at first but will disappear.
- Recommend that patient wear a medical identification bracelet or necklace identifying him as having a seizure disorder and listing drug.
- Tell patient to shake oral suspension well before use.

probenecid

Benemid, Probalan

Pharmacologic classification: sulfonamide-derivative
Therapeutic classification: uricosuric
Pregnancy risk category NR

How supplied

Available by prescription only
Tablets: 500 mg
Tablets (film-coated): 500 mg

Indications and dosages

Adjunct to penicillin therapy
Adults and children over age 14 or weighing more than 110 lb (50 kg): 500 mg P.O. q.i.d.
Children age 2 to 14 or weighing less than 110 lb: Initially, 25 mg/kg or 700 mg/m^2 daily, then 40 mg/kg or 1.2 g/m^2 divided q.i.d.
Single-dose penicillin treatment of gonorrhea
Adults: 1 g P.O. given together with penicillin treatment, or 1 g P.O. 30 minutes before I.M. dose of penicillin.
Hyperuricemia associated with gout
Adults: 250 mg P.O. b.i.d. for first week, then 500 mg b.i.d., to maximum of 2 to 3 g daily.
◇ ***To diagnose parkinsonian syndrome or mental depression***
Adults: 500 mg P.O. q 12 hours for five doses.

Pharmacodynamics

Uricosuric action: Probenecid competitively inhibits the active reabsorption of uric acid at the proximal convoluted tubule, increasing urinary excretion of uric acid.
Adjunctive action in antibiotic therapy: Probenecid competitively inhibits secretion of weak organic acids, including penicillins, cephalosporins, and other beta-lactam antibiotics, increasing serum levels of these drugs.

Pharmacokinetics

Absorption: Completely absorbed after oral administration.
Distribution: Distributed throughout the body; drug is about 75% protein-bound. CSF levels are about 2% of serum levels.
Metabolism: Metabolized in the liver to active metabolites, with some uricosuric effect.
Excretion: Drug and metabolites are excreted in urine; probenecid (but not metabolites) is actively reabsorbed.

Route	Onset	Peak	Duration
P.O.	Unknown	2-4 hr	Unknown

Contraindications and precautions

Contraindicated in patients with hypersensitivity to drug, uric acid kidney stones, or blood dyscrasias; in acute gout attack; and in children under age 2. Use cautiously in patients with impaired renal function or peptic ulcer.

Interactions

Drug-drug. *Aminosalicylic acid, dapsone, methotrexate, nitrofurantoin:* Increased serum levels, which increase risk of toxicity. Altered doses may be needed.
Cephalosporins, penicillins, and other beta-lactam antibiotics, sulfonamides, and possibly ketamine and thiopental: Probenecid significantly increases or prolongs effects of these drugs. Use together cautiously.
Chlorpropamide and other oral sulfonylureas: Enhanced hypoglycemic effects. Monitor blood glucose levels.
Diuretics and pyrazinamide: Decrease uric acid levels of probenecid; increased doses of probenecid may be required.
Indomethacin, naproxen: Decreased excretion of these drugs. Use of lower doses may be possible.
Salicylates: Inhibit the uricosuric effect of probenecid only in doses that achieve levels of 50 mcg/ml or more. Don't use together.
Zidovudine: Cutaneous eruptions accompanied by systemic symptoms, including malaise, myalgia, or fever. Monitor patient.
Drug-lifestyle. *Alcohol use:* Decreases uric acid levels of probenecid; increased doses of probenecid may be required.

Effects on diagnostic tests

Probenecid causes false-positive test results for urinary glucose with tests using cupric sulfate reagent (Benedict's reagent, Clinitest, and Fehling's test); perform tests with glucose oxidase reagent (Diastix, Chemstrip uG, or glucose enzymatic test strip) instead.

Adverse reactions

CNS: *headache,* dizziness.
GI: anorexia, nausea, vomiting, sore gums, ***hepatic necrosis.***
GU: urinary frequency, renal colic, nephrotic syndrome.
Hematologic: ***hemolytic anemia, aplastic anemia,*** anemia.
Skin: dermatitis, pruritus.
Other: flushing, fever, exacerbation of gout, hypersensitivity reactions (including ***anaphylaxis).***

Overdose and treatment

Signs and symptoms include nausea, copious vomiting, stupor, coma, and tonic-clonic seizures. Treat supportively, using mechanical ventilation, if needed; induce emesis or use gastric lavage, as appropriate. Control seizures with I.V. phenobarbital and phenytoin.

Clinical considerations

- When used for hyperuricemia associated with gout, probenecid has no analgesic or anti-inflammatory actions, and no effect on acute attacks; start therapy after attack subsides. Because drug may increase the frequency of acute attacks during the first 6 to 12 months of therapy, prophylactic doses of colchicine or an NSAID should be administered during the first 3 to 6 months of probenecid therapy.
- Give with food, milk, or prescribed antacids to lessen GI upset.
- Maintain adequate hydration with high fluid intake to prevent formation of uric acid stones. Also maintain alkalinization of urine.
- Drug has been used in the diagnosis of parkinsonian syndrome and mental depression.

Therapeutic monitoring

- Monitor BUN and serum creatinine levels closely; drug is ineffective in severe renal insufficiency.
- Monitor uric acid levels and adjust dose to the lowest dose that maintains normal uric acid levels.

Special populations

Breast-feeding patients. It's unknown if drug is excreted in breast milk. An alternative feeding method is recommended during therapy.
Pediatric patients. Drug is contraindicated in infants under age 2.
Geriatric patients. Lower doses are indicated in geriatric patients.

Patient counseling

- Instruct patient not to discontinue drug without medical approval.
- Warn patient not to use drug for pain or inflammation and not to increase dose during gouty attack.
- Tell patient to drink 8 to 10 glasses of fluid daily and to take drug with food to minimize GI upset.

procainamide hydrochloride

Procanbid, Promine, Pronestyl, Pronestyl-SR

Pharmacologic classification: procaine derivative
Therapeutic classification: ventricular antiarrhythmic, supraventricular antiarrhythmic
Pregnancy risk category C

How supplied

Available by prescription only
Tablets (film-coated): 250 mg, 375 mg, 500 mg
Tablets (extended-release, film-coated): 250 mg, 500 mg, 750 mg, 1 g
Capsules: 250 mg, 375 mg, 500 mg
Injection: 100 mg/ml, 500 mg/ml

Indications and dosages

Symptomatic PVCs; life-threatening ventricular tachycardia; ◇atrial fibrillation and flutter unresponsive to quinidine; ◇paroxysmal atrial tachycardia
Adults: 50 to 100 mg q 5 minutes by slow I.V. push, no faster than 25 to 50 mg/minute, until arrhythmias disappear, adverse effects develop, or 500 mg has been given. When arrhythmias disappear, give continuous infusion of 1 to 6 mg/minute. Usual effective loading dose is 500 to 600 mg. If arrhythmias recur, repeat bolus as above and increase infusion rate. For I.M. administration, give 50 mg/kg divided q 3 to 6 hours; during surgery, 100 to 500 mg I.M. For oral therapy, initiate dosage at 50 mg/kg P.O. in divided doses q 3 hours until therapeutic levels are reached. Once patient is stable, may substitute sustained-release form q 6 hours or extended-release form at dose of 50 mg/kg in two divided doses q 12 hours.
◇Loading dose to prevent atrial fibrillation or paroxysmal atrial tachycardia
Adults: 1 to 1.25 g P.O. If arrhythmias persist after 1 hour, give additional 750 mg. If no change occurs, give 500 mg to 1 g q 2 hours until arrhythmias disappear or adverse effects occur.
Loading dose to prevent ventricular tachycardia
Adults: 1 g P.O. Maintenance dosage is 50 mg/kg/day given at 3-hour intervals; average is 250 to 500 mg q 4 hours but may require 1 to 1.5 g q 4 to 6 hours.
◇Treatment of malignant hyperthermia
Adults: 200 to 900 mg I.V., followed by an infusion.

Pharmacodynamics

Antiarrhythmic action: A class IA antiarrhythmic agent, procainamide depresses phase 0 of the action potential. It's considered a myocardial depressant because it decreases myocardial excitability and conduction velocity and may depress myocardial contractility. It also possesses anticholinergic activity, which may modify its direct myocardial effects. In therapeutic doses, it reduces conduction velocity in the atria, ventricles, and His-Purkinje system. Its effectiveness in controlling atrial tachyarrhythmias stems from its ability to prolong the effective refractory period (ERP) and increase the action potential duration in the atria, ventricles, and His-Purkinje system. Because ERP prolongation exceeds action potential duration, tissue remains refractory even after returning to resting membrane potential (membrane-stabilizing effect).

Procainamide shortens the effective refractory period of the AV node. Anticholinergic action of drug also may increase AV node conductivity. Suppression of automaticity in the His-Purkinje system and ectopic pacemakers accounts for effectiveness of drug in treating ventricular premature beats. At therapeutic doses, procainamide prolongs the PR and QT intervals. (This effect may be used as an index of drug effectiveness and toxicity.) The QRS interval usually isn't prolonged beyond normal range; the QT interval isn't prolonged to the extent achieved with quinidine.

Procainamide exerts a peripheral vasodilatory effect; with I.V. administration, it may cause hypotension, which limits the administration rate and amount of drug deliverable.

Pharmacokinetics

Absorption: Rate and extent of absorption from the intestines vary; usually, 75% to 95% of an orally administered dose is absorbed. Extended-release tablets are formulated to provide a sustained and relatively constant rate of release and absorption throughout the small intestine. After release of drug, extended wax matrix isn't absorbed and may appear in feces after 15 minutes to 1 hour.
Distribution: Distributed widely in most body tissues, including CSF, liver, spleen, kidneys, lungs, muscles, brain, and heart. Only about 15% binds to plasma proteins. Usual therapeutic range for serum procainamide levels is 4 to 8 mcg/ml. Some experts suggest that a range of 10 to 30 mcg/ml for the sum of procainamide and N-acetyl procainamide (NAPA) serum levels are therapeutic.
Metabolism: Acetylated in the liver to form NAPA. Acetylation rate is determined genetically and affects NAPA formation. NAPA also exerts antiarrhythmic activity.
Excretion: Procainamide and NAPA metabolite are excreted in the urine. Half-life of procainamide is about 2½ to 4¾ hours. Half-life of NAPA is about 6 hours. In patients with heart failure or renal dysfunction, half-life increases; therefore, in such patients, dosage reduction is required to avoid toxicity.

Route	Onset	Peak	Duration
P.O.	1-2 hr	½-1½ hr	Unknown
I.V.	Immediate	Immediate	Unknown
I.M.	10-30 min	15-60 min	Unknown

Contraindications and precautions

Contraindicated in patients with hypersensitivity to procaine and related drugs; in those with complete, second-, or third-degree heart block in the absence of an artificial pacemaker; and in patients with myasthenia gravis or systemic lupus erythematosus. Also contraindicated in patients with atypical ventricular tachycardia (torsades de pointes) because procainamide may aggravate this condition.

Use cautiously in patients with ventricular tachycardia during coronary occlusion; heart failure or other conduction disturbances, such as bundle-branch heart block, sinus bradycardia, and cardiac glycoside intoxication; impaired renal or hepatic function; preexisting blood dyscrasia; or bone marrow suppression.

Interactions

Drug-drug. *Anticholinergic agents, such as atropine, diphenhydramine, and tricyclic antidepressants:* May cause additive anticholinergic effects. Monitor patient closely.
Antihypertensives: May cause additive hypotensive effects (most common with I.V. procainamide). Monitor blood pressure closely.
Cholinergic agents, such as neostigmine and pyridostigmine: May negate the effects of these agents, requiring increased dosage.
Cimetidine: May result in impaired renal clearance of procainamide and NAPA, with elevated serum drug levels. Monitor patient for toxicity.
Neuromuscular blocking agents, such as decamethonium bromide, gallium triethiodide, metocurine iodide, pancuronium bromide, succinylcholine chloride, and tubocurarine chloride: May potentiate the effects of the neuromuscular blocking agents. Monitor patient closely.
Other antiarrhythmics: May result in additive or antagonistic cardiac effects and with possible additive toxic effects. Use cautiously.
Drug-herb. *Jimsonweed:* May adversely affect the function of the cardiovascular system. Avoid use together.
Licorice: May prolong the QT interval and be potentially additive. Use together cautiously.
Drug-lifestyle. *Alcohol use:* Reduced drug levels. Advise patient to avoid use.

Effects on diagnostic tests

Procainamide invalidates bentiromide test results; discontinue at least 3 days before bentiromide test. Procainamide may alter edrophonium test results.

Adverse reactions

CNS: hallucinations, confusion, ***seizures,*** depression, dizziness.
CV: *hypotension,* ***ventricular asystole,*** *bradycardia,* AV block, ***ventricular fibrillation*** (after parenteral use).
GI: nausea, vomiting, anorexia, diarrhea, bitter taste.
Hematologic: ***thrombocytopenia, neutropenia*** (especially with sustained-release forms), ***agranulocytosis, hemolytic anemia.***
Hepatic: increased liver function test.
Skin: *maculopapular rash, urticaria, pruritus, flushing, angioneurotic edema.*
Other: *fever, lupuslike syndrome* (especially after prolonged administration) positive antinuclear antibody (ANA) titers, positive direct antiglobulin (Coombs') tests.

Overdose and treatment

Effects of overdose include severe hypotension, widening QRS complex, junctional tachycardia, intraventricular conduction delay, ventricular fibrillation, oliguria, confusion and lethargy, and nausea and vomiting.

Treatment involves general supportive measures, including respiratory and CV support, with hemodynamic and ECG monitoring. After recent ingestion of oral form, gastric lavage, emesis, and activated charcoal may be used to decrease absorption. Phenylephrine or norepinephrine may be used to treat hypotension after adequate hydration has been ensured. Hemodialysis may be effective in removing procainamide and NAPA. A 1/6 M solution of sodium lactate may reduce cardiotoxic effect of procainamide.

Clinical considerations

- In treating atrial fibrillation and flutter, ventricular rate may accelerate due to vagolytic effects on the AV node; to prevent this effect, a cardiac glycoside may be administered before procainamide therapy begins.
- Monitor patient receiving infusions at all times.
- Use infusion pump or microdrip system and timer to monitor infusion precisely.
- Baseline and periodic determinations of ANA titers, lupus erythematosus cell preparations, and CBCs may be indicated because procainamide therapy (usually long-term) has been associated with syndrome resembling systemic lupus erythematosus.
- For initial oral therapy, use conventional capsules and tablets; use extended-release tablets only for maintenance therapy.
- I.V. drug form is more likely to cause adverse cardiac effects, possibly resulting in severe hypotension.
- In prolonged use of oral form, perform ECGs occasionally to determine continued need for drug.

Therapeutic monitoring

- Monitor blood pressure and ECG continuously during I.V. administration. Watch for prolonged QT and QRS intervals (50% or greater widening), heart block, or increased arrhythmias. When these ECG signs appear, procainamide should be discontinued and the patient monitored closely.
- Monitor therapeutic serum levels of procainamide: 3 to 10 mcg/ml (most patients are controlled at 4 to 8 mcg/ml); may exhibit toxicity at levels greater than 16 mcg/ml). Monitor NAPA levels as well; some clinicians believe that procainamide and NAPA levels should be 10 to 30 mcg/ml.

Special populations

Breast-feeding patients. Because procainamide and NAPA are distributed into breast milk, an alternative feeding method is recommended for women receiving procainamide.
Pediatric patients. Manufacturer hasn't established dosage guidelines for pediatric patients because safety in children hasn't been established. For treating arrhythmias, the suggested dosage is 40 to 60 mg/kg of standard tablets or capsules, P.O. daily, given in four to six divided doses; or 3 to 6 mg/kg I.V. over 5 minutes, followed by a drip of 0.02 to 0.08 mg/kg/minute.
Geriatric patients. Geriatric patients may require reduced dosage. Because of highly variable metabolism, monitoring of serum levels is recommended.

Patient counseling

- Stress importance of taking drug exactly as prescribed.
- Instruct patient to report fever, rash, muscle pain, diarrhea, bruises, or pleuritic chest pain.

procarbazine hydrochloride

Matulane, Natulan*

Pharmacologic classification: antibiotic antineoplastic (cell cycle-phase specific, S phase)
Therapeutic classification: antineoplastic
Pregnancy risk category D

How supplied

Available by prescription only
Capsules: 50 mg

Indications and dosages

Dosage and indications may vary. Check current literature for recommended protocol.
Hodgkin's disease, lymphomas, brain and lung cancer
Adults: 2 to 4 mg/kg/day P.O. in single or divided doses for the first week, followed by 4 to 6 mg/kg/day until response or toxicity occurs. Maintenance dosage is 1 to 2 mg/kg/day.
Children: 50 mg/m^2 daily P.O. for first week, then 100 mg/m^2 daily until response or toxicity occurs. Maintenance dosage is 50 mg/m^2 P.O. daily after bone marrow recovery.

Pharmacodynamics

Antineoplastic action: Exact mechanism of cytotoxic activity of procarbazine is unknown. Drug appears to have several sites of action; the result is inhibition of DNA, RNA, and protein synthesis. Procarbazine has also been reported to damage DNA directly and to inhibit the mitotic S phase of cell division.

Pharmacokinetics

Absorption: Rapidly and completely absorbed following oral administration.
Distribution: Distributed widely into body tissues, with the highest levels found in the liver, kidneys, intestinal wall, and skin. Drug crosses the blood-brain barrier.
Metabolism: Extensively metabolized in the liver. Some metabolites have cytotoxic activity.
Excretion: Excreted primarily in urine.

Route	Onset	Peak	Duration
P.O.	Unknown	Unknown	Unknown

Contraindications and precautions

Contraindicated in patients hypersensitive to drug and in those with inadequate bone marrow reserve as shown by bone marrow aspiration. Use cautiously in patients with impaired renal or hepatic function.

Interactions

Drug-drug. *CNS depressants:* Enhanced CNS depression through an additive mechanism. Avoid use together.
Digoxin: Serum digoxin levels may be decreased. Monitor patient closely.
Levodopa: May cause flushing and a significant increase in blood pressure. Monitor patient closely.
MAO inhibitors, selective serotonin reuptake inhibitors, sympathomimetics, or tricyclic antidepressants: Can cause a hypertensive crisis, tremors, excitation, and cardiac palpitations. Monitor patient closely.
Meperidine: May result in severe hypotension and death. Avoid use together.
Drug-food. *Tyramine-containing foods:* Can cause a hypertensive crisis, tremors, excitation, and cardiac palpitations. Don't give together.
Drug-lifestyle. *Alcohol use:* Can cause a disulfiram-like reaction. Advise patient to avoid alcohol use.
Sun exposure: May cause photosensitivity reactions. Advise patient to take precautions.

Effects on diagnostic tests

None reported.

Adverse reactions

CNS: nervousness, depression, headache, dizziness, ***coma, seizures,*** insomnia, nightmares, paresthesia, neuropathy, *hallucinations,* confusion.
CV: hypotension, tachycardia, syncope.
EENT: retinal hemorrhage, nystagmus, photophobia.
GI: *nausea, vomiting,* anorexia, stomatitis, dry mouth, dysphagia, diarrhea, constipation.
GU: hematuria, urinary frequency, nocturia.
Hematologic: ***bleeding tendency, thrombocytopenia, leukopenia, anemia,*** hemolytic anemia.
Respiratory: ***pleural effusion,*** pneumonitis, cough.
Skin: dermatitis, pruritus, rash.
Other: reversible alopecia, allergic reactions, gynecomastia.

Overdose and treatment

Signs and symptoms of overdose include myalgia, arthralgia, fever, weakness, dermatitis, alopecia, paresthesia, hallucinations, tremors, seizures, coma, myelosuppression, nausea, and vomiting.

Treatment is usually supportive and includes transfusion of blood components, antiemetics, antipyretics, and appropriate antianxiety agents.

Clinical considerations

- Nausea and vomiting may be decreased if drug is taken at bedtime and in divided doses.
- Use cautiously in inadequate bone marrow reserve, leukopenia, thrombocytopenia, anemia, and impaired hepatic or renal function.
- Store capsules in dry environment.

Therapeutic monitoring

- Observe for signs of bleeding.
- Monitor CBC and platelet counts.

Special populations

Pregnant patients. Drug causes fetal toxicity and teratogenicity in laboratory studies. Advise patient not to become pregnant while on drug therapy and to consult doctor before becoming pregnant.
Breast-feeding patients. It isn't known if drug is distributed in breast milk. However, because of potential for serious adverse reactions, mutagenicity, and carcinogenicity in the infant, breast-feeding isn't recommended.
Pediatric patients. Severe reactions, such as tremors, seizures, and coma, have occurred in children after administration of procarbazine.

Patient counseling

- Emphasize importance of continuing medication despite nausea and vomiting.
- Advise patient to immediately report if vomiting occurs shortly after taking dose.
- Warn patient that drowsiness may occur, so patient should avoid hazardous activities that require alertness until effect of drug is established.
- Instruct patient to stop medication and immediately report disulfiram-like reactions, such as chest pains, rapid or irregular heartbeat, severe headache, or stiff neck, that may occur.
- Tell patient to avoid exposure to people with infections.
- Tell patient to contact health care provider if a sore throat or fever or unusual bruising or bleeding occurs.

prochlorperazine
Compazine, Stemetil*

prochlorperazine edisylate
Compazine

prochlorperazine maleate
Compazine, Compazine Spansule, Stemetil*

Pharmacologic classification: phenothiazine (piperazine derivative)
Therapeutic classification: antipsychotic, antiemetic, antianxiety
Pregnancy risk category C

How supplied

Available by prescription only
prochlorperazine edisylate
Spansules (sustained-release): 10 mg, 15 mg
Syrup: 5 mg/ml
Injection: 10 mg/2 ml
prochlorperazine maleate
Tablets: 5 mg, 10 mg
Suppositories: 2.5 mg, 5 mg, 25 mg

Indications and dosages

Preoperative nausea control
Adults: 5 to 10 mg I.M. 1 to 2 hours before induction of anesthesia, repeated once in 30 minutes, if necessary; or 5 to 10 mg I.V. 15 to 30 minutes before induction of anesthesia, repeated once, if necessary; or 20 mg/L D_5W and normal saline solution by I.V. infusion, added to infusion 15 to 30 minutes before induction. Maximum parenteral dose is 40 mg daily.
Severe nausea, vomiting
Adults: 5 to 10 mg P.O. t.i.d. or q.i.d.; or 15 mg of sustained-release form P.O. on arising; or 10 mg of sustained-release form P.O. q 12 hours; or 25 mg P.R. b.i.d.; or 5 to 10 mg I.M. injected deeply into upper outer quadrant of gluteal region. Repeat q 3 to 4 hours, p.r.n. May be given I.V. Maximum parenteral dose, 40 mg daily.
Children weighing 39 to 86 lb (18 to 39 kg): 2.5 mg P.O. or rectally t.i.d.; or 5 mg P.O. or P.R. b.i.d.; or 0.132 mg/kg deep I.M. injection (control usually obtained with one dose). Maximum dose is 15 mg daily.

Children weighing 31 to 38 lb (14 to 17 kg): 2.5 mg P.O. or P.R. b.i.d. or t.i.d.; or 0.132 mg/kg deep I.M. injection (control usually is obtained with one dose). Maximum dose, 10 mg daily.
Children weighing 20 to 30 lb (9 to 14 kg): 2.5 mg P.O. or P.R. daily or b.i.d.; or 0.132 mg/kg deep I.M. injection (control usually is obtained with one dose). Maximum dose, 7.5 mg daily.
Anxiety
Adults: 5 mg P.O. t.i.d. or q.i.d.
Psychotic disorders
Adults: 5 to 10 mg P.O. or 10 to 20 mg I.M. t.i.d. or q.i.d.; up to 150 mg daily P.O. for hospitalized patients.

Pharmacodynamics

Antipsychotic action: Prochlorperazine is thought to exert its antipsychotic effects by postsynaptic blockade of CNS dopamine receptors, inhibiting dopamine-mediated effects.
Antiemetic action: Antiemetic effects are attributed to dopamine receptor blockade in the medullary chemoreceptor trigger zone.

Prochlorperazine has many other central and peripheral effects: It produces alpha and ganglionic blockade and counteracts histamine- and serotonin-mediated activity. Its most prevalent adverse reactions are extrapyramidal. It's used primarily as an antiemetic, and is ineffective against motion sickness.

Pharmacokinetics

Absorption: Rate and extent of absorption vary with administration route.
Distribution: Distributed widely into the body, including breast milk. Drug is 91% to 99% protein-bound. Peak effect occurs at 2 to 4 hours; steady-state serum levels are achieved within 4 to 7 days.
Metabolism: Metabolized extensively by the liver, but no active metabolites are formed; duration of action is about 3 to 4 hours and 10 to 12 hours for the extended-release form.
Excretion: Mostly excreted in urine via the kidneys; some is excreted in feces via the biliary tract.

Route	Onset	Peak	Duration
P.O.	30-40 min	Unknown	3-12 hr
I.V.	Unknown	Unknown	Unknown
I.M.	10-20 min	Unknown	3-4 hr
P.R.	1 hr	Unknown	3-4 hr

Contraindications and precautions

Contraindicated in patients hypersensitive to phenothiazines and in those with CNS depression including coma; during pediatric surgery; when using spinal or epidural anesthetic, adrenergic blockers, or ethanol; and in infants under age 2.

Use cautiously in patients with impaired CV function, glaucoma, or seizure disorders; in those who have been exposed to extreme heat; and in children with acute illness.

Interactions

Drug-drug. *Aluminum- and magnesium-containing antacids and antidiarrheals:* Decreased absorption. Don't administer together.
Anesthetics (general, spinal, epidural), CNS depressants, parenteral magnesium sulfate: Additive effects are likely. Avoid use together.
Antiarrhythmic agents, disopyramide, procainamide, quinidine: Increased incidence of arrhythmias and conduction defects. Monitor patient closely.
Appetite suppressants; sympathomimetics, such as ephedrine, epinephrine, phenylephrine, and phenylpropanolamine: May decrease their stimulatory and pressor effects and may cause epinephrine reversal (hypotensive response to epinephrine). Use cautiously.
Atropine, other anticholinergic drugs, antihistamines, antiparkinson agents, MAO inhibitors, meperidine, phenothiazines: Oversedation, paralytic ileus, visual changes, and severe constipation: Monitor patient closely.
Beta blockers: May inhibit prochlorperazine metabolism, increasing plasma levels and toxicity. Monitor for toxicity.
Bromocriptine: Prochlorperazine may antagonize therapeutic effect of bromocriptine on prolactin secretion. Monitor patient closely.
Clonidine, guanabenz, guanadrel, guanethidine, methyldopa, reserpine: Prochlorperazine may inhibit blood pressure response. Monitor patient closely.
High-dose dopamine: Decreases the vasoconstricting effects of dopamine. Monitor patient.
Levodopa: Decreases effectiveness and increases toxicity (by dopamine blockade). Monitor patient closely.
Lithium: May result in severe neurologic toxicity with an encephalitis-like syndrome and in decreased therapeutic response to prochlorperazine. Monitor patient closely.
Metrizamide: Increased risk of seizures. Patient requires careful observation.
Nitrates: Can cause hypotension. Monitor blood pressure.
Phenobarbital: Enhanced renal excretion. Monitor for lack of drug effect.
Phenytoin: Prochlorperazine may inhibit metabolism and increase toxicity of phenytoin. Monitor patient closely.
Propylthiouracil: Increases risk of agranulocytosis. Monitor CBC.
Drug-food. *Caffeine:* Increases prochlorperazine metabolism. Discourage use together.
Drug-lifestyle. *Alcohol use:* Additive effects are likely. Advise patient to avoid alcohol use.
Heavy smoking: Increases prochlorperazine metabolism. Advise patient to avoid smoking while on medication.
Sun exposure: May cause photosensitivity reactions. Advise patient to take precautions.

Effects on diagnostic tests

Prochlorperazine causes false-positive test results for urinary porphyrins, urobilinogen, amylase, and 5-hydroxyindoleacetic acid because of darkening of urine by metabolites; it also causes false-positive urine pregnancy results in tests using human chorionic gonadotropin as the indicator.

Adverse reactions

CNS: *extrapyramidal reactions,* sedation, pseudoparkinsonism, EEG changes, dizziness.
CV: *orthostatic hypotension,* tachycardia, ECG changes.
EENT: *ocular changes, blurred vision.*
GI: *dry mouth, constipation,* ileus.
GU: *urine retention,* dark urine, menstrual irregularities, inhibited ejaculation.
Hematologic: *transient leukopenia,* ***agranulocytosis, thrombocytopenia, hemolytic anemia.***
Hepatic: *cholestatic jaundice.*
Skin: mild photosensitivity, allergic reactions, ***exfoliative dermatitis.***
Other: hyperprolactinemia, gynecomastia, weight gain, increased appetite, hyperglycemia or hypoglycemia.

Overdose and treatment

CNS depression is characterized by deep, unarousable sleep and possible coma, hypotension or hypertension, extrapyramidal symptoms, dystonia, abnormal involuntary muscle movements, agitation, seizures, arrhythmias, ECG changes, hypothermia or hyperthermia, and autonomic nervous system dysfunction.

Treatment is symptomatic and supportive and includes maintaining vital signs, airway, stable body temperature, and fluid and electrolyte balance.

Don't induce vomiting: Drug inhibits cough reflex, and aspiration may occur. Use gastric lavage, then activated charcoal and saline cathartics; dialysis doesn't help. Regulate body temperature as needed. Treat hypotension with I.V. fluids: Don't give epinephrine. Treat seizures with parenteral diazepam or barbiturates; arrhythmias with parenteral phenytoin (1 mg/kg with rate titrated to blood pressure); and extrapyramidal reactions with benztropine or parenteral diphenhydramine 2 mg/kg/minute.

Clinical considerations

Consider the recommendations relevant to all phenothiazines as well as the following:

- Liquid and injectable formulations may cause a rash after contact with skin.
- Drug is associated with a high incidence of extrapyramidal effects.
- Dilute the concentrate in 60 to 120 ml (2 to 4 oz) of water. Store the suppository form in a cool place.
- Give I.V. dose slowly (5 mg/minute). I.M. injection may cause skin necrosis; take care to prevent extravasation. Don't mix with other medications in the syringe. Don't administer S.C.
- Administer I.M. injection deep into the upper outer quadrant of the buttock. Massaging the area after administration may prevent formation of abscesses.
- Solution for injection may be slightly discolored. Don't use if excessively discolored or if a precipitate is evident.
- Drug is ineffective in treating motion sickness.
- Protect the liquid formulation from light.

Therapeutic monitoring

- Monitor patient's blood pressure before and after parenteral administration.
- Advise patient that drug may cause a pink to brown discoloration of urine.

Special populations

Breast-feeding patients. Drug is distributed in breast milk; use with caution. Potential benefits to the woman should outweigh potential harm to the infant.
Pediatric patients. Prochlorperazine is contraindicated in infants under age 2 or weighing less than 20 lb (9 kg). Don't give sustained-release form to children.
Geriatric patients. Geriatric patients tend to require lower doses, adjusted to individual effects. These patients are at greater risk for adverse reactions, especially tardive dyskinesia, other extrapyramidal effects, and hypotension.

Patient counseling

- Explain risks of dystonic reactions and tardive dyskinesia. Tell patient to report abnormal body movements promptly.
- Tell patient to avoid spilling the liquid form. Contact with skin may cause rash and irritation.
- Warn patient to avoid extremely hot or cold baths and exposure to temperature extremes, sunlamps, or tanning beds; drug may cause thermoregulatory changes.
- Advise patient to take drug exactly as prescribed, not to double the doses after missing one, and not to share drug with others.
- Oral formulations may cause stomach upset. Administer with food or fluid.
- Tell patient to dilute the concentrate in water; explain the dropper technique of measuring dose; teach correct use of suppository.
- Tell patient that hard candy, chewing gum, or ice chips can alleviate dry mouth.
- Warn patient not to stop taking drug suddenly and to promptly report difficulty urinating, sore throat, dizziness, or fainting. Reassure patient that most reactions can be relieved by reducing dose.
- Caution patient to avoid hazardous activities that require alertness until effect of drug is es-

tablished. Reassure patient that sedative effects subside and become tolerable in several weeks.

progesterone

Crinone, Gesterol 50, Progestasert, Prometrium

Pharmacologic classification: progestin
Therapeutic classification: progestin, contraceptive
Pregnancy risk category X

How supplied

Available by prescription only
Capsules: 100 mg
Gel: 4% (45 mg), 8% (90 mg)
Injection: 25 mg, 50 mg, and 100 mg/ml (in oil); 25 mg and 50 mg/ml (aqueous)
Intrauterine device: 38 mg (with barium sulfate, dispersed in silicone fluid)

Indications and dosages

Amenorrhea
Adults: 5 to 10 mg I.M. daily for 6 to 8 days. Or, for secondary amenorrhea, one application of 4% gel vaginally every other day up to a total of six doses. If no response, may use Crinone 8% every other day up to a total of six doses.
Secondary amenorrhea
Adults: 400 mg (Prometrium) P.O. daily, in the evening, for 10 days.
Dysfunctional uterine bleeding
Adults: 5 to 10 mg I.M. daily for 6 days. Alternatively, a single 50- to 100-mg I.M. dose.
Corpus luteum insufficiency
Adults: 12.5 mg I.M. initiated within several days of ovulation and continuing for 2 weeks. May continue for up to 11th week of gestation. Or, for infertility, one application of 8% gel vaginally, daily or twice daily. If pregnancy occurs, treatment may be continued until placental autonomy is achieved up to 10 to 12 weeks.
Contraception (as an intrauterine device [IUD])
Adults: Progestasert system inserted into uterine cavity; replaced after 1 year.

Pharmacodynamics

Contraceptive action: Progesterone suppresses ovulation, thickens cervical mucus, and induces sloughing of the endometrium.

Pharmacokinetics

Absorption: Must be administered parenterally because it's inactivated by the liver after oral administration.
Distribution: Little information available.
Metabolism: Reduced to pregnanediol in the liver, then conjugated with glucuronic acid. Plasma half-life of progesterone is short (several minutes).
Excretion: Glucuronide-conjugated pregnanediol is excreted in urine.

Route	Onset	Peak	Duration
I.M., P.O.	Unknown	Unknown	Unknown
Intrauterine	Unknown	Unknown	Unknown
Vaginally	Unknown	Unknown	Unknown

Contraindications and precautions

Contraindicated in patients with thromboembolic disorders or cerebral apoplexy (or history of these conditions), hypersensitivity to drug, breast cancer, undiagnosed abnormal vaginal bleeding, severe hepatic disease, missed abortion, and in breast-feeding women.

Use cautiously in patients with diabetes mellitus, seizures, migraines, cardiac or renal disease, asthma, or mental depression.

Interactions

Drug-drug. *Bromocriptine:* Progesterone may cause amenorrhea or galactorrhea, interfering with the action of bromocriptine. Concurrent use isn't recommended. Use IUD with caution in patients receiving anticoagulants.

Effects on diagnostic tests

None reported.

Adverse reactions

CNS: depression, somnolence, headache (Crinone).
CV: thrombophlebitis, ***thromboembolism, CVA, pulmonary embolism,*** edema.
GI: nausea, constipation, diarrhea, vomiting (Crinone).
GU: breakthrough bleeding, dysmenorrhea, amenorrhea, cervical erosion, abnormal secretions, nocturia (Crinone).
Hepatic: cholestatic jaundice.
Skin: melasma, rash, acne, pruritus, pain at injection site.
Other: breast tenderness, enlargement, or secretion; pregnanediol excretion may decrease; serum alkaline phosphatase and amino acid levels may increase.

Overdose and treatment

No information available.

Clinical considerations

Consider the recommendations relevant to all progestins as well as the following:
- Parenteral form for I.M. administration only. Inject deep into large muscle mass, preferably the gluteal muscle. Check sites for irritation.
- Large doses of progesterone may cause a moderate catabolic effect and a transient increase in sodium and chloride excretion.

Therapeutic monitoring

Be alert for signs and symptoms of increased depression.

Special populations

Breast-feeding patients. Drug is contraindicated in breast-feeding women.
Pregnant patients. Potential exists for fetal harm, especially during first 4 months of pregnancy. Instruct patient to promptly report if she suspects pregnancy while receiving progestin therapy.

Patient counseling

- Advise patient that withdrawal bleeding usually occurs 2 to 3 days after discontinuing drug.

For patient using Progestasert

- Inform patient that bleeding and cramping may occur for a few weeks after insertion.
- Advise patient to contact health care provider if abnormal or excessive bleeding, severe cramping, abnormal vaginal discharge, fever, or flulike syndrome occurs.
- Teach patient how to check for proper placement of IUD.
- Tell patient with Progestasert IUD that the progesterone supply is depleted in 1 year and the device must be changed at that time. Pregnancy risk increases after 1 year if patient relies on progesterone-depleted device for contraception.
- Inform patient of adverse effects, including uterine perforation, increased risk of infection, pelvic inflammatory disease, ectopic pregnancy, abdominal cramping, increased menstrual flow, and expulsion of the device.

For patient using Crinone gel

- Inform patient not to use the gel concurrently with other local intravaginal therapy. If other local intravaginal therapy is used concurrently, there should be at least a 6-hour period before or after gel administration.

promethazine hydrochloride

Histantil*, Pentazine, Phencen-50, Phenergan, Phenergan Fortis, Phenergan Plain, Phenoject-50, Prorex-25, Prorex-50, Prothazine, Prothazine Plain, V-Gan-25, V-Gan-50

Pharmacologic classification: phenothiazine derivative
Therapeutic classification: antiemetic antivertigo, antihistamine (H_1-receptor antagonist), preoperative, postoperative, or obstetric sedative and adjunct to analgesics
Pregnancy risk category NR

How supplied

Available by prescription only
Tablets: 12.5 mg, 25 mg, 50 mg
Syrup: 6.25 mg/5 ml, 25 mg/5 ml
Suppositories: 12.5 mg, 25 mg, 50 mg
Injection: 25 mg/ml, 50 mg/ml

Indications and dosages

Motion sickness
Adults: 25 mg P.O. b.i.d.
Children: 12.5 to 25 mg P.O., I.M., or P.R. b.i.d.
Nausea
Adults: 12.5 to 25 mg P.O., I.M., or P.R. q 4 to 6 hours, p.r.n.
Children: 0.25 to 0.5 mg/kg I.M. or P.R. q 4 to 6 hours, p.r.n.
Rhinitis, allergy symptoms
Adults: 12.5 to 25 mg P.O. before meals and h.s.; or 25 mg P.O. h.s.
Children: 6.25 to 12.5 mg P.O. t.i.d., or 25 mg P.O. or P.R. h.s.
Sedation
Adults: 25 to 50 mg P.O. or I.M. h.s., or P.R., p.r.n.
Children: 12.5 to 25 mg P.O., I.M., or P.R. h.s.
Routine preoperative or postoperative sedation or as an adjunct to analgesics
Adults: 25 to 50 mg I.M., I.V., or P.O.
Children: 12.5 to 25 mg I.M., I.V., or P.O.
Obstetric sedation
25 to 50 mg I.M. or I.V. in early stages of labor, and 25 to 75 mg after labor is established; repeat q 2 to 4 hours, p.r.n. Maximum daily dose, 100 mg.

Pharmacodynamics

Antiemetic and antivertigo actions: The central antimuscarinic actions of antihistamines probably are responsible for their antivertigo and antiemetic effects; promethazine also is believed to inhibit the medullary chemoreceptor trigger zone.
Antihistamine action: Promethazine competes with histamine for the H_1-receptor, thereby suppressing allergic rhinitis and urticaria; drug doesn't prevent the release of histamine.
Sedative action: CNS depressant mechanism of promethazine is unknown; phenothiazines probably cause sedation by reducing stimuli to the brain-stem reticular system.

Pharmacokinetics

Absorption: Well absorbed from the GI tract.
Distribution: Distributed widely throughout the body; it crosses the placenta.
Metabolism: Metabolized in the liver.
Excretion: Metabolites are excreted in urine and feces.

Route	Onset	Peak	Duration
P.O.	15-60 min	Unknown	< 12 hr
I.V.	3-5 min	Unknown	< 12 hr
I.M., P.R.	20 min	Unknown	< 12 hr

Contraindications and precautions

Contraindicated in patients with hypersensitivity to drug; in those with intestinal obstruction, prostatic hyperplasia, bladder neck obstruction, seizure disorders, coma, CNS depression, and stenosing peptic ulcerations; in newborns, premature neonates, and breast-feeding women; and in acutely ill or dehydrated children.

Use cautiously in patients with asthma or cardiac, pulmonary, or hepatic disease.

Interactions

Drug-drug. *CNS depressants, such as antianxiety agents, barbiturates, sleeping aids, and tranquilizers; other antihistamines:* Additive CNS depression may occur. Use together cautiously.
Epinephrine: Use may result in partial adrenergic blockade, producing further hypotension. Don't give together.
Levodopa: Promethazine may block the antiparkinsonian action of levodopa. Avoid use together.
MAO inhibitors: Interfere with the detoxification of antihistamines and phenothiazines and thus prolong and intensify their sedative and anticholinergic effects. Don't use together.
Drug-lifestyle. *Alcohol use:* Additive CNS depression may occur. Advise patient to avoid alcohol use.
Sun exposure: May cause photosensitivity reactions. Advise patient to take precautions.

Effects on diagnostic tests

Discontinue drug 4 days before diagnostic skin tests to avoid preventing, reducing, or masking test response. Promethazine may cause either false-positive or false-negative pregnancy test results. It also may interfere with blood grouping in the ABO system.

Adverse reactions

CNS: *sedation,* confusion, sleepiness, dizziness, disorientation, extrapyramidal symptoms, *drowsiness.*
CV: hypotension, hypertension.
EENT: blurred vision.
GI: nausea, vomiting, *dry mouth.*
GU: urine retention.
Hematologic: leukopenia, ***agranulocytosis, thrombocytopenia.***
Other: photosensitivity, rash, hyperglycemia.

Overdose and treatment

Signs and symptoms of overdose may include either CNS depression (sedation, reduced mental alertness, apnea, and CV collapse) or CNS stimulation (insomnia, hallucinations, tremors, or seizures). Atropine-like signs and symptoms, such as dry mouth, flushed skin, fixed and dilated pupils, and GI symptoms, are common, especially in children.

Empty stomach by gastric lavage; don't induce vomiting. Treat hypotension with vasopressors, and control seizures with diazepam or phenytoin; correct acidosis and electrolyte imbalance. Urinary acidification promotes excretion of drug. Don't give stimulants.

Clinical considerations

Consider the recommendations relevant to all phenothiazines as well as the following:

- Pronounced sedative effects may limit use in some ambulatory patients.
- The 50-mg/ml concentration is for I.M. use only; inject deep into large muscle mass. Don't administer drug S.C.; this may cause chemical irritation and necrosis. Drug may be administered I.V., in concentrations not to exceed 25 mg/ml and at a rate not to exceed 25 mg/minute; when using I.V. drip, wrap in aluminum foil to protect drug from light.
- Promethazine and meperidine (Demerol) may be mixed in the same syringe.

Therapeutic monitoring

- Monitor CBC.
- There may be a pronounced sedative effect. Take precautions for patient's safety.

Special populations

Breast-feeding patients. Antihistamines such as promethazine shouldn't be used during breast-feeding. Many of these drugs are excreted in breast milk, exposing the infant to risks of unusual excitability, especially premature infants and other neonates, who may experience seizures.
Pediatric patients. Use cautiously in children with respiratory dysfunction. Safety and efficacy in children under age 2 haven't been established; don't give promethazine to infants under age 3 months.
Geriatric patients. Geriatric patients are usually more sensitive to adverse effects of antihistamines and are especially likely to experience a greater degree of dizziness, sedation, hyperexcitability, dry mouth, and urine retention than younger patients. Symptoms usually respond to a decrease in dosage.

Patient counseling

- When treating motion sickness, tell patient to take first dose 30 to 60 minutes before travel; on succeeding days, he should take dose upon arising and with evening meal.
- Tell patient that coffee or tea may reduce drowsiness.
- Suggest sugarless gum, sugarless sour hard candy, or ice chips to relieve dry mouth.
- Tell patient to take oral form with food or milk.

propafenone hydrochloride

Rythmol

Pharmacologic classification: sodium channel antagonist
Therapeutic classification: antiarrhythmic
Pregnancy risk category C

How supplied

Available by prescription only
Tablets: 150 mg, 225 mg, 300 mg

Indications and dosages

Suppression of documented life-threatening ventricular arrhythmias
Adults: Initially, 150 mg P.O. q 8 hours. Dosage may be increased to 225 mg q 8 hours after 3 or 4 days; if necessary, increase dosage to 300 mg q 8 hours. Maximum daily dose, 900 mg.
≡ ***Dosage adjustment.*** Reduce dosage in patients with hepatic failure to 20% to 30% of usual dosage.

Pharmacodynamics

Antiarrhythmic action: Propafenone reduces the inward sodium current in myocardial cells and Purkinje fibers; it also has weak beta blocking effects. It slows the upstroke velocity of the action potential (phase 0 depolarization) and slows conduction in the AV node, His-Purkinje system, and intraventricular conduction system and prolongs the refractory period in the AV node.

Pharmacokinetics

Absorption: Well absorbed from the GI tract; absorption isn't affected by food. Because of a significant first-pass effect, bioavailability is limited; however, it increases with dosage. Absolute bioavailability is 3.4% with the 150-mg tablet and 10.6% with the 300-mg tablet.
Distribution: Peak plasma levels occur about 3½ hours after administration.
Metabolism: Metabolized in the liver, with a significant first-pass effect. Two active metabolites have been identified: 5-hydroxypropafenone and N-depropylpropafenone. A few patients (10% of all patients and patients receiving quinidine) metabolize drug more slowly. Little (if any) 5-hydroxypropafenone is present in the plasma.
Excretion: Elimination half-life is 2 to 10 hours in normal metabolizers (about 90% of patients); it can be as long as 10 to 32 hours in slow metabolizers.

Route	Onset	Peak	Duration
P.O.	Unknown	3½ hr	Unknown

Contraindications and precautions

Contraindicated in patients with hypersensitivity to drug and in those with severe or uncontrolled heart failure; cardiogenic shock; SA, AV, or intraventricular disorders of impulse conduction in the absence of a pacemaker; bradycardia; marked hypotension; bronchospastic disorders; and electrolyte imbalance.

Use cautiously in patients with renal or hepatic failure or heart failure, and in those receiving other cardiac depressant drugs.

Interactions

Drug-drug. *Beta blockers, including metoprolol, propranolol, and warfarin:* May increase plasma levels of these drugs, resulting in increased INR. Monitor appropriately.
Cimetidine: May increase plasma levels of propafenone. Monitor patient closely.
Digoxin: Propafenone causes a dose-related increase in plasma digoxin levels, ranging from 35% at 450 mg/day to 85% at 900 mg/day. Monitor plasma digoxin levels closely and dosage adjustment of digoxin may be necessary.
Local anesthetics: May increase the risk of CNS toxicity. Avoid use together.
Quinidine: Competitively inhibits one of the metabolic pathways for propafenone, increasing its half-life. Use together isn't recommended.

Effects on diagnostic tests

None reported.

Adverse reactions

CNS: anxiety, ataxia, *dizziness,* drowsiness, fatigue, headache, insomnia, syncope, tremor.
CV: atrial fibrillation, bradycardia, bundle-branch block, angina, chest pain, edema, first-degree AV block, hypotension, increased QRS duration, intraventricular conduction delay, palpitations, ***heart failure, proarrhythmic events (ventricular tachycardia, PVCs, ventricular fibrillation).***
EENT: blurred vision.
GI: abdominal pain or cramps, constipation, diarrhea, dyspepsia, anorexia, flatulence, *nausea, vomiting,* dry mouth, unusual taste.
Musculoskeletal: joint pain.
Respiratory: dyspnea.
Skin: diaphoresis, rash.

Overdose and treatment

Symptoms usually develop within 3 hours of ingestion. Hypotension, somnolence, bradycardia, conduction disturbances, ventricular arrhythmias, and seizures have been reported. Provide supportive treatment and assist respirations as necessary. Rhythm and blood pressure may be controlled with dopamine and isoproterenol; seizures may respond to I.V. diazepam.

Clinical considerations

- Propafenone pharmacokinetics are complex; studies have shown that a threefold increase in daily dosage (from 300 to 900 mg/day) may produce a tenfold increase in plasma levels. Dosage must be individualized for each patient.
- Administer drug with food to minimize adverse GI effects.

Therapeutic monitoring
Continuous cardiac monitoring is recommended during initiation of therapy and during dose adjustments. If PR interval or QRS complex increases by more than 23%, a reduction in dosage may be necessary.

Special populations
Breast-feeding patients. It isn't known if drug is excreted in breast milk. Because of potential for serious toxicity in the infant, consider alternative feeding methods during therapy.
Geriatric patients. In geriatric patients and patients with substantial heart disease, increase dosage more gradually during the initial phase of treatment.

Patient counseling
- Instruct patient to report signs and symptoms of infection, such as sore throat, chills, or fever.
- Stress importance of taking drug exactly as prescribed.

propantheline bromide
Pro-Banthine, Propanthel*

Pharmacologic classification: anticholinergic
Therapeutic classification: antimuscarinic, GI antispasmodic
Pregnancy risk category C

How supplied
Available by prescription only
Tablets: 7.5 mg, 15 mg

Indications and dosages
Adjunctive treatment of peptic ulcer, irritable bowel syndrome, and other GI disorders; to reduce duodenal motility during diagnostic radiologic procedures
Adults: 15 mg P.O. t.i.d. before meals, and 30 mg h.s. up to 60 mg q.i.d.
Geriatric patients: 7.5 mg P.O. t.i.d. before meals.
Children: Antispasmodic dose 2 to 3 mg/kg/day P.O. divided q 4 hours to q 6 hours and h.s. Antisecretory dose 1.5 mg/kg/day P.O. divided q 6 hours to q 8 hours.

Pharmacodynamics
Anticholinergic action: Propantheline competitively blocks actions of acetylcholine at cholinergic neuroeffector sites, decreasing GI motility and inhibiting gastric acid secretion.

Pharmacokinetics
Absorption: Only about 10% to 25% is absorbed (absorption varies among patients).
Distribution: Doesn't cross the blood-brain barrier; little else is known about its distribution.
Metabolism: Appears to undergo considerable metabolism in the upper small intestine and liver.
Excretion: Absorbed drug is excreted in urine as metabolites and unchanged drug.

Route	Onset	Peak	Duration
P.O.	1½ hr	2-6 hr	6 hr

Contraindications and precautions
Contraindicated in patients with angle-closure glaucoma, obstructive uropathy, obstructive disease of the GI tract, severe ulcerative colitis, myasthenia gravis, hypersensitivity to anticholinergics, paralytic ileus, intestinal atony, unstable CV status in acute hemorrhage, or toxic megacolon.

Use cautiously in patients with impaired renal or hepatic function, autonomic neuropathy, hyperthyroidism, coronary artery disease, arrhythmias, heart failure, hypertension, hiatal hernia associated with gastric reflux, or ulcerative colitis and in those living in a hot or humid environment.

Interactions
Drug-drug. *Antacids:* Decrease oral absorption of anticholinergics. Administer propantheline at least 1 hour before antacids.
Atenolol: Propantheline may increase atenolol absorption, thereby enhancing effects of atenolol. Monitor patient closely.
Digoxin (slowly dissolving tablets): May yield higher serum digoxin levels when administered with anticholinergics. Monitor patient closely for digitalis toxicity.
Drugs with anticholinergic effects: May cause additive toxicity. Avoid use together.
Ketoconazole, levodopa: Decreased GI absorption. Separate administration times by 2 to 3 hours.
Oral potassium supplements, especially wax-matrix formulations: Incidence of potassium-induced GI ulcerations may be increased. Avoid use together.

Effects on diagnostic tests
None reported.

Adverse reactions
CNS: headache, insomnia, drowsiness, dizziness, *confusion or excitement in geriatric patients,* nervousness, weakness.
CV: *palpitations,* tachycardia.
EENT: *blurred vision,* mydriasis, increased intraocular pressure, cycloplegia, drying of salivary secretions.
GI: *dry mouth,* constipation, loss of taste, nausea, vomiting, paralytic ileus, bloated feeling.
GU: *urinary hesitancy, urine retention,* impotence.
Skin: urticaria, decreased sweating or possible anhidrosis, other dermal signs and symptoms.

Other: allergic reactions ***(anaphylaxis)***.

Overdose and treatment

Signs and symptoms of overdose include curare-like symptoms, such as respiratory paralysis, and such peripheral effects as headache; dilated, nonreactive pupils; blurred vision; flushed, hot, dry skin; dryness of mucous membranes; dysphagia; decreased or absent bowel sounds; urine retention; hyperthermia; tachycardia; hypertension; and increased respirations.

Treatment is primarily symptomatic and supportive, as needed. If patient is alert, induce emesis (or use gastric lavage) and follow with a NaCl cathartic and activated charcoal to prevent further drug absorption. In severe cases, physostigmine may be administered to block antimuscarinic effects of propantheline. Give fluids, as needed, to treat shock. If urine retention develops, catheterization may be necessary.

Clinical considerations

- Consider the recommendations relevant to all anticholinergics.
- Drug may be used with histamine-2 receptor to treat Zollinger-Ellison syndrome as an unlabeled use.

Therapeutic monitoring

- Adjust drug until therapeutic effect is obtained or adverse effects become intolerable.
- Monitor urine output and vital signs carefully.

Special populations

Breast-feeding patients. Drug may be excreted in breast milk, possibly resulting in infant toxicity. Don't use in breast-feeding women. Propantheline may decrease milk production.
Geriatric patients. Administer drug cautiously to geriatric patients. Lower doses are recommended.

Patient counseling

- Instruct patient to swallow tablets whole rather than chewing or crushing them.
- Advise patient to avoid driving and other activities that require alertness if drowsiness, dizziness, or blurred vision occur.
- Encourage patient to increase fluid intake to avoid constipation.

propofol

Diprivan

Pharmacologic classification: phenol derivative
Therapeutic classification: anesthetic
Pregnancy risk category B

How supplied

Available by prescription only
Injection: 10 mg/ml in 20-ml ampules and 50-ml and 100-ml infusion vials

Indications and dosages

Induction and maintenance of sedation in mechanically ventilated intensive care unit patients
Adults: Initially, 5 mcg/kg/minute I.V. for 5 minutes (0.3 mg/kg/hour). Subsequent increments of 5 to 10 mcg/kg/minute (0.3 to 0.6 mg/kg/hour) over 5 to 10 minutes until desired level of sedation is achieved. Maintenance rates of 5 to 50 mcg/kg/minute (0.3 to 3 mg/kg/hour) or higher may be required. Use minimum amount necessary. Lower dosages are required for patients over age 55.
Induction of anesthesia
Adults: Individualize doses based on patient's condition and age. Most patients classified as American Society of Anesthesiologists (ASA) Physical Status category (PS) I or II under age 55 require 2 to 2.5 mg/kg I.V. Drug is usually administered in a 40-mg bolus q 10 seconds until desired response is obtained.
Children age 3 and over: 2.5 to 3.5 mg/kg I.V. over 20 to 30 seconds.
Geriatric, debilitated, or hypovolemic patients or patients in ASA PS III or IV: Half of the usual induction dose (20-mg bolus q 10 seconds).
Maintenance of anesthesia
Adults: May give as a variable rate infusion, titrated to clinical effect. Most patients may be maintained with 0.1 to 0.2 mg/kg/minute (6 to 12 mg/kg/hour).
Geriatric, debilitated, or hypovolemic patients or patients in ASA PS III or IV: Half the usual maintenance dosage (0.05 to 0.1 mg/kg/minute or 3 to 6 mg/kg/hour).
Children age 3 and older: 125 to 300 mcg/kg/minute I.V.

Pharmacodynamics

Anesthetic action: Propofol produces a dose-dependent CNS depression similar to benzodiazepines and barbiturates. However, it can be used to maintain anesthesia through careful titration of infusion rate.

Pharmacokinetics

Absorption: Must be administered I.V.
Distribution: Terminal half-life of 1 to 3 days.
Metabolism: Metabolized within liver and tissues. Metabolites aren't fully characterized.
Excretion: Excreted through the kidneys. However, termination of drug action is probably caused by redistribution out of the CNS as well as metabolism.

Route	Onset	Peak	Duration
I.V.	< 40 sec	Unknown	10-15 min

Contraindications and precautions

Contraindicated in patients hypersensitive to propofol or components of the emulsion, including soybean oil, egg lecithin, and glycerol. Don't use drug in obstetric anesthesia because safety to fetus hasn't been established. Also avoid in patients with increased intracranial pressure or impaired cerebral circulation because the reduction in systemic arterial pressure caused by drug may substantially reduce cerebral perfusion pressure. Don't use drug in children under age 3 and in those in intensive care units or under monitored anesthesia care sedation.

Because drug is administered as an emulsion, administer with caution to patients with a disorder of lipid metabolism, such as pancreatitis, primary hyperlipoproteinemia, and diabetic hyperlipidemia. Use cautiously if patient is receiving lipids as part of a total parenteral nutrition infusion; I.V. lipid dose may need to be reduced. Use cautiously in geriatric or debilitated patients and in those with circulatory disorders. Although the hemodynamic effects of drug can vary, its major effect in patients maintaining spontaneous ventilation is arterial hypotension (arterial pressure can decrease as much as 30%) with little or no change in heart rate and cardiac output. However, significant depression of cardiac output may occur in patients undergoing assisted or controlled positive pressure ventilation.

Administer drug under direct medical supervision by persons familiar with airway management and the administration of I.V. anesthetics.

Interactions

Drug-drug. *Inhalational anesthetics, such as enflurane, halothane and isoflurane; supplemental anesthetics, such as nitrous oxide and opiates:* May be expected to enhance the anesthetic and CV actions of propofol. Monitor patient closely.
Opiate analgesics or sedatives: May intensify the reduction of systolic, diastolic, mean arterial pressure, and cardiac output and may decrease induction dose requirements. Monitor patient closely.

Effects on diagnostic tests

None reported.

Adverse reactions

CNS: *movement,* headache, dizziness, twitching, clonic-myoclonic movement.
CV: *hypotension,* bradycardia, hypertension.
GI: nausea, vomiting, abdominal cramping.
GU: discolored urine
Respiratory: ***apnea,*** cough, hiccups.
Skin: flushing.
Other: fever, *injection site burning or stinging, pain,* tingling or numbness, coldness, hyperlipidemia.

Overdose and treatment

Specific information not available. However, treatment of overdose may include support of respiration and administration of fluids, pressor agents, and anticholinergics as indicated.

Clinical considerations

□ ***ALERT*** Don't mix propofol with other drugs or blood products. If it's to be diluted before infusion, use only D_5W and don't dilute to a concentration less than 2 mg/ml. After dilution, drug appears to be more stable in glass containers than in plastic.

- Drug has no vagolytic activity. Premedication with anticholinergics, such as glycopyrrolate or atropine, may help manage potential increases in vagal tone caused by other drugs or surgical manipulations.
- When administered into a running I.V. catheter, emulsion is compatible with D_5W, lactated Ringer's injection, lactated Ringer's and 5% dextrose injection, 5% dextrose and 0.45% saline injection, and 5% dextrose and 0.2% saline injection.
- Store emulsion in temperatures more than 40° F (4° C) and less than 72° F (22° C). Refrigeration isn't recommended.
- If used for sedation of mechanically ventilated patients, wake patient every 24 hours.
- Use strict aseptic technique when administering drug; discard unused drug after 12 hours.

Therapeutic monitoring

Monitor patients receiving drug for signs of significant hypotension or bradycardia. Treatment may include increased rate of fluid administration, pressor agents, elevation of lower extremities, or atropine. Apnea may occur during induction and may persist for longer than 60 seconds. Ventilatory support may be required.

Special populations

Breast-feeding patients. Propofol is excreted in breast milk and shouldn't be used by breast-feeding women.
Pediatric patients. Safety in children hasn't been established.
Geriatric patients. Pharmacokinetics of propofol aren't influenced by chronic hepatic cirrhosis, chronic renal failure, or gender.

Patient counseling

Advise patient that performance of activities that require mental alertness, such as operating a motor vehicle or hazardous machinery, may be impaired for some time after drug use.

propoxyphene hydrochloride, propoxyphene hydrochloride with acetaminophen, propoxyphene with aspirin and caffeine

Darvon, Dolene, Wygesic, Darvon Compound-65

propoxyphene napsylate

Darvon-N, Propocet 100 (with acetaminophen)

Pharmacologic classification: opioid
Therapeutic classification: analgesic
Controlled substance schedule IV
Pregnancy risk category NR

How supplied

Available by prescription only
propoxyphene hydrochloride
Tablets: 65 mg
Capsules: 65 mg
propoxyphene hydrochloride and acetaminophen
Tablets: 65 mg propoxyphene hydrochloride, 650 mg acetaminophen
propoxyphene hydrochloride, aspirin, and caffeine
Capsules: 65 mg propoxyphene hydrochloride, 389 mg aspirin, 32.4 mg caffeine
propoxyphene napsylate
Tablets: 50 mg, 100 mg
Capsules: 50 mg, 100 mg
Suspension: 50 mg/5 ml
propoxyphene napsylate and acetaminophen
Tablets: 50 mg propoxyphene napsylate, 325 mg acetaminophen; 100 mg propoxyphene napsylate, 650 mg acetaminophen

Indications and dosages

Mild to moderate pain
Adults: 65 mg (hydrochloride) P.O. q 4 hours, p.r.n., or 100 mg (napsylate) P.O. q 4 hours, p.r.n.

Pharmacodynamics

Analgesic action: Propoxyphene exerts its analgesic effect by way of opiate agonist activity and alters the patient's response to painful stimuli, particularly those causing mild to moderate pain.

Pharmacokinetics

Absorption: After oral administration, drug is absorbed primarily in the upper small intestine. Equimolar doses of the hydrochloride and napsylate salts provide similar plasma levels.
Distribution: Enters the CSF. It's assumed that it crosses the placental barrier; however, placental fluid and fetal blood levels haven't been determined.
Metabolism: Degraded mainly in the liver; about one-fourth of a dose is metabolized to norpropoxyphene, an active metabolite.
Excretion: Excreted in the urine. Duration of effect is 4 to 6 hours.

Route	Onset	Peak	Duration
P.O.	15-60 min	2-2½ hr	4-6 hr

Contraindications and precautions

Contraindicated in patients with hypersensitivity to drug. Use cautiously in patients with impaired renal or hepatic function, emotional instability, or history of drug or alcohol abuse.

Interactions

Drug-drug. *Antagonists:* Patients who become physically dependent on propoxyphene may experience acute withdrawal syndrome when given a single dose of an antagonist. Use with caution and monitor patient closely.
Antidepressants: Propoxyphene may inhibit the metabolism of these drugs. A lower dose of antidepressant may be necessary.
Carbamazepine: Increased effects of carbamazepine. Monitor serum carbamazepine levels.
Cimetidine: May enhance respiratory and CNS depression. Avoid use together.
CNS depressants, such as antidepressants, antihistamines, barbiturates, benzodiazepines, general anesthetics, narcotic analgesics, muscle relaxants, phenothiazines, and sedative-hypnotics: Potentiation of adverse effects (respiratory depression, sedation, hypotension). Reduced doses of propoxyphene are usually needed.
Digitoxin, phenytoin, rifampin: Accumulation of either drug may occur. Withdrawal symptoms may result if used together. Avoid use together.
General anesthetics: Severe CV depression may result from use with these drugs. Monitor patient closely and use with caution.
Drug-lifestyle. *Alcohol use:* Potentiated CNS depressant effects of propoxyphene. Advise patient to avoid alcohol use.
Smoking: Increased metabolism of propoxyphene. Monitor patient closely.

Effects on diagnostic tests

Drug may cause false decrease in test results for urinary steroid excretion.

Adverse reactions

CNS: *dizziness, sedation,* headache, euphoria, light-headedness, weakness, hallucinations.
GI: *nausea, vomiting,* constipation, abdominal pain, abnormal liver function tests.
Respiratory: ***respiratory depression.***
Other: psychological and physical dependence.

Overdose and treatment

The most common signs and symptoms of overdose are CNS depression, respiratory depression, and miosis (pinpoint pupils). Others include hypotension, bradycardia, hypothermia, shock, apnea, cardiopulmonary arrest, circulatory collapse, pulmonary edema, and seizures.

Drug is known to cause ECG changes (prolonged QRS complex) and nephrogenic diabetes insipidus in acute toxic doses. Death from an acute overdose is most likely to occur within the first hour. Signs and symptoms of overdose with propoxyphene combination products may include salicylism from aspirin or acetaminophen toxicity.

To treat an acute overdose, first establish adequate respiratory exchange by way of a patent airway and ventilation as needed; administer a narcotic antagonist (naloxone) to reverse respiratory depression. (Because the duration of action of drug is longer than naloxone, repeated dosing is necessary.) Don't give naloxone in the absence of clinically significant respiratory or CV depression. Monitor vital signs closely.

If patient shows symptoms within 2 hours of ingestion of an oral overdose, empty the stomach immediately by inducing emesis (ipecac syrup) or gastric lavage. Use caution to avoid risk of aspiration. Administer activated charcoal via nasogastric tube for further removal of drug in an oral overdose.

Provide symptomatic and supportive treatment (continued respiratory support, correction of fluid or electrolyte imbalance). Anticonvulsants may be needed; monitor laboratory parameters, vital signs, and neurologic status closely. Dialysis may be helpful in the treatment of overdose with propoxyphene combination products containing aspirin or acetaminophen.

Clinical considerations

Consider the recommendations relevant to all opioids as well as the following:

- Propoxyphene may obscure the signs and symptoms of an acute abdominal condition or worsen gallbladder pain.
- Don't prescribe drug maintenance purposes in narcotic addiction.
- Propoxyphene can be considered a mild narcotic analgesic, but pain relief is equivalent to that of aspirin.

Therapeutic monitoring

Closely monitor patient's response to pain relief.

Special populations

Breast-feeding patients. Drug is excreted in breast milk; use with caution in breast-feeding women.

Geriatric patients. Lower doses are usually indicated for geriatric patients because they may be more sensitive to therapeutic and adverse effects of drug.

Patient counseling

- Advise patient not to exceed recommended dosage.
- Warn patient of additive depressant effect that can occur if drug is prescribed for medical conditions requiring use of sedatives, tranquilizers, muscle relaxants, antidepressants, or other CNS-depressant drugs.
- Tell patient to take drug with food if GI upset occurs.

propranolol hydrochloride

Inderal, Inderal LA

Pharmacologic classification: beta blocker
Therapeutic classification: antihypertensive, antianginal, antiarrhythmic, adjunctive therapy of migraine, adjunctive therapy of MI
Pregnancy risk category C

How supplied

Available by prescription only
Tablets: 10 mg, 20 mg, 40 mg, 60 mg, 80 mg
Capsules (extended-release): 60 mg, 80 mg, 120 mg, 160 mg
Injection: 1 mg/ml
*Solution:*4mg/ml, 8mg/ml, 80 mg/ml (concentrated)

Indications and dosages

Hypertension

Adults: Initially, 20 to 40 mg P.O. b.i.d. or 60 to 80 mg once daily (extended-release). Increase at 3- to 7-day intervals until optimum blood pressure response is achieved. Usual maintenance dosage is 160 to 480 mg daily. Or, 120 to 160 mg P.O. once daily (extended release). Maximum daily dose 640 mg.

◇ *Children:* 1 mg/kg P.O. daily (maximum daily dose is 16 mg/kg).

Management of angina pectoris

Adults: 10 to 20 mg P.O. t.i.d. or q.i.d., or one 80-mg extended-release capsule daily. Dosage may be increased at 3- to 7-day intervals. Average optimum dose is 160 to 240 mg daily.

Supraventricular, ventricular, and atrial arrhythmias; tachyarrhythmias caused by excessive catecholamine action during anesthesia, hyperthyroidism, and pheochromocytoma

Adults: 1 to 3 mg I.V. diluted in 50 ml D_5W or normal saline solution infused slowly, not to exceed 1 mg/minute. After 3 mg have been infused, another dose may be given in 2 minutes; subsequent doses no sooner than q 4 hours. Usual maintenance dosage is 10 to 30 mg P.O. t.i.d. or q.i.d.

Prevention of frequent, severe, uncontrollable, or disabling migraine or vascular headache
Adults: Initially, 80 mg P.O. daily in divided doses or one extended-release capsule once daily. Usual maintenance dosage is 160 to 240 mg daily, divided t.i.d. or q.i.d.
To reduce risk of death after MI
Adults: 180 to 240 mg P.O. daily in divided doses. Usually given in three to four doses daily, beginning 5 to 21 days after infarct.
Hypertrophic subaortic stenosis
Adults: 20 to 40 mg P.O. t.i.d. or q.i.d. Or, 80 to 160 mg once daily (extended release).
Preoperative pheochromocytoma
Adults: 60 mg P.O. daily in divided doses in conjunction with alpha blocker for 3 days before surgery.
◊ ***Adjunctive treatment of anxiety***
Adults: 10 to 80 mg P.O. 1 hour before anxiety-provoking activity.
◊ ***Treatment of essential, familial, or senile movement tremors***
Adults: 40 mg P.O. b.i.d., as needed.

Pharmacodynamics
Antihypertensive action: Exact mechanism of antihypertensive effect is unknown; drug may reduce blood pressure by blocking adrenergic receptors (decreasing cardiac output), by decreasing sympathetic outflow from the CNS, and by suppressing renin release.
Antianginal action: Propranolol decreases myocardial oxygen consumption by blocking catecholamine access to beta-adrenergic receptors, relieving angina.
Antiarrhythmic action: Propranolol decreases heart rate and prevents exercise-induced increases in heart rate. It also decreases myocardial contractility, cardiac output, and SA and AV nodal conduction velocity.
Migraine prophylactic action: Migraine-preventive effect of propranolol is thought to result from inhibition of vasodilation.
MI prophylactic action: Mechanism by which drug reduces risk of death after MI is unknown.

Pharmacokinetics
Absorption: Absorbed almost completely from the GI tract, especially when given with food.
Distribution: Distributed widely throughout the body; drug is more than 90% protein-bound.
Metabolism: Hepatic metabolism is almost total; oral dosage form undergoes extensive first-pass metabolism.
Excretion: About 96% to 99% of a given dose of propranolol is excreted in urine as metabolites; remainder is excreted in feces as unchanged drug and metabolites. Biologic half-life is about 4 hours.

Route	Onset	Peak	Duration
P.O.	30 min	1-1½ hr	12 hr
I.V.	1 min	Immediate	5 min

Contraindications and precautions
Contraindicated in patients with bronchial asthma, sinus bradycardia and heart block greater than first-degree, cardiogenic shock, and heart failure (unless failure is secondary to a tachyarrhythmia that can be treated with propranolol).

Use cautiously in the elderly; in patients with impaired renal or hepatic function, nonallergic bronchospastic diseases, diabetes mellitus, or thyrotoxicosis; and in those receiving other antihypertensive medications.

Interactions
Drug-drug. *Aluminum hydroxide antacid:* Decreases GI absorption. Don't give together.
Antihypertensive agents: Propranolol may potentiate antihypertensive effects. Monitor patient closely.
Atropine, tricyclic antidepressants, and other drugs with anticholinergic effects: May antagonize propranolol-induced bradycardia. Monitor ECG.
Calcium channel blockers, especially I.V. verapamil: May depress myocardial contractility or AV conduction. Use together cautiously.
Cimetidine: May decrease clearance of propranolol. Monitor for increased beta-blocking effects.
Epinephrine: causes severe vasoconstriction. Monitor blood pressure and patient closely.
Insulin or antidiabetic agents: Can alter dosage requirements in previously stable diabetic patients. Monitor for hypoglycemia.
NSAIDs: May antagonize hypotensive effects. Monitor blood pressure closely.
Phenytoin, rifampin: Accelerate clearance of propranolol. Monitor patient closely.
Sympathomimetic agents, such as isoproterenol and MAO inhibitors: Propranolol may antagonize beta-adrenergic-stimulating effects. Monitor patient closely. May be used therapeutically and in emergencies.
Tubocurarine: High doses of propranolol may potentiate neuromuscular blocking effect. Monitor patient closely.
Drug-herb. *Betel palm:* Reduces temperature-elevating effects and enhanced CNS effects of arecoline in betel palm. Don't use together.
Drug-lifestyle. *Cocaine use:* Increased angina-inducing potential of cocaine. Monitor patient closely.

Effects on diagnostic tests
None reported.

Adverse reactions
CNS: *fatigue, lethargy,* vivid dreams, hallucinations, mental depression, light-headedness, insomnia.
CV: *bradycardia, hypotension,* ***heart failure,*** intermittent claudication, intensification of AV block.

GI: nausea, vomiting, diarrhea, abdominal cramping.
Respiratory: ***bronchospasm.***
Skin: rash.
Other: fever, ***agranulocytosis,*** elevated serum transaminase, alkaline phosphatase, and LD levels and BUN levels.

Overdose and treatment

Signs of overdose include severe hypotension, bradycardia, heart failure, and bronchospasm.

After acute ingestion, induce emesis or empty stomach by gastric lavage; follow with activated charcoal to reduce absorption, and administer symptomatic and supportive care. Treat bradycardia with atropine (0.25 to 1 mg); if no response, administer isoproterenol cautiously. Treat cardiac failure with cardiac glycosides and diuretics, and treat hypotension with glucagon, vasopressors, or both; epinephrine is preferred. Treat bronchospasm with isoproteronol and aminophylline.

Clinical considerations

Consider the recommendations relevant to all beta blockers as well as the following:

- Propranolol also has been used to treat aggression and rage, stage fright, recurrent GI bleeding in cirrhotic patients, and menopausal symptoms.
- Never administer propranolol as an adjunct in treatment of pheochromocytoma unless patient has had pretreatment with alpha blockers.

Therapeutic monitoring

Always check patient's apical rate before giving drug. If extremes in pulse rates are detected, withhold drug and contact doctor immediately.

Special populations

Breast-feeding patients. Drug is distributed into breast milk; an alternative feeding method is recommended during therapy.
Pediatric patients. Safety and efficacy of propranolol in children haven't been established; use only if potential benefit outweighs risk.
Geriatric patients. Geriatric patients may require lower maintenance dosages of propranolol because of increased bioavailability or delayed metabolism; they also may experience enhanced adverse effects.

Patient counseling

- Warn patient not to abruptly stop taking propranolol because this can exacerbate angina and precipitate MI.
- Instruct patient on proper use, dosage, and potential adverse effects of propranolol.
- Tell patient to contact health care provider before taking OTC drugs that may interact with propranolol, such as nasal decongestants or cold preparations.

propylthiouracil (PTU)

Propyl-Thyracil*

Pharmacologic classification: thyroid hormone antagonist
Therapeutic classification: antihyperthyroid
Pregnancy risk category D

How supplied

Available by prescription only
Tablets: 50 mg

Indications and dosages

Hyperthyroidism
Adults: 300 to 450 mg P.O. daily in divided doses. Continue until patient is euthyroid; then start maintenance dosage of 100 mg daily to t.i.d.
Neonates and children: 5 to 7 mg/kg P.O. daily in divided doses q 8 hours. Alternatively, give according to age.
Children age 6 to 10: 50 to 150 mg P.O. daily in divided doses q 8 hours.
Children over age 10: 100 mg P.O. t.i.d. Continue until patient is euthyroid; then start maintenance dosage of 25 mg t.i.d. to 100 mg b.i.d.

Pharmacodynamics

Antithyroid action: Used to treat hyperthyroidism, PTU inhibits synthesis of thyroid hormone by interfering with the incorporation of iodine into thyroglobulin; it also inhibits the formation of iodothyronine. Besides blocking hormone synthesis, it also inhibits the peripheral deiodination of thyroxine to triiodothyronine (liothyronine). Clinical effects become evident only when the preformed hormone is depleted and circulating hormone levels decline.

As preparation for thyroidectomy, PTU inhibits synthesis of the thyroid hormone and causes a euthyroid state, reducing surgical problems during thyroidectomy; as a result, the risk of death for a single-stage thyroidectomy is low. Iodide reduces the vascularity of the gland and makes it less friable.

Used in treating thyrotoxic crisis, PTU inhibits peripheral deiodination of thyroxine to triiodothyronine. Theoretically, it's preferred over methimazole in thyroid storm because of its peripheral action.

Pharmacokinetics

Absorption: Absorbed rapidly and readily (about 80%) from the GI tract.
Distribution: PTU appears to be concentrated in the thyroid gland. PTU readily crosses the placenta and is distributed into breast milk. Drug is 75% to 80% protein-bound.

Metabolism: Metabolized rapidly in the liver.
Excretion: About 35% of a dose is excreted in urine. Half-life is 1 to 2 hours in patients with normal renal function and 8½ hours in anuric patients.

Route	Onset	Peak	Duration
P.O.	Unknown	1-1½ hr	Unknown

Contraindications and precautions
Contraindicated in patients with hypersensitivity to drug and in breast-feeding women. Use cautiously in pregnant women.

Interactions
Drug-drug. *Adrenocorticoids, corticotropin:* May require a dosage adjustment of the steroid when thyroid status changes.
Bone marrow depressant agents: Increases the risk of agranulocytosis. Monitor patient closely.
Hepatotoxic agents: Increased risk of hepatotoxicity. Monitor patient closely.
Iodinated glycerol, lithium, potassium iodide: May potentiate hypothyroid effects. Dosage adjustment may be necessary.
Oral anticoagulants: May be potentiated by the anti-vitamin K activity attributed to PTU. Monitor PT and INR.

Effects on diagnostic tests
PTU therapy alters selenomethionine levels and INR; it also alters AST, ALT, and LD levels, as well as liothyronine uptake.

Adverse reactions
CNS: headache, drowsiness, vertigo, paresthesia, neuritis, neuropathies, CNS stimulation, depression.
CV: vasculitis.
EENT: visual disturbances.
GI: diarrhea, *nausea, vomiting* (may be dose-related), epigastric distress, salivary gland enlargement, loss of taste.
GU: nephritis.
Hematologic: ***agranulocytosis, thrombocytopenia, aplastic anemia,*** leukopenia.
Hepatic: jaundice, ***hepatotoxicity.***
Musculoskeletal: arthralgia, myalgia.
Skin: rash, urticaria, skin discoloration, pruritus, erythema nodosum, exfoliative dermatitis, lupuslike syndrome.
Other: fever, lymphadenopathy; dose-related hypothyroidism (mental depression; hypoprothrombinemia and bleeding; cold intolerance; hard, nonpitting edema).

Overdose and treatment
Signs and symptoms of overdose include nausea, vomiting, epigastric distress, fever, headache, arthralgia, pruritus, edema, and pancytopenia.

Treatment includes withdrawal of drug in the presence of agranulocytosis, pancytopenia, hepatitis, fever, or exfoliative dermatitis. For depression of bone marrow, treatment may require antibiotics and transfusions of fresh whole blood. For hepatitis, treatment includes rest, adequate diet, and symptomatic support, including analgesics, gastric lavage, I.V. fluids, and mild sedation.

Clinical considerations
- Best response occurs when drug is administered around the clock and given at the same time each day in respect to meals.
- A beta blocker, usually propranolol, commonly is given to manage the peripheral signs of hyperthyroidism, which are primarily cardiac related (tachycardia).

Therapeutic monitoring
- Observe for signs and symptoms of hypothyroidism (mental depression; cold intolerance; hard, nonpitting edema; hair loss).
- Discontinue drug if severe rash or enlarged cervical lymph nodes develop.

Special populations
Pregnant patients. Potential exists for harm to the fetus. If drug must be used, administer the lowest possible dose.
Breast-feeding patients. Because PTU is excreted in breast milk, avoid breast-feeding during treatment. However, if it's necessary, PTU is the preferred antithyroid agent.

Patient counseling
- Warn patient to avoid using self-prescribed cough medicines; many contain iodine.
- Suggest taking drug with meals to reduce GI adverse effects.
- Instruct patient to store drug in a light-resistant container. Warn patient not to store medication in the bathroom; heat and humidity may cause drug to deteriorate.
- Tell patient to promptly report fever, sore throat, malaise, unusual bleeding, yellowing of eyes, nausea, or vomiting.
- Advise patient to have medical review of thyroid status before undergoing surgery, including dental surgery.
- Teach patient how to recognize the signs of hyperthyroidism and hypothyroidism and what to do if they occur.

protamine sulfate

Pharmacologic classification: antidote
Therapeutic classification: heparin antagonist
Pregnancy risk category C

How supplied
Available by prescription only
Injection: 10 mg/ml in 5-ml ampule, 25-ml ampule, 5-ml vial, 10-ml vial, 25-ml vial

Indications and dosages

Heparin overdose

Adults and children: Dosage based on venous blood coagulation studies, usually 1 mg for each 90 units of heparin derived from lung tissue or 1 mg for each 115 units of heparin derived from intestinal mucosa. Give by slow I.V. injection over 1 to 3 minutes. Maximum dose, 50 mg in any 10-minute period.

Pharmacodynamics

Heparin antagonism: Protamine has weak anticoagulant activity; however, when given in the presence of heparin, it forms a salt that neutralizes anticoagulant effects of both drugs.

Pharmacokinetics

Absorption: Heparin-neutralizing effect of protamine occurs rapidly.
Distribution: Unknown.
Metabolism: Fate of the heparin-protamine complex is unknown; however, it appears to be partially degraded, with release of some heparin.
Excretion: Binding action lasts about 2 hours.

Route	Onset	Peak	Duration
I.V.	30-60 sec	Unknown	2 hr

Contraindications and precautions

Contraindicated in patients with hypersensitivity to drug. Use cautiously after cardiac surgery.

Interactions

None significant.

Effects on diagnostic tests

Drug shortens heparin-prolonged PTT.

Adverse reactions

CV: decrease in blood pressure, bradycardia, ***circulatory collapse.***
GI: nausea, vomiting.
Respiratory: dyspnea, ***pulmonary edema, acute pulmonary hypertension.***
Other: transitory flushing, feeling of warmth, ***anaphylaxis, anaphylactoid reactions,*** lassitude.

Overdose and treatment

Overdose may cause bleeding secondary to interaction with platelets and proteins including fibrinogen. Replace blood loss with blood transfusions or fresh frozen plasma. If hypotension occurs, consider treating with fluids, epinephrine, dobutamine, or dopamine.

Clinical considerations

- Check for possible fish allergy.
- Don't mix protamine with any other medication.
- Reconstitute powder by adding 5 ml sterile water to 50-mg vial (25 ml to 250-mg vial); discard unused solution.
- Slow I.V. administration (over 1 to 3 minutes) decreases adverse effects; have antishock equipment available.

Therapeutic monitoring

- Monitor patient continually, and check vital signs frequently; blood pressure may fall suddenly.
- Dosage is based on blood coagulation studies as well as on route of administration of heparin and time elapsed since heparin was administered.

Special populations

Pregnant patients. Use only when clearly needed; it isn't known if drug will cause harm to the fetus.
Pediatric patients. Safety and efficacy haven't been established for children.

Patient counseling

Advise patient that he may experience transitory flushing or feel warm after I.V. administration.

pseudoephedrine hydrochloride

pseudoephedrine sulfate

Cenafed, Decofed, Efidac 24, Myfedrine, Novafed, PediaCare Infants' Decongestant Drops, Pseudogest, Sinufed Timecelles, Sudafed

Pharmacologic classification: adrenergic
Therapeutic classification: decongestant
Pregnancy risk category B

How supplied

Available without a prescription
Oral solution: 7.5 mg/0.8 ml, 15 mg/5 ml, 30 mg/5 ml
Tablets: 30 mg, 60 mg
Tablets (extended-release): 120 mg, 240 mg
Tablets (extended-release, film-coated): 120 mg
Tablets (chewable): 15 mg
Capsules: 60 mg

Indications and dosages

Nasal and eustachian tube decongestant

Adults and children age 12 and older: 60 mg P.O. q 4 to 6 hours. Maximum dose, 240 mg daily, or 120 mg P.O. extended-release tablet q 12 hours.

Children age 6 to 11: Administer 30 mg P.O. q 4 to 6 hours. Maximum dose, 120 mg daily.
Children age 2 to 5: 15 mg P.O. q 4 to 6 hours. Maximum dose, 60 mg/day, or 4 mg/kg or 125 mg/m² P.O. divided q.i.d.

Pharmacodynamics
Decongestant action: Pseudoephedrine directly stimulates alpha-adrenergic receptors of respiratory mucosa to produce vasoconstriction; shrinkage of swollen nasal mucous membranes; reduction of tissue hyperemia, edema, and nasal congestion; an increase in airway (nasal) patency and drainage of sinus excretions; and opening of obstructed eustachian ostia. Relaxation of bronchial smooth muscle may result from direct stimulation of beta-adrenergic receptors. Mild CNS stimulation may also occur.

Pharmacokinetics
Absorption: Nasal decongestion occurs within 30 minutes and persists 4 to 6 hours after oral dose of 60-mg tablet or oral solution. Effects persist 8 hours after 60-mg dose and up to 12 hours after 120-mg dose of extended-release form.
Distribution: Widely distributed throughout the body.
Metabolism: Incompletely metabolized in liver by N-demethylation to inactive compounds.
Excretion: 55% to 75% of a dose is excreted unchanged in urine; remainder is excreted as unchanged drug and metabolites.

Route	Onset	Peak	Duration
P.O.	½ hr	½-1 hr	4-12 hr

Contraindications and precautions
Contraindicated in patients with severe hypertension or severe coronary artery disease; in those receiving MAO inhibitors; and in breast-feeding women. Extended-release preparations are contraindicated in children under age 12.

Use cautiously in the elderly and in patients with hypertension, cardiac disease, diabetes, glaucoma, hyperthyroidism, or prostatic hyperplasia.

Interactions
Drug-drug. *Beta blockers:* May increase pressor effects of pseudoephedrine. Monitor patient closely.
MAO inhibitors: Potentiate pressor effects of pseudoephedrine. Avoid use together.
Methyldopa, reserpine: May reduce their anithypertensive effects. Monitor patient closely.
Sympathomimetics: May produce additive effects and toxicity. Monitor patient closely; give with extreme caution.
Tricyclic antidepressants: May antagonize effects of pseudoephedrine. Use cautiously.

Effects on diagnostic tests
None reported.

Adverse reactions
CNS: *anxiety,* transient stimulation, tremor, dizziness, headache, insomnia, *nervousness.*
CV: ***arrhythmias,*** *palpitations,* tachycardia.
GI: anorexia, nausea, vomiting, dry mouth.
GU: difficulty urinating.
Respiratory: respiratory difficulties.
Skin: pallor.

Overdose and treatment
Signs and symptoms of overdose include exaggeration of common adverse reactions, particularly seizures, arrhythmias, and nausea and vomiting.

Treatment may include an emetic and gastric lavage within 4 hours of ingestion. Charcoal is effective only if administered within 1 hour, unless extended-release form was used. If renal function is adequate, forced diuresis will increase elimination. Don't force diuresis in severe overdose. Monitor vital signs, cardiac state, and electrolyte levels. I.V. propranolol may control cardiac toxicity; I.V. diazepam may be helpful to manage delirium or seizures; dilute I.V. potassium chloride solutions may be given for hypokalemia.

Clinical considerations
Consider the recommendations relevant to all adrenergics as well as the following:
- Administer last daily dose several hours before bedtime to minimize insomnia.
- If symptoms persist longer than 5 days or fever is present, reevaluate therapy.

Therapeutic monitoring
- Observe patient for complaints of headache or dizziness.
- Monitor blood pressure.

Special populations
Breast-feeding patients. Drug may be excreted in breast milk; avoid use in breast-feeding women.
Pediatric patients. Don't use extended-release form in children under age 12.
Geriatric patients. Geriatric patients may be sensitive to effects of drug; lower dose may be needed. Overdose may cause hallucinations, CNS depression, seizures, and death in patients over age 60. Use extended-release preparations with caution in geriatric patients.

Patient counseling
- If it's difficult for patient to swallow medication, suggest opening capsules and mixing contents with applesauce, jelly, honey, or syrup. Mixture must be swallowed without chewing.
- Suggest using ice chips, sugarless gum, or hard candy for relief of dry mouth.

■ Instruct patient to take missed dose if remembered within 1 hour. If beyond 1 hour, patient should skip dose and resume regular schedule; patient shouldn't double the dose.
■ Tell patient to store drug away from heat and light (not in bathroom medicine cabinet) and safely out of reach of children.
■ Caution patient that many OTC preparations may contain sympathomimetics, which can cause additive, hazardous reactions.
■ Advise patient to take last dose at least 2 to 3 hours before bedtime to avoid insomnia.

psyllium

Cillium, Fiberall, Hydrocil Instant, Konsyl, Konsyl-D, Metamucil, Naturacil, Reguloid, Serutan, Syllact, V-Lax

Pharmacologic classification: adsorbent
Therapeutic classification: bulk laxative
Pregnancy risk category C

How supplied

Available without a prescription
Powder: 3.3 g/teaspoon, 3.4 g/teaspoon, 3.5 g/teaspoon, 4.94 g/teaspoon
Powder (effervescent): 3.4 g/packet, 3.7 g/packet
Granules: 2.5 g/teaspoon, 4.03 g/teaspoon
Wafers: 1.7 g/wafer, 3.4 g/wafer

Indications and dosages

Constipation, bowel management, irritable bowel syndrome
Adults: 1 to 2 rounded tsp P.O. in full glass of liquid daily, b.i.d. or t.i.d., followed by second glass of liquid; or 1 packet P.O. dissolved in water daily; or 2 wafers b.i.d., or t.i.d.
Children over age 6: 1 level tsp P.O. in ½ glass of liquid h.s.

Pharmacodynamics

Laxative action: Psyllium adsorbs water in the gut; it also serves as a source of indigestible fiber, increasing stool bulk and moisture, stimulating peristaltic activity and bowel evacuation.

Pharmacokinetics

Absorption: None; onset of action varies from 12 hours to 3 days.
Distribution: Distributed locally in the gut.
Metabolism: Not metabolized.
Excretion: Excreted in feces.

Route	Onset	Peak	Duration
P.O.	12-24 hr	3 days	Variable

Contraindications and precautions

Contraindicated in patients with hypersensitivity to drug, abdominal pain, nausea, vomiting, or other symptoms of appendicitis and in those with intestinal obstruction or ulceration, disabling adhesions, or difficulty swallowing.

Interactions

None reported.

Effects on diagnostic tests

None reported.

Adverse reactions

GI: nausea, vomiting, diarrhea (with excessive use); esophageal, gastric, small intestinal, and rectal obstruction when drug is taken in dry form; abdominal cramps, especially in severe constipation.

Overdose and treatment

No cases of overdose have been reported; probable clinical effects include abdominal pain and diarrhea.

Clinical considerations

■ Before administering drug, add at least 8 oz (240 ml) of water or juice and stir for a few seconds to improve taste. Have patient drink mixture immediately to prevent it from congealing; then have him drink another glass of fluid.
■ Separate administration of psyllium and oral anticoagulants, cardiac glycosides, and salicylates by at least 2 hours.
■ Drug may reduce appetite if administered before meals.
■ Psyllium and other bulk laxatives most closely mimic natural bowel function and don't cause laxative dependence; they're especially useful for patients with postpartum constipation or diverticular disease, for debilitated patients, for irritable bowel syndrome, and for chronic laxative users.

Therapeutic monitoring

Inform patient that laxative effect usually occurs in 12 to 24 hours but may be delayed 3 days.

Special populations

Breast-feeding patients. Because drug isn't absorbed, it presumably is safe for use in breast-feeding women.

Patient counseling

■ Warn patient not to swallow drug in dry form; he should mix it with at least 8 oz (240 ml) of fluid, stir briefly, drink immediately (to prevent mixture from congealing), and follow it with another 8 oz of fluid.
■ Explain that drug may reduce appetite if taken before meals; recommend taking drug 2

hours after meals and any other oral medication.

- Advise diabetic patients and those with restricted sodium or sugar intake to avoid psyllium products containing salt or sugar. Advise patients who must restrict phenylalanine intake to avoid psyllium products containing aspartame.

pyrantel pamoate

Antiminth, Combantrin*, Pin-X, Reese's Pinworm

Pharmacologic classification: pyrimidine derivative
Therapeutic classification: anthelmintic
Pregnancy risk category C

How supplied

Available by prescription only
Oral suspension: 250 mg/5ml
Tablets: 62.5 mg

Indications and dosages

Roundworm and pinworm infections
Adults and children over age 2: Single dose of 11 mg/kg P.O. Maximum dose is 1 g. For pinworm infection, dosage should be repeated in 2 weeks.

Pharmacodynamics

Anthelmintic action: Pyrantel causes the release of acetylcholine and inhibits cholinesterases, paralyzing the worms. It's active against *Ancylostoma duodenale, Ascaris lumbricoides, Enterobius vermicularis, Necator americanus,* and *Trichostrongylus orientalis.*

Pharmacokinetics

Absorption: Absorbed poorly.
Distribution: Little is known.
Metabolism: Small amount of absorbed drug is metabolized partially in the liver.
Excretion: More than 50% of an oral dose is excreted unchanged in feces; about 7% is excreted in urine as unchanged drug or known metabolites.

Route	Onset	Peak	Duration
P.O.	Variable	1-3 hr	Variable

Contraindications and precautions

Contraindicated in patients with hypersensitivity to drug. Use cautiously in patients with hepatic dysfunction or severe malnutrition or anemia.

Interactions

Drug-drug. *Piperazine:* Pyrantel pamoate antagonizes the effects of piperazine. Don't give together.

Effects on diagnostic tests

None reported.

Adverse reactions

CNS: headache, dizziness, drowsiness, insomnia.
GI: anorexia, nausea, vomiting, gastralgia, abdominal cramps, diarrhea, tenesmus.
Hepatic: transient elevation of AST.
Skin: rash.
Other: fever, weakness.

Overdose and treatment

Treatment of overdose is largely supportive, particularly of CV and respiratory functions. After recent ingestion (within 4 hours), empty stomach by induced emesis or gastric lavage. Follow with activated charcoal to decrease absorption. Osmotic cathartics may be helpful.

Clinical considerations

- Shake suspension well before measuring, to ensure accurate dosage.
- Drug may be given with milk, fruit juice, or food.
- Protect drug from light.
- Treat all family members.

Therapeutic monitoring

Be alert for signs of reinfection.

Special populations

Pregnant patients. Use drug during pregnancy only when clearly needed, because no adequate and controlled studies have been done in pregnant women.
Breast-feeding patients. Safety in breast-feeding women hasn't been established.
Pediatric patients. Safety and efficacy for children under age 2 haven't been established.

Patient counseling

- Tell patient to wash perianal area daily and to change undergarments and bedclothes daily.
- To help prevent reinfection, instruct patient and family members in personal hygiene, including sanitary disposal of feces as well as hand washing and nail cleaning after defecation and before handling, preparing, or eating food.
- Explain routes of transmission and tell patient to encourage other household members and suspected contacts to be tested.

pyrazinamide

pms-Pyrazinamide*, Tebrazid*

Pharmacologic classification: synthetic pyrazine analogue of nicotinamide
Therapeutic classification: antituberculotic
Pregnancy risk category C

How supplied

Available by prescription only
Tablets: 500 mg

Indications and dosages

Adjunctive treatment of tuberculosis (when primary and secondary antitubercular drugs can't be used or have failed)
Adults: 15 to 30 mg/kg P.O. daily, in one or more doses. Maximum dose is 3 g daily. Alternatively, a twice-weekly dose of 50 to 70 mg/kg (based on lean body weight) has been developed to promote patient compliance. Lower dosage is recommended in decreased renal function.

Pharmacodynamics

Antibiotic action: Mechanism of action is unknown; drug may be bactericidal or bacteriostatic depending on organism susceptibility and drug concentration at infection site. Pyrazinamide is active only against *Mycobacterium tuberculosis.* Pyrazinamide is considered adjunctive in tuberculosis therapy and is given with other drugs to prevent or delay development of resistance to pyrazinamide by *M. tuberculosis.*

Pharmacokinetics

Absorption: Well absorbed after oral administration.
Distribution: Distributed widely into body tissues and fluids, including lungs, liver, and CSF; drug is 50% protein-bound. It isn't known if it crosses the placenta.
Metabolism: Hydrolyzed in the liver; some hydrolysis occurs in stomach.
Excretion: Excreted almost completely in urine by glomerular filtration. It isn't known if drug is excreted in breast milk. Elimination half-life in adults is 9 to 10 hours. Half-life is prolonged in renal and hepatic impairment.

Route	Onset	Peak	Duration
P.O.	Unknown	1-2 hr	Unknown

Contraindications and precautions

Contraindicated in patients with hypersensitivity to drug, severe hepatic disease, or acute gout. Use cautiously in patients with diabetes mellitus, renal failure, or gout.

Interactions

Drug-lifestyle. *Sun exposure:* May cause photosensitivity reactions; advise patient to take precautions.

Effects on diagnostic tests

Pyrazinamide may interfere with urine ketone determinations. Systemic effects of drug may temporarily decrease 17-ketosteroid levels; it may increase protein-bound iodine and urate levels and results of liver enzyme tests.

Adverse reactions

GI: anorexia, nausea, vomiting.
GU: dysuria.
Hematologic: sideroblastic anemia, ***thrombocytopenia.***
Skin: rash, urticaria, pruritus, photosensitivity.
Other: malaise, fever, porphyria, hyperuricemia and gout, interstitial nephritis, *arthralgia, myalgia,* ***hepatitis.***

Overdose and treatment

No specific recommendations are available. Treatment is supportive. After recent ingestion (4 hours or less), empty stomach by induced emesis or gastric lavage. Follow with activated charcoal to decrease absorption.

Clinical considerations

- In patients with diabetes mellitus, pyrazinamide therapy may hinder stabilization of serum glucose levels.
- In many cases, drug elevates serum uric acid levels. Although usually asymptomatic, a uricosuric agent, such as probenecid or allopurinol, may be necessary.
- Patients with concomitant infection HIV may require a longer course of treatment.

Therapeutic monitoring

Recommend monitoring liver function, especially enzyme and bilirubin levels, and renal function, especially serum uric acid levels, before therapy and thereafter at 2- to 4-week intervals; observe patient for signs of liver damage or decreased renal function.

Special populations

Breast-feeding patients. Safety in breast-feeding women hasn't been established. Alternative feeding method is recommended during therapy.
Pediatric patients. Drug isn't recommended for use in children.
Geriatric patients. Because geriatric patients commonly have diminished renal function, which decreases drug excretion, use pyrazinamide with caution.

Patient counseling

- Explain disease process and rationale for long-term therapy.

- Teach signs and symptoms of hypersensitivity and other adverse reactions, and emphasize need to report them; urge patient to report unusual reactions, especially signs of gout.
- Be sure patient understands how and when to take drugs; urge patient to complete entire prescribed regimen, to comply with instructions for around-the-clock dosage, and to keep follow-up appointments.

pyridostigmine bromide

Mestinon, Regonol

Pharmacologic classification: cholinesterase inhibitor
Therapeutic classification: muscle stimulant
Pregnancy risk category NR

How supplied

Available by prescription only
Tablets: 60 mg
Tablets (sustained-release): 180 mg
Syrup: 60 mg/5 ml
Injection: 5 mg/ml in 2-ml ampule or 5-ml vial

Indications and dosages

Reversal of the effects of nondepolarizing agents, curariform antagonist (postoperatively)
Adults: 10 to 20 mg I.V. preceded by atropine sulfate 0.6 to 1.2 mg I.V.
Myasthenia gravis
Adults: 60 to 180 mg P.O. b.i.d. or q.i.d. Usual dose 600 mg daily, but higher doses may be needed (up to 1,500 mg daily). Give one-thirtieth of oral dose I.M. or I.V. Adjust dosage based on patient response and tolerance of adverse effects. Sustained-release and rapid-release forms are often used together depending on patient's symptoms.
Children: 7 mg/kg/24 hours P.O. divided into five or six doses.
Neonates of myasthenic mothers: 0.05 to 0.15 mg/kg I.M.

Pharmacodynamics

Muscle stimulant action: Pyridostigmine blocks hydrolysis of acetylcholine by cholinesterase, resulting in acetylcholine accumulation at cholinergic synapses, increasing stimulation of cholinergic receptors at the myoneural junction.

Pharmacokinetics

Absorption: Poorly absorbed from the GI tract.
Distribution: Little is known; however, drug may cross the placenta, especially when administered in large doses.
Metabolism: Exact metabolic fate is unknown. Duration of effect is usually 3 to 6 hours after oral dose and 2 to 3 hours after I.V. dose, depending on patient's physical and emotional status and disease severity. Pyridostigmine is hydrolyzed by cholinesterase.
Excretion: Excreted in urine.

Route	Onset	Peak	Duration
P.O.	20-30 min	1-2 hr	3-6 hr
P.O. (extended)	30-60 min	1-2 hr	6-12 hr
I.V.	2-5 min	Unknown	2-4 hr
I.M.	15 min	Unknown	2-4 hr

Contraindications and precautions

Contraindicated in patients with hypersensitivity to anticholinesterase agents and in those with mechanical obstruction of the intestine or urinary tract. Use cautiously in patients with bronchial asthma, bradycardia, and arrhythmias.

Interactions

Drug-drug. *Aminoglycoside antibiotics:* Have a mild but definite nondepolarizing blocking action that may accentuate neuromuscular block. Use together cautiously.
Corticosteroids: May decrease cholinergic effect of pyridostigmine; when corticosteroids are stopped, this effect may increase, possibly affecting muscle strength. Monitor patient closely.
Ganglionic blockers: May critically decrease blood pressure; effect is usually preceded by abdominal symptoms. Monitor patient closely.
Magnesium: Has a direct depressant effect on skeletal muscle and may antagonize beneficial effects of pyridostigmine. Use together cautiously. Monitor patient closely.
Procainamide, quinidine: May reverse cholinergic effect of pyridostigmine on muscle. Monitor for drug effect.
Succinylcholine: May result in prolonged respiratory depression from plasma esterase inhibition, delaying succinylcholine hydrolysis. Use together cautiously.

Effects on diagnostic tests

None reported.

Adverse reactions

CNS: headache (with high doses), weakness.
CV: bradycardia, hypotension, thrombophlebitis.
EENT: miosis.
GI: abdominal cramps, nausea, vomiting, diarrhea, excessive salivation, increased peristalsis.
Musculoskeletal: muscle cramps, muscle fasciculations.
Respiratory: ***bronchospasm, bronchoconstriction,*** increased bronchial secretions.
Skin: rash, diaphoresis.

Overdose and treatment
Clinical effects of overdose include nausea, vomiting, diarrhea, blurred vision, miosis, excessive tearing, bronchospasm, increased bronchial secretions, hypotension, incoordination, excessive sweating, muscle weakness, cramps, fasciculations, paralysis, bradycardia or tachycardia, excessive salivation, and restlessness or agitation.

Support respiration; bronchial suctioning may be performed. Discontinue drug immediately. Atropine may be given to block muscarinic effects of pyridostigmine; however, it won't counter skeletal muscle paralysis. Avoid atropine overdose because it may lead to bronchial plug formation.

Clinical considerations
Consider the recommendations relevant to all cholinesterase inhibitors, including the following:
- If muscle weakness is severe, determine whether this effect stems from drug toxicity or exacerbation of myasthenia gravis. A test dose of edrophonium I.V. will aggravate drug-induced weakness but will temporarily relieve weakness that results from the disease.
- Avoid giving large doses to patients with decreased GI motility because toxicity may result once motility has been restored.
- Give drug with food or milk to reduce risk of muscarinic adverse effects.
- Atropine sulfate should always be readily available as an antagonist for the muscarinic effects of pyridostigmine.

Therapeutic monitoring
Patients may develop resistance to drug. Monitor patient closely.

Special populations
Breast-feeding patients. It isn't known if drug is excreted in breast milk. Because of the potential for serious adverse reactions in the breast-fed infant, either breast-feeding or drug should be discontinued, taking into account the importance of drug to the woman.

Patient counseling
- When drug is used in patient with myasthenia gravis, stress importance of taking drug exactly as ordered, on time, and in evenly spaced doses.
- If patient is taking sustained-release tablets, explain how these work and instruct him to take them at the same time each day and to swallow these tablets whole rather than crushing them.
- Teach patient how to evaluate muscle strength; instruct him to observe changes in muscle strength and to report muscle cramps, rash, or fatigue.

pyridoxine hydrochloride (vitamin B_6)
Nestrex

Pharmacologic classification: water-soluble vitamin
Therapeutic classification: nutritional supplement
Pregnancy risk category A (C if greater than RDA)

How supplied
Available by prescription only
Injection: 10-ml vial (100 mg/ml), 30-ml vial (100 mg/ml), 10-ml vial (100 mg/ml, with 1.5% benzyl alcohol), 30-ml vial (100 mg/ml, with 1.5% benzyl alcohol), 10-ml vial (100 mg/ml, with 0.5% chlorobutanol), 1-ml vial (100 mg/ml)
Available without a prescription
Tablets: 10 mg, 25 mg, 50 mg, 100 mg, 200 mg, 250 mg, 500 mg, 500 mg timed-release

Indications and dosages
RDA
Neonates and infants to age 6 months: 0.3 mg daily.
Infants age 6 months to 1 year: 0.6 mg daily.
Children age 1 to 3: 1 mg daily.
Children age 4 to 6: 1.1 mg daily.
Children age 7 to 10: 1.4 mg daily.
Girls age 11 to 14: 1.4 mg daily.
Girls age 15 to 18: 1.5 mg daily.
Women age 19 and older: 1.6 mg daily.
Women during pregnancy: 2.2 mg daily.
Breast-feeding women: 2.1 mg daily.
Boys age 11 to 14: 1.7 mg daily.
Men age 15 and older: 2 mg daily.
Dietary vitamin B_6 deficiency
Adults: 2.5 to 10 mg P.O. daily until signs of deficiency are corrected, then 2 to 5 mg daily as a multivitamin preparation for several weeks.
Drug-induced deficiency anemia or neuritis
Adults: 100 to 200 mg P.O. daily for 3 weeks. Then 25 to 100 mg daily.
Pyridoxine-dependent seizures
Neonates and infants: 10 to 100 mg I.M. or I.V.
◇***Premenstrual syndrome***
Adults: 40 to 500 mg P.O., I.M., or I.V. daily.

◇ ***Hyperoxaluria type I***
Adults: 25 to 300 mg P.O., I.M., or I.V. daily.
Seizures secondary to isoniazid overdose
Adults and children: A dose of pyridoxine hydrochloride equal to the amount of isoniazid ingested is usually given; generally, 1 to 4 g I.V. initially and then 1 g I.M. every 30 minutes until the entire dose has been given.

Pharmacodynamics
Metabolic action: Natural vitamin B_6 contained in plant and animal foodstuffs is converted to physiologically active forms of vitamin B_6, pyridoxal phosphate, and pyridoxamine phosphate. Exogenous forms of the vitamin are metabolized. Vitamin B_6 acts as a coenzyme in protein, carbohydrate, and fat metabolism and participates in the decarboxylation of amino acids in protein metabolism. Vitamin B_6 also helps convert tryptophan to niacin as well as facilitate the deamination, transamination, and transulfuration of amino acids. Finally, vitamin B_6 is responsible for the breakdown of glycogen to glucose-1-phosphate in carbohydrate metabolism. The total adult body store consists of 16 to 27 mg of pyridoxine. The need for pyridoxine increases with the amount of protein in the diet.

Pharmacokinetics
Absorption: After oral administration, pyridoxine and its substituents are absorbed readily from the GI tract. GI absorption may be diminished in patients with malabsorption syndromes or following gastric resection. Normal serum levels of pyridoxine are 30 to 80 ng/ml.
Distribution: Stored mainly in the liver. The total body store is about 16 to 27 mg. Pyridoxal and pyridoxal phosphate are the most common forms found in the blood and are highly protein-bound. Pyridoxal crosses the placenta; fetal plasma levels are five times greater than maternal plasma levels. After maternal intake of 2.5 to 5 mg/day of pyridoxine, the level of the vitamin in breast milk is about 240 ng/ml.
Metabolism: Degraded to 4-pyridoxic acid in the liver.
Excretion: In erythrocytes, pyridoxine is converted to pyridoxal phosphate, and pyridoxamine is converted to pyridoxamine phosphate. The phosphorylated form of pyridoxine is transaminated to pyridoxal and pyridoxamine, which is phosphorylated rapidly. The conversion of pyridoxine phosphate to pyridoxal phosphate requires riboflavin. Biologic half-life is 15 to 20 days.

Route	Onset	Peak	Duration
P.O., I.V., I.M.	Unknown	Unknown	Unknown

Contraindications and precautions
Contraindicated in patients hypersensitive to pyridoxine.

Interactions
Drug-drug. *Cycloserine, hydralazine, isoniazid, oral contraceptives, penicillamine:* May increase pyridoxine requirements. Monitor patient closely.
Levodopa: Pyridoxine reverses the therapeutic effects of levodopa. Avoid use together.
Phenobarbital, phenytoin: May cause a 50% decrease in serum levels of these anticonvulsants. Avoid use together.

Effects on diagnostic tests
Pyridoxine therapy alters determinations for urobilinogen in the spot test using Ehrlich's reagent, resulting in a false-positive reaction.

Adverse reactions
CNS: paresthesia, unsteady gait, numbness, somnolence.

Overdose and treatment
Signs of overdose include ataxia and severe sensory neuropathy after chronic consumption of high daily doses of pyridoxine (2 to 6 g). These neurologic deficits usually resolve after pyridoxine is discontinued.

Clinical considerations
- Prepare a dietary history. A single vitamin deficiency is unusual; lack of one vitamin often indicates a deficiency of others.
- Don't mix with sodium bicarbonate in the same syringe.
- Store in a tight, light-resistant container.
- Don't use injection solution if it contains precipitate. Slight darkening is acceptable.
- Pyridoxine is sometimes useful for treating nausea and vomiting during pregnancy.

Therapeutic monitoring
- Monitor protein intake; excessive protein intake increases pyridoxine requirements.
- A dosage of 25 mg/kg/day is well tolerated. Adults consuming 200 mg/day for 33 days and on a normal dietary intake develop vitamin B_6 dependency.

Special populations
Breast-feeding patients. It's unknown if drug is excreted in breast milk. Use caution when administering to breast-feeding women. Pyridoxine may inhibit lactation by suppression of prolactin.
Pediatric patients. Safety and efficacy in children haven't been established. The use of large doses of pyridoxine during pregnancy has been implicated in pyridoxine-dependency seizures in neonates.

Patient counseling
Teach patient about dietary sources of vitamin B_6, such as yeast, wheat germ, liver, whole grain cereals, bananas, and legumes.

pyrimethamine

Daraprim

Pharmacologic classification: aminopyrimidine derivative (folic acid antagonist)
Therapeutic classification: antimalarial
Pregnancy risk category C

How supplied

Available by prescription only
Tablets: 25 mg

Indications and dosages

Chemoprophylaxis of malaria
Adults and children over age 10: 25 mg P.O. weekly.
Children age 4 to 10: 12.5 mg P.O. weekly.
Children under age 4: 6.25 mg P.O. weekly.

Dosage should be continued for all age-groups for at least 10 weeks after leaving endemic areas.

Treatment of acute malaria
Not recommended alone for treatment. 25 mg P.O. once daily for 2 days with a sulfonamide to initiate transmission control and suppression of non-*falciparum* malaria. If drug must be used alone in semi-immune patients:
Adults: 50 mg P.O. daily for 2 days followed by 25 mg once weekly for at least 10 weeks.
Children age 4 to 10: 25 mg P.O. once daily for 2 days followed by 12.5 mg once weekly for at least 10 weeks.

Toxoplasmosis
Adults: Initially, 50 to 75 mg P.O. daily with sulfonamide 1 to 4 g P.O. daily for 1 to 3 weeks. Then may decrease dose of each drug 50% and continue for an additional 4 to 5 weeks.
Children: 1 mg/kg/day P.O. divided in 2 equal doses. After 2 to 4 days may decrease dose 50% to 0.5 mg/kg/day and continue treatment for 1 month.

◊ ***Primary prophylaxis against toxoplasmosis in patients with HIV infection***
Adults and adolescents: 50 mg P.O. once weekly with leucovorin and dapsone. Or, 25 mg P.O. once daily with leucovorin and atovaquone.

◊ ***Secondary prophylaxis of toxoplasmosis in patients with HIV infection***
Adults and adolescents: 25 to 75 mg P.O. once daily with leucovorin and sulfadiazine. Or, 25 mg P.O. daily with leucovorin and atovaquone.

◊ ***Isosporiasis***
Adults: 50 to 75 mg P.O. daily.

Pharmacodynamics

Antimalarial action: Pyrimethamine inhibits the reduction of dihydrofolate to tetrahydrofolate, blocking folic acid metabolism needed for survival of susceptible organisms. This mechanism is distinct from sulfonamide-induced folic acid antagonism. Pyrimethamine is active against the asexual erythrocytic forms of susceptible plasmodia and against *Toxoplasma gondii.*

Pharmacokinetics

Absorption: Well absorbed from the intestinal tract.
Distribution: Distributed to the kidneys, liver, spleen, and lungs; drug is about 80% bound to plasma proteins.
Metabolism: Metabolized to several unidentified compounds.
Excretion: Excreted in the urine and in breast milk; elimination half-life is 2 to 6 days. Its half-life isn't changed in end-stage renal disease.

Route	Onset	Peak	Duration
P.O.	Unknown	1½-8 hr	2 wk

Contraindications and precautions

Contraindicated in patients with hypersensitivity to drug and in those with megaloblastic anemia caused by folic acid deficiency.

Use cautiously in patients with impaired renal or hepatic function, severe allergy or bronchial asthma, G6PD deficiency, or seizure disorders and in those following treatment with chloroquine.

Interactions

Drug-drug. *Co-trimoxazole, sulfonamides:* Act synergistically against some organisms because each inhibits folic acid synthesis at a different level. Don't use together.
Folic acid, para-aminobenzoic acid: Reduce the antitoxoplasmic effects of pyrimethamine and may require higher dosage of the latter drug.
Lorazepam: Mild hepatotoxicity has been reported in patients who were also given lorazepam. Monitor patient closely.

Effects on diagnostic tests

None reported.

Adverse reactions

GI: anorexia, vomiting, atrophic glossitis.
Hematologic: ***aplastic anemia,*** megaloblastic anemia, leukopenia, ***thrombocytopenia, pancytopenia.***

Note: Adverse drug reactions related to sulfadiazine are similar to those related to sulfonamides.

Overdose and treatment

Overdose is marked by anorexia, vomiting, and CNS stimulation, including seizures. Megaloblastic anemia, thrombocytopenia, leukopenia, glossitis, and crystalluria may also occur.

Treatment of overdose consists of gastric lavage followed by a cathartic; barbiturates may help to control seizures. Leucovorin (folinic acid) in a dosage of 5 to 15 mg/day P.O.,

I.M., or I.V. for 3 days or longer is used to restore decreased platelet or leukocyte counts.

Clinical considerations

- No longer considered a first-line antimalarial agent. Other antimalarial drugs, such as mefloquine, chloroquine, and sulfadoxine, are generally preferred.
- Give drug with meals to minimize GI distress.
- Because severe reactions may occur, give pyrimethamine with sulfadoxine only in unusual situations in which the recommended agents cannot be used.

Therapeutic monitoring

- Monitor CBC, including platelet counts twice weekly.
- Monitor patient for signs of folate deficiency or bleeding when platelet count is low; if abnormalities appear, decrease dosage or discontinue drug. Leucovorin (folinic acid) may be prescribed to raise blood counts during reduced dosage or after drug is discontinued.

Special populations

Breast-feeding patients. Pyrimethamine and sulfadoxine combination is contraindicated in breast-feeding women because it contains a sulfonamide.
Pediatric patients. Use with caution in children.

Patient counseling

- Teach patient how to recognize signs and symptoms of adverse blood reactions and tell him to report them immediately. Teach emergency measures to control overt bleeding.
- Teach patient signs and symptoms of folate deficiency.
- Counsel patient about need to report adverse effects and to keep follow-up medical appointments.
- Tell patient to keep drug out of reach of children.

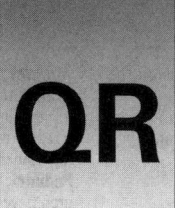

quetiapine fumarate

Seroquel

Pharmacologic classification: dibenzothiazepine derivative
Therapeutic classification: antipsychotic
Pregnancy risk category C

How supplied

Available by prescription only
Tablets: 25 mg, 100 mg, 200 mg

Indications and dosages

Management of signs and symptoms of psychotic disorders
Adults: Initially, 25 mg P.O. b.i.d., with increases in increments of 25 to 50 mg b.i.d. or t.i.d. on days 2 and 3, as tolerated to a target dosage range of 300 to 400 mg daily by day 4, divided into two or three doses. Further dosage adjustments, if indicated, should generally occur at intervals of not less than 2 days. Dosages can be increased or decreased by 25 to 50 mg b.i.d. Antipsychotic efficacy is generally in dosage range of 150 to 750 mg/day. Safety of doses above 800 mg/day hasn't been evaluated.
≡ ***Dosage adjustment.*** In geriatric or debilitated patients or those who have hepatic impairment or a predisposition to hypotensive reactions, consider lower doses, slower dosage adjustment, and careful monitoring during initial dosing period. No specific dosing recommendations are given.

Pharmacodynamics

Antipsychotic action: Exact mechanism of action is unknown. Quetiapine is a dibenzothiazepine derivative that is thought to exert antipsychotic activity through antagonism of dopamine type 2 (D_2) and serotonin type 2 (5-HT_2) receptors. Antagonism at serotonin 5-HT_{1A}, D_1, H_1, and alpha$_1$- and alpha$_2$-adrenergic receptors may explain other effects.

Pharmacokinetics

Absorption: Rapidly absorbed after oral administration. Absorption is affected by food, with maximum level increasing 25% and bioavailability increasing 15%.
Distribution: Apparent volume of distribution is 10 ± 4 L/kg. Drug is 83% plasma-protein bound. Steady-state levels are reached within 2 days.
Metabolism: Extensively metabolized by the liver via sulfoxidation and oxidation. Cytochrome P-450 3A4 is the major isoenzyme involved.
Excretion: Less than 1% of dose is excreted as unchanged drug. About 73% is recovered in urine and 20% in feces. Mean terminal half-life is about 6 hours.

Route	Onset	Peak	Duration
P.O.	Unknown	1½ hr	Unknown

Contraindications and precautions

Contraindicated in patients hypersensitive to drug or its ingredients.

Use cautiously in patients with known CV or cerebrovascular disease or conditions that would predispose patient to hypotension, in patients with history of seizures or with conditions that potentially lower the seizure threshold, and in those at risk for aspiration pneumonia because of associated esophageal dysmotility and aspiration. Also use with caution in patients with conditions that may contribute to an elevation in core body temperature.

Interactions

Drug-drug. *Antihypertensives:* May potentiate the hypotensive effect of both drugs. Monitor blood pressure.
Cimetidine, phenytoin, thioridazine: Increase the mean oral clearance of quetiapine. Quetiapine dose may need adjustment.
CNS depressants: Increased CNS effects. Use cautiously.
Dopamine agonists, levodopa: Quetiapine may antagonize the effect of these drugs. Monitor patient closely.
Erythromycin, fluconazole, itraconazole, ketoconazole: Decreased quetiapine clearance. Use with caution.
Lorazepam: Reduced clearance when coadministered with quetiapine. Monitor patient.
Drug-lifestyle. *Alcohol use:* May cause potentiated cognitive and motor effects. Advise patient to avoid use of alcohol during quetiapine therapy.

Effects on diagnostic tests

None reported.

Adverse reactions

CNS: *dizziness, headache, somnolence,* hypertonia, asthenia, dysarthria.

CV: orthostatic hypotension, tachycardia, palpitations, peripheral edema.
EENT: pharyngitis, rhinitis, ear pain.
GI: dry mouth, dyspepsia, abdominal pain, constipation, anorexia.
Hematologic: ***leukopenia.***
Metabolic: *weight gain.*
Musculoskeletal: back pain.
Respiratory: increased cough, dyspnea.
Skin: rash, diaphoresis.
Other: fever, flulike syndrome.

Overdose and treatment

Usually exaggeration of pharmacologic effects of drug is seen (drowsiness, sedation, tachycardia, hypotension). Hypokalemia and first-degree heart block may also occur.

For acute overdose, treatment includes establishing and maintaining an airway to ensure adequate oxygenation and ventilation. Consider gastric lavage and administration of activated charcoal or a laxative. Begin CV monitoring, including ECG monitoring, immediately. Avoid use of disopyramide, procainamide, quinidine, and bretylium if antiarrhythmic therapy is indicated. Administer I.V. fluids or sympathomimetic agents (not epinephrine or dopamine) to treat hypotension and circulatory collapse. For severe extrapyramidal symptoms, administer anticholinergic agents.

Clinical considerations

- A decrease in total and free T_4 may occur; this is usually not clinically significant. Although rare, some patients experience increased thyroid-stimulating hormone and require thyroid replacement.
- Increases in cholesterol and triglycerides have been observed.
- Asymptomatic, transient, and reversible increases in serum transaminases (primarily ALT) have been reported. These elevations usually occur within the first 3 weeks of therapy and promptly return to pretreatment levels with continued use.
- Neuroleptic malignant syndrome, a potentially fatal syndrome, has been reported with use of antipsychotic drugs. Signs and symptoms include hyperpyrexia, muscle rigidity, altered mental status, and evidence of autonomic instability. Carefully monitor at-risk patients.
- Use smallest effective dose for shortest duration to minimize risk of tardive dyskinesia.

Therapeutic monitoring

- Recommend examining the lens before therapy begins or shortly thereafter, and at 6-month intervals during chronic treatment for possible cataract formation.
- Closely supervise schizophrenic patient during drug therapy because of the inherent risk of a suicide attempt.

Special populations

Pregnant patients. Instruct women to report if pregnancy is being planned or is suspected.
Breast-feeding patients. Breast-feeding isn't recommended during quetiapine therapy.
Pediatric patients. Safety and efficacy in children haven't been established.
Geriatric patients. There appears to be no difference in tolerability in patients age 65 or older. However, factors that may decrease pharmacokinetic clearance, increase pharmacodynamic response to the drug, or cause poorer tolerance or orthostasis should indicate use of a lower starting dose, slower dosage adjustment, and careful monitoring during the initial dosing period.

Patient counseling

- Advise patient of risk of orthostatic hypotension, especially during the 3- to 5-day period of initial dose adjustment and when dose is increased or treatment reinitiated.
- Tell patient to avoid becoming overheated or dehydrated.
- During initial dose adjustment period or dosage increases, warn patient to avoid activities that require mental alertness such as driving a car or operating hazardous machinery until CNS effects of drug are known.
- Remind patient to have an initial eye examination at beginning of drug therapy and every 6 months during treatment period to monitor for cataract formation.
- Tell patient to contact his health care provider before taking other prescription or OTC drugs.

quinapril hydrochloride

Accupril

Pharmacologic classification: ACE inhibitor
Therapeutic classification: antihypertensive
Pregnancy risk category C (D second and third trimesters)

How supplied

Available by prescription only
Tablets: 5 mg, 10 mg, 20 mg, 40 mg

Indications and dosages

Heart failure
Adults: Initially, 5 mg P.O. b.i.d., given in conjunction with a cardiac glycoside, diuretic, and a beta blocker. Adjust dosage weekly based on response. Usual dose is 20 to 40 mg P.O. daily in two equally divided doses.
Hypertension in patients not receiving a diuretic
Adults: Initially, 10 mg P.O. daily. Adjust dosage based on response at intervals of about 2 weeks. Most patients are controlled at 20, 40, or 80

mg daily, as a single dose or in two divided doses.

≡ ***Dosage adjustment.*** In adults with renal impairment, initial dose is 10 mg P.O. daily if creatinine clearance exceeds 60 ml/minute; 5 mg if it's 30 to 60 ml/minute; and 2.5 mg if it's 10 to 30 ml/minute. No dose recommendations are available for creatinine clearance less than 10 ml/minute.

Pharmacodynamics

Antihypertensive action: Quinapril and its active metabolite, quinaprilat, inhibit angiotensin-converting enzyme (ACE), preventing conversion of angiotensin I to angiotensin II, a potent vasoconstrictor. Reduced formation of angiotensin II decreases peripheral arterial resistance, decreases aldosterone secretion, reduces sodium and water retention, and lowers blood pressure. Quinapril also has antihypertensive activity in patients with low-renin hypertension.

Pharmacokinetics

Absorption: At least 60% of drug is absorbed. Rate and extent of absorption are decreased 25% to 30% when drug is administered during a high-fat meal.
Distribution: About 97% of drug and active metabolite are bound to plasma proteins.
Metabolism: About 38% of an oral dose is deesterified in the liver to quinaprilat, the active metabolite.
Excretion: Primarily excreted in urine; terminal elimination half-life is about 25 hours.

Route	Onset	Peak	Duration
P.O.	1 hr	2-6 hr	24 hr

Contraindications and precautions

Contraindicated in patients with hypersensitivity to ACE inhibitors or who have a history of angioedema related to treatment with an ACE inhibitor. Use cautiously in patients with impaired renal function. Also contraindicated in patients at immediate risk for cardiogenic shock.

Interactions

Drug-drug. *Diuretics, other antihypertensives:* Increase risk of excessive hypotension. Discontinue diuretic or lower dose of quinapril as needed.
Lithium: Increased serum lithium levels and lithium toxicity. Monitor serum lithium levels.
Potassium-sparing diuretics and potassium supplements: May increase risk of hyperkalemia. Don't use together.
Tetracycline: Significantly impairs absorption of tetracycline. Avoid use together.
Drug-food. *Potassium-containing salt-substitutes:* Can cause hyperkalemia. Don't use together.

Effects on diagnostic tests

None reported.

Adverse reactions

CNS: somnolence, vertigo, nervousness, headache, dizziness, fatigue, depression.
CV: palpitations, tachycardia, angina, hypertensive crisis, orthostatic hypotension, chest pain, *rhythm disturbances.*
GI: dry mouth, abdominal pain, constipation, vomiting, nausea, hemorrhage.
Hematologic: thrombocytopenia, agranulocytosis.
Hepatic: elevated liver enzymes.
Respiratory: *dry, persistent, tickling, nonproductive cough.*
Skin: pruritus, ***exfoliative dermatitis,*** *photosensitivity,* diaphoresis.
Other: ***angioedema,*** hyperkalemia.

Overdose and treatment

No information is available regarding overdose. The most likely symptom is hypotension.

Peritoneal dialysis or hemodialysis isn't beneficial. No data are available to support use of certain physiologic maneuvers such as acidification of urine. Treat symptomatically. Infusions of normal saline solution have been suggested to treat hypotension.

Clinical considerations

- Because administration with diuretics is associated with risk of excessive hypotension, discontinue diuretic therapy 2 to 3 days before start of quinapril, if possible. If quinapril alone doesn't adequately control blood pressure, a diuretic may be carefully added to the regimen.
- Like other ACE inhibitors, drug may cause a dry, persistent, tickling cough; it's reversible when therapy is discontinued.
- Each tablet of quinapril contains magnesium carbonate and magnesium stearate.

Therapeutic monitoring

- Blood pressure measurements should be made when drug levels are at their peak (2 to 6 hours after dosing) and at their trough (just before a dose) to verify adequate blood pressure control.
- Assess renal and hepatic function before and periodically throughout therapy. Also monitor CBC and serum potassium levels.

Special populations

Breast-feeding patients. It's unknown if drug is excreted in breast milk. Use with caution in breast-feeding women.
Pediatric patients. Safety and efficacy in children haven't been established.

Geriatric patients. Geriatric patients have demonstrated higher peak plasma levels and slower elimination of drug; these changes were related to decreased renal function that often occurs in geriatric patients. No overall differences in safety or efficacy have been seen in geriatric patients.

Patient counseling

- Tell patient that drug should be taken on an empty stomach because meals, particularly high-fat meals, can impair absorption.
- Advise patient to immediately report signs or symptoms of angioedema: swelling of face, eyes, lips, tongue, or difficulty in breathing. If these occur, patient should stop taking drug and seek immediate medical attention.
- Warn patient that light-headedness may occur, especially during first few days of therapy. Tell him to arise slowly to minimize this effect and to report persistent or severe symptoms. If syncope (fainting) occurs, patient should stop taking drug and report immediately.
- Inadequate fluid intake, vomiting, diarrhea, and excessive perspiration can lead to light-headedness and syncope. Patient should take care in hot weather and during periods of exercise to avoid dehydration and overheating.
- Tell patient to report immediately signs or symptoms of infection (sore throat, fever) or of easy bruising or bleeding. Other ACE inhibitors have been associated with development of agranulocytosis and neutropenia.

quinidine gluconate

Quinaglute Dura-Tabs, Quinalan

quinidine polygalacturonate

Cardioquin

quinidine sulfate

Apo-Quinidine*, Quinidex Extentabs

Pharmacologic classification: cinchona alkaloid
Therapeutic classification: ventricular antiarrhythmic, supraventricular antiarrhythmic, atrial antitachyarrhythmic
Pregnancy risk category C

How supplied

Available by prescription only
Tablets: 275 mg (polygalacturonate); 200 mg, 300 mg (sulfate); 300 mg (extended-release, sulfate); 324 mg (extended-release, gluconate)
Injection: 80 mg/ml (gluconate)

Indications and dosages

Atrial flutter or fibrillation
Adults: 200 mg (sulfate or equivalent base) P.O. q 2 to 3 hours for five to eight doses with subsequent daily increases until sinus rhythm is restored or toxic effects develop. Administer quinidine only after digitalization, to avoid increasing AV conduction. Maximum dose, 3 to 4 g daily.

Maintenance dosage, 200 to 400 mg P.O. t.i.d. or q.i.d., or 600 mg P.O. q 8 to 12 hours daily (extended-release).

Paroxysmal supraventricular tachycardia
Adults: 400 to 600 mg (sulfate) P.O. q 2 to 3 hours until toxic effects develop or arrhythmia subsides.

Premature atrial contractions, PVCs, paroxysmal AV junctional rhythm or atrial or ventricular tachycardia, maintenance of cardioversion
Adults: Give test dose of 50 to 200 mg P.O. of sulfate (or 200 mg gluconate I.M.); then monitor vital signs before beginning therapy: 200 to 400 mg P.O. sulfate or equivalent base q 4 to 6 hours; or initially, 600 mg of gluconate I.M., then up to 400 mg q 2 hours, p.r.n.; or 800 mg I.V. gluconate diluted in 40 ml of D_5W, infused at 16 mg (1 ml)/minute. Alternatively, give 300 to 600 mg of sulfate (extended-release), or 324 to 648 mg of gluconate (extended-release), q 8 to 12 hours.
Children: Give test dose of 2 mg/kg, then 30 mg/kg/day P.O. or 900 mg/m^2/day P.O. in five divided doses.

◇***Malaria (when quinine dihydrochloride is unavailable)***
Adults: Administer quinidine gluconate by continuous I.V. infusion. Initial loading dose of 10 mg/kg diluted in 250 ml of normal saline injection and infused over 1 to 2 hours, followed by a continuous maintenance infusion of 0.02 mg/kg/minute (20 mcg/kg/minute) for 72 hours or until parasitemia is reduced to less than 1% or oral therapy can be started; or 10 mg/kg quinidine sulfate P.O. q 8 hours for 5 to 7 days. Contact the Centers for Disease Control and Prevention (CDC) Malaria Branch for protocol instructions for recommendations at (707) 488-7760 (weekdays) or (707) 639-2888 (evenings, weekends, holidays), if using regimen.

Pharmacodynamics

Antiarrhythmic action: A class IA antiarrhythmic, quinidine depresses phase O of the action potential. It's considered a myocardial depressant because it decreases myocardial excitability and conduction velocity and may depress myocardial contractility. It also exerts anticholinergic activity, which may modify its direct myocardial effects. In therapeutic doses, quinidine reduces conduction velocity in the atria, ventricles, and His-Purkinje system. It helps control atrial tachyarrhythmias by prolonging the effective refractory period (ERP) and increasing the action potential duration in the atria, ventricles, and His-Purkinje system. Because ERP prolongation exceeds action potential duration, tissue remains refractory even after returning to resting membrane potential (membrane-stabilizing effect).

Quinidine shortens the effective refractory period of the AV node. Because anticholinergic action of quinidine may increase AV node conductivity, a cardiac glycoside should be administered for atrial tachyarrhythmias before quinidine therapy begins, to prevent ventricular tachyarrhythmias. Quinidine also suppresses automaticity in the His-Purkinje system and ectopic pacemakers, making it useful in treating PVCs. At therapeutic doses, quinidine prolongs the QRS complex and QT interval; these ECG effects may be used as an index of drug effectiveness and toxicity.

Pharmacokinetics

Absorption: Although all quinidine salts are well absorbed from the GI tract, individual serum drug levels vary greatly. For extended-release forms, onset of action may be slightly slower but duration of effect is longer because drug delivery system allows longer-than-usual dosing intervals.

Distribution: Well distributed in all tissues except the brain, and concentrates in the heart, liver, kidneys, and skeletal muscle. Distribution volume decreases in patients with heart failure, possibly requiring reduction in maintenance dosage. About 80% of drug is bound to plasma proteins; the unbound (active) fraction may increase in patients with hypoalbuminemia from various causes, including hepatic insufficiency. Usual therapeutic serum levels depend on assay method and ranges as follows:

—Specific assay (enzyme multiplied immunoassay technique, high-performance liquid chromatography, fluorescence polarization): 2 to 5 mcg/ml.

—Nonspecific assay (fluorometric): 4 to 8 mcg/ml.

Metabolism: About 60% to 80% of drug is metabolized in the liver to two metabolites that may have some pharmacologic activity.

Excretion: About 10% to 30% of administered dose is excreted in the urine within 24 hours as unchanged drug. Urine acidification increases quinidine excretion; alkalinization decreases excretion. Most of an administered dose is eliminated in the urine as metabolites; elimination half-life ranges from 5 to 12 hours (usual half-life is about 6½ hours). Duration of effect ranges from 6 to 8 hours.

Route	Onset	Peak	Duration
P.O.	1-3 hr	1-6 hr	6-8 hr
I.V.	Immediate	Immediate	Unknown
I.M.	½-1½ min	Unknown	Unknown

Contraindications and precautions

Contraindicated in patients with idiosyncrasy or hypersensitivity to quinidine or related cinchona derivatives, intraventricular conduction defects, cardiac glycoside toxicity when AV conduction is grossly impaired, abnormal rhythms due to escape mechanisms, and history of drug-induced torsades de pointes or QT syndrome.

Use cautiously in patients with impaired renal or hepatic function, asthma, muscle weakness, or infection accompanied by a fever because hypersensitivity reactions may be masked.

Interactions

Drug-drug. *Antacids, sodium bicarbonate, thiazide diuretics:* May decrease quinidine elimination when urine pH increases, requiring close monitoring of therapy.

Anticholinergic agents: May lead to additive anticholinergic effects. Use with caution.

Anticonvulsants, such as phenobarbital and phenytoin: Increases the rate of quinidine metabolism; this leads to decreased quinidine levels. Monitor drug levels closely.

Cholinergic agents: May fail to terminate paroxysmal supraventricular tachycardia Also, anticholinergic effects of quinidine may negate the effects of these drugs when these agents are used to treat myasthenia gravis. Use with caution.

Coumarin: May potentiate anticoagulant effect of coumarin, possibly leading to hypoprothrombinemic hemorrhage. Monitor closely.

Digitoxin or digoxin: May cause increased (possibly toxic) serum digoxin levels. Some experts recommend a 50% reduction in digoxin dosage when quinidine therapy is initiated, with subsequent monitoring of serum levels.

Hypotensive agents: May cause additive hypotensive effects, mainly when administered I.V. Monitor blood pressure closely.

Neuromuscular blocking agents, such as metocurine iodide, pancuronium bromide, succinylcholine chloride, and tubocurarine chloride: May potentiate anticholinergic effects. Use of quinidine should be avoided immediately after use of these agents; if quinidine must be used, respiratory support may be needed.

Other antiarrhythmic agents, such as amiodarone, lidocaine, phenytoin, procainamide, and propranolol: May cause additive or antagonistic cardiac effects and additive toxic effects. Use together cautiously.

Phenothiazines, reserpine: May cause additive cardiac depressant effects. Avoid use together.

Rifampin: May increase quinidine metabolism and decrease serum quinidine levels, possibly necessitating dosage adjustment when rifampin therapy is initiated or discontinued.

Rifedipine: May result in decreased quinidine levels. Monitor closely.

Verapamil: May result in significant hypotension in some patients with hypertrophic cardiomyopathy. Monitor closely.

Drug-herb. *Jimsonweed:* May adversely affect cardiovascular function. Avoid using together.
Licorice: May prolong the QT interval and be potentially additive. Use cautiously together.

Effects on diagnostic tests
None reported.

Adverse reactions
CNS: *vertigo, headache, light-headedness,* confusion, ataxia, depression, dementia.
CV: *PVCs;* ***ventricular tachycardia; atypical ventricular tachycardia (torsades de pointes);*** *hypotension;* ***complete AV block,*** *tachycardia; ECG changes (particularly widening of QRS complex, widened QT and PR intervals).*
EENT: *tinnitus,* excessive salivation, blurred vision, diplopia, photophobia.
GI: *diarrhea, nausea, vomiting,* anorexia, abdominal pain.
Hematologic: ***hemolytic anemia, thrombocytopenia, agranulocytosis.***
Hepatic: ***hepatotoxicity.***
Respiratory: acute asthmatic attack, ***respiratory arrest.***
Skin: rash, petechial hemorrhage of buccal mucosa, pruritus, urticaria, lupus erythematosus, photosensitivity.
Other: angioedema, *fever, cinchonism.*

Overdose and treatment
The most serious clinical effects of overdose include severe hypotension, ventricular arrhythmias (including torsades de pointes), and seizures. QRS complexes and QT and PR intervals may be prolonged, and ataxia, anuria, respiratory distress, irritability, and hallucinations may develop. If ingestion was recent, gastric lavage, emesis, and activated charcoal may be used to decrease absorption. Urine acidification may be used to help increase quinidine elimination.

Treatment involves general supportive measures (including CV and respiratory support) with hemodynamic and ECG monitoring. Metaraminol or norepinephrine may be used to reverse hypotension (after adequate hydration has been ensured). Avoid CNS depressants because CNS depression may occur, possibly with seizures. Cardiac pacing may be necessary. Isoproterenol or ventricular pacing possibly may be used to treat torsades de pointes tachycardia.

I.V. infusion of 1/6 M sodium lactate solution reduces cardiotoxic effect of quinidine. Hemodialysis, although rarely warranted, also may be effective.

Clinical considerations
☐ ***ALERT*** When changing route of administration or oral salt form, be aware that dosage needs to be altered to compensate for variations in quinidine base content.

☐ ***ALERT*** Don't confuse drug with Quinamm, quinine, or clonidine.

- When drug is used to treat atrial tachyarrhythmias, ventricular rate may be accelerated from anticholinergic effects of drug on AV node. This can be prevented by previous treatment with a digitalis glycoside.
- Because conversion of chronic atrial fibrillation may be associated with embolism, administer anticoagulant for several weeks before quinidine therapy begins.
- Use I.V. route for acute arrhythmias only; it's generally avoided because of the potential for severe hypotension.
- Don't use discolored (brownish) quinidine solution.
- For maintenance, give only by oral or I.M. route. Dosage requirements vary. Some patients may require drug q 4 hours, others q 6 hours. Titrate dose by both clinical response and blood levels.
- When changing administration route, alter dosage to compensate for variations in quinidine base content.
- Decrease dosage in patients with heart failure and hepatic disease.
- Drug may increase toxicity of cardiac glycoside derivatives. Use cautiously in patients receiving cardiac glycosides. Monitor digoxin levels and expect to reduce dosage of cardiac glycoside derivatives. Many clinicians recommend that digoxin dosage be reduced by 50% when quinidine therapy is initiated.
- Lidocaine may be effective in treating quinidine-induced arrhythmias because it increases AV conduction.
- Quinidine may cause hemolysis in patients with G6PD deficiency.
- Small amounts of quinidine are removed by hemodialysis; drug isn't removed by peritoneal dialysis.
- Amount of quinidine in the various salt forms varies as follows:

—Gluconate: 62% quinidine (324 mg of gluconate, 202 mg sulfate)
—Polygalacturonate: 60% quinidine (275 mg polygalacturonate, 166 mg sulfate)
—Sulfate: 83% quinidine. The sulfate form is considered the standard dosage preparation.

- Quinidine gluconate is reported to be as or more active in vitro against *Plasmodium falciparum* than quinine dihydrochloride. Because the latter drug is only available through the CDC, quinidine gluconate may be useful in the treatment of severe malaria when delay of therapy may be life-threatening. The current CDC protocol involves follow-up treatment with either tetracycline or sulfadoxine and pyrimethamine.

Therapeutic monitoring
- Check apical pulse rate, blood pressure, and ECG tracing, before starting therapy.

■ Monitor ECG, especially when large doses of drug are being administered. Quinidine-induced cardiotoxicity is evidenced by conduction defects (50% widening of the QRS complex), ventricular tachycardia or flutter, frequent PVCs, and complete AV block. When these ECG signs appear, discontinue drug and monitor patient closely.
■ Monitor liver function tests during first 4 to 8 weeks of therapy.
■ GI adverse effects, especially diarrhea, are signs of toxicity. Check quinidine blood levels; suspect toxicity when they exceed 8 mcg/ml. GI symptoms may be minimized by giving drug with meals.

Special populations

Pregnant patients. The drug has some oxytocic properties. Safety for use during pregnancy and labor and delivery hasn't been established.
Breast-feeding patients. Because drug is excreted in breast milk, alternative feeding method is recommended during therapy with quinidine.
Pediatric patients. Safety and efficacy haven't been established for use in children.
Geriatric patients. Dosage reduction may be necessary in geriatric patients. Because of highly variable metabolism, monitor serum levels.

Patient counseling

■ Instruct patient to report rash, fever, unusual bleeding, bruising, ringing in ears, or visual disturbance.
■ Stress importance of taking drug exactly as prescribed.

quinine sulfate

Pharmacologic classification: cinchona alkaloid
Therapeutic classification: antimalarial
Pregnancy risk category D

How supplied

Available by prescription only
Tablets: 260 mg, 325 mg
Capsules: 260 mg

Indications and dosages

Malaria (chloroquine-resistant)
Adults: 650 mg P.O. q 8 hours for 10 days, with 25 mg pyrimethamine q 12 hours for 3 days and with 500 mg sulfadiazine q.i.d. for 5 days.
Children: 25 mg/kg/day P.O. divided into three doses for 10 days.
Babesia microti *infections*
Adults: 650 mg P.O. q 6 to 8 hours for 7 days.
Children: 25 mg/kg/day P.O. divided into three doses for 7 days.
◇***Nocturnal recumbency leg muscle cramps***
Adults: 200 to 300 mg P.O. h.s. Discontinue if leg cramps don't occur after several days to determine if continued therapy is necessary.

Pharmacodynamics

Antimalarial action: Quinine intercalates into DNA, disrupting the parasite's replication and transcription; it also depresses its oxygen uptake and carbohydrate metabolism. It's active against the asexual erythrocytic forms of *Plasmodium falciparum, P. malariae, P. ovale,* and *P. vivax* and is used for chloroquine-resistant malaria.
Skeletal muscle relaxant action: Quinine increases the refractory period, decreases excitability of the motor end plate, and affects calcium distribution within muscle fibers.

Pharmacokinetics

Absorption: Almost completely absorbed.
Distribution: Distributed widely into the liver, lungs, kidneys, and spleen; CSF levels reach 2% to 5% of serum levels. Quinine is about 70% bound to plasma proteins and readily crosses the placenta.
Metabolism: Metabolized in the liver.
Excretion: Less than 5% of a single dose is excreted unchanged in the urine; small amounts of metabolites appear in the feces, gastric juice, bile, saliva, and breast milk. Half-life is 7 to 21 hours in healthy or convalescing persons; it's longer in patients with malaria. Urine acidification hastens elimination.

Route	Onset	Peak	Duration
P.O.	Unknown	1-3 hr	Unknown

Contraindications and precautions

Contraindicated during pregnancy and in patients with known hypersensitivity to drug, G6PD deficiency, optic neuritis, tinnitus, or history of blackwater fever or thrombocytopenic purpura associated with previous quinine ingestion.

Use cautiously in patients with arrhythmias and in those taking sodium bicarbonate together.

Interactions

Drug-drug. *Acetazolamide or sodium bicarbonate:* May increase the level of quinine by decreasing urinary excretion. Monitor closely.
Aluminum-containing antacids: May delay or decrease absorption of quinine. Avoid use together.
Digitoxin and digoxin: Increased plasma levels of these drugs. Monitor levels closely.
Mefloquine: May cause additive cardiac effects. Don't use together.
Neuromuscular blocking agents: May potentiate the effects of these drugs. Monitor closely.

Warfarin: May potentiate the action by depressing synthesis of vitamin K–dependent clotting factors. Monitor PT and INR closely.

Effects on diagnostic tests
Drug causes false elevations of urinary catecholamines and may interfere with 17-hydroxycorticosteroid and 17-ketogenic steroid tests.

Adverse reactions
CNS: severe headache, apprehension, excitement, confusion, delirium, syncope, hypothermia, vertigo, ***seizures*** (with toxic doses).
CV: hypotension, ***CV collapse*** (with overdose or rapid I.V. administration), conduction disturbances.
EENT: altered color perception, photophobia, blurred vision, night blindness, amblyopia, scotoma, diplopia, mydriasis, optic atrophy, tinnitus, impaired hearing.
GI: epigastric distress, diarrhea, nausea, vomiting.
GU: renal tubular damage, anuria.
Hematologic: hemolytic anemia, ***thrombocytopenia, agranulocytosis,*** hypoprothrombinemia, thrombosis at infusion site.
Respiratory: asthma, dyspnea.
Skin: rash, pruritus.
Other: flushing, fever, facial edema, hypoglycemia.

Overdose and treatment
Signs and symptoms of overdose include tinnitus, vertigo, headache, fever, rash, CV effects, GI distress (including vomiting), blindness, apprehension, confusion, and seizures.

Treatment includes gastric lavage followed by supportive measures, which may include fluid and electrolyte replacement, artificial respiration, and stabilization of blood pressure and renal function.

Anaphylactic reactions may require epinephrine, corticosteroids, or antihistamines. Urinary acidification may increase elimination of quinine but will also augment renal obstruction. Hemodialysis or hemoperfusion may be helpful. Vasodilator therapy or stellate blockage may relieve visual disturbances.

Clinical considerations
- Administer quinine after meals to minimize gastric distress; don't crush tablets, as drug irritates gastric mucosa.
- Quinine is no longer used for acute malarial attack by *P. vivax* or for suppression of malaria from resistant organisms.

Therapeutic monitoring
- Discontinue drug if signs of idiosyncrasy or toxicity occur.
- Serum levels of 10 mcg/ml or more may confirm toxicity as the cause of tinnitus or hearing loss.

Special populations
Breast-feeding patients. Before drug is given to a breast-feeding woman, evaluate the infant for possible G6PD deficiency.
Geriatric patients. Use with caution in patients with conduction disturbances.

Patient counseling
- Teach patient about adverse reactions and need to report these immediately, especially tinnitus and hearing impairment.
- Tell patient to avoid concurrent use of aluminum-containing antacids because these may alter drug absorption.
- Instruct patient to keep drug out of reach of children.

quinupristin/dalfopristin
Synercid

Pharmacologic classification: streptogramin
Therapeutic classification: antibiotic
Pregnancy risk category B

How supplied
Available by prescription only
Injection: 500mg/10ml (150 mg quinupristin and 350 mg dalfopristin)

Indications and dosages
Serious or life-threatening infections associated with vancomycin-resistant* Enterococcus faecium *(VREF) bacteremia
Adults and adolescents age 16 and older: 7.5 mg/kg I.V. infusion over 1 hour q 8 hours. Treatment duration should be determined by the site and severity of the infection.
***Complicated skin and skin structure infections caused by* Staphylococcus aureus *(methicillin susceptible) or* Streptococcus pyogenes**
Adults and adolescents age 16 and older: 7.5 mg/kg by I.V. infusion over 1 hour q 12 hours for at least 7 days.

Pharmacodynamics
Antibiotic action: The two antibacterial agents that make up quinopristin/dalfopristin work synergistically to inhibit or destroy susceptible bacteria through combined inhibition on protein synthesis in bacterial cells. Dalfopristin has been shown to inhibit the early phase of protein synthesis in the bacterial ribosome while quinupristin inhibits the late phase of protein synthesis. Without the ability to manufacture new proteins, the bacterial cells are inactivated or die.

Pharmacokinetics
Absorption: Quinupristin and dalfopristin have different pharmacokinetic profiles. Following multiple infusion doses of 7.5 mg/kg every 8

hours, peak concentrations of quinupristin and metabolites are 3.2 mcg/ml; peak dalfopristin concentrations are 8.0 mcg/ml.
Distribution: Protein binding is moderate.
Metabolism: Quinupristin and dalfopristin are converted to several active major metabolites by nonenzymatic reactions.
Excretion: Biliary excretion with resultant fecal elimination accounts for about 75% of elimination of both drugs and their metabolites. Urinary excretion accounts for about 15% of a quinupristin dose and 19% of a dalfopristin dose. The elimination half-lives of quinupristin and dalfopristin are about 0.85 and 0.70 hours, respectively.

Route	Onset	Peak	Duration
I.V.	Unknown	Variable	Unknown

Contraindications and precautions
Contraindicated in patients with known hypersensitivity to drug or other streptogramin antibiotics.

Interactions
Drug-drug: *Calcium channel blockers, such as diltiazem, nifedipine, or verapamil; carbamazepine; diazepam; disopyramide; docetaxel; drugs metabolized by cytochrome P-450 3A4, including protease inhibitors such as delavirdine, indinavir, lidocaine; nevirapine, and ritonavir; lovastatin; methylprednisolone; midazolam; paclitaxel, tacrolimus; vinblastine:* Increased plasma concentrations of these drugs that could increase their therapeutic effects and adverse reactions. Use together cautiously.
Cyclosporine: Metabolism is reduced and concentrations may be increased. Monitor cyclosporine levels.
Drugs metabolized by cytochrome P-450 3A4 that increase the QT_c interval on the ECG (quinidine, cisapride, and others): Decreased metabolism of these drugs resulting in QT_c prolongation. Avoid use together.

Effects on diagnostic tests
None reported.

Adverse reactions
CNS: headache, pain.
CV: thrombophlebitis.
GI: nausea, diarrhea, vomiting.
Hepatic: *elevated total and conjugated bilirubin,* altered liver function studies.
Musculoskeletal: arthralgia, myalgia.
Skin: rash, pruritus.
Other: *inflammation, pain, edema at infusion site, infusion site reaction.*

Overdose and treatment
Patients given an overdose should be observed and given supportive care. Drug isn't removed by peritoneal or hemodialysis.

Clinical considerations
- Quinupristin/dalfopristin isn't active against *Enterococcus faecalis.* Appropriate blood cultures are needed to avoid misidentifying *E. faecalis* as *E. faecium.*
- Because mild to life-threatening pseudomembranous colitis has been reported with use of quinupristin/dalfopristin, consider this diagnosis in patients who develop diarrhea during or following therapy with drug.
- Adverse reactions, such as arthralgia and myalgia, may be reduced by decreasing dosage interval to every 12 hours.
- Reconstitute powder for injection by adding 5 ml of either sterile water for injection or D_5W and gently swirling vial by manual rotation to ensure dissolution; avoid shaking to limit foaming. Reconstituted solutions must be further diluted within 30 minutes.
- The appropriate dose, according to patient's weight, of reconstituted solution should be added to 250 ml of D_5W to make a final concentration of no more than 2 mg/ml. This diluted solution is stable for 5 hours at room temperature or 54 hours if refrigerated.
- Fluid-restricted patients with a central venous catheter may receive dose in 100 ml of D_5W. This concentration isn't recommended for peripheral venous administration.
- If moderate to severe peripheral venous irritation occurs, consider increasing infusion volume to 500 or 750 ml, changing injection site, or infusing by a central venous catheter.
- Administer all doses by I.V. infusion over 1 hour. An infusion pump or device may be used to control rate of infusion.
- Quinupristin/dalfopristin is incompatible with saline and heparin solutions. Don't dilute drug with saline-containing solutions or infuse into lines that contain saline or heparin. Flush line with D_5W before and after each dose.

Therapeutic monitoring
- Monitor I.V. site closely.
- Monitor blood work and vital signs frequently.
- Because overgrowth of nonsusceptible organisms may occur, monitor patient closely for signs and symptoms of superinfection.
- Monitor liver function tests during therapy.

Special populations
Pregnant patients. Safety hasn't been established for use during pregnancy.
Breast-feeding patients. It isn't known if drug is excreted in breast milk. Use caution in breast-feeding women.
Pediatric patients. Safety and efficacy in patients under age 16 haven't been established. Limited clinical trials in pediatric patients used a dosage of 7.5 mg every 8 or 12 hours.
Geriatric patients. No dosage adjustment is required in the elderly.

Patient counseling
- Advise patient to report irritation at I.V. site, pain in joints or muscles, and diarrhea immediately.
- Tell patient about the importance of reporting persistent or worsening symptoms of infection, such as pain or erythema.

rabeprazole sodium
Aciphex

Pharmacologic classification: proton pump inhibitor
Therapeutic classification: antiulcerative
Pregnancy risk category B

How supplied
Available by prescription only
Tablets (delayed-release): 20 mg

Indications and dosages
Healing of erosive or ulcerative gastroesophageal reflux disease (GERD)
Adults: 20 mg P.O. daily for 4 to 8 weeks. Additional 8-week course may be considered, if necessary.
Maintenance of healing of erosive or ulcerative GERD
Adults: 20 mg P.O. daily.
Healing of duodenal ulcers
Adults: 20 mg P.O. daily after morning meal for up to 4 weeks.
Treatment of pathological hypersecretory conditions including Zollinger-Ellison syndrome
Adults: 60 mg P.O. daily; may be increased, as needed, to 100 mg P.O. daily or 60 mg P.O. twice daily.

Pharmacodynamics
Antiulcerative action: Rabeprazole blocks activity of the acid (proton) pump by inhibiting gastric hydrogen-potassium adenosine triphosphatase at the secretory surface of the gastric parietal cell, blocking gastric acid secretion.

Pharmacokinetics
Absorption: Drug is acid labile because enteric coating allows it to pass through the stomach relatively intact.
Distribution: 96.3% plasma protein-bound.
Metabolism: Extensively metabolized by the liver to inactive compounds.
Excretion: 90% is eliminated in urine as metabolites. Remaining 10% of metabolites are eliminated in feces. Plasma half-life is 1 to 2 hours.

Route	Onset	Peak	Duration
P.O.	Unknown	2-5 hr	> 24 hr

Contraindications and precautions
Contraindicated in patients with known hypersensitivity to rabeprazole, other benzimidazoles (lansoprazole, omeprazole), or components in these formulations. Use cautiously in patients with severe hepatic impairment.

Interactions
Drug-drug. *Cyclosporine:* May inhibit cyclosporine metabolism. Use together cautiously.
Digoxin, ketoconazole, other gastric pH-dependent drugs: Decreased or increased drug absorption at increased pH values. Monitor patient closely during use with rabeprazole.

Effects on diagnostic tests
None reported.

Adverse reactions
CNS: headache, dizziness, malaise, asthenia, migraine, syncope, insomnia, anxiety, depression, nervousness, somnolence, neuralgia, vertigo, ***seizures,*** abnormal dreams, neuropathy, paresthesia, tremor.
CV: substernal chest pain, hypertension, ***myocardial infarction,*** electrocardiogram abnormalities, angina, bundle-branch block, palpitations, ***sinus bradycardia,*** tachycardia, edema.
EENT: epistaxis, cataracts, amblyopia, glaucoma, dry eyes, abnormal vision, tinnitus, otitis media.
GI: diarrhea, nausea, abdominal pain, vomiting, dyspepsia, flatulence, constipation, dry mouth, eructation, gastroenteritis, rectal hemorrhage, melena, anorexia, cholelithiasis, mouth ulceration, stomatitis, dysphagia, gingivitis, cholecystitis, increased appetite, abnormal stools, colitis, esophagitis, glossitis, ***pancreatitis,*** proctitis.
GU: cystitis, urinary frequency, dysmenorrhea, dysuria, renal calculi, metrorrhagia, polyuria.
Hematologic: anemia.
Metabolic: hyperthyroidism, hypothyroidism, weight gain, weight loss.
Musculoskeletal: neck rigidity, myalgia, arthritis, leg cramps, bone pain, arthrosis, bursitis, hypertonia.
Respiratory: bronchitis, dyspnea, asthma, laryngitis, hiccups, hyperventilation.
Skin: rash, pruritus, sweating, urticaria, alopecia, photosensitivity reaction.
Other: infection, fever, allergic reaction, chills, lymphadenopathy, dehydration, decreased libido, ecchymosis, gout.

Overdose and treatment
Treatment is supportive and symptomatic. There's no specific antidote for rabeprazole overdose, and drug isn't dialyzable because of extensive protein-binding.

Clinical considerations

- Consider additional courses of therapy when duodenal ulcers or GERD isn't healed after first course of therapy.
- Symptomatic response to therapy doesn't preclude presence of GI cancer.

Therapeutic monitoring

Monitor patient's response to drug therapy.

Special populations

Breast-feeding patients. It's unknown if drug is excreted in breast milk. Taking into account importance of drug to woman, either discontinue drug or advise patient to discontinue breast-feeding.
Pediatric patients. Safety and efficacy haven't been established in pediatric patients.
Geriatric patients. No differences in safety and efficacy have been observed in geriatric patients.

Patient counseling

- Explain importance of taking drug exactly as prescribed for treatment course.
- Advise patient that rabeprazole delayed-release tablets should be swallowed whole. Tablets shouldn't be crushed, chewed, or split.
- Advise patient that drug may be taken without regard to meals.

rabies immune globulin, human (RIG)

Hyperab, Imogam Rabies Immune Globulin

Pharmacologic classification: immune serum
Therapeutic classification: rabies prophylaxis
Pregnancy risk category C

How supplied

Available by prescription only
Injection: 150 IU/ml in 2-ml and 10-ml vials

Indications and dosages

Rabies exposure
Adults and children: 20 IU/kg at time of first dose of rabies vaccine. Use half dose to infiltrate wound area. Give remainder I.M. (gluteal area preferred). Don't give rabies vaccine and RIG in same syringe or at same site.

Pharmacodynamics

Postexposure rabies prophylaxis: RIG provides passive immunity to rabies.

Pharmacokinetics

Absorption: After slow I.M. absorption, rabies antibody appears in serum within 24 hours and peaks within 2 to 13 days.
Distribution: Probably crosses the placenta and is distributed into breast milk.
Metabolism: No information available.
Excretion: Serum half-life for rabies antibody titer is about 24 days.

Route	Onset	Peak	Duration
I.M.	24 hr	Unknown	Unknown

Contraindications and precautions

Don't give repeated doses once vaccine treatment has been started.

Use cautiously in patients with immunoglobulin A deficiency or history of prior systemic allergic reactions following administration of human immunoglobulin preparations and in those with known hypersensitivity to thimerosal.

Interactions

Drug-drug. *Corticosteroids, immunosuppressant agents:* May interfere with the immune response to RIG. Whenever possible, avoid using these agents during the postexposure immunization period. Because antirabies serum may partially suppress the antibody response to rabies vaccine, use only the recommended dose of antirabies vaccine.
Live virus vaccine, such as measles, mumps, and rubella: RIG may interfere with the immune response to these live viruses. Don't administer live virus vaccines within 3 months after administration of RIG.

Effects on diagnostic tests

None reported.

Adverse reactions

GU: ***nephrotic syndrome.***
Skin: ***rash,*** pain, redness, induration at injection site.
Other: slight fever, ***anaphylaxis, angioedema.***

Overdose and treatment

No information available.

Clinical considerations

☐ ***ALERT*** Don't confuse drug with rabies vaccine, which is a suspension of attenuated or killed microorganisms used to confer active immunity. These two drugs are commonly given together prophylactically after exposure to known or suspected rabid animals.

- Obtain a thorough history of the animal bite, allergies, and reactions to immunizations.
- Epinephrine solution 1:1,000 should be available to treat allergic reactions.
- Don't administer more than 5 ml I.M. at one injection site; divide I.M. doses exceeding 5 ml and administer them at different sites.
- Ask patient when he received his last tetanus immunization; a booster may be indicated.
- Patients previously immunized with a tissue culture-derived rabies vaccine and those who

have confirmed adequate rabies antibody titers should receive only the vaccine.

- RIG hasn't been associated with an increased frequency of AIDS. The immune globulin is devoid of HIV. Immune globulin recipients don't develop antibodies to HIV.
- Store between 36° and 46° F (2° and 8° C). Don't freeze.

Therapeutic monitoring

- Repeated doses of RIG shouldn't be given after rabies vaccine is started.
- Reactions to antirabies serum may occur up to 12 days after product is given.

Special populations

Pregnant patients. Because rabies can be fatal if untreated, use of RIG during pregnancy appears justified. No fetal risk from RIG use has been reported to date.

Breast-feeding patients. Safety in breast-feeding women hasn't been established. RIG is probably excreted in breast milk. An alternative feeding method is recommended.

Patient counseling

- Explain that the body needs about 1 week to develop immunity to rabies after vaccine is administered. Therefore, patients receive RIG to provide antibodies in their blood for immediate protection against rabies.
- Advise patient to report skin changes, difficulty breathing, or headache.
- Tell patient that local pain, swelling, and tenderness at injection site may occur. Recommend acetaminophen to alleviate these minor effects.

rabies vaccine, adsorbed

Pharmacologic classification: vaccine
Therapeutic classification: viral vaccine
Pregnancy risk category C

How supplied

Available by prescription only
Injection: 1 ml single-dose vial

Indications and dosages

Preexposure prophylaxis rabies immunization for patients in high-risk groups
Adults and children: 1 ml I.M. at 0, 7, and 21 or 28 days for a total of three injections. Patients at increased risk for rabies should be checked every 6 months and given a booster vaccination, 1 ml I.M., p.r.n., to maintain adequate serum titer.

Postexposure rabies prophylaxis
Adults and children not previously vaccinated against rabies: 20 IU/kg of human rabies immune globulin (HRIG) I.M. and five 1-ml injections of rabies vaccine, adsorbed, I.M. given one each on days 0, 3, 7, 14, and 28.
Adults and children previously vaccinated against rabies: Two 1-ml injections of rabies vaccine, adsorbed, I.M. given one each on days 0 and 3. HRIG shouldn't be given.

Pharmacodynamics

Vaccine action: Promotes active immunity to rabies.

Pharmacokinetics

Absorption: People at high risk should be retested for rabies antibody titer every 6 months.
Distribution: No information available.
Metabolism: No information available.
Excretion: No information available.

Route	Onset	Peak	Duration
I.M.	Unknown	2 wk after 3 doses	Unknown

Contraindications and precautions

Contraindicated in patients who have experienced life-threatening allergic reactions to previous injections of vaccine or its components, including thimerosal. Use cautiously in patients with history of nonlife-threatening allergic reactions to previous injections of vaccine or hypersensitivity to monkey proteins.

Interactions

Drug-drug. *Antimalarial drugs, corticosteroids, and immunosuppressive agents:* Decrease response to rabies vaccine. Don't use together.

Effects on diagnostic tests

None reported.

Adverse reactions

CNS: *headache, dizziness.*
GI: *abdominal pain, nausea.*
Musculoskeletal: aching of injected muscle, *myalgia.*
Other: ***anaphylaxis,*** *fatigue, slight fever,* serum sickness-like reactions; transient pain, erythema, swelling, itching, mild inflammatory reaction at injection site.

Overdose and treatment

No information available.

Clinical considerations

- Keep epinephrine 1:1,000 readily available.
- Administer I.M. into deltoid region in adults and older children; midanterolateral aspect of the thigh is acceptable for younger children. Vaccine shouldn't be used by intradermal route. Don't inject vaccine in close approximation to a peripheral nerve or in adipose and subcutaneous tissue.

■ Vaccine is normally a light pink color because of presence of phenol red in the suspension.
■ Delay preexposure immunization in patient with acute intercurrent illness.

Therapeutic monitoring
■ If patient experiences a serious adverse reaction to the vaccine, report this promptly to the manufacturer: Michigan Department of Public Health, (517) 335-8050 during working hours or (517) 335-9030 at other times.

Special populations
Pregnant patients. Administration isn't contraindicated because of the potential harm from rabies exposure.
Pediatric patients. Use caution when administering vaccine because of limited experience in children.

Patient counseling
■ Tell patient that pain, swelling, and itching at injection site, headache, stomach upset, or fever may occur.
■ Recommend acetaminophen to alleviate headache, fever, and muscle aches.

rabies vaccine, human diploid cell (HDCV)
Imovax Rabies I.D. Vaccine (inactivated whole virus), Imovax Rabies Vaccine

Pharmacologic classification: vaccine
Therapeutic classification: viral vaccine
Pregnancy risk category C

How supplied
Available by prescription only
I.M. injection: 2.5 IU of rabies antigen/ml, in single-dose vial with diluent
I.D. injection: 0.25 IU rabies antigen per dose

Indications and dosages
Preexposure prophylaxis immunization for persons in high-risk groups
Adults and children: Three 0.1-ml injections intradermally or three 1-ml injections I.M. Give first dose on day 0 (first day vaccination), second dose on day 7, and third dose on day 21 or 28.
Booster: Persons exposed to rabies virus at their workplace should have antibody titers checked q 6 months. Those persons with continued risk of exposure should have antibody titers checked q 2 years. When the titers are inadequate, administer a booster dose.
Primary postexposure dosage
Adults and children: Five 1-ml doses I.M. on days 3, 7, 14, and 28 (in conjunction with rabies immune globulin on day 0). A sixth dose may be given on day 90. For patients who previously received the full HDCV vaccination regimen or who have demonstrated rabies antibody, give two 1-ml doses I.M. Give first dose on day 0 and the second 3 days later. Rabies immune globulin (RIG) shouldn't be given.

Pharmacodynamics
Rabies prophylaxis: Vaccine promotes active immunity to rabies.

Pharmacokinetics
Absorption: After I.D. injection, rabies antibodies appear in the serum within 7 to 10 days.
Distribution: No information available.
Metabolism: No information available.
Excretion: No information available.

Route	Onset	Peak	Duration
I.M., Intradermal	1 wk	1-2 mo	>2 yr

Contraindications and precautions
No contraindications reported for persons after exposure. An acute febrile illness contraindicates use of vaccine for persons previously exposed. Use cautiously in patients with history of hypersensitivity.

Interactions
Drug-drug. *Corticosteroids, immunosuppressants:* May interfere with the development of active immunity to rabies vaccine. Avoid use whenever possible.

Effects on diagnostic tests
None reported.

Adverse reactions
CNS: *headache,* dizziness, *fatigue.*
GI: abdominal pain, diarrhea, *nausea.*
Musculoskeletal: muscle aches.
Other: ***anaphylaxis,*** *fever, serum sickness; pain, erythema, swelling, itching at injection site.*

Overdose and treatment
No information available.

Clinical considerations
□ ***ALERT*** I.D. form is for preexposure use only.
■ Obtain a thorough history of allergies, especially to antibiotics, and of reactions to immunizations.
■ Epinephrine solution 1:1,000 should be available to treat allergic reactions.
■ I.M. injections should be made in the deltoid or upper outer quadrant of the gluteus muscle in adults and children. In infants and young children, use the midlateral aspect of the thigh.
■ Reconstitute with diluent provided. Gently shake vial until vaccine is completely dissolved.

- Store vaccine at 36° to 46° F (2° to 8° C). Don't freeze.

Therapeutic monitoring
Watch for signs of serum sickness-like hypersensitivity reactions. Antihistamine treatment may be needed in these patients.

Special populations
Pregnant patients. It's recommended that treatment be given to pregnant women, due to the possible harm of rabies exposure. Preexposure immunization may also be indicated for a pregnant woman at high exposure risk for rabies.
Breast-feeding patients. It's unknown if HDCV is distributed in breast milk or if transmission to breast-feeding infant presents risk. Breast-feeding women should choose an alternative feeding method.

Patient counseling
- Tell patient that pain, swelling, and itching at injection site as well as headache, stomach upset, or fever may occur after vaccination.
- Recommend acetaminophen to alleviate headache, fever, and muscle aches.

raloxifene hydrochloride
Evista

Pharmacologic classification: selective estrogen receptor modulator (SERM)
Therapeutic classification: antiosteoporotic
Pregnancy risk category X

How supplied
Available by prescription only
Tablets: 60 mg

Indications and dosages
Prevention and treatment of osteoporosis in postmenopausal women
Adults: One 60-mg tablet P.O. once daily.

Pharmacodynamics
Antiosteoporotic action: Decreases bone turnover and reduces bone resorption, manifested as reduced serum and urine levels of bone turnover markers and increased bone mineral density. Biologic actions of drug are mediated through binding to estrogen receptors resulting in differential expression of multiple estrogen-regulated genes in different tissues.

Pharmacokinetics
Absorption: Rapidly absorbed. Peak levels depend upon systemic interconversion and enterohepatic cycling of drug and its metabolites. Following oral administration, about 60% of raloxifene is absorbed. Absolute bioavailability is 2%.
Distribution: Apparent volume of distribution is 2,348 L/kg and doesn't depend on dose administered. Drug is highly bound to plasma proteins, both albumin and alpha-1 acid glycoprotein, but it doesn't appear to interact with the binding of warfarin, phenytoin, or tamoxifen to plasma proteins.
Metabolism: Undergoes extensive first-pass metabolism to glucuronide conjugates.
Excretion: Primarily excreted in the feces with less than 6% of dose eliminated as glucuronide conjugates in the urine. Less than 0.2% of dose is excreted unchanged in urine.

Route	Onset	Peak	Duration
P.O.	Unknown	Unknown	24 hr

Contraindications and precautions
Contraindicated in patients hypersensitive to drug or constituents of tablet. Also contraindicated in pregnant women or those planning pregnancy and in women with past history of or currently active venous thromboembolic events including pulmonary embolism, retinal vein thrombosis, and deep vein thrombosis. Use with hormone replacement therapy or systemic estrogen hasn't been evaluated and isn't recommended. Use with caution in patients with severe hepatic impairment. Potential risk/benefit should be assessed in women at righ risk for thromboembolic disease secondary to heart failure, superficial thrombophlebitis, or active malignancy.

Interactions
Drug-drug. *Cholestyramine:* Causes a significant reduction in absorption of raloxifene; don't use these drugs together.
Other highly protein-bound drugs, such as clofibrate, diazepam, diazoxide, ibuprofen, indomethacin, and naproxen: May interfere with binding sites. Use together cautiously .
Warfarin: Decreases PT. Monitor PT and INR.

Effects on diagnostic tests
None reported.

Adverse reactions
CNS: depression, insomnia, headache.
CV: *hot flashes,* chest pain, migraine.
EENT: *sinusitis,* pharyngitis, laryngitis.
GI: nausea, dyspepsia, vomiting, flatulence, GI disorder, gastroenteritis, diarrhea, abdominal pain.
GU: vaginitis, urinary tract infection, cystitis, leukorrhea, endometrial disorder, vaginal bleeding, breast pain.
Metabolic: weight gain.
Musculoskeletal: *arthralgia,* myalgia, arthritis, leg cramps.
Respiratory: increased cough, pneumonia.
Skin: rash, sweating.
Other: *infection, flu syndrome,* fever, peripheral edema; increased apolipoprotein A-I and

reduced serum total cholesterol, low-density lipoprotein cholesterol, fibrinogen, apolipoprotein B, and lipoprotein; increased hormone-binding globulin levels.

Overdose and treatment
There have been no reports of overdose. No specific antidote for raloxifene overdose exists. In one study, a dose of 600 mg/day was safely tolerated.

Clinical considerations
- Discontinue drug at least 72 hours before prolonged immobilization.
- Endometrial proliferation hasn't been associated with drug use. Evaluate unexplained uterine bleeding.
- A decrease in total and low-density lipoprotein cholesterol by 6% and 11% respectively has been reported. No effect on high-density lipoprotein or triglycerides has been shown.
- There are no data to support drug use in premenopausal women; avoid use in this population.
- Safety and efficacy haven't been evaluated in men.
- Effect on bone mineral density beyond 2 years of drug treatment isn't known. Safety and efficacy haven't been established beyond 2 years.

Therapeutic monitoring
- The greatest risk for thromboembolic events (deep vein thrombosis, pulmonary embolism, retinal vein thrombosis) occurs during first 4 months of treatment.
- No association between breast enlargement, breast pain, or an increased risk of breast cancer has been shown. Evaluate breast abnormalities that occur during treatment.

Special populations
Breast-feeding patients. It's unknown if drug is excreted in breast milk. Don't use in breast-feeding women.
Pediatric patients. Drug hasn't been evaluated in children; don't use in this population.
Geriatric patients. No age-related differences have been observed in patients age 42 to 84.

Patient counseling
- Tell patient to avoid long periods of restricted movement (such as during traveling) because of an increased risk of venous thromboembolic events, such as deep vein thrombosis and pulmonary embolism.
- Inform patient that hot flashes or flushing may occur and don't disappear with drug use.
- Tell patient to take supplemental calcium and vitamin D if dietary intake is inadequate.
- Encourage patient to perform weight-bearing exercises. Also advise her to stop alcohol consumption and smoking.
- Tell patient that drug may be taken without regard for food.

ramipril
Altace

Pharmacologic classification: ACE inhibitor
Therapeutic classification: antihypertensive
Pregnancy risk category C (D second and third trimesters)

How supplied
Available by prescription only
Capsules: 1.25 mg, 2.5 mg, 5 mg, 10 mg

Indications and dosages
Treatment of hypertension either alone or in combination with thiazide diuretics
Adults: Initially, 2.5 mg P.O. daily in patients not receiving concomitant diuretic therapy. Adjust dose based on blood pressure response. Usual maintenance dosage is 2.5 to 20 mg daily as a single dose or in two equal doses.

In patients receiving diuretic therapy, symptomatic hypotension may occur. To minimize this, discontinue diuretic, if possible, 2 to 3 days before starting ramipril. When this isn't possible, initial dose of ramipril should be 1.25 mg.

≡ ***Dosage adjustment.*** In renally impaired patients with creatinine clearance below 40 ml/minute (serum creatinine above 2.5 mg/dl), recommended initial dose is 1.25 mg daily, adjusted upward to maximum dose of 5 mg based on blood pressure response.

Heart failure post-MI
Adults: Initially, 2.5 mg P.O. b.i.d. Adjust to target dose of 5 mg P.O. b.i.d.

Pharmacodynamics
Antihypertensive action: Ramipril and its active metabolite, ramiprilat, inhibit ACE, preventing conversion of angiotensin I to angiotensin II, a potent vasoconstrictor. Reduced formation of angiotensin II decreases peripheral arterial resistance and, in turn, decreases aldosterone secretion, reduces sodium and water retention, and lowers blood pressure. Ramipril also has antihypertensive activity in patients with low-renin hypertension.

Pharmacokinetics
Absorption: 50% to 60% is absorbed after oral administration.
Distribution: Ramipril is 73% serum protein-bound; ramiprilat, 56%.
Metabolism: Ramipril is almost completely metabolized to ramiprilat, which has six times more ACE inhibitory effects than parent drug.

Excretion: 60% is excreted in urine; 40% in feces. Less than 2% of administered dose is excreted in urine as unchanged drug.

Route	Onset	Peak	Duration
P.O.	1-2 hr	1-3 hr	24 hr

Contraindications and precautions
Contraindicated in patients with hypersensitivity to ACE inhibitors or history of angioedema related to treatment with an ACE inhibitor. Use cautiously in patients with impaired renal function.

Interactions
Drug-drug. *Diuretics:* Excessive hypotension may result if used together. Discontinue diuretic or lower dosage of ramipril as needed.
Lithium: Increased serum lithium levels and lithium toxicity have been reported when used together. Monitor levels closely.
Potassium-sparing diuretics or potassium supplements: May result in hyperkalemia. Monitor serum potassium levels.
Drug-food. *Potassium-containing salt substitutes:* May cause hyperkalemia. Don't use together.
Drug-lifestyle. *Sun exposure:* May cause photosensitivity reaction. Advise patient to take precautions.

Effects on diagnostic tests
None reported.

Adverse reactions
CNS: asthenia, dizziness, fatigue, headache, malaise, light-headedness, anxiety, amnesia, ***seizures,*** depression, insomnia, nervousness, neuralgia, neuropathy, paresthesia, somnolence, tremor, vertigo.
CV: orthostatic hypotension, syncope, angina, ***arrhythmias, MI,*** chest pain, palpitations.
EENT: epistaxis, tinnitus.
GI: nausea, vomiting, abdominal pain, anorexia, constipation, diarrhea, dyspepsia, dry mouth, gastroenteritis, ***hepatitis.***
GU: impotence, increased BUN and creatinine levels.
Hematologic: hemolytic anemia, ***pancytopenia, neutropenia, thrombocytopenia.***
Musculoskeletal: arthralgia, arthritis, myalgia.
Respiratory: *dry, persistent, tickling, nonproductive cough;* dyspnea.
Skin: hypersensitivity reactions, rash, dermatitis, pruritus, photosensitivity.
Other: ***angioedema,*** edema, hyperkalemia, increased diaphoresis, weight gain; decreased hemoglobin levels and hematocrit, and elevations of liver enzymes, serum bilirubin, uric acid, and blood glucose.

Overdose and treatment
The most common sign is expected to be hypotension. No cases of overdose have been reported; specific management of ramipril overdose hasn't been established. Provide supportive care.

Clinical considerations
Like other ACE inhibitors, ramipril may cause a dry, persistent, tickling, nonproductive cough, which is reversible when drug is stopped.

Therapeutic monitoring
- Monitor blood pressure regularly.
- Monitor CBC and differential counts before and during therapy.
- Assess renal and hepatic function before and periodically throughout therapy.
- Monitor serum potassium levels.

Special populations
Breast-feeding patients. Drug shouldn't be administered to breast-feeding women.
Pediatric patients. Safety and efficacy in children haven't been established.
Geriatric patients. No age-related differences in safety or efficacy have been observed.

Patient counseling
- Tell patient to report signs or symptoms of angioedema immediately: swelling of face, eyes, lips or tongue or difficulty in breathing. Tell him to stop taking drug and seek medical attention.
- Warn patient that light-headedness can occur, especially during first few days of therapy. Tell him to change positions slowly to reduce hypotensive effect and to report these symptoms. If syncope (fainting) occurs, instruct patient to stop taking drug and call doctor immediately.
- Warn patient that inadequate fluid intake, vomiting, diarrhea, or excessive perspiration can lead to light-headedness and syncope. Advise caution in excessive heat and during exercise.
- Tell patient to immediately report signs of infection, such as sore throat or fever.

ranitidine
Zantac, Zantac 75, Zantac EFFERdose, Zantac GELdose

Pharmacologic classification:
H_2-receptor antagonist
Therapeutic classification: antiulcer
Pregnancy risk category B

How supplied
Available by prescription only
Tablets: 150 mg, 300 mg
Tablets (effervescent): 150 mg
Capsules: 150 mg, 300 mg

Granules (effervescent): 150 mg
Injection: 25 mg/ml
Injection (premixed): 50 mg/50 ml, 50 mg/100 ml
Syrup: 15 mg/ml
Available without a prescription
Tablets: 75 mg

Indications and dosages

Duodenal and gastric ulcer (short-term treatment); pathologic hypersecretory conditions such as Zollinger-Ellison syndrome
Adults: 150 mg P.O. b.i.d. or 300 mg h.s. Doses up to 6 g/day may be given in patients with Zollinger-Ellison syndrome. May give drug parenterally: 50 mg I.V. or I.M. q 6 to 8 hours.
Maintenance therapy in duodenal ulcer
Adults: 150 mg P.O. h.s.
Prophylaxis of stress ulcer
Adults: Continuous I.V. infusion of 150 mg in 250 ml compatible solution delivered at a rate of 6.25 mg/ hour using an infusion pump.
Gastroesophageal reflux disease
Adults: 150 mg P.O. b.i.d.
Erosive esophagitis
Adults: 150 mg or 10 ml (2 teaspoonfuls equivalent to 150 mg of ranitidine) P.O. q.i.d.
Self-medication for relief of occasional heartburn, acid indigestion, and sour stomach
Adults and adolescents age 12 and older: 75 mg P.O. once or twice daily; maximum dose, 150 mg in 24 hours.

Pharmacodynamics

Antiulcer action: Ranitidine competitively inhibits action of histamine at H_2-receptors in gastric parietal cells. This reduces basal and nocturnal gastric acid secretion as well as that caused by histamine, food, amino acids, insulin, and pentagastrin.

Pharmacokinetics

Absorption: About 50% to 60% of an oral dose is absorbed; food doesn't significantly affect absorption. After I.M. injection, drug is absorbed rapidly from parenteral sites.
Distribution: Distributed to many body tissues and appears in CSF and breast milk. Drug is about 10% to 19% protein-bound.
Metabolism: Metabolized in the liver.
Excretion: Excreted in urine and feces. Half-life is 2 to 3 hours.

Route	Onset	Peak	Duration
P.O.	1 hr	1-3 hr	13 hr
I.V., I.M.	Unknown	Unknown	Unknown

Contraindications and precautions

Contraindicated in patients hypersensitive to drug or in those with history of acute porphyria. Use cautiously in patients with impaired renal or hepatic function.

Interactions

Drug-drug. *Antacids:* Decrease ranitidine absorption. Give drugs at least 1 hour apart.
Diazepam: Concurrent use decreases diazepam absorption. Monitor closely.
Glipizide: May increase hypoglycemic effect. Dosage adjustment of glipizide may be necessary.
Procainamide: Drug may decrease renal clearance of procainamide. Monitor patient closely for toxicity.
Warfarin: May interfere with clearance of warfarin. Monitor closely.

Effects on diagnostic tests

Ranitidine may cause false-positive results in urine protein tests using Multistix.

Adverse reactions

CNS: malaise, vertigo.
EENT: blurred vision.
Hematologic: reversible leukopenia, ***pancytopenia, granulocytopenia, thrombocytopenia.***
Hepatic: elevated liver enzymes, jaundice.
Other: burning, itching (at injection site); ***anaphylaxis;*** angioneurotic edema, increased serum creatinine.

Overdose and treatment

No cases of overdose have been reported. However, treatment would involve emesis or gastric lavage and supportive measures as needed. Drug is removed by hemodialysis.

Clinical considerations

- When administering I.V. push, dilute to a total volume of 20 ml and inject over 5 minutes. No dilution necessary when administering I.M. Drug may also be administered by intermittent I.V. infusion. Dilute 50 mg ranitidine in 100 ml of D_5W and infuse over 15 to 20 minutes.
- Dosage adjustment may be required in patients with impaired renal function.
- Dialysis removes ranitidine; administer drug after treatment.

Therapeutic monitoring

Assess for abdominal pain. Note presence of blood in emesis, stool, or gastric aspirate.

Special populations

Breast-feeding patients. Drug is excreted in breast milk; use cautiously in breast-feeding women.
Geriatric patients. Geriatric patients may experience more adverse reactions because of reduced renal clearance. Debilitated patients may experience reversible confusion, agitation, depression, and hallucinations.

Patient counseling

- Instruct patient to take drug as directed, even after pain subsides, to ensure proper healing.

- If patient is taking a single daily dose, advise him to take it at bedtime.
- Instruct patient not to take OTC preparations continuously for longer than 2 weeks without medical supervision.
- Tell patient to swallow oral medication whole with water and not to chew tablets.

ranitidine bismuth citrate

Tritec

Pharmacologic classification:
H_2-receptor antagonist, antimicrobial
Therapeutic classification: antiulcer
Pregnancy risk category C

How supplied

Available by prescription only
Tablets: 400 mg

Indications and dosages

In combination with clarithromycin for treatment of active duodenal ulcer associated with* Helicobacter pylori *infection
Adults: 400 mg P.O. b.i.d for 28 days in conjunction with clarithromycin 500 mg P.O. t.i.d. for first 14 days.

Pharmacodynamics

Antiulcer activity: Ranitidine reduces gastric acid secretion by competitively inhibiting histamine at the H_2-receptor of the gastric parietal cells. Bismuth is a topical agent that disrupts the integrity of bacterial cell walls, prevents adhesion of *H. pylori* to gastric epithelium, decreases the development of resistance, and inhibits *H. pylori's* urease, phospholipase and proteolytic activity.

Pharmacokinetics

Absorption: Dissociates to ranitidine and bismuth following ingestion. Oral bioavailability of bismuth is variable.
Distribution: Volume of distribution of ranitidine is 1.7 L/kg. Ranitidine and bismuth are 15% and 98% protein-bound, respectively.
Metabolism: Metabolized by the liver. It's unknown if bismuth undergoes biotransformation.
Excretion: Primarily eliminated by the kidney. Elimination half-life of ranitidine is about 3 hours. Bismuth is excreted primarily in feces. Bismuth also undergoes minor excretion in the bile and urine. Terminal elimination half-life of bismuth is 11 to 28 days.

Route	Onset	Peak	Duration
P.O.	Unknown	Variable	Variable

Contraindications and precautions

Contraindicated in patients with known hypersensitivity to drug or its components.

Interactions

Drug-drug. *Clarithromycin:* Combination of these drugs shouldn't be used in patients with history of acute porphyria. Also, this combination isn't recommended in patients with creatinine clearance below 25 ml/minute.
Diazepam: Decreased absorption. Separate administration times.
Glipizide: Ranitidine may increase the hypoglycemic effects of glipizide. Monitor glucose levels.
High-dose antacids (170 mEq): May decrease plasma level of ranitidine and bismuth. Monitor closely.
Procainamide: Ranitidine may increase plasma levels of procainamide. Monitor closely.
Warfarin: May increase hypoprothrombinemic effects. Monitor PT and INR and adjust dose as needed.

Effects on diagnostic tests

Drug may cause false-positive results in urine protein tests using Multistix; test with sulfosalicylic acid if necessary.

Adverse reactions

CNS: headache.
GI: constipation, diarrhea.

Overdose and treatment

There has been limited experience with overdose. If overdose occurs, take measures to remove unabsorbed drug from GI tract. Monitor symptoms and use other supportive measures if necessary.

Clinical considerations

- Drug shouldn't be prescribed alone for treatment of active duodenal ulcers.
- If drug therapy in combination with clarithromycin isn't successful, patient is considered to have clarithromycin-resistant *H. pylori* and shouldn't be retreated with another regimen containing clarithromycin.
- Dialysis removes ranitidine; administer drug after treatment.

Therapeutic monitoring

Monitor patient for abdominal pain, and blood in stool, or emesis. Drug may cause a temporary and harmless darkening of the tongue or stool.

Special populations

Breast-feeding patients. Ranitidine has been shown to be excreted in breast milk; use caution when administering drug to breast-feeding women.
Pediatric patients. Safety and efficacy haven't been established in children.
Geriatric patients. Serum drug levels may be increased in geriatric patients.

Patient counseling
- Inform patient that drug may be administered without regard to food.
- Instruct patient to take drug as directed, even after pain has subsided.
- Stress importance of taking clarithromycin with drug for specified length of time.

rapacuronium bromide
Raplon

Pharmacologic classification: nondepolarizing neuromuscular blocker
Therapeutic classification: skeletal muscle relaxant
Pregnancy risk category C

How supplied
Available by prescription only
Injection: 20 mg/ml

Indications and dosages
Adjunct to general anesthesia to facilitate tracheal intubation and to provide skeletal muscle relaxation during short surgical procedures
Dosage is highly individualized. The following doses should serve as a guide only.
Adults: Initially, 1.5 mg/kg I.V. bolus. In most patients, tracheal intubation may be performed within 60 to 90 seconds and muscle paralysis should last about 15 minutes. Following an intubating dose of 1.5 mg/kg, up to three maintenance dosages of 0.5 mg/kg I.V. bolus may be administered. Repeat dosing based on the clinical duration of the previous dose; this shouldn't be administered until recovery of neuromuscular function is evident.
Adults undergoing Cesarean section with thiopental induction: 2.5 mg/kg I.V. bolus.
Children age 13 to 17: Individualize dosage considering physical maturity, height, and weight.
Children age 1 month to 12 years: 2 mg/kg I.V. bolus will produce acceptable intubating conditions within 60 to 90 seconds and muscle paralysis should last about 15 minutes.

Pharmacodynamics
Skeletal muscle relaxant action: Rapacuronium bromide acts by competing with acetylcholine for cholinergic receptors at the motor end plate, blocking depolarization. This action can be reversed by neostigmine, an acetylcholinesterase inhibitor.

Pharmacokinetics
Absorption: After I.V. administration, the onset occurs rapidly. The duration of action is about 15 minutes for the recommended adult dose of 1.5 mg/kg.
Distribution: About 50% to 88% protein-bound.
Metabolism: Undergoes hydrolysis to the 3-hydroxy metabolite, the major and active metabolite.
Excretion: Of the administered dose, about 28% is excreted in both urine and feces.

Route	Onset	Peak	Duration
I.V.	Rapid	90 sec	15 min

Contraindications and precautions
Contraindicated in patients with a known hypersensitivity to rapacuronium bromide.

Use cautiously in patients with myasthenia gravis, myasthenic syndrome, renal or hepatic dysfunction, acid-base abnormalities, electrolyte disturbances, burns, disuse atrophy, cachexia, and carcinomatosis. Also use cautiously in debilitated patients and in patients with neuromuscular disease.

Interactions
Drug-drug. *Anticonvulsants such as carbamazepine and phenytoin:* May reduce the duration of action of rapacuronium bromide, resulting in higher infusion rates and the development of resistance. Use with extreme caution. *Certain antibiotics, such as aminoglycosides, vancomycin, tetracyclines, bacitracin, polymyxin, and colistin; inhalation anesthetics, such as desflurane, enflurane, halothane, isoflurane, and sevoflurane; lithium; local anesthetics; magnesium salts; procainamide; quinidine:* May enhance the neuromuscular blocking action of rapacuronium bromide. Use cautiously together; consider lower doses of bromide.

Effects on diagnostic tests
None reported.

Adverse reactions
CV: hypotension, tachycardia, ***bradycardia.***
GI: vomiting, nausea.
Respiratory: *bronchospasm.*
Skin: rash.

Overdose and treatment
Overdose of rapacuronium bromide may result in neuromuscular block extending beyond the time needed for surgery and anesthesia. The primary treatment is maintenance of a patent airway and controlled ventilation until recovery of neuromuscular function is assured. Neostigmine may reverse the effects of the drug. Use a peripheral nerve stimulator to monitor recovery and to evaluate neuromuscular blockade.

Clinical considerations
☐ ***ALERT:*** Rapacuronium bromide shouldn't be administered as a continuous infusion, particularly during long surgical procedures or in an ICU setting.
- Use only under direct medical supervision by experienced clinicians skilled with the use

of neuromuscular blockers and techniques in airway management. Don't administer unless facilities and equipment for artificial respiration, oxygen therapy, and intubation and an antagonist are within reach.

- Administration of rapacuronium bromide must be accompanied by adequate anesthesia or sedating agents because it has no effect on consciousness or pain.
- Reconstitute drug with sterile water for injection or other compatible I.V. solutions such as normal saline, 5% dextrose in water, 5% dextrose in saline, lactated Ringers, and bacteriostatic water for injection.
- Use within 24 hours of reconstitution with solution. Prepared solutions may be stored at room temperature or refrigerated at 36° to 77° F (2° to 25° C). Don't use if particulate matter is present in solution.
- Use a peripheral nerve stimulator to measure neuromuscular function during administration in order to monitor drug effect, determine the need for additional doses, and confirm recovery from neuromuscular block.
- Additional doses shouldn't be administered until there's a definite response to nerve stimulation.
- In morbidly obese (body mass index over 40 kg/m^2) patients, dose should be based on ideal body weight. In all other patients, the initial dose is based on actual body weight.
- In patients with end stage renal disease, monitor closely for return of neuromuscular function because the condition increases the clearance time of the drug.
- Profound neuromuscular blockade can be reversed by neostigmine.

Therapeutic monitoring

- Assess baseline electrolyte determinations; electrolyte imbalance can potentiate neuromuscular blocking effects.
- Monitor vital signs, especially respirations and heart rate.

Special populations

Breast-feeding patients. It isn't known if drug is excreted in breast milk. Use with caution in breast-feeding women.
Pediatric patients. Safety and efficacy haven't been established in infants under age 1 month.
Geriatric patients. No dosage adjustment is recommended for geriatric patients.

Patient counseling

- Explain all events and procedures to the patient.
- Reassure the patient and his family that he'll be monitored at all times.

remifentanil hydrochloride

Ultiva

Pharmacologic classification: µ-opioid agonist
Therapeutic classification: analgesic, anesthetic
Controlled substance schedule II
Pregnancy risk category C

How supplied

Available by prescription only
Injection: 1 mg/3 ml, 2 mg/5 ml, 5 mg/10 ml vials

Indications and dosages

Induction of anesthesia through intubation
Adults: 0.5 to 1 mcg/kg/minute with hypnotic or volatile agent; may load with 1 mcg/kg over 30 to 60 seconds if endotracheal intubation is to occur less than 8 minutes after start of remifentanil infusion.
Maintenance of anesthesia
Adults: 0.25 to 0.4 mcg/kg/minute, based on concurrent anesthetic agents (nitrous oxide, isoflurane, propofol). Increase doses by 25% to 100% and decrease by 25% to 50% q 2 to 5 minutes, p.r.n. If rate exceeds 1 mcg/kg/minute, consider increases in concurrent anesthetics. May supplement with 1 mcg/kg boluses over 30 to 60 seconds q 2 to 5 minutes, p.r.n.
Continuation as analgesic immediately postoperatively
Adults: 0.1 mcg/kg/minute, followed by infusion rate of 0.025 to 0.2 mcg/kg/minute. Adjust rate by 0.025-mcg/kg/minute increments q 5 minutes. Rates over 0.2 mcg/kg/minute are associated with respiratory depression (under 8 breaths/minute).
Dosing for monitored anesthesia care
Adults: As single I.V. dose: administer 0.5 to 1 mcg/kg over 30 to 60 seconds starting 90 seconds before placement of local or regional anesthetic. Decrease dose by 50% if given with 2 mg midazolam.

As continuous I.V. infusion: 0.1 mcg/kg/minute beginning 5 minutes before local anesthetic given; after placement of local anesthetic, adjust rate to 0.05 mcg/kg/minute. Adjust rate by 0.025 mcg/kg/minute q 5 minutes, p.r.n. Rates over 0.2 mcg/kg/minute are associated with respiratory depression (less than 8 breaths/minute). Decrease dose by 50% if given with 2 mg midazolam. Bolus doses administered simultaneously with continuously infusing remifentanil to spontaneously breathing patients aren't recommended.

≡ ***Dosage adjustment.*** In obese patients, base starting dose on ideal body weight.

In patients over age 65, decrease starting dose by 50%. Cautiously titrate to effect.

Pharmacodynamics

Analgesic action: Drug binds to μ-opiate receptors throughout the CNS, resulting in analgesia.

Pharmacokinetics

Absorption: After I.V. administration, drug is rapidly absorbed.
Distribution: Initially, drug is distributed throughout the blood and rapidly perfused tissues; then moves into peripheral tissues. Drug is about 70% bound to plasma proteins, of which two-thirds is bound to alpha$_1$-acid-glycoprotein.
Metabolism: Rapidly metabolized by hydrolysis via blood and tissue esterases, resulting in an inactive carboxylic acid metabolite. Drug isn't metabolized by plasma cholinesterase and isn't appreciably metabolized by the liver or lungs.
Excretion: After hydrolysis, inactive metabolite is excreted by the kidneys with an elimination half-life of about 90 minutes. Clearance of active drug is high; elimination half-life is 3 to 10 minutes.

Route	Onset	Peak	Duration
I.V.	Immediate	Unknown	5-10 min

Contraindications and precautions

Don't use via epidural or intrathecal routes because of presence of glycine in preparation. Contraindicated in patients with known hypersensitivity to fentanyl analogues.

Interactions

Drug-drug. *Inhaled anesthetics, benzodiazepines, and hypnotics:* Produce a synergistic effect. Monitor patient closely.

Effects on diagnostic tests

None reported.

Adverse reactions

CNS: agitation, chills, dizziness, *headache.*
CV: ***bradycardia,*** hypertension, *hypotension,* tachycardia.
EENT: visual disturbances.
GI: *nausea, vomiting.*
Musculoskeletal: *muscle rigidity.*
Respiratory: ***apnea,*** *hypoxia, respiratory depression.*
Skin: flushing, pain at injection site, *pruritus.*
Other: chills, fever, postoperative pain, shivering, sweating, warm sensation.

Overdose and treatment

Signs of overdose include apnea, chest wall rigidity, hypoxemia, hypotension, seizures, or bradycardia. If these signs occur, discontinue drug, maintain patent airway, initiate assisted or controlled ventilation with oxygen, and maintain CV function. Administer a neuromuscular blocker or opioid antagonist if decreased respiration is associated with muscle rigidity. Administer I.V. fluids and vasopressors for hypotension and glycopyrrolate or atropine for bradycardia. Naloxone may be used to manage severe respiratory depression. Use other supportive measures as needed.

Clinical considerations

- Don't use as a single agent in general anesthesia.
- Effects of long-term (over 16 hours) use in intensive care settings isn't known.
- Bradycardia has been reported and is responsive to ephedrine, atropine, and glycopyrrolate.
- Continuous infusions of drug must be administered by infusion device; use I.V. bolus administration only during maintenance of general anesthesia. In nonintubated patients, administer single doses over 30 to 60 seconds. Interruption of drug infusion results in rapid reversal (no residual opioid effects within 5 to 10 minutes of infusion discontinuation) of effects; first establish adequate postoperative anesthesia. Upon discontinuation of drug, I.V. clear tubing to avoid inadvertent administration of drug at a later time.
- Drug shouldn't be used outside the monitored anesthesia care setting.
- Drug is incompatible with blood products; don't mix with lactated Ringer's solution or dextrose 5% lactated Ringer's solutions, but can coadminister with these two diluents into a running I.V. administration set.
- Obtain history from patient regarding previous adverse anesthesia reactions in patient or patient's family.

Therapeutic monitoring

- Monitor vital signs and oxygenation continually throughout drug administration.
- If respiratory depression occurs in a spontaneously breathing patient, decrease infusion rate by 50% or temporarily discontinue infusion.
- If skeletal muscle rigidity occurs in a spontaneously breathing patient, stop or decrease rate of infusion.
- If hypotension occurs, treat by decreasing administration rate, I.V. fluids, or catecholamine administration.

Special populations

Breast-feeding patients. Because fentanyl analogues are excreted in breast milk, use with caution in breast-feeding women.
Pediatric patients. Use in children under age 2 hasn't been studied.
Geriatric patients. Decrease initial doses by 50% in the elderly and titrate to desired effect.

Patient counseling

Reassure patient that appropriate monitoring will occur during anesthesia administration.

repaglinide

Prandin

Pharmacologic classification: meglitinide
Therapeutic classification: antidiabetic
Pregnancy risk category C

How supplied

Available by prescription only
Tablets: 0.5 mg, 1 mg, 2 mg

Indications, and dosages

Adjunct to diet and exercise in lowering blood glucose in patients with type 2 diabetes mellitus whose hyperglycemia can't be controlled by diet and exercise alone

Adults: For patients not previously treated or whose HbA_{1c} is below 8%, starting dose is 0.5 mg P.O. with each meal given 15 minutes before meal; however, time may vary from immediately before to as long as 30 minutes before meal. For patients previously treated with glucose-lowering drugs and whose HbA_{1c} is 8% or more, initial dose is 1 to 2 mg P.O. with each meal. Recommended dosage range is 0.5 to 4 mg with meals b.i.d., t.i.d., or q.i.d. Maximum daily dose is 16 mg.

Dosage should be determined by blood glucose response. May double dosage up to 4 mg with each meal until satisfactory blood glucose response is achieved. At least 1 week should elapse between dosage adjustments to assess response to each dose.

Metformin may be added if repaglinide monotherapy is inadequate.

Pharmacodynamics

Antidiabetic action: Stimulates the release of insulin from the beta cells in the pancreas. Repaglinide closes ATP-dependent potassium channels in the beta cell membrane, which causes depolarization of the B-cell and opening of the calcium channels. The increased calcium influx induces insulin secretion; the overall effect is to lower the blood glucose level.

Pharmacokinetics

Absorption: Rapidly and completely absorbed with oral administration.

Distribution: Mean volume of distribution after I.V. administration is 31 L; protein binding to albumin exceeds 98%.

Metabolism: Completely metabolized by oxidative biotransformation and conjugation with glucuronic acid. The P-450 isoenzyme system (specifically CYP 3A4) has also been shown to be involved in N-dealkylation of repaglinide. All metabolites are inactive and don't contribute to the blood glucose-lowering effect.

Excretion: About 90% of dose occurs in the feces as metabolites. About 8% of a dose is recovered in the urine as metabolites and less than 0.1% as parent drug. Half-life is about 1 hour.

Route	Onset	Peak	Duration
P.O.	Unknown	1 hr	Unknown

Contraindications and precautions

Contraindicated in patients with hypersensitivity to drug or its inactive ingredients and in those with insulin-dependent diabetes mellitus or ketoacidosis. Use cautiously in patients with hepatic insufficiency in whom reduced metabolism could cause elevated blood levels of repaglinide and hypoglycemia.

Interactions

Drug-drug. *Barbiturates, carbamazepine, rifampin, and troglitazone:* May increase the metabolism of repaglinide. Monitor glucose levels.

Beta blockers, chloramphenicol, coumarin, MAO inhibitors, NSAIDs, other drugs that are highly protein-bound, probenecid, salicylates, and sulfonamides: May potentiate the hypoglycemic action of repaglinide. Monitor glucose levels.

Calcium channel blockers, corticosteroids, estrogens, isoniazid, nicotinic acid, oral contraceptives, phenothiazines, phenytoin, sympathomimetics, thiazides and other diuretics, thyroid products: May produce hyperglycemia. Monitor glucose levels.

Erythromycin, ketoconazole, miconazole, and similar inhibitors of the P-450 cytochrome system 3A4: Repaglinide metabolism may be inhibited. Monitor glucose levels.

Effects on diagnostic tests

None reported.

Adverse reactions

CNS: *headache.*
CV: chest pain, angina.
EENT: tooth disorder, rhinitis.
GI: nausea, diarrhea, constipation, vomiting, dyspepsia.
GU: urinary tract infection.
Metabolic: HYPOGLYCEMIA.
Musculoskeletal: arthralgia, back pain.
Respiratory: bronchitis, sinusitis, *upper respiratory infection.*

Overdose and treatment

Overdose is associated with few adverse effects other than those associated with the intended effect of lowering blood glucose. Treat hypoglycemic symptoms without loss of consciousness or neurologic findings aggressively with oral glucose and dosage or meal pattern adjustments. Monitor patient closely for minimum of 24 to 48 hours because hypoglycemia may recur after apparent clinical recovery. Treat severe hypoglycemic reactions with coma, seizure, or other neurologic impairment immediately with I.V. dextrose 50% solution followed by a continuous infusion of glucose 10% solution. Careful blood sugar monitoring must occur.

Clinical considerations

- Be aware that administration of other oral antidiabetic agents has been reported to be associated with increased CV mortality compared with diet treatment alone. Although not specifically evaluated for repaglinide, this warning may also apply.
- Loss of glycemic control can occur during stress, such as fever, trauma, infection, or surgery. If this occurs, discontinue drug and administer insulin.
- Be aware that hypoglycemia may be difficult to recognize in the elderly and in patients taking beta blockers.

Therapeutic monitoring

- Use caution when increasing drug dosage in patients with impaired renal function or renal failure requiring dialysis.
- Monitor patient's blood glucose periodically to determine minimum effective dose.
- Monitor long-term efficacy by measuring HbA_{1c} levels every 3 months.

Special populations

Breast-feeding patients. Although it isn't known if drug is excreted in breast milk, studies in animals have indicated excretion similar to other glucose-lowering agents. Because the potential for hypoglycemia in a breast-fed infant exists, a decision should be made as to whether to discontinue drug or breast-feeding.
Pediatric patients. No studies have been performed in pediatric patients to determine safety and efficacy.
Geriatric patients. In clinical studies there was no increase in the frequency or severity of hypoglycemia in older patients.

Patient counseling

- Instruct patient on importance of diet and exercise in combination with drug therapy.
- Discuss symptoms of hypoglycemia with patient and family.
- Tell patient to take drug before meals, usually 15 minutes before start of meal; however, time can vary from immediately preceding meal to up to 30 minutes before meal.
- Tell patient that if a meal is skipped or an extra meal added, he should skip the dose or add an extra dose of drug for that meal.

reteplase, recombinant

Retavase

Pharmacologic classification: tissue-plasminogen activator
Therapeutic classification: thrombolytic enzyme
Pregnancy risk category C

How supplied

Available by prescription only
Injection: 10.8 units (18.8 mg)/vial (supplied in kit with components for reconstitution and administration of two single-use vials)

Indications and dosages

Management of acute MI
Adults: Double-bolus injection of 10 + 10 units. Give each bolus I.V. over 2 minutes. If no complications occur after first bolus, such as serious bleeding or anaphylactoid reactions, give second bolus 30 minutes after start of first bolus. Initiate treatment soon after onset of symptoms of acute MI. There's no experience of repeat courses with reteplase.

Pharmacodynamics

Thrombolytic action: Drug catalyzes the cleavage of plasminogen to generate plasmin, which leads to fibrinolysis.

Pharmacokinetics

Absorption: Given I.V.
Distribution: Cleared from plasma at a rate of 250 to 450 ml/minute.
Metabolism: Metabolized primarily by the liver and kidney.
Excretion: Plasma half-life of drug is 13 to 16 minutes.

Route	Onset	Peak	Duration
I.V.	Unknown	Unknown	Unknown

Contraindications and precautions

Contraindicated in patients with active internal bleeding, known bleeding diathesis, history of CVA, recent intracranial or intraspinal surgery or trauma, severe uncontrolled hypertension, intracranial neoplasm, arteriovenous malformation, or aneurysm.

Use cautiously in patients with recent (within 10 days) major surgery, obstetric delivery, organ biopsy, or trauma; previous puncture of noncompressible vessels; cerebrovascular disease; recent GI or GU bleeding; hypertension (systolic pressure 180 mm Hg or more or diastolic pressure 110 mm Hg or more); likelihood of left-sided heart thrombus; subacute bacterial endocarditis; acute pericarditis; hemostatic defects; diabetic hemorrhagic retinopathy; septic thrombophlebitis; other conditions in which bleeding would be difficult to manage; pregnancy; and in patients age 75 or older.

Interactions

Drug-drug. *Heparin, oral anticoagulants, platelet inhibitors, such as abciximab, aspirin, and dipyridamole, and vitamin K antagonists:* May increase risk of bleeding. Use together cautiously.

Effects on diagnostic tests

Drug may alter coagulation studies; it remains active in vitro and can lead to degradation of fibrinogen in sample. Collect blood samples in the presence of PPACK (chloromethylketone) at 2-μM concentrations.

Adverse reactions

CNS: ***intracranial hemorrhage.***
CV: ***arrhythmias, cholesterol embolization.***
GI: *hemorrhage.*
GU: hematuria.
Hematologic: *anemia,* ***bleeding tendency.***
Other: *bleeding* (at puncture site), ***hemorrhage.***

Overdose and treatment

No information available. Monitor for increased bleeding.

Clinical considerations

- Drug is administered I.V. as a double-bolus injection. If bleeding or anaphylactoid reactions occur after first bolus; second bolus may be withheld.
- Reconstitute drug according to manufacturer's instructions using items provided in the kit.
- Don't administer drug with other I.V. medications through same I.V. line. Heparin and reteplase are incompatible in solution.
- Be aware that potency is expressed in terms of units specific for reteplase and not comparable to other thrombolytic agents.
- Avoid use of noncompressible pressure sites during therapy. If an arterial puncture is needed, use an upper extremity vessel. Apply pressure for at least 30 minutes; then apply a pressure dressing. Check site frequently.

Therapeutic monitoring

- Carefully monitor ECG during treatment. Coronary thrombolysis may result in arrhythmias associated with reperfusion. Be prepared to treat bradycardia or ventricular irritability.
- Monitor for bleeding. Avoid I.M. injections, invasive procedures, and nonessential handling of patient. Bleeding is the most common adverse reaction and may occur internally or at external puncture sites. If local measures don't control serious bleeding, discontinue concurrent anticoagulation therapy. Withhold second bolus of reteplase.

Special populations

Breast-feeding patients. It's unknown if drug is excreted in the breast milk. Exercise caution if administered.
Pediatric patients. Safety and efficacy in children haven't been established.
Geriatric patients. Use cautiously in geriatric patients. Risk of intracranial hemorrhage increases with age.

Patient counseling

- Explain to patient and family about use and administration of reteplase.
- Tell patient to report adverse reactions such as signs and symptoms of bleeding or allergic reaction immediately.
- Advise patient about proper dental care to avoid excessive gum trauma.

ribavirin

Virazole

Pharmacologic classification: synthetic nucleoside
Therapeutic classification: antiviral
Pregnancy risk category X

How supplied

Available by prescription only
Powder to be reconstituted for inhalation: 6 g in 100-ml glass vial

Indications and dosages

Treatment of hospitalized infants and young children infected by respiratory syncytial virus (RSV)
Infants and young children: Solution in concentration of 20 mg/ml delivered via the Viratek Small Particle Aerosol Generator (SPAG-2) results in a mist with a concentration of 190 mcg/L. Treatment is carried out for 12 to 18 hours/day for at least 3, and no more than 7, days with a flow rate of 12.5 L of mist per minute.

For ventilated patients, use same dose with a pressure- or volume-cycled ventilator in conjunction with SPAG-2. Patient should be suctioned q 1 to 2 hours and pulmonary pressures checked q 2 to 4 hours.

Pharmacodynamics

Antiviral action: Drug action probably involves inhibition of RNA and DNA synthesis, inhibition of RNA polymerase, and interference with completion of viral polypeptide coat.

Pharmacokinetics

Absorption: Some ribavirin is absorbed systemically.
Distribution: Concentrates in bronchial secretions; plasma levels are subtherapeutic for plaque inhibition.

Metabolism: Metabolized to 1,2,4-triazole-3-carboxamide (deribosylated ribavirin).
Excretion: Mostly excreted renally. First phase of drug's plasma half-life is 9½ hours; second phase has extended half-life of 40 hours (from slow drug release from RBC binding sites).

Route	Onset	Peak	Duration
Inhalation	Unknown	Unknown	Unknown

Contraindications and precautions
Contraindicated in patients with hypersensitivity to drug and in women who are or may become pregnant during treatment. Contraindicated in women of childbearing age and their male partners when used in combination with interferon alfa-2b. Women of childbearing age and men must use two forms of contraception during therapy and 6 months after.

Interactions
None reported.

Effects on diagnostic tests
None reported.

Adverse reactions
CV: ***cardiac arrest,*** hypotension.
EENT: conjunctivitis, erythema of eyelids.
Hematologic: anemia, reticulocytosis.
Respiratory: worsening respiratory state, ***apnea,*** bacterial pneumonia, pneumothorax, ***bronchospasm.***
Skin: rash.

Overdose and treatment
Unknown in humans; high doses in animals have produced GI symptoms.

Clinical considerations
- Ribavirin aerosol is indicated for use only for lower respiratory tract infection caused by RSV. Although treatment may begin before test results are available, RSV infection must eventually be confirmed.
- Administer ribavirin aerosol only by SPAG-2. Don't use other aerosol-generating devices.
- Reconstitute solution with USP sterile water for injection or inhalation, then transfer aseptically to sterile 500-ml Erlenmeyer flask. Dilute further with sterile water to 300 ml to yield final level of 20 mg/ml. Solution remains stable for 24 hours at room temperature.
- Don't use bacteriostatic water (or any other water containing antimicrobial agent) to reconstitute drug.
- Discard unused solution in SPAG-2 unit before adding newly reconstituted solution. Change solution at least every 24 hours.

Therapeutic monitoring
- Monitor ventilator-dependent patients carefully because drug may precipitate in ventilatory apparatus. Change heated wire connective tubing and bacteria filters in series in expiratory limb of the system frequently (such as every 4 hours).
- Drug is most useful for infants with most severe RSV form, typically premature infants and those with underlying disorders such as cardiopulmonary disease. Most other infants and children with RSV infection don't require treatment because disease is self-limiting.
- Drug therapy must be accompanied by appropriate respiratory and fluid therapy.

Special populations
Pregnant patients. May cause fetal toxicity.
Breast-feeding patients. It's unknown if drug is excreted in breast milk. Not recommended for use in breast-feeding women.

Patient counseling
- Inform parents of need for drug and answer any questions they may have.
- Parents should report any change in child immediately.
- Inform patient that drug may be taken without regard to meals but should be administered in a consistent manner.

riboflavin (vitamin B_2)

Pharmacologic classification: water-soluble vitamin
Therapeutic classification: vitamin B complex vitamin
Pregnancy risk category A (C if more than the RDA)

How supplied
Available without a prescription
Tablets: 25 mg, 50 mg, 100 mg

Indications and dosages
Riboflavin deficiency or adjunct to thiamine treatment for polyneuritis or cheilosis secondary to pellagra
Adults and adolescents over age 12: 5 to 30 mg P.O. daily, depending on severity.
Children under age 12: 3 to 10 mg P.O. daily, depending on severity.
Microcytic anemia associated with splenomegaly and glutathione reductase deficiency
Adults: 10 mg P.O. daily for 10 days.
Dietary supplementation
Adults: 1 to 4 mg P.O. daily. For maintenance, increase nutritional intake and supplement with vitamin B complex.

Pharmacodynamics
Metabolic action: Riboflavin, a coenzyme, functions in the forms of flavin adenine dinucleotide (FAD) and flavin mononucleotide (FMN) and plays a vital metabolic role in numerous tissue respiration systems. FAD and

FMN act as hydrogen-carrier molecules for several flavoproteins involved in intermediary metabolism. Riboflavin is also directly involved in maintaining erythrocyte integrity.

Riboflavin deficiency causes a clinical syndrome with the following symptoms: cheilosis, angular stomatitis, glossitis, keratitis, scrotal skin changes, ocular changes, and seborrheic dermatitis. In severe deficiency, normochromic, normocytic anemia and neuropathy may occur. Clinical signs may become evident after 3 to 8 months of inadequate riboflavin intake. Administration of riboflavin reverses signs of deficiency. Riboflavin deficiency rarely occurs alone and is commonly associated with deficiency of other B vitamins and protein.

Pharmacokinetics

Absorption: Although riboflavin is absorbed readily from the GI tract, extent of absorption is limited. Absorption occurs at a specialized segment of the mucosa; drug absorption is limited by duration of drug's contact with this area. Before being absorbed, riboflavin-5-phosphate is rapidly dephosphorylated in the GI lumen. GI absorption increases when drug is administered with food and decreases when hepatitis, cirrhosis, biliary obstruction, or probenecid administration is present.
Distribution: FAD and FMN are distributed widely to body tissues. Free riboflavin is present in the retina. Riboflavin is stored in limited amounts in the liver, spleen, kidneys, and heart, mainly in the form of FAD. FAD and FMN are about 60% protein-bound in blood. Drug crosses the placenta, and breast milk contains about 400 ng/ml.
Metabolism: Metabolized in the liver.
Excretion: After a single oral dose, biologic half-life is about 66 to 84 minutes in healthy individuals. Drug is metabolized to FMN in erythrocytes, GI mucosal cells, and the liver; FMN is converted to FAD in the liver. About 9% of drug is excreted unchanged in the urine after normal ingestion. Excretion involves renal tubular secretion and glomerular filtration. Amount renally excreted unchanged is directly proportional to the dose. Drug removal by hemodialysis is slower than by natural renal excretion.

Route	Onset	Peak	Duration
P.O.	Unknown	Unknown	Unknown

Contraindications and precautions

No known contraindications.

Interactions

Drug-drug. *Oral contraceptives:* Riboflavin dose may need to be increased.
Propantheline bromide: Delays absorption rate of riboflavin but increases total amount absorbed. Monitor closely.

Drug-lifestyle. *Alcohol use:* Impairs intestinal absorption of riboflavin. Advise patient to avoid alcohol use.

Effects on diagnostic tests

Riboflavin therapy alters urinalysis based on spectrophotometry or color reactions. Riboflavin produces fluorescent substances in urine and plasma, which can falsely elevate fluorometric determinations of catecholamines and urobilinogen.

Adverse reactions

GU: bright yellow urine with high doses.

Overdose and treatment

No information available.

Clinical considerations

- RDA of riboflavin is 0.4 to 1.8 mg/day in children, 1.2 to 1.7 mg/day in adults, and 1.6 to 1.8 mg/day in pregnant and breast-feeding women.
- Give oral preparation of riboflavin with food to increase absorption.

Therapeutic monitoring

Obtain patient's dietary history because other vitamin deficiencies may coexist.

Special populations

Breast-feeding patients. Drug crosses the placenta; during pregnancy and lactation, riboflavin requirements are increased. Increased food intake during this time usually provides adequate amounts of the vitamin. The National Research Council recommends daily intake of 1.8 mg/day during first 6 months of breast-feeding.

Patient counseling

- Teach patient about good dietary sources of riboflavin, such as whole grain cereals and green vegetables. Liver, kidney, heart, eggs, and dairy products are also dietary sources but may not be appropriate, based on patient's serum cholesterol and triglyceride levels.
- Advise patient to store riboflavin in a tight, light-resistant container.

rifabutin

Mycobutin

Pharmacologic classification: semisynthetic ansamycin
Therapeutic classification: antibiotic
Pregnancy risk category B

How supplied

Available by prescription only
Capsules: 150 mg

Indications and dosages

Primary prevention of disseminated* Mycobacterium avium *complex (MAC) in patients with advanced HIV infection
Adults: 300 mg P.O. daily as a single dose or divided b.i.d. with food.

Pharmacodynamics

Antibiotic action: Rifabutin inhibits DNA-dependent RNA polymerase in susceptible strains of *Escherichia coli* and *Bacillus subtilis,* but not in mammalian cells. It isn't known whether rifabutin inhibits this enzyme in *M. avium* or in *M. intracellulare,* which compose MAC.

Pharmacokinetics

Absorption: Readily absorbed from the GI tract.
Distribution: Because of its high lipophilicity, rifabutin demonstrates a high propensity for distribution and intracellular tissue uptake. About 85% of drug is bound in a concentration-independent manner to plasma proteins.
Metabolism: Metabolized in the liver to five identified metabolites. The 25-0-desacetyl metabolite has an activity equal to parent drug and contributes up to 10% of total antimicrobial activity.
Excretion: Less than 10% is excreted in urine as unchanged drug. About 53% of the oral dose is excreted in urine, primarily as metabolites. About 30% is excreted in feces.

Route	Onset	Peak	Duration
P.O.	Unknown	2-4 hr	Unknown

Contraindications and precautions

Contraindicated in patients with hypersensitivity to drug or other rifamycin derivatives such as rifampin, and in patients with active tuberculosis because single-agent therapy with rifabutin increases the risk of inducing bacterial resistance to both rifabutin and rifampin.

Use cautiously in patients with preexisting neutropenia and thrombocytopenia.

Interactions

Drug-drug. *Drugs metabolized by the liver, zidovudine:* Rifabutin may decrease the serum levels, although it doesn't affect zidovudine's inhibition of HIV. Dosage adjustments may be necessary.
Oral contraceptives: Rifabutin decreases the effectiveness. Instruct patient to use nonhormonal forms of birth control.

Effects on diagnostic tests

None reported.

Adverse reactions

CNS: headache, insomnia.
GI: dyspepsia, eructation, flatulence, diarrhea, nausea, vomiting, abdominal pain, altered taste.
GU: *discolored urine* (brown-orange).
Hematologic: **NEUTROPENIA, LEUKOPENIA,** ***thrombocytopenia,*** eosinophilia.
Skin: *rash.*
Other: fever, myalgia.

Overdose and treatment

Although there's no experience in the treatment of drug overdose, clinical experience with rifamycins suggests that gastric lavage to evacuate gastric contents (within a few hours of overdose), followed by instillation of an activated charcoal slurry into the stomach, may help absorb any remaining drug from the GI tract. Hemodialysis or forced diuresis isn't expected to enhance systemic elimination of unchanged rifabutin.

Clinical considerations

□ ***ALERT*** Don't confuse similar-sounding drugs like rifabutin, rifampin, and rifapentine.

- High-fat meals slow rate but not extent of drug absorption.

Therapeutic monitoring

- Evaluate patient who develops complaints consistent with active tuberculosis during rifabutin prophylaxis immediately, so active disease may be given an effective combination regimen of antituberculosis medications. Administration of single-agent rifabutin to patients with active tuberculosis likely leads to development of tuberculosis that is resistant to rifabutin and rifampin.
- Because rifabutin may be associated with neutropenia, and more rarely thrombocytopenia, consider obtaining hematologic studies periodically in patients receiving rifabutin prophylaxis.

Special populations

Breast-feeding patients. It's unknown if drug is excreted in breast milk. Because of potential for serious adverse effects in breast-fed infants, either breast-feeding or drug should be discontinued, depending on importance of drug to woman.
Pediatric patients. Although safety and efficacy in children haven't been fully established, several studies indicate that drug may be helpful in children at maximum daily dose of 5 mg/kg.

Patient counseling

- Tell patient with swallowing difficulty to mix drug with soft foods such as applesauce.
- Advise patient with nausea, vomiting, or other GI upset to take drug with food, in two divided doses.
- Warn patient that urine and other body fluids may become discolored (brown-orange). Clothes and soft contact lenses may become permanently discolored.

rifampin

Rifadin, Rimactane

Pharmacologic classification: semisynthetic rifamycin B derivative (macrocyclic antibiotic)
Therapeutic classification: antituberculotic
Pregnancy risk category C

How supplied

Available by prescription only
Capsules: 150 mg, 300 mg
Injection: 600 mg/vial

Indications and dosages

Primary treatment in pulmonary tuberculosis
Adults: 600 mg P.O. or I.V. daily as a single dose (give P.O. dose 1 hour before or 2 hours after meals).
Children: 10 to 20 mg/kg P.O. or I.V. daily as a single dose (give P.O. dose 1 hour before or 2 hours after meals). Maximum daily dose, 600 mg. Concurrent administration of other effective antitubercular drugs is recommended. Treatment usually lasts 6 to 9 months.
Asymptomatic meningococcal carriers
Adults: 600 mg P.O. b.i.d. for 2 days.
Infants and children over age 1 month: 10 mg/kg P.O. b.i.d. for 2 days.
Neonates under age 1 month: 5 mg/kg P.O. b.i.d. for 2 days.
≡ ***Dosage adjustment.*** Reduce dosage in patients with hepatic dysfunction.
Prophylaxis of* Haemophilus influenzae *type B
Adults and children: 20 mg/kg (up to 600 mg) once daily for 4 consecutive days.
◊ ***Leprosy***
Adults: 600 mg P.O. once monthly, usually used in combination with other agents.

Pharmacodynamics

Antibiotic action: Rifampin impairs RNA synthesis by inhibiting DNA-dependent RNA polymerase. Rifampin may be bacteriostatic or bactericidal, depending on organism susceptibility and drug level at infection site.

Rifampin acts against *Mycobacterium bovis, M. kansasii, M. marinum, and M. tuberculosis,* some strains of *M. avium, M. avium-intracellulare and M. fortuitum,* and many gram-positive and some gram-negative bacteria. Resistance to rifampin by *M. tuberculosis* can develop rapidly; rifampin is usually given with other antituberculosis drugs to prevent or delay resistance.

Pharmacokinetics

Absorption: Absorbed completely from the GI tract after oral administration. Food delays absorption.
Distribution: Distributed widely into body tissues and fluids, including ascitic, pleural, seminal, and cerebrospinal fluids, tears, and saliva; and into liver, prostate, lungs, and bone. Drug crosses the placenta, and is 84% to 91% protein-bound.
Metabolism: Metabolized extensively in the liver by deacetylation. It undergoes enterohepatic circulation.
Excretion: Undergoes enterohepatic circulation, and drug and metabolite are excreted primarily in bile; drug, but not metabolite, is reabsorbed. From 6% to 30% of rifampin and metabolite appear unchanged in urine in 24 hours; about 60% is excreted in feces. Some drug is excreted in breast milk. Plasma half-life in adults is 1½ to 5 hours; serum levels rise in obstructive jaundice. Dosage adjustment isn't necessary for patients with renal failure. Rifampin isn't removed by either hemodialysis or peritoneal dialysis.

Route	Onset	Peak	Duration
P.O.	Unknown	2-4 hr	Unknown
I.V.	Unknown	Unknown	Unknown

Contraindications and precautions

Contraindicated in patients with hypersensitivity to drug. Use cautiously in patients with hepatic disease.

Interactions

Drug-drug. *Anticoagulants, barbiturates, beta blockers, cardiac glycoside derivatives, chloramphenicol, clofibrate, corticosteroids, cyclosporine, dapsone, disopyramide, estrogens, methadone, oral contraceptives, oral sulfonylureas, phenytoin, quinidine, tocainide, and verapamil:* Decreased effectiveness of these drugs. Monitor patient closely; may need dosage adjustment.
Isoniazid: Increased hazard of isoniazid hepatotoxicity. Monitor closely.
Oral contraceptives: Rifampin inactivates such drugs and may alter menstrual patterns. Advise oral contraceptive users to substitute other methods.
Para-aminosalicylate: May decrease oral absorption of rifampin, lowering serum levels. Administer drugs 8 to 12 hours apart.
Drug-lifestyle. *Alcohol use:* May increase risk of hepatotoxicity. Advise patient to avoid alcohol use during drug therapy.

Effects on diagnostic tests

Rifampin alters standard serum folate and vitamin B_{12} assays.

Rifampin may cause temporary retention of sulfobromophthalein in the liver excretion test; it may also interfere with contrast material in gallbladder studies and urinalysis based on spectrophotometry.

Adverse reactions

CNS: headache, fatigue, drowsiness, behavioral changes, dizziness, ataxia, mental confusion, generalized numbness.
EENT: visual disturbances, exudative conjunctivitis.
GI: epigastric distress, anorexia, nausea, vomiting, abdominal pain, diarrhea, flatulence, sore mouth and tongue, pseudomembranous colitis, pancreatitis.
GU: hemoglobinuria, hematuria, menstrual disturbances, ***acute renal failure.***
Hematologic: eosinophilia, ***thrombocytopenia,*** transient leukopenia, hemolytic anemia.
Hepatic: ***hepatotoxicity,*** *transient abnormalities in liver function tests.*
Respiratory: shortness of breath, wheezing.
Skin: pruritus, urticaria, rash.
Other: flulike syndrome, discoloration of body fluids, hyperuricemia, ***shock,*** osteomalacia, porphyria exacerbation.

Overdose and treatment

Signs of overdose include lethargy, nausea, and vomiting; hepatotoxicity from massive overdose includes hepatomegaly, jaundice, elevated liver function studies and bilirubin levels, and loss of consciousness. Red-orange discoloration of the skin, urine, sweat, saliva, tears, and feces may occur.

Treat by gastric lavage, followed by activated charcoal; if necessary, force diuresis. Perform bile drainage if hepatic dysfunction persists beyond 24 to 48 hours.

Clinical considerations

□ ***ALERT*** Don't confuse similar-sounding drugs like rifabutin, rifampin, and rifapentine.
- Give drug 1 hour before or 2 hours after meals for maximum absorption; capsule contents may be mixed with food or fluid to enhance swallowing.
- Specimens for culture and sensitivity testing will be obtained before giving first dose but don't delay therapy; repeat periodically to detect drug resistance.
- Reconstituted solution is stable for 24 hours at room temperature. Use infusion solutions of 100 to 500 ml within 4 hours.
- Increased liver enzyme activity inactivates certain drugs, especially warfarin, corticosteroids, and oral hypoglycemics, requiring dosage adjustments.

Therapeutic monitoring

- Observe patient for adverse reactions and monitor hematologic, renal and liver function studies, and serum electrolytes to minimize toxicity. Watch for signs and symptoms of hepatic impairment, such as anorexia, fatigue, malaise, jaundice, dark urine, and liver tenderness.

Special populations

Breast-feeding patients. Drug may be excreted in breast milk. Use with caution in breast-feeding women.
Pediatric patients. Safety in children under age 5 hasn't been established.
Geriatric patients. Usual dose in geriatric and debilitated patients is 10 mg/kg once daily. Monitor renal function closely, as geriatric patients may be more susceptible to toxic effects.

Patient counseling

- Explain disease process and rationale for long-term therapy.
- Teach signs and symptoms of hypersensitivity and other adverse reactions, and emphasize need to call if these occur; urge patient to report any unusual reactions.
- Urge patient to comply with prescribed regimen, not to miss doses, and not to discontinue drug without medical approval. Explain importance of follow-up appointments.
- Encourage patient to report promptly any flulike signs or symptoms, weakness, sore throat, loss of appetite, unusual bruising, rash, itching, tea-colored urine, clay-colored stools, or yellow discoloration of eyes or skin.
- Explain that drug turns all body fluids red-orange color; advise patient of possible permanent stains on clothes and soft contact lenses.

rifapentine

Priftin

Pharmacologic classification: cyclopentyl rifamycin
Therapeutic classification: antibiotic
Pregnancy risk category C

How supplied

Available by prescription only
Tablets (film-coated): 150 mg

Indications and dosages

Pulmonary tuberculosis, in conjunction with at least one other antitubercular agent to which the isolate is susceptible
Adults: During the intensive phase of short-course therapy, 600 mg P.O. twice weekly for 2 months, with an interval between doses of not less than 3 days (72 hours).

During the continuation phase of short-course therapy, 600 mg P.O. once weekly for 4 months in combination with isoniazid or another agent to which the isolate is susceptible.

Pharmacodynamics

Antibiotic action: Rifapentine inhibits DNA-dependent RNA polymerase in susceptible strains of *Mycobacterium tuberculosis*. It has bactericidal activity against the organism both intra- and extracellularly. Rifapentine and rifampin share similar antimicrobial action.

Pharmacokinetics

Absorption: Relative bioavailablity after oral absorption is 70%.
Distribution: Bound primarily to albumin.
Metabolism: Unknown.
Excretion: Appears to be excreted through the urine and feces.

Route	Onset	Peak	Duration
P.O.	Unknown	5-6 hr	Unknown

Contraindications and precautions

Contraindicated in patients with history of hypersensitivity to a rifamycin (rifapentine, rifampin, or rifabutin). Use drug cautiously and with frequent monitoring in patients with liver disease.

Interactions

Drug-drug. *Anticonvulsants such as phenytoin; antiarrhythmics, such as disopyramide, mexiletine, quinidine, and tocainide; antibiotics, such as chloramphenicol, clarithromycin, dapsone, doxycycline, or fluoroquinolones; antifungals, such as fluconazole, itraconazole, and ketoconazole; barbiturates; benzodiazepines such as diazepam; beta blockers; calcium channel blockers, such as diltiazem, nifedipine, and verapamil; cardiac glycosides; corticosteroids; clofibrate; haloperidol; HIV protease inhibitors, such as indinavir, nelfinavir, ritonavir, and saquinavir; oral anticoagulants such as warfarin; immunosuppressants, such as cyclosporine and tacrolimus; levothyroxine; narcotic analgesics such as methadone; oral or other systemic hormonal contraceptives; oral hypoglycemics such as sulfonylureas; progestins; quinine; reverse transcriptase inhibitors, such as delavirdine and zidovudine; sildenafil; theophylline; tricyclic antidepressants, such as amitriptyline and nortriptyline:* Rifapentine decreases the activity of these drugs. Dosage adjustments may be needed.

Effects on diagnostic tests

None reported.

Adverse reactions

CNS: headache, dizziness.
CV: hypertension.
GI: anorexia, nausea, vomiting, dyspepsia, diarrhea.
GU: pyuria, proteinuria, hematuria, urinary casts.
Hematologic: ***neutropenia,*** lymphopenia, anemia, ***leukopenia,*** thrombocytosis.
Hepatic: elevated AST and ALT.
Respiratory: hemoptysis.
Skin: rash, pruritus, acne, maculopapular rash.
Other: *hyperuricemia*, arthralgia, pain.

Overdose and treatment

Use of gastric lavage followed by activated charcoal may help after rifapentine overdose. Neither hemodialysis or forced diuresis is suggested. Supportive care and close monitoring of the patient should be initiated.

Clinical considerations

☐ ***ALERT*** Don't confuse similar-sounding drugs like rifabutin, rifampin, and rifapentine.

- Coadministration of pyridoxine (vitamin B_6) is recommended in malnourished patients, in those predisposed to neuropathy (alcoholics, diabetics), and in adolescents.
- Drug must be given with appropriate daily companion drugs. Compliance with all medications, especially with daily companion drugs on the days when rifapentine isn't given, is crucial for early sputum conversion and protection from relapse of tuberculosis.
- Rifapentine can turn body tissues and fluids red-orange. This can lead to permanent staining of contact lenses.

Therapeutic monitoring

- Rifamycin antibiotics have been associated with hepatotoxicity. Monitor liver function test results before beginning drug therapy.
- Drug therapy may affect liver function test results, CBC, and platelet counts; monitor carefully.
- Notify doctor of persistent or severe diarrhea.

Special populations

Pregnant patients. Administration of drug during the last 2 weeks of pregnancy may lead to postnatal hemorrhage in the woman or infant. Monitor clotting parameters closely if drug is given.
Breast-feeding patients. Because rifapentine may be excreted in breast milk, it isn't recommended for breast-feeding women.
Pediatric patients. Safety and efficacy in children under age 12 haven't been established.

Patient counseling

- Stress importance of strict compliance with drug and daily companion medications, as well as necessary follow-up visits and laboratory tests.
- Advise patient to use nonhormonal methods of birth control.
- Tell patient to take drug with food if nausea, vomiting, or GI upset occurs.
- Instruct patient to notify doctor if the following occur: fever, loss of appetite, malaise, nausea, vomiting, darkened urine, yellowish discoloration of the skin and eyes, pain or swelling of the joints, and excessive loose stools or diarrhea.
- Instruct patient to protect pills from excessive heat.

riluzole

Rilutek

Pharmacologic classification: benzothiazole
Therapeutic classification: neuroprotector
Pregnancy risk category C

How supplied

Available by prescription only
Tablets: 50 mg

Indications and dosages

Amyotrophic lateral sclerosis (ALS)
Adults: 50 mg P.O. q 12 hours on an empty stomach.

Pharmacodynamics

Neuroprotector action: It isn't known how riluzole improves signs and symptoms of ALS.

Pharmacokinetics

Absorption: Well absorbed from GI tract (about 90%) with average absolute oral bioavailability of about 60%. A high-fat meal decreases absorption.
Distribution: 96% protein-bound.
Metabolism: Extensively metabolized in the liver to six major and several minor metabolites, not all of which have been identified.
Excretion: Excreted primarily in urine and a small amount in feces. Half-life is 12 hours with repeated doses.

Route	Onset	Peak	Duration
P.O.	Unknown	Unknown	Unknown

Contraindications and precautions

Contraindicated in patients with history of severe hypersensitivity reactions to drug or components in its tablets.

Use cautiously in patients with hepatic or renal dysfunction and in the elderly. Also use cautiously in women and Japanese patients who may possess a lower metabolic capacity to eliminate drug compared with men and white patients, respectively.

Interactions

Drug-drug. *Allopurinol, methyldopa, or sulfasalazine:* Increased potential for hepatotoxicity. Use caution when administering together.
Drug-food. *Any food:* Decreased bioavailability. Give drug 1 hour before or 2 hours after meals.
Charbroiled foods: May increase riluzole elimination. Advise patient to avoid charbroiled foods.
Drug-lifestyle. *Alcohol use:* May increase risk of hepatotoxicity. Advise patient to avoid alcohol use.
Smoking: May increase riluzole elimination. Advise patient to avoid smoking.

Effects on diagnostic tests

None reported.

Adverse reactions

CNS: headache, aggravation reaction, hypertonia, malaise, depression, dizziness, insomnia, somnolence, vertigo, circumoral paresthesia.
CV: hypertension, tachycardia, palpitation, orthostatic hypotension.
GI: abdominal pain, *nausea,* vomiting, dyspepsia, anorexia, diarrhea, flatulence, stomatitis, tooth disorder, oral moniliasis, dry mouth.
GU: urinary tract infection, dysuria.
Musculoskeletal: *asthenia,* back pain, arthralgia.
Respiratory: *decreased lung function,* rhinitis, increased cough, sinusitis.
Skin: pruritus, eczema, alopecia, exfoliative dermatitis.
Other: phlebitis, weight loss, peripheral edema.

Overdose and treatment

No information available. In the event of an overdose, discontinue therapy immediately and implement supportive measures.

Clinical considerations

Use cautiously in patients with hepatic or renal dysfunction; in geriatric patients, women, and Japanese patients who may have a lower metabolic capacity to eliminate drug.

Therapeutic monitoring

- Baseline elevations in liver function studies, especially elevated bilirubin, should preclude riluzole use.
- Perform liver function studies periodically during therapy. In many patients, drug may cause serum aminotransferase elevations; discontinue drug if levels exceed 10 times upper limit of normal range or if clinical jaundice develops.

Special populations

Breast-feeding patients. It's unknown if drug is excreted in breast milk. Because of potential for serious adverse reactions in infants, use of drug in breast-feeding women isn't recommended.
Pediatric patients. Safety and efficacy in children haven't been established.
Geriatric patients. Age-related decreased renal and hepatic function may cause a decrease in clearance of riluzole. Administer drug cautiously to this age group.

Patient counseling

- Tell patient or caregiver that drug must be taken regularly and at the same time each day. If a dose is missed, tell patient to take the next tablet as originally planned.

- Instruct patient to report febrile illness; the patient's WBC count should be checked.
- Warn patient to avoid hazardous activities until CNS effects of drug are known.
- Tell patient to store drug at room temperature and protect it from bright light.
- Stress importance of keeping drug out of reach of children.

rimantadine hydrochloride
Flumadine

Pharmacologic classification: adamantine
Therapeutic classification: antiviral
Pregnancy risk category C

How supplied
Available by prescription only
Tablets: 100 mg
Syrup: 50 mg/5 ml

Indications and dosages
Prophylaxis against influenza A virus
Adults and children age 10 and older: 100 mg P.O. b.i.d.; for patients with severe hepatic dysfunction or renal failure (creatinine clearance 10 ml/minute or less) and for geriatric nursing home patients, a dose reduction to 100 mg P.O. daily is recommended.
Children under age 10: 5 mg/kg P.O. once daily. Maximum dose, 150 mg.
Treatment of illness caused by various strains of influenza A virus
Adults: 100 mg P.O. b.i.d. for 7 days from initial onset of symptoms; for patients with severe hepatic dysfunction or renal failure (creatinine clearance 10 ml/minute or less) and for geriatric nursing home patients, a dose reduction to 100 mg P.O. daily is recommended.

Note: If seizures develop, discontinue rimantadine.

Pharmacodynamics
Antiviral action: Mechanism of action isn't fully understood. It appears to exert its inhibitory effect early in the viral replicative cycle, possibly inhibiting the uncoating of the virus. Genetic studies suggest that a virus protein specified by the virion M^2 gene plays an important role in the susceptibility of influenza A virus to inhibition by rimantadine.

Pharmacokinetics
Absorption: Tablet and syrup formulations are equally absorbed after oral administration.
Distribution: Plasma protein-binding is about 40% for rimantadine.
Metabolism: Extensively metabolized in the liver.
Excretion: Less than 25% is excreted in urine as unchanged drug. Elimination half-life of drug is about 25½ to 32 hours. Hemodialysis doesn't contribute to drug clearance.

Route	Onset	Peak	Duration
P.O.	Unknown	6 hr	Unknown

Contraindications and precautions
Contraindicated in patients with hypersensitivity to drug or to amantadine. Use cautiously during pregnancy and in patients with impaired renal or hepatic function or seizure disorders (especially epilepsy).

Interactions
Drug-drug. *Acetaminophen, aspirin:* Reduced concentration of rimantadine. Monitor for drug effect.
Cimetidine: May decrease total rimantadine clearance by about 16%. Monitor for adverse effects.

Effects on diagnostic tests
None reported.

Adverse reactions
CNS: insomnia, headache, dizziness, nervousness, fatigue, asthenia.
GI: nausea, vomiting, anorexia, dry mouth, abdominal pain.

Overdose and treatment
Information specific to rimantadine overdose isn't available. As with any overdose, administer supportive therapy as indicated. Overdoses of a related drug, amantadine, have been reported, with reactions ranging from agitation to hallucinations, cardiac arrhythmia, and death. Administration of I.V. physostigmine (1 to 2 mg in adults and 0.5 mg in children; repeated as needed but not to exceed 2 mg/hour) has been reported anecdotally to benefit patients with CNS effects from overdose of amantadine.

Clinical considerations
☐ ***ALERT*** Don't confuse this drug with amantadine.
- For illnesses associated with various strains of influenza A, treatment should begin as soon as possible, preferably within 48 hours after onset of signs and symptoms, to reduce duration of fever and systemic symptoms.
- An increased incidence of seizures has been observed in some patients with history of seizures who weren't taking anticonvulsant medication during rimantadine therapy. If seizures develop, discontinue drug.
- Influenza A-resistant strains can emerge during therapy. Patients taking drug may still be able to spread the disease.

Therapeutic monitoring
Because of risk of drug metabolites accumulation during multiple dosing, monitor patient

with any degree of renal insufficiency for adverse effects, and adjust dosage as necessary.

Special populations

Breast-feeding patients. Drug shouldn't be administered to breast-feeding women because of the potential adverse effects to the infant.
Pediatric patients. Drug is recommended for prophylaxis of influenza A. Safety and efficacy of drug in treating symptomatic influenza infection in children haven't been established. Prophylaxis studies with rimantadine haven't been performed in those under age 1.
Geriatric patients. Adverse reactions associated with drug occur more frequently in geriatric patients than in general population. Monitor these patients closely.

Patient counseling

- Advise patient to take drug several hours before bedtime to prevent insomnia.
- Inform patient that taking drug doesn't prevent him from spreading the disease and that he should limit contact with others until fully recovered.
- Warn patient that drug may cause adverse CNS effects; he shouldn't drive or perform activities that require mental alertness until these effects are known.

risperidone

Risperdal

Pharmacologic classification: benzisoxazole derivative
Therapeutic classification: antipsychotic
Pregnancy risk category C

How supplied

Available by prescription only
Tablets: 0.25 mg, 0.5 mg, 1 mg, 2 mg, 3 mg, 4 mg
Solution: 1 mg/mL

Indications and dosages

Psychosis
Adults: Initially, 1 mg P.O. b.i.d. Increase in increments of 1 mg b.i.d. on days 2 and 3 of treatment to a target dose of 3 mg b.i.d. Wait at least 1 week before adjusting dosage further. Doses above 6 mg/day weren't more effective than lower doses and were associated with more extrapyramidal reactions.
≡ ***Dosage adjustment.*** Geriatric or debilitated patients, hypotensive patients, or patients with severe renal or hepatic impairment should initially receive 0.5 mg P.O. b.i.d. Increase dosage in increments of 0.5 mg b.i.d. on second and third days of treatment to target dose of 1.5 mg P.O. b.i.d. Wait at least 1 week before increasing dosage further.

Pharmacodynamics

Antipsychotic action: Exact mechanism of action is unknown. Its antipsychotic activity may be mediated through a combination of dopamine type 2 (D_2) and serotonin type 2 ($5\text{-}HT_2$) antagonism. Antagonism at receptors other than D_2 and $5\text{-}HT_2$ may explain other effects of drug.

Pharmacokinetics

Absorption: Well absorbed after oral administration. Absolute oral bioavailability is 70%. Food doesn't affect rate or extent of absorption.
Distribution: Plasma protein binding is about 90% for drug and 77% for its major active metabolite, 9-hydroxyrisperidone.
Metabolism: Extensively metabolized in the liver to 9-hydroxyrisperidone, which is the predominant circulating species and appears about equi-effective with risperidone with respect to receptor binding activity. About 6% to 8% of whites and a low percentage of Asians show little or no receptor binding activity and are "poor metabolizers."
Excretion: Metabolite is excreted by the kidney. Clearance of drug and its metabolite is reduced in renally impaired patients.

Route	Onset	Peak	Duration
P.O.	Unknown	1 hr	Unknown

Contraindications and precautions

Contraindicated in patients hypersensitive to drug and in breast-feeding women. Use cautiously in patients with prolonged QT interval, CV disease, cerebrovascular disease, dehydration, hypovolemia, history of seizures, or exposure to extreme heat or conditions that could affect metabolism or hemodynamic responses.

Interactions

Drug-drug. *Antihypertensive agents:* May enhance the effects of certain antihypertensive agents. Monitor closely.
Carbamazepine: May increase risperidone clearance, decreasing the effectiveness of carbamazepine. Monitor patient closely.
Clozapine: May decrease risperidone clearance, increasing the risk of toxicity. Monitor patient closely.
CNS depressants: May cause additive CNS depression when administered together. Administer together with caution.
Levodopa and dopamine agonists: Risperidone may antagonize the effects of these drugs. Avoid use together.
Drug-lifestyle. *Alcohol use:* Additive CNS depression. Avoid use together.
Sun exposure: May cause photosensitivity reactions. Advise patient to take precautions.

Effects on diagnostic tests

None reported.

Adverse reactions

CNS: *somnolence, extrapyramidal reactions, headache, insomnia, agitation, anxiety,* tardive dyskinesia, aggressiveness.
CV: tachycardia, chest pain, orthostatic hypotension, prolonged QT interval.
EENT: *rhinitis,* sinusitis, pharyngitis, abnormal vision.
GI: *constipation, nausea, vomiting, dyspepsia.*
Musculoskeletal: arthralgia, back pain.
Respiratory: coughing, upper respiratory infection.
Skin: rash, dry skin, photosensitivity.
Other: fever, ***neuroleptic malignant syndrome*** (rare); increase serum prolactin levels.

Overdose and treatment

Signs and symptoms of overdose result from an exaggeration of the known pharmacologic effects of risperidone, such as drowsiness and sedation, tachycardia and hypotension, and extrapyramidal symptoms. Hyponatremia, hypokalemia, prolonged QT interval, widened QRS complex, and seizures also have been reported.

There's no specific antidote to risperidone overdose; institute appropriate supportive measures. Consider gastric lavage (after intubation, if patient is unconscious) and administration of activated charcoal with a laxative. CV monitoring is essential to detect possible arrhythmias. If antiarrhythmic therapy is administered, disopyramide, procainamide, and quinidine carry a theoretical hazard of QT-prolonging effects that might be additive to those of risperidone. Similarly, it's reasonable to expect that the alpha-blocking properties of bretylium might be additive to those of risperidone, resulting in problematic hypotension.

Clinical considerations

- Risperidone and 9-hydroxyrisperidone appear to lengthen the QT interval in some patients, although there's no average increase in treated patients, even at 12 to 16 mg/day (well above recommended dose). Other drugs that prolong the QT interval have been associated with torsades de pointes, a life-threatening arrhythmia. Bradycardia, electrolyte imbalance, use with other drugs that prolong the QT interval, or congenital prolongation of the QT interval can increase risk for occurrence of this arrhythmia.
- Drug has an antiemetic effect in animals; this may occur in humans, masking signs and symptoms of overdose or of such conditions as intestinal obstruction, Reye's syndrome, and brain tumor.
- When restarting drug therapy for patients who have been off drug, follow initial 3-day dose initiation schedule.
- When switching patient from another antipsychotic agent to risperidone, immediately discontinue other antipsychotic agent on initiation of risperidone therapy when medically appropriate.

Therapeutic monitoring

- Tardive dyskinesia may occur after prolonged risperidone therapy. It may not appear until months or years later and may disappear spontaneously or persist for life despite discontinuation of drug.
- Neuroleptic malignant syndrome is rare, but in many cases fatal. It isn't necessarily related to length of drug use or type of neuroleptic. Monitor patient closely for symptoms, including hyperpyrexia, muscle rigidity, altered mental status, irregular pulse, alteration in blood pressure, and diaphoresis.

Special populations

Pregnant patients. Instruct women to call doctor if pregnancy is being planned or is suspected.
Breast-feeding patients. Discontinue breast-feeding while patient is receiving drug.
Pediatric patients. Safety and efficacy in children haven't been established.
Geriatric patients. A lower starting dose is recommended for geriatric patients because they have decreased pharmacokinetic clearance; a greater incidence of hepatic, renal, or cardiac dysfunction; and a greater tendency toward orthostatic hypotension.

Patient counseling

- Advise patient to rise slowly from a recumbent or seated position to minimize light-headedness.
- Warn patient not to operate hazardous machinery, including driving a car, until effects of drug are known.
- Tell patient to call before taking new medications, including OTC drugs, because of potential for interactions.

ritodrine hydrochloride

Yutopar

Pharmacologic classification: beta-receptor agonist
Therapeutic classification: adjunct in suppression of preterm labor
Pregnancy risk category B

How supplied

Available by prescription only
Injection (ampule): 10 mg/ml, 15 mg/ml
Injection (pre-mixed): 0.3 mg/ml

Indications and dosages

Management of preterm labor
Adults: Initially, 0.05 mg/minute I.V. infusion; increase q 10 minutes, p.r.n., or until maternal heart rate is 130 beats/minute, in 0.05-mg increments to effective dose (usually, 0.15 to 0.35

mg/minute). Continue for at least 12 hours after uterine contractions cease. Dose shouldn't exceed 0.35 mg/minute. Initiate oral 10 mg 30 minutes before I.V. infusion is discontinued, then 10 mg q 2 hours for 24 hours. Maintenance dosage of 10 to 20 mg orally q 4 to 6 hours until term or until medical judgment dictates.

Pharmacodynamics

Tocolytic action: Ritodrine is a beta-receptor agonist that exerts a preferential effect on $beta_2$-adrenergic receptors (such as uterine smooth muscle). Stimulation of the $beta_2$-receptors inhibits contractility of the uterine smooth muscle. Ritodrine also may act to affect directly the interaction between actin and myosin in muscle to decrease the intensity and frequency of contractions.

Pharmacokinetics

Absorption: 100% absorbed by I.V. route.
Distribution: Peak ritodrine serum levels are 32 to 50 ng/ml after an I.V. infusion of 60 minutes. I.V. dose has a distribution half-life of 6 to 9 minutes.
Metabolism: Metabolized in the liver, primarily to inactive sulfate and glucuronide conjugates.
Excretion: About 70% to 90% of I.V. dose is excreted in urine in 10 to 12 hours as unchanged drug and its conjugates. Drug can be removed by dialysis.

Route	Onset	Peak	Duration
I.V.	5 min	60 min	Unknown

Contraindications and precautions

Contraindicated in pregnant women before 20th week of pregnancy and in women with antepartum hemorrhage, eclampsia, intrauterine fetal death, chorioamnionitis, maternal cardiac disease, pulmonary hypertension, maternal hyperthyroidism, or uncontrolled maternal diabetes mellitus. Also contraindicated in patients hypersensitive to drug or with preexisting maternal medical conditions that would seriously be affected by the known pharmacologic properties of drug, such as hypovolemia, pheochromocytoma, or uncontrolled hypertension.

Use cautiously in patients with sulfite allergies.

Interactions

Drug-drug. *Atropine:* May worsen hypertension. Monitor blood pressure.
Beta blockers such as propranolol: May inhibit action of ritodrine. Avoid use together.
Corticosteroids: May produce additive diabetogenic effects, pulmonary edema, and possibly death in women. Discontinue drugs if pulmonary edema occurs. Monitor patient closely during concurrent use.
Diazoxide, magnesium sulfate, or meperidine: May potentiate CV effects. Monitor patient's heart rate and blood pressure closely.
Sympathomimetic amines: May produce an additive effect, especially CV. Use together with caution.

Effects on diagnostic tests

None reported.

Adverse reactions

CNS: nervousness; anxiety, *headache,* emotional upset, malaise (with I.V. administration); *tremor* (with oral administration).
CV: *palpitation; dose-related alterations in blood pressure, tachycardia,* ***pulmonary edema*** (with I.V. administration).
GI: *nausea, vomiting.*
Hematologic: leukopenia, ***agranulocytosis.***
Skin: rash.
Other: *erythema, hyperglycemia,* hypokalemia, *anaphylactic shock.*

Overdose and treatment

Overdose produces signs and symptoms similar to those of excessive beta-adrenergic stimulation, such as maternal and fetal tachycardia, palpitations, cardiac arrhythmia, hypotension, nervousness, tremor, nausea, and vomiting.

Treat I.V. overdose by stopping infusion and administering appropriate beta blocker such as propranolol as an antidote. Treat oral overdose by emptying stomach and administering activated charcoal. Subsequent treatment is supportive and symptomatic.

Clinical considerations

- Because CV responses are common, especially during I.V. administration, CV effects, including maternal pulse rate and blood pressure and fetal heart rate, must be closely monitored. A maternal tachycardia of over 140 beats/minute or persistent respiratory rate of over 20 breaths/minute may be signs of impending pulmonary edema.
- Discontinue drug if pulmonary edema occurs.
- Monitor amount of I.V. fluid administered, to prevent circulatory overload.
- Don't use drug I.V. if solution is discolored or contains a precipitate. Don't use more than 48 hours after preparation.
- Control infusion rate by use of a microdrip chamber I.V. infusion set or an infusion control device.
- Prepare I.V. solution by diluting 150 mg ritodrine in 500 ml of D_5W to produce a solution containing 300 mcg (0.3 mg) of ritodrine per milliliter. Reserve use of saline diluents, such as normal saline, Ringer's solution, and Hartmann's solution, for cases in which dextrose solution is medically undesirable due to increased probability of pulmonary edema.

Therapeutic monitoring

- Place patient in left lateral recumbent position to reduce risk of hypotension.
- Drug may uncover previously unknown cardiac pathology. Sinus bradycardia may follow drug withdrawal.
- Maternal tachycardia or decreased diastolic blood pressure usually reverses with a dosage reduction but requires discontinuation of drug in 1% of patients.
- Monitor blood glucose levels during ritodrine infusions, especially in mothers predisposed to diabetes mellitus.

Special populations

Pregnant patients. Drug is contraindicated in pregnant women before the 20th week of gestation.

Patient counseling

- Advise patient to keep scheduled follow-up appointments and to report adverse reactions immediately.
- Explain use and administration of drug to patient.

ritonavir

Norvir

Pharmacologic classification: HIV protease inhibitor
Therapeutic classification: antiviral
Pregnancy risk category B

How supplied

Available by prescription only
Capsules: 100 mg
Oral solution: 80 mg/ml

Indications and dosages

Treatment of HIV infection when antiretroviral therapy is warranted
Adults: 600 mg P.O. b.i.d. with meals. If nausea occurs, this schedule may provide some relief: 300 mg b.i.d., increased at 2- to 3-day intervals by 100 mg b.i.d., up to 600 mg b.i.d.
Children age 2 and older: 400 mg/m^2 P.O. b.i.d. in combination with other antiretroviral agents. To minimize nausea, initially 250 mg/m^2 b.i.d. May increase by 50 mg/m^2 b.i.d. at 2- to 3-day intervals.

Pharmacodynamics

Antiviral action: Ritonavir is an HIV protease inhibitor. HIV protease is an enzyme required for the proteolytic cleavage of the viral polyprotein precursors into the individual functional proteins found in infectious HIV. Ritonavir binds to the protease active site and inhibits the activity of the enzyme. This inhibition prevents cleavage of the viral polyproteins, resulting in the formation of immature noninfectious viral particles.

Pharmacokinetics

Absorption: Absorbed better when taken with food; its absolute bioavailability hasn't been determined.
Distribution: 98% to 99% bound to plasma proteins.
Metabolism: Metabolized in the liver; P-450 3A (CYP3A) is the major isoform involved in ritonavir metabolism.
Excretion: Primarily excreted in feces, although a small amount has been found in the urine. Half-life is 3 to 5 hours.

Route	Onset	Peak	Duration
P.O.	Unknown	2-4 hr	Unknown

Contraindications and precautions

Contraindicated in patients with hypersensitivity to any components of drug. Use cautiously in patients with hepatic insufficiency.

Interactions

Drug-drug. *Agents that increase CYP3A activity, such as carbamazepine, dexamethasone, phenobarbital, phenytoin, rifabutin, and rifampin:* Increase ritonavir clearance resulting in decreased ritonavir plasma levels. Monitor patient closely.
Alprazolam, clorazepate, diazepam, estazolam, flurazepam, midazolam, triazolam, and zolpidem: Potential for extreme sedation and respiratory depression from these agents. Don't co-administer with ritonavir.
Alprazolam, methadone: Decreased levels of these drugs. Use together cautiously.
Amiodarone, bepridil, bupropion, cisapride, clozapine, encainide, flecainide, meperidine, piroxicam, propafenone, propoxyphene, quinidine, rifabutin: Significant increases in the plasma levels of these drugs, thus increasing the patient's risk of arrhythmias, hematologic abnormalities, seizures, or other potentially serious adverse effects. Don't administer together.
Clarithromycin: Reduced creatinine clearance. Patients with impaired renal function receiving drug with ritonavir require a 50% reduction in their clarithromycin if creatinine clearance is 30 to 60 ml/minute and a 75% reduction if it's below 30 ml/minute.
Desipramine: Increased overall serum concentrations of desipramine. May require dosage adjustment when administered with ritonavir.
Disopyramide: Cardiac and neurologic events may occur. Use together with caution.
Disulfiram or other drugs that produce disulfiram-like reactions, such as metronidazole: Increased risk of disulfiram-like reactions. Ritonavir formulations contain alcohol that can produce reactions when co-administered. Monitor patient.
Glucuronosyltransferases, including oral anticoagulants or immunosuppressants: Loss of therapeutic effects from directly glucuronidated agents. May need dosage alteration of these

agents; monitor drug levels and drug effects. A dosage reduction greater than 50% may be required for those agents extensively metabolized by CYP3A.
Ketoconazole: Increased level of ritonavir. Use together cautiously and monitor patient carefully.
Ketoconazole, sildenafil: Increased levels of these drugs. Use together cautiously.
Oral contraceptives: Decreased overall serum levels of the contraceptive. May require a dosage increase in the oral contraceptive or alternate contraceptive measures.
Theophylline: Decreased overall serum levels of theophylline. Increased dosage may be required when co-administered with ritonavir.
Drug-food. *Any food:* Increased absorption. Drug should be taken with food.
Drug-lifestyle. *Smoking:* Decrease in serum levels of ritonavir. Discourage alcohol use.

Effects on diagnostic tests
None reported.

Adverse reactions
CNS: *asthenia,* headache, malaise, circumoral paresthesia, dizziness, insomnia, paresthesia, peripheral paresthesia, somnolence, thinking abnormality, *taste perversion,* migraine headache, syncope, abnormal dreams, abnormal gait, agitation, amnesia, anxiety, aphasia, ataxia, confusion, depression, diplopia, emotional lability, euphoria, ***generalized tonic-clonic seizure,*** hallucinations, hyperesthesia, incoordination, decreased libido, nervousness, neuralgia, neuropathy, paralysis, peripheral neuropathy, peripheral sensory neuropathy, personality disorder, tremor, vertigo.
CV: vasodilation, hemorrhage, hypertension, palpation, peripheral vascular disorder, orthostatic hypotension, tachycardia.
EENT: abnormal electrooculogram, abnormal electroretinogram, abnormal vision, amblyopia, blurred vision, blepharitis, ear pain, epistaxis, eye pain, hearing impairment, increased cerumen, iritis, parosmia, pharyngitis, photophobia, rhinitis, taste loss, tinnitus, uveitis, visual field defect.
GI: abdominal pain, anorexia, constipation, *diarrhea, nausea, vomiting,* dyspepsia, flatulence, enlarged abdomen, abnormal stools, bloody diarrhea, cheilitis, cholangitis, colitis, dry mouth, dysphagia, eructation, esophagitis, gastritis, gastroenteritis, GI disorder, GI hemorrhage, gingivitis, hepatitis, hepatomegaly, ileitis, liver damage, liver function tests abnormality, mouth ulcer, oral moniliasis, pancreatitis, periodontal abscess, rectal disorder, tenesmus, thirst.
GU: kidney pain, dysuria, hematuria, impotence, kidney calculus, kidney failure, nocturia, penis disorder, polyuria, pyelonephritis, urethritis, urine retention, urinary frequency.
Hematologic: anemia, ecchymosis, leukopenia, lymphadenopathy, lymphocytosis, ***thrombocytopenia.***
Metabolic: altered hormonal levels, diabetes mellitus, avitaminosis, glycosuria, gout, hyperlipidemia, hypercholesteremia.
Musculoskeletal: arthralgia, arthrosis, joint disorder, muscle cramps, muscle weakness, myalgia, myositis, and twitching.
Respiratory: asthma, dyspnea, hiccups, hypoventilation, increased cough, interstitial pneumonia, lung disorder.
Skin: rash, sweating, photosensitivity reaction, acne, contact dermatitis, dry skin, eczema, folliculitis, maculopapular rash, molluscum contagiosum, pruritus, psoriasis, seborrhea, urticaria, vesiculobullous rash.
Other: fever, local throat irritation, increased CK level, allergic reaction, back pain, cachexia, chest pain, chills, facial edema, facial pain, flu syndrome, hypothermia, neck pain, neck rigidity, pain (unspecified, substernal chest pain, peripheral edema, dehydration, edema).

Overdose and treatment
Information is limited to one patient who reported paresthesia, which resolved after the dose was decreased. Treatment consists of general supportive measures. Emesis or gastric lavage may be used as well as activated charcoal. Dialysis isn't likely to be beneficial.

Clinical considerations
- Drug may be administered alone or in combination with nucleoside analogues.
- GI tolerance may be improved in patients initiating combination regimens with ritonavir and nucleosides by initiating ritonavir alone and subsequently adding nucleosides before completing 2 weeks of ritonavir monotherapy.

Therapeutic monitoring
- Monitor patient's response to drug therapy.
- Measure plasma HIV-1 RNA levels and CD4+ T-cell counts to determine disease progression and when to modify therapy.

Special populations
Breast-feeding patients. It's unknown if ritonavir is excreted in breast milk. However, HIV-positive women shouldn't breast-feed to prevent transmission of infection.
Pediatric patients. Safety and efficacy in children under age 12 haven't been established.

Patient counseling
- Inform patient that drug isn't a cure for HIV infection. He may continue to develop opportunistic infections and other complications associated with HIV infection. Drug has also not been shown to reduce risk of transmitting HIV to others through sexual contact or blood contamination.

- Caution patient not to adjust dosage or discontinue ritonavir therapy without medical approval.
- Tell patient that he may improve taste of oral solution by mixing with chocolate milk, Ensure, or Advera within 1 hour of dosing.
- Tell patient that if a dose is missed, he should take the next dose as soon as possible. However, if a dose is skipped, he shouldn't double the next dose.
- Advise patient to report use of other medications, including OTC drugs, because of drug interactions.

rizatriptan benzoate

Maxalt, Maxalt-MLT

Pharmacologic classification: selective 5-hydroxytryptamine (5-$HT_{1b/1d}$) receptor agonist
Therapeutic classification: antimigraine
Pregnancy risk category C

How supplied

Available by prescription only
Tablets: 5 mg, 10 mg
Tablets (orally disintegrating): 5 mg, 10 mg

Indications and dosages

Treatment of acute migraine headaches with or without aura

Adults: Initially, 5 or 10 mg P.O. If first dose is ineffective, another dose can be given at least 2 hours after first dose. Maximum dose is 30 mg within a 24-hour period. For patients receiving propranolol, 5 mg P.O. up to maximum of three doses (15 mg) in 24 hours.

Pharmacodynamics

Vasoconstricting action: Rizatriptan is believed to exert its effect by acting as an agonist at serotonin receptors on the extracerebral intracranial blood vessels, which results in vasoconstriction of the affected vessels, inhibition of neuropeptide release, and reduction of pain transmission in the trigeminal pathways.

Pharmacokinetics

Absorption: Bioavailablity after oral administration is 45%.
Distribution: Minimally plasma bound.
Metabolism: Primary metabolism takes place via oxidative deamination by monoamine oxidase-A to the indole acetic acid metabolite.
Excretion: 82% excreted in urine, 12% in feces, after oral administration.

Route	Onset	Peak	Duration
P.O.	Unknown	1-1½ hr	Unknown

Contraindications and precautions

Use cautiously in patients with hepatic or renal impairment. Use with caution in patients with risk factors for coronary artery disease, such as hypertension, hypercholesterolemia, smoking, obesity, diabetes, strong family history of coronary artery disease, women with surgical or physiologic menopause, or men over 40 years, unless a cardiac evaluation provides evidence that patient is free from cardiac disease.

Contraindicated in patients with ischemic heart disease (angina pectoris, history of MI, or documented silent ischemia) or in those with symptoms or findings consistent with ischemic heart disease, coronary artery vasospasm (Prinzmetal's variant angina), or other significant underlying CV disease. Also contraindicated in patients with uncontrolled hypertension or within 24 hours of treatment with another 5-HT agonist, or an ergotamine-containing or ergot-type medication like dihydroergotamine or methysergide. Don't use within 2 weeks of discontinuation of MAO inhibitor. Also contraindicated in patients hypersensitive to drug or its inactive ingredients.

Interactions

Drug-drug. *Ergot-containing or ergot-type drugs, such as dihydroergotamine and methysergide; other 5-HT_1 agonists:* May cause prolonged vasospastic reactions. Shouldn't be used within 24 hours of rizatriptan.
MAO inhibitors (moclobemide), nonselective MAO inhibitors (types A and B; isocarboxazid, pargyline, phenelzine, tranylcypromine): May cause increased plasma levels of rizatriptan. Avoid use together and allow at least 14 days to elapse between discontinuation of an MAO inhibitor and administration of rizatriptan.
Propranolol: May cause increased rizatriptan levels. Dose reduction may be needed.
Selective serotonin reuptake inhibitors, such as fluoxetine, fluvoxamine, paroxetine, and sertraline: May cause weakness, hyperreflexia, and incoordination. Monitor patient closely.

Effects on diagnostic tests

None reported.

Adverse reactions

CNS: dizziness, headache, somnolence, paresthesia, asthenia, fatigue, hypesthesia, decreased mental acuity, euphoria, tremor.
CV: chest pain, pressure or heaviness, palpitations.
EENT: neck, throat and jaw pain, pressure or heaviness.
GI: dry mouth, nausea, diarrhea, vomiting.
Respiratory: dyspnea.
Skin: flushing.
Other: pain, warm or cold sensations, hot flashes.

Clinical considerations

- Drug should be used only after a definite diagnosis of migraine is established.

- Don't use for prophylactic therapy of migraines or in patients with hemiplegic or basilar migraine or cluster headaches.
- Safety of treating, on average, more than four headaches in a 30-day period hasn't been established.
- Remember that the orally disintegrating tablets contain phenylalanine.

Therapeutic monitoring
- For patients with risk factors that have a satisfactory cardiac evaluation, monitor closely after first dose.
- Assess CV status in patients who develop risk factors for coronary artery disease during treatment.

Special populations
Pregnant patients. Advise women to notify doctor if pregnancy occurs or is suspected.
Breast-feeding patients. Instruct women not to breast-feed because the effects on infants are unknown.
Pediatric patients. Safety and efficacy in children under age 18 haven't been established.

Patient counseling
- Inform patient that drug doesn't prevent migraine headache from occurring.
- For Maxalt-MLT, tell patient to remove blister pack from pouch, then remove drug from blister pack immediately before use. Tablet shouldn't be popped out of blister pack, but pack should be carefully peeled away with dry hands, and tablet placed on tongue and allowed to dissolve. Tablet is then swallowed with the saliva. No water is necessary or recommended. Tell patient that orally dissolving tablet doesn't provide more rapid headache relief.
- Advise patient that if headache returns after initial dose, a second dose may be taken with medical approval at least 2 hours after the first dose. Don't take more than 30 mg in a 24-hour period.
- Inform patient that drug may cause somnolence and dizziness and warn him to avoid hazardous activities until effects are known.
- Tell patient that food may delay onset of action of drug.

rocuronium bromide
Zemuron

Pharmacologic classification: nondepolarizing neuromuscular blocker
Therapeutic classification: skeletal muscle relaxant
Pregnancy risk category B

How supplied
Available by prescription only
Injection: 10 mg/ml

Indications and dosages
Adjunct to general anesthesia, facilitation of endotracheal intubation, or skeletal muscle relaxation during surgery or mechanical ventilation
Adults and children age 3 months or older: Initially, 0.6 to 1.2 mg/kg I.V. bolus. In most patients, tracheal intubation may be performed within 2 minutes; muscle paralysis should last about 31 minutes. Maintenance dosage of 0.1 mg/kg should provide an additional 12 minutes of muscle relaxation (0.15 mg/kg will add 17 minutes; 0.2 mg/kg will add 24 minutes).

Note: Dosage depends on anesthetic used, individual needs, and response. Dosages are representative and must be adjusted.

Pharmacodynamics
Skeletal muscle relaxation action: Rocuronium acts by competing for cholinergic receptors at the motor end plate. This action is antagonized by acetylcholinesterase inhibitors, such as neostigmine and edrophonium.

Pharmacokinetics
Absorption: Given I.V.
Distribution: Rapid distribution half-life is 1 to 2 minutes; slower distribution half-life is 14 to 18 minutes. Drug is about 30% bound to plasma proteins.
Metabolism: No information available, but hepatic clearance could be significant. The rocuronium analogue 17-desacetyl-rocuronium, a metabolite, has rarely been observed in plasma or urine.
Excretion: About 33% of administered dose is recovered in urine within 24 hours.

Route	Onset	Peak	Duration
I.V.	1 min	2 min	22-67 min

Contraindications and precautions
Contraindicated in patients with hypersensitivity to bromides. Use cautiously in patients with hepatic disease, severe obesity, bronchogenic carcinoma, electrolyte disturbances, neuromuscular disease, or altered circulation time caused by CV, age, or edematous states.

Interactions
Drug-drug. *Antibiotics, such as aminoglycosides, bacitracin, colistimethate sodium, colistin, polymyxins, tetracylines, and vancomycin:* May enhance neuromuscular blocking action of rocuronium. Use cautiously.
Anticonvulsant therapy, such as carbamazepine or phenytoin: May develop a form of diminished magnitude of neuromuscular block or shortened clinical duration. Use cautiously.
Enflurane, isoflurane: May prolong duration of action of initial and maintenance dosages of rocuronium. Use cautiously during surgical and postoperative periods.

Quinidine: An injection of quinidine during recovery from rocuronium may cause recurrent paralysis. Avoid use together.

Effects on diagnostic tests
None reported.

Adverse reactions
CV: tachycardia, abnormal ECG, ***arrhythmias*** (rare), transient hypotension and hypertension.
GI: nausea, vomiting.
Respiratory: asthma.
Skin: rash, edema, pruritus.
Other: hiccups.

Overdose and treatment
No cases of rocuronium overdose have been reported. Overdose with neuromuscular blocking agents may result in neuromuscular block beyond the time needed for surgery and anesthesia. Primary treatment is maintenance of a patent airway and controlled ventilation until patient recovers normal neuromuscular function. After initial evidence of such recovery is observed, further recovery may be facilitated by administration of an anticholinesterase agent, such as neostigmine or edrophonium, in conjunction with an appropriate anticholinergic agent.

Clinical considerations
- Drug should be used only by personnel experienced in airway management.
- Keep airway clear. Have emergency respiratory support equipment (endotracheal equipment, ventilator, oxygen, atropine, edrophonium, epinephrine, and neostigmine) available.
- Neuromuscular blockers don't obtund consciousness or alter the pain threshold. Patients should receive sedatives or general anesthetics before neuromuscular blockers are administered.
- Drug is well tolerated in patients with renal failure.
- In obese patients, base initial dose on patient's actual body weight.
- Drug, which has an acid pH, shouldn't be mixed with alkaline solutions such as barbiturate solutions in same syringe or administered simultaneously during I.V. infusion through same needle.
- Store reconstituted solution in refrigerator. Discard after 24 hours.

Therapeutic monitoring
A peripheral nerve stimulator should be used to measure neuromuscular function during drug administration to monitor drug effect, determine need for additional doses, and confirm recovery from neuromuscular block. Once spontaneous recovery starts, drug-induced neuromuscular blockade may be reversed with an anticholinesterase agent.

Special populations
Pediatric patients. Use of rocuronium in children under age 3 months hasn't been studied.

Patient counseling
Explain all events and procedures to patient because he can still hear.

rofecoxib
Vioxx

Pharmacologic classification: cyclooxygenase-2 (COX-2) inhibitor
Therapeutic classification: nonnarcotic analgesic, anti-inflammatory
Pregnancy risk category C

How supplied
Available by prescription only
Tablets: 12.5 mg, 25 mg
Oral suspension: 12.5 mg/5 ml, 25 mg/5 ml

Indications and dosages
Relief of signs and symptoms of osteoarthritis
Adults: Initially, 12.5 mg P.O. once daily, increased as needed to a maximum of 25 mg P.O. once daily.
Management of acute pain and treatment of primary dysmenorrhea
Adults: 50 mg P.O. once daily as needed for up to 5 days.

Pharmacodynamics
Analgesic and anti-inflammatory actions: The exact mechanism of action of rofecoxib is unknown. Its anti-inflammatory and analgesic effects along with its antipyretic activity may come from its ability to inhibit prostaglandin synthesis, which it does by inhibiting the COX-2 isoenzyme. At therapeutic serum levels, rofecoxib doesn't inhibit the cyclooxygenase-1 (COX-1) isoenzyme.

Pharmacokinetics
Absorption: Well absorbed, with a mean bioavailability of 93%. The median time for serum levels to peak is 2 to 3 hours.
Distribution: About 87% binds to proteins.
Metabolism: The liver metabolizes the drug to inactive metabolites.
Excretion: Eliminated predominantly through hepatic metabolism. Less than 1% of the drug is eliminated from the kidneys as unchanged drug. Half-life is about 17 hours.

Route	Onset	Peak	Duration
P.O.	Unknown	2-9 hr	Unknown

Contraindications and precautions
Contraindicated in patients with known hypersensitivity to rofecoxib or any of its components, and in patients who have experienced

asthma, urticaria, or allergic-type reactions after taking aspirin or other NSAIDs. Avoid use in patients with advanced kidney disease or moderate or severe hepatic insufficiency and in pregnant women because it may cause the ductus arteriosus to close prematurely.

Use cautiously in patients with preexisting asthma, renal disease, liver dysfunction, or abnormal liver function tests. Also use cautiously in patients with a history of ulcer disease or GI bleeding. Use cautiously in patients being treated with oral corticosteroids or anticoagulants, in patients with a history of smoking or alcoholism, and in geriatric or debilitated patients because of the increased risk of GI bleeding.

Use cautiously in patients with considerable dehydration. Rehydration is recommended before therapy begins. Use cautiously, and initiate therapy at the lowest recommended dose, in patients with fluid retention, hypertension, or heart failure.

Interactions

Drug-drug. *Angiotensin-converting enzyme (ACE) inhibitors:* Decreased antihypertensive effects of ACE inhibitors. Monitor patient closely.
Aspirin: Increased rate of GI ulceration and other complications. Don't use together, if possible. If used together, monitor patient closely for GI bleeding.
Furosemide, thiazide diuretics: Potentially reduced efficacy of these drugs. Monitor patient closely.
Lithium: Increased plasma lithium levels and decreased lithium clearance. Monitor patient closely for toxic reaction to lithium.
Methotrexate: Increased plasma methotrexate levels. Monitor patient closely for toxic reaction to methotrexate.
Rifampin: Decreased rofecoxib levels by about 50%. Initiate therapy with a higher dosage of rofecoxib.
Warfarin: Increased effects of warfarin. Monitor INR frequently in the first few days after therapy with rofecoxib is initiated or changed.
Drug-lifestyle. *Long-term alcohol use, smoking:* Increased risk of GI bleeding. Monitor patient closely.

Effects on diagnostic tests

None reported.

Adverse reactions

CNS: headache, asthenia, fatigue, dizziness.
CV: hypertension, lower-extremity edema.
EENT: sinusitis.
GI: diarrhea, dyspepsia, epigastric discomfort, heartburn, nausea, abdominal pain.
GU: urinary tract infection.
Musculoskeletal: back pain.
Respiratory: bronchitis, upper respiratory tract infection.
Other: flulike syndrome.

Overdose and treatment

In an overdose, remove unabsorbed drug from GI tract, monitor patient, and institute supportive therapy as needed. Hemodialysis doesn't remove drug; it's unknown if peritoneal dialysis removes it.

Clinical considerations

□ ***ALERT*** Patient may be allergic to rofecoxib if he has an allergy to aspirin or other NSAIDs.

- Rehydrate patients who are dehydrated before starting treatment with rofecoxib.
- Rofecoxib may be hepatotoxic. Monitor patient for signs and symptoms of hepatotoxicity. Discontinue the drug, as ordered, if any signs and symptoms consistent with liver disease develop.
- Fluid retention and edema have occurred in patients taking rofecoxib. Use the lowest recommended dose cautiously in patients with fluid retention, hypertension, or heart failure.

Therapeutic monitoring

- NSAIDs may cause serious GI toxicity. Signs and symptoms include bleeding, ulceration, and perforation of the stomach, small intestine, and large intestine. Such toxicity can occur any time, with or without warning. To minimize the risk of an adverse GI event, use the lowest effective dosage of rofecoxib for the shortest possible duration. Monitor patient closely for GI bleeding.
- Patients undergoing long-term treatment should have their hemoglobin level and hematocrit checked if they experience signs or symptoms of anemia or blood loss.

Special populations

Pregnant patients. Instruct women to inform doctor if pregnancy is suspected or planned while taking this drug.
Breast-feeding patients. It's unknown if rofecoxib is excreted in breast milk. However, because breast-fed infants are at risk for serious adverse reactions, women taking this drug shouldn't breast-feed.
Pediatric patients. The safety and efficacy of rofecoxib in pediatric patients under age 18 haven't been evaluated.
Geriatric patients. No substantial differences in safety and effectiveness exist between geriatric and younger patients. Although dosage doesn't need to be adjusted in geriatric patients, rofecoxib should be initiated at the lowest recommended dosage.

Patient counseling

- Warn patient that he may experience GI bleeding. Signs and symptoms include bloody vomitus, blood in urine and stool, and black, tarry stools. Advise patient to seek medical advice if he experiences any of these signs or symptoms.

- Advise patient to report rash, unexplained weight gain, or edema.
- Tell patient that drug may be taken without regard to food, though taking the drug with food may decrease GI upset.
- Tell patient that the most common minor adverse effects are dyspepsia, epigastric discomfort, heartburn, and nausea. Taking drug with food may help minimize these effects.
- Tell patient to avoid aspirin and aspirin-containing products unless his doctor has instructed him otherwise.
- Inform patient to avoid OTC anti-inflammatories such as ibuprofen (Advil) unless his doctor has instructed him otherwise.
- Tell patient that all NSAIDs, including rofecoxib, may adversely affect the liver. Signs and symptoms of liver toxicity include nausea, fatigue, lethargy, itching, jaundice, right upper quadrant tenderness, and flulike symptoms. Advise patient to stop therapy and seek immediate medical advice if he experiences any of these signs or symptoms.

ropinirole hydrochloride

Requip

Pharmacologic classification: nonergoline dopamine agonist
Therapeutic classification: antiparkinsonian
Pregnancy risk category C

How supplied

Available by prescription only
Tablets: 0.25 mg, 0.5 mg, 1 mg, 2 mg, 5 mg

Indications and dosages

Treatment of signs and symptoms of idiopathic Parkinson's disease
Adults: Initially, 0.25 mg P.O. t.i.d. Based on patient response, dosage should then be adjusted at weekly intervals: 0.5 mg t.i.d. after week 1, 0.75 mg t.i.d. after week 2, and 1 mg t.i.d. after week 3. After week 4, dosage may be increased by 1.5 mg/day on a weekly basis up to a dose of 9 mg/day and then increased weekly by up to 3 mg/day to maximum dose of 24 mg/day.

Pharmacodynamics

Antiparkinsonian action: Exact mechanism of action is unknown. Ropinirole is a nonergoline dopamine agonist thought to stimulate postsynaptic dopamine D_2 receptors within the caudate-putamen in the brain.

Pharmacokinetics

Absorption: Rapidly absorbed. Absolute bioavailability is 55%.
Distribution: Widely distributed throughout the body, with an apparent volume of distribution of 7.5 L/kg. Up to 40% is bound to plasma proteins.
Metabolism: Extensively metabolized by cytochrome P-450 CYP1A2 isoenzyme to inactive metabolites.
Excretion: Less than 10% of the administered dose is excreted unchanged in the urine. Elimination half-life is 6 hours.

Route	Onset	Peak	Duration
P.O.	Unknown	1-2 hr	6 hr

Contraindications and precautions

Contraindicated in patients with known hypersensitivity to drug or its components. Use cautiously in patients with severe renal or hepatic impairment.

Interactions

Drug-drug. *CNS depressants, including antipsychotics and benzodiazepines:* Increase CNS effects. Use cautiously.
Dopamine antagonists, including butyrophenones, metoclopramide, phenothiazines, and thioxanthenes: May decrease effectiveness of ropinirole when administered together. Avoid use together.
Estrogens: Reduce clearance of ropinirole. Dose adjustment of ropinirole may be needed.
Inhibitors or substrates of cytochrome P-450 CYP1A2, such as ciprofloxacin, fluvoxamine, mexiletine, and norfloxacin: Alter clearance. Dosage adjustment of ropinirole may be required.
Drug-lifestyle. *Alcohol use:* Increases CNS effects. Use cautiously.
Smoking: May increase clearance of ropinirole. Monitor closely.

Effects on diagnostic tests

None reported.

Adverse reactions

Early Parkinson's disease (without levodopa)
CNS: asthenia, hallucinations, *dizziness,* aggravated Parkinson's disease, *somnolence, fatigue,* headache, confusion, hyperkinesia, hypesthesia, vertigo, amnesia, impaired concentration, malaise.
CV: orthostatic hypotension, orthostatic symptoms, hypertension, *syncope,* edema, chest pain, extrasystoles, ***atrial fibrillation,*** palpitation, tachycardia.
EENT: pharyngitis, dry mouth, abnormal vision, eye abnormality, xerophthalmia, rhinitis, sinusitis.
GI: *nausea, vomiting, dyspepsia,* flatulence, abdominal pain, anorexia, abdominal pain.
GU: urinary tract infection, impotence.
Respiratory: bronchitis; dyspnea.
Skin: flushing, increased sweating.
Other: *viral infection,* pain, yawning, peripheral ischemia.
Advanced Parkinson's disease (with levodopa)
CNS: *dizziness,* aggravated parkinsonism, *somnolence, headache,* insomnia, *hallucinations,*

abnormal dreaming, confusion, tremor, *dyskinesia*, anxiety, nervousness, amnesia, hypokinesia, paresthesia, paresis.
CV: hypotension, syncope.
EENT: diplopia, dry mouth.
GI: *nausea*, abdominal pain, vomiting, constipation, diarrhea, dysphagia, flatulence, increased saliva.
GU: urinary tract infection, pyuria, urinary incontinence.
Hematologic: anemia.
Metabolic: weight decrease.
Musculoskeletal: arthralgia, arthritis.
Respiratory: upper respiratory infection, dyspnea.
Skin: increased sweating.
Other: injury, *falls*, viral infection, increased drug level, pain.

Overdose and treatment

There are reports of 10 patients ingesting more than 24 mg/day. Symptoms of overdose include mild or facial dyskinesia, agitation, increased dyskinesia, grogginess, sedation, orthostatic hypotension, chest pain, confusion, vomiting, and nausea.

Treatment involves general supportive measures and removal of unabsorbed drug.

Clinical considerations

- Dosage adjustment isn't needed in patients with mild to moderate renal impairment.
- Adjust drug with caution in patients with severe renal or hepatic impairment.
- Although not reported with ropinirole, a symptom complex resembling neuroleptic malignant syndrome (elevated temperature, muscular rigidity, altered consciousness, and autonomic instability) has been reported with rapid dose reduction or withdrawal of antiparkinsonian agents. If this occurs, stop drug gradually over 7 days and reduce frequency of administration to twice daily for 4 days and then once daily over the remaining 3 days.
- Other adverse events reported with dopaminergic therapy may occur with ropinirole, including withdrawal emergent hyperpyrexia and confusion, and fibrotic complications.
- Ropinirole can potentiate the dopaminergic adverse effects of levodopa and may cause or exacerbate existing dyskinesia. If this occurs, the levodopa dose may need to be decreased.

Therapeutic monitoring

- Drug may cause increased alkaline phosphatase and BUN levels. Monitor these levels.
- Symptomatic hypotension may occur due to dopamine agonists impairment of systemic regulation of blood pressure. Monitor patient carefully for orthostatic hypotension, especially during dose escalation.
- Syncope, with or without bradycardia, has been reported. Monitor patient carefully, especially after 4 weeks of initiation of therapy and with dosage increases.

Special populations

Breast-feeding patients. Drug inhibits prolactin secretion and could potentially inhibit lactation. It's unknown if drug is excreted in breast milk. A decision should be made whether to discontinue the drug or breast-feeding, taking into account the importance of drug to the woman.
Pediatric patients. Safety and efficacy in children haven't been established.
Geriatric patients. Dosage adjustments aren't necessary.

Patient counseling

- Inform patient to take drug with food to reduce nausea.
- Advise patient that hallucinations may occur. Geriatric patients are at greater risk than younger patients with Parkinson's disease.
- Instruct patient to rise slowly after sitting or lying down because of risk of orthostatic hypotension, which may occur during initial therapy or after a dosage increase.
- Advise patient to use caution when driving or operating machinery until CNS effects of drug are known.

ropivacaine hydrochloride

Naropin

Pharmacologic classification: aminoamide
Therapeutic classification: local anesthetic
Pregnancy risk category B

How supplied

Available by prescription only
E-Z off single-dose vials: 7.5 mg/ml, 10 mg/ml in 10-ml vials
Single-dose vials: 2 mg/ml, 7.5 mg/ml, 10 mg/ml in 20-ml vials; 5 mg/ml in 30-ml vials
Single-dose ampules: 2 mg/ml, 7.5 mg/ml, 10 mg/ml in 20-ml ampules; 5 mg/ml in 30-ml ampules
Infusion bottles: 2 mg/ml in 100-ml and 200-ml bottles
Sterile-pak single-dose vials: 2 mg/ml, 7.5 mg/ml, 10 mg/ml in 20-ml vials; 5 mg/ml in 30-ml vials

Indications and dosages

Surgical anesthesia

Adults: Lumbar epidural administration in surgery: 75 to 200 mg doses (duration, 2 to 6 hours). Lumbar epidural administration for cesarean section: 100 to 150 mg (duration, 2 to 4 hours). Thoracic epidural administration: 25 to 75 mg doses to establish block for postoperative pain relief. Major nerve block (for example, brachial plexus block): 175 to 250 mg (duration, 5 to 8 hours). Field block (such as minor nerve blocks and infiltration): 5 to 200 mg (duration, 2 to 6 hours).

Labor pain management

Adults: Lumbar epidural administration: Initially, 20 to 40 mg (duration, ½ to 1½ hours), then 12 to 28 mg/hour as continuous infusion or 20 to 30 mg/hour as incremental "top-up" injections.

Postoperative pain management

Adults: Lumbar epidural administration: 12 to 20 mg/hour as continuous infusion. Thoracic epidural administration: 8 to 16 mg/hour as continuous infusion. For infiltration (minor nerve block): 2 to 200 mg (duration, 2 to 6 hours).

Pharmacodynamics

Anesthetic action: Drug blocks the generation and conduction of nerve impulses, presumably by increasing the threshold for electrical excitation in the nerve by slowing the propagation of the nerve impulse and by reducing the rate of the action potential. Generally, progression of anesthesia is related to the diameter, myelination and conduction velocity of affected nerve fibers. Clinically, the order of loss of nerve function is as follows: pain, temperature, touch, proprioception, and skeletal muscle tone.

Pharmacokinetics

Absorption: Absorption depends on total dose and concentration of administered drug, route of administration, patient's hemodynamic or circulatory condition, and vascularity of administration site. From the epidural space, drug shows complete and biphasic absorption; mean half-lives of two phases are 14 minutes and 4 ¼ hours, respectively. The slow absorption is a rate-limiting factor in elimination of drug. Terminal half-life is longer after epidural than after I.V. administration.

Distribution: After intravascular infusion, drug has steady-state volume of distribution of 41 ± 7 L. Drug is 94% protein-bound, mainly to $alpha_1$ acid glycoprotein. An increase in total plasma levels during continuous epidural infusion has been observed, secondary to a postoperative increase in $alpha_1$ acid glycoprotein.

Metabolism: Extensively metabolized in the liver, via cytochrome P-4501A to 3-hydroxy ropivacaine. About 37% of dose is excreted in the urine as free drug and as a conjugated metabolites. Urinary excretion of metabolites accounts for only 3% of dose.

Excretion: Primarily excreted by the kidneys; 86% of the dose appears in urine after I.V. administration, of which only 1% relates to unchanged drug.

Route	Onset	Peak	Duration
Epidural	Unknown	Unknown	Unknown

Contraindications and precautions

Contraindicated in patients with known hypersensitivity to drug or local anesthetics of amide type.

Use with caution in debilitated, geriatric, and acutely ill patients because accumulation may result. Also use cautiously in patients with hypotension, hypovolemia, impaired CV function, or heart block and in those with hepatic disease, especially repeat doses of drug.

Interactions

Drug-drug. *Amide-type anesthetics:* Effects are additive if given with ropivacaine. Use with caution.

Fluvoxamine, imipramine, theophylline, verapamil: May result in competitive inhibition of ropivacaine. Use with caution.

Effects on diagnostic tests

None reported.

Adverse reactions

CNS: anxiety, dizziness, headache, hypesthesia, pain, paresthesia.

CV: *bradycardia*, chest pain, *hypotension*, hypertension, tachycardia.

GI: *nausea*, neonatal vomiting, vomiting.

GU: oliguria, urine retention.

Hematologic: anemia.

Hepatic: neonatal jaundice.

Respiratory: ***neonatal tachypnea, respiratory distress.***

Skin: pruritus.

Other: back pain, **FETAL BRADYCARDIA,** ***fetal tachycardia,*** **FETAL DISTRESS,** fever, neonatal fever, postoperative complications, rigors.

Overdose and treatment

Treatment should be supportive and symptomatic. Discontinue drug. In case of unintentional subarachnoid injection of drug, establish a patent airway and administer 100% oxygen. This may prevent seizures if they haven't already occurred. Administer medication to control seizures as appropriate.

Clinical considerations

□ ***ALERT*** Don't inject drug rapidly. Have emergency equipment and personnel immediately available.

- Drug should only be used by personnel familiar with its use.
- Increase doses in incremental steps.
- Don't use in emergency situations where a rapid onset of surgical anesthesia is necessary. Drug shouldn't be used for production of obstetric paracervical block anesthesia, retrobulbar block, or spinal anesthesia (subarachnoid block) because of insufficient data to support use. I.V. regional anesthesia (bier block) shouldn't be performed because of lack of clinical experience and risk of obtaining toxic blood levels of ropivacaine.

- To reduce risk of potentially serious adverse reactions, attempts should be made to optimize patient who may be at risk, such as those with complete heart block, and hepatic or renal impairment.
- Use an adequate test dose (3 to 5 ml of short-acting local anesthetic solution containing epinephrine) before induction of complete block.
- Don't use drug in ophthalmic surgery.

Therapeutic monitoring

- Early signs of CNS toxicity include restlessness, anxiety, incoherent speech, lightheadedness, numbness and tingling of mouth and lips, metallic taste, tinnitus, dizziness, blurred vision, tremors, twitching, depression, or drowsiness.

Special populations

Breast-feeding patients. Excretion of drug in breast milk hasn't been studied; use with caution.
Pediatric patients. Don't use in children under age 12.

Patient counseling

Tell patient that he may experience a temporary loss of sensation and motor activity in the anesthetized body part following proper administration of lumbar epidural anesthesia. Also explain adverse reactions that may occur.

rosiglitazone maleate

Avandia

Pharmacologic classification: thiazolidinedione
Therapeutic classification: antidiabetic
Pregnancy risk category C

How supplied

Available by prescription only
Tablets: 2 mg, 4 mg, 8 mg

Indications and dosages

Monotherapy adjunct to diet and exercise to improve glycemic control in patients with type 2 diabetes mellitus or combination therapy with metformin when diet, exercise, and rosiglitazone alone or diet, exercise, and metformin alone don't provide adequate glycemic control in patients with type 2 diabetes mellitus
Adults: Initially, 4 mg P.O. daily in the morning or in divided doses b.i.d. in the morning and evening. Dosage may be increased to 8 mg P.O. daily or in divided doses b.i.d. if fasting plasma glucose level doesn't improve after 12 weeks of treatment.

Pharmacodynamics

Antidiabetic action: Rosiglitazone lowers blood glucose levels by improving insulin sensitivity. Rosiglitazone is a highly selective and potent agonist for the receptors, which are found in key target areas for insulin action, such as adipose tissue, skeletal muscle, and liver.

Pharmacokinetics

Absorption: Plasma levels peak about 1 hour after dosing. The absolute bioavailability is 99%.
Distribution: About 99.8% binds to plasma proteins, primarily albumin.
Metabolism: Extensively metabolized, with no unchanged drug excreted in the urine. Primarily metabolized through *N*-demethylation and hydroxylation.
Excretion: Following oral administration, about 64% and 23% of dose is eliminated in urine and feces, respectively. The elimination half-life is 3 to 4 hours.

Route	Onset	Peak	Duration
P.O.	Unknown	1 hr	Unknown

Contraindications and precautions

Contraindicated in patients with known hypersensitivity to rosiglitazone or any of its components and in patients with New York Heart Association Class III and IV cardiac status unless the expected benefits outweigh the potential risks. Don't use in patients with active liver disease, increased baseline liver enzyme levels (ALT level is greater than 2½ times the upper limit of normal), type 1 diabetes, or diabetic ketoacidosis or in patients who experienced jaundice while taking troglitazone. Because metformin is contraindicated in patients with renal impairment, combination therapy with metformin and rosiglitazone is also contraindicated in such patients.

Rosiglitazone can be used as monotherapy in patients with renal impairment. Use cautiously in patients with edema or heart failure.

Interactions

None reported.

Effects on diagnostic tests

None reported.

Adverse reactions

CNS: headache, fatigue.
CV: edema.
EENT: sinusitis.
GI: diarrhea.
Hematologic: anemia.
Metabolic: hyperglycemia.
Musculoskeletal: back pain.
Respiratory: upper respiratory tract infection.
Other: injury.

Overdose and treatment

In an overdose, initiate supportive treatment appropriate to patient's condition.

Clinical considerations

- Management of type 2 diabetes should include diet control. Because caloric restriction, weight loss, and exercise help improve insulin sensitivity and help make drug therapy effective, these measures are essential to proper diabetes treatment.
- Patients with normal hepatic enzyme levels who are switched from troglitazone to rosiglitazone should undergo a 1-week washout before starting rosiglitazone.
- For patients whose blood glucose levels are inadequately controlled with metformin, rosiglitazone should be added to—not substituted for—metformin.

Therapeutic monitoring

- Liver enzyme levels should be checked before therapy starts, every 2 months for the first 12 months of treatment, and then periodically afterward. If ALT level is elevated during treatment, recheck levels as soon as possible. Discontinue drug if levels remain elevated.
- Hemoglobin level and hematocrit may decrease while patient is receiving this drug, usually during the first 4 to 8 weeks of therapy. Increases in total cholesterol, low-density lipoprotein, and high-density lipoprotein levels and decreases in free fatty acid levels may also occur.

Special populations

Breast-feeding patients. It's unknown if rosiglitazone is excreted in breast milk. Rosiglitazone shouldn't be administered to breast-feeding women.
Pediatric patients. The safety and efficacy of rosiglitazone in pediatric patients haven't been established.
Geriatric patients. No substantial differences in safety and efficacy exist between patients over age 65 and younger patients. No dosage adjustments are required for geriatric patients.

Patient counseling

- Advise patient that rosiglitazone can be taken with or without food.
- Tell patient to immediately report unexplained signs and symptoms, such as nausea, vomiting, abdominal pain, fatigue, anorexia, or dark urine, to his doctor because these may indicate potential liver problems.
- Inform premenopausal, anovulatory women with insulin resistance that ovulation may resume and contraceptive measures may need to be considered.
- Advise patient that management of diabetes should include diet control. Because caloric restriction, weight loss, and exercise help improve insulin sensitivity and help make drug therapy effective, these measures are essential to proper diabetes treatment.

rubella and mumps virus vaccine, live

Biavax II

Pharmacologic classification: vaccine
Therapeutic classification: viral vaccine
Pregnancy risk category C

How supplied

Available by prescription only
Injection: Single-dose vial containing not less than 1,000 $TCID_{50}$ (tissue culture infective doses) of the Wistar RA 27/3 rubella virus (propagated in human diploid cell culture) and not less than 20,000 $TCID_{50}$ of the Jeryl Lynn mumps strain (grown in chick embryo cell culture)

Indications and dosages

Rubella (German measles) and mumps immunization
Adults and children over age 1: 1 vial (0.5 ml) S.C. in outer aspect of the upper arm.

Pharmacodynamics

Live rubella and mumps prophylaxis: Vaccine promotes active immunity to rubella and mumps viruses by inducing production of antibodies.

Pharmacokinetics

Absorption: Antibodies are usually detectable within 2 to 6 weeks; duration of vaccine-induced immunity is expected to be lifelong.
Distribution: No information available.
Metabolism: No information available.
Excretion: No information available.

Route	Onset	Peak	Duration
S.C.	Unknown	Unknown	10½ yr

Contraindications and precautions

Contraindicated in pregnant women or immunosuppressed patients; in those with cancer, blood dyscrasia, gamma globulin disorders, fever, active untreated tuberculosis, or history of anaphylaxis or anaphylactoid reactions to neomycin or eggs; and in those receiving corticosteroids (except those receiving corticosteroids as replacement therapy) or radiation therapy.

Interactions

Drug-drug. *Immune serum globulin or transfusions of blood and blood products:* May impair the immune response to the vaccine. Defer vaccination for 3 months in these situations.
Immunosuppressive agents: May interfere with the response to vaccine. Monitor closely.

Effects on diagnostic tests

Rubella and mumps vaccine may temporarily decrease the response to tuberculin skin testing. Should a tuberculin skin test be necessary, administer it either before or simultaneously with rubella and mumps vaccine.

Adverse reactions

Musculoskeletal: arthritis, arthralgia.
Other: polyneuritis, rash, thrombocytopenic purpura, urticaria, fever, diarrhea, ***anaphylaxis,*** lymphadenopathy; pain, erythema, induration (at injection site).

Overdose and treatment

No information available.

Clinical considerations

- Obtain a thorough history of allergies (especially to antibiotics, eggs, chicken, or chicken feathers) and of reactions to immunizations.
- Perform skin testing first to assess vaccine sensitivity (against a control of normal saline solution in the opposite arm) in patients with history of anaphylactoid reactions to egg ingestion. Administer I.D. or scratch test with a 1:10 dilution. Read results after 5 to 30 minutes. Positive reaction is a wheal with or without pseudopodia and surrounding erythema.
- Epinephrine solution 1:1,000 should be available to treat allergic reactions.
- Rubella and mumps vaccine shouldn't be given less than 1 month before or after immunization with other live virus vaccines, except for monovalent or trivalent live poliovirus vaccine or live, attenuated measles virus vaccine, which may be administered simultaneously.
- Use only the diluent supplied. Discard reconstituted vaccine after 8 hours.
- Inject S.C. (not I.M.) into the outer aspect of the upper arm.
- Women who have rubella antibody titers of 1:8 or greater (by hemagglutination inhibition) need not be vaccinated with the rubella vaccine component.
- Although rubella vaccine administration should be deferred in patients with febrile illness, it may be administered to susceptible children with mild illness such as upper respiratory infection.
- According to Centers for Disease Control and Prevention recommendations, measles, mumps, and rubella is the preferred vaccine.
- Women who aren't immune to rubella are at risk for congenital rubella injury to the fetus if exposed to it during pregnancy.
- Store vaccine at 36° to 46° F (2° to 8° C) and protect from light. Solution may be used if red, pink, or yellow, but it must be clear.

Therapeutic monitoring

- Revaccination or booster isn't required if patient was previously vaccinated at age 1 or older; however, there's no conclusive evidence of an increased risk of adverse reactions for persons who are already immune when vaccinated.
- Vaccine won't offer protection when given after exposure to natural rubella or mumps, but there's no evidence that it would be harmful.

Special populations

Pregnant patients. Tell women of childbearing age to avoid pregnancy for 3 months after immunization. Provide contraceptive information if necessary.
Breast-feeding patients. Some reports have demonstrated transfer of rubella virus or virus antigen into breast milk in about 68% of patients. Few adverse effects have been associated with breast-feeding after immunization with rubella-containing vaccines. Use caution when administering vaccine to breast-feeding women.
Pediatric patients. Live rubella and mumps virus vaccine isn't recommended for children under age 1 because retained maternal antibodies may interfere with immune response.

Patient counseling

- Tell patient that tingling sensations in the extremities or joint aches and pains that may resemble arthritis, may occur beginning several days to several weeks after vaccination. These symptoms usually resolve within 1 week. Pain and inflammation at injection site and low-grade fever, rash, or breathing difficulties may also occur. Encourage patient to report distressing adverse reactions.
- Recommend acetaminophen to relieve fever or other minor discomfort.

rubella virus vaccine, live

Meruvax II

Pharmacologic classification: vaccine
Therapeutic classification: viral vaccine
Pregnancy risk category C

How supplied

Available by prescription only
Injection: Single-dose vial containing not less than 1,000 $TCID_{50}$ (tissue culture infective doses) of the Wistar RA 27/3 strain of rubella virus propagated in human diploid cell culture

Indications and dosages

Rubella (German measles) immunization
Adults and children over age 1: 1 vial (0.5 ml) S.C.

Pharmacodynamics

Rubella prophylaxis: Vaccine promotes active immunity to rubella by inducing production of antibodies.

Pharmacokinetics

Absorption: Antibodies are usually detectable 2 to 6 weeks after injection; duration of vaccine-induced immunity is expected to be lifelong.

Distribution: No information available.
Metabolism: No information available.
Excretion: No information available.

Route	Onset	Peak	Duration
S.C.	2-6 wk	Unknown	> 10 yr

Contraindications and precautions
Contraindicated in pregnant women or immunosuppressed patients; in those with cancer, blood dyscrasia, gamma globulin disorders, fever, active untreated tuberculosis, or history of hypersensitivity to neomycin; and in patients receiving corticosteroids (except those receiving corticosteroids as replacement therapy) or radiation therapy.

Interactions
Drug-drug. *Immune serum globulin or transfusions of blood and blood products:* May impair the immune response to the vaccine. If possible, defer vaccination for 3 months in these situations.
Immunosuppressants: May have reduced response to vaccine. Monitor closely. Defer vaccination until immunosuppressant is discontinued, if possible.

Effects on diagnostic tests
Rubella vaccine may temporarily decrease response to tuberculin skin testing. If a tuberculin test is necessary, administer it either before, simultaneously with, or at least 8 weeks after rubella vaccine.

Adverse reactions
Musculoskeletal: arthralgia, arthritis.
Other: polyneuritis, rash, thrombocytopenic purpura, urticaria, malaise, headache, sore throat, fever, ***anaphylaxis,*** lymphadenopathy; pain, erythema, induration (at injection site).

Overdose and treatment
No information available.

Clinical considerations
- Obtain a thorough history of allergies, especially to antibiotics, and of reactions to immunizations.
- Epinephrine solution 1:1,000 should be available to treat allergic reactions.
- Don't give rubella vaccine less than 1 month before or after immunization with other live virus vaccines, except for monovalent or trivalent live poliovirus vaccine; live, attenuated measles virus vaccine; or live mumps virus vaccine, which may be administered simultaneously.
- Don't inject I.M. Inject S.C. into the outer aspect of the upper arm.
- Use only diluent supplied. Discard 8 hours after reconstituting.
- Store vaccine at 36° to 46° F (2° to 8° C), and protect from light. Solution may be used if red, pink, or yellow, but it must be clear.
- Vaccine won't offer protection when given after exposure to natural rubella, although there's no evidence that it would be harmful.
- Although rubella vaccine administration should be deferred in patients with febrile illness, it may be administered to susceptible children with mild illnesses such as upper respiratory tract infection.

Therapeutic monitoring
- Women who have rubella antibody titers of 1:8 or greater (by hemagglutination inhibition) need not be vaccinated with rubella virus vaccine.
- Revaccination or booster dose is required if patient was previously vaccinated under age 1. The Advisory Committee on Immunization Practices and the American Academy of Pediatrics currently recommend that a second dose be routinely given at ages 4 to 6 or 11 to 12. It may be given at any other time provided at least 1 month has elapsed since the first dose. There's no conclusive evidence of an increased risk of adverse reactions for persons who are already immune when revaccinated.

Special populations
Pregnant patients. Women who aren't immune to rubella are at risk for congenital rubella injury to the fetus if exposed to rubella during pregnancy. Tell women of childbearing age to avoid pregnancy for 3 months after rubella immunization. Provide contraceptive information if necessary.
Breast-feeding patients. Although early studies failed to show evidence of attenuated rubella virus in breast milk, subsequent reports showed transfer of rubella virus or virus antigen into breast milk in about 68% of patients. Few adverse effects have been associated with breast-feeding after immunization with rubella-containing vaccines. Risk-benefit ratio suggests that breast-feeding women may be immunized, if necessary.
Pediatric patients. Live, attenuated rubella virus vaccine isn't recommended for children under age 1 because retained maternal antibodies may impair immune response.

Patient counseling
- Tell patient to expect tingling sensations in the extremities or joint aches and pains that may resemble arthritis, to occur beginning several days to several weeks after vaccination. The symptoms usually resolve within 1 week. Pain and inflammation at injection site and low-grade fever, rash, or breathing difficulties may also occur. Encourage patient to report distressing reactions.
- Recommend acetaminophen to relieve fever or other minor discomfort after vaccination.

S

salmeterol xinafoate

Serevent

Pharmacologic classification: selective beta$_2$-adrenergic stimulating agonist
Therapeutic classification: bronchodilator
Pregnancy risk category C

How supplied

Available by prescription only
Inhalation aerosol: 25 mcg per activation in 6.5-g canister (60 activations), 25 mcg per activation in 13-g canister (120 activations)
Inhalation powder: 50 mcg/blister

Indications and dosages

Long-term maintenance treatment of asthma; prevention of bronchospasm in patients with nocturnal asthma or reversible obstructive airway disease who require regular treatment with short-acting beta agonists
Adults and children over age 12: Two inhalations b.i.d. in the morning and evening.
Prevention of exercise-induced bronchospasm
Adults and children over age 12: Two inhalations at least 30 to 60 minutes before exercise.

Note: Paradoxical bronchospasms (which can be life-threatening) have been reported after use of salmeterol. If they occur, discontinue salmeterol immediately and institute alternative therapy.

◊ ***COPD or emphysema***
Adults and children over age 12: Single oral inhalation of 42 to 63 mcg.

Pharmacodynamics

Bronchodilator action: Salmeterol selectively stimulates beta$_2$-adrenergic receptors, resulting in bronchodilation. Drug also blocks the release of histamine from mast cells lining the respiratory tract, which produces vasodilation and increases ciliary motility.

Pharmacokinetics

Absorption: Because of the low therapeutic dose, systemic levels of salmeterol are low or undetectable after inhalation.
Distribution: Highly bound to human plasma proteins (94% to 99%).
Metabolism: Extensively metabolized by hydroxylation.
Excretion: Excreted primarily in the feces.

Route	Onset	Peak	Duration
Inhalation	10-20 min	3 hr	12 hr

Contraindications and precautions

Contraindicated in patients with hypersensitivity to drug or its formulation. Use cautiously in patients with coronary insufficiency, arrhythmias, hypertension, other CV disorders, thyrotoxicosis, or seizure disorders and in those unusually responsive to sympathomimetics.

Interactions

Drug-drug. *Beta-adrenergic agonists, theophylline, or other methylxanthines:* May result in possible adverse cardiac effects with excessive use of salmeterol. Monitor patient closely.
MAO inhibitors or tricyclic antidepressants: Risk of severe adverse CV effects. Avoid use of salmeterol within 14 days of MAO therapy.

Effects on diagnostic tests

None reported.

Adverse reactions

CNS: *headache,* sinus headache, tremor, nervousness, giddiness.
CV: tachycardia, palpitations, ***ventricular arrhythmias.***
EENT: *upper respiratory infection, nasopharyngitis,* nasal cavity or sinus disorder.
GI: nausea, vomiting, diarrhea, heartburn.
Musculoskeletal: joint and back pain, myalgia.
Respiratory: cough, lower respiratory infection, ***bronchospasm.***
Other: hypersensitivity reactions (rash, urticaria).

Overdose and treatment

Overdose may result in exaggerated pharmacologic adverse effects associated with beta-adrenoceptor agonists: tachycardia, arrhythmias, tremor, headache, and muscle cramps. Overdose can lead to clinically significant prolongation of the QT interval, which can produce ventricular arrhythmias. Cardiac arrest and death may be associated with abuse of salmeterol. Other signs of overdose may include hypokalemia and hyperglycemia.

In these cases, stop therapy with salmeterol and all beta-adrenergic-stimulant drugs, provide supportive therapy, and consider judicious use of a beta blocker, bearing in mind the possibility that such agents can produce bronchospasm. Cardiac monitoring is recommended in cases of salmeterol overdose. Dialysis isn't appropriate treatment.

Clinical considerations

- Don't use drug in patients whose asthma can be managed by occasional use of a short-acting, inhaled beta$_2$-agonist such as albuterol.
- Salmeterol inhalation shouldn't be used more than twice daily (morning and evening) at the recommended dose. Provide patient with a short-acting inhaled beta$_2$-agonist for treatment of symptoms that occur despite regular twice-daily use of salmeterol.
- Patients taking a short-acting inhaled beta$_2$-agonist daily should be advised to use it only as needed if they develop asthma symptoms while taking salmeterol.
- Salmeterol isn't a substitute for oral or inhaled corticosteroids.

Therapeutic monitoring

- Monitor patient's response to drug therapy.
- Tell patient to call if the short-acting agonist no longer provides sufficient relief or if more than four inhalations are being used daily. This may be a sign that asthma symptoms are worsening.
- Patients receiving drug twice daily shouldn't use additional doses for prevention of exercise-induced bronchospasm.

Special populations

Breast-feeding patients. Give drug cautiously to breast-feeding women because it isn't known if drug is excreted in breast milk.
Pediatric patients. Safety and efficacy in children under age 12 haven't been established.
Geriatric patients. As with other beta$_2$-agonists, use with extreme caution when using drug in geriatric patients who have CV disease and who could be adversely affected by this class of drugs.

Patient counseling

- Instruct patient on the proper use of the salmeterol inhalation device and tell him to review the illustrated instructions in the package insert.
- Tell patient to shake the container well before using.
- Remind patient to take drug at 12-hour intervals for optimum effect and to take it even when he's feeling better.
- Inform patient that drug isn't meant to relieve acute asthmatic symptoms. Instead, acute symptoms should be treated with an inhaled, short-acting bronchodilator that has been prescribed for symptomatic relief.
- Instruct patient already receiving short-acting beta$_2$-agonist to discontinue the regular daily-dosing regimen for drug and to use the short-acting agent only if asthma symptoms are experienced while taking salmeterol.
- Tell patient taking an inhaled corticosteroid to continue to use it regularly. Warn patient not to take other medications without medical approval.
- If drug is being used to prevent exercise-induced bronchospasm, tell patient to take it 30 to 60 minutes before exercise.

saquinavir
Fortovase

saquinavir mesylate
Invirase

Pharmacologic classification: HIV-1 and HIV-2 proteinase inhibitor
Therapeutic classification: antiviral
Pregnancy risk category B

How supplied

Available by prescription only
saquinavir
Capsules (soft gelatin): 200 mg
saquinavir mesylate
Capsules (hard gelatin): 200 mg

Indications and dosages

Adjunct treatment of advanced HIV infection in selected patients
Adults: 600 mg (Invirase, three 200-mg capsules) P.O. t.i.d. taken within 2 hours after a full meal and in combination with a nucleoside analogue such as zalcitabine at a dose of 0.75 mg P.O. t.i.d. or 200 mg zidovudine P.O. t.i.d. Or, 1,200 mg (Fortovase, six 200-mg capsules) t.i.d. within 2 hours after a full meal in combination with a nucleoside analogue.
≡ ***Dosage adjustment.*** If toxicity develops with saquinavir or saquinavir mesylate, interrupt drug therapy. In combination therapy with nucleoside analogues, base dosage adjustments of the nucleoside analogue on the known toxicity profile of specific drug.

Pharmacodynamics

Antiviral action: Saquinavir inhibits the activity of HIV protease and prevents the cleavage of HIV polyproteins, which are essential for the maturation of HIV.

Pharmacokinetics

Absorption: Poorly absorbed from the GI tract. Higher saquinavir levels are achieved with Fortovase compared with Invirase. Fortovase has a relative bioavailability of 331% of Invirase.
Distribution: About 98% bound to plasma proteins.

Metabolism: Rapidly metabolized.
Excretion: Excreted mainly in feces.

Route	Onset	Peak	Duration
P.O.	Unknown	Unknown	Unknown

Contraindications and precautions
Contraindicated in patients with hypersensitivity to drug or the components contained in the capsule. Safety of drug hasn't been established in pregnant women.

Interactions
Drug-drug. *Amprenavir:* Decreased plasma levels of amprenavir. Use together cautiously.
Cisapride: May cause serious CV events. Avoid use with these drugs.
Delavirdine: Increased saquinavir plasma concentration. Use cautiously and monitor hepatic enzymes.
Indinavir, nelfinavir, ritonavir: Increased plasma levels of saquinavir. Use together cautiously.
Macrolide antibiotics such as clarithromycin: Increased plasma levels of both drugs. Use together cautiously.
Rifabutin, rifampin: Reduce the steady-state concentration of saquinavir.Use rifabutin and saquinavir together cautiously. Don't use with rifampin.
Sildenafil: Increased peak plasma levels and AUC of sildenafil. Reduce initial dose of sildenafil to 25 mg when given with saquinavir.
Drug-food. *Any food:* Increases drug absorption. Advise patient to take drug with food.

Effects on diagnostic tests
None reported.

Adverse reactions
CNS: paresthesia, headache.
GI: diarrhea, ulcerated buccal mucosa, abdominal pain, nausea, increased liver function tests (rare), ***pancreatitis*** (may be fatal).
Musculoskeletal: asthenia, musculoskeletal pain.
Respiratory: bronchitis, dyspnea, hemoptysis, pharyngitis, rhinitis, upper respiratory tract disorder, cough, epistaxis.
Skin: rash.

Overdose and treatment
Limited information available. One patient in clinical studies ingested 8 g as a single dose without showing evidence of acute toxicity. Emesis was induced in the patient within 2 to 4 hours after ingestion.

Clinical considerations
- If a serious or severe toxicity occurs during treatment, discontinue drug until the cause is identified or the toxicity resolves. Dose modification isn't needed when drug is resumed.
- Invirase will be phased out and replaced by Fortovase. Be aware of the dosing differences.

Therapeutic monitoring
- Evaluate CBC, platelets, electrolytes, uric acid, liver enzymes, and bilirubin before therapy is begun and then at appropriate intervals during therapy.
- Monitor plasma HIV-1 RNA levels and CD4+ T-cell counts to determine risk of disease progression and when to modify antiretroviral therapy.

Special populations
Breast-feeding patients. Although safety of drug hasn't been established in breast-feeding women, women with HIV infection shouldn't breast-feed to avoid transmitting virus to infant.
Pediatric patients. Safety and efficacy in children under age 16 haven't been established.

Patient counseling
- Warn patient of adipogenic effects such as redistribution or accumulation of body fat.
- Inform patient that drug should be taken within 2 hours following a full meal.
- Tell patient to report adverse reactions.
- Inform patient that drug is usually administered together with other AIDS-related antiviral agents.
- Tell patient to use Fortovase within 3 months when stored at room temperature or refer to expiration date on the label if capsules are refrigerated.

sargramostim (granulocyte macrophage-colony stimulating factor, GM-CSF)
Leukine

Pharmacologic classification: biologic response modifier
Therapeutic classification: colony stimulating factor
Pregnancy risk category C

How supplied
Available by prescription only
Injection (preservative-free): 250 mcg, 500 mcg (as lyophilized powder) in single-dose vials

Indications and dosages
Acceleration of hematopoietic reconstitution after autologous bone marrow transplantation in patients with malignant lymphoma, acute lymphoblastic leukemia, or Hodgkin's disease
Adults: 250 mcg/m^2 daily for 21 consecutive days given as a 2-hour I.V. infusion daily, beginning 2 to 4 hours after the bone marrow transplant. Don't administer within 24 hours of last dose of chemotherapy or within 12 hours after last dose of radiotherapy because of po-

tential sensitivity of rapidly dividing progenitor cells to cytotoxic chemotherapeutic or radiologic therapies.

≡ *Dosage adjustment.* Reduce dosage by half or temporarily discontinue if severe adverse reactions occur. Therapy may be resumed when reaction abates. If blast cells appear or increase to 10% or more of the WBC count or if progression of the underlying disease occurs, discontinue therapy. If absolute neutrophil count is more than 20,000 cells/mm^3 or if WBC counts are more than 50,000 cells/mm^3, discontinue therapy temporarily or reduce the dose by half.

Bone marrow transplantation failure or engraftment delay

Adults: 250 mcg/m^2 daily for 14 days as a 2-hour I.V. infusion. Same course may be repeated after 7 days off therapy if engraftment hasn't occurred. Third course of 500 mcg/m^2 daily for 14 days may be given after another 7 days off therapy if engraftment hasn't occurred.

Acute myelogenous leukemia

Adults: 250 mcg/m^2 daily by I.V. infusion over 4 hours. Start therapy about day 11 or 4 days following completion of induction therapy. Use only if bone marrow is hypoplastic (fewer than 5% blasts on day 10). Continue until absolute neutrophil count exceeds 1,500/mm^3 for 3 consecutive days or for a maximum of 42 days.

◊ ***Myelodysplastic syndromes***

Adults: 15 to 500 mcg/m^2 daily by I.V. infusion over 1 to 12 hours.

◊ ***Aplastic anemia***

Adults: 15 to 480 mcg/m^2 daily by I.V. infusion over 1 to 12 hours.

Pharmacodynamics

Immunostimulant action: Sargramostim is a 127-amino acid glycoprotein manufactured by recombinant DNA technology in a yeast expression system. It differs from the natural human granulocyte-macrophage colony stimulating factor by the substitution of leucine for arginine at position 23. The carbohydrate moiety may also be different. Sargramostim induces cellular responses by binding to specific receptors on cell surfaces of target cells. Blood counts return to normal or baseline levels within 2 to 10 days after stopping treatment.

Pharmacokinetics

Absorption: Blood levels detectable within 5 minutes after S.C. administration.

Distribution: Bound to specific receptors on target cells.

Metabolism: Unknown.

Excretion: Unknown.

Route	Onset	Peak	Duration
I.V., S.C.	15 min	2-4 hr	Unknown

Contraindications and precautions

Contraindicated in patients with excessive leukemic myeloid blasts in bone marrow or peripheral blood and in those with hypersensitivity to drug or its components or to yeast-derived products. Also contraindicated in patients receiving chemotherapy or radiotherapy.

Use cautiously in patients with impaired renal or hepatic function, preexisting cardiac disease or fluid retention, hypoxia, pulmonary infiltrates, or heart failure.

Interactions

Drug-drug. *Corticosteroids, lithium:* May potentiate the myeloproliferative effects of sargramostim. Use with caution.

Effects on diagnostic tests

None reported.

Adverse reactions

CNS: *malaise, CNS disorders, asthenia.*

CV: *blood dyscrasias, edema,* hemorrhage, supraventricular arrhythmia, pericardial effusion, *peripheral edema.*

GI: *nausea, vomiting, diarrhea, anorexia, hemorrhage, GI disorders, stomatitis.*

GU: *urinary tract disorder,* abnormal kidney function.

Hematologic: stimulation of hematopoiesis.

Hepatic: *liver damage.*

Musculoskeletal: *bone pain.*

Respiratory: *dyspnea, lung disorders,* pleural effusion.

Skin: *alopecia, rash.*

Other: *fever, mucous membrane disorder,* **SEPSIS.**

Overdose and treatment

Doses up to 16 times the recommended dose have been administered with the following reversible adverse reactions: WBC counts up to 200,000/mm^3, dyspnea, malaise, nausea, fever, rash, sinus tachycardia, headache, and chills. The maximum dose that can be administered safely has yet to be determined. If overdose is suspected, monitor WBC count increase and respiratory symptoms.

Clinical considerations

- To prepare, reconstitute with 1 ml sterile water for injection. Don't reenter or reuse the single-dose vial. Discard unused portion. Direct stream of sterile water against side of vial and gently swirl contents to minimize foaming. Avoid excessive or vigorous agitation or shaking. Dilute in normal saline. If final concentration is less than 10 mcg/ml, add albumin (human) at a final concentration of 0.1% to the saline before addition of sargramostim to prevent adsorption to components of the delivery system. For a final concentration of 0.1% human albumin, add 1 mg human albumin per milliliter normal saline. Administer as soon as possible after admixture, because sargramostim has no preservative, and within 6 hours of reconstitution or dilution. Don't add other medications to infusion solution without compatibility and stability data. Discard unused solution after 6 hours. Don't infuse drug using an in-line membrane filter because absorption of drug could occur.

- Transient rash and local injection site reactions may occur; no serious allergic or anaphylactic reactions have been reported.
- Drug can act as a growth factor for any tumor type, particularly myeloid malignancies.
- Unlabeled indications include use to increase WBC counts in patients with myelodysplastic syndromes and in patients with AIDS on zidovudine; to decrease nadir of leukopenia secondary to myelosuppressive chemotherapy; to decrease myelosuppression in preleukemic patients; to correct neutropenia in patients with aplastic anemia; and to decrease transplant-associated organ system damage, particularly of the liver and kidneys.
- Drug is effective in accelerating myeloid recovery in patients receiving bone marrow purged from monoclonal antibodies.
- Refrigerate the sterile powder, reconstituted solution, and diluted solution for injection. Don't freeze or shake. Don't use after expiration date.

Therapeutic monitoring

- Stimulation of marrow precursors may result in rapid elevation of WBC count; biweekly monitoring of CBC count with differential, including examination for blast cells, is recommended.
- The effect of drug may be limited in patients who have received extensive radiotherapy to hematopoietic sites for treatment of primary disease in the abdomen or chest or have been exposed to several agents (alkylating agents, anthracycline antibiotics, antimetabolites) before autologous bone marrow transplant.

Special populations

Breast-feeding patients. It isn't known if drug is excreted in breast milk; use with caution.
Pediatric patients. Safety and efficacy in children haven't been established; however, available data suggest that no differences in toxicity exist. The type and frequency of adverse reactions were comparable with those seen in adults.

Patient counseling

- Review administration schedule with patient and caregivers. Answer any questions and address concerns.

scopolamine hydrobromide

Isopto Hyoscine, Scopace, Transderm-Scop

Pharmacologic classification: anticholinergic
Therapeutic classification: antimuscarinic, cycloplegic mydriatic
Pregnancy risk category C

How supplied

Available by prescription only
Injection: 0.3 and 1 mg/ml in 1-ml vials; 0.4 mg/ml, 0.86 mg/ml in 0.5-ml ampules
Topical: Transdermal system 1.5 mg
Ophthalmic solution: 0.25%
Oral: soluble tablets 0.4 mg

Indications and dosages

Antimuscarinic, adjunct to anesthesia, prevention of nausea and vomiting
Adults: 0.3 to 0.6 mg I.M., S.C., or I.V. (after dilution with sterile water for injection) as a single dose. Apply transdermal system the evening before surgery. In cesarean section, apply 1 hour before surgery.
Children: 0.006 mg/kg I.M., S.C., or I.V. (after dilution with sterile water for injection) as a single daily dose; maximum dose, 0.3 mg.
Prevention of nausea and vomiting associated with motion sickness
Adults: 1 transdermal patch applied behind the ear 4 hours before anticipated exposure to motion, or 0.25 to 0.8 mg P.O. 1 hour before exposure to motion, then t.i.d., as needed.
Cycloplegic refraction
Adults: 1 to 2 drops 0.25% solution in eye 1 hour before refraction.
Children: 1 drop 0.25% solution b.i.d. for 2 days before refraction.
Iritis, uveitis
Adults: 1 to 2 drops of 0.25% solution daily or up to t.i.d.
Children: 1 drop of 0.25% solution up to t.i.d.

Pharmacodynamics

Antimuscarinic action: Scopolamine inhibits muscarinic action of acetylcholine on autonomic effectors, decreasing secretions and GI motility; blocks vagal inhibition of SA node.
Mydriatic action: Scopolamine competitively blocks acetylcholine at cholinergic neuroeffector sites, antagonizing effects of acetylcholine on the sphincter muscle and ciliary body, producing mydriasis and cycloplegia.

Pharmacokinetics

Absorption: Rapidly absorbed when administered I.M. or S.C. Systemic drug absorption may occur from drug passage through the nasolacrimal duct.

Distribution: Distributed widely throughout body tissues. Drug crosses the placenta and probably the blood-brain barrier.
Metabolism: Probably metabolized completely in the liver; however, its exact metabolic fate is unknown. Mydriatic and cycloplegic effects persist for 3 to 7 days.
Excretion: Probably in urine as metabolites.

Route	Onset	Peak	Duration
P.O.	Unknown	1 hr	Unknown
I.M., I.V., S.C.	Varies	Varies	Varies
Ophthalmic	Rapid	15-45 min	< 1 wk
Transdermal	4 hr	24 hr	72 hr

Contraindications and precautions

Scopolamine is contraindicated in patients hypersensitive to the drug, to any other belladonna alkaloid, or to any ingredient or component in the formulation or administration system.

Systemic form is contraindicated in patients with angle-closure glaucoma, obstructive uropathy, obstructive disease of the GI tract, asthma, chronic pulmonary disease, myasthenia gravis, paralytic ileus, intestinal atony, unstable CV status in acute hemorrhage, or toxic megacolon. Ophthalmic form is contraindicated in patients with shallow anterior chamber and angle-closure glaucoma.

Soluble tablets are contraindicated in patients with prostatic hyperplasia or impaired renal or hepatic function, and should be used cautiously in patients with cardiac disease.

Use systemic form cautiously in patients with autonomic neuropathy, hyperthyroidism, coronary artery disease, arrhythmias, heart failure, hypertension, hiatal hernia associated with reflux esophagitis, hepatic or renal disease, or ulcerative colitis; or in patients in a hot or humid environment. Use ophthalmic form cautiously in the elderly, in infants and children, and in those with cardiac disease.

Use transdermal form cautiously in patients with history of seizures or psychosis.

Interactions

Drug-drug. *Anticholinergics, such as ketoconazole and levodopa:* Decreased GI absorption has been reported. Separate administration times by 2 to 3 hours.
CNS depressants, including sedative-hypnotics and tranquilizers: May increase CNS depression. Monitor patient closely.
Digoxin: Higher serum digoxin levels when administered with anticholinergics. Monitor for digitalis toxicity.
Drugs having anticholinergic effects: May cause additive toxicity. Avoid use together.
Oral potassium supplements, especially wax-matrix formulations: Potassium-induced GI ulcerations may be increased. Use cautiously.
Drug-herb. *Jaborandi tree and pill-bearing spurge:* May have decreased effects. Monitor patient closely.
Squaw vine: Tannic acid may decrease metabolic breakdown. Monitor patient.
Drug-lifestyle. *Alcohol use:* May increase the incidence of CNS depression. Advise patient to avoid alcohol use.
Sun exposure: With ophthalmic form, photophobia may occur. Take precautions.

Effects on diagnostic tests

Scopolamine may interfere with the gastric secretion test.

Adverse reactions

CNS: disorientation, restlessness, irritability, dizziness, drowsiness, headache, confusion, hallucinations, delirium.
CV: tachycardia; palpitations, paradoxical bradycardia (with systemic form).
EENT: blurred vision, photophobia, increased intraocular pressure; dilated pupils, difficulty swallowing (with systemic form); ocular congestion (with prolonged use), conjunctivitis, eye dryness, eye pruritus, transient stinging and burning, edema (with ophthalmic form).
GI: dry mouth; *constipation, nausea, vomiting, epigastric distress* (with systemic form).
GU: urinary hesitancy, urine retention (with systemic form).
Respiratory: bronchial plugging, depressed respirations (with systemic form).
Skin: rash, flushing (with systemic form); dryness or contact dermatitis (with ophthalmic form).
Other: fever (with systemic form).

Overdose and treatment

Effects of overdose include excitability, seizures, CNS stimulation followed by depression, and such psychotic symptoms as disorientation, confusion, hallucinations, delusions, anxiety, agitation, delirium, and restlessness. Peripheral effects include dilated, nonreactive pupils; blurred vision; flushed, hot, dry skin; dryness of mucous membranes; dysphagia; decreased or absent bowel sounds; urine retention; hyperthermia; tachycardia; hypertension; and increased respiration.

Treatment is primarily symptomatic and supportive, as needed. Maintain patent airway. Remove transdermal system. If patient is awake and alert, induce emesis (or use gastric lavage) and follow with a sodium chloride cathartic and activated charcoal to prevent further drug absorption. In severe life-threatening cases, physostigmine may be administered to block the antimuscarinic effects of scopolamine. Give fluids, as needed, to treat shock; diazepam to control psychotic symptoms; and pilocarpine (instilled into the eyes) to relieve mydriasis. If urine retention develops, catheterization may be necessary.

Clinical considerations
Consider the recommendations relevant to all anticholinergics as well as the following:
- Intermittent and continuous I.V. infusions aren't recommended.
- Some patients, especially the elderly, may experience transient excitement or disorientation.

Ophthalmic
- Apply pressure to the lacrimal sac for 1 minute after instillation to reduce the risk of systemic drug absorption.
- Have patient lie down, tilt head back, or look at ceiling to aid instillation.

Therapeutic monitoring
Therapeutic doses may produce amnesia, drowsiness, and euphoria (desired effects for use as an adjunct to anesthesia). As necessary, reorient patient.

Special populations
Breast-feeding patients. Scopolamine is distributed in breast milk. Use cautiously in nursing women.
Pediatric patients. Safety and efficacy of soluble tablets or transdermal system have not been established in children. Use ophthalmic form cautiously, if at all, in infants and young children.
Geriatric patients. Use caution when administering drug to geriatric patients. Lower doses are indicated.

Patient counseling
Ophthalmic
- Instruct patient to apply pressure to bridge of nose for about 1 minute after instillation.
- Advise patient not to close eyes tightly or blink for about 1 minute after instillation.

Topical
- Tell patient to wash hands after applying the patch.
- Instruct patient to use only one patch at a time.
- Patch delivers about 1 mg in 72 hours. Remove the patch when antiemetic effect is no longer required.

secobarbital sodium
Novosecobarb*, Seconal

Pharmacologic classification: barbiturate
Therapeutic classification: sedative-hypnotic, anticonvulsant
Controlled substance schedule II
Pregnancy risk category D

How supplied
Available by prescription only
Capsules: 50 mg, 100 mg
Injection: 50 mg/ml in 2-ml disposable syringe

Indications and dosages
Preoperative sedation
Adults: 200 to 300 mg P.O. 1 to 2 hours before surgery or 1 mg/kg I.M. 15 minutes before procedure.
Children: 2 to 6 mg/kg P.O. (maximum dose, 100 mg) or 4 to 5 mg/kg I.M.
Insomnia
Adults: 100 mg P.O., 100 to 200 mg I.M., or 50 to 250 mg I.V.
Status epilepticus
Adults: 250 to 350 mg I.M. or I.V.
Children: 15 to 20 mg/kg I.V. over 15 minutes.
Note: No more than 250 mg (5 ml) should be injected in any one site.

Pharmacodynamics
Sedative-hypnotic action: Secobarbital acts throughout the CNS as a nonselective depressant with a rapid onset and short duration of action. Particularly sensitive to this drug is the reticular activating system, which controls CNS arousal. Secobarbital decreases both presynaptic and postsynaptic membrane excitability by facilitating the action of gamma-aminobutyric acid. The exact cellular site and mechanisms of action are unknown.

Pharmacokinetics
Absorption: After oral administration, 90% is absorbed rapidly. Levels of 1 to 5 mcg/ml are needed to produce sedation; 5 to 15 mcg/ml are needed for hypnosis.
Distribution: Distributed rapidly throughout body tissues and fluids; about 30% to 45% is protein-bound.
Metabolism: Oxidized in the liver to inactive metabolites. Duration of action is 3 to 4 hours.
Excretion: About 95% of a dose is eliminated as glucuronide conjugates and other metabolites in urine. Drug has an elimination half-life of about 30 hours.

Route	Onset	Peak	Duration
P.O.	15 min	15-30 min	1-4 hr
I.V.	Immediate	1-3 min	15 min
I.M.	Unknown	7-10 min	Unknown

Contraindications and precautions
Contraindicated in patients with respiratory disease in which dyspnea or obstruction is evident, or there's hypersensitivity to barbiturates or porphyria.

Use cautiously in patients with acute or chronic pain, depression, suicidal tendencies, history of drug abuse, or impaired hepatic or renal function.

Interactions
Drug-drug. *Antidepressants, antihistamines, narcotics, sedative-hypnotics, tranquilizers:* Secobarbital may add to or potentiate CNS and

respiratory depressant effects. Use together cautiously.
Corticosteroids, digitoxin (not digoxin), doxycycline, oral contraceptives and other estrogens, theophylline and other xanthines, warfarin and other oral anticoagulants: Secobarbital enhances the metabolism of these drugs. Monitor for lack of effect.
Disulfiram, MAO inhibitors, valproic acid: Decrease the metabolism of secobarbital and can increase its toxicity. Reduce barbiturate dosage.
Griseofulvin: Secobarbital impairs the effectiveness of griseofulvin by decreasing absorption from the GI tract. Monitor effectiveness of griseofulvin.
Rifampin: May decrease secobarbital levels by increasing metabolism. Monitor for decreased effect.
Drug-lifestyle. *Alcohol use:* May potentiate CNS depressant effects. Advise patient to avoid alcohol use.

Effects on diagnostic tests

Secobarbital may cause a false-positive phentolamine test. The physiologic effects of the drug may impair the absorption of cyanocobalamin C57.

Adverse reactions

CNS: *drowsiness, lethargy, hangover,* paradoxical excitement in geriatric patients, somnolence, change in EEG patterns.
CV: hypotension (with I.V. use).
GI: nausea, vomiting.
Hematologic: exacerbation of porphyria.
Hepatic: decreased serum bilirubin levels.
Respiratory: ***respiratory depression.***
Skin: rash, urticaria, ***Stevens-Johnson syndrome,*** tissue reactions, injection-site pain.
Other: ***angioedema,*** physical and psychological dependence.

Overdose and treatment

Signs and symptoms of overdose include unsteady gait, slurred speech, sustained nystagmus, somnolence, confusion, respiratory depression, pulmonary edema, areflexia, and coma. Typical shock syndrome with tachycardia and hypotension, jaundice, hypothermia followed by fever, and oliguria may occur.

Maintain and support ventilation and pulmonary function as necessary; support cardiac function and circulation with vasopressors and I.V. fluids as needed. If patient is conscious and gag reflex is intact, induce emesis (if ingestion was recent) by administering ipecac syrup. If emesis is contraindicated, perform gastric lavage while a cuffed endotracheal tube is in place to prevent aspiration. Follow with administration of activated charcoal or sodium chloride cathartic. Measure intake and output, vital signs, and laboratory parameters; maintain body temperature. Roll patient from side to side every 30 minutes to avoid pulmonary congestion.

Alkalinization of urine may be helpful in removing drug from the body; hemodialysis may be useful in severe overdose.

Clinical considerations

Consider the recommendations relevant to all barbiturates as well as the following:
- Use I.V. route of administration only in emergencies or when other routes are unavailable.
- Dilute secobarbital injection with sterile water for injection solution, normal saline injection, or Ringer's injection solution. Total I.V. dose shouldn't exceed 500 mg. Don't use if solution is discolored or if a precipitate forms.
- Avoid I.V. administration at a rate greater than 50 mg/15 seconds to prevent hypotension and respiratory depression. Have emergency resuscitative equipment on hand.
- Administer I.M. dose deep into large muscle mass to prevent tissue injury.
- Secobarbital sodium injection, diluted with lukewarm tap water to a concentration of 10 to 15 mg/ml, may be administered rectally in children. A cleaning enema should be administered before secobarbital enema.

Therapeutic monitoring

- Watch for signs of barbiturate toxicity: coma, pupillary constriction, cyanosis, clammy skin, and hypotension. Overdose can be fatal.
- Monitor hepatic and renal studies frequently to prevent possible toxicity.

Special populations

Breast-feeding patients. Because drug is excreted in breast milk, don't administer to breast-feeding women.
Pediatric patients. Drug may cause paradoxical excitement in children; use cautiously.
Geriatric patients. Geriatric patients are more susceptible to effects of drug and usually require lower doses. Confusion, disorientation, and excitability may occur in geriatric patients.

Patient counseling

- Inform patient the morning "hangover" is common after hypnotic dose which suppresses REM sleep.
- Caution patient about performing activities that require mental alertness or physical coordination.

selegiline hydrochloride (L-deprenyl hydrochloride)

Eldepryl

Pharmacologic classification: MAO inhibitor
Therapeutic classification: antiparkinsonian
Pregnancy risk category C

How supplied

Available by prescription only
Capsules: 5 mg
Tablets: 5mg

Indications and dosages

Adjunctive treatment to carbidopa-levodopa in the management of symptoms associated with Parkinson's disease
Adults: 10 mg P.O. daily, taken as 5 mg at breakfast and 5 mg at lunch. After 2 or 3 days of therapy, begin gradual decrease of carbidopa-levodopa dose.

Pharmacodynamics

Antiparkinsonian action: Probably acts by selectively inhibiting MAO type B (found mostly in the brain). At higher-than-recommended doses, it's a nonselective inhibitor of MAO, including MAO type A found in the GI tract. It may also directly increase dopaminergic activity by decreasing the reuptake of dopamine into nerve cells. It has pharmacologically active metabolites (amphetamine and methamphetamine) that may contribute to this effect.

Pharmacokinetics

Absorption: Rapidly absorbed; about 73% of dose is absorbed.
Distribution: After a single dose, plasma levels are below detectable levels (less than 10 ng/ml).
Metabolism: Three metabolites have been detected in the serum and urine: N-desmethyldeprenyl, amphetamine, and methamphetamine.
Excretion: About 45% appears as a metabolite in urine after 48 hours.

Route	Onset	Peak	Duration
P.O.	Unknown	½-2 hr	Unknown

Contraindications and precautions

Contraindicated in patients with hypersensitivity to drug and in those receiving meperidine and other opioids.

Interactions

Drug-drug. *Adrenergic agents:* May increase the pressor response. Use together cautiously.
Meperidine: Fatal interactions have been reported. Don't use together.
Drug-herb. *Ginseng:* May cause headache, tremors, mania. Avoid use together.
Drug-food. *Cacao:* May cause potential vasopressor effects if used together. Avoid use together.
Foods high in tyramine: May cause possible hypertensive crisis. Monitor blood pressure.
Drug-lifestyle. *Alcohol use:* Excessive depressant effect is possible. Advise patient to avoid alcohol.

Effects on diagnostic tests

None reported.

Adverse reactions

CNS: malaise, *dizziness,* increased tremor, chorea, loss of balance, restlessness, increased bradykinesia, facial grimacing, stiff neck, dyskinesia, involuntary movements, twitching, increased apraxia, behavioral changes, fatigue, headache, confusion, hallucinations, vivid dreams, anxiety, insomnia, lethargy.
CV: orthostatic hypotension, hypertension, hypotension, ***arrhythmias,*** palpitations, new or increased anginal pain, tachycardia, peripheral edema, syncope.
EENT: blepharospasm.
GI: dry mouth, *nausea,* vomiting, constipation, weight loss, abdominal pain, anorexia or poor appetite, dysphagia, diarrhea, heartburn.
GU: slow urination, transient nocturia, prostatic hyperplasia, urinary hesitancy, urinary frequency, urine retention, sexual dysfunction.
Skin: rash, hair loss.
Other: diaphoresis.

Overdose and treatment

Limited experience with overdose suggests that symptoms may include hypotension and psychomotor agitation. Because selegiline becomes a nonselective MAO inhibitor in high doses, consider the possibility of symptoms of MAO inhibitor poisoning: drowsiness, dizziness, hyperactivity, agitation, seizures, coma, hypertension, hypotension, cardiac conduction disturbances, and CV collapse. These symptoms may not develop immediately after ingestion; delays of 12 hours or more are possible.

Provide supportive treatment and closely monitor the patient for worsening of symptoms. Emesis or lavage may be helpful in the early stages of overdose treatment. Avoid phenothiazine derivatives and CNS stimulants; adrenergic agents may provoke an exaggerated response. Diazepam may be useful in treating seizures.

Clinical considerations

In some patients who experience an increase of adverse reactions associated with levodopa (including dyskinesias), reduction of carbidopa-levodopa is necessary. Most of these patients require a carbidopa-levodopa dose reduction of 10% to 30%.

Therapeutic monitoring
Monitor patient's response to drug therapy.

Special populations
Breast-feeding patients. It isn't known if drug is excreted in breast milk. Use with caution in breast-feeding women.

Patient counseling
- Advise patient not to take more than 10 mg daily. There's no evidence that higher doses improve efficacy and it may increase adverse reactions.
- Tell patient to move about cautiously at the start of therapy because dizziness may occur, which can cause falls.
- Because drug is an MAO inhibitor, tell patient about the possibility of an interaction with tyramine-containing foods. Tell patient to immediately report signs or symptoms of hypertension, including severe headache. Reportedly, however, this interaction doesn't occur at the recommended dose; at 10 mg daily, drug inhibits only MAO type B. Therefore, dietary restrictions appear unnecessary, provided that patient doesn't exceed the recommended dose.
- Advise patient to take second dose with lunch to avoid nighttime sedation.

senna
Black-Draught, Fletcher's Castoria, Nytilax, Senexon, Senokot, Senolax, X-Prep

Pharmacologic classification: anthraquinone derivative
Therapeutic classification: stimulant laxative
Pregnancy risk category C

How supplied
Available without a prescription
(Dosages expressed as sennosides [active principle])
Tablets: 6 mg, 8.6 mg, 17 mg
Granules: 15 mg/tsp, 20 mg/5 ml
Liquid: 3 mg/ml
Suppositories: 30 mg
Syrup: 8.8 mg/5 ml

Indications and dosages
Acute constipation, preparation for bowel examination
Black-Draught
Adults: 2 tablets or ¼ to ½ level tsp of granules mixed with water. Not for children.
Other preparations
Adults and children age 12 and older: Usual dose is 2 tablets, 1 tsp of granules dissolved in water, 1 suppository, or 10 to 15 ml syrup h.s. Maximum dose varies with preparation used.
Children age 6 to 11: 1 tablet, ½ tsp of granules dissolved in water, ½ suppository h.s., or 5 to 10 ml syrup. Maximum dose is 2 tablets b.i.d. or 1 tsp of granules b.i.d.
Children age 2 to 5: ½ tablet, ¼ tsp of granules dissolved in water. Maximum dose is 1 tablet b.i.d. or ½ tsp of granules b.i.d.
Children age 1 to 5: 2.5 to 5 ml syrup h.s.
Children age 1 to 12 months: Consult doctor.

Pharmacodynamics
Laxative action: Senna has a local irritant effect on the colon, which promotes peristalsis and bowel evacuation. It also enhances intestinal fluid accumulation, thereby increasing the moisture content of the stool.

Pharmacokinetics
Absorption: Absorbed minimally.
Distribution: May be distributed in bile, saliva, the colonic mucosa, and breast milk.
Metabolism: Absorbed portion is metabolized in the liver.
Excretion: Unabsorbed senna is excreted mainly in feces; absorbed drug is excreted in urine and feces.

Route	Onset	Peak	Duration
P.O.	6-10 hr	Variable	Variable
P.R.	½-2 hr	Unknown	Unknown

Contraindications and precautions
Contraindicated in patients with ulcerative bowel lesions; nausea, vomiting, abdominal pain, or other symptoms of appendicitis or acute surgical abdomen; fecal impaction; or intestinal obstruction or perforation.

Interactions
None reported.

Effects on diagnostic tests
None reported.

Adverse reactions
GI: *nausea,* vomiting, diarrhea, loss of normal bowel function with excessive use, *abdominal cramps* (especially in severe constipation), malabsorption of nutrients, "cathartic colon" (syndrome resembling ulcerative colitis radiologically) with chronic misuse, possible constipation after catharsis, yellow or yellow-green cast to feces, diarrhea in breast-feeding infants of mothers receiving senna, darkened pigmentation of rectal mucosa with long-term use (usually reversible within 4 to 12 months after stopping drug), laxative dependence with excessive use.
GU: red-pink discoloration in alkaline urine; yellow-brown color to acidic urine.
Metabolic: protein-losing enteropathy, electrolyte imbalance such as hypokalemia.

Overdose and treatment
No information available.

Clinical considerations

- Protect drug from excessive heat or light.
- Drug is for short-term treatment.

Therapeutic monitoring

Before giving drug, determine whether patient has adequate fluid intake, exercise, and diet. Also, stress importance of maintaining these during drug therapy as well.

Special populations

Breast-feeding patients. Senna is excreted in breast milk; diarrhea has been reported in breast-feeding infants.
Pediatric patients. Senna and other stimulant laxatives are used infrequently in children.
Geriatric patients. Geriatric patients often overuse laxatives and may be more susceptible to laxative dependency.

Patient counseling

- In the phenolsulfonphthalein excretion test, senna may turn urine pink to red, red to violet, or red to brown.
- Instruct patient that laxative use shouldn't exceed 1 week. Excessive use may result in dependence or electrolyte imbalance.
- Tell patient that bowel movement may have a yellow or yellow-green cast.
- Teach patient about dietary sources of bulk, including bran and other cereals, fresh fruit and vegetables.

sertraline hydrochloride

Zoloft

Pharmacologic classification: serotonin uptake inhibitor
Therapeutic classification: antidepressant
Pregnancy risk category C

How supplied

Available by prescription only
Tablets (film-coated): 25 mg, 50 mg, 100 mg

Indications and dosages

Post-traumatic stress disorder or panic disorder
Adults: 25 mg P.O. daily. Increase to 50 mg P.O. daily after 1 week. If no improvement, dose may be increased up to a maximum of 200 mg P.O. daily.
Depression, obsessive-compulsive disorder
Adults: 50 mg P.O. daily. Adjust dose as needed and tolerated; clinical trials involved doses of 50 to 200 mg daily. Dosage adjustments should be made at intervals of no less than 1 week.
≡ ***Dosage adjustment.*** Use a lower or less-frequent dosage in patients with hepatic impairment. Use particular care in patients with renal failure.

Pharmacodynamics

Antidepressant action: Sertraline probably acts by blocking the reuptake of serotonin (5-hydroxy-tryptamine; 5-HT) into presynaptic neurons in the CNS, prolonging the action of 5-HT.

Pharmacokinetics

Absorption: Well absorbed after oral administration; absorption rate and extent are enhanced when taken with food.
Distribution: In vitro studies indicate that drug is highly protein-bound (more than 98%).
Metabolism: Metabolism is probably hepatic; drug undergoes significant first-pass metabolism. N-desmethylsertraline is substantially less active than the parent compound.
Excretion: Excreted mostly as metabolites in the urine and feces. Mean elimination half-life is 26 hours. Steady-state levels are reached within 1 week of daily dosing in young, healthy patients.

Route	Onset	Peak	Duration
P.O.	Unknown	4½-8½ hr	Unknown

Contraindications and precautions

Contraindicated in patients receiving MAO inhibitors. Use cautiously in patients at risk for suicide and in those with seizure disorders, major affective disorder, or diseases or conditions that affect metabolism or hemodynamic responses.

Interactions

Drug-drug. *Cimetidine:* Increased sertraline bioavailability, peak plasma levels, and half-life. Monitor patient closely.
Diazepam, tolbutamide: Clearance of these drugs is decreased by sertraline. Monitor patient for increased drug effects.
MAO inhibitors: Serious mental status changes, hyperthermia, autonomic instability, rapid fluctuations of vital signs, delirium, coma, and death. Drug must not be given within 14 days of an MAO inhibitor.
Warfarin, other highly protein-bound drugs: May cause interactions, increasing the plasma levels of sertraline or the other highly bound drug. Monitor patient closely.

Effects on diagnostic tests

None reported.

Adverse reactions

CNS: *headache, tremor, dizziness, insomnia, somnolence,* paresthesia, hypoesthesia, *fatigue,* nervousness, anxiety, agitation, hypertonia, twitching, confusion.
CV: palpitations, chest pain, hot flashes.
GI: *dry mouth, nausea, diarrhea, loose stools, dyspepsia,* vomiting, constipation, thirst, flatulence, anorexia, abdominal pain, increased appetite.

GU: *male sexual dysfunction,* polyuria, nocturia, dysuria.
Hepatic: elevated liver enzymes.
Metabolic: minor increases in serum cholesterol and triglycerides; decreased uric acid.
Musculoskeletal: myalgia.
Skin: rash, pruritus.
Other: *diaphoresis.*

Overdose and treatment
Clinical experience with sertraline overdose is limited. Treatment is supportive. Establish an airway and maintain adequate ventilation. Because recent studies question the value of forced emesis or lavage, consider the use of activated charcoal in sorbitol to bind drug in the GI tract.

There's no specific antidote for sertraline. Monitor vital signs closely. Because drug has a large volume of distribution, hemodialysis, peritoneal dialysis, or forced diuresis probably isn't useful.

Clinical considerations
Drug may activate mania or hypomania in patients with cyclic disorders.

Therapeutic monitoring
- Patients who respond during the first 8 weeks of therapy will probably continue to respond to drug, although there are limited studies of drug in depressed patients for periods longer than 16 weeks. If patients are continued on drug for prolonged therapy, periodically monitor the effectiveness of drug. It's unknown if periodic dose adjustments are necessary to maintain effectiveness.
- Record mood changes and monitor for suicidal tendencies.

Special populations
Breast-feeding patients. It isn't known if drug is excreted in breast milk. Use with caution in breast-feeding women.
Pediatric patients. Safety and efficacy in children haven't been established.
Geriatric patients. Plasma clearance of drug is slower in geriatric patients. Studies indicate that it may take 2 to 3 weeks of daily dosing before steady-state levels are reached. Monitor patient closely for dose-related side effects.

Patient counseling
- Tell patient to take drug once daily, either in the morning or evening, with or without food.
- Advise patient to avoid use of alcohol while taking drug and to call before taking OTC medications.
- Although problems haven't been reported to date, advise patient to use caution when performing hazardous tasks that require alertness, such as driving and operating heavy machinery. Drugs that influence the CNS may impair judgment.

sibutramine hydrochloride monohydrate
Meridia

Pharmacologic classification: norepinephrine, serotonin, and dopamine reuptake inhibitor
Therapeutic classification: antiobesity
Controlled substance schedule IV
Pregnancy risk category C

How supplied
Available by prescription only
Capsules: 5 mg, 10 mg, 15 mg

Indications and dosages
Management of obesity, including weight loss and maintenance of weight loss; should be used in conjunction with a reduced-calorie diet
Adults: 10 mg P.O. once daily with or without food. May increase dose to 15 mg daily after 4 weeks if there is inadequate weight loss. Patients who don't tolerate the 10-mg dose may receive 5 mg daily. Doses above 15 mg daily aren't recommended.

Pharmacodynamics
Antiobesity action: Sibutramine produces its therapeutic effects by inhibiting the reuptake of norepinephrine, serotonin, and dopamine.

Pharmacokinetics
Absorption: Rapidly absorbed from the GI tract. On average, at least 77% of a single oral dose of sibutramine is absorbed.
Distribution: Distributed extensively into tissues, especially the liver and kidney with relatively low transfer to the fetus. In vitro, sibutramine, M_1, and M_2 are extensively bound (97%, 94%, and 94%, respectively) to human plasma proteins.
Metabolism: Undergoes extensive first-pass metabolism by the cytochrome P-450 3A4 isoenzyme to active desmethyl metabolites M_1 and M_2; elimination half-lives of M_1 and M_2 are 14 and 16 hours, respectively.
Excretion: About 77% of a single oral dose is excreted in the urine.

Route	Onset	Peak	Duration
P.O.	Unknown	3-4 hr	Unknown

Contraindications and precautions
Contraindicated in patients taking MAO inhibitors or other centrally acting appetite-suppressant drugs. Also contraindicated in patients with known hypersensitivity to drug or its inactive ingredients and in those with anorexia nervosa. Don't use drug in patients with history of coronary artery disease, heart failure,

arrhythmias, stroke, severe renal failure, hepatic dysfunction, or a history of seizures.

Use cautiously in patients with narrow angle glaucoma.

Interactions

Drug-drug. *CNS depressants:* May enhance CNS depression. Use with caution.

Dextromethorphan, dihydroergotamine, fentanyl, fluoxetine, fluvoxamine, lithium, MAO inhibitors, meperidine, paroxetine, pentazocine, sertraline, sumatriptan, tryptophan, venlafaxine: May cause hyperthermia, tachycardia, and loss of consciousness. Don't use together. At least 2 weeks should elapse between stopping an MAO inhibitor and starting sibutramine, and vice versa.

Drugs that inhibit cytochrome P-450 3A4 metabolism, such as erythromycin and ketoconazole: Dose of sibutramine may need to be reduced when given together.

Ephedrine, phenylpropanolamine, pseudoephedrine: May increase blood pressure or heart rate. Monitor patient carefully.

Drug-lifestyle. *Alcohol use:* May enhance CNS depression. Discourage use.

Effects on diagnostic tests

None reported.

Adverse reactions

CNS: *headache*, *insomnia*, dizziness, nervousness, anxiety, depression, paresthesia, somnolence, CNS stimulation, emotional lability, migraine.

CV: tachycardia, vasodilation, hypertension, palpitation, chest pain. generalized edema.

EENT: thirst, *dry mouth, rhinitis, pharyngitis,* laryngitis, sinusitis, taste perversion, ear disorder, ear pain.

GI: *anorexia, constipation,* increased appetite, nausea, dyspepsia, gastritis, vomiting, abdominal pain, rectal disorder.

GU: dysmenorrhea, urinary tract infection, vaginal monilia, metrorrhagia.

Hepatic: elevated liver function tests.

Musculoskeletal: arthralgia, myalgia, asthenia, tenosynovitis, joint disorder, neck or back pain.

Respiratory: cough increase, laryngitis.

Skin: rash, sweating, herpes simplex, acne.

Other: flu syndrome, ***allergic reaction.***

Overdose and treatment

There's no specific antidote to sibutramine. Treatment should consist of general measures used in the management of overdose: Establish an airway, monitor cardiac and vital signs, and institute general symptomatic and supportive measures. Cautious use of beta blockers may be indicated to control elevated blood pressure or tachycardia. The benefits of forced diuresis and hemodialysis are unknown.

Clinical considerations

- Drug is recommended for obese patients with an initial body mass index of 30 kg/m^2 or more or 27 kg/m^2 or more in the presence of other risk factors, such as hypertension, diabetes, or dyslipidemia.
- Rule out organic causes of obesity before starting therapy.
- Weight loss can precipitate or exacerbate gallstone formation.
- Although not reported with sibutramine, some centrally acting weight-loss agents have been associated with a rare but fatal condition known as primary pulmonary hypertension.

Therapeutic monitoring

- Measure blood pressure and heart rate before starting therapy, with dose changes, and at regular intervals during therapy because drug is known to increase both blood pressure and heart rate.
- If a patient has not lost at least 4 lb in the first 4 weeks of treatment, reevaluate therapy to consider dose increase or discontinuation of drug.

Special populations

Breast-feeding patients. It isn't known whether drug or its metabolites are excreted in breast milk. Avoid use of drug in breast-feeding women.

Pediatric patients. Safety and efficacy in children under age 16 haven't been established.

Geriatric patients. Dose selection for a geriatric patient should be cautious, reflecting the greater frequency of decreased hepatic, renal, or cardiac function, and of concomitant disease or other drug therapy.

Patient counseling

- Advise patient to read the package insert before starting therapy and to review again each time the prescription is renewed.
- Instruct patient to report rash, hives, or other allergic reactions immediately.
- Inform patient to inform doctor of other prescription or OTC drugs being taken, especially other weight-reducing agents, decongestants, antidepressants, cough suppressants, lithium, dihydroergotamine, sumatriptan, or tryptophan, as there is a potential for drug interactions.
- Emphasize importance of regular follow-up visits with doctor.
- Advise patient to use drug with a reduced-calorie diet.

sildenafil citrate

Viagra

Pharmacologic classification: selective inhibitor of cyclic guanosine monophosphate-specific phosphodiesterase type 5
Therapeutic classification: therapy for erectile dysfunction
Pregnancy risk category B

How supplied

Available by prescription only
Tablets: 25 mg, 50 mg, 100 mg

Indications and dosages

Treatment of erectile dysfunction
Adults: 50 mg P.O. as a single dose, p.r.n., 1 hour before sexual activity. However, may take drug 30 minutes to 4 hours before sexual activity. Based on effectiveness and tolerance by patient, may increase dose to maximum single dose of 100 mg or decrease dose to 25 mg. A maximum recommended dosing frequency is once daily.
≡ ***Dosage adjustment.*** Elderly patients with hepatic impairment or severe renal impairment, and those concurrently taking potent cytochrome P-450 3A4 inhibitors, consider a starting dose of 25 mg.

Pharmacodynamics

Erectile action: Sildenafil has no direct relaxant effect on isolated human corpus cavernosum, but enhances the effect of nitric oxide (NO) by inhibiting phosphodiesterase type 5 (PDE5), which is responsible for degradation of cyclic guanosine monophosphate (cGMP) in the corpus cavernosum. When sexual stimulation causes local release of NO, inhibition of PDE5 by sildenafil causes increased levels of cGMP in the corpus cavernosum, resulting in smooth muscle relaxation and inflow of blood to the corpus cavernosum.

Pharmacokinetics

Absorption: Rapidly absorbed after oral administration. A high-fat meal delays the rate of absorption by about 1 hour and reduces peak levels by one third. Absolute bioavailability of sildenafil is about 40%.
Distribution: Widely distributed to body tissues with a mean steady-state volume of distribution of 105 L. Both drug and its major active metabolite are 96% bound to plasma proteins. Protein binding is independent of drug levels.
Metabolism: The primary pathway for sildenafil elimination is metabolism by the CYP 3A4 and CYP 2C9 hepatic microsomal isoenzymes. N-desmethylation converts sildenafil into the major circulating metabolite, which accounts for about 20% of the pharmacologic effects of sildenafil.
Excretion: About 80% of an oral dose is metabolized and excreted in the feces, and about 13% is excreted in the urine.

Route	Onset	Peak	Duration
P.O.	Unknown	½-2 hr	4 hr

Contraindications and precautions

Contraindicated in patients also using organic nitrates and in those with known hypersensitivity to drug or its components.

Use with caution in patients who have had an MI, stroke, or life-threatening arrhythmias within the past 6 months; have a history of cardiac failure, coronary artery disease, or uncontrolled high or low blood pressure; in those with anatomic deformation of the penis; and in those predisposed to priapism (sickle cell anemia, multiple myeloma, leukemia), retinitis pigmentosa, bleeding disorders, or active peptic ulcers.

Interactions

Drug-drug. *Inhibitors of cytochrome P-450 isoforms 3A4, such as cimetidine, erythromycin, itraconazole and ketoconazole:* May reduce the clearance of sildenafil. Avoid use together.
Nitrates: Sildenafil enhances the hypotensive effects of nitrates. Don't use together.
Rifampin: May reduce sildenafil plasma levels. Monitor effect closely.
Drug-food. *High-fat meals:* Can delay absorption of drug and onset of action by 1 hour. Separate administration time from meals.

Effects on diagnostic tests

None reported.

Adverse reactions

CNS: *headache,* dizziness.
CV: *flushing.*
EENT: nasal congestion, abnormal vision (photophobia, color blindness).
GI: dyspepsia, diarrhea.
GU: urinary tract infection.
Skin: rash.

Overdose and treatment

In healthy volunteers, doses up to 800 mg produced adverse events similar to those seen at lower doses, but at an increased rate. Use standard supportive measures to treat overdose. Renal dialysis isn't expected to increase clearance.

Clinical considerations

- Because cardiac risk is associated with sexual activity, evaluate patient's CV status before initiating therapy.
- Drug seems to have favorable teratogenic, embryotoxic, and fetotoxic profiles, and isn't

readily distributed into semen; it isn't expected to be harmful to pregnant women.

Therapeutic monitoring

Monitor patient's compliance with drug regimen.

Special populations

Breast-feeding patients. Drug isn't indicated for use in women.
Pediatric patients. Drug shouldn't be used in children or neonates.
Geriatric patients. Reduced drug clearance is seen in healthy geriatric patients age 65 or older. This reduction results in plasma levels about 40% greater than those in younger subjects.

Patient counseling

- Tell patient that drug doesn't protect against sexually transmitted diseases and that he should use protective measures to prevent infection.
- Advise patient that drug is most rapidly absorbed if taken on an empty stomach.
- Tell patient to notify physician of visual changes.
- Urge patient to seek medical attention if erection persists for more than 4 hours.
- Advise patient that drug has no effect in the absence of sexual stimulation.

silver nitrate

Silver Nitrate

Pharmacologic classification: heavy metal (silver compound)
Therapeutic classification: ophthalmic antiseptic; topical cauterizing agent
Pregnancy risk category C

How supplied

Available by prescription only
Ophthalmic solution: 1%
Topical ointment: 10%
Topical solution: 10%, 25%, 50%

Indications and dosages

Prevention of gonorrheal ophthalmia neonatorum
Neonates: Clean lids thoroughly; instill 2 drops of 1% solution into lower conjunctival sac of each eye and ensure that solution contacts the entire conjunctival sac for 30 seconds or longer.
To treat indolent wounds, destroy exuberant granulations, freshen the edges of ulcers and fissures, provide styptic action, and treat vesicular bullous or aphthous lesions
Adults: Apply ointment on a pad to lesion for 5 days; or a cotton applicator dipped in solution to affected area two to three times a week for 2 to 3 weeks.

Pharmacodynamics

Antiseptic action: Liberated silver ions precipitate bacterial proteins, resulting in germicidal activity. Drug is effective mainly in preventing gonorrheal ophthalmia neonatorum.
Cauterizing action: Denatures protein, producing a caustic or corrosive effect.

Pharmacokinetics

Absorption: Not readily absorbed from mucous membranes or other tissues.
Distribution: Unknown.
Metabolism: Unknown.
Excretion: Unknown.

Route	Onset	Peak	Duration
Ophthalmic	Unknown	Unknown	Unknown

Contraindications and precautions

No known contraindications.

Interactions

Drug-drug. *Alkalies, benzalkonium chloride, halogenated acids or salts, phosphates, and thimerosal:* Silver nitrate is incompatible with these. Don't use together.

Effects on diagnostic tests

None reported.

Adverse reactions

EENT: periorbital edema, temporary staining of lids and surrounding tissue, *conjunctivitis*.

Overdose and treatment

Signs and symptoms of overdose are extremely rare with ophthalmic use.

Toxicity is highly dependent on the concentration of silver nitrate and extent of exposure. Oral overdose is treated by dilution with 4 to 8 oz (120 to 240 ml) of water. To remove the chemical, administer saline (10 g/L) by lavage to precipitate silver chloride. Activated charcoal or a cathartic can be used. Treat eye overexposure initially by irrigation with tepid water for at least 15 minutes. Treat dermal overexposure by washing with soap and water twice. Dizziness, seizures, mucous membrane irritation, nausea, vomiting, stomach ache and diarrhea, methemoglobinemia, dermatitis, rash, and hypochloremia with associated hyponatremia may occur. Treat seizures with diazepam. Depending on the extent of exposure, evaluate for methemoglobinemia; treat with methylene blue.

Clinical considerations

- Silver nitrate is bacteriostatic, germicidal, and astringent.
- Don't use repeatedly.
- If solution stronger than 1% is accidentally used in eye, promptly irrigate with isotonic saline to prevent eye irritation.

- Handle drug carefully; solution may stain skin and utensils.
- Don't use solution if it's discolored or contains a precipitate.
- Moisten silver nitrate pencils with water before use.
- In low levels (0.125% to 0.5%) as a wet dressing, silver nitrate is used as a local anti-infective to treat burns and skin wounds or ulcers.
- Drug may be painful when administered topically in higher levels.

Therapeutic monitoring
Topical use of solutions above 1% concentration may cause burns. Avoid contact with skin and eyes. If accidental contact with skin occurs, flush with water for at least 15 minutes; for accidental contact with eyes, irrigate with sterile water or normal saline immediately.

Special populations
Pediatric patients. Instillation may be briefly delayed to allow neonate to bond with mother; however, application should occur within 1 hour after delivery. Most states require instillation by law at birth; don't irrigate eyes after instillation. Store wax ampules away from light and heat.

Patient counseling
- Explain that preparations may stain skin and clothing. Teach parents that silver nitrate may discolor neonate's eyelids temporarily.
- Inform parents that instillation at birth is required by law in most states.

simethicone
Gas-X, Mylicon, Phazyme

Pharmacologic classification: dispersant
Therapeutic classification: antiflatulent
Pregnancy risk category C

How supplied
Available without a prescription
Tablets (delayed-release; enteric-coated core): 60 mg, 95 mg
Tablets (chewable): 40 mg, 80 mg, 125 mg
Capsules: 125 mg
Drops: 40 mg/0.6 ml

Indications and dosages
Flatulence, functional gastric bloating
Adults and children over age 12: 40 to 125 mg P.O. after each meal and h.s.
Children age 2 to 12: 40 mg (drops) P.O. q.i.d.
Children under age 2: 20 mg (drops) P.O. q.i.d., up to 240 mg/day.

Pharmacodynamics
Antiflatulent action: Simethicone acts as a defoaming agent by decreasing the surface tension of gas bubbles, preventing the formation of mucous-coated gas bubbles.

Pharmacokinetics
Absorption: None.
Distribution: None.
Metabolism: None.
Excretion: Excreted in feces.

Route	Onset	Peak	Duration
P.O.	Immediate	Unknown	Unknown

Contraindications and precautions
Contraindicated in patients hypersensitive to drug.

Interactions
Drug-drug. *Alginic acid:* Decreased effectiveness of alginic acid. Monitor patient closely.

Effects on diagnostic tests
None reported.

Adverse reactions
GI: expulsion of excessive liberated gas as belching, rectal flatus.

Overdose and treatment
No information available.

Clinical considerations
- Simethicone is found in many combination antacid products.
- This medication doesn't prevent formation of gas.

Therapeutic monitoring
Monitor patient's response to drug therapy.

Special populations
Pediatric patients. Simethicone isn't recommended as treatment for infant colic; it has limited use in children.

Patient counseling
- Tell patient to chew tablets thoroughly or to shake suspension well before using.
- Encourage patient to change positions frequently and ambulate to aid flatus passage.

simvastatin
Zocor

Pharmacologic classification: HMG-CoA reductase inhibitor
Therapeutic classification: antilipemic, cholesterol-lowering agent
Pregnancy risk category X

How supplied
Available by prescription only
Tablets: 5 mg, 10 mg, 20 mg, 40 mg, 80 mg

Indications and dosages

Reduction of low-density lipoprotein (LDL) and total cholesterol levels in patients with primary hypercholesterolemia (types IIa and IIb)

Adults: Initially, 5 to 10 mg daily in the evening. Adjust dose q 4 weeks based on patient tolerance and response; maximum daily dose, 40 mg. Maximum daily dose for geriatric patients, 20 mg.

≡ ***Dosage adjustment.*** For patients receiving immunosuppressants, start with 5 mg/day; maximum daily dose, 10 mg. For patients with mild to moderate renal insufficiency, give usual daily dose; in those with severe renal impairment, start therapy with 5 mg P.O. daily and closely monitor patient.

Pharmacodynamics

Antilipemic action: Simvastatin inhibits the enzyme 3-hydroxy-3-methylglutaryl-coenzyme A (HMG-CoA) reductase. This hepatic enzyme is an early (and rate-limiting) step in the synthetic pathway of cholesterol.

Pharmacokinetics

Absorption: Readily absorbed; however, extensive hepatic extraction limits the plasma availability of active inhibitors to 5% of a dose or less. Individual absorption varies considerably.

Distribution: Parent drug and active metabolites are more than 95% bound to plasma proteins.

Metabolism: Hydrolysis occurs in the plasma; at least three major metabolites have been identified.

Excretion: Excreted primarily in bile.

Route	Onset	Peak	Duration
P.O.	Unknown	1⅓-2½ hr	Unknown

Contraindications and precautions

Contraindicated in patients with hypersensitivity to drug and in those with active hepatic disease or conditions that cause unexplained persistent elevations of serum transaminase; in pregnant and breast-feeding women; and in women of childbearing age unless there's no risk of pregnancy.

Use cautiously in patients with history of liver disease or who consume excessive amounts of alcohol.

Interactions

Drug-drug. *Cimetidine, ketoconazole, spironolactone:* May increase the risk of development of endocrine dysfunction. No intervention appears necessary; obtain complete drug history in patients in whom endocrine dysfunction develops.

Digoxin: Simvastatin may slightly elevate levels. Closely monitor plasma digoxin levels at the start of simvastatin therapy.

Erythromycin; fibric acid derivatives such as clofibrate and gemfibrozil; high doses of niacin (nicotinic acid; 1 g or more daily); immunosuppressive agents such as cyclosporine: May increase risk of rhabdomyolysis. Monitor patient closely if use together can't be avoided. Limit daily dose of simvastatin to 10 mg if patient must take cyclosporine.

Hepatotoxic drugs: Increased risk for hepatotoxicity. Avoid use together.

Warfarin: Simvastatin may slightly enhance the anticoagulant effect. Monitor PT at the start of therapy and during dose adjustment.

Drug-lifestyle. *Alcohol use:* May increase the risk of hepatotoxicity. Advise patient to avoid alcohol use.

Effects on diagnostic tests

None reported.

Adverse reactions

CNS: headache, asthenia.

GI: abdominal pain, constipation, diarrhea, dyspepsia, flatulence, nausea, vomiting.

Hepatic: elevated liver enzymes.

Respiratory: upper respiratory tract infection.

Overdose and treatment

There has been no experience with simvastatin overdose. No specific antidote is known. Treat symptomatically.

Clinical considerations

Initiate simvastatin only after diet and other nonpharmacologic therapies have proved ineffective. Patient should continue a cholesterol-lowering diet during therapy.

Therapeutic monitoring

- Dose adjustments should be made about every 4 weeks. If the cholesterol levels decrease below the target range, dose may be reduced.
- Perform liver function tests frequently at the start of therapy and periodically thereafter.

Special populations

Pregnant patients. Safety hasn't been established. Patient should immediately notify doctor if pregnancy occurs or is suspected.

Breast-feeding patients. It isn't known if drug is excreted in breast milk. Because of the risk to infants, avoid breast-feeding during therapy.

Pediatric patients. Safety and efficacy in children haven't been established.

Geriatric patients. Most geriatric patients respond to daily dose of 20 mg or less.

Patient counseling

- Tell patient that drug should be taken in the evening and may be taken without regard to meals.
- Tell patient to report adverse reactions, particularly muscle aches and pains.
- Explain importance of controlling serum lipids to CV health. Teach appropriate dietary

management (restricting total fat and cholesterol intake), weight control, and exercise.

sodium bicarbonate

Bell/ans, Neut, Soda Mint

Pharmacologic classification: alkalinizer
Therapeutic classification: systemic and urinary alkalinizer, systemic hydrogen ion buffer, oral antacid
Pregnancy risk category C

How supplied

Available by prescription only
Injection: 4% (2.4 mEq/5 ml), 4.2% (5 mEq/10 ml), 5% (297.5 mEq/500 ml), 7.5% (8.92 mEq/10 ml and 44.6 mEq/50 ml), 8.4% (10 mEq/10 ml and 50 mEq/50 ml)
Available without a prescription
Tablets: 325 mg, 500 mg, 520 mg, 650 mg

Indications and dosages

Adjunct to advanced cardiac life support
Adults and children over age 2: Although no longer routinely recommended, inject either 300 to 500 ml of a 5% solution or 200 to 300 mEq of a 7.5% or 8.4% solution as rapidly as possible. Base further doses on subsequent blood gas values.
Children age 2 or under: 1 mEq/kg I.V. bolus of a 4.2% solution. Dose may be repeated q 10 minutes depending on blood gas values. Don't exceed daily dose of 8 mEq/kg.
Metabolic acidosis
Adults and children: Dose depends on blood carbon dioxide content, pH, and patient's clinical condition. Generally, administer 90 to 180 mEq/L I.V. during first hour, then adjust, p.r.n.
Urinary alkalization
Adults: 325 mg to 2 g P.O., up to q.i.d. Don't exceed 17 g in patients under age 60 or 8 g in patients over age 60.
Children: 1 to 10 mEq (84 to 840 mg)/kg daily.
Antacid
Adults: 300 mg to 2 g P.O. one to four times daily.

Pharmacodynamics

Alkalizing buffering action: Sodium bicarbonate is an alkalinizing agent that dissociates to provide bicarbonate ion. Bicarbonate in excess of that needed to buffer hydrogen ions causes systemic alkalinization and, when excreted, urinary alkalinization as well.
Oral antacid action: Taken orally, sodium bicarbonate neutralizes stomach acid by the above mechanism.

Pharmacokinetics

Absorption: Well absorbed after oral administration as sodium ion and bicarbonate.
Distribution: Occurs naturally and is confined to the systemic circulation.
Metabolism: None.
Excretion: Filtered and reabsorbed by the kidney; less than 1% of filtered bicarbonate is excreted.

Route	Onset	Peak	Duration
P.O.	Unknown	Unknown	Unknown
I.V.	Immediate	Immediate	Unknown

Contraindications and precautions

Contraindicated in patients with metabolic or respiratory alkalosis; in those who are losing chlorides by vomiting or from continuous GI suction; in those receiving diuretics known to produce hypochloremic alkalosis; and in patients with hypocalcemia in which alkalosis may produce tetany, hypertension, seizures, or heart failure. Orally administered sodium bicarbonate is contraindicated in patients with acute ingestion of strong mineral acids.

Use with extreme caution in patients with heart failure, renal insufficiency, or other edematous or sodium-retaining conditions.

Interactions

Drug-drug. *Amphetamines, ephedrine, pseudoephedrine, quinidine:* If urinary alkalinization occurs, sodium bicarbonate increases half-life of these drugs. Monitor patient closely.
Chlorpropamide, lithium, salicylates, tetracyclines: Increased urinary excretion of these drugs. Monitor patient closely.
Corticosteroids: May increase sodium retention. Monitor patient closely.

Effects on diagnostic tests

None reported.

Adverse reactions

GI: gastric distention, belching, flatulence.
Metabolic: ***metabolic alkalosis,*** hypernatremia, increased serum lactate levels, hyperosmolarity (with overdose).
Other: local pain and irritation at injection site.

Overdose and treatment

Signs of overdose include depressed consciousness and obtundation from hypernatremia, tetany from hypocalcemia, arrhythmias from hypokalemia, and seizures from alkalosis. Correct fluid, electrolyte, and pH abnormalities. Monitor vital signs and fluid and electrolytes closely.

Clinical considerations

◻ ***ALERT*** Sodium bicarbonate isn't routinely recommended for use in cardiac arrest because it may produce a paradoxical acidosis from carbon dioxide production.
- Avoid extravasation of I.V. solutions. Addition of calcium salts may cause precipitate; bicarbonate may inactivate catecholamines in so-

lution (epinephrine, phenylephrine, and dopamine).
- Discourage use as an oral antacid because of hazardous excessive systemic absorption.
- Drug may be used as an adjunct to treat hyperkalemia (with dextrose and insulin).

Therapeutic monitoring
- Monitor blood pH, partial pressure of arterial oxygen, partial pressure of arterial carbon dioxide and serum electrolytes.
- Assess patient for milk-alkali syndrome if drug use is long-term.
- Monitor vital signs regularly; when drug is used as urinary alkalinizer, monitor urine pH.

Special populations
Pregnant patients. Safety hasn't been established for use during pregnancy.
Breast-feeding patients. It isn't known if sodium bicarbonate is excreted in breast milk. Use cautiously when administering to breast-feeding women.
Pediatric patients. Avoid rapid infusion (10 ml/minute) of hypertonic solutions in children under age 2.
Geriatric patients. Geriatric patients with heart failure or other fluid-retaining conditions are at greater risk for increased fluid retention; therefore, use drug with caution.

Patient counseling
- Advise patient not to take drug with milk. Drug may cause hypercalcemia, alkalosis, and possibly renal calculi.
- If patient takes an oral dose form, tell patient to take drug 1 hour before or 2 hours after taking enteric-coated medications because drug may cause enteric-coated products to dissolve in the stomach.

sodium ferric gluconate complex
Ferrlecit

Pharmacologic classification: macromolecular iron complex
Therapeutic classification: hematinic
Pregnancy risk category B

How supplied
Available by prescription only
Injection: 62.5 mg elemental iron (12.5 mg/ml) in 5-ml ampules

Indications and dosages
Treatment of iron deficiency anemia in patients undergoing chronic hemodialysis who are receiving supplemental erythropoietin therapy
Adults: Before initiating therapeutic doses, administer a test dose of 2 ml sodium ferric gluconate complex (25 mg elemental iron) diluted in 50 ml normal saline and given I.V. over 1 hour. If test dose is tolerated, give therapeutic dose of 10 ml (125 mg elemental iron) diluted in 100 ml normal saline and given I.V. over 1 hour. Most patients require a minimum cumulative dose of 1 g elemental iron administered at more than eight sequential dialysis treatments to achieve a favorable hemoglobin or hematocrit response.

Pharmacodynamics
Hematinic action: Sodium ferric gluconate complex restores total body iron content, which is critical for normal hemoglobin synthesis and oxygen transport. Iron deficiency in hemodialysis patients can be due to increased iron utilization (such as from erythropoietin therapy), blood loss (such as from fistula, retention in dialyzer, hematologic testing, menses), decreased dietary intake or absorption, surgery, iron sequestration resulting from inflammatory process, and malignancy.

Sodium ferric gluconate complex restores total body iron content, which is critical for normal hemoglobin synthesis and oxygen transport.

Pharmacokinetics
No information available.

Route	Onset	Peak	Duration
I.V.	Unknown	Unknown	Unknown

Contraindications and precautions
Contraindicated in patients with hypersensitivity to sodium ferric gluconate complex or its components (such as benzyl alcohol). Also contraindicated in patients with anemias not associated with iron deficiency. Don't administer to patients with iron overload. Use cautiously in geriatric patients.

Interactions
None reported.

Effects on diagnostic tests
None reported.

Adverse reactions
CNS: asthenia, headache, fatigue, malaise, dizziness, paresthesia, agitation, insomnia, somnolence, syncope.
CV: hypotension, hypertension, tachycardia, ***bradycardia,*** angina, chest pain, ***myocardial infarction,*** edema, flushing.
EENT: conjunctivitis, abnormal vision, rhinitis.
GI: nausea, vomiting, diarrhea, rectal disorder, dyspepsia, eructation, flatulence, melena, abdominal pain.
GU: urinary tract infection.
Hematologic: abnormal erythrocytes, anemia.
Metabolic: hyperkalemia, hypoglycemia, hypokalemia, hypervolemia.

Musculoskeletal: myalgia, arthralgia, back pain, arm pain, cramps.
Respiratory: dyspnea, coughing, upper respiratory tract infections, pneumonia, pulmonary edema.
Skin: pruritus, increased sweating, rash.
Other: injection site reaction, pain, fever, infection, rigors, chills, flulike syndrome, sepsis, ***carcinoma, hypersensitivity reactions,*** lymphadenopathy.

Overdose and treatment

Serum iron levels greater than 300 mcg/dl (with transferrin oversaturation) may indicate iron poisoning. Symptoms include abdominal pain, diarrhea, or vomiting that progresses to pallor or cyanosis; lassitude; drowsiness; hyperventilation resulting from acidosis; and cardiovascular collapse. Treatment consists of supportive measures. Drug isn't dialyzable.

Clinical considerations

☐ ***ALERT*** Dosage is expressed in milligrams of elemental iron.
- Drug shouldn't be administered to patients with iron overload, which generally occurs in hemoglobinopathies and other refractory anemias.

☐ ***ALERT*** Potentially life-threatening hypersensitivity reactions, characterized by cardiovascular collapse, cardiac arrest, bronchospasm, oral or pharyngeal edema, dyspnea, angioedema, urticaria, or pruritus sometimes associated with pain and muscle spasm of chest or back, may occur during infusion. Have adequate supportive measures readily available. Monitor patient closely during infusion.
- Some adverse reactions in hemodialysis patients may be related to dialysis itself or to chronic renal failure.
- Dilute test dose of sodium ferric gluconate complex in 50 ml normal saline and administer over 1 hour. Dilute therapeutic doses of drug in 100 ml normal saline and give over 1 hour.
- Don't mix sodium ferric gluconate complex with other drugs, or add to parenteral nutrition solutions for I.V. infusion. Use immediately after dilution in normal saline.
- Profound hypotension associated with flushing, light-headedness, malaise, fatigue, weakness, or severe chest, back, flank, or groin pain has been reported following rapid I.V. administration of iron. These reactions aren't associated with hypersensitivity reactions and may be due to too rapid administration of drug. Don't exceed recommended rate of administration (2.1 mg/min). Monitor patient closely during infusion.

Therapeutic monitoring

- Monitor hematocrit and hemoglobin, serum ferritin, and iron saturation levels during therapy, as ordered.
- Check with patient about other potential sources of iron, such as nonprescription iron preparations and iron-containing multiple vitamins with minerals.

Special populations

Breast-feeding patients. It's unknown if drug is excreted in breast milk. Use caution when administering drug to breast-feeding women.
Pediatric patients. Safety and efficacy of drug haven't been established in children.
Geriatric patients. It's unknown if patients age 65 and older respond differently than younger patients. In general, use cautiously in geriatric patients because they may be taking other drugs or may have concomitant disease or decreased hepatic, renal, or cardiac function.

Patient counseling

Abdominal pain, diarrhea, vomiting, drowsiness, or hyperventilation may indicate iron poisoning. Advise patient to report any of these symptoms immediately.

sodium fluoride

ACT, Fluorigard, Fluorinse, Fluoritab, Flura-Drops, Flura-Loz, Karidium, Karigel, Karigel-N, Listermint with Fluoride, Luride, Luride Lozi-Tabs, Luride-SF Lozi-Tabs, Pediaflor, Phos-Flur, Point-Two, Prevident, Thera-Flur, Thera-Flur-N

Pharmacologic classification: trace mineral
Therapeutic classification: dental caries prophylactic
Pregnancy risk category C

How supplied

Available by prescription only
Tablets: 1 mg (sugar-free)
Tablets (chewable): 0.5 mg, 1 mg (sugar-free)
Drops: 0.125 mg/drop (30 ml), 0.125 mg/drop (60 ml, sugar-free), 0.25 mg/drop (19 ml), 0.25 mg/drop (24 ml, sugar-free), 0.5 mg/ml (50 ml)
Rinse: 0.09% (240 ml, 480 ml), 0.09% (480 ml, sugar-free)
Gel: 0.1% (65 g, 105 g, 122 g), 0.5% (24 g, 30 g, 60 g, 120 g, 130 g, 250 g), 1.23% (480 ml)
Gel drops: 0.5% (24 ml)
Available without a prescription
Rinse: 0.02%; 0.04%; 0.08%; 0.2%
Gel: 0.1%

Indications and dosages

Aid in the prevention of dental caries
Oral
Children age 6 months to 3 years: 0.25 mg daily.
Children age 3 to 6: 0.5 mg daily.
Children age 6 to 16: 1 mg daily.

≡ *Dosage adjustment.* If fluoride in the drinking water is less than 0.3 ppm, use dosage listed; if fluoride content is 0.3 to 0.7 ppm, use one half of dosage; if fluoride content exceeds 0.7 ppm, don't use.

Topical

Adults and children over age 12: 10 ml of 0.09% (0.2% fluoride ion) rinse. Use once daily after thoroughly brushing teeth and rinsing mouth. Rinse around and between teeth for 1 minute, then spit out.

Children age 6 to 12: 5 ml of 0.09% (0.2% fluoride ion) solution.

Pharmacodynamics

Dental caries prophylactic action: Sodium fluoride acts systemically before tooth eruption and topically afterward by increasing tooth resistance to acid dissolution, by promoting remineralization, and by inhibiting the cariogenic microbial process. Acidulation provides greater topical fluoride uptake by dental enamel than neutral solutions. When topical fluoride is applied to hypersensitive exposed dentin, the formation of insoluble materials within the dentinal tubules blocks transmission of painful stimuli.

Pharmacokinetics

Absorption: Absorbed readily and almost completely from the GI tract. A large amount of an oral dose may be absorbed in the stomach; rate of absorption may depend on the gastric pH. Normal total plasma fluoride levels range from 0.14 to 0.19 mcg/ml.

Distribution: Stored in bones and developing teeth after absorption. Skeletal tissue also has a high storage capacity for fluoride ions. Because of the storage-mobilization mechanism in skeletal tissue, a constant fluoride supply may be provided. Fluoride has been found in all organs and tissues with a low accumulation in noncalcified tissues. Fluoride is distributed into sweat, tears, hair, and saliva. Fluoride crosses the placenta and is distributed into breast milk. Fluoride levels in milk range from about 0.05 to 0.13 ppm and remain fairly constant.

Metabolism: Not metabolized.

Excretion: Excreted rapidly, mainly in urine. About 90% of fluoride is filtered by the glomerulus and reabsorbed by the renal tubules.

Route	Onset	Peak	Duration
P.O.	Unknown	30-60 min	Unknown

Contraindications and precautions

Contraindicated in patients hypersensitive to fluoride or when intake from drinking water exceeds 0.6 ppm.

Interactions

Drug-drug. *Aluminum hydroxide or magnesium:* May impair the absorption of sodium fluoride. Administer drugs at separate times.

Drug-food. *Dairy foods:* Incompatibility may occur due to formation of calcium fluoride, which is poorly absorbed. Avoid use together.

Effects on diagnostic tests

None reported.

Adverse reactions

CNS: headache, weakness.
GI: gastric distress.
Skin: hypersensitivity reactions (atopic dermatitis, eczema, urticaria).
Other: staining of teeth.

Overdose and treatment

In children, acute ingestion of 10 to 20 mg of sodium fluoride may cause excessive salivation and GI disturbances; 500 mg may be fatal. GI disturbances include salivation, nausea, abdominal pain, vomiting, and diarrhea. CNS disturbances include CNS irritability, paresthesia, tetany, hyperactive reflexes, seizures, and respiratory or cardiac failure (from the calcium-binding effect of fluoride). Hypoglycemia and hypocalcemia are frequent laboratory findings.

By using gastric lavage with 1% to 5% calcium chloride solution, the fluoride may be precipitated. Administer glucose I.V. in saline solution; parenteral calcium administration may be indicated for tetany. Maintain adequate urine output.

Clinical considerations

- Recommended doses are currently under study. Some evidence suggests that considerably less fluoride is needed for adequate supplementation.
- Tablets can be dissolved in the mouth, chewed, swallowed whole, added to drinking water or fruit juice, or added to water in infant formula or other foods.
- Drops may be administered orally undiluted or added to fluids or food.
- Sodium fluoride may be preferred to stannous fluoride to avoid staining tooth surfaces. Neutral sodium fluoride may also be preferred to acidulated fluoride to avoid dulling of porcelain and ceramic restorations.
- Prolonged intake of drinking water containing a fluoride ion concentration of 0.4 to 0.8 ppm may result in increased density of bone mineral and fluoride osteosclerosis.
- An oral sodium fluoride dose of 40 to 65 mg/day has resulted in adverse rheumatic effects.
- Drug is used investigationally to treat osteoporosis.

Therapeutic monitoring

- Fluoride supplementation must be continuous from infancy to age 14 to be effective.
- Review dietary history with the family. A diet that includes large amounts of fish, min-

eral water, and tea provides about 5 mg/day of fluoride.

Special populations

Breast-feeding patients. Very little sodium fluoride is distributed into breast milk. The fluoride levels in breast milk increase only when daily intake exceeds 1.5 mg.
Pediatric patients. Young children usually can't perform the rinse process necessary with oral solutions. Because prolonged ingestion or improper techniques may result in dental fluorosis and osseous changes, the dose must be carefully adjusted according to the amount of fluoride ion in drinking water.

Patient counseling

- Tell patient that sodium fluoride tablets and drops should be taken with meals, but not with dairy products.
- Advise patient that rinse and gel are most effective if used immediately after brushing or flossing and when taken just before retiring to bed.
- Tell patient to expectorate (and not swallow) excess liquid or gel.
- Warn patient not to eat, drink, or rinse mouth for 15 to 30 minutes after application. Tell patient to use a plastic container—not glass—to dilute drops or rinse, because the fluoride interacts with glass.
- Encourage patient to notify dentist if mottling of teeth occurs.
- Advise patient that if there is a change in water supply or if the patient moves to another area, then a dentist should be contacted because excessive fluoride causes mottled tooth enamel. If patient uses a private well, the water should be tested for fluoride.
- Warn parents to treat fluoride tablets as a drug and to keep them away from children.

sodium phosphates (sodium phosphate and sodium biphosphate)

Fleet Phospho-soda

Pharmacologic classification: acid salt
Therapeutic classification: NaCl laxative
Pregnancy risk category C

How supplied

Available without a prescription
Solution: 18 g sodium phosphate and 48 g sodium biphosphate/100 ml

Indications and dosages

Constipation
Adults: 20 to 30 ml solution mixed with 4 oz (120 ml) cold water.
Children age 10 to 12: 10 ml solution mixed with 4 oz cold water.
Children age 5 to 10: 5 ml solution mixed with 4 oz cold water.
Purgative action
Adults: 45 ml solution mixed with 4 oz cold water.

Pharmacodynamics

Laxative action: Sodium phosphate and sodium biphosphate exert an osmotic effect in the small intestine by drawing water into the intestinal lumen, producing distention that promotes peristalsis and bowel evacuation.

Pharmacokinetics

Absorption: About 1% to 20% of an oral dose of sodium and phosphate is absorbed. With oral administration, action begins in 3 to 6 hours.
Distribution: Unknown.
Metabolism: Unknown.
Excretion: Unknown; probably in feces and urine.

Route	Onset	Peak	Duration
P.O.	Variable	Variable	Variable

Contraindications and precautions

Contraindicated in patients with abdominal pain, nausea, vomiting, or other symptoms of appendicitis or acute surgical abdomen; intestinal obstruction or perforation; edema; heart failure; megacolon; or impaired renal function and in patients on sodium-restricted diets. Use cautiously in patients with large hemorrhoids or anal excoriations.

Interactions

Drug-drug. *Antacids:* May cause inactivation of both. Don't use together.

Effects on diagnostic tests

None reported.

Adverse reactions

GI: *abdominal cramping.*
Metabolic: fluid and electrolyte disturbances (hypernatremia, hyperphosphatemia) with daily use.
Other: laxative dependence with long-term or excessive use.

Overdose and treatment

No information available; probable clinical effects include abdominal pain and diarrhea.

Clinical considerations

- Dilute drug with water before giving orally (add 30 ml of drug to 120 ml of water). Follow drug administration with full glass of water.
- Drug isn't routinely used to treat constipation but is commonly used to evacuate the bowel.

Therapeutic monitoring
Monitor serum electrolyte levels; when drug is given as NaCl laxative, up to 10% of sodium content may be absorbed.

Special populations
Breast-feeding patients. It's not known if drug is excreted in human milk. Use cautiously in nursing women.

Patient counseling
- Instruct patient on how to mix the drug.
- Instruct patient on dose schedule.
- Warn patient that frequent or prolonged use of drug may lead to laxative dependence.
- Teach patient about dietary sources of bulk, which include bran and other cereals, fresh fruit, and vegetables.
- Tell patient to drink 8 oz of cool water after taking Fleet Phospho-soda.
- For children under age 5, parent should contact doctor.

sodium polystyrene sulfonate
Kayexalate, SPS

Pharmacologic classification: cation-exchange resin
Therapeutic classification: potassium-removing resin
Pregnancy risk category C

How supplied
Available by prescription only
Oral powder: 1.25 g/5 ml suspension
Powder for oral or rectal administration: 454 g in 1-lb jar
Rectal administration: 1.25 g/5 ml, 15 g/60 ml suspension

Indications and dosages
Hyperkalemia
Adults: 15 g P.O. daily to q.i.d. in water or sorbitol. Alternatively, give 30 to 50 g q.i.d. or q 6 hours as a retention enema.

Pharmacodynamics
Potassium-removing action: Sodium polystyrene sulfonate is a cation-exchange resin that releases sodium in exchange for other cations in the GI tract. High levels of potassium ion are found in the large intestine and therefore are exchanged and eliminated.

Pharmacokinetics
Absorption: Not absorbed. The onset of action varies from hours to days.
Distribution: None.
Metabolism: None.
Excretion: Excreted unchanged in feces.

Route	Onset	Peak	Duration
P.O., P.R.	Unknown	Unknown	Unknown

Contraindications and precautions
Contraindicated in patients with hypokalemia or hypersensitivity to drug. Use cautiously in patients with marked edema or severe heart failure or hypertension.

Interactions
Drug-drug. *Cardiac glycosides:* Toxic effects are exaggerated by hypokalemia, even when serum digoxin levels are in the normal range. Don't use together.
Magnesium- and calcium-containing antacids: Metabolic alkalosis in patients with renal impairment. Don't use together.

Effects on diagnostic tests
None reported.

Adverse reactions
GI: *constipation,* fecal impaction (in elderly patients), anorexia, gastric irritation, nausea, vomiting, *diarrhea* (with sorbitol emulsions).
Metabolic: ***hypokalemia,*** hypocalcemia, sodium retention, altered serum magnesium level.

Overdose and treatment
Signs and symptoms of overdose include signs and symptoms of hypokalemia, such as irritability, confusion, arrhythmias, ECG changes, severe muscle weakness, and sometimes paralysis; and digitalis toxicity in digitalized patients. Drug may be discontinued or dose lowered when serum potassium level decreases to the 4 to 5 mEq/L range.

Clinical considerations
- For oral administration: mix resin only with water or sorbitol; never mix with orange juice because of its high potassium content.
- Chill oral suspension to increase palatability; don't heat because that inactivates resin.
- Use P.R. route when vomiting, P.O. restrictions, or upper GI tract problems are present.
- Fecal impaction can be prevented in geriatric patients by administering resin P.R. Cleaning enema should precede rectal administration.
- For rectal administration, mix polystyrene resin only with water and sorbitol for rectal use. Don't use other vehicles such as mineral oil for rectal administration to prevent impactions. Ion exchange requires aqueous medium. Sorbitol content prevents impaction. Prepare rectal dose at room temperature. Stir emulsion gently during administration.
- Constipation is more likely when drug is given with phosphate binders such as aluminum hydroxide. Monitor patient's bowel habits.

Therapeutic monitoring
- Monitor serum potassium at least once daily. Watch for other signs of hypokalemia.

- Monitor for symptoms of other electrolyte deficiencies (magnesium, calcium) because drug is nonselective. Monitor serum calcium determination in patients receiving sodium polystyrene therapy for more than 3 days. Supplementary calcium may be needed.
- If hyperkalemia is severe, more drastic modalities should be added; for example, dextrose 50% with regular insulin I.V. push. Don't depend solely on polystyrene resin to lower serum potassium levels in severe hyperkalemia.

Special populations

Pediatric patients. Adjust dose in children based on a calculation of 1 mEq of potassium bound for each 1 g of resin.
Geriatric patients. Fecal impaction is more likely in geriatric patients.

Patient counseling

- Instruct patient in the importance of following a prescribed low-potassium diet.
- Explain necessity of retaining enema to patient. Retention for 6 to 10 hours is ideal, but 30 to 60 minutes is acceptable.

somatropin

Humatrope, Nutropin

Pharmacologic classification: anterior pituitary hormone
Therapeutic classification: purified growth hormone (GH)
Pregnancy risk category C

How supplied

Available by prescription only
Injection: 10 mg (30 IU)/2-ml vial
Powder for injection: 5 mg (15 IU)/vial with 5-ml diluent

Indications and dosages

Long-term treatment of growth failure in children with inadequate secretion of endogenous growth hormone (GH)
Children: 0.18 mg/kg of body weight of Humatrope S.C. or I.M. weekly divided equally and given on either three alternate days or 6 times per week; or 0.3 mg/kg of body weight of Nutropin S.C. weekly in daily divided doses.
Growth failure in children associated with chronic renal insufficiency up to time of renal transplantation
Children: Administer 0.35 mg/kg of body weight of Nutropin S.C. weekly in daily divided doses.

Pharmacodynamics

Growth-stimulating action: Somatropin is a purified GH of recombinant DNA origin that stimulates skeletal, linear bone, muscle, and organ growth.

Pharmacokinetics

Absorption: Absorbed from the injection site in a similar fashion as somatrem (human growth hormone).
Distribution: Localizes to highly perfused organs, notably the liver and kidney.
Metabolism: Metabolized in the liver.
Excretion: Returned to the systemic circulation as amino acids.

Route	Onset	Peak	Duration
I.M., S.C.	Unknown	3-5 hr	12-48 hr

Contraindications and precautions

Contraindicated in patients with closed epiphyses or an active underlying intracranial lesion. Humatrope shouldn't be reconstituted with the supplied diluent for patients with known sensitivity to either m-Cresol or glycerin.

Use cautiously in children with hypothyroidism and in those whose GH deficiency results from an intracranial lesion; these children should be examined frequently for progression or recurrence of underlying disease.

Interactions

None reported.

Effects on diagnostic tests

None reported.

Adverse reactions

CNS: headache, weakness.
CV: mild, transient edema.
Hematologic: ***leukemia.***
Metabolic: mild hyperglycemia, hypothyroidism; inorganic phosphorus, alkaline phosphatase, and parathyroid hormone levels may increase.
Other: injection site pain, localized muscle pain, antibody formation to GH.

Overdose and treatment

Long-term overdose may result in signs and symptoms of gigantism or acromegaly consistent with the known effects of excess human GH.

Clinical considerations

- To prepare solution, inject the supplied diluent into the vial containing the drug by aiming the stream of the liquid against the glass wall of the vial. Swirl the vial with a gentle rotary motion until the contents are completely dissolved. Don't shake the vial.
- After reconstitution, vial solution should be clear. Don't use if it's cloudy or contains particles.
- Store reconstituted vial in refrigerator; use within 14 days.
- If sensitivity to diluent occurs, vial may be reconstituted with sterile water for injection. When drug is reconstituted in this manner, use only one reconstituted dose per vial and refrig-

erate the solution if it isn't used immediately after reconstitution. Use reconstituted dose within 24 hours, and discard unused portion.

Therapeutic monitoring

- Monitor child's height regularly. Regular monitoring of blood and radiologic studies is also necessary.
- Monitor patient's blood glucose levels regularly because GH may induce a state of insulin resistance.
- Excessive glucocorticoid therapy inhibits the growth-promoting effect of somatropin. Adjust glucocorticoid replacement dose in patients with a coexisting corticotropin deficiency to avoid an inhibitory effect on growth.
- Periodically monitor thyroid function tests for hypothyroidism, which may require treatment with a thyroid hormone.

Patient counseling

- Inform parents that children with endocrine disorders including GH deficiency are more likely to develop slipped capital epiphyses. Tell them to call if they notice their child limping.
- Stress to parents importance of close follow-up care.

sotalol

Betapace

Pharmacologic classification: beta blocker
Therapeutic classification: antiarrhythmic
Pregnancy risk category B

How supplied

Available by prescription only
Tablets: 80 mg, 120 mg, 160 mg, 240 mg

Indications and dosages

Documented, life-threatening ventricular arrhythmias

Adults: Initially, 80 mg P.O. b.i.d. Increase dose q 2 to 3 days as needed and tolerated. Most patients respond to daily dose of 160 to 320 mg. A few patients with refractory arrhythmias have received as much as 640 mg daily.

≡ ***Dosage adjustment.*** For adults with renal failure and creatinine clearance above 60 ml/minute, no adjustment in dose interval is necessary. If creatinine clearance is 30 to 60 ml/minute, give q 24 hours; 10 to 30 ml/minute, q 36 to 48 hours; and if it is less than 10 ml/minute, individualize dosage.

Pharmacodynamics

Antiarrhythmic action: Sotalol is a nonselective beta blocker that depresses sinus heart rate, slows AV conduction, increases AV nodal refractoriness, prolongs the refractory period of atrial and ventricular muscle and AV accessory pathways in anterograde and retrograde directions, decreases cardiac output, and lowers systolic and diastolic blood pressure.

Pharmacokinetics

Absorption: Well absorbed after oral administration, with a bioavailability of 90% to 100%. After oral administration, steady-state plasma levels are attained in 2 to 3 days (after five to six doses when administered twice daily).
Distribution: Doesn't bind to plasma proteins and crosses the blood-brain barrier poorly.
Metabolism: Not metabolized.
Excretion: Excreted primarily in urine unchanged.

Route	Onset	Peak	Duration
P.O.	Unknown	2½-4 hr	Unknown

Contraindications and precautions

Contraindicated in patients with hypersensitivity to drug, severe sinus node dysfunction, sinus bradycardia, second- and third-degree AV block in the absence of an artificial pacemaker, congenital or acquired long QT syndrome, cardiogenic shock, uncontrolled heart failure, and bronchial asthma.

Use cautiously in patients with impaired renal function or diabetes mellitus.

Interactions

Drug-drug. *Antacids:* Decreased effects of sotalol. Advise patient to take 2 hours apart.
Antiarrhythmic agents: Cause additive effects when administered with sotalol. Avoid use together.
Calcium channel antagonists: Enhance myocardial depression. Don't give with sotalol.
Catecholamine-depleting drugs, such as guanethidine and reserpine: Enhance the hypotensive effects of sotalol. Monitor patient closely.
Clonidine: Sotalol may enhance the rebound hypertensive effect seen after withdrawal of clonidine. Discontinue sotalol several days before withdrawing clonidine.
Insulin, oral antidiabetic agents: Increase blood glucose levels; may mask symptoms of hypoglycemia. Sotalol may require dose adjustments with these drugs.
Drug-food. *Any food:* Decreases absorption. Give drug on an empty stomach.

Effects on diagnostic tests

None reported.

Adverse reactions

CNS: asthenia, light-headedness, headache, dizziness, weakness, fatigue, sleep problems.
CV: ***bradycardia,*** *palpitations, chest pain,* ***arrhythmias, heart failure, AV block, proarrhythmic events (ventricular tachycardia, PVCs, ventricular fibrillation),*** edema, ECG abnormalities, hypotension.

GI: *nausea, vomiting,* diarrhea, dyspepsia.
Hepatic: elevated liver enzyme levels.
Metabolic: increased serum glucose.
Respiratory: *dyspnea, bronchospasm.*

Overdose and treatment

The most common signs of overdose are bradycardia, heart failure, hypotension, bronchospasm, and hypoglycemia. If overdose occurs, discontinue sotalol and the observe patient closely. Because of the lack of protein binding, hemodialysis is useful in reducing sotalol plasma levels. Observe patient carefully until QT intervals are normalized.

Atropine, another anticholinergic drug, a beta-adrenergic agonist, or transvenous cardiac pacing may also be used to treat bradycardia; transvenous cardiac pacing to treat second- or third-degree heart block; epinephrine to treat hypotension (depending on associated factors); aminophylline or an aerosol $beta_2$-receptor stimulant to treat bronchospasm; and DC cardioversion, transvenous cardiac pacing, epinephrine, or magnesium sulfate to treat torsades de pointes.

Clinical considerations

- Because proarrhythmic events, such as sustained ventricular tachycardia or ventricular fibrillation, may occur at start of therapy and during dose adjustments, patient should be hospitalized. Facilities and personnel should be available for cardiac rhythm monitoring and ECG interpretation.
- Although patients receiving I.V. lidocaine have begun sotalol therapy without ill effect, other antiarrhythmic drugs should be withdrawn before sotalol therapy begins. Sotalol therapy typically is delayed until two or three half-lives of the withdrawn drug have elapsed. After withdrawal of amiodarone, sotalol shouldn't be administered until the QT interval normalizes.

Therapeutic monitoring

- Make dose adjustments slowly, allowing 2 to 3 days between dose increments for adequate monitoring of QT intervals and for drug plasma levels to reach steady state.
- Monitor serum electrolytes regularly, especially if patient is receiving diuretics. Electrolyte imbalances, such as hypokalemia or hypomagnesemia, may enhance QT prolongation and increase risk of serious arrhythmias, such as torsades de pointes.

Special populations

Pregnant patients. Safety hasn't been established. Use only when potential benefits outweigh the risks to the fetus.
Breast-feeding patients. Because drug may be excreted in breast milk, either breast-feeding or sotalol may be discontinued depending on importance of drug to woman's health.
Pediatric patients. Safety and efficacy in children haven't been established.

Patient counseling

- Explain importance of taking sotalol as prescribed, even when feeling well.
- Caution patient not to discontinue drug suddenly.
- Tell patient not to take antacids within 2 hours of taking sotalol.

sparfloxacin

Zagam

Pharmacologic classification: fluorinated quinolone
Therapeutic classification: broad-spectrum antibacterial
Pregnancy risk category C

How supplied

Available by prescription only
Tablets: 200 mg

Indications and dosages

***Acute bacterial exacerbation of chronic bronchitis caused by* Staphylococcus aureus, Streptococcus pneumoniae, Chlamydia pneumoniae, Enterobacter cloacae, Klebsiella pneumoniae, Moraxella catarrhalis, Haemophilus influenzae, *or* H. parainfluenzae**
Adults over age 18: 400 mg P.O. on first day as a loading dose, then 200 mg daily for total of 10 days of therapy (total, 11 tablets).
***Community-acquired pneumonia caused by* S. pneumoniae, M. catarrhalis, H. influenzae, H. parainfluenzae, C. pneumoniae, *or* Mycoplasma pneumoniae**
Adults over age 18: 400 mg P.O. on first day as a loading dose, then 200 mg daily for total of 10 days of therapy (total, 11 tablets).
≡ ***Dosage adjustment.*** In patients with renal impairment, if creatinine clearance is less than 50 ml/minute, give a loading dose of 400 mg P.O.; thereafter, 200 mg P.O. q 48 hours for a total of 9 days of therapy (total, six tablets).

Pharmacodynamics

Antibactericidal action: Inhibits bacterial DNA gyrase and prevents DNA replication, transcription, repair, and deactivation in susceptible bacteria.

Pharmacokinetics

Absorption: Well absorbed following oral administration with an absolute bioavailability of 92%.
Distribution: Volume of distribution is about 3.9 L/kg, indicating distribution well into the tissues. Level of drug in respiratory tissues at 2 to 6 hours following dosing is about three to six times greater than plasma.

Metabolism: Metabolized by the liver, primarily by phase II glucuronidation. Its metabolism doesn't interfere with or use the cytochrome P-450 system.
Excretion: Excreted in both the urine (50%) and feces (50%). Terminal elimination half-life varies between 16 and 30 hours; mean, 20 hours.

Route	Onset	Peak	Duration
P.O.	Unknown	3-6 hr	Unknown

Contraindications and precautions
Contraindicated in patients with history of hypersensitivity or photosensitivity reactions to drugs and those who can't stay out of the sun. Don't use in patients with cardiac conditions that predispose them to arrhythmias. Contraindicated in patients taking drugs that prolong the QT_c interval.

Use with caution in patients with known or suspected CNS disorders, such as seizures, toxic psychoses, or tremors.

Interactions
Drug-drug. *Antacids containing aluminum or magnesium, iron salts, zinc, or sucralfate:* May interfere with GI absorption of sparfloxacin. Administer at least 4 hours apart.
Drugs that prolong the QTc interval, including amiodarone, bepridil, disopyramide, class Ia antiarrhythmics (procainamide, quinidine), class III drugs (sotalol); cisapride, erythromycin, pentamidine, tricyclic antidepressants, and some antipsychotics including phenothiazines: May cause torsades de pointes. Don't administer together.
Drug-lifestyle. *Sun exposure:* May cause photosensitivity reactions. Advise patient to take precautions.

Effects on diagnostic tests
Drug may produce false-negative culture results for *Mycobacterium tuberculosis.*

Adverse reactions
CNS: asthenia, dizziness, headache, insomnia, ***seizures,*** somnolence.
CV: ***QT interval prolongation,*** vasodilatation.
EENT: dry mouth, taste perversion.
GI: abdominal pain, diarrhea, dyspepsia, flatulence, nausea, pseudomembranous colitis, vomiting.
GU: vaginal moniliasis.
Hematologic: elevated WBC.
Hepatic: elevated liver enzymes.
Musculoskeletal: tendon rupture.
Skin: photosensitivity, pruritus, rash.
Other: ***hypersensitivity reactions.***

Overdose and treatment
If overdose is suspected, have patient avoid sunlight exposure for 5 days. Monitor ECG for possible QTc prolongation. It isn't known if drug is dialyzable.

Clinical considerations
- Use cautiously in patients with a history of seizure disorder or other CNS diseases, such as cerebral arteriosclerosis.
- Acute hypersensitivity reactions may require treatment with epinephrine, oxygen, I.V. fluids, antihistamines, corticosteroids, pressor amines, and airway management.

Therapeutic monitoring
- Monitor renal function.
- Obtain specimen for culture and sensitivity before starting therapy and as needed and ordered to determine whether bacterial resistance has occurred.

Special populations
Breast-feeding patients. Because drug is excreted in breast milk, discontinue either breast-feeding or drug.
Pediatric patients. Safety and efficacy of children and adolescents under age 18 haven't been established. Quinolones, including sparfloxacin, cause arthropathy and osteochondrosis in juvenile animals of several species.
Geriatric patients. Pharmacokinetics of drug aren't altered in the elderly with normal renal function. Monitor renal function carefully and adjust doses as recommended.

Patient counseling
- Inform patient that drug may be taken with food, milk, or products that contain caffeine.
- Tell patient to take drug as prescribed, even if symptoms disappear.
- Advise patient to take drug with plenty of fluids and to avoid antacids, sucralfate, and products containing iron or zinc for at least 4 hours after each dose.
- Warn patient to avoid hazardous tasks until adverse CNS effects of drug are known.
- Tell patient to discontinue drug and report pain or inflammation; tendon rupture can occur with drug. Tell patient to rest and refrain from exercise until a diagnosis is made.

spectinomycin hydrochloride
Trobicin

Pharmacologic classification: aminocyclitol
Therapeutic classification: antibiotic
Pregnancy risk category NR

How supplied
Available by prescription only
Injection: 2-g vial with 3.2-ml diluent; 4-g vial with 6.2-ml diluent

Indications and dosages

Uncomplicated gonorrhea in patients who are hypersensitive to penicillins or cephalosporins

Adults: 2 to 4 g I.M. single dose injected deeply into upper outer quadrant of the buttocks (divide 4-g dose into two sites).

◊***Disseminated gonorrhea***

Adults: 2 g I.M. b.i.d. for 3 to 7 days. Inject deeply into upper outer quadrant of the buttocks.

Pharmacodynamics

Antibacterial action: Bacteriostatic effect results from binding of drug to 30S ribosomal subunits, thus inhibiting protein synthesis. Although drug is effective against many gram-positive and gram-negative organisms, it's used mostly against penicillin-resistant *Neisseria gonorrhoeae*.

Pharmacokinetics

Absorption: Not absorbed orally. I.M. injection results in rapid absorption

Distribution: Unknown.

Metabolism: Unknown.

Excretion: Most of dose is excreted unchanged in the urine. Elimination half-life ranges from 1 to 3 hours. Drug dose is unchanged in renal failure.

Route	Onset	Peak	Duration
I.M.	Unknown	1-2 hr	Unknown

Contraindications and precautions

Contraindicated in patients with hypersensitivity to drug.

Interactions

None reported.

Effects on diagnostic tests

None reported.

Adverse reactions

CNS: insomnia, dizziness.

GI: nausea.

GU: decreased urine output and creatinine clearance, increased BUN.

Hematologic: decreased hemoglobin and hematocrit levels.

Hepatic: transient increases in liver enzymes.

Skin: urticaria.

Other: fever, chills (may mask or delay symptoms of incubating syphilis), pain at injection site.

Overdose and treatment

No information available.

Clinical considerations

- Drug is usually reserved for patients with penicillin-resistant gonorrhea strains or for whom other drugs are contraindicated. Ceftriaxone is considered drug of choice for uncomplicated gonorrhea.
- To prepare drug, add supplied diluent to vial and shake until completely dissolved. Use reconstituted solution within 24 hours.
- Inject deep I.M. into upper outer quadrant of gluteal muscle. Give 2-g dose at single site; divide 4-g dose into two equal injections and give at two sites.
- Drug is ineffective against syphilis and may mask symptoms of incubating syphilis infection; it is also not effective in pharyngeal gonococcal infections.

Therapeutic monitoring

- Obtain specimen for culture and sensitivity tests before starting therapy.
- Lack of response to drug usually results from reinfection.

Special populations

Breast-feeding patients. Because it isn't known if drug is excreted in breast milk, an alternative feeding method is recommended during therapy.

Pediatric patients. Because its safety in infants and children hasn't been established, drug isn't first choice in treatment of these patients. However, drug may be used in children for the treatment of gonococcal infections in those hypersensitive to penicillins. A single dose of 40 mg/kg is recommended by the Centers for Disease Control and Prevention. Drug shouldn't be used in neonates because of the benzyl alcohol preservative.

Patient counseling

- Tell patient that sexual partners must be treated.
- Patient should have all infection sites cultured 7 days posttreatment to confirm eradication of organism.

spironolactone

Aldactone

Pharmacologic classification: potassium-sparing diuretic

Therapeutic classification: management of edema; antihypertensive; diagnosis of primary hyperaldosteronism; treatment of diuretic-induced hypokalemia

Pregnancy risk category NR

How supplied

Available by prescription only

Tablets (film-coated): 25 mg, 50 mg, 100 mg

Tablets: 25 mg

Indications and dosages

Edema

Adults: 25 to 200 mg P.O. daily in divided doses.

Children: Initially, 3.3 mg/kg or 60 mg/m^2 P.O. daily in divided doses.
Hypertension
Adults: 50 to 100 mg P.O. daily in divided doses.
Diuretic-induced hypokalemia
Adults: 25 to 100 mg P.O. daily when oral potassium supplements are considered inappropriate.
Detection of primary hyperaldosteronism
Adults: 400 mg P.O. daily for 4 days (short test) or for 3 to 4 weeks (long test). If hypokalemia and hypertension are corrected, a presumptive diagnosis of primary hyperaldosteronism is made.
◇***Hirsutism***
Adults: 50 to 200 mg P.O. daily.
◇***Premenstrual syndrome***
Adults: 25 mg q.i.d. P.O. on day 14 of menstrual cycle.
◇***Heart failure in patients receiving an ACE inhibitor and a loop diuretic with or without a cardiac glycoside***
Adults: Initially, 12.5 to 25 mg P.O. daily.
◇***To decrease risk of metrorrhagia***
Adults: 50 mg b.i.d. P.O. on days 4 through 21 of menstrual cycle.
◇***Acne vulgaris***
Adults: 100 mg P.O. daily.

Pharmacodynamics

Diuretic and potassium-sparing actions: Spironolactone competitively inhibits aldosterone effects on the distal renal tubules, increasing sodium and water excretion and decreasing potassium excretion.
Spironolactone is used to treat edema associated with excessive aldosterone secretion, such as that associated with hepatic cirrhosis, nephrotic syndrome, and heart failure. It's also used to treat diuretic-induced hypokalemia.
Antihypertensive action: The mechanism of action is unknown; spironolactone may block the effect of aldosterone on arteriolar smooth muscle.
Diagnosis of primary hyperaldosteronism: Spironolactone inhibits the effects of aldosterone; therefore, correction of hypokalemia and hypertension is presumptive evidence of primary hyperaldosteronism.

Pharmacokinetics

Absorption: About 90% is absorbed after oral administration.
Distribution: Drug and its major metabolite, canrenone, are more than 90% plasma protein-bound.
Metabolism: Rapidly and extensively metabolized to canrenone.
Excretion: Canrenone and other metabolites are excreted primarily in urine, and a small amount is excreted in feces via the biliary tract; half-life of canrenone is 13 to 24 hours. Half-life of parent compound is 1 to 2 hours.

Route	Onset	Peak	Duration
P.O.	1-2 days	2-3 days	2-3 days

Contraindications and precautions

Contraindicated in patients with anuria, acute or progressive renal insufficiency, or hyperkalemia. Use cautiously in patients with impaired renal function, hepatic disease, or fluid and electrolyte imbalances.

Interactions

Drug-drug. *Anesthetics, norepinephrine:* Reduced response to these drugs. Use together cautiously.
Aspirin: May slightly decrease the clinical response to spironolactone. Watch for diminished effect.
Cardiac glycosides: Increased serum digoxin levels and subsequent toxicity. Monitor drug levels of digoxin.
NSAIDs, such as ibuprofen or indomethacin: May impair renal function and thus affect potassium excretion. Avoid use together.
Other antihypertensive agents: Spironolactone may potentiate the hypotensive effects. May be used to therapeutic advantage.
Other potassium-sparing diuretics, ACE inhibitors, potassium supplements, potassium-containing medications such as parenteral penicillin G: Spironolactone increases the risk of hyperkalemia when administered with these drugs. Use together cautiously, especially in patients with renal impairment.
Drug-herb. *Licorice:* Antiulcer and aldosterone-like effects of herb may be blocked. Avoid use together.
Drug-food. *Potassium-containing salt substitutes, potassium-rich foods, such as citrus fruit and tomatoes:* Increase the risk of hyperkalemia. Low-potassium salt substitutes and high-potassium foods should be ingested cautiously.

Effects on diagnostic tests

Spironolactone therapy alters fluorometric determinations of plasma and urinary 17-hydroxycorticosteroid levels and may cause false elevations on radioimmunoassay of serum digoxin.

Adverse reactions

CNS: headache, drowsiness, lethargy, confusion, ataxia.
GI: diarrhea, gastric bleeding, ulceration, cramping, gastritis, vomiting.
GU: inability to maintain erection, hirsutism, gynecomastia, breast soreness and menstrual disturbances in women.
Hematologic: ***agranulocytosis.***
Metabolic: ***hyperkalemia,*** dehydration, hyponatremia, transient elevation in BUN, metabolic acidosis.

Skin: urticaria, maculopapular eruptions.
Other: drug fever.

Overdose and treatment
Signs of overdose are consistent with dehydration and electrolyte disturbance.

Treatment is supportive and symptomatic. In acute ingestion, empty stomach by emesis or lavage. In severe hyperkalemia (more than 6.5 mEq/L), reduce serum potassium levels with I.V. sodium bicarbonate or glucose with insulin. A cation exchange resin, sodium polystyrene sulfonate (Kayexalate), given orally or as a retention enema, may also reduce serum potassium levels.

Clinical considerations
Consider the recommendations relevant to all potassium-sparing diuretics as well as the following:
- Give drug with meals to enhance absorption.
- Protect drug from light.
- Spironolactone is antiandrogenic and has been used to treat hirsutism in doses of 200 mg/day.
- Avoid unnecessary use of drug. Drug has been shown to induce tumors in laboratory animals.

Therapeutic monitoring
- Diuretic effect may be delayed 2 to 3 days if drug is used alone; maximum antihypertensive effect may be delayed 2 to 3 weeks.
- Adverse reactions are related to dose levels and duration of therapy and usually disappear with withdrawal of drug; however, gynecomastia may persist.
- Watch for hyperchloremic metabolic acidosis.

Special populations
Breast-feeding patients. Safety during breast-feeding hasn't been established. Canrenone, a metabolite, is distributed into breast milk. Alternative feeding method is recommended during therapy with spironolactone.
Pediatric patients. When administering drug to children, crush tablets and administer them in cherry syrup as an oral suspension.
Geriatric patients. Geriatric patients are more susceptible to diuretic effects and may require lower doses to prevent excessive diuresis.

Patient counseling
- Instruct patient to report mental confusion or lethargy immediately.
- Explain that adverse reactions usually disappear after drug is discontinued; gynecomastia, however, may persist.
- Caution patient to avoid such hazardous activities as driving until response to drug is known.

stavudine (d4T)
Zerit

Pharmacologic classification: synthetic thymidine nucleoside analogue
Therapeutic classification: antiviral
Pregnancy risk category C

How supplied
Available by prescription only
Capsules: 15 mg, 20 mg, 30 mg, 40 mg
Oral solution: 1 mg/ml

Indications and dosages
Treatment of patients with HIV infection who have received prolonged prior zidovudine therapy
Adults: For patients weighing 132 lb (60 kg) or more, 40 mg P.O. q 12 hours; for patients weighing less than 132 lb, 30 mg P.O. q 12 hours.
Children weighing less than 66 lb (30 kg): 1 mg/kg q 12 hours.
≡***Dosage adjustment.*** For adults with renal impairment, refer to the table below.

Creatine clearance (ml/min)	Dosage for patients weighing ≥ 60 kg	Dosage for patients weighing < 60 kg
> 50	40 mg q 12 hours	30 mg q 12 hours
26 to 50	20 mg q 12 hours	15 mg q 12 hours
10 to 25	20 mg q 24 hours	15 mg q 24 hours

In adults undergoing hemodialysis: 20 mg q 24 hours for patients weighing 132 lb or more and 15 mg q 24 hours for patients weighing less than 132 lb.

Pharmacodynamics
Antiviral action: Stavudine is phosphorylated by cellular kinases to stavudine triphosphate, which retards HIV replication by inhibiting HIV reverse transcriptase and inhibiting viral DNA synthesis. The triphosphate also inhibits cellular DNA polymerase beta and gamma and reduces mitochondrial DNA synthesis.

Pharmacokinetics
Absorption: Rapidly absorbed with a mean absolute bioavailability of 86.4%.
Distribution: Mean volume of distribution is 58 L, suggesting distribution into extravascular space. Drug is distributed equally between RBCs and plasma. It binds poorly to plasma proteins.
Metabolism: Not clearly defined.
Excretion: Renal elimination accounts for about 40% of overall clearance, regardless of

administration route; there's active tubular secretion in addition to glomerular filtration.

Contraindications and precautions
Contraindicated in patients with hypersensitivity to drug. Use cautiously in patients with impaired renal function or history of peripheral neuropathy and in pregnant women.

Interactions
None significant.

Effects on diagnostic tests
None reported.

Adverse reactions
CNS: *peripheral neuropathy, headache, malaise, insomnia, anxiety, depression, nervousness,* dizziness.
CV: chest pain.
EENT: conjunctivitis.
GI: *abdominal pain, diarrhea, nausea, vomiting, anorexia,* dyspepsia, constipation, weight loss.
Hematologic: ***neutropenia, thrombocytopenia,*** anemia.
Hepatic: elevated liver enzymes, ***hepatotoxicity.***
Musculoskeletal: *myalgia, asthenia, back pain, arthralgia.*
Respiratory: *dyspnea.*
Skin: *rash, diaphoresis, pruritus,* maculopapular rash.
Other: *chills, fever,* lactic acidosis.

Overdose and treatment
Experience with adults who had received 12 to 24 times the recommended daily dose revealed no acute toxicity. Complications of chronic overdose include peripheral neuropathy and hepatic toxicity. It isn't known if drug is eliminated by peritoneal dialysis or hemodialysis.

Clinical considerations
☐ ***ALERT*** Don't confuse this drug with other antivirals that may use initials for identification.
- Use cautiously in patients with renal impairment or history of peripheral neuropathy. Dosage adjustment may be necessary.
- Monitor patient for development of peripheral neuropathy, usually characterized by numbness, tingling, or pain in the feet or hands. If symptoms develop, interrupt drug therapy. Symptoms may resolve if therapy is withdrawn promptly. Sometimes symptoms may worsen temporarily after drug discontinuation. If symptoms resolve completely, resume treatment using the following dosage schedule: patients weighing 132 lb or more should receive 20 mg twice daily; patients weighing less than 132 lb should receive 15 mg twice daily. Manage clinically significant elevations of hepatic transaminase levels in same way.
- If neruopathy recurs after restarting drug, consideration should be given to permanently discontinuing drug.
- Use in combination with other antiretroviral agents.

Therapeutic monitoring
Monitor CBC and serum levels of creatinine, AST, ALT, and alkaline phosphatase.

Special populations
Breast-feeding patients. It isn't known if drug is excreted in breast milk. Because of the potential for adverse reactions from stavudine in breast-fed infants, breast-feeding should be discontinued during therapy.

Patient counseling
- Inform patient that stavudine isn't a cure for HIV infection and that the patient may continue to acquire illnesses associated with AIDS or AIDS-related complex, including opportunistic infections.
- Inform patient that drug doesn't reduce risk of transmitting HIV to others through sexual contact or blood contamination.
- Instruct patient to report signs of peripheral neuropathy, such as tingling, burning, pain, or numbness in the hands or feet, because dose adjustments may be necessary.
- Advise patient not to use other medications, including OTC preparations, without contacting health care provider first.
- Explain that long-term effects of drug are currently unknown.

streptokinase
Kabikinase, Streptase

Pharmacologic classification: plasminogen activator
Therapeutic classification: thrombolytic enzyme
Pregnancy risk category C

How supplied
Available by prescription only
Injection: 250,000 IU, 750,000 IU, 1,500,000 IU in vials for reconstitution

Indications and dosages
Lysis of coronary artery thrombi after acute MI
Adults: 1,500,000 IU by I.V. infusion over 60 minutes; intracoronary loading dose of 20,000 IU via coronary catheter, followed by a maintenance dosage of 2,000 IU/minute for 60 minutes as an infusion.
Venous thrombosis, pulmonary embolism, and arterial thrombosis and embolism
Adults: Loading dose of 250,000 IU I.V. infusion over 30 minutes. Sustaining dose: 100,000 IU/hour I.V. infusion for 72 hours for deep vein

thrombosis and 100,000 IU/hour over 24 hours by I.V. infusion pump for pulmonary embolism.
◇***Arteriovenous cannula occlusion***
Adults: 250,000 IU in 2 ml I.V. solution by I.V. infusion pump into each occluded limb of the cannula over 25 to 35 minutes. Clamp off cannula for 2 hours, then aspirate contents of cannula, flush with saline solution, and reconnect. The manufacturer doesn't recommend using drug to restore patency of occluded I.V. catheters.

Pharmacodynamics

Thrombolytic action: Streptokinase promotes thrombolysis by activating plasminogen in two steps. First, plasminogen and streptokinase form a complex, exposing plasminogen-activating site, and second, cleavage of peptide bond converts plasminogen to plasmin.

In treatment of acute MI, streptokinase prevents primary or secondary thrombus formation in microcirculation surrounding the necrotic area.

Pharmacokinetics

Absorption: Plasminogen activation begins promptly after infusion or instillation of streptokinase.
Distribution: Doesn't cross placenta, but antibodies do.
Metabolism: Insignificant.
Excretion: Removed from circulation by antibodies and reticuloendothelial system. Half-life is biphasic; initially it's 18 minutes (from antibody action) and then extends up to 83 minutes. Anticoagulant effect may persist for 12 to 24 hours after infusion is discontinued.

Route	Onset	Peak	Duration
I.V.	Immediate	20 min-2 hr	4 hr

Contraindications and precautions

Contraindicated in patients with ulcerative wounds, active internal bleeding, and recent CVA; recent trauma with possible internal injuries; visceral or intracranial malignant neoplasms; ulcerative colitis; diverticulitis; severe hypertension; acute or chronic hepatic or renal insufficiency; uncontrolled hypocoagulation; chronic pulmonary disease with cavitation; subacute bacterial endocarditis or rheumatic valvular disease; or recent cerebral embolism, thrombosis, or hemorrhage.

Also contraindicated within 10 days after intra-arterial diagnostic procedure or any surgery, including liver or kidney biopsy, lumbar puncture, thoracentesis, paracentesis, or extensive or several cutdowns. I.M. injections and other invasive procedures are contraindicated during streptokinase therapy.

Use cautiously in patients with arterial embolism that originates from the left side of the heart.

Not recommended by manufacturer to restore patency of occluded I.V. catheters, because of the risk of life-threatening reactions.

Interactions

Drug-drug. *Aminocaproic acid:* Inhibits streptokinase-induced activation of plasminogen. Don't use together.
Anticoagulants: May cause hemorrhage. It may also be necessary to reverse effects of oral anticoagulants before beginning therapy. Monitor patient closely.
Aspirin, indomethacin, phenylbutazone, or other drugs affecting platelet activity: Increases risk of bleeding. Monitor patient closely.

Effects on diagnostic tests

None reported.

Adverse reactions

CNS: polyradiculoneuropathy, headache.
CV: reperfusion arrhythmias, *hypotension,* vasculitis.
EENT: periorbital edema.
GI: nausea.
Hematologic: ***bleeding.***
Musculoskeletal: musculoskeletal pain.
Respiratory: minor breathing difficulty, ***bronchospasm, apnea.***
Skin: urticaria, pruritus, flushing.
Other: phlebitis at injection site, hypersensitivity reactions ***(anaphylaxis),*** delayed hypersensitivity reactions (interstitial nephritis, serum sickness-like reactions), ***angioedema,*** *fever.*

Overdose and treatment

Symptoms of overdose include signs of potentially serious bleeding: bleeding gums, epistaxis, hematoma, spontaneous ecchymoses, oozing at catheter site, increased pulse, and pain from internal bleeding. Discontinue drug and restart when bleeding stops.

Clinical considerations

Consider the recommendations relevant to all thrombolytic enzymes as well as the following:
- Reconstitute vial with 5 ml normal saline injection, and further dilute to 45 ml; roll gently to mix. Don't shake. Use immediately; refrigerate remainder and discard after 8 hours. Store powder at room temperature.
- Rate of I.V. infusion depends on thrombin time and streptokinase resistance; higher loading dose may be necessary in patients with recent streptococcal infection or recent treatment with streptokinase, to compensate for antibody drug neutralization.
- Don't discontinue therapy for minor allergic reactions that can be treated with antihistamines or corticosteroids; about one third of patients experience a slight temperature elevation, and some have chills. Symptomatic treatment with acetaminophen (but not aspirin or other salicylates) is indicated if temperature

reaches 104° F (40° C). Patients may be pretreated with corticosteroids, repeating doses during therapy, to minimize pyrogenic or allergic reactions.

Therapeutic monitoring

- Monitor pulse, color, and sensation of extremities every hour.
- If minor bleeding can be controlled by local pressure, don't decrease dose so more plasminogen is available for conversion to plasmin.
- Antibodies to streptokinase can persist for 3 to 6 months or longer after the initial dose; if further thrombolytic therapy is needed, consider urokinase.

Special populations

Pediatric patients. Safety and efficacy in children haven't been established.
Geriatric patients. Patients age 75 or older have a greater risk of cerebral hemorrhage because they're likely to have preexisting cerebrovascular disease.

Patient counseling

- Explain use and administration to patient and family.

streptomycin sulfate

Pharmacologic classification: aminoglycoside
Therapeutic classification: antibiotic
Pregnancy risk category D

How supplied

Available by prescription only
Injection: 400 mg/ml

Indications and dosages

Primary and adjunctive treatment in tuberculosis
Adults with normal renal function: 1 g or 15 mg/kg I.M. daily for 2 to 3 months, then 1 g two or three times weekly. Inject deeply into upper outer quadrant of buttocks or midlateral thigh. Maximum daily dose, 1 g.
Children with normal renal function: 20 to 40 mg/kg I.M. daily in divided doses injected deeply into large muscle mass, preferably in the midlateral muscles of the thigh. Give with other antitubercular agents, but not with capreomycin, and continue until sputum specimen becomes negative. Maximum daily dose, 1 g.
Enterococcal endocarditis
Adults: 1 g I.M. q 12 hours for 2 weeks, then 500 mg I.M. q 12 hours for 4 weeks with penicillin.
Tularemia
Adults: 1 to 2 g I.M. daily in divided doses injected deep into upper outer quadrant of buttocks. Continue until patient is afebrile for 5 to 7 days.
Plague
Adults: 2 g I.M. daily in divided doses injected deep into upper outer quadrant of buttocks for a minimum of 10 days.
≡ ***Dosage adjustment.*** In adults and children with renal failure, initial dose is same as for those with normal renal function. Subsequent doses and frequency determined by renal function study results and blood serum levels; peak serum levels shouldn't exceed 20 to 25 mcg/ml, and trough levels should be 5 mcg/ml or less. Patients with a creatinine clearance of more than 50 ml/minute usually can tolerate drug daily; if creatinine clearance is 10 to 50 ml/minute, increase administration interval to q 24 to 72 hours. Patients with a creatinine clearance less than 10 ml/minute may require 72 to 96 hours between doses.

Pharmacodynamics

Antibiotic action: Streptomycin is bactericidal; it binds directly to the 30S ribosomal subunit, inhibiting bacterial protein synthesis. Its spectrum of activity includes many aerobic gram-negative organisms and some aerobic gram-positive organisms. Streptomycin is generally less active against many gram-negative organisms than is tobramycin, gentamicin, amikacin, or netilmicin. Streptomycin is also active against *Mycobacterium* and *Brucella.*

Pharmacokinetics

Absorption: Absorbed poorly after oral administration and usually is given by deep I.M. injection.
Distribution: Widely distributed after parenteral administration; intraocular penetration is poor. CSF penetration is low, even in patients with inflamed meninges. Streptomycin crosses the placenta, and is 36% protein-bound.
Metabolism: Not metabolized.
Excretion: Excreted primarily in urine by glomerular filtration; small amounts may be excreted in bile and breast milk. Elimination half-life in adults is 2 to 3 hours. In severe renal damage, half-life may extend to 110 hours.

Route	Onset	Peak	Duration
I.M.	Unknown	1-2 hr	Unknown

Contraindications and precautions

Contraindicated in patients with hypersensitivity to drug or other aminoglycosides and in those with labyrinthine disease. Never administer I.V. Use cautiously in patients with impaired renal function or neuromuscular disorders and in the elderly.

Interactions

Drug-drug. *Amphotericin B, capreomycin, cephalosporins, cisplatin, methoxyflurane, polymyxin B, vancomycin, and other aminoglycosides:* Use with these drugs may increase

the hazard of nephrotoxicity, ototoxicity, and neurotoxicity. Use together cautiously.
Bumetanide, ethacrynic acid, furosemide, mannitol, urea: Hazard of ototoxicity is increased during use together. Use together cautiously.
Dimenhydrinate, other antiemetic and antivertigo drugs: May mask streptomycin-induced ototoxicity. Use together cautiously.
General anesthetics or neuromuscular blocking agents, such as succinylcholine and tubocurarine: Streptomycin may potentiate neuromuscular blockade. Monitor patient closely.
Penicillin: Results in synergistic bactericidal effect against *Pseudomonas aeruginosa, Escherichia coli, Klebsiella, Citrobacter, Enterobacter, Proteus mirabilis,* and *Serratia;* however, the drugs are physically and chemically incompatible and are inactivated when mixed or given together. Don't use together.

Effects on diagnostic tests
Streptomycin may cause false-positive reaction in copper sulfate test for urine glucose (Benedict's reagent or Clinitest).

Adverse reactions
CNS: ***neuromuscular blockade.***
EENT: *ototoxicity.*
GI: vomiting, nausea.
GU: some ***nephrotoxicity*** (not as frequently as with other aminoglycosides).
Hematologic: eosinophilia, ***leukopenia, thrombocytopenia.***
Respiratory: ***apnea.***
Skin: ***exfoliative dermatitis.***
Other: hypersensitivity reactions (rash, fever, urticaria, ***angioedema***), ***anaphylaxis.***

Overdose and treatment
Signs of overdose include ototoxicity, nephrotoxicity, and neuromuscular toxicity. Remove drug by hemodialysis or peritoneal dialysis. Treatment with calcium salts or anticholinesterases reverses neuromuscular blockade.

Clinical considerations
Consider the recommendations relevant to all aminoglycosides as well as the following:
- Protect hands when preparing drug; drug irritates skin.
- In primary tuberculosis therapy, discontinue streptomycin when sputum culture is negative.
- Because streptomycin is dialyzable, patients undergoing hemodialysis may need dose adjustments.

Therapeutic monitoring
Check blood for peak streptomycin level 1 to 2 hours after I.M. injection; for trough levels, blood should be drawn just before next dose. Heparinized tube shouldn't be used because heparin is incompatible with aminoglycosides.

Special populations
Pregnant patients. Aminoglycosides have caused fetal harm.
Pediatric patients. Use with caution and at reduced doses in premature and full-term neonates because of renal immaturity.

Patient counseling
- Instruct patient to report adverse reactions promptly.
- Encourage adequate fluid intake.
- Emphasize the need for blood tests to monitor streptomycin levels and determine the effectiveness of therapy.

streptozocin
Zanosar

Pharmacologic classification: antibiotic antineoplastic nitrosourea (cell cycle-phase nonspecific)
Therapeutic classification: antineoplastic
Pregnancy risk category C

How supplied
Available by prescription only
Injection: 1-g vials

Indications and dosages
Dosage and indications may vary. Check current literature for recommended protocol.
Metastatic islet cell carcinoma of the pancreas
Adults and children: 500 mg/m² I.V. for 5 consecutive days q 6 weeks until maximum benefit or toxicity is observed. Alternatively, 1,000 mg/m² at weekly intervals for first 2 weeks; may be increased to a maximum single dose of 1,500 mg/m². Usual course of therapy is 4 to 6 weeks.
≡ ***Dosage adjustment.*** In patients with impaired renal function, give 75% of dose if creatinine clearance is 10 to 50 ml/minute and 50% of dose if it's less than 10 ml/minute.

Pharmacodynamics
Antineoplastic action: Streptozocin exerts its cytotoxic activity by selectively inhibiting DNA synthesis. The drug also causes cross-linking of DNA strands through an alkylation mechanism.

Pharmacokinetics
Absorption: Not active orally; it must be given I.V.
Distribution: After an I.V. dose, drug and its metabolites distribute mainly into the liver, kidneys, intestines, and pancreas. Drug hasn't been shown to cross the blood-brain barrier; however, its metabolites achieve levels in the CSF equivalent to the level in the plasma.

Metabolism: Extensively metabolized in the liver and kidneys.
Excretion: Elimination of drug from the plasma is biphasic, with an initial half-life of 5 minutes and a terminal phase half-life of 35 to 40 minutes. Plasma half-life of metabolites is longer than parent drug. Drug and its metabolites are excreted primarily in urine and a small amount of dose may also be excreted in expired air.

Route	Onset	Peak	Duration
I.V.	Unknown	Unknown	Unknown

Contraindications and precautions

No known contraindications. Use cautiously in patients with preexisting renal and hepatic disease.

Interactions

Drug-drug. *Doxorubicin:* Prolongs elimination half-life of doxorubicin. Reduced dose of doxorubicin is necessary.
Other nephrotoxic drugs: May potentiate nephrotoxicity caused by streptozocin. Use cautiously.
Phenytoin: May decrease effects of streptozocin on the pancreas. Monitor carefully.

Effects on diagnostic tests

None reported.

Adverse reactions

CNS: confusion, lethargy, depression.
GI: *nausea, vomiting,* diarrhea.
GU: ***renal toxicity*** (evidenced by azotemia, glycosuria, and renal tubular acidosis), mild proteinuria.
Hematologic: *anemia,* ***leukopenia, thrombocytopenia.***
Hepatic: elevated liver enzyme levels, jaundice, *liver dysfunction,* ***hepatotoxicity.***
Metabolic: hyperglycemia, hypoglycemia, diabetes mellitus.

Overdose and treatment

Signs and symptoms of overdose include myelosuppression, nausea, and vomiting. Treatment is usually supportive and includes transfusion of blood components and antiemetics.

Clinical considerations

- To reconstitute drug, use 9.5 ml of normal saline injection to yield a level of 100 mg/ml.
- Use drug within 12 hours of reconstitution. Reconstituted solution is a golden color that changes to dark brown upon decomposition.
- Product contains no preservatives and isn't intended as a multiple-dose vial.
- Drug may be administered by rapid I.V. push injection.
- Drug may be further diluted in 10 to 200 ml of D_5W to infuse over 10 to 15 minutes. It can also be infused over 6 hours.
- Wear gloves to protect the skin from contact during preparation or administration. If contact occurs, wash solution off immediately with soap and water. Follow recommended procedures for the safe preparation, administration, and disposal of chemotherapeutic agents.
- Extravasation may cause ulceration and tissue necrosis.
- Keep dextrose 50% at bedside because of risk of hypoglycemia from sudden release of insulin.
- Drug has also been used in the treatment of colon cancer, pancreatic adenocarcinoma, and carcinoid tumors. These uses are unlabeled and dosing schedules and protocols vary.

Therapeutic monitoring

- Nausea and vomiting occur in almost all patients within 1 to 4 hours. Make sure patient is being treated with an antiemetic.
- Mild proteinuria is one of the first signs of renal toxicity and may necessitate dose reduction.
- Test urine regularly for protein and glucose.
- Monitor CBC and liver function studies at least weekly.
- Renal toxicity resulting from therapy is dose related and cumulative. Monitor renal function before and after each course of therapy. Obtain urinalysis, BUN levels, and creatinine clearance before therapy and at least weekly during drug administration. Continue weekly monitoring for 4 weeks after each course.

Special populations

Breast-feeding patients. It isn't known if drug is excreted in breast milk. However, because of the potential for serious adverse reactions, mutagenicity, and carcinogenicity in the infant, breast-feeding isn't recommended.

Patient counseling

- Encourage adequate fluid intake to increase urine output and reduce potential for renal toxicity.
- Remind diabetic patients that intensive monitoring of blood glucose levels is necessary.
- Tell patient to report symptoms of anemia, infection, or bleeding immediately.
- Warn patient that bruising may occur easily because of effect of drug on blood count.

succimer

Chemet

Pharmacologic classification: heavy metal
Therapeutic classification: chelating agent
Pregnancy risk category C

How supplied

Available by prescription only
Capsules: 100 mg

Indications and dosages

Treatment of lead poisoning in children with blood lead levels greater than 45 mcg/dl

Children: Initially, 10 mg/kg or 350 mg/m² P.O. q 8 hours for 5 days. Higher starting doses aren't recommended. Frequency of administration may be reduced to 10 mg/kg or 350 mg/m² q 12 hours for an additional 2 weeks of therapy. A course of treatment lasts 19 days and repeated courses may be necessary if indicated by weekly monitoring of blood lead levels. A minimum of 2 weeks between courses is recommended unless blood lead levels mandate more prompt action.

≡ ***Dosage adjustment.*** Dose is to be administered q 8 hours for 5 days, followed by same dose q 12 hours for 14 days.

PEDIATRIC DOSES

Weight (lb)	Weight (kg)	Dose (mg)	No. of Capsules
18 to 35	8 to 15	100	1
36 to 55	16 to 23	200	2
56 to 75	24 to 34	300	3
76 to 100	35 to 44	400	4
> 100	> 45	500	5

Pharmacodynamics

Antidote action: Succimer forms water-soluble chelates and increases the urinary excretion of lead.

Pharmacokinetics

Absorption: Rapidly but variably absorbed after oral administration.

Distribution: Unknown.

Metabolism: Rapidly and extensively metabolized.

Excretion: Excreted 39% in feces as nonabsorbed drug; 9% in urine; 1% as carbon dioxide from the lungs. About 90% of absorbed drug is excreted in urine.

Route	Onset	Peak	Duration
P.O.	Unknown	1-2 hr	Unknown

Contraindications and precautions

Contraindicated in patients with hypersensitivity to drug. Use cautiously in patients with impaired renal function.

Interactions

Drug-drug. *Other chelating agents:* Concurrent administration of succimer with other chelating agents isn't recommended. Interactions haven't been systematically studied. Avoid use together.

Effects on diagnostic tests

False-positive results for ketones in urine using nitroprusside reagents (Ketostix) and false decreased levels of serum uric acid and CK have been reported.

Adverse reactions

CNS: *drowsiness, dizziness, sensory motor neuropathy, sleepiness, paresthesia, headache.*
CV: ***arrhythmias.***
EENT: plugged ears, cloudy film in eyes, otitis media, watery eyes, sore throat, rhinorrhea, nasal congestion.
GI: *nausea, vomiting, diarrhea, loss of appetite, abdominal cramps, hemorrhoidal symptoms, metallic taste in mouth, loose stools.*
GU: decreased urination, difficult urination, proteinuria, moniliasis.
Hematologic: increased platelet count, intermittent eosinophilia.
Hepatic: *elevated serum AST, ALT, alkaline phosphatase.*
Metabolic: *elevated cholesterol levels.*
Musculoskeletal: *leg, kneecap, back, stomach, rib, or flank pain.*
Respiratory: cough, head cold.
Skin: papular rash, herpetic rash, mucocutaneous eruptions, pruritus.
Other: *flu-like symptoms.*

Overdose and treatment

No cases of overdose have been reported. In cases of acute overdose, induce vomiting with ipecac syrup or perform gastric lavage, followed by administration of activated charcoal slurry and appropriate supportive therapy.

Clinical considerations

- Identification and abatement of lead sources in child's environment are critical to successful therapy. Chelation therapy isn't a substitute for preventing further exposure and shouldn't be used to permit continued exposure.
- Don't use drug for treatment of lead poisoning.
- Patients who have received ethylenediaminetetraacetic acid, with or without dimercaprol, may use succimer as subsequent therapy after an interval of 4 weeks. Use with other chelating agents isn't recommended.
- Consider the possibility of allergic or other mucocutaneous reactions each time drug is used, including during the initial course.

Therapeutic monitoring

- Monitor serum transaminase levels before and at least weekly during therapy. Patients with a history of hepatic disease should be monitored more closely.
- Elevated blood lead levels and associated symptoms may return rapidly after drug is discontinued because of redistribution of lead from bone to soft tissues and blood. Monitor patients

at least once weekly for rebound blood lead levels.

- The severity of lead intoxication should be used as a guide for more frequent blood lead monitoring. This is measured by the initial blood lead level and the rate and degree of rebound of blood lead.

Special populations

Pediatric patients. For young children who can't swallow capsules, succimer capsule may be opened and sprinkled on a small amount of soft food, or medicated beads from the capsules may be poured onto a spoon for administration and followed with a fruit drink.

Patient counseling

- Instruct parents to maintain child's adequate fluid intake.
- Tell parents to report rash.
- Urge parents to identify and remove source of lead in environment.
- Tell parents to store capsules at room temperature, out of reach of children.

succinylcholine chloride (suxamethonium chloride)

Anectine, Anectine Flo-Pack, Quelicin, Sucostrin

Pharmacologic classification: depolarizing neuromuscular blocker
Therapeutic classification: skeletal muscle relaxant
Pregnancy risk category C

How supplied

Available by prescription only
Injection: 20 mg/ml, 50 mg/ml, 100 mg/ml (parenteral); 500 mg, 1 g (sterile for I.V. infusion)

Indications and dosages

To induce skeletal muscle relaxation; facilitate intubation, ventilation, or orthopedic manipulations; and lessen muscle contractions in induced seizures

Dosage depends on the anesthetic used, patient's needs, and response. Doses are representative and must be adjusted. Paralysis is induced after inducing hypnosis with thiopental or other appropriate agent.

Adults: For short procedures, 0.6 mg/kg (range, 0.3 to 1.1 mg/kg) I.V. over 10 to 30 seconds; additional doses may be given if needed. For long procedures, 2.5 mg/minute (range, 0.5 to 10 mg/minute) continuous I.V. infusion, or alternatively, 0.3 to 1.1 mg/kg by intermittent I.V. injection, followed by additional doses of 0.04 to 0.07 mg/kg, p.r.n.

Children: Administer 2 mg/kg I.V. for infants; for older children and adolescents, give 1 mg/kg I.V. or 3 to 4 mg/kg I.M. Don't exceed 150 mg.

Pharmacodynamics

Skeletal muscle relaxant action: Similar to acetylcholine (ACh), succinylcholine produces depolarization of the motor end-plate at the myoneural junction. Drug has a high affinity for ACh receptor sites and is resistant to acetylcholinesterase, producing a more prolonged depolarization at the motor end-plate. It also possesses histamine-releasing properties and reportedly stimulates the cardiac vagus and sympathetic ganglia.

A transient increase in intraocular pressure occurs immediately after injection and may persist after the onset of complete paralysis.

Pharmacokinetics

Absorption: After I.V. administration, drug has a rapid onset of action.
Distribution: After I.V. administration, drug is distributed in extracellular fluid and rapidly reaches its site of action. It crosses the placenta.
Metabolism: Rapidly metabolized by plasma pseudocholinesterase.
Excretion: About 10% is excreted unchanged in urine.

Route	Onset	Peak	Duration
I.V.	½-1 sec	1-2 min	4-10 min
I.M.	2-3 min	Unknown	10-30 min

Contraindications and precautions

Contraindicated in patients with hypersensitivity to drug and in those with abnormally low plasma pseudocholinesterase, angle-closure glaucoma, malignant hyperthermia, or penetrating eye injuries.

Use cautiously in geriatric or debilitated patients; in those receiving quinidine or cardiac glycoside therapy; in those undergoing a cesarean section; and in patients with respiratory depression, severe burns or trauma, electrolyte imbalances, hyperkalemia, paraplegia, spinal neuraxis injury, CVA, degenerative or dystrophic neuromuscular disease, myasthenia gravis, myasthenic syndrome of lung or bronchiogenic cancer, dehydration, thyroid disorders, collagen diseases, porphyria, fractures, muscle spasms, eye surgery, pheochromocytoma, or impaired renal, pulmonary, or hepatic function.

Interactions

Drug-drug. *Aminoglycoside antibiotics, including amikacin, gentamicin, kanamycin, neomycin, and streptomycin; polymyxin antibiotics, such as colistin and polymyxin B sulfate; clindamycin, lincomycin; general anesthetics; local anesthetics; antimalarial agents; cholinesterase inhibitors, such as demecarium, echothiophate and isofluran; cyclophos-*

phamide; oral contraceptives; nondepolarizing neuromuscular blocking agents; parenteral magnesium salts; lithium, phenelzine; quinidine; quinine; pancuronium; phenothiazines; thiotepa; and exposure to neurotoxic insecticides: Enhance or prolong neuromulcular blocking effects of succinylcholine. Use drugs cautiously during surgical and postoperative periods.
Cardiac glycosides: Produces possible arrhythmias. Use together cautiously.
Drug-herb. *Melatonin:* Potentiates blocking properties of succinylcholine. Don't use together.

Effects on diagnostic tests
None reported.

Adverse reactions
CV: ***bradycardia,*** tachycardia, hypertension, hypotension, ***arrhythmias,*** flushing, ***cardiac arrest.***
EENT: increased intraocular pressure.
Hematologic: myoglobinemia.
Metabolic: hyperkalemia.
Musculoskeletal: muscle fasciculation, *postoperative muscle pain.*
Respiratory: ***prolonged respiratory depression, apnea,*** bronchostriction.
Other: ***malignant hyperthermia,*** allergic or idiosyncratic hypersensitivity reactions ***(anaphylaxis).***

Overdose and treatment
Signs and symptoms of overdose include apnea or prolonged muscle paralysis, which may be treated with controlled respiration. Use a peripheral nerve stimulator to monitor effects and degree of blockade.

Clinical considerations
- Succinylcholine is drug of choice for short procedures (less than 3 minutes) and for orthopedic manipulations; use cautiously in fractures or dislocations.
- Duration of action is prolonged to 20 minutes with continuous I.V. infusion or when given with hexafluorenium bromide.
- Some clinicians advocate pretreating adult patients with tubocurarine (3 to 6 mg) to minimize muscle fasciculations.
- Repeated fractional doses of succinylcholine alone aren't advised; they may cause reduced response or prolonged apnea.
- Store injectable form in refrigerator. Store powder form at room temperature and keep tightly closed. Use immediately after reconstitution.
- Don't mix drug with alkaline solutions, such as thiopental, sodium bicarbonate, and barbiturates.
- Administration requires direct medical supervision by trained anesthesia personnel.
- Usually administered I.V., succinylcholine may be administered I.M. if suitable vein is inaccessible. Give deep I.M., preferably high into the deltoid muscle.

Therapeutic monitoring
- Monitor baseline electrolyte determinations and vital signs; check respirations every 5 to 10 minutes during infusion.
- Keep airway clear. Have emergency respiratory support (endotracheal equipment, ventilator, oxygen, atropine, neostigmine) on hand.
- Tachyphylaxis may occur.

Special populations
Breast-feeding patients. Use cautiously in breast-feeding women because it isn't known if drug is excreted in breast milk.
Geriatric patients. Use with caution in geriatric patients.

Patient counseling
- Reassure patient that postoperative stiffness is normal and will soon subside. Monitor for residual muscle weakness.
- Explain all procedures and events to patient because he can still hear.

sucralfate
Carafate

Pharmacologic classification: pepsin inhibitor
Therapeutic classification: antiulcer agent
Pregnancy risk category B

How supplied
Available by prescription only
Tablets: 1 g
Suspension: 1 g/10 ml

Indications and dosages
Short-term (up to 8 weeks) treatment of duodenal ulcer, ◇aspirin-induced gastric erosion
Adults: 1 g P.O. q.i.d. 1 hour before meals and h.s.
Maintenance therapy of duodenal ulcer
Adults: 1 g P.O. b.i.d.

Pharmacodynamics
Antiulcer action: Sucralfate has a unique mechanism of action. It adheres to proteins at the ulcer site, forming a protective coating against gastric acid, pepsin, and bile salts. It also inhibits pepsin, exhibits a cytoprotective effect, and forms a viscous, adhesive barrier on the surface of the intact intestinal mucosa and the stomach.

Pharmacokinetics

Absorption: Only about 3% to 5% of a dose is absorbed. Drug activity isn't related to the amount absorbed.
Distribution: Acts locally, at the ulcer site. Absorbed drug is distributed to many body tissues, including the liver and kidneys.
Metabolism: None.
Excretion: About 90% of a dose is excreted in feces; absorbed drug is excreted unchanged in urine.

Route	Onset	Peak	Duration
P.O.	Unknown	Unknown	6 hr

Contraindications and precautions

No known contraindications. Use cautiously in patients with chronic renal failure.

Interactions

Drug-drug. *Antacids:* May decrease binding of drug to gastroduodenal mucosa, impairing effectiveness. Separate dosing of sucralfate and antacids by 30 minutes.
Cimetidine, digoxin, phenytoin, quinidine, quinolones, ranitidine, tetracycline, theophylline, and fat-soluble vitamins A, D, E, and K: Sucralfate decreases absorption of these drugs. Separate administration times by at least 2 hours.

Effects on diagnostic tests

None reported.

Adverse reactions

CNS: dizziness, sleepiness, headache, vertigo.
GI: *constipation,* nausea, gastric discomfort, diarrhea, bezoar formation, vomiting, flatulence, dry mouth, indigestion.
Musculoskeletal: back pain.
Skin: rash, pruritus.

Overdose and treatment

No information available.

Clinical considerations

- Drug is poorly water-soluble. For administration by nasogastric tube, prepare water-sorbitol suspension of sucralfate. Alternatively, place tablet in 60-ml syringe; add 20 ml water. Let stand with tip up for about 5 minutes, occasionally shaking gently. The resultant suspension may be administered from the syringe. After administration, flush tube several times to ensure that the patient receives the entire dose.
- Patients who have difficulty swallowing tablet may place it in 15 to 30 ml of water at room temperature, allow it to disintegrate, and then ingest the resulting suspension. This is particularly useful for patients with esophagitis and painful swallowing.
- Some experts believe that 2 g given b.i.d. is as effective as the standard regimen.
- Drug treats ulcers as effectively as H_2-receptor antagonists.

Therapeutic monitoring

- Monitor patient for constipation.
- Therapy exceeding 8 weeks isn't recommended.

Special populations

Breast-feeding patients. The risks to breast-feeding infants must be weighed against benefits.
Pediatric patients. Safety and efficacy in children haven't been established.

Patient counseling

- Remind patient to take drug on an empty stomach and at least 1 hour before meals.
- Advise patient to continue taking drug as directed, even after pain begins to subside, to ensure adequate healing.
- Warn patient not to take drug for more than 8 weeks.

sufentanil citrate

Sufenta

Pharmacologic classification: opioid
Therapeutic classification: analgesic, adjunct to anesthesia, anesthetic
Controlled substance schedule II
Pregnancy risk category C

How supplied

Available by prescription only
Injection: 50 mcg/ml

Indications and dosages

Adjunct to general anesthetic
Adults: 1 to 8 mcg/kg I.V. administered with nitrous oxide and oxygen. Maintenance dosage, 10 to 50 mcg.
Primary anesthetic
Adults: 8 to 30 mcg/kg I.V. administered with 100% oxygen and a muscle relaxant. Maintenance dosage, 25 to 50 mcg.
Children: 10 to 25 mcg/kg I.V. administered with 100% oxygen and a muscle relaxant. Maintenance dosage, up to 25 to 50 mcg.

Pharmacodynamics

Analgesic action: Sufentanil has a high affinity for the opiate receptors, exerting an agonistic effect to provide analgesia. It's also used as an adjunct to anesthesia or as a primary anesthetic because of its potent CNS depressant effects.

Pharmacokinetics

Absorption: Has a more rapid onset of action than morphine or fentanyl.
Distribution: Highly lipophilic and is rapidly and extensively distributed in animals. It's high-

ly protein-bound (greater than 90%) and redistributed rapidly.
Metabolism: Appears to be metabolized mainly in the liver and small intestine. Relatively little accumulation occurs. Drug has an elimination half-life of about 2½ hours.
Excretion: Drug and its metabolites are excreted primarily in urine.

Route	Onset	Peak	Duration
I.V.	1 min	1 min	5 min

Contraindications and precautions
Contraindicated in patients with hypersensitivity to drug. Use cautiously in geriatric or debilitated patients and in those with decreased respiratory reserve, head injuries, or renal, pulmonary, or hepatic disease.

Interactions
Drug-drug. *Anticholinergics:* Use together may cause paralytic ileus. Monitor patient closely.
Beta blockers: If beta blockers have been used preoperatively, decrease dose of sufentanil.
Cimetidine: Increased respiratory and CNS depression. Reduced dose of sufentanil is usually necessary.
Digitoxin, phenytoin, rifampin: Drug accumulation and enhanced effects may result from use together. Monitor patient closely.
General anesthetics: Severe CV depression may result from use together. Monitor patient closely.
Narcotic agonist-antagonist or a single dose of an antagonist: Patient who becomes physically dependent on drug may experience acute withdrawal syndrome if given high doses of these drugs. Avoid this use.
Nitrous oxide: May produce CV depression when given with high doses of sufentanil. Monitor patient closely.
Other CNS depressants, such as antihistamines, barbiturates, benzodiazepines, general anesthetics, muscle relaxants, narcotic analgesics, phenothiazines, sedative-hypnotics, and tricyclic antidepressants: Additive CNS depression. Use together cautiously.
Pancuronium: May produce a dose-dependent elevation in heart rate during sufentanil and oxygen anesthesia. Use moderate doses of pancuronium or a less vagolytic neuromuscular blocking agent. The vagolytic effect of pancuronium may be reduced in patients administered nitrous oxide with sufentanil.
Drug-lifestyle. *Alcohol use:* May cause additive effects. Discourage use together.

Effects on diagnostic tests
None reported.

Adverse reactions
CNS: chills, somnolence.
CV: *hypotension, **bradycardia,*** hypertension, ***arrhythmias,*** tachycardia.
GI: nausea, vomiting.
Metabolic: increased plasma amylase, lipase and serum prolactin levels.
Musculoskeletal: intraoperative muscle movement.
Respiratory: ***chest wall rigidity, apnea, bronchospasm.***
Skin: *pruritus,* erythema.

Overdose and treatment
There's no clinical experience with acute overdose of sufentanil, but signs and symptoms are expected to be similar to those occurring with other opioids, with less CV toxicity. The most common signs and symptoms of acute opiate overdose are CNS depression, respiratory depression, and miosis (pinpoint pupils). Other acute toxic effects include hypotension, bradycardia, hypothermia, shock, apnea, cardiopulmonary arrest, circulatory collapse, pulmonary edema, and seizures.

To treat acute overdose, establish adequate respiratory exchange via a patent airway and ventilation, as needed; administer a narcotic antagonist (naloxone) to reverse respiratory depression. (Because the duration of action of sufentanil is longer than that of naloxone, repeated naloxone dosing is necessary.) Don't give naloxone unless the patient has clinically significant respiratory or CV depression. Monitor vital signs closely.

Provide symptomatic and supportive treatment (continued respiratory support, correction of fluid or electrolyte imbalance). Monitor laboratory parameters, vital signs, and neurologic status closely.

Clinical considerations
Consider the recommendations relevant to all opioids as well as the following:
- Sufentanil should only be administered by persons specifically trained in the use of I.V. anesthetics.
- Compared with fentanyl, sufentanil has a more rapid onset and shorter duration of action.

Therapeutic monitoring
- When used at doses exceeding 8 mcg/kg, postoperative mechanical ventilation and observation are essential because of extended postoperative respiratory depression.
- Sufentanil may produce muscle rigidity involving all the skeletal muscles (incidence and severity are dose-related). Choose a neuromuscular blocker appropriate for the patient's CV status.
- In patients weighing more than 20% above ideal body weight, determine dose based on ideal body weight.

Special populations
Pediatric patients. Safety and efficacy in children under age 2 have been documented in only a limited number of patients (who were undergoing CV surgery).
Geriatric patients. Lower doses are usually indicated for geriatric patients, who may be more sensitive to the therapeutic and adverse effects of drug.

Patient counseling
- Assure patient and family that he'll be monitored continuously.
- Answer questions and concerns regarding drug.

sulfadiazine

Pharmacologic classification: sulfonamide
Therapeutic classification: antibiotic
Pregnancy risk category NR

How supplied
Available by prescription only
Tablets: 500 mg

Indications and dosages
Urinary tract infection
Adults: Initially, 2 to 4 g P.O.; then 2 to 4 g/day in three to six divided doses.
Children age 2 months or older: Initially, 75 mg/kg or 2 g/m^2 P.O.; then 150 mg/kg/day P.O. in four to six divided doses. Maximum daily dose, 6 g.
Rheumatic fever prophylaxis, as an alternative to penicillin
Children weighing more than 66 lb (30 kg): 1 g P.O. daily.
Children weighing less than 66 lb: 500 mg P.O. daily.
Adjunctive treatment in toxoplasmosis
Adults: 1 to 1.5 g P.O. q.i.d. for 3 to 4 weeks; given with pyrimethamine.
Children: 100 to 200 mg/kg P.O. daily in divided doses q 6 hours for 3 to 4 weeks; given with pyrimethamine.
Nocardiasis
Adults: 4 to 8 g P.O. daily in divided doses q 6 hours for 6 weeks.
Asymptomatic meningococcal carrier
Adults: 1 g P.O. b.i.d. for 2 days.
Children age 1 to 12: 500 mg P.O. b.i.d. for 2 days.
Children age 2 to 12 months: 500 mg P.O. daily for 2 days.

Pharmacodynamics
Antibacterial action: Sulfadiazine is bacteriostatic. It inhibits formation of tetrahydrofolic acid from para-aminobenzoic acid (PABA), preventing bacterial cell synthesis of folic acid. Sulfadiazine is active against many gram-positive bacteria, *Chlamydia trachomatis,* many Enterobacteriaceae, and some strains of *Toxoplasma gondii* and *Plasmodium falciparum.*

Pharmacokinetics
Absorption: Absorbed from the GI tract after oral administration.
Distribution: Distributed widely into most body tissues and fluids, including synovial, pleural, amniotic, prostatic, peritoneal, and seminal fluids; CSF penetration, however, is poor. Drug crosses the placenta, and is 32% to 56% protein-bound.
Metabolism: Metabolized partially in the liver.
Excretion: Both unchanged drug and metabolites are excreted primarily in urine by glomerular filtration and, to a lesser extent, renal tubular secretion; some drug is excreted in breast milk. Urine solubility of unchanged drug increases as urine pH increases.

Route	Onset	Peak	Duration
P.O.	Unknown	4-6 hr	Unknown

Contraindications and precautions
Contraindicated in patients with hypersensitivity to sulfonamides, in those with porphyria, in infants under age 2 months (except in congenital toxoplasmosis), in pregnant women at term, and during breast-feeding.

Use cautiously in patients with impaired renal or hepatic function, bronchial asthma, multiple allergies, G6PD deficiency, or blood dyscrasia.

Interactions
Drug-drug. *Oral anticoagulants:* Sulfadiazine may inhibit hepatic metabolism of these drugs and enhance anticoagulant effects. Monitor PT, INR blood levels, and patient for bleeding.
PABA: Antagonizes effects of sulfonamides. Don't use together.
Oral antidiabetic agents including sulfonylureas: Enhances their hypoglycemic effects. Monitor blood glucose levels.
Trimethoprim or pyrimethamine (folic acid antagonists with different mechanisms of action): Results in synergistic antibacterial effects and delays or prevents bacterial resistance. Don't use together.
Drug-lifestyle. *Sun exposure:* May cause photosensitivity reactions. Advise patient to take precautions.

Effects on diagnostic tests
Sulfadiazine alters urine glucose tests using cupric sulfate (Benedict's reagent or Clinitest).

Adverse reactions
CNS: headache, mental depression, ***seizures,*** hallucinations.

GI: *nausea, vomiting, diarrhea,* abdominal pain, anorexia, stomatitis.
GU: elevated serum creatinine, ***toxic nephrosis*** with oliguria and anuria, crystalluria, hematuria.
Hematologic: ***agranulocytosis, aplastic anemia, hemolytic anemia, thrombocytopenia,*** megaloblastic anemia, ***leukopenia.***
Hepatic: elevated liver enzymes, jaundice.
Skin: ***erythema multiforme (Stevens-Johnson syndrome),*** generalized skin eruption, ***epidermal necrolysis, exfoliative dermatitis,*** photosensitivity, urticaria, pruritus.
Other: hypersensitivity reactions (*serum sickness, drug fever,* ***anaphylaxis***), local irritation, extravasation.

Overdose and treatment

Signs and symptoms of overdose include dizziness, drowsiness, headache, unconsciousness, anorexia, abdominal pain, nausea, and vomiting. More severe complications, including hemolytic anemia, agranulocytosis, dermatitis, acidosis, sensitivity reactions, and jaundice, may be fatal.

Treatment includes gastric lavage if ingestion has occurred within the preceding 4 hours followed by correction of acidosis, forced fluids, and urinary alkalinization to enhance solubility and excretion. Treatment of renal failure as well as transfusion of appropriate blood products (in severe hematologic toxicity) may be required.

Clinical considerations

Consider the recommendations relevant to all sulfonamides as well as the following:
□ ***ALERT*** Beware of sound-alikes: sulfadiazine and sulfasalazine. Don't confuse the sulfonamide drugs.
- Sulfadiazine is a less soluble sulfonamide; therefore, it's more likely to cause crystalluria. Avoid using drug with urine acidifiers and ensure adequate fluid intake. If adequate fluid intake can't be ensured, recommend sodium bicarbonate to reduce risk of crystalluria.

Therapeutic monitoring

- Monitor renal and liver function tests.
- Monitor for signs of blood dyscrasia.
- Monitor urine cultures and CBCs, and conduct urinalyses before and during therapy.

Special populations

Breast-feeding patients. Drug is excreted in breast milk and shouldn't be used in breast-feeding women.
Pediatric patients. Contraindicated in children under age 2 months.

Patient counseling

- Instruct patient to report adverse reactions promptly.
- Patient should drink a glass of water with each dose and extra water daily as tolerated to prevent crystalluria.

sulfamethoxazole

Gantanol

Pharmacologic classification: sulfonamide
Therapeutic classification: antibiotic
Pregnancy risk category C

How supplied

Available by prescription only
Tablets: 500 mg

Indications and dosages

Urinary tract and systemic infections
Adults: Initially, 2 g P.O.; then 1 g P.O. b.i.d., up to t.i.d. for severe infections.
Children and infants over age 2 months: Initially, 50 to 60 mg/kg P.O., then 25 to 30 mg/kg b.i.d. Maximum dose shouldn't exceed 75 mg/kg daily.

Pharmacodynamics

Antibacterial action: Sulfamethoxazole is bacteriostatic. It acts by inhibiting formation of tetrahydrofolic acid from para-aminobenzoic acid (PABA), thus preventing bacterial cell synthesis of folic acid.

Spectrum of action includes some gram-positive bacteria, *Chlamydia trachomatis,* many Enterobacteriaceae, and some strains of *Toxoplasma* and *Plasmodium.*

Pharmacokinetics

Absorption: Absorbed from the GI tract after oral administration.
Distribution: Distributed widely into most body tissues and fluids, including cerebrospinal, synovial, pleural, amniotic, prostatic, peritoneal, and seminal fluids. Sulfamethoxazole crosses the placenta, and is 50% to 70% protein-bound.
Metabolism: Metabolized partially in the liver.
Excretion: Both unchanged drug and metabolites are excreted primarily in urine by glomerular filtration and, to a lesser extent, renal tubular secretion; some drug is excreted in breast milk. Urinary solubility of unchanged drug increases as urine pH increases. Elimination half-life in patients with normal renal function is 7 to 12 hours.

Route	Onset	Peak	Duration
P.O.	Unknown	2 hr	Unknown

Contraindications and precautions

Contraindicated in patients with porphyria or hypersensitivity to sulfonamides, in infants under age 2 months (except in congenital toxoplasmosis), in pregnant women at term, and during breast-feeding. Use cautiously in patients with renal or hepatic impairment, bronchial asthma, severe allergies, G6PD deficiency, or blood dyscrasia.

Interactions

Drug-drug. *Oral anticoagulants:* Enhanced anticoagulant effects. Monitor for bleeding.
Oral antidiabetic agents including sulfonylureas: Enhanced hypoglycemic effects. Monitor blood sugar.
PABA: Antagonizes sulfonamide effects. Don't use together.
Trimethoprim or pyrimethamine (folic acid antagonists with different mechanisms of action): Results in synergistic antibacterial effects and delays or prevents bacterial resistance. Don't use together.
Drug-lifestyle. *Sun exposure:* May cause photosensitivity reactions. Advise patient to take precautions.

Effects on diagnostic tests

Sulfamethoxazole alters results of urine glucose tests using cupric sulfate (Benedict's reagent or Clinitest.)

Adverse reactions

CNS: headache, mental depression, ***seizures,*** hallucinations, aseptic meningitis, tinnitus, apathy.
GI: *nausea, vomiting, diarrhea,* abdominal pain, anorexia, stomatitis, ***pancreatitis,*** pseudomembranous colitis.
GU: ***toxic nephrosis*** *with oliguria and anuria,* crystalluria, hematuria, interstitial nephritis.
Hematologic: ***agranulocytosis, hemolytic anemia, aplastic anemia,*** megaloblastic anemia, ***thrombocytopenia, leukopenia.***
Hepatic: elevated liver enzymes, *jaundice.*
Skin: ***erythema multiforme (Stevens-Johnson syndrome),*** generalized skin eruption, ***epidermal necrolysis, exfoliative dermatitis,*** photosensitivity, urticaria, pruritus.
Other: hypersensitivity reactions *(serum sickness, drug fever,* ***anaphylaxis).***

Overdose and treatment

Signs and symptoms of overdose include dizziness, drowsiness, headache, unconsciousness, anorexia, abdominal pain, nausea, and vomiting. More severe complications, including hemolytic anemia, agranulocytosis, dermatitis, acidosis, sensitivity reactions, and jaundice, may be fatal.

Treat by gastric lavage if ingestion has occurred within the preceding 4 hours, followed by correction of acidosis, forced fluids, and I.V. fluids if urine output is low and renal function is normal. Treatment of renal failure and transfusion of appropriate blood products (in severe hematologic toxicity) may be required.

Clinical considerations

Consider the recommendations relevant to all sulfonamides as well as the following:
☐ ***ALERT*** Beware of sound-alikes: sulfamethoxazole and sulfamethizole. Don't confuse the combination products with sulfamethoxazole alone (such as Azo-gantanol and Gantanol)

Therapeutic monitoring

- Monitor urine cultures and CBCs, and conduct urinalyses before and during therapy.
- Monitor fluid intake and output.

Special populations

Breast-feeding patients. Sulfamethoxazole is excreted in breast milk and shouldn't be administered to breast-feeding women.
Pediatric patients. Sulfamethoxazole is contraindicated in children under age 2 months.

Patient counseling

- Instruct patient to take drug exactly as prescribed, even if he feels better.
- Tell patient to drink a glass of water with each dose, and extra water daily as tolerated to prevent crystalluria.
- Advise patient to use precautions and avoid sun exposure if possible.

sulfasalazine

Azulfidine, Azulfidine En-tabs

Pharmacologic classification: sulfonamide
Therapeutic classification: antibiotic
Pregnancy risk category B

How supplied

Available by prescription only
Tablets (with or without enteric coating): 500 mg
Suspension: 250 mg/5 ml

Indications and dosages

Mild to moderate ulcerative colitis, adjunctive therapy in severe ulcerative colitis
Adults: Initially, 3 to 4 g P.O. daily in evenly divided doses. Maintenance dosage is 2 g P.O. daily in divided doses q 6 hours. May need to start with 1 to 2 g initially, with a gradual increase in dose to minimize adverse reactions.
Children over age 2: Initially, 40 to 60 mg/kg P.O. daily, divided into three to six doses; then 30 mg/kg daily in four doses. Maximum daily dose, 2 g. May need to start at lower dose if GI intolerance occurs.

Pharmacodynamics

Antibacterial action: Exact mechanism of action of drug in ulcerative colitis is unknown; it's believed to be a prodrug metabolized by intestinal flora in the colon. One metabolite (5-

aminosalicylic acid or mesalamine) is responsible for the anti-inflammatory effect; the other metabolite (sulfapyridine) may be responsible for antibacterial action and for some adverse effects.

Pharmacokinetics

Absorption: Absorbed poorly from the GI tract after oral administration; 70% to 90% is transported to the colon where intestinal flora metabolize drug to its active ingredients—sulfapyridine (antibacterial) and 5-aminosalicylic acid (anti-inflammatory)—which exert their effects locally. Sulfapyridine is absorbed from the colon, but only a small portion of 5-aminosalicylic acid is absorbed.
Distribution: Human data on sulfasalazine distribution is lacking; animal studies have identified drug and metabolites in sera, liver, and intestinal walls. Parent drug and both metabolites cross the placenta.
Metabolism: Cleaved by intestinal flora in the colon.
Excretion: Systemically absorbed sulfasalazine is excreted chiefly in urine; some parent drug and metabolites are excreted in breast milk. Plasma half-life is about 6 to 8 hours.

Route	Onset	Peak	Duration
P.O.	Unknown	3-12 hr	Unknown

Contraindications and precautions

Contraindicated in patients with known hypersensitivity to salicylates or sulfonamides or to other drugs containing sulfur, such as thiazides, furosemide, or oral sulfonylureas; in those with porphyria or severe renal or hepatic dysfunction; during pregnancy and at term; in breast-feeding women; and in infants and children under age 2. Sulfasalazine is also contraindicated in patients with intestinal or urinary tract obstructions because of the risk of local GI irritation and crystalluria.

Use cautiously in patients with mild to moderate renal or hepatic dysfunction, severe allergies, asthma, blood dyscrasia, or G6PD deficiency.

Interactions

Drug-drug. *Antacids:* Increased systemic absorption and hazard of toxicity. Monitor patient closely.
Antibiotics that alter intestinal flora: May interfere with conversion of sulfasalazine to sulfapyridine and 5-aminosalicylic acid, decreasing its effectiveness. Monitor closely.
Digoxin and folic acid: Sulfasalazine may reduce GI absorption of these drugs. Monitor patient closely.
Oral anticoagulants: Enhanced anticoagulant effects. Monitor patient for bleeding.
Oral antidiabetic agents including sulfonylureas: Enhanced hypoglycemic effects. Monitor blood glucose levels.
Urine acidifying agents, such as ammonium chloride and ascorbic acid: Increasing risk of crystalluria. Monitor closely.
Drug-lifestyle. *Sun exposure:* Photosensitivity may occur. Advise patient to take precautions.

Effects on diagnostic tests

Sulfasalazine alters results of urine glucose tests using cupric sulfate (Benedict's reagent or Clinitest).

Adverse reactions

CNS: headache, mental depression, ***seizures,*** hallucinations, tinnitus.
GI: *nausea, vomiting, diarrhea, abdominal pain, anorexia,* stomatitis.
GU: toxic nephrosis with oliguria and anuria, crystalluria, hematuria, oligospermia, infertility.
Hematologic: ***agranulocytosis, aplastic anemia,*** megaloblastic anemia, ***thrombocytopenia, leukopenia, hemolytic anemia.***
Hepatic: jaundice, elevated liver enzymes.
Skin: ***erythema multiforme (Stevens-Johnson syndrome),*** generalized skin eruption, ***epidermal necrolysis, exfoliative dermatitis,*** photosensitivity, urticaria, pruritus.
Other: *hypersensitivity reactions,* serum sickness, drug fever, ***anaphylaxis,*** bacterial and fungal superinfection.

Overdose and treatment

Signs and symptoms of overdose include dizziness, drowsiness, headache, unconsciousness, anorexia, abdominal pain, nausea, and vomiting. More severe complications, including hemolytic anemia, agranulocytosis, dermatitis, acidosis, sensitivity reactions, and jaundice, may be fatal.

Treat by gastric lavage, if ingestion has occurred within the preceding 4 hours, followed by correction of acidosis, forced fluids, and urinary alkalinization to enhance solubility and excretion. Treatment of renal failure and transfusion of appropriate blood products (in severe hematologic toxicity) may be required.

Clinical considerations

Consider the recommendations relevant to all sulfonamides as well as the following:

- Most adverse effects involve the GI tract; minimize reactions and facilitate absorption by spacing doses evenly and administering drug after food.
- Drug colors urine orange-yellow; may also color patient's skin orange-yellow.
- Don't give antacids together with enteric-coated sulfasalazine; they may alter absorption.

Therapeutic monitoring

Drug should be discontinued if signs of toxicity or hypersensitivity occur; if hematologic abnormalities are accompanied by sore throat, pallor, fever, jaundice, purpura, or weakness; if crystalluria is accompanied by renal colic, hematuria, oliguria, proteinuria, urinary obstruction, urolithiasis, increased BUN levels, or anuria; if severe diarrhea indicates pseudomembranous colitis; or if severe nausea, vomiting, or diarrhea persists.

Special populations

Breast-feeding patients. Drug is excreted in breast milk; use with caution.
Pediatric patients. Contraindicated in patients under age 2 months.

Patient counseling

- Tell patient that sulfasalazine normally turns urine orange-yellow. Warn him that skin may also turn orange-yellow and that drug may permanently stain soft contact lenses yellow.
- Advise patient to take drug after meals to reduce GI distress and to facilitate passage into intestines.

sulfinpyrazone

Anturane

Pharmacologic classification: uricosuric
Therapeutic classification: renal tubular-blocking agent, platelet aggregation inhibitor
Pregnancy risk category NR

How supplied

Available by prescription only
Tablets: 100 mg
Capsules: 200 mg

Indications and dosages

Chronic gouty arthritis and intermittent gouty arthritis, or hyperuricemia associated with gout
Adults: initially, 200 to 400 mg P.O. daily in two divided doses, gradually increasing to maintenance dosage in 1 week. Maintenance dosage is 400 mg P.O. daily in two divided doses; may increase to 800 mg daily or decrease to 200 mg daily.
◊ ***Prophylaxis of thromboembolic disorders, including angina, MI, and transient (cerebral) ischemic attacks, and in patients with prosthetic heart valves***
Adults: 600 to 800 mg P.O. daily in divided doses to decrease platelet aggregation.

Pharmacodynamics

Uricosuric action: Sulfinpyrazone competitively inhibits renal tubule reabsorption of uric acid. Sulfinpyrazone inhibits adenosine diphosphate and 5-HT, resulting in decreased platelet adhesiveness and increased platelet survival time.

Pharmacokinetics

Absorption: Absorbed completely after oral administration.
Distribution: 98% to 99% protein-bound.
Metabolism: Metabolized rapidly in the liver.
Excretion: Drug and its metabolites are eliminated in urine; about 50% is excreted unchanged.

Route	Onset	Peak	Duration
P.O.	Unknown	1-2 hr	4-6 hr

Contraindications and precautions

Contraindicated in patients with hypersensitivity to pyrazolone derivatives (including oxyphenbutazone and phenylbutazone), blood dyscrasia, active peptic ulcer, or symptoms of GI inflammation or ulceration.

Use cautiously in patients with healed peptic ulcer and during pregnancy.

Interactions

Drug-drug. *Cholestyramine:* Decreases absorption of sulfinpyrazone. Sulfinpyrazone should be taken 1 hour before or 4 to 6 hours after cholestyramine.
Diazoxide, diuretics, pyrazinamide: Increase serum uric acid. Increased sulfinpyrazone dose requirements.
Oral antidiabetic agents: Increased effects. Monitor blood glucose levels.
Penicillin, other beta-lactam antibiotics, nitrofurantoin, and sulfonylureas: Reduced excretion of nitrofurantoin, decreasing the efficacy of sulfinpyrazone in urinary tract infections and increasing systemic toxicity; may cause hypoglycemia. Monitor closely.
Probenecid: Inhibits renal excretion of sulfinpyrazone. Use together cautiously.
Salicylates: Block the uricosuric effects of sulfinpyrazone only in high doses. Avoid use together.
Warfarin: Enhanced hypoprothrombinemic effect and risk of bleeding; increased bleeding in these patients also may result from the antiplatelet effect of sulfinpyrazone. Use together cautiously.
Drug-lifestyle. *Alcohol use*: May decrease effectiveness of drug. Advise patient to avoid alcohol use.

Effects on diagnostic tests

None reported.

Adverse reactions

GI: *nausea, dyspepsia,* epigastric pain, reactivation of peptic ulcerations.
GU: altered renal function test results, decreased urinary excretion of aminohippuric acid and phenolsulfonphthalein.
Hematologic: ***blood dyscrasia*** (such as anemia, ***leukopenia, agranulocytosis, thrombocytopenia, aplastic anemia***).

Respiratory: ***bronchoconstriction*** in patients with aspirin-induced asthma.
Skin: rash.

Overdose and treatment
Signs and symptoms of overdose include nausea, vomiting, epigastric pain, ataxia, labored breathing, seizures, and coma. Treat supportively; induce emesis or use gastric lavage as appropriate. Treat seizures with diazepam or phenytoin or both.

Clinical considerations
- Drug doesn't accumulate and tolerance to it doesn't develop; it's suitable for long-term use.
- Drug has no analgesic or anti-inflammatory actions
- Give with food, milk, or prescribed antacids to lessen GI upset.
- Sulfinpyrazone is used investigationally to increase platelet survival time, to treat thromboembolic phenomena, and to prevent MI recurrence.

Therapeutic monitoring.
- Drug may not be effective and should be avoided when creatinine clearance is less than 50 ml/minute.
- Monitor renal function and CBC routinely.
- Monitor serum uric acid levels and adjust dose accordingly.
- Maintain adequate hydration with high fluid intake to prevent formation of uric acid kidney stones.

Special populations
Breast-feeding patients. Safety in breast-feeding women hasn't been established. An alternative feeding method is recommended during therapy.
Geriatric patients. Geriatric patients are more likely to have glomerular filtration rates less than 50 ml/minute; sulfinpyrazone may be ineffective.

Patient counseling
- Explain that gouty attacks may increase during first 6 to 12 months of therapy; patient shouldn't discontinue drug without medical approval.
- Encourage patient to comply with dose regimen and to keep scheduled follow-up visits.
- Tell patient to drink 8 to 10 glasses of fluid each day and to take drug with food to minimize GI upset; warn patient to avoid alcoholic beverages, which decrease the therapeutic effect of sulfinpyrazone.

sulfisoxazole
Gantrisin

sulfisoxazole diolamine
Gantrisin (Ophthalmic Solution)

Pharmacologic classification: sulfonamide
Therapeutic classification: antibiotic
Pregnancy risk category C

How supplied
Available by prescription only
Tablets: 500 mg
Liquid: 500 mg/5 ml (sulfisoxazole acetyl)
Ophthalmic solution: 4%

Indications and dosages
Urinary tract and systemic infections
Adults: Initially, 2 to 4 g P.O. then 4 to 8 g P.O. daily in divided doses q 4 to 6 hours.
Children and infants over age 2 months: Initially, 75 mg/kg P.O., then 150 mg/kg (or 4 g/m^2) P.O. daily in divided doses q 4 to 6 hours. Maximum dose shouldn't exceed 6 g/24 hours.
Conjunctivitis, corneal ulcer, superficial ocular infections; adjunct in systemic treatment of trachoma
Adults: Instill 1 to 2 drops in the lower conjuctival sac of affected eye daily q 1 to 4 hours.

Pharmacodynamics
Antibacterial action: Sulfisoxazole is bacteriostatic. It acts by inhibiting formation of tetrahydrofolic acid from para-aminobenzoic acid (PABA), preventing bacterial cell synthesis of folic acid. It acts synergistically with folic acid antagonists such as trimethoprim, which block folic acid synthesis at a later stage, thus delaying or preventing bacterial resistance.

Sulfisoxazole is active against some gram-positive bacteria, *Chlamydia trachomatis,* many Enterobacteriaceae, and some strains of *Toxoplasma* and *Plasmodium.*

Pharmacokinetics
Absorption: Absorbed readily from the GI tract after oral administration.
Distribution: Distributed into extracellular compartments; CSF penetration is 8% to 57% of blood levels in uninflamed meninges. Sulfisoxazole crosses the placenta, and is 85% protein-bound.
Metabolism: Metabolized partially in the liver.
Excretion: Both unchanged drug and metabolites are excreted primarily in urine by glomerular filtration and, to a lesser extent, renal tubular secretion; some drug is excreted in breast milk. Urinary solubility of unchanged drug increases as urine pH increases. Plasma half-life

in patients with normal renal function is about 4½ to 8 hours.

Route	Onset	Peak	Duration
P.O.	Unknown	1-4 hr	Unknown
Ophthalmic	Unknown	Unknown	Unknown

Contraindications and precautions

Contraindicated in patients with hypersensitivity to sulfonamines, in infants under age 2 months (except in congenital toxoplasmosis [with oral form only]), in pregnant women at term, and during breast-feeding.

Use oral form cautiously in patients with impaired renal or hepatic function, severe allergies, bronchial asthma, or G6PD deficiency. Use ophthalmic form cautiously in patients with severely dry eyes.

Interactions

Drug-drug. *Oral anticoagulants:* Exaggerated anticoagulant effects. Monitor for bleeding.
Oral antidiabetic agents including sulfonylureas: Enhance hypoglycemic effects. Monitor blood glucose levels.
PABA: Antagonizes effects of sulfonamides. Don't use together.
Trimethoprim or pyrimethamine (folic acid antagonists with different mechanisms of action): Results in synergistic antibacterial effects and delays or prevents bacterial resistance. Don't use together.
Urine acidifying agents, such as ammonium chloride and ascorbic acid: Increased risk of crystalluria. Monitor closely.
Drug-lifestyle. *Sun exposure:* Photosensitivity reaction may occur. Advise patient to take precautions.

Effects on diagnostic tests

Sulfisoxazole alters results of urine glucose tests using cupric sulfate (Benedict's reagent or Clinitest).

Adverse reactions

CNS: headache; mental depression, hallucinations, ***seizures*** (with oral administration).
CV: tachycardia, palpitations, syncope, cyanosis (with oral administration).
EENT: *ocular irritation, itching, chemosis, periorbital edema* (with ophthalmic form).
GI: *nausea, vomiting, diarrhea,* abdominal pain, anorexia, stomatitis, pseudomembranous colitis (with oral administration).
GU: *toxic nephrosis with oliguria and anuria, acute renal failure,* crystalluria, hematuria (with oral administration).
Hematologic: ***agranulocytosis, aplastic anemia, thrombocytopenia, hemolytic anemia,*** megaloblastic anemia, ***leukopenia*** (with oral administration).
Hepatic: elevated liver enzymes, jaundice (with oral administration), ***hepatitis.***
Skin: ***erythema multiforme, epidermal necrolysis, exfoliative dermatitis,*** *generalized skin eruption,* photosensitivity, urticaria, pruritus (with oral administration).
Other: hypersensitivity reactions (*serum sickness, drug fever,* ***anaphylaxis***), ***Stevens-Johnson syndrome,*** overgrowth of nonsusceptible organisms (with ophthalmic form).

Overdose and treatment

Signs and symptoms of overdose include dizziness, drowsiness, headache, unconsciousness, anorexia, abdominal pain, nausea, and vomiting. More severe complications, including hemolytic anemia, agranulocytosis, dermatitis, acidosis, sensitivity reactions, and jaundice, may be fatal.

Treatment requires gastric lavage, if ingestion has occurred within the preceding 4 hours, followed by correction of acidosis, and forced fluids and urinary alkalinization to enhance solubility and excretion. Treatment of renal failure and transfusion of appropriate blood products (in severe hematologic toxicity) may be required.

Clinical considerations

Consider the recommendations relevant to all sulfonamides:

□ ***ALERT*** Don't confuse the combination products with sulfamethoxazole alone (such as Azo-gantrisin and Gantrisin). Beware of sound-alike names, such as sulfisoxazole and sulfasalazine.
- Sulfisoxazole-pyrimethamine is used to treat toxoplasmosis.

Therapeutic monitoring

- Monitor urine cultures, CBCs, and PT, and conduct urinalyses before and during therapy.
- Monitor renal and liver function tests.

Special populations

Breast-feeding patients. Drug is excreted in breast milk and shouldn't be administered to breast-feeding women.
Pediatric patients. Contraindicated in children under age 2 months.

Patient counseling

- Tell patient to drink 8 oz (240 ml) of water with each oral dose and to take drug on an empty stomach.
- Tell patient to complete prescribed medication.
- Teach patient how to use ophthalmic preparations. Warn patient not to touch tip of dropper or tube to any surface.
- Warn patient that ophthalmic solution may cause blurred vision immediately after application. Tell patient to gently close eyes and keep closed for 1 to 2 minutes.

sulindac

Clinoril

Pharmacologic classification: NSAID
Therapeutic classification: nonnarcotic analgesic, antipyretic, anti-inflammatory
Pregnancy risk category NR

How supplied

Available by prescription only
Tablets: 150 mg, 200 mg

Indications and dosages

Osteoarthritis, rheumatoid arthritis, ankylosing spondylitis
Adults: 150 mg P.O. b.i.d. initially; may increase to 200 mg P.O. b.i.d.
Acute subacromial bursitis or supraspinatus tendinitis, acute gouty arthritis
Adults: 200 mg P.O. b.i.d. for 7 to 14 days. Dose may be reduced as symptoms subside.

Pharmacodynamics

Analgesic, antipyretic, and anti-inflammatory actions: Mechanisms of action are unknown but are thought to inhibit prostaglandin synthesis.

Pharmacokinetics

Absorption: Rapidly and completely absorbed from the GI tract.
Distribution: Highly protein-bound.
Metabolism: Inactive and metabolized hepatically to the active sulfide metabolite.
Excretion: Excreted in urine. Half-life of parent drug is about 8 hours; half-life of active metabolite is about 16 hours.

Route	Onset	Peak	Duration
P.O.	Unknown	2-4 hr	Unknown

Contraindications and precautions

Contraindicated in patients with hypersensitivity to drug or in whom acute asthmatic attacks, urticaria, or rhinitis is precipitated by use of aspirin or NSAIDs. Avoid use during pregnancy.

Use cautiously in patients with history of ulcer or GI bleeding, renal dysfunction, compromised cardiac function, hypertension, or conditions predisposing to fluid retention.

Interactions

Drug-drug. *Antacids:* Delay and decrease the absorption of sulindac. Give drugs at separate times.
Anticoagulants, thrombolytic agents: May be potentiated by the platelet-inhibiting effect of sulindac. Monitor PT closely.
Diflunisal, aspirin: Cause decreased plasma levels of the active sulfide metabolite. Don't use together.
Dimethyl sulfoxide: May cause decreased plasma levels of the active sulfide metabolite. Peripheral neuropathies have also been reported with this combination. Monitor closely.
GI-irritating drugs, including antibiotics, NSAIDs, and steroids: May potentiate the adverse GI effects of sulindac. Use together with caution.
Highly protein-bound drugs, such as phenytoin, sulfonylureas and warfarin: May cause displacement of either drug, and adverse effects. Monitor therapy closely for both drugs.
Lithium carbonate: NSAIDs are known to decrease renal clearance of this drug, thus increasing lithium serum levels and risks of adverse effects. Avoid use together.
Probenecid: Increases plasma levels of sulindac; sulindac may decrease the uricosuric effect of probenecid. Monitor for toxicity.

Effects on diagnostic tests

None reported.

Adverse reactions

CNS: dizziness, headache, nervousness, psychosis.
CV: hypertension, ***heart failure,*** palpitations, edema.
EENT: tinnitus, transient visual disturbances.
GI: *epigastric distress,* ***peptic ulceration, GI bleeding, pancreatitis,*** occult blood loss, nausea, constipation, dyspepsia, flatulence, anorexia, vomiting, diarrhea.
GU: increased BUN, serum creatinine; interstitial nephritis, ***nephrotic syndrome, renal failure.***
Hematologic: prolonged bleeding time, ***aplastic anemia, thrombocytopenia, agranulocytosis, neutropenia, hemolytic anemia.***
Hepatic: elevated liver enzymes.
Metabolic: hyperkalemia.
Skin: *rash,* pruritus.
Other: drug fever, ***anaphylaxis, hypersensitivity syndrome, angioedema.***

Overdose and treatment

Signs and symptoms of overdose include dizziness, drowsiness, mental confusion, disorientation, lethargy, paresthesias, numbness, vomiting, gastric irritation, nausea, abdominal pain, headache, stupor, coma, and hypotension.

To treat overdose of sulindac, empty stomach immediately by inducing emesis with ipecac syrup or by gastric lavage. Administer activated charcoal via nasogastric tube. Provide symptomatic and supportive measures (respiratory support and correction of fluid and electrolyte imbalances). Dialysis is thought to be of minimal value because sulindac is highly protein-bound. Monitor laboratory parameters and vital signs closely.

Clinical considerations

Consider the recommendations relevant to all NSAIDs as well as the following:

- Sulindac may be the safest NSAID for patients with mild renal impairment. It may also be less likely to cause further renal toxicity.
- Impose safety measures to prevent injury, such as using raised side rails and supervised ambulation.

Therapeutic monitoring

- Assess cardiopulmonary status frequently. Monitor vital signs, especially heart rate and blood pressure, to detect abnormalities.
- Assess fluid balance status. Monitor intake and output and daily weight. Observe for presence and amount of edema.
- Symptomatic improvement may take 7 days or longer.

Special populations

Breast-feeding patients. Safe use of sulindac during breast-feeding hasn't been established. Avoid use of drug in breast-feeding women.
Pediatric patients. Safety of long-term drug use in children hasn't been established.
Geriatric patients. Patients over age 60 are more sensitive to the adverse effects of sulindac. Use with caution. Because of its effect on renal prostaglandins, drug may cause fluid retention and edema. This may be significant in geriatric patients and those with heart failure.

Patient counseling

- Caution patient to avoid use of OTC medications unless medically approved.
- Teach patient how to recognize signs and symptoms of possible adverse reactions; instruct patient to report such adverse reactions.
- Instruct patient to check weight two or three times weekly and to report weight gain of 3 lb (1.4 kg) or more within 1 week, to doctor.
- Advise patient to report edema and have blood pressure checked routinely.
- Instruct patient in safety measures; advise him to avoid hazardous activities that require alertness until CNS effects of drug are known.

sumatriptan succinate

Imitrex

Pharmacologic classification: selective 5-hydroxytryptamine ($5HT_1$)-receptor agonist
Therapeutic classification: antimigraine agent
Pregnancy risk category C

How supplied

Available by prescription only
Tablets: 25 mg, 50 mg
Injection: 12 mg/ml (0.5 ml in 1-ml prefilled syringe), 6-mg single-dose (0.5 ml in 2 ml) vial, and stat dose system.
Nasal spray: 5 mg/0.1 ml, 20 mg/0.1 ml

Indications and dosages

Acute migraine attacks (with or without aura)
Adults: 6 mg S.C. Maximum recommended dose is two 6-mg injections in 24 hours, separated by at least 1 hour, or 25 to 100 mg P.O. initially. If response isn't achieved in 2 hours, may give second dose of 25 to 100 mg. Additional doses may be used in at least 2-hour intervals. Maximum daily dose, 300 mg.

For nasal spray, administer single dose of 5 mg, 10 mg, or 20 mg once in one nostril; may repeat once after 2 hours under doctor's guidance for maximum daily dose of 40 mg. A 10-mg dose may be achieved by the administration of a single 5-mg dose in each nostril.

Pharmacodynamics

Antimigraine action: Sumatriptan selectively binds to a $5\text{-}HT_1$ receptor subtype found in the basilar artery and vasculature of dura mater, where it presumably exerts its antimigraine effect. In these tissues, sumatriptan activates the receptor to cause vasoconstriction, an action correlating with the relief of migraine.

Pharmacokinetics

Absorption: Bioavailability via S.C. injection is 97% of that obtained via I.V. injection.
Distribution: Has a low protein-binding capacity (about 14% to 21%).
Metabolism: About 80% is metabolized in the liver, primarily to an inactive indoleacetic acid metabolite.
Excretion: Excreted primarily in urine, partly (20%) as unchanged drug and partly as the indoleacetic acid metabolite. Elimination half-life is about 2 hours.

Route	Onset	Peak	Duration
P.O.	½ hr	1½ hr	Unknown
S.C.	10-20 min	12 min	Unknown
Nasal	Unknown	Unknown	Unknown

Contraindications and precautions

Contraindicated in patients with hypersensitivity to drug; in those with uncontrolled hypertension; ischemic heart disease, such as angina pectoris, Prinzmetal's angina, history of MI, or documented silent ischemia; or hemiplegic or basilar migraine; within 14 days of MAO therapy; and in patients taking ergotamine.

Use cautiously in patients who may be at risk for coronary artery disease (CAD) (such as postmenopausal women or men over age 40) or those with risk factors such as hypertension, hypercholesterolemia, obesity, diabetes, smoking, or family history. Use cautiously in women of childbearing age and during pregnancy.

Interactions

Drug-drug. *Ergot and ergot derivatives:* Prolong vasospastic effects when given with sumatriptan. These drugs shouldn't be used within 24 hours of sumatriptan therapy.
MAO inhibitors: Increased effects of sumatriptan. Avoid use within 2 weeks of discontinuing MAO inhibitor therapy.
Drug-herb. *Horehound:* May enhance serotonergic effects. Don't use together.

Effects on diagnostic tests

None reported.

Adverse reactions

CNS: *dizziness, vertigo,* drowsiness, headache, anxiety, malaise, fatigue.
CV: ***atrial fibrillation, ventricular fibrillation, ventricular tachycardia, MI,*** *ECG changes such as ischemic ST-segment elevation* (rare), pressure or tightness in chest.
EENT: discomfort of throat, nasal cavity or sinus, mouth, jaw, or tongue; altered vision.
GI: abdominal discomfort, dysphagia.
Musculoskeletal: myalgia, muscle cramps, neck pain.
Skin: flushing.
Other: *tingling; warm or hot sensation; burning sensation; heaviness, pressure or tightness;* anxious feeling; tight feeling in head; cold sensation; diaphoresis; *injection site reaction.*

Overdose and treatment

No specific information available. However, it would be expected to cause seizures, tremor, inactivity, erythema of the extremities, reduced respiratory rate, cyanosis, ataxia, mydriasis, injection site reactions, and paralysis. Continue monitoring of patient while signs and symptoms persist and for at least 10 hours thereafter. Effect of hemodialysis or peritoneal dialysis on serum levels of sumatriptan is unknown.

Clinical considerations

- Don't use drug for management of hemiplegic or basilar migraine. Safety and effectiveness also haven't been established for cluster headache, which occurs in an older, predominantly male population.
- Don't give drug I.V. because coronary vasospasm may occur.
- Nasal spray is generally well tolerated, however adverse reactions seen with the other forms of the drug can still occur.
- Clinical data on sumatriptan injection include rare reports of serious or life-threatening arrhythmias, such as atrial and ventricular fibrillation, ventricular tachycardia, MI, and marked ischemic ST elevations. Data also include rare, but more frequent, reports of chest and arm discomfort thought to represent angina pectoris. Because such coronary events can occur, consider administering first dose in an outpatient setting to patients in whom unrecognized coronary artery disease (CAD) is comparatively likely (postmenopausal women; men over age 40; and patients with risk factors for CAD, such as hypertension, hypercholesterolemia, obesity, diabetes, smoking, and strong family history of CAD).

Therapeutic monitoring

Patient response to nasal spray may be varied. The choice of dose should be made individually, weighing the possible benefit of the 20-mg dose with the potential for a greater risk of adverse events.

Special populations

Pregnant patients. Potential for harm to fetus. Use only when benefits outweigh risks to fetus. Tell pregnant women or those who intend to become pregnant during therapy to consult doctor and discuss risks and benefits of drug use.
Breast-feeding patients. Drug is excreted in breast milk. Use caution when administering to breast-feeding women.
Pediatric patients. Safety and efficacy in children haven't been established.

Patient counseling

- Tell patient that drug may be given at any time during a migraine attack, but preferably as soon as symptoms begin. A second injection may be given if symptoms recur. Tell patient not to use more than two injections in 24 hours and to allow at least 1 hour between doses. Pain or redness at the injection site may occur but usually lasts less than 1 hour.
- Explain that drug is intended to relieve migraine, not to prevent or reduce the number of attacks.
- Tell patient not to use a second nasal spray dose if there was no response to the initial dose unless the health care provider is first contacted.
- Explain that drug is available in a spring-loaded injector system that facilitates self-administration. Review detailed information with patient. Be sure he understands how to load the injector, administer the injection, and dispose of the used syringes.
- Tell patient who feels persistent or severe chest pain to call the health care provider immediately. Tell patient who experiences pain or tightness in the throat, wheezing, heart throbbing, rash, lumps, hives, or swollen eyelids, face, or lips to stop using the drug and call at once.

T

tacrine hydrochloride

Cognex

Pharmacologic classification: centrally acting reversible cholinesterase inhibitor
Therapeutic classification: psychotherapeutic agent (for Alzheimer's disease)
Pregnancy risk category C

How supplied

Available by prescription only
Capsules: 10 mg, 20 mg, 30 mg, 40 mg

Indications and dosages

Mild to moderate dementia of the Alzheimer's type
Adults: Initially, 10 mg P.O. q.i.d. Maintain dose for at least 4 weeks, with every-other-week monitoring of transaminase levels beginning at week 4 of therapy. If patient tolerates treatment and transaminase levels remain normal, increase to 20 mg P.O. q.i.d. After 4 weeks, adjust dosage to 30 mg P.O. q.i.d. If still tolerated, increase to 40 mg P.O. q.i.d. after another 4 weeks.
≡ ***Dosage adjustment.*** In patients with ALT level two to three times the upper limit of normal, monitor ALT level weekly. If ALT level is three to five times the upper normal limit, reduce daily dose by 40 mg/day and monitor ALT level weekly. Resume dose adjustment and every-other-week monitoring when ALT level returns to normal. If ALT level is above five times upper normal limit, stop treatment and monitor ALT level. Monitor for signs and symptoms associated with hepatitis. Rechallenge when ALT level is normal and monitor weekly.

Pharmacodynamics

Psychotherapeutic action: Tacrine presumably slows degradation of acetylcholine released by still-intact cholinergic neurons, thereby elevating acetylcholine levels in the cerebral cortex. If this theory is correct, the effects of tacrine may lessen as the disease process advances and fewer cholinergic neurons remain functionally intact. No evidence suggests that tacrine alters the course of the underlying dementia.

Pharmacokinetics

Absorption: Rapidly absorbed after oral administration. Absolute bioavailability of tacrine is about 17%. Food reduces tacrine bioavailability by about 30% to 40% if taken less than 1 hour before a meal.
Distribution: About 55% bound to plasma proteins.
Metabolism: Undergoes first-pass metabolism, which is dose dependent. It's extensively metabolized by the cytochrome P-450 system to multiple metabolites, not all of which have been identified.
Excretion: Elimination half-life is about 2 to 4 hours.

Route	Onset	Peak	Duration
P.O.	Unknown	½-3 hr	Unknown

Contraindications and precautions

Contraindicated in patients hypersensitive to drug or acridine derivatives. Also contraindicated in patients with tacrine-related jaundice that's been confirmed with an elevated total bilirubin level of more than 3 mg/dl, and in patients with hypersensitivity reactions associated with ALT elevations.

Use cautiously in patients with sick sinus syndrome, bradycardia, history of hepatic disease, renal disease, Parkinson's disease, asthma, prostatic hyperplasia, or other urinary outflow impairment and in those at risk for peptic ulcer.

Interactions

Drug-drug. *Agents that undergo extensive metabolism via cytochrome P-450:* Drug interactions may occur. Use cautiously.
Anticholinergics: Decreased effectiveness of anticholinergics. Monitor patient closely.
Cholinergics, cholinesterase inhibitors: Additive effects. Monitor patient for signs of toxicity.
Cimetidine: Increases the plasma level of tacrine. Monitor patient.
NSAIDs: May contribute to GI irritation and gastric bleeding. Monitor patient carefully.
Theophylline: Increased theophylline elimination half-life and average plasma levels. Monitor plasma theophylline level.
Drug-food. *Any food:* Can delay absorption of drug. Give drug 1 hour before meals.
Drug-lifestyle. *Smoking:* Decreases plasma levels of drug. Advise patient to avoid smoking.

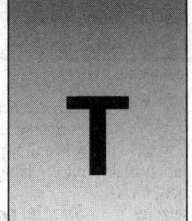

Effects on diagnostic tests
None reported.

Adverse reactions
CNS: agitation, ataxia, insomnia, abnormal thinking, somnolence, depression, anxiety, *headache, dizziness,* fatigue, confusion, seizures.
CV: *bradycardia*, hypertension, palpitations, chest pain.
GI: *nausea, vomiting, diarrhea,* dyspepsia, loose stools, changes in stool color, anorexia, abdominal pain, flatulence, constipation.
Hepatic: elevated liver enzymes.
Metabolic: weight loss.
Musculoskeletal: myalgia.
Respiratory: rhinitis, upper respiratory tract infection, cough.
Skin: rash, jaundice, facial flushing.
Other: increased sweating.

Overdose and treatment
Overdose with cholinesterase inhibitors can cause a cholinergic crisis characterized by severe nausea, vomiting, salivation, sweating, bradycardia, hypotension, and seizures. Increasing muscle weakness may occur and can result in death if respiratory muscles are involved.

Use general supportive measures. Tertiary anticholinergics, such as atropine, may be used as an antidote for tacrine overdose. I.V. atropine sulfate titrated to effect is recommended (initial dose of 1 to 2 mg I.V., with subsequent doses based on clinical response). It isn't known if tacrine or its metabolites can be eliminated by dialysis.

Clinical considerations
- Tacrine as a cholinesterase inhibitor is likely to exaggerate succinylcholine-type muscle relaxation during anesthesia.
- Drug may have vagotonic effects on the heart rate, such as bradycardia. Use with caution in patients with sick sinus syndrome.
- Rate of dose escalation may be slowed if patient is intolerant to recommended titration schedule. Acceleration of titration schedule is never recommended.
- Cognitive function can worsen after abrupt discontinuation of tacrine or after a reduction in total daily dose of 80 mg/day or more.
- If drug is discontinued for 4 weeks or more, restart full dose titration and monitoring schedule.
- The incidence of transaminase elevations is higher among women. There are no other known predictors of risk of hepatocellular injury.

Therapeutic monitoring
- Monitor serum ALT levels every other week from at least week 4 to week 16 following initiation of therapy, after which monitoring may be decreased to every 3 months if ALT is less than or equal to 2 times the upper limit of normal. After each dose adjustment, resume monitoring schedule.
- Monitor patient for dose tolerance and cognitive changes.

Special populations
No information available.

Patient counseling
- Instruct caregiver to give drug between meals. If GI upset occurs, drug may be taken with food but plasma levels may be reduced.
- Inform caregiver that drug can alleviate symptoms but doesn't alter the underlying degenerative disease.
- Inform caregiver that effectiveness of therapy depends on drug administration at regular intervals.
- Caution caregiver that dose adjustment is an integral part of the safe use of drug. Abrupt discontinuation or a large reduction in daily dose (80 mg/day or more) may precipitate behavioral disturbances and a decline in cognitive function.
- Advise caregiver to promptly report significant adverse effects or changes in status.

tamoxifen citrate
Nolvadex, Nolvadex-D*, Tamofen*

Pharmacologic classification: nonsteroidal antiestrogen
Therapeutic classification: antineoplastic
Pregnancy risk category D

How supplied
Available by prescription only
Tablets: 10 mg, 20 mg
Tablets (enteric-coated): 20 mg*

Indications and dosages
Dosage and indications may vary. Check current literature for recommended protocol.

Advanced breast cancer (men and postmenopausal women)
Adults: 10 to 20 mg P.O. b.i.d.

Adjunct treatment for breast cancer
Adults: 10 mg P.O. b.i.d. to t.i.d. for no more than 2 years.

Reduction of breast cancer incidence in high risk women
Adults: 20 mg P.O. daily for 5 years.

◊***Mastalgia***
Adults: 10 mg P.O. daily for 4 months.

◊***Stimulation of ovulation***
Adults: 5 to 40 mg P.O. b.i.d. for 4 days.

Pharmacodynamics
Antineoplastic action: Exact mechanism of action is unclear. Tamoxifen may exert its cytotoxic action by blocking estrogen receptors

within tumor cells that require estrogen to thrive. The estrogen receptor-tamoxifen complex may be translocated into the nucleus of the tumor cell, where it inhibits DNA synthesis.

Pharmacokinetics

Absorption: Appears to be well absorbed across the GI tract after oral administration. Steady-state serum levels are generally attained after 3 to 4 weeks.
Distribution: Distribution of drug and its metabolites into body tissues and fluids hasn't been fully established.
Metabolism: Metabolized extensively in the liver to several metabolites.
Excretion: Excreted primarily in feces, mostly as metabolites. Drug has a distribution phase half-life of 7 to 14 hours. Half-life of the terminal elimination phase is more than 7 days.

Route	Onset	Peak	Duration
P.O.	1 to several months	Unknown	Unknown

Contraindications and precautions

Contraindicated in patients hypersensitive to drug and during pregnancy. Also contraindicated in women who are also taking coumarin-type anticoagulants or in women with a history of deep vein thrombosis (DVT) or pulmonary edema (PE).

Use cautiously in patients with existing leukopenia or thrombocytopenia.

Interactions

Drug-drug. *Antacids:* May affect absorption of enteric-coated tablet. Give drugs 2 hours apart.
Bromocriptine: Increased tamoxifen levels. Dosage adjustment may be needed. Monitor patient closely.
Coumadin: Significant increase in anticoagulation effect. Monitor PT and INR. Dose adjustment may be needed.
Cytotoxic agents: Increased thromboembolic events. Avoid use together.
Estrogens: Decreased therapeutic effect of drug. Dose adjustment may be needed. Monitor patient closely.

Effects on diagnostic tests

Variations on karyopyknotic index in vaginal smears and various degrees of estrogen effect on Papanicolaou smears have been seen in some postmenopausal patients.

Adverse reactions

GI: *nausea, vomiting, diarrhea.*
GU: *vaginal discharge* and bleeding, *irregular menses, increased BUN and creatinine, amenorrhea.*
Hematologic: ***leukopenia, thrombocytopenia.***
Hepatic: elevated liver enzymes.
Metabolic: hypercalcemia, increased serum triglycerides and cholesterol, increased thyroxine level, *weight gain or loss.*
Musculoskeletal: temporary bone or tumor pain, brief exacerbation of pain from osseous metastases.
Skin: *skin changes.*
Other: *hot flashes, fluid retention.*

Overdose and treatment

Acute overdose hasn't been reported. No specific treatment is known. Treatment should include supportive measures.

Clinical considerations

- Tamoxifen acts as an antiestrogen. Best results occur in patients with positive estrogen receptors.
- Adverse reactions are usually minor and well tolerated. They can usually be controlled by dose reduction.
- Clotting factor abnormalities may occur with prolonged tamoxifen therapy at usual doses.

Therapeutic monitoring

- Monitor WBC and platelet counts and periodic liver function tests.
- Monitor serum calcium levels; hypercalcemia may occur during initial therapy in patients with bone metastases.
- Initial adverse reactions (increased bone pain) may be associated with a good tumor response shortly after starting tamoxifen therapy.

Special populations

Pregnant patients. Drug isn't to be used during pregnancy or for a period of at least 2 months before pregnancy because of potential risks to fetus.
Breast-feeding patients. It isn't known if drug is excreted in breast milk. However, because of the potential for serious adverse reactions and carcinogenicity in the infant, breast-feeding isn't recommended.
Pediatric patients. Safety and efficacy haven't been established for use in children.
Geriatric patients. The risk of serious adverse effects for women age 65 and older is the same as for women age 50 and older (the group identified in one study as being at highest risk for serious adverse effects).

Patient counseling

- Stress importance of swallowing enteric-coated tablets without crushing or breaking them.
- Emphasize importance of continuing drug despite occurrence of nausea and vomiting.
- Tell patient to promptly report vomiting if it occurs shortly after dose ingestion.
- Reassure patient that acute exacerbation of bone pain during tamoxifen therapy usually indicates drug will produce good response.

- Advise women to avoid becoming pregnant during drug therapy. Also recommend barrier or nonhormonal contraceptive measures for sexually active patients during treatment period.

tamsulosin hydrochloride

Flomax

Pharmacologic classification: alpha$_{1a}$-antagonist
Therapeutic classification: BPH agent
Pregnancy risk category B

How supplied

Available by prescription only
Capsules: 0.4 mg

Indications and dosages

Benign prostatic hyperplasia (BPH)
Adult men: 0.4 mg P.O. once daily, administered 30 minutes after same meal each day. For those who fail to respond after 2 to 4 weeks, increase dose to 0.8 mg P.O. once daily. If either dosing regimen is interrupted for several days, restart therapy with the 0.4-mg once-daily dose.

Pharmacodynamics

Anti-BPH action: Drug selectively blocks alpha$_1$-receptors in the prostate, leading to relaxation of smooth muscles in the bladder neck and prostate, improving urine flow, and reducing BPH symptoms.

Pharmacokinetics

Absorption: Completely absorbed following oral administration under fasting conditions.
Distribution: Studies suggest distribution into extracellular fluids and most tissues, including kidney, prostate, gallbladder, heart, aorta, and brown fat, with minimal distribution into brain, spinal cord, and testes. Drug is extensively bound to plasma proteins but isn't thought to affect other highly bound drugs.
Metabolism: Metabolized by cytochrome P-450 in the liver, with less than 10% excreted unchanged; however, pharmacokinetic profile of metabolites hasn't been established. Metabolites undergo extensive conjugation to glucuronide or sulfate before renal excretion.
Excretion: Excreted primarily in urine (76%); about 21% excreted in feces. Elimination half-life is 5 to 7 hours, with apparent half-life from 9 to 15 hours secondary to rate-controlled absorption pharmacokinetics.

Route	Onset	Peak	Duration
P.O.	Unknown	4-7 hr	9-15 hr

Contraindications and precautions

Contraindicated in patients with hypersensitivity to drug or its components.

Interactions

Drug-drug. *Alpha blockers:* Presumed to interact with drug. Avoid use together.
Cimetidine: Decreased clearance of tamsulosin. Use together with caution.

Effects on diagnostic tests

None reported.

Adverse reactions

CNS: *dizziness, headache,* insomnia, somnolence.
CV: chest pain, syncope.
EENT: amblyopia, pharyngitis, *rhinitis,* sinusitis.
GI: diarrhea, nausea.
GU: abnormal ejaculation, decrease in libido.
Musculoskeletal: asthenia, back pain.
Respiratory: increased cough.
Other: *infection,* tooth disorder, allergic reactions (rash, pruritus, urticaria, ***angioedema***).

Overdose and treatment

Overdose can lead to hypotension. Treatment is with support of CV system. Keep patient in supine position, and administer I.V. fluids if necessary. Initiate vasopressors, if needed, and monitor renal function, supporting as needed. Dialysis is unlikely to be beneficial.

Clinical considerations

- Symptoms of BPH and carcinoma of the prostate are similar; rule out carcinoma before initiating therapy with tamsulosin.
- If treatment is interrupted for several days or more, restart therapy at 1 capsule daily.

Therapeutic monitoring

Monitor patient for decreased blood pressure.

Special populations

Breast-feeding patients. Drug isn't indicated for use in women.
Pediatric patients. Drug isn't indicated for use in children.

Patient counseling

- Instruct patient not to crush, chew, or open capsules and to take drug at the same time each day 30 minutes after eating.
- Tell patient to get up slowly from chair or bed during initiation of therapy and to avoid situations in which injury could occur as a result of syncope.
- Instruct patient not to drive or perform hazardous tasks during initiation of therapy and for 12 hours following the initial dose or changes in dose until response can be monitored.

telmisartan

Micardis

Pharmacologic classification: angiotensin II antagonist
Therapeutic classification: antihypertensive
Pregnancy risk category C (D in second and third trimesters)

How supplied

Available by prescription only
Tablets: 40 mg, 80 mg

Indications and dosages

Hypertension (used alone or in combination with other antihypertensive agents)
Adults: 40 mg P.O. once daily. Blood pressure response is dose-related over a range of 20 to 80 mg daily.

Pharmacodynamics

Antihypertensive action: Inhibits vasoconstriction and aldosterone production by selectively blocking the binding of angiotensin II to its receptors.

Pharmacokinetics

Absorption: Absolute bioavailability is about 42% for a 40-mg dose. Peak plasma levels are reached in ½ to 1 hour following oral administration.
Distribution: Extensively bound to plasma proteins (more than 99.5%).
Metabolism: Metabolized by glucuronide conjugation to an inactive metabolite.
Excretion: Half-life is about 24 hours. Majority is excreted unchanged in the feces via biliary excretion.

Route	Onset	Peak	Duration
P.O.	Unknown	½-1 hr	24 hr

Contraindications and precautions

Contraindicated in patients hypersensitive to drug or its components and during pregnancy.

Use cautiously in patients with biliary obstruction disorders, renal stenosis, or renal or hepatic insufficiency and in those with an activated renin-angiotensin system, such as volume- or salt-depleted patients (such as those receiving high doses of diuretics).

Interactions

Drug-drug. *Digoxin:* Increased digoxin plasma levels. Monitor digoxin levels closely.
Warfarin: Decreased plasma warfarin levels. Monitor patient closely.
Drug-lifestyle. *Alcohol use:* Enhanced hypotensive effects of the drug. Avoid use together.

Effects on diagnostic tests

None reported.

Adverse reactions

CNS: dizziness, pain, fatigue, headache.
CV: chest pain, hypertension, peripheral edema.
EENT: pharyngitis, sinusitis.
GI: abdominal pain, diarrhea, dyspepsia, nausea.
GU: urinary tract infection.
Hepatic: elevated liver enzymes.
Musculoskeletal: back pain, myalgia.
Respiratory: cough, upper respiratory tract infection.
Other: flulike symptoms.

Overdose and treatment

Limited data exist. Most likely, symptoms include hypotension, tachycardia, dizziness, and possibly bradycardia. Treatment should involve supportive care. Telmisartan isn't removed by hemodialysis.

Clinical considerations

- Blood pressure response in black patients is less than in white patients.
- Most of the antihypertensive effect is present within 2 weeks. Maximal blood pressure reduction is generally attained after 4 weeks.
- Diuretic may be added if blood pressure isn't controlled by drug alone.
- Drug isn't removed by hemodialysis. Orthostatic hypotension may develop in patients undergoing dialysis.

Therapeutic monitoring

- Monitor for hypotension following initiation of drug. Place patient in supine position if hypotension occurs and administer I.V. normal saline if necessary, as indicated.
- Closely monitor blood pressure.

Special populations

Pregnant patients. Use of drug is contraindicated during pregnancy because of potential risk of fetal and neonatal morbidity and death.
Breast-feeding patients. It isn't known if drug is excreted in breast milk. Assess risks and benefits before continuing drug in breast-feeding women.
Pediatric patients. Safety and efficacy in children haven't been established.
Geriatric patients. No significant difference has been reported compared to younger patients.

Patient counseling

- Inform patient that drug shouldn't be removed from blister-sealed packet until immediately before use.
- Inform women of childbearing age of the consequences of second- and third-trimester exposure to drug.
- Inform patient that transient hypotension may occur.

temazepam

Restoril

Pharmacologic classification: benzodiazepine
Therapeutic classification: sedative-hypnotic
Controlled substance schedule IV
Pregnancy risk category X

How supplied

Available by prescription only
Capsules: 7.5 mg, 15 mg, 30 mg

Indications and dosages

Insomnia
Adults: 7.5 to 30 mg P.O. 30 minutes before bedtime.
Elderly: Initiate at 7.5 mg P.O. h.s. until individual response is determined.
≡***Dosage adjustment.*** In debilitated patients, 7.5 mg P.O. h.s. until individual response is determined.

Pharmacodynamics

Sedative-hypnotic action: Temazepam depresses the CNS at the limbic and subcortical levels of the brain. It produces a sedative-hypnotic effect by potentiating the effect of the neurotransmitter gamma-aminobutyric acid on its receptor in the ascending reticular activating system, which increases inhibition and blocks both cortical and limbic arousal.

Pharmacokinetics

Absorption: Well absorbed through the GI tract when administered orally.
Distribution: Widely distributed throughout the body. Drug is 96% protein-bound.
Metabolism: Metabolized in the liver primarily to inactive metabolites.
Excretion: Metabolites are excreted in urine as glucuronide conjugates. Half-life of drug is 4 to 20 hours.

Route	Onset	Peak	Duration
P.O.	½-1 hr	1¼-1½ hr	Unknown

Contraindications and precautions

Contraindicated in patients with hypersensitivity to drug or other benzodiazepines and during pregnancy.

Use cautiously in patients with impaired renal or hepatic function, chronic pulmonary insufficiency, severe or latent mental depression, suicidal tendencies, or history of drug abuse.

Interactions

Drug-drug. *Antidepressants, antihistamines, barbiturates, general anesthetics, MAO inhibitors, narcotics, and phenothiazines:* Enhanced CNS depressant effects. Use together cautiously.
Haloperidol: Increased serum haloperidol level. Monitor patient closely.
Levodopa: Reduced levodopa therapeutic effect. Use together cautiously.
Drug-lifestyle. *Alcohol use:* Increased CNS depression. Avoid use together.
Smoking: Accelerated temazepam metabolism, which lowers clinical effectiveness. Advise patient to avoid smoking.

Effects on diagnostic tests

None reported.

Adverse reactions

CNS: *drowsiness, dizziness, lethargy,* disturbed coordination, daytime sedation, confusion, nightmares, vertigo, euphoria, weakness, headache, fatigue, nervousness, anxiety, depression, minor changes in EEG patterns.
EENT: blurred vision.
GI: diarrhea, nausea, dry mouth.
Hepatic: elevated liver enzymes.
Other: physical and psychological dependence.

Overdose and treatment

Signs and symptoms of overdose include somnolence, confusion, hypoactive or absent reflexes, dyspnea, labored breathing, hypotension, bradycardia, slurred speech, unsteady gait or impaired coordination and, ultimately, coma.

Support blood pressure and respiration until drug effects subside; monitor vital signs. Mechanical ventilatory assistance via endotracheal tube may be required to maintain a patent airway and support adequate oxygenation. Flumazenil, a specific benzodiazepine antagonist, may be useful. Use I.V. fluids and vasopressors, such as dopamine and phenylephrine, to treat hypotension as needed. If patient is conscious, induce emesis. Use gastric lavage if ingestion was recent, but only if an endotracheal tube is present to prevent aspiration. After emesis or lavage, administer activated charcoal with a cathartic as a single dose. Don't use barbiturates if excitation occurs. Dialysis is of limited value.

Clinical considerations

Consider the recommendations relevant to all benzodiazepines as well as the following:
- Prolonged use isn't recommended; however, drug has proved effective for up to 4 weeks of continuous use.
- After long-term use, avoid abrupt withdrawal and follow a gradual tapering dose schedule.
- Drug is useful for patients who have difficulty falling asleep or who awaken frequently in the night.

Therapeutic monitoring

Monitor hepatic function studies to prevent toxicity; lower doses are indicated in patients with hepatic dysfunction.

Special populations

Pregnant patients. Use is contraindicated during pregnancy because of potential risk of harm to fetus.
Breast-feeding patients. Drug is excreted in breast milk. A breast-fed infant may become sedated, have feeding difficulties, or lose weight. Avoid use in breast-feeding women.
Pediatric patients. Safe use in patients under age 18 hasn't been established.
Geriatric patients. Geriatric patients are more susceptible to the CNS depressant effects of temazepam. Use with caution.

Patient counseling

- Instruct patient to seek medical approval before making changes in medication regimen.
- Inform patient of the risk for physical and psychological dependence with chronic use.
- Caution women of risks to fetus.
- Warn patient about potential CNS depression with alcohol use and the decreased therapeutic benefits associated with heavy smoking.

temozolomide

Temodar

Pharmacologic classification: alkylating agent
Therapeutic classification: antineoplastic
Pregnancy risk category D

How supplied

Available by prescription only
Capsules: 5 mg, 20 mg, 100 mg, 250 mg

Indications and dosages

Refractory anaplastic astrocytoma that has relapsed following chemotherapy regimen containing a nitrosourea and procarbazine
Adults: Initial cycle: 150 mg/m² by mouth once daily for first 5 days of 28-day treatment cycle. Subsequent cycles: 100 to 200 mg/m² by mouth once daily for first 5 days of subsequent 28-day treatment cycles. Timing and dosage of subsequent cycles must be adjusted according to the absolute neutrophil count (ANC) and platelet count measured on cycle day 22 (expected nadir) and cycle day 29 (initiation of next cycle).

Dosage adjustments are based on the lowest of these ANC and platelet results. For ANC less than 1,000/mm³ or platelets less than 50,000/mm³: Hold therapy until ANC is greater than 1,500/mm³ and platelets greater than 100,000/mm³. Reduce dose by 50 mg/m² for subsequent cycle. Minimum dose is 100 mg/m².

For ANC 1,000 to 1,500/mm³ or platelets 50,000 to 100,000/mm³: Hold therapy until ANC is greater than 1,500/mm³ and platelets greater than 100,000/mm³. Maintain prior dose for subsequent cycle.

For ANC greater than 1,500/mm³ and platelets greater than 100,000/mm³: Increase dose to, or maintain at, 200 mg/m² for first 5 days of subsequent cycle.

Pharmacodynamics

Antineoplastic action: Temozolomide is a prodrug that's rapidly hydrolyzed to the active agent. It's thought to interfere with DNA replication in rapidly dividing tissues, primarily through alkylation (methylation) of guanine nucleotides in the DNA structure.

Pharmacokinetics

Absorption: Rapidly and completely absorbed from the GI tract following oral administration, with plasma levels peaking in 1 hour.
Distribution: 15% bound to plasma proteins.
Metabolism: Undergoes spontaneous hydrolysis to its active form and other metabolites. After 7 days, 38% of administered dose is recovered in urine and 0.8% in feces.
Excretion: Rapidly eliminated, with an elimination half-life of 1¾ hours.

Route	Onset	Peak	Duration
P.O.	Unknown	Unknown	Unknown

Contraindications and precautions

Contraindicated in patients with hypersensitivity to temozolomide or its components; also in those allergic to dacarbazine, which is structurally similar to temozolomide. Also contraindicated in pregnancy.

Interactions

Drug-drug. *Valproic acid:* Decreases oral clearance of temozolomide by about 5%. Use cautiously.
Drug-food. *Any food:* Reduces rate and extent of drug absorption; however, there are no dietary restrictions with drug administration. Give drug on an empty stomach to reduce nausea and vomiting.

Effects on diagnostic tests

None reported.

Adverse reactions

CNS: *amnesia,* anxiety, *asthenia,* ataxia, confusion, *seizures, coordination abnormality,* depression, *dizziness,* dysphasia, *fatigue,* gait abnormality, *headache, hemiparesis, insomnia,* local seizures, paresis, *paresthesia, somnolence.*
EENT: abnormal vision, diplopia, pharyngitis, sinusitis.
GI: *abdominal pain, anorexia, constipation, diarrhea, nausea, vomiting.*
GU: increased urinary frequency, urinary incontinence, urinary tract infection.

Hematologic: anemia, ***leukopenia, neutropenia, thrombocytopenia.***
Musculoskeletal: back pain, myalgia.
Respiratory: coughing, upper respiratory tract infection.
Skin: pruritus, rash.
Other: breast pain (female), *fever,* hyperadrenocorticism, *peripheral edema, viral infection.* weight increase.
Drug-food. *Any food:* Reduces rate and extent of drug absorption; however, there are no dietary restrictions with drug administration. Give drug on an empty stomach to reduce nausea and vomiting.

Overdose and treatment
Neutropenia and thrombocytopenia occurred following a single dose of 1,000 mg/m². Closely monitor patient's hematologic status and administer supportive therapies, as needed.

Clinical considerations
- Avoid skin contact with, or inhalation of, capsule contents if capsule is accidentally opened or damaged. Follow procedures for safe handling and disposal of antineoplastics.
- Store capsules at room temperature (59° to 86° F [15° to 30° C]).

Therapeutic monitoring
A complete blood count (CBC) should be drawn on day 22 and then weekly until ANC is greater than 1,500/mm³ and platelet count greater than 100,000/mm³.

Special populations
Pregnant patients. Drug shouldn't be used during pregnancy because of risk of harm to the fetus, unless potential benefit outweighs fetal risk.
Breast-feeding patients. It's unknown if temozolomide is excreted in breast milk; patient should discontinue breast-feeding while receiving drug.
Pediatric patients. Safety and efficacy haven't been evaluated in children.
Geriatric patients. Severe neutropenia and thrombocytopenia are more common following first treatment cycle in patients age 70 and older.

Patient counseling
- Emphasize importance of taking dose exactly as prescribed, to swallow capsules, and to take drug on an empty stomach or at bedtime.
- Stress importance of continuing medication even when suffering nausea and vomiting.
- Tell patient to call prescriber immediately if vomiting (dose loss) occurs shortly after a dose is taken.
- Tell patient to promptly report sore throat, fever, unusual bruising or bleeding, rash, or seizures.
- Advise patient to avoid exposure to people with infections.
- Advise patient that drug may cause birth defects.

teniposide (VM-26)
Vumon

Pharmacologic classification: podophyllotoxin (cell cycle-phase specific, G_2 and late S phase)
Therapeutic classification: antineoplastic
Pregnancy risk category D

How supplied
Available by prescription only
Injection: 50 mg/5 ml ampules

Indications and dosages
Dosage and indications may vary. Check current literature for recommended protocol.
Acute lymphoblastic leukemia induction therapy in childhood
Children: Optimum dose hasn't been established. One protocol reported by manufacturer is 165 mg/m² I.V. teniposide with cytarabine 300 mg/m² I.V. twice weekly for eight or nine doses.

Pharmacodynamics
Antineoplastic action: Teniposide causes single- and double-stranded breaks in DNA and DNA protein cross-links, preventing cells from entering mitosis.

Pharmacokinetics
Absorption: Not administered orally.
Distribution: Highly bound to plasma proteins (more than 99%). Teniposide crosses the blood-brain barrier to a limited extent.
Metabolism: Metabolized extensively in the liver.
Excretion: About 4% to 12% of a dose is eliminated through the kidneys as unchanged drug or metabolites. Terminal half-life of drug is 5 hours.

Route	Onset	Peak	Duration
I.V.	Unknown	Unknown	Unknown

Contraindications and precautions
Contraindicated in patients hypersensitive to drug or to polyoxyethylated castor oil, an injection vehicle.

Interactions
Drug-drug. *Heparin:* Incompatible. Don't mix together.
Methotrexate: May increase clearance and intracellular levels of methotrexate. Avoid use together.

Sodium salicylate, sulfamethizole, tolbutamide: May displace teniposide from protein-binding sites and increase toxicity. Don't administer together.

Effects on diagnostic tests
None reported.

Adverse reactions
CV: hypotension from rapid infusion.
GI: *nausea, vomiting, mucositis, diarrhea.*
Hematologic: **LEUKOPENIA, NEUTROPENIA, THROMBOCYTOPENIA, MYELOSUPPRESSION** (dose-limiting), *anemia.*
Metabolic: elevated uric acid levels in blood and urine.
Skin: rash.
Other: alopecia (rare), ***anaphylaxis*** (rare), *infection,* bleeding, ***hypersensitivity reactions*** (chills, fever, urticaria, tachycardia, ***bronchospasm,*** dyspnea, hypotension, flushing); *phlebitis and extravasation* (at injection site).

Overdose and treatment
Signs and symptoms of overdose include myelosuppression, nausea, and vomiting. Treatment is usually supportive and includes transfusion of blood components, antiemetics, and antibiotics for infections that may develop.

Clinical considerations
- Use glass or polyolefin plastic bags or containers for infusion. Don't use polyvinyl chloride containers.
- Use caution when handling and preparing solution. The use of gloves is recommended.
- Dilute with 5% dextrose injection USP or normal saline injection USP to give final teniposide levels of 0.1 mg/ml, 0.2 mg/ml, 0.4 mg/ml, or 1 mg/ml.
- Solutions containing levels of 0.1 mg/ml, 0.2 mg/ml, or 0.4 mg/ml are stable at room temperature for 24 hours. Solutions with a final level of 1 mg/ml should be administered within 4 hours of preparation.
- If teniposide solution contacts skin, immediately wash with soap and water. If drug makes contact with mucous membranes, immediately flush with water.
- Don't administer drug through a membrane-type in-line filter because the diluent may dissolve the filter.

□ ***ALERT*** Have diphenhydramine, hydrocortisone, epinephrine, and oral airway available in case of an anaphylactic reaction.

- Administer I.V. infusion over 30 to 60 minutes to prevent hypotension. Avoid I.V. push because of increased risk of hypotension.
- Decrease dose in patients with renal or hepatic insufficiency and in patients with Down syndrome.

Therapeutic monitoring
- Monitor for chemical phlebitis at injection site.
- Monitor blood pressure before infusion and at 30-minute intervals during infusion. If systolic blood pressure decreases below 90 mm Hg, stop infusion.
- Monitor CBC. Observe patient for signs of bone marrow depression.
- Monitor renal and hepatic function during therapy.

Special populations
Pregnant patients. Use of drug during pregnancy can cause fetal harm. Use during pregnancy only when expected benefits justify risk to fetus.
Breast-feeding patients. It isn't known if drug is excreted in breast milk. However, because of the risk of serious adverse reactions, mutagenicity, and carcinogenicity in the infant, breast-feeding isn't recommended.

Patient counseling
- Encourage adequate fluid intake to increase urine output and facilitate excretion of uric acid.
- Caution patient to avoid exposure to people with infections.
- Caution patient of potential for harm to fetus.
- Advise patient that hair should grow back after treatment is discontinued.
- Tell patient to call promptly if a sore throat or fever develops or if unusual bruising or bleeding occur.

terazosin hydrochloride
Hytrin

Pharmacologic classification: selective $alpha_1$ blocker
Therapeutic classification: antihypertensive
Pregnancy risk category C

How supplied
Available by prescription only
Capsules: 1 mg, 2 mg, 5 mg, 10 mg

Indications and dosages
Mild to moderate hypertension
Adults: Initially, 1 mg P.O. h.s. Adjust dose and schedule according to patient response. Recommended range, 1 to 5 mg daily or divided b.i.d.

If therapy is discontinued for several days or longer, reinstitute using the initial dosing regimen of 1 mg P.O. h.s. Slowly increase dose until desired blood pressure is attained. Doses of more than 20 mg don't appear to further affect blood pressure.

Benign prostatic hyperplasia
Adults: Initially, 1 mg P.O. h.s. Dose may be adjusted upward based on patient response. Increase in a stepwise manner to 2 mg, 5 mg, and 10 mg. A daily dose of 10 mg may be required.

Pharmacodynamics

Antihypertensive action: Terazosin reduces blood pressure by selectively inhibiting $alpha_1$ receptors in vascular smooth muscle, reducing peripheral vascular resistance. Because of its selectivity for $alpha_1$ receptors, heart rate increases minimally. Significant decreases in serum cholesterol, low-density lipoprotein, and very-low-density lipoprotein cholesterol fractions occur during therapy; the significance of these changes is unknown, as is the mechanism by which they occur.

Terazosin administration doesn't significantly alter potassium or glucose levels; it has been used successfully with diuretics, beta blockers, and a combination of other antihypertensive regimens.
Hypertrophic action: Alpha-blockade in nonvascular smooth muscle causes relaxation, notably in prostatic tissue, reducing urinary symptoms in men with BPH.

Pharmacokinetics

Absorption: Rapidly absorbed after oral administration. About 90% of oral dose is bioavailable; ingestion of food doesn't appear to alter bioavailability.
Distribution: About 90% to 94% is plasma protein-bound.
Metabolism: Metabolized in the liver. Pharmacokinetics of drug don't appear to be affected by hypertension, heart failure, or age.
Excretion: About 40% is excreted in urine, 60% in feces, mostly as metabolites. Up to 30% may be excreted unchanged. Elimination half-life is about 12 hours.

Route	Onset	Peak	Duration
P.O.	15 min	2-3 hr	24 hr

Contraindications and precautions

Contraindicated in patients with hypersensitivity to drug.

Interactions

Drug-drug. *Antihypertensives:* Excessive hypotension. Use together cautiously.
Clonidine: Decreased antihypertensive effect of clonidine. Monitor patient closely.
Drug-herb. *Butcher's broom:* May cause a possible reduction in effects. Don't use together.

Effects on diagnostic tests

Terazosin therapy causes small but significant decreases in hematocrit, WBC count, and hemoglobin, total protein, and albumin levels; the magnitude of these decreases hasn't been shown to worsen with time, suggesting the possibility of hemodilution.

Adverse reactions

CNS: *asthenia, dizziness, headache,* nervousness, paresthesia, somnolence.
CV: *palpitations, peripheral edema,* postural hypotension, tachycardia, syncope.
EENT: *nasal congestion,* sinusitis, blurred vision.
GI: *nausea.*
GU: impotence.
Musculoskeletal: back pain, muscle pain.
Respiratory: dyspnea.

Overdose and treatment

Signs of overdose are exaggerated adverse reactions, particularly hypotension and shock. In case of overdose, treatment is symptomatic and supportive. Dialysis may not be helpful because drug is highly protein-bound.

Clinical considerations

- Consider the recommendations relevant to all alpha blockers.
- Terazosin can cause marked hypotension, especially postural hypotension, and syncope with the first dose or during the first few days of therapy. A similar response occurs if therapy is interrupted for more than a few doses.

Therapeutic monitoring

Monitor blood pressure closely.

Special populations

Pregnant patients. Safety during pregnancy hasn't been established.
Breast feeding patients. It isn't known if drug is excreted in breast milk. Avoid use in breast-feeding women.
Pediatric patients. Safety and efficacy in patients under age 21 haven't been established.
Geriatric patients. Patients over age 65 may be particularly susceptible to adverse reactions of drug.

Patient counseling

- Instruct patient to take first dose at bedtime.
- Warn patient to avoid hazardous tasks that require alertness for 12 hours following the first dose, dose increases, or when restarting dose after interruption of therapy.
- Caution patient to rise carefully and slowly from sitting and supine positions and to report dizziness, light-headedness, or palpitations. Dose adjustment may be necessary.

terbinafine hydrochloride

Lamisil, Lamisil AT

Pharmacologic classification: synthetic allylamine derivative
Therapeutic classification: antifungal
Pregnancy risk category B

How supplied

Available by prescription only
Tablets: 250 mg
Available without a prescription
Cream: 1%

Indications and dosages

***Interdigital tinea pedis (athlete's foot), tinea cruris (jock itch), or tinea corporis (ringworm) caused by* Epidermophyton floccosum, Trichophyton mentagrophytes, *or* T. rubrum**

Adults and children over age 12: For interdigital tinea pedis, apply to cover the affected and immediately surrounding areas b.i.d. until signs and symptoms are significantly improved (for most patients this occurs by day 7 of drug therapy); for tinea cruris or tinea corporis, apply to cover the affected and immediately surrounding areas once or twice daily until signs and symptoms are significantly improved (for most patients this occurs by day 7 of drug therapy). Treatment duration should be at least 1 week and no longer than 4 weeks.

Onychomycosis of fingernails or toenails caused by dermatophytes (tinea unguium)

Adults and children over age 12: For treatment of fingernails, give 250 mg/day P.O. for 6 weeks; for toenails, give 250 mg/day P.O. for 12 weeks.

Pharmacodynamics

Antifungal action: Terbinafine exerts its antifungal effect by inhibiting squalene epoxidase, a key enzyme in sterol biosynthesis in fungi. This action results in a deficiency in ergosterol and a corresponding accumulation of squalene within the fungal cell and causes fungal cell death.

Pharmacokinetics

Topical

Absorption: Systemic absorption of terbinafine is highly variable.
Distribution: None reported.
Metabolism: None reported.
Excretion: About 75% of cutaneously absorbed terbinafine is eliminated in urine, predominantly as metabolites.

Oral

Absorption: More than 70% of drug is absorbed; food enhances absorption.
Distribution: Distributed to serum and skin. Plasma half-life is about 36 hours; half-life in tissue is 200 to 400 hours. More than 99% of drug is bound to plasma proteins.
Metabolism: First-pass metabolism is about 40%.
Excretion: About 70% of dose is eliminated in urine; clearance is decreased by 50% in patients with hepatic cirrhosis and impaired renal function.

Route	Onset	Peak	Duration
P.O.	Unknown	2 hr	Unknown
Topical	Unknown	Unknown	Unknown

Contraindications and precautions

Contraindicated in patients hypersensitive to drug. Oral form is also contraindicated in patients with preexisting hepatic disease or impaired renal function (creatinine clearance of 50 ml/minute or less) and during pregnancy.

Interactions

None reported for topical form.
Drug-drug. *I.V. caffeine:* Decreases caffeine clearance. Monitor patient closely.
Cimetidine: Decreases terbinafine clearance by 33%. Avoid use together.
Cyclosporine: Increases cyclosporine clearance. Monitor levels carefully.
Rifampin: Increases terbinafine clearance by 100%. Monitor patient closely.

Effects on diagnostic tests

None reported.

Adverse reactions

CNS: *headache.*
EENT: taste disturbances, visual disturbances.
GI: diarrhea, dyspepsia, abdominal pain, nausea, flatulence.
Hematologic: decreased absolute lymphocyte count, ***neutropenia***.
Hepatic: elevated liver enzymes.
Skin: ***Stevens-Johnson syndrome, toxic epidermal necrolysis,*** irritation, burning, pruritus, dryness.

Overdose and treatment

Acute overdose with topical application is unlikely because of the limited absorption of topically applied drug and wouldn't be expected to lead to a life-threatening situation.

Clinical considerations

□ ***ALERT*** Be aware of sound-alikes: terbinafine and terbutaline.

- Diagnosis should be confirmed either by direct microscopic examination of scrapings from infected tissue mounted in a solution of potassium hydroxide or by culture.
- Topical form of drug is for topical use only; it isn't for oral, ophthalmic, or intravaginal use.

Therapeutic monitoring

- Many patients given shorter durations of therapy (1 to 2 weeks) continue to improve during the 2 to 4 weeks after drug therapy has been completed. As a consequence, patients shouldn't be considered therapeutic failures until they've been observed for a period of 2 to 4 weeks off therapy. If successful outcome isn't achieved during the post-treatment observation period, review the diagnosis.
- Monitor patient for irritation or sensitivity to drug. Discontinue therapy if irritation or sensitivity is present and institute appropriate treatment measures.
- Perform liver function tests for patients receiving oral treatment for more than 6 weeks.

Special populations

Pregnant patients. Not recommended for use during pregnancy.
Breast-feeding patients. Drug is excreted in breast milk. A decision to either discontinue breast-feeding or drug must be made, taking into account the importance of drug to the woman. Women who are breast-feeding should avoid application of terbinafine cream to the breast.
Pediatric patients. Safety and efficacy in children under age 12 haven't been established.

Patient counseling

- Advise patient to use drug as directed and to avoid contact with eyes, nose, mouth, or other mucous membranes.
- Stress importance of using drug for recommended treatment time.
- Tell patient to call his doctor if the area of application shows signs or symptoms of increased irritation or possible sensitization, such as redness, itching, burning, blistering, swelling, or oozing.
- Instruct patient not to use occlusive dressings unless directed.

terbutaline sulfate

Brethaire, Brethine, Bricanyl

Pharmacologic classification: adrenergic ($beta_2$ agonist)
Therapeutic classification: bronchodilator, premature labor inhibitor (tocolytic)
Pregnancy risk category B

How supplied

Available by prescription only
Tablets: 2.5 mg, 5 mg
Aerosol inhaler: 200 mcg/metered spray
Injection: 1 mg/ml parenteral

Indications and dosages

Relief of bronchospasm in patients with reversible obstructive airway disease
Adults and adolescents age 15 or older: Administer 5 mg P.O. t.i.d. at 6-hour intervals. Reduce dose to 2.5 mg P.O. t.i.d. if side effects occur. Maximum daily dose, 15 mg. Alternatively, 0.25 mg S.C. may be repeated in 15 to 30 minutes; maximum, 0.5 mg q 4 hours. Alternatively, 2 inhalations may be given q 4 to 6 hours with 1 minute between inhalations.
Children age 12 to 15: 2.5 mg P.O. t.i.d. Maximum daily dose, 7.5 mg. Alternatively, 2 inhalations may be given q 4 to 6 hours with 1 minute between inhalations.
◇***Premature labor***
Adults: Initially, 10 mcg/minute I.V. Titrate to maximum dose of 80 mcg/minute. Maintain I.V. dosage at minimum effective dose for 4 hours. Maintainance therapy until term is 2.5 mg P.O. q 4 to 6 hours.

Pharmacodynamics

Bronchodilator action: Terbutaline acts directly on $beta_2$-adrenergic receptors to relax bronchial smooth muscle, relieving bronchospasm and reducing airway resistance. Cardiac and CNS stimulation may occur with high doses.
Tocolytic action: When used in premature labor, terbutaline relaxes uterine smooth muscle, which inhibits uterine contractions.

Pharmacokinetics

Absorption: About 33% to 50% of an oral dose is absorbed through the GI tract.
Distribution: Distributed widely throughout the body.
Metabolism: Partially metabolized in liver to inactive compounds.
Excretion: After parenteral administration, 60% of drug is excreted unchanged in urine, 3% in feces through bile, and the remainder in urine as metabolites. After oral administration, most drug is excreted as metabolites.

Route	Onset	Peak	Duration
P.O.	30 min	2-3 hr	4-8 hr
S.C.	15 min	½ hr	1½-4 hr
Inhalation	5-30 min	1-2 hr	3-6 hr

Contraindications and precautions

Contraindicated in patients with hypersensitivity to drug or sympathomimetic amines. Use cautiously in patients with CV disorders, hyperthyroidism, diabetes, or seizure disorders.

Interactions

Drug-drug. *Cardiac glycosides, cyclopropane, halogenated inhalation anesthetics, levodopa:* Increased risk of arrhythmias. Monitor patient closely. Avoid use with levodopa.
CNS stimulants: Increased CNS stimulation. Avoid use together.

MAO inhibitors: Potential for hypertensive crisis. Avoid use together.
Propranolol, other beta blockers: Blocked bronchodilation effects of terbutaline. Avoid use together.

Effects on diagnostic tests
Terbutaline may reduce the sensitivity of spirometry for diagnosis of bronchospasm.

Adverse reactions
CNS: *nervousness, tremor, drowsiness, dizziness, headache,* weakness.
CV: *palpitations,* tachycardia, ***arrhythmias,*** flushing.
EENT: dry and irritated nose and throat (with inhaled form).
GI: *vomiting, nausea,* heartburn.
Metabolic: hypokalemia (with high doses).
Respiratory: ***paradoxical bronchospasm with prolonged usage,*** dyspnea.
Other: diaphoresis.

Overdose and treatment
Signs and symptoms of overdose include exaggeration of common adverse reactions, particularly arrhythmias, seizures, nausea, and vomiting.

Treatment requires supportive measures. If patient is conscious and ingestion was recent, induce emesis and follow with gastric lavage. If patient is comatose, after endotracheal tube is in place with cuff inflated, perform gastric lavage; then administer activated charcoal to reduce drug absorption. Maintain adequate airway, provide cardiac and respiratory support, and monitor vital signs closely.

Clinical considerations
□ ***ALERT*** Be aware of sound-alikes: terbinafine and terbutaline.
Consider the recommendations relevant to all adrenergics as well as the following:
- Store injection solution away from light. Don't use if discolored.
- CV effects are more likely with S.C. route and when patient has arrhythmias.
- Most adverse reactions are transient; however, tachycardia may persist for a relatively long time.
- Patient may use tablets and aerosol together.
- Aerosol terbutaline produces minimal cardiac stimulation and tremors.

Therapeutic monitoring
- Carefully monitor patient for toxicity.
- When drug is used for tocolytic therapy, monitor patient for CV effects, including tachycardia, for 12 hours after discontinuation of drug. Monitor intake and output; fluid restriction may be necessary. Muscle tremor is common but may subside with continued use.
- Monitor neonate for hypoglycemia if the mother used terbutaline during pregnancy.

Special populations
Pregnant patients. Manufacturers state that drug shouldn't be used to treat preterm labor. Use drug during pregnancy only when expected benefits justify risk to fetus.
Breast-feeding patients. Distributed into breast milk in minute amounts. Use drug with caution in breast-feeding women.
Pediatric patients. Drug isn't recommended for use in children under age 12.
Geriatric patients. Geriatric patients are more sensitive to the effects of terbutaline; a lower dose may be required.

Patient counseling
- Instruct patient to avoid simultaneous administration with adrenocorticoid aerosol. Separate administration time by 15 minutes.
- Instruct patient on proper inhalation administration.
- Instruct patient to use terbutaline only as directed. If drug produces no relief or if condition worsens, call prescriber promptly.
- Advise patient to take a missed dose within 1 hour, and if remembered longer than 1 hour after missed dose, to skip and not double the dose.
- Caution patient that many OTC cold and allergy remedies contain a sympathomimetic agent that may be harmful when combined with terbutaline.

terconazole
Terazol 3, Terazol 7

Pharmacologic classification: triazole derivative
Therapeutic classification: antifungal
Pregnancy risk category C

How supplied
Available by prescription only
Vaginal cream: 0.4% in 45-g tube, 0.8% in 20-g tube with applicator
Vaginal suppositories: 80 mg

Indications and dosages
Local treatment of vulvovaginal candidiasis (moniliasis)
Adults: 0.4%: 1 full applicator (5 g) intravaginally once daily h.s. for 7 consecutive days. 0.8%: 1 full applicator (5 g) intravaginally once daily h.s. for 3 consecutive days. Alternatively, insert 1 suppository vaginally h.s. for 3 consecutive days.

Pharmacodynamics
Exact mechanism of action is unknown. Terconazole may disrupt fungal cell membrane permeability.

Pharmacokinetics

Absorption: Minimally absorbed, about 5% to 16%.
Distribution: Effect is mainly local.
Metabolism: Metabolized mainly by oxidative *N*- and *O*-dealkylation, dioxolane ring cleavage, and conjugation pathways.
Excretion: Following oral administration of terconazole, 32% to 56% of dose is excreted in urine and 47% to 52% is excreted in feces within 24 hours.

Route	Onset	Peak	Duration
Intravaginal	Unknown	Unknown	Unknown

Contraindications and precautions

Contraindicated in patients with known sensitivity to terconazole or any inactive ingredients in drug.

Interactions

None reported.

Effects on diagnostic tests

None reported.

Adverse reactions

CNS: *headache.*
GU: dysmenorrhea, pain of the female genitalia, vulvovaginal burning.
Skin: irritation, *pruritus,* photosensitivity.
Other: fever, chills, body aches.

Overdose and treatment

None reported.

Clinical considerations

- Drug is only effective against vulvovaginitis caused by *Candida.* Confirm diagnosis by cultures or potassium hydroxide smears.
- A persistent infection may be caused by reinfection. Evaluate patient for possible sources.
- Intractable candidiasis may be a sign of diabetes mellitus. Perform blood and urine glucose determinations to rule out undiagnosed diabetes mellitus.

Therapeutic monitoring

None reported.

Special populations

Pregnant patients. There are no adequate and controlled studies regarding use of drug during first trimester. Drug was used during second and third trimesters in at least 100 women without adverse effects on the outcome of pregnancy.
Breast-feeding patients. Safety isn't established. Breast-feeding isn't recommended during therapy with terconazole.

Patient counseling

- Instruct patient to insert cream high into the vagina.
- Tell patient to complete full course of therapy and to use it continuously, even during menstrual period. The therapeutic effect of terconazole isn't affected by menstruation.
- Inform patient to report if drug causes burning or irritation.

testosterone

Histerone 100, Malogen in Oil*, Tesamone, Testandro, Testaqua

testosterone cypionate

depAndro 100, depAndro 200, Depotest 100, Depotest 200, Depo-Testosterone, Duratest-100, Duratest-200, T-Cypionate, Testred Cypionate 200, Virilon IM

testosterone enanthate

Andro L.A. 200, Andropository 200, Delatestryl, Durathate-200, Everone 200, Testrin-P.A.

testosterone propionate

Malogen in Oil*, Testex

Pharmacologic classification: androgen
Therapeutic classification: androgen replacement, antineoplastic
Controlled substance schedule III
Pregnancy risk category X

How supplied

Available by prescription only
testosterone
Injection (aqueous suspension): 25 mg/ml, 50 mg/ml, 100 mg/ml
testosterone cypionate (in oil)
Injection: 100 mg/ml, 200 mg/ml
testosterone enanthate (in oil)
Injection: 100 mg/ml, 200 mg/ml
testosterone propionate (in oil)
Injection: 50 mg/ml, 100 mg/ml

Indications and dosages

Male hypogonadism
testosterone or testosterone propionate
Adults: 10 to 25 mg I.M. two or three times weekly.
testosterone cypionate or enanthate
Adults: 50 to 400 mg I.M. q 2 to 4 weeks.
Delayed puberty in males
testosterone or testosterone propionate
Children: 25 to 50 mg I.M. two or three times weekly for up to 6 months.
testosterone cypionate or enanthate
Children: 50 to 200 mg I.M. q 2 to 4 weeks for up to 6 months.
Postpartum breast pain and engorgement
testosterone or testosterone propionate
Adults: 25 to 50 mg I.M. daily for 3 to 4 days.

Inoperable breast cancer
testosterone propionate
Adults: 50 to 100 mg I.M. three times weekly.
testosterone cypionate or enanthate
Adults: 200 to 400 mg I.M. q 2 to 4 weeks.
testosterone
Adults: 100 mg I.M. three times weekly.
Postpubertal cryptorchidism
testosterone or testosterone propionate
Adults: 10 to 25 mg I.M. two or three times weekly.
Growth stimulation in Turner's syndrome
testosterone propionate
Adults: 40 to 50 mg/m^2 I.M. once monthly for 6 months.

Pharmacodynamics

Androgenic action: Testosterone is the endogenous androgen that stimulates receptors in androgen-responsive organs and tissues to promote growth and development of male sexual organs and secondary sexual characteristics.
Antineoplastic action: Testosterone exerts inhibitory, antiestrogenic effects on hormone-responsive breast tumors and metastases.

Pharmacokinetics

Absorption: Testosterone and its esters must be administered parenterally because they're inactivated rapidly by the liver when given orally. The onset of action of cypionate and enanthate esters of testosterone is somewhat slower than that of testosterone itself.
Distribution: Normally 98% to 99% plasma protein-bound, primarily to the testosterone-estradiol binding globulin.
Metabolism: Metabolized to several 17-ketosteroids by two main pathways in the liver. A large portion of these metabolites then form glucuronide and sulfate conjugates. Plasma half-life of testosterone ranges from 10 to 100 minutes. The cypionate and enanthate esters of testosterone have longer durations of action than testosterone.
Excretion: Very little unchanged testosterone appears in urine or feces. About 90% of metabolized testosterone is excreted in urine in the form of sulfate and glucuronide conjugates.

Route	Onset	Peak	Duration
I.M.	Unknown	10-100 min	Unknown

Contraindications and precautions

Contraindicated in men with breast or prostate cancer; in patients with hypercalcemia or cardiac, hepatic, or renal decompensation; during pregnancy; and in breast-feeding women.

Use cautiously in the elderly and in women of childbearing age.

Interactions

Drug-drug. *Hepatotoxic medication:* Increased risk of hepatotoxicity. Monitor patient closely.
Insulin, oral antidiabetic agents: Decreased serum glucose; altered glucose levels in diabetic patients. Monitor patient closely. Dose may require adjustment.
Oral anticoagulants: Prolonged PT and INR. Monitor patient closely.
Oxyphenbutazone: May increase serum oxyphenbutazone levels. Monitor patient closely.

Effects on diagnostic tests

None reported.

Adverse reactions

CNS: headache, anxiety, depression, paresthesia, sleep apnea syndrome.
CV: edema.
GI: nausea.
GU: hypoestrogenic effects in women (flushing; diaphoresis; vaginitis, including itching, drying, and burning; vaginal bleeding; menstrual irregularities); androgenic effects in women *(acne, edema, oily skin, weight gain, hirsutism, hoarseness,* clitoral enlargement, deepening voice, decreased or increased libido); excessive hormonal effects in men (prepubertal—premature epiphyseal closure, *acne,* priapism, *growth of body and facial hair,* phallic enlargement; postpubertal—testicular atrophy, oligospermia, decreased ejaculatory volume, impotence, gynecomastia, epididymitis), increased serum creatinine.
Hematologic: elevated PT and INR; polycythemia; suppression of clotting factors.
Hepatic: reversible jaundice, cholestatic hepatitis, abnormal liver enzyme levels.
Metabolic: hypercalcemia; hypernatremia; hyperkalemia; hyperphosphatemia; hypercholesteremia; abnormal results of glucose tolerance tests; decreased thyroid function tests and serum 17-ketosteroid levels.
Skin: pain and induration at injection site, local edema, hypersensitivity manifestations.

Overdose and treatment

None reported.

Clinical considerations

Consider the recommendations relevant to all androgens, as well as the following:
- When used to treat male hypogonadism, initiate therapy with full therapeutic doses and taper according to patient tolerance and response. Administering long-acting esters (enanthate or cypionate) at intervals greater than every 2 to 3 weeks may cause hormone levels to fall below those found in normal adults.
- Testosterone enanthate has been used for postmenopausal osteoporosis and to stimulate erythropoiesis.

Therapeutic monitoring

Carefully observe women for signs of excessive virilization. If possible, discontinue therapy at first sign of virilization because some adverse effects, such as deepening of voice and clitoral enlargement, are irreversible. Patients with metastatic breast cancer should have regular determinations of serum calcium levels to avoid serious hypercalcemia.

Special populations

Pregnant patients. Drug isn't indicated for use during pregnancy.
Breast-feeding patients. It's unknown if drug is excreted in breast milk. An alternative feeding method is recommended because of potential for severe adverse effects of androgens on the infant.
Pediatric patients. Use with extreme caution in children to avoid precocious puberty and premature closure of the epiphyses. Obtain X-ray examinations every 6 months to assess skeletal maturation.
Geriatric patients. Observe elderly men for prostatic hyperplasia. Development of symptomatic prostatic hyperplasia or prostatic carcinoma mandates the discontinuation of drug.

Patient counseling

- Explain to women that virilization may occur and to report androgenic effects immediately. Stopping drug prevents further androgenic changes but probably won't reverse those already present.
- Tell women to report menstrual irregularities; drug may be discontinued pending determination of the cause.
- Inform men to report too frequent or persistent penile erections.
- Advise patient to report persistent GI distress, diarrhea, or the onset of jaundice.

testosterone transdermal system

Androderm, Testoderm

Pharmacologic classification: androgen
Therapeutic classification: androgen replacement
Controlled substance schedule III
Pregnancy risk category X

How supplied

Available by prescription only
Transdermal system: 2.5 mg/day (Androderm), 4 mg/day (Testoderm), 6 mg/day (Testoderm)

Indications and dosages

Primary or hypogonadotropic hypogonadism
Androderm
Adult men age 18 and older: Two systems applied nightly for 24 hours, providing a total dose of 5 mg/day. Apply on dry area of skin on back, abdomen, upper arms, or thighs. Don't apply to scrotum.
Testoderm
Adult men age 18 and older: Apply one 6-mg/day patch to scrotal area daily for 22 to 24 hours. If scrotal area is too small for 6-mg/day patch, start therapy with 4-mg/day patch.

Note: Discontinue testosterone transdermal system if edema occurs.

Pharmacodynamics

Androgenic action: Testosterone transdermal system releases testosterone, the endogenous androgen that stimulates receptors in androgen-responsive organs and tissues to promote growth and development of male sex organs and secondary sex characteristics.

Pharmacokinetics

Absorption: After placement of a testosterone transdermal system on scrotal skin. Daily application of two Androderm systems at bedtime results in a serum testosterone concentration profile that mimics the normal circadian variation observed in healthy young men.
Distribution: Circulating testosterone is chiefly bound in the serum to sex hormone-binding globulin and albumin.
Metabolism: Metabolized to various 17-ketosteroids through two different pathways; the major active metabolites are estradiol and dihydrotestosterone.
Excretion: Little unchanged testosterone appears in urine or feces.

Route	Onset	Peak	Duration
Transdermal	Unknown	2-4 hr	2 hr after removal

Contraindications and precautions

Contraindicated in patients hypersensitive to drug, in women, and in men with known or suspected breast or prostate cancer.

Use cautiously in patients with preexisting renal, cardiac, or hepatic disease and in elderly men.

Interactions

Drug-drug. *Hepatotoxic medications:* Increased risk of hepatotoxicity. Monitor patient closely.
Insulin, oral antidiabetic agents: Decreased serum glucose; altered glucose levels in diabetic patients. Monitor patient closely. Dose may require adjustment.
Oral anticoagulants: Prolonged PT and INR. Monitor patient closely.
Oxyphenbutazone: May increase serum oxyphenbutazone levels. Monitor patient closely.

Effects on diagnostic tests

None reported.

Adverse reactions

CNS: *CVA.*
GU: *gynecomastia,* prostatitis, urinary tract infection, breast tenderness.
Metabolic: altered thyroid function tests.
Skin: acne, *pruritus.*
Other: discomfort, irritation.

Overdose and treatment

Testosterone levels of up to 11,400 ng/dl have been implicated in CVA. No other information is available.

Clinical considerations

- Testoderm form of testosterone transdermal system doesn't produce adequate serum testosterone level if applied to nongenital skin.
- Gynecomastia commonly develops and occasionally persists in patients receiving treatment for hypogonadism.
- Topical adverse reactions decrease with duration of use.
- Store testosterone transdermal system at room temperature.

Therapeutic monitoring

- Check hemoglobin levels and hematocrit periodically (to detect polycythemia) in patients on long-term androgen therapy.
- Check liver function, prostatic acid phosphatase, prostatic specific antigen, cholesterol, and high-density lipoproteins periodically.
- After 3 to 4 weeks of daily system use in patients receiving Testoderm, draw blood 2 to 4 hours after system application for determination of serum total testosterone. For patients receiving Androderm, monitor serum testosterone the morning following regular evening application. Because of variability in analytical values among diagnostic laboratories, this laboratory work and later analyses for assessing the effect of testosterone transdermal system should be performed at the same laboratory.
- If patient hasn't achieved desired results within 8 weeks, consider another form of testosterone replacement therapy.

Special populations

Pediatric patients. Testosterone transdermal system hasn't been evaluated clinically in males under age 18.
Geriatric patients. Geriatric patients given androgens may be at increased risk for development of prostatic hyperplasia and prostatic carcinoma. Cautious use of testosterone transdermal system is required in this age-group.

Patient counseling

- Instruct patient regarding proper administration technique.
- Advise patient to report if nausea, vomiting, skin color changes, ankle edema, too-frequent or persistent penile erections occur.
- Inform patient that topical testosterone preparations used by men have caused virilization in female partners. Changes in body hair distribution or significant increase in acne of the female partner should be reported.

tetanus immune globulin, human (TIG)

Bay-Tet

Pharmacologic classification: immune serum
Therapeutic classification: tetanus prophylaxis
Pregnancy risk category C

How supplied

Available by prescription only
Injection: 250 units/ml in 1 ml vial or syringe

Indications and dosages

Tetanus prophylactic dose
Adults and children over age 7: 250 units I.M.
Children under age 7: 4 units/kg I.M.
Tetanus treatment
Adults and children: Although optimal therapeutic doses have not been established, single doses of 3,000 to 6,000 units I.M. have been used. Dosages should be adjusted based on severity of the infection. Don't give at same site as toxoid.

Pharmacodynamics

Antitetanus action: TIG provides passive immunity to tetanus. Antibodies remain at effective levels for 3 weeks or longer. TIG protects the patient for the incubation period of most tetanus cases.

Pharmacokinetics

Absorption: Absorbed slowly.
Distribution: None reported.
Metabolism: None reported.
Excretion: Serum half-life is about 28 days.

Route	Onset	Peak	Duration
I.M.	Unknown	2-3 days	4 wk

Contraindications and precautions

Contraindicated in patients with thrombocytopenia or any coagulation disorder that contraindicates I.M. injection unless potential benefits outweigh risks. Contraindicated for use in patients with hypersensitivity to thimerosal or TIG. Not recommended for use in immunoglobulin A deficiency. Don't give I.V.

Interactions
None reported.

Effects on diagnostic tests
None reported.

Adverse reactions
GU: ***nephrotic syndrome.***
Other: slight fever, ***hypersensitivity reactions, anaphylaxis, angioedema,*** pain, stiffness, erythema at injection site.

Overdose and treatment
None reported.

Clinical considerations
- Don't confuse drug with tetanus toxoid, which should be given at the same time (but at different sites) to produce active immunization.
- Have epinephrine solution 1:1,000 available to treat allergic reactions.
- TIG is used for prophylaxis in patients with dirty wounds if patient has had fewer than three previous tetanus toxoid injections or if the immunization history is unknown or uncertain.
- Tetanus increases risks of severe morbidity and mortality in both mother and fetus if untreated. No fetal risk from the use of immune globulin has been reported to date.
- TIG hasn't been associated with an increase of AIDS cases. The immune globulin is devoid of HIV. Immune globulin recipients don't develop antibodies to HIV.
- Store TIG between 36° and 46° F (2° and 8° C). Don't freeze.

Therapeutic monitoring
Monitor for hypersensitivity reactions and site injection reactions.

Special populations
Pregnant patients. No fetal risk from the use of immune globulin has been reported to date.
Breast-feeding patients. It's unknown if TIG is excreted in breast milk. Use with caution in breast-feeding women.

Patient counseling
- Tell patient that available data indicate that TIG administration doesn't cause AIDS or hepatitis.
- Inform patient that he may experience some local pain, swelling, and tenderness at the injection site. Recommend acetaminophen to alleviate these minor effects.
- Instruct patient to report headache, skin changes, or difficulty breathing.

tetanus toxoid, adsorbed
tetanus toxoid, fluid

Pharmacologic classification: toxoid
Therapeutic classification: tetanus prophylaxis
Pregnancy risk category C

How supplied
Available by prescription only
Adsorbed toxoid
Injection: 5 to 10 Lf units of inactivated tetanus/0.5-ml dose, in 0.5-ml syringes and 5-ml vials
Fluid toxoid
Injection: 4 to 5 Lf units of inactivated tetanus/0.5-ml dose, in 0.5-ml syringes and 7.5-ml vials

Indications and dosages
Primary immunization (adsorbed formulation)
Adults and children age 1 and older: 0.5 ml I.M. 4 to 8 weeks apart for two doses, then a third dose 6 to 12 months after the second dose.
Children age 2 to 12 months: 0.5 ml I.M. 4 to 8 weeks apart for three doses, followed by a fourth dose of 0.5 ml, 6 to 12 months after the third dose. Booster dosage, 0.5 ml I.M. q 5 to 10 years.
Primary immunization (fluid formulation)
Adults and children: 0.5 ml I.M. or S.C. 4 to 8 weeks apart for three doses, then a fourth dose 6 to 12 months after the third dose. Booster dosage, 0.5 ml I.M. or S.C. q 10 years.

Pharmacodynamics
Tetanus prophylaxis action: Tetanus toxoid promotes active immunity by inducing production of tetanus antitoxin.

Pharmacokinetics
Absorption: Absorbed slowly. Fluid formulation provides quicker booster effect.
Distribution: Unknown.
Metabolism: Unknown.
Excretion: Unknown. Active immunity usually persists for 10 years. Adsorbed tetanus toxoid usually produces more persistent antitoxin titers than fluid tetanus toxoid.

Route	Onset	Peak	Duration
I.M., S.C.	2 doses	Unknown	>10 yr

Contraindications and precautions
Contraindicated in immunosuppressed patients and in those with immunoglobulin abnormalities or severe hypersensitivity or neurologic reactions to the toxoid or its ingredients such as thimerosal.

Also contraindicated in patients with thrombocytopenia or any coagulation disorder that would contraindicate I.M. injection unless the potential benefits outweigh the risks. Defer vaccination in patients with acute illness and during polio outbreaks, except in emergencies.

Use absorbed form cautiously in infants or children with cerebral damage, neurologic disorders, or history of febrile seizures.

Interactions

Drug-drug. *Chloramphenicol, corticosteroids, immunosuppressants:* May impair the immune response to tetanus toxoid. Avoid concomitant elective immunization.

Effects on diagnostic tests

None reported.

Adverse reactions

CV: *tachycardia, hypotension.*
Skin: urticaria, pruritus, erythema, induration, nodule (at injection site).
Other: slight fever, chills, headache, ***seizure,*** malaise, aches and pains, flushing, ***anaphylaxis.***

Overdose and treatment

None reported.

Clinical considerations

- Adsorbed toxoids induce higher antitoxin titers and more persistent antitoxin levels. Therefore, adsorbed tetanus toxoid is strongly recommended over fluid tetanus toxoid for primary and booster immunizations.
- Have epinephrine 1:1,000 solution available to treat allergic reactions.
- Don't confuse drug with tetanus immune globulin.
- Store at 36° to 46° F (2° to 8° C). Don't freeze.

Therapeutic monitoring

Monitor for hypersensitivity reactions, seizures and injection site reactions.

Special populations

Pregnant patients. Although there's no evidence of teratogenicity, it's recommended that administration be deferred until second trimester.

Breast-feeding patients. It isn't known if tetanus toxoid is excreted in breast milk. Use with caution in breast-feeding women.

Geriatric patients. Geriatric patients develop lower to normal antitoxin levels following tetanus immunization than younger patients. Therefore, skin test responsiveness may be delayed or reduced in the population.

Patient counseling

- Inform patient of possible adverse reactions.
- Encourage patient to report distressing adverse reactions.
- Tell patient that immunization requires a series of injections. Stress the importance of keeping scheduled appointments for subsequent doses.

tetracycline hydrochloride

Achromycin, Ala-Tet, Novotetra*, Robitet, Sumycin, Teline, Tetralan*, Topicycline

Pharmacologic classification: tetracycline
Therapeutic classification: antibiotic
Pregnancy risk category D (B for topical form)

How supplied

Available by prescription only
Capsules: 100 mg, 250 mg, 500 mg
Tablets: 250 mg, 500 mg
Suspension: 125 mg/5 ml
Available without a prescription
Topical ointment: 3%

Indications and dosages

Infections caused by sensitive organisms
Adults: 1 to 2 g P.O. divided into two to four doses.
Children over age 8: 25 to 50 mg/kg P.O. daily, divided into two to four doses.
***Uncomplicated urethral, endocervical, or rectal infection caused by* Chlamydia trachomatis**
Adults: 500 mg P.O. q.i.d. for at least 7 days.
Brucellosis
Adults: 500 mg P.O. q 6 hours for 3 weeks with streptomycin 1 g I.M. q 12 hours week 1, then once daily during week 2.
Gonorrhea in patients sensitive to penicillin
Adults: Initially, 1.5 g P.O.; then 500 mg q 6 hours for 4 days.
Syphilis in nonpregnant patients sensitive to penicillin
Adults: 500 mg P.O. q.i.d. for 14 days.
Acne
Adults and adolescents: Initially, 500 to 1,000 mg P.O. divided q.i.d.; then 125 to 500 mg P.O. daily or every other day; apply topical ointment generously to affected areas b.i.d. until skin is thoroughly wet.
◇***Lyme disease***
Adults: 250 to 500 mg P.O. q.i.d. for 10 to 30 days.
◇***Acute transmitted epididymitis (children over age 9);*** ◇***pelvic inflammatory disease;*** ◇***infection with* Helicobacter pylori *(all these indications use tetracycline as adjunctive therapy)***
Adults: 500 mg P.O. q.i.d. for 10 to 14 days.

Infection prophylaxis in minor skin abrasions and treatment of superficial infections caused by susceptible organisms
Adults and children: Apply topical ointment to infected area one to five times daily.

Pharmacodynamics

Antibacterial action: Tetracycline is bacteriostatic; it binds reversibly to ribosomal subunits, inhibiting bacterial protein synthesis. Its spectrum of action includes many gram-negative and gram-positive organisms, *Mycoplasma, Rickettsia, Chlamydia,* and spirochetes.

Tetracycline is useful against brucellosis, glanders, mycoplasma pneumonia infections (some clinicians prefer erythromycin), leptospirosis, early stages of Lyme disease, rickettsial infections (such as Rocky Mountain spotted fever, Q fever, and typhus fever), and chlamydial infections. It's an alternative to penicillin for infection with *Neisseria gonorrhoeae,* but because of a high level of resistance in the United States, other alternative agents should be considered.

Pharmacokinetics

Absorption: 75% to 80% absorbed after oral administration. Food or milk products significantly reduce oral absorption.
Distribution: Widely distributed into body tissues and fluids, including synovial, pleural, prostatic, and seminal fluids, bronchial secretions, saliva, and aqueous humor; CSF penetration is poor. Drug crosses the placenta, and is 20% to 67% protein-bound.
Metabolism: Not metabolized.
Excretion: Excreted primarily unchanged in urine by glomerular filtration; plasma half-life is 6 to 12 hours in adults with normal renal function. Some drug is excreted in breast milk. Only minimal amounts of tetracycline are removed by hemodialysis or peritoneal dialysis.

Route	Onset	Peak	Duration
P.O.	Unknown	2-4 hr	Unknown
Topical	Unknown	Unknown	Unknown

Contraindications and precautions

Contraindicated in patients with hypersensitivity to tetracyclines. Use cautiously in patients with impaired renal or hepatic function. Use oral form cautiously in last half of pregnancy and in children under age 8.

Interactions

Drug-drug. *Antacids containing aluminum, calcium, magnesium; laxatives containing magnesium, oral iron, sodium bicarbonate:* Decreased absorption of tetracycline. Avoid use together.
Anticoagulants: Enhanced anticoagulation effects; monitor effects closely. Dose adjustment may be needed.
Cimetidine: May decrease GI absorption of tetracycline. Avoid use together.
Digoxin: Because of increased bioavailability, dose adjustment may be needed. Monitor patient closely.
Methoxyflurane: Increases risk of nephrotoxicity. Avoid use together.
Oral contraceptives: Decreased contraceptive effect. Advise patient to use another contraceptive method.
Penicillin: Inhibited cell growth from bacteriostatic action. Give penicillin 2 to 3 hours before tetracycline.
Drug-food. *Milk, dairy products, and other foods:* Decreased antibiotic absorption. Give antibiotic 1 hour before or 2 hours after ingesting such foods.
Drug-lifestyle. *Sun exposure:* Enhanced photosensitivity reactions. Advise patient to take precautions.

Effects on diagnostic tests

Tetracycline causes false-negative results in urine tests using glucose oxidase reagent (Diastix, Chemstrip uG, or glucose enzymatic test strip) and false elevations in fluorometric tests for urinary catecholamines.

Adverse reactions

Unless otherwise noted, the following adverse reactions refer to oral form of drug.
CNS: dizziness, headache, ***intracranial hypertension (pseudotumor cerebri).***
CV: ***cardiac arrest, arrhythmias,*** pericarditis.
EENT: sore throat, glossitis, dysphagia.
GI: anorexia, *epigastric distress, nausea,* vomiting, *diarrhea,* esophagitis, oral candidiasis, stomatitis, enterocolitis, inflammatory lesions in anogenital region.
GU: elevated BUN levels.
Hematologic: ***neutropenia,*** eosinophilia, ***thrombocytopenia.***
Hepatic: elevated liver enzymes.
Skin: *candidal superinfection, maculopapular and erythematous rashes, urticaria, photosensitivity, increased pigmentation;* temporary stinging or burning on application; slight yellowing of treated skin, especially in patients with light complexions; severe dermatitis (with topical administration).
Other: ***anaphylactoid reactions, status asthmaticus, respiratory arrest,*** *hypersensitivity reactions, permanent discoloration of teeth, enamel defects,* and *retardation of bone growth* when used in children under age 8.

Overdose and treatment

Signs of overdose are usually limited to GI tract; give antacids or empty stomach by gastric lavage if ingestion occurs within the preceding 4 hours.

Clinical considerations

Consider the recommendations relevant to all tetracyclines as well as the following:

□ ***ALERT*** Check expiration date. Outdated or deteriorated tetracyclines have been associated with reversible nephrotoxicity (Fanconi's syndrome).

Topical use

- Avoid contact with eyes, nose, and mouth.

Therapeutic monitoring

- Monitor patient for hypersensitivity reactions.
- Monitor for resolution of symptoms.
- Discontinue use if condition persists or worsens.

Special populations

Pregnant patients. Drug causes fetal harm and should be administered during pregnancy only when expected benefits justify risk to fetus.

Breast-feeding patients. Because drug is excreted in breast milk, don't use in breast-feeding women.

Pediatric patients. Don't use in children under age 8.

Patient counseling

- Inform patient using topical form that normal use of cosmetics may continue.
- Tell patient that stinging may occur with topical use but resolves quickly.
- Inform patient that tetracycline may stain clothing.
- Warn patient to avoid prolonged exposure to sunlight.
- Tell patient to report persistent nausea or vomiting, or yellowing of skin or eyes.

tetrahydrozoline hydrochloride

Collyrium Fresh, Eyesine, Geneye, Mallazine Eye Drops, Murine Plus, Optigene 3, Tetrasine, Tyzine, Tyzine Pediatric, Visine

Pharmacologic classification: sympathomimetic
Therapeutic classification: vasoconstrictor, decongestant
Pregnancy risk category C

How supplied

Available by prescription only
Nasal solution: 0.05%, 0.1%
Available without a prescription
Ophthalmic solution: 0.05%

Indications and dosages

Nasal congestion

Adults and children over age 6: Apply 2 to 4 drops in each nostril t.i.d. or q.i.d., p.r.n., or 3 to 4 sprays of 0.1% nasal solution in each nostril q.i.d., p.r.n.

Children age 2 to 6: Apply 2 or 3 drops of 0.05% solution in each nostril q 4 to 6 hours, p.r.n.

Conjunctival congestion

Adults: 1 or 2 drops of ophthalmic solution in each eye b.i.d. to q.i.d.

Pharmacodynamics

Decongestant action: In ocular use, vasoconstriction is produced by local adrenergic action on the blood vessels of the conjunctiva. After nasal application, drug acts on alpha-adrenergic receptors in nasal mucosa to produce constriction, decreasing blood flow and nasal congestion.

Pharmacokinetics

None reported.

Route	Onset	Peak	Duration
Ophthalmic	Few min	Unknown	1-4 hr

Contraindications and precautions

Contraindicated in patients hypersensitive to drug or its components and in those with angle-closure glaucoma or other serious eye diseases and in patients on MAO inhibitor therapy. Nasal solution is contraindicated in children under age 2; 0.1% solution is contraindicated in children under age 6.

Use cautiously in patients with hyperthyroidism, hypertension, and diabetes mellitus. Use ophthalmic form cautiously in patients with cardiac disease.

Interactions

Drug-drug. *Guanethidine, MAO inhibitors, tricyclic antidepressants:* Increased adrenergic response and hypertensive crisis. Avoid use together.

Effects on diagnostic tests

None reported.

Adverse reactions

CNS: headache, drowsiness, insomnia, dizziness, tremor (with ophthalmic form).
CV: ***arrhythmias*** (with ophthalmic form), tachycardia, palpitations.
EENT: transient eye stinging, pupillary dilation, increased intraocular pressure, keratitis, lacrimation, eye irritation (with ophthalmic form); transient burning, stinging; sneezing, rebound nasal congestion with excessive or long-term use (with nasal form).

Overdose and treatment

Signs and symptoms of accidental overdose include bradycardia, decreased body temperature, shocklike hypotension, apnea, drowsiness, CNS depression, and coma.

Because of rapid onset of sedation, emesis isn't recommended unless induced early. Activated charcoal or gastric lavage may be used initially. Monitor vital signs and ECG. Treat seizures with I.V. diazepam.

Clinical considerations

- Excessive use of either preparation may cause rebound effect.
- Drug shouldn't be used for more than 3 to 4 days.
- Don't use in geriatric patients to treat redness and inflammation, which may represent more serious eye conditions.
- Use in glaucoma requires close medical supervision.

Therapeutic monitoring

- Monitor cardiac status (ophthalmic solution only).
- Monitor for resolution of symptoms.

Special populations

Pregnant patients. It isn't known if drug causes fetal harm. Administer drug during pregnancy only when clearly indicated.
Pediatric patients. The 0.1% nasal solution is contraindicated in children under age 6. All uses are contraindicated in children under age 2.
Geriatric patients. Geriatric patients are more likely to experience adverse reactions to sympathomimetics.

Patient counseling

- Instruct patient on proper administration technique.
- Advise patient not to exceed recommended dose and to use drug only when needed.
- Tell patient to remove contact lenses before using drug.

thalidomide

Thalomid

Pharmacologic classification: immunomodulator
Therapeutic classification: leprosy agent
Pregnancy risk category X

How supplied

Available by prescription only
Capsules: 50 mg

Indications and dosages

Acute treatment of cutaneous manifestations of moderate-to-severe erythema nodosum leprosum (ENL)
Adults: 100 to 300 mg P.O. daily h.s. If patient weighs less than 110 lb (50 kg), start dosing at the lower end of range.

Maintenance therapy for prevention and suppression of the cutaneous manifestations of ENL recurrence
Adults: Up to 400 mg P.O. daily h.s. or in divided doses at least 1 hour after meals.

Pharmacodynamics

An immunomodulatory agent whose mechanism of action in patients with ENL isn't fully elucidated.

Pharmacokinetics

Absorption: Slowly absorbed from GI tract.
Distribution: Not reported.
Metabolism: Exact metabolic fate isn't known.
Excretion: Mean half-life is 5 to 7 hours. Route of elimination isn't fully understood.

Route	Onset	Peak	Duration
P.O.	Unknown	3-6 hr	Unknown

Contraindications and precautions

Contraindicated in patients hypersensitive to drug or its components; in pregnant women, and in those capable of becoming pregnant, except when alternative therapies are inappropriate and patient meets all conditions listed in the System for Thalidomide Education and Prescribing Safety (S.T.E.P.S.) program.

Interactions

Drug-drug. *Barbiturates, chlorpromazine, reserpine:* Can enhance sedative activity. Use together with caution.
Medications associated with peripheral neuropathy: Pose an increased risk of peripheral neuropathy. Use together cautiously.
Drug-food. *Any food:* Decreases absorption of drug. Give drug at least 1 hour after meals at h.s.
Drug-lifestyle. *Alcohol use:* Increased sedation. Caution patient against using together.

Effects on diagnostic tests

None reported.

Adverse reactions

CNS: *asthenia, drowsiness, somnolence, dizziness,* peripheral neuropathy, *headache,* agitation, insomnia, malaise, nervousness, *paresthesia,* tremor, vertigo.
CV: orthostatic hypotension, *bradycardia,* peripheral edema.
EENT: dry mouth, oral candidiasis, pharyngitis, sinusitis.
GI: abdominal pain, anorexia, constipation, *diarrhea,* flatulence, *nausea.*
GU: albuminuria, *hematuria,* impotence.
Hematologic: ***neutropenia, increased HIV viral load,*** anemia, *lymphadenopathy,* LEUKOPENIA.
Hepatic: abnormal liver function tests, increased AST.

Musculoskeletal: back pain, neck pain, neck rigidity.
Skin: acne, fungal dermatitis, nail disorder, pruritus, *rash*, ***maculopapular rash***, *sweating*.
Other: ***human teratogenicity, hypersensitivity reactions,*** facial edema, hyperlipidemia, lymphadenopathy, fever, chills, accidental injury, infection, pain.

Overdose and treatment

There have been three reported cases of overdose, none of which resulted in fatality.

Clinical considerations

☐ ***ALERT*** Thalidomide must only be administered in compliance with all of the terms outlined in the S.T.E.P.S. program; may only be prescribed by doctors registered with the S.T.E.P.S. program; and may only be dispensed by pharmacists registered with the S.T.E.P.S. program.

- All sexually mature patients, men or women, capable of reproduction must meet rigid S.T.E.P.S. program requirements including ability to understand and carry out instructions, ability and willingness to comply with mandatory contraceptive measures (concurrent use of at least two highly effective means of contraception), and a written acknowledgment of understanding of all warnings concerning the hazards of fetal exposure to thalidomide and the risk of contraception failure.
- Sexually mature women who haven't undergone a hysterectomy or who haven't been postmenopausal for at least 24 consecutive months (who have had menses at some time in the preceding 24 consecutive months) are considered to be women of childbearing potential even with history of infertility.
- Pregnancy test is mandatory within 24 hours before thalidomide therapy for women of childbearing potential, then weekly during first month of therapy, then monthly for women with regular menstrual cycles. If menstrual cycles are irregular, pregnancy testing continues every 2 weeks during therapy. Retesting is performed if menstrual changes occur, including missed menses.
- Corticosteroids may be administered with drug in patients with moderate-to-severe neuritis associated with severe ENL reaction. Corticosteroids can be tapered and discontinued when neuritis improves.
- A patient with a history of requiring prolonged treatment to prevent recurrence of cutaneous ENL or who experiences flare during tapering, should use minimum effective dose. Tapering should be attempted every 3 to 6 months at a dose reduction rate of 50 mg every 2 to 4 weeks.

Therapeutic monitoring

- Report immediately suspected fetal exposure to FDA via MedWATCH at 1-800-FDA-1088 and report to manufacturer.
- Perform CBC and differential before initiating therapy and periodically thereafter, as ordered. Patients with an absolute neutrophil count going below 750/mm^2 while on treatment should be reevaluated.
- Monitor patient for signs and symptoms of neuropathy, such as numbness, tingling, or pain in hands or feet, at least once monthly during first 3 months of drug therapy, then periodically.

Special populations

Pregnant patients. Drug is highly dangerous to fetus in any amount. At least two highly reliable means of contraception must be used simultaneously and continuously from at least 1 month before thalidomide therapy until 1 month following completion of therapy.
Breast-feeding patients. It isn't known if drug is excreted in breast milk. Either the drug or nursing should be discontinued, depending on the importance of the drug to the woman.
Pediatric patients. Safety and efficacy in children under age 12 aren't known.
Geriatric patients. Safety and efficacy in geriatric patients aren't significantly different from use in younger patients.

Patient counseling

- Warn patient of dangers of fetal exposure to any amount of thalidomide and that blood and sperm donations are prohibited while taking thalidomide.
- Explain that at least two highly reliable means of contraception must be used simultaneously and continuously from at least 1 month before thalidomide therapy until 1 month following completion of therapy.
- Instruct patient to report signs or symptoms of pregnancy immediately without regard to probability or improbability of pregnancy.
- Inform women with childbearing potential of mandatory pregnancy testing schedule.
- Inform patient that if pregnancy occurs, drug must be discontinued immediately.
- Caution patient that it isn't known if drug is present in ejaculate of men receiving drug, and that men receiving thalidomide must always use a latex condom when engaging in sexual activity with women of childbearing potential.
- Advise patient to read package insert carefully.
- Caution patient about potential for dizziness and orthostatic hypotension; instruct patient to change position slowly when rising.
- Inform patient that drug frequently causes drowsiness and somnolence. Advise patient to avoid hazardous activities and the use of alcohol or other medications that might cause drowsiness.
- Tell patient to take drug at bedtime with a glass of water, at least 1 hour after the evening meal.

■ Tell patient drug has caused hypersensitivity reactions and to notify his doctor if erythematous macular rash, fever, tachycardia, and hypotension, or any other adverse reactions occur.

theophylline

Accurbron, Aerolate, Aquaphyllin, Asmalix, Bronkodyl, Constant-T, Elixophyllin, Lanophyllin, Quibron-T, Respbid, Slo-bid Gyrocaps, Slo-Phyllin, Sustaire, Theobid Duracaps, Theochron, Theoclear-80, Theo-Dur, Theolair, Theo-Sav, Theo-24, Theospan-SR, Theostat 80, Theovent, Theo-X, T-Phyl, Uniphyl

Pharmacologic classification: xanthine derivative
Therapeutic classification: bronchodilator
Pregnancy risk category C

How supplied

Available by prescription only
Capsules: 100 mg, 200 mg
Capsules (extended-release): 50 mg, 60 mg, 65 mg, 75 mg, 100 mg, 125 mg, 130 mg, 200 mg, 250 mg, 260 mg, 300 mg
Tablets: 100 mg, 125 mg, 200 mg, 250 mg, 300 mg
Tablets (extended-release): 100 mg, 200 mg, 250 mg, 300 mg, 400 mg, 450 mg, 500 mg
Elixir: 50 mg/5 ml, 80 mg/15 ml
Syrup: 50 mg/5 ml, 80 mg/15 ml, 150 mg/15 ml
Dextrose 5% injection: 200 mg in 50 ml or 100 ml; 400 mg in 100 ml, 250 ml, 500 ml, or 1,000 ml; 800 mg in 500 ml or 1,000 ml

Indications and dosages

Symptomatic relief of bronchospasm in patients not currently receiving theophylline who require rapid relief of acute symptoms
Loading dose: 6 mg/kg anhydrous theophylline, then:
Adults (nonsmokers): 3 mg/kg P.O. q 6 hours for two doses; then 3 mg/kg q 8 hours.
Older adults with cor pulmonale: 2 mg/kg P.O. q 6 hours for two doses; then 2 mg/kg q 8 hours.
Adults with heart failure: 2 mg/kg P.O. q 8 hours for two doses; then 1 to 2 mg/kg q 12 hours.
Children and adolescents age 9 to 16 and young adult smokers: 3 mg/kg P.O. q 4 hours for three doses; then 3 mg/kg q 6 hours.
Neonates and children age 6 months to 9 years: 4 mg/kg P.O. q 4 hours for three doses; then 4 mg/kg q 6 hours.
◇*Neonates and infants under age 6 months:* Dose highly individualized. Serum theophylline levels should be maintained at less than 10 mcg/ml in neonates and less than 20 mcg/ml in older infants.
Loading dose: 1 mg/kg P.O. or I.V. for each 2 mcg/ml increase in theophylline level, then:
Infants age 8 weeks to 6 months: 1 to 3 mg/kg q 6 hours.
Infants age 4 to 8 weeks: 1 to 2 mg/kg q 8 hours.
Neonates up to age 4 weeks: 1 to 2 mg/kg q 12 hours.
Premature neonates (less than 40 weeks' gestational age): 1 mg/kg q 12 hours.
Parenteral theophylline for patients not currently receiving theophylline
Loading dose: 4.7 mg/kg (equivalent to 6 mg/kg anhydrous aminophylline) I.V. slowly; then maintenance infusion.
Adults (nonsmokers): 0.55 mg/kg/hour (equivalent to 0.7 mg/kg/hour anhydrous aminophylline) for 12 hours, then 0.39 mg/kg/hour (equivalent to 0.5 mg/kg/hour anhydrous aminophylline).
Older adults with cor pulmonale: 0.47 mg/kg/hour (equivalent to 0.6 mg/kg/hour anhydrous aminophylline) for 12 hours; then 0.24 mg/kg/hour (equivalent to 0.3 mg/kg/hour anhydrous aminophylline).
Adults with heart failure or liver disease: 0.39 mg/kg/hour (equivalent to 0.5 mg/kg/hour anhydrous aminophylline) for 12 hours; then 0.08 to 0.16 mg/kg/hour (equivalent to 0.1 to 0.2 mg/kg/ hour anhydrous aminophylline).
Children age 9 to 16: 0.79 mg/kg/hour (equivalent to 1 mg/kg/hour anhydrous aminophylline) for 12 hours; then 0.63 mg/kg/hour (equivalent to 0.8 mg/kg/hour anhydrous aminophylline).
Infants and children age 6 months to 9 years: 0.95 mg/kg/hour (equivalent to 1.2 mg/kg/hour anhydrous aminophylline) for 12 hours; then 0.79 mg/kg/hour (equivalent to 1 mg/kg/hour anhydrous aminophylline).
Switch to oral theophylline as soon as patient shows adequate improvement.
Symptomatic relief of bronchospasm in patients currently receiving theophylline
Adults and children: Each 0.5 mg/kg I.V. or P.O. (loading dose) increases plasma levels by 1 mcg/ml. Ideally, dose is based on current theophylline level and lean body weight. In emergency situations, may use a 2.5 mg/kg P.O. dose of rapidly absorbed form if no obvious signs of theophylline toxicity are present.
Prophylaxis of bronchial asthma, bronchospasm of chronic bronchitis, and emphysema
Adults and children: Using rapidly absorbed dose forms, initial dose is 16 mg/kg or 400 mg P.O. daily (whichever is less) divided q 6 to 8 hours; dose may be increased in approximate increments of 25% at 2- to 3-day intervals. Using extended-release dose forms, initial dose is 12 mg/kg or 400 mg P.O. daily (whichever is less) divided q 8 to 12 hours; dose may be increased, if tolerated, by 2 to 3 mg/kg daily at 3-

day intervals. Regardless of dose form used, dose may be increased, if tolerated, up to the following maximum daily doses, without measurements of serum theophylline level.
Adults and adolescents age 16 and older: 13 mg/kg P.O. or 900 mg P.O. daily in divided doses.
Adolescents age 12 to 16: 18 mg/kg P.O. daily in divided doses.
Children age 9 to 12: 20 mg/kg P.O. daily in divided doses.
Children under age 9: 24 mg/kg P.O. daily in divided doses.

Note: Dose individualization is required. Use peak plasma and trough levels to estimate dose. Therapeutic range is 10 to 20 mcg/ml. All doses are based on theophylline anhydrous and lean body weight.

◇ Cystic fibrosis
Infants: 10 to 20 mg/kg I.V. daily.
◇ Promotion of diuresis; ◇ treatment of Cheyne-Stokes respirations; ◇ paroxysmal nocturnal dyspnea
Adults: 200 to 400 mg I.V. bolus (single dose).

Pharmacodynamics

Bronchodilator action: Drug may act by inhibiting phosphodiesterase, elevating cellular cyclic AMP levels, or antagonizing adenosine receptors in the bronchi, resulting in relaxation of the smooth muscle.

Drug also increases sensitivity of the medullary respiratory center to carbon dioxide, to reduce apneic episodes. It prevents muscle fatigue, especially that of the diaphragm. It also causes diuresis and cardiac and CNS stimulation.

Pharmacokinetics

Absorption: Well absorbed. Rate and onset of action depend on the dose form; food may further alter rate of absorption, especially of some extended release preparations.
Distribution: Distributed throughout the extracellular fluids; equilibrium between fluid and tissues occurs within an hour of an I.V. loading dose. Therapeutic plasma levels are 10 to 20 mcg/ml, but many patients respond to lower levels.
Metabolism: Metabolized in the liver to inactive compounds. Half-life is 7 to 9 hours in adults, 4 to 5 hours in smokers, 20 to 30 hours in premature infants, and 3 to 5 hours in children.
Excretion: About 10% of dose is excreted in urine unchanged. The other metabolites include 1,3-dimethyluric acid, 1-methyluric acid, and 3-methylxanthine.

Route	Onset	Peak	Duration
P.O.	15-60 min	1-2 hr	Unknown
P.O. (extended)	15-60 min	4-7 hr	Unknown
I.V.	15 min	15-30 min	Unknown

Contraindications and precautions

Contraindicated in patients with hypersensitivity to xanthine compounds, such as caffeine and theobromine, and in those with active peptic ulcer and seizure disorders.

Use cautiously in the elderly; in neonates, infants under age 1, and young children; and in patients with COPD, cardiac failure, cor pulmonale, renal or hepatic disease, peptic ulcer, hyperthyroidism, diabetes mellitus, glaucoma, severe hypoxemia, hypertension, compromised cardiac or circulatory function, angina, acute MI, or sulfite sensitivity.

Interactions

Drug-drug. *Allopurinol (high dose), calcium channel blockers, cimetidine, corticosteroids, erythromycin, interferon, mexiletine, oral contraceptives, propranolol, quinolones, troleandomycin:* May increase serum levels of theophylline. Monitor patient closely. Dose adjustment may be needed if use together can't be avoided.
Activated charcoal, barbiturates, ketoconazole, phenytoin, rifampin: Decreased plasma theophylline levels. Monitor patient closely. Dose adjustment may be needed if use together can't be avoided.
Beta blockers: Exert an antagonistic pharmacologic effect. Avoid use together.
Carbamazapine, isoniazid, loop diuretics: May increase or decrease theophylline levels. Monitor patient closely. Dose adjustment may be needed if use together can't be avoided.
Lithium: Increased excretion of lithium. Lithium dose may require adjustment. Monitor patient carefully.
Drug-herb. *Cacao tree:* Possible inhibition of theophylline metabolism. Patient should avoid ingesting large amounts of cocoa when using theophylline.
Guarana, caffeine: Additive CNS and CV effects. Avoid use together.
Drug-food. *Any food:* Accelerates absorption. Advise patient to take drug on an empty stomach.
Drug-lifestyle. *Smoking (cigarettes, marijuana):* Increases elimination of theophylline. Monitor theophylline response and serum levels. Dose adjustment may be required.

Effects on diagnostic tests

Depending on assay used, theophylline levels may be falsely elevated in the presence of furosemide, phenylbutazone, probenecid, theobromine, caffeine, tea, chocolate, cola beverages, and acetaminophen.

Adverse reactions

CNS: *restlessness, dizziness, insomnia,* headache, irritability, ***seizures,*** muscle twitching.
CV: *palpitations, sinus tachycardia, extrasystoles,* flushing, marked hypotension, ***arrhythmias.***

GI: *nausea, vomiting,* diarrhea, epigastric pain.
Respiratory: tachypnea, ***respiratory arrest.***

Overdose and treatment
Signs and symptoms of overdose include nausea, vomiting, insomnia, irritability, tachycardia, extrasystoles, tachypnea, or tonic-clonic seizures. The onset of toxicity may be sudden and severe, with arrhythmias and seizures as the first signs. Induce emesis except in convulsing patients, then use activated charcoal and cathartics. Treat arrhythmias with lidocaine and seizures with I.V. diazepam; support respiratory and CV systems.

Clinical considerations
- Theophylline has a low therapeutic index.
- Dosage is determined by monitoring response, tolerance, pulmonary function, and serum theophylline levels. Target range is 10 to 20 mcg/ml.
- Use cautiously in young children, infants, neonates and the elderly.

Therapeutic monitoring
- Monitor vital signs and observe for signs and symptoms of toxicity.
- Obtain serum theophylline measurements in patients receiving long-term therapy. Ideal levels are between 10 and 20 mcg/ml, although some patients may respond adequately with lower serum levels. Check every 6 months. If levels are less than 10 mcg/ml, increase dose by about 25% each day. If levels are 20 to 25 mcg/ml, decrease dose by about 10% each day. If levels are 25 to 30 mcg/ml, skip next dose and decrease by 25% each day. If levels are more than 30 mcg/ml, skip next two doses and decrease by 50% each day. Repeat serum level determination.

Special populations
Breast-feeding patients. Drug is excreted in breast milk and may cause irritability, insomnia, or fretfulness in the breast-fed infant. A decision must be made to stop either breast-feeding or drug therapy.
Pediatric patients. Use with caution in neonates. Children usually require higher doses (on a mg/kg basis) than adults. Maximum recommended doses are 24 mg/kg/day in children under age 9; 20 mg/kg/day in children age 9 to 12; 18 mg/kg/day in adolescents age 12 to 16; 13 mg/kg/day or 900 mg (whichever is less) in adolescents and adults age 16 or older.

Patient counseling
- Instruct patient regarding medications and dosing schedule; if a dose is missed, he should take it as soon as possible, but he shouldn't double the dose.
- Advise patient to take drug at regular intervals as instructed, around the clock.
- Inform patient of adverse effects and possible signs of toxicity.
- Tell patient to take drug with food if GI upset occurs with liquid preparations or nonsustained release forms.
- Instruct patient to continue to use the same brand of theophylline.

thiabendazole
Mintezol

Pharmacologic classification: benzimidazole
Therapeutic classification: anthelmintic
Pregnancy risk category C

How supplied
Available by prescription only
Tablets (chewable): 500 mg
Oral suspension: 500 mg/5 ml

Indications and dosages
Systemic infections with pinworm, roundworm, threadworm, whipworm, visceral larva migrans, trichinosis
Adults and children weighing 30 to 154 lb (14 to 70 kg): 25 mg/kg P.O. q 12 hours for 2 successive days.
Adults and children weighing more than 154 lb: 1.5 g P.O. q 12 hours for 2 successive days. Maximum dose, 3 g daily.
Trichinosis—Two doses daily for 2 to 4 successive days.
Visceral larva migrans—Two doses daily for 7 successive days.
Cutaneous infestations with larva migrans (creeping eruption)
Adults and children: 25 mg/kg P.O. b.i.d. for 2 to 5 days. Maximum dose, 3 g daily. If lesions persist after 2 days, repeat course.
◇***Dracunculiasis;*** ◇***infections caused by* Angiostrongylus costaricensis**
Adults: 25 to 37.5 mg/kg P.O. b.i.d. (25 mg t.i.d. for *A. costaricensis*) for 3 successive days.
◇***Capillariasis***
Adults: 25 mg/kg P.O. q 12 hours for 30 days.

Pharmacodynamics
Anthelmintic action: Thiabendazole kills susceptible helminths by inhibiting fumarate reductase. It's the drug of choice for *Strongyloides stercoralis* (threadworm) infections and may be useful in disseminated strongyloidiasis. It's also preferred for oral and topical therapy of *Ancylostoma braziliense*, *Toxocara canis*, and *T. cati.* It has shown activity in certain other nematode infections, but other agents are preferred for the treatment of ascariasis, tricuriasis, uncinariasis, and enterobiasis.

Pharmacokinetics
Absorption: Absorbed readily; peak serum levels occur at 1 to 2 hours.

Distribution: Unknown.
Metabolism: Metabolized almost completely by hydroxylation and conjugation.
Excretion: About 90% of dose is excreted in urine as metabolites within 48 hours; about 5% is excreted in feces.

Route	Onset	Peak	Duration
P.O.	Unknown	1-2 hr	Unknown

Contraindications and precautions

Contraindicated in patients with hypersensitivity to drug. Use cautiously in patients with renal or hepatic dysfunction, severe malnutrition, or anemia and in those who are vomiting.

Interactions

Drug-drug. *Theophylline:* Increased risk of theophylline toxicity. Monitor patient closely.

Effects on diagnostic tests

None reported.

Adverse reactions

CNS: impaired mental alertness, impaired coordination, numbness, ***seizures,*** *drowsiness, fatigue, headache,* giddiness, dizziness.
CV: *hypotension.*
EENT: tinnitus, blurry or yellow vision, dry mouth and eyes, xanthopsia.
GI: *anorexia, nausea, vomiting,* diarrhea, epigastric distress, cholestasis.
GU: hematuria, enuresis, crystalluria, malodorous urine.
Hematologic: ***leukopenia.***
Hepatic: *jaundice,* ***parenchymal liver damage,*** elevations of AST levels.
Metabolic: hyperglycemia.
Skin: *rash, pruritus,* ***erythema multiforme, Stevens-Johnson syndrome.***
Other: lymphadenopathy, fever, flushing, chills, ***angioedema, anaphylaxis.***

Overdose and treatment

Signs of overdose may include visual disturbances and altered mental status. Treatment includes induced emesis or gastric lavage if ingested within 4 hours, followed by supportive and symptomatic treatment.

Clinical considerations

- Drug may be given with milk, fruit juice, or food.
- Assess patient and review laboratory reports for signs of anemia, dehydration, or malnutrition before starting therapy.

Therapeutic monitoring

Monitor patient for adverse reactions, which usually occur 3 to 4 hours after drug is administered. Adverse effects are usually mild and related to dose and duration of therapy.

Special populations

Pregnant patients. Use drug during pregnancy only when potential benefit justifies risk to fetus.
Breast-feeding patients. Safety in breast-feeding women hasn't been established.

Patient counseling

- Warn patient that drug causes drowsiness or dizziness and to avoid driving or other hazardous activities during therapy.
- Instruct patient to promptly report adverse reactions.

thiamine hydrochloride (vitamin B_1)

Biamine, Thiamilate

Pharmacologic classification: water-soluble vitamin
Therapeutic classification: nutritional supplement
Pregnancy risk category A (C if more than RDA)

How supplied

Available by prescription only
Injection: 1-ml ampules (100 mg/ml), 1-ml vials (100 mg/ml), 2-ml vials (100 mg/ml), 10-ml vials (100 mg/ml), 30-ml vials (100 mg/ml).
Available without a prescription
Tablets: 25 mg, 50 mg, 100 mg, 250 mg, 500 mg
Tablets (enteric-coated): 20 mg

Indications and dosages

Beriberi
Adults: 10 to 20 mg I.M., depending on severity (can receive up to 100 mg I.M. or I.V. for severe cases), t.i.d. for 2 weeks, followed by dietary correction and multivitamin supplement containing 5 to 30 mg thiamine daily in single or three divided doses for 1 month.
Children: 10 to 25 mg, depending on severity, I.M. daily for several weeks with adequate dietary intake.
Anemia secondary to thiamine deficiency; polyneuritis secondary to alcoholism, pregnancy, or pellagra
Adults and children: P.O. dosage is based on RDA for age group.
Wernicke's encephalopathy
Adults: Initially, 100 mg I.V., followed by 50 to 100 mg I.M. or I.V. daily.
"Wet beriberi" with heart failure
Adults and children: 10 to 30 mg I.V. for emergency treatment.

Pharmacodynamics

Metabolic action: Exogenous thiamine is required for carbohydrate metabolism. Thiamine combines with ATP to form thiamine pyrophosphate, a coenzyme in carbohydrate metabolism and transketolation reactions. This coenzyme is also necessary in the hexose monophosphate shunt during pentose utilization. One sign of thiamine deficiency is an increase in pyruvic acid. The body's need for thiamine is greater when the carbohydrate content of the diet is high. Within 3 weeks of total absence of dietary thiamine, significant vitamin depletion can occur. Thiamine deficiency can cause beriberi.

Pharmacokinetics
Absorption: Absorbed readily after oral administration of small doses; after oral administration of a large dose, the total amount absorbed is limited to 4 to 8 mg. In alcoholics and in patients with cirrhosis or malabsorption, GI absorption of thiamine is decreased. When given with meals, GI rate of drug absorption decreases, but total absorption remains the same. After I.M. administration, drug is absorbed rapidly and completely.
Distribution: Distributed widely into body tissues. When intake exceeds the minimal requirements, tissue stores become saturated. About 100 to 200 mcg/day of thiamine is distributed into the milk of breast-feeding women on a normal diet.
Metabolism: Metabolized in the liver.
Excretion: Excess thiamine is excreted in urine. After administration of large doses (more than 10 mg), both unchanged thiamine and metabolites are excreted in urine after tissue stores become saturated.

Route	Onset	Peak	Duration
P.O., I.V., I.M.	Unknown	Unknown	Unknown

Contraindications and precautions
Contraindicated in patients hypersensitive to thiamine products.

Interactions
Drug-drug. *Alkaline solutions, such as carbonates, citrates and bicarbonates:* Thiamine shouldn't be used in combination with these agents.
Neuromuscular-blocking agents: May enhance their effects.
Neutral or alkaline solutions: Thiamine is unstable in these solutions.
Sulfites: Solutions containing sulfites are incompatible with thiamine.

Effects on diagnostic tests
Drug therapy may produce false-positive results in the phosphotungstate method for determination of uric acid and in urine spot tests with Ehrlich's reagent for urobilinogen.

Large doses of thiamine interfere with the Schack and Waxler spectrophotometric determination of serum theophylline levels.

Adverse reactions
CNS: restlessness.
CV: ***angioedema, CV collapse,*** cyanosis.
EENT: tightness of throat (allergic reaction).
GI: nausea, ***hemorrhage.***
Respiratory: pulmonary edema.
Skin: feeling of warmth, pruritus, urticaria, diaphoresis.
Other: weakness; tenderness and induration following I.M. administration.

Overdose and treatment
Very large doses of thiamine administered parenterally may produce neuromuscular and ganglionic blockade and neurologic symptoms. Treatment is supportive.

Clinical considerations
- The RDA of thiamine is as follows:

Neonates and infants up to age 6 months: 0.3 mg daily.
Infants age 6 months to 1 year: 0.4 mg daily.
Children age 1 to 3: 0.7 mg daily.
Children age 4 to 6: 0.9 mg daily.
Children age 7 to 10: 1 mg daily.
Males age 11 to 14: 1.3 mg daily.
Males age 15 to 50: 1.5 mg daily.
Men age 51 and older: 1.2 mg daily.
Females age 11 to 50: 1.1 mg daily.
Women age 51 and older: 1 mg daily.
Pregnant women: 1.5 mg daily.
Breast-feeding women: 1.6 mg daily.

- An intradermal skin test should be performed before I.V. thiamine administration if sensitivity is suspected.
- Keep epinephrine available when administering large parenteral doses.
- I.M. injection may be painful. Injection site rotation is recommended.
- Total absence of dietary thiamine can produce a deficiency state in about 3 weeks.
- Accurate dietary history is important during vitamin replacement therapy.
- Store thiamine in light-resistant, nonmetallic container.

Therapeutic monitoring
- Monitor patient for adverse reactions including injection site reactions.
- Monitor patient for symptom relief.

Special populations
Breast-feeding patients. Thiamine, in amounts that don't exceed the RDA, is safe to use in breast-feeding women. It's excreted in breast milk and fulfills a nutritional requirement of the infant.

Patient counseling
Inform patient of potential adverse reactions.

thioguanine (6-thioguanine, 6-TG)

Lanvis*

Pharmacologic classification: antimetabolite (cell cycle-phase specific, S phase)
Therapeutic classification: antineoplastic
Pregnancy risk category D

How supplied

Available by prescription only
Tablets (scored): 40 mg

Indications and dosages

Dosage and indications may vary. Check current literature for recommended protocol.
Acute nonlymphocytic leukemias
Adults and children: Initially, 2 mg/kg/day P.O. (usually calculated to nearest 20 mg); then, if no toxic effects occur, increase dose gradually over 3 to 4 weeks to 3 mg/kg/day. Maintenance dosage, 2 to 3 mg/kg/day P.O.

Pharmacodynamics

Antineoplastic action: Thioguanine requires conversion intracellularly to its active form to exert its cytotoxic activity. Acting as a false metabolite, thioguanine inhibits purine synthesis. Cross-resistance exists between mercaptopurine and thioguanine.

Pharmacokinetics

Absorption: After an oral dose, absorption is incomplete and variable. The average bioavailability is 30%.
Distribution: Well distributed into bone marrow cells. It doesn't cross the blood-brain barrier to any appreciable extent.
Metabolism: Extensively metabolized to a less active form in the liver and other tissues.
Excretion: Plasma levels of thioguanine decrease in a biphasic manner, with a half-life of 15 minutes in the initial phase and 11 hours in the terminal phase. Drug is excreted in the urine, mainly as metabolites.

Route	Onset	Peak	Duration
P.O.	Unknown	Unknown	Unknown

Contraindications and precautions

Contraindicated in patients whose disease has shown resistance to drug and in those who have a known hypersensitivity to drug or mercaptopurine. Use cautiously in patients with renal or hepatic dysfunction.

Interactions

Drug-drug. *Busulfan:* Risk of hepatotoxicity, esophageal varices, portal hypertension. Avoid prolonged use together.

Effects on diagnostic tests

None reported.

Adverse reactions

GI: nausea, vomiting, stomatitis, diarrhea, anorexia.
Hematologic: ***leukopenia, anemia, thrombocytopenia*** (occurs slowly over 2 to 4 weeks).
Hepatic: ***hepatotoxicity,*** jaundice.
Metabolic: hyperuricemia.
Skin: rash.

Overdose and treatment

Signs and symptoms of overdose include myelosuppression, nausea, vomiting, malaise, hypertension, and diaphoresis.

Treatment is usually supportive and includes transfusion of blood components and antiemetics. Induction of emesis may be helpful if performed soon after ingestion.

Clinical considerations

- Total daily dose can be given at one time.
- Dose modification may be required in renal or hepatic dysfunction.
- Drug is sometimes ordered as 6-thioguanine.
- Avoid all I.M. injections when platelet count is less than 100,000/mm^3.

Therapeutic monitoring

- Monitor serum uric acid levels. Alkalinize urine if serum uric acid levels are elevated.
- Monitor liver function tests.
- Watch for jaundice, which may reverse if drug is stopped promptly.
- Conduct CBC daily during induction, then weekly during maintenance therapy.

Special populations

Pregnant patients. Use drug during pregnancy only in life-threatening situations or severe disease for which safer drugs can't be used or are ineffective.
Breast-feeding patients. It isn't known if drug is excreted in breast milk. However, because of risk of serious adverse reactions, mutagenicity, and carcinogenicity in the infant, breast-feeding isn't recommended.

Patient counseling

- Emphasize importance of continuing medication despite occurrence of nausea and vomiting.
- Tell patient to report promptly if vomiting (dose loss) occurs shortly after a dose is taken.
- Advise avoiding exposure to people with infections and to promptly report signs of infection or unusual bleeding.
- Encourage adequate fluid intake to increase urine output and facilitate excretion of uric acid.

thiopental sodium

Pentothal

Pharmacologic classification: barbiturate
Therapeutic classification: anesthetic
Controlled substance schedule III
Pregnancy risk category C

How supplied

Available by prescription only
Injection: 250-mg (2.5%), 400-mg (2% or 2.5%), 500-mg (2.5%) syringes; 500-mg (2.5%), 1-g (2.5%), 2.5-g (2.5%), 5-g (2.5%), 1-g (2%), 2.5-g (2%), 5-g (2%) kits
Rectal suspension: 2-g disposable syringe (400 mg/g of suspension)

Indications and dosages

General anesthetic for short-term procedures
Adults and children: 2 to 4 ml 2.5% solution (50 to 100 mg) administered I.V. for induction and repeated as a maintenance dosage; dose is individualized.
Convulsive states following anesthesia
Adults: 50 to 125 mg (2 to 5 ml 2.5% solution) I.V.
Basal anesthesia by rectal administration
Adults and children: 30 mg/kg P.R.

Pharmacodynamics

Anesthetic action: Thiopental produces anesthesia by direct depression of the polysynaptic midbrain reticular activating system. Thiopental decreases presynaptic (by way of decreased neurotransmitter release) and postsynaptic excitation. These effects may be subsequent to increased gamma-aminobutyric acid (GABA) levels, enhancement of GABA effects, or a direct effect on GABA receptor sites.

Pharmacokinetics

Absorption: Depth of anesthesia may increase for up to 40 seconds. Consciousness returns in 20 to 30 minutes.
Distribution: Distributed throughout the body; highest initial level occurs in vascular areas of the brain, primarily gray matter; drug is 80% protein-bound. Redistribution of drug is primarily responsible for its short duration of action.
Metabolism: Metabolized extensively but slowly in the liver.
Excretion: Unchanged thiopental isn't excreted in significant amounts; duration of action depends on tissue redistribution.

Route	Onset	Peak	Duration
I.V., P.R.	Immediate	10-20 sec	Unknown

Contraindications and precautions

Contraindicated in patients with acute intermittent or variegate porphyria but not in other porphyrias; in those with known hypersensitivity to drug; and whenever general anesthesia is contraindicated. Don't use rectal form in patients with ulcerative, bleeding rectal lesions, or neoplasms of the lower bowel or in those undergoing rectal surgery.

Use with extreme caution in patients with respiratory, cardiac, circulatory, renal, or hepatic dysfunction; severe anemia; shock; myxedema; and status asthmaticus because drug may worsen these conditions. Also use cautiously in patients with hypotension, Addison's disease, myasthenia gravis, or increased intracranial pressure and in breast-feeding women.

Interactions

Drug-drug. *Antihistamines, benzodiazepines, hypnotics, narcotics, phenothiazines, sedatives:* Increased CNS effect. Monitor patient closely.
Drug-lifestyle. *Alcohol use:* Increased CNS depressant effects. Avoid use together.

Effects on diagnostic tests

None reported.

Adverse reactions

CNS: anxiety, restlessness, retrograde amnesia, prolonged somnolence, dose-dependent alteration in EEG patterns.
CV: thrombophlebitis, hypotension, tachycardia, peripheral vascular collapse, ***myocardial depression, arrhythmias.***
GI: nausea and vomiting, abdominal pain; diarrhea, cramping, rectal bleeding (with rectal form).
Respiratory: coughing, sneezing, ***respiratory depression, apnea, laryngospasm, bronchospasm.***
Other: pain, swelling, ulceration, necrosis on extravasation (unlikely at levels less than 2.5%), gangrene after intra-arterial injection, *allergic reactions,* hiccups, shivering, local irritation.

Note: Discontinue drug if peripheral vascular collapse, respiratory arrest, or hypersensitivity occurs.

Overdose and treatment

Signs of overdose include respiratory depression, respiratory arrest, hypotension, and shock. Treat supportively, using mechanical ventilation if needed; give I.V. fluids or vasopressors (dopamine, phenylephrine) for hypotension. Monitor vital signs closely.

Clinical considerations

- Solutions of succinylcholine, tubocurarine, or atropine shouldn't be mixed with thiopental but can be given to the patient at the same time.

▪ A small test dose of 25 to 75 mg may be administered to assess tolerance or unusual sensitivity.

Therapeutic monitoring
Monitor cardiac and respiratory status.

Special populations
Pediatric patients. Use cautiously in children.
Geriatric patients. Lower doses may be indicated in geriatric patients.

thioridazine
Mellaril-S

thioridazine hydrochloride
Apo-Thioridazine*, Mellaril, Novo-Ridazine*, PMS Thioridazine*

Pharmacologic classification: phenothiazine (piperidine derivative)
Therapeutic classification: antipsychotic
Pregnancy risk category C

How supplied
Available by prescription only
Tablets: 10 mg, 15 mg, 25 mg, 50 mg, 100 mg, 150 mg, 200 mg
Oral concentrate: 30 mg/ml, 100 mg/ml (3% to 4.2% alcohol)
Suspension: 25 mg/5 ml, 100 mg/5 ml

Indications and dosages
Psychosis
Adults: Initially, 50 to 100 mg P.O. t.i.d., with gradual increments up to 800 mg daily in divided doses, if needed. Dosage varies.
Dysthymic disorder (neurotic depression), dementia in geriatric patients, behavioral problems in children
Adults: Initially, 25 mg P.O. t.i.d. Maintenance dosage is 20 to 200 mg daily.
Children over age 2: Usually, 0.5 to 3 mg/kg/day P.O. in divided doses. Give 10 mg b.i.d. or t.i.d. to children with moderate disorders and 25 mg b.i.d. or t.i.d. to hospitalized children.

Pharmacodynamics
Antipsychotic action: Thioridazine is thought to exert its antipsychotic effects by postsynaptic blockade of CNS dopamine receptors, inhibiting dopamine-mediated effects.

Thioridazine has many other central and peripheral effects: It produces both alpha and ganglionic blockade and counteracts histamine- and serotonin-mediated activity. Its most prevalent adverse reactions are antimuscarinic and sedative; it causes fewer extrapyramidal effects than other antipsychotics.

Pharmacokinetics
Absorption: Rate and extent of absorption vary with administration route. Oral tablet absorption is erratic and variable, with onset ranging from ½ to 1 hour. Oral concentrates and suspensions are much more predictable.
Distribution: Distributed widely into the body, including breast milk. Steady-state serum level is achieved within 4 to 7 days. Drug is 91% to 99% protein-bound.
Metabolism: Metabolized extensively by the liver and forms the active metabolite mesoridazine.
Excretion: Mostly excreted as metabolites in urine; some is excreted in feces by way of the biliary tract.

Route	Onset	Peak	Duration
P.O.	Unknown	2-4 hr	4-6 hr

Contraindications and precautions
Contraindicated in patients with hypersensitivity to drug or in those experiencing coma, CNS depression, or severe hypertensive or hypotensive cardiac disease.

Use cautiously in geriatric or debilitated patients and in those with hepatic or CV disease, respiratory or seizure disorders, hypocalcemia, severe reactions to insulin or electroconvulsive therapy, and exposure to extreme cold or heat or to organophosphate insecticides.

Interactions
Drug-drug. *Aluminum- and magnesium-containing antacids and antidiarrheals, phenobarbital:* Decreased therapeutic effect. Avoid use together.
Antiparkinsonian agents: Oversedation, paralytic ileus, visual changes, and severe constipation. Monitor patient closely.
Beta blockers: Increased thioridazine plasma levels and toxicity.
Bromocriptine: Antagonized therapeutic effect on prolactin secretion. Monitor patient closely. Dose adjustment may be needed.
Centrally acting antihypertensive drugs, clonidine, guanabenz, guanadrel, guanethidine, methyldopa, reserpine: Inhibited blood pressure response. Monitor patient; dose adjustment may be needed.
CNS depressants, analgesics, barbiturates, narcotics, tranquilizers, anesthetics (general, spinal, or epidural), parenteral magnesium, antiarrhythmic agents, including atropine, disopyramide, quinidine, other anticholinergic drugs, antidepressants, antihistamines, MAO inhibitors, meperidine, phenothiazines: Additive effect. Avoid use together.
Dopamine (high dose): Decreased vasoconstricting effects. Dose may need adjustment; monitor patient closely.
Levodopa: Decreased effectiveness and increased toxicity. Monitor patient carefully.

Lithium: Severe neurologic toxicity with an encephalitis-like syndrome may occur. Avoid use together.
Metrizamide: Increased risk of seizures. Avoid use together.
Nitrates: Hypotension. Monitor patient closely.
Phenytoin: Increased toxicity. Avoid use together.
Procainamide: Increased incidence of arrhythmias and conduction defects. Avoid use together.
Propylthiouracil: Increased risk of agranulocytosis. Monitor patient closely.
Sympathomimetics, epinephrine, ephedrine (commonly found in nasal sprays), phenylephrine, phenylpropanolamine, appetite suppressants: Decreased stimulatory and pressor effects. Monitor patient closely.
Drug-food. *Caffeine:* Increased metabolism of drug. Avoid use together.
Drug-lifestyle. *Alcohol use:* Increased CNS depression. Avoid use together.
Sun exposure: Potentiation of photosensitivity reactions. Advise patient to avoid prolonged or unprotected sun exposure.
Smoking (heavy): Increases metabolism of drug. Advise patient to avoid or limit smoking.

Effects on diagnostic tests
Thioridazine causes false-positive test results for urinary porphyrins, urobilinogen, amylase, and 5-hydroxyindoleacetic acid because of darkening of urine by metabolites; it also causes false-positive urine pregnancy results in tests using human chorionic gonadotropin as the indicator.

Adverse reactions
CNS: extrapyramidal reactions (low incidence), *tardive dyskinesia, sedation* (high incidence), EEG changes, dizziness.
CV: *orthostatic hypotension,* tachycardia, ECG changes.
EENT: *ocular changes, blurred vision,* retinitis pigmentosa.
GI: *dry mouth, constipation.*
GU: *urine retention,* dark urine, menstrual irregularities, gynecomastia, inhibited ejaculation.
Hematologic: ***transient leukopenia, agranulocytosis,*** hyperprolactinemia.
Hepatic: cholestatic jaundice, elevated liver enzymes.
Skin: *mild photosensitivity,* allergic reactions.
Other: weight gain; increased appetite; ***neuroleptic malignant syndrome*** (rare).
After abrupt withdrawal of long-term therapy: gastritis, nausea, vomiting, dizziness, tremor, feeling of warmth or cold, diaphoresis, tachycardia, headache, insomnia.

Overdose and treatment
CNS depression is characterized by deep, unarousable sleep and possible coma, hypotension or hypertension, extrapyramidal symptoms, abnormal involuntary muscle movements, agitation, seizures, arrhythmias, ECG changes, hypothermia or hyperthermia, and autonomic nervous system dysfunction.

Treatment is symptomatic and supportive and includes maintaining vital signs, airway, stable body temperature, and fluid and electrolyte balance.

Don't induce vomiting: Drug inhibits cough reflex, and aspiration may occur. Use gastric lavage, then activated charcoal and sodium chloride cathartics; dialysis doesn't help. Regulate body temperature as needed. Treat hypotension with I.V. fluids: Don't give epinephrine. Treat seizures with parenteral diazepam or barbiturates; arrhythmias with parenteral phenytoin (1 mg/kg with rate adjusted to blood pressure); and extrapyramidal reactions with benztropine at 1 to 2 mg or parenteral diphenhydramine at 10 to 50 mg. Contact local or regional poison information center for specific instructions.

Clinical considerations
Consider the recommendations relevant to all phenothiazines as well as the following:
☐ ***ALERT*** Different liquid formulations have different concentrations. Check dosage carefully.
- Doses of more than 300 mg/day are usually reserved for adults with severe psychosis. Don't exceed 800 mg daily because ophthalmic toxicity may result.
- Liquid formulations may cause a rash if skin contact occurs.
- Drug can cause pink to brown discoloration of patient's urine.
- Thioridazine is associated with a high incidence of sedation, anticholinergic effects, orthostatic hypotension, photosensitivity reactions, and delayed or absent ejaculation. It has the lowest potential for extrapyramidal reactions of all phenothiazines.
- Oral formulations may cause stomach upset. Administer with food or fluid.
- Concentrate must be diluted in 2 to 4 oz (60 to 120 ml) of liquid, preferably water, carbonated drinks, fruit juice, tomato juice, milk, or pudding.
- All liquid formulations must be protected from light.

Therapeutic monitoring
Check patient regularly for abnormal body movements (at least once every 6 months).

Special populations
Breast-feeding patients. Thioridazine may enter breast milk. Potential benefits to the woman should outweigh the potential harm to the infant.

Pediatric patients. Drug isn't recommended for children under age 2. For children over age 2, dosage is 1 mg/kg/day in divided doses.
Geriatric patients. Geriatric patients tend to require lower doses, adjusted to individual response. Such patients also are more likely to develop adverse reactions, especially tardive dyskinesia and other extrapyramidal effects.

Patient counseling

- Explain risks of dystonic reactions and tardive dyskinesia, and tell patient to report abnormal body movements.
- Tell patient to avoid sun exposure and to wear sunscreen when going outdoors to prevent photosensitivity reactions. (Heat lamps and tanning beds also may cause burning of the skin or skin discoloration.)
- Warn patient not to spill the liquid on the skin; rash and irritation may result.
- Warn patient to avoid extremely hot or cold baths or exposure to temperature extremes, sunlamps, or tanning beds; drug may cause thermoregulatory changes.
- Advise patient to take drug exactly as prescribed and not to double doses that are missed.
- Explain that many drug interactions are possible. Patient should seek medical approval before taking any self-prescribed medication.
- Tell patient not to stop taking drug suddenly; most adverse reactions may be relieved by dose reduction. However, patient should call his doctor if difficulty urinating, sore throat, dizziness or fainting, or if visual changes develop.
- Warn patient to avoid hazardous activities that require alertness until the effect of drug is established. Reassure patient that excessive sedation usually subsides after several weeks.
- Tell patient not to drink alcohol or take other medications that may cause excessive sedation.
- Advise patient to maintain adequate hydration.
- Explain which fluids are appropriate for diluting the concentrate and the dropper technique of measuring dose.
- Tell patient to store drug safely away from children.

thiotepa

Thioplex

Pharmacologic classification: alkylating (cell cycle-phase nonspecific)
Therapeutic classification: antineoplastic
Pregnancy risk category D

How supplied

Available by prescription only
Injection: 15-mg vials

Indications and dosages

Dosage and indications may vary. Check current literature for recommended protocol.
Breast and ovarian cancer, Hodgkin's disease, lymphomas
Adults and adolescents age 12 and older: 0.2 mg/kg I.V. daily for 4 to 5 days, repeated q 2 to 4 weeks; or 0.3 to 0.4 mg/kg I.V. q 1 to 4 weeks.
Bladder tumor
Adults and adolescents age 12 and older: 60 mg in 30 to 60 ml of normal saline solution (thiotepa in distilled water) instilled in bladder once weekly for 4 weeks.
Neoplastic effusions
Adults and adolescents age 12 and over: 0.6 to 0.8 mg/kg intracavity or intratumor q 1 to 4 weeks.
◇***Malignant meningeal neoplasm***
Adults: 1 to 10 mg/m^2 intrathecally, once to twice weekly.

Pharmacodynamics

Antineoplastic action: Thiotepa exerts its cytotoxic activity as an alkylating agent, cross-linking strands of DNA and RNA and inhibiting protein synthesis, resulting in cell death.

Pharmacokinetics

Absorption: Incompletely absorbed across the GI tract; absorption from the bladder is variable, ranging from 10% to 100% of an instilled dose. Absorption is increased by certain pathologic conditions. I.M. and pleural membrane absorption of thiotepa is also variable.
Distribution: It isn't known if drug or its metabolites are distributed into breast milk.
Metabolism: Metabolized extensively in the liver.
Excretion: Drug and its metabolites are excreted in urine. Half-life is 2½ hours.

Route	Onset	Peak	Duration
I.V., Intrathecal, Intracavitary	Unknown	Unknown	Unknown

Contraindications and precautions

Contraindicated in patients with hypersensitivity to drug and in those with severe bone marrow, hepatic, or renal dysfunction. Use cautiously in patients with impaired renal or hepatic function or bone marrow suppression.

Interactions

Drug-drug. *Anticoagulants, aspirin:* Increased risk of bleeding. Avoid use together.
Myelosuppressive agents: Additive myelosuppression. Monitor patient closely.
Neuromuscular blocking agents: Prolonged muscular paralysis. Monitor patient closely.
Other alkylating agents, irradiation therapy: Toxicity. Avoid use together.

Succinylcholine: Causes prolonged respirations and apnea. Monitor patient closely. Avoid use together.

Effects on diagnostic tests
None reported.

Adverse reactions
CNS: headache, dizziness, blurred vision, fatigue, weakness.
EENT: *laryngeal edema,* conjunctivitis.
GI: *nausea, vomiting,* abdominal pain, anorexia.
GU: amenorrhea, decreased spermatogenesis, dysuria, urine retention, hemorrhagic cystitis.
Hematologic: leukopenia (begins within 5 to 10 days), thrombocytopenia, neutropenia, anemia.
Metabolic: hyperuricemia, decreased plasma pseudocholinesterase levels.
Respiratory: asthma.
Skin: hives, rash, dermatitis.
Other: fever, alopecia, ***hypersensitivity, anaphylactic shock.***

Overdose and treatment
Signs and symptoms of overdose include nausea, vomiting, and precipitation of uric acid in the renal tubules. Treatment is usually supportive and includes transfusion of blood components, antiemetics, hydration, and allopurinol.

Clinical considerations
- Refrigerate dry powder; protect from light.
- Use only sterile water for injection to reconstitute. Refrigerated solution is stable for 8 hours.
- Drug can be given by all parenteral routes, including direct injection into the tumor.
- Drug may be mixed with procaine 2% or epinephrine 1:1,000, or both, for local use.
- Drug may be further diluted to larger volumes with normal saline solution, D_5W, or lactated Ringer's solution for administration by I.V. infusion, intracavitary injection, or perfusion therapy.
- Filter solutions through a 0.22-micron filter before administration. Don't use solutions that are opaque or precipitate after filtration.
- To prevent hyperuricemia with resulting uric acid nephropathy, allopurinol may be given; keep patient well hydrated.
- Avoid all I.M. injections when platelet count is less than $100,000/mm^3$.
- Toxicity may be delayed and prolonged because drug binds to tissues and stays in body several hours.

Therapeutic monitoring
- Stop drug or decrease dose if WBC count decreases to less than $4,000/mm^3$ or if platelet count decreases to less than $150,000/mm^3$.
- Monitor uric acid.
- Monitor CBC weekly for at least 3 weeks after last dose. Warn patient to report even mild infections.

Special populations
Pregnant patients. Drug shouldn't be used during pregnancy.
Breast-feeding patients. It isn't known if drug is excreted in breast milk. However, because of risk of serious adverse reactions, mutagenicity, and carcinogenicity in the infant, breast-feeding isn't recommended.

Patient counseling
- Encourage patient to maintain an adequate fluid intake to facilitate the excretion of uric acid.
- Instruct patient to avoid OTC products containing aspirin.
- Tell patient to avoid exposure to people with infections.
- Advise patient that hair should grow back after therapy has ended.
- Tell patient to report sore throat, fever, or unusual bruising or bleeding.
- Instruct patient to use effective contraception measures; if patient becomes pregnant, she should notify prescriber immediately.

thiothixene

thiothixene hydrochloride
Navane

Pharmacologic classification: thioxanthene
Therapeutic classification: antipsychotic
Pregnancy risk category C

How supplied
Available by prescription only
Capsules: 1 mg, 2 mg, 5 mg, 10 mg, 20 mg
Oral concentrate: 5 mg/ml (7% alcohol)
Injection: 2 mg/ml, 5 mg/ml

Indications and dosages
Acute agitation
Adults: 4 mg I.M. b.i.d. to q.i.d.; maximum dose, 30 mg I.M. daily. Change to P.O. form as soon as possible; I.M. dosage form is irritating.
Mild to moderate psychosis
Adults: Initially, 2 mg P.O. t.i.d.; may increase gradually to 15 mg daily.
Severe psychosis
Adults: Initially, 5 mg P.O. b.i.d.; may increase gradually to 20 to 30 mg daily. Maximum recommended daily dose, 60 mg.

Pharmacodynamics
Antipsychotic action: Thiothixene is thought to exert its antipsychotic effects by postsynaptic blockade of CNS dopamine receptors, thereby inhibiting dopamine-mediated effects.

Thiothixene has many other central and peripheral effects; it also acts as an alpha blocker. Its most prominent adverse reactions are extrapyramidal.

Pharmacokinetics

Absorption: Rapidly absorbed.
Distribution: Widely distributed into the body. Drug is 91% to 99% protein-bound.
Metabolism: Metabolized in the liver.
Excretion: Mostly excreted as parent drug in feces by way of the biliary tract.

Route	Onset	Peak	Duration
P.O., I.M.	10-30 min	1-6 hr	Unknown

Contraindications and precautions

Contraindicated in patients with hypersensitivity to drug and in those experiencing circulatory collapse, coma, CNS depression, or blood dyscrasia.

Use cautiously in geriatric or debilitated patients; in those with history of seizure disorders, CV disease, heat exposure, glaucoma, or prostatic hyperplasia; and in those in a state of alcohol withdrawal.

Interactions

Drug-drug. *CNS depressants:* Increased CNS depression. Avoid use together.
Drug-herb. *Nutmeg:* May cause a loss of symptom control. Avoid use together.
Drug-food. *Caffeine:* Increases metabolism of drug. Advise patient to avoid caffeine.
Drug-lifestyle. *Alcohol use:* Increased CNS depression. Advise patient to avoid alcohol use.
Sun exposure: Can potentiate photosensitivity reactions. Advise patient to avoid prolonged or unprotected sun exposure.
Heavy smoking: Increases metabolism of drug. Advise patient to avoid or limit smoking.

Effects on diagnostic tests

Drug causes false-positive test results for urinary porphyrins, urobilinogen, amylase, and 5-hydroxyindoleacetic acid because of darkening of urine by metabolites; it also causes false-positive urine pregnancy results in tests using human chorionic gonadotropin as the indicator.

Adverse reactions

CNS: *extrapyramidal reactions,* drowsiness, restlessness, agitation, insomnia, *tardive dyskinesia,* sedation, pseudoparkinsonism, EEG changes, dizziness.
CV: *hypotension,* tachycardia, ECG changes.
EENT: ocular changes, *blurred vision,* nasal congestion.
GI: *dry mouth, constipation.*
GU: *urine retention,* menstrual irregularities, gynecomastia, inhibited ejaculation.
Hematologic: ***transient leukopenia, leukocytosis, agranulocytosis.***
Hepatic: jaundice, elevated liver enzymes.
Skin: *mild photosensitivity,* allergic reactions, pain at I.M. injection site, sterile abscess.
Other: weight gain, ***neuroleptic malignant syndrome.***
After abrupt withdrawal of long-term therapy: gastritis, nausea, vomiting, dizziness, tremor, feeling of warmth or cold, diaphoresis, tachycardia, headache, insomnia.

Overdose and treatment

CNS depression is characterized by deep, unarousable sleep and possible coma, hypotension or hypertension, extrapyramidal symptoms, abnormal involuntary muscle movements, agitation, seizures, arrhythmias, ECG changes, hypothermia or hyperthermia, and autonomic nervous system dysfunction.

Treatment is symptomatic and supportive and includes maintaining vital signs, airway, stable body temperature, and fluid and electrolyte balance.

Don't induce vomiting: Drug inhibits cough reflex, and aspiration may occur. Use gastric lavage, then activated charcoal and sodium chloride cathartics; dialysis doesn't help. Regulate body temperature as needed. Treat hypotension with I.V. fluids: Don't give epinephrine. Seizures may be treated with parenteral diazepam or barbiturates; arrhythmias with parenteral phenytoin (1 mg/kg with rate titrated to blood pressure); and extrapyramidal reactions with benztropine at 1 to 2 mg or parenteral diphenhydramine at 10 to 50 mg.

Clinical considerations

- Drug is associated with a high incidence of extrapyramidal effects.
- Liquid and injectable formulations may cause a rash if skin contact occurs.
- Because stomach upset may occur, administer oral form with food or fluid.
- Dilute the concentrate in 2 to 4 oz (60 to 120 ml) of liquid, preferably water, carbonated drinks, fruit juice, tomato juice, milk, or pudding.
- Photosensitivity reactions may occur; advise patient to avoid exposure to sunlight or heat lamps.
- Administer I.M. injection may cause skin necrosis.
- Solution for injection may be slightly discolored. Don't use if excessively discolored or if a precipitate is evident.
- Drug is stable after reconstitution for 48 hours at room temperature.
- Protect liquid formulation from light.

Therapeutic monitoring

- Monitor blood pressure before and after parenteral administration.
- Check patient regularly for abnormal body movements (at least once every 6 months).

Special populations

Pregnant patients. Hyperreflexia has been reported in infants following in utero exposure. Use drug during pregnancy only when potential benefit justifies risk to fetus.
Pediatric patients. Drug isn't recommended for children under age 12.
Geriatric patients. Geriatric patients tend to require lower doses, adjusted to individual response. Adverse reactions are more likely to develop in such patients, especially tardive dyskinesia and other extrapyramidal effects.

Patient counseling

- Explain risks of dystonic reactions and tardive dyskinesia, and tell patient to report abnormal body movements.
- Tell patient to avoid sun exposure and to wear sunscreen when going outdoors to prevent photosensitivity reactions. Remind him that heat lamps and tanning beds also may cause burning of the skin or skin discoloration.
- Instruct patient not to spill the liquid on skin. Contact with skin may cause rash and irritation.
- Tell patient to take drug exactly as prescribed, not to double doses for missed doses, and not to share drug with others.
- Explain that many drug interactions are possible. He should seek medical approval before taking any self-prescribed medication.
- Tell patient not to stop taking drug suddenly; most adverse reactions may be relieved by reducing the dose. However, patient should call if difficulty urinating, sore throat, dizziness, or fainting develops.
- Warn patient against hazardous activities that require alertness until effect of drug is established. Reassure patient that sedation usually subsides after several weeks.
- Tell patient not to drink alcohol or take other medications that may cause excessive sedation.
- Explain which fluids are appropriate for diluting the concentrate and the dropper technique of measuring dose.
- Tell patient to shake concentrate before administration.
- Instruct patient to store drug away from children.

tiagabine hydrochloride

Gabitril

Pharmacologic classification: gamma aminobutyric acid (GABA) enhancer
Therapeutic classification: anticonvulsant
Pregnancy risk category C

How supplied

Available by prescription only
Tablets: 4 mg, 12 mg, 16 mg, 20 mg

Indications and dosages

Adjunctive therapy in the treatment of partial seizures

Adults: Initially, 4 mg P.O. once daily. May increase total daily dose by 4 to 8 mg at weekly intervals until clinical response occurs or up to maximum of 56 mg/day. Give total daily dose in divided doses b.i.d. to q.i.d.
Adolescents age 12 to 18: Initially, 4 mg P.O. once daily. May increase total daily dose by 4 mg beginning of week 2 and thereafter by 4 to 8 mg/week at weekly intervals until clinical response is seen or up to maximum of 32 mg/day. Give total daily dose in divided doses b.i.d. to q.i.d.

≡ ***Dosage adjustment.*** In patients with impaired liver function, initial and maintenance dosages may be reduced or dosing intervals increased.

Pharmacodynamics

Anticonvulsant action: Exact mechanism unknown. Tiagabine is thought to act by enhancing the activity of GABA, the major inhibitory neurotransmitter in the CNS. It binds to recognition sites associated with the GABA uptake carrier and may thus permit more GABA to be available for binding to receptors on postsynaptic cells.

Pharmacokinetics

Absorption: Rapidly and nearly completely absorbed (more than 95%). Absolute bioavailability is about 90%.
Distribution: About 96% is bound to human plasma proteins, mainly to serum albumin and alpha-1 acid glycoprotein.
Metabolism: Likely to be metabolized by the cytochrome P-450 3A isoenzymes.
Excretion: About 2% is excreted unchanged, with 25% and 63% of dose excreted into urine and feces, respectively. Half-life is about 7 to 9 hours.

Route	Onset	Peak	Duration
P.O.	Rapid	45 min	7-9 hr

Contraindications and precautions

Contraindicated in patients with hypersensitivity to drug or its ingredients. Use cautiously in breast-feeding women.

Interactions

Drug-drug. *Carbamazepine, phenobarbital, phenytoin:* Increased tiagabine clearance. Monitor patient closely.
CNS depressants: Enhanced CNS effects. Use cautiously.
Valproate: Decreased valproate level. Monitor patient closely.
Drug-lifestyle. *Alcohol use:* Enhanced CNS effects. Advise patient to avoid alcohol use.

Effects on diagnostic tests

None reported.

Adverse reactions

CNS: *dizziness, asthenia, somnolence, nervousness,* tremor, difficulty with concentration and attention, insomnia, ataxia, confusion, speech disorder, difficulty with memory, paresthesia, depression, emotional lability, abnormal gait, hostility, language problems, agitation.
CV: vasodilation.
EENT: amblyopia, nystagmus, pharyngitis.
GI: abdominal pain, *nausea,* diarrhea, vomiting, increased appetite, mouth ulceration.
GU: urinary tract infection.
Musculoskeletal: myalgia, myasthenia.
Respiratory: increased cough.
Skin: rash, pruritus.
Other: flulike syndrome.

Overdose and treatment

Common symptoms reported after an overdose include somnolence, impaired consciousness, impaired speech, agitation, confusion, speech difficulty, hostility, depression, weakness, and myoclonus. There's no specific antidote for tiagabine. If indicated, elimination of unabsorbed drug should be achieved by emesis or gastric lavage. Observe usual precautions to maintain the airway, and provide general supportive care.

Clinical considerations

- A therapeutic range for plasma drug levels hasn't been established.
- Status epilepticus and sudden unexpected death in epilepsy have occurred in patients receiving tiagabine. Patients who aren't receiving at least one other enzyme-inducing antiepilepsy drug at the time of tiagabine initiation may require lower doses or a slower dose adjustment.
- Never withdraw drug suddenly because seizure frequency may increase. Withdraw tiagabine gradually unless safety concerns require a more rapid withdrawal.

Therapeutic monitoring

Because of the potential for pharmacokinetic interactions between tiagabine and drugs that induce or inhibit hepatic metabolizing enzymes, obtain plasma levels of tiagabine before and after changes are made in the therapeutic regimen.

Special populations

Pregnant patients. Drug shouldn't be used during pregnancy unless potential benefit justifies potential risk.
Breast-feeding patients. Tiagabine and its metabolites are excreted in breast milk. Use in breast-feeding women only if the benefits clearly outweigh the risks.
Pediatric patients. Drug hasn't been investigated in adequate and well-controlled trials in patients under age 12.
Geriatric patients. Because few patients over age 65 were exposed to tiagabine hydrochloride during its clinical evaluation, safety or efficacy in this age group isn't clear.

Patient counseling

- Advise patient to take drug only as prescribed and to take tiagabine with food.
- Warn patient that drug may cause dizziness, somnolence, and other symptoms and signs of CNS depression.
- Advise patient to avoid driving and other potentially hazardous activities that require mental alertness until CNS effects of drug are known.

ticarcillin disodium/ clavulanate potassium

Timentin

Pharmacologic classification: extended-spectrum penicillin, beta-lactamase inhibitor
Therapeutic classification: antibiotic
Pregnancy risk category B

How supplied

Available by prescription only
Injection: 3 g ticarcillin and 100 mg clavulanic acid

Indications and dosages

Infections of the lower respiratory tract, urinary tract, bones and joints, skin and skin structure, and septicemia when caused by susceptible organisms
Adults: 3.1 g (contains 3 g ticarcillin and 0.1 g clavulanate potassium) diluted in 50 to 100 ml D_5W, saline, or lactated Ringer's injection and administered by I.V. infusion over 30 minutes q 4 to 6 hours.
Children 3 months to 16 years weighing less than 132 lb (60 kg): For mild to moderate infections, 200 mg/kg/day (contains 3 g ticarcillin and 0.1 g clavulanate potassium) I.V. infusion given in divided doses q 6 hours. For severe infections, 300 mg/kg/day (contains 3 g ticarcillin and 0.1 g clavulanate potassium) I.V. given in divided doses q 4 hours.
≡ ***Dosage adjustment.*** In patients with renal failure, loading dose is 3.1 g (3 g ticarcillin with 100 mg clavulanate).

Creatinine clearance (ml/min)	Adult dosage
> 60	3.1 g I.V. q 4 hours
30 to 60	2 g I.V. q 4 hours
10 to 30	2 g I.V. q 8 hours
< 10	2 g I.V. q 12 hours
< 10 with hepatic failure	2 g I.V. q 24 hours

Pharmacodynamics

Antibiotic action: Ticarcillin is bactericidal; it adheres to bacterial penicillin-binding proteins, inhibiting bacterial cell wall synthesis. Extended-spectrum penicillins are more resistant to inactivation by certain beta-lactamases, especially those produced by gram-negative organisms, but are still liable to inactivation by certain others.

Clavulanic acid has only weak antibacterial activity and doesn't affect the action of ticarcillin. However, clavulanic acid has a beta-lactam ring and is structurally similar to penicillin and cephalosporins; it binds irreversibly with certain beta-lactamases, preventing inactivation of ticarcillin and broadening its bactericidal spectrum.

Spectrum of activity of ticarcillin includes many gram-negative aerobic and anaerobic bacilli, many gram-positive and gram-negative aerobic cocci, and some gram-positive aerobic and anaerobic bacilli. The combination of ticarcillin and clavulanate potassium is also effective against many beta-lactamase-producing strains, including *Staphylococcus aureus, Haemophilus influenzae, Neisseria gonorrhoeae, Escherichia coli, Klebsiella, Providencia,* and *Bacteroides fragilis,* but not *Pseudomonas aeruginosa.*

Pharmacokinetics

Absorption: Only administered I.V.
Distribution: Distributed widely. It penetrates minimally into CSF with uninflamed meninges; clavulanic acid penetrates into pleural fluid, lungs, and peritoneal fluid. Ticarcillin sodium achieves high levels in urine. Protein-binding is 45% to 65% for ticarcillin and 22% to 30% for clavulanic acid; both cross the placenta.
Metabolism: About 13% of a ticarcillin dose is metabolized by hydrolysis to inactive compounds; clavulanic acid is thought to undergo extensive metabolism, but its fate is as yet unknown.
Excretion: Ticarcillin is excreted primarily (83% to 90%) in urine by renal tubular secretion and glomerular filtration; it's also excreted in bile and in breast milk. Metabolites of clavulanate are excreted in urine by glomerular filtration and in breast milk. Elimination half-life of ticarcillin in adults is about 1 hour and that of clavulanate is about 1 hour; in severe renal impairment, half-life of ticarcillin is extended to about 8 hours and that of clavulanate to about 3 hours. Both drugs are removed by hemodialysis but only slightly by peritoneal dialysis.

Route	Onset	Peak	Duration
I.V.	Unknown	Immediate	Unknown

Contraindications and precautions

Contraindicated in patients with hypersensitivity to drug or other penicillins. Use cautiously in patients with other drug allergies, especially to cephalosporins, impaired renal function, hemorrhagic conditions, hypokalemia, or sodium restrictions.

Interactions

Drug-drug. *Aminoglycoside antibiotics:* Chemically incompatible. Don't mix in the same I.V. container.
Oral contraceptives: Decreased efficacy of contraceptive. Advise patient to use another contraceptive method.
Probenecid: Elevated serum ticarcillin level. Monitor patient carefully.

Effects on diagnostic tests

Ticarcillin disodium/clavulanate potassium alters tests for urinary or serum proteins; it interferes with turbidimetric methods that use sulfosalicylic acid, trichloroacetic acid, acetic acid, or nitric acid. Ticarcillin disodium/clavulanate potassium doesn't interfere with tests using bromophenol blue (Albustix, Albutest, MultiStix). It may falsely decrease serum aminoglycoside level.

Adverse reactions

CNS: ***seizures,*** neuromuscular excitability, headache, giddiness.
GI: nausea, diarrhea, stomatitis, vomiting, epigastric pain, flatulence, pseudomembranous colitis, taste and smell disturbances.
Hematologic: ***leukopenia, neutropenia,*** eosinophilia, ***thrombocytopenia,*** hemolytic anemia, anemia, positive Coombs' test, prolonged PT and INR.
Hepatic: elevated liver enzymes.
Metabolic: hypokalemia, hypernatremia.
Other: hypersensitivity reactions (rash, pruritus, urticaria, chills, fever, edema, ***anaphylaxis***), overgrowth of nonsusceptible organisms, pain at injection site, vein irritation, phlebitis.

Overdose and treatment

Signs of overdose include neuromuscular hypersensitivity or seizures; ticarcillin and clavulanate potassium can be removed by hemodialysis.

Clinical considerations

Consider the recommendations relevant to all penicillins as well as the following:

- Ticarcillin disodium/clavulanate potassium is almost always used with another antibiotic such as an aminoglycoside in life-threatening situations.
- Administer aminoglycosides 1 hour before or after administration of ticarcillin disodium/clavulanate potassium.
- Ticarcillin contains 5.2 mEq of sodium per gram of drug. Use with caution in patients with sodium restriction.

■ Because ticarcillin disodium/clavulanate potassium is dialyzable, patients undergoing hemodialysis may need dose adjustments.

Therapeutic monitoring

■ Monitor serum electrolytes. Observe for signs of hypernatremia and hypokalemia.
■ Monitor neurologic status. High blood levels may cause seizures.

Special populations

Pregnant patients. Use drug during pregnancy only when clearly needed.
Breast-feeding patients. Ticarcillin and clavulanate potassium are excreted in breast milk; use with caution in breast-feeding women.
Geriatric patients. Half-life may be prolonged in geriatric patients because of impaired renal function.

Patient counseling

Advise patient of adverse experiences and advise limiting salt intake during drug therapy.

ticlopidine hydrochloride

Ticlid

Pharmacologic classification: platelet aggregation inhibitor
Therapeutic classification: antithrombotic
Pregnancy risk category B

How supplied

Available by prescription only
Tablets (film-coated): 250 mg

Indications and dosages

Reduction of risk of thrombotic stroke in patients with history of stroke, in those who have experienced stroke precursors, or in those who are intolerant to aspirin therapy
Adults: 250 mg P.O. b.i.d. with meals.

Pharmacodynamics

Antithrombotic action: Ticlopidine blocks adenosine diphosphate-induced platelet-fibrinogen and platelet-platelet binding.

Pharmacokinetics

Absorption: Rapidly and extensively (more than 80%) absorbed after oral administration. Absorption is enhanced by food.
Distribution: 98% bound to serum proteins and lipoproteins.
Metabolism: Extensively metabolized by the liver. It's unknown whether parent drug or active metabolites are responsible for pharmacologic activity.
Excretion: About 60% is excreted in urine and 23% in feces; only trace amounts of intact drug are found in urine. After one dose, half-life is 12½ hours; with repeat dosing, half-life increases to 4 to 5 days.

Route	Onset	Peak	Duration
P.O.	Unknown	2 hr	Unknown

Contraindications and precautions

Contraindicated in patients with hypersensitivity to drug; hematopoietic disorders, such as neutropenia, thrombocytopenia, or disorders of hemostasis; active pathologic bleeding from peptic ulceration or active intracranial bleeding; or severe liver dysfunction.

Interactions

Drug-drug. *Antacids:* Decreased plasma levels of ticlopidine. Separate administration times by at least 2 hours.
Aspirin: Potentiates effects of aspirin on platelets. Avoid use together.
Cimetidine: Decreased clearance of ticlopidine; increased toxicity risk. Don't use together.
Digoxin: Causes slightly decreased serum digoxin levels. Monitor serum digoxin levels.
Theophylline: Increased risk of theophylline toxicity. Monitor patient closely; adjust theophylline dose as needed.
Drug-herb. *Red clover:* Increased risk of bleeding. Don't use together.

Effects on diagnostic tests

None reported.

Adverse reactions

CNS: dizziness, *intracerebral bleeding,* peripheral neuropathy.
CV: vasculitis.
EENT: epistaxis, conjunctival hemorrhage.
GI: *diarrhea, nausea, dyspepsia, abdominal pain,* anorexia, vomiting, flatulence, bleeding, light-colored stools.
GU: hematuria, ***nephrotic syndrome,*** dark-colored urine.
Hematologic: prolonged bleeding time, ***neutropenia, pancytopenia, agranulocytosis, immune thrombocytopenia.***
Hepatic: hepatitis, cholestatic jaundice, abnormal liver function tests.
Metabolic: ***hyponatremia,*** *increased serum cholesterol levels.*
Musculoskeletal: arthropathy, myositis.
Respiratory: ***allergic pneumonitis.***
Skin: *rash,* pruritus, ecchymoses, maculopapular rash, urticaria, ***thrombocytopenic purpura.***
Other: *hypersensitivity reactions,* postoperative bleeding, systemic lupus erythematosus, ***serum sickness.***

Overdose and treatment

Only one case of overdose has been reported. The patient, who ingested more than 6 g of drug, showed increased bleeding time and increased ALT levels. The patient recovered with supportive therapy alone.

Clinical considerations

- If drug is being substituted for a fibrinolytic or anticoagulant drug, discontinue previous agent before starting ticlopidine therapy.
- If necessary, methylprednisolone 20 mg I.V. has been shown to normalize the bleeding time within 2 hours. Platelet transfusions may also be necessary.
- Drug has been used investigationally for many conditions, including intermittent claudication, chronic arterial occlusion, subarachnoid hemorrhage, primary glomerulonephritis, sickle cell disease, and uremic patients with AV shunts. When used preoperatively, it may decrease incidence of graft occlusion in patients receiving coronary artery bypass grafts and reduce severity of decreased platelet count in patients receiving extracorporeal hemoperfusion during open heart surgery.

Therapeutic monitoring

- Perform baseline liver function tests and repeat whenever liver dysfunction is suspected. Monitor patient closely, especially during the first 4 months of treatment.
- Monitor CBC and WBC differential every 2 weeks for the first 3 months of therapy. Severe hematologic adverse events can occur with ticlopidine.
- After the first 3 months of therapy, perform CBC and WBC differential determinations in patients showing signs of infection.

Special populations

Pregnant patients. Use drug during pregnancy only when clearly needed.
Breast-feeding patients. Although drug has been found in breast milk in animals, it isn't known if it's excreted in human milk. Breastfeeding isn't recommended.
Pediatric patients. Safety and efficacy in children under age 18 haven't been established.

Patient counseling

- Tell patient to take drug with meals because food substantially increases bioavailability and improves GI tolerance.
- Emphasize that drug prolongs bleeding time. Tell patient to report unusual bleeding and to inform dentists and other health care providers that he's taking ticlopidine.
- Be sure patient understands the need to report for regular blood tests. Neutropenia can result in an increased risk of infection. Tell patient to report signs and symptoms of infection, such as fever, chills, or sore throat, immediately.
- Warn patient to avoid aspirin and aspirin-containing products, which may prolong bleeding. Instruct him to call before taking OTC medications because many contain aspirin.
- Tell patient to report yellow skin or sclera, severe or persistent diarrhea, rash, subcutaneous bleeding, light-colored stools, dark urine.

tiludronate disodium

Skelid

Pharmacologic classification: bisphosphonate analogue
Therapeutic classification: antihypercalcemic
Pregnancy risk category C

How supplied

Available by prescription only
Tablets: 200 mg

Indications and dosages

Paget's disease
Adults: 400 mg P.O. once daily taken with 6 to 8 oz (180 to 240 ml) of water for 3 months, given 2 hours before or after meals.

Pharmacodynamics

Antihypercalcemic action: Tiludronate is thought to suppress bone resorption by reducing osteoclastic activity through inhibition of the osteoclastic proton pump and through disruption of the cytoskeletal ring structure, possibly by inhibiting protein-tyrosine-phosphatase, leading to detachment of osteoclasts from the bone surface.

Pharmacokinetics

Absorption: Bioavailability of drug on an empty stomach is 8%. Food and beverages other than water can reduce bioavailability by up to 90%.
Distribution: Widely distributed in bone and soft tissue. Protein binding is about 90% (mainly albumin).
Metabolism: Probably not metabolized.
Excretion: Principally excreted in urine. Mean plasma half-life is 150 hours.

Route	Onset	Peak	Duration
P.O.	Unknown	2 hr	Unknown

Contraindications and precautions

Contraindicated in patients with known hypersensitivity to any component of drug and in patients with creatinine clearance below 30 ml/minute. Use cautiously in patients with upper GI disease, such as dysphagia, esophagitis, esophageal ulcer, or gastric ulcer.

Interactions

Drug-drug. *Aspirin, calcium supplements, aluminum antacids, indomethacin, magnesium antacids:* Reduced bioavailability of tiludronate.

Monitor patient closely and adjust dose as needed.
Drug-food. *Any food:* Delayed drug absorption. Don't give drug within 2 hours of meals. *Beverages other than plain water:* Reduced drug absorption. Don't give with drug.

Effects on diagnostic tests
None reported.

Adverse reactions
CNS: anxiety, dizziness, headache, insomnia, involuntary muscle contractions, paresthesia, somnolence, vertigo.
CV: chest pain, hypertension.
EENT: cataracts, conjunctivitis, glaucoma, pharyngitis, sinusitis, rhinitis.
Endocrine: hyperparathyroidism.
GI: anorexia, constipation, diarrhea, dry mouth, dyspepsia, flatulence, gastritis, nausea, tooth disorder, vomiting.
Metabolic: vitamin D deficiency.
Musculoskeletal: arthralgia, arthrosis, back pain.
Respiratory: bronchitis, coughing, crackles.
Skin: pruritus.
Other: edema, sweating, *whole body pain.*

Overdose and treatment
No specific information available. Use standard treatment for hypocalcemia or renal insufficiency, if they occur. Dialysis isn't beneficial.

Clinical considerations
- Use drug in patients with Paget's disease who have serum alkaline phosphatase level at least twice the upper limit of normal or who are symptomatic or at risk for future complications of disease.
- Administer drug for 3 months to assess response.
- Hypocalcemia and other disturbances of mineral metabolism such as vitamin D deficiency should be corrected before initiating therapy.

Therapeutic monitoring
- Monitor symptom control.
- Monitor for adverse reaction.

Special populations
Breast-feeding patients. It isn't known if drug is excreted in breast milk. Use cautiously in breast-feeding women.
Pediatric patients. Safety and efficacy in children haven't been established.
Geriatric patients. Plasma levels may be higher in the elderly. However, dose adjustment isn't necessary.

Patient counseling
- Instruct patient to take drug with 6 to 8 oz (180 to 240 ml) of water and not to take it within 2 hours of food.
- Advise patient to maintain adequate vitamin D and calcium intake.
- Inform patient that calcium supplements, aspirin, and indomethacin shouldn't be taken within 2 hours before or after tiludronate.
- Tell patient that aluminum- and magnesium-containing antacids can be taken 2 hours after taking tiludronate.

timolol maleate
Blocadren, Timoptic, Timoptic-XE

Pharmacologic classification: beta blocker
Therapeutic classification: antihypertensive, adjunct in MI, antiglaucoma
Pregnancy risk category C

How supplied
Available by prescription only
Tablets: 5 mg, 10 mg, 20 mg
Ophthalmic gel: 0.25%, 0.5%
Ophthalmic solution: 0.25%, 0.5%

Indications and dosages
Hypertension
Adults: Initially, 10 mg P.O. b.i.d. Usual maintenance dosage, 20 to 40 mg/day. Maximum dose, 60 mg/day. There should be an interval of at least 7 days between dose increases.
Reduction of risk of CV mortality and reinfarction after MI
Adults: 10 mg P.O. b.i.d. initiated within 1 to 4 weeks after infarction.
Migraine headache
Adults: 10 mg P.O. daily b.i.d., then increase up to 20 mg; or 30-mg dose (10 mg P.O. in the morning and 20 mg P.O. in the evening).
Glaucoma
Adults: 1 drop of 0.25% or 0.5% solution to the conjunctiva once or twice daily; or 1 drop of 0.25% or 0.5% gel to the conjunctiva once daily.
◊***Angina***
Adults: 15 to 45 mg P.O. daily given in three divided doses.

Pharmacodynamics
Antihypertensive action: Exact mechanism of antihypertensive effect of timolol is unknown. Timolol may reduce blood pressure by blocking adrenergic receptors (decreasing cardiac output), by decreasing sympathetic outflow from the CNS, and by suppressing renin release.
MI prophylactic action: Exact mechanism by which timolol decreases risk of mortality after MI is unknown. Timolol produces a negative chronotropic and inotropic activity. This decrease in heart rate and myocardial contractility results in reduced myocardial oxygen consumption.

Antiglaucoma action: Beta-blocking action of timolol decreases the production of aqueous humor, decreasing intraocular pressure.

Pharmacokinetics

Absorption: About 90% of an oral dose is absorbed from the GI tract.
Distribution: After oral administration, timolol is distributed throughout the body; depending on assay method, drug is 10% to 60% protein-bound.
Metabolism: About 80% of a given dose is metabolized in the liver to inactive metabolites.
Excretion: Drug and its metabolites are excreted primarily in urine; half-life is about 4 hours.

Route	Onset	Peak	Duration
P.O.	15-30 min	1-2 hr	6-12 hr
Ophthalmic	30 min	1-2 hr	12-24 hr

Contraindications and precautions

Contraindicated in patients with bronchial asthma, severe COPD, sinus bradycardia and heart block greater than first degree, cardiogenic shock, heart failure, or hypersensitivity to drug.

Use cautiously in patients with diabetes, hyperthyroidism, or respiratory disease (especially nonallergic bronchospasm or emphysema). Use oral form cautiously in patients with compensated heart failure and hepatic or renal disease. Use ophthalmic form cautiously in patients with cerebrovascular insufficiency.

Interactions

Drug-drug. *Cardiac glycosides, diltiazem, verapamil:* Excessive bradycardia and increased depressant effect on myocardium. Use together cautiously.
Indomethacin: Decreased antihypertensive effect. Monitor patient closely; dose may need adjustment.
Insulin, oral antidiabetic agents: Altered requirements for these drugs. Monitor glucose levels; dose may need adjustment.
Other antihypertensive agents, general anesthetics, fentanyl, NSAIDs: Hypotension. Monitor patient closely.

Effects on diagnostic tests

Drug therapy may slightly increase BUN, serum potassium, uric acid, and blood glucose levels and may slightly decrease hemoglobin levels and hematocrit.

Adverse reactions

CNS: fatigue, lethargy, dizziness; depression, hallucinations, confusion (with ophthalmic form).
CV: *arrhythmias, bradycardia,* hypotension, ***heart failure,*** peripheral vascular disease, *pulmonary edema* (with oral administration); *CVA, cardiac arrest, heart block,* palpitations (with ophthalmic form).
EENT: minor eye irritation, decreased corneal sensitivity with long-term use, conjunctivitis, blepharitis, keratitis, visual disturbances, diplopia, ptosis (with ophthalmic form).
GI: nausea, vomiting, diarrhea (with oral administration).
GU: increased BUN.
Hematologic: decreased hemoglobin levels and hematocrit.
Metabolic: hyperkalemia, hyperuricemia, hyperglycemia.
Respiratory: dyspnea, ***bronchospasm,*** increased airway resistance (with oral administration); *asthmatic attacks in patients with history of asthma* (with ophthalmic form).
Skin: pruritus (with oral administration).

Overdose and treatment

Signs of overdose include severe hypotension, bradycardia, heart failure, and bronchospasm.

After acute ingestion, empty stomach by induced emesis or gastric lavage and give activated charcoal to reduce absorption. Subsequent treatment is usually symptomatic and supportive.

Clinical considerations

Consider the recommendations relevant to all beta blockers as well as the following:
- Dose adjustment may be necessary for patient with renal or hepatic impairment.
- Although controversial, drug may need to be discontinued 48 hours before surgery in patients receiving ophthalmic timolol because systemic absorption occurs.

Therapeutic monitoring

Monitor for cardiac and respiratory symptoms.

Special populations

Pregnant patients. Use drug during pregnancy only when potential benefits justify possible risk to fetus.
Breast-feeding patients. Timolol is distributed into breast milk. Because of the potential for serious adverse reactions in breast-fed infants, an alternative feeding method is recommended during therapy.
Pediatric patients. Safety and efficacy in children haven't been established; use only if potential benefit outweighs risk.
Geriatric patients. Geriatric patients may require lower oral maintenance dosages of timolol because of increased bioavailability or delayed metabolism; they also may experience enhanced adverse effects. Use cautiously because half-life may be prolonged in geriatric patients.

Patient counseling

- For ophthalmic form of timolol, teach patient proper method of eye drop administration. Warn patient not to touch dropper to eye or surrounding tissue; lightly press lacrimal sac with finger after administration to decrease systemic absorption.

- Instruct patient to invert ophthalmic gel container once before each use.
- Instruct patient to administer other ophthalmic drugs at least 10 minutes before the ophthalmic gel.

tioconazole

Vagistat-1

Pharmacologic classification: imidazole derivative
Therapeutic classification: antifungal
Pregnancy risk category C

How supplied

Available by prescription only
Vaginal ointment: 6.5%

Indications and dosages

Vulvovaginal candidiasis
Adults: Insert 1 full applicator (about 4.6 g) intravaginally h.s. as a single dose.

Pharmacodynamics

Antifungal action: Tioconazole is a fungicidal imidazole that alters cell wall permeability.

Pharmacokinetics

Absorption: Negligible.
Distribution: Unknown.
Metabolism: Unknown.
Excretion: Unknown.

Route	Onset	Peak	Duration
Intravaginal	Unknown	Unknown	Unknown

Contraindications and precautions

Contraindicated in patients hypersensitive to drug or other imidazole antifungal agents (miconazole, ketoconazole) and in breast-feeding women.

Interactions

None reported.

Effects on diagnostic tests

None reported.

Adverse reactions

GU: *burning, pruritus,* discharge, vaginal pain, dysuria, dyspareunia, vulvar edema, irritation.

Overdose and treatment

None reported.

Clinical considerations

Because drug is useful only for candidial vulvovaginitis, the diagnosis should be confirmed by potassium hydroxide smears or cultures before treatment with tioconazole.

Therapeutic monitoring

- Monitor for relief of symptoms.
- Monitor for adverse reactions.

Special populations

Pregnant patients. Limit course of treatment to 7 days during pregnancy.
Breast-feeding patients. Instruct patient to temporarily stop breast-feeding during therapy.

Patient counseling

- Review correct use of drug with patient.
- Tell patient to avoid sexual intercourse during therapy or advise partner to use a condom to prevent reinfection.
- Tell patient to promptly report irritation or symptoms of sensitivity.
- Emphasize need for patient to continue therapy for the full course, even if symptoms have improved, and during menstrual period.

tirofiban hydrochloride

Aggrastat

Pharmacologic classification: GP IIb/IIIa receptor antagonist
Therapeutic classification: Platelet aggregation inhibitor
Pregnancy risk category B

How supplied

Available by prescription only
Injection: 50-ml vials (250 mcg/ml), 500-ml premixed vials (50 mcg/ml)

Indications and dosages

Treatment of acute coronary syndrome, in combination with heparin, including patients who are to be managed medically and those undergoing percutaneous transluminal coronary angioplasty (PTCA) or atherectomy
Adults: I.V. loading dose of 0.4 mcg/kg/minute for 30 minutes followed by a continuous I.V. infusion of 0.1 mcg/kg/minute. Continue infusion through angiography and for 12 to 24 hours after angioplasty or atherectomy.
≡ ***Dosage adjustment.*** In patients with renal insufficiency (creatinine clearance less than 30 ml/minute), use a loading dose of 0.2 mcg/kg/minute for 30 minutes followed by a continuous infusion of 0.05 mcg/kg/minute. Continue infusion through angiography and for 12 to 24 hours after angioplasty or atherectomy.

Pharmacodynamics

Platelet-inhibiting action: Drug is a reversible antagonist of fibrinogen binding to the GP IIb/IIIa receptor on human platelets producing a dose-dependent inhibition of platelet aggregation.

Pharmacokinetics

Absorption: Not reported.
Distribution: 65% protein bound. Volume of distribution ranges from 22 to 42 liters.
Metabolism: Metabolism is limited. Half-life is about 2 hours
Excretion: Renal clearance accounts for 39% to 69% of elimination; feces accounts for 25%.

Route	Onset	Peak	Duration
I.V.	Immediate	Immediate	4-8 hrs after end of infusion

Contraindications and precautions

Contraindicated in patients with a known hypersensitivity to drug or its components; active internal bleeding or history of bleeding diathesis within the previous 30 days, or past history of intracranial hemorrhage, intracranial neoplasm, arteriovenous malformation, or aneurysm; thrombocytopenia following prior exposure to drug, stroke within 30 days or history of hemorrhagic stroke; symptoms or findings suggestive of aortic dissection; severe hypertension (systolic blood pressure over 180 mm Hg or diastolic blood pressure greater than 110 mm Hg); acute pericarditis; major surgical procedure or severe physical trauma within previous month; and use with another parenteral GP IIb/IIIa inhibitor. Use with caution in patients with platelet count less than 150,000 mm^3 and in patients with hemorrhagic retinopathy.

Interactions

Drug-drug. *Anticoagulants such as warfarin, clopidogrel, dipyridamole, NSAIDs, thrombolytics, ticlopidine:* Increased risk of bleeding. Monitor patient closely.
Levothyroxine, omeprazole: Increased renal clearance of tirofiban. Monitor patient carefully.

Effects on diagnostic tests

None reported.

Adverse reactions

CNS: dizziness, fever, headache.
CV: ***bradycardia, coronary artery dissection,*** edema, vasovagal reaction.
GI: nausea, *occult bleeding.*
GU: pelvic pain.
Hematologic: *bleeding,* ***thrombocytopenia,*** decreased hemoglobin and hematocrit.
Musculoskeletal: leg pain.
Skin: sweating.
Other: bleeding at arterial access site.

Overdose and treatment

Treat overdose by assessing patient's clinical condition and by stopping or adjusting infusion. Drug is removed by dialysis.

Clinical considerations

- Don't infuse at levels greater than 50 mcg/ml.
- Minimize use of arterial and venous punctures, I.M. injections, urinary catheters, nasotracheal intubation, and nasogastric tubes. Avoid noncompressible I.V. access sites, such as subclavian or jugular veins.

Therapeutic monitoring

- Drug is associated with increases in bleeding rates, particularly at the site of arterial access for femoral sheath placement. Before pulling the sheath, discontinue heparin for 3 to 4 hours and document activated clotting time less than 180 seconds or APTT less than 45 seconds. Sheath hemostasis should be achieved at least 4 hours before hospital discharge.
- Monitor hemoglobin, hematocrit, and platelet counts before starting therapy, 6 hours following loading dose, and at least daily during therapy.

Special populations

Pregnant patients. Use drug during pregnancy only if expected benefit justifies potential risk.
Breast-feeding patients. It isn't known if drug is excreted in breast milk. Depending on the importance of the drug to the woman, either nursing or the drug should be discontinued.
Pediatric patients. Safety and efficacy in patients under age 18 haven't been established.

Patient counseling

- Instruct patient to report chest discomfort or other adverse events immediately.
- Inform patient that frequent blood sampling may be needed to evaluate therapy.

tobramycin

tobramycin ophthalmic

Tobrex

tobramycin sulfate

Nebcin

tobramycin solution for inhalation

TOBI

Pharmacologic classification: aminoglycoside
Therapeutic classification: antibiotic
Pregnancy risk category D

How supplied

Available by prescription only
Injection: 40 mg/ml, 10 mg/ml (pediatric)
Ophthalmic solution: 0.3%
Ophthalmic ointment: 0.3%
Nebulizer solution for inhalation: Single-use 5-ml (300-mg) ampule

Indications and dosages

***Serious infections caused by sensitive* Escherichia coli, Proteus, Klebsiella, Enterobacter, Serratia, Staphylococcus aureus, Pseudomonas, Citrobacter, *or* Providencia**

Adults and children with normal renal function: 3 mg/kg I.M. or I.V. daily, divided q 8 hours. Up to 5 mg/kg I.M. or I.V. daily, divided q 6 to 8 hours for life-threatening infections.
Neonates under age 1 week: Up to 4 mg/kg I.M. or I.V. daily, divided q 12 hours. For I.V. use, dilute in 50 to 100 ml normal saline solution or D_5W for adults and in less volume for children. Infuse over 20 to 60 minutes.

≡ ***Dosage adjustment.*** In patients with impaired renal function, initial dosage is same as for those with normal renal function. Subsequent doses and frequency are determined by renal function study results and blood levels; keep peak serum levels between 4 and 10 mcg/ml and trough serum levels between 1 and 2 mcg/ml. Several methods have been used to calculate dosage in renal failure.

After a 1 mg/kg loading dose, adjust subsequent dosage by reducing doses administered at 8-hour intervals or by prolonging the interval between normal doses. Both of these methods are useful when serum levels of tobramycin can't be measured directly. They're based on either creatinine clearance (preferred) or serum creatinine because these values correlate with half-life of drug.

To calculate reduced dosage for 8-hour intervals, use available nomograms; or, if patient's steady-state serum creatinine values are known, divide the normally recommended dose by patient's serum creatinine value. To determine frequency in hours for normal dosage (if creatinine clearance rate isn't available), divide the normal dose by patient's serum creatinine value. Dosage schedules derived from either method require careful clinical and laboratory observations of patient and should be adjusted as appropriate. These methods of calculation may be misleading in geriatric patients and in those with severe wasting; neither should be used when dialysis is performed.

Hemodialysis removes 50% to 75% of a dose in 6 hours. In anephric patients maintained by dialysis, 1.5 to 2 mg/kg after each dialysis usually maintains therapeutic, nontoxic serum levels. Patients receiving peritoneal dialysis twice a week should receive a 1.5 to 2 mg/kg loading dose followed by 1 mg/kg q 3 days. Those receiving dialysis q 2 days should receive a 1.5 mg/kg loading dose after first dialysis and 0.75 mg/kg after each subsequent dialysis.

◇ Intrathecally or intraventricularly, in conjunction with I.M. or I.V. administration
Adults: 3 to 8 mg q 18 to 48 hours.

Management of cystic fibrosis patients with* Pseudomonas aeruginosa *infection
Adults and children over age 6: 1 single-use ampule (300 mg) administered q 12 hours for 28 days, then off for 28 days, then on for 28 days as advised by prescriber. There's no dose adjustment for age or renal failure.

Treatment of external ocular infection caused by susceptible gram-negative bacteria
Adults and children: In mild to moderate infections, instill 1 or 2 drops into affected eye q 4 to 6 hours. In severe infections, instill 2 drops into affected eye hourly or apply a small amount of ointment into conjunctival sac t.i.d. or q.i.d.

Pharmacodynamics

Antibiotic action: Tobramycin is bactericidal; it binds directly to the 30S ribosomal subunit, thereby inhibiting bacterial protein synthesis. Its spectrum of activity includes many aerobic gram-negative organisms, including most strains of *P. aeruginosa* and some aerobic gram-positive organisms. Tobramycin may act against some bacterial strains resistant to other aminoglycosides; many strains resistant to tobramycin are susceptible to amikacin, gentamicin, or netilmicin.

Pharmacokinetics

Absorption: Absorbed poorly after oral administration and usually is given parenterally. Inhaled drug remains concentrated in the airway, with serum level after 20 weeks of therapy being 1.05 mcg/ml 1 hour after dosing.
Distribution: Distributed widely after parenteral administration; intraocular penetration is poor. CSF penetration is low, even in patients with inflamed meninges. Protein binding is minimal; tobramycin crosses the placenta. Inhaled drug remains primarily concentrated in the airway.
Metabolism: Not metabolized.
Excretion: Excreted primarily in urine by glomerular filtration; small amounts may be excreted in bile and breast milk. Elimination half-life in adults is 2 to 3 hours. In severe renal damage, half-life may extend to 24 to 60 hours. With inhalation use, unabsorbed tobramycin is probably eliminated in the sputum.

Route	Onset	Peak	Duration
I.V.	Immediate	Immediate	8 hr
I.M.	Unknown	30-90 min	8 hr
Ophthalmic, Inhalation	Unknown	Unknown	Unknown

Contraindications and precautions

Contraindicated in patients with hypersensitivity to drug or other aminoglycosides. Use injectable form cautiously in patients with impaired renal function or neuromuscular disorders and in the elderly.

Interactions

Drug-drug. *Bumetanide, ethacrynic acid, furosemide, mannitol, urea:* Increased hazard of ototoxicity. Monitor patient closely.
Dimenhydrinate, antiemetic and antivertigo drugs: May mask tobramycin-induced ototoxicity. Monitor patient closely.
General anesthetics, neuromuscular blocking agents, succinylcholine, tubocurarine: Potentiate neuromuscular blockade. Monitor patient closely.
Methoxyflurane, polymyxin B, vancomycin, capreomycin, cisplatin, cephalosporins, amphotericin B, and other aminoglycosides: Increased hazard of nephrotoxicity, ototoxicity, and neurotoxicity. Monitor patient carefully.
Penicillins: Physically and chemically incompatible. Don't mix in same I.V. line.

Effects on diagnostic tests

None reported.

Adverse reactions

CNS: headache, lethargy, confusion, ***seizures,*** disorientation (with injectable form).
EENT: *ototoxicity* (with injectable form); blurred vision (with ophthalmic ointment); burning or stinging on instillation, lid itching or swelling, conjunctival erythema (with ophthalmic administration).
GI: vomiting, nausea, diarrhea (with injectable form).
GU: elevated BUN, nonprotein nitrogen, and serum creatinine levels; increased urinary excretion of casts; ***nephrotoxicity*** (with injectable form).
Hematologic: anemia, eosinophilia, ***leukopenia, thrombocytopenia, granulocytopenia*** (with injectable form).
Respiratory: *bronchospasm* (with inhalation form).
Skin: rash, urticaria, pruritus (with injectable form).
Other: fever, ***hypersensitivity reactions,*** overgrowth of nonsusceptible organisms (with ophthalmic administration).

Overdose and treatment

Signs of overdose include ototoxicity, nephrotoxicity, and neuromuscular toxicity. Remove drug by hemodialysis or peritoneal dialysis. Treatment with calcium salts or anticholinesterases reverses neuromuscular blockade.

Clinical considerations

☐ ***ALERT*** Don't confuse tobramycin with Trobicin.
Consider the recommendations relevant to all aminoglycosides as well as the following:

- For I.V. administration, the usual volume of diluent (normal saline injection or 5% dextrose injection) for adult doses is 50 to 100 ml. For children, the volume should be proportionately less. Infusion should be over 20 to 60 minutes.
- Don't premix tobramycin with other drugs; administer separately at least 1 hour apart.
- Discontinue ophthalmic preparation if keratitis, erythema, lacrimation, edema, or lid itching occurs.
- Because tobramycin is dialyzable, patients undergoing hemodialysis may need dose adjustments.
- Inhalation form of tobramycin is an orphan drug used specifically for management of cystic fibrosis patients with *P. aeruginosa* infection.

Therapeutic monitoring

Monitor for symptoms of toxicity.

Special populations

Pregnant patients. Use drug during pregnancy only when clearly indicated.
Breast-feeding patients. A decision should be made between discontinuing medication or discontinuing breast-feeding.

Patient counseling

- Advise patient that inhalation doses should be taken as close to 12 hours apart as possible and no less than 6 hours apart.
- Instruct patient on proper administration (inhalation).

tocainide hydrochloride

Tonocard

Pharmacologic classification: local anesthetic (amide type)
Therapeutic classification: ventricular antiarrhythmic
Pregnancy risk category C

How supplied

Available by prescription only
Tablets: 400 mg, 600 mg

Indications and dosages

Suppression of symptomatic ventricular arrhythmias, including frequent PVC
Dosage must be individualized based on antiarrhythmic response and tolerance.
Adults: Initially, 400 mg P.O. q 8 hours. Usual dose is between 1,200 and 1,800 mg/day, divided into three doses. Drug may be administered on a twice-daily regimen if patient is able to tolerate the t.i.d. regimen.
≡ ***Dosage adjustment.*** Patients with impaired renal or hepatic function may be adequately treated with less than 1,200 mg/day.
◇ ***Myotonic dystrophy***
Adults: 800 to 1,200 mg P.O. daily.
◇ ***Trigeminal neuralgia***
Adults: 20 mg/kg/day P.O. t.i.d.

Pharmacodynamics

Antiarrhythmic action: Tocainide is structurally similar to lidocaine and possesses similar electrophysiologic and hemodynamic effects. A class IB antiarrhythmic, it suppresses automaticity and shortens the effective refractory period and action potential duration of His-Purkinje fibers and suppresses spontaneous ventricular depolarization during diastole. Conductive atrial tissue and AV conduction aren't affected significantly at therapeutic levels. Unlike quinidine and procainamide, tocainide doesn't significantly alter hemodynamics when administered in usual doses. Tocainide exerts its effects on the conduction system, causing inhibition of reentry mechanisms and cessation of ventricular arrhythmias; these effects may be more pronounced in ischemic tissue. Tocainide doesn't cause a significant negative inotropic effect. Its direct cardiac effects are less potent than those of lidocaine.

Pharmacokinetics

Absorption: Rapidly and completely absorbed from the GI tract; unlike lidocaine, it undergoes negligible first-pass effect in the liver. Bioavailability is nearly 100%.
Distribution: Distribution is only partially known; however, it appears to be distributed widely and apparently crosses the blood-brain barrier and placenta in animals (it is, however, less lipophilic than lidocaine). Only about 10% to 20% is bound to plasma protein.
Metabolism: Apparently metabolized in the liver to inactive metabolites.
Excretion: Excreted in urine as unchanged drug and inactive metabolites. About 30% to 50% of an orally administered dose is excreted in urine as metabolites. Elimination half-life is about 11 to 23 hours, with an initial biphasic plasma level decline similar to that of lidocaine. Half-life may be prolonged in patients with renal or hepatic insufficiency. Urine alkalinization may substantially decrease the amount of unchanged drug excreted in urine.

Route	Onset	Peak	Duration
P.O.	Unknown	½-2 hr	8 hr

Contraindications and precautions

Contraindicated in patients with hypersensitivity to lidocaine or other amide-type local anesthetics and in those with second- or third-degree AV block in the absence of an artificial pacemaker.

Use cautiously in patients with heart failure, diminished cardiac reserve, preexisting bone marrow failure, cytopenia, or impaired renal or hepatic function.

Interactions

Drug-drug. *Allopurinol:* Increased effects of this drug. Monitor carefully.
Lidocaine: May cause CNS toxicity. Monitor patient closely.
Metoprolol: Decreased myocardial contractility and bradycardia. Monitor cardiac status.
Other antiarrhythmics: Additive, synergistic, or antagonistic effects. Monitor cardiac status closely.
Rifampin, cimetidine: Decrease elimination half-life and bioavailability of tocainide. Monitor patient carefully. Dose adjustment may be needed.

Effects on diagnostic tests

None reported.

Adverse reactions

CNS: *light-headedness, tremor,* paresthesia, *dizziness, vertigo,* drowsiness, fatigue, confusion, headache.
CV: hypotension, ***new or worsened arrhythmias, heart failure, bradycardia,*** palpitations.
EENT: blurred vision, tinnitus.
GI: *nausea, vomiting,* diarrhea, anorexia.
Hematologic: ***blood dyscrasia.***
Hepatic: abnormal liver function tests, hepatitis.
Respiratory: ***respiratory arrest,*** *pulmonary fibrosis, pneumonitis,* ***pulmonary edema.***
Skin: rash, diaphoresis.

Overdose and treatment

Effects of overdose include extensions of common adverse reactions, particularly those associated with the CNS or GI tract.

Treatment generally involves symptomatic and supportive care. In acute overdose, perform gastric emptying by way of emesis induction or gastric lavage. Respiratory depression necessitates immediate attention and maintenance of a patent airway with ventilatory assistance, if required. Seizures may be treated with small incremental doses of a benzodiazepine, such as diazepam or a short or ultrashort-acting barbiturate, such as pentobarbital or thiopental.

Clinical considerations

- Drug is considered an oral lidocaine and may be used to ease transition from I.V. lidocaine to oral antiarrhythmic therapy.
- Use cautiously and with lower doses in patients with hepatic or renal impairment.
- A chest radiograph should be obtained if pulmonary symptoms exist.
- Adverse effects tend to be frequent and problematic.

Therapeutic monitoring

- Monitor blood levels; therapeutic levels range from 4 to 10 mcg/ml.
- Monitor periodic blood counts for the first 3 months of therapy and frequently thereafter. Perform CBC promptly if signs of infection develop.

■ Observe patient for tremors, a possible sign that maximum safe dose has been reached.

Special populations

Pregnant patients. Use drug during pregnancy only when potential benefits justify possible risks to fetus.
Breast-feeding patients. Safety in breast-feeding women hasn't been established. An alternative feeding method is recommended.
Geriatric patients. Use with caution in geriatric patients; increased serum drug levels and toxicity are more likely. Monitor patient carefully. Geriatric patients are more likely to experience dizziness and may require assistance while walking.

Patient counseling

■ Instruct patient to report unusual bleeding or bruising; signs or symptoms of infection, such as fever, sore throat, stomatitis, or chills; or pulmonary symptoms, such as cough, wheezing, or exertional dyspnea.
■ Tell patient he may take tocainide with food to lessen GI upset.
■ Tell patient that tocainide may cause drowsiness or dizziness, and he should be careful while performing tasks that require alertness.

tolazamide

Tolinase

Pharmacologic classification: sulfonylurea
Therapeutic classification: antidiabetic
Pregnancy risk category C

How supplied

Available by prescription only
Tablets: 100 mg, 250 mg, 500 mg

Indications and dosages

Adjunct to diet to lower blood glucose levels in patients with non-insulin-dependent diabetes mellitus (type 2)
Adults: Initially, 100 mg P.O. daily with breakfast if fasting blood sugar (FBS) is less than 200 mg/dl; or 250 mg P.O. daily if FBS is more than 200 mg/dl. May adjust dose at weekly intervals in increments of 100 to 250 mg based on blood glucose response. Maximum dose is 500 mg P.O. b.i.d. before meals.
Elderly: Initially, 100 mg P.O. daily.
≡ ***Dosage adjustment.*** Initially, malnourished or underweight patients may be given 100 mg P.O. daily.

Pharmacodynamics

Antidiabetic action: Tolazamide lowers blood glucose levels by stimulating insulin release from functioning beta cells of the pancreas. After prolonged administration, the hypoglycemic effects of drug appear to reflect extrapancreatic effects, possibly including reduction of basal hepatic glucose production and enhanced peripheral sensitivity to insulin.

Pharmacokinetics

Absorption: Absorbed well from the GI tract.
Distribution: Probably distributed into the extracellular fluid.
Metabolism: Metabolized probably by the liver to several mildly active metabolites.
Excretion: Excreted in urine primarily as metabolites, with small amounts excreted as unchanged drug. Half-life is 7 hours.

Route	Onset	Peak	Duration
P.O.	Unknown	3-4 hr	Unknown

Contraindications and precautions

Contraindicated in patients with hypersensitivity to drug or other sulfonylureas; type 1 diabetes (insulin-dependent) or diabetes that can be adequately controlled by diet; in patients with type 2 diabetes complicated by ketosis, acidosis, coma, or other acute complications such as major surgery, severe infection, or severe trauma; in patients with uremia; and in pregnant or breast-feeding women.

Use cautiously in geriatric, debilitated, or malnourished patients and in those with impaired renal or hepatic function or those with adrenal or pituitary insufficiency.

Interactions

Drug-drug. *Beta blockers, including ophthalmics:* Increase risk of hypoglycemia, mask its symptoms (increasing pulse rate and blood pressure), and prolong it by blocking gluconeogenesis. Use together cautiously.
Corticosteroids, phenothiazines, sympathomimetics, calcium channel blockers, isoniazid, estrogens, oral contraceptives, phenytoin, thiazide diuretics, triamterene, thyroid hormones: Decreased hypoglycemic effect. Monitor blood glucose level and adjust dose accordingly.
NSAIDs, chloramphenicol, insulin, MAO inhibitors, probenecid, salicylates, sulfonamides: Enhanced hypoglycemic effect. Monitor blood glucose level closely.
Oral anticoagulants: May increase hypoglycemic activity or enhance anticoagulant effect. Monitor blood glucose level and PT and INR.
Drug-lifestyle. *Alcohol use:* Disulfiram-like reaction (nausea, vomiting, abdominal cramps, headaches). Advise patient to avoid alcohol use.

Effects on diagnostic tests

None reported.

Adverse reactions

CNS: weakness, fatigue, dizziness, vertigo, malaise, headache.

GI: nausea, vomiting, epigastric distress, heartburn.
Hematologic: *leukopenia,* hemolytic anemia, ***thrombocytopenia, aplastic anemia, agranulocytosis,*** pancytopenia.
Metabolic: *hyponatremia, hypoglycemia.*
Other: photosensitivity reactions.

Overdose and treatment

Signs and symptoms of overdose include low blood glucose levels, tingling of lips and tongue, hunger, nausea, decreased cerebral function (lethargy, yawning, confusion, agitation, nervousness), increased sympathetic activity (tachycardia, sweating, tremor), and ultimately, seizures, stupor, and coma.

Mild hypoglycemia, without loss of consciousness or neurologic findings, responds to treatment with oral glucose and adjustments in drug doses and meal patterns. If patient loses consciousness or neurologic findings develop, he should receive rapid injection of dextrose 50%, followed by a continuous infusion of dextrose 10% at a rate to maintain blood glucose levels greater than 100 mg/dl. Monitor for 24 to 48 hours.

Clinical considerations

Consider the recommendations relevant to all sulfonylureas as well as the following:
- Over time, patients may become unresponsive (uncontrolled blood sugar) to therapy with this agent as well as other sulfonylureas; monitor appropriately.
- To avoid GI intolerance for those patients receiving doses of 500 mg/day or more and to improve control of hyperglycemia, divided doses are recommended; these are given before the morning and evening meals.
- Tablets may be crushed to ease administration.
- Use with caution in women of childbearing age. Tolazamide isn't recommended for treatment of diabetes associated with pregnancy.
- Oral antidiabetic agents have been associated with an increased risk of CV mortality as compared with diet or diet and insulin therapy.

To change from insulin to oral therapy with tolazamide:
- If insulin dose is less than 20 units daily, insulin may be stopped and oral therapy started at 100 mg P.O. daily in the morning. If insulin dose is 20 to 40 units daily, insulin may be stopped and oral therapy started at 250 mg P.O. daily in the morning. If insulin dose is more than 40 units daily, decrease insulin dose by 50% and start oral therapy at 250 mg P.O. daily with breakfast. Increase doses as appropriate based on blood glucose response.

Therapeutic monitoring

When substituting tolazamide for chlorpropamide therapy, monitor patient closely for 1 to 2 weeks because of prolonged retention of chlorpropamide in the body, which may result in hypoglycemia.

Special populations

Pregnant patients. Use with caution in pregnant women.
Breast-feeding patients. Because of the risk of hypoglycemia in the breast-fed infant, a risk/benefit decision should be made to discontinue the drug or to discontinue breast-feeding.
Pediatric patients. Tolazamide is ineffective in insulin-dependent (type 1, juvenile-onset) diabetes. Safety and efficacy in children haven't been established.
Geriatric patients. Geriatric patients may be more sensitive to the effects of drug because of reduced metabolism and elimination. Hypoglycemia causes more neurologic symptoms in these patients. Geriatric patients usually require a lower initial dose.

Patient counseling

- Advise patient to take drug at the same time each day. If a dose is missed, it should be taken immediately, unless it's almost time to take the next dose; he shouldn't double the doses.
- Warn patient to avoid alcohol when taking tolazamide.
- Recommend that patient take the drug with food if it causes GI upset.

tolazoline hydrochloride

Priscoline

Pharmacologic classification: peripheral vasodilator, alpha blocker
Therapeutic classification: antihypertensive
Pregnancy risk category C

How supplied

Available by prescription only
Injection: 25 mg/ml in 4-ml ampules

Indications and dosages

Persistent pulmonary vasoconstriction and hypertension of the neonate (persistent fetal circulation)
Neonates: Initially, 1 to 2 mg/kg I.V. by way of a scalp vein over 10 minutes, followed by an I.V. infusion of 1 to 2 mg/kg/hour.
◇ ***Peripheral vasospastic disorders***
Adults: 10 to 50 mg S.C., I.M., or I.V. q.i.d.
◇ ***To improve visualization of vasculature***
Adults: 12.5 to 50 mg intra-arterially before angiography.

Pharmacodynamics

Antihypertensive action: Tolazoline, by direct relaxation of vascular smooth muscle, causes peripheral vasodilation and decreased peripheral resistance. Tolazoline inhibits responses to adrenergic stimuli by competitively blocking alpha-adrenergic receptors; however, at usual doses, this effect is relatively transient and incomplete.

Pharmacokinetics

Absorption: Absorbed rapidly and almost completely after parenteral administration.
Distribution: Concentrates primarily in kidneys and liver.
Metabolism: None.
Excretion: Excreted in urine, primarily as unchanged drug; half-life is inversely related to urine output and can range from 1½ to 41 hours.

Route	Onset	Peak	Duration
I.V.	½ hr	Unknown	Unknown
S.C., I.M.	Unknown	Unknown	Unknown

Contraindications and precautions

Contraindicated in patients with hypersensitivity to drug, known or suspected coronary artery disease, or after CVA. Use cautiously in patients with known or suspected mitral stenosis.

Interactions

Drug-drug. *Epinephrine, norepinephrine:* Causes "epinephrine reversal," a paradoxical decrease in blood pressure followed by exaggerated rebound hypertension. Monitor patient closely.
Drug-food. *Alcohol use:* May cause disulfiram-type reaction. Advise patient to avoid use of products containing alcohol.

Effects on diagnostic tests

None reported.

Adverse reactions

CV: ***arrhythmias,*** pain, *hypertension, flushing, hypotension,* tachycardia.
GI: *nausea, vomiting, diarrhea,* ***GI hemorrhage.***
GU: edema, oliguria, hematuria.
Hematologic: *leukopenia,* ***thrombocytopenia.***
Respiratory: ***pulmonary hemorrhage.***
Skin: increased pilomotor activity with tingling and chilliness, rash.

Overdose and treatment

Signs and symptoms of overdose include flushing, hypotension, and shock.

Treat overdose symptomatically and supportively; if vasopressor is necessary, use ephedrine, which has both central and peripheral actions. Avoid epinephrine or norepinephrine because epinephrine reversal may occur from the alpha-blocking effects of tolazoline.

Clinical considerations

- Keeping patient warm increases the effect of drug.
- Pretreatment of infants with antacids may prevent GI bleeding.
- Appearance of flushing usually indicates maximum tolerable dose.
- Response should be evident within 30 minutes.

Therapeutic monitoring

- Monitor blood pH for acidosis, which may reduce the effect of drug.
- Monitor patient closely for hypotension and arrhythmias.
- Monitor for adverse reactions, including overdose and hemorrhage (GI and pulmonary).

Special populations

Pregnant patients. Use drug during pregnancy only when clearly needed.
Breast-feeding patients. Use drug with caution in breast-feeding women.

Patient counseling

Inform patient of potential therapeutic benefits and potential adverse reactions.

tolbutamide

Orinase

Pharmacologic classification: sulfonylurea
Therapeutic classification: antidiabetic
Pregnancy risk category C

How supplied

Available by prescription only
Tablets: 500 mg

Indications and dosages

Adjunct to diet to lower blood glucose levels in patients with non-insulin-dependent diabetes mellitus (type 2)
Adults: Initially, 1 to 2 g P.O. daily as single dose or divided b.i.d. or t.i.d. May adjust dosage to maximum of 3 g P.O. daily.

Pharmacodynamics

Antidiabetic action: Tolbutamide lowers blood glucose levels by stimulating insulin release from functioning beta cells of the pancreas. After prolonged administration, the hypoglycemic effects of the drug appear to reflect extrapancreatic effects, possibly including reduction of basal hepatic glucose production and enhanced peripheral sensitivity to insulin.

Pharmacokinetics

Absorption: Absorbed readily from the GI tract with peak levels occurring at 3 to 4 hours.
Distribution: Probably distributed into extracellular fluid. Drug is 95% bound to plasma proteins.
Metabolism: Metabolized in the liver to inactive metabolites.

Excretion: Drug and its metabolites are excreted in urine and feces. Half-life is 4½ to 6½ hours.

Route	Onset	Peak	Duration
P.O.	½-1 hr	3-5 hr	24 hr

Contraindications and precautions

Contraindicated in patients with hypersensitivity to drug or other sulfonylureas; in patients with type 1 diabetes (insulin-dependent) or diabetes that can be adequately controlled by diet; in patients with type 2 diabetes complicated by fever, ketosis, acidosis, coma, or other acute complications such as major surgery, severe infection, or severe trauma; in patients with severe renal insufficiency; and in pregnant or breast-feeding women.

Use cautiously in geriatric, debilitated, or malnourished patients and in those with impaired renal or hepatic function or porphyria.

Interactions

Drug-drug. *Anticoagulants:* Increased hypoglycemic activity, enhanced anticoagulant effect. Monitor blood glucose levels, PT, and INR. Doss may need adjustment.
Beta blockers, including ophthalmics: Mask symptoms of hypogylcemia and may prolong hypoglycemia.. Use together cautiously.
Corticosteroids, calcium channel blockers, estrogens, isoniazid, oral contraceptives, phenothiazines, phenytoin, sympathomimetics, thyroid products, thiazide diuretics, triamterene: Decreased hypoglycemic effect. Monitor blood glucose level; dose may need adjustment.
NSAIDs, chloramphenicol, insulin, MAO inhibitors, probenecid, salicylates, sulfonamides: Enhanced hypoglycemic effect. Monitor blood glucose levels closely.
Drug-lifestyle. *Alcohol use:* May produce a disulfiram-like reaction with nausea, vomiting, abdominal cramps, and headaches. Advise patient to avoid alcohol use.

Effects on diagnostic tests

Tolbutamide may give a false-positive reading for albumin in urine if measured by the acidification-after-boiling test. There's no interference with the sulfosalicylic acid test.

Adverse reactions

CNS: headache.
GI: nausea, heartburn, epigastric distress.
Hematologic: ***leukopenia,*** hemolytic anemia, ***thrombocytopenia, aplastic anemia, agranulocytosis,*** pancytopenia.
Hepatic: hepatic porphyria.
Metabolic: ***hypoglycemia, dilutional hyponatremia,*** SIADH secretion.
Skin: rash, pruritus, erythema, urticaria.
Other: ***hypersensitivity reactions,*** taste alterations, *disulfiram-like reactions.*

Overdose and treatment

Signs and symptoms of overdose include low blood glucose levels, tingling of lips and tongue, hunger, nausea, decreased cerebral function (lethargy, yawning, confusion, agitation, nervousness), increased sympathetic activity (tachycardia, sweating, tremor), and ultimately, seizures, stupor, and coma.

Mild hypoglycemia, without loss of consciousness or neurologic findings, responds to treatment with oral glucose and dose adjustments. If patient loses consciousness or develops neurologic findings, the patient should receive rapid injection of dextrose 50%, followed by a continuous infusion of dextrose 10% at a rate to maintain blood glucose levels greater than 100 mg/dl. Monitor for 24 to 48 hours.

Clinical considerations

Consider the recommendations relevant to all sulfonylureas as well as the following:

- To avoid GI intolerance for those patients on larger doses and to improve control of hyperglycemia, divided doses given before the morning and evening meals are recommended.
- Patients should avoid taking tolbutamide at bedtime because of the potential for nocturnal hypoglycemia.

To change from insulin to oral therapy with tolbutamide:

- If insulin dose is less than 20 units daily, insulin may be stopped and oral therapy started at 1 to 2 g daily. If insulin dose is 20 to 40 units daily, insulin dose is reduced 30% to 50% and oral therapy started as above. If insulin dose is more than 40 units daily, insulin dose is decreased 20% and oral therapy started as above. Further reductions in insulin dose are based on patient's response to oral therapy.

Therapeutic monitoring

When substituting tolbutamide for chlorpropamide therapy, monitor patient closely for the first 2 weeks because of prolonged retention of chlorpropamide in the body, which may result in hypoglycemia.

Special populations

Pregnant patients. Use with caution in women of childbearing age. Tolbutamide isn't recommended for treatment of diabetes associated with pregnancy.
Breast-feeding patients. Tolbutamide is excreted in breast milk. Because of the risk of hypoglycemia in the breast-fed infant, a decision should be made whether to discontinue the drug or to discontinue breast-feeding.
Pediatric patients. Tolbutamide is ineffective in insulin-dependent and type 1, juvenile-onset diabetes. Safety and efficacy in children haven't been established.
Geriatric patients. Geriatric patients may be more sensitive to the effects of drug because

of reduced metabolism and elimination. Hypoglycemia causes more neurologic symptoms in these patients. Geriatric patients usually require a lower initial dose.

Patient counseling

- Emphasize to patient the importance of following prescribed diet, exercise, and medical regimen.
- Instruct patient to take drug at the same time each day.
- Inform patient that, if a dose is missed, it should be taken immediately, unless it's almost time to take the next dose. Patient shouldn't double the doses.
- Advise patient to avoid products containing alcohol while taking tolbutamide because of prolonged hypoglycemic effect.

tolcapone

Tasmar

Pharmacologic classification: catechol-*O*-methyltransferase (COMT) inhibitor
Therapeutic classification: antiparkinsonian
Pregnancy risk category C

How supplied

Available by prescription only
Tablets: 100 mg, 200 mg

Indications and dosages

Adjunct to levodopa and carbidopa for treatment of signs and symptoms of idiopathic Parkinson's disease
Adults: Recommended initial dose is 100 mg (preferred) or 200 mg P.O. t.i.d. If initiating treatment with 200 mg t.i.d. and dyskinesias occur, then a decrease in dose of levodopa may be necessary. Maximum daily dose is 600 mg daily. Always give in combination with levodopa/carbidopa. The first tolcapone dose of the day should always be taken with the first levodopa/carbidopa dose of the day.
≡ ***Dosage adjustment.*** Don't use doses over 100 mg t.i.d. in patients with severe hepatic or renal dysfunction.

Pharmacodynamics

Antiparkinsonian action: Exact mechanism of action isn't known. It's thought to reversibly inhibit human erythrocyte COMT when given in combination with levodopa/carbidopa, resulting in a decrease in the clearance of levodopa and a two-fold increase in the bioavailability of levodopa. The decrease in clearance of levodopa prolongs the elimination half-life of levodopa from 2 to 3½ hours.

Pharmacokinetics

Absorption: Rapidly absorbed and reaches peak plasma levels within 2 hours. Following oral administration, absolute bioavailability is 65%. Onset of effect occurs following administration of first dose. Absorption of tolcapone decreases when given within 1 hour before or 2 hours after food; however, drug can be administered without regard to meals.
Distribution: Highly bound to plasma proteins (greater than 99.9%), primarily to albumin. The steady-state volume of distribution is small.
Metabolism: Completely metabolized before excretion. The main mechanism of metabolism is glucuronidation.
Excretion: Only 0.5% of dose is found unchanged in urine. Tolcapone is a low-extraction-ratio drug with a systemic clearance of 7 L/hour. Elimination half-life is 2 to 3 hours. Dialysis isn't expected to effect clearance because of the high protein binding.

Route	Onset	Peak	Duration
P.O.	Unknown	2 hr	Unknown

Contraindications and precautions

Contraindicated in patients with known hypersensitivity to drug or its components; in those with liver disease or ALT or AST values exceeding the upper limit of normal; patients withdrawn from therapy because of drug-induced hepatocellular injury; and in patients with history of nontraumatic rhabdomyolysis or hyperpyrexia and confusion, possibly related to drug.

Use cautiously in patients with Parkinson's disease because syncope and orthostatic hypotension may worsen.

Interactions

Drug-drug. *Desipramine:* Increased incidence of adverse effects. Use together cautiously.
MAO inhibitors: Hypertensive crisis may occur. Avoid use together.

Effects on diagnostic tests

None reported.

Adverse reactions

CNS: *dyskinesia, sleep disorder, dystonia, excessive dreaming, somnolence, dizziness, confusion, headache, hallucinations,* hyperkinesia, fatigue, falling, syncope, balance loss, depression, tremor, speech disorder, paresthesia.
CV: *orthostatic complaints,* chest pain, chest discomfort, palpitation, hypotension.
EENT: pharygitis, tinnitus.
GI: *nausea, anorexia, diarrhea,* flatulence, *vomiting,* constipation, abdominal pain, dyspepsia, dry mouth.
GU: urinary tract infection, urine discoloration, hematuria, urinary incontinence, impotence.
Musculoskeletal: *muscle cramps,* myalgia, stiffness, arthritis, neck pain.
Respiratory: bronchitis, dyspnea, upper respiratory infections.
Skin: increased sweating, rash.

Overdose and treatment
The highest dose used is 800 mg t.i.d.; nausea, vomiting, and dizziness were noted. Provide supportive care and hospitalize, if indicated.

Clinical considerations
- Because of the risk of potentially fatal, acute fulminant liver failure, use drug only in patients on levodopa/carbidopa who don't respond to or who aren't suitable for other adjunctive therapy.
- Diarrhea occurs commonly in patients taking tolcapone. It may occur 2 weeks after therapy begins or after 6 to 12 weeks. Although it usually resolves with discontinuation of drug, hospitalization may be required in rare cases.
- Dose adjustments aren't needed in patients with mild to moderate renal dysfunction; use cautiously in patients with severe renal impairment.
- Withdraw drug in patients who fail to show clinical benefit within 3 weeks of treatment.

Therapeutic monitoring
- Monitor liver enzymes every 2 weeks for the first year of therapy, and then every 8 weeks. Stop drug if hepatic transaminases exceed the upper limits of normal or if patient appears jaundiced.
- Monitor for clinical improvement, which should occur within 3 weeks.

Special populations
Pregnant patients. Use drug during pregnancy only when potential benefits justify risk to fetus.
Breast-feeding patients. Because of the risk that drug may be excreted in breast milk, use with caution in breast-feeding women.
Pediatric patients. There's no identified potential use in children.

Patient counseling
- Advise patient to take drug exactly as prescribed.
- Warn patient about risk of orthostatic hypotension; tell him to use caution when rising from a seated or recumbent position.
- Caution patient to avoid hazardous activities until CNS effects of drug are known.
- Tell patient that nausea may occur and to report signs of liver injury immediately.
- Advise patient about risk of increased dyskinesia or dystonia.
- Inform patient that hallucinations may occur.
- Tell patient to report if pregnancy is being planned or suspected during therapy.

tolmetin sodium
Tolectin, Tolectin DS

Pharmacologic classification: NSAID
Therapeutic classification: nonnarcotic analgesic, anti-inflammatory
Pregnancy risk category C

How supplied
Available by prescription only
Tablets: 200 mg, 600 mg
Capsules: 400 mg

Indications and dosages
Rheumatoid arthritis and osteoarthritis, juvenile rheumatoid arthritis
Adults: Initially, 400 mg P.O. t.i.d.; maximum dose is 1,800 mg/day; usual dose ranges from 600 to 1,800 mg daily in three divided doses.
Children age 2 or older: Initially, 20 mg/kg/day P.O. in three or four divided doses; usual dose ranges from 15 to 30 mg/kg/day in three or four divided doses.

Pharmacodynamics
Analgesic and anti-inflammatory actions: Although the exact mechanism of action is unknown, inhibition of prostaglandin synthesis may be responsible for the anti-inflammatory effects of tolmetin. Drug also seems to possess analgesic and antipyretic activity.

Pharmacokinetics
Absorption: Absorbed rapidly from GI tract.
Distribution: Highly protein-bound.
Metabolism: Metabolized in the liver.
Excretion: Excreted in urine as an inactive metabolite or conjugates of tolmetin. Elimination is biphasic, consisting of a rapid phase with a half-life of 1 to 2 hours followed by a slower phase with a half-life of about 5 hours.

Route	Onset	Peak	Duration
P.O.	Unknown	½-1½ hr	24 hr

Contraindications and precautions
Contraindicated in patients with hypersensitivity to drug or in whom acute asthmatic attacks, urticaria, or rhinitis is precipitated by aspirin or NSAIDs and in breast-feeding women. Use cautiously in patients with renal or cardiac disease, GI bleeding, history of peptic ulcer, hypertension, and conditions predisposing to fluid retention.

Interactions
Drug-drug. *Anticoagulants, thrombolytics:* Increased risk of bleeding. Use together cautiously.
Aspirin: Decreased plasma levels of tolmetin. Monitor patient closely. Dose adjustment may be required.

Highly protein-bound drugs, such as phenytoin, salicylates, sulfonamides, sulfonylureas, and warfarin: Increased adverse effects. Monitor patient closely.
Methotrexate: Increased risk of methotrexate toxicity. Avoid use together. If given together, monitor patient closely.
Other GI irritating drugs, such as antibiotics, corticosteroids, and NSAIDs: Potentiate adverse GI effects. Use together cautiously.
Drug-food. *Any food:* Delayed and decreased absorption of tolmetin. Separate administration times.

Effects on diagnostic tests
Tolmetin falsely elevates results of urinary protein (pseudoproteinuria) in tests that rely on acid precipitation, such as those using sulfosalicylic acid.

Adverse reactions
CNS: headache, dizziness, drowsiness, asthenia, depression.
CV: chest pain, hypertension, edema.
EENT: tinnitus, visual disturbances.
GI: epigastric distress, peptic ulceration, occult blood loss, *nausea,* vomiting, abdominal pain, diarrhea, constipation, dyspepsia, flatulence, anorexia.
GU: urinary tract infection
Hematologic: elevated BUN, decreased hemoglobin and hematocrit.
Skin: irritation.
Other: ***anaphylaxis,*** weight gain, weight loss.

Overdose and treatment
Signs and symptoms of overdose include dizziness, drowsiness, mental confusion, and lethargy. To treat tolmetin overdose, empty stomach immediately by inducing emesis or by gastric lavage followed by administration of activated charcoal. Provide symptomatic and supportive measures (respiratory support and correction of fluid and electrolyte imbalances). Monitor laboratory parameters and vital signs closely. Alkalinization of urine by sodium bicarbonate ingestion may enhance renal excretion of tolmetin.

Clinical considerations
Consider the recommendations relevant to all NSAIDs as well as the following:
- Assess cardiopulmonary status closely.
- Therapeutic effect usually occurs within a few days to 1 week of therapy. Evaluate patient's response to drug as evidenced by relief of symptoms.
- Administer drug on empty stomach for maximum absorption. However, it may be administered with meals to lessen GI upset.

Therapeutic monitoring
- Monitor vital signs closely, especially heart rate and blood pressure.
- Assess renal function periodically during therapy; monitor fluid intake and output and daily weight.
- Monitor for presence and amount of edema.

Special populations
Pregnant patients. Use drug during pregnancy only when clearly needed.
Breast-feeding patients. Because drug is excreted in breast milk, it may adversely affect neonates. Avoid use in breast-feeding women.
Pediatric patients. Safety and efficacy in children under age 2 haven't been established.

Patient counseling
- Explain that therapeutic effects may occur in 1 week but could take 2 to 4 weeks.
- Advise patient to avoid use of OTC medications such as NSAIDs, unless medically approved.
- Instruct patient to follow prescribed regimen and recommended schedule of follow-up.
- Advise patient to report any signs of edema or other adverse reactions.

tolterodine tartrate
Detrol

Pharmacologic classification: muscarinic receptor antagonist
Therapeutic classification: anticholinergic
Pregnancy risk category C

How supplied
Available by prescription only
Tablets: 1 mg, 2 mg

Indications and dosages
Treatment of patients with overactive bladder with symptoms of urinary frequency, urgency, or urge incontinence
Adults: Initial dosage is 2 mg P.O. b.i.d. May lower to 1 mg b.i.d. based on response and tolerance.
≡ ***Dosage adjustment.*** In patients who have significantly reduced hepatic function or who are currently taking a drug that inhibits the cytochrome P-450 3A4 isoenzyme system, recommended dose is 1 mg b.i.d.

Pharmacodynamics
Anticholinergic action: Tolterodine is a competitive muscarinic receptor antagonist. Both urinary bladder contraction and salivation are mediated by way of cholinergic muscarinic receptors.

Pharmacokinetics
Absorption: Well absorbed with about 77% bioavailability. Food increases bioavailability by 53%.

Distribution: Volume of distribution is about 113 L. Tolterodine is 96% protein-bound.
Metabolism: Metabolized by the liver primarily by oxidation by the cytochrome P-450 2D6 pathway; leads to formation of a pharmacologically active 5-hydroxymethyl metabolite.
Excretion: Mostly via urine; the rest in feces. Less than 1% of a dose is recovered as unchanged drug and 5% to 14% is recovered as the active metabolite. Half-life is 2 to 3½ hours.

Route	Onset	Peak	Duration
P.O.	Unknown	1-2 hr	Unknown

Contraindications and precautions
Contraindicated in patients with urine or gastric retention and uncontrolled narrow-angle glaucoma. Also contraindicated in patients hypersensitive to tolterodine or its ingredients.

Use with caution in patients with significantly reduced hepatic or renal function.

Interactions
Drug-drug. *Antifungal agents, such as itraconazole, ketoconazole, and miconazole; cytochrome P-450 3A4 inhibitors such as macrolide antibiotics, including clarithromycin and erythromycin:* Haven't been studied. However, tolterodine doses of more than 1 mg b.i.d. shouldn't be given together.
Drug-food. *Food:* Increases tolterodine absorption. May be used for this effect.

Effects on diagnostic tests
None reported.

Adverse reactions
CNS: paresthesia, vertigo, dizziness, *headache,* nervousness, somnolence, fatigue.
CV: hypertension, chest pain.
EENT: abnormal vision (including accommodation), xerophthalmia, pharyngitis, rhinitis, sinusitis.
GI: *dry mouth,* abdominal pain, constipation, diarrhea, dyspepsia, flatulence, nausea, vomiting.
GU: dysuria, micturition frequency, urine retention, urinary tract infection.
Musculoskeletal: arthalgia, back pain.
Respiratory: bronchitis, coughing, upper respiratory infection.
Skin: pruritis, rash, erythema, dry skin.
Other: flulike symptoms, weight gain.

Overdose and treatment
Overdoses can potentially result in severe central anticholinergic effects and should be treated accordingly. Perform ECG monitoring if an overdose occurs.

Clinical considerations
- Food increases the absorption of tolterodine, but no dose adjustment is needed.
- Dry mouth is the most frequently reported adverse event.

Therapeutic monitoring
Monitor for urinary symptoms and adverse reactions.

Special populations
Pregnant patients. Use drug during pregnancy only when clearly needed.
Breast-feeding patients. Excretion in breast milk is unknown. Drug isn't recommended for use in breast-feeding women.
Pediatric patients. Safety and efficacy in children haven't been established.
Geriatric patients. No overall differences in safety have been observed between older and younger patients.

Patient counseling
- Inform patient that antimuscarinics such as tolterodine may produce blurred vision.
- Caution patient to avoid hazardous activities until effects of drug are known.

topiramate
Topamax

Pharmacologic classification: sulfamate-substituted monosaccharide
Therapeutic classification: anticonvulsant
Pregnancy risk category C

How supplied
Available by prescription only
Capsules: 15, 25 mg
Tablets: 25, 100, 200 mg

Indications and dosages
Adjunctive therapy of partial onset seizures or primary generalized tonic-clonic seizures
Adults: Adjust up to maximum daily dose of 400 mg in two divided doses. Adjustment schedule is as follows.

Week	A.M. dose	P.M. dose
1	None	50 mg
2	50 mg	50 mg
3	50 mg	100 mg
4	100 mg	100 mg
5	100 mg	150 mg
6	150 mg	150 mg
7	150 mg	200 mg
8	200 mg	200 mg

Children age 2 to 16 years: 5 to 9 mg/kg P.O. daily in 2 divided doses. Dosage titration should begin at 1 to 3 mg/kg daily for 1 week. Then increase at 1- to 2-week intervals by 1 to 3 mg/kg daily to achieve optimal clinical response. Dosage titration should be guided by clinical outcome.

≡***Dosage adjustment.*** In patients with moderate to severe renal impairment, reduce dose by 50%. A supplemental dose may be required during hemodialysis.

Pharmacodynamics

Anticonvulsant action: Mechanism of action is unknown. Thought to block action potential, suggestive of a sodium channel-blocking action. Drug may potentiate activity of gamma-aminobutyric acid (GABA) and antagonize the ability of kainate to activate the kainate/AMPA subtype of excitatory amino acid (glutamate) receptor. Topiramate also has weak carbonic anhydrase inhibitor activity, which is unrelated to its anticonvulsant properties.

Pharmacokinetics

Absorption: Rapidly absorbed. Relative bioavailability of drug is about 80% compared with a solution and isn't affected by food.
Distribution: Plasma levels increase proportionately with dose; mean elimination half-life is 21 hours. Steady state is reached in 4 days in patients with normal renal function. Drug is 13% to 17% bound to plasma proteins.
Metabolism: Not extensively metabolized.
Excretion: Primarily eliminated unchanged in urine (about 70% of an administered dose). Mean plasma half-life is 21 hours.

Route	Onset	Peak	Duration
P.O.	Unknown	2 hr	Unknown

Contraindications and precautions

Contraindicated in patients with history of hypersensitivity to any component of the preparation.

Interactions

Drug-drug. *Carbamazepine, phenytoin:* Decreased topiramate levels. Monitor patient closely.
Carbonic anhydrase inhibitors, such as acetazolamide and dichlorphenamide: May increase the risk of renal stone formation. Avoid use together.
CNS depressants: Haven't been evaluated, because of the risk of topiramate-induced CNS depression and other adverse cognitive and neuropsychiatric events. Use together cautiously.
Oral contraceptives: Decreased contraceptive effect. Advise patient to use another method of contraception.
Phenobarbital, primidone, valproic acid: Increased phenytoin levels. Monitor closely.
Drug-food. *Alcohol use:* CNS depression, as well as other adverse cognitive and neuropsychiatric events. Advise avoiding alcohol use.

Effects on diagnostic tests

None reported.

Adverse reactions

CNS: abnormal coordination; agitation; apathy; asthenia; *ataxia; confusion;* depression; difficulty with concentration, attention, language, or memory; *dizziness;* emotional liability; euphoria; ***generalized tonic-clonic seizures;*** hallucination; hyperkinesia; hypertonia; hypoaesthesia; hypokinesia; insomnia; mood problems; *nervousness; nystagmus; paresthesia;* personality disorder; *psychomotor slowing;* psychosis; *somnolence; speech disorders;* stupor; ***suicide attempts;*** *tremor;* vertigo.
CV: chest pain, palpitations.
EENT: *abnormal vision,* conjunctivitis, *diplopia,* eye pain, epistaxis, hearing or vestibular problems, pharyngitis, sinusitis, taste perversion, tinnitus.
GI: abdominal pain, anorexia, constipation, diarrhea, dry mouth, dyspepsia, flatulence, gastroenteritis, gingivitis, *nausea,* vomiting.
GU: amenorrhea, dysuria, dysmenorrhea, leukorrhea, hematuria, impotence, intermenstrual bleeding, menstrual disorder, menorrhagia, micturition frequency, renal calculus, urinary incontinence, urinary tract infection, vaginitis.
Hematologic: anemia, ***leukopenia.***
Metabolic: increased or decreased weight.
Musculoskeletal: back pain, leg pain, myalgia.
Respiratory: bronchitis, coughing, dyspnea, *upper respiratory infection.*
Skin: acne, alopecia, aggressive reaction, increased sweating, pruritus, rash.
Other: body odor, edema, *fatigue,* fever, flu-like symptoms, hot flashes, malaise, rigors.

Overdose and treatment

In acute overdose after recent ingestion, institute gastric lavage or emesis. Activated charcoal isn't recommended. Institute supportive treatment. Hemodialysis is an effective means of removing drug.

Clinical considerations

- Because of the bitter taste, tablets shouldn't be broken.
- Capsules can be opened and contents sprinkled on soft food.
- If necessary, withdraw anticonvulsant drugs gradually to minimize risk of increased seizure activity.

Therapeutic monitoring

- Monitor CBC.
- Monitor for seizure activity.

Special populations
Breast-feeding patients. It isn't known if drug is excreted in breast milk. Use with caution in breast-feeding women.
Pediatric patients. Safety and efficacy in children under age 2 haven't been established.
Geriatric patients. No age-related problems were seen in the elderly; however, age-related renal abnormalities should be considered.

Patient counseling
- Carefully review dosing schedule with patient to avoid undermedication or overmedication.
- Tell patient to maintain adequate fluid intake during therapy because of potential to form renal stones.
- Advise patient to avoid hazardous activities until effects of drug are known.

topotecan hydrochloride
Hycamtin

Pharmacologic classification: semisynthetic camptothecin derivative
Therapeutic classification: antineoplastic
Pregnancy risk category D

How supplied
Available by prescription only
Injection: 4-mg single-dose vial

Indications and dosages
Metastatic carcinoma of the ovary after failure of initial or subsequent chemotherapy
Adults: 1.5 mg/m²/day as an I.V. infusion given over 30 minutes for 5 consecutive days, starting on day 1 of a 21-day cycle. Minimum of four cycles should be given.
≡ ***Dosage adjustment.*** In adults with renal impairment and creatinine clearance of 20 to 39 ml/minute, adjust dosage to 0.75 mg/m². In patients with mild renal impairment (creatinine clearance, 40 to 60 ml/minute), adjustment isn't required. There are insufficient data available for a dosage recommendation for patients with creatinine clearance less than 20 ml/minute. In the event of severe neutropenia occurring during any course, reduce the dose by 0.25 mg/m² for subsequent courses. Alternatively, administer granulocyte-colony stimulating factor (G-CSF) starting from day 6 of subsequent courses (24 hours after completion of topotecan) before resorting to dosage reduction.
Treatment of small-cell lung cancer sensitive disease after failure of first-line chemotherapy
Adults: 1.5 mg/m² I.V. infusion given over 30 minutes daily for 5 consecutive days, followed by a 16-day rest period for a 21-day treatment course. Minimum of four cycles should be given.
≡ ***Dosage adjustment.*** In patients with creatinine clearance of 20 to 39 ml/minute, dosage is decreased to 0.75 mg/m². If severe neutropenia occurs, dosage is decreased by 0.25 mg/m² for subsequent courses. Alternatively, if severe neutropenia occurs, G-CSF may be administered following the subsequent course (before resorting to dosage reduction) starting from day 6 of course (24 hours after completion of topotecan administration).

Pharmacodynamics
Antineoplastic action: Topotecan relieves torsional strain in DNA by inducing reversible single-strand breaks. It binds to the topoisomerase I-DNA complex and prevents religation of these single-strand breaks. The cytotoxicity of topotecan is thought to be due to double-strand DNA damage produced during DNA synthesis when replication enzymes interact with the ternary complex formed by topotecan, topoisomerase I, and DNA.

Pharmacokinetics
Absorption: Given only I.V.
Distribution: About 35% is bound to plasma protein.
Metabolism: Undergoes a reversible pH-dependent hydrolysis of its lactone moiety; the lactone form is pharmacologically active.
Excretion: About 30% is excreted in the urine. Terminal half-life is 2 to 3 hours.

Route	Onset	Peak	Duration
I.V.	Unknown	Unknown	Unknown

Contraindications and precautions
Contraindicated in patients hypersensitive to drug or its components, in those with severe bone marrow depression, and in pregnant or breast-feeding women.

Interactions
Drug-drug. *Cisplatin:* Increased severity of myelosuppression. Use together with extreme caution.
G-CSF: Prolonged duration of neutropenia. Don't initiate G-CSF until day 6 of the course of therapy, 24 hours after completion of treatment with topotecan.

Effects on diagnostic tests
None reported.

Adverse reactions
CNS: *fatigue, asthenia, headache,* paresthesia.
GI: *nausea, vomiting, diarrhea, constipation, abdominal pain, stomatitis, anorexia.*
Hematologic: NEUTROPENIA, LEUKOPENIA, THROMBOCYTOPENIA, *anemia.*
Hepatic: transient elevations of liver enzymes.

Respiratory: *dyspnea.*
Skin: *alopecia.*
Other: *sepsis,* fever.

Overdose and treatment

The primary adverse effect associated with topotecan overdose is thought to be bone marrow suppression. Treatment should be supportive. There's no known antidote.

Clinical considerations

- Before administration of the first course, baseline neutrophil count should exceed 1,500 cells/mm^3 and platelet count of more than 100,000 cells/mm^3.
- Protect unopened vials of drug from light. Reconstituted vials are stable at about 68° to 77° F (20° to 25° C) with ambient lighting conditions for 24 hours.
- Prepare drug under a vertical laminar flow hood wearing gloves and protective clothing. If drug solution contacts the skin, wash the skin immediately and thoroughly with soap and water. If mucous membranes are affected, flush areas thoroughly with water.
- Reconstitute each 4-mg vial with 4 ml sterile water for injection. Then dilute appropriate volume of reconstituted solution in either normal saline solution or D_5W before use.
- Bone marrow suppression (primarily neutropenia) is the dose-limiting toxicity of topotecan. The nadir occurs at about 11 days. If severe neutropenia occurs during therapy, reduce dose by 0.25 mg/m^2 for subsequent courses. Alternatively, administer G-CSF after the subsequent course (before dose is reduced) starting from day 6 (24 hours after completion of topotecan administration). Neutropenia isn't cumulative over time.
- Thrombocytopenia occurred with a median duration of 5 days and platelet nadir at a medium of 15 days; anemia occurred with a median nadir at day 15. Blood or platelet (or both) transfusions may be necessary.
- Inadvertent extravasation with topotecan has been associated with only mild local reactions, such as erythema and bruising.

Therapeutic monitoring

Frequent monitoring of peripheral blood cell counts is necessary. Don't give patients subsequent courses of topotecan until neutrophil counts exceed 1,000 cells/mm^3, platelet counts are more than 100,000 cells/mm^3, and hemoglobin levels are 9 mg/dl (with transfusion if needed).

Special populations

Pregnant patients. Contraindicated during pregnancy.
Breast-feeding patients. Because it isn't known if drug is excreted in breast milk, avoid use of drug in breast-feeding women.
Pediatric patients. Safety and efficacy in children haven't been established.

Patient counseling

- Instruct patient to promptly report sore throat, fever, chills, bruising or unusual bleeding.
- Inform patient of need for frequent blood work to monitor for potential bone marrow suppression.

toremifene citrate

Fareston

Pharmacologic classification: nonsteroidal antiestrogen
Therapeutic classification: antineoplastic
Pregnancy risk category D

How supplied

Available by prescription only
Tablets: 60 mg

Indications and dosages

For treatment of metastatic breast cancer in postmenopausal women with estrogen-receptor positive or unknown tumors
Adults: 60 mg P.O. once daily. Treatment is usually continued until disease progression is observed.

Pharmacodynamics

Antineoplastic action: Toremifene is a nonsteroidal triphenylethylene derivative that exerts its antitumor effect by competing with estrogen for binding sites in the tumor. This blocks the growth-stimulating effects of endogenous estrogen in the tumor, causing an antiestrogenic effect.

Pharmacokinetics

Absorption: Well absorbed after oral administration and not influenced by food. Peak plasma levels are obtained within 3 hours. Steady-state levels are reached in about 4 to 6 weeks.
Distribution: Apparent volume of distribution is 580 L; drug binds extensively (greater than 99.5%) to serum proteins, mainly albumin.
Metabolism: Extensively metabolized in liver, mainly by CYP3A4, to *N*-demethyltoremifene, which is also antiestrogenic but with weak in vivo antitumor potency. Elimination half-life is about 5 days.
Excretion: Eliminated in feces, with about 10% excreted unchanged in urine. Elimination is slow because of enterohepatic circulation.

Route	Onset	Peak	Duration
P.O.	Unknown	3 hr	Unknown

Contraindications and precautions

Contraindicated in patients with known hypersensitivity to drug. Avoid use in patients with history of thromboembolic diseases. Don't use drug long-term in patients with preexisting endometrial hyperplasia.

Interactions

Drug-drug. *Drugs that decrease renal calcium excretion such as thiazide diuretics:* Increased risk of hypercalcemia. Monitor calcium levels closely.
Coumarin-like anticoagulants such as warfarin: Prolonged PT and INR. Monitor PT and INR closely.
Cytochrome P-450 3A4 enzyme inducers, such as carbamazepine, phenobarbital, and phenytoin: Increased toremifene metabolism. Monitor patient closely; dose adjustment may be needed.
Cytochrome P-450 3A4-6 enzyme inhibitors, such as erythromycin and ketoconazole: Decreased toremifene metabolism. Monitor patient closely; dose adjustment may be needed.

Effects on diagnostic tests

None reported.

Adverse reactions

CNS: dizziness, fatigue, depression.
CV: edema, ***thromboembolism, heart failure, MI, pulmonary embolism.***
EENT: visual disturbances, glaucoma, ocular changes (such as dry eyes), *cataracts, abnormal visual fields.*
GI: *nausea,* vomiting.
GU: *vaginal discharge,* vaginal bleeding.
Hepatic: *elevated levels of AST, alkaline phosphatase,* and bilirubin.
Metabolic: hypercalcemia.
Skin: *sweating.*
Other: *hot flashes.*

Overdose and treatment

Theoretically, overdose may be manifested as an increase of antiestrogenic effects (hot flashes), estrogenic effects (vaginal bleeding), or nervous system disorders (vertigo, dizziness, ataxia, and nausea). There's no specific antidote; treatment is symptomatic.

Clinical considerations

- Disease flare-up may occur during first weeks of therapy. This doesn't indicate treatment failure.
- Drug causes fetal harm; indicated only for postmenopausal women.

Therapeutic monitoring

- Obtain periodic CBC, calcium levels, and liver function tests.
- Monitor calcium levels closely for first weeks of treatment in patients with bone metastases because of increased risk of hypercalcemia and tumor flare.

Special populations

Pregnant patients. Drug is contraindicated during pregnancy because of potential for fetal harm.
Breast-feeding patients. Presence of drug in breast milk isn't known.
Geriatric patients. No significant age-related differences in drug's efficacy or safety were noted.

Patient counseling

- Instruct patient to take drug exactly as prescribed.
- Warn patient not to discontinue therapy without consulting with health care provider.
- Inform patient to report vaginal bleeding and other adverse effects.
- Warn patient that a disease flare-up may occur during first weeks of therapy. Reassure patient that this doesn't indicate treatment failure.

torsemide

Demadex

Pharmacologic classification: loop diuretic
Therapeutic classification: diuretic/antihypertensive
Pregnancy risk category B

How supplied

Available by prescription only
Tablets: 5 mg, 10 mg, 20 mg, 100 mg
Solution: 2-ml ampule (10 mg/ml), 5-ml ampule (10 mg/ml)

Indications and dosages

Diuresis in patients with heart failure
Adults: Initially, 10 to 20 mg P.O. or I.V. once daily. If response is inadequate, double the dose until response is obtained. Maximum dose, 200 mg daily.
Diuresis in patients with chronic renal failure
Adults: Initially, 20 mg P.O. or I.V. once daily. If response is inadequate, double the dose until response is obtained. Maximum dose, 200 mg daily.
Diuresis in patients with hepatic cirrhosis
Adults: Initially, 5 to 10 mg P.O. or I.V. once daily with an aldosterone antagonist or a potassium-sparing diuretic. If response is inadequate, double the dose until response is obtained. Maximum dose, 40 mg daily.
Hypertension
Adults: Initially, 5 mg P.O. daily. Increase to 10 mg once daily in 4 to 6 weeks, if needed and tolerated. If response is still inadequate, add another antihypertensive agent.

Pharmacodynamics

Diuretic and antihypertensive actions: Loop diuretics such as torsemide enhance excretion of sodium, chloride, and water by acting on the ascending portion of the loop of Henle. Torsemide doesn't significantly alter glomerular filtration rate, renal plasma flow, or acid-base balance.

Pharmacokinetics

Absorption: Absorbed with little first-pass metabolism; serum level reaches its peak within 1 hour after oral administration.
Distribution: Volume of distribution is 12 to 15 L in healthy patients and in those with mild to moderate renal failure or heart failure. In patients with hepatic cirrhosis, volume of distribution is about doubled. Drug is extensively bound (97% to 99%) to plasma protein.
Metabolism: Metabolized in the liver to an inactive major metabolite and to two lesser metabolites that have some diuretic activity; for practical purposes, metabolism terminates action of drug. Duration of action is 6 to 8 hours after oral or I.V. use.
Excretion: From 22% to 34% of dose is excreted unchanged in urine via active secretion of drug by the proximal tubules.

Route	Onset	Peak	Duration
P.O.	1 hr	1-2 hr	6-8 hr
I.V.	10 min	1 hr	6-8 hr

Contraindications and precautions

Contraindicated in patients with anuria or hypersensitivity to drug or other sulfonylurea derivatives. Use cautiously in patients with hepatic disease and associated cirrhosis and ascites.

Interactions

Drug-drug. *Aminoglycosides and other ototoxic drugs:* Auditory toxicity. Monitor patient carefully.
Cholestyramine: Decreased torsemide absorption. Separate administration by at least 3 hours.
Lithium: Lithium toxicity. Monitor patient closely.
NSAIDs: Renal dysfunction. Use together cautiously.
Probenecid, indomethacin: Decreased diuretic effect. Avoid use together.
Salicylates: Reduced excretion of salicylate. Avoid use together.

Effects on diagnostic tests

None reported.

Adverse reactions

CNS: asthenia, dizziness, headache, nervousness, insomnia, syncope.
CV: ECG abnormalities, chest pain, edema, ***dehydration.***
EENT: rhinitis, cough, sore throat.
GI: diarrhea, constipation, nausea, dyspepsia, ***hemorrhage.***
GU: *excessive urination,* altered renal function tests.
Metabolic: altered electrolyte balance.
Musculoskeletal: arthralgia, myalgia.

Overdose and treatment

Although data specific to torsemide overdose are lacking, signs and symptoms would probably reflect excessive pharmacologic effect: dehydration, hypovolemia, hypotension, hyponatremia, hypokalemia, hypochloremic alkalosis, and hemoconcentration. Treatment should consist of fluid and electrolyte replacement.

Clinical considerations

- Tinnitus and hearing loss (usually reversible) have been observed after rapid I.V. injection of other loop diuretics and have been noted after oral torsemide administration. Inject drug slowly over 2 minutes; single doses shouldn't exceed 200 mg.
- CV disease (especially in patients receiving cardiac glycosides) and diuretic-induced hypokalemia may be risk factors for the development of arrhythmias.
- The risk of hypokalemia is greatest in patients with hepatic cirrhosis, brisk diuresis, inadequate oral intake of electrolytes, or concurrent therapy with corticosteroids or corticotropin. Perform periodic monitoring of serum potassium and other electrolytes.
- Excessive diuresis may cause dehydration, blood-volume reduction, and possibly thrombosis and embolism, especially in geriatric patients.

Therapeutic monitoring

Monitor fluid intake and output, serum electrolyte levels, blood pressure, weight, and pulse rate during rapid diuresis and routinely with chronic use. If fluid and electrolyte imbalances occur, discontinue drug until the imbalances are corrected. Drug may then be restarted at a lower dose.

Special populations

Breast-feeding patients. It isn't known if drug is excreted in breast milk. Use caution when administering drug to breast-feeding women.
Pediatric patients. Safety and efficacy in children under age 18 haven't been established.
Geriatric patients. Special dose adjustment usually isn't necessary. However, geriatric patients are at greater risk for dehydration, blood-volume reduction, and possibly thrombosis and embolism with excessive diuresis.

Patient counseling

- Instruct patient to take torsemide in the morning to prevent nocturia and to change positions slowly to prevent dizziness.
- Instruct patient to report ringing in ears immediately because this may indicate toxicity.

tramadol hydrochloride

Ultram

Pharmacologic classification: synthetic derivative
Therapeutic classification: analgesic
Pregnancy risk category C

How supplied

Available by prescription only
Tablets: 50 mg

Indications and dosages

Moderate to moderately severe pain
Adults: 50 to 100 mg P.O. q 4 to 6 hours, p.r.n. Maximum dose, 400 mg/day.
≡ ***Dosage adjustment.*** In patients with creatinine clearance less than 30 ml/minute, increase dosing interval to q 12 hours; maximum daily dose, 200 mg.

In patients with cirrhosis, recommended dosage is 50 mg q 12 hours.

Pharmacodynamics

Analgesic action: Mechanism of action is unknown. It's a centrally acting synthetic analgesic compound that isn't chemically related to opiates but is thought to bind to opioid receptors and inhibit reuptake of norepinephrine and serotonin.

Pharmacokinetics

Absorption: Almost completely absorbed. Mean absolute bioavailability of a 100-mg dose is about 75%.
Distribution: About 20% bound to plasma protein; it may cross the blood-brain barrier.
Metabolism: Extensively metabolized.
Excretion: About 30% of a dose is excreted unchanged in urine and 60% as metabolites. Half-life of drug is about 6 to 7 hours.

Route	Onset	Peak	Duration
P.O.	Unknown	2 hr	Unknown

Contraindications and precautions

Contraindicated in patients with hypersensitivity to drug or acute intoxication with alcohol, hypnotics, centrally acting analgesics, opioids, or psychotropic drugs.

Use cautiously in patients at risk for seizures or respiratory depression; in those with increased intracranial pressure or head injury, acute abdominal conditions, impaired renal or hepatic function; and in patients physically dependent on opioids.

Interactions

Drug-drug. *Carbamazepine:* Increases tramadol metabolism. Monitor patient closely. Dose adjustment may be needed.
CNS depressants: Additive effects. Use together cautiously. Tramadol dose may need to be reduced.
MAO inhibitors, neuroleptic drugs: Increased risk of seizures. Monitor patient closely.
Drug-food. *Alcohol use:* Increased CNS depression. Advise patient to avoid alcohol use.

Effects on diagnostic tests

None reported.

Adverse reactions

CNS: *dizziness, vertigo, headache, somnolence, CNS stimulation, asthenia,* anxiety, confusion, coordination disturbance, euphoria, nervousness, sleep disorder, ***seizures,*** malaise.
CV: vasodilation.
EENT: visual disturbances.
GI: *nausea, constipation, vomiting,* dyspepsia, dry mouth, diarrhea, abdominal pain, anorexia, flatulence.
GU: urine retention, urinary frequency, increased creatinine clearance, proteinuria, menopausal symptoms.
Hematologic: decreased hemoglobin levels.
Hepatic: elevated liver enzymes.
Musculoskeletal: hypertonia.
Respiratory: ***respiratory depression.***
Skin: *pruritus,* diaphoresis, rash.

Overdose and treatment

Serious potential consequences are respiratory depression and seizures. Because naloxone will reverse some, but not all, of the symptoms caused by tramalol overdose, supportive therapy is recommended. Hemodialysis removes only a small percentage of drug.

Clinical considerations

- Drug has been reported to reduce seizure threshold.
- Serious and rarely fatal anaphylactoid reactions have been reported (less than 1%).

Therapeutic monitoring

- Monitor patient closely for seizures.
- Monitor patient's CV and respiratory status and stop dose if respirations decrease or rate is less than 12 breaths/minute or if patient exhibits signs of respiratory depression.
- Monitor patient for drug dependence. Because drug dependence similar to codeine or dextropropoxyphene can occur, the potential for abuse exists.

Special populations

Pregnant patients. Safe use during pregnancy hasn't been established.
Breast-feeding patients. Use of drug in breast-feeding women isn't recommended.

Pediatric patients. Safety and efficacy in children under age 16 haven't been established.
Geriatric patients. Use cautiously in geriatric patients because serum levels are slightly elevated and the elimination half-life of drug is prolonged. Don't exceed daily dose of 300 mg in patients over age 75.

Patient counseling

- Instruct patient to take drug only as prescribed.
- Caution patient to avoid potentially hazardous activities that require mental alertness until adverse CNS effects of drug are known.

trandolapril

Mavik

Pharmacologic classification: ACE inhibitor
Therapeutic classification: antihypertensive
Pregnancy risk category C (D second and third trimesters)

How supplied

Available by prescription only
Tablets: 1 mg, 2 mg, 4 mg

Indications and dosages

Hypertension
Adults: In patient not taking a diuretic, initially 1 mg for the nonblack patient and 2 mg for the black patient P.O. once daily. If control isn't adequate, dose can be increased at intervals of at least 1 week. Maintenance dosage ranges from 2 to 4 mg daily for most patients; there's little experience with doses of more than 8 mg. Patients receiving once-daily dosing at 4 mg may use b.i.d. dosing.

For patient receiving a diuretic, initially 0.5 mg P.O. once daily. Subsequent dose adjustment made based on blood pressure response.
Heart failure post-MI or left ventricular dysfunction post-MI
Adults: Initially, 1 mg P.O. daily, adjusted to 4 mg P.O. daily. If patient can't tolerate 4 mg, continue at highest tolerated dose.

Pharmacodynamics

Antihypertensive action: Unknown. Drug action is thought to result primarily from inhibition of circulating and tissue ACE activity, reducing angiotensin II formation, decreasing vasoconstriction, decreasing aldosterone secretion, and increasing plasma renin. Decreased aldosterone secretion leads to diuresis, natriuresis, and a small increase in serum potassium.

Pharmacokinetics

Absorption: Absolute bioavailability after oral administration of trandolapril is about 10% for trandolapril and 70% for its metabolite, trandolaprilat.
Distribution: About 80% protein-bound.
Metabolism: Metabolized by the liver to the active metabolite, trandolaprilat, and at least seven other metabolites.
Excretion: About 66% excreted in feces; 33% in urine. Elimination half-lives of trandolapril and trandolaprilat are about 6 and 10 hours, respectively, but like all ACE inhibitors, trandolaprilat also has a prolonged terminal elimination phase.

Route	Onset	Peak	Duration
P.O.	Unknown	1-10 hr	24 hr

Contraindications and precautions

Contraindicated in patients with hypersensitivity to drug and history of angioedema related to previous treatment with an ACE inhibitor. Drug isn't recommended for use in pregnant women.

Use cautiously in patients with impaired renal function, heart failure, or renal artery stenosis.

Interactions

Drug-drug. *Diuretics:* Increased risk of excessive hypotension. Stop diuretic or lower dose of trandolapril.
Lithium: Lithium toxicity. Don't use together.
Potassium-sparing diuretics, potassium supplements: Increased risk of hyperkalemia. Monitor serum potassium closely.
Drug-food. *Salt substitutes containing potassium:* Increased risk of hyperkalemia. Monitor serum potassium closely.

Effects on diagnostic tests

None reported.

Adverse reactions

CNS: dizziness, headache, fatigue, drowsiness, insomnia, paresthesia, vertigo, anxiety.
CV: chest pain, *AV first-degree block, bradycardia,* edema, flushing, hypotension, palpitations.
EENT: epistaxis, throat inflammation, upper respiratory tract infection.
GI: diarrhea, dyspepsia, abdominal distention, abdominal pain or cramps, constipation, vomiting, *pancreatitis.*
GU: urinary frequency, increased creatinine clearance and BUN, impotence, decreased libido.
Hepatic: elevated liver enzymes.
Hematologic: ***neutropenia, leukopenia.***
Metabolic: hyperkalemia, hyponatremia, hyperuricemia.
Respiratory: dry, persistent, tickling, nonproductive cough; dyspnea.
Skin: rash, pruritus, pemphigus.
Other: ***anaphylactoid reactions, angioedema.***

Overdose and treatment
It's thought that the effects of overdose are similar to other ACE inhibitor overdose, with hypotension being the main adverse reaction. Because the hypotensive effect of trandolapril is achieved through vasodilation and effective hypovolemia, it's reasonable to treat trandolapril overdose by infusion of normal saline solution. In addition, renal function and serum potassium should be monitored. Trandolaprilat is removed by hemodialysis.

Clinical considerations
- Other ACE inhibitors have been associated with agranulocytosis and neutropenia.
- Angioedema associated with involvement of the tongue, glottis, or larynx may be fatal because of airway obstruction. Appropriate therapy, such as S.C. epinephrine 1:1,000 (0.3 to 0.5 ml) and equipment to ensure a patent airway, should be readily available.
- Obtain baseline CBC with differential counts before therapy, especially in patients who have collagen vascular disease with impaired renal function.
- If jaundice develops, discontinue drug; although rare, ACE inhibitors have been associated with a syndrome of cholestatic jaundice, fulminant hepatic necrosis, and death.

Therapeutic monitoring
- Assess patient's renal function before and periodically throughout therapy. Monitor serum potassium levels.
- Monitor for hypotension. Excessive hypotension can occur when drug is given with diuretics. If possible, discontinue diuretic therapy 2 to 3 days before starting trandolapril to decrease potential for excessive hypotensive response. If trandolapril doesn't adequately control blood pressure, diuretic therapy may be reinstituted with care.

Special populations
Pregnant patients. Drug is contraindicated for use during pregnancy.
Breast-feeding patients. It isn't known if drug is excreted in breast milk; avoid use in breast-feeding women.
Pediatric patients. Safety and efficacy in children haven't been established.

Patient counseling
- Advise patient to report signs of infection, easy bruising or bleeding; swelling of tongue, lips, face, eyes, mucous membranes, or extremities; difficulty swallowing or breathing; and hoarseness.
- Instruct patient to avoid products containing potassium, such as sodium substitutes.
- If syncope occurs, instruct patient to stop taking drug and notify prescriber immediately.

trastuzumab
Herceptin

Pharmacologic classification: monoclonal antibody to human epidermal growth factor receptor 2 protein (HER2)
Therapeutic classification: antineoplastic
Pregnancy risk category B

How supplied
Available by prescription only
Injection: lyophilized sterile powder containing 440 mg per vial

Indications and dosages
Single-agent treatment of metastatic breast cancer in patients whose tumors overexpress the HER2 protein and who have received one or more chemotherapy regimens for their metastatic disease, or in combination with paclitaxel for metastatic breast cancer in patients whose tumors overexpress the HER2 protein and who haven't received chemotherapy for their metastatic disease
Adults: Initial loading dose 4 mg/kg I.V. over 90 minutes. Maintenance dosage is 2 mg/kg I.V. weekly as a 30-minute I.V. infusion if initial loading dose is well tolerated.

Pharmacodynamics
Antineoplastic action: Protein overexpression is observed in 25% to 30% of primary breast cancers. Drug is a recombinant DNA-derived monoclonal antibody that selectively binds to HER2, inhibiting the proliferation of human tumor cells that overexpress HER2.

Pharmacokinetics
Absorption: Not reported.
Distribution: Volume of distribution is about that of serum volume (44 ml/kg). Between weeks 16 and 32, serum levels reach steady state with a mean trough of 79 mcg/ml and peak of 123 mcg/ml.
Metabolism: Not reported.
Excretion: Half-life and clearance are dose dependent. At the recommended dose, a mean half-life of 5¾ days (range 1 to 32 days) has been observed.

Route	Onset	Peak	Duration
I.V.	Unknown	Unknown	Unknown

Contraindications and precautions
Use with caution in a patient with a known hypersensitivity to drug, or any of its components. Use cautiously in patients with preexisting cardiac dysfunction or in those with known hypersensitivity to drug or its components and in the elderly.

Interactions
Drug-drug. *Anthracyclines:* Increased risk of cardiotoxicity. Avoid use together.
Paclitaxel: Increased trastuzumab serum levels. Monitor patient closely.

Effects on diagnostic tests
None reported.

Adverse reactions
CNS: depression, *headache, dizziness, insomnia, asthenia,* neuropathy, paresthesia, peripheral neuritis.
CV: ***heart failure,*** *peripheral edema,* tachycardia, paroxysmal nocturnal dyspnea, cardiomyopathy, decreased ejection fraction.
EENT: *rhinitis, pharyngitis,* sinusitis.
GI: *anorexia, abdominal pain, diarrhea, nausea, vomiting.*
GU: urinary tract infection.
Hematologic: ***leukopenia,*** anemia.
Musculoskeletal: arthralgia, *back pain,* bone pain.
Respiratory: *dyspnea, increased cough.*
Skin: acne, herpes simplex, rash.
Other: *allergic reaction,* chills, edema, *fever, flu syndrome, infection, pain.*

Overdose and treatment
None reported.

Clinical considerations
- Before beginning therapy, patients should undergo a thorough baseline cardiac assessment, including history and physical examination and other evaluation methods to identify those at risk of cardiotoxicity development.
- Drug should only be used in patients with metastatic breast cancer whose tumors have HER2 protein overexpression.
- A first-infusion symptom complex (chills or fever) was observed in about 40% of patients. Treat with acetaminophen, diphenhydramine, and meperidine (with or without reducing infusion rate). Other signs or symptoms may include nausea, vomiting, pain, rigors, headache, dizziness, dyspnea, hypotension, rash, and asthenia. These symptoms occur infrequently with subsequent infusions.
- Stopping drug should be strongly considered in patients in whom a clinically significant decrease in left ventricular function develops.

Therapeutic monitoring
Monitor for dyspnea, increased cough, paroxysmal nocturnal dyspnea, peripheral edema, or S_3 gallop, especially if patient is receiving drug with anthracyclines and cyclophosphamide.

Special populations
Breast-feeding patients. Because IgG is excreted in milk and because the potential for absorption harm to the infant is unknown, advise women to discontinue breast-feeding during and for 6 months following therapy.
Pediatric patients. Safety and efficacy in children haven't been established
Geriatric patients. Risk of cardiac dysfunction may be increased in geriatric patients.

Patient counseling
- Tell patient about risk of first-dose infusion-associated adverse effects.
- Instruct patient to notify health care provider immediately if signs or symptoms of cardiac dysfunction occur, such as shortness of breath, increased cough, or peripheral edema.

trazodone hydrochloride
Desyrel

Pharmacologic classification: triazolopyridine derivative
Therapeutic classification: antidepressant
Pregnancy risk category C

How supplied
Available by prescription only
Tablets (film-coated): 50 mg, 100 mg
Dividose tablets: 150 mg, 300 mg

Indications and dosages
Depression
Adults: Initial dose is 150 mg daily in divided doses, which can be increased by 50 mg/day q 3 to 4 days. Average dose ranges from 150 mg to 400 mg/day. Maximum dose, 400 mg/day in outpatients; 600 mg/day in hospitalized patients.
◇***Aggressive behavior***
Adults: 50 mg P.O. b.i.d.
◇***Panic disorder***
Adults: 300 mg P.O. daily.

Pharmacodynamics
Antidepressant action: Trazodone is thought to exert its antidepressant effects by inhibiting reuptake of norepinephrine and serotonin in CNS nerve terminals (presynaptic neurons), which results in increased level and enhanced activity of these neurotransmitters in the synaptic cleft. Trazodone shares some properties with tricyclic antidepressants: It has antihistaminic, alpha-blocking, analgesic, and sedative effects as well as relaxant effects on skeletal muscle. Unlike tricyclic antidepressants, however, trazodone counteracts the pressor effects of norepinephrine, has limited effects on the CV system and, in particular, has no direct quinidine-like effects on cardiac tissue; it also causes relatively fewer anticholinergic effects. Trazodone has been used in patients with alcohol dependence to decrease tremors and to alleviate anxiety and depression. Adverse reactions

somewhat dose-related; incidence increases with higher dose levels.

Pharmacokinetics

Absorption: Well absorbed from GI tract after oral administration. Taking drug with food delays absorption and increases amount absorbed by 20%.
Distribution: Widely distributed in the body; drug doesn't concentrate in any particular tissue, but small amounts may appear in breast milk. About 90% is protein-bound. Proposed therapeutic drug levels haven't been established. Steady-state plasma levels are reached in 3 to 7 days, and onset of therapeutic activity occurs in 7 days.
Metabolism: Metabolized by the liver; more than 75% of metabolites are excreted within 3 days.
Excretion: Mostly excreted in urine; the rest is excreted in feces via the biliary tract.

Route	Onset	Peak	Duration
P.O.	Unknown	1-2 hr	Unknown

Contraindications and precautions

Contraindicated during initial recovery phase of MI or in patients with hypersensitivity to drug. Use cautiously in patients with cardiac disease and in those at risk for suicide.

Interactions

Drug-drug. *Antihypertensive drugs, CNS depressants:* Additive effects of antihypertensives and CNS depressants. Monitor patient closely. Dose adjustment may be needed.
Digoxin, phenytoin: Increased serum levels of digoxin and phenytoin. Monitor patient closely.
Drug-herb. *St. John's wort:* Serotonin syndrome. Avoid use together.
Drug-lifestyle. *Alcohol use:* Exacerbated CNS depression. Advise patient to avoid alcohol use.

Effects on diagnostic tests

None reported.

Adverse reactions

CNS: *drowsiness, dizziness,* nervousness, fatigue, confusion, tremor, weakness, hostility, anger, nightmares, vivid dreams, headache, insomnia, *generalized tonic-clonic seizures.*
CV: orthostatic hypotension, tachycardia, hypertension, prolonged conduction time on ECG, syncope, shortness of breath.
EENT: blurred vision, tinnitus, nasal congestion.
GI: dry mouth, dysgeusia, constipation, nausea, vomiting, anorexia.
GU: urine retention; priapism, possibly leading to impotence; decreased libido; hematuria.
Hematologic: anemia, decreased WBC counts.
Hepatic: elevated liver function tests.
Metabolic: altered serum glucose levels.
Skin: rash, urticaria.
Other: diaphoresis.

Overdose and treatment

The most common signs and symptoms of drug overdose are drowsiness and vomiting; other signs and symptoms include orthostatic hypotension, tachycardia, headache, shortness of breath, dry mouth, and incontinence. Coma may occur.

Treatment is symptomatic and supportive and includes maintaining airway and stabilizing vital signs and fluid and electrolyte balance. Induce emesis if gag reflex is intact; follow with gastric lavage (begin with lavage if emesis is unfeasible) and activated charcoal to prevent further absorption. Forced diuresis may aid elimination. Dialysis is usually ineffective.

Clinical considerations

- Drug has fewer adverse cardiac and anticholinergic effects than tricyclic antidepressants.
- Consider the inherent risk of suicide until significant improvement of depressive state occurs.
- Tolerance to adverse effects (especially sedative effects) usually develops after 1 to 2 weeks of treatment.
- Drug may cause prolonged painful erections that may require surgical correction. An involuntary erection lasting more than 1 hour should be considered a medical emergency.
- Adverse effects are more common when doses exceed 300 mg/day.
- Don't withdraw drug abruptly.
- Discontinue drug at least 48 hours before surgical procedures.

Therapeutic monitoring

- Closely monitor patients at high risk for suicide, especially during initial stage of drug therapy.
- Monitor blood pressure because hypotension may occur.

Special populations

Pregnant patients. Use drug during pregnancy only when potential benefits justify risk to fetus.
Breast-feeding patients. Drug is excreted in breast milk; use with caution in breast-feeding women.
Pediatric patients. Drug isn't recommended for children under age 18.
Geriatric patients. Geriatric patients usually require lower initial doses; because adverse reactions are more likely to develop. However, it may be preferred in geriatric patients because it has fewer adverse cardiac effects.

Patient counseling

- Tell patient that full effects of drug may not become apparent for up to 2 weeks after therapy begins.

- Tell patient to take drug exactly as prescribed.
- Instruct patient not to participate in activities that require mental alertness until full effects of drug are known.
- Tell patient to avoid alcoholic beverages and medicinal elixirs while taking drug.
- Advise patient to promptly report adverse reactions including prolonged, painful erections, sexual dysfunction, dizziness, fainting, or rapid heartbeat.

tretinoin (systemic)

Vesanoid

Pharmacologic classification: retinoid
Therapeutic classification: antineoplastic
Pregnancy risk category D

How supplied

Available by prescription only
Capsules: 10 mg

Indications and dosages

Induction of remission in patients with acute promyelocytic leukemia (APL), French-American-British classification M^3 (including the M^3 variant), characterized by the presence of the t(15,17) translocation or the presence of PML/RAR alpha gene, who are refractory to, or who have relapsed from, anthracycline chemotherapy or for whom anthracycline-based chemotherapy is contraindicated

Adults and children age 1 and older: 45 mg/m^2/day P.O. administered as two evenly divided doses until complete remission is documented. Discontinue therapy 30 days after achievement of complete remission or after 90 days of treatment, whichever occurs first.

Pharmacodynamics

Antineoplastic action: Exact mechanism of action of tretinoin is unknown. Tretinoin produces an initial maturation of primitive promyelocytes derived from the leukemic clone, followed by a repopulation of bone marrow and peripheral blood by normal, polyclonal hematopoietic cells.

Pharmacokinetics

Absorption: Well absorbed from the GI tract.
Distribution: About 95% is bound to plasma protein.
Metabolism: May induce its own metabolism.
Excretion: Excreted in urine and feces.

Route	Onset	Peak	Duration
P.O.	Unknown	1-2 hr	Unknown

Contraindications and precautions

Contraindicated in patients with known hypersensitivity to retinoids or parabens, which are used as preservatives in the gelatin capsule. Don't use in pregnant or breast-feeding women.

Interactions

Drug-drug. *Ketoconazole:* Increased tretinoin plasma level. Use together cautiously.

Effects on diagnostic tests

None reported.

Adverse reactions

CNS: *malaise,* cerebral hemorrhage, dizziness, *paresthesia, headache, anxiety, insomnia, depression, confusion,* ***cerebral hemorrhage,*** intracranial hypertension, agitation, hallucination, abnormal gait, agnosia, aphasia, asterixis, cerebellar edema, cerebellar disorders, ***seizures, coma,*** CNS depression, dysarthria, encephalopathy, facial paralysis, hemiplegia, hyporeflexia, hypotaxia, no light reflex neurologic reaction, spinal cord disorder, tremor, leg weakness, unconsciousness, dementia, forgetfulness, somnolence, slow speech.
CV: *chest discomfort,* ***arrhythmias, heart failure,*** *hypotension, hypertension, peripheral edema, phlebitis, edema,* ***cardiac failure, cardiac arrest, MI,*** enlarged heart, heart murmur, ischemia, ***stroke,*** myocarditis, pericarditis, secondary cardiomyopathy.
EENT: *ear fullness, visual disturbances, ocular disorders,* hearing loss, *mucositis.*
GI: *GI hemorrhage, nausea, vomiting, anorexia, abdominal pain, GI disorders, diarrhea, constipation, dyspepsia, abdominal distention,* hepatosplenomegaly, ulcer, unspecified liver disorder.
GU: *renal insufficiency,* ***acute renal failure,*** micturition frequency, dysuria, renal tubular necrosis, enlarged prostate.
Hematologic: leukocytosis, ***hemorrhage, DIC.***
Hepatic: elevated liver function study results, *hepatitis.*
Metabolic: acidosis, hypothermia, fluid imbalance, hypercholesterolemia, hypertriglyceridemia, *weight increase, weight decrease.*
Musculoskeletal: flank pain, *myalgia, bone pain,* bone inflammation.
Respiratory: *pneumonia, upper respiratory tract disorders, dyspnea, respiratory insufficiency, pleural effusion, crackles, expiratory wheezing,* lower respiratory tract disorders, pulmonary infiltrate, bronchial asthma, pulmonary or larynx edema, unspecified pulmonary disease, pulmonary hypertension.
Skin: *flushing, skin mucous membrane dryness, pruritus, decreased sweating, alopecia, skin changes.*
Other: *fever, infections, shivering, pain, injection site reactions,* ***retinoic acid-APL syndrome, septicemia, multiorgan failure,*** cellulitis, facial edema, pallor, lymph disorder, ascites.

Overdose and treatment
None reported. Overdose with other retinoids has been associated with transient headache, facial flushing, cheilosis, abdominal pain, dizziness, and ataxia. These signs and symptoms have quickly resolved without apparent residual effects.

Clinical considerations
- Drug must be administered in a facility with laboratory and supportive services sufficient to monitor drug tolerance and protect and maintain patients compromised by drug toxicity.
- For women, a pregnancy test is required within 1 week before tretinoin therapy. When possible, therapy is delayed until a negative result is obtained.
- Patients with high WBC counts at diagnosis are at greater risk for rapid increases in WBC counts. Rapidly evolving leukocytosis is associated with a higher risk of life-threatening complications.
- About 25% of patients given drug during clinical studies have experienced retinoic acid-APL syndrome, characterized by fever, dyspnea, weight gain, radiographic pulmonary infiltrates, and pleural or pericardial effusions. This syndrome has occasionally been accompanied by impaired myocardial contractility and episodic hypotension with or without leukocytosis. Some patients have died because of progressive hypoxemia and multiorgan failure. The syndrome generally occurs during the first month of therapy. Treatment with high-dose steroids at the first signs of the syndrome appear to reduce morbidity and mortality risk.

Therapeutic monitoring
- Monitor CBC and platelet counts regularly.
- Monitor patient, especially children, for symptoms of pseudotumor cerebri, such as papilledema, headache, nausea, vomiting, and visual disturbances.
- Monitor cholesterol and triglyceride levels and liver function studies.

Special populations
Pregnant patients. Drug use is contraindicated during pregnancy.
Breast-feeding patients. It isn't known if drug is excreted in breast milk. Because of the potential for serious adverse reactions in breast-fed infants, drug shouldn't be given to breast-feeding women.
Pediatric patients. Safety and efficacy in children under age 1 haven't been established.

Patient counseling
- Instruct patient to report signs or symptoms of infection, (fever, sore throat, fatigue) or bleeding (easy bruising, nosebleeds, bleeding gums, melena).
- Tell patient to record his temperature daily.

tretinoin (topical)
Renova, Retin-A, Retin-A Micro

Pharmacologic classification: vitamin A derivative
Therapeutic classification: antiacne
Pregnancy risk category C

How supplied
Available by prescription only
Cream: 0.01%, 0.025%, 0.05%, 0.1%
Gel: 0.025%, 0.01%
Solution: 0.05%
Microsphere gel: 0.1%

Indications and dosages
Acne vulgaris (especially grades I, II, and III)
Adults and children: Clean affected area and lightly apply solution once daily h.s. or as directed.
◇ ***Treatment of photodamaged skin (wrinkles)***
Adults: 0.05% solution or 0.025% to 0.1% cream applied daily for at least 4 months.

Pharmacodynamics
Antiacne action: Mechanism of action of tretinoin hasn't been determined; however, it appears that tretinoin acts as a follicular epithelium irritant, preventing horny cells from sticking together and inhibiting the formation of additional comedones.

Pharmacokinetics
Absorption: Limited with topical use.
Distribution: None.
Metabolism: None.
Excretion: Minimal amount is excreted in the urine.

Route	Onset	Peak	Duration
Topical	Unknown	Unknown	Unknown

Contraindications and precautions
Contraindicated in patients with known hypersensitivity to vitamin A or retinoic acid, and in pregnancy.

Use cautiously in patients with eczema. Avoid contact of drug with eyes, mouth, angles of the nose, mucous membranes, or open wounds. Avoid use of topical preparations containing high levels of alcohol, menthol, spices, or lime because they may cause skin irritation. Avoid use of medicated cosmetics on treated skin.

Interactions
Drug-drug. *Topical agents:* risk of skin irritation. Avoid use together.
Drug-lifestyle. *Abrasive cleaners, medicated cosmetics, and skin preparations containing*

alcohol: Increased risk of skin irritation. Avoid use together.
Sun exposure: Potentiation of photosensitivity reactions. Advise patient to avoid prolonged or unprotected exposure to the sun.

Effects on diagnostic tests
None reported.

Adverse reactions
Skin: peeling, erythema, blisters, crusting, hyperpigmentation and hypopigmentation, contact dermatitis.

Note: Discontinue drug if sensitization or extreme redness and blistering of skin occur.

Overdose and treatment
None reported. Stop use and rinse area thoroughly. Oral ingestion of drug may lead to the same adverse effects as those associated with excessive oral intake of vitamin A.

Clinical considerations
- Don't use drug in patients who can't or won't minimize sun exposure.
- Although tretinoin microsphere gel was developed to minimize dermal irritation, the skin of some individuals may become excessively dry, red, swollen, blistered, or crusted.

Therapeutic monitoring
Therapeutic effect normally occurs in 2 to 3 weeks but may take 6 weeks or more. Relapses generally occur within 3 to 6 weeks of stopping medication.

Special populations
Pregnant patients. Drug use is contraindicated during pregnancy.
Breast-feeding patients. It isn't known if drug is excreted in breast milk. Because of the potential for serious adverse reactions in breastfed infants, drug shouldn't be given to breastfeeding women.
Pediatric patients. Safety and efficacy in children under age 1 haven't been established.

Patient counseling
- Advise patient on proper application technique. Stress importance of thorough removal of dirt and makeup before application and of hand washing after each use.
- Inform patient that application of medication may cause a temporary feeling of warmth and, if discomfort occurs, to promptly report to prescriber.
- Advise patient that initial exacerbation of inflammatory lesions is common and that redness and scaling (usually occurring in 7 to 10 days) are normal skin responses which disappear when therapy is discontinued.
- Caution patient to minimize exposure to sunlight or ultraviolet rays.
- Advise patient to keep medication away from eyes, mouth, angles of nose, and mucous membranes or open wounds.

triamcinolone (systemic)
Aristocort, Kenacort

triamcinolone acetonide
Kenalog, Triam-A

triamcinolone diacetate
Amcort, Aristocort, Aristocort Forte, Aristocort Intralesional, Articulose-L.A., Cenocort Forte, Kenacort, Triam-Forte, Triamolone 40, Tristoject

triamcinolone hexacetonide
Aristospan Intra-articular, Aristospan Intralesional

Pharmacologic classification: glucocorticoid
Therapeutic classification: anti-inflammatory, immunosuppressant
Pregnancy risk category C

How supplied
Available by prescription only
triamcinolone
Tablets: 1 mg, 2 mg, 4 mg, 8 mg
Syrup: 2 mg/ml, 4 mg/ml
triamcinolone acetonide
Injection: 10 mg/ml, 40 mg/ml suspension
triamcinolone diacetate
Injection: 25 mg/ml, 40 mg/ml suspension
triamcinolone hexacetonide
Injection: 5 mg/ml, 20 mg/ml suspension

Indications and dosages
Adrenal insufficiency
triamcinolone
Adults: 4 to 12 mg P.O. daily, in single or divided doses.
Children: 117 mcg/kg or 3.3 mg/m^2 P.O. daily, in single or divided doses.
Severe inflammation or immunosuppression
triamcinolone
Adults: 8 to 16 mg P.O. daily, in single or divided doses.
Children: 416 mcg to 1.7 mg/kg or 12.5 to 50 mg/m^2 P.O. daily, in single or divided doses.
triamcinolone acetonide
Adults: Initially, 60 mg I.M. Additional doses of 20 to 100 mg may be given, p.r.n., at 6-week intervals. Alternatively, administer 2.5 to 15 mg intra-articularly, or up to 1 mg intralesionally, p.r.n.
Children age 6 to 12: 0.03 to 0.2 mg/kg I.M. at 1- to 7-day intervals.

triamcinolone diacetate
Adults: 40 mg I.M. once weekly; or 2 to 40 mg intra-articularly, intrasynovially, or intralesionally q 1 to 8 weeks; or 4 to 48 mg P.O. divided q.i.d.
Children: 0.117 to 1.66 mg/kg/day P.O. divided q.i.d.
triamcinolone hexacetonide
Adults: 2 to 20 mg intra-articularly q 3 to 4 weeks, p.r.n.; or up to 0.5 mg intralesionally per square inch of skin.
Tuberculous meningitis
triamcinolone
Adults: 32 to 48 mg P.O. daily.
Edematous states
triamcinolone
Adults: 16 to 48 mg P.O. daily.
Collagen diseases
triamcinolone
Adults: 30 to 48 mg P.O. daily.
Dermatologic disorders
triamcinolone
Adults: 8 to 16 mg P.O. daily.
Allergic states
triamcinolone
Adults: 8 to 12 mg P.O. daily.
Ophthalmic diseases
triamcinolone
Adults: 12 to 40 mg P.O. daily.
Respiratory diseases
triamcinolone
Adults: 16 to 48 mg P.O. daily.
Hematologic diseases
triamcinolone
Adults: 16 to 60 mg P.O. daily.
Neoplastic diseases
triamcinolone
Adults: 16 to 100 mg P.O. daily.

Pharmacodynamics

Anti-inflammatory action: Triamcinolone stimulates the synthesis of enzymes needed to decrease the inflammatory response. It suppresses the immune system by reducing activity and volume of the lymphatic system, producing lymphocytopenia (primarily of T lymphocytes), decreasing immunoglobulin and complement levels, decreasing passage of immune complexes through basement membranes, and possibly depressing reactivity of tissue to antigen-antibody interactions.

Triamcinolone is an intermediate-acting glucocorticoid. The addition of a fluorine group in the molecule increases the anti-inflammatory activity, which is five times more potent than an equal weight of hydrocortisone. It has essentially no mineralocorticoid activity.

Triamcinolone may be administered orally. The diacetate and acetonide salts may be administered by I.M., intra-articular, intrasynovial, intralesional or sublesional, and soft-tissue injection. The diacetate suspension is slightly soluble, providing a prompt onset of action and a longer duration of effect (1 to 2 weeks). Triamcinolone acetonide is relatively insoluble and slowly absorbed. Its extended duration of action lasts for several weeks. Triamcinolone hexacetonide is relatively insoluble, is absorbed slowly, and has a prolonged action of 3 to 4 weeks. Don't administer any of the parenteral suspensions I.V.

Pharmacokinetics

Absorption: Absorbed readily after oral administration. After oral and I.V. administration, peak effects occur in about 1 to 2 hours. The suspensions for injection have variable onset and duration of action, depending on whether they're injected into an intra-articular space or a muscle, and on the blood supply to that muscle.
Distribution: Removed rapidly from the blood and distributed to muscle, liver, skin, intestines, and kidneys. Drug is extensively bound to plasma proteins (transcortin and albumin). Only the unbound portion is active. Adrenocorticoids are distributed into breast milk and through the placenta.
Metabolism: Metabolized in the liver to inactive glucuronide and sulfate metabolites.
Excretion: The inactive metabolites and small amounts of unmetabolized drug are excreted by the kidneys. Insignificant quantities of drug are also excreted in feces. Biologic half-life of triamcinolone is 18 to 36 hours.

Route	Onset	Peak	Duration
P.O., I.V., I.M., Intralesion, Intra-articular	Variable	Variable	Variable

Contraindications and precautions

Contraindicated in patients with hypersensitivity to any component of the formulation or systemic fungal infections.

Use cautiously in patients with GI ulcer, renal disease, hypertension, osteoporosis, diabetes mellitus, hypothyroidism, cirrhosis, diverticulitis, nonspecific ulcerative colitis, recent intestinal anastomosis, thromboembolic disorders, seizures, myasthenia gravis, heart failure, tuberculosis, ocular herpes simplex, emotional instability, or psychotic tendencies.

Interactions

Drug-drug. *Antacids, cholestyramine, colestipol:* Decreased effect of triamcinolone. Dose may need adjustment.
Oral anticoagulants: Decreased anticoagulation. Monitor patient closely; dose may need adjustment.
Barbiturates, phenytoin, rifampin: Decreased corticosteroid effects. Dose may need adjustment.
Cardiac glycosides: Increased toxicity. Monitor patient closely.
Diuretic, amphotercin B: Enhanced hypokalemia. Monitor patient closely.

Estrogens: Reduces the metabolism of triamcinolone. Dose may need adjustment.
Isoniazid and salicylates: Hyperglycemia. Dose may need adjustment.
Ulcerogenic drugs, NSAIDs: Increased risk of GI ulceration. Avoid use together.

Effects on diagnostic tests
Triamcinolone suppresses reactions to skin tests; causes false-negative results in the nitroblue tetrazolium test for systemic bacterial infections; and decreases ^{131}I uptake and protein-bound iodine levels in thyroid function tests.

Adverse reactions
Most adverse reactions to corticosteroids are dose- or duration-dependent.
CNS: *euphoria, insomnia,* psychotic behavior, pseudotumor cerebri, vertigo, headache, paresthesia, ***seizures.***
CV: ***heart failure, thromboembolism,*** hypertension, edema, ***arrhythmias,*** thrombophlebitis.
EENT: cataracts, glaucoma.
Endocrine: menstrual irregularities, cushingoid state (moonface, buffalo hump, central obesity).
GI: *peptic ulceration,* GI irritation, increased appetite, *pancreatitis,* nausea, vomiting.
GU: increased urine glucose and calcium levels.
Metabolic: hypokalemia, hyperglycemia, hypocalcemia, decreased T_3 and T_4 levels, hypercholesterolemia, and carbohydrate intolerance.
Musculoskeletal: muscle weakness, osteoporosis.
Skin: delayed wound healing, acne, various skin eruptions.
Other: hirsutism, susceptibility to infections; growth suppression in children; ***acute adrenal insufficiency with increased stress (infection, surgery, or trauma) or abrupt withdrawal after long-term therapy.***
After abrupt withdrawal: rebound inflammation, fatigue, weakness, arthralgia, fever, dizziness, lethargy, depression, fainting, orthostatic hypotension, dyspnea, anorexia, hypoglycemia. ***After prolonged use, sudden withdrawal may be fatal.***

Overdose and treatment
Acute ingestion, even in massive doses, is rarely a clinical problem. Toxic signs and symptoms rarely occur if drug is used for less than 3 weeks, even at large doses. However, chronic use causes adverse physiologic effects, including suppression of the hypothalamic-pituitary-adrenal axis, cushingoid appearance, muscle weakness, and osteoporosis.

Clinical considerations
Recommendations for use of triamcinolone and for care and teaching of patients during therapy are the same as those for all systemic adrenocorticoids.

Therapeutic monitoring
- Monitor for allergic reactions, adrenal insufficiency and seizure activity.
- Monitor cardiac status.

Special populations
Breast-feeding patients. Use drug with caution in breast-feeding women.
Pediatric patients. Chronic use of drug in children and adolescents may delay growth and maturation.

Patient counseling
- Instruct patient to take exactly as prescribed and not to suddenly discontinue drug.
- Instruct patient to promptly report any adverse reactions or unusual symptoms.

triamcinolone acetonide (oral and nasal inhalant)
Azmacort, Nasacort

Pharmacologic classification: glucocorticoid
Therapeutic classification: anti-inflammatory, antiasthmatic
Pregnancy risk category C

How supplied
Available by prescription only
Oral inhalation aerosol: 100 mcg/metered spray, 240 doses/inhaler
Nasal aerosol: 55 mcg/metered spray

Indications and dosages
Steroid-dependent asthma
Adults: 2 inhalations t.i.d. or q.i.d. Maximum dose, 16 inhalations daily.
Children age 6 to 12: 1 or 2 inhalations t.i.d. or q.i.d. Maximum dose, 12 inhalations daily.
Rhinitis, allergic disorders, inflammatory conditions, nasal polyps
Adults: 2 sprays in each nostril daily; may increase dose to maximum of 4 sprays per nostril daily, if needed.

Pharmacodynamics
Anti-inflammatory action: Glucocorticoids stimulate the synthesis of enzymes needed to decrease the inflammatory response. Triamcinolone acetonide is used as an oral inhalant to treat bronchial asthma in patients who require corticosteroids to control symptoms.

Pharmacokinetics
Absorption: Systemic absorption from the lungs is similar to oral administration.
Distribution: After oral inhalation, 10% to 25% is distributed to the lungs; the rest is swallowed

or deposited within the mouth. After nasal use, only a small amount reaches systemic circulation.
Metabolism: Metabolized mainly by the liver. Some that reaches the lungs may be metabolized locally.
Excretion: The major portion of a dose is eliminated in feces. Biologic half-life of triamcinolone is 18 to 36 hours.

Route	Onset	Peak	Duration
Inhalation	Unknown	1-2 hours	Unknown

Contraindications and precautions
Oral form is contraindicated in patients hypersensitive to any component of the formulation and in those with status asthmaticus. Nasal form is contraindicated in patients with hypersensitivity or untreated localized infections.

Use oral form cautiously in patients with tuberculosis of the respiratory tract; untreated fungal, bacterial, or systemic viral infections; or ocular herpes simplex and in those receiving corticosteroids. Use both forms with caution in breast-feeding women.

Interactions
None reported.

Effects on diagnostic tests
None reported.

Adverse reactions
Most adverse reactions to corticosteroids are dose- or duration-dependent.
EENT: *oral candidiasis,* dry or irritated tongue or mouth, dry or irritated nose or throat, hoarseness.
Respiratory: cough, wheezing (with oral form).
Other: facial edema (with oral form).

Overdose and treatment
None reported.

Clinical considerations
Recommendations for use of triamcinolone and for care and teaching of patients during therapy are the same as those for all inhalant adrenocorticoids.

Therapeutic monitoring
- Monitor for symptom resolution.
- Monitor respiratory status.

Special populations
Breast-feeding patients. Use drug with caution in breast-feeding women.
Pediatric patients. Safety and efficacy haven't been established for children under age 12 for nasal aerosol and under age 6 for oral aerosol.

Patient counseling
- Instruct patient to rinse mouth or gargle after inhaler use.
- Instruct patient to report lack of therapeutic effect or any adverse events.

triamcinolone acetonide (topical)
Aristocort, Flutex, Kenalog, Kenalog in Orabase, Triacet, Triaderm*

Pharmacologic classification: topical adrenocorticoid
Therapeutic classification: anti-inflammatory
Pregnancy risk category C

How supplied
Available by prescription only
Cream, ointment: 0.025%, 0.1%, 0.5%
Lotion: 0.025%, 0.1%
Paste: 0.1%

Indications and dosages
Inflammation of corticosteroid-responsive dermatoses
Adults and children: Apply cream, ointment, or lotion sparingly once to four times daily. Apply paste to oral lesions by pressing a small amount into lesion without rubbing until thin film develops. Apply b.i.d. or t.i.d. after meals and h.s.

Pharmacodynamics
Anti-inflammatory action: Glucocorticoids stimulate the synthesis of enzymes needed to decrease the inflammatory response. Triamcinolone acetonide is a synthetic fluorinated corticosteroid. The 0.5% cream and ointment are recommended only for dermatoses refractory to treatment with lower levels.

Pharmacokinetics
Absorption: Absorption depends on potency of preparation, amount applied, and nature of skin at application site. It ranges from about 1% in areas with a thick stratum corneum, such as the palms, soles, elbows, and knees, to as high as 36% in areas of the thinnest stratum corneum, such as the face, eyelids, and genitals. Absorption increases in areas of skin damage, inflammation, or occlusion. Some systemic absorption of steroids occurs, especially through the oral mucosa.
Distribution: After topical application, drug is distributed throughout the local skin layer. Drug absorbed into circulation is rapidly distributed into muscle, liver, skin, intestines, and kidneys.
Metabolism: After topical administration, drug is metabolized primarily in the skin. The small amount that's absorbed into systemic circula-

tion is metabolized primarily in the liver to inactive compounds.
Excretion: Inactive metabolites are excreted by the kidneys, primarily as glucuronides and sulfates, but also as unconjugated products. Small amounts of the metabolites are also excreted in feces.

Route	Onset	Peak	Duration
Topical	Unknown	Unknown	Unknown

Contraindications and precautions
Contraindicated in patients hypersensitive to drug.

Interactions
None reported.

Effects on diagnostic tests
None reported.

Adverse reactions
Metabolic: *hyperglycemia, glycosuria.*
Skin: *burning, pruritus, irritation, dryness, erythema, folliculitis, hypertrichosis, hypopigmentation, acneiform eruptions, perioral dermatitis, allergic contact dermatitis, maceration, secondary infection, atrophy, striae, miliaria* (with occlusive dressings).
Other: *hypothalamic-pituitary-adrenal axis suppression,* Cushing's syndrome.

Overdose and treatment
None reported.

Clinical considerations
Recommendations for use of triamcinolone acetonide and for care and teaching of patients during therapy are the same as those for all topical adrenocorticoids.

Therapeutic monitoring
- Monitor for symptom resolution.
- Monitor respiratory status.

Special populations
Recommendations for use of triamcinolone in breast-feeding women, children, and geriatric patients are the same as those for all topical adrenocorticoids.

Patient counseling
- Advise patient or family members of proper administration technique.
- If an occlusive dressing is ordered, advise patient not to leave it in place longer than 12 hours each day and not to use occlusive dressings on infected or exudative lesions.
- Tell patient to promptly report signs of systemic absorption, skin irritation or ulceration, hypersensitivity, infection, or no improvement.

triamterene
Dyrenium
Pharmacologic classification: potassium-sparing diuretic
Therapeutic classification: diuretic
Pregnancy risk category B

How supplied
Available by prescription only
Capsules: 50 mg, 100 mg

Indications and dosages
Edema
Adults: Initially, 100 mg P.O. b.i.d. after meals. Total daily dose shouldn't exceed 300 mg.

Pharmacodynamics
Diuretic action: Triamterene acts directly on the distal renal tubules to inhibit sodium reabsorption and potassium excretion, reducing the potassium loss associated with other diuretic therapy.

Triamterene is commonly used with other more effective diuretics to treat edema associated with excessive aldosterone secretion, hepatic cirrhosis, nephrotic syndrome, and heart failure.

Pharmacokinetics
Absorption: Absorbed rapidly after oral administration, but the extent varies. Diuretic effect may be delayed 2 to 3 days if used alone; maximum antihypertensive effect may be delayed 2 to 3 weeks.
Distribution: About 67% protein-bound.
Metabolism: Metabolized by hydroxylation and sulfation.
Excretion: Excreted in urine; half-life of triamterene is 100 to 150 minutes.

Route	Onset	Peak	Duration
P.O.	2-4 hr	2-4 hr	7-9 hr

Contraindications and precautions
Contraindicated in patients receiving other potassium-sparing agents, such as spirolactone or amiloride hydrochloride, and in those with hypersensitivity to drug, anuria, severe or progressive renal disease or dysfunction, severe hepatic disease, or hyperkalemia.

Use cautiously in patients with impaired hepatic function or diabetes mellitus and in geriatric or debilitated patients.

Interactions
Drug-drug. *Antihypertensive agents:* Enhanced hypoglycemia. Monitor patient closely. May be a therapeutic advantage.
Cimetidine: Increased bioavailability of triamterene. Monitor patient closely.
Lithium: Decreased lithium clearance. Avoid use together.

Other potassium-sparing diuretics; ACE inhibitors, such as captopril and enalapril; potassium supplements; potassium-containing medications such as parenteral penicillin G: Increased risk of hyperkalemia. Monitor patient closely.
NSAIDs: Altered potassium excretion. Monitor patient closely.
Drug-food. *Potassium-containing salt substitutes, potassium-rich foods:* Increased risk of hyperkalemia. Avoid use together.
Drug-lifestyle. *Sun exposure:* May cause photosensitivity reactions. Advise patient to avoid excessive sun exposure.

Effects on diagnostic tests

Drug therapy may interfere with enzyme assays that use fluorometry, such as serum quinidine determinations.

Adverse reactions

CNS: dizziness, weakness, fatigue, headache.
CV: hypotension.
GI: dry mouth, nausea, vomiting, diarrhea.
GU: transient elevation in BUN or creatinine levels, interstitial nephritis.
Hematologic: megaloblastic anemia related to low folic acid levels, ***agranulocytosis, thrombocytopenia.***
Hepatic: jaundice, increased liver enzyme abnormalities.
Metabolic: ***hyperkalemia,*** acidosis, hypokalemia, azotemia.
Musculoskeletal: muscle cramps.
Skin: photosensitivity, rash.
Other: ***anaphylaxis.***

Overdose and treatment

Signs include those indicative of dehydration and electrolyte disturbance. Treatment is supportive and symptomatic. For recent ingestion (less than 4 hours), empty stomach by induced emesis or gastric lavage. In severe hyperkalemia (more than 6.5 mEq/L), reduce serum potassium levels with I.V. sodium bicarbonate or glucose with insulin. A cation exchange resin, sodium polystyrene sulfonate (Kayexalate), given orally or as a retention enema, may also reduce serum potassium levels.

Clinical considerations

Consider the recommendations relevant to all potassium-sparing diuretics as well as the following:

- Drug is less potent than thiazides and loop diuretics and is useful as an adjunct to other diuretic therapy. Usually used with potassium-wasting diuretics. Full effect is delayed 2 to 3 days when used alone.
- To minimize excessive rebound potassium excretion, withdraw drug gradually.

Therapeutic monitoring

- Monitor blood pressure, blood uric acid, CBC, blood glucose, BUN, and serum electrolyte levels.
- Watch for blood dyscrasia.

Special populations

Pregnant patients. Use drug during pregnancy only when potential benefits justify possible risk to fetus.
Breast-feeding patients. Drug may be excreted in breast milk; safety during breast-feeding hasn't been established.
Pediatric patients. Use with caution; children are more susceptible to hyperkalemia.
Geriatric patients. Geriatric and debilitated patients require close observation because they're more susceptible to drug-induced diuresis and hyperkalemia. Reduced doses may be indicated.

Patient counseling

- Warn patient to avoid excessive ingestion of potassium-rich foods, such as citrus fruits, tomatoes, bananas, dates, and apricots; potassium-containing salt substitutes; and potassium supplements to prevent serious hyperkalemia.
- Advise patient to avoid direct sunlight, wear protective clothing, and use a sunblock to prevent photosensitivity reactions.
- Tell patient his urine may turn blue.
- Tell patient to promptly report weakness, sore throat, headache, fever, bruising, bleeding, mouth sores, nausea, vomiting, and/or dry mouth.

triazolam

Halcion

Pharmacologic classification: benzodiazepine
Therapeutic classification: sedative-hypnotic
Controlled substance schedule IV
Pregnancy risk category X

How supplied

Available by prescription only
Tablets: 0.125 mg, 0.25 mg

Indications and dosages

Insomnia
Adults: 0.125 to 0.25 mg P.O. h.s. (0.5 mg P.O. h.s. only in exceptional patients; maximum dose, 0.5 mg).
Elderly: 0.125 mg P.O. h.s. May give up to 0.25 mg.

Pharmacodynamics

Sedative-hypnotic action: Triazolam depresses the CNS at the limbic and subcortical levels of the brain. It produces a sedative-hypnotic effect by potentiating the effect of the neurotransmitter gamma-aminobutyric acid on its receptor in the ascending reticular activating system, which increases inhibition and blocks both cortical and limbic arousal.

Pharmacokinetics

Absorption: Well-absorbed through the GI tract after oral administration.
Distribution: Distributed widely throughout the body. Drug is 90% protein-bound.
Metabolism: Metabolized in the liver primarily to inactive metabolites.
Excretion: Metabolites are excreted in urine. Half-life of triazolam ranges from about 1½ to 5½ hours.

Route	Onset	Peak	Duration
P.O.	15-20 min	1-2 hr	Unknown

Contraindications and precautions

Contraindicated in patients with hypersensitivity to benzodiazepines and during pregnancy. Also, contraindicated in patients taking ketoconazole, itraconazole, nefazodone, or any other medications that impair the oxidative metabolism of triazolam by cytochrome P-450 3A.

Use cautiously in patients with impaired renal or hepatic function, chronic pulmonary insufficiency, sleep apnea, mental depression, suicidal tendencies, or history of drug abuse.

Interactions

Drug-drug. *Antidepressants, antihistamines, barbiturates, general anesthetics, MAO inhibitors, narcotics, phenothiazines:* Enhanced CNS depressant effects. Avoid use together.
Cimetidine, isoniazid, oral contraceptives, disulfiram: Increased plasma triazolam concentration. Monitor patient carefully.
Erythromycin: Decreased triazolam clearance. Monitor patient closely.
Haloperidol: Decreased serum levels of haloperidol. Monitor patient closely.
Levodopa: Decreased therapeutic effects of levodopa. Avoid use together.
Drug-food. *Grapefruit juice:* Increases triazolam levels. Use with caution. Monitor patient closely.
Drug-lifestyle. *Alcohol use:* Enhanced amnesia, excessive CNS depression. Advise patient to avoid alcohol use.
Smoking (heavy): Lowered triazolam effectiveness. Advise patient to avoid smoking.

Effects on diagnostic tests

None reported.

Adverse reactions

CNS: *drowsiness, dizziness, headache,* rebound insomnia, amnesia, light-headedness, lack of coordination, mental confusion, depression, nervousness, ataxia, minor changes in EEG patterns.
GI: nausea, vomiting.
Hepatic: elevated liver enzymes.
Other: physical or psychological dependence.

Overdose and treatment

Signs and symptoms of overdose include somnolence, confusion, hypoactive reflexes, dyspnea, labored breathing, hypotension, bradycardia, slurred speech, unsteady gait or impaired coordination and, ultimately, coma.

Support blood pressure and respiration until drug effects subside; monitor vital signs. Flumazenil, a specific benzodiazepine antagonist, may be useful. Mechanical ventilatory assistance via endotracheal tube may be required to maintain a patent airway and support adequate oxygenation. Use I.V. fluids and vasopressors, such as dopamine and phenylephrine, to treat hypotension as needed. If patient is conscious, induce emesis. Use gastric lavage if ingestion was recent, but only if an endotracheal tube is present to prevent aspiration. After emesis or lavage, administer activated charcoal with a cathartic as a single dose. Don't use barbiturates if excitation occurs. Dialysis is of limited value.

Clinical considerations

- Consider the recommendations relevant to all benzodiazepines.
- Onset of sedation or hypnosis is rapid; patient should be in bed when taking triazolam.

Therapeutic monitoring

Monitor hepatic function studies to prevent toxicity.

Special populations

Breast-feeding patients. Triazolam is excreted in breast milk. A breast-fed infant may become sedated, have feeding difficulties, or lose weight. Avoid use in breast-feeding women.
Pediatric patients. Safety in children under age 18 hasn't been established.
Geriatric patients. Geriatric patients are more susceptible to CNS depressant effects of drug and require supervision during initiation and after dose increases.

Patient counseling

- Advise patient of the potential for physical and psychological dependence.
- Instruct patient not to take OTC drugs or to change medication regimen without medical approval.
- Advise patient that rebound insomnia may occur after stopping drug.
- Advise women to report suspected pregnancy immediately.
- Advise patient not to take triazolam when a full night's sleep and clearance of the drug from the body isn't possible before normal daily activities resume.

trifluoperazine hydrochloride

Apo-Trifluoperazine*, Novo-Flurazine*, Solazine*, Stelazine, Terfluzine*

Pharmacologic classification: phenothiazine (piperazine derivative)
Therapeutic classification: antipsychotic, antiemetic
Pregnancy risk category C

How supplied

Available by prescription only
Tablets (regular and film-coated): 1 mg, 2 mg, 5 mg, 10 mg
Oral concentrate: 10 mg/ml
Injection: 2 mg/ml

Indications and dosages

Anxiety states
Adults: 1 to 2 mg P.O. b.i.d. Increase dosage, p.r.n., but don't exceed 6 mg/day.
Schizophrenia and other psychotic disorders
Adults: For outpatients, 1 to 2 mg P.O. b.i.d., increased, p.r.n. For hospitalized patients, 2 to 5 mg P.O. b.i.d.; may increase gradually to 40 mg daily. For I.M. injection, 1 to 2 mg q 4 to 6 hours, p.r.n.
Children age 6 to 12 (hospitalized or under close supervision): 1 mg P.O. daily or b.i.d.; may increase dosage gradually to 15 mg daily. Alternatively, administer 1 mg I.M. once or twice daily.

Pharmacodynamics

Antipsychotic action: Trifluoperazine is thought to exert its antipsychotic effects by postsynaptic blockade of CNS dopamine receptors, inhibiting dopamine-mediated effects; antiemetic effects are attributed to dopamine receptor blockade in the medullary chemoreceptor trigger zone. Trifluoperazine has many other central and peripheral effects; it produces alpha and ganglionic blockade and counteracts histamine- and serotonin-mediated activity. Its most prevalent adverse reactions are extrapyramidal; it has less sedative and autonomic activity than aliphatic and piperidine phenothiazines.

Pharmacokinetics

Absorption: Rate and extent of absorption vary with route of administration: Oral tablet absorption is erratic and variable, with onset of action ranging from ½ to 1 hour; oral concentrate absorption is much more predictable. I.M. drug is absorbed rapidly.
Distribution: Distributed widely in the body, including breast milk. Drug is 91% to 99% protein-bound; steady-state serum levels are achieved within 4 to 7 days.
Metabolism: Metabolized extensively by the liver, but no active metabolites are formed.
Excretion: Mostly excreted in urine via the kidneys; some is excreted in feces by way of the biliary tract.

Route	Onset	Peak	Duration
P.O., I.M.	Unknown	2-4 hr	4-6 hr

Contraindications and precautions

Contraindicated in patients with hypersensitivity to phenothiazines or in patients experiencing coma, CNS depression, bone marrow suppression, or liver damage.

Use cautiously in geriatric or debilitated patients; in those exposed to extreme heat; and in patients with CV disease, seizure disorders, glaucoma, or prostatic hyperplasia.

Interactions

Drug-drug. *Barbiturates, lithium:* Decreased phenothiazine effect. Monitor patient closely.
Beta blockers: Increased trifluoperazine levels and toxicity. Monitor patient closely.
Centrally acting antihypertensive drugs, such as clonidine, guanabenz, guanadrel, guanethidine, methyldopa, and reserpine: Inhibition of blood pressure response.
CNS depressants: Enhanced CNS depression. Avoid use together.
Epinephrine: Further lowering of blood pressure. Monitor patient closely. Dose adjustment may be necessary.
Lithium: Severe neurologic toxicity with an encephalitis-like syndrome, decreased therapeutic response to trifluoperazine. Avoid use together.
Propylthiouracil: Increased risk of agranulocytosis. Monitor patient closely.
Sympathomimetics: Decreased stimulatory and pressor effects. Monitor patient carefully.
Drug-food. *Caffeine:* Decreased therapeutic effects. Dose adjustment may be necessary.
Drug-lifestyle. *Alcohol use:* Additive effects. Advise patient to avoid alcohol.
Smoking: Decreased therapeutic effects. Avoid use together.
Sun exposure: Increased photosensitivity reactions. Advise patient to avoid sun exposure.

Effects on diagnostic tests

Drug causes false-positive test results for urine porphyrins, urobilinogen, amylase, and 5-hydroxyindoleacetic acid levels from darkening of urine by metabolites; it also causes false-positive urine pregnancy results in tests using human chorionic gonadotropin as the indicator.

Adverse reactions

CNS: *extrapyramidal reactions, tardive dyskinesia,* pseudoparkinsonism, dizziness, drowsiness, insomnia, fatigue, headache.

CV: *orthostatic hypotension,* tachycardia, ECG changes.
EENT: ocular changes, *blurred vision.*
GI: *dry mouth, constipation,* nausea.
GU: *urine retention,* menstrual irregularities, gynecomastia, inhibited lactation.
Hematologic: transient leukopenia, ***agranulocytosis.***
Hepatic: cholestatic jaundice, elevated tests for liver function.
Skin: *photosensitivity,* allergic reactions, pain at I.M. injection site, sterile abscess, rash.
Other: weight gain; rarely, ***neuroleptic malignant syndrome*** (fever, tachycardia, tachypnea, profuse diaphoresis).
After abrupt withdrawal of long-term therapy: gastritis, nausea, vomiting, dizziness, tremor, feeling of warmth or cold, diaphoresis, tachycardia, headache, insomnia, anorexia, muscle rigidity, altered mental status, and evidence of autonomic instability.

Overdose and treatment

CNS depression is characterized by deep, unarousable sleep and possible coma, hypotension or hypertension, extrapyramidal symptoms, dystonia, abnormal involuntary muscle movements, agitation, seizures, arrhythmias, ECG changes, hypothermia or hyperthermia, and autonomic nervous system dysfunction.

Treatment is symptomatic and supportive and includes maintaining vital signs, airway, stable body temperature, and fluid and electrolyte balance.

Don't induce vomiting. Drug inhibits cough reflex, and aspiration may occur. Use gastric lavage, then activated charcoal and sodium chloride cathartics; dialysis is usually ineffective. Regulate body temperature as needed. Treat hypotension with I.V. fluids. Don't give epinephrine. Treat seizures with parenteral diazepam or barbiturates; arrhythmias with parenteral phenytoin (1 mg/kg with rate titrated to blood pressure); extrapyramidal reactions with benztropine at 1 to 2 mg or parenteral diphenhydramine at 10 to 50 mg.

Clinical considerations

Consider the recommendations relevant to all phenothiazines as well as the following:

- Other agents such as benzodiazepines are preferred for the treatment of anxiety. When drug is given for anxiety, don't exceed 6 mg daily for longer than 12 weeks.
- Drug is associated with a high incidence of extrapyramidal symptoms and photosensitivity reactions.
- Worsening anginal pain has been reported in patients receiving trifluoperazine; however, ECG reactions are less common with drug than with other phenothiazines.
- Liquid and injectable formulations may cause a rash after contact with skin.
- Drug may cause pink to brown discoloration of urine or blue-gray skin.

Therapeutic monitoring

- Monitor blood pressure before and after parenteral administration.
- Monitor regularly for abnormal body movements (at least once every 6 months).

Special populations

Breast-feeding patients. Drug may enter breast milk. Potential benefits to the woman should outweigh the potential harm to the infant.
Pediatric patients. Not recommended for children under age 6.
Geriatric patients. Geriatric patients tend to require lower doses, adjusted to effect. Adverse effects, especially tardive dyskinesia and other extrapyramidal effects and hypotension, are more likely to develop in such patients.

Patient counseling

- Explain risks of dystonic reactions, akathisia, and tardive dyskinesia, and tell patient to report abnormal body movements.
- Explain that many drug interactions are possible. Tell patient to seek medical approval before taking any self-prescribed medication.
- Warn patient against hazardous activities that require alertness until the effect of drug is established.
- Tell patient to avoid sun exposure and to avoid exposure to temperature extremes because drug may cause thermoregulatory changes.
- Tell patient to take drug exactly as prescribed and to avoid alcohol and other medications that may cause excessive sedation.

trihexyphenidyl hydrochloride

Apo-Trihex*, Artane, Artane Sequels, Trihexane, Trihexy-2, Trihexy-5

Pharmacologic classification: anticholinergic
Therapeutic classification: antiparkinsonian
Pregnancy risk category C

How supplied

Available by prescription only
Tablets: 2 mg, 5 mg
Capsules (sustained-release): 5 mg
Elixir: 2 mg/5 ml

Indications and dosages

Idiopathic parkinsonism
Adults: 1 mg P.O. on first day, 2 mg on second day, then increase 2 mg q 3 to 5 days until total of 6 to 10 mg is given daily. Usually given t.i.d. with meals and, if needed, q.i.d. (last dose

should be before bedtime). Postencephalitic parkinsonism may require 12 to 15 mg total daily dose. Patients receiving levodopa may need 3 to 6 mg daily. Sustained-release capsules shouldn't be used as initial therapy, but after the patient has been stabilized on the conventional dose forms. Sustained-release capsules can be dosed on a mg per mg of total daily dose and administered as a single dose after breakfast or in two divided doses 12 hours apart.

Drug-induced parkinsonism
Adults: 5 to 15 mg daily.

Pharmacodynamics
Antiparkinsonian action: Trihexyphenidyl blocks central cholinergic receptors, helping to balance cholinergic activity in the basal ganglia. It may also prolong the effects of dopamine by blocking dopamine reuptake and storage at central receptor sites.

Pharmacokinetics
Absorption: Rapidly absorbed after oral administration.
Distribution: Crosses the blood-brain barrier; little else is known about its distribution.
Metabolism: Exact metabolic fate is unknown.
Excretion: Excreted in urine as unchanged drug and metabolites.

Route	Onset	Peak	Duration
P.O.	1 hr	Unknown	6-12 hr

Contraindications and precautions
Contraindicated in patients hypersensitive to drug. Use cautiously in patients with impaired renal, cardiac, or hepatic function, glaucoma, obstructive disease of the GI or GU tract, or prostatic hyperplasia.

Interactions
Drug-drug. *Amantadine:* Amplified anticholinergic adverse effects including confusion and hallucinations. Reduce trihexyphenidyl dose before giving amantadine.
Antacids and antidiarrheals: May decrease absorption of trihexyphenidyl. Monitor patient closely. Dose adjustment may be needed.
CNS depressants, including tranquilizers and sedative-hypnotics: Increase sedative effects. Avoid use together.
Haloperidol, phenothiazines: Decreased antipsychotic effectiveness. Dose adjustment may be needed.
Levodopa: Synergistic anticholinergic effects, enhanced GI metabolism of levodopa. Monitor patient closely. Dose adjustment may be needed
Phenothiazine: Increased risk of anticholinergic adverse effects.
Drug-lifestyle. *Alcohol use:* Increased sedative effects. Advise patient to avoid alcohol use.

Effects on diagnostic tests
None reported.

Adverse reactions
CNS: nervousness, dizziness, headache, hallucinations, drowsiness, weakness.
CV: tachycardia.
EENT: blurred vision, mydriasis, increased intraocular pressure.
GI: *dry mouth, nausea,* constipation, vomiting.
GU: urinary hesitancy, urine retention.

Overdose and treatment
Clinical effects of overdose include central stimulation followed by depression, with such psychotic symptoms as disorientation, confusion, hallucinations, delusions, anxiety, agitation, and restlessness. Peripheral effects may include dilated, nonreactive pupils; blurred vision; flushed, dry, hot skin; dry mucous membranes; dysphagia; decreased or absent bowel sounds; urine retention; hyperthermia; headache; tachycardia; hypertension; and increased respiration.

Treatment is primarily symptomatic and supportive, as needed. Maintain patent airway. If the patient is alert, induce emesis (or use gastric lavage) and follow with sodium chloride cathartic and activated charcoal to prevent further drug absorption. In severe cases, physostigmine may be administered to block antimuscarinic effects of trihexyphenidyl. Give fluids, as needed, to treat shock; diazepam to control psychotic symptoms; and pilocarpine (instilled into the eyes) to relieve mydriasis. If urine retention occurs, catheterization may be necessary.

Clinical considerations
Consider the recommendations relevant to all anticholinergics as well as the following:
- Tolerance may develop to drug, necessitating higher doses.
- Use drug with caution in hot weather due to the increased risk of heat prostration.

Therapeutic monitoring
- Monitor patient for urinary hesitancy.
- Obtain gonioscopic evaluation and close intraocular pressure monitoring, especially in patients over age 40.

Special populations
Breast-feeding patients. Drug may be excreted in breast milk, possibly resulting in infant toxicity. It may also decrease milk production.
Geriatric patients. Use caution when administering drug to geriatric patients. Lower doses are indicated.

Patient counseling
- Tell patient to avoid activities that require alertness until CNS effects of drug are known.

- Advise patient to report signs of urinary hesitation or urine retention.
- Tell patient to take drug with food if GI upset occurs.

trimethobenzamide hydrochloride

Arrestin, Tebamide, T-Gen, Ticon, Tigan, Tiject-20, Trimazide

Pharmacologic classification: ethanolamine-related antihistamine
Therapeutic classification: antiemetic
Pregnancy risk category C

How supplied

Available by prescription only
Capsules: 100 mg, 250 mg
Suppositories: 100 mg, 200 mg
Injection: 100 mg/ml

Indications and dosages

Nausea and vomiting (treatment)
Adults: 250 mg P.O. t.i.d. or q.i.d.; or 200 mg I.M. or P.R. t.i.d. or q.i.d.
Children weighing 30 to 90 lb (14 to 41 kg): 100 to 200 mg P.O. or P.R. t.i.d. or q.i.d.
Children weighing less than 30 lb: 100 mg P.R. t.i.d. or q.i.d.

Pharmacodynamics

Antiemetic action: Trimethobenzamide is a weak antihistamine with limited antiemetic properties. Its exact mechanism of action is unknown. Drug effects may occur in the chemoreceptor trigger zone of the brain; however, drug apparently doesn't inhibit direct impulses to the vomiting center.

Pharmacokinetics

Absorption: About 60% of an oral dose is absorbed.
Distribution: Unknown.
Metabolism: About 50% to 70% of dose is metabolized, probably in the liver.
Excretion: Excreted in urine and feces.

Route	Onset	Peak	Duration
P.O.	10-20 min	Unknown	3-4 hr
I.M.	15-35 min	Unknown	2-3 hr
P.R.	Unknown	Unknown	Unknown

Contraindications and precautions

Contraindicated in patients with hypersensitivity to drug. Suppositories are contraindicated in patients hypersensitive to benzocaine hydrochloride or similar local anesthetic. Parenteral form is contraindicated in children and suppositories are contraindicated in premature infants and neonates. Use cautiously in children.

Interactions

Drug-drug. *Other CNS depressants, including tricyclic antidepressants, antihypertensives, phenothiazines, and belladonna alkaloids:* Increased trimethobenzamide toxicity. Avoid use together.
Drug-lifestyle. *Alcohol use:* Increased sedative effects. Avoid use together.

Effects on diagnostic tests

None reported.

Adverse reactions

CNS: *drowsiness,* dizziness (in large doses), headache, disorientation, depression, parkinsonian-like symptoms, ***coma, seizures.***
CV: hypotension.
EENT: blurred vision.
GI: diarrhea.
Hepatic: jaundice.
Musculoskeletal: muscle cramps.
Other: *hypersensitivity reactions* (pain, stinging, burning, redness, swelling at I.M. injection site).

Overdose and treatment

Signs and symptoms of overdose may include severe neurologic reactions, such as opisthotonos, seizures, coma, and extrapyramidal reactions. Discontinue drug and provide supportive care.

Clinical considerations

- Drug may be less effective against severe vomiting than other agents.
- Drug has little or no value in treating motion sickness.

Therapeutic monitoring

- Monitor for hypersensitivity reactions.
- Monitor for relief of symptoms.

Special populations

Pregnant patients. Safety during pregnancy hasn't been established.
Breast-feeding patients. Safety in breast-feeding women hasn't been established.
Pediatric patients. Use drug with caution in children. Don't administer to children with viral illness because drug may contribute to development of Reye's syndrome. Don't use in newborn or premature infants.
Geriatric patients. Use drug with caution in geriatric patients because they may be more susceptible to adverse CNS effects.

Patient counseling

- Warn patient to avoid hazardous activities that require alertness because drug may cause drowsiness, and to avoid consuming alcohol to prevent additive sedation.
- Instruct patient to report persistent vomiting.
- Instruct patient on proper administration and storage of suppositories.

trimethoprim

Proloprim, Trimpex

Pharmacologic classification: synthetic folate antagonist
Therapeutic classification: antibiotic
Pregnancy risk category C

How supplied

Available by prescription only
Tablets: 100 mg, 200 mg

Indications and dosages

Treatment of uncomplicated urinary tract infections
Adults: 100 mg P.O. q 12 hours or 200 mg q 24 hours for 10 days. Drug isn't recommended for children under age 12.
◇ ***Prophylaxis of chronic and recurrent urinary tract infections***
Adults: 100 mg P.O. h.s. for 6 weeks to 6 months.
◇ ***Traveler's diarrhea***
Adults: 200 mg P.O. b.i.d. for 3 to 5 days.
◇ **Pneumocystis carinii** ***pneumonia***
Adults: 5 mg/kg P.O. t.i.d. in conjunction with dapsone 100 mg daily for 21 days.
≡ ***Dosage adjustment.*** If creatinine clearance is 15 to 30 ml/minute, give 50 mg every 12 hours. If creatinine clearance is less than 15 ml/minute, manufacturer doesn't recommend use of this drug.

Pharmacodynamics

Antibacterial action: By interfering with action of dihydrofolate reductase, drug inhibits bacterial synthesis of folic acid. Drug is effective against many gram-positive and gram-negative organisms, including most Enterobacteriaceae organisms (except *Pseudomonas), Proteus mirabilis, Klebsiella,* and *Escherichia coli.* Trimethoprim is usually bactericidal.

Pharmacokinetics

Absorption: Absorbed quickly and completely.
Distribution: Widely distributed. About 42% to 46% of dose is plasma protein-bound.
Metabolism: Less than 20% of dose is metabolized in the liver.
Excretion: Most of dose is excreted in urine via filtration and secretion. In patients with normal renal function, elimination half-life is 8 to 11 hours; in patients with impaired renal function, half-life is prolonged.

Route	Onset	Peak	Duration
P.O.	Unknown	1-4 hr	Unknown

Contraindications and precautions

Contraindicated in patients with hypersensitivity to drug and in those with documented megaloblastic anemia caused by folate deficiency. Use cautiously in patients with folate deficiency and impaired hepatic or renal function, especially those with creatinine clearance of 15 ml/minute or less.

Interactions

Drug-drug. *Phenytoin:* Increased serum phenytoin levels. Monitor patient closely.

Effects on diagnostic tests

None reported.

Adverse reactions

GI: *epigastric distress, nausea, vomiting,* glossitis.
GU: increased BUN and serum creatinine levels.
Hematologic: ***thrombocytopenia, leukopenia,*** megaloblastic anemia, methemoglobinemia.
Hepatic: elevated liver enzymes.
Skin: *rash, pruritus,* exfoliative dermatitis.
Other: fever.

Overdose and treatment

Clinical effects of acute overdose include nausea, vomiting, dizziness, headache, confusion, and bone marrow depression. Treatment includes gastric lavage and supportive measures. Urine may be acidified to enhance drug elimination.

Clinical effects of chronic toxicity caused by prolonged high-dose therapy include bone marrow depression, leukopenia, thrombocytopenia, and megaloblastic anemia. Treatment includes drug discontinuation and administration of leucovorin, 3 to 6 mg I.M. daily for 3 days or 5 to 15 mg P.O. daily until normal hematopoiesis returns.

Clinical considerations

□ ***ALERT*** Trimethoprim is also used in combination with sulfamethoxazole. Don't confuse the two products.
- Obtain urine specimen for culture and sensitivity tests before starting therapy.
- Drug is usually used with other antibiotics, especially sulfamethoxazole, because resistance develops rapidly when used alone.
- Advanced age, malnourishment, pregnancy, debilitation, renal impairment, and prolonged high-dose therapy increase risk of hematologic toxicity, as does use of drug with folate antagonistic drugs such as phenytoin.

Therapeutic monitoring

- If patient is receiving drug with phenytoin, monitor serum phenytoin levels.
- Sore throat, fever, pallor, and purpura may be early signs and symptoms of serious blood disorders. Monitor blood counts regularly.

Special populations

Pregnant patients. Use drug during pregnancy only when benefits justify risk to fetus.

Breast-feeding patients. Drug is excreted in breast milk; alternative feeding method is recommended during trimethoprim therapy.
Pediatric patients. Safety in children under age 2 months hasn't been established; efficacy in children under age 12 hasn't been established.
Geriatric patients. Geriatric patients may be more susceptible to hematologic toxicity.

Patient counseling

- Instruct patient to continue taking drug as directed, until course of therapy is completed.
- Advise patient to report signs or symptoms of blood disorders.

trimetrexate glucuronate

Neutrexin

Pharmacologic classification: dihydrofolate reductase inhibitor
Therapeutic classification: antimicrobial/antineoplastic
Pregnancy risk category D

How supplied

Available by prescription only
Injection: 25-mg vials

Indications and dosages

Treatment of patients with* Pneumocystis carinii *pneumonia who have exhibited serious (severe or life-threatening) intolerance to both cotrimoxazole and pentamidine (hospital use only)
Adults: Dosage and indication vary with protocol. Administer 45 mg/m^2 I.V. bolus daily for 21 days, with leucovorin (20 mg/m^2 I.V. or P.O. q 6 hours). Administer leucovorin with the last trimetrexate dose and for at least 72 hours after the last trimetrexate dose. Alternatively, patients weighing less than 110 lb (50 kg) may receive 1.5 mg/kg daily with leucovorin 0.6 mg/kg q.i.d.; those weighing 110 to 176 lb (50 to 80 kg) may receive 1.2 mg/kg daily with leucovorin 0.5 mg/kg q.i.d.; those weighing more than 80 kg may receive 1 mg/kg daily with leucovorin 0.5 mg/kg q.i.d. Course of treatment with trimetrexate is 21 days and leucovorin 24 days.

Dose modification or discontinuation is needed for patients with hematologic toxicity.

Pharmacodynamics

Dihydrofolate reductase inhibiting action: In vitro, the affinity of trimetrexate for pneumocystis dihydrofolate reductase is about 1,500 times that of trimethoprim. Trimetrexate is highly lipophilic and is passively taken up by and concentrated in protozoan cells.

Pharmacokinetics

Absorption: No data are available.
Distribution: Distributed rapidly after I.V. administration.
Metabolism: Probably metabolized by the liver; at least two metabolites (one active) have been identified.
Excretion: Excreted in bile and urine.

Route	Onset	Peak	Duration
I.V.	Unknown	Unknown	Unknown

Contraindications and precautions

Contraindicated during pregnancy, in breast-feeding patients, and in patients with hypersensitivity to trimetrexate, methotrexate, or leucovorin. Use cautiously in patients with impaired hematologic, renal, or hepatic function and in women of childbearing age.

Interactions

Drug-drug. *Acetaminophen, cimetidine, clotrimazole, erythromycin, miconazole, fluconazole, ketoconazole, rifabutin, rifampin:* Trimetrexate toxicity. Monitor patient closely.
Chloride-containing solutions, leucovorin: Precipitate formation. Must be given separately.
Hepatotoxic, myelosuppressive, nephrotoxic drugs: Enhanced toxicity. Use together cautiously.

Effects on diagnostic tests

None reported.

Adverse reactions

CNS: peripheral neuropathy.
GI: nausea, vomiting, stomatitis.
Hematologic: ***neutropenia, thrombocytopenia, anemia.***
Hepatic: ***hepatotoxicity.***
Skin: rash.

Overdose and treatment

Although no overdose information is available, clinical effects are expected to be similar to those of methotrexate. Methotrexate overdose produces myelosuppression, anemia, nausea, vomiting, dermatitis, alopecia, and melena.

Specific treatment information is unavailable, but calcium levocovorin would probably serve as an appropriate treatment. Contact the manufacturer for further information.

Clinical considerations

- Avoid I.M. injections in patients with thrombocytopenia.
- Store intact vials in refrigerator.
- Reconstitute with 5% dextrose injection or sterile water for injection to yield concentration of 12.5 mg/ml; solution should appear pale greenish yellow. Observe for particulate matter. Don't use if cloudiness or precipitate appears in the solution.
- Dilute further with 5% dextrose injection to yield concentration of 0.25 to 2 mg/ml. Administer over 60 minutes.

- Flush I.V. line with 10 ml 5% dextrose injection before and after administration.
- Drug is incompatible with chloride-containing solutions, including normal saline. Only D_5W is recommended for infusions.
- After reconstitution, solution is stable at room temperature for 2 days, under refrigeration for 5 days, and, when frozen, for 8 days.
- Dose adjustments may be necessary in patients with altered hepatic or renal function.
- Continue leucovorin for 72 hours after last dose of trimetrexate.

Therapeutic monitoring
- Monitor for signs of hepatotoxicity.
- Monitor for symptom relief.
- Monitor CBC.

Special populations
Pregnant patients. Drug use is contraindicated during pregnancy.
Breast-feeding patients. Drug use is contraindicated in breast-feeding women.

Patient counseling
- Instruct patient to promptly report signs of bleeding and infection.
- Advise patient of potential adverse reactions.

trimipramine maleate
Surmontil

Pharmacologic classification: tricyclic antidepressant
Therapeutic classification: antidepressant, antianxiety
Pregnancy risk category C

How supplied
Available by prescription only
Capsules: 25 mg, 50 mg, 100 mg

Indications and dosages
Depression
Adults: For outpatients, give 75 mg/day P.O. in divided doses and increase to 200 mg/day; maintenance dosage, 50 to 150 mg/day. Dosage for inpatients is 100 mg/day in divided doses and increased, p.r.n. Maximum daily dose, 300 mg.
Elderly: 50 to 100 mg/day P.O.
Adolescents: 50 to 100 mg/day P.O.

Pharmacodynamics
Antidepressant action: Trimipramine is thought to exert its antidepressant effects by equally inhibiting reuptake of norepinephrine and serotonin in CNS nerve terminals (presynaptic neurons), which results in increased concentration and enhanced activity of these neurotransmitters in the synaptic cleft. Trimipramine also has anxiolytic effects and inhibits gastric acid secretion.

Pharmacokinetics
Absorption: Absorbed rapidly from the GI tract after oral administration.
Distribution: Distributed widely in the body. Drug is 90% protein-bound; steady state occurs within 7 days.
Metabolism: Metabolized by the liver; a significant first-pass effect may explain variability of serum levels in different patients taking the same dose.
Excretion: Mostly excreted in urine; some is excreted in feces by way of the biliary tract.

Route	Onset	Peak	Duration
P.O.	Unknown	2 hr	Unknown

Contraindications and precautions
Contraindicated during acute recovery phase of MI, in patients with hypersensitivity to drug, or in those receiving MAO inhibitor therapy within 14 days.

Use cautiously in adolescents; in geriatric or debilitated patients; in those receiving thyroid medications; and in those with CV disease, increased intraocular pressure, hyperthyroidism, impaired hepatic function, or history of seizures, urine retention, or angle-closure glaucoma.

Interactions
Drug-drug. *Atropine and other anticholinergic drugs, including antihistamines, meperidine, phenothiazines, and antiparkinsonian agents:* May cause oversedation, paralytic ileus, visual changes, and severe constipation. Monitor patient.
Barbiturates: Decreased trimipramine therapeutic efficacy. Dose adjustment may be necessary.
Beta blockers, cimetidine, methylphenidate, oral contraceptives, propoxyphene: Increased trimipramine plasma levels and toxicity. Monitor patient closely.
Centrally acting antihypertensive drugs, including clonidine, guanabenz, guanadrel, guanethidine, methyldopa, and reserpine: Decreased hypotensive effects. Monitor patient carefully.
CNS depressants, including analgesics, barbiturates, narcotics, tranquilizers, and anesthetics: may cause oversedation. Monitor patient.
Disulfiram, ethchlorvynol: May cause delirium and tachycardia. Monitor patient carefully.
Haloperidol, phenothiazines: Decrease trimipramine metabolism, decreased therapeutic efficacy. Dose adjustment may be needed.
Metrizamide: Increased risk of seizures. Monitor patient closely.
SSRIs, including sertraline, paroxetine, and fluoxetine: Increased pharmacologic and toxic effects of trimipramine. Monitor patient closely. Dose adjustment may be needed.

Sympathomimetics, including epinephrine, phenylephrine, phenylpropanolamine, and ephedrine: Increased blood pressure. Monitor patient closely.
Thyroid medication, pimozide, and antiarrhythmic agents, such as disopyramide, procainamide, and quinidine: Increased incidence of cardiac arrhythmias and conduction defects. Monitor patient closely.
Warfarin: Increased PT and INR with resultant bleeding. Monitor PT and INR. Dose adjustment may be needed.
Drug-lifestyle. *Alcohol use:* Additive trimipramine effects. Advise patient to avoid alcohol use.
Smoking (heavy): Decreased therapeutic efficacy. Advise patient to avoid smoking.
Sun exposure: Increased risk of photosensitivity reactions. Advise patient to avoid sun exposure.

Effects on diagnostic tests
None reported.

Adverse reactions
CNS: *drowsiness, dizziness,* paresthesia, ataxia, hallucinations, delusions, anxiety, agitation, insomnia, tremor, weakness, confusion, headache, EEG changes, ***seizures,*** extrapyramidal reactions.
CV: *orthostatic hypotension,* tachycardia, hypertension, ***arrhythmias, heart block, MI, stroke,*** prolonged conduction time on ECG.
EENT: *blurred vision,* tinnitus, mydriasis.
GI: *dry mouth, constipation,* nausea, vomiting, anorexia, paralytic ileus.
GU: *urine retention.*
Hematologic: decreased WBC counts, altered PT and INR.
Hepatic: elevated liver function tests.
Metabolic: altered serum glucose.
Skin: rash, urticaria, photosensitivity.
Other: *diaphoresis,* ***hypersensitivity reaction.***
After abrupt withdrawal of long-term therapy: nausea, headache, malaise (doesn't indicate addiction).

Overdose and treatment
The first 12 hours after acute ingestion are a stimulatory phase characterized by excessive anticholinergic activity, including agitation, irritation, confusion, hallucinations, parkinsonian symptoms, seizure, urine retention, dry mucous membranes, pupillary dilation, constipation, and ileus. This is followed by CNS depressant effects, including hypothermia, decreased or absent reflexes, sedation, hypotension, cyanosis, and cardiac irregularities, including tachycardia, conduction disturbances, and quinidine-like effects on the ECG.

Severity of overdose is best indicated by prolongation of QRS interval beyond 100 milliseconds, which usually represents a serum level in excess of 1,000 ng/ml; serum levels are generally not helpful. Metabolic acidosis may follow hypotension, hypoventilation, and seizures.

Treatment is symptomatic and supportive and includes maintaining airway, stable body temperature, and fluid and electrolyte balance. Induce emesis with ipecac if patient is conscious; follow with gastric lavage and activated charcoal to prevent further absorption. Dialysis is of little use. Physostigmine given I.V. slowly has been used to reverse most CV and CNS effects of overdose. Treat seizures with parenteral diazepam or phenytoin; arrhythmias with parenteral phenytoin or lidocaine; and acidosis with sodium bicarbonate. Don't give barbiturates; these may enhance CNS and respiratory depressant effects.

Clinical considerations
Consider the recommendations relevant to all tricyclic antidepressants as well as the following:
- Consider the inherent risk of suicide until significant improvement of depressive state occurs.
- Tolerance generally develops to the sedative effects of drug.

Therapeutic monitoring
- Watch for bleeding because drug may cause alterations in PT and INR.
- Closely monitor high-risk patients during initial drug therapy.

Special populations
Geriatric patients. Geriatric patients may be more vulnerable to adverse cardiac effects.

Patient counseling
- Explain that full effects of drug may not become apparent for up to 4 to 6 weeks after therapy begins.
- Tell patient to take drug exactly as prescribed.
- Warn patient that drug may cause drowsiness or dizziness and to avoid activities that require mental alertness until the full effects of drug are known.
- Warn patient not to drink alcoholic beverages or medicinal elixirs while taking drug.
- Suggest taking drug with food or milk if it causes stomach upset and to ease dry mouth with sugarless chewing gum, hard candy, or ice.
- Tell patient to report adverse reactions promptly, especially confusion, movement disorders, rapid heartbeat, dizziness, fainting, or difficulty urinating.

troleandomycin
Tao

Pharmacologic classification: macrolide antibiotic
Therapeutic classification: antibiotic
Pregnancy risk category C

How supplied
Available by prescription only
Capsules: 250 mg

Indications and dosages
Pneumonia or respiratory tract infection caused by sensitive pneumococci or group A beta-hemolytic streptococci
Adults: 250 to 500 mg P.O. q 6 hours.
Children: 125 to 250 mg P.O. q 6 hours.

Pharmacodynamics
Antibacterial action: Drug inhibits bacterial protein synthesis by binding to 50S ribosomal subunit. It produces bacteriostatic effects on susceptible bacteria, including gram-positive cocci and bacilli and a few gram-negative organisms, including *Haemophilus influenzae, Neisseria gonorrhoeae,* and *N. meningitidis*.

Pharmacokinetics
Absorption: Absorbed rapidly but incompletely.
Distribution: Distributed widely to body fluids, except to CSF.
Metabolism: Metabolized in the liver.
Excretion: Excreted in bile, feces, and urine (10% to 25%).

Route	Onset	Peak	Duration
P.O.	Unknown	2 hr	Unknown

Contraindications and precautions
Contraindicated in patients with known hypersensitivity to drug. Use cautiously to patients with hepatic dysfunction.

Interactions
Drug-drug. *Carbamazepine, methylprednisolone, theophylline:* Increased toxicity of drugs. Avoid use together.
Cisapride: May cause serious cardiac arrhythmias. Monitor patient carefully.
Ergotamine: May precipitate severe ischemic reactions and peripheral vasospasms. Monitor patient closely.
Oral contraceptives: May cause marked cholestatic jaundice. Monitor patient closely.

Effects on diagnostic tests
None reported.

Adverse reactions
GI: *abdominal cramps, discomfort,* vomiting, diarrhea.
Hematologic: eosinophilia, leukocytosis.
Hepatic: elevated liver enzymes, cholestatic jaundice.
Skin: urticaria, rash.
Other: ***anaphylaxis.***

Overdose and treatment
None reported.

Clinical considerations
- Obtain culture and sensitivity tests before starting therapy.
- Repeated courses of therapy or therapy exceeding 2 weeks may lead to allergic cholestatic hepatitis, as indicated by jaundice, right upper abdominal quadrant pain, fever, nausea, vomiting, eosinophilia, and leukocytosis.
- Discontinue drug if liver function test values increase or if signs or symptoms of cholestatic hepatitis occur.

Therapeutic monitoring
- If patient is receiving drug with theophylline or carbamazepine, closely monitor serum theophylline or carbamazepine levels and assess patient frequently for signs and symptoms of theophylline or carbamazepine toxicity.
- Monitor total serum bilirubin and AST, ALT, and serum alkaline phosphatase levels.

Special populations
None reported.

Patient counseling
- Instruct patient to continue taking drug as prescribed, even if he's feeling better.
- Advise patient to take drug on an empty stomach for best absorption 1 hour before or 2 hours after meals, with full glass of water.
- Instruct patient to report abdominal pain or nausea immediately.

trovafloxacin mesylate
Trovan Tablets

alatrofloxacin mesylate
Trovan I.V.

Pharmacologic classification: fluoroquinolone derivative
Therapeutic classification: antibiotic
Pregnancy risk category C

How supplied
Available by prescription only
Tablets: 100 mg, 200 mg
Injection: 5 mg/ml, in 40 ml (200 mg) and 60 ml (300 mg) vials

Indications and dosages
For treatment of infections caused by susceptible microorganisms, the following dosages are administered once every 24 hours.

Gynecologic and pelvic infections, complicated intra-abdominal and postsurgical infections
Adults: 300 mg I.V. daily followed by 200 mg P.O. daily for 7 to 14 days.
Nosocomial pneumonia
Adults: 300 mg I.V. daily followed by 200 mg P.O. daily for 10 to 14 days.
Community-acquired pneumonia
Adults: 200 mg P.O. or I.V. daily followed by 200 mg P.O. daily for 7 to 14 days.
Complicated skin and diabetic foot infections
Adults: 200 mg P.O. or I.V. daily followed by 200 mg P.O. daily for 10 to 14 days.
≡***Dosage adjustment.*** Dosage adjustments are unnecessary when switching from I.V. to oral forms. An adjustment in dose isn't needed in patients with renal impairment; however, in patients with mild to moderate hepatic disease (cirrhosis), the following dose reductions are recommended: Reduce 300 mg I.V. to 200 mg I.V., reduce 200 mg I.V. or P.O. to 100 mg I.V. or P.O.; no reduction needed for 100 mg P.O.

Pharmacodynamics

Antibiotic action: Trovafloxacin is related to the fluoroquinolones with in vitro activity against a wide range of gram-positive and gram-negative aerobic and anaerobic microorganisms. The bactericidal action of trovafloxacin results from inhibition of DNA gyrase and topoisomerase IV, two enzymes involved in bacterial replication.

Pharmacokinetics

Absorption: Well absorbed after oral administration with an absolute bioavailability of about 88%. Steady-state levels are obtained by the third day of oral or I.V. administration.
Distribution: Widely and rapidly distributed throughout the body, resulting in significantly higher tissue levels than in plasma or serum. Mean plasma protein bound fraction is about 76%. Trovafloxacin is found in measurable levels in breast milk.
Metabolism: Primarily metabolized by conjugation although there is minimal oxidative metabolism by cytochrome P-450. About 13% of a dose is occurs in urine as the glucuronide ester and 9% as the *N*-acetyl metabolite.
Excretion: Primary route of elimination is fecal. About 50% of an oral dose (43% in feces and 6% in urine) is excreted as unchanged drug.

Route	Onset	Peak	Duration
P.O., I.V.	Unknown	1 hr	Unknown

Contraindications and precautions

Contraindicated in patients with hypersensitivity to trovafloxacin, alatrovafloxacin, or other quinolone antimicrobials. Use cautiously in patients with history of seizures, psychosis, or increased intracranial pressure.

Interactions

Drug-drug. *Aluminum-, magnesium-, and iron-containing preparations, such as antacids and vitamin-minerals, and divalent and trivalent cations such as didanosine:* Reduces P.O. bioavailability of drug. Separate administration times at least 2 hours apart.
Sucralfate and I.V. morphine: Reduced trovafloxacin plasma levels. Give I.V. morphine at least 2 hours after oral trovafloxacin in fasting state and at least 4 hours after oral trovafloxacin is taken with food.
Warfarin: Enhanced anticoagulation effect. Monitor PT/INR.
Drug-lifestyle. *Sun exposure:* Photosensitivity reaction. Advise patient to avoid sun exposure.

Effects on diagnostic tests

None reported.

Adverse reactions

CNS: *dizziness,* light-headedness, headache, ***seizures.***
GI: diarrhea, nausea, vomiting, abdominal pain, pseudomembranous colitis.
GU: vaginitis.
Hematologic: ***bone marrow aplasia (anemia, thrombocytopenia, leukopenia).***
Hepatic: elevated hepatic transaminases, ***hepatitis,*** jaundice, ***liver failure.***
Musculoskeletal: arthralgia, arthropathy, myalgia.
Skin: pruritis, rash, injection site reaction (I.V.), photosensitivity.

Overdose and treatment

Trovafloxacin has a low order of acute toxicity. Signs of overdose include decreased activity and respiration, ataxia, ptosis, tremors, and seizures.

Treat by emptying the stomach and providing symptomatic and supportive treatment. Drug isn't efficiently removed by hemodialysis.

Clinical considerations

- Oral form is more cost-effective and carries less risk; both forms have similar clinical efficacy and pharmacokinetics. Patients started with I.V. therapy may be switched to oral therapy when clinically indicated and at the discretion of the health care provider.
- Alatrofloxacin mesylate is supplied in single-use vials which must be further diluted with a compatible solution, such as D_5W or 0.45% saline, before administration. Don't dilute drug with normal saline solution or lactated Ringer's solution. Follow package insert for specific instructions regarding preparation of desired dose.

- After dilution, administer I.V. drug as a 60-minute infusion.
- Changes in laboratory values during trovafloxacin therapy didn't produce clinical abnormalities, and levels generally returned to normal 1 to 2 months after discontinuation of therapy.
- Duration of therapy should not exceed 2 weeks.

Therapeutic monitoring

- Perform periodic assessment of liver function because drug increases ALT, AST, and alkaline phosphatase levels.
- Monitor for neurologic complications.

Special populations

Breast-feeding patients. Drug is excreted in breast milk in measurable levels. Because of unknown effects in infants, the risks of therapy and breast-feeding should be evaluated.
Pediatric patients. Safety and efficacy in children under age 18 haven't been established.
Geriatric patients. At recommended doses, drug is as well tolerated and efficient in patients age 65 and older as in younger patients.

Patient counseling

- Inform patient that drug may be taken without regard to meals; however, tell him to take vitamins, minerals, and antacids at least 2 hours before or after a trovafloxacin dose.
- Warn patient to avoid excessive sunlight or artificial ultraviolet light.
- Instruct patient to discontinue treatment, refrain from exercise, and seek medical advice if pain, inflammation, or rupture of a tendon occurs.
- Advise patient to promptly report symptoms of allergic reaction or diarrhea.
- Advise patient to promptly report signs of liver dysfunction (nausea, vomiting, abdominal pain, jaundice, dark urine, anorexia, pale stools, or fatigue) to the health care provider and stop the medication.

tuberculosis skin test antigens

tuberculin purified protein derivative (PPD)

Aplisol, Tubersol

tuberculin cutaneous multiple-puncture device

Aplitest (PPD), Mono-Vacc Test (Old Tuberculin), Sclavo-Test PPD, Tine Test (Old Tuberculin), Tine Test PPD

Pharmacologic classification: Mycobacterium tuberculosis and *Mycobacterium bovis* antigen
Therapeutic classification: diagnostic skin test antigen
Pregnancy risk category C

How supplied

Available by prescription only
tuberculin PPD
Injection (intradermal): 1 tuberculin unit/0.1 ml, 5 tuberculin units/0.1 ml, 250 tuberculin units/0.1 ml
tuberculin cutaneous multiple-puncture device
Test: 25 devices/pack

Indications and dosages

Diagnosis of tuberculosis; evaluation of immunocompetence in patients with cancer or malnutrition
Adults and children: Intradermal injection of 5 tuberculin units/0.1 ml.

A single-use, multiple-puncture device is used for determining tuberculin sensitivity. All multiple-puncture tests are equivalent to or more potent than 5 tuberculin units of PPD.
Adults and children: Apply unit firmly and without any twisting to the upper one-third of the forearm for about 3 seconds; this ensures stabilizing the dried tuberculin B in the tissue lymph. Exert enough pressure to ensure that all four tines have entered the skin of the test area and a circular depression is visible.

Pharmacodynamics

Diagnosis of tuberculosis: Administration to a patient who is natural infected with *M. tuberculosis* usually results in sensitivity to tuberculin and a delayed hypersensitivity reaction (after administration of old tuberculin or PPD). The cell-mediated immune reaction to tuberculin in tuberculin-sensitive individuals, which results mainly from cellular infiltrates of the dermis of the skin, usually causes local edema.
Evaluation of immunocompetence in patients with cancer or malnutrition: PPD is given intradermally with three or more antigens to detect anergy, the absence of an immune response

to the test. The reaction may not be evident. Injection into a site subject to excessive exposure to sunlight may cause a false-negative reaction.

Pharmacokinetics
Absorption: Local.
Distribution: Local.
Metabolism: None reported.
Excretion: None reported.

Route	Onset	Peak	Duration
Intradermal	5-6 hr	48-72 hr	Unknown

Contraindications and precautions
Severe reactions to tuberculin PPD are rare and usually result from extreme sensitivity to the tuberculin. Inadvertent S.C. administration of PPD may result in a febrile reaction in highly sensitized patients. Old tubercular lesions aren't activated by administration of PPD.

Interactions
Drug-drug. *Live or inactivated viral vaccines:* Suppressed reaction. PPD antigen is used 4 to 6 weeks after immunization.
Systemic corticosteroids or aminocaproic acid: False-negative reactions may occur. Don't use together.
Topical alcohol: May inactivate the PPD antigen and invalidate the test. Avoid use together.
Drug-lifestyle. *Pregnancy:* Falsely insignificant reaction (Old Tuberculin multiple-puncture test). Avoid testing during pregnancy if possible.

Effects on diagnostic tests
None reported.

Adverse reactions
Other: Local pain, pruritus, vesiculation, ulceration, or necrosis, hypersensitivity, ***anaphylaxis,*** Arthus reaction (type III hypersensitivity reaction).

Overdose and treatment
None reported.

Clinical considerations
Positive reaction: Induration greater than 2 mm, but consider further diagnostic procedures.
Negative reaction: Induration less than 2 mm.
Tuberculin PPD
- Injection must be given intradermally or by skin puncture; an S.C. injection invalidates the test.

Multiple-puncture device
- Reaction may be depressed in patients with malnutrition, immunosuppression, or miliary tuberculosis.

Therapeutic monitoring
PPD
- Read test in 48 to 72 hours. An induration of 10 mm or greater is a significant reaction in patients who aren't suspected to have tuberculosis and who haven't been exposed to active tuberculosis, indicating present or past infection. An induration of 5 mm or more is significant in patients with AIDS or in those suspected to have tuberculosis or who have recently been exposed to active tuberculosis. An induration of 5 to 9 mm is inconclusive in patients not suspected of having been exposed or having tuberculosis infection; therefore, test should be repeated if there's more than 10 mm of erythema without induration. The amount of induration at the site, not the erythema, determines the significance of the reaction.

Multiple-puncture
- Read test at 48 to 72 hours.

Special populations
Pregnant patients. Use during pregnancy only when clearly needed and with the understanding that result can be falsely insignificant reaction (OT multiple-puncture test).
Breast-feeding patients. There appears to be no risk to breast-feeding infants.
Geriatric patients. Geriatric patients not having a cell-mediated immune reaction to the test may be anergic or they may test negative.

Patient counseling
- Advise patient that test must be read in 48 to 72 hours.
- Instruct patient to promptly report any unexpected adverse events.

tubocurarine chloride
Tubarine*

Pharmacologic classification: nondepolarizing neuromuscular blocker
Therapeutic classification: skeletal muscle relaxant
Pregnancy risk category C

How supplied
Available by prescription only
Injection: 3 mg/ml parenteral

Indications and dosages
Adjunct to general anesthesia to induce skeletal muscle relaxation, facilitate intubation, and reduce fractures and dislocations
Dose depends on anesthetic used, individual needs, and response. Doses listed are representative and must be adjusted. Dose may be calculated on the basis of 0.165 mg/kg.
Adults: Initially, 6 to 9 mg I.V. or I.M., followed by 3 to 4.5 mg in 3 to 5 minutes if needed. Additional doses of 3 mg may be given, if needed, during prolonged anesthesia.
To assist with mechanical ventilation
Adults: Initially, 0.0165 mg/kg I.V. or I.M. (average 1 mg), then adjust subsequent doses to patient's response.

To weaken muscle contractions in pharmacologically or electrically induced seizures
Adults: Initially, 0.165 mg/kg I.V. or I.M. slowly. As a precaution, 3 mg less than the calculated dose should be administered initially.
Diagnosis of myasthenia gravis
Adults: Single I.V. or I.M. dose of 0.004 to 0.033 mg/kg.

Pharmacodynamics
Skeletal muscle relaxant action: Tubocurarine prevents acetylcholine from binding to receptors on motor end-plate, blocking depolarization. Tubocurarine has histamine-releasing and ganglionic-blocking properties, and is usually antagonized by anticholinesterase agents.

Pharmacokinetics
Absorption: I.V. direct. I.M., none reported.
Distribution: After I.V. injection, drug is distributed in extracellular fluid and rapidly reaches its site of action. After tissue compartment is saturated, drug may persist in tissues for up to 24 hours; 40% to 45% is bound to plasma proteins, mainly globulins.
Metabolism: Undergoes *N*-demethylation in the liver.
Excretion: About 33% to 75% of a dose is excreted unchanged in urine in 24 hours; up to 11% is excreted in bile.

Route	Onset	Peak	Duration
I.V.	1 min	2-5 min	25-90 min (first dose, > for subsequent doses)
I.M.	10-25 min	Unknown	Unknown

Contraindications and precautions
Contraindicated in patients with hypersensitivity to drug and in those for whom histamine release is a hazard (asthmatic patients).

Use cautiously in geriatric or debilitated patients; in those with impaired hepatic or pulmonary function, hypothermia, respiratory depression, myasthenia gravis, myasthenic syndrome of lung cancer or bronchiogenic carcinoma, dehydration, thyroid disorders, collagen diseases, porphyria, electrolyte disturbances, fractures, or muscle spasms; and in women undergoing cesarean section.

Interactions
Drug-drug. *Aminoglycoside antibiotics, clindamycin, lincomycin, polymyxin antibiotics, general anesthetics, local anesthetics, beta blockers, calcium salts, furosemide, parenteral magnesium salts, depolarizing neuromuscular blocking agents, other nondepolarizing neuromuscular blocking agents, quinidine or quinine, thiazide diuretics, other potassium-depleting drugs:* Enhanced or prolonged tubocurarine-induced neuromuscular blockade. Use cautiously. Monitor patient closely.
Opioid analgesics, quinidine, quinine: Increased respiratory depression. Monitor patient closely. Use cautiously.

Effects on diagnostic tests
None reported.

Adverse reactions
CV: hypotension, ***arrhythmias, cardiac arrest, bradycardia.***
Musculoskeletal: profound and prolonged muscle relaxation, idiosyncrasy, residual muscle weakness.
Respiratory: ***respiratory depression or apnea, bronchospasm.***
Other: ***hypersensitivity reactions,*** increased salivation.

Overdose and treatment
Signs of overdose include apnea or prolonged muscle paralysis, which can be treated with controlled ventilation. Use a peripheral nerve stimulator to monitor effects and to determine nature and degree of blockade. Anticholinesterase agents may antagonize tubocurarine. Atropine given before or with the antagonist counteracts its muscarinic effects.

Clinical considerations
- The margin of safety between therapeutic dose and dose causing respiratory paralysis is small.
- Drug doesn't affect consciousness or relieve pain.
- Don't mix with barbiturates or other alkaline solutions in same syringe.
- I.V. administration requires direct medical supervision. Give drug I.V. slowly over 60 to 90 seconds or I.M. by deep injection in deltoid muscle. Tubocurarine is usually administered by I.V. injection, but if patient's veins are inaccessible, drug may be given I.M. in same dose as given I.V.
- Renal dysfunction prolongs drug action.

Therapeutic monitoring
- Assess baseline tests of renal function and serum electrolyte levels before drug administration. Electrolyte imbalance, particularly potassium and magnesium, can potentiate effects of drug.
- Monitor respirations closely for early symptoms of paralysis.
- A nerve stimulator may be used to evaluate recovery from neuromuscular blockade.
- Monitor blood pressure, vital signs, and airway until patient recovers from drug effects. Ganglionic blockade (hypotension), histamine liberation (increased salivation, bronchospasm), and neuromuscular blockade (respiratory depression) are known effects of tubocurarine.
- After neuromuscular blockade dissipates, watch for residual muscle weakness.

Special populations

Breast-feeding patients. It isn't known if drug is excreted in breast milk. Use with caution in breast-feeding women.
Pediatric patients. Administer cautiously to children.
Geriatric patients. Administer cautiously to geriatric patients.

typhoid vaccine

Vivotif Berna

Pharmacologic classification: vaccine
Therapeutic classification: bacterial vaccine
Pregnancy risk category C

How supplied

Available by prescription only
Oral vaccine: Enteric-coated capsules of 2 to 6×10^9 colony-forming units of viable *Salmonella typhi* Ty-21a and 5 to 10×10^9 bacterial cells of nonviable *S. typhi* Ty-21a
Injection: Suspension of killed Ty-2 strain of *S. typhi;* provides 8 units/ml in 5-ml, 10-ml, and 20-ml vials
Powder for suspension: Killed Ty-2 strain of *S. typhi;* provides 8 units/ml in 50-dose vial with 20 ml diluent/dose

Indications and dosages

Primary immunization (exposure to typhoid carrier or foreign travel planned to area endemic for typhoid fever)
Parenteral
Adults and children over age 9: 0.5 ml S.C.; repeat in 4 or more weeks.
Infants and children age 6 months to 9 years: 0.25 ml S.C.; repeat in 4 or more weeks.
Booster
Adults and children over age 10: 0.5 ml S.C. or 0.1 ml intradermally q 3 years.
Infants and children age 6 months to 10 years: 0.25 ml S.C. or 0.1 ml intradermally q 3 years.
Oral
Adults and children over age 6: Primary immunization—1 capsule on alternate days (such as days 1, 3, 5, 7) for four doses. Booster—repeat primary immunization regimen q 5 years.

Pharmacodynamics

Typhoid fever prophylaxis action: Vaccine promotes active immunity to typhoid fever in 70% to 90% of patients vaccinated.

Pharmacokinetics

None reported.

Route	Onset	Peak	Duration
P.O., S.C., Intradermal	After final dose	Unknown	3-5 years

Contraindications and precautions

Contraindicated in immunosuppressed patients and in those with hypersensitivity to vaccine. Defer vaccination in patients with acute illness. Oral vaccine shouldn't be given to patients with acute GI distress, such as diarrhea or vomiting.

Interactions

Drug-drug. *Corticosteroids, immunosuppressants, sulfonamides, other anti-infectives active against* S. typhi, *phenytoin:* May impair the immune response to this vaccine. Avoid use together.

Effects on diagnostic tests

None reported.

Adverse reactions

CNS: malaise, headache.
GI: nausea, abdominal cramps, vomiting.
Musculoskeletal: myalgia.
Skin: rash, urticaria, swelling, pain, inflammation (at injection site).
Other: *fever,* ***anaphylaxis.***

Overdose and treatment

None reported.

Clinical considerations

- Store injection at 36° to 50° F (2° to 10° C). Don't freeze.
- Store enteric-coated capsules at 36° to 46° F (2° to 8° C).
- It's essential that all four doses of oral vaccine be taken at the prescribed alternate-day interval to obtain a maximal protective immune response.

Therapeutic monitoring

Monitor for adverse reactions.

Special populations

Pregnant patients. Use in pregnancy only when clearly needed.
Breast-feeding patients. It isn't known if typhoid vaccine is excreted in breast milk. Use with caution in breast-feeding women.
Pediatric patients. Parenteral typhoid vaccine isn't indicated for children under age 6 months. Oral typhoid vaccine isn't indicated for children under age 6.

Patient counseling

- Advise patient that it's essential that all four doses of oral vaccine be taken at the prescribed alternate-day interval to obtain a maximal protective immune response.
- Tell patient to take oral vaccine capsule about 1 hour before a meal with a cold or lukewarm drink (not exceeding body temperature) and to swallow the capsule as soon as possible after placement in the mouth. Remind patient not to chew the capsule.

■ Tell patient what to expect after vaccination: pain and inflammation at the injection site, fever, malaise, headache, nausea, or difficulty breathing. These reactions occur in most patients within 24 hours and may persist for 1 to 2 days. Recommend acetaminophen for fever.
■ Encourage patient to report adverse reactions.
■ Inform patient that not all recipients of typhoid vaccine are fully protected. Travelers should take all necessary precautions to avoid infection.

typhoid Vi polysaccharide vaccine
Typhim Vi

Pharmacologic classification: vaccine
Therapeutic classification: bacterial vaccine
Pregnancy risk category C

How supplied
Available by prescription only
Injection: 0.5-ml syringe, 20-dose vial, 50-dose vial

Indications and dosages
Active immunization against typhoid fever
Adults and children age 2 and older: 0.5 ml I.M. as a single dose. Reimmunization is recommended q 2 years with 0.5 ml I.M. as a single dose, if needed.

Pharmacodynamics
Antibacterial vaccine action: Typhoid Vi polysaccharide vaccine promotes active immunity to typhoid fever.

Pharmacokinetics
Absorption: Antibody levels usually remain elevated for 12 months after vaccination. Because of the low incidence of typhoid fever in the United States, efficacy studies haven't been feasible.
Distribution: None reported.
Metabolism: None reported.
Excretion: None reported.

Route	Onset	Peak	Duration
I.M.	2 wk	Unknown	2 yr

Contraindications and precautions
Contraindicated in patients with hypersensitivity to any component of vaccine. Don't use to treat typhoid fever or give to those who are chronic typhoid carriers. Use cautiously in patients with thrombocytopenia or bleeding disorders and in those taking an anticoagulant because bleeding may occur following an I.M. injection in these individuals.

Interactions
None significant.

Effects on diagnostic tests
None reported.

Adverse reactions
CNS: *headache.*
GI: nausea, diarrhea, vomiting.
Musculoskeletal: myalgia.
Other: ***anaphylaxis,*** *local injection site pain or tenderness, induration, erythema* at injection site; *malaise,* fever.

Overdose and treatment
None reported.

Clinical considerations
■ Patients who should receive the vaccine include those traveling to or living in areas of higher endemicity for typhoid fever.
■ Although anaphylaxis is rare, keep epinephrine readily available to treat anaphylactoid reactions.
■ Delay administration of vaccine, if possible, in patients with febrile illnesses.
■ If vaccine is administered to immunosuppressed patients or those receiving immunosuppressive therapy, the expected immune response may not be obtained.

Therapeutic monitoring
Monitor for anaphylaxis and other adverse reactions.

Special populations
Pregnant patients. Use in pregnancy only when clearly needed.
Pediatric patients. Safety and efficacy in patients under age 2 haven't been established.

Patient counseling
■ Inform patient that immunization should be given at least 2 weeks before expected exposure. Although an optimal reimmunization schedule hasn't been established, reimmunization with a single dose for U.S. travelers every 2 years, if exposure to typhoid fever is possible, is recommended at this time.

urokinase

Abbokinase, Abbokinase Open-Cath

Pharmacologic classification: thrombolytic enzyme
Therapeutic classification: thrombolytic enzyme
Pregnancy risk category B

How supplied

Available by prescription only
Injection: 5,000 IU/ml unit-dose vial; 250,000-IU/vial

Indications and dosages

Lysis of acute massive pulmonary emboli and of pulmonary emboli accompanied by unstable hemodynamics
Adults: For I.V. infusion only by constant infusion pump; priming dose: 4,400 IU/kg over 10 minutes, followed with 4,400 IU/kg hourly for 12 hours.
Coronary artery thrombosis
Adults: 6,000 IU/minute of urokinase intra-arterial via a coronary artery catheter until artery is maximally opened, usually within 15 to 30 minutes; however, drug has been administered for up to 2 hours. Average total dose, 500,000 IU.
Venous catheter occlusion
Adults: Instill 5,000 IU into occluded line.

Pharmacodynamics

Thrombolytic action: Urokinase promotes thrombolysis by directly activating conversion of plasminogen to plasmin.

Pharmacokinetics

Absorption: Not absorbed from GI tract.
Distribution: Rapidly cleared from circulation; most drug accumulates in the kidneys and liver.
Metabolism: Rapidly metabolized by the liver.
Excretion: Small amount is eliminated in urine and bile. Half-life is 10 to 20 minutes; longer in patients with hepatic dysfunction.

Route	Onset	Peak	Duration
I.V.	Immediate	20 min-4 hr	4 hr

Contraindications and precautions

Contraindicated in patients with active internal bleeding, history of CVA, aneurysm, arteriovenous malformation, known bleeding diathesis, recent trauma with possible internal injuries, visceral or intracranial malignancy, ulcerative colitis, diverticulitis, severe hypertension, hemostatic defects including those resulting from severe hepatic or renal insufficiency, uncontrolled hypocoagulation, chronic pulmonary disease with cavitation, subacute bacterial endocarditis or rheumatic valvular disease, and recent cerebral embolism, thrombosis, or hemorrhage.

Also contraindicated during pregnancy and first 10 days postpartum; within 10 days after intra-arterial diagnostic procedure or any surgery (liver or kidney biopsy, lumbar puncture, thoracentesis, paracentesis, or extensive or multiple cutdowns); or within 2 months after intracranial or intraspinal surgery.

I.M. injections and other invasive procedures are contraindicated during urokinase therapy.

Interactions

Drug-drug. *Aminocaproic acid:* Inhibits urokinase-induced activation of plasminogen. Avoid use together.
Anticoagulants, including heparin and oral anticoagulants: Hemorrhage. Heparin must be stopped and its effects allowed to diminish. It may also be necessary to reverse effects of oral anticoagulants before beginning therapy.
Aspirin, indomethacin, phenylbutazone, other drugs affecting platelet activity: Increased risk of bleeding. Avoid use together.

Effects on diagnostic tests

None reported.

Adverse reactions

CV: ***reperfusion arrhythmias,*** tachycardia, transient hypotension or hypertension.
Hematologic: ***bleeding;*** increased thrombin time, activated partial thromboplastin time, and PT and INR; decreased hematocrit.
Respiratory: ***bronchospasm,*** minor breathing difficulties.
Other: phlebitis at injection site, fever, rash, ***anaphylaxis,*** chills, nausea, vomiting.

Overdose and treatment

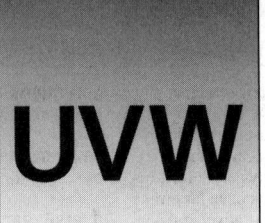

Signs and symptoms of overdose include signs of potentially serious bleeding: bleeding gums, epistaxis, hematoma, spontaneous ecchymoses, oozing at catheter site, increased pulse, and pain from internal bleeding. Discontinue drug and restart when bleeding stops.

Clinical considerations
Consider the recommendations relevant to all thrombolytic enzymes as well as the following:
- Don't use bacteriostatic water to reconstitute.
- Product contains no preservatives; discard unused portion.

Therapeutic monitoring
- Inform prescriber that drug may affect platelet function.
- Patient should be monitored for signs of hemorrhage.

Special populations
Pregnant patients. There are no adequate or controlled studies using urokinase in pregnant women. The drug shouldn't be used during pregnancy unless clearly needed.
Breast-feeding patients. It isn't known if drug is excreted in breast milk; use drug with caution in breast-feeding women.
Pediatric patients. Safety and efficacy in children haven't been established.
Geriatric patients. Patients age 75 or older have a greater risk of cerebral hemorrhage because they're more apt to have preexisting cerebrovascular disease.

Patient counseling
- Explain use and administration of urokinase to patient and family.
- Instruct patient to report adverse reactions promptly.

valacyclovir hydrochloride
Valtrex

Pharmacologic classification: synthetic purine nucleoside
Therapeutic classification: antiviral
Pregnancy risk category B

How supplied
Available by prescription only
Caplets: 500 mg

Indications and dosages
Treatment of herpes zoster in immunocompetent patients
Adults: 1 g P.O. t.i.d. daily for 7 days.
Treatment of initial episode of genital herpes
Adults: 1 g P.O. b.i.d. for 10 days.
Treatment of recurrent genital herpes in immunocompetent patients
Adults: 500 mg P.O. b.i.d. for 5 days.
Chronic suppressive therapy of recurrent genital herpes
Adults: 1 g P.O. once daily.
≡***Dosage adjustment.*** Base dosage adjustments in renally impaired patients on creatinine clearance levels.

Pharmacodynamics
Antiviral action: Valacyclovir rapidly becomes converted to acyclovir. Acyclovir becomes incorporated into viral DNA and inhibits viral DNA polymerase, inhibiting viral multiplication.

Pharmacokinetics
Absorption: Rapidly absorbed from GI tract. Absolute bioavailability of drug is about 54.5%.
Distribution: 13.5% to 17.9% protein-bound.
Metabolism: Rapidly and nearly completely converted to acyclovir and L-valine by first-pass intestinal or hepatic metabolism.
Excretion: Excreted in urine and feces. Half-life of drug is about 2½ to 3⅓ hours.

Route	Onset	Peak	Duration
P.O.	30 min	Unknown	Unknown

Contraindications and precautions
Contraindicated in patients with hypersensitivity or intolerance to valacyclovir, acyclovir, or any component of the formulation and in immunocompromised patients.

Use cautiously in patients with impaired renal function and in those receiving other nephrotoxic drugs.

Thrombotic thrombocytopenic purpura and hemolytic uremic syndrome have occurred, resulting in death in some patients with advanced HIV infection, and in bone marrow transplant and renal transplant recipients participating in clinical trials of valacyclovir.

Interactions
Drug-drug. *Cimetidine, probenecid:* Increased acyclovir blood levels. Monitor patient for possible toxicity.

Effects on diagnostic tests
None reported.

Adverse reactions
CNS: *headache,* dizziness, asthenia.
GI: *nausea,* vomiting, diarrhea, constipation, abdominal pain, anorexia.

Overdose and treatment
There is no report of overdose. However, precipitation of acyclovir in renal tubules may occur when the solubility (2.5 mg/ml) is exceeded in the intratubular fluid. If acute renal failure and anuria occur, hemodialysis may be helpful until renal function is restored.

Clinical considerations

Initiate treatment as soon as possible after symptoms appear. Drug is most effective when initiated within 48 hours of the onset of zoster rash.

Therapeutic monitoring

Symptoms should be monitored to determine success of therapeutic effect.

Special populations

Pregnant patients. Glaxo-Wellcome, the manufacturer, maintains an ongoing registry of women exposed to valacyclovir during pregnancy. Follow-up studies to date haven't shown an increased risk for birth defects in infants born to women exposed to this drug during pregnancy. Health care providers are encouraged to report such exposures to the registrar at 1-800-722-9292, extension 58465.
Breast-feeding patients. It isn't known if drug is excreted in breast milk. Use in breast-feeding women isn't recommended.
Pediatric patients. Safety and efficacy in children haven't been established.
Geriatric patients. Dose adjustment may be necessary in geriatric patients based on underlying renal status.

Patient counseling

- Tell patient that valacyclovir may be taken without regard to meals.
- Inform patient that valacyclovir isn't a cure for herpes but it may decrease the length and severity of symptoms.
- Instruct patient to report adverse events promptly.

valproic acid

Depakene, Epival*

divalproex sodium

Depakote, Depakote Sprinkle

valproate sodium

Depacon

Pharmacologic classification: carboxylic acid derivative
Therapeutic classification: anticonvulsant
Pregnancy risk category D

How supplied

Available by prescription only
valproic acid
Capsules: 250 mg
Syrup: 250 mg/5 ml
divalproex sodium
Tablets (enteric-coated): 125 mg, 250 mg, 500 mg
Capsules (sprinkle): 125 mg
valproate sodium
Injection: 5 ml single-dose vials

Indications and dosages

Simple and complex absence seizures and mixed seizure types, ◇tonic-clonic seizures
Adults and children: P.O.—initially, 15 mg/kg P.O. daily, divided b.i.d. or t.i.d.; may increase by 5 to 10 mg/kg daily at weekly intervals up to a maximum of 60 mg/kg daily, divided b.i.d. or t.i.d. The b.i.d. dose is recommended for the enteric-coated tablets.

Note: Doses of divalproex sodium (Depakote) are expressed as valproic acid.
Adults and children: I.V.—initially, 10 to 15 mg/kg/day as a 60-minute I.V. infusion (rate 20 mg/minute or less). The dose may increase by 5 to 10 mg/kg daily at weekly intervals up to a maximum of 60 mg/kg daily. Dilute drug in at least 50 ml of compatible diluent.
Mania
Adults: 750 mg P.O. in divided doses (divalproex sodium).
Migraine prophylaxis
Adults: 250 mg P.O. b.i.d. Some patients may benefit from doses up to 1 g daily.

Pharmacodynamics

Anticonvulsant action: Mechanism of action is unknown; effects may be from increased brain levels of gamma-aminobutyric acid (GABA), an inhibitory transmitter. Valproic acid also may decrease GABA's enzymatic catabolism. Onset of therapeutic effects may require a week or more. Valproic acid may be used with other anticonvulsants.

Pharmacokinetics

Absorption: Valproate sodium and divalproex sodium quickly convert to valproic acid after administration of oral dose; bioavailability of drug is same for all dose forms.
Distribution: Distributed rapidly throughout the body; drug is 80% to 95% protein-bound.
Metabolism: Metabolized by the liver.
Excretion: Excreted in urine; some drug is excreted in feces and exhaled air. Breast milk levels are 1% to 10% of serum levels.

Route	Onset	Peak	Duration
P.O.	Unknown	15 min-4 hr	Unknown
I.V.	Unknown	1 hr	Unknown

Contraindications and precautions

Contraindicated in patients with hypersensitivity to drug. Use cautiously in patients with history of hepatic dysfunction, and in children under age 2.

Don't administer valproate sodium injection to patients with hepatic disease or significant hepatic dysfunction.

Interactions

Drug-drug. *Clonazepam:* Absence seizures. Avoid use together.
Felbamate, salicylates, lamotrigine: Increased valproate levels. Monitor patient closely.
MAO inhibitors, other CNS antidepressants, and oral anticoagulants: Potentiated actions of these drugs. Monitor patient closely.
Phenobarbital, phenytoin, primidone: Excessive somnolence. Monitor patient closely.
Drug-lifestyle. *Alcohol use:* May decrease valproic acid effectiveness and increase CNS adverse effects. Monitor patient closely.

Effects on diagnostic tests

Valproic acid may cause false-positive test results for urinary ketones.

Adverse reactions

Because drug usually is used in combination with other anticonvulsants, adverse reactions reported may not be caused by valproic acid alone.
CNS: *sedation,* emotional upset, depression, psychosis, aggressiveness, hyperactivity, behavioral deterioration, muscle weakness, tremor, ataxia, headache, dizziness, incoordination.
EENT: nystagmus, diplopia.
GI: *nausea, vomiting, indigestion,* diarrhea, abdominal cramps, constipation, increased appetite and weight gain, anorexia, ***pancreatitis.***
Hematologic: ***thrombocytopenia,*** increased bleeding time, petechiae, bruising, eosinophilia, ***hemorrhage, leukopenia, bone marrow suppression.***
Hepatic: *elevated liver enzymes,* ***toxic hepatitis.***
Skin: rash, alopecia, pruritus, photosensitivity, erythema multiforme.

Overdose and treatment

Symptoms of overdose include somnolence and coma.

Treat overdose supportively; maintain adequate urinary output and monitor vital signs, fluid, and electrolyte balance carefully. Naloxone reverses CNS and respiratory depression but also may reverse anticonvulsant effects of valproic acid. Hemodialysis and hemoperfusion have been used.

Clinical considerations

- Therapeutic range of drug is 50 to 100 mcg/ml.
- Don't withdraw drug abruptly.
- Administer drug with food to minimize GI irritation. Enteric-coated formulation may be better tolerated.
- Use of valproate sodium injection for periods of more than 14 days hasn't been studied. Patients should be switched to oral products as soon as is clinically feasible. When switching from I.V. to oral therapy or from oral to I.V. therapy, the total daily dose should be equivalent and given with the same frequency.

Therapeutic monitoring

- Evaluate liver function, platelet count, and PT at baseline and monthly intervals, especially during first 6 months of therapy.
- Monitor plasma level and make dose adjustments as needed.
- Monitor for tremors, which may indicate need for dose reduction.

Special populations

Pregnant patients. Safe use during pregnancy hasn't been established; drug may cause teratogenic effects.
Breast-feeding patients. Valproic acid is excreted in breast milk in serum levels from 1% to 10%. Alternative feeding method is recommended during therapy.
Pediatric patients. Children under age 2 are at higher risk of development of fatal hepatotoxicity. Use drug with extreme caution in children; benefits should be weighed against the risks.
Geriatric patients. Geriatric patients eliminate drug more slowly; lower doses are recommended.

Patient counseling

- Tell patient to report promptly any adverse events.
- Instruct patient to take with food to reduce GI irritation.
- Advise patient to avoid activities requiring mental alertness.

valrubicin

Valstar

Pharmacologic classification: anthracycline
Therapeutic classification: antineoplastic
Pregnancy risk category C

How supplied

Available by prescription only
Solution for intravesical instillation: 200 mg/5 ml

Indication and dosages

Intravesical therapy of bacillus Calmette-Guérin carcinoma in situ (CIS) of the urinary bladder in patients for whom immediate cystectomy would be associated with unacceptable morbidity or mortality risks.
Adults: 800 mg intravesically once weekly for 6 weeks.

Pharmacodynamics

Antineoplastic action: Valrubicin is an anthracycline that exerts its cytotoxic activity by penetrating into cells, where it inhibits the incorporation of nucleosides into nucleic acids, causes extensive chromosomal damage, and arrests cell cycle in G_2. It also interferes with the normal DNA breaking-resealing action of DNA topoisomerase II, inhibiting DNA synthesis.

Pharmacokinetics

Absorption: Only small quantities are absorbed into the plasma after intravesical administration.
Distribution: Penetrates into the bladder wall after intravesical administration. Systemic exposure is dependent on the condition of the bladder wall.
Metabolism: Metabolites of valrubicin were found in the blood.
Excretion: After retention, drug is almost completely excreted by voiding the instillate.

Route	Onset	Peak	Duration
Intravesical	Unknown	Unknown	Unknown

Contraindications and precautions

Contraindicated in patients with known hypersensitivity to drug or other anthracyclines or Cremophor EL (polyoxyethyleneglycol triricinoleate). Also contraindicated in pregnant patients and in patients with concurrent urinary tract infections, patients with a small bladder capacity (patients unable to tolerate a 75-ml instillation), and patients with a perforated bladder or patients in whom the integrity of the bladder mucosa has been compromised.

Use cautiously in patients with severe irritable bladder symptoms.

Interactions

None reported.

Effects on diagnostic tests

None reported.

Adverse reactions

CNS: asthenia, headache, malaise, dizziness.
CV: vasodilation, chest pain, peripheral edema.
GI: diarrhea, flatulence, nausea, vomiting, abdominal pain.
GU: urinary retention, *urinary tract infection, urinary frequency*, *dysuria*, *urinary urgency, bladder spasm,* hematuria, *bladder pain, urinary incontinence,* pelvic pain, urethral pain, nocturia, *cystitis,* local burning symptoms.
Hematologic: anemia.
Metabolic: hyperglycemia.
Musculoskeletal: myalgia, back pain.
Respiratory: pneumonia.
Skin: rash.
Other: fever.

Overdose and treatment

There is no known antidote for overdoses of valrubicin. The primary anticipated complications of overdose associated with intravesical administration would be consistent with irritable bladder symptoms.

Clinical considerations

- Drug has been shown to induce complete response in only about 1 in 5 patients with refractory CIS.
- Use procedures for proper handling and disposal of antineoplastic drugs.
- Store unopened vials under refrigeration at 36° to 46° F (2° to 8° C). Diluted valrubicin is stable for 12 hours at temperatures up to 77° F (25° C).
- Prepare and store solution in glass, polypropylene, or polyolefin containers and tubing. It's recommended that polyethylene-lined administration sets be used. Don't use polyvinyl chloride I.V. bags and tubing.
- Administer drug intravesically only, and only under the supervision of clinicians experienced in the use of intravesical antineoplastic agents.
- Aseptic techniques must be used during administration to avoid introducing contaminants into the urinary tract or traumatizing the urinary mucosa.
- In patients with severe irritable bladder symptoms, bladder spasm and spontaneous discharge of the intravesical instillate may occur. Clamping of the urinary catheter isn't advised and, if performed, should be executed cautiously under medical supervision.

Therapeutic monitoring

- If there isn't a complete response of CIS to valrubicin treatment after 3 months or if CIS recurs, cystectomy must be reconsidered because delaying cystectomy could lead to the development of metastatic bladder cancer.
- Myelosuppression is possible if drug is inadvertently administered systemically or if significant systemic exposure occurs following intravesical administration, such as in patients with bladder rupture or perforation. If valrubicin is administered when bladder rupture or perforation is suspected, weekly monitoring of complete blood counts should be performed for 3 weeks. Myelosuppression begins during the first week, with the nadir by the second week, and recovery by the third week.
- Monitor patient closely for disease recurrence or progression by cystoscopy, biopsy, and urine cytology every 3 months.

Special populations

Pregnant patients. Women of childbearing age and men and their partners should be advised to avoid pregnancy during treatment. Effective contraception should be used during the treatment period.
Breast-feeding patients. It isn't known if valrubicin is excreted in breast milk, but because this drug is highly lipophilic and any exposure of infants to the drug could cause serious health risks, women should discontinue breast-feeding before the initiation of valrubicin therapy.
Pediatric patients. Safety and efficacy of valrubicin in children haven't been established.

Geriatric patients. There are no specific precautions regarding the use of valrubicin in geriatric patients who are otherwise in good health.

Patient counseling

- Inform patient that drug has been shown to induce complete response in only about 1 in 5 patients with refractory CIS. If there isn't a complete response of CIS to treatment after 3 months or if CIS recurs, tell patient to discuss with his doctor the risks for cystectomy versus the risks of metastatic bladder cancer.
- Advise patients to retain the drug for 2 hours before voiding, if possible. Instruct patient to void at the end of 2 hours.
- Instruct patient to maintain adequate hydration following treatment.
- Inform patients that the major adverse reactions are related to irritable bladder symptoms that may occur during instillation and retention of the drug and for a limited period following voiding. For the first 24 hours following administration, red-tinged urine is typical. Tell patient to report prolonged irritable bladder symptoms or prolonged passage of red-colored urine immediately.
- Advise women of childbearing age and men and their partners to avoid pregnancy during treatment. Effective contraception should be used during the treatment period.

valsartan

Diovan

Pharmacologic classification: angiotensin II antagonist
Therapeutic classification: antihypertensive
Pregnancy risk category C (D in second and third trimesters)

How supplied

Available by prescription only
Capsules: 80 mg, 160 mg

Indications and dosages

Hypertension, used alone or in combination with other antihypertensives
Adults: Initially, 80 mg P.O. once daily as monotherapy in patients who aren't volume-depleted. Blood pressure reduction should occur in 2 to 4 weeks. If additional antihypertensive effect is needed, dose may be increased to 160 or 320 mg daily or diuretic may be added. (Addition of diuretic has greater effect than dose increases beyond 80 mg.) Usual dose range, 80 to 320 mg daily.

Pharmacodynamics

Antihypertensive action: Blocks the binding of angiotensin II to receptor sites in vascular smooth muscle and the adrenal gland, which inhibits the pressor effects of the renin-angiotensin system.

Pharmacokinetics

Absorption: Absolute bioavailability is about 25%.
Distribution: Doesn't distribute extensively into tissues; drug is 95% bound to serum proteins, mainly to serum albumin.
Metabolism: Only about 20% is metabolized. The enzymes responsible for valsartan metabolism haven't been identified, but they don't appear to be cytochrome P-450 enzymes.
Excretion: Excreted primarily through feces (83% of dose) and about 13% in urine. Average elimination half-life is about 6 hours.

Route	Onset	Peak	Duration
P.O.	2 hr	2-4 hr	24 hr

Contraindications and precautions

Contraindicated in patients with known hypersensitivity to drug. Also contraindicated in the second and third trimesters of pregnancy. Use cautiously in patients with renal or hepatic disease.

Interactions

Drug-drug. *Diuretics:* Increased risk of excessive hypotension. Assess fluid status before using together; monitor patient carefully.

Effects on diagnostic tests

None reported.

Adverse reactions

CNS: fatigue, dizziness, headache.
GI: abdominal pain, diarrhea, nausea.
Hematologic: neutropenia.
Metabolic: hyperkalemia.
Musculoskeletal: arthralgia.
Respiratory: cough, pharyngitis, rhinitis, sinusitis, upper respiratory infection.
Other: edema, viral infection.

Overdose and treatment

Limited data are available. The most likely symptoms are hypotension and tachycardia; bradycardia could occur from parasympathetic (vagal) stimulation. If symptomatic hypotension occurs, institute supportive treatment.

Clinical considerations

- Excessive hypotension can occur when drug is given with high doses of diuretics.
- Volume depletion and salt depletion are to be corrected before initiating therapy.

Therapeutic monitoring

Monitor for therapeutic effect and for excessive hypotension.

Special populations

Pregnant patients. Drug can cause fetal or neonatal morbidity and death if administered during the second or third trimester.
Breast-feeding patients. Drug shouldn't be used in breast-feeding women.
Pediatric patients. Safety and efficacy in children haven't been established.
Geriatric patients. Although no overall difference in efficacy or safety was observed, greater sensitivity of some older individuals can't be ruled out.

Patient counseling

Inform women of fetal risk; advise informing prescriber immediately if pregnancy occurs.

vancomycin hydrochloride

Lyphocin, Vancocin, Vancoled

Pharmacologic classification: glycopeptide
Therapeutic classification: antibiotic
Pregnancy risk category C

How supplied

Available by prescription only
Pulvules: 125 mg, 250 mg
Powder for oral solution: 1-g, 10-g bottles
Powder for injection: 500-mg, 1-g, 5-g vials; 10-g pharmacy bulk package

Indications and dosages

Severe staphylococcal infections when other antibiotics are ineffective or contraindicated
Adults: 500 mg I.V. q 6 hours, or 1 g q 12 hours.
Children: 40 mg/kg I.V. daily, divided q 6 hours.
Neonates: Initially, 15 mg/kg; then 10 mg/kg I.V. q 12 hours for first week of life; then q 8 hours up to age 1 month.
Antibiotic-associated pseudomembranous and staphylococcal enterocolitis
Adults: 125 to 500 mg P.O. q 6 hours for 7 to 10 days.
Children: 40 mg/kg P.O. daily, divided q 6 to 8 hours for 7 to 10 days. Don't exceed 2 g/day in children.
Endocarditis prophylaxis for dental, GI, biliary, and GU instrumentation procedures; surgical prophylaxis in patients allergic to penicillin
Adults: 1 g I.V., given slowly over 1 hour, starting 1 hour before procedure. In high-risk patients, dose may be repeated in 8 to 12 hours.
Children: 20 mg/kg, if child weighs less than 60 lb (27 kg); adult dose, if child weighs more than 60 lb. In high-risk patients, dose may be repeated in 8 to 12 hours.
≡ ***Dosage adjustment.*** In patients with renal failure, adjust dosage based on degree of renal impairment, severity of infection, and susceptibility of causative organism. Base dosage on serum levels of drug.

Recommended initial dose is 15 mg/kg. Adjust subsequent doses, p.r.n. Some clinicians use the following schedule.

Serum creatinine level (mg/dl)	Adult dosage
< 1.5	1 g q 12 hours
1.5 to 5	1 g q 3 to 6 days
> 5	1 g q 10 to 14 days

Pharmacodynamics

Antibacterial action: Vancomycin is bactericidal by hindering cell-wall synthesis and blocking glycopeptide polymerization. Its spectrum of activity includes many gram-positive organisms, including those resistant to other antibiotics. It's useful for *Staphylococcus epidermidis* and methicillin-resistant *S. aureus.* It's also useful for penicillin-resistant *S. pneumococcus.*

Pharmacokinetics

Absorption: Minimal systemic absorption occurs with oral administration; however, drug may accumulate in patients with colitis or renal failure.
Distribution: Distributed widely in body fluids, including pericardial, pleural, ascitic, synovial, and placental fluid. It will achieve therapeutic levels in CSF in patients with inflamed meninges. Therapeutic drug levels are 18 to 26 mcg/ml for 2-hour, postinfusion peaks; 5 to 10 mcg/ml for preinfusion troughs (however, these values may vary, depending on laboratory and sampling time).
Metabolism: Unknown.
Excretion: When administered parenterally, drug is excreted renally, mainly by filtration. When administered orally, drug is excreted in feces. In patients with normal renal function, plasma half-life is 6 hours; in those with creatinine clearance of 10 to 30 ml/minute, plasma half-life is about 32 hours; if creatinine clearance is less than 10 ml/minute, plasma half-life is 146 hours.

Route	Onset	Peak	Duration
P.O.	Unknown	Unknown	Unknown
I.V.	Unknown	Immediate	Unknown

Contraindications and precautions

Contraindicated in patients with hypersensitivity to drug. Use cautiously in patients with impaired renal or hepatic function, preexisting hearing loss, or allergies to other antibiotics; in those receiving other neurotoxic, nephrotoxic, or ototoxic drugs; and in patients over age 60.

Interactions

Drug-drug. *Aminoglycosides, amphotericin B, capreomycin, cisplatin, colistin, methoxyflurane, polymyxin B:* Increased nephrotoxic effects. Monitor renal function.
Nondepolarizing muscle relaxants: Increased neuromuscular blockade. Avoid use together.

Effects on diagnostic tests

None reported.

Adverse reactions

CV: hypotension.
EENT: tinnitus, ototoxicity.
GI: nausea.
GU: increased BUN and serum creatinine levels, ***nephrotoxicity.***
Hematologic: ***neutropenia, leukopenia,*** eosinophilia.
Respiratory: wheezing, dyspnea.
Skin: maculopapular rash on face, neck, trunk, and extremities (with rapid I.V. infusion).
Other: chills, fever, ***anaphylaxis,*** superinfection, pain or thrombophlebitis at injection site.

Overdose and treatment

Little information is available on acute toxicity of vancomycin. Treatment includes providing supportive care and maintaining glomerular filtration rate. Hemodialysis and hemoperfusion have been used.

Clinical considerations

□ ***ALERT*** Oral administration is ineffective for systemic infections, and I.V. administration is ineffective for pseudomembranous (*Clostridium difficile*) diarrhea.

- Instruct prescriber to obtain culture and sensitivity tests before starting therapy (unless drug is being used for prophylaxis).
- I.M. administration is contraindicated because drug is highly irritating.
- Hemodialysis and peritoneal dialysis remove only minimal drug amounts. Patients receiving these treatments require usual dose only once every 5 to 7 days; however, some dialysis centers use high-flux hemodialysis, which can remove up to 50% of vancomycin, creating a need for supplemental doses. Dose should be based on serum level of drug.

Therapeutic monitoring

- Monitor blood counts and BUN, serum creatinine, and drug levels.
- If maculopapular rash develops on patient's face, neck, trunk, and upper extremities, slow infusion rate.
- If patient has preexisting auditory dysfunction or requires prolonged therapy, auditory function tests may be indicated before and during therapy.

Special populations

Pregnant patients. It isn't known if vancomycin can cause fetal harm; avoid use during pregnancy and use only when clearly needed.
Breast-feeding patients. Drug is excreted in breast milk. Use with caution in breast-feeding women.
Geriatric patients. Geriatric patients may be more susceptible to ototoxic effects of drug. Monitor serum levels closely and adjust dose as needed.

Patient counseling

- Instruct patient to take entire amount of drug, exactly as directed, for the full length of prescription.
- Inform patient that relief of symptoms shouldn't be used as a guide for discontinuing therapy.

varicella virus vaccine, live

Varivax

Pharmacologic classification: vaccine
Therapeutic classification: viral vaccine
Pregnancy risk category C

How supplied

Available by prescription only
Injection: Single-dose vial containing 1,350 plaque-forming units of Oka/Merck varicella virus

Indications and dosages

Prevention of varicella-zoster (chickenpox) infections
Adults and children age 13 and older: Administer 0.5 ml S.C. followed by a second dose of 0.5 ml 4 to 8 weeks later.
Children age 1 to 12: 0.5 ml S.C. as a single dose.

Pharmacodynamics

Antiviral vaccine action: Varicella virus vaccine prevents chickenpox by inducing the production of antibodies to varicella-zoster virus.

Pharmacokinetics

None reported.

Route	Onset	Peak	Duration
S.C.	4-6 wk	Unknown	> 2 yr

Contraindications and precautions

Contraindicated in patients hypersensitive to drug, in pregnant women, and in those with history of anaphylactoid reaction to neomycin, blood dyscrasia, leukemia, lymphomas, neoplasms affecting bone marrow or lymphatic system, primary and acquired immunosuppressive states, active untreated tuberculosis, or any febrile respiratory illness or other active febrile infection.

Interactions

Drug-drug. *Blood products, immune globulin:* Inactivate vaccine. Defer vaccination for at least 5 months following blood or plasma transfusions or administration of immune globulin or varicella-zoster immune globulin.
Immunosuppressants: Increased risk of severe reactions to live-virus vaccines. Postpone routine vaccination.
Salicylates: Reye's syndrome. Avoid use of salicylates for 6 weeks after varicella infections.

Effects on diagnostic tests

None reported.

Adverse reactions

Other: ***anaphylaxis,*** *fever, injection site reactions (swelling, redness, pain, rash),* varicella-like rash.

Overdose and treatment

None reported.

Clinical considerations

- Vaccine has been safely and effectively used with measles, mumps, and rubella vaccine.
- Vaccine appears to be less effective in adults compared with children.
- Vaccine contains live attenuated virus. Children in whom a rash develops may be capable of transmitting the virus.
- Have epinephrine available.

□ ***ALERT*** Administer immediately after reconstitution. Discard if not used within 30 minutes.

Therapeutic monitoring

Monitor patient for postadministration anaphylaxis.

Special populations

Pregnant patients. Pregnancy should be avoided for 3 months after receiving vaccine.
Breast-feeding patients. It isn't known if varicella vaccine virus is excreted in breast milk. Use cautiously in breast-feeding women.
Pediatric patients. A safety study protocol program is available for children and adolescents (age 12 to 17) with acute lymphocytic leukemia. Clinicians can enroll patients in this program by contacting Bio-Pharm Clinical Services at 1-215-283-0897. Safety and efficacy haven't been established for children under age 1.

Patient counseling

- Caution women of childbearing age to notify doctor of suspected pregnancy before administration and to avoid pregnancy for 3 months after administration.
- Instruct patient to avoid salicylate use for 6 weeks after administration to prevent Reye's syndrome.
- Warn patient to avoid close contact with susceptible high-risk individuals during postinjection period.

varicella-zoster immune globulin (VZIG)

Pharmacologic classification: immune serum
Therapeutic classification: varicella-zoster prophylaxis
Pregnancy risk category D

How supplied

Available by prescription only
Injection: 10% to 18% solution of the globulin fraction of human plasma containing 125 units of varicella-zoster virus antibody in 2.5 ml or less

Indications and dosages

Passive immunization of susceptible patients, primarily immunocompromised patients after exposure to varicella (chickenpox or herpes zoster)
Adults and children: 125 units per 10 kg of body weight I.M., to a maximum of 625 units. Higher doses may be needed in immunocompromised adults.

Pharmacodynamics

Postexposure prophylaxis: This agent provides passive immunity to varicella-zoster virus.

Pharmacokinetics

None reported.

Route	Onset	Peak	Duration
I.M.	Unknown	Unknown	1 mo

Contraindications and precautions

Contraindicated in patients with thrombocytopenia, coagulation disorders, IgA deficiency, or history of severe reaction to human immune serum globulin or thimerosal.

Interactions

Drug-drug. *Corticosteroids, immunosuppressants:* May interfere with the immune response to this immune globulin. Whenever possible, avoid using these agents during the postexposure immunization period.
Live virus vaccines, such as measles, mumps, and rubella: Reduced immune response. Don't administer live virus vaccines within 3 months after or 2 weeks before administering VZIG. If it becomes necessary to administer VZIG together with a live virus vaccine, confirm seroconversion with follow-up serologic testing.

Effects on diagnostic tests
False-positive results to serologic test for immunity to varicella-zoster virus may occur for a period of about 2 months after administration.

Adverse reactions
CV: chest tightness.
GI: GI distress.
GU: ***nephrotic syndrome.***
Musculoskeletal: myalgia.
Respiratory: respiratory distress.
Skin: rash.
Other: ***anaphylaxis,*** discomfort at injection site, malaise, headache, *angioedema, angioneurotic edema,* fever.

Overdose and treatment
None reported.

Clinical considerations
- VZIG is recommended primarily for immunodeficient children under age 15 and certain infants exposed in utero, although use in other patients (especially immunocompromised patients of any age, normal adults, pregnant women, and premature and full-term infants) should be considered on a case-by-case basis. It isn't routinely recommended for use in immunocompetent pregnant women because chickenpox is much less severe than in immunosuppressed patients. Moreover, it won't protect the fetus. VZIG isn't for use in immunodeficient patients with history of varicella, unless there's immunosuppression caused by bone marrow transplantation.
- For maximum benefit, administer VZIG within 96 hours of presumed exposure.
- The chance of AIDS or hepatitis developing from VZIG is very small.

◘ ***ALERT*** Have epinephrine solution 1:1,000 available to treat allergic reactions.

- Administer only by deep I.M. injection. Never administer I.V. Use the gluteal muscle in infants and small children and the deltoid or anterolateral thigh in adults and larger children. For patients weighing more than 22 lb (10 kg), give no more than 2.5 ml at a single injection site.

Therapeutic monitoring
Monitor for postadministration anaphylaxis, injection site reaction, and other adverse reactions.

Special populations
Pregnant patients. Use drug during pregnancy only when clearly indicated. Exposure to varicella has been associated with congenital abnormalities (congenital varicella syndrome). Postexposure administration of VZIG during pregnancy may prevent or suppress clinical disease in the woman without preventing fetal infection.

Breast-feeding patients. It's unknown if VZIG is distributed in breast milk. Use cautiously in breast-feeding women.

Patient counseling
- Warn patient about local adverse reactions associated with drug administration; discuss use of acetaminophen for fever reductions and cool compressses for injection site discomfort.
- Instruct patient to report serious adverse events promptly.

vasopressin (antidiuretic hormone [ADH])
Pitressin Synthetic

Pharmacologic classification: posterior pituitary hormone
Therapeutic classification: antidiuretic hormone, peristaltic stimulant, hemostatic
Pregnancy risk category C

How supplied
Available by prescription only
Injection: 0.5-ml and 1-ml ampules and vials, 20 units/ml

Indications and dosages
Nonnephrogenic, nonpsychogenic diabetes insipidus
Adults: 5 to 10 units I.M. or S.C. b.i.d. to q.i.d., p.r.n.
Children: 2.5 to 10 units I.M. or S.C. b.i.d. to q.i.d., p.r.n.
Postoperative abdominal distention
Adults: 5 units I.M. initially, then q 3 to 4 hours, increasing dose to 10 units, if needed. Reduce dose for children proportionately.
To expel gas before abdominal radiographic examination
Adults: Inject 5 to 15 units S.C. at 2 hours, then again at 30 minutes before x-ray study. Enema before first dose may also help to eliminate gas.
Upper GI tract hemorrhage
Adults: 0.2 to 0.4 units/minute I.V. or 0.1 to 0.5 units/minute intra-arterially.

Pharmacodynamics
Antidiuretic action: Vasopressin is used as an antidiuretic to control or prevent signs and complications of neurogenic diabetes insipidus. Acting primarily at the renal tubular level, vasopressin increases cAMP, which increases water permeability at the renal tubule and collecting duct, resulting in increased urine osmolality and decreased urinary flow rate.
Peristaltic stimulant action: Used to treat postoperative abdominal distention and to facilitate abdominal radiographic procedures, vasopressin induces peristalsis by directly stimulating contraction of smooth muscle in the GI tract.

Hemostatic action: In patients with GI hemorrhage, vasopressin, administered I.V. or intra-arterially into the superior mesenteric artery, controls bleeding of esophageal varices by directly stimulating vasoconstriction of capillaries and small arterioles.

Pharmacokinetics
Absorption: Destroyed by trypsin in the GI tract and must be administered intranasally or parenterally.
Distribution: Distributed throughout the extracellular fluid, with no evidence of protein-binding.
Metabolism: Most of dose is destroyed rapidly in the liver and kidneys.
Excretion: About 5% of an S.C. dose is excreted unchanged in urine after 4 hours.

Route	Onset	Peak	Duration
I.M., S.C.	2-8 hr	Unknown	Unknown

Contraindications and precautions
Contraindicated in patients with known anaphylaxis or hypersensitivity to vasopressin or its components. Also, contraindicated in patients with chronic nephritis accompanied by nitrogen retention.

Use cautiously in patients with seizure disorders, migraine headache, asthma, CV or renal disease, heart failure, goiter with cardiac complications, arteriosclerosis, or fluid overload; in children and geriatric patients, pregnant women; or in preoperative or postoperative patients who are polyuric.

Interactions
Drug-drug. *Carbamazepine, chlorpropamide, clofibrate:* May potentiate antidiuretic effect of vasopressin. Monitor fluid balance and renal function.
Demeclocycline, epinephrine, heparin, lithium, norepinephrine: Decreased antidiuretic effect. Monitor fluid balance and renal function.
Drug-lifestyle. *Alcohol use:* Reduced antidiuretic activity. Advise patient to avoid alcohol use.

Effects on diagnostic tests
None reported.

Adverse reactions
CNS: tremor, headache, vertigo.
CV: angina in patients with vascular disease; vasoconstriction, ***arrhythmias, cardiac arrest,*** myocardial ischemia, circumoral pallor, decreased cardiac output.
GI: abdominal cramps, nausea, vomiting, flatulence.
Skin: cutaneous gangrene.
Other: *water intoxication* (drowsiness, listlessness, headache, confusion, weight gain, ***seizures, coma***), hypersensitivity reactions (urticaria, *angioedema,* ***bronchoconstriction, anaphylaxis***), diaphoresis.

Overdose and treatment
Signs and symptoms of overdose include drowsiness, listlessness, headache, confusion, anuria, and weight gain (water intoxication). Treatment requires water restriction and temporary withdrawal of vasopressin until polyuria occurs. Severe water intoxication may require osmotic diuresis with mannitol, hypertonic dextrose, or urea, either alone or with furosemide.

Clinical considerations
- Administration during first stage of labor may cause ruptured uterus.
- Extravasation carries the risk of necrosis and gangrene.

Therapeutic monitoring
- Establish baseline vital signs and intake and output ratio at the initiation of therapy.
- Monitor patient's blood pressure twice daily. Watch for excessively elevated blood pressure or lack of response to drug, which may be indicated by hypotension. Also monitor fluid intake and output and daily weight.
- Monitor for signs of water intoxication and hypersensitivity reactions.

Special populations
Pregnant patients. Use drug during pregnancy only when clearly indicated because of its potential for producing tonic uterine contractions.
Breast-feeding patients. Use caution when administering to breast-feeding women.
Pediatric patients. Children show increased sensitivity to the effects of vasopressin. Use with caution.
Geriatric patients. Geriatric patients show increased sensitivity to the effects of vasopressin. Use with caution.

Patient counseling
- Advise patient that rotation of injection sites reduces risk of tissue damage.
- Instruct patient to report serious adverse events promptly.

vecuronium bromide
Norcuron

Pharmacologic classification: nondepolarizing neuromuscular blocker
Therapeutic classification: skeletal muscle relaxant
Pregnancy risk category C

How supplied
Available by prescription only
Injection: 10 mg (with or without diluent), 20 mg (without diluent)

Indications and dosages

Adjunct to anesthesia, to facilitate intubation, and to provide skeletal muscle relaxation during surgery or mechanical ventilation

Dose depends on anesthetic used, individual needs, and response. Doses are representative and must be adjusted.

Adults and children age 10 and older: Initially, 0.08 to 0.10 mg/kg I.V. bolus. Higher initial doses (up to 0.3 mg/kg) may be used for rapid onset. Maintenance dosages of 0.010 to 0.015 mg/kg within 25 to 40 minutes of initial dose should be administered during prolonged surgical procedures. Maintenance dosages may be given q 12 to 15 minutes in patients receiving balanced anesthetic.

Alternatively, after the initial dosing of 0.08 to 0.10 mg/kg, a continuous infusion of 1 mcg/kg/minute may be initiated 20 to 40 minutes later.

Pharmacodynamics

Skeletal muscle relaxant action: Vecuronium prevents acetylcholine from binding to receptors on motor end-plate, blocking depolarization. Vecuronium exhibits minimal CV effects and doesn't appear to alter heart rate or rhythm, systolic or diastolic blood pressure, cardiac output, systemic vascular resistance, or mean arterial pressure. It has little or no histamine-releasing properties.

Pharmacokinetics

Absorption: None reported.

Distribution: After I.V. administration, drug is distributed in extracellular fluid and rapidly reaches its site of action. It is 60% to 90% plasma protein-bound. Volume of distribution is decreased in children under age 1 and may be decreased in geriatric patients.

Metabolism: Undergoes rapid and extensive hepatic metabolism.

Excretion: Drug and its metabolites appear to be primarily excreted in feces by biliary elimination; it's also excreted in urine.

Route	Onset	Peak	Duration
I.V.	1 min	3-5 min	15-25 min

Contraindications and precautions

Contraindicated in patients with hypersensitivity to vecuronium and bromides. Use cautiously in patients with altered circulation caused by CV disease and edematous states, hepatic disease, severe obesity, bronchogenic carcinoma, electrolyte disturbances, or neuromuscular diseases and in the elderly.

Interactions

Drug-drug. *Aminoglycosides, clindamycin, lincomycin, polymyxin antibiotics, furosemide, parenteral magnesium salts, depolarizing neuromuscular blocking agents, other nondepolarizing neuromuscular blocking agents, quinidine or quinine, thiazide diuretics, other potassium-depleting drugs, general anesthetics (decrease dose by 15%, especially with enflurane and isoflurane):* Increased vecuronium-induced neuromuscular blockade. Use cautiously during and after surgery.

Anticholinesterase agents: Antagonize effects of vecuronium. Use with extreme caution. Monitor patient closely.

Narcotic (opioid) analgesics: Increased central respiratory depression. Use with extreme caution. Monitor patient closely.

Effects on diagnostic tests

None reported.

Adverse reactions

Other: skeletal muscle weakness, ***prolonged, dose-related respiratory insufficiency or apnea.***

Overdose and treatment

Signs and symptoms of overdose include prolonged duration of neuromuscular blockade, skeletal muscle weakness, decreased respiratory reserve, low tidal volume, and apnea. Treatment is supportive and symptomatic. Keep airway clear and maintain adequate ventilation.

Use peripheral nerve stimulator to determine and monitor the degree of blockade. Give an anticholinesterase agent, such as edrophonium, neostigmine, or pyridostigmine, to reverse neuromuscular blockade and atropine or glycopyrrolate to overcome muscarinic effects.

Clinical considerations

- Drug doesn't relieve pain or affect consciousness.

☐ ***ALERT*** Apply a bright label with WARNING: PARALYTIC AGENT if drug is prepared ahead of time as a premixed syringe. Store in a safe place. Be aware of careful drug calculation. Always verify with a second individual.

- Emergency respiratory support equipment should be immediately available.
- Reconstitute using diluent supplied by manufacturer (bacteriostatic water for injection) or a compatible solution, such as normal saline, D_5W, sterile water for injection, 5% dextrose in normal saline, or lactated Ringer's, to produce a solution containing 1 mg/ml or 2 mg/ml.
- Diluent supplied by manufacturer contains benzyl alcohol, which isn't intended for use in neonates.
- Protect solution from light.

☐ ***ALERT*** Drug must not be mixed in same syringe or given through same needle as barbiturates or other alkaline solutions.

- After reconstitution, store solution in refrigerator or at room temperature not exceeding 86° F (30° C). Don't use if discolored.

- Administer only by rapid I.V. injection or I.V. infusion and accompany by adequate anesthesia.

Therapeutic monitoring

- Assess baseline serum electrolyte levels, acid-base balance, and renal and hepatic function before administration.
- Peripheral nerve stimulator may be used to identify residual paralysis during recovery and is especially useful during administration to high-risk patients.
- After procedure, vital signs should be monitored at least every 15 minutes until patient is stable, then every 30 minutes for next 2 hours. Monitor airway and pattern of respirations until patient has recovered from drug effects. Anticipate problems with ventilation in obese patients and those with myasthenia gravis or other neuromuscular disease.
- Recovery from neuromuscular blockade is evaluated by checking strength of hard grip and by patient's ability to breathe naturally, to take deep breaths and cough, to keep eyes open, and to lift head, keeping mouth closed.

Special populations

Pregnant patients. Use drug during pregnancy only when clearly indicated.
Breast-feeding patients. It isn't known if drug is excreted in breast milk. Use with caution in breast-feeding women.
Pediatric patients. Safety and efficacy haven't been established in infants under age 7 weeks. Infants age 7 weeks to 1 year are more sensitive to neuromuscular blocking effects; less frequent administration may be necessary. Higher doses may be needed in children age 1 to 9.
Geriatric patients. Administer cautiously to geriatric patients.

venlafaxine hydrochloride

Effexor, Effexor XR

Pharmacologic classification: neuronal serotonin, norepinephrine, dopamine reuptake inhibitor
Therapeutic classification: antidepressant
Pregnancy risk category C

How supplied

Available by prescription only
Capsules (extended-release): 37.5 mg, 75 mg, 150 mg
Tablets: 25 mg, 37.5 mg, 50 mg, 75 mg, 100 mg

Indications and dosages

Depression
Adults: Initially, 75 mg P.O. daily, in two or three divided doses with food. Increase dosage as tolerated and needed in increments of 75 mg/day at intervals of no less than 4 days. For moderately depressed outpatients, usual maximum dose is 225 mg/day; in certain severely depressed patients, dose may be as high as 375 mg/day divided into three doses. For extended-release capsules, 75 mg P.O. daily, in a single dose. For some patients, it may be desirable to start at 37.5 mg P.O. daily for 4 to 7 days before increasing to 75 mg daily. Dose may be increased at increments of 75 mg/day q 4 days to a maximum of 225 mg/day.
≡ ***Dosage adjustment.*** Reduce dose by 50% in patients with impaired hepatic function. In patients with moderate renal impairment (glomerular filtration rate of 10 to 70 ml/minute), reduce total daily dose by 25%. In hemodialysis patients, reduce dose by 50% and withhold drug until after dialysis treatment.

Pharmacodynamics

Antidepressant action: Venlafaxine is thought to potentiate neurotransmitter activity in the CNS. Preclinical studies have shown that venlafaxine and its active metabolite, O-desmethylvenlafaxine (ODV), are potent inhibitors of neuronal serotonin and norepinephrine reuptake and weak inhibitors of dopamine reuptake.

Pharmacokinetics

Absorption: About 92% is absorbed after oral administration.
Distribution: 25% to 29% protein-bound in plasma.
Metabolism: Extensively metabolized in the liver, with ODV being the only major active metabolite.
Excretion: About 87% of dose is recovered in urine within 48 hours (5% as unchanged venlafaxine, 29% as unconjugated ODV, 26% as conjugated ODV, and 27% as minor inactive metabolites).

Route	Onset	Peak	Duration
P.O.	Unknown	Unknown	Unknown

Contraindications and precautions

Contraindicated in patients hypersensitive to drug and within 14 days of MAO inhibitor therapy. Use cautiously in patients with impaired renal or hepatic function, diseases or conditions that could affect hemodynamic responses or metabolism, or history of seizures or mania.

Interactions

Drug-drug. *Cimetidine:* Increased in venlafaxine concentration. Use with caution. Monitor patient closely.
MAO inhibitors: May precipitate a syndrome similar to neuroleptic malignant syndrome when used with venlafaxine. Don't start venlafaxine within 14 days of discontinuing ther-

apy with an MAO inhibitor, and don't start MAO inhibitor therapy within 7 days of stopping venlafaxine.
Drug-herb. *Yohimbe:* May cause additive stimulation. Use together cautiously.

Effects on diagnostic tests
None reported.

Adverse reactions
CNS: *headache, somnolence, dizziness, nervousness, insomnia,* anxiety, tremor, abnormal dreams, paresthesia, agitation, *asthenia.*
CV: hypertension, vasodilation.
EENT: blurred vision.
GI: *nausea, constipation,* vomiting, *dry mouth, anorexia,* diarrhea, dyspepsia, flatulence.
GU: *abnormal ejaculation,* impotence, urinary frequency, impaired urination.
Skin: *diaphoresis,* rash.
Other: weight loss, yawning, chills, infection.

Overdose and treatment
Symptoms may range from none (most commonly) to somnolence, generalized seizures, and prolongation of the QT interval.

Treatment should consist of general measures used in managing any antidepressant overdose (ensuring an adequate airway, providing oxygenation and ventilation, monitoring cardiac rhythm and vital signs). General supportive and symptomatic measures also are recommended. Use of activated charcoal, induction of emesis, or gastric lavage should be considered. No specific antidotes are known for venlafaxine overdose.

Clinical considerations
- Drug is associated with sustained increases in blood pressure.
- Drug may activate mania or hypomania.
- When discontinuing drug therapy after more than 1 week, taper dose; when discontinuing after at least 6 weeks, gradually taper dose over 2 weeks.
- Discontinue drug in patient in whom seizures develop.

Therapeutic monitoring
- Regular monitoring of blood pressure is recommended. For patients who experience a sustained increase in blood pressure while receiving venlafaxine, either dose reduction or discontinuation should be considered.
- Monitor for signs of mania or hypomania and for seizure activity.

Special populations
Pregnant patients. Use drug during pregnancy only when clearly indicated.
Breast-feeding patients. Use cautiously in breast-feeding women.
Pediatric patients. Safety and effectiveness in children under age 18 haven't been established.

Patient counseling
- Caution patient not to operate hazardous machinery until effects of drug are known.
- Advise women to call health care provider if pregnancy is planned or suspected during therapy.
- Instruct patient to call health care provider before taking other medications, including OTC preparations, because of potential interactions.
- Advise patient to avoid alcohol while taking venlafaxine.
- Instruct patient to report rash, hives, or a related allergic reaction.

verapamil hydrochloride
Calan, Calan SR, Covera-HS, Isoptin, Isoptin SR, Verelan

Pharmacologic classification: calcium channel blocker
Therapeutic classification: antianginal, antihypertensive, antiarrhythmic
Pregnancy risk category C

How supplied
Available by prescription only
Tablets: 40 mg, 80 mg, 120 mg
Tablets (sustained-release): 120 mg, 180 mg, 240 mg
Capsules (sustained-release): 120 mg, 180 mg, 240 mg, 360 mg
Injection: 2.5 mg/ml

Indications and dosages
Management of Prinzmetal's variant angina, unstable angina, and chronic stable angina pectoris
Adults: Initial dose of 80 to 120 mg P.O. t.i.d. Dosage may be increased at weekly intervals. Some patients may require up to 480 mg daily.
Supraventricular tachyarrhythmias
Adults: 0.075 to 0.15 mg/kg (5 to 10 mg) I.V. push over 2 minutes. If no response occurs, give a second dose of 10 mg (0.15 mg/kg) 15 to 30 minutes after the initial dose.
Children age 1 to 15: 0.1 to 0.3 mg/kg (2 to 5 mg) as I.V. bolus over 2 minutes. Dose shouldn't exceed 5 mg. Dose may be repeated in 30 minutes if no response occurs. Total dose shouldn't exceed 10 mg.
Children under age 1: 0.1 to 0.2 mg/kg (0.75 to 2 mg) as I.V. bolus over 2 minutes. Dose may be repeated in 30 minutes if no response occurs.

Control of ventricular rate in digitalized patients with chronic atrial flutter or fibrillation
Adults: 240 to 320 mg P.O. daily in three to four divided doses.
Prophylaxis of repetitive paroxysmal supraventricular tachycardia (PSVT)
Adults: 240 to 480 mg/day given in three to four divided doses.
Hypertension
Adults: Usual starting dose is 80 mg P.O. t.i.d. Daily dose may be increased to 360 to 480 mg.

Initiate therapy with sustained-release capsules at 180 mg (240 mg for Verelan) daily in the morning. A starting dose of 120 mg may be indicated in patients with an increased response to verapamil. Adjust dose based on clinical effectiveness 24 hours after dosing. Increase by 120 mg daily until a maximum dose of 480 mg daily is given. Sustained-release capsules should be given only once daily. Antihypertensive effects are usually seen within the first week of therapy. Most patients respond to 240 mg daily.

Pharmacodynamics

Antianginal action: Verapamil manages unstable and chronic stable angina by reducing afterload, both at rest and with exercise, decreasing oxygen consumption. It also decreases myocardial oxygen demand and cardiac work by exerting a negative inotropic effect, reducing heart rate, relieving coronary artery spasm (via coronary artery vasodilation), and dilating peripheral vessels. The net result of these effects is relief of angina-related ischemia and pain. In patients with Prinzmetal's variant angina, verapamil inhibits coronary artery spasm, resulting in increased myocardial oxygen delivery.
Antihypertensive action: Verapamil reduces blood pressure, mainly by dilating peripheral vessels. Its negative inotropic effect blocks reflex mechanisms that lead to increased blood pressure.
Antiarrhythmic action: Combined effects of verapamil on the SA and AV nodes help manage arrhythmias. Primary effect of drug is on the AV node; slowed conduction reduces the ventricular rate in atrial tachyarrhythmias and blocks reentry paths in paroxysmal supraventricular arrhythmias.

Pharmacokinetics

Absorption: Absorbed rapidly and completely from the GI tract after oral administration; however, only about 20% to 35% of drug reaches systemic circulation because of first-pass effect.
Distribution: Steady-state distribution volume in healthy adults ranges from about 4.5 to 7 L/kg but may increase to 12 L/kg in patients with hepatic cirrhosis. About 90% of circulating drug is bound to plasma proteins.
Metabolism: Metabolized in the liver.
Excretion: Excreted in urine as unchanged drug and active metabolites. Elimination half-life is normally 6 to 12 hours and increases to as much as 16 hours in patients with hepatic cirrhosis. In infants, elimination half-life may be 5 to 7 hours.

Route	Onset	Peak	Duration
P.O.	½ hr	1-2 hr	8-10 hr
P.O. (extended)	½ hr	5-9 hr	24 hr
I.V.	1-5 min	Immediate	1-6 hr

Contraindications and precautions

Contraindicated in patients with hypersensitivity to drug; severe left ventricular dysfunction; cardiogenic shock; second- or third-degree AV block or sick sinus syndrome except in presence of functioning pacemaker; atrial flutter or fibrillation and accessory bypass tract syndrome; severe heart failure (unless secondary to verapamil therapy); and severe hypotension. In addition, I.V. verapamil is contraindicated in patients receiving I.V. beta blockers and in those with ventricular tachycardia.

Use cautiously in the elderly and in patients with impaired renal or hepatic function or increased intracranial pressure.

Interactions

Drug-drug. *Antihypertensives, quinidine:* May result in hypotension. Monitor blood pressure closely.
Carbamazepine, cardiac glycosides, cyclosporine: May increase serum levels of these drugs; monitor serum levels. Cut digoxin dose by 50%.
Disopyramide, flecainide, propranolol, other beta blockers, including ophthalmic timolol: May cause heart failure. Use together cautiously.
Lithium: May decrease or increase serum lithium levels. Monitor patient closely.
Rifampin: May decrease oral bioavailability of verapamil. Monitor patient for lack of effect.
Drug-herb. *Black catechu:* May cause additive effects. Don't use together.
Yerba maté: May decrease clearance of yerba maté methylxanthines and cause toxicity. Use together cautiously.
Drug-food. *Any food:* Helps increase absorption. Advise patient to take drug with food.
Drug-lifestyle. *Alcohol use:* Verapamil may prolong intoxicating effects of alcohol. Advise patient to avoid alcohol use.

Effects on diagnostic tests

None reported.

Adverse reactions

CNS: dizziness, headache, asthenia.

CV: *transient hypotension,* ***heart failure,*** *pulmonary edema, bradycardia, AV block,* ***ventricular asystole, ventricular fibrillation,*** peripheral edema.
GI: *constipation,* nausea.
Hepatic: elevated liver enzymes.
Skin: rash.

Overdose and treatment

Clinical effects of overdose are primarily extensions of adverse reactions. Heart block, asystole, and hypotension are the most serious reactions and require immediate attention.

Treatment may include administering I.V. isoproterenol, norepinephrine, epinephrine, atropine, or calcium gluconate in usual doses. Ensure adequate hydration.

In patients with hypertrophic cardiomyopathy, use alpha-adrenergic agents, including methoxamine, phenylephrine, and metaraminol, to maintain blood pressure. (Avoid isoproterenol and norepinephrine.) Inotropic agents, including dobutamine and dopamine, may be used if necessary.

If severe conduction disturbances, such as heart block and asystole, occur with hypotension that doesn't respond to drug therapy, initiate cardiac pacing immediately, with CPR measures as indicated.

In patients with Wolff-Parkinson-White or Lown-Ganong-Levine syndrome and a rapid ventricular rate caused by hemodynamically significant antegrade conduction, synchronized cardioversion may be used. Lidocaine and procainamide may be used as adjuncts.

Clinical considerations

- Generic sustained-release verapamil tablets may be substituted only for Isoptin SR and Calan SR, not Verelan capsules. The capsule formulation should be given only once daily. When using sustained-release tablets, doses of more than 240 mg should be given b.i.d.
- Discontinue disopyramide 48 hours before starting verapamil therapy and don't reinstitute until 24 hours after verapamil has been discontinued.
- Reduce dose in patients with renal or hepatic impairment.
- Use reduced doses in patients with severely compromised cardiac function and those receiving beta blockers.

Therapeutic monitoring

- Monitor patient closely for signs of toxicity.
- If patient is receiving I.V. verapamil, monitor ECG and blood pressure continuously.
- During long-term combination therapy with verapamil and digoxin, monitor ECG periodically to observe for AV block and bradycardia.
- Obtain periodic liver function tests.

Special populations

Pregnant patients. Use drug during pregnancy only when clearly indicated.
Breast-feeding patients. Drug is excreted in breast milk. To avoid possible adverse effects in infants, discontinue breast-feeding during therapy.
Pediatric patients. Currently, only the I.V. form is indicated for use in children to treat supraventricular tachyarrhythmias.
Geriatric patients. Geriatric patients may require lower doses. Administer I.V. doses over at least 3 minutes to minimize risk of adverse effects.

Patient counseling

Instruct patient to report signs of heart failure, such as swelling of hands and feet or shortness of breath.

vidarabine (adenine arabinoside)

Vira-A

Pharmacologic classification: purine nucleoside
Therapeutic classification: antiviral
Pregnancy risk category C

How supplied

Available by prescription only
Ophthalmic ointment: 3% in 3.5-g tube (equivalent to 2.8% vidarabine)

Indications and dosages

Acute keratoconjunctivitis and recurrent epithelial keratitis caused by herpes simplex virus types 1 and 2
Adults and children: Administer ½" (1.3 cm) ointment into lower conjunctival sac five times daily at 3-hour intervals.

Pharmacodynamics

Antiviral action: Vidarabine is an adenine analogue. Its exact mechanism of action is unknown; presumably it involves inhibition of DNA polymerase and viral replication by incorporation into viral DNA.

Pharmacokinetics

Absorption: No systemic absorption occurs with ophthalmic use.
Distribution: Only trace amounts are detected in the aqueous humor if the cornea is intact.
Metabolism: Metabolized into the active metabolite arabinosyl-hypoxanthine.
Excretion: Unknown.

Route	Onset	Peak	Duration
Ophthalmic	Unknown	Unknown	Unknown

Contraindications and precautions
Contraindicated in patients with hypersensitivity to drug or with sterile trophic ulcers. Use cautiously in patients receiving corticosteroids.

Interactions
None reported.

Effects on diagnostic tests
None reported.

Adverse reactions
EENT: temporary burning, itching, mild irritation, pain, lacrimation, foreign body sensation, conjunctival injection, punctal occlusion, sensitivity, superficial punctate keratitis, photophobia.
Other: ***hypersensitivity reactions.***

Overdose and treatment
None reported.

Clinical considerations
- Drug is effective only if patient has at least minimal immunocompetence.
- If there are no signs of improvement after 7 days or if re-epithelialization hasn't occurred in 21 days, consider other forms of therapy. However, severe cases may require longer treatment. Continue drug for 5 to 7 days, b.i.d., to prevent recurrence.
- Definitive diagnosis of herpes simplex conjunctivitis should be made before administration of ophthalmic form.

Therapeutic monitoring
Monitor for signs of improvement and reepithelialization.

Special populations
Pregnant patients. Use drug during pregnancy only when potential benefits justify possible risks to the fetus.
Breast-feeding patients. Because vidarabine has been shown to be tumorigenic, breastfeeding should be discontinued during drug therapy.

Patient counseling
- Warn patient who is receiving ophthalmic ointment not to exceed recommended frequency or duration of therapy. Instruct him to wash hands before and after applying ointment.
- Warn patient against allowing tip of tube to touch eye or surrounding area.
- Advise patient to wear sunglasses if photosensitivity occurs.
- Instruct patient to store ophthalmic ointment in tightly sealed, light-resistant container.

vinblastine sulfate (VLB)
Velban, Velbe*

Pharmacologic classification: vinca alkaloid (cell cycle-phase specific, M phase)
Therapeutic classification: antineoplastic
Pregnancy risk category D

How supplied
Available by prescription only
Injection: 10-mg vials (lyophilized powder), 10 mg/10 ml vials

Indications and dosages
Dosage and indications may vary. Check current literature for recommended protocol.
Breast or testicular cancer, Hodgkin's and malignant lymphomas, choriocarcinoma, lymphosarcoma, neuroblastoma, lung cancer, mycosis fungoides, histiocytosis, Kaposi's sarcoma
Adults: 0.1 mg/kg or 3.7 mg/m^2 I.V. weekly or q 2 weeks. May be increased in weekly increments of 50 mcg/kg or 1.8 to 1.9 mg/m^2 to maximum dose of 0.5 mg/kg or 18.5 mg/m^2 I.V. weekly, based on response. Dose shouldn't be repeated if WBC count goes to less than 4,000/mm^3.
Children: 2.5 mg/m^2 I.V. as a single dose every week, increased weekly in increments of 1.25 mg/m^2 to maximum of 7.5 mg/m^2.

Pharmacodynamics
Antineoplastic action: Vinblastine exerts its cytotoxic activity by arresting the cell cycle in the metaphase portion of cell division, resulting in a blockade of mitosis. Drug also inhibits DNA-dependent RNA synthesis and interferes with amino acid metabolism, inhibiting purine synthesis.

Pharmacokinetics
Absorption: Absorbed unpredictably across the GI tract after oral administration and must be given I.V.
Distribution: Distributed widely into body tissues. Drug crosses the blood-brain barrier but doesn't achieve therapeutic levels in the CSF.
Metabolism: Metabolized partially in the liver to an active metabolite.
Excretion: Excreted primarily in bile as unchanged drug. A smaller portion is excreted in urine. Plasma elimination of vinblastine is described as triphasic, with half-lives of 3½ minutes, 1½ hours, and 24¾ hours for the alpha, beta, and terminal phases, respectively.

Route	Onset	Peak	Duration
I.V.	Unknown	Unknown	Unknown

Contraindications and precautions
Contraindicated in patients with severe leukopenia, granulocytopenia (unless result of disease being treated), or bacterial infection. Use cautiously in patients with hepatic dysfunction.

Interactions
Drug-drug. *Erythromycin:* Vinblastine toxicity. Use with caution; monitor for signs of toxicity.
Mitomycin: Acute shortness of breath and severe bronchospasm. Monitor respiratory status closely.
Phenytoin: May lower plasma phenytoin levels, requiring increased doses of phenytoin. Monitor phenytoin plasma level.

Effects on diagnostic tests
None reported.

Adverse reactions
CNS: depression, *paresthesia, peripheral neuropathy and neuritis, numbness, loss of deep tendon reflexes, muscle pain and weakness,* ***seizures, CVA,*** headache.
CV: hypertension, ***MI.***
EENT: pharyngitis.
GI: *nausea, vomiting,* ulcer, bleeding, *constipation, ileus, anorexia,* diarrhea, *weight loss,* abdominal pain, *stomatitis.*
Hematologic: *anemia,* ***leukopenia*** (nadir occurs days 4 to 10 and lasts another 7 to 14 days), ***thrombocytopenia.***
Metabolic: hyperuricemia.
Respiratory: ***acute bronchospasm,*** shortness of breath.
Skin: vesiculation.
Other: reversible alopecia, *irritation, phlebitis,* cellulitis, necrosis with extravasation.

Overdose and treatment
Signs and symptoms of overdose include stomatitis, ileus, mental depression, paresthesia, loss of deep reflexes, permanent CNS damage, and myelosuppression.

Treatment is usually supportive and includes transfusion of blood components and appropriate symptomatic therapy.

Clinical considerations
- Peripheral infusion increases risk of extravasation. Drug may be administered as an I.V. infusion through a central venous catheter.
- Drug may be administered by I.V. push injection over 1 minute through the tubing of a freely flowing I.V. infusion.
- Drug shouldn't be administered more frequently than every 7 days to allow for review of effect on leukocytes.
- Reduced doses may be required in patients with liver disease.
- Risk of uric acid nephropathy can be reduced with generous oral fluid intake and administration of allopurinol.
- Drug is less neurotoxic than vincristine.

Therapeutic monitoring
- Review effect on leukocytes before administration of each dose.
- Monitor for life-threatening acute bronchospasm reaction. This reaction is most likely to occur in patients also receiving mitomycin.

Special populations
Pregnant patients. Drug may cause fetal toxicity when administered during pregnancy.
Breast-feeding patients. It isn't known if drug is excreted in breast milk. However, because of risk of serious adverse reactions, mutagenicity, and carcinogenicity in infants, breast-feeding isn't recommended.
Geriatric patients. Patients with cachexia or ulceration of the skin (which is more common in geriatric patients) may be more susceptible to leukopenic effect of drug.

Patient counseling
- Inform women of childbearing age of the potential risks to fetus.
- Encourage adequate fluid intake to increase urine output and facilitate excretion of uric acid.
- Reassure patient that therapeutic response isn't immediate. Adequate trial is 12 weeks.
- Advise patient to avoid exposure to people with infections and to report signs of infection or unusual bleeding immediately.
- Reassure patient that hair should grow back after treatment has ended.

vincristine sulfate
Oncovin, Vincasar PFS

Pharmacologic classification: vinca alkaloid (cell cycle-phase specific, M phase)
Therapeutic classification: antineoplastic
Pregnancy risk category D

How supplied
Available by prescription only
Injection: 1 mg/1 ml, 2 mg/2 ml, 5 mg/5 ml multiple-dose vials; 1 mg/1 ml, 2 mg/2 ml preservative-free vials

Indications and dosages
Dosage and indications may vary. Check current literature for recommended protocol.
Acute lymphoblastic and other leukemias; Hodgkin's disease; lymphosarcoma; reticulum cell, osteogenic, and other sarcomas; neuroblastoma; rhabdomyosarcoma; Wilms' tumor; lung and ◇breast cancer
Adults: 10 to 30 mcg/kg I.V. or 0.4 to 1.4 mg/m^2 I.V. weekly.

Children: 1.5 to 2 mg/m^2 I.V. weekly. Maximum single dose (adults and children), 2 mg. *Children weighing less than 22 lb (10 kg) or body surface area less than 1 m^2:* 0.05 mg/kg once weekly.

≡ ***Dosage adjustment.*** Reduce dose by 50% in patients with direct serum bilirubin concentration exceeding 3 ml/dl or other evidence of significant hepatic impairment.

Pharmacodynamics

Antineoplastic action: Vincristine exerts its cytotoxic activity by arresting the cell cycle in the metaphase portion of cell division, resulting in a blockade of mitosis. Drug also inhibits DNA-dependent RNA synthesis and interferes with amino acid metabolites, inhibiting purine synthesis.

Pharmacokinetics

Absorption: Absorbed unpredictably across the GI tract after oral administration and must be given I.V.

Distribution: Rapidly and widely distributed into body tissues and is bound to erythrocytes and platelets. Drug crosses blood-brain barrier but doesn't achieve therapeutic levels in CSF.

Metabolism: Largely metabolized in the liver.

Excretion: Drug and its metabolites are primarily excreted into bile. A smaller portion is eliminated through the kidneys. The plasma elimination of vincristine is described as triphasic, with half-lives of about 4 minutes, 2¼ hours, and 85 hours for the distribution, second, and terminal phases, respectively.

Route	Onset	Peak	Duration
I.V.	Unknown	Unknown	Unknown

Contraindications and precautions

Contraindicated in patients hypersensitive to drug or who have the demyelinating form of Charcot-Marie-Tooth syndrome. Don't give to patients who are also receiving radiation therapy through ports that include the liver.

Use cautiously in patients with hepatic dysfunction, neuromuscular disease, or infection.

Interactions

Drug-drug. *Asparaginase:* Decreases the hepatic clearance of vincristine. Monitor for toxicity.

Calcium channel blockers: Enhance vincristine accumulation in cells. Monitor patient closely.

Digoxin: Decreases digoxin levels. Monitor serum digoxin levels.

Methotrexate: Increases therapeutic effect of methotrexate. This interaction may be used to therapeutic advantage; it allows a lower dose of methotrexate, reducing the potential for methotrexate toxicity. Monitor closely.

Mitomycin: May increase frequency of bronchospasm and acute pulmonary reactions. Monitor respiratory status.

Other neurotoxic drugs: Increases neurotoxicity through an additive effect. Use with caution. Monitor for toxicity.

Phenytoin: May decrease plasma phenytoin levels; dose adjustments may be needed. Monitor patient closely.

Effects on diagnostic tests

None reported.

Adverse reactions

CNS: *peripheral neuropathy,* sensory loss, *loss of deep tendon reflexes, paresthesia, wristdrop and footdrop,* ***seizures, coma,*** headache, ataxia, cranial nerve palsies, *jaw pain,* hoarseness, vocal cord paralysis, *muscle weakness and cramps* (some neurotoxicities may be permanent).

CV: hypotension, hypertension.

EENT: diplopia, optic and extraocular neuropathy, hearing impairment, ptosis, photophobia, transient cortical blindness, optical atrophy.

GI: diarrhea, *constipation, cramps,* ileus that mimics surgical abdomen, paralytic ileus, *nausea, vomiting,* anorexia, weight loss, dysphagia, ***intestinal necrosis,*** *stomatitis.*

GU: urine retention, syndrome of inappropriate antidiuretic hormone, dysuria, acute uric acid neuropathy, polyuria.

Hematologic: anemia, ***leukopenia, thrombocytopenia.***

Metabolic: *hyperuricemia,* hyponatremia.

Respiratory: ***acute bronchospasm,*** dyspnea.

Other: *reversible alopecia,* fever, severe local reaction with extravasation, *phlebitis,* cellulitis at injection site.

Overdose and treatment

Signs and symptoms of overdose include alopecia, myelosuppression, paresthesia, neuritic pain, motor difficulties, loss of deep tendon reflexes, nausea, vomiting, and ileus.

Treatment is usually supportive and includes transfusion of blood components, antiemetics, enemas for ileus, phenobarbital for seizures, and other appropriate symptomatic therapy. Administration of calcium leucovorin at a dosage of 15 mg I.V. every 3 hours for 24 hours, then every 6 hours for 48 hours may help protect cells from the toxic effects of vincristine.

Clinical considerations

- Necrosis may result from extravasation.
- Drug may be administered by I.V. push injection over 1 minute into the tubing of a freely flowing I.V. infusion.
- Neurotoxicity is dose-related and usually reversible.
- Risk of uric acid nephropathy is reduced with generous oral fluid intake and administration of allopurinol. Alkalinization of urine may be required if serum uric acid concentration is increased.

- Reduced dose may be required in patients with obstructive jaundice or liver disease.
- Drug may cause SIADH secretion.

Therapeutic monitoring

- Monitor for neurotoxicity.
- Monitor for life-threatening bronchospasm reaction.
- Monitor for leukopenia and thrombocytopenia.

Special populations

Pregnant patients. Vincristine can cause fetal toxicity and should be used during pregnancy only in life-threatening situations or in severe circumstances in which safer drugs aren't available.
Breast-feeding patients. It isn't known if drug is distributed into breast milk. However, because of risk of serious adverse reactions, mutagenicity, and carcinogenicity in the infant, breast-feeding isn't recommended.
Geriatric patients. Geriatric patients who are weak or bedridden may be more susceptible to neurotoxic effects. Use cautiously.

Patient counseling

- Inform women of the potential for fetal harm.
- Encourage adequate fluid intake to increase urine output and facilitate excretion of uric acid.
- Assure patient that hair growth should resume after treatment is discontinued.

vinorelbine tartrate

Navelbine

Pharmacologic classification: semisynthetic vinca alkaloid
Therapeutic classification: antineoplastic
Pregnancy risk category D

How supplied

Available by prescription only
Injection: 10 mg/ml in 1-ml and 5-ml single-use vials

Indications and dosages

Alone or as adjunct therapy with cisplatin for first-line treatment of ambulatory patients with nonresectable advanced non-small cell lung cancer (NSCLC); alone or with cisplatin in stage IV of NSCLC; with cisplatin in stage III of NSCLC
Adults: 30 mg/m² I.V. weekly. In combination treatment, same dosage used along with 120 mg/m² of cisplatin, given on days 1 and 29, then q 6 weeks.
≡ ***Dosage adjustment.*** Adjust dose based on hematologic toxicity or hepatic insufficiency.

Pharmacodynamics

Antineoplastic action: Vinorelbine exerts its antineoplastic effect by disrupting microtubule assembly, which disrupts spindle formation and prevents mitosis.

Pharmacokinetics

Absorption: Only given I.V.
Distribution: Binding to plasma constituents ranges from 79.6% to 91.2%. It demonstrates high binding to human platelets and lymphocytes.
Metabolism: Undergoes substantial hepatic metabolism.
Excretion: About 18% is excreted in urine and 46% is excreted in feces. Terminal phase half-life averages 27½ to 43½ hours.

Route	Onset	Peak	Duration
I.V.	Unknown	Unknown	Unknown

Contraindications and precautions

Contraindicated in patients with pretreatment granulocyte counts less than 1,000 cells/m³. Use with extreme caution in patients whose bone marrow may have been compromised by previous exposure to radiation or chemotherapy or whose bone marrow is still recovering from previous chemotherapy. Also use cautiously in patients with impaired hepatic function. Use in pregnancy only if benefit outweighs risk to fetus.

Interactions

Drug-drug. *Cisplatin:* Increased risk of bone marrow depression. Monitor hematologic status closely.
Mitomycin: May cause pulmonary reactions. Monitor respiratory status closely.

Effects on diagnostic tests

None reported.

Adverse reactions

CNS: *fatigue, peripheral neuropathy, asthenia.*
CV: chest pain.
GI: *nausea, vomiting, anorexia, diarrhea, constipation, stomatitis.*
Hematologic: ***bone marrow suppression (agranulocytosis,*** **LEUKOPENIA,** ***thrombocytopenia,*** anemia).
Hepatic: *abnormal liver function tests, bilirubinemia.*
Musculoskeletal: jaw pain, myalgia, arthralgia.
Respiratory: dyspnea.
Skin: *alopecia,* rash, *injection pain or reaction.*
Other: SIADH.

Overdose and treatment

The primary anticipated complications of overdose are bone marrow suppression and peripheral neurotoxicity. Treatment includes general supportive measures and appropriate blood transfusions and antibiotics as needed. There's no known antidote.

Clinical considerations

- Drug can cause considerable irritation, localized tissue necrosis, and thrombophlebitis.
- Drug may be a contact irritant and the solution must be handled and administered with care. Use gloves. Avoid inhalation of vapors and contact with skin or mucous membranes, especially the eyes. If contact occurs, wash with copious amounts of water for at least 15 minutes.
- Adjust dose based on hematologic toxicity or hepatic insufficiency, whichever results in a lower dose. Reduce dose by 50% if patient's granulocyte count goes to less than 1,500 cells/mm^3 but exceeds 1,000 cells/mm^3. If three consecutive doses are skipped because of granulocytopenia, discontinue drug therapy.

Therapeutic monitoring

- Check patient's granulocyte count before initiating therapy. It should be 1,000 cells/mm^3 or more for drug to be administered.
- Monitor patient closely for hypersensitivity reactions.
- Monitor patient's peripheral blood count and bone marrow to guide effects of therapy.

Special populations

Pregnant patients. Drug can cause fetal toxicity and should be used during pregnancy only in life-threatening situations or severe conditions for which safer drugs aren't available.
Breast-feeding patients. It isn't known if drug is excreted in breast milk. Because of risk of adverse effects in the breast-fed infant, don't use drug in breast-feeding women.
Pediatric patients. Safety and effectiveness in children haven't been established.

Patient counseling

- Instruct patient not to take other drugs, including OTC preparations, unless instructed.
- Tell patient to report signs and symptoms of infection (fever, chills, malaise) because drug has immunosuppressive activity.
- Inform the patient of the risk of fetal toxicity.

vitamin A (retinol)

Aquasol A, Del-Vi-A, Palmitate-A 5000

Pharmacologic classification: fat-soluble vitamin
Therapeutic classification: vitamin
Pregnancy risk category A (X if dose exceeds RDA)

How supplied

Available by prescription only
Tablets: 10,000 IU
Capsules: 25,000 IU, 50,000 IU
Injection: 2-ml vials (50,000 IU/ml with 0.5% chlorobutanol, polysorbate 80, butylated hydroxyanisole, and butylated hydroxytoluene)
Available without a prescription, as appropriate
Drops: 30 ml with dropper (5,000 IU/0.1 ml)
Capsules: 10,000 IU
Tablets: 5,000 IU

Indications and dosages

Severe vitamin A deficiency with xerophthalmia
Adults and children over age 8: 500,000 IU P.O. daily for 3 days, then 50,000 IU P.O. daily for 14 days, then maintenance dosage of 10,000 to 20,000 IU P.O. daily for 2 months, followed by adequate dietary nutrition and RDA vitamin A supplements.
Severe vitamin A deficiency
Adults and children over age 8: 100,000 IU P.O. or I.M. daily for 3 days, then 50,000 IU P.O. or I.M. daily for 14 days, then maintenance dosage of 10,000 to 20,000 IU P.O. daily for 2 months, followed by adequate dietary nutrition and RDA vitamin A supplements.
Children age 1 to 8: 17,500 to 35,000 IU I.M. daily for 10 days.
Infants under age 1: 7,500 to 15,000 IU I.M. daily for 10 days.

Note: The RDA for vitamin A is as follows:

	Vitamin A RDA	Vitamin A and beta carotene RDA
Infants		
birth to 12 months	375 RE	1,875 IU
Children		
age 1 to 3	400 RE	2,000 IU
age 4 to 6	500 RE	2,500 IU
age 7 to 10	700 RE	3,500 IU
Males		
age 11 and over	1,000 RE	5,000 IU
Females		
age 11 and over	800 RE	4,000 IU
Pregnant	800 RE	4,000 IU
Breast-feeding	1,300 RE (1st 6 months)	6,500 IU
	1,200 RE (2nd 6 months)	6,000 IU

RE = retinol equivalents; IU = combination of retinol and beta-carotene.

Pharmacodynamics

Metabolic action: One IU of vitamin A is equivalent to 0.3 mcg of retinol or 0.6 mcg of beta-carotene. Beta-carotene, or provitamin A, yields retinol after absorption from the intestinal tract. Use of retinol with opsin, the red pigment in the retina, helps form rhodopsin, which is needed for visual adaptation to darkness. Vitamin A prevents growth retardation and preserves the integrity of the epithelial cells. Vitamin A deficiency is characterized by nyctalopia (night blindness), keratomalacia (necrosis of the cornea), keratinization and drying of the skin, low resistance to infection, growth retardation, bone thickening, diminished cortical steroid production, and fetal malformations.

Pharmacokinetics

Absorption: Absorbed readily and completely in normal doses if fat absorption is normal. Larger doses, or regular doses in patients with fat malabsorption, low protein intake, or hepatic or pancreatic disease, may be absorbed incompletely. Because vitamin A is fat-soluble, absorption requires bile salts, pancreatic lipase, and dietary fat.
Distribution: Stored (primarily as palmitate) in Kupffer's cells of the liver. Normal adult liver stores are sufficient to provide vitamin A requirements for 2 years. Lesser amounts of retinyl palmitate are stored in the kidneys, lungs, adrenal glands, retinas, and intraperitoneal fat. Vitamin A circulates bound to a specific $alpha_1$ protein, retinol-binding protein (RBP). Blood level assays may not reflect liver storage of vitamin A because serum levels depend partly on circulating RBP. Liver storage should be adequate before discontinuing therapy. Vitamin A is distributed into breast milk. It doesn't readily cross the placenta.
Metabolism: Vitamin A is metabolized in the liver.
Excretion: Retinol (fat-soluble) is conjugated with glucuronic acid and then further metabolized to retinal and retinoic acid. Retinoic acid is excreted in feces via biliary elimination. Retinal, retinoic acid, and other water-soluble metabolites are excreted in urine and feces. Normally, no unchanged retinol is excreted in urine, except in patients with pneumonia or chronic nephritis.

Route	Onset	Peak	Duration
P.O.	Unknown	3-5 hr	Unknown
I.M.	Unknown	Unknown	Unknown

Contraindications and precautions

Oral form is contraindicated in patients with malabsorption syndrome; if malabsorption is from inadequate bile secretion, oral route may be used with concurrent administration of bile salts (dehydrocholic acid). Also contraindicated in those with hypervitaminosis A and hypersensitivity to any ingredient in product. I.V. route is contraindicated except for special water-miscible forms intended for infusion with large parenteral volumes. I.V. push of vitamin A of any type is also contraindicated; anaphylaxis or anaphylactoid reactions and death have resulted.

Use cautiously in pregnant women.

Interactions

Drug-drug. *Cholestyramine:* May decrease the absorption of vitamin A by decreasing bile acids and preventing the micellar phase in the GI lumen. Daily vitamin A supplements are recommended during long-term cholestyramine therapy.
Mineral oil (prolonged use): May interfere with the intestinal absorption of vitamin A. Avoid use together.
Neomycin: Mmay decrease vitamin A absorption. Avoid use together.
Orlistat: May decrease vitamin A absorption. Give drugs at least 2 hours apart.
Oral contraceptives: Significantly increase vitamin A plasma levels. Monitor patient closely.
Retinoids, such as etretinate or isotretinoin: Increased risk of adverse drug events resulting from potentiation. Avoid use together.
Warfarin: Decreased anticoagulation effect. Monitor PT and INR closely.

Effects on diagnostic tests

Vitamin A therapy may falsely increase serum cholesterol level readings by interfering with the Zlatkis-Zak reaction. Vitamin A has also been reported to falsely elevate bilirubin determinations.

Adverse reactions

Adverse reactions usually occur only with toxicity.
CNS: irritability, headache, ***increased intracranial pressure,*** fatigue, lethargy, malaise.
EENT: papilledema, exophthalmos.
GI: anorexia, epigastric pain, vomiting, polydipsia.
GU: hypomenorrhea, polyuria.
Hepatic: jaundice, hepatomegaly, ***cirrhosis,*** elevated liver enzymes.
Musculoskeletal: slow growth, decalcification, hypercalcemia, periostitis, premature closure of epiphyses, migratory arthralgia, cortical thickening over the radius and tibia.
Skin: alopecia; dry, cracked, scaly skin; pruritus; lip fissures; erythema; inflamed tongue, lips, and gums; massive desquamation; increased pigmentation; night sweats.
Other: splenomegaly, ***anaphylactic shock, death*** (reported with I.V. use).

Overdose and treatment

In cases of acute toxicity, increased intracranial pressure develops within 8 to 12 hours; cutaneous desquamation follows in a few days.

Toxicity can follow a single dose of 25,000 IU/kg, which in infants would represent about 75,000 IU and in adults over 2 million IU.

Chronic toxicity results from administration of 4,000 IU/kg for 6 to 15 months. In infants (age 3 to 6 months), this represents about 18,500 IU/day for 1 to 3 months; in adults, 1 million IU/day for 3 days, 50,000 IU/day for more than 18 months, or 500,000 IU/day for 2 months.

To treat toxicity, discontinue vitamin A administration if hypercalcemia persists; administer I.V. saline solution, prednisone, and calcitonin, if indicated. Perform liver function tests to detect possible liver damage.

Clinical considerations

- In any dietary deficiency, multiple vitamin deficiency should be suspected.
- It's recommended that vitamin A be given with bile salts to patients with malabsorption caused by inadequate bile secretion.
- Vitamin A given by I.V. push is contraindicated because of the risk of anaphylaxis and death.
- Special water-miscible forms of vitamin A are available for use when adding to large parenteral volumes.

Special populations

Pregnant patients. Safety of amounts exceeding 5,000 IU/day (oral) or 6,000 IU/day (parenteral) during pregnancy isn't known.

Breast-feeding patients. Vitamin A is excreted in breast milk. The RDA of vitamin A for breast-feeding women in the United States is 1,300 and 1,200 retinol equivalents (RE) for the first 6 months and second 6 months, respectively. Unless the maternal diet is grossly inadequate, infants can usually obtain sufficient vitamin A from breast-feeding. The effect of large maternal doses of vitamin A on breast-fed infants is unknown.

Patient counseling

- Instruct patient to avoid prolonged use of mineral oil while taking drug because mineral oil reduces vitamin A absorption in the intestine.
- Tell patient not to exceed recommended dose.
- Instruct patient to report promptly symptoms of overdose, such as nausea, vomiting, anorexia, malaise, drying or cracking of skin or lips, irritability, headache, or loss of hair.
- Inform patient of the need to consume adequate protein, vitamin E, and zinc, which, along with bile, are necessary for vitamin A absorption.

vitamin E (alpha tocopherol)

Amino-Opti-E, Aquasol E, E-200 IU Softgels, E-400 IU in a water-soluble base, E-1000 IU Softgels, E-Complex-600, E-Vitamin Succinate, Vita-Plus E

Pharmacologic classification: fat-soluble vitamin
Therapeutic classification: vitamin
Pregnancy risk category A (C if greater than RDA)

How supplied

Available without a prescription, as appropriate
Capsules: 100 IU, 200 IU, 400 IU, 500 IU, 600 IU, 1,000 IU
Tablets: 100 IU, 200 IU, 400 IU, 500 IU, 600 IU, 1,000 IU
Oral solution: 50 IU/ml

Indications and dosages

Vitamin E deficiency in premature infants and in patients with impaired fat absorption (including patients with cystic fibrosis); biliary atresia
Adults: 60 to 75 IU P.O. daily, depending on severity. Maximum dose, 300 IU/day.
Children: 1 unit/kg P.O. daily.
Premature neonates: 5 units P.O. daily.
Full-term neonates: 5 units P.O. per liter of formula.

Note: The RDA for vitamin E is as follows:
Infants up to age 6 months: 3 α-TE or 4 IU.
Children age 6 months to 1 year: 4 α-TE or 6 IU.
Children age 1 to 3: 6 α-TE or 9 IU.
Children age 4 to 10: 7 α-TE or 10 IU.
Males over age 11: 10 α-TE or 15 IU.
Females over age 11: 8 α-TE or 12 IU.
Pregnant women: 10 α-TE or 15 IU.
Breast-feeding women: First 6 months, 12 α-TE or 18 IU, over 6 months, 11 α-TE or 16 IU.

TE is alpha tocopherol equivalent (equal to 1 mg d-alpha-tocopherol or 1.49 IU).

Pharmacodynamics

Nutritional action: As a dietary supplement, the exact biochemical mechanism is unclear, although it's believed to act as an antioxidant. Vitamin E protects cell membranes, vitamin A, vitamin C (ascorbic acid), and polyunsaturated fatty acids from oxidation. It also may act as a cofactor in enzyme systems, and some evidence exists that it decreases platelet aggregation.

Pharmacokinetics

Absorption: GI absorption depends on the presence of bile. Only 20% to 60% of the vitamin

obtained from dietary sources is absorbed. As dose increases, the fraction of vitamin E absorbed decreases.
Distribution: Distributed to all tissues and is stored in adipose tissue.
Metabolism: Metabolized in the liver by glucuronidation.
Excretion: Excreted primarily in bile. Some enterohepatic circulation may occur. Small amounts of the metabolites are excreted in urine.

Route	Onset	Peak	Duration
P.O.	Unknown	Unknown	Unknown

Contraindications and precautions
No known contraindications. Use cautiously in patients with liver or gallbladder disease.

Interactions
Drug-drug. *Cholestyramine, colestipol, mineral oil, or sucralfate:* May increase vitamin E requirements. Use together cautiously.
Oral anticoagulants: May be at risk for hemorrhage after large doses of vitamin E. Monitor patient closely for bleeding.
Orlistat: May decrease absorption of vitamin E. Give drugs at least 2 hours apart.
Vitamin K: Decreased therapeutic effect of vitamin K. Avoid use together.

Effects on diagnostic tests
None reported.

Adverse reactions
None reported with recommended doses. Hypervitaminosis E symptoms include fatigue, weakness, nausea, headache, blurred vision, flatulence, diarrhea.

Overdose and treatment
Signs of overdose include a possible increase in blood pressure. Treatment is generally supportive.

Clinical considerations
Give drug with bile salts if patient has malabsorption caused by lack of bile.

Therapeutic monitoring
Monitor for adverse drug events and for therapeutic effect.

Special populations
None reported.

Patient counseling
- Tell patient to store vitamin E in a tight, light-resistant container.
- Instruct patient to swallow capsules whole and not to crush or chew them.

vitamin K derivatives

phytonadione
AquaMEPHYTON, Mephyton

Pharmacologic classification: vitamin K
Therapeutic classification: blood coagulation modifier
Pregnancy risk category C

How supplied
Available by prescription only
Tablets: 5 mg
Injection (aqueous colloidal solution): 2 mg/ml, 10 mg/ml
Injection (aqueous dispersion): 2 mg/ml, 10 mg/ml

Indications and dosages
Hypoprothrombinemia secondary to vitamin K malabsorption or drug therapy, or when oral administration is desired and bile secretion is inadequate
Adults: 5 to 10 mg P.O. daily, or titrated to patient's requirements.
Hypoprothrombinemia secondary to vitamin K malabsorption, drug therapy, or excess vitamin A
Adults: 2 to 25 mg P.O. or parenterally, repeated and increased up to 50 mg, if necessary.
Children: 5 to 10 mg P.O. or parenterally.
Infants: 2 mg P.O. or parenterally.
Hypoprothrombinemia secondary to effect of oral anticoagulants
Adults: 2.5 to 10 mg P.O., S.C., or I.M., based on PT and INR, repeated, if necessary, 12 to 48 hours after oral dose or 6 to 8 hours after parenteral dose. In emergency, give 10 to 50 mg slow I.V., rate not to exceed 1 mg/minute, repeated q 6 to 8 hours, p.r.n.
Prevention of hemorrhagic disease in neonates
Neonates: 0.5 to 1 mg S.C. or I.M. immediately after birth, repeated in 2 to 3 weeks, if needed, especially if mother received oral anticoagulants or long-term anticonvulsant therapy during pregnancy.
Prevention of hypoprothrombinemia related to vitamin K deficiency in long-term parenteral nutrition
Adults: 5 to 10 mg I.M. weekly.
Children: 2 to 5 mg I.M. weekly.

Note: The RDA for vitamin K is as follows:
Infants up to age 6 months: 5 mcg.
Children age 6 months to 1 year: 10 mcg.
Children age 1 to 3: 15 mcg.
Children age 4 to 6: 20 mcg.
Children age 7 to 10: 30 mcg.
Males age 11 to 14: 45 mcg.
Males age 15 to 18: 65 mcg.
Men age 19 to 24: 70 mcg.
Men over age 24: 80 mcg.

Females age 11 to 14: 45 mcg.
Females age 15 to 18: 55 mcg.
Women age 19 to 24: 60 mcg.
Women over age 24: 65 mcg.
Pregnant or breast-feeding women: 65 mcg.

Pharmacodynamics

Coagulation modifying action: Vitamin K is a lipid-soluble vitamin that promotes hepatic formation of active prothrombin and several other coagulation factors (specifically factors II, VII, IX, and X).

Phytonadione (vitamin K_1) is a synthetic form of vitamin K and is also lipid-soluble. Vitamin K doesn't counteract the action of heparin.

Pharmacokinetics

Absorption: Phytonadione requires the presence of bile salts for GI tract absorption. Once absorbed, vitamin K enters the blood directly. Onset of action after I.V. injection is more rapid, but of shorter duration, than that occurring after S.C. or I.M. injection.
Distribution: Concentrates in the liver for a short time. Hemorrhage is usually controlled within 3 to 6 hours, and normal prothrombin levels are achieved in 12 to 14 hours.
Metabolism: Metabolized rapidly by the liver; little tissue accumulation occurs.
Excretion: Data are limited. High concentrations occur in feces; however, intestinal bacteria can synthesize vitamin K.

Route	Onset	Peak	Duration
P.O.	6-12 hr	Unknown	Unknown
I.V., I.M., S.C.	1-2 hr	Unknown	Unknown

Contraindications and precautions

Contraindicated in patients with hypersensitivity to drug.

Interactions

Drug-drug. *Broad-spectrum antibiotics, especially cefamandole, cefoperazone, and cefotetan:* May interfere with the actions of vitamin K, producing hypoprothrombinemia. Use together cautiously.
Mineral oil: Inhibits absorption of oral vitamin K. Give drugs at well-spaced intervals, and monitor result.
Oral anticoagulants: Antagonizes anticoagulant therapeutic effect. Use vitamin K only for severe hypoprothrombinemia.
Orlistat: May decrease absorption of vitamin K. Give drugs at least 2 hours apart.

Effects on diagnostic tests

Phytonadione can falsely elevate urine steroid levels.

Adverse reactions

CNS: headache, dizziness, convulsive movements.
CV: transient hypotension after I.V. administration, rapid and weak pulse, *arrhythmias.*
GI: nausea, vomiting.
Respiratory: *bronchospasm,* dyspnea.
Skin: diaphoresis, flushing, erythema, urticaria, pruritus, allergic rash.
Other: cramplike pain, ***anaphylaxis and anaphylactoid reactions,*** (usually after too-rapid I.V. administration), pain, swelling, hematoma at injection site; hyperbilirubinemia, ***fatal kernicterus,*** *severe hemolytic anemia* in neonates.

Overdose and treatment

Excessive doses of vitamin K may cause hepatic dysfunction in adults; in neonates, and in premature infants; large doses may cause hemolytic anemia, kernicterus, and death. Treatment is supportive.

Clinical considerations

- Excessive use of vitamin K may temporarily defeat oral anticoagulant therapy; higher doses of oral anticoagulant or interim use of heparin may be required.
- Phytonadione for hemorrhagic disease in infants causes fewer adverse reactions than do other vitamin K analogues; phytonadione is the vitamin K analogue of choice to treat an oral anticoagulant overdose.
- Patients receiving phytonadione who have bile deficiency require concurrent use of bile salts to ensure adequate absorption.
- When I.V. administration is considered unavoidable, the drug should be injected very slowly, not exceeding 1 mg/minute.
- Discontinue drug if allergic or severe CNS reactions appear.

Therapeutic monitoring

- With I.V. administration, monitor for flushing, weakness, tachycardia, and hypotension. Shock may follow. Deaths have occurred.
- Monitor PT and INR to determine effectiveness.
- Monitor patient response, and watch for adverse effects; failure to respond to vitamin K may indicate coagulation defects or irreversible hepatic damage.

Special populations

Pediatric patients. Don't exceed recommended dose. Hemolysis, jaundice, and hyperbilirubinemia in neonates, particularly premature infants, may be related to vitamin K administration.
Breast-feeding patients. It isn't known if vitamin K is excreted in breast milk. Use with caution in breast-feeding women.

Patient counseling

- Explain rationale for drug therapy; stress importance of complying with medical regimen and keeping follow-up appointments.

■ Instruct patient to take a missed dose as soon as possible, but not if it's almost time for next dose, and to report missed doses.

warfarin sodium

Coumadin, Panwarfin

Pharmacologic classification: coumarin derivative
Therapeutic classification: anticoagulant
Pregnancy risk category X

How supplied

Available by prescription only
Tablets: 1 mg, 2 mg, 2.5 mg, 3 mg, 4 mg, 5 mg, 6 mg, 7.5 mg, 10 mg
Injection: 5 mg/vial

Indications and dosages

Pulmonary emboli, deep vein thrombosis, MI, rheumatic heart disease with heart valve damage, atrial arrhythmias
Adults: Initially, 2 to 5 mg P.O. or I.V.; then daily. PT and INR are used to establish optimal dose. Usual maintenance dosage, 2 to 10 mg P.O. daily.

Pharmacodynamics

Anticoagulant action: Warfarin inhibits vitamin K-dependent activation of clotting factors II, VII, IX, and X, which are formed in the liver; it has no direct effect on established thrombi and can't reverse ischemic tissue damage. However, warfarin may prevent additional clot formation, extension of formed clots, and secondary complications of thrombosis.

Pharmacokinetics

Absorption: Rapidly and completely absorbed from GI tract.
Distribution: Highly bound to plasma protein, especially albumin; it crosses placenta but doesn't appear to accumulate in breast milk.
Metabolism: Warfarin is hydroxylated by liver into inactive metabolites.
Excretion: Metabolites are reabsorbed from bile and excreted in urine. Half-life of parent drug is 1 to 3 days, but is highly variable. Because therapeutic effect is relatively more dependent on clotting factor depletion (factor X has half-life of 40 hours).

Route	Onset	Peak	Duration
P.O.	½-3 days	Unknown	2-5 days
I.V.	Unknown	Unknown	Unknown

Contraindications and precautions

Contraindicated in pregnant women; in patients with bleeding or hemorrhagic tendencies, GI ulcerations, severe hepatic or renal disease, severe uncontrolled hypertension, subacute bacterial endocarditis, aneurysm, ascorbic acid deficiency, history of warfarin-induced necrosis, threatened abortion, eclampsia, preeclampsia, regional or lumbar block anesthesia, polycythemia vera, and vitamin K deficiency; in those in whom diagnostic tests or therapeutic procedures have potential for uncontrolled bleeding; in unsupervised patients with senility, alcoholism, psychosis, or lack of cooperation; and after recent eye, brain, or spinal cord surgery.

Use cautiously in patients with diverticulitis, colitis, hypertension, hepatic or renal disease, drainage tubes in any orifice, infectious disease or disturbance of intestinal flora, trauma, surgery resulting in large exposed surface, indwelling catheters, known or suspected deficiency in protein C or S, heart failure, severe diabetes, vasculitis, polycythemia vera, concurrent use of NSAIDs, or risk of hemorrhage and during lactation.

Interactions

Drug-drug. *Acetaminophen:* May increase bleeding with use of acetaminophen longer than 2 weeks and doses higher than 2 g/day. Monitor patient closely.
Allopurinol, amiodarone, anabolic steroids, cephalosporins, chloramphenicol, cimetidine, ciprofloxacin, clofibrate, danazol, diazoxide, diflunisal, disulfiram, erythromycin, glucagon, heparin, ibuprofen, influenza virus vaccine, isoniazid, itraconazole, ketoprofen, lovastatin, metronidazole, methimazole, miconazole, neomycin (oral), norfloxacin, ofloxacin, omeprazole, pentoxifylline, propafenone, propoxyphene, propylthiouracil, quinidine, salicylates, simvastatin, streptokinase, sulfinpyrazone, sulfonamides, sulindac, tamoxifen, tetracyclines, thiazides, thyroid drugs, tricyclic antidepressants, urokinase, vitamin E: Increase PT. Monitor patient closely for bleeding. Dose reduction of warfarin may be necessary.
Anticonvulsants: Increased serum levels of phenytoin and phenobarbital. Monitor patient closely.
Barbiturates: May inhibit anticoagulant effect for several weeks after barbiturate withdrawal, and fatal hemorrhage can occur after cessation of barbiturate effect. Monitor patient closely. If barbiturates are withdrawn, reduce anticoagulant dose.
Carbamazepine, corticosteroids, ethchlorvynol, glutethimide, griseofulvin, oral contraceptives, rifampin, vitamin K: Decreased anticoagulant effect. Avoid use together.
Chloral hydrate: May increase or decrease anticoagulant effect of warfarin. Avoid use together.
Ethacrynic acid, indomethacin, mefenamic acid, phenylbutazone, sulfinpyrazone: Increase anticoagulant effect of warfarin and cause severe GI irritation (may be ulcerogenic). Avoid use together.

Cholestyramine: Decreases anticoagulant effect of warfarin when used together. Administer 6 hours after warfarin.
Drug-herb. *Angelica sinensis:* May significantly prolong PT. Avoid use together.
Motherwort and red clover: Increase the risk for bleeding. Avoid use together.
Drug-food. *Foods or enteral products containing vitamin K:* May impair anticoagulation. Advise patient to maintain a consistent daily intake of leafy green vegetables.
Drug-lifestyle. *Alcohol use*: Enhanced anticoagulant effects may occur. Advise patient to avoid alcohol use.

Effects on diagnostic tests
Warfarin causes false-negative serum theophylline levels.

Adverse reactions
GI: anorexia, nausea, vomiting, cramps, *diarrhea,* mouth ulcerations, sore mouth.
GU: hematuria.
Hematologic: prolongs both PT and INR and partial thromboplastin time, ***hemorrhage*** (with excessive dosage).
Hepatic: hepatitis, elevated liver function tests, jaundice.
Skin: dermatitis, urticaria, necrosis, gangrene, alopecia, *rash.*
Other: *fever,* enhanced uric acid excretion.

Overdose and treatment
Signs and symptoms of overdose vary with severity and may include internal or external bleeding or skin necrosis of fat-rich areas, but most common sign is hematuria. Excessive prolongation of PT and INR or minor bleeding mandates withdrawal of therapy; withholding one or two doses may be adequate in some cases.

Treatment to control bleeding may include oral or I.V. phytonadione (vitamin K_1) and, in severe hemorrhage, fresh frozen plasma or whole blood. Use of phytonadione may interfere with subsequent oral anticoagulant therapy.

Clinical considerations
- Store drug in light-resistant containers at controlled room temperature (59° to 86° F [15° to 30° C]).
- After reconstitution, warfarin injection is stable for 4 hours at controlled room temperature.
- I.V. warfarin provides an alternative for patients who can't tolerate or receive oral medication.
- PT and INR are used to determine optimal dose.

Therapeutic monitoring
- Monitor PT and INR closely.
- Monitor for signs of bleeding.

Special populations
Pregnant patients. Drug use is contraindicated during pregnancy.
Breast-feeding patients. Although drug doesn't appear to accumulate in breast milk, use with caution in breast-feeding women.
Pediatric patients. Infants, especially neonates, may be more susceptible to anticoagulants because of vitamin K deficiency. Safety and efficacy haven't been established in children under age 18.
Geriatric patients. Geriatric patients are more susceptible to effects of anticoagulants and are at increased risk of hemorrhage; this may be caused by altered hemostatic mechanisms or age-related deterioration of hepatic and renal functions.

Patient counseling
- Tell patient to promptly report any unusual bruising or bleeding.
- Warn patient to avoid taking OTC products containing aspirin, other salicylates, or drugs that may interact with the anticoagulant, causing an increase or decrease in action of drug, and to seek medical approval before stopping or starting medication.
- Advise patient not to substantially alter daily intake of leafy green vegetables, such as asparagus, broccoli, cabbage, lettuce, turnip greens, spinach, or watercress, or of fish, pork or beef liver, green tea, or tomatoes. These foods contain vitamin K and widely varying daily intake may alter anticoagulant effect of warfarin.
- Instruct patient to inform all health care providers (including dentists) about use of warfarin.

XYZ

xylometazoline hydrochloride

Otrivin, Otrivin Pediatric Nasal Drops

Pharmacologic classification: sympathomimetic
Therapeutic classification: decongestant, vasoconstrictor
Pregnancy risk category C

How supplied

Available without a prescription
Nasal drops: 0.05%, 0.1% (pediatric use)
Nasal spray: 0.1%

Indications and dosages

Nasal congestion

Adults and children over age 12: Apply 2 or 3 drops or sprays of 0.1% solution to nasal mucosa q 8 to 10 hours, not to exceed three times in 24 hours.
Infants and children age 6 months to 12 years: Apply 2 or 3 drops of 0.05% solution to nasal mucosa q 8 to 10 hours, not to exceed three times in 24 hours.
Infants under age 6 months: 1 drop of 0.05% solution in each nostril q 6 hours, p.r.n., under medical direction.

Pharmacodynamics

Decongestant action: Acts on alpha-adrenergic receptors in nasal mucosa to produce constriction, decreasing blood flow and nasal congestion.

Pharmacokinetics

None reported.

Route	Onset	Peak	Duration
Nasal	5-10 min	Unknown	5-6 hr

Contraindications and precautions

Contraindicated in patients with hypersensitivity to drug or acute-closure glaucoma. Use cautiously in patients with hyperthyroidism, cardiac disease, hypertension, diabetes mellitus, and advanced arteriosclerosis.

Interactions

Drug-drug. *Tricyclic antidepressants, xylometazoline:* May potentiate the pressor effects of tricyclic antidepressants if significant systemic absorption occurs. Monitor patient closely.

Effects on diagnostic tests

None reported.

Adverse reactions

EENT: transient burning, stinging; dryness or ulceration of nasal mucosa; sneezing; rebound nasal congestion, irritation (with excessive or long-term use).

Overdose and treatment

Signs and symptoms of overdose include somnolence, sedation, sweating, CNS depression with hypertension, bradycardia, decreased cardiac output, rebound hypotension, CV collapse, depressed respirations, coma.

Because of rapid onset of sedation, emesis isn't recommended in therapy unless given early. Activated charcoal or gastric lavage may be used initially. Monitor vital signs and ECG. Treat seizures with I.V. diazepam.

Clinical considerations

Systemic absorption is less likely and drug is more effective if 3 to 5 minutes elapse between sprays and nose is cleared before next spray.

Therapeutic monitoring

Monitor carefully for adverse effects in patients with CV disease, diabetes mellitus, or hyperthyroidism.

Special populations

Pediatric patients. Children may be prone to greater systemic absorption, with resultant increase in adverse effects.
Geriatric patients. Use with caution in geriatric patients with cardiac disease, diabetes mellitus, or poorly controlled hypertension.

Patient counseling

- Inform patient that drug should only be used for short-term relief of symptoms (3 to 5 days maximum).
- Instruct patient on correct method of administration.
- Caution patient not to exceed recommended dose to avoid rebound congestion.
- Instruct patient to promptly report insomnia, dizziness, weakness, tremor, or irregular heartbeat.

zafirlukast

Accolate

Pharmacologic classification: leukotriene receptor antagonist
Therapeutic classification: antiasthmatic
Pregnancy risk category B

How supplied

Available by prescription only
Tablets: 10 mg, 20 mg

Indications and dosages

Prophylaxis and chronic treatment of asthma
Adults and children age 12 and older: 20 mg P.O. b.i.d. taken 1 hour before or 2 hours after meals.
Children age 7 to 11: 10 mg P.O. b.i.d., 1 hour before or 2 hours after meals.
◊ ***Prophylaxis for seasonal allergic rhinitis***
Adults: 20 to 40 mg P.O. single dose before environmental exposure.

Pharmacodynamics

Antiasthma action: Selectively competes for leukotriene receptor (LTD_4 and LTE_4) sites, blocking inflammatory action.

Pharmacokinetics

Absorption: Rapidly absorbed.
Distribution: Over 99% is protein-bound to plasma proteins, predominantly albumin.
Metabolism: Extensively metabolized via cytochrome P-450 2C9 (CYP 2C9) system. Also inhibits CYP 3A4 and CYP 2C9 isoenzymes.
Excretion: Primarily excreted in feces. Mean terminal half-life is about 10 hours.

Route	Onset	Peak	Duration
P.O.	Rapid	3 hr	Unknown

Contraindications and precautions

Contraindicated in patients with known hypersensitivity to drug or its components. Use cautiously in patients with hepatic impairment and in the elderly.

Interactions

Drug-drug. *Aspirin:* Increased plasma levels of zafirlukast. Monitor patient closely.
Erythromycin, theophylline: Decreased plasma levels of zafirlukast. Monitor patient closely.
Warfarin: Increased PT and INR. Monitor PT and INR; dose adjustment may be necessary.

Effects on diagnostic tests

None reported.

Adverse reactions

CNS: asthenia, dizziness, *headache.*
GI: abdominal pain, diarrhea, dyspepsia, nausea, vomiting.
Hepatic: elevated liver enzymes.
Musculoskeletal: back pain, myalgia.
Other: accidental injury, fever, infection, pain.

Overdose and treatment

There is no experience with zafirlukast overdose. If an overdose occurs, treat patient symptomatically and provide supportive measures, as required. If indicated, remove unabsorbed drug from GI tract.

Clinical considerations

- Drug isn't indicated for the reversal of bronchospasm in acute asthma attacks.
- Food reduces bioavailability; drug should be taken on an empty stomach.

Therapeutic monitoring

Monitor for adverse reactions.

Special populations

Pregnant patients. Use during pregnancy only if clearly indicated.
Breast-feeding patients. Drug is excreted in breast milk and shouldn't be used by breast-feeding women because of potential risk to infant.
Pediatric patients. Safety and efficacy in children under age 7 haven't been established.
Geriatric patients. Drug clearance is reduced in the elderly; use with caution.

Patient counseling

- Instruct patient to continue taking drug as prescribed even if symptoms resolve.
- Advise patient to continue taking other antiasthma drugs as prescribed.
- Instruct patient to take drug 1 hour before or 2 hours after meals.

zalcitabine (dideoxycytidine, ddC)

Hivid

Pharmacologic classification: nucleoside analogue
Therapeutic classification: antiviral
Pregnancy risk category C

How supplied

Available by prescription only
Tablets (film-coated): 0.375 mg, 0.75 mg

Indications and dosages

Patients with advanced HIV infection (CD4 count less than 300 cells/mm³) who have demonstrated significant clinical or immunologic deterioration
Adults weighing 66 lb (30 kg) or more: 0.75 mg P.O. q 8 hours. Can be taken with zidovudine (200 mg P.O. q 8 hours).

≡*Dosage adjustment.* Dosage adjustment may be necessary in patients with impaired renal function (creatinine clearance less than 55 ml/minute). In adults with renal failure, refer to following dosing chart.

Creatinine clearance (ml/min)	Adult dosage
> 40	0.75 mg P.O. q 8 hours
10 to 40	0.75 mg P.O. q 12 hours
< 10	0.75 mg P.O. q 24 hours

Pharmacodynamics

Antiviral action: Zalcitabine is active against HIV. Within cells, it's converted by cellular enzymes into its active metabolite, dideoxycytidine 5′-triphosphate. It inhibits the replication of HIV by blocking viral DNA synthesis. The drug inhibits reverse transcriptase by acting as an alternative for the enzyme's substrate, deoxycytidine triphosphate.

Pharmacokinetics

Absorption: Well absorbed, however, absorption has considerable interindividual variation. Average oral bioavailability is 70% to 88%.
Distribution: Steady-state volume of distribution is 0.534 ± 0.127 L/kg. Drug enters the CNS.
Metabolism: Doesn't appear to undergo significant hepatic metabolism; phosphorylation to the active form occurs within cells.
Excretion: Primarily excreted by the kidneys; about 70% of a dose appears in urine within 24 hours. Mean elimination half-life is 2 hours.

Route	Onset	Peak	Duration
P.O.	Unknown	½-2 hr	Unknown

Contraindications and precautions

Contraindicated in patients with hypersensitivity to drug or any component of the formulation. Use cautiously in patients with preexisting peripheral neuropathy, impaired renal function, hepatic failure, and history of pancreatitis, heart failure, or cardiomyopathy.

Interactions

Drug-drug. *Aminoglycosides, amphotericin, foscarnet:* Increased risk of nephrotoxicity. Monitor renal function closely. Avoid use together when possible.
Chloramphenicol, cisplatin, dapsone, didanosine, disulfiram, ethionamide, glutethimide, gold salts, hydralazine, iodoquinol, isoniazid, metronidazole, nitrofurantoin, phenytoin, ribavirin, vincristine: Increased risk of peripheral neuropathy. Monitor closely and avoid use together when possible.
Cimetidine, probenecid: Increased serum zalcitabine level. Monitor closely.
Pentamidine: Increased risk of pancreatitis. Avoid use together.

Effects on diagnostic tests

None reported.

Adverse reactions

CNS: *peripheral neuropathy, headache, fatigue,* dizziness, confusion, ***seizures,*** impaired concentration, amnesia, insomnia, mental depression, tremor, hypertonia, anxiety.
CV: cardiomyopathy, ***heart failure,*** chest pain.
EENT: pharyngitis, cough, ocular pain, abnormal vision, ototoxicity, nasal discharge.
GI: nausea, vomiting, diarrhea, abdominal pain, anorexia, constipation, stomatitis, esophageal ulcer, glossitis, *pancreatitis.*
Hematologic: anemia, ***neutropenia, leukopenia, thrombocytoenia.***
Hepatic: AST, ALT and alkaline phosphatase levels elevated.
Skin: pruritus, night sweats, *erythematous, maculopapular, or follicular rash,* urticaria.
Other: myalgia, arthralgia, fever, hypoglycemia.

Overdose and treatment

Inadvertent overdose in children has been treated with gastric lavage and activated charcoal, without sequelae. Acute overdose associated with high doses hasn't been reported; sequelae are unknown. Treat by emptying stomach (gastric lavage or induced emesis) and providing supportive and symptomatic treatment. There's no known antidote; it isn't known whether drug is removed by hemodialysis or peritoneal dialysis.

Clinical considerations

☐ ***ALERT*** Don't confuse this drug with other antivirals that may use initials for identification.
- The main dose-limiting toxicity is peripheral neuropathy, initially characterized by numbness and burning in the extremities. If drug isn't withdrawn, symptoms can progress to sharp, shooting pain or severe, continuous burning pain requiring narcotic analgesics and may or may not be reversible.
- Discontinue drug if symptoms indicating peripheral neuropathy are bilateral and persist beyond 72 hours. When symptoms subside, drug may be reintroduced at 0.375 mg P.O. every 8 hours. If symptoms worsen or persist beyond 1 week, permanently withdraw drug.
- If drug is discontinued because of toxicity, resume recommended dose for zidovudine alone, which is 100 mg every 4 hours.

Therapeutic monitoring

- Monitor closely for signs of toxicity, CNS and cardiovascular symptoms.
- Complete blood count should be performed before drug therapy and periodically thereafter.

Special populations

Pregnant patients. Use drug in pregnancy only when potential benefits justify possible risks to fetus.
Breast-feeding patients. It isn't known if drug is excreted in breast milk. Because of risk of transmitting the virus, HIV-positive women shouldn't breast-feed.
Pediatric patients. Safety and efficacy in children under age 13 haven't been established. Drug has been used in children 6 months to 13 years of age (0.015-0.04 mg/kg every 6 hours) with adverse reactions similar to those reported for adults.

Patient counseling

- Inform patient that drug doesn't cure HIV infection and that HIV can still be transmitted.
- Instruct patient to promptly report symptoms of peripheral neuropathy and pancreatitis.

zaleplon

Sonata

Pharmacologic classification: pyrazolopyrimidine
Therapeutic classification: hypnotic
Controlled substance schedule IV
Pregnancy risk category C

How supplied

Available by prescription only
Capsules: 5 mg, 10 mg

Indications and dosages

Short-term treatment for insomnia
Adults: 10 mg P.O. daily immediately before bedtime; may increase dose to 20 mg if needed. Low-weight adults may respond to 5-mg dose.
Elderly: Initially, 5 mg P.O. daily immediately before bedtime; doses over 10 mg aren't recommended.
≡ ***Dosage adjustment.*** For debilitated patients: Initially, 5 mg P.O. daily immediately before bedtime; doses over 10 mg aren't recommended.
≡ ***Dosage adjustment.*** For patients with mild to moderate hepatic failure or those also receiving cimetidine: 5 mg P.O. daily immediately before bedtime.

Pharmacodynamics

Hypnotic action: Although zaleplon is a hypnotic with a chemical structure unrelated to benzodiazepines, it interacts with the gamma-aminobutyric acid-BZ receptor complex in the CNS. Modulation of this complex is hypothesized to be responsible for sedative, anxiolytic, muscle relaxant, and anticonvulsant effects of benzodiazepines.

Pharmacokinetics

Absorption: Rapidly and almost completely absorbed.
Distribution: Distributed substantially into extravascular tissues. Plasma protein-binding is about 60%.
Metabolism: Extensively metabolized, primarily by aldehyde oxidase and, to a lesser extent, CYP3A4 to inactive metabolites. Less than 1% of dose is excreted unchanged in urine.
Excretion: Rapidly excreted, with a mean half-life of about 1 hour.

Route	Onset	Peak	Duration
P.O.	Rapid	1-2 hr	Unknown

Contraindications and precautions

Don't use in patients with severe hepatic impairment. Use cautiously in geriatric and debilitated patients, in those with compromised respiratory function, and in those with signs and symptoms of depression.

Interactions

Drug-drug. *Carbamazepine, phenobarbital, phenytoin, rifampin, other CYP3A4:* May reduce bioavailability and peak levels of zaleplon by about 80%. Consider an alternative hypnotic.
CNS depressants, such as imipramine and thioridazine: May produce additive CNS effects. Use cautiously together.
Cimetidine: Increases zaleplon bioavailability and peak levels by 85%. For patient taking cimetidine, use initial zaleplon dose of 5 mg.
Drug-food. *High-fat foods, heavy meals:* Prolong absorption, delaying peak zaleplon levels by about 2 hours; sleep onset may be delayed. Drug shouldn't be given with meals.
Drug-lifestyle. *Alcohol use:* May increase CNS effects. Advise patient to avoid alcohol use.

Effects on diagnostic tests

None reported.

Adverse reactions

CNS: *headache,* amnesia, dizziness, somnolence, depression, hypertonia, nervousness, depersonalization, hallucinations, vertigo, difficulty concentrating, anxiety, paresthesia, hypoesthesia, tremor, asthenia, migraine, malaise.
CV: chest pain, peripheral edema.
EENT: abnormal vision, conjunctivitis, eye pain, ear pain, hyperacusis, epistaxis, parosmia.
GI: constipation, dry mouth, anorexia, dyspepsia, nausea, abdominal pain, colitis.
GU: dysmenorrhea.
Musculoskeletal: arthritis, myalgia, back pain.
Respiratory: bronchitis.

Skin: pruritus, rash, photosensitivity reaction.
Other: fever.

Overdose and treatment:

Signs and symptoms usually include exaggerated CNS depressant effects of drug, ranging from drowsiness to coma. Use immediate gastric lavage when appropriate and general supportive measures for symptomatic management.

Clinical considerations

- Limit hypnotics use to 7 to 10 days.
- Potential for drug abuse and dependence exists.
- Because zaleplon works rapidly, it should only be ingested immediately before bedtime or after patient has gone to bed and has experienced difficulty falling asleep.
- Adverse reactions are usually dose-related. Use the lowest effective dose.

Therapeutic monitoring

- Closely monitor patients with compromised respiratory function caused by preexisting illness.
- Closely monitor geriatric or debilitated patients.
- Reevaluate patient if hypnotics are to be taken for more than 2 to 3 weeks.

Special populations

Pregnant patients. Drug isn't recommended for use during pregnancy.
Breast-feeding patients. A small amount of drug is excreted in breast milk. Breast-feeding women shouldn't take this drug because its effects on infants aren't known.
Pediatric patients. Safety and efficacy in children haven't been established.
Geriatric patients. Geriatric patients appear to be more sensitive to the effects of hypnotics. Monitor patient closely.

Patient counseling

- Inform patient that dependence can occur, and that drug is recommended for short-term use only.
- Advise patient that insomnia may recur for a few nights after stopping drug, but should resolve on its own.
- Advise patient that zaleplon works rapidly and should only be taken when a 4-hour period of undisturbed sleep is possible.
- Advise patient to avoid alcohol while taking drug and to notify his doctor before taking any prescription or OTC drugs.
- Inform patient that a high fat or heavy meal may delay onset of drug action.
- Instruct patient to promptly report adverse events.

zanamivir

Relenza

Pharmacologic classification: neuraminidase inhibitor
Therapeutic classification: antiviral
Pregnancy risk category B

How supplied

Available by prescription only
Powder for inhalation: 5 mg per blister

Indications and dosages

Treatment of uncomplicated acute illness due to influenza virus in patients who have been symptomatic for no more than 2 days
Adults and adolescents age 12 and older: Two oral inhalations (one 5-mg blister per inhalation for a total dose of 10 mg) twice daily using the Diskhaler inhalation device for 5 days. Two doses should be taken on the 1st day of treatment as long as there's at least 2 hours between doses. Subsequent doses should be about 12 hours apart (in the morning and evening) at about the same time each day.

Pharmacodynamics

Antiviral action: Zanamivir most likely inhibits neuraminidase on the surface of the influenza virus, potentially altering virus particle aggregation and release. With the inhibition of neuraminidase, the virus can't escape from its host cell to attack others, inhibiting the process of viral proliferation.

Pharmacokinetics

Absorption: About 4% to 17% of orally inhaled drug is systemically absorbed.
Distribution: Limited (less than 10%) plasma protein binding.
Metabolism: Not metabolized and excreted by the kidneys as unchanged drug.
Excretion: Excreted unchanged in urine. Unabsorbed drug is excreted in feces. The serum half-life of zanamivir ranges from 2½ to 5 hours.

Route	Onset	Peak	Duration
Oral inhalation	Unknown	1-2 hr	< 24 hr

Contraindications and precautions

Contraindicated in patients with known hypersensitivity to zanamivir or its components. Use cautiously in patients with severe or decompensated chronic obstructive pulmonary disease, asthma, or other underlying respiratory disease.

Interactions

None reported.

Effects on diagnostic tests
None reported.

Adverse reactions
CNS: headache, dizziness.
EENT: nasal signs and symptoms; sinusitis; ear, nose, and throat infections.
GI: diarrhea, nausea, vomiting.
Respiratory: bronchitis, ***bronchospasm,*** cough.

Overdose and treatment
No reports of overdose from administration of zanamivir exist. Signs and symptoms of overdose include exaggeration of adverse reactions of drug.

Clinical considerations
- Patients with underlying respiratory disease should have a fast-acting bronchodilator available in case of wheezing while taking zanamivir. Patients scheduled to use an inhaled bronchodilator for asthma should use their bronchodilator before taking zanamivir.
- Safety and efficacy of zanamivir haven't been established for influenza prophylaxis.
- Use of zanamivir shouldn't affect the evaluation of patients for their annual influenza vaccination.

Therapeutic monitoring
Monitor patient for bronchospasm and decline in lung function. Discontinue drug if this occurs.

Special populations
Pregnant patients. Use drug during pregnancy only when the potential benefits justify possible risk to fetus.
Breast-feeding patients. It isn't known if drug is excreted in breast milk. Use cautiously in breast-feeding women.
Pediatric patients. Safety and efficacy of zanamivir in children under age 12 haven't been established.
Geriatric patients. No overall differences in safety and efficacy were observed in clinical trials involving the elderly and younger patients.

Patient counseling
- Advise patient that zanamivir hasn't been shown to reduce the risk of transmitting influenza virus to others.
- Advise patient with underlying respiratory disease who is scheduled to use an inhaled bronchodilator to do so before taking zanamivir. Tell patient to have a fast-acting bronchodilator available if wheezing occurs while taking zanamivir.
- Advise patient to always check inside the mouthpiece of the Diskhaler before each use to make sure it's free of foreign objects.
- Instruct patient on proper administration technique and demonstrate when possible.
- Advise patient to finish the entire 5-day course of treatment, even if symptoms improve before the fifth day.

zidovudine (AZT)
Retrovir

Pharmacologic classification: thymidine analogue
Therapeutic classification: antiviral
Pregnancy risk category C

How supplied
Available by prescription only
Capsules: 100 mg
Syrup: 50 mg/5 ml
Injection: 10 mg/ml

Indications and dosages
Symptomatic HIV, AIDS, or advanced AIDS-related complex
Adults and children over age 12: 200 mg P.O. q 8 hours or 300 mg P.O. q 12 hours (600 mg daily dose). Or I.V. infusion 1 mg/kg (at a constant rate over 1 hour) q 4 hours for total of 6 mg/kg/day.
Children age 3 months to 12 years: 180 mg/m^2 q 6 hours (720 mg/m^2/day). Don't exceed 200 mg q 6 hours.
Asymptomatic HIV infection (CD4 count less than 500/mm^3)
Adults and children over age 12: 100 mg P.O. q 4 hours while awake (for total of five doses or 500 mg daily). Alternatively, administer 1 mg/kg I.V. over 1 hour q 4 hours while awake (5 mg/kg daily).
Children age 3 months to 12 years: 180 mg/m^2 q 6 hours (720 mg/m^2 P.O. daily) in divided doses q 6 hours. Don't exceed 200 mg q 6 hours.
Maternal-fetal transmission of HIV
Adults: Maternal dosing: Give 100 mg P.O. q 4 hours while awake (for total of five doses daily) until onset of labor. During labor and delivery, administer 2 mg/kg I.V. over 1 hour followed by a continuous infusion of 1 mg/kg/hour until clamping of the umbilical cord. Infant dosing: 2 mg/kg P.O. q 6 hours starting 12 hours after birth and continuing until 6 weeks of age; alternatively, administer 1.5 mg/kg via I.V. infusion over 30 minutes q 6 hours.
≡***Dosage adjustment.*** Because drug is partially removed by dialysis, dosage adjustment may be required in affected patients. Dosage adjustment may also be warranted in patients with decreased liver function.

Pharmacodynamics
Antiviral action: Zidovudine is converted intracellularly to an active triphosphate compound that inhibits reverse transcriptase (an

enzyme essential for retroviral DNA synthesis), inhibiting viral replication. When used in vitro, drug inhibits certain other viruses and bacteria; however, this has undetermined clinical significance.

Pharmacokinetics

Absorption: Absorbed rapidly from GI tract. Average systemic bioavailability is 65% of dose; drug undergoes first-pass metabolism.
Distribution: Preliminary data reveal good CSF penetration. About 36% of dose is plasma protein-bound.
Metabolism: Metabolized rapidly to an inactive compound.
Excretion: Parent drug and metabolite are excreted by glomerular filtration and tubular secretion in the kidneys. Urine recovery of parent drug and metabolite is 14% and 74%, respectively. Elimination half-life of these compounds is 1 hour.

Route	Onset	Peak	Duration
P.O., I.V.	Unknown	½-1½ hr	Unknown

Contraindications and precautions

Contraindicated in patients with hypersensitivity to drug. Use cautiously in patients in advanced stages of HIV and in those with severe bone marrow suppression, renal insufficiency, or hepatomegaly, hepatitis, or other risk factors for hepatic disease.

Interactions

Drug-drug. *Acetaminophen, aspirin, indomethacin:* May impair hepatic metabolism of zidovudine. Monitor patient closely.
Acyclovir: Possible seizures, lethargy, and fatigue. Use together cautiously.
Amphotericin B, dapsone, flucytosine, ganciclovir, pentamidine: Increased risk of nephrotoxicity and bone marrow suppression. Monitor patient closely.
Fluconazole, methadone, valproic acid: Increased zidovudine concentration. Monitor for toxicity.
Ganciclovir, interferon-alpha: Increased risk of hematologic toxicity. Monitor patient closely.
Other cytotoxic drugs: Additive adverse effects on bone marrow. Avoid use together.
Probenecid: Impaired elimination of zidovudine. Monitor for toxicity.
Ribavirin: Antagonized antiviral activity of zidovudine against HIV. Avoid use together.

Effects on diagnostic tests

None reported.

Adverse reactions

CNS: *headache, seizures,* paresthesia, *malaise, asthenia,* insomnia, *dizziness,* somnolence.
GI: *nausea, anorexia, abdominal pain, vomiting,* constipation, *diarrhea,* dyspepsia.
Hematologic: ***severe bone marrow suppression (resulting in anemia), agranulocytosis, thrombocytopenia.***
Musculoskeletal: myalgia.
Skin: *rash.*
Other: diaphoresis, *fever,* taste perversion.

Overdose and treatment

None reported.

Clinical considerations

- Optimum duration of treatment, as well as dose for optimum effectiveness and minimum toxicity, isn't known.
- Drug doesn't cure HIV infection or AIDS but may reduce morbidity resulting from opportunistic infections.
- Significant anemia (hemoglobin less than 7.5 g/dl or reduction of less than 25% of baseline) or significant neutropenia (granulocyte count less than 750 cells/mm^3 or reduction of less than 50% from baseline) may require suspension of zidovudine therapy until occurrence of bone marrow recovery. With less severe anemia or neutropenia, a reduction in zidovudine dose may be adequate.

Therapeutic monitoring

- Monitor CBC and platelet count at least every 2 weeks.
- Monitor for adverse events.

Special populations

Pregnant patients. Drug is given antepartum and intrapartum.
Pediatric patients. Drug is given to children of all ages.

Patient counseling

- Inform patient that drug frequently causes low RBC count possibly requiring blood transfusions or epoetin alfa therapy during treatment.
- Stress importance of following prescribed dose schedule.
- Instruct patient to promptly report adverse drug effects.
- Inform patient that drug therapy doesn't reduce ability to transmit HIV infection.

zileuton

Zyflo Filmtab

Pharmacologic classification: 5-lipoxygenase inhibitor
Therapeutic classification: antiasthmatic
Pregnancy risk category C

How supplied

Available by prescription only
Tablets: 600 mg

Indications and dosages

Prophylaxis and chronic treatment of asthma

Adults and children age 12 and older: 600 mg P.O. q.i.d.

Pharmacodynamics

Antiasthmatic action: Inhibits enzyme responsible for the formation of leukotrienes, reducing inflammatory response.

Pharmacokinetics

Absorption: Rapidly absorbed with oral administration.
Distribution: Apparent volume of distribution is 1.2 L/kg. Drug is 93% bound to plasma proteins, primarily albumin.
Metabolism: Oxidatively metabolized by the cytochrome P-450 system. Several active and inactive metabolites of zileuton have been identified.
Excretion: Elimination is predominantly via metabolism with a mean terminal half-life of 2½ hours.

Route	Onset	Peak	Duration
P.O.	Rapid	2 hr	Unknown

Contraindications and precautions

Contraindicated in patients with known hypersensitivity to drug or its components and in those with active hepatic disease or transaminase elevations at least three times the normal upper limit. Use with caution in patients with hepatic impairment or history of heavy alcohol use.

Interactions

Drug-drug. *Propranolol and other beta blockers:* Increased beta-blocker effect. Monitor patient; beta-blocker dose may need to be reduced.
Theophylline: Decreased theophylline clearance; serum theophylline levels may double. Reduce theophylline dose and monitor serum levels.
Warfarin: Increased PT and INR. Monitor PT, INR; adjustment of anticoagulant dose may be necessary.

Effects on diagnostic tests

None reported.

Adverse reactions

CNS: malaise, asthenia, dizziness, *headache*, insomnia, nervousness, somnolence.
CV: chest pain.
EENT: conjunctivitis.
GI: abdominal pain, constipation, dyspepsia, flatulence, nausea.
GU: urinary tract infection, vaginitis.
Hematologic: ***leukopenia.***
Hepatic: elevated liver enzymes.
Musculoskeletal: arthralgia, hypertonia, myalgia, neck pain and rigidity.
Skin: pruritus.
Other: accidental injury, fever, lymphadenopathy, pain.

Overdose and treatment

Acute overdose with zileuton is limited. Drug isn't removed by dialysis. If overdose occurs, treat patient symptomatically and provide supportive measures. If indicated, eliminate unabsorbed drug by emesis or gastric lavage.

Clinical considerations

Drug isn't indicated for use in the reversal of bronchospasm in acute asthma attacks.

Therapeutic monitoring

Obtain liver enzyme levels at baseline and then once a month for the first 3 months, then every 2 to 3 months for the remainder of the first year and periodically thereafter.

Special populations

Breast-feeding patients. It isn't known if drug is excreted in breast milk. Use with caution in breast-feeding women.
Pediatric patients. Safety and efficacy in children under age 12 haven't been studied.

Patient counseling

- Caution patient that drug isn't a bronchodilator and shouldn't be used to treat an acute asthma attack.
- Advise patient to continue taking all other antiasthmatic drugs.
- Tell patient to promptly report adverse drug events.

zinc

Orazinc, Verazinc, Zinc 15, Zinc-220, Zincate

zinc sulfate (ophthalmic)

Eye-Sed

Pharmacologic classification: trace element, miscellaneous anti-infective
Therapeutic classification: nutritional supplement, topical anti-infective
Pregnancy risk category C

How supplied

Available by prescription only
Injection: 10 ml (1 mg/ml), 30 ml (1 mg/ml with 0.9% benzyl alcohol), 5 ml (5 mg/ml); 10 ml (5 mg/ml), 50 ml (1 mg/ml)
Capsules: 220 mg (50 mg zinc)
Available without a prescription, as appropriate
Tablets: 66 mg (15 mg zinc), 110 mg (25 mg zinc), 200 mg (47 mg zinc)

Capsules: 110 mg (25 mg zinc), 220 mg (50 mg zinc)
Solution: 15 ml (0.25%)

Indications and dosages

RDA of zinc is 15 mg/day P.O. for adults and 0.3 mg/kg/day P.O. for children.
Metabolically stable zinc deficiency
Adults: 2.5 to 4 mg/day I.V.; add 2 mg/day for acute catabolic states.
Stable zinc deficiency with fluid loss from the small bowel
Adults: Add 12.2 mg/L of total parenteral nutrition solution or 17.1 mg/kg of stool output.
Zinc deficiency
Children under age 5: 100 mcg/kg/day I.V.
Premature infants: 300 mcg/kg/day I.V.
Dietary supplementation
Adults: 25 to 50 mg P.O. daily.
For relief of minor eye irritation
Adults: 1 to 2 drops ophthalmic solution into the eye b.i.d. to q.i.d. Patients are advised to report irritation that persists for more than 3 days.

Pharmacodynamics

Metabolic action: Zinc serves as a cofactor for more than 70 different enzymes. It facilitates wound healing, normal growth rates, and normal skin hydration and helps maintain the senses of taste and smell.

Adequate zinc provides normal growth and tissue repair. In patients receiving total parenteral nutrition with low plasma levels of zinc, dermatitis has been followed by alopecia. Zinc is an integral part of many enzymes important to carbohydrate and protein mobilization of retinal-binding protein.

Zinc sulfate ophthalmic solution exhibits astringent and weak antiseptic activity, which may result from precipitation of protein by the zinc ion and by clearing mucous from the outer surface of the eye. Drug has no decongestant action and produces mild vasodilation.

Pharmacokinetics

Absorption: Absorbed poorly from GI tract; only 20% to 30% of dietary zinc is absorbed. After administration, zinc resides in muscle, bone, skin, kidney, liver, pancreas, retina, prostate, and, particularly, RBCs and WBCs. Zinc binds to plasma albumin, alpha-2 macroglobulin, and some plasma amino acids including histidine, cysteine, threonine, glycine, and asparagine.
Distribution: Major zinc stores are in the skeletal muscle, skin, bone, and pancreas.
Metabolism: Zinc is a cofactor in many enzymatic reactions. It's required for the synthesis and mobilization of retinal binding protein.
Excretion: After parenteral administration, 90% is excreted in stool, urine, and sweat. After oral use, the major route of excretion is secretion into the duodenum and jejunum. Small amounts are also excreted in urine (0.3 to 0.5 mg/day) and sweat (1.5 mg/day).

Route	Onset	Peak	Duration
P.O.	Unknown	Unknown	Unknown
I.V.	Immediate	Immediate	Unknown
Ophthalmic	Unknown	Unknown	Unknown

Contraindications and precautions

Parenteral use of zinc sulfate is contraindicated in patients with renal failure or biliary obstruction (and requires caution in all patients); monitor zinc plasma levels frequently. Don't exceed prescribed doses. In patients with renal dysfunction or GI malfunction, trace metal supplements may need to be reduced, adjusted, or omitted. Hypersensitivity may result. Routine use of zinc supplementation during pregnancy isn't recommended.

Administering copper in the absence of zinc or administering zinc in the absence of copper may result in decreased serum levels of either element. When only one trace element is needed, it should be added separately and serum levels monitored closely. To avoid overdose, administer multiple trace elements only when clearly needed. In patients with extreme vomiting or diarrhea, extreme amounts of trace element replacement may be needed. Excessive intake in healthy persons may be deleterious.

Interactions

Drug-drug. *Fluoroquinolones and tetracycline:* Impaired antibiotic absorption. Avoid use together.
Sodium borate (ophthalmic preparation): Precipitation of zinc borate may occur. Avoid use together; glycerin may prevent this interaction.
Methylcellulose suspensions (ophthalmic preparation): Precipitation of methylcellulose. Avoid use together.
Drug-food. *Dairy products:* May reduce zinc absorption. Advise patient to avoid dairy products during therapy.

Effects on diagnostic tests

None reported.

Adverse reactions

CNS: restlessness.
GI: distress and irritation, nausea, vomiting with high doses, gastric ulceration, diarrhea.
Skin: rash.
Other: dehydration.

Overdose and treatment

Signs and symptoms of severe toxicity include hypotension, pulmonary edema, diarrhea, vomiting, jaundice, and oliguria. Discontinue dose and begin support measures.

Clinical considerations

- Results may not appear for 6 to 8 weeks in zinc-depleted patients.
- Calcium supplements may confer a protective effect against zinc toxicity.
- Because of potential for infusion phlebitis and tissue irritation, an undiluted direct injection must not be administered into a peripheral vein.

Therapeutic monitoring

- Monitor for signs of toxicity.
- Monitor for eye irritation (ophthalmic solution).

Special populations

None reported.

Patient counseling

- Instruct patient on proper ophthalmic solution administration technique.
- Caution patient about self-medication with zinc sulfate ophthalmic solution, which shouldn't continue longer than 3 days.
- Warn patient that GI upset may occur after oral administration but may be diminished if zinc is taken with food.

zolmitriptan

Zomig

Pharmacologic classification: selective 5-hydroxytryptamine receptor agonist
Therapeutic classification: antimigraine
Pregnancy risk category C

How supplied

Available by prescription only
Tablets: 2.5 mg, 5 mg

Indications and dosages

Treatment of acute migraine headaches with or without aura

Adults: Initially, 2.5 mg P.O. or lower. A dose lower than 2.5 mg can be achieved by manually breaking a 2.5-mg tablet in half. If headache returns after initial dose, a second dose may be given after 2 hours. Maximum dose is 10 mg in 24-hour period.

≡ ***Dosage adjustment.*** In patients with liver disease, use doses less than 2.5 mg.

Pharmacodynamics

Antimigraine action: Zolmitriptan binds with high affinity to human recombinant 5-HT_{1D} and 5-HT_{1B} receptors, aborting migraine headaches by causing constriction of cranial blood vessels and inhibition of pro-inflammatory neuropeptide release.

Pharmacokinetics

Absorption: Well absorbed after oral administration. Mean absolute bioavailability is about 40%.

Distribution: Apparent volume of distribution is 7 L/kg. Plasma protein binding is 25%.

Metabolism: Converted to an active *N*-desmethyl metabolite. Time to maximum concentration for the metabolite is 2 to 3 hours. Mean elimination half-life of zolmitriptan and the active *N*-desmethyl metabolite is 3 hours.

Excretion: Mean total clearance is 31.5 ml/minute/kg, of which one-sixth is renal clearance. The renal clearance is greater than the glomerular filtration rate, suggesting renal tubular secretion. About 65% of dose is excreted in urine and 30% in feces.

Route	Onset	Peak	Duration
P.O.	Unknown	2 hr	3 hr

Contraindications and precautions

Contraindicated in patients with hypersensitivity to drug or its components; in those with uncontrolled hypertension, ischemic heart disease (angina pectoris, history of MI or documented silent ischemia), or other significant heart disease (including Wolff-Parkinson-White syndrome).

Avoid use within 24 hours of other 5-HT_1 agonists, ergot-containing medications, or within 2 weeks of discontinuing MAO inhibitor therapy. Also avoid use in patients with hemiplegic or basilar migraine.

Use cautiously in patients with liver disease and in pregnant or breast-feeding women.

Interactions

Drug-drug. *Cimetidine:* Doubles the half-life of zolmitriptan. Monitor patient closely.
Ergot-containing drugs: Additive vasospastic reactions. Avoid use together.
Fluoxetine, fluvoxamine, paroxetine, sertraline: Weakness, hyperreflexia, and incoordination. Use together cautiously.
MAO inhibitors, oral contraceptives: Increased plasma levels of zolmitriptan. Avoid use together.

Effects on diagnostic tests

None reported.

Adverse reactions

CNS: somnolence, vertigo, *dizziness,* hyperesthesias, paresthesia, asthenia.
CV: ***arrhythmias,*** hypotension, palpitations, pain or heaviness in chest, *pain, tightness, or pressure in the neck, throat, or jaw.*
GI: dry mouth, dyspepsia, dysphagia, nausea.
Musculoskeletal: myalgia.
Skin: sweating.
Other: warm or cold sensations.

Overdose and treatment
No specific antidote exists. If severe intoxication occurs, intensive care procedures are recommended including establishing and maintaining a patent airway ensuring adequate oxygenation and ventilation, and monitoring and support of the CV system. The effect of hemodialysis or peritoneal dialysis on the plasma levels of zolmitriptan is unknown.

Clinical considerations
- Drug isn't intended for prophylactic therapy of migraine headaches or for use in hemiplegic or basilar migraines.
- Safety hasn't been established for cluster headaches.
- Although not reported in clinical trials, serious cardiac events, including some that have been fatal, have occurred rarely following use of 5-HT_1 agonists. Events reported have included coronary artery vasospasm, transient myocardial ischemia, MI, ventricular tachycardia, and ventricular fibrillation.

Therapeutic monitoring
Monitor blood pressure in patients with liver disease.

Special populations
Pregnant patients. Use cautiously during pregnancy.
Breast-feeding patients. It isn't known if drug is excreted in breast milk. Use caution when administering to breast-feeding women.
Pediatric patients. Safety and efficacy in children haven't been established.
Geriatric patients. Although the pharmacokinetic disposition is similar to that seen in younger adults, there's no information in this population because patients over age 65 were excluded from clinical trials.

Patient counseling
- Advise patient to take drug only as prescribed.
- Advise patient to report pain or tightness in the chest or throat, heart throbbing, rash, skin lumps, or swelling of the face, lips, or eyelids at once.
- Caution patient not to take drug with other migraine agents.

zolpidem tartrate
Ambien

Pharmacologic classification: imidazopyridine
Therapeutic classification: hypnotic
Controlled substance schedule IV
Pregnancy risk category B

How supplied
Available by prescription only
Tablets: 5 mg, 10 mg

Indications and dosages
Short-term management of insomnia
Adults: 10 mg P.O. immediately before bedtime.
≡***Dosage adjustment.*** In geriatric or debilitated patients or patients with hepatic insufficiency, 5 mg P.O. immediately before bedtime. Maximum daily dose, 10 mg.

Pharmacodynamics
Hypnotic action: While zolpidem is a hypnotic agent with a chemical structure unrelated to benzodiazepines, barbiturates, or other drugs with known hypnotic properties, it interacts with a gamma-aminobutyric acid (GABA)-benzodiazepine or omega-receptor complex and shares some of the pharmacologic properties of the benzodiazepines. It exhibits no muscle relaxant or anticonvulsant properties.

Pharmacokinetics
Absorption: Absorbed rapidly from GI tract. Food delays drug absorption.
Distribution: Protein-binding is about 92.5%.
Metabolism: Converted to inactive metabolites in the liver.
Excretion: Primarily eliminated in urine; elimination half-life is about 2½ hours.

Route	Onset	Peak	Duration
P.O.	Rapid	½-2 hr	Unknown

Contraindications and precautions
No known contraindications. Use cautiously in patients with conditions that could affect metabolism or hemodynamic response and in those with decreased respiratory drive, depression, or history of alcohol or drug abuse.

Interactions
Drug-drug. *Other CNS depressants:* Enhanced CNS depression. Don't use together.
Drug-lifestyle. *Alcohol use:* May cause excessive CNS depression. Advise patient to avoid alcohol use.

Effects on diagnostic tests
None reported.

Adverse reactions
CNS: daytime drowsiness, light-headedness, abnormal dreams, amnesia, dizziness, *headache,* hangover, sleep disorder, lethargy, depression.
CV: palpitations, chest pain.
EENT: sinusitis, pharyngitis, dry mouth.
GI: nausea, vomiting, diarrhea, dyspepsia, constipation, abdominal pain.
Musculoskeletal: back pain, myalgia, arthralgia.
Skin: rash.
Other: flulike symptoms, ***hypersensitivity reactions.***

Overdose and treatment

Symptoms may range from somnolence to light coma. CV and respiratory compromise also may occur. Use general symptomatic and supportive measures, along with immediate gastric lavage when appropriate. Administer I.V. fluids as needed. Flumazenil may be useful. Monitor and treat hypotension and CNS depression. Withhold sedatives after zolpidem overdose even if excitation occurs.

Clinical considerations

- Be aware of potential for hoarding or self-overdosing by hospitalized patients who are depressed, suicidal, or known to abuse drugs.
- Limit drug therapy to 7 to 10 days; reevaluate patient if drug is to be taken for more than 2 weeks.
- Zolpidem has CNS-depressant effects similar to other sedative-hypnotic drugs. Because of its rapid onset of action, drug should be taken immediately before going to bed.
- Dose adjustments may be necessary when drug is given with other CNS-depressant agents because of the potentially additive effects.

Therapeutic monitoring

Observe patients with history of addiction to or abuse of drugs or alcohol because they're at risk of habituation and dependence.

Special populations

Breast-feeding patients. Use of drug in breast-feeding women isn't recommended.
Pediatric patients. Safety and efficacy in children under age 18 haven't been established.
Geriatric patients. Impaired motor or cognitive performance after repeated exposure or unusual sensitivity to sedative-hypnotics may occur in geriatric patients. Recommended dose is 5 mg rather than 10 mg.

Patient counseling

- Stress importance of taking drug only as prescribed; inform patient of potential drug dependency associated with hypnotics taken for long periods.
- Inform patient that tolerance may occur if drug is taken for more than a few weeks.
- Warn patient against use of alcohol or other sleep medications during therapy to avoid serious adverse effects.
- Caution patient to avoid activities that require alertness, such as driving a car, until adverse CNS effects of drug are known.

Subcutaneous, intramuscular, and intravenous injection techniques

Subcutaneous administration

S.C. injection allows slower, more sustained drug administration than I.M. injection. Drugs and solutions for S.C. injections are injected through a relatively short needle, using meticulous sterile technique.

Equipment and preparation

Gather the patient's medication record and chart, gloves, prescribed drug, needle of appropriate gauge and length, gloves, 1- to 3-ml syringe, and alcohol sponges. Other materials may include an antiseptic cleaning agent, filter needle, insulin syringe, and insulin pump.

Inspect the drug to make sure its appearance is within normal limits. Wash your hands. Select a needle of the proper gauge and length. An average adult patient requires a 25G ⅝" needle; an infant, child, or elderly or thin patient usually requires a 25G to 27G ⅛" needle.

For single-dose ampules

Wrap the neck of the ampule in an alcohol sponge and snap off the top. If desired, attach a filter needle to the needle and withdraw the drug. Tap the syringe to clear air from it. Cover the needle with the needle sheath. Before discarding the ampule, check the label against the patient's medication record. Discard the filter needle and the ampule. Attach the appropriate needle to the syringe.

For single-dose or multidose vials

Reconstitute powdered drugs according to the instructions on the label. Clean the vial's rubber stopper with an alcohol sponge. Pull the syringe plunger back until the volume of air in the syringe equals the volume of drug to be withdrawn from the vial. Insert the needle into the vial. Inject the air, invert the vial, and keep the bevel tip of the needle below the level of the solution as you withdraw the prescribed amount of drug. Cover the needle with the needle sheath. Tap the syringe to clear any air from it. Check the drug label against the patient's medication record before returning the multidose vial to the shelf or drawer or before discarding the single-dose vial.

Implementation

- Select the injection site from those shown, and tell the patient where you'll be giving the injection.

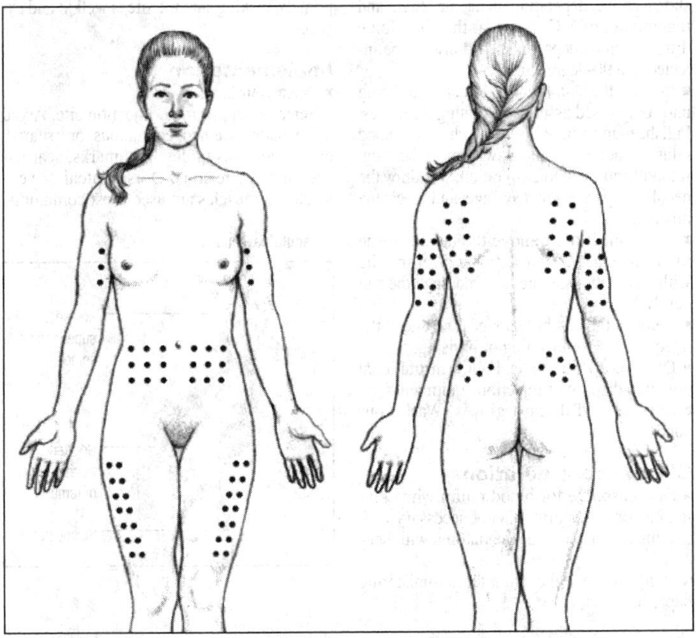

- Put on gloves. Position and drape the patient if necessary.
- Clean the injection site with an alcohol sponge. Loosen the protective needle sheath.
- With your nondominant hand, pinch the skin around the injection site firmly to elevate the S.C. tissue, forming a 1" (2.5 cm) fat fold, as shown.

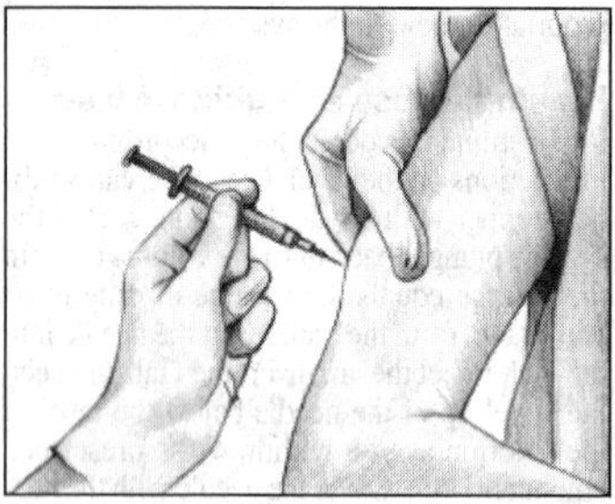

- Holding the syringe in your dominant hand (while pinching the skin around the injection site with the index finger and thumb of your nondominant hand), grip the needle sheath between the fourth and fifth fingers of your nondominant hand, and pull back to uncover the needle. Don't touch the needle.
- Position the needle with its bevel up.
- Tell the patient she'll feel a prick as the needle is inserted. Insert the needle quickly in one motion at a 45-degree or 90-degree angle, as shown above, depending on needle length and the amount of S.C. tissue at the site. Some drugs, such as heparin, should always be injected at a 90-degree angle.
- Release the skin to avoid injecting the drug into compressed tissue and irritating the nerves. Pull the plunger back slightly to check for blood return. If none appears, slowly inject the drug. If blood appears upon aspiration, withdraw the needle, prepare another syringe, and repeat the procedure.
- After injection, remove the needle at the same angle used for insertion. Cover the site with an alcohol sponge, and massage the site gently.
- Remove the alcohol sponge, and check the injection site for bleeding or bruising.
- Don't recap the needle. Follow institutional policy to dispose of injection equipment.
- Remove and discard gloves. Wash your hands.

Clinical considerations

- Don't aspirate for blood return when giving insulin or heparin. It's not necessary with insulin and may cause a hematoma with heparin.
- Don't massage the site after administering heparin.
- Repeated injections in the same site can cause lipodystrophy, a natural immune response. This complication can be minimized by rotating injection sites.

Intramuscular administration

I.M. injections deposit the drug deep into well-vascularized muscle for rapid systemic action and absorption of up to 5 ml.

Equipment and preparation

Gather the patient's medication record and chart, prescribed drug, diluent or filter needle (if needed), 3- to 5-ml syringe, 20G to 25G 1" to 3" needle, gloves, and alcohol sponges.

The prescribed drug must be sterile. The needle may be packaged separately or already attached to the syringe. Needles used for I.M. injections are longer than S.C. needles because they reach deep into the muscle. Needle length also depends on the injection site, the patient's size, and the amount of S.C. fat covering the muscle. A larger needle gauge accommodates viscous solutions and suspensions.

Check the drug for abnormal changes in color and clarity.

Wipe the vial stopper with alcohol, and draw up the prescribed amount of drug.

Provide privacy and explain the procedure to the patient. Position and drape him appropriately, making sure the site is well lit and exposed.

Implementation

- Wash your hands.
- Select an appropriate injection site. Avoid a site that's inflamed, edematous, or irritated, or that contains moles, birthmarks, scar tissue, or other lesions. Dorsogluteal or ventrogluteal muscles are used most commonly.

Dorsogluteal muscle

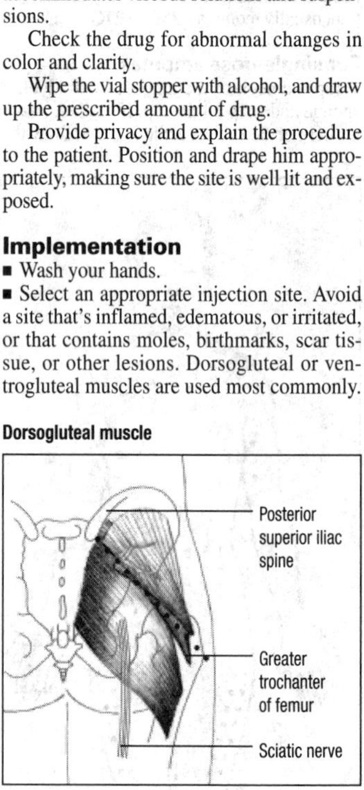

Ventrogluteal muscle

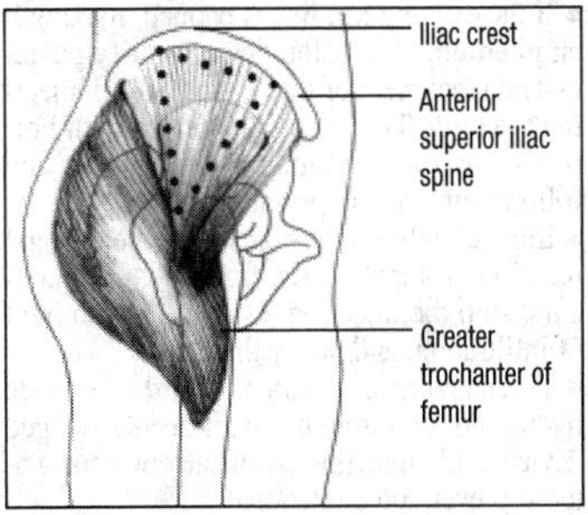

Deltoid muscle

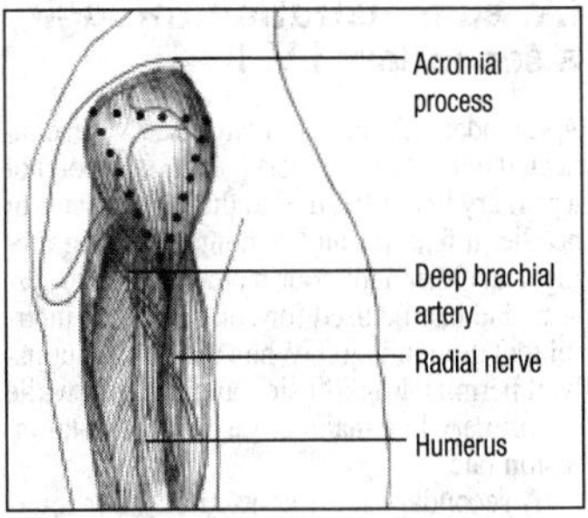

Vastus lateralis and rectus femoris muscles

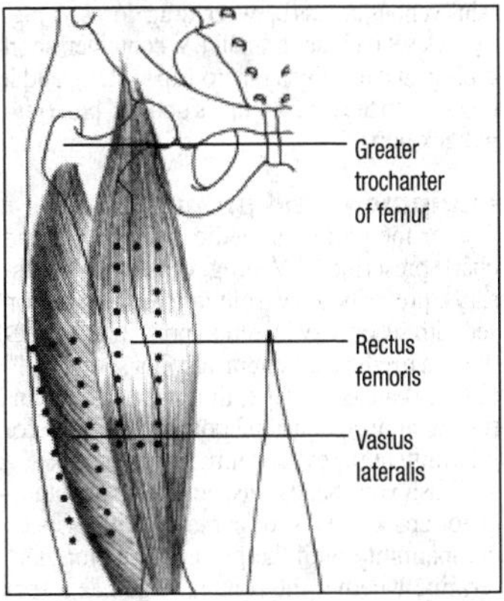

- The deltoid muscle may be used for injections of 2 ml or less, as shown.
- The vastus lateralis is used most often in children; the rectus femoris may be used in infants, as shown.
- Rotate injection sites for patients who require repeated injections.
- Position and drape the patient appropriately.
- Loosen, but don't remove, the needle sheath.
- Gently tap the site to stimulate nerve endings and minimize pain.
- Clean the site by moving an alcohol sponge in circles increasing in diameter to about 2" (5 cm). Allow the skin to dry; alcohol stings in the puncture.
- Put on gloves.
- With the thumb and index finger of your nondominant hand, gently stretch the skin.
- With the syringe in your dominant hand, remove the needle sheath with the free fingers of your other hand.
- Position the syringe perpendicular to the skin surface and a couple of inches from the skin. Tell the patient that he'll feel a prick. Then quickly and firmly thrust the needle into the muscle.
- Pull back slightly on the plunger to aspirate for blood. If none appears, inject the drug slowly and steadily to let the muscle distend gradually. You should feel little or no resistance. Gently but quickly remove the needle at a 90-degree angle.
- If blood appears, the needle is in a blood vessel. Withdraw it, prepare a fresh syringe, and inject another site.
- Using a gloved hand, apply gentle pressure to the site with an alcohol sponge. Massage the relaxed muscle, unless contraindicated, to distribute the drug and promote absorption.
- Inspect the site for bleeding or bruising. Apply pressure as necessary.
- Discard all equipment properly. Don't recap needles; put them in an appropriate biohazard container to avoid needle-stick injuries.
- Remove and discard gloves. Wash your hands.

Clinical considerations

- To slow absorption, some drugs are dissolved in oil. Mix them well before use.
- Never inject into the gluteal muscles of a child who has been walking for less than 1 year.
- If the patient must have repeated injections, consider numbing the area with ice before cleaning it. If you must inject more than 5 ml, divide the solution and inject it at two sites.
- Urge the patient to relax the muscle to reduce pain and bleeding.
- I.M. injections can damage local muscle cells and elevate serum enzyme levels (creatine kinase), which can be confused with elevated levels caused by MI. Diagnostic tests can be used to differentiate between them.

I.V. bolus administration

This method allows rapid I.V. drug administration to quickly achieve peak levels in the bloodstream. It may also be used for drugs that can't be given I.M. because they're toxic or the patient has reduced ability to absorb them, or to deliver drugs that can't be diluted.

Bolus doses may be injected directly into a vein or through an existing I.V. line.

Equipment and preparation
Gather the patient's medication record and chart, prescribed drug, 20G needle and syringe, diluent (if necessary), tourniquet, povidone-iodine sponge, alcohol sponge, sterile 2" × 2" gauze pad, gloves, adhesive bandage, and tape. Other materials may include a steel needle-winged device primed with normal saline solution and a second syringe (and needle) filled with normal saline solution.

Draw the drug into the syringe, and dilute it if necessary.

Implementation
To give a direct injection:
- Wash your hands and put on gloves.
- Select the largest vein suitable to dilute the drug and minimize irritation.
- Apply a tourniquet above the site to distend the vein, and clean the site with an alcohol or povidone-iodine sponge, working outward in a circle.
- If you're using the needle of the drug syringe, insert it at a 30-degree angle with the bevel up. The bevel should reach ¼" (0.6 cm) into the vein. Insert a steel needle-winged device bevel up, tape the wings in place when you see blood return, and attach the syringe containing the drug.
- Check for blood backflow.
- Remove the tourniquet, and inject the drug at the ordered rate.
- Check for blood backflow to ensure that the needle remained in place and all of the injected drug entered the vein.
- For a steel needle-winged device, flush the line with normal saline solution from the second syringe to ensure complete delivery.
- Withdraw the needle, and apply pressure to the site with a sterile gauze pad for at least 3 minutes to prevent hematoma.
- Apply an adhesive bandage when the bleeding stops.
- Remove and discard gloves. Wash your hands.

To give an injection through an existing I.V. line:
- Wash your hands and put on gloves.
- Check the compatibility of the drug.
- Close the flow clamp, wipe the injection port with an alcohol sponge, and inject the drug as you would a direct injection.
- Open the flow clamp and readjust the flow rate.
- Remove and discard gloves. Wash hands.
- If the drug isn't compatible with the I.V. solution, flush the line with normal saline solution before and after the injection.

Clinical considerations
- If the existing I.V. line is capped, making it an intermittent infusion device, verify patency and placement of the device before injecting the drug. Then flush the device with normal saline solution, administer the drug, and follow with the appropriate flush.
- Immediately report signs of acute allergic reaction or anaphylaxis. If extravasation occurs, stop the injection, estimate the amount of infiltration, and notify the doctor.
- When giving diazepam or chlordiazepoxide hydrochloride through a steel needle-winged device or I.V. line, flush with bacteriostatic water to prevent precipitation.

I.V. administration through a secondary I.V. line

A secondary I.V. line is a complete I.V. set connected to the lower Y-port (secondary port) of a primary line instead of to the I.V. catheter or needle. It features an I.V. container, long tubing, and either a microdrip or a macrodrip system, and can be used for continuous or intermittent drug infusion. When used continuously, it permits drug infusion and titration while the primary line maintains a constant total infusion rate.

A secondary I.V. line used only for intermittent drug administration is called a piggyback set. In this case, the primary line maintains venous access between drug doses. A piggyback set includes a small I.V. container, short tubing, and usually a macrodrip system, and it connects to the primary line's upper Y-port (piggyback port).

Equipment and preparation
Gather the patient's medication record and chart, prescribed I.V. drug, diluent (if necessary), prescribed I.V. solution, administration set with secondary injection port, 22G 1" needle or a needleless system, alcohol sponges, 1" (2.5 cm) adhesive tape, time tape, labels, infusion pump, extension hook, and solution for intermittent piggyback infusion.

Wash your hands. Inspect the I.V. container for cracks, leaks, or contamination. Check compatibility with the primary solution. Determine whether the primary line has a secondary injection port.

If necessary, add the drug to the secondary I.V. solution. To do so, remove any seals from the secondary container and wipe the main port with an alcohol sponge. Inject the prescribed drug and agitate the solution to mix the drug. Label the I.V. mixture. Insert the administration set spike, and attach the needle or needleless system. Open the flow clamp and prime the line. Then close the flow clamp.

Some drugs come in vials for hanging directly on an I.V. pole. In this case, inject diluent directly into the drug vial. Then spike the vial, prime the tubing, and hang the set.

Implementation

- If the drug is incompatible with the primary I.V. solution, replace the primary solution with a fluid that's compatible with both solutions, and flush the line before starting the drug infusion.
- Hang the container of the secondary set and wipe the injection port of the primary line with an alcohol sponge.
- Insert the needle or needleless system from the secondary line into the injection port, and tape it securely to the primary line.
- To run the container of the secondary set by itself, lower the primary set's container with an extension hook. To run both containers simultaneously, place them at the same height.
- Open the clamp and adjust the drip rate.
- For continuous infusion, set the secondary solution to the desired drip rate; then adjust the primary solution to the desired total infusion rate.
- For intermittent infusion, wait until the secondary solution is completely infused; then adjust the primary drip rate, as required.
- If the secondary solution tubing is being reused, close the clamp on the tubing and follow your institution's policy: Either remove the needle or needleless system and replace it with a new one, or leave it taped in the injection port and label it with the time it was first used.
- Leave the empty container in place until you replace it with a new drug dose at the prescribed time. If the tubing won't be reused, discard it appropriately with the I.V. container.

Clinical considerations

- If institutional policy allows, use a pump for drug infusion. Put a time tape on the secondary container to help prevent an inaccurate administration rate.
- When reusing secondary tubing, change it according to institutional policy, usually every 48 to 72 hours. Inspect the injection port for leakage with each use; change it more often if needed.
- Except for lipids, don't piggyback a secondary I.V. line to a total parenteral nutrition line because it risks contamination.

Therapeutic drug monitoring guidelines

Drug	Laboratory test monitored	Therapeutic ranges of test
aminoglycoside antibiotics (amikacin, gentamicin, tobramycin)	Serum amikacin peak trough Serum gentamicin/tobramycin peak trough Serum creatinine	20 to 25 mcg/ml 5 to 10 mcg/ml 4 to 8 mcg/ml 1 to 2 mcg/ml 0.6 to 1.3 mg/dl
amphotericin B	Serum creatinine BUN Serum electrolytes (especially potassium and magnesium) Liver function tests CBC with differential and platelets	0.6 to 1.3 mg/dl 7 to 18 mg/dl Potassium: 3.5 to 5 mEq/L Magnesium: 1.7 to 2.1 mEq/L Sodium: 135 to 145 mEq/L Chloride: 98 to 106 mEq/L * *****
antibiotics	WBC with differential Cultures and sensitivities	*****
biguanides (metformin)	Serum creatinine Fasting serum glucose Glycosylated hemoglobin CBC	0.6 to 1.3 mg/dl 65 to 110 mg/dl 5.5 to 8.5% of total hemoglobin *****
clozapine	WBC with differential	*****
digoxin	Serum digoxin Serum electrolytes (especially potassium, magnesium, and calcium) Serum creatinine	0.5 to 2 ng/ml Potassium: 3.5 to 5 mEq/L Magnesium: 1.7 to 2.1 mEq/L Sodium: 135 to 145 mEq/L Chloride: 98 to 106 mEq/L Calcium: 8.6 to 10 mg/dl 0.6 to 1.3 mg/dl
diuretics	Serum electrolytes Serum creatinine BUN Uric acid Fasting serum glucose	Potassium: 3.5 to 5 mEq/L Magnesium: 1.7 to 2.1 mEq/L Sodium: 135 to 145 mEq/L Chloride: 98 to 106 mEq/L Calcium: 8.6 to 10 mg/dl 0.6 to 1.3 mg/dl 7 to 18 mg/dl 2 to 7 mg/dl 65 to 110 mg/dl
erythropoietin	Hematocrit	Female: 36% to 48% Male: 42% to 52%
ethosuximide	Serum ethosuximide	40 to 75 mcg/ml
gemfibrozil	Serum lipids	Total cholesterol: < 200 mg/dl LDL: < 130 mg/dl HDL: female: 40 to 85 mg/dl male: 37 to 70 mg/dl Triglycerides: 40 to 160 mg/dl

Note: ***** For those areas marked with asterisks, the following values can be used:

Hemoglobin: Female: 12 to 16 g/dl
Male: 14 to 18 g/dl
Hematocrit: Female: 37% to 48%
Male: 42% to 52%
RBCs: 4 to 5.5 x 10^6/mm^3
WBCs: 5 to 10 x 10^3/mm^3

Differential: Neutrophils: 45% to 74%
Bands: 0% to 4%
Lymphocytes: 16% to 45%
Monocytes: 4% to 10%
Eosinophils: 0% to 7%
Basophils: 0% to 2%

Monitoring guidelines
Wait until the administration of the third dose to check drug levels. Obtain blood for peak level 30 minutes after I.V. infusion or 60 minutes after I.M. administration. For trough levels, draw blood just before next dose. Notify doctor of drug levels so that dosage may be adjusted accordingly. Recheck after three doses. Montior serum creatinine, BUN, and urine output for signs of decreasing renal function.
Monitor serum creatinine, BUN, and serum electrolytes at least weekly during therapy. Blood counts and liver function tests should also be monitored regularly during therapy.
Specimen cultures and sensitivities will determine the causative agent of the infection and the best treatment. Monitor WBC with differential weekly during therapy.
Check renal function and hematologic parameters before initiation of therapy and at least annually thereafter. In the presence of impaired renal function, metformin may cause lactic acidosis and should not be used. Monitor response to therapy with periodic evaluations of fasting glucose and glycosylated hemoglobin. Home glucose monitoring by the patient can also be very useful.
Obtain WBC with differential before initiating therapy, weekly during therapy, and 4 weeks after discontinuation.
Serum digoxin levels should be checked at least 12 hours after the administration of the last dose, preferably 24 hours after the last dose. For monitoring maintenance therapy, levels should be checked at least 1 to 2 weeks after the initiation or a change of therapy. Adjustments in therapy should be made based on entire clinical picture, not solely on drug levels. Electrolytes and renal function should also be checked periodically during therapy.
Baseline and periodic determinations of serum electrolytes, serum calcium, BUN, uric acid, and serum glucose should be performed to monitor fluid and electrolyte balance.
With the initiation of therapy and after any dosage change, monitor the hematocrit twice weekly for 2 to 6 weeks until stabilized in the target range and a maintenance dose determined. The hematocrit should be monitored at regular intervals thereafter.
Check level 10 to 13 days after initiation or change in therapy.
Therapy is usually withdrawn after 3 months if response is not adequate. Patient must be fasting to measure triglycerides.

(continued)

* For those areas marked with one asterisk, the following values can be used:

ALT: 7 to 56 U/L
AST: 5 to 40 U/L
Alkaline phosphatase: 17 to 142 U/L
LD: 60 to 220 U/L
GGTP: < 40 U/L
Total bilirubin: 0.2 to 1 mg/dl

Drug	Laboratory test monitored	Therapeutic ranges of test
heparin	Activated partial thromboplastin time (APTT)	1.5 to 2 times control
HMG-CoA reductase inhibitors (fluvastatin, lovastatin, pravastatin, simvastatin)	Serum lipids	Total cholesterol: < 200 mg/dl LDL: < 130 mg/dl HDL: female: 40 to 85 mg/dl male: 37 to 70 mg/dl Triglycerides: 40 to 160 mg/dl
	Liver function tests	*
insulin	Fasting serum glucose Glycosylated hemoglobin	65 to 110 mg/dl 5.5% to 8.5% of total hemoglobin
lithium	Serum lithium Serum creatinine CBC	0.8 to 1.2 mEq/L 0.6 to 1.3 mg/dl *****
	Serum electrolytes (especially potassium and sodium)	Potassium: 3.5 to 5 mEq/L Magnesium: 1.7 to 2.1 mEq/L Sodium: 135 to 145 mEq/L Chloride: 98 to 106 mEq/L
	Fasting serum glucose	65 to 110 mg/dl
	Thyroid function tests	TSH: 0.2 to 5.4 microU/mL T3: 80 to 200 ng/dl T4: 5.4 to 11.5 mcg/dl
methotrexate	Serum methotrexate	Normal elimination: < 10 micromol 24 hours post dose < 1 micromol 48 hours post dose < 0.2 micromol 72 hours post dose
	CBC with differential Platelet count Liver function tests Serum creatinine	***** 140 to 400 x 10^3/mm^3 * 0.6 to 1.3 mg/dl
phenytoin	Serum phenytoin CBC	10 to 20 mcg/ml *****
potassium chloride	Serum potassium	3.5 to 5 mEq/L
procainamide	Serum procainamide Serum N-acetylprocainamide	4 to 8 mcg/ml (procainamide) 5 to 30 mcg/ml (combined procainamide and NAPA)
	CBC	*****
quinidine	Serum quinidine CBC Liver function tests Serum creatinine	2 to 6 mcg/ml ***** * 0.6 to 1.3 mg/dl
	Serum electrolytes (especially potassium)	Potassium: 3.5 to 5 mEq/L Magnesium: 1.7 to 2.1 mEq/L Sodium: 135 to 145 mEq/L Chloride: 98 to 106 mEq/L
sulfonylureas	Fasting serum glucose Glycosylated hemoglobin	65 to 110 mg/dl 5.8% to 8.5% of total hemoglobin

Note: ***** For those areas marked with asterisks, the following values can be used:

Hemoglobin: Female: 12 to 16 g/dl
Male: 14 to 18 g/dl
Hematocrit: Female: 37% to 48%
Male: 42% to 52%
RBCs: 4 to 5.5 x 10^6/mm^3
WBCs: 5 to 10 x 10^3/mm^3

Differential: Neutrophils: 45% to 74%
Bands: 0% to 4%
Lymphocytes: 16% to 45%
Monocytes: 4% to 10%
Eosinophils: 0% to 7%
Basophils: 0% to 2%

Monitoring guidelines
When given by continuous I.V. infusion, check APTT every 4 hours in the early stages of therapy. When given by deep S.C. injection, check APTT 4 to 6 hours after injection.
Know that liver function tests should be determined at baseline, 6 to 12 weeks after the initiation of therapy or any increase in dose, and periodically thereafter. If adequate response is not achieved within 6 weeks, a change in therapy should be considered.
Monitor response to therapy with evaluations of serum glucose and glycosylated hemoglobin. Glycosylated hemoglobin is a good measure of long-term control. Home glucose monitoring by the patient is also useful for measuring compliance and response.
Determination of lithium blood concentration is crucial to the safe use of the drug. Obtain serum lithium levels immediately before next dose. Levels should be monitored twice weekly until stable. Once at steady state, levels may be obtained weekly; when the patient is on the appropriate maintenance dose, levels may be monitored every 2 to 3 months. Monitor serum creatinine, CBC, serum electrolytes, fasting serum glucose, and thyroid function tests, as ordered, before the initiation of therapy and periodically during therapy.
Monitor methotrexate levels according to dosing protocol. CBC with differential and platelet, liver, and renal function tests should be monitored more frequently during initial or changing dosing and times when methotrexate levels may be elevated (such as in dehydration).
Monitor serum phenytoin levels immediately before next dose, 2 to 4 weeks after initiation of therapy or dosage adjustment. Obtain a CBC at baseline and monthly early in therapy. Notify doctor if toxic effects appear at therapeutic levels. The measured level should be adjusted for hypoalbuminemia or renal impairment, which can increase free drug levels.
Check level weekly after initiation of oral replacement therapy until stable, and every 3 to 6 months thereafter.
Measure procainamide levels 6 to 12 hours after the start of a continuous infusion, or immediately prior to the next oral dose. Combined (procainamide and NAPA) levels can be used as an index of toxicity when renal impairment exists. CBC should be obtained periodically during longer-term therapy.
Obtain levels immediately before next oral dose, 30 to 35 hours after initiation of therapy or dosage change. Obtain periodic blood counts, liver and kidney function tests, and serum electrolytes.
Monitor response to therapy with periodic evaluations of fasting glucose and glycosylated hemoglobin. Home glucose monitoring by the patient is a good measure of compliance and response.

(continued)

* For those areas marked with one asterisk, the following values can be used:

ALT: 7 to 56 U/L
AST: 5 to 40 U/L
Alkaline phosphatase: 17 to 142 U/L
LD: 60 to 220 U/L
GGTP: < 40 U/L
Total bilirubin: 0.2 to 1 mg/dl

Drug	Laboratory test monitored	Therapeutic ranges of test
theophylline	Serum theophylline	10 to 20 mcg/ml
thyroid hormone	Thyroid function tests	TSH: 0.2 to 5.4 microU/ml T3: 80 to 200 ng/dl T4: 5.4 to 11.5 mcg/dl
vancomycin	Serum vancomycin Serum creatinine	20 to 40 mcg/ml (peak) 5 to 10 mcg/ml (trough) 0.6 to 1.3 mg/dl
warfarin	INR	For acute MI, atrial fibrillation, treatment of pulmonary embolism, prevention of systemic embolism, tissue heart valves, valvular heart disease, or prophylaxis or treatment of venous thrombosis: INR of 2 to 3 For mechanical prosthetic valves or recurrent systemic embolism: INR of 3 to 4.5

Note: ***** For those areas marked with asterisks, the following values can be used:

Hemoglobin: Female: 12 to 16 g/dl
Male: 14 to 18 g/dl
Hematocrit: Female: 37% to 48%
Male: 42% to 52%
RBCs: 4 to 5.5 x 10^6/mm^3
WBCs: 5 to 10 x 10^3/mm^3

Differential: Neutrophils: 45% to 74%
Bands: 0% to 4%
Lymphocytes: 16% to 45%
Monocytes: 4% to 10%
Eosinophils: 0% to 7%
Basophils: 0% to 2%

Monitoring guidelines
Obtain serum quinidine levels immediately before next dose of sustained-release oral product, at least 2 days after initiation or change of therapy.
Monitor thyroid function tests every 2 to 3 weeks until appropriate maintenance dose is determined.
Serum vancomycin levels may be checked with the third dose administered (at the earliest). Peak levels should be drawn ½ hour after the completion of an I.V. infusion. Trough levels should be drawn immediately before the administration of the next dose. Renal function can be used to adjust dosing and intervals.
Obtain daily INR beginning 3 days after initiation of therapy, continue until therapeutic goal is achieved, monitor periodically thereafter. Also check levels 7 days after any change in warfarin dose or concomitant, potentially interacting therapy.

* For those areas marked with one asterisk, the following values can be used:

ALT: 7 to 56 U/L
AST: 5 to 40 U/L
Alkaline phosphatase: 17 to 142 U/L
LD: 60 to 220 U/L
GGTP: < 40 U/L
Total bilirubin: 0.2 to 1 mg/dl

Guidelines for use of selected antimicrobials

The following chart provides guidelines for the first-line (denoted by the numeral 1) and second-line (numeral 2) management of specific selected organisms and should be used as a general reference only. Use patient condition, sensitivities, institutional policies, and recent research when initiating new therapy.

	Aminoglycosides				Cephalosporins									
	Amikacin	Gentamicin	Netilmicin	Tobramycin	Cefazolin	Cefepime	Cefixime	Cefoperazone	Cefotaxime	Cefoxitin	Ceftazidime	Ceftizoxime	Ceftriaxone	Cefuroxime
Acinetobacter	1	1	1	1							2			
Bacillus anthracis														
Bacteroides fragilis										2		2		
Borrelia burgdorferi (skin)													1	2
Campylobacter jejuni														
Chlamydia pneumoniae														
Chlamydia psittaci														
Chlamydia trachomatis														
Citrobacter fruendii		1		1										
Clostridium difficile														
Clostridium perfringens					2				2	2		2	2	
Enterobacter sp.	1	1	1	1		2		2	2		2		2	
Enterococcus faecalis														
Enterococcus faecium														
Escherichia coli	2	2	2	2	1		1	1	1	1	1	1	1	1
*Haemophilus influenzae**	1	1	1	1					1			1	1	
Haemophilus influenzae†							2							2
Klebsiella pneumoniae (UTI)					1		1		1	1		1	1	1
Klebsiella pneumoniae (pneumonia)	2	2	2	2			1	1	1	1	1	1	1	1
Legionella pneumophila														
Listeria monocytogenes		1		1										
Moraxella catarrhalis					2	2	2	2	2	2	2	2	2	2
Mycoplasma pneumoniae														
Neisseria gonorrhoeae							1						1	
Nocardia asteroides														
Pneumocystis carinii														
Proteus mirabilis					2	2	2	2	2	2	2	2	2	2
Proteus vulgaris							1	1	1		1	1	1	
Pseudomonas aeruginosa	2	2	2	1		2		1			1			
Serratia marcescens	2	2	2	2				2	1		2	2	1	
Shigella sp.														
Staphylococcus aureus					1									
Staphylococcus saprophyticus														
Streptococcus pneumoniae									2				2	
Streptococcus pyogenes (group A)					1	1	1		1	1		1	1	1
Streptococcus (anaerobic sp.)														
Streptococcus (viridans group)		1											2	
Vibrio cholerae														

* Life-threatening † Non-life-threatening

	Miscellaneous											Penicillins								
	Azithromycin	Aztreonam	Clarithromycin	Clindamycin	Erythromycin	Imipenem/Cilastatin	Meropenem	Metronidazole	Quinupristin/ Dalfopristin	Trimethoprim/Sulfa- methoxazole	Vancomycin	Amoxicillin	Ampicillin	Mezlocillin	Nafcillin	Oxacillin	Penicillin G	Piperacillin	Piperacillin/ Tazobactam	Ticarcillin
						1	1			2										
			2		2															
				2				1				1							2	
	2		2		2									2						
					1															
	2		2		2															
	1				2															
	2	2				1	1											2		2
								1			2									
				2													1			
		2				1	1			1								2	2	2
											2	1	1				1			
						1			2		1	1	1							
		2				2	2			2				2				2		2
		2				2	2													
	2		2							1										
		2								1									2	
		2				2	2			2									2	
	2		2		1															
				2						2			1				1			
	2			2						1										
	2		2		1															
										1										
										1										
					1					1			1							
						2	2			1										
		2				2	2							1				1	1	1
		2				2	2			1										
										1			2							
			2	2	1	1				2	1				1	1			2	
				2																
											1	1	1				1			
	2		2	2	2							1	1				1			
				2													1			
	2		2	2	2												1			
										2										

(continued)

	Combination with β-lactamase inhibitors			Tetracyclines		Fluoroquinolones					
	Amoxicillin/ Clavulanic acid	Ampicillin/ Sulbactam	Ticarcillin/ Clavulanic acid	Doxycyline	Minocycline	Ciprofloxacin	Levofloxacin	Ofloxacin	Norfloxacin	Sparfloxacin	Trovafloxacin
Acinetobacter						2	2	2		2	2
Bacillus anthracis				1		1		2			
Bacteroides fragilis	2	2	2								2
Borrelia burgdorferi (skin)				1							
Campylobacter jejuni						2	2	2		2	2
Chlamydia pneumoniae				1			2			2	2
Chlamydia psittaci				1							
Chlamydia trachomatis				1			2	2			2
Citrobacter freundii						1	2	2		2	2
Clostridium difficile											
Clostridium perfringens				2							
Enterobacter sp.			2			1					
Enterococcus faecalis											
Enterococcus faecium				2							
Escherichia coli	1	1				2	2	2		2	2
*Haemophilus influenzae**	1	1	1			1	1	1	1	1	1
Haemophilus influenzae†	1	1		1					2		
Klebsiella pneumoniae (UTI)	2	2	2			1	1	1	1	1	1
Klebsiella pneumoniae (pneumonia)	2	2	2			2	2	2	2	2	2
Legionella pneumophila						2	1	2	2	1	1
Listeria monocytogenes											
Moraxella catarrhalis	1			2							
Mycoplasma pneumoniae				1							
Neisseria gonorrhoeae						2	2	2			2
Nocardia asteroides					2						
Pneumocystis carinii											
Proteus mirabilis											
Proteus vulgaris	2					1	1	1	1	1	1
Pseudomonas aeruginosa			1			2					
Serratia marcescens						2	2	2	2	2	2
Shigella sp.				2		1	1	1	1	1	1
Staphylococcus aureus	2	2	2			2	2	2		2	2
Staphylococcus saprophyticus						2	2	2	1	2	2
Streptococcus pneumoniae				1			1			1	1
Streptococcus pyogenes (group A)											
Streptococcus (anaerobic sp.)											
Streptococcus (viridans group)											
Vibrio cholerae				1		1	1	1		1	1

* Life-threatening † Non-life-threatening

Selected analgesic combination products

Many common analgesics are combinations of two or more generic drugs. This table gives you the components of common nonnarcotic analgesics and narcotic and opioid analgesic products.

Nonnarcotic analgesics

Trade name	Generic combination
Allerest No-Drowsiness Tablets, Coldrine, Ornex No Drowsiness Caplets, Sinus-Relief Tablets, Sinutab Without Drowsiness	▪ acetaminophen 325 mg ▪ pseudoephedrine hydrochloride 30 mg
Amaphen, Anoquan, Butace, Endolor, Esgic, Femcet, Fioricet, Fiorpap, Isocet, Medigesic, Repan	▪ acetaminophen 325 mg ▪ caffeine 40 mg ▪ butalbital 50 mg
Anacin, Gensan	▪ aspirin 400 mg ▪ caffeine 32 mg
Arthritis Foundation Nighttime, Extra Strength Tylenol PM, Midol PM	▪ acetaminophen 500 mg ▪ diphenhydramine 25 mg
Ascriptin	▪ aspirin 325 mg ▪ magnesium hydroxide 50 mg ▪ aluminum hydroxide 50 mg ▪ calcium carbonate 50 mg
Ascriptin A/D	▪ aspirin 325 mg ▪ magnesium hydroxide 75 mg ▪ aluminum hydroxide 75 mg ▪ calcium carbonate 75 mg
Cama Arthritis Pain Reliever	▪ aspirin 500 mg ▪ magnesium oxide 150 mg ▪ aluminum hydroxide 125 mg
COPE	▪ aspirin 421 mg ▪ caffeine 32 mg ▪ magnesium hydroxide 50 mg ▪ aluminum hydroxide 25 mg
Doan's P.M. Extra Strength	▪ magnesium salicylate 500 mg ▪ diphenhydramine 25 mg
Esgic-Plus	▪ acetaminophen 500 mg ▪ caffeine 40 mg ▪ butalbital 50 mg
Excedrin Extra Strength	▪ aspirin 250 mg ▪ acetaminophen 250 mg ▪ caffeine 65 mg
Excedrin P.M. Caplets	▪ acetaminophen 500 mg ▪ diphenhydramine citrate 38 mg
Fiorinal†, Fiortal†, Lanorinal†	▪ aspirin 325 mg ▪ caffeine 40 mg ▪ butalbital 50 mg
Midrin	▪ isometheptene mucate 65 mg ▪ dichloralphenazone 100 mg ▪ acetaminophen 325 mg
Phrenilin	▪ acetaminophen 325 mg ▪ butalbital 50 mg
Phrenilin Forte, Sedapap	▪ acetaminophen 650 mg ▪ butalbital 50 mg

(continued)

* Available in Canada only. † Controlled substance schedule III.

Nonnarcotic analgesics *(continued)*

Trade name	*Generic combination*
Sinus Excedrin Extra Strength	■ acetaminophen 500 mg ■ pseudoephedrine hydrochloride 30 mg
Sinutab Regular*	■ acetaminophen 325 mg ■ chlorpheniramine maleate 2 mg ■ pseudoephedrine hydrochloride 30 mg
Sinutab Maximum Strength	■ acetaminophen 500 mg ■ pseudoephedrine hydrochloride 30 mg ■ chlorpheniramine maleate 2 mg
Tecnal*	■ aspirin 330 mg ■ caffeine 40 mg ■ butalbital 50 mg
Vanquish	■ aspirin 227 mg ■ acetaminophen 194 mg ■ caffeine 33 mg ■ aluminum hydroxide 25 mg ■ magnesium hydroxide 50 mg

Narcotic and opioid analgesics

Trade name	*Controlled substance schedule*	*Generic combination*
Aceta with Codeine	III	■ acetaminophen 300 mg ■ codeine phosphate 30 mg
Anexsia 7.5/650, Lorcet Plus	III	■ acetaminophen 650 mg ■ hydrocodone bitartrate 7.5 mg
Azdone, Damason-P	III	■ acetaminophen 500 mg ■ hydrocodone bitartrate 5 mg
Capital with Codeine, Tylenol with Codeine Elixir	V	■ acetaminophen 120 mg ■ codeine phosphate 12 mg/5 ml
Darvocet-N 50	IV	■ acetaminophen 325 mg ■ propoxyphene napsylate 50 mg
Darvocet-N 100, Propacet 100	IV	■ acetaminophen 650 mg ■ propoxyphene napsylate 100 mg
E-Lor, Genagesic, Wygesic	IV	■ acetaminophen 650 mg ■ propoxyphene hydrochloride 65 mg
Empirin With Codeine No. 3	III	■ aspirin 325 mg ■ codeine phosphate 30 mg
Empirin With Codeine No. 4	III	■ aspirin 325 mg ■ codeine phosphate 60 mg
Fioricet With Codeine	III	■ acetaminophen 325 mg ■ butalbital 50 mg ■ caffeine 40 mg ■ codeine phosphate 30 mg
Fiorinal With Codeine	III	■ aspirin 325 mg ■ butalbital 50 mg ■ caffeine 40 mg ■ codeine phosphate 30 mg
Innovar Injection	II	■ droperidol 2.5 mg ■ fentanyl citrate 0.05 mg/ml
Lorcet 10/650	III	■ acetaminophen 650 mg ■ hydrocodone bitartrate 10 mg

* Available in Canada only.

Narcotic and opioid analgesics *(continued)*

Trade name	Controlled substance schedule	Generic combination
Lortab 2.5/500	III	■ acetaminophen 500 mg ■ hydrocodone bitartrate 2.5 mg
Lortab 5/500	III	■ acetaminophen 500 mg ■ hydrocodone bitartrate 5 mg
Lortab 7.5/500	III	■ acetaminophen 500 mg ■ hydrocodone bitartrate 7.5 mg
Percocet 2.5/325	II	■ acetaminophen 325 mg ■ oxycodone hydrochloride 2.5 mg
Percocet 5/325	II	■ acetaminophen 325 mg ■ oxycodone hydrochloride 5 mg
Percocet 7.5/500	II	■ acetaminophen 500 mg ■ oxycodone hydrochloride 7.5 mg
Percocet 10/650	II	■ acetaminophen 650 mg ■ oxycodone hydrochloride 10 mg
Percodan-Demi	II	■ aspirin 325 mg ■ oxycodone hydrochloride 2.25 mg ■ oxycodone terephthalate 0.19 mg
Percodan, Roxiprin	II	■ aspirin 325 mg ■ oxycodone hydrochloride 4.5 mg ■ oxycodone terephthalate 0.38 mg
Phenaphen/Codeine No. 3	III	■ acetaminophen 325 mg ■ codeine phosphate 30 mg
Phenaphen/Codeine No. 4	III	■ acetaminophen 325 mg ■ codeine phosphate 60 mg
Propoxyphene Napsylate/ Acetaminophen	IV	■ propoxyphene napsylate 100 mg ■ acetaminophen 650 mg
Roxicet	II	■ acetaminophen 325 mg ■ oxycodone hydrochloride 5 mg
Roxicet 5/500	II	■ acetaminophen 500 mg ■ oxycodone hydrochloride 5 mg
Roxicet Oral Solution	II	■ acetaminophen 325 mg ■ oxycodone hydrochloride 5 mg/5 ml
Talacen	IV	■ acetaminophen 650 mg ■ pentazocine hydrochloride 25 mg
Talwin Compound	IV	■ aspirin 325 mg ■ pentazocine hydrochloride 12.5 mg
Tylenol With Codeine No. 2	III	■ acetaminophen 300 mg ■ codeine phosphate 15 mg
Tylenol With Codeine No. 3	III	■ acetaminophen 300 mg ■ codeine phosphate 30 mg
Tylenol With Codeine No. 4	III	■ acetaminophen 300 mg ■ codeine phosphate 60 mg
Tylox	II	■ acetaminophen 500 mg ■ oxycodone hydrochloride 5 mg
Vicodin, Zydone	III	■ acetaminophen 500 mg ■ hydrocodone bitartrate 5 mg
Vicodin ES	III	■ acetaminophen 750 mg ■ hydrocodone bitartrate 7.5 mg

* Available in Canada only.

Cancer chemotherapy: Acronyms

Acronym and indication	Generic drug name	Trade drug name
ABVD (Hodgkin's disease)	doxorubicin	Adriamycin
	bleomycin	Blenoxane
	vinblastine	Velban
	dacarbazine	DTIC-Dome
AC (Bony sarcoma)	doxorubicin	Adriamycin
	cisplatin	Platinol
AC (Breast cancer)	doxorubicin	Adriamycin
	cyclophosphamide	Cytoxan
ACE (CAE) (Small-cell lung cancer)	doxorubicin	Adriamycin
	cyclophosphamide	Cytoxan
	etoposide (VP-16)	VePesid
AP (Endometrial cancer)	doxorubicin	Adriamycin
	cisplatin	Platinol
BEP (Testicular cancer)	bleomycin	Blenoxane
	etoposide (VP-16)	VePesid
	cisplatin	Platinol
CAF (FAC) (Breast cancer)	cyclophosphamide	Cytoxan
	doxorubicin	Adriamycin
	fluorouracil (5-FU)	Adrucil
CAP (Non-small-cell lung cancer)	cyclophosphamide	Cytoxan
	doxorubicin	Adriamycin
	cisplatin	Platinol
CAV (VAC) (Small-cell lung cancer)	cyclophosphamide	Cytoxan
	doxorubicin	Adriamycin
	vincristine	Oncovin
CC (Ovarian cancer, epithelial)	carboplatin	Paraplatin
	cyclophosphamide	Cytoxan
CF (Head and neck cancer)	cisplatin	Platinol
	fluorouracil (5-FU)	Adrucil
or	carboplatin	Paraplatin
	fluorouracil (5-FU)	Adrucil
CFM (CNF, FNC) (Breast cancer)	cyclophosphamide	Cytoxan
	fluorouracil (5-FU)	Adrucil
	mitoxantrone	Novantrone
CHOP (Malignant lymphoma)	cyclophosphamide	Cytoxan
	doxorubicin	Adriamycin
	vincristine	Oncovin
	prednisone	Deltasone

Acronym and indication	Generic drug name	Trade drug name
CHOP-Bleo (Malignant lymphoma)	cyclophosphamide	Cytoxan
	doxorubicin	Adriamycin
	vincristine	Oncovin
	prednisone	Deltasone
	bleomycin	Blenoxane
CISCA (Genitourinary cancer)	cisplatin	Platinol
	cyclophosphamide	Cytoxan
	doxorubicin	Adriamycin
CMF (Breast cancer)	cyclophosphamide	Cytoxan
	methotrexate	Folex
	fluorouracil (5-FU)	Adrucil
COP (Malignant lymphoma)	cyclophosphamide	Cytoxan
	vincristine	Oncovin
	prednisone	Deltasone
COPP (Hodgkin's disease and malignant lymphoma)	cyclophosphamide	Cytoxan
	vincristine	Oncovin
	procarbazine	Matulane
	prednisone	Deltasone
CP (Ovarian cancer)	cyclophosphamide	Cytoxan
	cisplatin	Platinol
CVP (Leukemia—CLL)	cyclophosphamide	Cytoxan
	vincristine	Oncovin
	prednisone	Deltasone
CVPP (Hodgkin's disease)	lomustine (CCNU)	CeeNU
	vinblastine	Velban
	procarbazine	Matulane
	prednisone	Deltasone
CYVADIC (Soft-tissue sarcoma)	cyclophosphamide	Cytoxan
	vincristine	Oncovin
	doxorubicin	Adriamycin
	dacarbazine	DTIC-Dome
DCBT (Dartmouth regimen) (Melanoma)	dacarbazine	DTIC-Dome
	cisplatin	Platinol
	carmustine (BCNU)	BiCNU
	tamoxifen	Nolvadex
DVP (Leukemia—ALL, adult induction)	daunorubicin	Cerubidine
	vincristine	Oncovin
	prednisone	Deltasone
EP (Small-cell or non-small-cell lung cancer)	cisplatin	Platinol
	etoposide (VP-16)	VePesid

(continued)

Acronym and indication	Generic drug name	Trade drug name
FAC (CAF) (Breast cancer)	fluorouracil (5-FU)	Adrucil
	doxorubicin	Adriamycin
	cyclophosphamide	Cytoxan
FAM (Adenocarcinoma, gastric cancer)	fluorouracil (5-FU)	Adrucil
	doxorubicin	Adriamycin
	mitomycin	Mutamycin
F-CL (Colorectal cancer)	fluorouracil (5-FU)	Adrucil
	leucovorin calcium	Wellcovorin
5 + 2 (Leukemia—AML, induction)	cytarabine (ara-C)	Cytosar-U
	daunorubicin	Cerubidine
FL (Prostate cancer)	flutamide	Eulexin
	leuprolide acetate	Lupron
FLe (Colorectal cancer)	levamisole	Ergamisol
	fluorouracil (5-FU)	Adrucil
FZ (Genitourinary, prostate cancer)	flutamide	Eulexin
	goserelin acetate	Zoladex
HDMTX (Bony sarcoma)	methotrexate	Folex
	leucovorin calcium	Wellcovorin
MACOP-B (Malignant lymphoma)	methotrexate	Folex
	leucovorin calcium	Wellcovorin
	doxorubicin	Adriamycin
	cyclophosphamide	Cytoxan
	vincristine	Oncovin
	bleomycin	Blenoxane
	prednisone	Deltasone
MAID (Soft-tissue sarcoma)	mesna	Mesnex
	doxorubicin	Adriamycin
	ifosfamide	Ifex
	dacarbazine	DTIC-Dome
MBC (Head and neck cancer)	methotrexate	Folex
	bleomycin	Blenoxane
	cisplatin	Platinol
MC (Leukemia—AML, induction)	mitoxantrone	Novantrone
	cytarabine (ara-C)	Cytosar-U
MICE (ICE) (Non-small-cell lung cancer)	mesna	Mesnex
	ifosfamide	Ifex
	carboplatin	Paraplatin
	etoposide (VP-16)	VePesid
MOPP (Hodgkin's disease)	mechlorethamine (nitrogen mustard)	Mustargen
	vincristine	Oncovin
	procarbazine	Matulane
	prednisone	Deltasone

Acronym and indication	Generic drug name	Trade drug name
MOPP (ABV hybrid) (Hodgkin's disease)	mechlorethamine (nitrogen mustard)	Mustagen
	vincristine	Oncovin
	procarbazine	Matulane
	prednisone	Deltasone
	doxorubicin	Adriamycin
	bleomycin	Blenoxane
	vinblastine	Velban
MP (Multiple myeloma)	melphalan (l-phenylalanine mustard)	Alkeran
	prednisone	Deltasone
MVAC (Genitourinary cancer)	methotrexate	Folex
	vinblastine	Velban
	doxorubicin	Adriamycin
	cisplatin	Platinol
MVPP (Hodgkin's disease)	mechlorethamine (nitrogen mustard)	Mustargen
	vinblastine	Velban
	procarbazine	Matulane
	prednisone	Deltasone
PCV (Brain tumors)	procarbazine	Matulane
	lomustine (CCNU)	CeeNu
	vincristine	Oncovin
ProMACE (Malignant lymphoma)	prednisone	Deltasone
	methotrexate	Folex
	leucovorin calcium	Wellcovorin
	doxorubicin	Adriamycin
	cyclophosphamide	Cytoxan
	etoposide (VP-16)	VePesid
ProMACE/cytaBOM (Malignant lymphoma)	cyclophosphamide	Cytoxan
	doxorubicin	Adriamycin
	etoposide (VP-16)	VePesid
	prednisone	Deltasone
	cytarabine (ara-C)	Cytosar-U
	bleomycin	Blenoxane
	vincristine	Oncovin
	methotrexate	Folex
	leucovorin calcium	Wellcovorin
7 + 3 (A + D) (Leukemia—AML, induction)	cytarabine (ara-C)	Cytosar-U
	daunorubicin	Cerubidine
VAC Standard (Soft-tissue sarcoma)	vincristine	Oncovin
	dactinomycin (actinomycin D)	Cosmegen
	cyclophosphamide	Cytoxan

(continued)

Acronym and indication	Generic drug name	Trade drug name
VAD (Multiple myeloma)	vincristine	Oncovin
	doxorubicin	Adriamycin
	dexamethasone	Decadron
VBP (Genitourinary, testicular cancer)	vinblastine	Velban
	bleomycin	Blenoxane
	cisplatin	Platinol
VC (Non-small-cell lung cancer)	vinorelbine	Navelbine
	cisplatin	Platinol
VDP (Malignant melanoma)	vinblastine	Velban
	dacarbazine	DTIC-Dome
	cisplatin	Platinol
VIP (Genitourinary, testicular cancer)	vinblastine	Velban
	ifosfamide	Ifex
	cisplatin	Platinol
	mesna	Mesnex
or	etoposide (VP-16)	VePesid
	ifosfamide	Ifex
	cisplatin	Platinol
	mesna	Mesnex

Immunization schedule

The current childhood immunization schedule as approved by the American Academy of Family Physicians, the American Academy of Pediatrics, and the Advisory Committee on Immunization Practices encompasses recent changes in recommendations. These guidelines were developed so the recommended immunization schedule would minimize adverse reactions while preserving effectiveness and maximizing patient compliance. The schedule may be appropriately altered wtih the use of currently licensed combination vaccines.

The following includes important information to consider when immunizing children.

<table>
<tr><th rowspan="2">Vaccine</th><th colspan="11">Age</th></tr>
<tr><th>Birth</th><th>1 mo.</th><th>2 mos.</th><th>4 mos.</th><th>6 mos.</th><th>12 mos.</th><th>15 mos.</th><th>18 mos.</th><th>4-6 yrs.</th><th>11-12 yrs.</th><th>14-16 yrs.</th></tr>
<tr><td rowspan="2">Hepatitis B[1]</td><td colspan="3">Hep B-1</td><td></td><td></td><td></td><td></td><td></td><td></td><td></td><td></td></tr>
<tr><td></td><td colspan="3">Hep B-2</td><td colspan="4">Hep B-3</td><td></td><td>Hep B</td><td></td></tr>
<tr><td>Diphtheria and tetanus toxoids and acellular pertussis[2] (DTaP, DTP)</td><td></td><td></td><td>DTaP or DTP</td><td>DTaP or DTP</td><td>DTaP or DTP</td><td></td><td colspan="2">DTaP or DTP</td><td>DTaP or DTP</td><td colspan="2">Td</td></tr>
<tr><td>Haemophilus influenzae type b[3]</td><td></td><td></td><td>Hib</td><td>Hib</td><td>Hib</td><td colspan="2">Hib</td><td></td><td></td><td></td><td></td></tr>
<tr><td>Poliovirus[4]</td><td></td><td></td><td>IPV</td><td>IPV</td><td colspan="4">IPV</td><td>IPV</td><td></td><td></td></tr>
<tr><td>Measles, mumps, rubella[5]</td><td></td><td></td><td></td><td></td><td></td><td colspan="2">MMR</td><td></td><td>MMR</td><td>MMR</td><td></td></tr>
<tr><td>Varicella virus[6]</td><td></td><td></td><td></td><td></td><td></td><td colspan="3">Var</td><td></td><td>Var</td><td></td></tr>
</table>

Range of acceptable ages for vaccination.

"Catch-up" vaccination.

[1]**Hepatitis B:** Children and adolescents who were not immunized against hepatits B in infancy may begin the series at any time. The series should be initiated or completed at age 11 or 12 in any child who has not previously received three doses of hepatitis B. The second dose should be administered at least 1 month after the first dose, and the third dose should be given at least 4 months after the first dose and at least 2 months after the second dose.

Infants born to hepatitis B surface antigen (HBsAg)-negative mothers should receive hepatitis B vaccine by age 2 months.The second dose is given at least 1 month after the first. The third dose is given at least 4 months after the first dose and at least 2 months after the second dose, but not before 6 months of age for infants.

Infants born to HBsAg-positive mothers should receive 0.5 ml of hepatitis B immune globulin (HBIG) within 12 hours of birth, and either 5 mcg of Recombivax HB (Merck) or 10 mcg of Engerix-B (SmithKline Beecham) at a separate site. The second dose is given at age 1 to 2 months and the third dose at age 6 months.

Infants born to mothers with unknown HBsAg status should receive 5 mcg of Recombivax HB (Merck) or 10 mcg of Engerix-B (SmithKline Beecham) within 12 hours of birth. Blood should be drawn at the time of delivery to determine the mother's HBsAg status. If positive, the baby should receive 0.5 ml of HBIG as soon as possible and no later than age 1 week. The dosage and timing of subsequent vaccine doses should be based upon the mother's HBsAg status.

[2]**DTP:** DTaP is the recommended vaccine for all doses in the series. Children who have received one or more doses of the whole-cell DTP may complete the series with DTaP. To combat compliance issues in patients who are unlikely to return at age 15 to 18 months, the fourth dose of the vaccine may be given as early as age 12 months, as long as 6 months have elapsed since the third dose. Td is recommended at age 11 to 12 provided at least 5 years have elapsed since last dose of DTP, DTaP, or DT. Routine Td boosters are recommended every 10 years for adults.

[3]***H. influenzae* type B:** Three *H. influenzae* type b (Hib) vaccines are licensed for use in infants. They are given at age 2, 4, 6, and 12 to 15 months unless the PRP-OMP (PedvaxHIB [Merck]) is used, in which case a dose at age 6 months is not necessary. Any Hib conjugate vaccine may be used as a booster dose at age 12 to 15 months.

[4]**Poliovirus:** Inactivated poliovirus vaccine (IVP) is given at age 2, 4, 6 to 18 months, and 4 to 6 years.

Oral polio vaccine (OPV) is no longer recommended for routine immunizations. However, OPV may still be appropriate in special circumstances, such as when parents do not accept the number of injections the child receives, late immunization would call for too many injections, or for imminent travel to polio-endemic areas and in mass vaccination campaigns to control outbreaks. OPV should not be used in immunocompromised children or those in close contact with immunocompromised persons.

[5]**Measles, Mumps, Rubella:** The second dose is recommended at age 4 to 6 before school entry, but may be administered at any visit, as long as both doses are given at or after age 12 months, and at least 1 month has elapsed between the first and second doses. Those who have not received the second dose should complete the schedule by age 11 or 12.

[6]**Varicella virus:** Varicella vaccine may be administered on or after age 12 months to any child who lacks a reliable history of varicella and who has not been previously vaccinated. Children age 13 or older must be given two doses of the vaccine at least 1 month apart.

Cytochrome P-450 enzymes and common drug interactions

Cytochrome P-450 enzymes, identified by "CYP" followed by numbers and letters identifying the enzyme families and subfamilies, are found throughout the body (primarily in the liver), and are important in the metabolism of many drugs. The following table lists potential drug-drug interactions based on the substrates, inducers, and inhibitors that can influence drug metabolism. The table includes common drug interactions, and the absence of a drug from the table doesn't necessarily imply that it isn't metabolized by one of the CYP enzymes.

CYP enzyme	Substrates
1A2	Amitriptyline, caffeine, chlordiazepoxide, clomipramine, clozapine, cyclobenzaprine, desipramine, diazepam, haloperidol, imipramine, olanzapine, ropinisole, tacrine, theophylline, warfarin, zileuton
2C9	Amitriptyline, carvedilol, clomipramine, dapsone, diazepam, diclofenac, flurbiprofen, fluvastatin, glimepiride, ibuprofen, imipramine, indomethacin, losartan, mirtazapine, naproxen, omeprazole, phenytoin, piroxicam, ritonavir, sildenafil, tolbutamide, torsemide, S-warfarin, zafirlukast, zileuton
2C19	Amitriptyline, carisoprodol, clomipramine, diazepam, imipramine, lansoprazole, mephenytoin, omeprazole, pentamidine, R-warfarin
2D6	Amitriptyline, carvedilol, chlorpheniramine, chlorpromazine, clomipramine, clozapine, codeine, cyclobenzaprine, desipramine, dextromethorphan, donepezil, doxepin, fentanyl, flecainide, fluoxetine, fluphenazine, fluvoxamine, haloperidol, hydrocodone, imipramine, loratadine, maprotiline, meperidine, methadone, metoprolol, mexiletine, morphine, methamphetamine, nortriptyline, oxycodone, paroxetine, perphenazine, propafenone, propoxyphene, propranolol, risperidone, thioridazine, timolol, tramadol, trazodone, venlafaxine
3A4	Alfentanil, alprazolam, amiodarone, amitriptyline, amlodipine, atorvastatin, bromocriptine, buspirone, carbamazepine, cisapride, clarithromycin, clomipramine, clonazepam, cocaine, corticosteroids, cyclophosphamide, cyclosporine (neural), dapsone, delavirdine, doxorubicin, dexamethasone, diazepam, diltiazem, disopyramide, ergotamine, erythromycin, ethosuximide, etoposide, felodipine, fentanyl, fexofenadine, finasteride, flutamide, fluvastatin, ifosfamide, imipramine, indinavir, isradipine, itraconazole, ketoconazole, lidocaine, loratadine, losartan, lovastatin, midazolam, methadone, methylprednisolone, miconazole, nefazodone, nicardipine, nifedipine, nimodipine, nisoldipine, paclitaxel, pravastatin, prednisone, quinidine, quinine, rifabutin, ritonavir, saquinavir, sertraline, sildenafil, simvastatin, tacrolimus, tamoxifen, teniposide, testosterone, triazolam, troleandomycin, verapamil, vinca alkaloids, warfarin, zileuton, zolpidem

Inducers	Inhibitors
Cigarette smoking, phenobarbital, phenytoin, primidone, rifampin, ritonavir	Ciprofloxacin, cimetidine, clarithromycin, enoxacin, erythromycin, fluvoxamine, grapefruit juice, isoniazid, ketoconazole, levofloxacin, mexiletine, norethindrone, norfloxacin, omeprazole, paroxetine, tacrine, zileuton
Carbamazepine, phenobarbital, phenytoin, primidone, rifampin	Amiodarone, chloramphenicol, cimetidine, co-trimoxazole, disulfiram, fluconazole, fluoxetine, fluvastatin, fluvoxamine, isoniazid, itraconazole, ketoconazole, metronidazole, omeprazole, ritonavir, sulfinpyrazone, ticlopidine, zafirlukast
No information available.	Felbamate, fluconazole, fluoxetine, fluvoxamine, omeprazole, ticlopidine
Carbamazepine, phenobarbital, phenytoin, primidone	Amiodarone, chloroquine, cimetidine, fluoxetine, fluphenazine, fluvoxamine, haloperidol, paroxetine, perphenazine, propafenone, propoxyphene, quinidine, ritonavir, sertraline, thioridazine
Barbiturates, carbamazepine, glucocorticoids, griseofulvin, nafcillin, phenytoin, primidone, rifabutin, rifampin, troglitazone	Clarithromycin, cyclosporine (neural), danazol, delavirdine, diltiazem, erythromycin, fluconazole, fluoxetine, fluvoxamine, grapefruit juice, indinavir, isoniazid, itraconazole, ketoconazole, metronidazole, miconazole, nefazodone, nelfinavir, nicardipine, nifedipine, norfloxacin, omeprazole, prednisone, quinidine, quinine, rifabutin, ritonavir, saquinavir, sertraline, troleandomycin, verapamil, zafirlukast

Guide to selected antidotes

This table summarizes the major uses and dosage recommendations for selected antidotes. For more information about specific antidotes, contact your local poison information center.

Antidote	Type of poisoning or overdose	General considerations
acetylcysteine (Mucomyst, Mucosil) *Adults:* 140 mg/kg P.O. diluted to a 5% concentration in soft drinks or juice, given within 16 to 24 hr after ingestion. Follow loading dose with 17 additional doses of 70 mg/kg q 4 hr unless acetaminophen assay reveals a nontoxic level (repeat if dose is vomited within 1 hr).	acetaminophen	▪ Activated charcoal will adsorb the antidote if both are present in the gut. If charcoal is used, it must be aspirated before the antidote is given. ▪ If patient is unable to retain the oral dose, administer by duodenal intubation.
activated charcoal (Actidose-Aqua, Liqui-Char) *Adults and children:* 5 to 10 times the weight of the ingested poison. Minimum dose is 20 to 30 g (½ cup of lightly packed powder) in 250 ml of water (to make a slurry); repeat as soon as possible. Most adults can tolerate doses of 120 g. For best results, use within 30 min of ingestion.	all oral poisonings except those caused by iron, cyanide, organic solvents, mineral acids, or corrosive agents	▪ After ipecac-induced vomiting, patient may be intolerant of activated charcoal for 1 to 2 hr. ▪ Repeated doses may not provide additional benefit unless the poison undergoes enterohepatic recycling. ▪ Activated charcoal may adsorb other orally administered antidotes. ▪ Contraindicated in patients at risk for aspiration.
amyl nitrite inhalants (Step I) *Adults:* Inhale for 30 sec q min until an I.V. sodium nitrite infusion is available. **sodium nitrite** (Step II) *Adults:* 300 mg in 10-ml solution given I.V. at a rate of 2.5 to 5 ml/min (if symptoms reappear, administer half the original dose in 2 hr). *Children:* Depends on hemoglobin level. **sodium thiosulfate** (Step III) *Adults:* 12.5 g in 50-ml solution given I.V. over 10 min (if symptoms reappear, give half the original dose of sodium nitrite again in 2 hr). *Children:* Depends on hemoglobin level.	cyanide	▪ Nitrites cause vasodilation. Hypotension is a common adverse reaction.
atropine sulfate *Adults:* 1 to 6 mg I.V. for pesticides (may repeat q 5 to 60 min until signs of atropinization appear). *Children:* 0.05 mg/kg for pesticides (may repeat q 10 to 30 min until signs of atropinization appear).	anticholinesterase substances, organophosphate pesticides, carbamate pesticides	▪ Large doses (up to 2,000 mg over several days) may be required to maintain full atropinization. ▪ Sudden cessation of atropine may cause pulmonary edema. ▪ Maintain adequate ventilation to prevent cardiac arrhythmias. ▪ A cholinesterase reactivator, such as pralidoxime, is also given in organophosphate poisoning; a cholinesterase reactivator is also given in carbamate poisoning when severe respiratory depression and severe muscle weakness exist.

Antidote	Type of poisoning or overdose	General considerations
calcium disodium edetate (Calcium Disodium Versenate, EDTA) *Adults and Children:* 1,000 mg/m2/day I.M or I.V. for 5 days. Infuse I.V. dose over 8 to 12 hr. I.M. dose should be divided into equal doses spaced 8 to 12 hr apart. Give second course after 2 to 4 days' rest.	chromium, lead, manganese, nickel, zinc, cadmium, cobalt	■ Most experts recommend that calcium disodium edetate be used in conjunction with dimercaprol for the treatment of severe lead poisoning. ■ Rapid injection may precipitate renal failure. ■ I.M. route is recommended in small children.
deferoxamine mesylate (Desferal) *Adults and children:* 1,000 mg I.M. or I.V. (<15 mg/kg/hr initially, then 500 mg q 4 hr for two doses. Subsequent doses of 500 mg q 4 to 12 hr may be given, depending on patient response; maximum dosage 6,000 mg daily.	iron	■ Renal excretion of compound will cause the urine to turn reddish pink.
digoxin immune Fab (Digibind) *Adults:* Depends on amount of digoxin or digitoxin to be neutralized. If unable to determine dosage using manufacturer-supplied dosage formulas, 760 mg I.V. may be infused over 30 min.	digoxin, digitoxin	■ Use is reserved for severe overdose only. ■ If possible, first obtain serum digoxin and digitoxin concentrations. ■ If cardiac arrest seems imminent, give dose as a bolus injection. ■ Monitor serum potassium levels carefully. ■ Monitor cardiac rate and rhythm.
dimercaprol (BAL in oil) *Adults:* For arsenic or gold poisoning, 3 mg/kg I.M. q 4 hr for first 2 days, then q 6 hr on day 3, followed by 3 mg/kg q 12 hr for 10 days or until recovery; for mercury poisoning, 5 mg/kg I.M. initially, followed by 2.5 mg/kg once or twice daily for 10 days.	mercury, arsenic, gold, lead (in conjunction with calcium disodium edetate)	■ Dimercaprol must be given promptly to be effective. ■ Contraindicated in iron, cadmium, selenium, and uranium poisoning. ■ Use requires that patient has adequate renal and hepatic function to excrete toxins.
flumazenil (Romazicon) *Adults:* Initially, give 0.2 mg I.V. over 30 sec. If patient does not reach the desired level of consciousness after 30 sec, give 0.3 mg over 30 sec. If response is inadequate, give 0.5 mg over 30 sec; repeat doses of 0.5 mg at 1-min intervals until 3 mg has been given.	benzodiazepines	■ Most patients respond to cumulative doses between 1 and 3 mg; rarely, patients who partially respond after 3 mg may require more. Don't give more than 5 mg in a 5-min period initially, and don't give more than 3 mg/hr. ■ Contraindicated in patients who also have severe cyclic antidepressant overdose. ■ Use with caution in cases of mixed overdose.
naloxone hydrochloride (Narcan) *Adults:* 0.4 to 2 mg I.V. bolus to reverse the narcotic effect (may need to repeat dose q 2 to 3 min). *Children:* 0.01 mg/kg I.V. bolus. Give subsequent dose of 0.1 mg/kg if needed.	opiates: morphine, heroin, methadone, meperidine, oxycodone, codeine, diphenoxylate, fentanyl, propoxyphene	■ Time of action is shorter than that of narcotic; observe patient for recurring narcosis. Repeat doses or a continuous infusion may be necessary. ■ If no response occurs after 10 mg has been administered, depression may be caused by a drug or disease that does not respond to naloxone.
penicillamine (Cuprimine) *Adults:* 500 mg to 1,500 mg/day for 1 to 2 months. *Children:* 30 to 40 mg/kg/day P.O. for 1 to 6 months. Doses above 500 mg should be divided b.i.d.	heavy metals	■ Penicillamine should be used in patients with minimal signs and symptoms and positive serum lead levels.

(continued)

Antidote	Type of poisoning or overdose	General considerations
physostigmine salicylate (Antilirium) *Adults:* 0.5 to 2 mg I.V. slowly over 2 to 3 min (repeat with a 1-mg to 2-mg dose in 20 min if symptoms are still present; repeat with a 1-mg to 4-mg dose if life-threatening symptoms reappear). *Children:* 0.02 mg/kg slow I.V. over 2 to 3 min (repeat within 5 min if symptoms recur); maximum dosage is 2 mg.	anticholinergics; tricyclics (amitriptyline, doxepin, imipramine, nortriptyline); antihistamines; some antiemetics, antiparkinsonian agents, and phenothiazines	▪ Use is reserved for severe poisoning (coma, hallucinations, delirium, tachycardia, arrhythmias, and hypertension). ▪ Rapid I.V. injection may cause bradycardia and hypersalivation with respiratory difficulties and convulsions. ▪ Physostigmine can produce a cholinergic crisis. If so, atropine should be used as an antidote.
pralidoxime chloride (Pralidoxime Chloride, Protopam Chloride) *Adults:* 1 to 2 g I.V. as 15- to 30-min infusion in 100 ml of normal saline solution; repeat dose in 1 hr if muscle weakness persists. Additional doses may be needed q 3 to 8 hr in severe cases. *Children:* 20 to 40 mg/kg/dose, administer as above.	organophosphate pesticides	▪ Best if given within 24 hr after exposure; is still effective within 36 to 48 hr. ▪ Pesticide absorption through the skin is possible—wash patient and remove contaminated clothing, or symptoms may reappear within 48 to 72 hr. ▪ Drug has no anticholinergic effects. ▪ Use with atropine.
protamine sulfate *Adults:* 5 ml of a 1% solution slow I.V. over 10 min (give 1 to 1.5 mg protamine for each 100 units of heparin consumed).	heparin	▪ Maximum dosage is 50 mg (as a single dose).
vitamin K analogue (AquaMEPHYTON) *Adults:* Usual initial dose is 2.5 to 10 mg I.M., S.C., or P.O. (if patient is not vomiting); it may be as high as 25 mg, or, rarely, 50 mg. Monitor patient response or PT to determine need for subsequent doses. If results unsatisfactory 6 to 8 hr after parenteral dose or 12 to 48 hr after P.O. dose, repeat.	warfarin	▪ Fresh whole blood may be necessary to stop bleeding.

Creatinine clearance calculations

In adults with stable renal function, the following formulas will provide a reliable estimate of creatinine clearance (Cl_{Cr}) except:

Patients with falsely low serum creatinine (such as paraplegic patients with muscle wasting) will give an artificially high predicted creatinine clearance.

Patients with rapidly increasing serum creatinine (over 0.5 to 0.7 mg/dl/day) will give an unreliable estimate of creatinine clearance.

Adults (age 18 and older)

Method 1*:

Estimated creatinine clearance, Cl_{Cr} (ml/minute):

$$\text{Male } Cl_{Cr} = \frac{(140 - \text{age})\ (\text{IBW})}{(72)\ (\text{SrCr})}$$

Female Cl_{Cr} = (Estimated male Cl_{Cr}) (0.85)

where age = in years
IBW = ideal body weight in kilograms:
IBW (Male) = 50 + [(2.3) (height in inches over 5 feet)]
IBW (Female) = 45.5 + [(2.3) (height in inches over 5 feet)]

Note: The use of the patient's IBW is recommended except when the patient's actual body weight is less than IBW.

SrCr = Serum creatinine in mg/dl

Method 2†:

Estimated creatinine clearance, Cl_{Cr} (ml/minute/1.73 m^2):

$$\text{Male } Cl_{Cr} = \frac{98 - [(0.8)\ (\text{age} - 20)]}{\text{SrCr}}$$

Female Cl_{Cr} = (Estimated male Cl_{Cr}) (0.90)

where age is in years, SrCr is serum creatinine in mg/dl.

*Cockroft, D.W., and Gault, M.H. "Prediction of Creatinine Clearance From Serum Creatinine," *Nephron* 16:31, 1976.
†Jelliffe, R.W. "Creatinine Clearance: Bedside Estimate," *Ann Intern Med* 79:604, 1973.

Herbal medicines

Plants have been used to cure disease for thousands of years, but the recent popularity of herbal medicines means that many patients need reliable information on using these substances appropriately. Most botanical products, vitamins, minerals, amino acids, and mammalian tissue abstracts are currently regulated only under the federal Dietary Supplement Health and Education Act of 1994. This act limits the FDA's authority to require proof of efficacy, safety, or quality before these products are sold commercially. And that means that herbal medicines have many unknown and undocumented risks. With these warnings in mind, you need to teach patients who use herbal medicines. Remind a patient to disclose all

Names	Reported uses	Forms and dosages
Aloe (aloe vera, burn plant, plant of immortality)	External: burns/sunburn, cuts, skin irritations, wounds, abrasions Internal: constipation	External: gels, creams, lotions Internal: not recommended
Angelica (dong-quai, tang-kuei)	Gynecologic disorders, postmenopausal symptoms, menstrual discomfort	Fluidextract, tablets, capsules, injection; no consistently reported dosage
Cayenne pepper (Capsicum, capsaicin, chili pepper, pepper sauce, hot pepper)	External: pain, including shingles, stump pain, diabetic neuropathy, cluster headache, arthritis Internal: stimulation of stomach secretions	External: creams, gels, ointment, lotion, 0.025%-0.075% Internal: diet as tolerated; supplements not recommended
Chamomile	Treatment of stomach maladies including GI spasms and inflammatory conditions of the GI tract, sedation	Teas most common; also capsules and liquid. For tea, dose is 2-3 grams (1 tablespoon) of dried flowers t.i.d. or q.i.d.
Cranberry (marsh apple, mountain cranberry)	Prevention of urinary tract infections (UTIs), possible antitumor effects	Capsules: 475-500 mg, 1-2 capsules per day P.O. Juices: 10-16 oz per day Powdered concentrates
Echinacea (American cone flower, coneflower, hedgehog, snakeroot)	Wound-healing agent and nonspecific immunostimulant for upper respiratory infections and UTIs	Capsules: 125, 355, and 500 mg P.O. t.i.d. Tablets: 335 mg P.O. t.i.d. Tincture: 0.75-1.5 ml P.O. 2-5 times per day
Feverfew (bachelors' buttons, febrifuge plant)	Prophylaxis of migraine headache, antipyretic for treating fever, toothache, psoriasis, insect bites, asthma, rheumatism and menstrual problems	Capsules: 380 mg (pure leaf); 250 mg (leaf extract) P.O. Liquid Tablets No consensus for dosage exists.
Flax (flaxseed, linseed, lint bells, linium)	External: inflammation Internal: constipation, irritable bowel, diverticulitis, functional disorders of the colon, hypercholesterolemia	External: 30-50 grams of flax meal applied as a poultice Internal: 1-2 tablespoons of oil or seeds daily in 2 or 3 divided doses P.O.
Garlic (allium, stinking rose, nectar of the gods, camphor of the poor)	Antimicrobial, lowers cholesterol and blood pressure, antiplatelet agent	600-900 mg daily P.O.

medications she takes to her health care provider at each visit. Inform her that herbal medicines may interact adversely with her existing medications, and make her aware of the variable quality of products produced in the "alternative care" industry. She should agree to monitor the goals of therapy along with her health care provider; if she hasn't achieved those goals after a sufficient time, suggest she consider conventional pharmacotherapy. Be sure to tell her to watch for any unusual reactions to any medications, particularly alternative ones, and to report them to her health care provider.

Considerations	Patient counseling
Internal use produces a cathartic action and has resulted in painful intestinal contractions, electrolyte imbalance, hemorrhagic diarrhea, and kidney damage.	Tell patient with a history of allergy to aloe, garlic, onion, or tulips not to use aloe. Warn against internal use. Can cause severe burning in patients undergoing dermabrasion or chemical peel.
Avoid in pregnancy and during breast-feeding because of possible uterine stimulation. Prolongs PT. Avoid use with anticoagulants. Human study data are lacking.	Tell diabetic patient she may exhibit poor glycemic control; instruct patient to monitor for signs of bleeding and warn of potential carcinogenic risk.
Topical application as a counterirritant produces a "heat" sensation. Repeated applications produce analgesia due to neuronal depletion of substance P, a mediator of pain transmission between periphery and spinal cord. Burning and itching diminish with continued use. Commercially available capsaicin preparations proved effective topical analgesics for some pain syndromes.	Pain relief may take up to 28 days. Avoid contact with eyes, mucous membranes, or nonintact skin. If contact occurs, flush area with cool running water as long as needed until burning sensation subsides. Used orally, capsicum has the potential to reduce the effectiveness of antihypertensives and may promote hypertensive crisis when used with MAO inhibitors.
Theoretical potential exists for decreased absorption of certain medications from antispasmodic activity. Excessive anticoagulation may occur when used with other anticoagulants.	Avoid use in pregnancy because of potential abortifacient and teratogenic effects. Instruct atopic patients to avoid use because of potential allergic reactions.
Has the potential to enhance the elimination of some drugs normally excreted in urine. Consumption of large quantities may cause diarrhea. Cranberry, which prevents bacteria from embedding in bladder walls, may be an important agent for prophylaxis in patients prone to UTIs.	Counsel diabetic patient to use sugar-free juices. Encourage patient to drink sufficient fluids and to notify his doctor if urinary symptoms worsen or don't resolve.
Activity shown against influenza, herpes, and *Candida*. Adverse effects, except possible allergy, are uncommon. No documented drug interactions. Prolonged use may lead to overstimulation of the immune system and possible immune suppression.	Instruct patient not to use echinacea for more than 8 weeks; therapy for 10-14 days probably is sufficient. Advise patient with HIV/AIDS, collagen disease, multiple sclerosis, tuberculosis, and other autoimmune diseases not to use echinacea.
Adverse effects include allergic reactions, mouth ulcers, and postfeverfew syndrome (withdrawal symptoms of aches, pains, and joint and muscle stiffness). Avoid use during pregnancy and lactation.	Instruct patient to taper off the agent on doctor's advice and to use proven therapies for migraine before using feverfew.
Adverse effects include diarrhea, nausea, and flatulence. May diminish absorption of other medications. Contraindicated in pregnancy, breast-feeding, ileus, and prostate cancer.	Instruct patient to refrigerate the oil and to never ingest immature seed because of potential toxicity. Overdose signs and symptoms include tachypnea, paralysis, and convulsions.
Adverse effects include contact dermatitis, dizziness, garlic odor, hypothyroidism, GI irritation, nausea, and vomiting. Potential drug interactions exist with antiplatelet therapy or anticoagulants. Avoid use in pregnant women and patients with GI disorders.	Advise patient that chronic or excessive use might cause decreased hemoglobin production or lysis of blood cells. Also advise patient using garlic to lower cholesterol that proven regimens should be part of his plan.

(continued)

Names	Reported uses	Forms and dosages
Ginger (Zingiber)	Antiemetic for morning sickness, motion sickness, postoperative nausea; anti-inflammatory, antitumor, antioxidant, antimicrobial agent	Varies with disease Antiemetic: 500-1,000 mg in 4 divided doses P.O.
Ginkgo biloba (EGB 761, GBE, GBX, Rokan, Tebonin, Ginkogink)	Cerebrovascular disease and peripheral vascular insufficiency resulting in short-term memory loss, vertigo, tinnitus, intermittent claudication; dementia	Vascular: 120-160 mg daily in 2 or 3 divided doses P.O. Dementia: 120-240 mg daily in 2 or 3 divided doses P.O.
Ginseng (five fingers, tartar root, Western ginseng, seng, sang, Asian Ginseng)	Improvement of stamina, concentration, healing, work efficiency, and well-being; aphrodisiac; sleep aid; antidepressant; antistress agent	200-600 mg ginseng extract daily P.O.
Green tea (tea, matsu-cha)	Prevention of cancer, dental caries, hypercholesterolemia, atherosclerosis; diuretic; stimulant; astringent; antibacterial	6-10 cups of tea per day
Kava (sakau, kawa, awa, kava-kava, tonga)	Treatment of anxiety, stress, and restlessness	90-110 mg dried kava extract P.O. t.i.d.
Ma huang (ephedra, Chinese ephedra, Teamster's tea, desert tea, popotillo, natural ecstasy)	CNS stimulant, appetite suppressant, treatment of asthma, colds, flu, nasal congestion	Tablets: 7 mg P.O. Teas: Unknown
Milk thistle (Mary thistle, Marian thistle, Lady's thistle, Holy thistle, silymarin)	Liver disease, including cirrhosis and chronic hepatitis; gallstones; liver protectant from toxins (death cap mushroom, halothane, psychotropic drugs)	420-800 mg P.O. daily as a single dose or in 2 or 3 divided doses
Nettle (stinging nettle, common nettle, greater nettle)	Diuretic, BPH, allergic rhinitis, bladder irrigation, gout	Tincture: ¼-1 teaspoon b.i.d. P.O. Capsules: 150-300 mg b.i.d. P.O.
Passion flower (passion fruit, granadilla, water lemon, maypop)	Sedative	4-8 g (3-6 teaspoons) as a tea daily in divided doses
Peppermint (brandy mint, balm mint, menthol)	External: Common cold, arthritis, other musculoskeletal problems Internal: Irritable bowel syndrome, dyspepsia	External: 3 or 4 times per day as menthol in creams, rubs, and similar preparations Internal: Teas—1 tablespoon in 160 ml 3 or 4 times per day P.O.
Saw palmetto (sabal, American dwarf palm tree, Serenoa repens, LSESR)	BPH	320 mg daily in divided doses (160 mg b.i.d.) P.O.

Considerations	Patient counseling
Overdose may produce CNS depression and arrhythmias. Ginger may enhance the effect of anticoagulants.	Advise patient considering ginger for morning sickness that the teratogenic potential is largely unstudied and to avoid ginger in large doses in pregnancy. Also advise her to monitor for signs of bleeding and that no consensus exists for dosing or monitoring.
Studies have shown that ginkgo extract produces arterial and venous vasoactive changes that increase tissue perfusion and cerebral blood flow. Adverse reactions are uncommon, but there have been reports of seizures in children and bleeding complications. Potential drug interactions may exist with antiplatelet therapy or anticoagulants.	Avoid use in children and pregnancy. Warn patient to monitor for unusual bleeding or bruising. If applied externally, gingko may cause irritation or blistering of the skin or mucous membranes. Results may not be evident for 6-8 weeks.
Avoid in pregnancy or during breast-feeding. Patients with CV disease, hypertension, hypotension, diabetes, or concurrent steroid therapy should avoid use. Drug interactions may exist with agents that inhibit MAO (phenelzine, St. John's wort, selegeline).	Counsel patient that large doses may be fatal and not to use for long periods. Use of coffee or tea may enhance CNS effects. Patient should monitor for signs of ginseng toxicity, which include diarrhea, hypertension, restlessness, insomnia, and skin eruptions.
Administration with milk may inhibit the antioxidant effect. A patient taking doxorubicin may experience enhanced antitumor activity.	Patient with "green-tea asthma" should avoid use due to immunoglobulin E–mediated allergic reactions.
Kava doesn't appear to cause physiologic dependence. Expect enhanced sedative effects if combined with other CNS depressants (alcohol, benzodiazepines, and opioid analgesics). Heavy use may cause nutritional deficiencies, skin dermopathy, blood dyscrasias, pulmonary hypertension, and dopamine antagonism.	Counsel patient to avoid in pregnancy and during breast-feeding and not to use in children under age 12. Advise patient to avoid alcohol while using. Kava is generally well tolerated except in high doses or for long-term use.
Adverse reactions appear to be dose-related and include anxiety, cardiac arrhythmia and infarction, insomnia, psychosis, stroke, urine retention, and uterine contractions. Avoid use in individuals with hypertension, diabetes, cardiac disease, prostatic enlargement, cerebrovascular disease, or pregnancy.	Caution patient to beware of such signs and symptoms as chest pain or shortness of breath. Advise patient not to exceed 24 mg/day or more than 8 mg in 6 hours or to use ephedra for more than 7 days. Avoid use with other CNS stimulants such as caffeine.
Historic use and clinical trials indicate a promising role for milk thistle in acute and chronic liver disease. Because there are no allopathic alternatives, a trial of milk thistle may be warranted in life-threatening situations.	Advise patient that concentrations of 70%-80% are necessary because of poor bioavailability. Patient with liver disease should seek advice of a specialist before pursuing this therapy.
Adverse reactions are rare but include edema, oliguria, and stomach irritation. Avoid in pregnancy and during breast-feeding. Treat for heart failure and BPH only under a doctor's supervision. Only proven action is diuresis.	Tell patient that the plant causes intense burning if it rubs against the skin. Advise her to eat food high in potassium to replenish electrolytes lost through diuresis.
Adverse effects and drug interactions are unknown. Avoid in pregnancy and during breast-feeding.	Warn patient of the potential for oversedation.
Patients with gastroesophageal reflux disease should avoid because peppermint may exacerbate it. Peppermint teas and mentholated ointment shouldn't be used in infants and small children. Menthol can cause sensitization and allergic reactions.	Advise patient not to apply topical mentholated products to broken skin. Menthol is generally recognized as safe when used externally. Internal use of peppermint for purposes other than flavoring isn't recommended.
Adverse events include minor GI reactions, decreased libido, hypertension, back pain, dysuria, and headache. Appears to be well tolerated and has demonstrated greater efficacy than placebo and equal efficacy to finasteride in improving symptoms of BPH.	Advise patient to take with morning and evening meals to minimize GI disturbances. Those seeking to use saw palmetto for BPH should do so only after diagnosis and on the advice of their health care professional.

(continued)

Names	Reported uses	Forms and dosages
St. John's wort (Hypericum, amber, chassediable, devil's scourge, goat weed)	Mild to moderate depression; anxiety; viral infection	300 mg (standardized to 0.3% Hypericum) t.i.d. for 4-6 weeks P.O.
Tea tree oil (Australian tea tree oil, melaleuca alternifolia, melaleuca oil, tea tree)	Local antiseptic; treatment of burns, cuts, athlete's foot, and various other cutaneous conditions	Topical application in various concentrations (0.4%-100%)

By Christine K. O'Neil, PharmD, Assistant Professor, Duquesne University Mylan School of Pharmacy, Pittsburgh; Juan R. Avila, PharmD, Medical Therapeutics Liaison, Sanofi-Synthelabo Pharmaceuticals, New York; C.W. Fetrow, PharmD, Coordinator, Pharmacokinetics, Outpatient Anticoagulation, and Drug Evaluation Services, St. Francis Medical Center, Pittsburgh.

Considerations	Patient counseling
There are numerous case reports and clinical trials evaluating the efficacy and safety of St. John's wort. Most trials contain design flaws, but overall suggest that St. John's wort may be beneficial for depression. Adverse reactions are uncommon but include photosensitivity, constipation, dizziness, dry mouth, restlessness, and sleep disturbances.	Advise patient to take precautions against sun exposure. Caution that the possibility of serotonin syndrome exists when this herb is used with other serotoninergic drugs such as serotonin reuptake inhibitors, trazodone, tricyclic antidepressants, and amphetamines. Avoid use with MAO inhibitors, alcoholic beverages, opioids, sympathomimetics, OTC cold and flu medications, and tyramine-containing foods such as chocolate, aged cheeses, and beer. Avoid in pregnancy and during breast-feeding; don't use in children.
Topical application hasn't been shown to be toxic, but ingesting the oil can produce CNS depression and GI irritation. The oil's antimicrobial activity has been well documented, but only anecdotal evidence exists for its efficacy in treating skin maladies.	Advise patient of the various product concentrations. Those with a propensity for contact dermatitis should probably avoid the use of tea tree oil.

Acknowledgments

We would like to thank the following companies for granting us permission to include their drugs in the full-color photoguide.

Abbott Laboratories
Biaxin®
Depakote®
Depakote® Sprinkle
E.E.S.®
Ery-Tab®
Erythrocin Stearate Filmtab®
Erythromycin Base Filmtab®
Hytrin®
PCE®

AstraZeneca LP
Nolvadex®
Prilosec®
Tenormin®
Toprol XL®
Zestril®

Aventis Pharmaceuticals
Allegra®
Carafate®
Cardizem®
Cardizem® CD
DiaBeta®
Lasix®
Slo-BidTM Gyrocaps®
Trental®

Bayer Corporation
Adalat CC®
Cipro®

Bristol-Myers Squibb Company
BuSpar®
Capoten®
Cefzil®
Duricef®
Estrace®
Glucophage®
Monopril®
Pravachol®
Serzone®
Sumycin®
Trimox®
Veetids®

DuPont Pharmaceuticals Company
Coumadin®

Eli Lilly and Company
Axid®
Ceclor®
Darvocet-N® 100
Prozac®

Endo Pharmaceuticals, Inc.
Percocet® 5/325

ESI Lederle Division of American Home Products
atenolol

Ethex Corporation
potassium chloride

Forest Pharmaceuticals, Inc.
Lorcet® 10/650

Glaxo Wellcome, Inc.
Ceftin®
Lanoxin®
Zantac®
Zantac® EFFERdose®
Zovirax®

Janssen Pharmaceutica, Inc.
Risperdal®

Jones Pharma
Levoxyl®

King Pharmaceuticals, Inc.
Altace®
Lorabid®

KV Pharmaceutical Company
Micro-K Extencaps®

McNeil-PPC, Inc.
Motrin®

Medeva Pharmaceuticals
methylphenidate hydrochloride

Merck & Co., Inc.
Cozaar®
Fosamax®
Mevacor®
Pepcid®
Prinivil®
Sinemet®
Sinemet® CR
Vasotec®
Vioxx®
Zocor®

Mylan Pharmaceuticals, Inc.
amitriptyline hydrochloride
cimetidine
cyclobenzaprine hydrochloride
doxepin hydrochloride
furosemide
glipizide
naproxen
propoxyphene napsylate with acetaminophen

Novartis Pharmaceuticals Corporation
Fiorinal® with Codeine
Lotensin®
Pamelor®

Novopharm USA, Inc., Division of Novopharm
Limited
amoxicillin trihydrate

Ortho-McNeil Pharmaceutical
Floxin®
Levaquin®
Tylenol® with Codeine No. 3
Ultram®

Pfizer, Inc.
Cardura®
Diflucan®
Glucotrol®
Glucotrol XL®
Norvasc®
Procardia XL®
Viagra®
Zithromax®
Zoloft®
Zyrtec®

Pharmacia & Upjohn
Deltasone®
Glynase®
Micronase®
Provera®
Xanax®

Procter and Gamble Pharmaceuticals, Inc.
Macrobid®

Roche Laboratories, Inc.
Bumex®
Klonopin®
Naprosyn®
Ticlid®
Toradol®
Valium®

Roxane Laboratories, Inc.
Roxicet™

Schein Pharmaceutical, Inc.
nortriptyline hydrochloride

Schering-Plough Corporation/Key Pharmaceuticals, Inc.
Claritin®
K-Dur®
Theo-Dur®

Schwarz Pharma
Verelan®

G.D. Searle & Company
Ambien®
Calan®
Celebrex®
Daypro®

SmithKline Beecham Pharmaceuticals
Amoxil®
Augmentin®
Compazine®
Coreg®
Dyazide®
Paxil®
Relafen®
Tagamet®

Tap Pharmaceuticals, Inc.
Prevacid®

Teva Pharmaceuticals USA
cephalexin

Warner-Lambert Company
Accupril®
Dilantin® Infatabs
Dilantin® Kapseals®
Lipitor®
Lopid®
Nitrostat®

Watson Pharma Inc.
Dilacor XR®
hydrocodone bitartrate and acetaminophen

Wyeth-Ayerst Laboratories
Ativan®
Cordarone®
Effexor®
Inderal®
Lodine®
Oruvail®
Premarin®

Zenith Goldline Pharmaceuticals
verapamil hydrochloride

Index

C

t refers to a table; **boldface** refers to full-color photographs.

t refers to a table; **boldface** refers to full-color photographs.

H

J

K

L

Q

R

t refers to a table; **boldface** refers to full-color photographs.

S

T